2011

Bi̶̶ ̶ ̶College ̶
Te̶

D0320897

39

reference

reference

Equine
Clinical Medicine, Surgery, and Reproduction

Graham A Munroe

BVSc (Hons), PhD, DipECVS, CertEO, DESM, FRCVS
Cowrig Cottage
Greenlaw, Duns
Berwickshire
Scotland, UK

J Scott Weese

DVM, DVSc, DipACVIM
Associate Professor
Department of Pathobiology
Ontario Veterinary College
University of Guelph
Guelph
Ontario, Canada

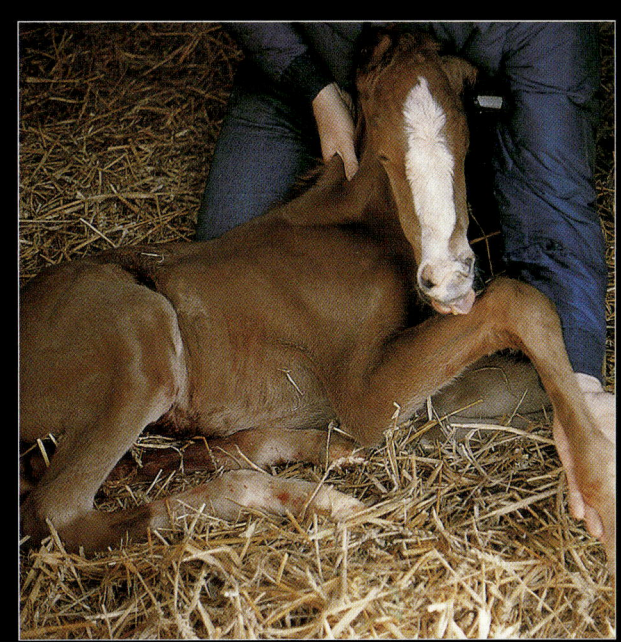

Copyright © 2011 Manson Publishing Ltd
ISBN: 978-1-84076-119-1

All rights reserved. No part of this publication may be reproduced, stored in a retrieval system or transmitted in any form or by any means without the written permission of the copyright holder or in accordance with the provisions of the Copyright Act 1956 (as amended), or under the terms of any licence permitting limited copying issued by the Copyright Licensing Agency, 33–34 Alfred Place, London WC1E 7DP, UK.

Any person who does any unauthorized act in relation to this publication may be liable to criminal prosecution and civil claims for damages.

A CIP catalogue record for this book is available from the British Library.

For full details of all Manson Publishing Ltd titles please write to:
Manson Publishing Ltd, 73 Corringham Road, London NW11 7DL, UK.
Tel: +44(0)20 8905 5150
Fax: +44(0)20 8201 9233
Email: manson@mansonpublishing.com
Website: www.mansonpublishing.com

Commissioning editor: Jill Northcott
Project manager and book design: Ayala Kingsley
Copy editor: Peter Beynon
Layout: Diacritech, Chennai, India
Illustration: Cactus Design
Index: Jill Dormon
Proofreader: John Forder
Colour reproduction: Tenon & Polert Colour Scanning, Ltd, Hong Kong
Printed by: Grafos Sa, Barcelona, Spain

Contents

Contributors   5

Preface   7

Abbreviations   8

1 Musculoskeletal system ———————————— 11

   1.1   **Approach to the lame horse**   12
        Cedric Chan and Graham Munroe

   1.2   **The foal and developing animal**   40
        Cedric Chan and Graham Munroe

   1.3   **The foot**   62
        Andrew Parks

   1.4   **The forelimb**   102
        Peter Milner

   1.5   **The hindlimb**   136
        Ehud Eliashar

   1.6   **The head**   166
        Martin Weaver

   1.7   **The axial skeleton**   174
        Martin Weaver

   1.8   **Soft-tissue injuries**   186
        Eddy Cauvin

2 Reproductive system ———————————— 241

   2.1   **Female reproductive tract**   242
        Graham Munroe, Madeleine Campbell,
        Zoë Munroe, and Matthew Hanks

   2.2   **Male reproductive tract**   326
        Theresa Burns, Tracey Chenier,
        and Graham Munroe

   2.3   **Equine castration**   374
        Luis Lamas and Graham Munroe

3 Respiratory system ———————————— 381

   3.1   **Introduction**   382
        Josh Slater

   3.2   **Surgical conditions of the upper respiratory tract**   392
        Bruce Bladon and Graham Munroe

   3.3   **Medical conditions of the upper respiratory tract**   450
        Josh Slater

   3.4   **Medical conditions of the lower respiratory tract**   458
        Joanne Hewson, Luis Arroyo, and Josh Slater

4 Gastrointestinal system ———————————— 481

    4.1 **Upper gastrointestinal tract**   482
        Henry Tremaine

    4.2 **Lower gastrointestinal tract**   516
        Scott Weese, Ludovic Boure, Simon Pearce,
        and Nathalie Cote

5 Liver ———————————— 598
    Thomas Koch, Anthony Knight, and Scott Weese

6 Endocrine system ———————————— 620
    Babetta Breuhaus

7 Urinary system ———————————— 637
    Modest Vengust

8 Cardiovascular system ———————————— 671
    Kim McGurrin

9 Hemolymphatic system ———————————— 709
    Darren Wood and Sonya Keller

10 Nervous system ———————————— 745
    Siobhan McAuliffe and Nathan Slovis

11 Eyes ———————————— 809
    Heather Gray

12 Skin ———————————— 873
    Reginald Pascoe

13 Wound management
and infections of synovial structures ———— 939
    Antonio Cruz and Graham Munroe

14 The foal ———————————— 966
    Sarah Stoneham and Graham Munroe

15 Behavioral problems ———————————— 995
    Katherine Houpt

Further reading   1012

Index   1020

Contributors

Luis G Arroyo DVM, DVSc
Department of Clinical Studies
Ontario Veterinary College
University of Guelph
Guelph, Ontario, Canada

Bruce Bladon BVM&S, CertEP, DESTS, DipECVS, MRCVS
Donnington Grove Veterinary Surgery
Newbury, Berkshire, UK

Ludovic Boure DVM, MSc, DipACVS, Dip ECVS
Head of Experimental Surgery
AO Research Institute
Davos, Switzerland

Babetta Breuhaus DVM, PhD, DACVIM
Department of Clinical Sciences
North Carolina State University
Raleigh, North Carolina, USA

Theresa Burns DVM, MSc, DipACT
Yarrow Station
Chilliwack, British Columbia, Canada

Madeleine L H Campbell BVetMed(Hons), MA(Oxon), PhD, DipECAR, MRCVS
Hobgoblins Stud and Equine Reproduction Centre
Duddleswell, Ashdown Forest, East Sussex, UK

Eddy R J Cauvin DrVétérinaire, MVM, PhD, HDR, CertVR, CertES(Ortho), DipECVS
Azurvet
Hippodrome de la Côte d'Azur,
Cagnes sur Mer, France

Cedric C-H Chan BVSc, DipECVS, CertES(Orth), MRCVS
Northwest Equine Referrals
Putney, London, UK

Tracey Chenier DVM, DVSc DipACT
Assistant Professor, Large Animal Theriogenology
Ontario Veterinary College
University of Guelph
Guelph, Ontario, Canada

Nathalie Cote DVM, DVSc, DipACVS
Milton Equine Hospital
Milton, Ontario, Canada

Antonio Cruz DVM, MVM, MSc, DrMedVet, DipACVS, DipECVS
Hospital Director,
Paton and Martin Veterinary Services,
Aldergrove, British Columbia, Canada

Ehud Eliashar DVM, DipECVS, MRCVS
Lecturer in Equine Surgery,
Department of Clinical Veterinary Sciences
Royal Veterinary College
North Mymms, Hatfield, Hertfordshire, UK

Heather E Gray DVM, DipACVO
Oak Ridges Veterinary Professional Corporation
Claremont, Ontario, Canada

Matthew L Hanks BVSc, MRCVS
Lecturer in Reproduction
Division of Veterinary Clinical Studies
Royal (Dick) School of Veterinary Studies
Easter Bush, Midlothian, Scotland, UK

Joanne Hewson DVM, PhD, DipACVIM
Department of Clinical Studies
Ontario Veterinary College
University of Guelph
Guelph, Ontario, Canada

Katherine A Houpt VMD, PhD, DACVB
James Law Professor of Animal Behavior
Department of Clinical Sciences
College of Veterinary Medicine
Cornell University
Ithaca, New York, USA

Sonya Keller DVM, DVSc, DipACVP
Clinical Pathologist
IDEXX Reference Laboratories
Markham, Ontario, Canada

Anthony P Knight BVSc, MS, MRCVS, DACVIM
Professor, Department of Clinical Sciences
College of Veterinary Medicine & Biomedical Sciences
Colorado State University
Fort Collins, Colorado, USA

Thomas G Koch DVM, PhD Candidate
Department of Clinical Studies
Ontario Veterinary College
University of Guelph
Guelph, Ontario, Canada

Luis RGP Lamas DVM, CertES(Orth), MRCVS
Rua de Junqueira 148,
1300–1345 Lisbon, Portugal

Siobhan McAuliffe MVB, MRCVS, DipACVIM
Dreamland Farm Rehabilitation Center
Lexington, Kentucky, USA

M Kim J McGurrin DVM, DVSc, DipACVIM
Department of Clinical Studies
Ontario Veterinary College
University of Guelph
Guelph, Ontario, Canada

Peter I Milner BVetMed, BSc, PhD, CertES(Orth), MRCVS
Lecturer, Equine Division
Department of Veterinary Clinical Science
Faculty of Veterinary Science
University of Liverpool
Neston, Wirral, UK

Graham Munroe BVSc (Hons), PhD, DipECVS, CertEO, DESM, FRCVS
Flanders Veterinary Services
Greenlaw, Duns. Berwickshire, Scotland, UK

Zoë J Munroe BVSc, MRCVS
Flanders Veterinary Services
Greenlaw, Duns, Berwickshire, Scotland, UK

Andrew H Parks MA, Vet MB, MRCVS, CertVR, DipACVS
Professor, Large Animal Surgery
Department of Large Animal Medicine
College of Veterinary Medicine
University of Georgia
Athens, Georgia, USA

Reginald R Pascoe AM, BVSc, DVSc, FRCVS, FACVSc
Adjunct Professor, Veterinary School Queensland
Consultant, Oakey Veterinary Hospital
Oakey, Queensland, Australia

Simon Pearce BVSc, PhD, DipACVS
Bio Innovation SA
Adelaide, South Australia, Australia

Josh D Slater BVM&S, PhD, DipECEVIM, MRCVS
Professor of Equine Clinical Studies
Royal Veterinary College
North Mimms, Hatfield, Hertfordshire, UK

Nathan Slovis DVM, DipACVIM, CHT (Certified Hyperbaric Technologist)
Hagyard Equine Medical Insititute
Director McGee Critical Care and Medical Center
Lexington, Kentucky, USA

Sarah J Stoneham BVSc, CertESM, MRCVS
Lone Oak Stud
Hilborough, Norfolk, UK

W Henry Tremaine BVet Med, MPhil, Cert ES, DipECVS, MRCVS
Department of Clinical Veterinary Science
School of Veterinary Science
University of Bristol, Langford, Bristol, UK

Modest Vengust DVM, DVSc, DipACVIM
Assistant Professor
Veterinary Faculty
University of Ljubljana,
Ljubljana, Slovenia

Martin P Weaver BVMS, DrMedVet, PhD, DVR, MRCVS
Senior Lecturer
Division of Veterinary Clinical Studies
Royal (Dick) School of Veterinary Studies
University of Edinburgh
Easter Bush, Roslin, Midlothian, Scotland, UK

J Scott Weese DVM, DVSc, DipACVIM
Associate Professor, Department of Pathobiology
Ontario Veterinary College
University of Guelph
Guelph, Ontario, Canada

Darren Wood DVM, DVSc, DipACVP
Associate Professor, Department of Pathobiology
Ontario Veterinary College
University of Guelph
Guelph, Ontario, Canada

Preface

THE FIELDS of equine medicine, surgery, and reproduction have developed massively over the last 25–30 years and new knowledge and techniques for the diagnosis and treatment of all sorts of conditions and diseases continues to be added. This new knowledge is presented initially in scientific papers and congresses around the world and gradually is distilled down to appear in new editions of textbooks. There continues to be published an increasing number of equine-based textbooks, often concentrating on one body system and written from a specialist point of view. Very few have been produced in the last 10 years that specifically address the needs of the clinician who is not a full-time equine specialist or the equine-interested undergraduate or postgraduate veterinary student. This textbook is designed and written with these colleagues very much in mind.

The breadth of content in this book is large, covering a comprehensive range of topics in equine medicine, surgery, and reproduction, and it is organized into chapters using a systems-based approach. Each individual system is introduced with precise information on the relevant basic anatomy and physiology, standard clinical examination techniques, and useful differential diagnostic aids. The remainder of the chapter is split up into diseases and disorders that are pertinent to that system. The diseases and disorders are grouped together, either anatomically or based on presenting clinical signs, into sections where specific problems or diseases are presented in a strict format that is common to the whole book. Thus each disorder is presented under the individual headings of definition/overview, etiology/pathophysiology, clinical presentation, differential diagnosis, diagnosis, management, and prognosis. These systems-based chapters are complemented by additional chapters on specific areas such as behavioral problems and wounds. The focus is on providing clinically relevant information that is required for good case management, but with enough concise information about etiology and pathophysiology to enable readers to understand the conditions and the rationale for diagnostic and treatment options. Some conditions that produce multisystem manifestations may be discussed in more than one chapter, with each chapter providing a different emphasis, thereby ensuring a complete overall content, but with less duplication.

The scope of equine veterinary medicine makes it impossible for any one book to act as the sole resource for all areas. With this in mind and considering the target readership of this book, complicated or advanced diagnostic and treatment techniques are mentioned, but not covered in detail; however, further reading lists are provided to guide the reader to additional information. These include material such as reviews deemed to be of particularly high quality by chapter authors, as well as selected primary scientific reports and websites.

Patterns of disease can be highly variable between different geographic regions, and while no book can provide a comprehensive overview of all geographical differences, the editors and authors have endeavored to make the chapters in this book useful and relevant to a broad international audience. It is hoped that in the future this aim will be enhanced by the translation of the text into several of the major languages of the world.

A unique feature of this book is the inclusion of a large number of images, including color photographs, radiographic and ultrasound images, and diagrams. Images are provided for the majority of topics and are intended to complement the text on the basis that a 'picture speaks a thousand words'. The inclusion of clinical images can be useful in further understanding the pathogenesis and pathophysiology of certain conditions, helping the pattern recognition of some diseases and disorders, and visualizing the surgical pathology or procedures that general clinicians and students rarely see. It is also anticipated that the number and quality of images will be a valuable educational tool for horse owners, enabling veterinarians to explain more easily certain aspects of disease pathogenesis, diagnosis, and management.

Finally, it is intended that this textbook, although it is large and, hopefully, comprehensive, will not stay gathering dust on a shelf in a practice library or student's study, but will be in a vehicle with a busy practitioner or on the desk of a student, well thumbed and constantly open, helping educate and assist each individual in his or her daily life. If it does this some of the time, it will have achieved its goal.

Graham Munroe
Scott Weese

Abbreviations

AA	aplastic anemia
ACB	accessory carpal bone
ACE	angiotensin converting enzyme
ACS	autologous conditioned serum
ACTH	adrenocorticotropic hormone
ADAF	axial deviation of the aryepiglottic folds
ADH	antidiuretic hormone
AF	atrial fibrillation
AHF	anovulatory hemorrhagic follicle
AHS	African horse sickness
AI	artificial insemination
AID	anemia of inflammatory disease
ALD	angular limb deformitiy
ALDDFT	accessory ligament of the deep digital flexor tendon
ALP	alkaline phosphatase
ALSDFT	accessory ligament of the superficial digital flexor tendon
AM	atypical myopathy
ANA	antinuclear antibody
AP	alkaline phosphatase
APC	atrial premature contraction
ARAS	ascending reticular activating system
ARF	acute renal failure
ASD	atrial septal defect
ASIT	allergen-specific immunotherapy
AST	aspartate aminotransferase
AV	atrioventricular
BAB	blood–aqueous barrier
4-BAD	fourth branchial arch defect
BAL	bronchoalveolar lavage
BAP	bone-specific alklaline phosphatase
BCG	Bacillus Calmette–Guérin
BOB	blood–ocular barrier
bpm	beats per minute
BPV	bovine papillomavirus
BSE	breeding soundness examination
BSP	bromsulphalein
C1/C2/C3	first/second/third carpal (bone)
CARS	compensatory anti-inflammatory response syndrome
CASA	computer-assisted sperm motion analysis
CBC	complete blood count
CDI	*C. difficile* infection
CDE	common digital extensor (tendon)
CEM	contagious equine metritis
CFT	complement fixation test
CFU	colony forming unit
CK	creatine kinase

CL	corpus luteum/corpora lutea
CLE	cutaneous lupus erythematosus
CMA	cranial mesenteric artery
CN	cranial nerve
CNS	central nervous system
COMP	cartilage oligomeric protein
COPD	chronic obstructive pulmonary disease
CPII	carboxypropetides of type II collagen
CPE	*C. perfringens* enterotoxin
CPG	conjunctival pedicle graft
CPK	creatinine phosphokinase
CRF	chronic renal failure
CRT	capillary refill time
CsA	cyclosporine A
CSF	cerebrospinal fluid
CSNB	congenital stationary night blindness
CT	computed tomography
CTUP	combined thickness of uterus and placenta
cTnT/I	cardiac troponin T and I
CTXs	type I collagen C telopeptides
CUI	chronic uterine infection
D	diopter(s)
DCP	dynamic compression plate
DCS	dynamic condylar screw (plate)
DDFT	deep digital flexor tendon
DDSL	short (deep) distal sesamoidean ligament
DDSP	dorsal displacement of the soft palate
DHS	dynamic hip screw (plate)
DIC	disseminated intravascular coagulation
DIP	distal interphalangeal (joint)
DIT	distal intertarsal (centrodistal) (joint)
DJD	degenerative joint disease
DMSO	dimethyl sufoxide
DOD	developmental orthopedic disease
DP	dorsopalmar/plantar
DPJ	duodenitis/proximal jejunitis
DSP	dorsal spinous process
DSS	dioctyl sodium succinate
DV	dorsoventral
ECE	equine coital exanthema
eCG	equine chorionic gonadotropin
ECG	electrocardiogram/electrocardiography
ECR	extensor carpi radialis (tendon)
EDM	equine degenerative myeloencephalopathy
EDTA	ethylenediaminetetraacetic acid
EE	eosinophilic enterocolitis
EED	early embryonic death
EEE	Eastern equine encephalitis
EGE	equine granulocytic ehrlichiosis

EGS	equine grass sickness		KCS	keratoconjunctivitis sicca
EHM	equine herpesvirus myeloencephalopathy			
EHV-1	equine herpesvirus-1		L1/2/3/4/5	first/second/third/fourth/fifth stage (larvae)
EIA	equine infectious anemia		LCP	locking compression plate
EIAV	equine infectious anemia virus		LDE	lateral digital extensor (tendon)
EIPH	exercise-induced pulmonary hemorrhage		LDF	lateral digital flexor (tendon)
ELEM	equine leukoencephalomalacia		LDH	lactate dehydrogenase
ELISA	enzyme-linked immunosorbent assay		LE	lupus erythematosus
EMG	electromyogram/electromyography		LH	luteinizing hormone
EMND	equine motor neuron disease		LMN	lower motor neuron
EPF	early pregnancy factor		LPL	long plantar ligament (of the tarsus)
epg	eggs per gram		LRT	lower respiratory tract
EPH	equine purpura hemorrhagica		LSA	lymphosarcoma
EPM	equine protozoal myeloencephalitis			
ERG	electroretinogram/electroretinography		MC/MT	metacarpal/metatarsal
ERU	equine recurrent uveitis		MCH	mean corpuscular hemoglobin
ESFD	external skeletal fixation device		MCHC	mean corpuscular hemoglobin concentration
ETRs	excessive transverse ridges		MCP	metacarpophalangeal
EVA	equine viral arteritis		MCV	mean corpuscular volume
			MDF	medial digital flexor (tendon)
FDPs	fibrin(ogen) degradation products		MDP	methyl diphosphonate
FFAs	free fatty acids		MEED	multisystemic eosinophilic epitheliotropic disease
FFD	film focal distance			
FNA	fine-needle aspirate		MIA	monoiodoacetic acid
FPT	failure of passive transfer		MMP	matrix metalloproteinase
FSH	follicle-stimulating hormone		MPD	myeloproliferative disorder
			MPICL	medial palmar intercarpal ligament
GABA	gamma aminobutyric acid		MPV	mean platelet volume
GCT	granulosa (thecal) cell tumor		MRI	magnetic resonance imaging
GFR	glomerular filtration rate		MRLS	mare reproductive loss syndrome
GGT	gamma-glutamyltransferase		α-MSH	α-melanophore-stimulating hormone
GI	gastrointestinal		MTP	metatarsophalangeal (joint)
GLDH	glutamate dehydrogenase			
GnRH	gonadotropin-releasing hormone		NI	neonatal isoerythrolysis
			NLS	nasolacrimal system
H2	histamine		NMD	nutritional myodegeneration
hCG	human chorionic gonadotropin		NSAID	nonsteroidal anti-inflammatory drug
HYPP	hyperkalemic periodic paralysis			
			OA	osteoarthritis
IAD	inflammatory airway disease		OAMM	occipitoatlantoaxial malformation
ICA	iridocorneal angle		OC	osteocalcin
ICP	intracranial pressure		OCD	osteochondrosis
ICS	intercostal space		OCLL	osseous cyst-like lesions
ICSI	intracytoplasmic sperm injection		ODSL	oblique distal sesamoidean ligament
IFA	immunofluorescent antibody (test)		OIE	World Organization for Animal Health
Ig	immunoglobulin		OMO	open-mouthed oblique
IGF-1	insulin-like growth factor-1		ONH	optic nerve head
IL-1	interleukin-1			
i/m	intramuscular, intramuscularly		p/o	per os, orally
IMHA	immune-mediated hemolytic anemia		P1/P2	first/second phalanx
IRAP	interleukin receptor antagonist protein		PA	pyrrolizidine alkaloid
ITP	immune-mediated thrombocytopenia		PaO2	arterial partial pressure of oxygen
i/v	intravenous, intravenously		PAL	palmar/plantar annular ligament
			PAS	periodic acid–Schiff (stain)

PCR	poylmer chain reaction	SSPL	single-entry subpalpebral lavage (tube)
PCV	packed cell volume	STT	Schirmer tear test
PDA	patent ductus arteriosus		
PG	prostaglandin	T4	thyroxine
PGF2α	prostaglandin F2 alpha	T3	tri-iodothyronine
PHF	Potomac horse fever	TAT	tetanus antitoxin
PIFM	preiridal fibrovascular membrane	TC	tarsocrural
PIP	proximal interphalangeal (joint)	TD	testicular degeneration
PIT	proximal intertarsal (talocalcaneal–centroquatral) joint	TENS	transcutaneous electrical nerve stimulation
PLK	posterior lamellar keratoplasty	TIBC	total iron-binding capacity
PLR	pupillary light reflex	TL	tracheal lavage
PMI	point of maximal intensity	TMJ	temporomandibular joint
PMIE	persistent mating-induced endometritis	TMT	tarsometatarsal (joint)
PMMA	polymethylmethacrylate	TNF	tumor necrosis factor
PMMN	progressively motile morphologically normal (sperm)	TPA	tissue plasminogen activator
		TPK	therapeutic penetrating keratoplasty
PMN	polymorphonuclear (cell)	TRH	thyrotropin-releasing hormone
POMC	proopiomelanocortin	TSH	thyroid-stimulating hormone
PRCA	pure red cell aplasia		
PRNT	plaque reduction neutralization test	UMN	upper motor neuron
PSB	proximal sesamoid bone	UP/UC	protein:creatinine ratio
PSSM	polysaccharide storage myopathy	URT	upper respiratory tract
PT	prothrombin time	UV	ultraviolet
PTT	partial thromboplastin time		
PTH	parathyroid hormone	VC	vulval conformation
PU/PD	polyuria/polydipsia	VD	ventrodorsal
		VEE	Venezuelan equine encephalitis
RAO	recurrent airway obstruction	VLDLs	very low-density lipoproteins
RAST	radioallergosorbent test	VSD	ventricular septal defect
RBC	red blood cell		
RDPPA	rostral displacement of the palatopharyngeal arch	WBC	white blood cell
		WEE	Western equine encephalitis
RDW	red cell distribution width	WNV	West Nile virus
REM	rapid eye movement		
RPE	retinal pigment-epithelium		
RT-PCR	reverse transcriptase-polymerase chain reaction		
RTA	renal tubular acidosis		
s/c	subcutaneous, subcutaneously		
SCC	squamous cell carcinoma		
SCID	severe combined immunodeficiency		
SDFT	superficial digital flexor tendon		
SDH	sorbitol dehydrogenase		
SDSL	straight distal sesamoidean ligament		
SFT	Society of Fertility and Theriogenology (USA)		
SG	specific gravity		
SIRS	systemic inflammatory response syndrome		
SLE	systemic lupus erythematosus		
SPL	subpalpebral lavage (system)		
SRH	single radial hemolysis		
SRID	serial radial immunodiffusion (assay)		

Musculoskeletal system

1   Approach to the lame horse
Cedric Chan and Graham Munroe

2   The foal and developing animal
Cedric Chan and Graham Munroe

3   The foot
Andrew Parks

4   The forelimb
Peter Milner

5   The hindlimb
Ehud Eliashar

6   The head
Martin Weaver

7   The axial skeleton
Martin Weaver

8   Soft-tissue injuries
Eddy Cauvin

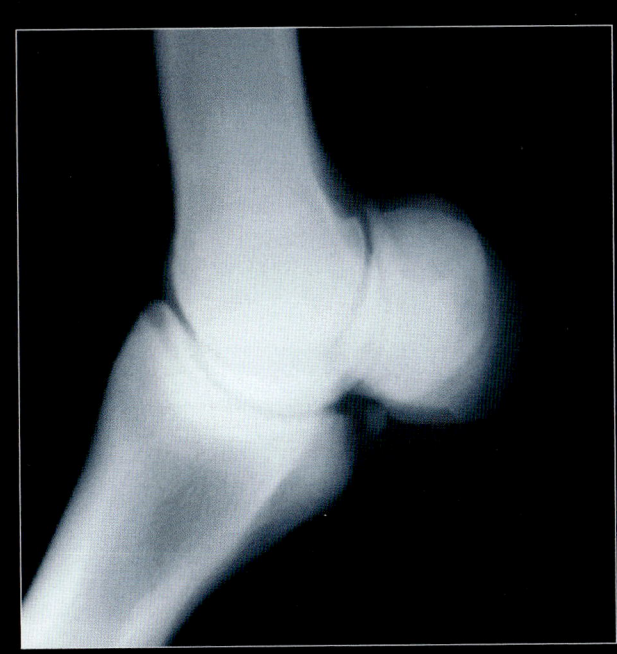

1 Approach to the lame horse

Lameness is common in all types of horse and is defined as an alteration in the animal's normal stance and/or mode of progression caused by pain or neural or mechanical dysfunction. The approach to the lame horse should ideally be carried out in a logical sequence in order to a) define which limb or limbs are involved and b) find the exact site of pain. Only then can other techniques such as radiography or more advanced imaging (e.g. bone scintigraphy or MRI) be used to determine a specific pathologic process and make a diagnosis. Once a provisional or accurate diagnosis is made, a management plan can be formulated and a prognosis given to the owner. In practice, many factors may alter this sequence slightly (e.g. environment where the examination is taking place, financial considerations, impending competition).

History

Obtaining an accurate history is essential and this requires careful questioning, as some of the information supplied can be quite subjective. It should begin with the signalment of the case. Age, sex, breed, and use of the horse can suggest certain particular conditions. For example, developmental orthopedic conditions are seen in young horses, tibial stress fractures are seen in young racing Thoroughbreds in training, and navicular syndrome is usually seen in adult horses used for general riding and sport horse activities. The length of ownership or training, as well as the type and amount of work the horse has been given, is useful basic information.

Previous lameness problems should be noted. A history of previous arthroscopic surgery for an apical chip sesamoid fracture 1 year ago may be significant in a horse that is still lame in the operated limb due to, for example, associated chronic suspensory branch desmitis.

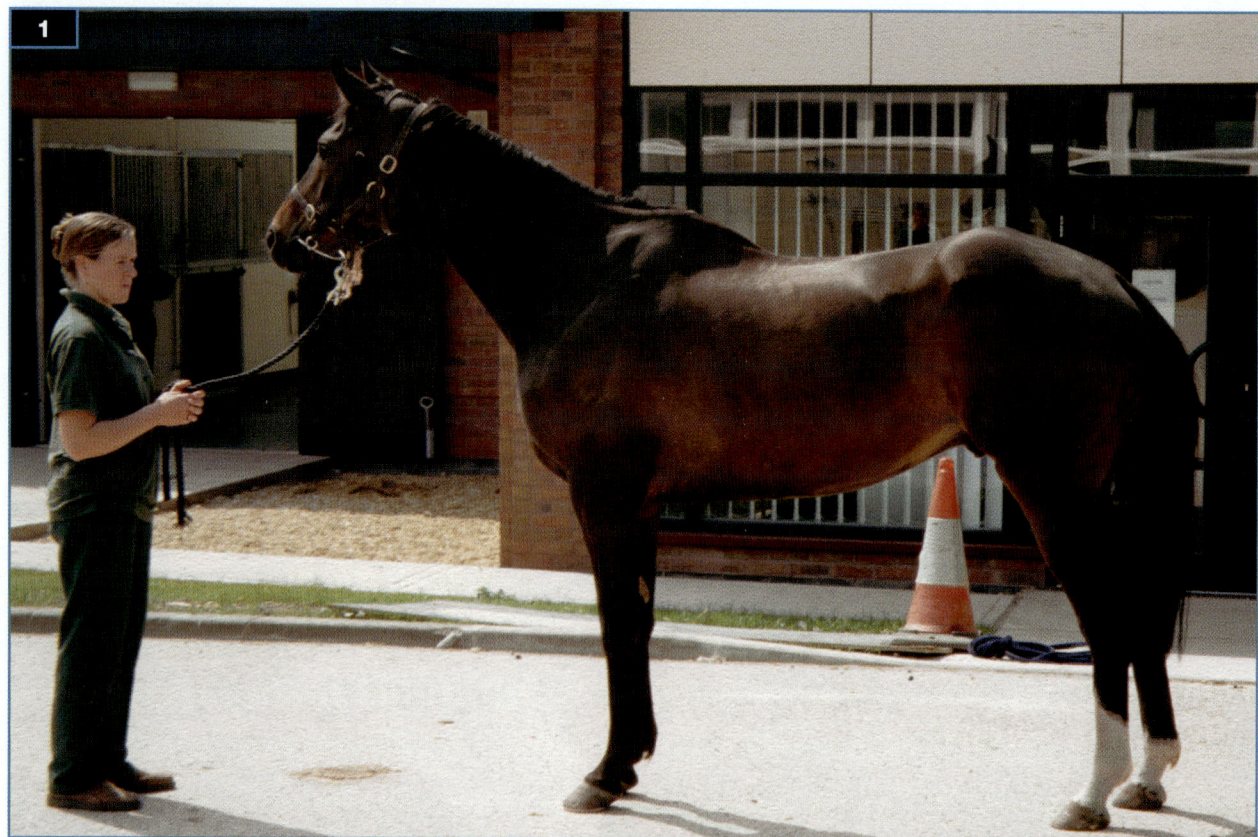

Musculoskeletal system

To discuss the present lameness problem, questions should include when (duration of lameness) and where (at pasture or in competition) the lameness was first noted; has the lameness improved or worsened with rest; which limb do the owners think is affected or what are they noticing when the horse is ridden; were any traumatic episodes associated (kick injury or striking a fence on jumping) with onset of lameness; any other associations (e.g. recent change in shoeing for nail-bind, turn out to lush pasture for a high-risk laminitic pony); and any obvious regions of heat or swellings noted by the owner. The owner should be asked if the lameness improves or deteriorates with exercise. It is prudent to ascertain if any treatment or shoeing has been tried by the owner before examination that might change or mask the current presentation (e.g. the administration of pain killers to a possible synovial sepsis from a small penetrating injury).

Clinical examination

At rest

The horse should be visually inspected, ideally standing square on a level surface, from both sides, front and behind for overall conformation, signs of asymmetry of the muscles and bones, swelling, sites of trauma, foot conformation, and stance (1–3). The conformation of a horse affects the way it moves at all gaits and there are certain types of conformation in certain breeds and disciplines of horse that may predispose to lameness (e.g. straight hindlimb conformation may predispose a horse to upward fixation of the patella or proximal suspensory ligament desmitis). Foot conformation is important in the incidence of foot lameness. Evaluation of pastern and foot angle (dorsopalmar/plantar hoof balance), mediolateral foot balance, and foot symmetry/shape is important because it

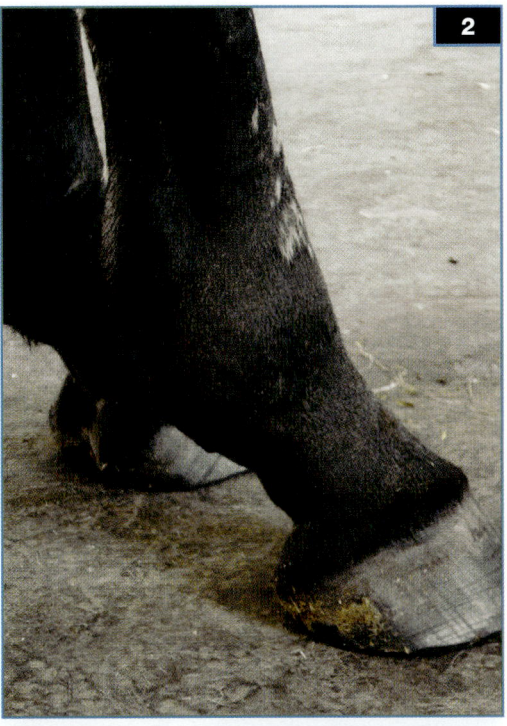

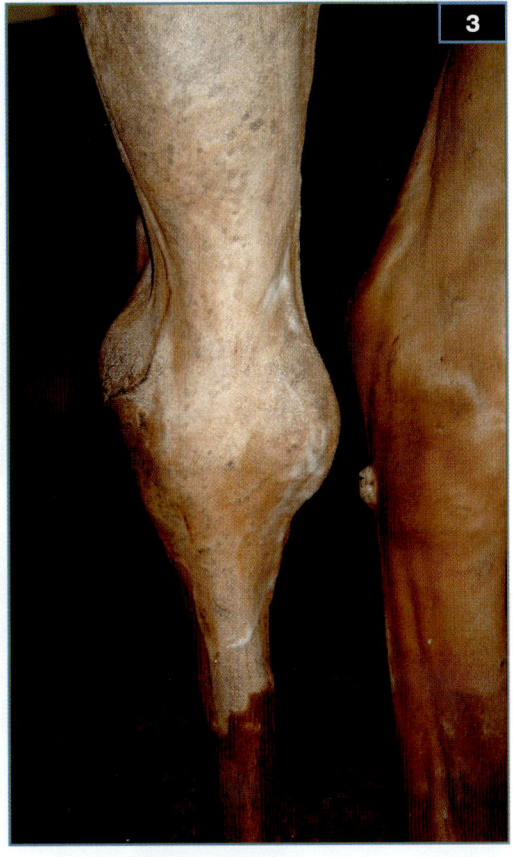

1 Initial examination of a Thoroughbred racehorse with hindlimb and back problems. The horse is stood squarely on a hard surface and is examined from each side, behind, and in front for stance, swellings, muscle wastage, and conformation.

2 Observation of a right hindlimb fetlock illustrating a markedly distended digital sheath. A diagnosis of chronic digital tenosynovitis and annular ligament syndrome was made after the results of diagnostic analgesia, radiography, and ultrasonography.

3 A distended tarsocrural joint in the right hindlimb of a horse with lameness, which was localized to the joint by intra-articular analgesia.

13

determines the load distribution of the structures in the foot and elsewhere within the limb (4–7). For example, a broken-back foot pastern axis and low heel conformation are commonly associated with palmar foot pain and conditions of the DIP joint (8). Comparing sizes of opposite feet is important; a smaller foot compared with the contralateral foot may indicate chronic lameness in that limb. Any hoof horn defects (e.g. hoof cracks) should be noted (9).

The posture or stance may indicate the horse's response to acute or chronic pain in one or more limbs (10) (e.g. a non-weight-bearing lameness due to a simple foot abscess or a long-bone fracture, or subtle unloading of the limb in chronic intertarsal joint pain of the hindlimb). More specifically, a dropped elbow posture is indicative of a loss of function of the triceps apparatus, most likely due to radial paralysis or olecranon fractures (11).

4–7 Observation of both forefeet at rest from both sides (4, 5), the front (6), and behind (7) for conformation. Note the contracted right forefoot and the long toe/low heel conformation of both forefeet. A diagnosis of chronic palmar hoof pain of navicular bone origin was made after the results of diagnostic analgesia and radiography.

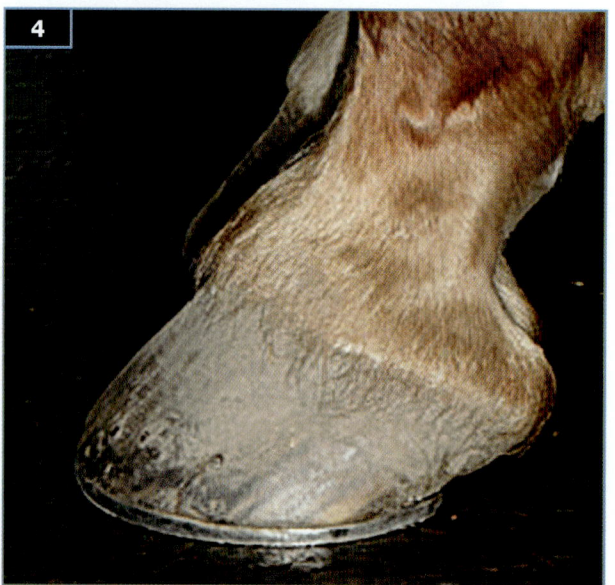
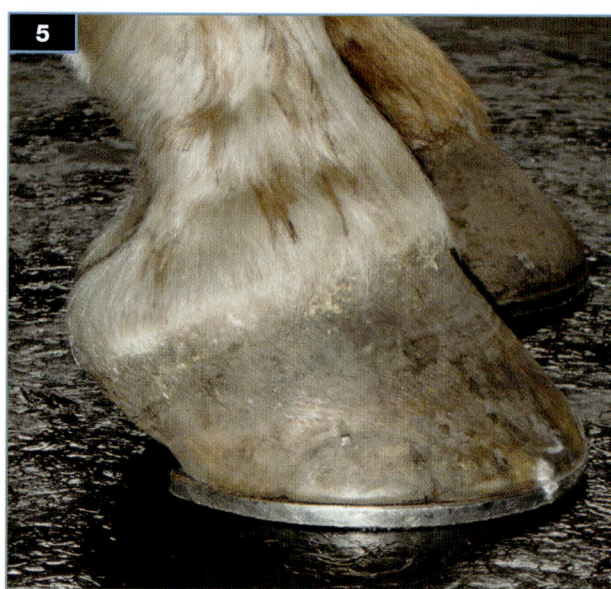
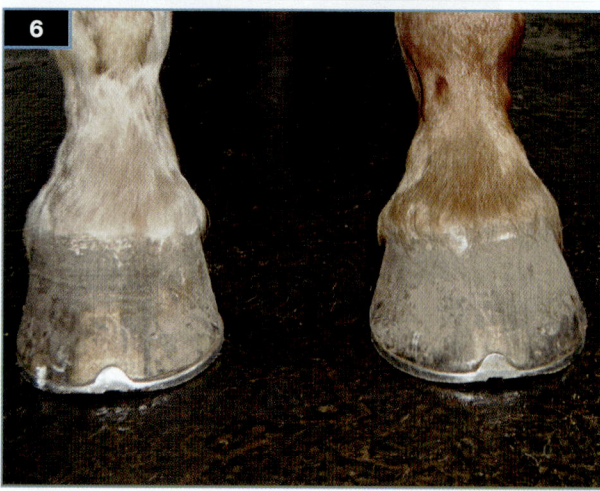
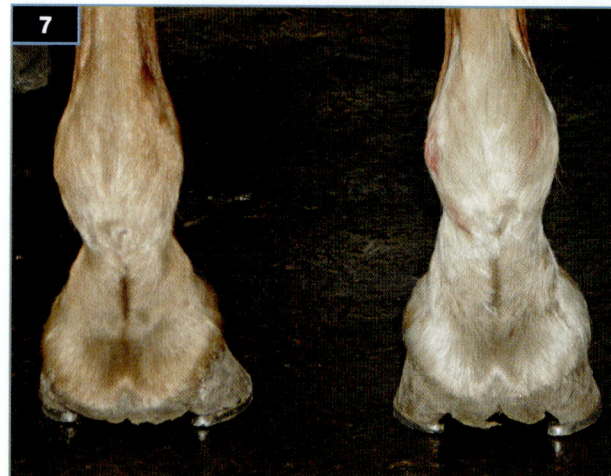

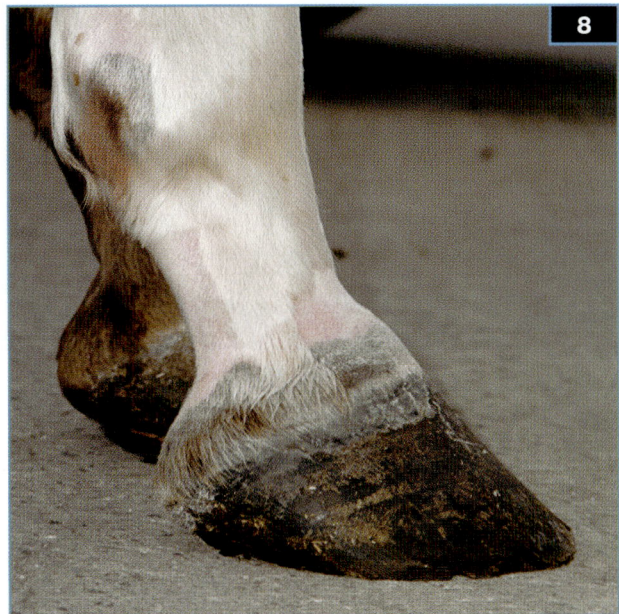

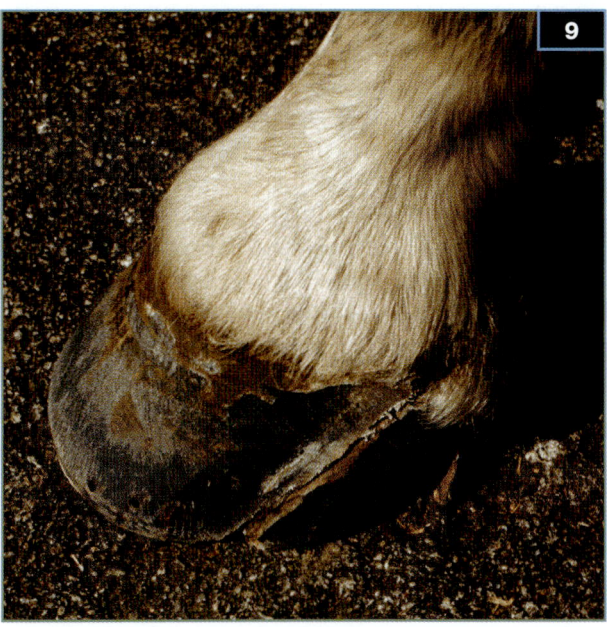

8 A long-toed, low-heeled front foot conformation leading to a broken-back hoof pastern axis. Note the distal interphalangeal joint distension dorsally above the coronary band.

9 This horse suffered a severe trauma to the coronary band and hoof of this foot several years ago. It is now left with a permanent injury to the coronary band, which is leading to a crack in the quarter of the hoof.

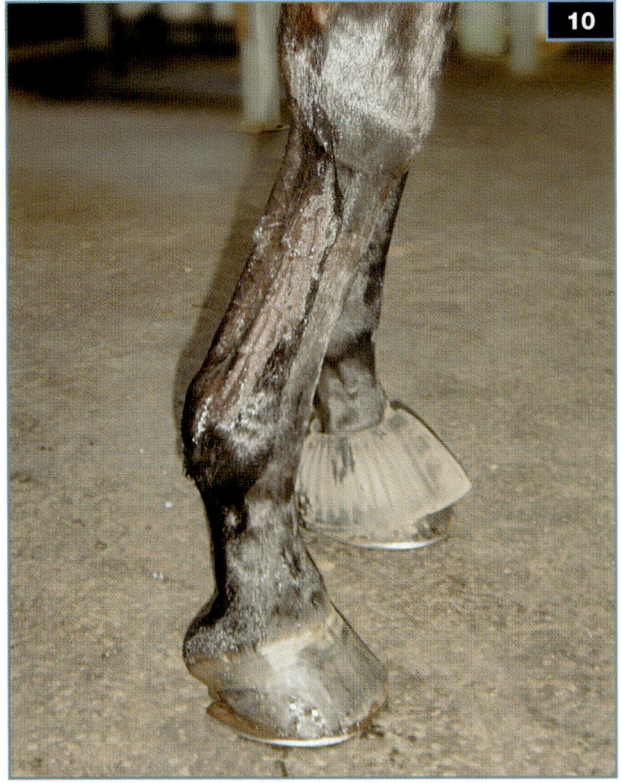

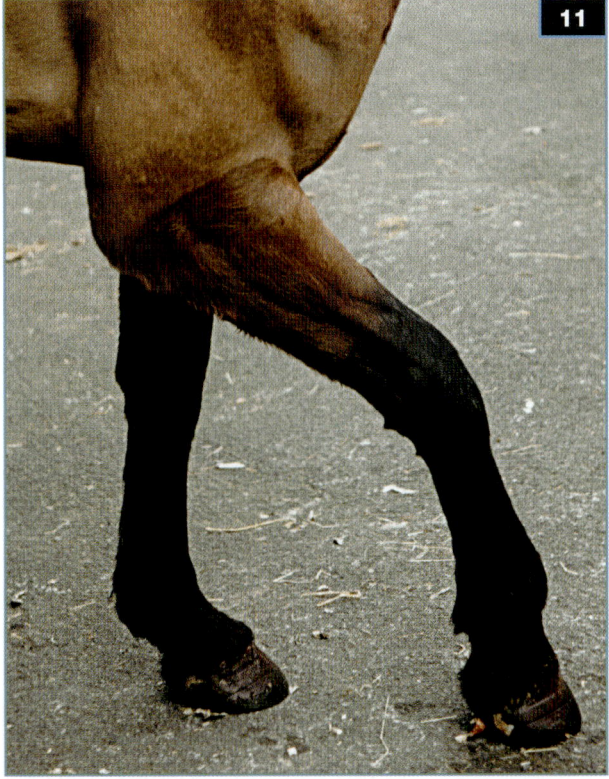

10 Observation of the forelimb stance of a horse from the right side. Note the acquired carpal contracture of the right forelimb in this case of a chronic proximal suspensory ligament insertional desmitis of over 2-years' duration.

11 Note the dropped elbow with flexed carpus and fetlock seen in this horse, which is exhibiting temporary radial nerve paresis post a general anesthesia in right lateral recumbency.

Approach to the lame horse

Palpation of the affected limb(s) adds information to the visual appraisal. A knowledge of normal musculoskeletal anatomy is a prerequisite, although comparison with the contralateral limb may be useful, unless the condition is bilateral (e.g. osteochondrosis dissecans of both tarsocrural joints might exhibit bilateral tarsocrural joint distension). If time permits, all the limbs, both weight-bearing and held off the ground, the neck, and the back should be palpated sequentially regardless of the suspected lame limb suggested by the owner, unless an obvious reason merits further inspection (e.g. a recent wound). The cardinal signs of inflammation of heat, swelling, and pain are noted. Normal reaction to gentle digital pressure versus that of flinching to pain should be assessed. It is common in Thoroughbreds for there to be excessive reaction to palpation of the distal suspensory ligaments without evidence of any pathology. Careful repeat examination of the area, or palpation in the same area of the contralateral limb, will help differentiate the significance of findings. The ground bearing surface of the foot is inspected carefully for any abnormalities (e.g. underrun heels) when the limb is off the ground. If the horse is shod, the shoe is inspected for type, wear, and nail placement. Hoof testers can be used to assess solar reaction and their application across the frog and heels may reveal sites of pain. The shoe should be removed and the foot inspected further if there is evidence of a foot-related condition. The digital pulse to the feet should be palpated. Bounding pulses are commonly felt in acute laminitis, subsolar abscesses, or bruising (12), and pedal bone fractures.

At exercise

Lameness is generally assessed from in front (for forelimbs) (13) and behind (for hindlimbs) (14) at the walk and trot, in-hand, and in a straight line on a level, hard, even surface. The movement of the whole horse and individual limbs should be evaluated, including foot placement and breakover, and examination from the side of the horse can reveal a shortened stride length and a lowered foot flight arc in a lame limb. Additionally, if lameness is subtle or there is multiple limb involvement, watching the horse move in circles on the lunge at the trot is useful. A comparison between movement on a circle on a soft and hard surface is also helpful, particularly in increasing the degree of lameness in some cases (15). Examination of the horse at higher speeds, such as the canter and gallop, and when ridden/driven are necessary if the lameness has only been noticed in those situations (16).

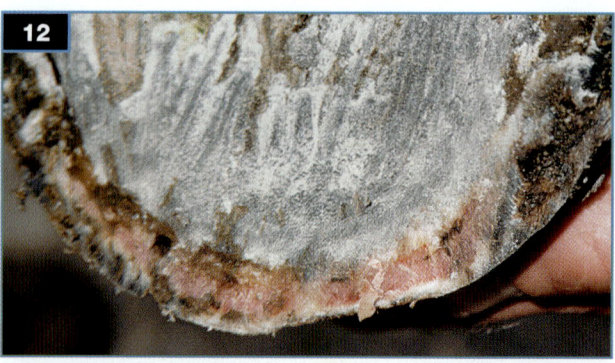

12 This horse presented with an acute-onset, moderate lameness of a forelimb, which was localized to the foot by hoof tester reaction, and a strong digital pulse. After removal of the shoe, clear areas of fresh subsolar and white line hemorrhage are visible at the toe underneath where the shoe was placed.

Symmetrical movement is the normal situation in the sound horse and appreciating a change in this is the key to starting to identify the lameness and the limb(s) involved. In general, with a weight-bearing forelimb lameness, a 'head nod' is appreciated with the head being raised when the lame limb strikes the ground. In the hindlimbs, a 'hip hike' (also termed 'pelvic hike') is present in the lame hindlimb. The pelvis 'hikes' upward when the lame hindlimb hits the ground and moves downward when the sound limb hits the ground. It is easier for some clinicians to see a downward movement of the pelvis on the side of the lame limb as it leaves the ground. 'Fetlock drop' or extension of the fetlock joint may also be helpful in recognition of the lame limb. Generally, the fetlock joint of the sound limb drops farther when weight bearing than does the fetlock joint of the lame limb. In some instances of more severe unilateral hindlimb lameness it may appear that the ipsilateral forelimb is lame due to the horse shifting its weight forward in compensation. Video recording of a lame horse in motion, particularly when later evaluation of the recording is made in slow motion, can provide a good baseline for visualizing lameness.

Lameness is graded to indicate severity, commonly on a scale of 0–5 or 0–10, where 0 is sound and 5 out of 5 or 10 out of 10 is non-weight-bearing.

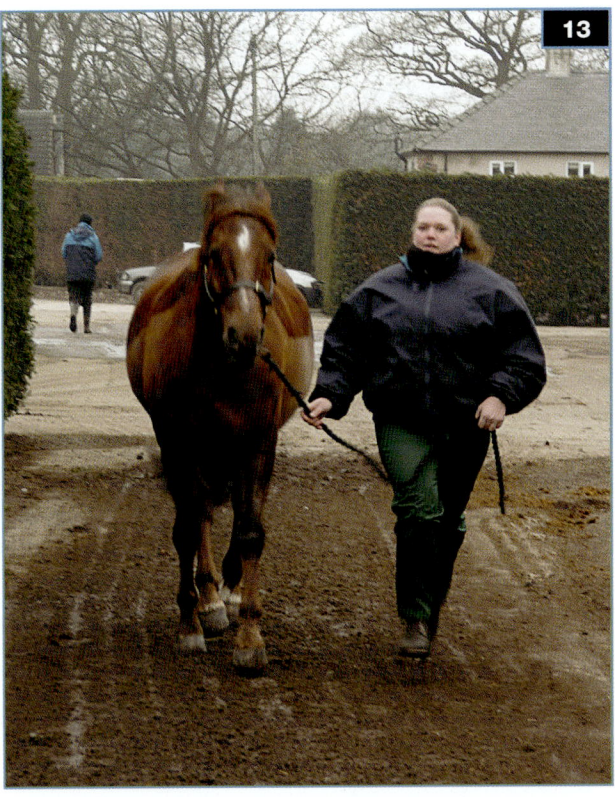

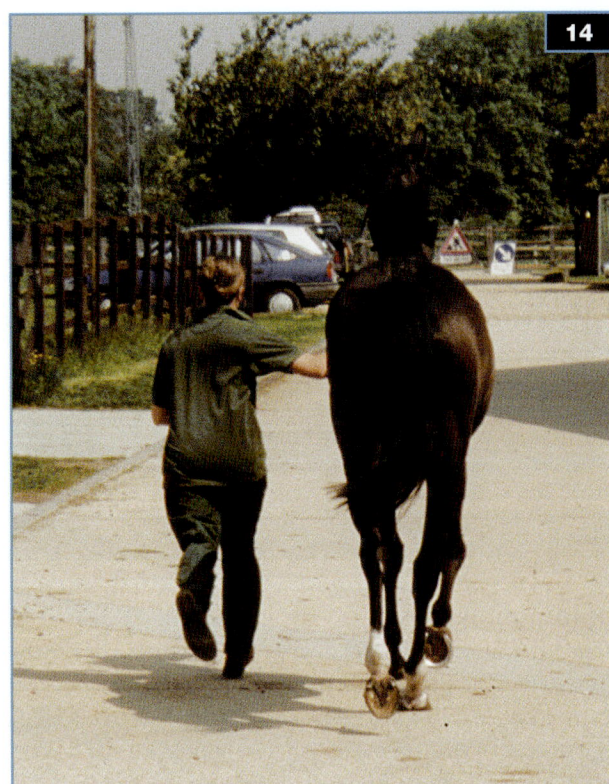

13, 14 Trotting a horse towards the examining veterinarian on a firm level gravel surface (13). Note the loose way the horse is led to allow any movement of the head to be clearly seen. Horses that are lame should always be examined from in front, behind, and the side (14).

15 Lungeing exercise on a soft and/or hard surface can be useful to give a further baseline lameness to record before embarking on diagnostic analgesia as part of a full lameness examination.

16 Examination of a dressage horse under saddle to assess all movements and to discuss with the rider what they can feel in relation to what the veterinarian observes.

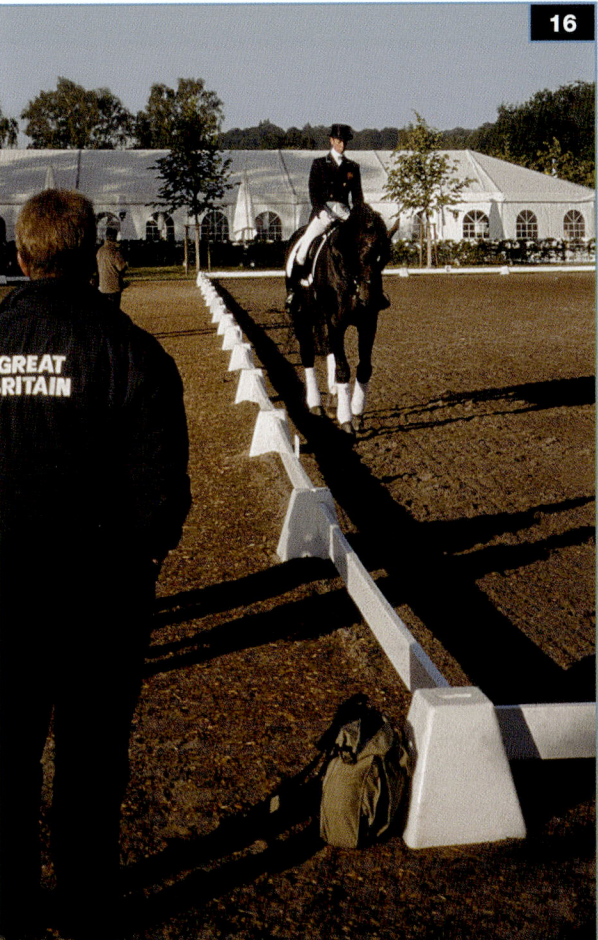

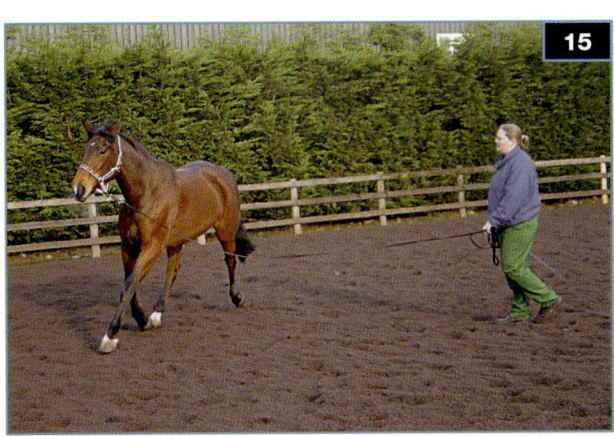

Approach to the lame horse

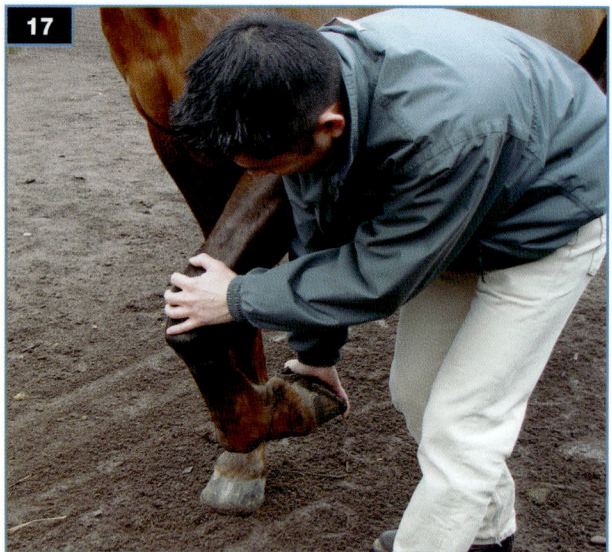

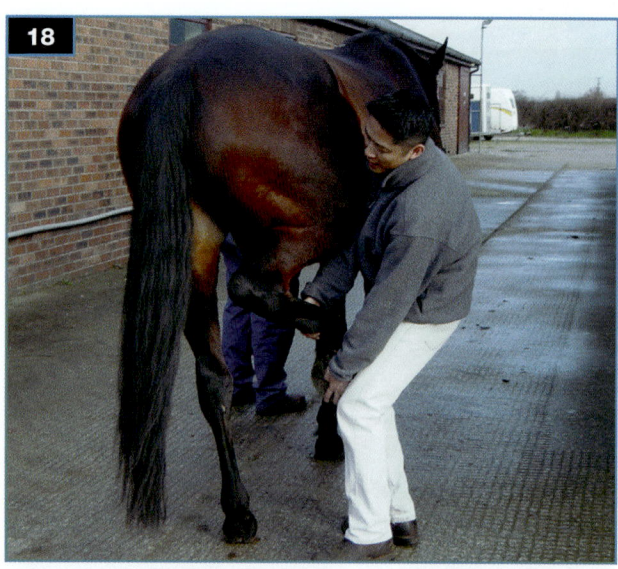

Manipulative tests

Once the lame limb and degree of lameness have been ascertained, identification of the site(s) of the lameness is carried out. Manipulative tests aim to exacerbate temporarily the degree of lameness. Flexion tests should ideally be performed on all pairs of limbs for comparison, but lastly on the lame limb. Any increase in severity is noted. The time and force required to carry out flexion tests are personal, but should be consistent. Generally 45–60 seconds with mild force is used. The horse is trotted away from, and back to, the examiner immediately after the test for 10–15 meters. A persistent increase in lameness over baseline is positive. (Note that it may not be appropriate to carry out flexion tests on severely lame horses such as suspect fracture cases.)

Forelimb flexion tests may be divided into full, distal/lower (**17**), carpal, and proximal/upper limb depending on the joints flexed:

✦ A full forelimb flexion test aims to flex all the joints by supporting the limb at the toe with the cannon and radius parallel to the ground.
✦ A distal forelimb flexion test aims to flex the foot and fetlock by supporting the limb at the toe with the carpus at around 90 degrees, and with minimum flexion of the elbow and shoulder joints.
✦ A carpal flexion test aims to flex mainly the carpus by holding the cannon parallel to the ground, and allowing the distal joints to remain unflexed.
✦ A proximal forelimb flexion test flexes mainly the shoulder joint, and involves holding the limb at the radius and pulling the entire limb caudally and slightly proximally.

17 Right forelimb distal limb flexion test. Note how the carpus is kept as minimally flexed as possible.

18 Full right hindlimb flexion test. Note how all the joints are flexed, with the limb directly underneath the horse.

Similarly, hindlimb flexion tests can also be divided in this way into full, distal/lower, and proximal/upper (also called hock or 'spavin' test):

✦ In a full flexion test the limb is supported at the toe with the cannon and tibia parallel to the ground (**18**).
✦ A distal hindlimb flexion test consists of flexing the foot and fetlock by supporting the limb at the toe with the cannon perpendicular to the ground and the hock and stifle at 90 degrees.
✦ A proximal hindlimb flexion test involves supporting the limb at the cannon parallel to the ground and held fully flexed at the hock and stifle.
✦ A hip abduction test is used by some clinicians to abduct the hindlimb away from the horse in order to test the hip region, but it can be dangerous and must be used with care.

Due to the reciprocal apparatus of the hindlimb, flexion tests may not be as specific as in the forelimb.

Extension tests may also be carried out to exacerbate a degree of lameness in a certain region. For example, placement of a reverse heel wedge under a foot is used by some clinicians to evaluate suspected caudal hoof pain.

Evaluation at the trot after direct digital pressure to a painful region (e.g. over a collateral ligament insertion) or after hoof tester application to a suspicious region of the solar surface of the foot may sometimes be useful manipulative tests.

Diagnosis

Diagnostic analgesia

Diagnostic analgesia (perineural nerve blocks, local infiltration, and intrasynovial joint/sheath/bursa blocks) is used to abolish lameness temporarily in the limb being investigated and thereby further isolate a site of pain. The most commonly used local anesthetics are mepivicaine and prilocaine. Only lameness due to pain (i.e. not mechanical or neurologic types of lameness) are suitable for this approach to lameness diagnosis. The blocks should ideally be carried out sequentially, starting distally and progressing proximally (19). The selection of blocks is based on the previous clinical examination. For example, if a forelimb foot lameness is suspected, a palmar digital nerve block may be carried out first. If marked joint distension is present in the metacarpophalangeal (MCP) joint, and a markedly positive fetlock flexion test is observed, intrasynovial analgesia of the MCP joint may be appropriate. If no apparent signs for a particular region are identified from previous examinations, it is prudent to start as distally as possible and work proximally with perineural analgesia techniques. Note that in suspected fracture cases, diagnostic analgesia may be contraindicated and examination should continue with survey radiographs of the region under suspicion.

A partial or complete response to diagnostic analgesia warrants further investigation of that region by appropriate diagnostic imaging such as radiography. If a contralateral limb lameness is revealed, this limb should be examined with diagnostic analgesia, starting distally as before. Imaging is then carried out after the site of lameness in this limb is confirmed (e.g. bilateral forefoot lameness).

The sites for perineural nerve blocks should be cleaned and can be clipped if identification of anatomic landmarks is difficult or the coat is dirty. For all intrasynovial blocks, aseptic precautions, after clipping the hair, are a prerequisite for this technique. Physical restraint and consideration of personnel safety are advisable in the majority of horses. The authors routinely place a nose twitch if the horse tolerates this and may have an assistant lift a contralateral limb for forelimb blocks or ipsilateral forelimb for hindlimb blocks. Chemical restraint is occasionally required for intractable horses, and the use of intravenous acepromazine or shorter-acting alpha-2 agonists (e.g. xylazine) is advised. The dosage required depends on the individual animal's behavior. The horse is re-examined once the sedation has worn off, usually after 20–45 minutes. If this approach is necessary, it may be advisable to use longer-acting local anesthetics such as bupivacaine. Horses are usually re-examined 10 minutes after blocking, at the trot in a straight line and/or on the lunge. This minimum

19 This horse has had sequential regional and intra-articular analgesia carried out up to the level of the stifle joints in an effort to localize the source of the hindlimb lameness.

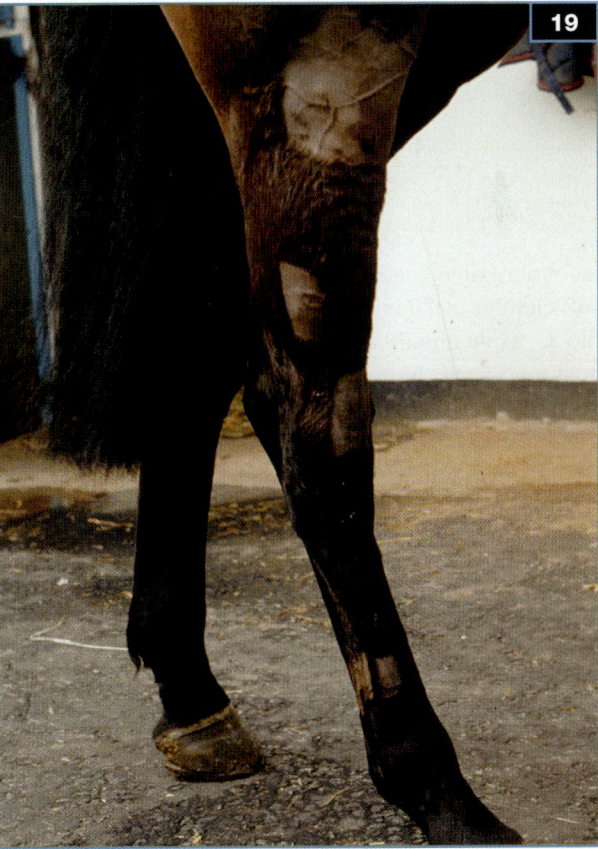

TABLE 1 More commonly used perineural nerve blocks, local infiltration, and intrasynovial blocks for the forelimb and hindlimb

	FORELIMB	HINDLIMB
Perineural blocks	Palmar digital	Plantar digital
	Abaxial sesamoid	Abaxial sesamoid
	Low 4-point	Low 6-point
	High 4-point (subcarpal)	Deep branch of the lateral plantar nerve
	Lateral palmar	High 6-point
	Median/ulnar/musculocutaneous	Tibial/superficial and deep fibular (peroneal) (21)
Local infiltration	Painful exostoses including 'splints'	Painful exostoses including 'splints'
	Origin of the suspensory ligament	Origin of the suspensory ligament
		Dorsal spinous processes (22)
		Sacroiliac region
Intrasynovial blocks	Navicular bursa (20)	Navicular bursa
	Distal interphalangeal joint	Distal interphalangeal joint
	Proximal interphalangeal joint	Proximal interphalangeal joint
	Metacarpophalangeal joint	Metatarsophalangeal joint
	Digital sheath	Digital sheath
	Intercarpal joint (communicates with the carpometacarpal joint)	Tarsometatarsal joint
	Antebrachiocarpal joint	Central tarsal joint
	Carpal sheath	Tarsocrural joint
	Humeroradial joint	Tarsal sheath
	Bicipital bursa	Femoropatellar joint
	Scapulohumeral joint	Medial femorotibial joint
		Lateral femorotibial joint
		Coxofemoral joint

amount of time generally allows the nerve targeted to be sufficiently anesthetized to allow interpretation of the block, while minimizing the spread of the drug to other anatomic sites. Intrasynovial blocks such as the large scapulohumeral and stifle joints are re-examined after a longer period of time (30–60 minutes) by some clinicians. Certain perineural nerve blocks may be tested for efficacy by loss of skin sensation prior to re-examination (e.g. lightly pressing a pen into the bulbs of the heel is normally strongly resented by the horse, but is not felt after successful palmar digital nerve block). Interpretation of the results of diagnostic analgesia are based on a knowledge of which region the block desensitizes (*Table 1*).

Synovial fluid collection and analysis

Sites for diagnostic intrasynovial (joint/sheath/bursa) analgesia may also be used for synovial fluid collection for analysis if this is indicated (e.g. suspicion of a synovial septic process). Clipping the hair and aseptic preparation of the collection site are mandatory (23). The fluid is aspirated and placed in EDTA and plain tubes for analysis.

Visual assessment of normal joint fluid reveals it to be slightly viscous and a clear, straw color. Fluid from inflamed joints tends to be less viscous due to a depletion of hyaluronan, but a similar color to normal. Degrees of hemorrhage will be present depending on sampling technique or the presence of a hemarthrosis. Septic fluid is also less viscous and often cloudy and discolored (24). Small amounts of fibrin may be present. Parameters routinely measured include cytology and total protein concentration. Cytologic analysis is most useful for identifying and

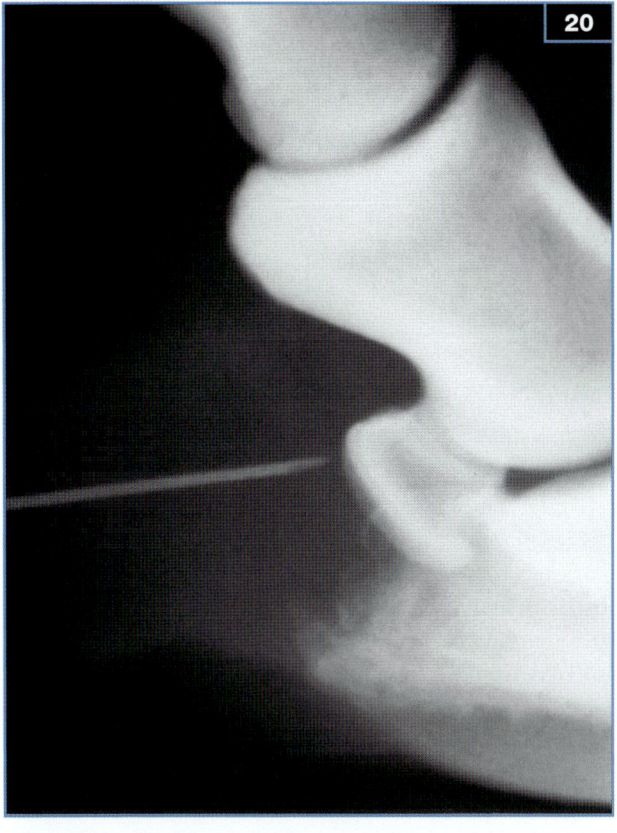

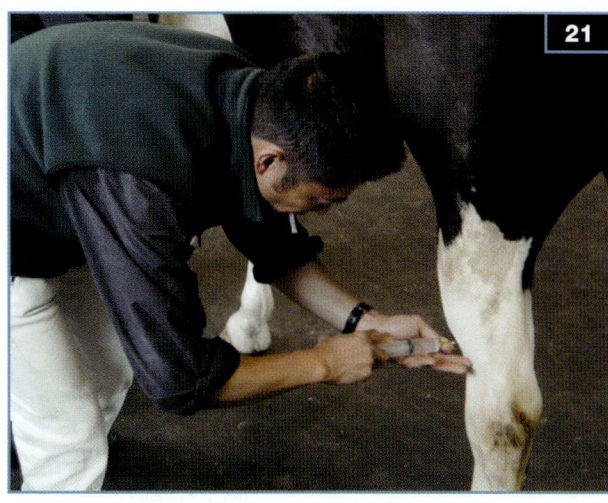

20 Lateromedial radiograph of the foot confirming the correct placement of a needle into the navicular bursa before the local anesthetic is injected.

21 An example of diagnostic analgesic technique. The left hindlimb superficial and deep peroneal (fibular) nerves are being injected with local anesthetic as part of analgesia of the tarsus and entire distal hindlimb. This nerve block is routinely combined with a tibial nerve block.

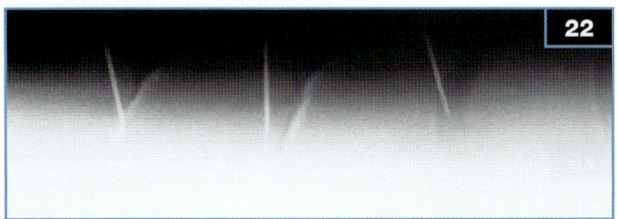

22 Lateromedial radiograph of the dorsal spinous processes of a horse with back pain showing needles in the interspinous spaces prior to the injection of local anesthetic. The horse responded very clearly to the local infiltration.

23 Synoviocentesis of a septic fetlock joint in a foal under general anesthesia prior to regional antibiotic perfusion.

24 A syringe of synovial fluid aspirated from the distended metacarpo-phalangeal joint of a very lame Thoroughbred yearling that had sustained a wound in the region of the fetlock 48 hours earlier. Note the very turbid and discolored synovial fluid that had a WBC count of $> 100 \times 10^9/1$.

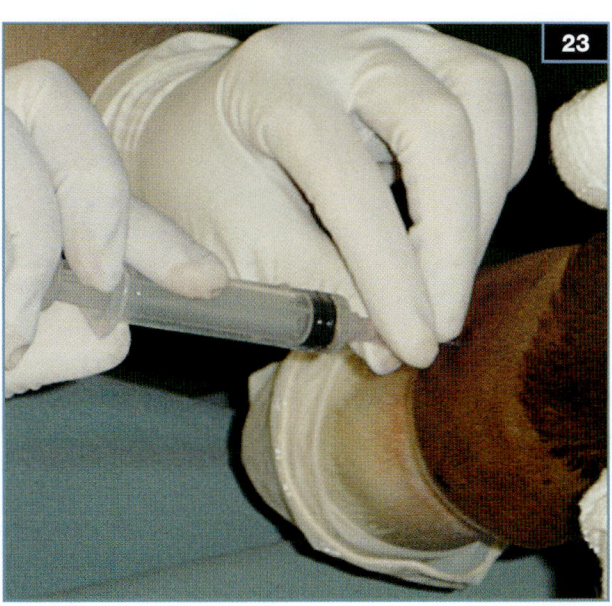

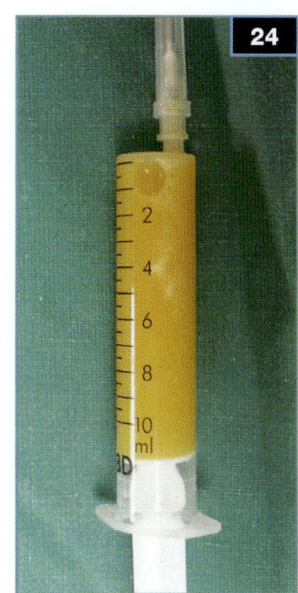

Approach to the lame horse

TABLE 2	**Synovial fluid cytology reference ranges**			
	APPEARANCE	TOTAL WBCS (x 10^9/l)	NEUTROPHILS	TOTAL PROTEIN (g/l)
Normal	Clear Straw colored	≤0.5	<10%	<20
Sepsis	Turbid Degenerate	15–150	>90%	30–60
OA	Pale yellow	≤1.0	10–15%	<25
OCD	Pale yellow	0.5–1.0	10–30%	<25
Acute trauma (e.g. intra-articular fracture)	Serosanguineous	3–10	<10%	<30

monitoring sepsis or postinjection reactions. Total protein concentrations normally tend to be higher in the larger joints. Hyaluronan concentration is not normally measured since there is a large variation between individual horses. Polymerase chain reaction (PCR) analysis may be useful in the near future to reveal bacterial DNA in suspected septic joint samples where cytology is equivocal. The normal parameters of synovial fluid and ranges for certain conditions are shown in *Table 2*.

Radiography

Radiography is the most common diagnostic imaging modality used for the musculoskeletal system. Images are produced by X-rays that are attenuated by the different tissues in the region of interest onto film inside a lightproof cassette lined with a special screen that intensifies the image. The film is then processed to give the final black and white radiographic image for interpretation. The total number of X-rays produced (mAs) and ability of the X-ray

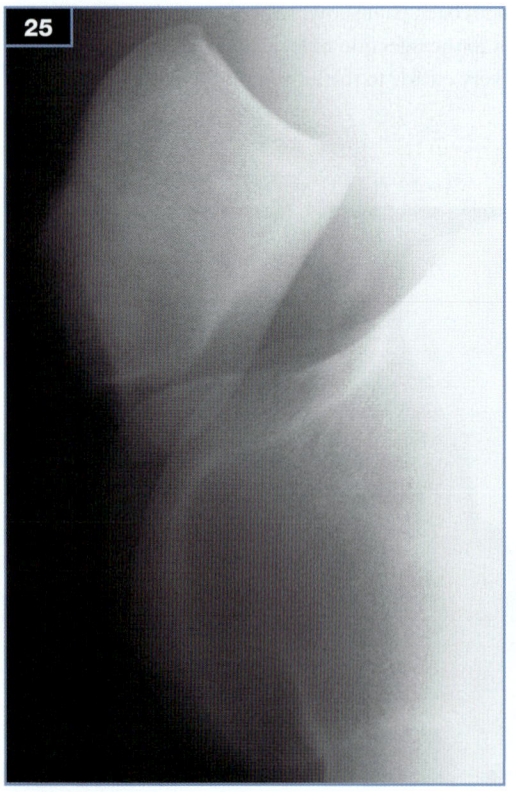

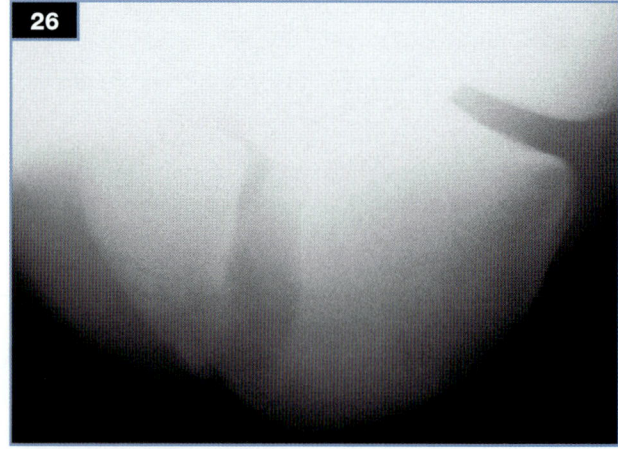

25 Lateromedial radiograph of the stifle of a horse with an acute and severe lameness. There was swelling of the femoropatellar joint and patella. Although the craniodistal aspect of the patella appears abnormal, it is not clear what has happened in this horse.

26 This flexed cranioproximal/craniodistal oblique (skyline) view of the stifle of the horse in 25 clearly shows a parasagittal fracture of the patella.

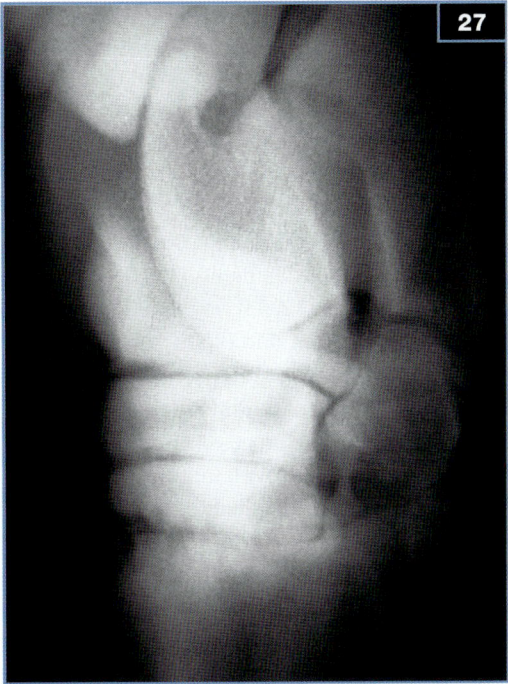

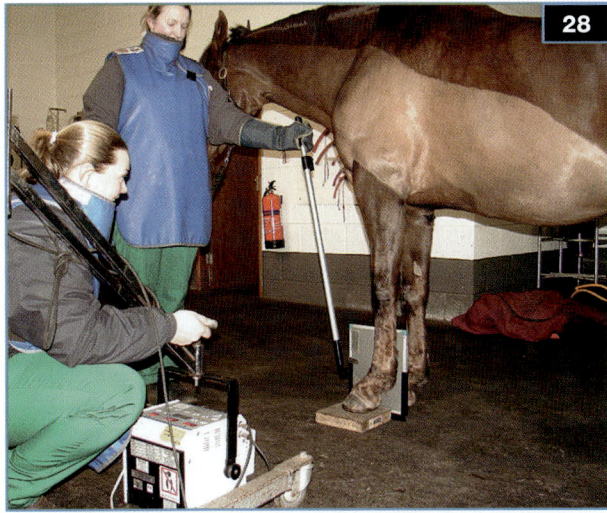

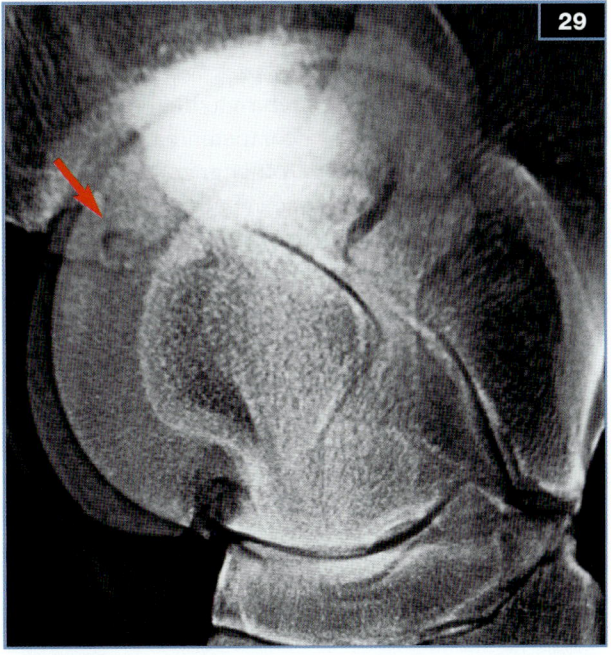

27 Standard radiograph of a dorsolateral/plantaromedial oblique projection of a tarsus illustrating degenerative joint disease of the small tarsal joints ('bone spavin'). Note the joint collapse, periarticular new bone formation, and subchondral bone lysis and surrounding sclerosis.

28 Lateral radiograph of the foot is being taken. Note the radiation safety measures and that the foot is raised off the ground to assist in correct positioning.

29 Digital radiograph of a lateromedial projection of a tarsus showing osteochondral fragmentation of the distal intermediate ridge of the tibia in a young horse. (Photo courtesy Clinique Vétérinaire Equine, Falaise, France)

to penetrate tissue (kV), which are set on the radiographic unit, combined with the film focal distance (FFD) determine the exposure and quality of the film. Different film/screen combinations can be used to provide different detail. Mineralized structures are radiodense and absorb many of the X-rays of the primary beam, whereas soft tissues are more radiolucent, and these differences are reflected on the final film.

Multiple projections are necessary since a 2-D image of a 3-D structure is produced (**25, 26**). Plain radiography refers to a standard radiograph and is used routinely (**27**). Contrast radiography refers to the placement of a metallic probe or radiodense contrast material (e.g. nonionic, water-soluble compounds such as iohexol) into a specific region to highlight certain pathology. More specifically,

contrast arthrography refers to injection of contrast material into a joint space (carried out in an aseptic manner). For example, contrast radiography can be useful for confirming synovial wound penetration where the results of clinical examination are equivocal. Note that contrast material can also be injected into tendon sheaths, bursae, and fistulous tracts. Radiography is conveniently carried out in an ambulatory or clinic situation and a range of mobile and fixed gantry machines are available (**28**). Recently, digital radiography (CR and DR systems) using computer processing hard and software has become available, allowing the veterinarian to collect the radiograph digitally and further edit afterwards (**29**). This allows better image collection and manipulation, reduces the number of exposures needed to completely examine

Approach to the lame horse

the targeted area, and allows easier image storage on CD and digital image transfer (e.g. by email to colleagues in other locations). Note that X-rays are a radiation hazard and radiation safety is essential to protect personnel and to comply with health and safety regulations. These include using long-handled cassette holders where possible, reducing the number of personnel present during radiographic examination to the minimum required to obtain the radiograph required, collimation of the primary X-ray beam to reduce scatter, and the routine wearing of lead-lined protective gowns, gloves and thyroid shields (see **28**). Film badges should be worn and checked regularly to monitor personnel X-ray total exposure.

Ultrasonography

Ultrasonography relies on the emission of high-frequency sound waves by electrically stimulated piezoelectric crystals in a transducer that are transmitted through the region of interest via a probe. The sound waves are attenuated by the different tissues and reflected back to the transducer as echoes. The reflected waves return to the probe and are electronically passed on to a computer that formulates a visual image of the tissues. A 2-D gray scale real-time image representing the acoustic impedance of the tissues scanned is produced for interpretation. Different frequencies determine the detail and depth of the image acquired. The higher the frequency (mHz) rating the better the

resolution (detail) but the less the penetration (depth). A 7.5 Mhz linear probe is the most common probe used in equine musculoskeletal ultrasound examinations. The term hypoechoic denotes a decreased echogenicity of the tissue (darker image), anechoic denotes no echogenicity (i.e. fluid [black image]), and hyperechoic denotes an increased echogenicity (brighter image).

Ultrasonography is most commonly used to image soft tissue structures (e.g. tendons, ligaments [30, 31], joint capsules, and synovial linings [32, 33], localized soft tissue swellings [34], muscles, nerves, and blood vessels). Transverse and longitudinal images are essential in order to allow complete examination of tendinous tissue in particular. Monitoring of the healing process is routinely carried out with ultrasonography and provides information to help recommend an appropriate rehabilitation. It is also useful for imaging bone and joint contours (e.g. ilium for ilial wing fractures) and articular cartilage in articulations such as the femoropatellar joint for osteochondrosis. It can guide biopsy or injection techniques such as interspinous anti-inflammatory injections for impingement of the dorsal spinous processes. A high skill factor for accurate interpretation of images is required, since artifact production (e.g. through probe contact and positioning) is common. Ultrasonography represents a safe, noninvasive imaging technique.

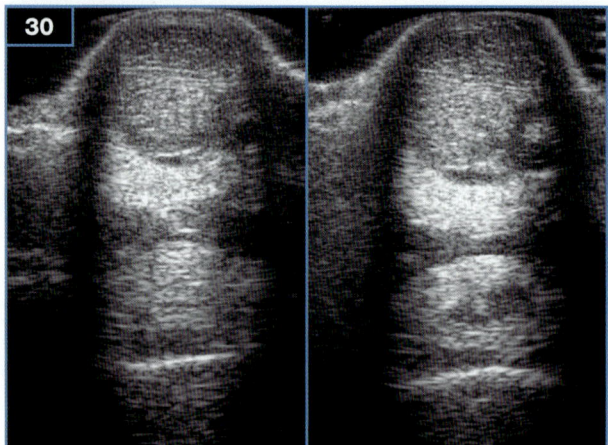

30 Transverse ultrasonogram of the upper palmar metacarpus of a racehorse with acute-onset lameness and soft tissue swelling of the area. Note the core lesion in the right upper midbody of the suspensory ligament.

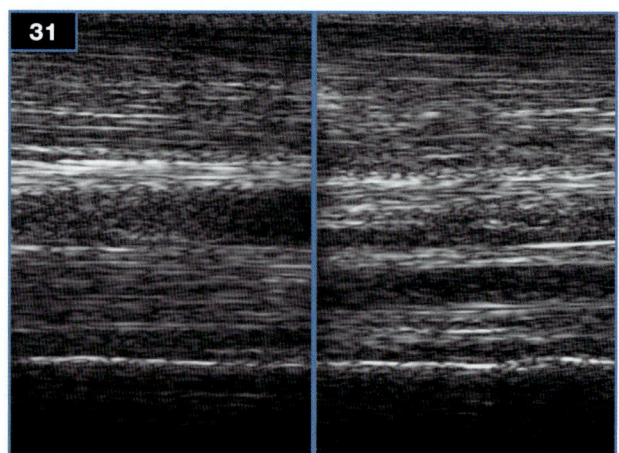

31 Sagittal longitudinal ultrasonogram of the case in 30 demonstrating the lesion in the right limb and confirming the length of ligament that is injured.

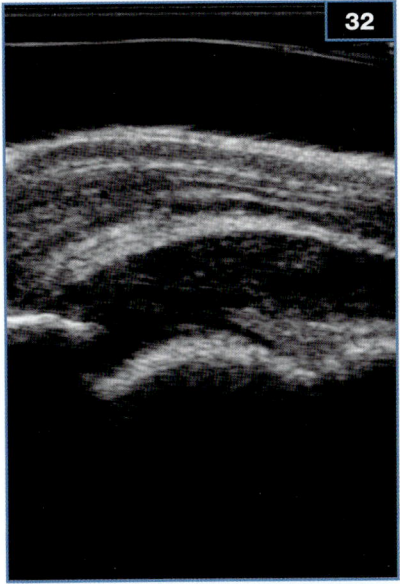
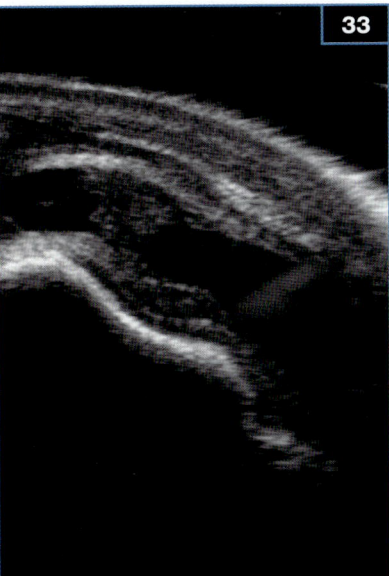
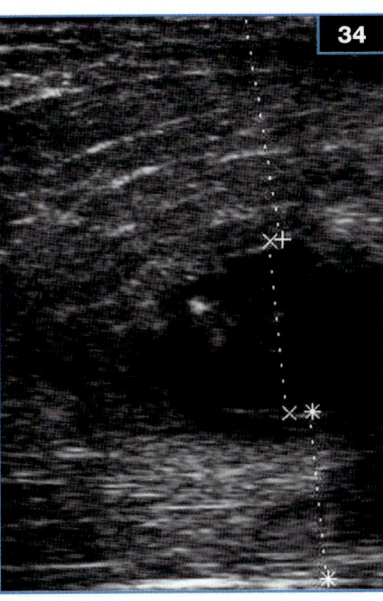

32, 33 Sagittal (32) and oblique (33) ultrasonograms of the dorsal fetlock region of the case described in 24. Note the distended dorsal metacarpophalangeal joint filled with hyperechoic joint fluid and the hyperplasia of the dorsal synovial membrane.

34 Ultrasonogram of an injection abscess in the neck of a horse following vaccination. Note the oval shaped hypoechogenic abscess deep within the muscles of the neck.

Nuclear imaging

Nuclear imaging (gamma scintigraphy or 'bone scanning') involves the intravenous injection of a radioactive substance that is then distributed throughout the horse. A gamma camera is then placed alongside the horse and the energy emitted from radioactive decay of the substance is recorded, processed by a computer, and an image pattern produced for interpretation (35). Black and white, or various color combination pattern dot images, can be generated depending on the software used. Technetium (^{99m}Tc) is the radioactive substance most commonly used in equine musculoskeletal nuclear medicine. It is bound to methyl diphosphonate (MDP) as a carrier. This chemical complex rapidly distributes throughout the vascular space (phase I or vascular phase), then into the extravascular space by 5–7 minutes (phase II or soft tissue/pool phase), followed by binding to bone 2–4 hours plus later (phase III or bone phase). Bone scans are usually obtained at 3 hours post injection. Pooling occurs in the urine, so both the kidneys and bladder will show normal uptake distribution. Skeletal structures that are actively remodeling, both normally and abnormally, bind more ^{99m}Tc–MDP than

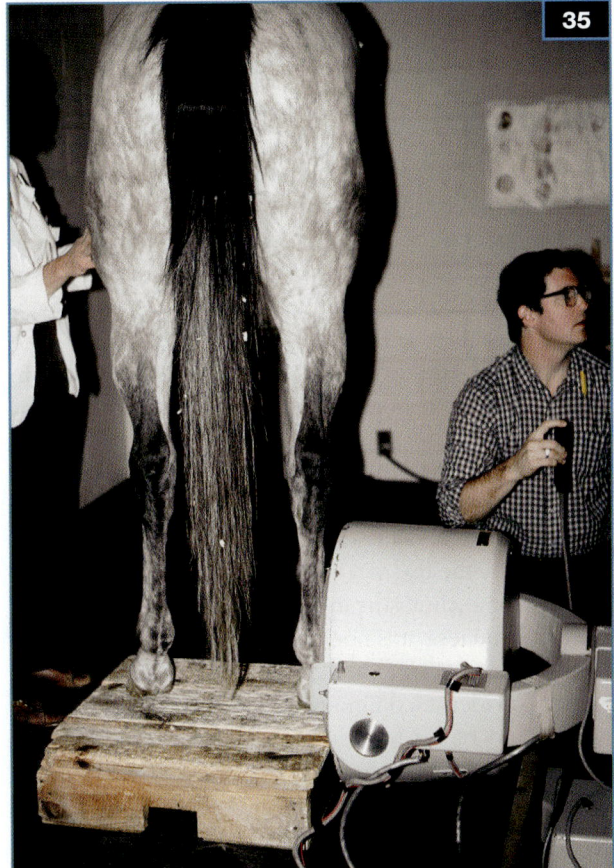

35 Bone scintigraphy being carried out on the distal hindlimb of a horse using a gamma camera.

25

Approach to the lame horse

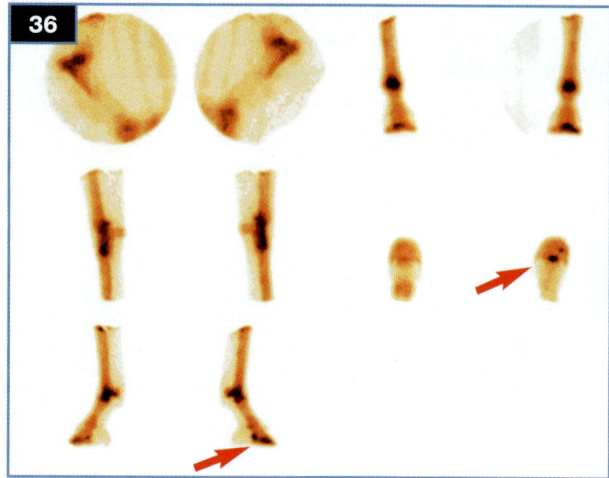

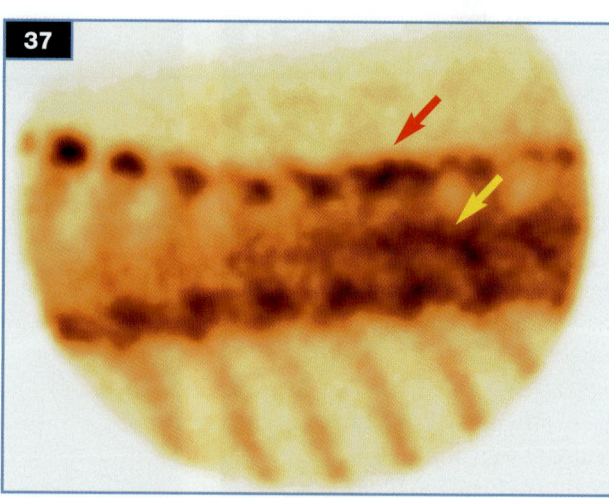

36 Bone scintigraphy results of a scan of the forelimb of a horse with pathology involving the right navicular bone.

37 Scintogram of the thoracic region of the back of a horse showing increased uptake in the dorsal spinal processes (red arrow) (this can be insignificant in some horses) and also the caudal thoracic intervertebral facet joints (yellow arrow). (Photo courtesy Alex Font)

surrounding bone. The abnormal intensity of increased uptake (so-called 'hot spot') in a particular site may indicate pathology within that osseous structure (36, 37). In contrast to other imaging modalities, nuclear images represent the metabolic state of the musculoskeletal system. It is more sensitive than radiography for actively remodeling areas, but not specific as to the exact diagnosis. Regions not easily radiographed and of large bulk (e.g. back and pelvis) are amenable to bone scanning (37). Pathology such as stress fractures (e.g. proximolateral cortex of the tibia in 2-year-old racing Thoroughbreds), or bone/joint remodeling (e.g. radiographically silent degenerative joint disease [DJD] of the intertarsal joints) lend themselves to the technique. Scanning is carried out in sedated, standing horses. Radiation safety precautions are mandatory.

Thermography

The surface temperature of an object can be measured and illustrated by the use of a thermographic camera, and it is used by some clinicians in the early diagnosis of certain types of lameness. It is noninvasive and can detect superficial inflammation, although there is very little serious scientific evidence confirming its efficacy. The circulatory pattern and blood flow in an area dictate the thermal pattern seen, and this forms the basis for thermographic interpretation. The examination must be carried out in a draft-free room and the hair of the horse must be uniform. Clipped areas, bandaged limbs, injection sites, or topical treatment areas produce erroneous results. Diagnoses made with thermography include laminitis, solar bruising and early abscessation, bucked shins, splints, early tendon injuries, proximal suspensory desmitis, and muscle strains. It is used in neck, back, and sacroiliac problems by some clinicians where injuries to the vertebral column have manifested themselves as areas of increased and decreased temperatures representing somatic dysfunction. Thermography results do not always correlate with those of other diagnostic techniques and at the present time its use is controversial.

Magnetic resonance imaging

MRI scans are produced by a complex process involving exciting hydrogen nuclei in the horse at specific resonance radio frequencies within a static magnetic field, and detecting the energy released. Water and fat contain the most hydrogen nuclei and the MRI signal created is built up from these. 2-D 'slices' or 3-D images can be achieved depending on the machine and computer software used. High-signal areas are depicted as white and low-signal areas are black.

At the present time, MRI in the horse is confined to the limbs (up to and including the carpus and tarsus usually) and head only. This is due to an inability to position other regions of interest in horses in human MRI machines. MRI can only be performed under general anesthesia, but in the last few years, specific veterinary machines have become available that can be used in sedated, standing horses (38–40). Generally, image quality obtained with standing machines is not as good as that obtained under general anesthesia, but recent improvements in the computer software of the former have improved this. Sequences of radio-frequency pulses are used to highlight different tissues and therefore different pathology. These include T1 and T2 weighted, STIR, and proton density images. T1 weighted images show regions with fat as high-signal areas (brightly), whereas T2 weighted images show regions with water and fat as high-signal areas. STIR (fat suppressed) images show regions with water as high-signal areas. The relative weighting of the image produces the contrast between tissues. In general, T1 images depict anatomy well and T2 and STIR images depict pathologic conditions better. STIR images allow pathologic conditions

in bone to be imaged more clearly. Proton density sequences are useful for evaluating ligaments and tendons in particular.

Knowledge of normal anatomy and MRI scans is essential in understanding and interpreting abnormalities. Sagittal, dorsal, and transverse sections are routinely taken of the region of interest. MRI has proven to be most useful for evaluating conditions of the foot, although recently, fetlocks, proximal cannon, and carpus/tarsus have been examined. Diagnoses are now being made that previously had not been recognized or accurately diagnosed. For example, collateral ligament desmitis of the coffin joint (39), deep digital flexor tendonitis (from proximal to the navicular bone to its insertion onto the pedal bone) (40), tendon adhesions at the level of the navicular bone, certain

38 Standing MRI being carried out on the distal right forelimb of a horse. (Photo courtesy A Font)

39 MRI scan of the foot in a transverse plane demonstrating an injury of the collateral ligament of the distal interphalangeal joint (left side of scan).

40 MRI scan in a transverse plane showing a lesion in the deep digital flexor tendon (right side of scan). (Photo courtesy A Font)

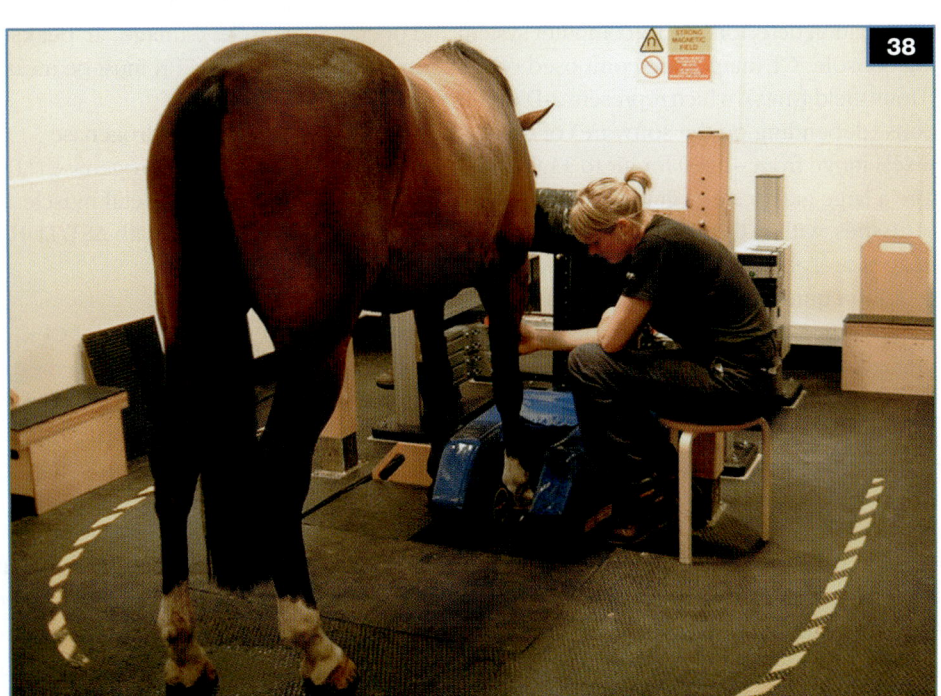

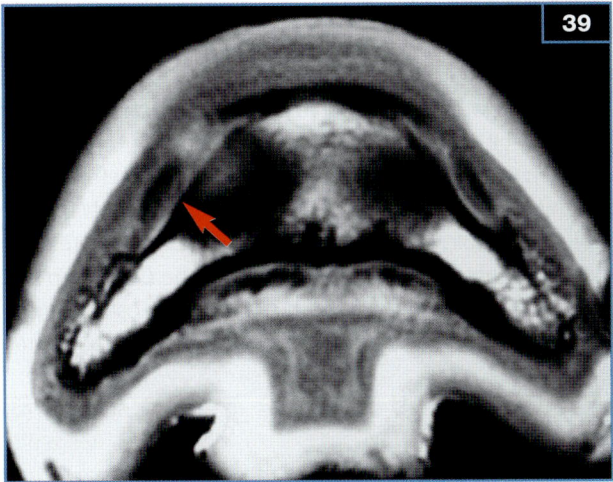

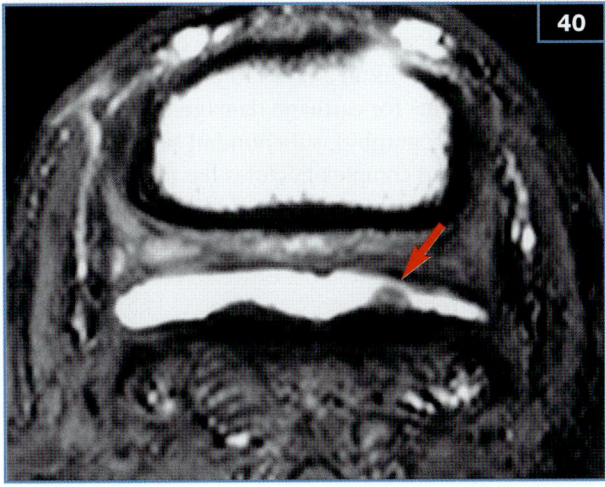

27

Approach to the lame horse

fractures, navicular bone degeneration and abnormalities of their supporting structures such as the proximal navicular suspensory and impar ligaments, navicular bursitis, articular cartilage damage of the coffin joint, and subchondral bone anomalies have been accurately diagnosed. Similarly, in the fetlock, subchondral bone injuries, osteochondral lesions, oblique distal sesamoidean ligament desmitis, small areas of suspensory ligament branch desmitis at their insertion onto the proximal sesamoid bones not recognized on ultrasound, and injuries to the collateral ligaments and cartilage have been recognized.

The availability of MRI as part of a lameness investigation is increasing as technology and software improve and more referral institutions gain experience with its use.

Computed tomography

CT scanning involves the use of advanced X-ray technology, radiation detectors, and a computer system and operating console. CT images are composed of numeric pixels (Hounsfield Units), which represent 2-D or 3-D representations (depending on the software) of tissue volume. The pixels range from –1,000 for air to +1,000 for bone, therefore a large gray scale of gradient is available for depiction of tissues within the region of interest. Cross-sectional images are obtained as required. General anesthesia is usually required, but new CT scanners for the limbs of standing horses are becoming increasingly available. At present only imaging up to the distal radius and tibia, or the head and neck, is attainable. As with MRI, knowledge of normal anatomy and CT images is essential for interpreting abnormalities. In general, MRI is most useful for soft tissue and CT for bone pathology. CT has shown that radiography can underestimate the degree of bone damage present. Navicular bone lesions imaged include prominent synovial invaginations along the distal border, cyst formation, and significant erosion of the flexor surface. 'Bone-bruising' (maladaptive bone disease or stress-related bone injury) affecting young Thoroughbred and Standardbred horses can be imaged before radiographic changes are seen. Cervical spinal cord CT scans can reveal sites of spinal cord and nerve compression. The examination by CT (as an adjunct to preoperative surgical planning) of joints for cartilage damage in osteoarthritis (OA) (with arthrography), subchondral bone anomalies, osseous cysts, and complex fractures has proven useful to date. As with MRI, the availability of CT as part of a lameness investigation will increase in the near future.

Laboratory tests

Muscle damage may be indicated from the results of measuring certain serum enzymes from a heparinized blood or serum sample.

Creatinine phosphokinase

Creatinine phosphokinase (CPK) is found in skeletal and cardiac muscle and in nervous tissue. It usually peaks at 4–6 hours post muscle damage and is specific for this. Normal ranges for CPK are laboratory specific, but in the first author's practice they are 110–250 IU/l. Mild elevations are seen in horses in training (<1,000 IU/l) and after heavy competition such as the cross country phase in 3-day eventing (<5,000 IU/l). A rapid return to normal is seen in these situations. Elevations of 7,000 to 100,000+ can be seen with rhabdomyolysis. Pathologic elevations are also seen in postanesthetic myopathies and recumbent horses.

Aspartate aminotransferase

Aspartate aminotransferase (AST) elevation indicates high activity in skeletal and cardiac muscle, liver, and RBCs. Unlike CPK, AST elevation is not specific for skeletal muscle damage. It peaks at 12–24 hours after muscle damage. CPK must be measured with AST.

Lactate dehydrogenase

Lactate dehydrogenase (LDH) is found in many organs as well as in skeletal muscle. Elevations are seen in rhabdomyolysis. As with AST, LDH should be measured with CPK.

Exercise test

The measurement of CPK, AST, and LDH at rest, 6 hours, and 24 hours after exercise can be useful as an aid to diagnosing chronic exertional rhabdomyolysis. A >4-fold increase on the first sample or persistently elevated levels of the three enzymes over the test period may indicate muscle damage.

Joint markers for osteoarthritis

Measuring the levels of the molecular products ('biomarkers') involved in joint turnover (both anabolic and catabolic products in joint fluid or serum) may be useful in the future to diagnose early, and monitor the progression of OA in the horse. Carboxypropetides of type II collagen (CPII), epitopes of chondroitin sulfate, the glycosaminoglycan keratan sulfate, and cartilage oligomeric matrix protein (COMP) are currently being investigated. Similarly, biomarkers of bone metabolism such as osteocalcin (OC), bone-specific alklaline phosphatase (BAP), and type I collagen C telopeptides (CTXs) may become useful.

Gene chip microarray represents the latest advance in molecular biology to provide a future diagnostic test for OA. Upregulation of different genes in the OA group has recently been identified from the serum of an osteoarthritic model.

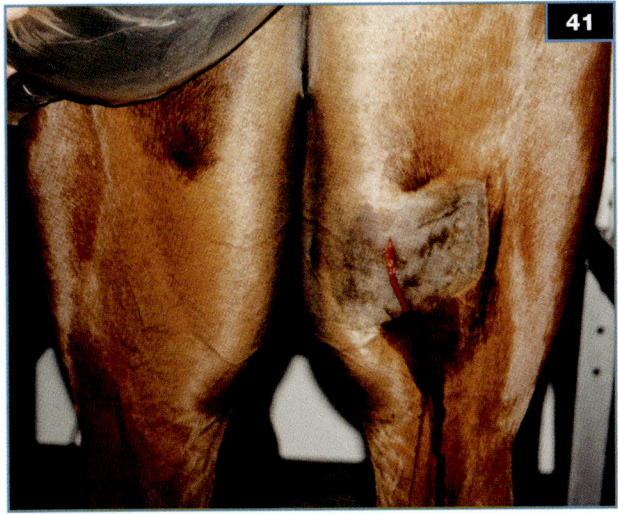

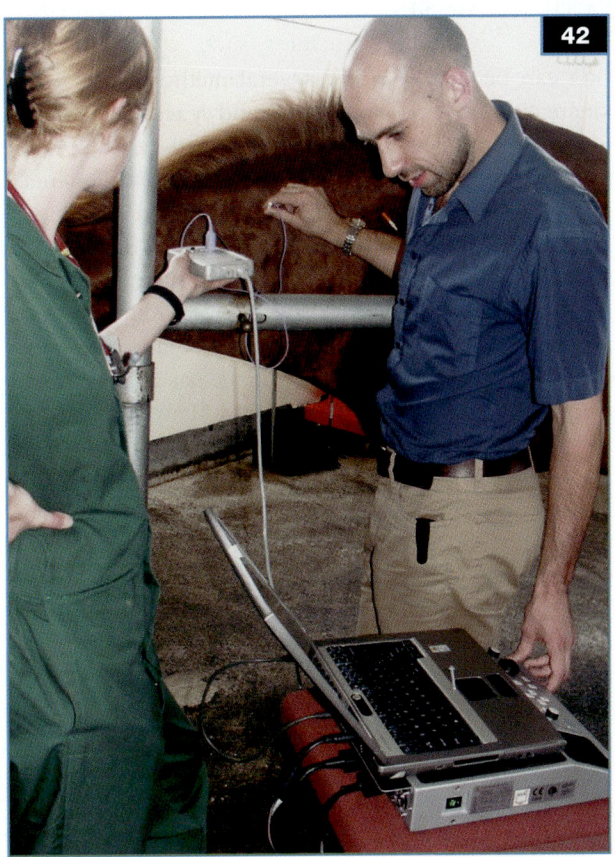

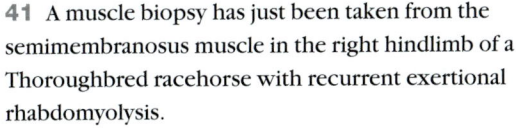
41 A muscle biopsy has just been taken from the semimembranosus muscle in the right hindlimb of a Thoroughbred racehorse with recurrent exertional rhabdomyolysis.

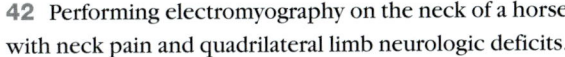
42 Performing electromyography on the neck of a horse with neck pain and quadrilateral limb neurologic deficits.

Tendon sheath markers for tendon pathology

COMP (measured in the synovial fluid of tendon sheaths) may in the future be a useful early indicator of tendon pathology in a tendon sheath.

Serology

High antibody titers to the tick-borne organism *Borrelia burgdorferi* may be seen in Lyme disease. Measurement of *Brucella* titers may be useful in the diagnosis of fistulous withers, vertebral osteomyelitis, or unexplained neck pain.

Muscle biopsy

Muscle biopsy can be useful for diagnosing specific muscle disorders such as polysaccharide storage myopathy (PSSM) and nutritional myodegeneration (NMD). Biopsy of the sacrocaudalis dorsalis muscle is also used for confirmation of equine motor neuron disease (EMND). The sample may be obtained under sedation and local anesthesia via a small, vertical skin incision over the muscle of interest by either using a 6 mm skin percutaneous biopsy needle or surgically excising a 2 cm cube of muscle (41). The skin is routinely closed with nonabsorbable suture material. Routine histopathologic biopsy samples are transported in formalin, whereas samples for histochemical analysis require fixation in methylbutane and chilling in liquid nitrogen. Placing such samples in saline-soaked gauze in a watertight container on ice is an alternative.

Electromyography

The diagnosis of neuromuscular problems such as specific areas of muscle atrophy or fasciculations can be helped by performing electromyography (EMG). This involves measuring electrical activity via needle electrodes placed in the affected muscles (42). Normal muscle exhibits little spontaneous electrical activity unless it contracts or the horse moves. Where there are abnormalities in the electrical conduction system of the muscle or denervation of motor units, spontaneous electrical activity in the form of fibrillation potentials, positive sharp waves, myotonic discharges, or complex repetitive discharges may be seen.

Approach to the lame horse

Gait analysis

Gait can be quantified by several methods that assess kinematics (limb position in time and space) and kinetics (direction and magnitude of forces on load-bearing). Kinematic analysis of gait looks at joint angles, stride length patterns, duration of stance phase, and head movement. Digital camera, computer, and light emitting or reflecting systems are used and specific data-acquisition software is installed to allow storage for later analysis. Although not a replacement for good visual appraisal of lameness by an experienced practitioner, the technique has been shown to identify subtle lameness consistently. Many variables are involved (e.g. the accurate, consistent placement of markers and analysing all four limbs simultaneously).

Kinetic analysis involves examining weight-bearing profiles that directly measure the direction and magnitude of force on loading or are extrapolated from these forces. These are obtained using hoof strain gauges, special instrumented shoes, or force plates. With the force plate, the horse is trotted up and the limb of interest must land squarely on the plate for a viable measurement. The parameters measured include peak force, average force, impulse, and loading and unloading rate, and variations in these 3D forces may be used to characterize the lameness. As with kinematic analysis, there are many variables and repeatability is critical. Instrumented shoes offer an advantage in that measurements can be made on successive strides or on a treadmill. Telemetric control is another development that means that data acquisition is not confined to the treadmill.

At the present time both methods of gait analysis are principally used in a research setting, although commercial gait-analysis programs have been produced.

Management

Arthroscopy, tenoscopy, and bursoscopy

Arthroscopic surgery ('key-hole' surgery) has revolutionized the treatment of joint diseases in the horse. Unlike arthrotomy it allows direct visualization of the majority of joints in the horse, thereby providing diagnostic information about the cartilage, joint capsule, menisci, and certain ligaments. Additionally, it is a surgical tool and can be used, for example, to remove chip fractures from the intercarpal joint, osteochondrosis fragments from the tarsocrural joint, and debride and lavage septic joints (43). Due to its minimally invasive technique, only small 'stab' incisions are needed, thereby reducing trauma, providing a better cosmetic effect, and allowing an earlier return to function in some cases. Arthroscopy requires specialized, expensive instrumentation and a high skill factor from the surgeon (44). It is not always possible to evaluate entire joint surfaces (e.g. the distal interphalangeal joint), so case selection is important.

Tenoscopy and bursoscopy are developments from arthroscopy, using the same techniques to evaluate tendon sheaths, in particular the digital tendon sheath, tarsal and carpal sheaths, and bursae, especially the navicular, calcaneal, and intertubercular (bicipital) bursae.

The use of these techniques has allowed new conditions to be diagnosed (e.g. desmitis of the intercarpal ligaments, cartilage lesions of the medial femoral condyle, longitudinal tears of the flexor tendons in the digital sheath, and meniscal and cruciate ligament injuries in the stifle joint). With further refinements in techniques, procedures such as cartilage resurfacing are now feasible.

43 Arthroscopic surgery of the right intercarpal joint being performed in dorsal recumbency under general anesthesia.

44 Intraoperative arthroscopic view of the distal aspect of the lateral trochlear ridge in a septic tarsus. Note the focal area of infective osteitis and cartilage loss.

45 Faradic stimulation of the lumbar musculature can be used in the investigation of back pain. Horses with back pathology may show resentment on stimulation of the muscles of the back or a decreased response to stimulation.

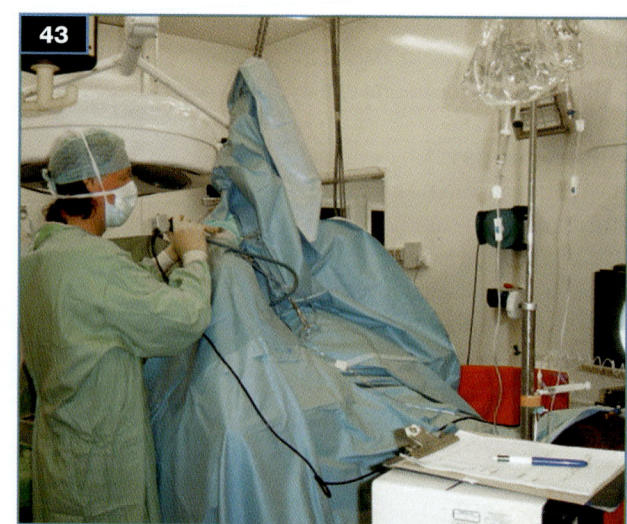

43

Physiotherapy

Physiotherapy forms an important part of rehabilitation for lame horses. Qualified physiotherapists undergo extensive training and certification programs in countries such as the UK and they work alongside veterinarians once an accurate diagnosis has been made. A variety of techniques are utilized depending on the lameness being treated, and combinations are often used.

Massage

Massage is used to promote muscle relaxation and good circulation. It is useful for relieving focal muscle spasm in longissimus dorsi and neck musculature.

Muscle ('Faradic') stimulation

Transcutaneous electrical nerve stimulation (TENS) can stimulate muscle groups and is used for neurogenic atrophy cases (e.g. supraspinatus and infraspinatus atrophy following suprascapular nerve damage ['Sweeney']). This technique is also useful for improving muscle tone and mass to atrophied muscles seen as a result of chronic back problems (after pain has been resolved) and contralateral limb disuse (e.g. after fracture repair or chronic poor/non-weight-bearing lameness). It has also been used as a diagnostic tool (45).

Controlled exercise

Controlled exercise can range from simply walking out in-hand through to schooling over poles or using a treadmill. It allows a graduated increase in strength and coordination and is timed to coincide with the natural healing processes of recovering tissues.

Swimming

Swimming exercises the cardiovascular system while reducing load on the limbs and allowing muscle groups to work. It can be carried out in a specially designed swimming pool environment, with or without a treadmill, or even in the sea in some countries.

Therapeutic ultrasound

Therapeutic ultrasound utilizes high-frequency sound waves to promote tissue healing, although the exact mechanisms of action are unknown. The sound energy is converted to thermal and vibrational energy on contact with tissue, and these may have biomechanical effects that produce positive healing processes in damaged tissue. The first author has had good results with adjunct ultrasound treatment of hematomas in various locations.

Therapeutic laser

Low-intensity lasers may have an effect on the local circulation and have biomodulation effects on the targeted tissue in order to trigger cell proliferation and provide analgesia, although the exact mechanisms within the tissue are unknown. Lasers have been used to aid the healing of wounds, superficial flexor tendonitis, and also for OA, but there are at present no objective data indicating their efficacy.

Magnetic and electromagnetic therapy

Magnets have been used to assist fracture healing and treat back problems due to the finding that bone has piezoelectrical properties. It is suggested that pulsed electromagnetic fields may stimulate bone healing and provide analgesia. Although widely used in equine practice, there are no objective data as to their efficacy.

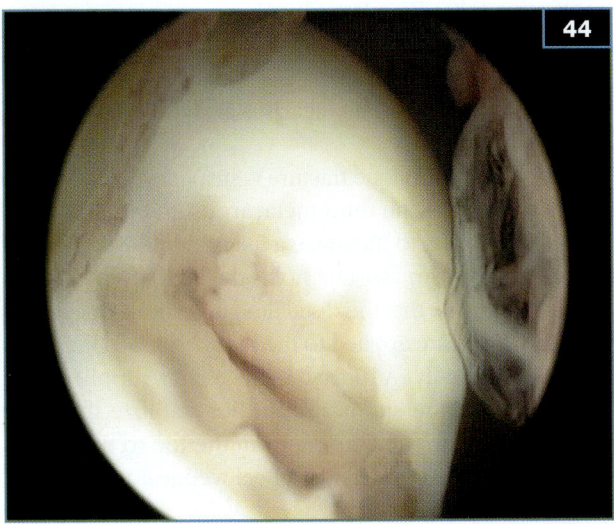

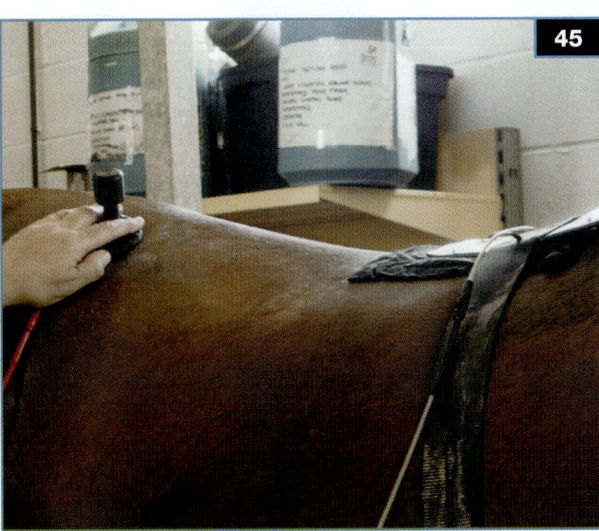

Extracorporeal shock-wave therapy

Shock-wave therapy was developed from the human technique of lithotripsy for the treatment of bladder and kidney stones. It has also been used for various human orthopedic injuries and has more recently been used in horses. High acoustic wave impulses are generated (either focused, where the waves are generated electrohydraulically, piezoelectrically, or electromagnetically and converge on a small point [46]; or radially, where the waves are generated pneumatically and expose surrounding tissues) and targeted at the tissue under treatment. It is suggested that shock-wave treatment may increase regional blood flow, have direct cellular effects, and activate osteogenic factors; it also has analgesic properties. Conditions treated with this technique in the horse are sore shins, insertional desmopathies (particularly proximal suspensory desmitis, suspensory branch insertions, and avulsion fractures at the proximal attachment of the suspensory ligament), and impinging dorsal spinous processes. Other conditions reported to be treated include tibial stress fractures, incomplete proximal phalangeal fractures, subchondral bone pain, OA of the distal hock joints, superficial digital flexor tendonitis, and deep digital flexor tendonitis (particularly at the palmar/plantar pastern region and at its insertion onto P3). Recently, treatment of angular limb deformities with shock-wave therapy to retard growth on the convex side of the deformity has also been reported. Many of the conditions where shock-wave therapy has been used have no or minimal scientific evidence basis and as such it should be prescribed with this in mind.

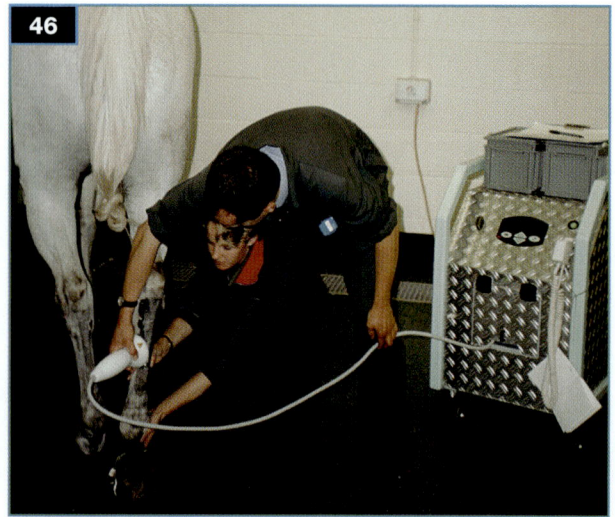

46 Extracorporeal shock-wave treatment of the right hindlimb of a horse with proximal suspensory ligament desmitis.

FIRST-AID TREATMENT OF THE FRACTURE PATIENT

Immediate fracture support with first-aid measures helps to relieve pain, minimizes further bony and soft tissue damage, stabilizes the limb, prevents further contamination if open, and renders the horse safer to travel. These factors allow the best possibility for appropriate treatment if this is achievable. A brief but thorough examination of the whole horse is necessary initially to ascertain that there are no life-threatening injuries present; these should be attended to first. Horses can (but not always) be extremely distressed and severely lame with fractures of the limb, so physical (e.g. a twitch) or chemical restraint may be needed before application of any splint support. Chemical restraint must be used with care since ataxia and collapse may occur in a compromised horse; small doses are advisable. Systemic analgesics such as NSAIDs can be given, and antibiotics should be prescribed if an open fracture is present. The horse's tetanus status should be checked.

First-aid fracture support is best achieved with the use of bandages and splints rather than casts. This is due to the difficulty in proper cast application in the standing horse and the fact that they do not accommodate post-injury swelling. Casts must also be removed and re-applied in order to re-adjust them, which is time consuming and unnecessarily expensive. A splint should ideally immobilize the joints proximal and distal to the fracture. It should be quick and easy to apply. Wood (45 mm × 20 mm) and/or PVC guttering cut lengthways to give a U-shape are suitable splint materials. The length of splint depends on the size of the horse and the injury. Snug padding at the proximal and distal ends of the splint before application lessens the incidence of pressure points. Commercial splints (e.g. the Kimsey splint) may also be used with certain fracture types. Sufficient bandaging materials for a half- or full-length Robert Jones bandage should be available depending on the fracture. It is useful to divide the fore and hindlimbs into regions for appropriate splint application (after Bramlage, 1983).

Forelimbs
Fractures of the distal metacarpus and the proximal and middle phalanges

If a transverse or oblique fracture is suspected, aligning the dorsal cortices of the third metacarpus and phalanges is advisable in order to minimize a fulcrum effect of the fracture on loading. An assistant holds the limb off the ground by the forearm so that the distal limb is vertical. One to two bandage layers are applied to the distal limb and the splint is applied dorsally. A further 1–2 layers are applied over this to protect the splint and further stabilize the limb. Heavy, tightly applied taping from the toe to the carpus prevents the splint loosening. A heel wedge is sometimes a useful addition.

Musculoskeletal system

47 A full-limb splinted Robert Jones bandage used in the hindlimb of a horse for the conservative treatment of a medial condylar fracture of the distal third metatarsus. Note the lateral and plantar splints.

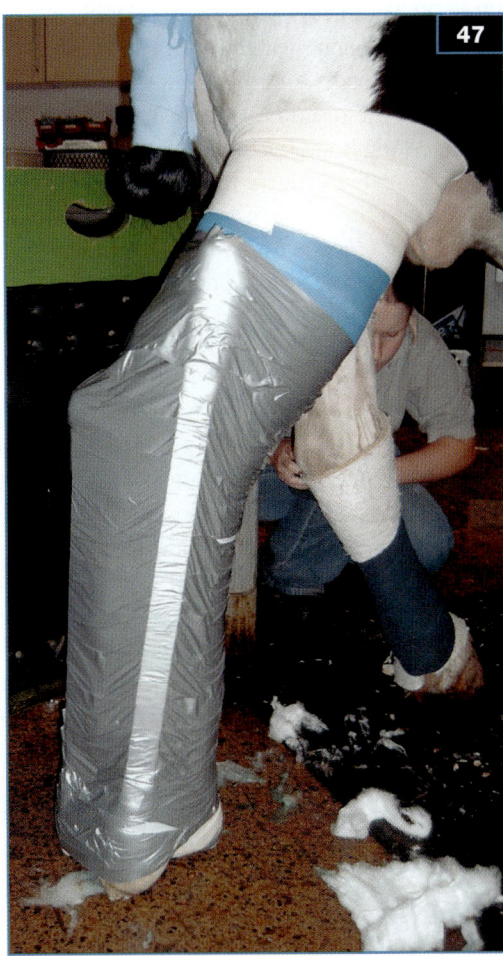

If a fracture in the sagittal plane is suspected, two splints on the lateral and medial aspects of the distal limb are applied over a half-limb Robert Jones bandage, with the limb weight-bearing.

Fractures from the mid-metacarpus to distal radius
A full Robert Jones bandage is applied from the toe to the elbow in the normal standing position. Splints are then taped tightly to the lateral and caudal aspects of the bandaged limb. The proximal ends of the splints must be padded to prevent rubbing.

Fractures of the mid and proximal radius
It is necessary to minimize abduction of the limb due to the lateral musculature of the forearm. A Robert Jones bandage is applied from the ground to the elbow. A splint is tightly applied laterally, extending from the foot to the mid-scapula level. The proximal end of the splint must be padded as previously.

Fractures of the ulna, humerus, and scapula
These fractures cannot be splinted and, therefore, supported, but their location disables the triceps muscles, which affects ambulation of the horse. A splint is applied caudally to fix the carpus in extension and allow the horse to move more easily. A Robert Jones bandage is applied from the foot to the elbow. The splint is tightly taped caudally from the fetlock to the elbow.

Hindlimbs
The reciprocal apparatus of the hindlimb presents problems with splinting and the splint can be less well tolerated than the forelimb. Further bandaging is often necessary after ambulation due to loosening of the splint.

Fractures of the distal metatarsus and below
As for the forelimb, but the splint is placed on the plantar rather than the dorsal aspect. An assistant should hold the limb above the hock so that the distal limb is vertical for application.

Fractures of the mid and proximal metatarsus
A Robert Jones bandage is applied from the toe up to and including the calcaneus, with the limb weight-bearing. Splints are tightly applied caudally and laterally to the level of the calcaneus (47).

Fractures of the tibia and tarsus
The splint must counteract the medial force of the lateral musculature of the tibia and the destabilizing effect of stifle flexion by the reciprocal apparatus. A full Robert Jones bandage is applied from the toe to the proximal tibia. A splint is tightly applied to the lateral aspect of the limb and should extend to the tuber coxae. In many textbooks it is suggested that a light steel rod (12 mm), shaped to form a loop proximally, can be used as a splint; however, this is rarely available and a long, thin wooden splint can be used instead.

Fractures of the stifle, femur and pelvis
These fractures are not amenable to external coaptation and should be cross-tied if possible to minimize further damage.

FRACTURE TREATMENT OPTIONS

Fractures can potentially occur in any of the bones of the musculoskeletal system and can range from a small chip fracture of the distal radial carpal bone to an open, comminuted long bone fracture. The range of treatments currently available reflects this diversity, but they can be divided into conservative and surgical treatments. The goal is to restore function to the affected limb so that the horse can either return to full work, become a breeding animal, or retire to pasture pain free.

Conservative

Box rest

All types of fracture require box rest whether treated by conservative or surgical means. Fractures that are amenable to box rest and bandaging as a sole treatment for a full return to function include certain splint fractures, incomplete nondisplaced fractures of long bones such as the radius and tibia, and some incomplete fractures of P1. The decision for this form of treatment alone must be based carefully on the individual case. The length of time required for complete healing will depend on the type of fracture and any complicating factors encountered, but it is often 10–12 weeks. Some cases may need cross-tying to prevent the horse lying down and getting up, which could be catastrophic. Additionally, the temperament of a horse is extremely important to the final outcome.

External coaptation

Splints. Splints are generally used for first-aid treatment of fractures to reduce further damage and allow safe transportation. In certain circumstances they can be used in fracture treatment (e.g. an adjunct after internal fixation immediately postoperatively or when a cast has just been removed).

Casts. Impregnated fiberglass casting materials have largely replaced the use of plaster of Paris in the horse (48, 49). Casts can be used as a primary treatment only for a limited number of fracture types (e.g. half- [distal/short] limb cast for an incompletely fractured pastern or a foot cast for a pedal bone wing fracture). The proper application of a cast requires careful preparation and positioning of the limb, cleaning of the foot, preplacement of suitable wound dressings, and a cast lining with stockinette, appropriate padding with orthopedic felt, and general limb padding such as Cast Support Foam prior to placement of the cast material itself (49).

Frequent cast changes due to loosening of the cast and cast-related soft tissue problems such as pressure sores is expensive and, if carried out under general anesthesia, puts the horse under unnecessary anesthetic and recovery risk. Casts are more commonly used to protect internal fixations during anesthetic recovery and until good fracture healing is well under way (e.g. a lateral condylar 3rd

48, 49 Hindlimb half-limb cast used for the postanesthetic recovery of a horse that had undertaken a surgical repair of a hindlimb first phalanx fracture (48). Note the layers of the cast, including the yellow cast foam, after it has been split prior to removal (49).

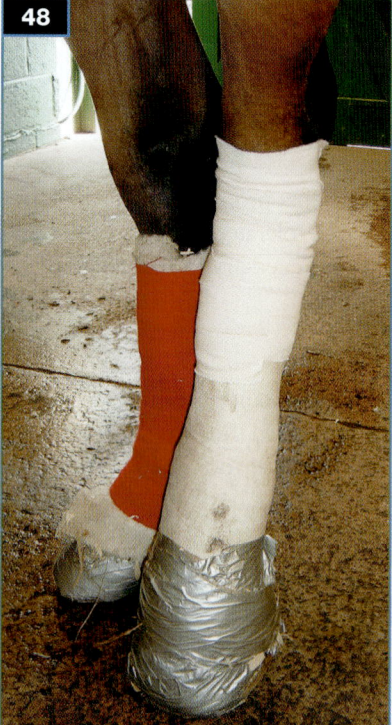
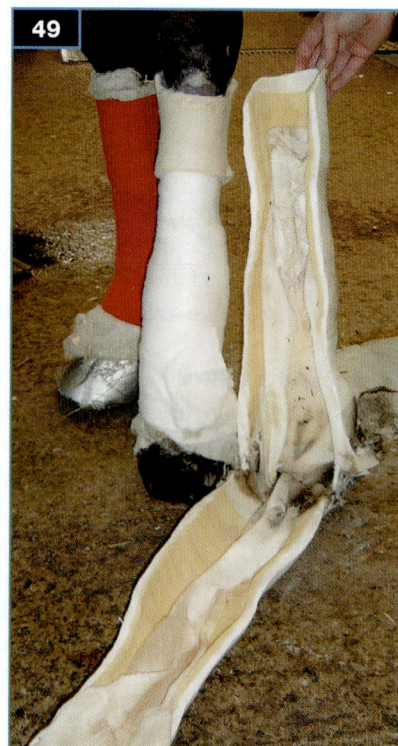

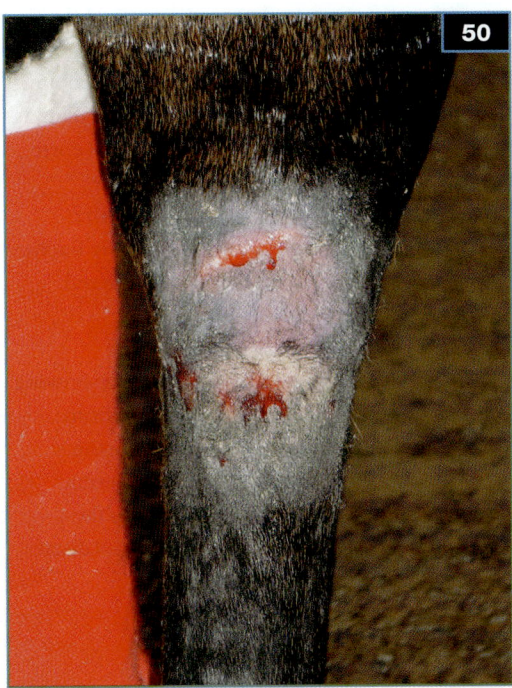

50 Healing dorsal proximal cannon skin pressure sores after the cast has been removed. The area was inadequately padded and the cast was not checked regularly enough.

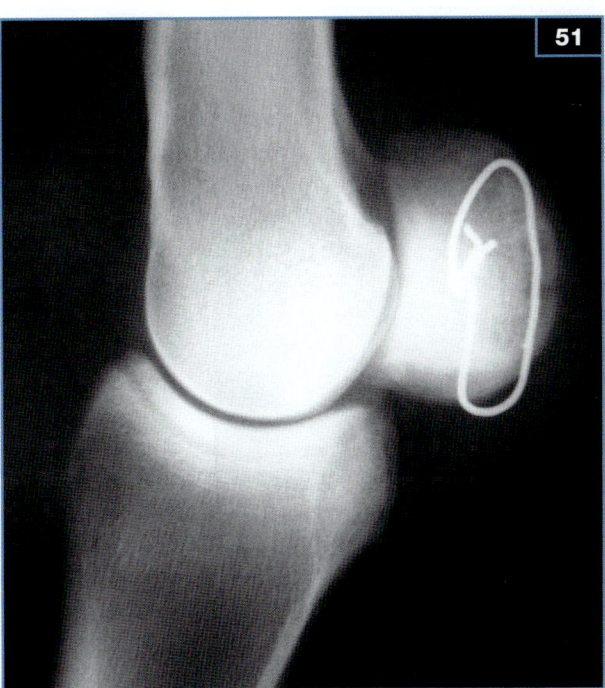

51 Postoperative lateromedial radiograph of a proximal sesamoid bone midbody fracture repaired by a cerclage wire.

metacarpal fracture repaired by lag screw fixation is protected with a half-limb cast). Long-term cast use can lead to DJD due to immobilization of joints, laxity of the soft tissue structures around the joints, and disuse osteoporosis if the treated limb remains non-weight-bearing for an excessive period of time.

Daily cast checks are necessary to prevent sores developing (especially dorsoproximally at the cannon, fetlock, and coronary band for a half-limb cast) (**50**). Casts should ideally be changed at 7–10 days post surgery to account for a decrease in soft-tissue swelling, and then at least every 4 weeks in adults and every 7–10 days in foals depending on the case.

Surgical
External fixation
Transfixation casting. The combination of two to three 4–6 mm positive-profile pins with a 30° divergence in a frontal plane through the 3rd metacarpus/metatarsus and a fiberglass cast provides a strong protection for comminuted fractures distal to the pins (i.e. of P1, P2, and distal 3rd metacarpus/metatarsus). The load of weight bearing is transferred away from the fracture site via the pins and cast and there is minimal distraction of fragments. These casts can be maintained for up to 6–8 weeks.

External fixator. Several small animal versions of these are infrequently used for severely comminuted fractures of P1, P2, and distal 3rd metacarpus/metatarsus. They have been used in foals with fractures, but many surgeons use positive-profile pins stabilized by gentamicin-impregnated polymethylmethacrylate (PMMA) placed in tubes as sidebars. An external skeletal fixation device (ESFD) is a special external fixator consisting of 2–3 transfixation pins placed proximal to the fracture and linked by sidebars to a base plate that has been designed for use in adult horses with distal limb comminuted fractures.

Internal fixation
Intramedullary implants
+ STEINMANN PINS. Infrequently used in the horse due to their lack of stability, but they can be used in foals for medullary stack pinning of humeral fractures, certain olecranon fractures, and femoral capital physeal fractures.
+ INTERLOCKING NAILS. Recently designed for use in foals for humeral and femoral fractures, but not commonly available.

Cerclage wire. Used in certain situations such as tension band wiring of midbody proximal sesamoid fractures (**51**), rostral fractures of the lower and upper mandibles, and certain olecranon fractures in foals.

Approach to the lame horse

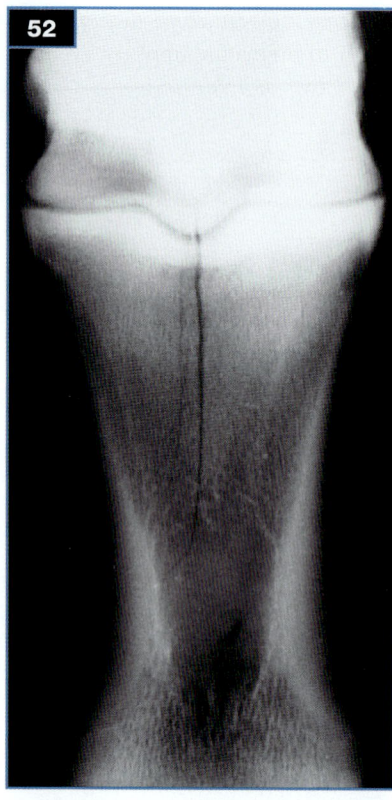

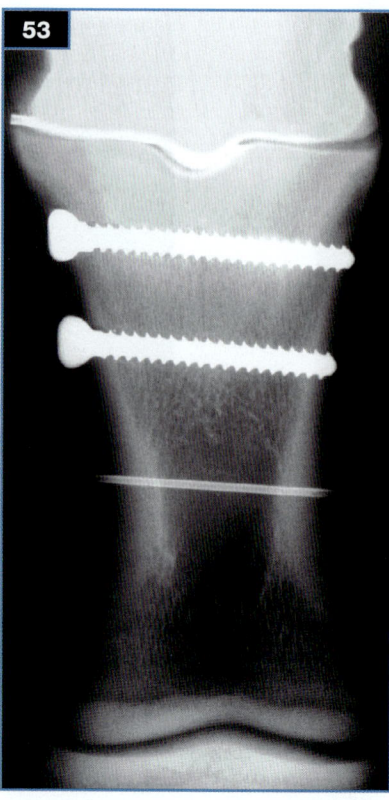

52 Dorsopalmar radiograph of the first phalanx of a Thoroughbred racehorse that has sustained a nondisplaced midline sagittal fracture during training. Note the two fracture lines that correspond to the dorsal and palmar cortices, the starting point at the sagittal groove, and the way the fracture turns and exits through the lateral cortex of the mid pastern.

53 Intraoperative radiograph showing placement of two lag screws from lateral to medial compressing the fracture line. Note the hypodermic needle markers at the level of the metacarpophalangeal joint and distal fracture line.

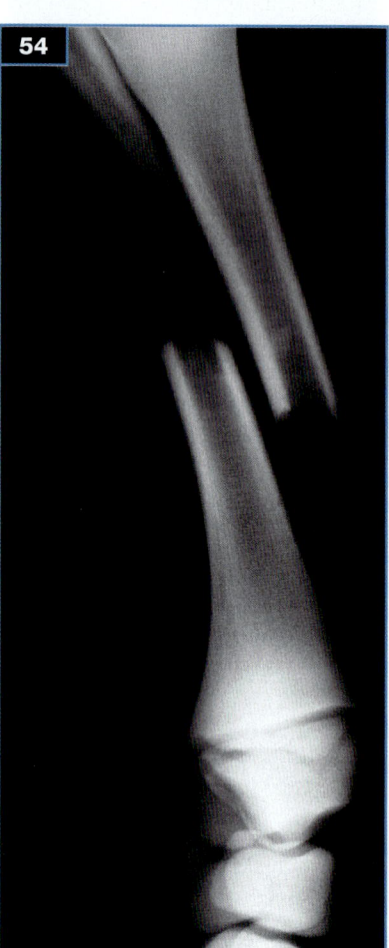

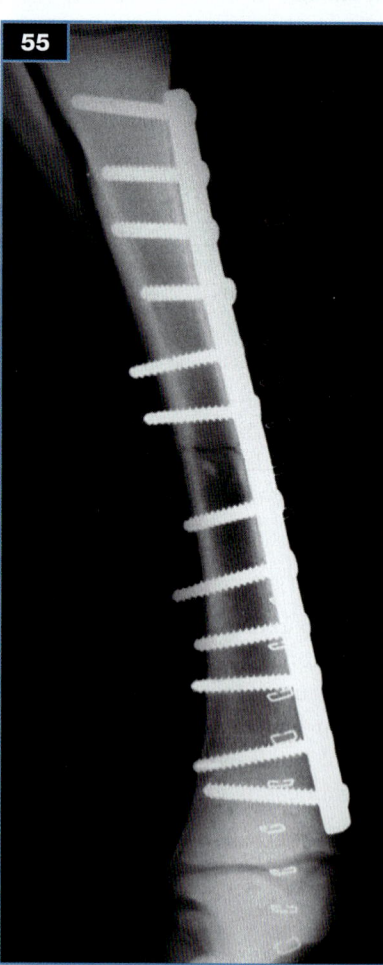

54 Lateral radiograph of a neonatal foal that sustained a mid-diaphyseal transverse fracture of the radius shortly after birth.

55 Postoperative radiograph showing placement of a single 4.5 mm broad DCP plate cranially, not crossing any physis. There is good anatomic reduction and the foal made a full recovery.

Screws and plating. If fracture fragments are placed under compression, they can heal without callus formation. Precise anatomic reduction of the fracture for primary union is critical. The AO/ASIF system of lag technique fixation and dynamic compression plates (DCP) are mainly used in the horse to achieve this effect. Cortical screw sizes commonly used in the horse are the 4.5 mm and 5.5 mm diameter screws. DCP plates can be narrow or broad and commonly 12 or 16 hole.

Fractures can be repaired with lag technique screw fixation (**52, 53**). Certain olecranon fractures can be repaired by using a caudally positioned narrow DCP to act as a tension band. Long-bone fractures such as simple oblique 3rd metacarpal bone fractures and radial and tibial fractures can be repaired using single or double broad DCP plates depending on the type of fracture configuration and the size of the animal (usually less than 300 kg) (**54, 55**). Other screws are used in certain circumstances (e.g. cancellous, cannulated, and self-tapping) and plates can also be used in a neutralization and buttress mode. The availability of special plates such as the dynamic condylar screw (DCS), dynamic hip screw (DHS) plates and PC-Fix system has improved the management of long-bone fractures. Additionally, the technique of plate luting has improved the plate–bone interface, strengthening the fracture repair in long bones. It must be noted that although fracture repair in the horse has advanced greatly in recent years, the size of adult horses and the quality of anesthetic recoveries are still major limiting factors for fracture repairs, particularly those of long bones.

Complications of fracture treatment

The most common and serious complication following fracture repair involves infection at the fracture site and surrounding soft tissues. Heat, local pain, and swelling are present and a discharging sinus and/or wound breakdown is common. Infective osteitis and osteomyelitis may be seen on postoperative radiographic evaluation if infection is present. The limb may be only poorly- or non-weight-bearing. This delays healing of the fracture, reduces weight bearing (which can lead to flexural limb deformities and/or contralateral laminitis and suspensory ligament breakdown), and significantly increases the cost. Chances of contamination are increased in open fractures and/or where the soft tissues are badly damaged and perfusion is altered at the outset. Mixed bacterial populations are usually present and include *Enterobacteriacae, Streptococcus, Staphylococcus, Pseudomonas,* and anaerobes. Treatment involves giving broad-spectrum or specific (based on bacterial culture and sensitivity testing) systemic and locally delivered antibiotics (such as using gentamicin-impregnated PMMA or regional limb local perfusion), drainage, debridement and lavage, and implant removal if this is possible.

Other complications include refracture through the original fracture plane due to premature implant removal or delayed healing. Spontaneous fracture at anesthetic recovery can be catastrophic and steps to prevent this include the use of external coaptation such as appropriate fiberglass casts, assisting recovery with head and tail ropes, and swimming pool recovery if this is available. Delayed healing can occur for a variety of other reasons where the healing environment is less than optimal (e.g. movement at the fracture repair site due to inadequate fixation or immobilization). Overloading of the opposite limb after fracture repair can lead to laminitis or suspensory ligament damage in the adult horse, which is potentially devastating. Prevention includes as early a return to normal weight bearing of the repaired limb as possible (dependent on the fracture type and complications encountered) and the use of prophylactic frog support bandaging. In foals, angular limb deformities and hyperextension of the fetlock can frequently result from limb overload and, occasionally, acquired contractural limb deformity of the carpus is seen. Prevention includes early return to normal weight bearing of the repaired limb and application of medial acrylic hoof extensions for acquired carpal valgus or heel extensions for fetlock hyperextension. Limb contractures may be treated with temporary caudally applied splints.

The owner must be made aware of these potential complications prior to fracture repair, since they may lead to euthanasia on humane and/or financial grounds.

Joint disease

Synovial joints are highly differentiated connective tissue structures composed of bone, articular cartilage, synovial membrane, and periarticular soft tissues. OA is characterized by degeneration and loss of articular cartilage. Clinically, the disease manifests itself as joint pain, reduction in joint movement, joint effusion, and variable degrees of localized inflammation. At a cellular and molecular level, research has shown that synoviocytes lining the joint synovium contribute to cartilage degeneration in OA by releasing a variety of inflammatory mediators and degradative enzymes against both collagen and proteoglycans. These include prostaglandins (PGs), cytokines such as interleukin-1 (IL-1) and tumor necrosis factor-alpha (TNF-α), and matrix metalloproteinases (MMPs) including collagenases, stromolysins (MMP-3), and gelatinases.

The exact pathogenesis of OA is still unclear and it may represent a common joint response to a number of potential causes. A single or repetitive traumatic event may produce mechanical damage directly to healthy cartilage, leading to the development of OA. Subsequent damage to the cartilage matrix and/or cellular injury results in metabolic release of proteolytic enzymes from chondrocytes, which in turn cause cartilage fibrillation and proteoglycan breakdown. Alternatively, the matrix of fundamentally defective cartilage with abnormal biomechanical properties may fail under normal loading. Subchondral and epiphyseal microfracture formation from normal mechanical stresses and resulting 'stiffening' of the subchondral bone plate may lead to eventual failure of the bone–cartilage interface, leading to OA.

Changes in the synovial fluid viscosity reflect the joint pathology in OA. A decrease in viscosity is common and is due to a depolymerization and reduction in concentration of the glycoprotein hyaluronan, which normally acts as a boundary lubricant in synovial joints. Cytologic and protein concentration changes are not dramatic in OA and are not routinely used as markers of OA. A distinction between OA in 'high-motion' joints and 'low-motion' joints has implications on clinical presentation, pathologic development, and progression and treatment. 'High-motion' joints include the distal interphalangeal, metacarpo/metatarsophalangeal, antebrachiocarpal and midcarpal, humeroradial, scapulohumeral, tarsocrural, femoropatellar, and coxofemoral joints, and they present with OA as above. The proximal interphalangeal and tarsometatarsal/centrotarsal joints represent the 'low-motion' joints (56). OA in these joints will not present with obvious joint effusion since the joint capsule allows less distension than 'high-motion' joints. Subchondral bone lysis and sclerosis of the bones making up the articulation contribute significantly to the overall disease process and progression towards joint ankylosis (partial or complete) via cartilage loss rather than reduced joint motion. Joint fibrosis only may occur. Treatment options for both types of joints will be discussed in the sections on conditions of the limbs.

Radiography of joints affected by OA may reveal narrowing of the joint space, subchondral bone sclerosis and/or lysis, periarticular osteophytosis (57), osteochondral intra-articular fractures, and finally joint ankylosis. Radiologic changes tend to reflect a later stage of pathologic events in OA and it is well recognized that a lack of correlation exists between arthroscopically evident cartilage degeneration and radiographic findings. Other imaging modalities such as ultrasonography, gamma scintigraphy, MRI, and CT are also useful in the diagnosis of OA.

Synovial and serum biomarkers and gene chip array represent new methods in the future of detecting early OA and monitoring progression (see Laboratory tests, p. 28).

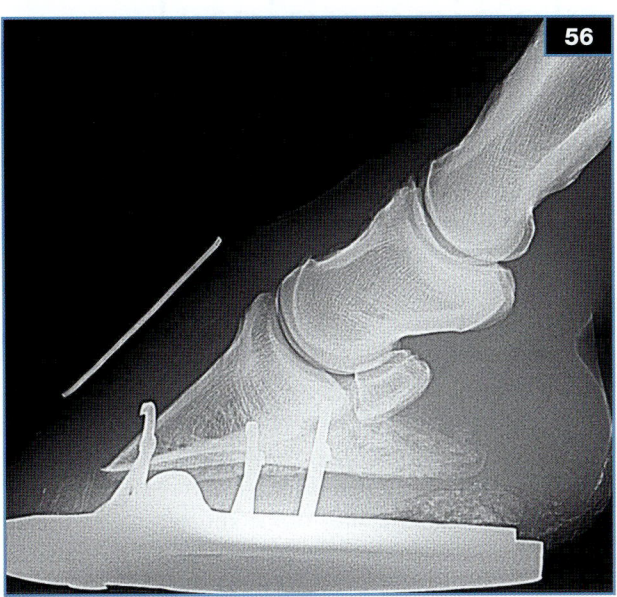

56 Lateromedial radiograph of the distal limb of a middle-aged riding horse with a unilateral forelimb lameness localized by intra-articular analgesia to the proximal inter-phalangeal joint. Note the periarticular osteophyte formation, change in joint contour, and extra-articular new bone formation typical of low-motion osteoarthritis in this joint.

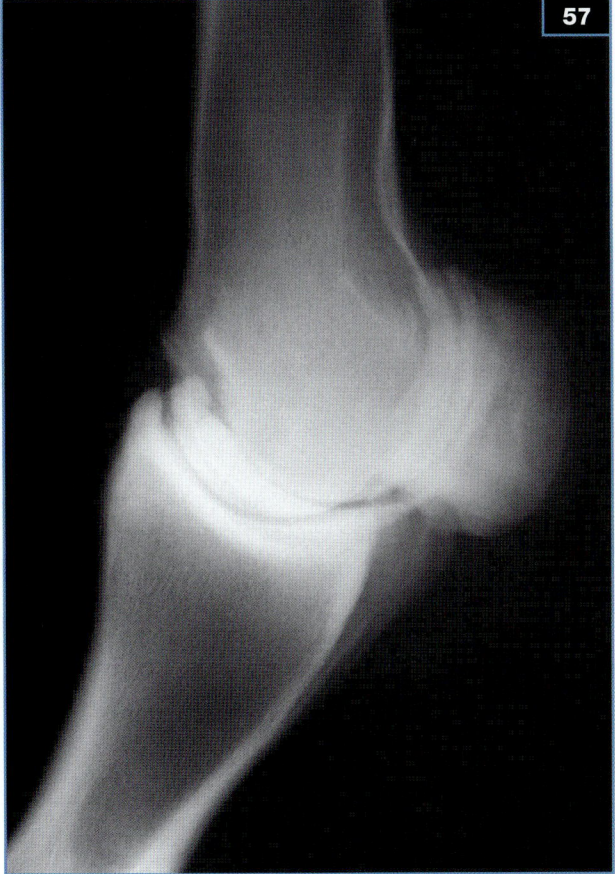

57 Lateromedial radiograph of a metacarpophalangeal joint of a horse suffering with persistent lameness localized to this joint. This joint has many of the radiographic changes of chronic high- motion degenerative joint disease with decreased joint space, large rounded marginal osteophytes on the proximal aspect of P1, subchondral sclerosis, modeling of the articular margins of the proximal sesamoid bones, and evidence of chronic enlargement of the joint capsule on the dorsal and palmar aspects of the distal third metacarpus.

Approach to the lame horse

The foal and developing animal

Congenital musculoskeletal abnormalities

Congenital defects are those abnormalities present at birth, either structural and/or functional, that result from abnormalities in embryogenesis. Theoretically, these abnormalities may be genetic or environmental in origin, but often no definitive cause is identified.

Congenital angular limb abnormalities
(See also page 52 for acquired deformities.)

Definition/overview
Congenital angular limb deformities are common, especially at the carpus (valgus) and fetlock (varus) joints. They refer to lateral (valgus) or medial (varus) deviations of the limb(s) distal to the joint that are present at birth (**58**). The forelimbs are most commonly affected and rotational deviation is also often present. They are usually seen in larger, faster growing breeds such as Thoroughbreds, and may be uni- or bilateral.

Etiology/pathophysiology
The etiology is multifactorial and not clearly understood, but possible cited factors include intrauterine malpositioning, overnutrition of the mare in the last third of pregnancy, joint laxity, and incomplete ossification of the cuboidal bones, with other hereditary (poor conformation), nutritional, and possibly hormonal influences also contributing.

The most common cause of congenital angular limb deformity is joint laxity. The majority of cases will resolve spontaneously over a few days as the muscles, tendons, and periarticular structures of the affected limb(s) gradually strengthen with gentle exercise. Defective or incomplete ossification of the cuboidal bones of the carpus or tarsus can also lead to congenital angular limb deformity (see below).

Clinical presentation
All four limbs should be examined for deformity in all planes, but particularly perpendicular to the frontal plane through the limb. Palpation and manipulation of affected limbs usually reveal gross joint instability medially to laterally without swelling, pain, or crepitus. Multiple limbs and joints can be involved and lameness is not usually a feature (**59,60**).

Differential diagnosis
Acquired angular limb deformities.

Diagnosis
The clinical history of a deformity present at birth, or shortly thereafter, and the clinical findings are diagnostic. Radiographs of the affected area will confirm the exact nature of the problem. Radiographs (lateromedial and dorsopalmar/plantar) with long plates to allow the visualization of the long bones proximal and distal to the deformity should be taken. Lines drawn on the radiographs through the mid-points of the long bones proximal and distal to the affected area should intersect within the affected joint and will allow the angle of deformity to be measured. In some cases there are hypoplastic bones present within the joint (**61**). Stressed views may be useful where joint laxity is suspected.

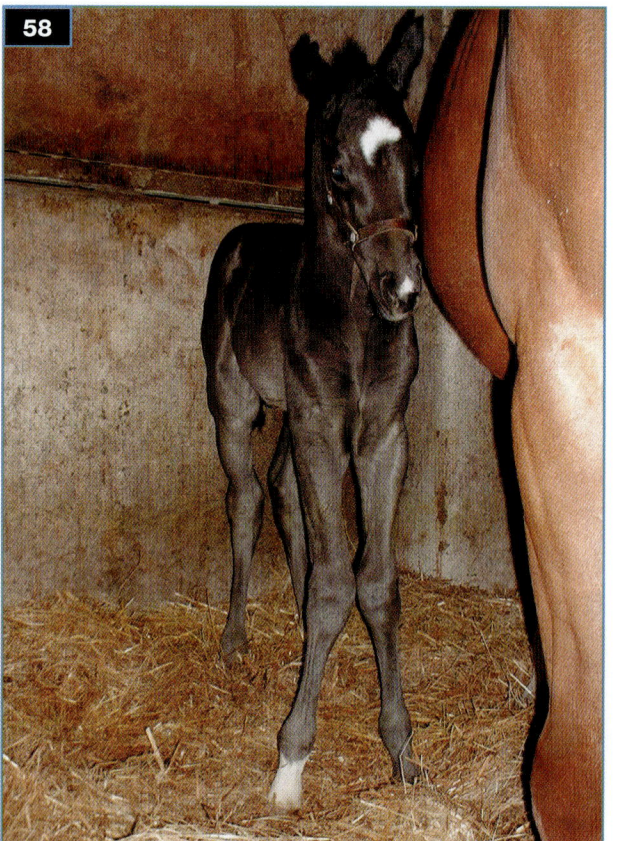

58 Bilateral congenital carpal valgus angular limb deformity in a neonatal foal.

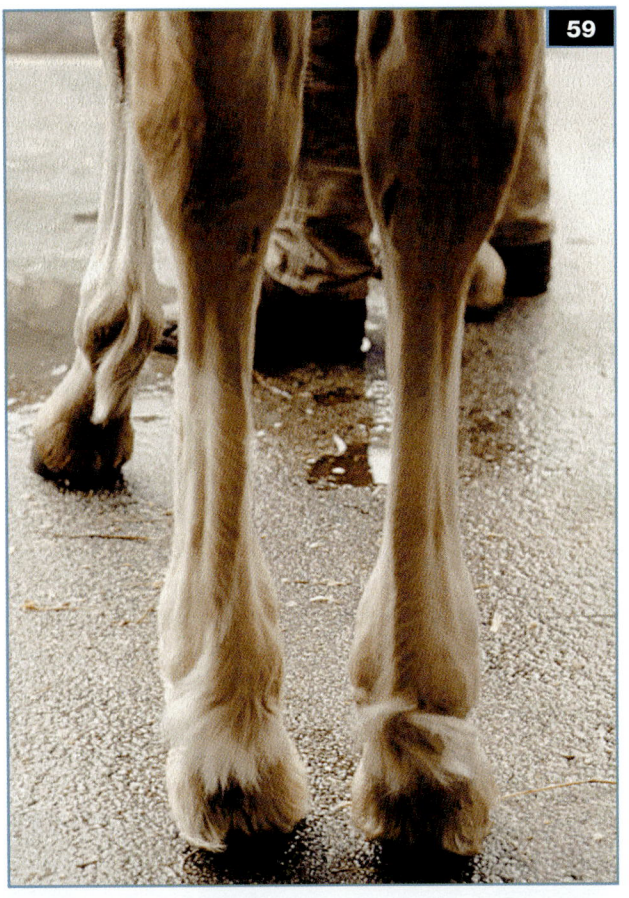

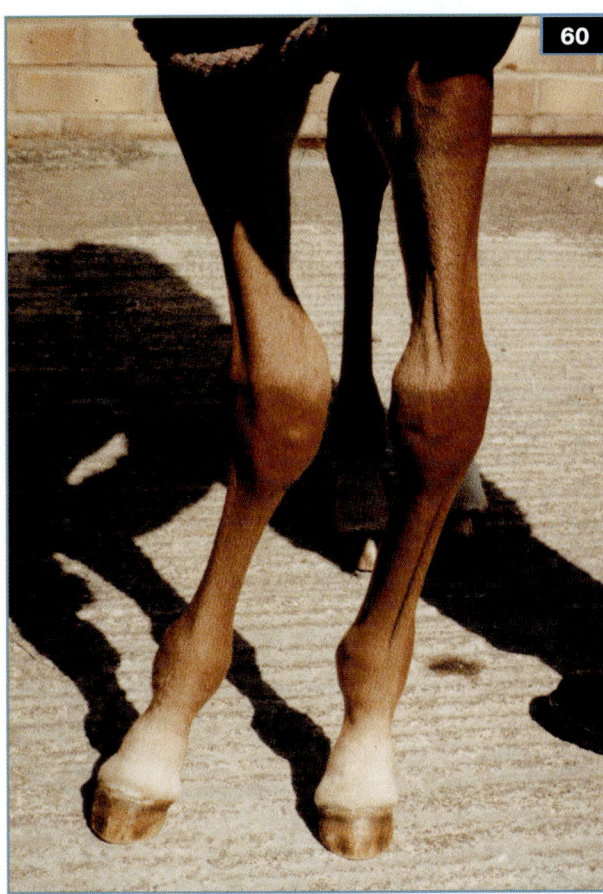

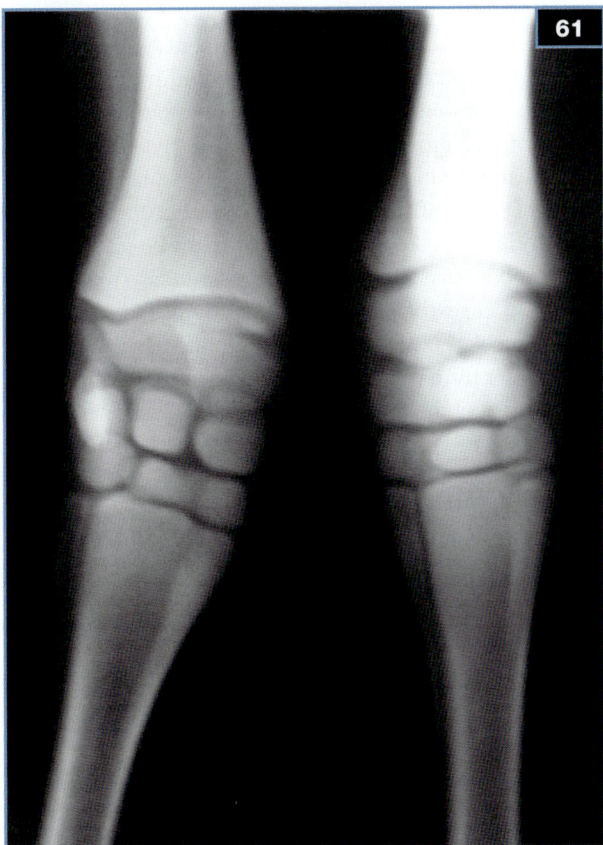

59 A 2-week-old Clydesdale foal with a left lindlimb fetlock varus that has been present since birth. Manipulation revealed marked mediolateral joint instability in the left fetlock compared with the right.

60 Neonatal dysmature Thoroughbred foal with 'windswept' appearance due to a right carpal valgus and a left carpal varus. There was carpal joint instability in all planes on manipulation and carpal bone hypoplasia on radiography.

61 Dorsopalmar radiograph of the foal in 58 showing carpal valgus (worse in right fore) and a rounded, slightly hypoplastic carpal bone shape.

Management

Treatment consists of immobilization in tube casts, custom-made braces, or large Robert Jones bandages and/or splints (e.g. for the carpus the bandage or cast should extend from the proximal radius to the distal metacarpus, allowing the foot to be exposed and the foal to walk on the limb). The unstable joint is supported, but the natural processes of stabilization are still encouraged by gentle exercise. The period of stabilization is determined by the individual case response, but may range from a few days to weeks. A gradual reduction in the degree of support over time encourages adaptive processes. Swimming is sometimes useful. Care should be taken to prevent pressure sore formation by regular bandage/cast changes (every 3–7 days). Corrective foot trimming and shoeing as for acquired angular limb deformities may also be used.

Defective ossification of the cuboidal bones of the carpus and tarsus

Defects in the ossification process can occur in any young foal, but premature and dysmature foals are most commonly affected. Fetal growth retardation due to placental disease, severe metabolic or parasitic disease in the mare, twin pregnancy, or poor mare nutrition may be involved. Carpal valgus is the most common presentation at birth; this either remains static or worsens over the first 2 weeks of life due to exercise deforming the soft cartilage structures. Clinical examination reveals no pain or swelling in the affected joint initially, and usually no lameness is present. An increased range of movement within the joint may be present both craniocaudally and mediolaterally, particularly if joint laxity is also present. Radiographs can reveal one or more abnormal carpal bones, but it is not possible to fully interpret the amount of cartilage precursor damage. Full ossification of these bones occurs at about 30 days and a more accurate prognosis can be given at this stage. Secondary DJD is a possible sequela. Treatment is similar to cases of joint laxity. Radiographic evaluation every 2 weeks is recommended to monitor ossification.

Another form of cuboidal bone defective ossification is the collapse of the third and/or central tarsal bone(s). This condition is usually bilateral and affected foals may present with excessive flexion of the hocks ('curby' conformation) leading to a characteristic bunny-hop gait (62). Tarsal valgus may also be present (63). Radiography reveals wedging of the central and third tarsal bones. Treatment is similar to cases of joint laxity to allow ossification to progress. DJD is a possible sequela.

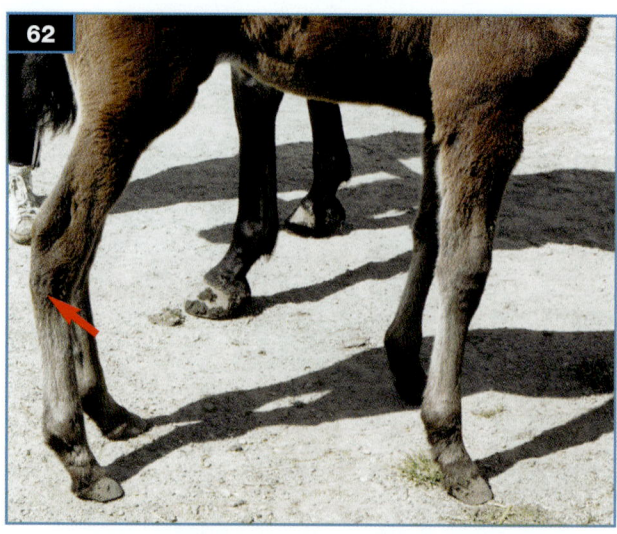

62 Three-week-old Warmblood foal with partial collapse of the small tarsal bones in a dorsal plantar plane, leading to a 'curby hock' appearance (arrow). (Plantar aspect from point of hock to plantar fetlock is not straight.)

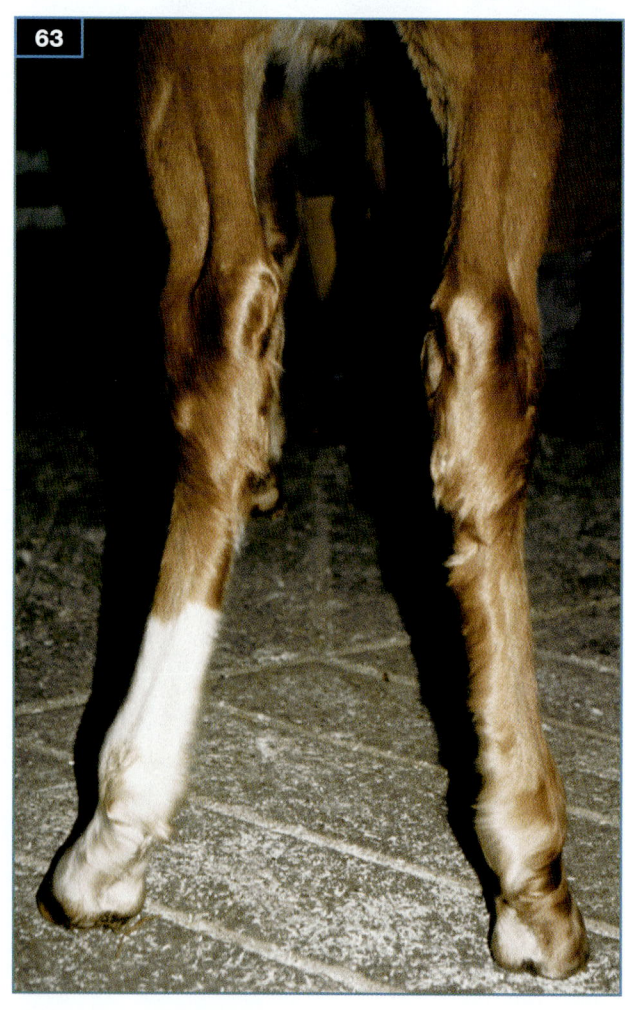

63 Older weanling Thoroughbred-type foal with tarsal valgus due to collapse of small tarsal bones in a medial to lateral plane as young foal.

Congenital flexural limb deformities
Definition/overview
Congenital flexural limb deformities by definition are present at birth and are of unknown etiology. Possible causes have been suggested and include intrauterine malpositioning, toxic insults during embryonic life (e.g. maternal ingestion of locoweed or hybrid Sudan grass), genetic factors, influenza virus infecting pregnant mares, dams fed goitrogenic diets, and neuromuscular disorders. They are not due to 'contracted tendons', but to a relative shortening of a tendon unit in relation to bony structures.

Clinical examination
Clinical examination should include careful palpation and manipulation of the affected joint(s) in a weight-bearing and nonweight-bearing position. Palpation of the flexor tendons, suspensory ligament, and inferior check ligament may further indicate those structures involved. Radiographic examination of affected joints is useful to determine the presence of specific bone or joint abnormalities, which may affect the prognosis of the case.

Congenital flexural deformity of the distal interphalangeal joint
Congenital flexural deformity of the distal interphalangeal (DIP) joint presents as varying degrees of DIP flexion so that the foal walks on its toe and the heel does not contact the ground ('ballerina foal') (64). Hoof shape does not alter in the early stages, unlike in acquired forms, although increased toe wear occurs. It is uncommon, can be uni- or bilateral, and be associated with other flexural deformities such as in the MCP joint. Increased tension in the inferior check ligament and deep digital flexor tendon may be present on palpation.

Treatment consists of a combination of regular exercise, passive manipulation, analgesics (beware of gastro-duodenal ulceration with the use of NSAID medication; use of anti-ulcer medication is advisable [e.g. omeprazole]), corrective foot trimming, splinting, or casting. Regular exercise on hard, even surfaces and specific exercises such as walking up inclines and 'hopping' on the affected limb are essential. NSAIDs help reduce pain and encourage use of the affected limb. Oxytetracycline may be useful (2–4 g in 500 ml saline slowly i/v once or twice in the first 48 hours post partum). The drug may chelate free calcium ions, prevent their influx into muscle fibers, and may lead to relaxation and passive lengthening of the muscle. Kidney function should be checked prior to using this form of treatment. Corrective foot trimming consists of mild heel rasping. A small toe extension with a glue-on plastic shoe or placing a hoof composite over the toe will prevent excessive toe wear and help to stretch affected periarticular soft-tissue structures. Casts can be very useful

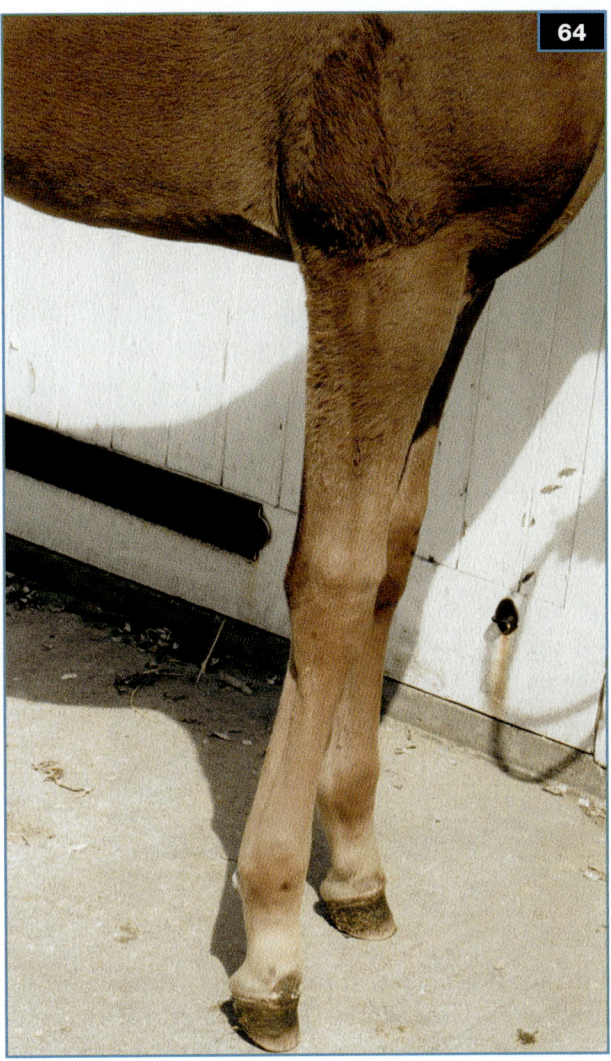

64 Young Thoroughbred foal with a right forelimb congenital flexural deformity of the distal interphalangeal joint. Note the typical 'ballerina' foal stance on the toe tip in the right fore.

in congenital DIP flexural deformities. Incorporation of the foot up to the carpus or tarsus for 7–14 days leads to a relaxation of the muscle–tendon unit. Care should be exercised with the use of casts in order to prevent the formation of pressure sores. In unresponsive cases, inferior check ligament desmotomy may be performed as for acquired cases, although the surgery is slightly more difficult due to the small size and less clear definition of the inferior check ligament.

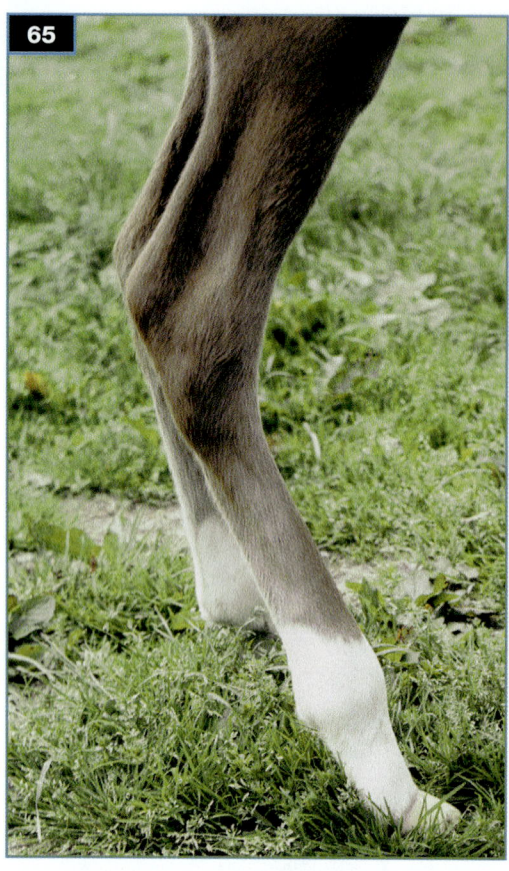

65

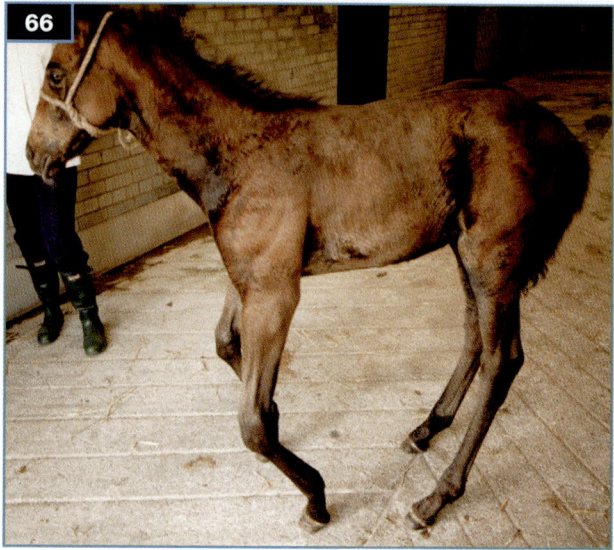

66

65 Newborn Thoroughbred foal with a congenital flexural deformity of the right hind metatarsophalangeal joint.

66 Older suckling Thoroughbred foal with history of a bilateral carpal flexural deformity at birth that was not corrected. The foal is shown at 9 weeks of age with bilateral severe carpal flexural and secondary varus angular limb deformities.

Congenital flexural deformity of the metacarpo/metatarsophalangeal joint

Congenital flexural deformity of the MCP/MTP joint may be uni- or bilateral and often involves the distal joints as well. The foal tends to knuckle over at the fetlock and may even walk on the dorsal aspect of the fetlock in severe cases. This is the most common congenital flexural deformity and the hindlimbs are mostly affected (**65**).

Treatment will vary according to the degree of the deformity. Since many cases also involve the DIP joint, treatment as described for this joint also needs to be initiated. Mild cases resolve with exercise, passive manipulation, and protective bandages. Casts and splints are very effective at treating this condition, as with congenital flexural deformity of the DIP joint. A PVC half-tubing splint, either bent or straight, placed on the palmar/plantar and dorsal aspect, respectively, of a well-padded limb allows forced extension of the limb, thereby facilitating stretching and relaxation of soft-tissue structures. Careful monitoring of splint bandages is essential to prevent pressure sores, and they should be changed every 3–5 days. Oxytetracycline may be useful as with congenital flexural deformity of the DIP joint. Surgical intervention with inferior check ligament desmotomy may be required in unresponsive or severe cases, where the distal joints are also involved.

Congenital flexural deformity of the carpal joint

Congenital flexural deformity of the carpal joint is usually bilateral with many cases exhibiting normal distal limb conformation. The condition is quite common, with affected foals either able to stand but 'buckling' forward at the carpus or, in severe cases, unable to stand (**66**). Careful examination of these foals is necessary since this presentation may be part of the 'contracted foal syndrome.'

Treatment with dorsal splint bandages or forelimb casts avoiding the phalangeal region can be effective. In severe cases, formation of pressure sores and rotation of the splints can be problematic, therefore frequent bandage changes are necessary. Many foals need assistance to suckle since they are unable to stand easily. Unilateral cases can rapidly develop overuse limb injuries in the contralateral limb and, sometimes, severe carpal valgus. Oxytetracycline may be useful as with congenital flexural deformity of the DIP joint. Surgical intervention for unresponsive or severe cases involves tenotomy of the insertions of the ulnaris lateralis and flexor carpi ulnaris muscles just proximal to the accessory carpal bone. Transection of the palmar ligament and capsule of the carpal joints has also been reported, but is rarely carried out. Euthanasia may be necessary in severe or unresponsive cases.

Congenital contracture of the peroneus tertius muscle

Congenital contracture of the peroneus tertius muscle is rare. The condition presents as a severe flexural deformity of the tarsus, often as part of the contracted foal syndrome. Treatment by resection of the muscle tendon unit has been reported.

Congenital hyperextension of newborn foals ('flaccid tendons')

Congenital hyperextension of newborn foals has an unknown etiology and pathogenesis and the condition may be a physiologic variant or a temporary failure of the agonist/antagonist muscle balance. It is common in premature (<320 days) or dysmature foals. The condition is more severe if there is accompanying systemic illness or inadequate exercise. The flaccidity of the flexor tendons is often accompanied by periarticular ligament laxity and joint instability. Commonly, both hindlimbs or all four limbs are affected. There appears to be a higher incidence in Thoroughbreds and heavy horse breeds. The MCP/MTP and/or interphalangeal joints are usually affected. There is often dropping of the fetlock and, in severe cases, the plantar/palmar aspect of the pastern and fetlock contacts the ground (67).

Many cases resolve spontaneously as muscle tone and ligament strength improves post partum. This process can be encouraged by careful exercise. Corrective foot trimming of the heel to provide a flat weight-bearing surface and eliminate a 'rocker heel' effect is useful. A light protective bandage to protect the heel/pastern/fetlock from trauma can be provided, but too much support exacerbates the condition.

Heel extension shoes should be used in unresolving or severe cases (68). Surgical management as a salvage procedure, with tendon shortening Z-plasties, has been described, but is rarely necessary or used.

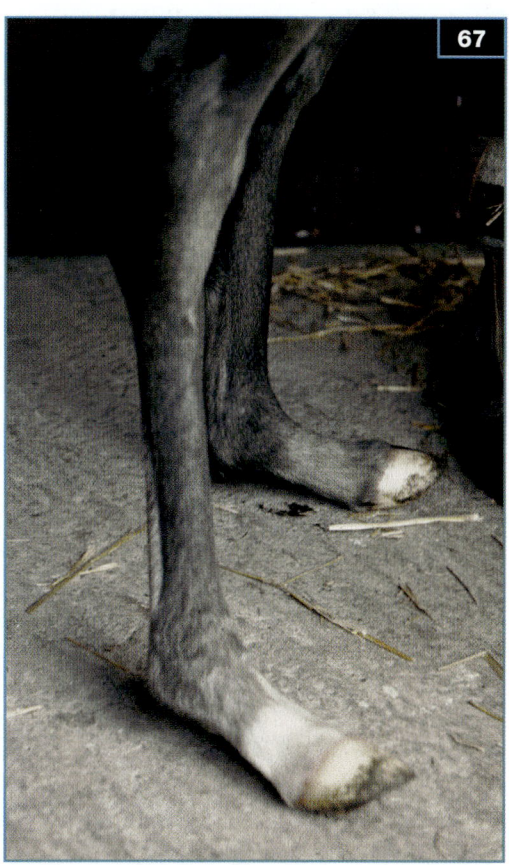

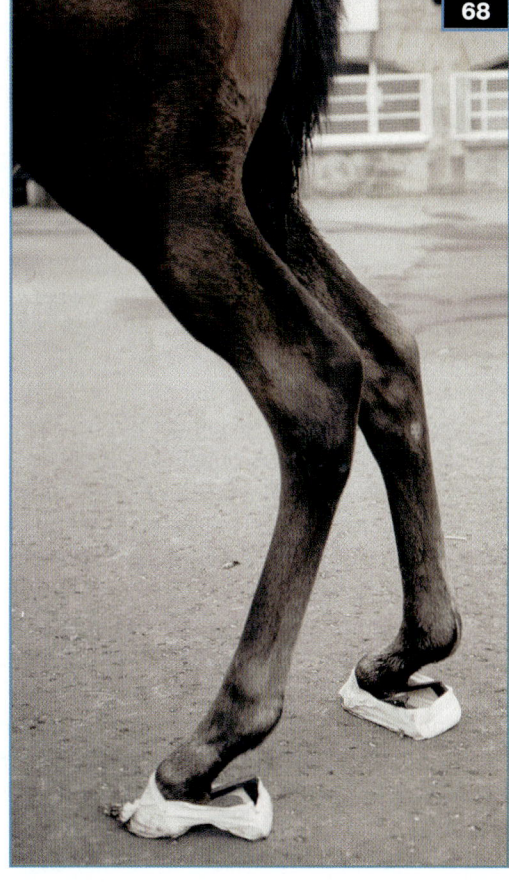

67 Neonatal foal with severe bilateral hyperextension of the distal limb joints (flaccid tendons).

68 Older Thoroughbred suckling foal with a history of bilateral hindlimb distal joint hyperextension that did not respond to conservative treatment and was eventually treated with heel extension shoes.

45

Rupture of the common digital extensor tendon

Rupture of the common digital extensor (CDE) tendon is relatively uncommon. It usually affects both forelimbs and is usually present in combination with other musculoskeletal defects, in particular carpal and metacarpophalangeal flexural deformities, hypoplasia of cuboidal bones, and underdeveloped pectoral muscles. The condition may be inheritable and a higher incidence has been reported in Arabs and Quarter horses.

Swelling of the tendon sheath over the dorsolateral surface of the carpus is present (69). Bilateral cases are common and affected foals adopt a slightly bowlegged, over at the knee stance. They may knuckle forward at the fetlock when walking. Palpation of the swelling may reveal tendon rupture. Radiography and ultrasonography can confirm the presence of hypoplastic carpal bones and partial/complete tendon rupture.

Treatment involves box rest and splint bandages or tube casts (changed every 3 days for up to 4–8 weeks) to maintain a normal limb axis and assist ossification of hypoplastic carpal bones. Concurrent treatment of any flexural deformity is essential. Spontaneous healing of the ruptured tendon occurs and surgical apposition is unnecessary. The prognosis is good provided concurrent flexural deformities are correctable.

Contracted foal/limb syndrome

Contracted foal/limb syndrome describes a variety of combinations of congenital appendicular and axial contractures and curvatures that are uncommon, but well recognized. The term includes arthrogryposis (deformity of the limbs characterized by curvature of the limbs, multiple articular rigidities, and dysplasia of the muscles), torticollis or 'wry neck' (lateral bending and rotation of the cervical spine), scoliosis (lateral deviation usually involving the last part of the thoracic and first part of the lumbar spine), and lordosis and kyphosis (ventral and dorsal curvature of usually the last part of the thoracic and first part of the lumbar spine). In addition, there may be varying degrees of flexural deformity involving the carpus, metacarpo/tarsophalangeal joints, and sometimes the tarsus, and asymmetric formation of the cranium or 'wry nose' (70, 71). Attenuation (thinning of the ventral abdominal wall or even visceral eventration) is present in some cases of severe scoliosis. The condition may be due to unfavorable, restrictive uterine conditions and no evidence of a genetic etiology has been described. If the deformities are mild, affected foals can develop normally given time and adequate nursing care. Combinations of conservative therapies should be utilized and surgery used in severe cases as appropriate (e.g. inferior check ligament desmotomy for severe MCP flexural deformity). Humane destruction may be necessary in severe cases.

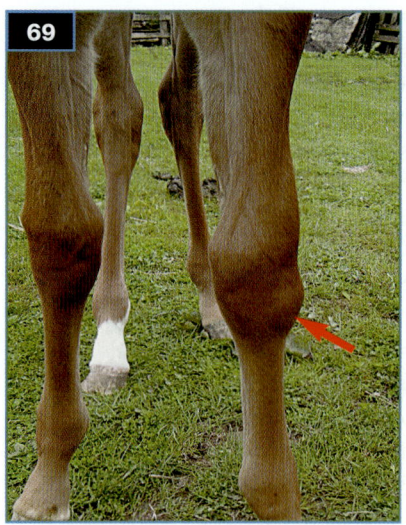

69 Two-week-old foal that presented with an acute onset of a dorsolateral distal radius fluid-filled swelling (arrow) due to rupture of the common digital extensor tendon. This was not associated in this foal with a flexural deformity.

70 A foal suffering with contracted foal syndrome, which was euthanized immediately after birth. There is a wry nose, neck torticollis, distal limb hyperextension, and carpal flexural deformity visible in this view.

71 Newborn pony foal with wry nose.

Polydactyly and adactyly

Polydactyly and adactyly are both rare. Polydactyly is defined as the occurrence of more digits than normal for a given species. A dominant hereditary transmission with incomplete penetrance has been postulated. The extra digit in horses can be teratologic where duplication is distal to the fetlock joint, resulting in two completely separate digits articulating with a third metacarpal bone, which may or may not be divided distally (72, 73). The more common atavistic ('developmental') form involves an extra digit on the medial aspect of the forelimb that fully articulates with a fully developed second metacarpal bone. Presentation is usually unilateral in a forelimb, but bilateral forelimb and involvement of all four limbs have been described. The atavistic form is managed successfully by surgical resection of the extra digit at its base, with no functional disturbance or cosmetic blemish.

Adactyly refers to absence of all or part of a normal digit and has been reported in the forelimb of a Welsh Mountain foal with a contralateral forelimb polydactyly.

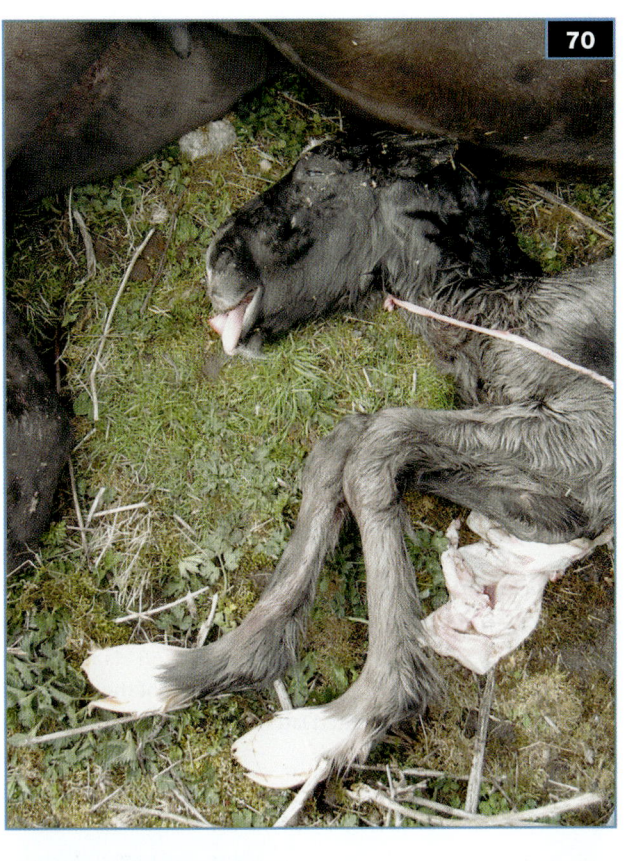

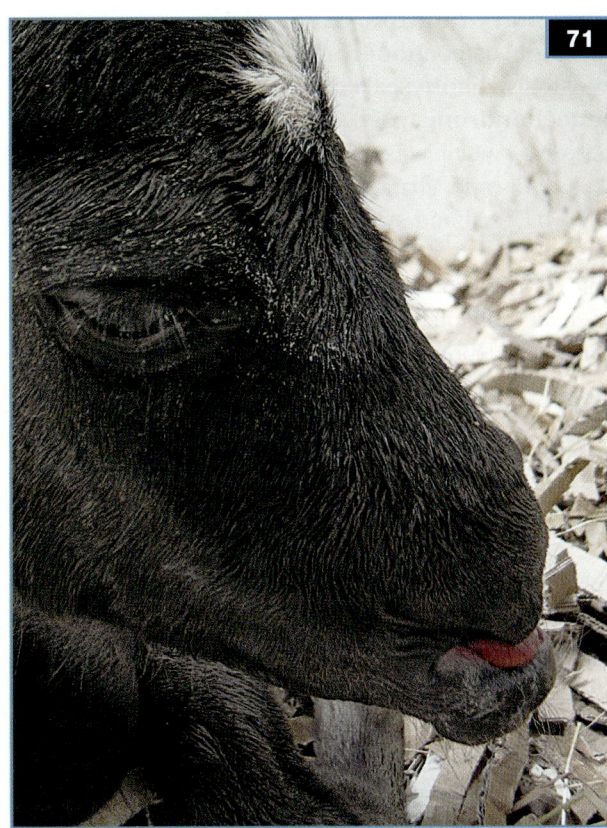

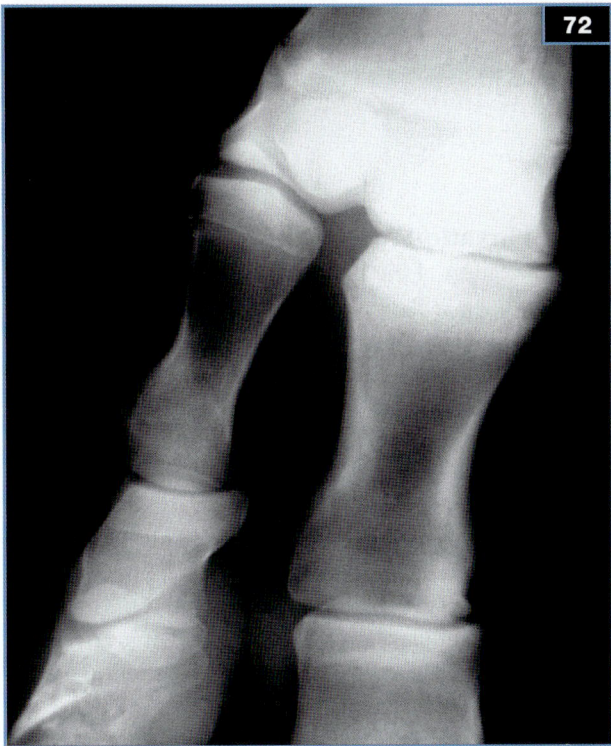

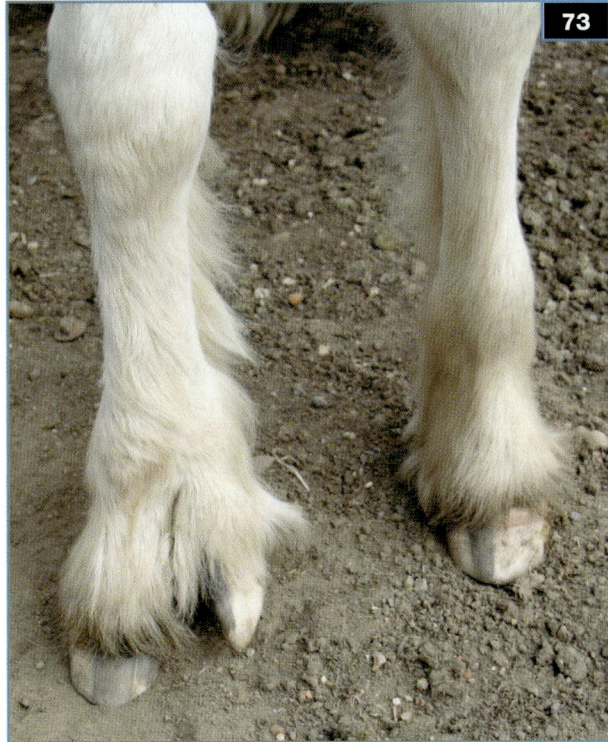

72 Dorsopalmar radiograph of the distal right forelimb of a foal with the teratologic form of polydactyly. Note the duplication of the distal end of the metacarpus and two formed digits.

73 Another case of teratologic polydactyly in the right forelimb of a Cob foal.

Hereditary multiple exostosis (multiple osteochondroma, multiple cartilaginous exostosis, diaphyseal aclasis, or endochondromatosis)

Hereditary multiple exostosis is an uncommon, hereditary, skeletal disorder characterized by many bony projections, often bilateral and symmetrical on the long bones, ribs (near the costochondral junctions), and pelvis. A single dominant autosomal gene has been cited as the cause, and affected individuals pass the trait to approximately half of their offspring. Histologically, the exostoses have cancellous bone capped by hyaline cartilage and appear to be osteochondromas. They remain benign and no transformation to malignancy has been reported.

The exostoses vary in morphology from smooth and rounded to 'spur-like'. As the foal matures, the swellings on the limbs tend not to enlarge, but those at other sites enlarge until maturity is attained. Lameness is present if the exostosis impinges on surrounding muscles or tendons. Radiography and ultrasonography can confirm the exact location and extent of the exostoses.

No treatment for the condition is known. The owner should be informed of the hereditary nature of the disease. Surgical excision of an individual exostosis may be indicated if it is shown to be causing lameness.

Solitary osteochondroma

Solitary osteochondromas may be abortive expressions of multiple exostosis, but unlike this condition they do not appear to be inheritable. This benign mass tends to be located at the caudomedial aspect of the radius and usually causes carpal sheath distension and subsequent lameness. Radiography and ultrasonography can confirm the extent of the lesion. Surgical excision is required and the prognosis for nonrecurrence of the tumor and restoration of normal limb function appears to be good.

Solitary osteochondromas have also been observed at the caudolateral aspect of the distal radius, on the nasal bone, and at the lateral aspect of the proximal calcaneus (74).

Unilateral phalangeal hypoplasia

Unilateral phalangeal hypoplasia is a rare condition where there are degrees of incomplete development and sometimes absence of the phalanges within an otherwise normal foot (although the foot is often contracted) (75). The condition occurs predominantly in the hindlimbs. Affected foals are lame on the affected limb. Radiography can confirm the condition. The prognosis for a long-term athletic future appears to be hopeless, although navicular agenesis was reported in a 2-year-old Thoroughbred in training.

74 Lateral radiograph of the hock of a Clydesdale foal with a developing firm swelling on the point of the hock. Note the mixed-pattern osseous density mass present on the point of the calcaneus, adjacent to the physis, and due to a solitary osteochondroma (arrow).

75 Postmortem specimens of the sagittal section of the feet of a foal that presented with unilateral lameness and a very small digit. The upper limb is affected by phalangeal hypoplasia, with a vestigial third phalanx (red arrow) and navicular bone and abnormal second phalanx (yellow arrow).

76 Postmortem specimen of the distal femur of a foal that presented with bilateral patellar luxation. Note the rather flattened hypoplastic lateral trochlear ridge (on the left) and shallow trochlear groove.

77 Typical squatting stance of a foal with bilateral patellar luxation.

78 Craniocaudal radiograph of the stifle joint of the foal in 77 showing the patella luxated laterally outside the plane of the femur (arrow).

Lateral luxation of the patella

Lateral luxation of the patella is a rare condition in most breeds, but it is commonly seen in Miniature Shetlands and oher small breeds. It can be uni- or bilateral. A hereditary mode of transmission involving a monogenic autosomal recessive gene in Shetland ponies is cited. The condition is usually due to hypoplasia of the lateral trochlear ridge of the femur (76). Bilaterally affected foals typically present with a 'squatting' stance, with hips, stifles, and hocks in extreme flexion (77). Lateromedial, caudocranial, and flexed skyline radiographs are useful to confirm the condition (78). Surgical repair can be attempted in unilateral cases where underlying bony development is adequate. The lateral patellar retinaculum is incised and the medial patellar retinaculum and fascia imbricated. Some surgeons also perform a trochleoplasty. The prognosis is guarded in unilateral cases and appears guarded to poor in bilateral cases, although miniature breeds can cope quite well with milder bilateral deformities.

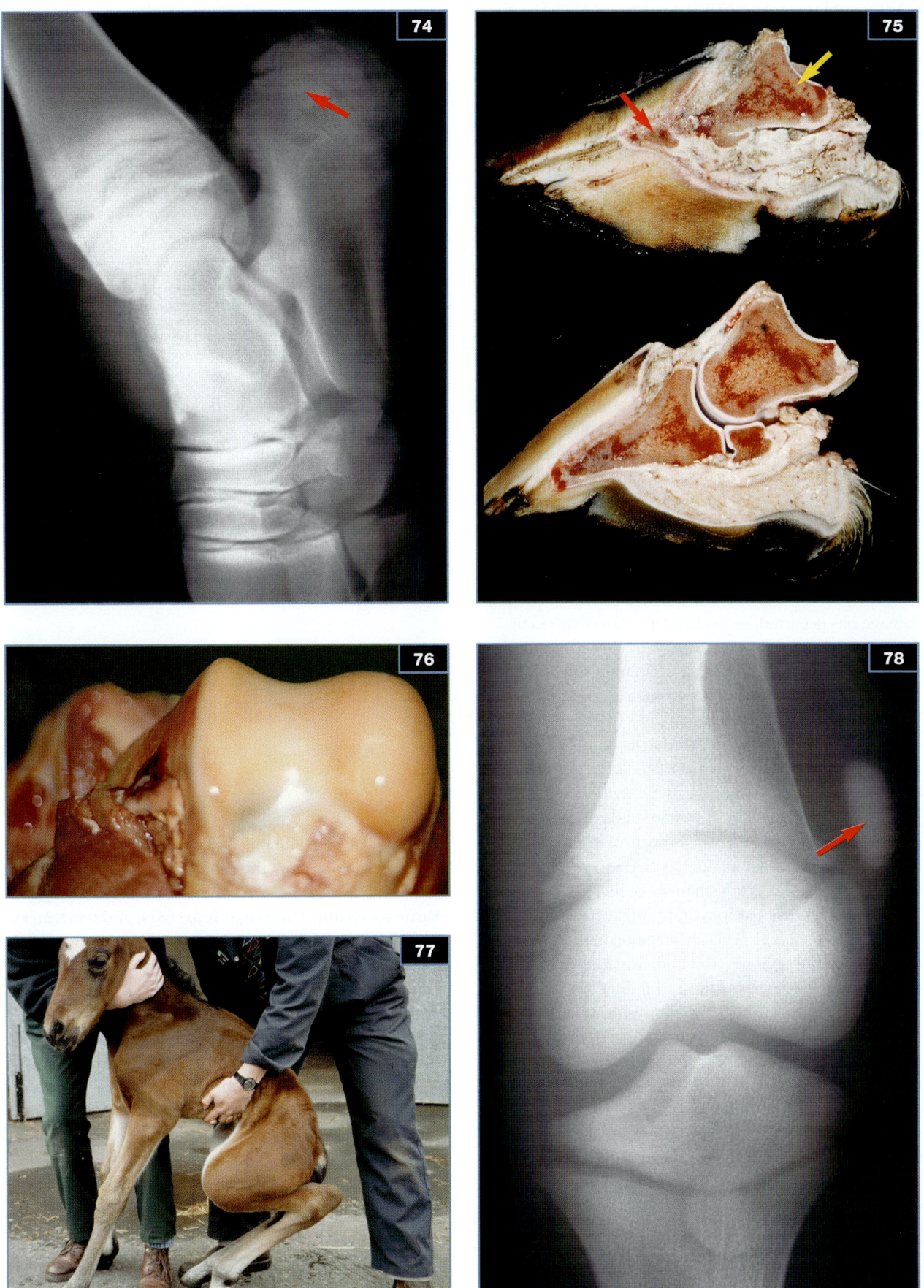

Osteochondrosis

Osteochondrosis (OCD) is a condition that is part of a group of orthopedic conditions affecting young, growing horses termed developmental orthopedic diseases (DODs) that also includes physitis, angular limb deformities, flexural limb deformities, and cervical vertebral malformation. OCD is defined as a 'failure of normal endochondral ossification'. There is a disturbance of the normal differentiation of cells in growing cartilage at the end of the long bones in the articular–epiphyseal growth plate; this leads to retention of cartilage or dyschondroplasia. These microscopic changes can either repair or develop into a clinical entity and lead to lameness. The manifestations of this disturbance in the horse are multiple. Necrosis of the affected cartilage may lead to cartilage fibrillation and fissuring at various depths. Osteochondral fragments ('joint mice') may detach to float free in the joint. Inflammation of the joint occurs in response to these changes, leading to the term 'osteochondritis'. Dissecting flaps of cartilage are specifically termed 'osteochondritis dissecans' (79). Cartilage infolding and subsequent resorption can result in the development of subchondral bone cysts, mainly of the medial femoral condyle. These are thought to be another manifestation of OCD by some clinicians. Once cartilage damage has occurred, secondary DJD (OA) may occur.

The etiology of OCD is not clear, but it is multifactorial. Various trigger factors have been implicated. Rapid growth rate in fast growing horses such as Thoroughbreds, Standardbreds, and Warmbloods is associated with the development of OCD, possibly due to bone growth outstripping blood supply. A genetic predisposition may also exist in these breeds and anecdotal evidence has been shown in some breed lines. Dietary imbalances and mismanagement are major factors. In particular, excessive carbohydrate and protein intake has been shown to induce OCD lesions. The exact mechanism of these factors is not known, but excess carbohydrate intake may influence chondrocyte metabolism via an alteration in insulin mediation. Excess phosphorus, calcium, and zinc and insufficient copper have been found to induce OCD. Copper deficiency may act via lysyl oxidase dysfunction, leading to decreased collagen cross-links and subsequent weakness of the cartilage. A recent scientific paper reported no relationship between copper and OCD, although it found a decreased ability of affected cartilage to repair if copper was low. The role of trauma is strongly implicated as a factor (whether primary or secondary is still controversial), although the stage of development when the articular–epiphyseal cartilage complex is vulnerable to damage is unknown at the present time, and early low-grade loading may actually promote adaptation of immature cartilage and prevent OCD lesions forming.

79 Large dissecting flap lesion of the mid-lateral trochlear ridge of the distal femur of a 6-month-old Warmblood foal, which represents the most common form of OCD lesion in the stifle joint.

80 Dorsomedial/plantarolateral oblique radiograph of the hock of an Irish Draught horse presenting with tarsocrural joint distension and lameness localized to this joint. There is a small OCD lesion of the distal intermediate ridge of the tibia (arrow).

81 Six-month-old Thoroughbred foal with marked bilateral stifle joint distension and hindlimb lameness. Note the enlarged femoropatellar joint in the left hindlimb just below the fold of the flank (arrow).

82 Lateral radiograph of the stifle joints of a yearling Warmblood showing an OCD lesion of the upper lateral trochlear ridge, with loss of the bony outline of the ridge and subchondral bone lysis.

OCD is more commonly encountered in the hindlimb joints. Depending on the breed, the tarsocrural joint (Warmbloods and Standardbreds) (80), the stifle joints (Warmbloods and Thoroughbreds) (81), and metacarpo/ tarsophalangeal joints (Thoroughbreds and Standardbreds) are the most commonly affected. OCD in other breeds is less common, but does occur. Bilateral lesions are common and radiography of the contralateral limb is always advisable. Multiple different joint lesions are not common. Lameness (from chronic, to mild to acute, to marked) and joint distension (81) are usually present. Radiography (82) and ultrasonography are most commonly used for imaging lesions. Treatment may be conservative or surgical (arthroscopy) depending on the type of lesion and age of the horse. The prognosis depends on the location, type, and severity of the lesion and age of the horse. The clinical signs, treatment, and prognosis of OCD in each joint are discussed in the relevant sections on the conditions of the forelimbs and hindlimbs.

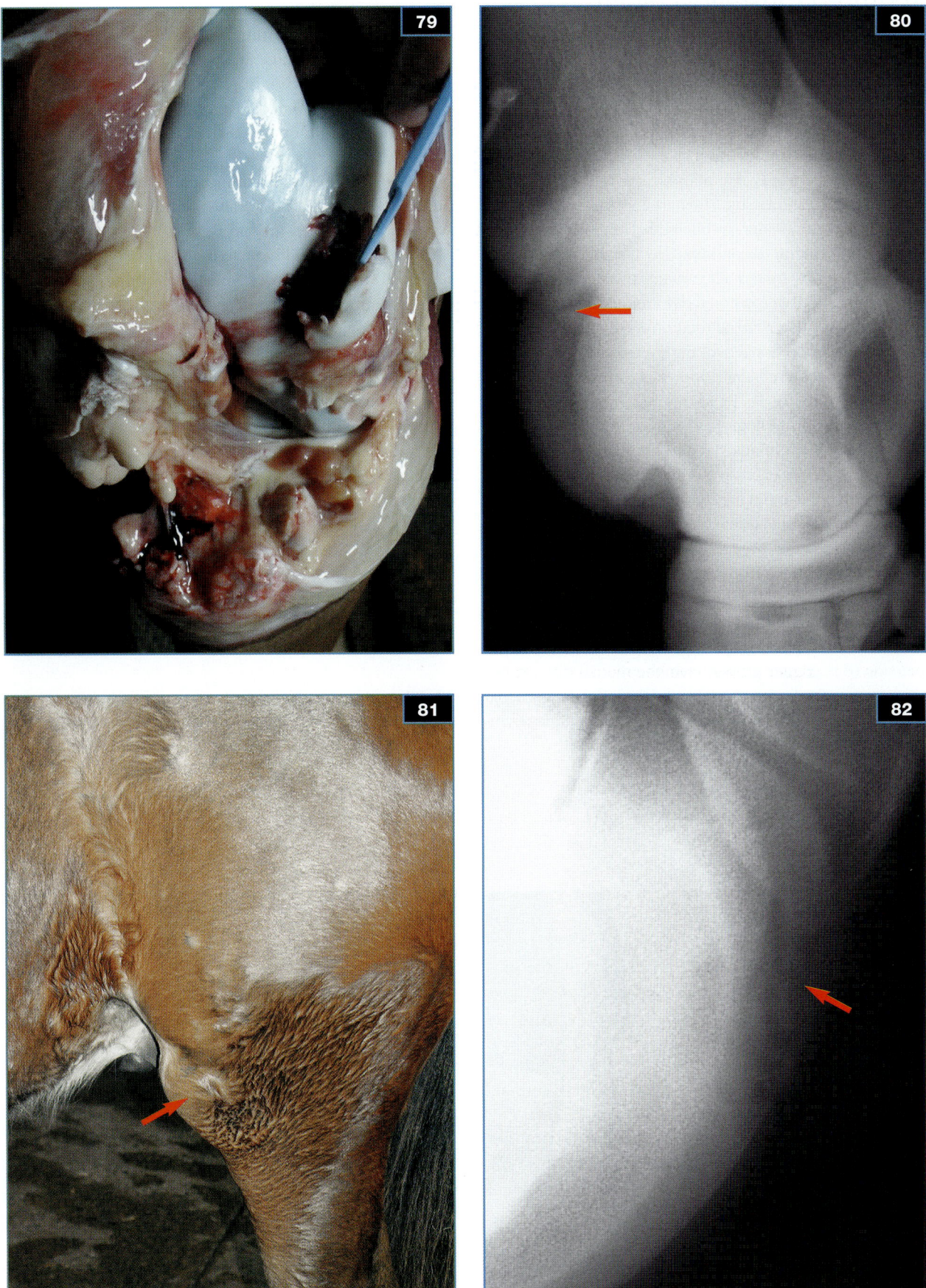

Acquired musculoskeletal abnormalities

Acquired angular limb deformities

Definition/overview

Acquired angular limb deformities (ALDs) usually manifest as a lateral or medial deviation to the long axis of the limb in the frontal or transverse plane, commonly seen at the carpus, fetlock, and tarsus. They are more common in the forelimb and can be uni- or bilateral. There is no sex predisposition. Lateral deviations are termed valgus and medial deviations are termed varus. Many ALDs are associated with postural or rotational deformities, especially with carpal valgus, when a lateral rotation is common. ALDs can be congenital (see Congenital musculoskeletal abnormalities, p. 40) or acquired/developmental (see below).

Etiology/pathophysiology

The etiology is multifactorial and includes genetics, fast growth rate and/or excessive bodyweight, over- or undernutrition, mineral and trace element imbalances, excessive exercise, internal or external trauma, and contralateral limb lameness. These factors, either individually or in combination, contribute to the development of acquired ALDs.

Asymmetric or imbalanced longitudinal bone growth occurs from a distal physis or epiphysis due to overload of the physis on one side, leading to decreased growth on that side (e.g. greater growth from the medial distal radial physis compared with the lateral physis leads to carpal valgus). Direct trauma to the physis can also lead to asymmetric damage and subsequent growth.

Clinical presentation

The history of a developing ALD is in two main periods: birth to 6–8 weeks of age and 6 weeks to 9 months of age. All breeds are affected, but it is particularly common in fast-growing larger breeds. Deformities are more common in the forelimb. Other types of developmental orthopedic disease may be present.

The foal should be examined at rest and walking. The site(s) and degree of angulation of affected joint(s) are assessed in the forelimbs from in front and in the hindlimbs from behind, with the foal standing as square as possible with the foot directly under the upper part of the limb. It is important that concurrent rotation from the chest is taken into account for forelimb evaluation by viewing the limb perpendicular to the frontal plane of the limb (83, 84). All limbs should be palpated and manipulated in a nonweight-bearing position for evidence of joint instability (mainly congenital forms), growth plate swelling, and heat/pain/swelling suggestive of external trauma. A full lameness examination is essential, including assessing foot placement. The presence of lameness is significant because foals with ALDs are not normally lame. Traumatically-induced cases usually present acutely with lameness and varying instability. Some bony swelling associated with the growth plate is quite common in longer standing cases.

83 Bilateral acquired carpal valgus angular limb deformity. In this detailed view of the left forelimb note the severe valgus deformity and very enlarged distal radial physis.

84 Left forelimb fetlock varus deformity.

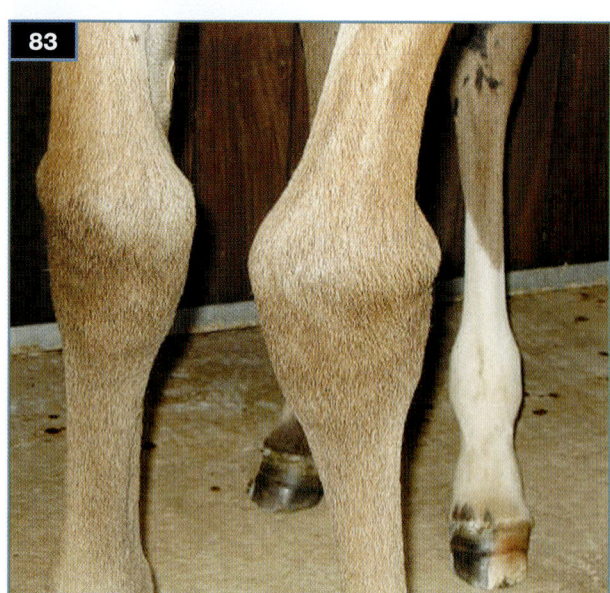

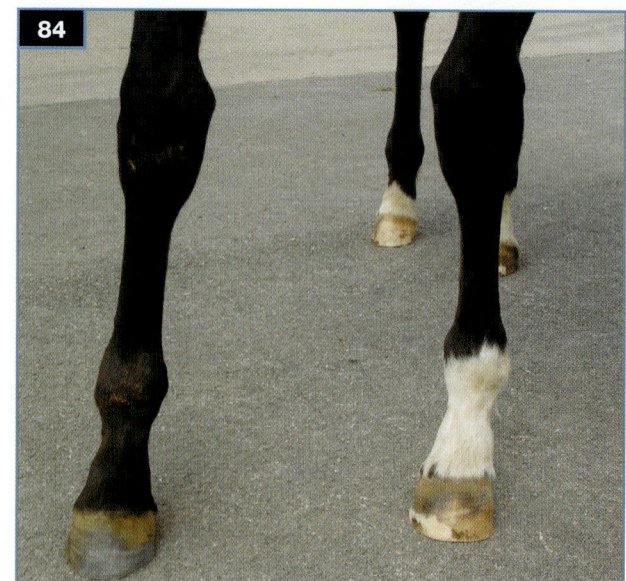

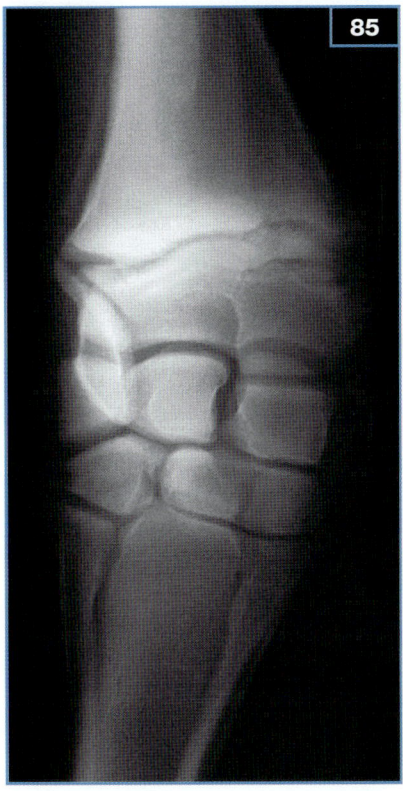

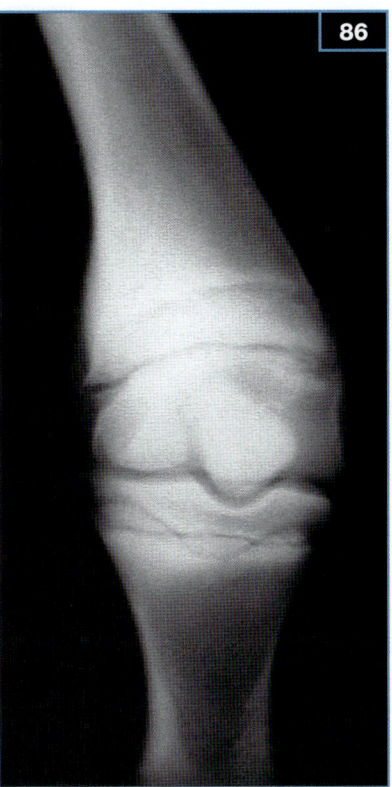

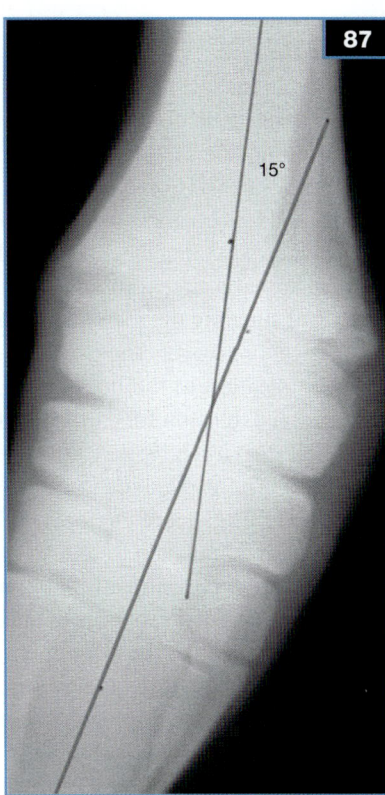

15°

Differential diagnosis

Concurrent flexural deformities and/or OCD; traumatic injuries.

Diagnosis

The clinical history and findings are diagnostic and the specific problem and subsequent management are confirmed by radiography. Dorsopalmar/plantar and latero-medial projections are taken using long plates, which allow the long bones proximal and distal to the deformity to be radiographed (85, 86). It is useful to assess objectively the angulation of the deformity by drawing a line joining proximal and distal points in the middle of the long bones, both above and below the affected joint, and measuring the angle of deviation from the vertical: a normal range of angulation of the carpus and tarsus can be expected to be from <5° through to mild/moderate (5–10°) and severe angulation (>10°) (87). In the fetlock joint the degree of angulation is more critical to the prognosis. Also evaluated are any concurrent malformation or injury to the distal physis and/or epiphysis and to bones making up the articulation. This can affect treatment option selection and prognosis (e.g. Salter–Harris type V or VI injury to the physis may lead to premature closure and loss of major growth potential on the affected side).

85 Dorsopalmar radiograph of the right forelimb of a foal with severe carpal valgus deformity showing the degree of angulation, wedging of the epiphysis, ectasia of the physis, and metaphyseal flaring often noted in such cases.

86 Severe varus angular limb deformity of the fetlock joint. Note the wedging of the epiphysis and severe tipping of the physis in the distal 3rd metacarpus.

87 Dorsopalmar radiograph of a foal with carpal valgus. Lines drawn between the mid points of the long bones proximal and distal to the carpus intersect at the level of the epiphysis, indicating that the source of the deformity may be imbalanced longitudinal bone growth. Note that the degree of deformity is measured as 15 degrees.

Management
Conservative

Conservative management is more effective in early cases, and exercise restriction (e.g. box rest and daily in-hand short walking, or small-yard rest [not a paddock]) is a crucial part of this. Corrective foot trimming to alter the mediolateral foot balance (e.g. lowering the lateral wall for carpal valgus, lowering the medial wall for fetlock varus) is essential in early cases. In addition, decreasing the toe length and squaring the toe of the hoof off will encourage symmetrical breakover. The use of glue-on shoes or composite application to the hoof for more advanced cases (e.g. medial extension for carpal valgus/lateral extension for fetlock varus) can be very effective, although contraction of the hoof capsule can occur if these are fitted for long periods. The diet of the foal and lactating broodmare will require manipulation to reduce excessive protein and decrease growth rate, and it is important to assess the diet for any deficiencies or excesses of trace elements and minerals, and to balance these by the use of supplements. Monitoring these cases frequently (e.g. every 7–10 days) is advisable to follow their progression and to respond with different treatments if the foal is not steadily improving.

The application of shock-wave therapy to retard growth on the convex side of various ALDs has recently been described, but is controversial. Three to five sessions at weekly intervals were used concurrently with the use of corrective farriery techniques, with comparable results to surgical correction.

Surgical

Surgical treatment is used when conservative treatment is unsuccessful, the condition is worsening, or the deviation is severe at the outset. Surgery is aimed at manipulating growth acceleration and/or growth retardation of the physis and epiphysis.

Hemicircumferential periosteal transection and elevation (periosteal stripping) aims to accelerate growth on the concave side of the affected limb (e.g. lateral distal radius for carpal valgus and medial distal third metacarpus for forelimb fetlock varus). Note that concurrent transection of the remnant ulna in the radius, or fibula in the tibia, is necessary to maximize the effect of this procedure for valgus deviations of the carpus and tarsus, respectively. Recently, it has been suggested that this procedure does not in fact lead to growth acceleration at the distal radial physis as previously described, and foals with mild carpal valgus receiving surgery and foals treated conservatively will correct equally well.

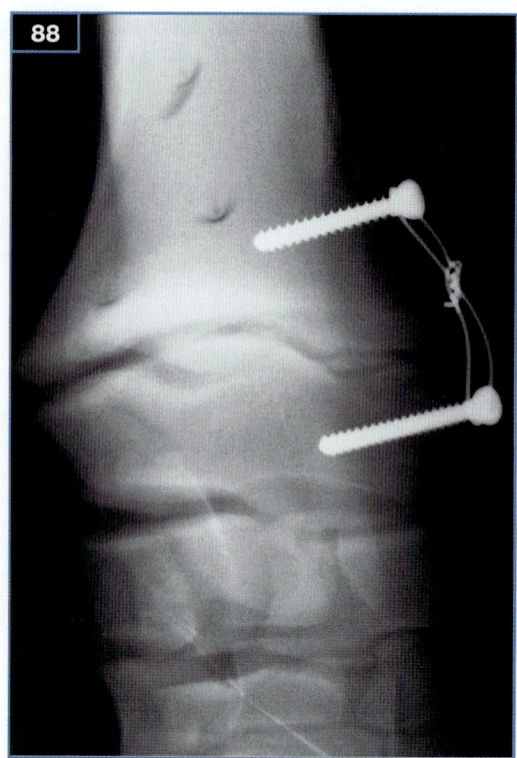

88 Intraoperative radiograph of the placement of two screws and wire in order to transphyseal bridge and compress the medial side of the distal radial physis for the treatment of an acquired valgus angular limb deformity of the carpus.

In unresponsive or severe ALDs, growth can be retarded by transphyseal bridging of the affected distal physis on the convex side (e.g. medial side for carpal valgus and lateral side for fetlock varus) using either cortical screws and wire, orthopedic staples, a single cortical screw from distal to proximal, or small bone compression plates (**88**).

Prognosis

The prognosis is good if cases are managed early and regularly monitored. It is guarded if there is a poor initial response to conservative treatment, if the condition is severe from the outset, concurrent problems are present (e.g. contralateral limb lameness), or if there is rapid deterioration.

Acquired flexural limb deformities

Definition/overview

Acquired flexural limb deformities are a deviation of the limb in a sagittal plane leading to persistent hyperflexion of a joint(s) region. They are either congenital (see Congenital musculoskeletal abnormalities, p. 40) or acquired (developmental) (see below). The condition is not due to contracted tendons, but to a relative shortening of a tendon unit in relation to bony structures.

Etiology/pathophysiology

The etiology is multifactorial and linked to overnutrition, genetics, excessive and rapid growth, and pain. Excessive feeding in predisposed individuals leads to excess and rapid growth. These factors plus mineral/trace element imbalances can lead to DOD and pain, which alter stance and loading of limbs.

During rapid bone growth the accompanying lengthening of the tendinous unit is limited due to the accessory ligaments, and a discrepancy may occur leading to the deformity. Pain during physeal dysplasia at rapid growth phases or for other reasons (e.g. OCD) may result in altered limb load bearing and initiate contraction and shortening of the musculoskeletal unit. In adults, true tendon contraction can occur post severe tendon injuries. In very painful limbs, chronic non-weight-bearing can lead to flexural deformities.

Clinical presentation

The condition develops after birth through to 2 years old and is commonly seen in the forelimbs at either the DIP (coffin) joint or MCP (fetlock) joint. There is no sex predisposition and unilateral and bilateral cases are seen. Acquired flexural deformity of the DIP joint is typically recognized between 3 and 18 months, and MCP flexural deformity between 9 and 18 months. Clinical signs of DIP deformity include a prominent bulge at the coronary band, 'dishing' of the dorsal hoof wall, an increase in heel length, and eventually a 'boxy' foot ('club foot') appearance (Stage I DIP deformity) (89). In severe cases the heel does not contact the ground and the dorsal hoof wall goes beyond the vertical (Stage II DIP deformity), with weight borne at the toe (90).

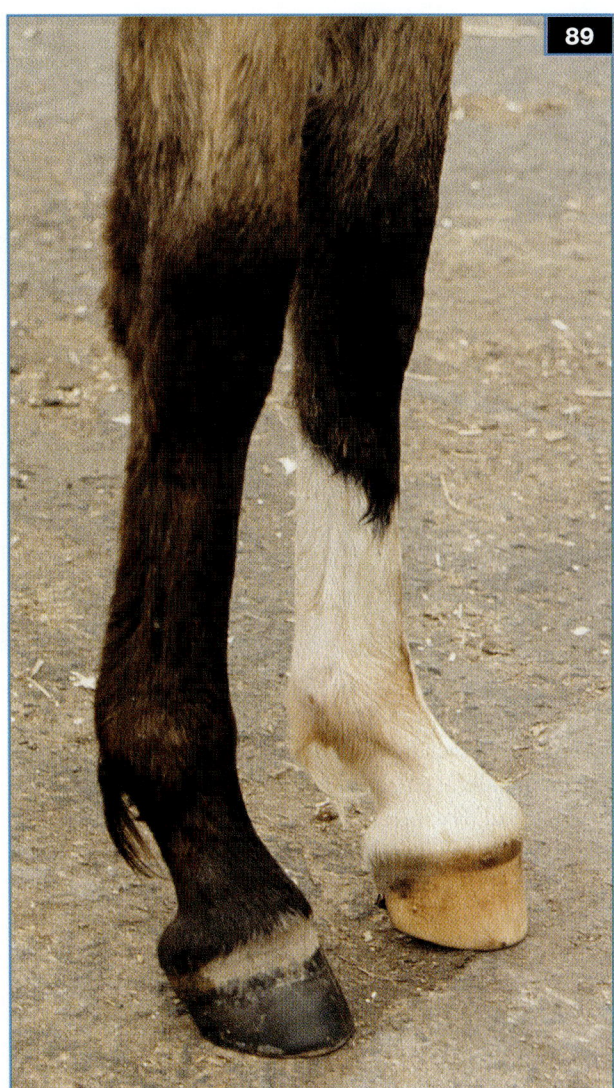

89 A yearling pony with an acquired flexural deformity of the left forelimb distal interphalangeal joint. Note the upright, boxy, and contracted left fore foot, with the heel raised just off the ground. Stage I deformity.

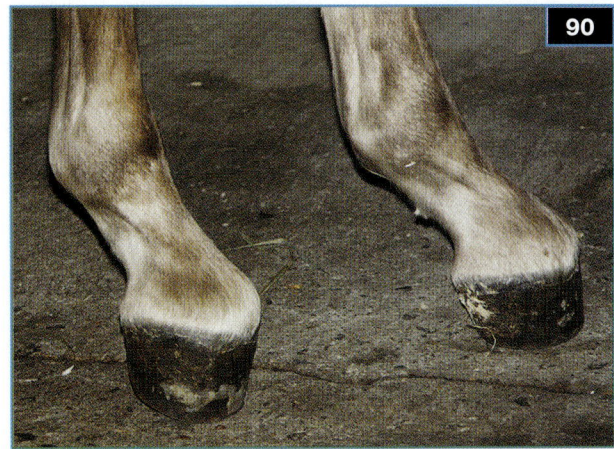

90 More severe case of bilateral acquired distal interphalangeal joint flexural deformity, with a Stage II deformity in the right forelimb.

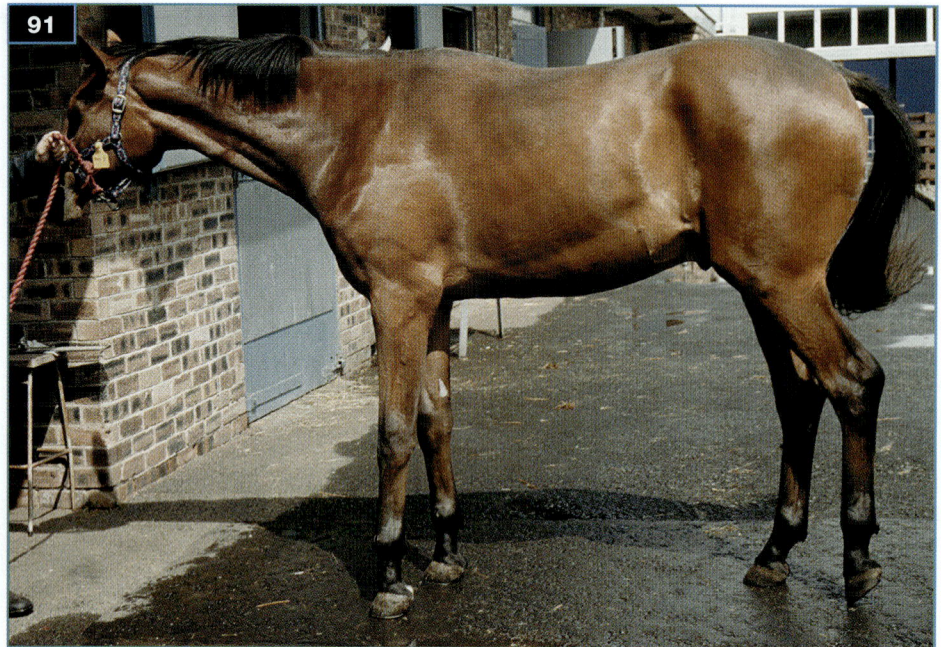

91 Yearling Thoroughbred with rapid onset of bilateral flexural deformity of the metacarpophalangeal joints of both forelimbs. Note the very good condition and size of the animal and the upright forelimb conformation through the fetlock. The left forelimb is intermittently knuckling forward.

Excessive wear at the toe of the hoof may allow infections to establish and further decrease weight bearing on the limb. Careful palpation of the accessory ligament of the deep digital flexor tendon (ALDDFT) (inferior check ligament), both weight- and non-weight-bearing, may reveal increased tension. MCP deformity is less common, mainly affects the forelimb, and presents after a period of compensatory growth as an upright conformation with intermittent dorsal knuckling in early or mild cases (91). The latter is persistent in advanced cases and 'knuckling over' and stumbling are sometimes seen at the walk in these cases. Palpation of the ALDDFT may reveal some DIP joint component. Acquired carpal flexural deformities are sometimes seen in adults in a chronic, non-weight-bearing limb.

Differential diagnoses
None.

Diagnosis
The clinical history and findings are diagnostic. Radiography of the foot of the affected limb may reveal bone remodeling at the tip of the pedal bone in severe cases of DIP deformity, which may affect the long-term prognosis in some cases. Infrequently, persistent infection in the hoof at the toe can be associated with damage and infection in the pedal bone.

Management
DIP flexural deformities

Conservative: A controlled exercise program on hard even surfaces (walking up small inclines and 'hopping' on the affected limb) can be useful. Placing the foal and mare into a small pen with an all-weather or dry surface for controlled but regular exercise is beneficial. Regular foot trimming (every 10 days) is important to lower the heels. Application of a plastic, glue-on, toe extension shoe (must be changed every 10–14 days to prevent further 'boxiness' developing) or placing a hoof composite cap over the toe is very effective. Both methods protect the toe and dorsal hoof capsule from bruising during exercise and act as a lever arm (92). Dietary restriction is necessary to lower the carbohydrate and protein intake for the mare and foal. Early weaning of the foal helps control feed intake in the fast growth phase and decrease growth rate.

NSAIDs can be used as analgesics to control any pain, but gastroduodenal ulceration is common in these foals and therefore consideration should be given to the use of prophylactic antiulcer medications.

Surgical: Surgical intervention with desmotomy of the ALDDFT (inferior check ligament desmotomy) is recommended if no improvement occurs in 4–6 weeks (93, 94). If the deformity is particularly severe, DDF tenotomy may be used, although it is emphasized that this is a salvage procedure only.

Postoperative management consists of continuing with the conservative management techniques outlined above. Note that it is not uncommon to have a cosmetic blemish at these incision sites.

Musculoskeletal system

MCP flexural deformities

CONSERVATIVE: A controlled exercise program (walking on level ground with secure footing) and small-area free exercise are less helpful than with DIP flexural deformity. The feet should be balanced in both planes and there are some reports of success using heel wedges in early cases. Application of a toe extension combined with a vertical bar ('fetlock brace') shoe can be useful. Dietary restriction to lower the carbohydrate and protein intake and decrease the growth rate is essential, as many of these cases are in a period of excessive compensatory growth. The use of supplements to ensure correct trace element and mineral intake is important. Pain control by addressing and treating any specific orthopedic disease as well as the careful use of NSAIDs as analgesics will help the animal to weight bear more normally on the affected limb(s).

SURGICAL: Desmotomy of the ALDDFT may be useful in cases where there is evidence of DIP joint involvement. It is important in the postoperative management to include the use of a palmar splint to help maintain the fetlock joint in an extended position. Desmotomy of the accessory ligament of the superficial digital flexor tendon ('superior check ligament'), either by the conventional open approach or via tenoscopy of the carpal sheath, may be useful if it appears that there is involvement of the superficial digital flexor tendon. In severe cases of MCP deformity, both accessory ligaments are transected. Desmotomy of the medial and lateral branches of the suspensory ligament is indicated as a salvage procedure only.

Prognosis

The prognosis is fair with Stage I DIP flexural deformities, guarded with Stage II DIP/MCP flexural deformities, and guarded to poor with carpal flexural deformities.

Other factors may worsen the prognosis (e.g. delay in appropriate treatment, severity at the outset, and any concurrent orthopedic problems in the affected limb).

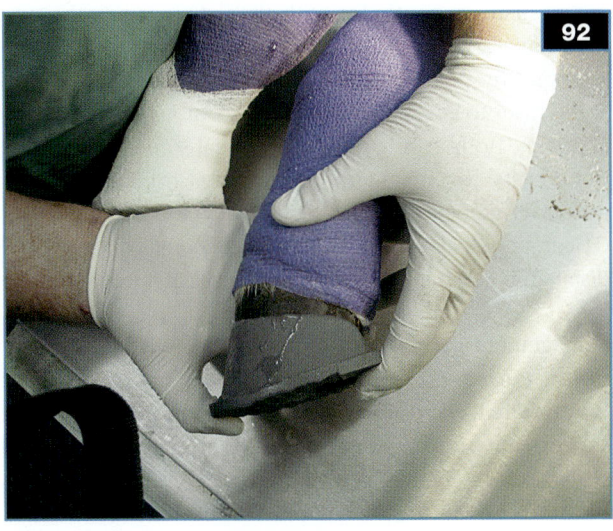

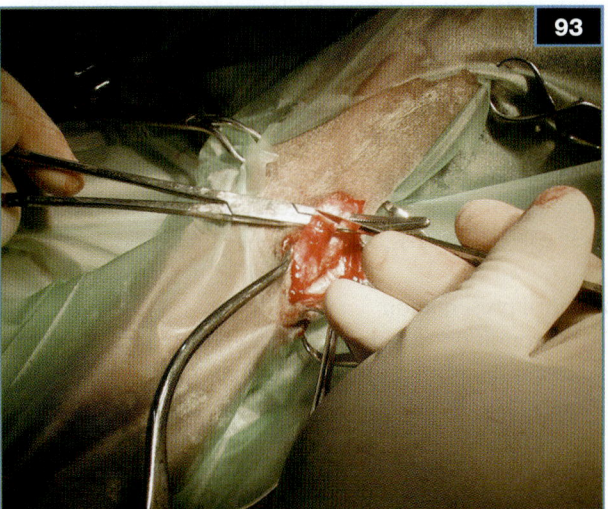

92 Fitting a plastic toe extension cuff shoe to the foot of a foal with bilateral flexural deformity of the distal interphalangeal joint.

93 Severing the inferior check ligament (accessory ligament of the deep digital flexor tendon) for treatment of the flexural deformity of the DIP joint in case 90.

94 Postoperative results of surgical treatment of the case in 90.

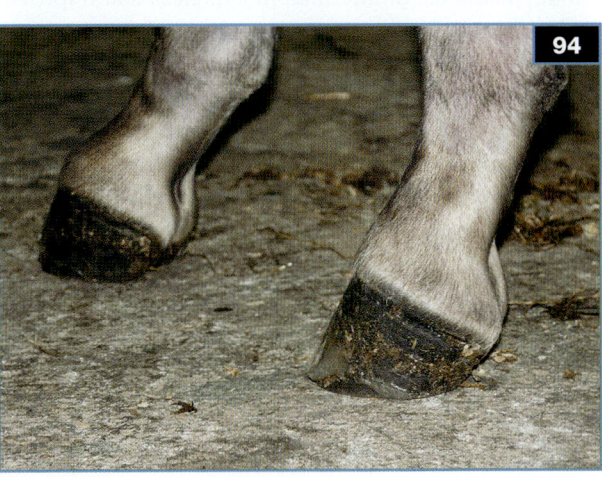

The foal and developing animal

Subchondral bone cysts

Definition/overview

Subchondral bone cysts are most commonly seen at the weight-bearing surface of the medial femoral condyle. They are also found less frequently at the distal epiphyses of the proximal phalanx, 3rd metacarpus/metatarsus, proximal epiphyses of the middle phalanx, radius and tibia, glenoid of the scapula, articular margin of the third phalanx, and occasionally the carpal and tarsal bones. The affected cartilage becomes infolded, creating an 'osseous cyst-like lesion'.

Etiology/pathophysiology

The etiology is not completely understood. Two main theories predominate:

✦ *OCD*: in the young horse a failure of endochondral ossification occurs focally and the thickened plug of cartilage invaginates to form a bone cyst. Necrosis and collapse with a secondary inflammatory response coupled with trauma are important factors in cyst formation.

✦ *Traumatic*: more frequently encountered in the adult horse, although some cysts seen in this age group may be subclinical forms of OCD that have become clinically relevant. Cysts in this group can be associated with concurrent soft-tissue damage such as ligament/meniscal damage.

Synovitis secondary to release of cystic inflammatory mediators into the synovial fluid and/or subchondral bone pain may cause lameness, although this is not well defined.

Clinical presentation

The condition is more common in younger horses (<4 years), although it can present well into adulthood. Mainly fast-growing larger breeds are affected, especially Thoroughbreds and Warmbloods, although the condition occasionally occurs in ponies. Lameness is usually seen when athletic work begins. Clinical signs are usually a subtle, insidious, or intermittent lameness that improves with rest only to recur once back in work. Acute-onset lameness is less common, but can occur. Mild joint distension may be present, but often is not, and flexion tests may increase lameness only slightly. Intra-articular analgesia is often required to identify the site of pain. Note that sufficient time should be allowed for the local anesthetic to diffuse into the cyst (e.g. up to 30–60 minutes in the medial femorotibial joint) and a partial improvement (50%) warrants radiographic evaluation.

Differential diagnoses

Subchondral lucencies primarily associated with advanced DJD, bone abscess.

Diagnosis

A full lameness examination should be carried out and systematic diagnostic analgesia is required to assess the relevance of any cystic structure within a joint.

A full radiographic series for the affected joint should be obtained. Certain views are more useful in depicting cysts at different locations (e.g. caudal cranial view [95] and flexed lateral medial of the femorotibial joints for subchondral bone cysts of the medial femoral condyle). Note that the condition can be bilateral, especially in the medial femorotibial joint, so the contralateral limb should always be radiographed for comparison. Different exposure settings and slightly different proximodistal obliquity of the radiographs are advisable to clarify fully the presence of a cyst, especially in the medial femoral condyle. Positive contrast arthrograms may also be useful in certain instances. Cysts vary in size from small indentations to a large radiolucent lucency depending on the stage of development of the cyst. They are often oval or rounded in shape, usually confluent with the articular margin, and may have a sclerotic peripheral margin (95, 96). Ultrasonography of the femorotibial joints may be useful in some cases to evaluate the cartilage contour of the femoral condyles. Bone scintigraphy may reveal some subchondral bone cysts, but this is not a consistent finding and may reflect different stages of the cyst's development. MRI and CT can help locate and define more accurately cysts of the distal limb and may be a useful presurgical intervention.

Management

Conservative

Box or small-paddock rest for up to 6 months has been successfully used in some medial femoral condyle bone cysts, but often it is only temporarily helpful in cysts located elsewhere. Many of the conservatively treated cases are placed on NSAIDs to control the pain and inflammation in the joint(s).

Various intra-articular medications have been used, including corticosteroids +/– sodium hyaluronate, with variable success. Polysulfated glycosaminoglycans used either intra-articularly or intramuscularly have also been used, often with a follow-up of long-term oral joint supplementation with chondroitin sulfate and glucosamine.

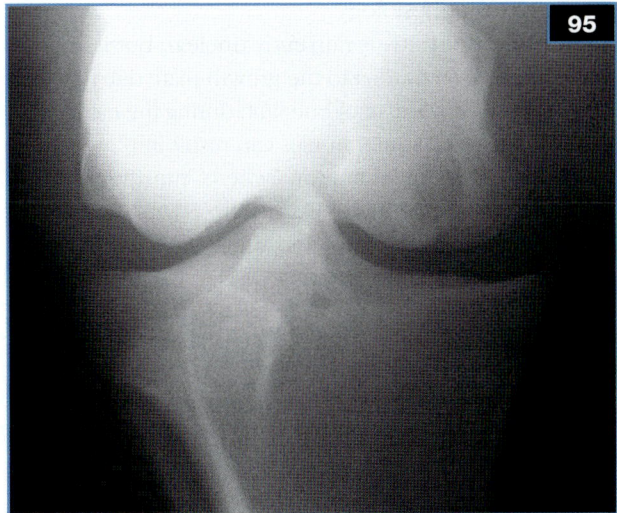

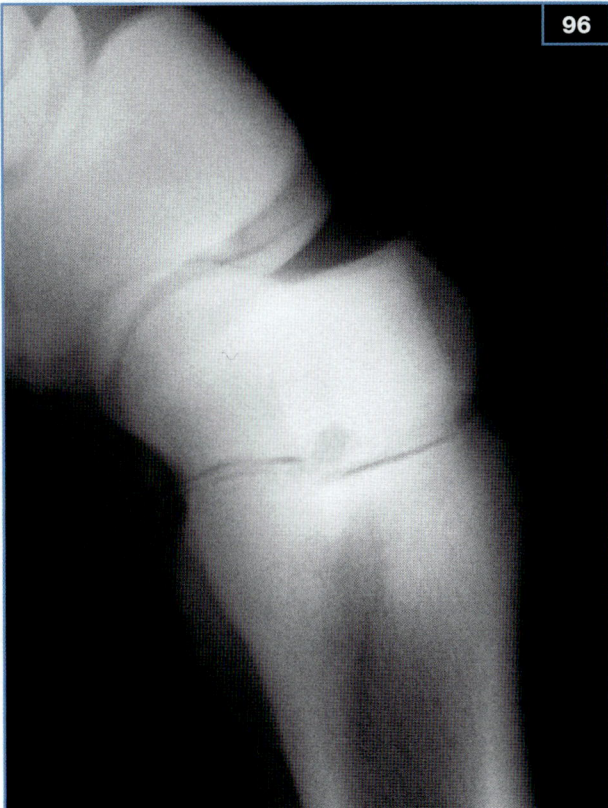

Surgical

Surgical treatment involves debridement of the cyst via arthroscopy, arthrotomy, or via a transosseous approach. The method used depends on the location of the cyst and surgeon preference. The cyst lining can be debrided and all debris removed. However, recently there has been a move away from aggressive debridement because enlargement of the cyst and worsening of lameness have been observed. Similarly, subchondral bone forage is currently contraindicated. Cancellous bone graft can be placed after debridement, but this does not appear to improve the outcome. Stem cell placement may offer a future treatment option. Intra- and postoperative intra-articular or intracyst steroids (particularly in medial femoral condyle bone cysts) are advocated to suppress the inflammatory mediators, and the above mentioned conservative therapy is used as postoperative management.

Prognosis

The prognosis depends on the joint affected, the severity of the lesion, associated DJD, intended use of the horse, and the treatment option selected. A 50% success rate with conservative treatment of medial femoral condylar subchondral bone cysts has been reported. Arthroscopic treatment carries a reported 70% success rate in horses under 3 years old. In general it appears that young horses with unilateral medial femoral condyle cysts are most likely to perform as intended. A much lower success rate is reported in horses over four years old (35%). Too few numbers of cysts treated in other locations are available to make definitive statements. Accompanying DJD worsens the prognosis.

Currently, the authors give an overall fair prognosis for young horses with unilateral medial femoral condyle subchondral cysts treated arthroscopically, but only a guarded prognosis in adult horses. A guarded prognosis is also given for all bone cysts for conservative treatment, bilateral presentation, and all other types of cyst.

95 Caudocranial radiograph of the stifle showing the femorotibial joint in a 4-year-old pony with lameness localized to this joint by intra-articular analgesia. Note the large subchondral bone cyst in the medial condyle of the distal femur and the large connection between the cyst and joint.

96 Incidental finding of an osseous cyst-like lesion in the third carpal bone adjacent to the carpometacarpal joint.

Physitis (epiphysitis, physeal dysplasia)
Definition/overview
Physitis is a form of DOD involving a disturbance of endochondral ossification at the peripheral or axial region of the metaphyseal growth plate, particularly at the distal radius/tibia and distal 3rd metacarpus/metatarsus of foals and young horses. It is mainly encountered in fast-growing breeds such as the Thoroughbred.

Etiology/pathophysiology
The cause of physitis is currently unclear, but it appears that compression trauma to the growth plate due to excessive exercise or overuse of one limb during the most active growth phases of young horses can result in physitis. The condition is more common where nutritional (lush pasture, high concentrates) and supplement excesses or deficiencies are implicated, and some clinicians believe it may be another manifestation of OCD in the horse.

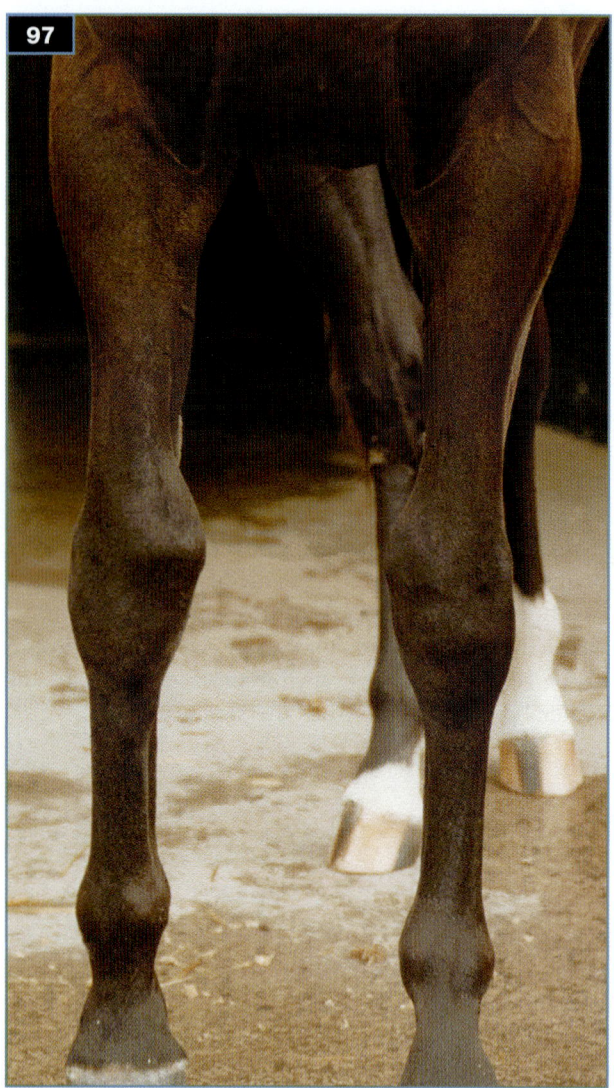

97 Yearling Warmblood colt with enlarged physis of both distal radii. The animal was being overfed and growing rapidly. This is a typical site for physitis.

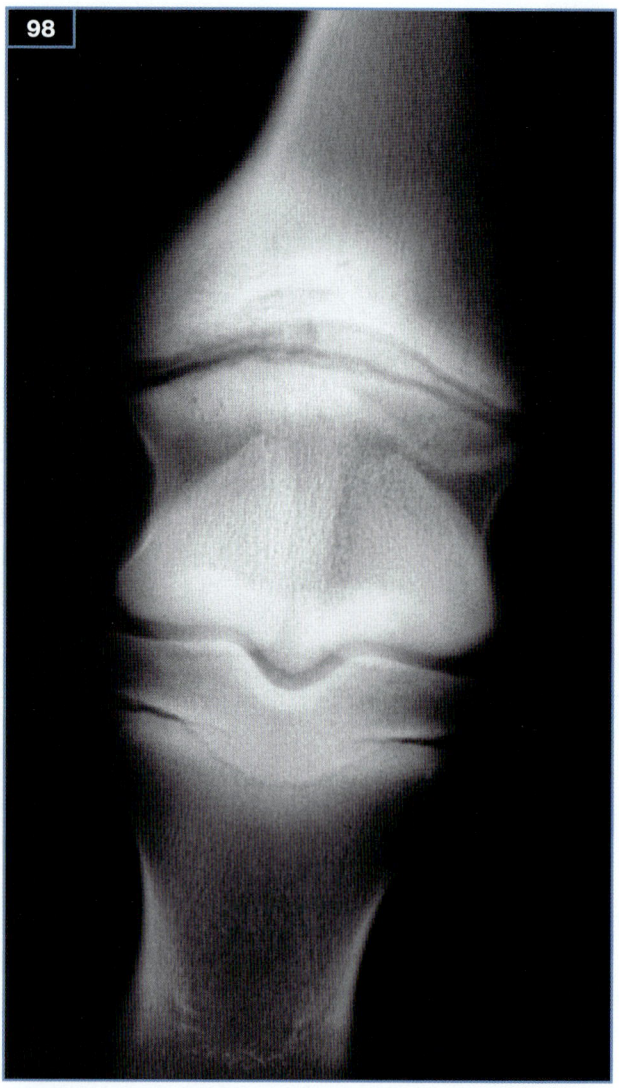

98 Dorsopalmar radiograph of a weanling foal with physitis showing changes within the physis and metaphyseal flaring and subchondral bone sclerosis.

Clinical presentation

Physitis is usually seen in the distal 3rd metacarpus/metatarsus from 3–6 months, the distal radius from 8 months to 2 years (97), and uncommonly in the distal tibia (from 9–18 months). The affected physes are usually enlarged, particularly on the medial aspect ('hourglass' appearance in the fetlock) and are firm, warm, and painful to palpation. Flexion of adjacent joints may be painful. Concurrent angular and/or flexural deformities may also be present in severe cases. Lameness can be overt or, more usually, show as a slight gait stiffness.

Differential diagnoses

Infectious physitis, Salter–Harris type V and type VI growth plate injuries.

Diagnosis

The clinical history and findings are suggestive, but radiography is necessary to reach a diagnosis. Lateral medial and dorsopalmar/plantar views are most useful (98). The metaphysis of the bone will appear widened and asymmetrical, with flaring and sclerosis of the metaphysis adjacent to the physis. The physis appears irregular and widened. ALDs may also be present along with overlying soft-tissue swelling.

Management

Restriction of exercise helps to reduce further physeal trauma and may include box rest (in severe cases) to small-yard rest, initially from 2 weeks to 2 months depending on the severity of the condition. NSAIDs should be used if the horse is very painful or lame in order to provide analgesia. Correction of any nutritional and supplement excesses and/or deficiencies is very important. A reduction in energy content (to decrease body weight) and correct balances of calcium, phosphorus, copper, and zinc are advisable. Corrective foot trimming should be aimed at balancing the feet generally, but also with regard to treating any angular and/or flexural deformity present.

Prognosis

The prognosis is good providing the condition does not lead to severe permanent conformational defects due to premature closure of growth plates. It is a self-limiting disease process that ceases when skeletal maturity is attained.

The foot as applied to the distal limb of a horse is not an anatomic term supported by the *Nomina Anatomica Veterinaria*, but from common usage it has evolved to mean that part of the distal limb surrounded by the hoof and all the structures contained within the hoof. The hoof is the integument of the foot and is composed of epidermis, dermis, and subcutaneous tissue. The stratum corneum of the hoof epidermis forms the hoof capsule. The wall of the hoof capsule is formed from three layers: the stratum externum, which is derived from the limbic (perioplic) epidermis; the stratum medium, which is derived from the coronary epidermis and forms the bulk of the thickness of the wall; and the stratum internum, which is thin and derived from the parietal (lamellar) epidermis.

The majority of the diseases of the foot are secondary to infection or trauma and to degeneration subsequent to recurrent low-grade trauma. Trauma to structures of the foot is primarily related to its proximity and interaction with the ground and internal stresses associated with exercise. Infection follows surface contamination, penetration of the integument through injury, or, rarely, hematogenous spread.

Clinical presentation

The most common presenting symptom for diseases affecting the horse's foot is lameness, usually caused by a focus of pain or, much less frequently, by a mechanical change in function. In more chronic cases the foot may present with a change in appearance, shape, or size. Diseases of the foot are the most common cause of lameness in the forelimbs. In the hindlimbs they are generally considered less common than diseases affecting the hock and fetlock joints, although this may lead to underdiagnosis.

The signalment is unlikely to be specific, but it is useful to compare it with the history and clinical signs when considering the likelihood of a specific diagnosis. The history for horses presenting with a disease affecting the foot is very variable. It is important to know when the horse was last shod, how frequently it is shod, and have there been any changes in the farriery management of the horse that might be related to the onset of symptoms.

The nature of the hoof capsule precludes palpation and manipulation of the distal digit in the same manner as the rest of the limb, but many basic elements of the examination are similar. Examination of the foot with the horse at rest involves visual inspection, palpation, application of hoof testers, paring the sole, and manipulation of the digit. Visual inspection of the foot rapidly identifies gross lesions such as hoof cracks or hoof-wall avulsions. Additionally, the size of the foot in relation to the size of the horse, the shape of each foot and the symmetry between the feet, and the relationship between the foot and the limb are evaluated. More subtle details such as the presence of flares and the circumferential patterns of the growth rings require closer observation. Palpation of the foot is the most practical way to determe if the foot is excessively warm, to identify soft areas in the sole, and also to identify moistness, particularly at the hairline, that was not identified on visual inspection. Paring of the sole, best performed without a shoe on the foot, will expose bruises and defects in the sole. Application of hoof testers elicits a withdrawal response when they are positioned over a focus of pain; however, this cannot be used to infer which of the tissues between their jaws is affected. Manipulation of the limb by flexion, extension, and rotation of the distal limb will determine restriction in range of motion and elicit a withdrawal response if structures associated with such motion are inflamed.

There are no characteristics of gait that conclusively identify lameness arising from the foot. Horses with bilateral disease frequently present with a stiff and short-strided gait, which in conjunction with the known incidence of diseases in the forefeet and the signalment are highly suggestive. The exception is the severely and acutely laminitic horse, whose extremely stilted gait is almost pathognomonic, particularly when associated with a shifting of weight from the forequarters to the hindquarters.

Ancillary diagnostic tests

When the physical examination fails to determine the source of the pain causing lameness, the diagnosis of diseases of the horse's foot requires, initially, localization to the foot using regional and/or intrasynovial analgesia. However, it is now known that local anesthetic deposited in one synovial structure can diffuse into an adjacent synovial structure or around an adjacent nerve, greatly decreasing the specificity of pain localization. An improvement in accuracy can be obtained by limiting the amount of anesthetic used and observing the response in relation to time.

Radiography of the foot is indicated whenever the physical examination and diagnostic regional analgesia do not provide a diagnosis. In horses with severe lameness, radiography should be performed before diagnostic analgesia in order to prevent exacerbation of a traumatic injury. The radiographic examination varies depending on the results of the physical examination, but typically either a series of three radiographic projections (i.e. lateral, dorsopalmar, and 45° dorsoproximal/palmarodistal oblique [upright pedal]) to examine the distal phalanx is performed, or a more extensive series to examine the whole foot is performed that requires an additional two projections (i.e. a 60° dorsoproximal/palmarodistal oblique and a palmaroproximal/palmarodistal oblique [skyline]). Specific additional obliques may be performed as necessary.

Scintigraphy is useful to detect disease that is occult on radiographs or to ascertain the significance of equivocal radiographic findings. To a lesser extent, ultrasound has also increased the clinician's ability to identify pathology. CT has greatly improved the ability to visualize the bones of the limb. MRI has vastly improved the clinician's ability to visualize soft tissue structures within the foot and previously unidentified pathology within the bones, joints, and soft tissues. Unfortunately, availability of these diagnostic tools, and hence the diagnosis itself, is limited by geographic availability and affordability. Additionally, these techniques are new and, consequently, while the interpretation of some new findings is obvious, the clinical significance of others will only become apparent with more experience.

Management

Treatment of diseases of the foot is in many ways similar to that of other parts of the limb, but its position at the distal end of the limb and the structure of the hoof capsule itself result in significant differences in treatment. Firstly, because the feet in working horses are usually shod, different shoeing techniques are used to achieve different ends: to protect the foot; to change the balance of the foot; to change the way the foot moves during the stride to prevent interference or enhance animation; to support the position of the foot on the ground; or to reduce the stress on an injured structure. Secondly, the structure of the hoof capsule alters the approach that can be used to treat surgically deeper structures because compromises have to be made between exposure and stability of the hoof. Additionally, defects created in the integument of the foot cannot be sutured in a comparable manner to skin.

Diseases of the feet

Foot wounds and infection

Foot wounds take many forms, from simple abscesses, to hoof-wall avulsions, to punctures of structures deep within the foot. Despite the varied appearance and presentation of these wounds, there are certain common features in the way they heal and are treated that warrant consideration in general terms to avoid repetition.

Abrasions to the coronary band and iatrogenic hoof-wall avulsions heal in a similar way to partial thickness skin wounds. Remnants of germinal epithelium are distributed across the surface of the wound, so healing is primarily by epithelialization. Defects that involve the full thickness of the coronary band, wall, sole, or frog follow the classical four phases of wound healing. Following an injury, however, the hoof wall does not retract nor, in the repair phase, do the wound margins contract. The epithelium that covers the wound may have diverse characteristics depending on whether it originated from the coronary band, wall, sole, frog, or pastern, and excessive granulation tissue on the surface of the foot is uncommon.

The tetanus vaccination history of all horses with wounds should be ascertained and if inadequate, tetanus antitoxin should be administered. The use of antimicrobial drugs depends on the nature of the wound. Wounds that only involve the superficial layers of the integument (e.g. abscesses) are usually satisfactorily treated with topical antibiotics or antiseptics and systemic antibiotics are seldom warranted. Topical antiseptics should be used at appropriate concentrations to inhibit bacterial growth without affecting fibroplasia and epithelialization. Systemic antibiotics are usually used in wounds that extend deep to the dermis in conjunction with topical antimicrobials. Systemic antibiotics should be continued until there is a healthy layer of granulation tissue across the surface of the wound; diffuse infection is unlikely after this occurs. In wounds that involve a synovial structure, antibiotics are continued until 1–2 weeks after the communication between the wound and the synovial structure has closed and the clinical signs have resolved. The choice of antibiotics is related to spectrum of activity, ease of administration, and cost. A combination of penicillin and trimethoprim-sulfonamide is commonly used for more superficial wounds, whereas combinations with a broader spectrum (e.g. penicillin and gentamicin) are frequently used when more vital structures are affected. Regional perfusion of the distal limb with antibiotics via a vein or intraosseous portal has been shown to be a very effective adjunct to systemic and topical antibiotics in treating wounds that involve deeper structures within the foot.

Bandaging for foot injuries requires two or three layers. The primary layer or surface dressing should be adherent if debridement is required and nonadherent if epithelialization and fibroplasia are to be encouraged. The secondary padding layer is frequently omitted, but is useful to protect and support the distal limb for heel-bulb lacerations and hoof wall avulsions. The tertiary layer holds the underlying layers in place, but care should be taken to avoid excessive pressure and contact with adhesive around the coronary band. Both dry-to-dry and wet-to-dry dressings are used. Wet-to-dry dressings containing antibiotic in physiologic solutions are excellent for maintaining an optimal environment on the surface of the wound for healing and controlling surface infection, but they may need to be replaced with dry-to-dry dressings if the adjacent hoof capsule shows evidence of maceration from excessive moisture.

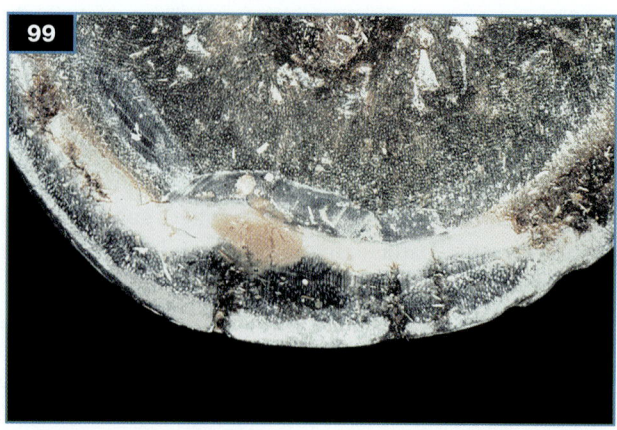

99 Abscess drainage immediately inside the white line after exposure with a hoof knife.

Abscesses

Definition/overview
Foot abscesses are a focal accumulation of purulent exudate that most commonly occurs between the germinal and keratinized layers of the hoof.

Etiology/pathophysiology
The cause is not usually specifically identifiable, but most cases of foot abscessation are presumed to follow small defects in the hoof capsule, such as microfractures or separation of the white line, which permit bacterial access to the underlying tissues. Less frequently, they follow puncture wounds or hoof cracks. Some horses are prone to recurrent abscess formation because of concurrent disease (e.g. laminitis) or poor hoof structure (e.g. dropped or thin soles) that predisposes to bruising. Abscesses within the foot are particularly painful because the low compliance of the hoof capsule results in a more rapid increase in pressure. The pressure will with time cause separation of the hoof capsule from the germinal layer of the epithelium to extend further under the sole or frog, or proximally under the wall. Abscesses that extend proximally deep to the wall and cause separation at the coronary band are called a 'gravel'. Abscesses may also extend through the germinal layers of the integument and dermis to affect deeper structures.

Clinical presentation
The clinical picture of a horse with a foot abscess is that of an acute, severely lame horse, sometimes becoming evident after exercise or turnout. Most horses with abscesses are found with a severe lameness, usually a 4–5/5, although the lameness may be seen to develop over 12–48 hours if they are observed closely. Distal limb swelling and/or cellulitis may be present in some cases. Swelling or a discharging sinus may occur at the coronary band.

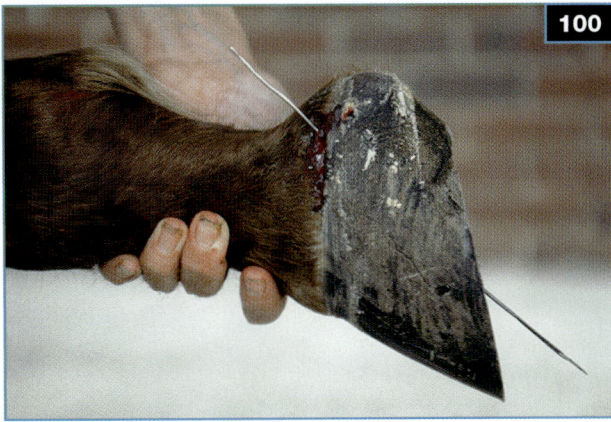

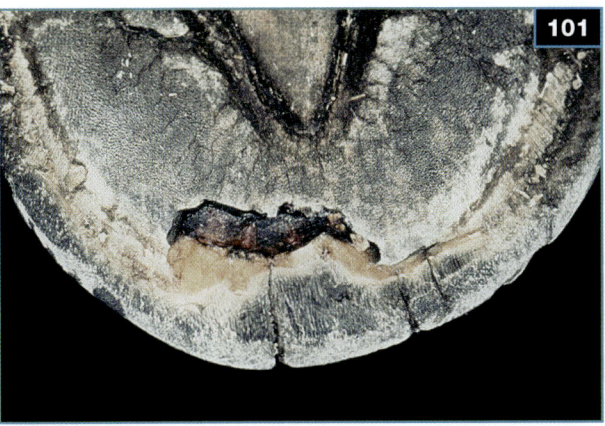

100 The probe demonstrates the tract created by an abscess that spontaneously drained at the coronet.

101 Cornified sole of the horse in 99 4–5 days after abscess drainage and dressing with povidone–iodine solution.

Differential diagnosis

Any disease of the foot associated with acute onset of severe lameness; fracture of the distal phalanx or distal sesamoid (navicular bone); sepsis of a deep digital structure; severe bruising; severe injury to a ligament or tendon within the foot.

Diagnosis

One foot may be palpably warmer than the others, and application of hoof testers nearly always induces a marked withdrawal response. Exploration of the ground surface of the foot may or may not reveal dark discoloration of the horn, indicating a track or injury site through which bacteria may have entered. Further exploration of the track should expose the abscess (99). Perineural analgesia with an abaxial sesamoid block is useful to facilitate exploration of the hoof. When no track is visible, but the symptoms are otherwise strongly suggestive of an abscess, further exploration may be warranted, although excessive paring of the foot is contraindicated. If exploration still fails to identify an abscess, the hoof capsule should be poulticed for 24–48 hours to soften the horn. The softer horn makes the capsule easier to explore, and the abscess may drain spontaneously, frequently at the coronary band (100). If the pain still persists and an abscess cannot be identified, the foot should be radiographed to exclude other acute foot lameness or detect gas/fluid pockets.

Management

Drainage is the primary treatment for hoof abscesses and may be facilitated in difficult horses by the use of regional nerve blocks and/or sedation. Usually, a small hole, approximately 1 cm in diameter, will suffice to drain the abscess regardless of the area of stratum corneum that has been underrun. If the abscess is adjacent to the white line, draining the abscess through a small notch in the distal wall is preferable to creating a hole in the sole because deficits in the latter are more difficult to manage. Bandaging the foot with an antiseptic dressing is required for a few days, but repeated poulticing or foot soaking is not usually indicated. Systemic antibiotics are not required unless the abscess has extended deep to the dermis, but tetanus prophylaxis is mandatory in horses without a recent history of vaccination. Once drainage is established, the clinical signs should decrease rapidly. The abscess wound should be dry within a few days (101). If the abscess was drained through the sole, the horse can return to athletic activity sooner by shoeing with a full pad or plate. If the clinical signs fail to improve or the abscess recurs, then radiography should be performed. If radiography does not indicate other pertinent pathology, further exploration is warranted, which may include further removal of any underrun sole or wall.

Prognosis

The prognosis is good for simple abscesses that are associated with neither a predisposing cause nor infection of the deeper structures of the foot. If the abscess is associated with a predisposing cause, then recurrent abscessation may be likely. If the infection involves a deeper structure, the prognosis varies with the structure affected.

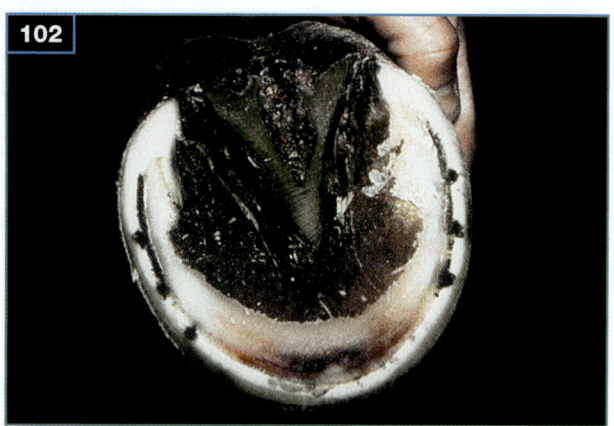

102

102 Bruise. Extensive bruising of the dorsal sole distal to the dorsal solar margin of the distal phalanx.

Bruising

Definition/overview
Bruises are an extravasation of blood from ruptured blood vessels into the surrounding tissues as a sequela to blunt trauma.

Etiology/pathophysiology
Most bruises occur in the sole or the lamellae, although bruising may occur at the coronary band and in the frog. Bruises may be caused by a single forceful contusion or recurrent lower-grade trauma. The former is likely to be an isolated incident. The latter is commonly associated with a conformational or pathologic predisposition such as flat feet or laminitis. Alternatively, bruising can be caused by pressure on the sole from poorly fitting shoes. Corns (bruises in the angle of the sole) are almost invariably associated with shoes that have been fitted too short or shoes that have been on for too long and migrated dorsally with toe growth. The extravasation of blood into the tissues gives a bruise its characteristic discoloration. In contrast to skin bruises, hemorrhage that occurs into the hoof capsule retains its red coloration. The hemorrhage penetrates a variable distance into the substance of the horn and appears stippled to reflect the tubular nature of the horn. It is not visible until the affected hoof reaches the surface through normal growth. Bruises can occasionally become infected through microfractures in the hoof capsule.

Clinical presentation
Foot bruises may or may not be a cause of lameness. They can be identified when a horse is being trimmed or shod and appear to be an incidental finding and may indicate an underlying problem with conformation or foot balance. The lameness can be acute or chronic, mild or severe, unilateral or bilateral. The latter is usually associated with a predisposing cause such as poor foot conformation.

Differential diagnosis
The clinical presentation is very varied and therefore overlaps with almost any other disease of the horse's foot.

Diagnosis
The site of a clinically significant bruise is usually identified by applying hoof testers to the affected area; this will elicit a withdrawal response. The bruise itself is identified when the foot has been cleaned and pared (after the shoe has been removed if necessary) and the blood staining of the hoof identified (**102**). Occult, but clinically significant, bruises may never be identified or may only be identified when the hemorrhage has become more superficial with hoof growth. Suppurative bruises are identified in a similar manner to abscesses. Bruising from the coronary band is visible in unpigmented horn of the wall as horizontal red stripes, but these are seldom clinically significant. Chronic bruising may lead to resorption of bone from the margins of the distal phalanx, which is radiographically identified as pedal osteitis.

Management
The treatment of foot bruising depends on the cause. Isolated stone bruises usually require nothing more than rest and NSAIDs to provide analgesia; these are titrated against the severity of discomfort experienced by the horse. Cold tubbing or icing the affected foot for 24 hours may decrease the inflammation. Partially paring the surface of the horn over the bruise may relieve pressure from the area as it heals. Recurrent bruising associated with flat soles requires protection of the sole, either with seated-out wide web shoes or full pads. Bruising in the sole and lamellae associated with laminitis will recur until corrective shoeing has eliminated sole pressure distal to the solar margin of the distal phalanx and stresses within the dorsal lamellae. Suppurative bruises should be treated as abscesses and the cause removed whenever possible.

Prognosis
The prognosis with bruising varies with the cause. When the bruising is an isolated event, a full recovery is probable, but when the bruising is secondary to conformation or concurrent disease, the prognosis for recovery without recurrence is guarded.

Thrush

Definition/overview
Thrush is a degenerative keratolytic condition of the frog and adjacent sulci.

Etiology/pathophysiology
Thrush is probably caused by an anaerobic bacterial infection, but the specific etiological agent has not been identified. The disease is frequently seen in horses standing in moist unhygienic conditions or subjected to poor daily foot management. Thrush usually starts superficially on the surface of the frog, particularly in the central and paracuneal sulci, before extending deeper into the stratum corneum of the frog and occasionally reaching the germinal layers of the epidermis and the dermis. Horses with deep and/or narrow sulci are more prone to developing thrush than those with wide and shallow sulci (**103**). The disease is common when the frog becomes too moist under a full pad.

Clinical presentation
Horses with thrush usually present because the affected foot has a characteristic foul odor and discharge, and the surface of the frog is ragged. Affected animals are often not lame, but deeper damage, especially between the bulbs of the heel, can be painful.

Differential diagnosis
Canker.

Diagnosis
The characteristic odor and appearance of the frog are usually sufficient to make a diagnosis of thrush, but it may need to be distinguished from early canker. The symptoms and progression of thrush differ from those of canker in several ways: 1) thrush is a degenerative condition of the superficial layers of the frog, whereas canker is a proliferative condition affecting the basal layers; 2) thrush is confined to the frog and paracuneal sulci, whereas canker may extend to any part of the hoof; 3) horses with thrush are less likely to be lame; and 4) remedies that usually cure cases of thrush frequently fail to improve canker.

Management
Thrush is effectively treated with debridement of ragged and undermined frog, transferring the horse to hygienic and dry conditions, improving daily foot management, and applying topical antiseptics and astringents (e.g. povidone–iodine, 2% tincture of iodine, or proprietary preparations of formalin [but formalin in its aldehyde state is best avoided]). Corrective trimming and shoeing are essential where there is poor foot conformation. Daily foot care should be considered and improved if necessary and the ground and stable bedding conditions changed if appropriate.

Prognosis
The prognosis is almost always good. Horses with narrow frogs and deep sulci are likely to experience recurrence if they have to stand on moist unhygienic surfaces.

103 A foot with severe thrush infection in the central sulci of the frog and midline of the bulbs of the heel. (Photo courtesy GA Munroe)

Canker

Definition/overview
Canker is defined histologically as a chronic proliferative pododermatitis.

Etiology/pathophysiology
The disease classically starts in the central or paracuneal (collateral) sulci and then rapidly spreads to the crura of the frog. It may extend to the sole or bulbs of the heel, and occasionally even to the walls of the hoof. Canker classically occurs in the hooves of horses that are standing for prolonged periods on a wet ground surface that is contaminated with feces. The etiology and pathogenesis of canker are unknown, but anaerobic bacterial infection affecting the germinal layer of the epithelium has been hypothesized in the literature. It has not yet been established whether canker in fact represents one or more disease processes or etiologic agents.

Clinical presentation
The duration of the disease is usually chronic, over several weeks to months. It may affect one or more feet. Canker has a characteristic proliferative appearance from which extend finger-like projections, and it is usually associated with a yellow, creamy exudate. The lesion is typically located on the frog, but may have extended to involve any other part of the hoof. Palpation of the affected area is likely to elicit a painful response. Early in the course of the disease the horse may be sound or slightly lame, but as the disease becomes more advanced the lameness becomes progressively worse.

Differential diagnosis
Thrush.

Diagnosis
Diagnosis is usually based on the physical appearance of the foot (104), but a biopsy and histopathology are required for confirmation. Canker is frequently mistaken for thrush early in the course of the disease, but is much less common. There are several features that help differentiate thrush from canker. In thrush the lesion is degenerative, whereas in canker it is proliferative. In thrush the disease is confined to the frog, whereas canker may spread to other parts of the hoof. Both may cause lameness, but this is more common in canker. Traditional topical medications that are effective against thrush are ineffective against canker.

Management
Treatment comprises a combination of surgical debridement and medical therapy. Prior to debridement the foot should be trimmed to ensure maximal width between the heels and, if necessary, part of the bars can be removed to

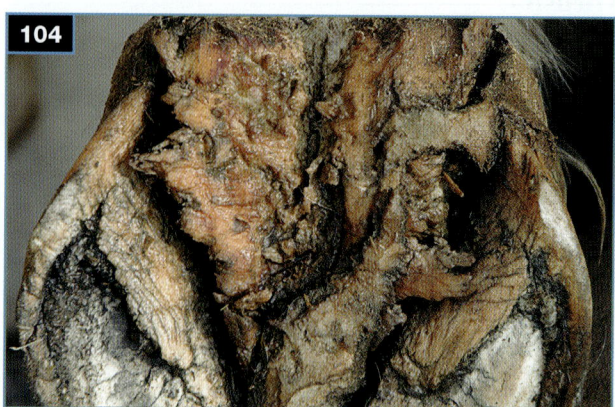

104 Canker. Extensive moist proliferation of the epidermis of the crura and sulci of the frog.

open up the sulci as much as possible. This maximizes drainage and limits the crevices in the sulci within which the causative agent can linger. Careful surgical excision of the proliferative tissue to preserve as much of the germinal layer of the epidermis as possible is best performed with a rongeur, but a scalpel or laser is also frequently used. More aggressive excision results in slower epithelialization of the wound without significantly improved results. Many topical medications have been used in the treatment of canker. A 2–5% suspension of metronidazole in saline or a paste made from crushed metronidazole tablets and saline applied as a wet-to-dry dressing after debridement is frequently effective. In refractory cases, 0.05% enrofloxacin or clindamycin in Tricide (Molecular Therapeutics LLC), applied either as a wet-to-dry dressing or as as a dry-to-dry dressing after the dressing has been soaked and dried, may be successful. Alternatively, topical dressings saturated with 10% benzoyl peroxide in acetone can be used. Systemic use of antibiotics with an anaerobic spectrum of activity (e.g. metronidazole or penicillin) are unlikely to be successful as a sole therapy, but may be useful as an adjunct to local therapy. Several other topical treatments have also been tried with varying success including chloramphenicol, fungicides, and sterile maggots.

In uncomplicated cases the lesion is dramatically improved within 2 weeks and resolved within 4 weeks. In complicated cases where there is a reservoir of the causative agent in a protected location in either the hoof or the environment, recurrence is common.

Prognosis
The response to treatment in this disease is highly variable and, therefore, the prognosis must always initially be guarded. A cautious long-term outlook is advised because it is not currently known whether individual animals may have a predisposition towards developing this disease.

Laminitis

Definition/overview
Laminitis is a syndrome in which a poorly defined series of pathophysiologic events cause injury to the dermal and epidermal lamellae, which weakens the attachment between the lamellae and, at its most extreme, causes separation of the hoof capsule from the underlying tissues. Laminitis is defined as acute if it is within 72 hours of onset of clinical signs and has not been accompanied by displacement of the distal phalanx. It is defined as chronic once the distal phalanx has displaced in relation to the hoof capsule (regardless of duration). Laminitis that is of >72 hours duration and is not accompanied by displacement is defined as subacute.

Etiology/pathophysiology
The etiology of acute laminitis is poorly defined, but risk factors that are associated with its development are primarily associated with toxemia, usually endotoxemia, including carbohydrate/grain overload, colic, colitis, pleuropneumonia, metritis, and renal failure. Grass-induced laminitis is common in some parts of the world, and is probably related to ingestion of water-soluble carbohydrates in the grass, similar to grain overload. Laminitis may also follow prolonged weight bearing on one limb or occur as a spontaneous event with no known cause. Anecdotal evidence implicates systemic or intra-articular steroid administration, particularly administration of triamcinolone, as a cause of laminitis, but this is not yet supported by controlled data in the literature. Horses with equine Cushing's disease and equine metabolic syndrome are more likely to have chronic laminitis than other horses, and it is postulated that this is associated with high levels of endogenous glucocorticoid activity generally or at the tissue level. Indiviual animal and breed susceptibility to predisposing factors may be relevant in certain cases. Several pathophysiologic processes have been identified in acute laminitis including endotoxemia, inflammation, coagulopathy, thrombosis, and ischemia. The most recent evidence suggests that early in acute laminitis there is an active systemic inflammatory process in which the foot is a target organ. Subsequent to the systemic inflammatory response, localization of neutrophils and expression of cytokines within the lamellae are observed. Metalloproteinase activation within the lamellae, secondary to production of either inflammatory mediators or a systemic toxin, is observed in conjunction with loss of the lamellar basement membrane, the prelude to separation of the dermal and epidermal lamellae. It is hypothesized that the ischemia and thrombus formation observed are downstream events. The net result is that there is a variable degree of cellular necrosis within the lamellae.

The pathophysiology of chronic laminitis is less well documented. Depending on the severity of the tissue necrosis within the lamellae, the stresses of weight bearing and movement cause displacement of the distal phalanx in relation to the hoof capsule. The necrotic tissue is repaired. In severe cases this forms a wedge of hyperplastic epidermal and dermal tissue between the parietal surface of the distal phalanx and the hoof capsule. In chronic laminitis the hoof wall grows faster at the heels than at the toe. The presence of the lamellar wedge and the abnormal growth give rise to the characteristically deformed hoof, with a concave dorsal wall, high heels, and flattened sole.

Clinical presentation
Horses with acute laminitis present with an acute lameness. Typically, the disease is bilateral. Both forefeet are most commonly affected, but any combination is possible (105). It may be difficult to tell whether forelimbs, hindlimbs, or all four limbs are affected. In horses with bilateral forelimb involvement, the lameness may manifest as an extremely stiff short-strided gait in which the forelimbs are placed out in front of the horse and the hindlimbs are thrust underneath the horse's body. Where all four limbs are affected the horse is less likely to thrust its hindlimbs under its body. More severely affected horses are reluctant to move or to pick up a foot that is contralateral to an affected limb; in the worst cases they become persistently recumbent.

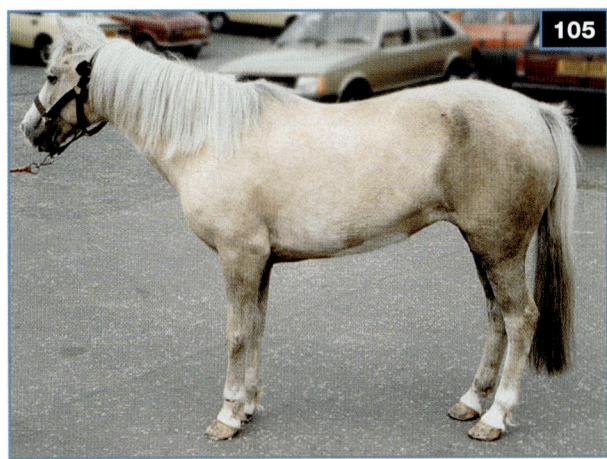

105 A pony with forelimb laminitis exhibiting the typical stance, with the forelimbs stretched out forwards and the hindlimbs placed underneath the body. (Photo courtesy GA Munroe)

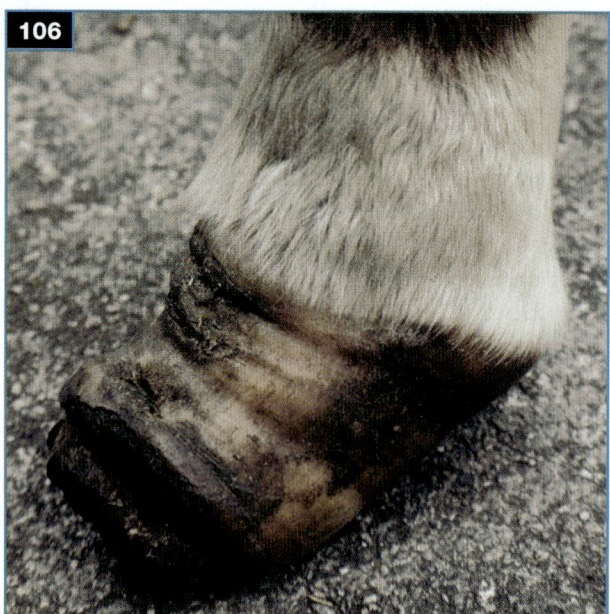

106

106 A chronic laminitic foot with long toe, dorsal compression of the hoof wall and hoof-ring formation. (Photo courtesy GA Munroe)

Horses with chronic laminitis present with either lameness of varying degree and/or hoof capsule deformation (106).

Differential diagnosis
Acute laminitis is almost unique, although it must be distinguished from diseases that make a horse move stiffly such as colic, pleuropneumonia, and rhabdomyolysis.

Chronic laminitis has to be differentiated from: 1) diseases causing bilateral chronic forelimb lameness (e.g. pedal osteitis, navicular disease, DJD); and 2) diseases that cause similar hoof-wall defects and displacement of the distal phalanx (e.g. white line disease).

Diagnosis
In acute lameness diagnosis is usually straightforward, based on the history, characteristic stilted gait, increased digital pulses, heat in the feet, withdrawal response to hoof testers, or reluctance to lift a limb. However, when the hindlimbs alone are affected acute laminitis may be hard to identify. Initially, radiographs indicate no changes except slight thickening of the dorsal hoof due to lamellar edema.

In horses with chronic laminitis the characteristic concavity of the dorsal hoof wall, convergence of growth rings dorsally (laminitic rings), dropped sole, widened white line, and coronary band depression may be sufficient to

make a diagnosis. Lightly paring the sole may indicate poor horn quality and demonstrate bruising distal to the solar margin of the distal phalanx, often seen as an arc just in front of the apex of the frog. Radiographs are useful to determine the severity of the disease. Prior to radiography the foot should be marked with a radiodense marker on the dorsal hoof wall in the median plane that extends from the coronary band distally, and a drawing pin is used to mark the apex of the frog. Lateral, horizontal dorsopalmar/plantar, and 45° dorsoproximal/palmarodistal oblique radiographs are necessary to evaluate the position of the distal phalanx in relation to the hoof capsule. The radiographs should be centered on the approximate location of the solar margin of the distal phalanx, approximately 1.5 cm from the ground surface of the foot, and exposed to permit evaluation of the surface of the hoof capsule. A 45° dorsoproximal/palmarodistal oblique view is useful to evaluate the solar margin of the distal phalanx for osteolysis and remodeling. In horses that develop capsular rotation the dorsal parietal surface of the distal phalanx diverges from the dorsal hoof wall, whereas in horses in which the distal phalanx displaces distally, the thickness of the dorsal hoof increases, the depth of sole decreases, and the extensor process of the distal phalanx moves distally in relation to the coronary band (**107**). In more chronically affected horses other changes occur, including remodeling of the distal phalanx, especially at the tip, and flexural deformity of the distal interphalangeal joint (also known as phalangeal rotation in laminitic horses) (**108**). Horses without gross morphologic changes of the hoof capsule may require regional analgesia to confirm that the lameness is in the foot; depending on whether most pain is arising from the sole or lamellae, the lameness should improve with palmar digital or abaxial sesamoid nerve blocks, respectively. Radiographic evidence of laminitis may also include lipping of the solar margin of the distal phalanx (**109**) and evidence of periosteal new bone formation on the dorsal parietal surface of the distal phalanx midway between the extensor process and the dorsal solar margin.

Management
The treatment of laminitis varies with the stage of the disease and can therefore be divided into prophylactic measures, treatment of acute laminitis, and treatment of chronic laminitis, although there is some gradation from the treatment of the acute, through the subacute, to the chronic stage of the disease.

Prophylactic measures are titrated against the risk of developing laminitis. The precipitating cause should be removed whenever possible (e.g. by taking the horse off lush pasture). Additionally, primary diseases frequently associated with endotoxemia and laminitis should be treated to limit systemic absorption and the effects of toxins that may precipitate the disease (e.g. horses that have ingested excessive amounts of grain should be treated with mineral oil and flunixin meglumine). Horses with endotoxemia should receive appropriate medical therapy including antibiotics, anti-inflammatory drugs, fluids, and anti-endotoxin hyperimmune serum as appropriate. When the risk of the disease is high it is also advisable to remove the shoes and provide some form of sole support (see treatment of acute laminitis).

Acute laminitis

The treatment of acute laminitis is a combination of medical therapy and supportive care, although the former is the mainstay. Medical therapy is aimed at limiting injury to the lamellae by intervention based on the pathophysiology of the disease. Although no medical therapy has been unequivocally proven to be of benefit, systemic treatment with phenylbutazone (2.2–4.4 mg/kg i/v or p/o q12h) or flunixin meglumine (0.25–1.0 mg/kg i/v q12h), acepromazine (0.01–0.02 mg/kg i/v or i/m q6–8h), and

dimethylsulfoxide (0.1–0.2 g/kg i/v or via a nasogastric tube q8–12h) is recommended. Other pharmacological interventions that are used include systemic administration of pentoxifylline, isoxsuprine, aspirin, and heparin. The primary objectives of supportive therapy are to decrease the likelihood that the distal phalanx will displace subsequent to lamellar injury and to control limb edema. This is achieved by strict stall rest, removing the shoes, bedding the stall with peat or sand, or packing the ground surface of the feet between the walls, typically with Styrofoam or silicone putty, moving the breakover back, and elevating the heels. Moving the breakover back and elevating the heels can be achieved simultaneously by applying a commercial cuff and wedge pad combination (Modified Redden Ultimates, Nanric Inc.). Some clinicians use homemade or commercially available frog pads to support the bony column within the foot. Limb edema should be controlled with stable bandages. Standing a horse in a slurry of ice and water during the developmental phases of the disease reduces the severity of the lamellar pathology.

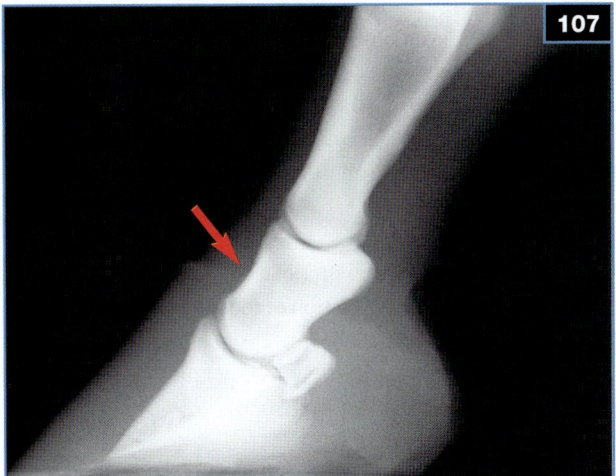

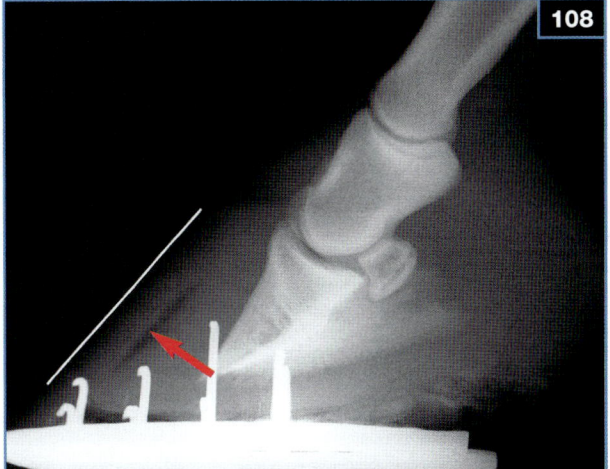

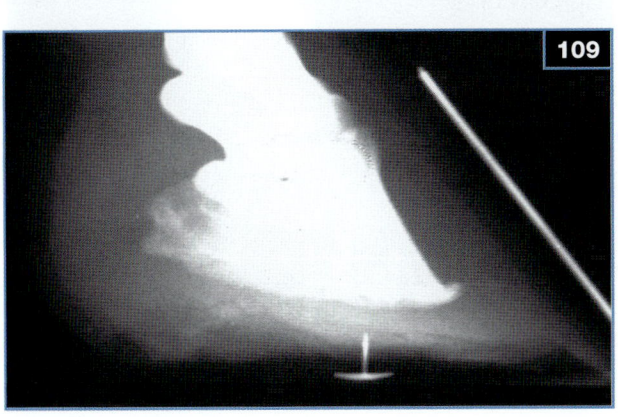

107 Laminitis. Distal displacement of the distal phalanx demonstrated by decreased depth of sole and a prominent 'sinker line' at the coronary band (arrow).

108 Laminitis. Radiograph after rotation of the distal phalanx. Note the gas line in the dorsal hoof wall (arrow), and the dorsal location of the original shoe in relation to the distal phalanx.

109 A lateral radiograph of a chronic laminitic foot with bony remodeling of the tip of P3. (Photo courtesy GA Munroe)

The foot

Chronic laminitis

The treatment of chronic laminitis is also a combination of medical therapy and supportive care; however, in contrast to acute laminitis, supportive care in the form of corrective shoeing is the mainstay. There have been many types of therapeutic shoes used in horses with chronic laminitis. Shoes should be positioned in relation to the distal phalanx using radiographic control that includes three specific objectives (110,111). The point of breakover is moved palmarly to decrease the length of the lever arm as a horse breaks over. The sole and frog are recruited to bear weight to decrease the stresses in the wall associated with weight bearing. The heels are elevated to decrease the tension in the deep digital flexor tendon, which decreases the tension in the dorsal lamellae caused by the movement opposing the pull of the tendon. Additionally, it is important to preserve the sole when its thickness has been reduced following displacement of the distal phalanx. These are titrated against the severity of the disease. The effectiveness of treatment is best gauged by the comfort of the horse and whether the horse's feet land flat. The techniques that are currently used most widely for shoeing are heart-bar shoes, egg-bar shoes in conjunction with silicone putty sole support, or one of two commercial shoes, the Aluminum Four Point Rail shoe (Nanric Inc.) and the Equine Digit Support System (Equine Digit Support System, Inc.). Pain is best controlled with phenylbutazone as needed. Rest must be balanced against the benefits of exercise. Occasionally, tenotomy is required to decrease the tension in the deep digital flexor tendon more than can be achieved with therapeutic shoeing. It is primarily indicated in horses that are showing progressive rotation of the distal phalanx, horses with rotation and thin soles that are displaying persistent pain despite all other attempts to control it, and in horses with secondary flexural deformities of the distal interphalangeal joint. Partial hoof-wall resections and hoof-wall grooving are used to try to correct the concavity that occurs in the dorsal hoof wall as the foot grows out by mechanically dissociating the new hoof growth at the coronary band from the stresses at the ground surface of the wall caused by weight bearing. Abscesses should be drained, preferably through distal wall rather than the sole, and the distal phalanx debrided if septic osteitis develops.

Prognosis

The prognosis for acute laminitis should always be guarded to poor because the course of the disease is highly unpredictable. The likelihood of survival and return to function is best correlated against the severity of the initial clinical signs. The prognosis for survival in horses with chronic laminitis is probably best correlated with the severity of the lameness, the degree of flexion of the distal interphalangeal joint (phalangeal rotation), and the thickness of the sole. The severity of rotation of the hoof capsule has also been used to predict the likelihood of survival, but is probably more useful in predicting the likelihood that the horse will need indefinite therapeutic hoof care.

110 Radiograph of the horse in 107 and 108 immediately after the first shoeing shows the position of the shoe in relation to the distal phalanx after the heels have been trimmed and the dorsal wall has been built up with a synthetic composite.

111 Radiograph 8 months after placement of first shoe. Note the greatly reduced rotation of the dorsal hoof wall and the thickness of the sole.

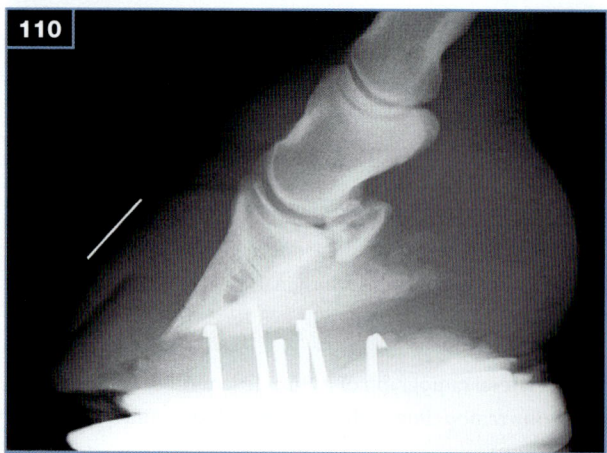

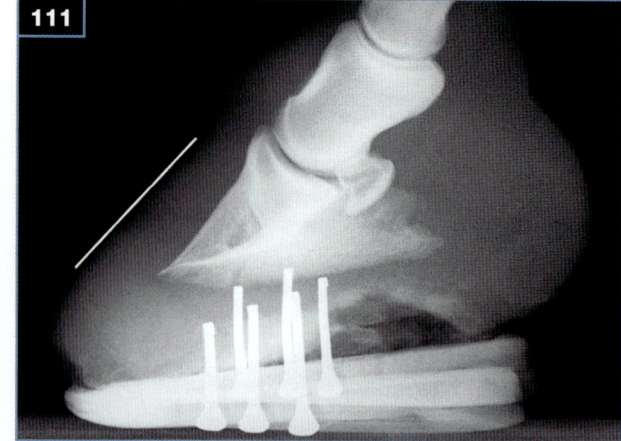

Musculoskeletal system

White line disease

Definition/overview

White line disease is a keratolytic syndrome of the deeper layers of the stratum medium of the hoof wall.

Etiology/pathophysiology

The etiology is presumed to be infectious, although the agent(s) is unknown. Both fungi and anaerobic bacteria have been implicated. The keratolytic process forms cavities within the hoof wall containing air and moist degenerating horn. Usually only one foot is affected, but multiple-foot cases do occur. The lesions are not associated with inflammation of the underlying tissues. If enough of the wall is affected, the distal phalanx is no longer adequately supported by the outer layers of the hoof wall and the distal phalanx displaces. Subsequent pressure on the sole may cause bruising and lameness of variable magnitude.

Clinical presentation

Early white line disease is often asymptomatic and only identified incidentally by the farrier when the foot is trimmed. It is seen as a discolored area or defect in the inner layers of the stratum medium on the ground surface of the wall. Alternatively, the horse presents with lameness associated with displacement of the distal phalanx and bruising. The sole may appear flattened and show the characteristic discoloration associated with bruising. The hoof feels warm and application of hoof testers to the sole elicits a withdrawal response.

Differential diagnosis

Laminitis; abscess.

Diagnosis

The size and appearance of the defect in the ground surface of the wall may not correlate with the degree or cause of cavitation within the wall. Radiographically, the cavitation is evident as radiolucent areas within the hoof wall, and displacement of the distal phalanx is determined by increased thickness of the wall, divergence of the parietal surface of the distal phalanx from the wall, and decreased thickness of the sole (112, 113). Radiographs taken in the horizontal plane at a tangent to the defect in the wall will identify the proximal extent of the cavitation. Multiple radiographs taken at various angles may be necessary to identify the extent of the circumference involved. The wall defect can also be explored with a flexible probe, although the true extent of the defect is frequently not physically identified until the overlying wall is removed during the course of treatment. The horn on the surface and at the margins of the defect is often chalky or moist and waxy.

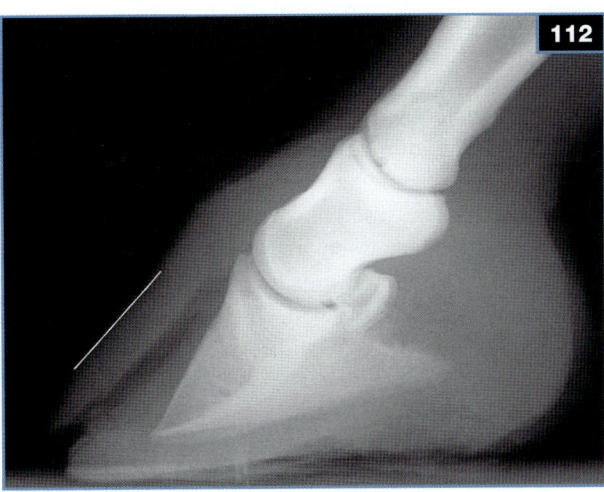

112 Lateral radiograph with a large radiolucent defect in the inner margin of the dorsal hoof wall indicative of white line disease, and secondary rotation of the hoof capsule.

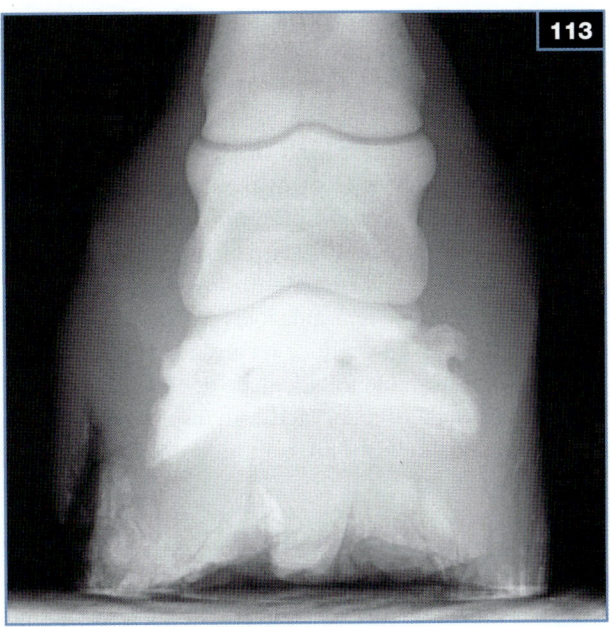

113 Dorsopalmar radiograph with a large radiolucent defect in the inner margin of the lateral hoof wall indicative of white line disease.

This disease is differentiated from laminitis and abscesses based on history, relatively superficial location, and appearance of horn in the defect. Horses with white line disease do not have the characteristic history of horses with chronic laminitis, and horses with white line disease that are severely lame have a more chronic history than horses with abscesses. The defect in the wall is more superficial than that seen in hooves with laminitis or abscesses, and there is no stretching of the lamellae as seen in the white line of hooves with chronic laminitis.

Management

The most important aspect of treatment is removal of all undermined hoof wall, which exposes the underlying surface to the air to dry. The affected hoof wall does not provide effective support to the distal phalanx and can therefore be removed without harm. If any affected wall is not debrided, the disease will continue to spread. Several topical medications have been used, but it has not been determined whether they provide additional benefit to the debridement. The horse is left barefoot and the lesion exposed to air during treatment if possible. If it is difficult to keep the surface clean, bandages may be applied, either dry or with a topical antiseptic such as 2% tincture of iodine. If it is essential that a horse returns to competition before the defect in the wall has grown out, and the surface has been free from evidence of disease for 2 weeks, then the defect can be patched with a synthetic composite. Any affected tissue still present under the reconstructed wall will spread, causing separation of the patch from the wall. Metronidazole incorporated into the synthetic polymer may reduce recurrence of the disease, but this is no substitute for adequate debridement. Those horses with lameness associated with displacement of the distal phalanx should be shod in the same manner as a laminitic horse.

Prognosis

Complete elimination of the disease may require persistence, but should be successful. Return to full work should be expected in those horses without displacement of the distal phalanx, and even in those horses with displacement the prognosis for return to work is much better than for laminitic horses with rotation.

Hoof cracks

Definition/overview

Hoof cracks are horizontal or vertical fissures within the hoof capsule.

Etiology/pathophysiology

Vertical hoof cracks are common. They are most commonly caused by poor mediolateral and/or dorsopalmar hoof balance. Additional causes include trauma to the coronary band, poor quality hoof horn, and inadequate/infrequent hoof trimming. Additionally, hoof cracks are more likely to occur if there is prior disease affecting the shape or mechanical properties of the hoof wall (e.g. laminitis). Hoof cracks are classified by location, depth, and whether they are complete or incomplete. They may occur at any point around the circumference of the hoof wall, including the bars. Partial and full thickness cracks extend through part of, or the entire thickness of, the hoof capsule, respectively. Blind hoof cracks that start deeper in the hoof capsule occur occasionally. Complete hoof cracks extend from the weight-bearing surface of the wall to the coronary band, whereas incomplete hoof cracks start either proximally or distally, but do not extend the full length of the wall. Toe cracks most frequently start at the ground surface, whereas quarter cracks are more likely to start at the coronary band. Hoof cracks become painful when they either are unstable and pinch the underlying tissues or become infected. Quarter cracks are more likely to be full thickness or become infected than toe cracks.

Horizontal hoof cracks are less common than vertical hoof cracks. They may spread around a variable amount of the circumference of the hoof wall. They most commonly occur following abscesses that drain at the coronary band. Much less common, but more severe, are horizontal fissures caused by selenium toxicity, which are likely to extend around a greater part of the circumference and to cause lameness.

Clinical presentation

The majority of hoof cracks are present on visual examination. Not all cracks are clinically significant, and regional and intrasynovial analgesia may be used to differentiate the cause of any lameness present. Lameness is usually associated with infection or hoof instability. Hoof testers can be used to assess instability and pain and to increase visibility of purulent or blood discharges.

Differential diagnosis

None.

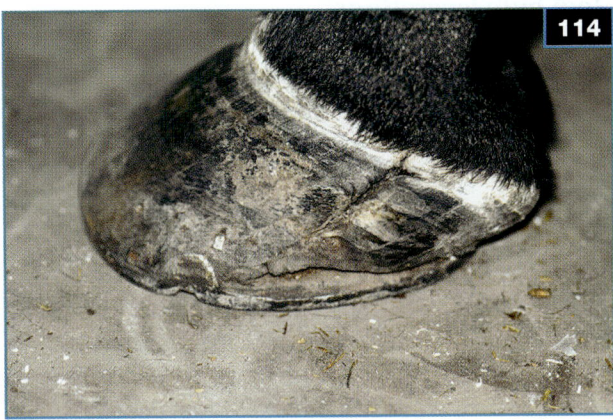

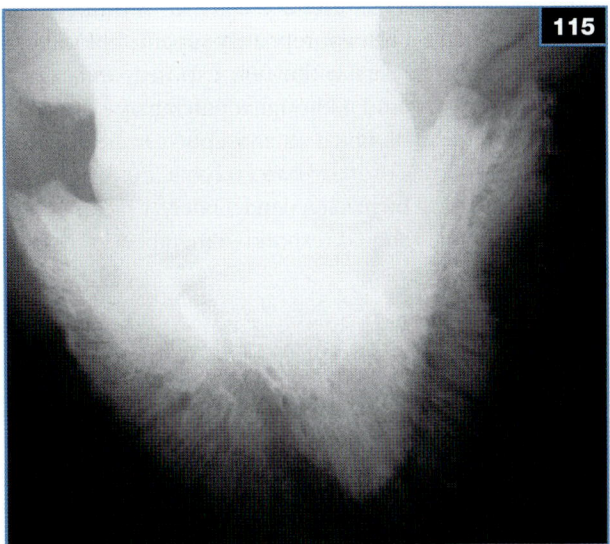

114–117 Hoof crack. Quarter crack (114). Radiograph of the foot showing chronic remodeling of the abaxial margin of P3 subsequent to a chronic quarter hoof crack (115). Quarter crack following debridement, floating of the heel, and shoeing with a heart-bar shoe (116, 117). (115 courtesy GA Munroe)

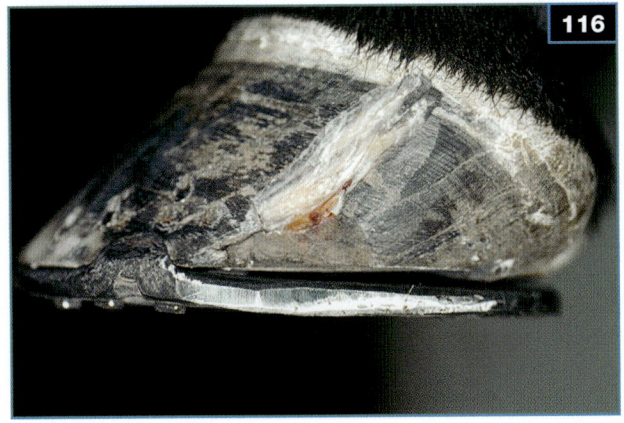

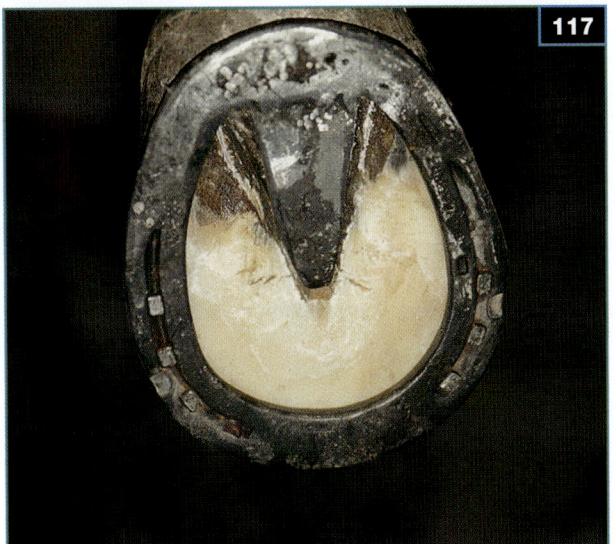

Diagnosis

Most hoof cracks are obvious (114), but careful inspection may be necessary to identify small cracks at the coronary band or cracks in the bars. Occult hoof cracks at the coronary band may be tentatively identified based on pain on palpation, particularly if there is an associated hoof imbalance. A definitive diagnosis is possible when it breaks through to the surface of the hoof. Foot radiographs may reveal changes in the distal phalanx associated with chronic cases (115).

Management

Not all hoof cracks need treatment. The nature of the crack and its relationship to hoof balance and prior trauma should be determined. The movement of toe cracks varies with conformation and as the animal moves. Toe cracks compress with weight bearing if the toe is short and squared off, and spread if it is too long. The treatment depends on the nature of the crack and the exercise expected of the horse in the near future. If rest from exercise is possible, most hoof cracks will respond to corrective trimming to restore the optimal balance with or without shoeing, and the crack will grow out (116, 117). For those horses that have to perform in the near future, a crack may need to be stabilized. Prior to stabilization the crack must be debrided to ensure no foreign, infected, or necrotic tissue is entrapped. Stabilization should prevent both compression and expansion of the crack, and is usually performed with synthetic polymer patches that incorporate sutures such as Kevlar or steel with or without sheet

75

metal screws (118, 119). The horse is then shod. Alternatives include shoes with appropriately placed clips or hoof staples. Infected cracks must be fully exposed, and cannot be completely covered, although a patch may be placed over a drain through which an antiseptic can be flushed. Cracks that follow coronary band trauma are unlikely to grow out and must be managed indefinitely. Cracks associated with laminitis should respond to therapeutic shoeing for the primary disease.

Prognosis

The prognosis varies with location, depth, balance of the foot, and the presence of other disease. The prognosis for elimination of cracks associated with poor conformation that can be corrected by trimming and shoeing is good. Those cracks associated with prior trauma, concurrent disease, or uncorrectable balance or conformation require indefinite therapeutic attention.

118, 119 Hoof crack. Filling of a toe crack with a thermoplastic compound after the crack has been debrided and thoroughly cleaned (118). Stabilization of the toe crack in 118 by application of a reinforced plastic patch, which is glued to the dorsal wall (119). (Photos courtesy GA Munroe)

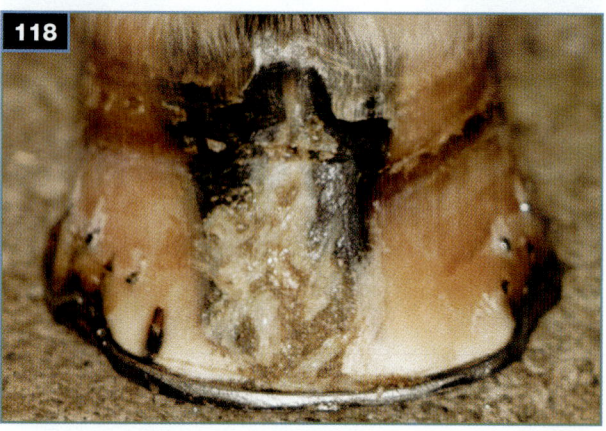

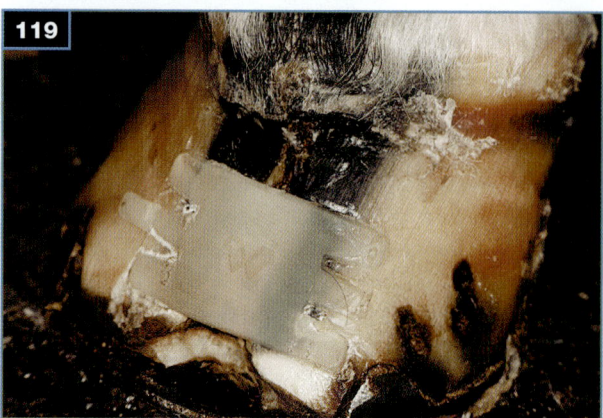

Heel-bulb lacerations

Definition/overview

Heel-bulb lacerations usually form an inverted U-shaped flap, with the apex of the U proximally. The distal extent of the wound margins is usually either just proximal to the coronary band or extending up to 1–2 cm into the coronary band.

Etiology/pathophysiology

The injury is caused by acute trauma. It is characterized by irregular margins and varying damage to the underlying tissues. If untreated, these wounds are prone to excessive granulation tissue formation and slow epithelialization because of the movement between the opposite margins of the wound. The prolonged healing delays the return to work, produces an unsightly scar when it has epithelialized, and if large enough, may impede function. Deeper structures that may be affected include the palmar digital vessels and nerves, the distal interphalangeal joint, the deep digital flexor tendon and sheath, the navicular bursa, and the ungual cartilage.

Clinical presentation

Heel-bulb lacerations present either soon after acute trauma or after excessive granulation tissue has delayed wound closure and caused an unsightly blemish. Lameness is variable, but is more likely in horses with acute wounds or wounds that are associated with injury and infection of deeper structures. The hemorrhage from lacerated palmar digital vessels can be profuse.

Differential diagnosis

None.

Diagnosis

Diagnosis is based on visual inspection. The wound should be examined to determine its full extent, the involvement of deeper structures, and the severity of contamination present (120). Additionally, the margins of the wound are assessed for viability and epithelialization, and the bed of the wound for evidence of granulation tissue formation (121). If excessive granulation exists, a biopsy may be necessary to exclude the development of a sarcoid or habronemiasis.

Management

In acute injuries in which there is persistent hemorrhage, this should be controlled by either ligating the affected vessel(s) or applying a pressure bandage before further treatment of the laceration is attempted. The systemic status of the horse should be assessed. The preferred treatment for heel-bulb lacerations is surgical closure followed by immobilization until the margins have heeled. If a deeper structure is affected, then that structure is treated as

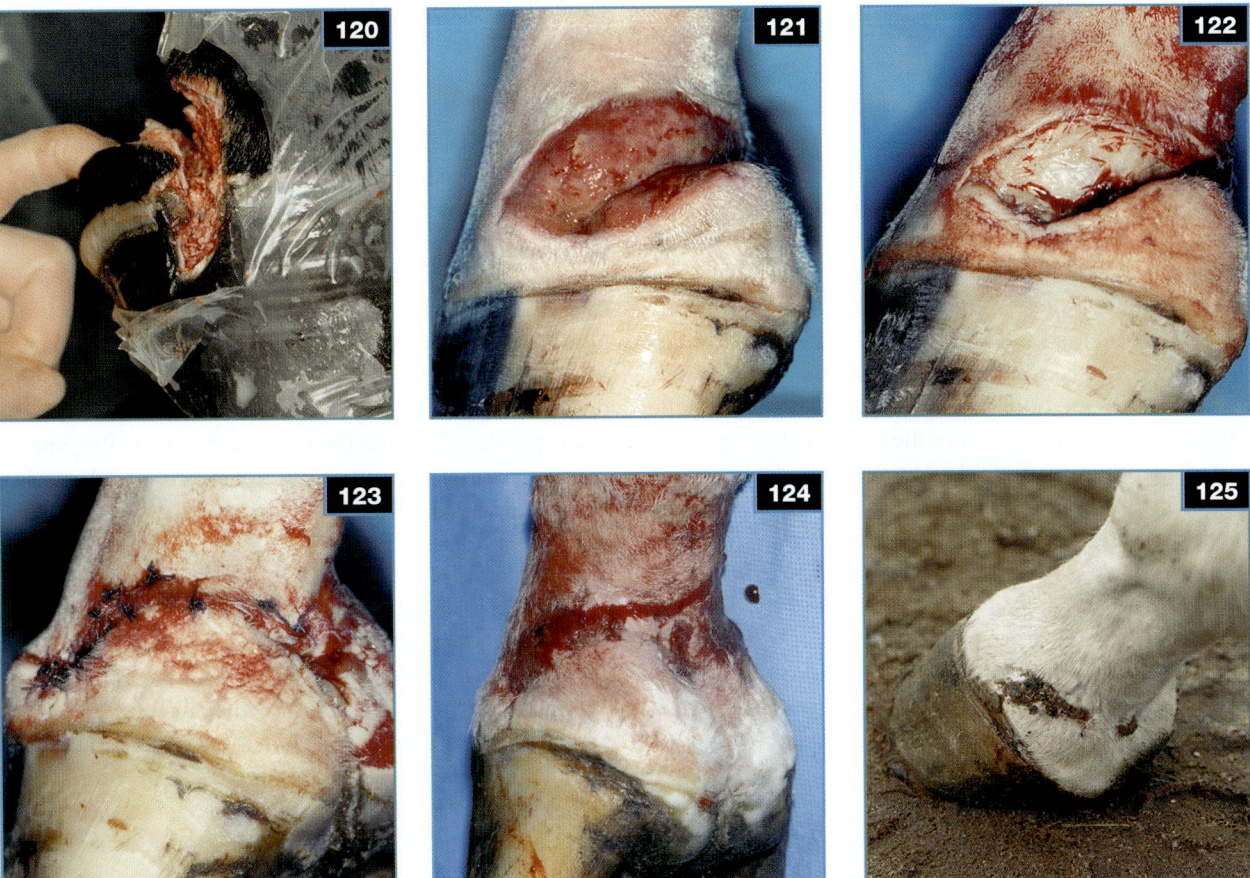

120 Heel-bulb laceration. A severe acute laceration of the heel bulb that has injured the lateral cartilages, coronary band, hoof and heel soft tissues. (Photo courtesy GA Munroe)

121 Heel-bulb laceration. Chronic heel-bulb wound with a healthy granulating surface.

122–125 Heel-bulb laceration. Laceration after excision of excess fibrogranulomatous tissue (122). Margins of laceration sutured together immediately prior to application of a phalangeal cast (123). Laceration three weeks after closure and immediately following cast removal (124). Residual scar after an additional 3–4 weeks (125).

if it is contaminated or infected. The treatment will vary with the age and contamination of the wound. Acute wounds with minimal contamination may be debrided, sutured, and immobilized with a cast for three weeks. Some clinicians use a phalangeal or short cast, while others prefer a half-limb form. Acute wounds with substantial contamination should be debrided and managed conservatively with topical antimicrobials, wound lavage and bandaging, until healthy granulation tissue is present across the surface of the wound. Once a healthy granulation bed is present, excessive granulation tissue is debrided, the wound margins opposed with sutures, and the foot immobilized in a phalangeal cast. Chronic heel-bulb lacerations should be treated conservatively until the surface is healthy and then treated with delayed secondary closure and immobilization (122–125). Such chronic wounds may require considerable excision of granulation tissue, and

complete closure of the wound may not be possible. That part of the wound not closed is then allowed to heal by secondary intention, often requiring prolonged casting. In those heel-bulb lacerations in which the coronary band is affected, the coronary band may be sutured in a similar manner to that used in the treatment of hoof-wall avulsions (see below). In all instances, tetanus prophylaxis and perioperative antibiotics are advisable.

Prognosis
The prognosis for most heel-bulb lacerations for return to athletic activity is good. There is usually a residual scar that varies in size with the original injury, the amount of granulation tissue that develop, and the success of the closure. The prognosis for wounds with involvement of deeper structures is dependent on which strucures are affected and how severely injured or contaminated they are.

Hoof-wall avulsions

Definition/overview

Hoof-wall avulsions occur when a segment of the hoof wall becomes separated from the underlying tissues.

Etiology/pathophysiology

Hoof-wall avulsions follow trauma to the wall that causes it to fracture and a segment to become elevated. Typically, this occurs in a distal to proximal direction. The avulsion is classified as complete if the avulsed wall is completely detached from the foot, and partial if the avulsed wall is still attached, usually along one border. The avulsion may be confined to the hoof capsule, but usually involves the coronary band and the skin of the pastern. The extent of underlying trauma is variable, but may include any of the underlying structures. The pattern of healing depends on the depth of the trauma. Superficial avulsions may heal in a manner comparable to partial-thickness skin wounds, whereas deeper avulsions heal as full-thickness wounds. Full-thickness avulsions epithelialize from the adjacent margin, so the nature of the new hoof wall varies accordingly. Occasionally, hoof integument grows up onto a pastern defect to create a horny spur.

Clinical presentation

Horses with hoof-wall avulsions present either acutely or chronically. Acute injuries demonstrate varying degrees of lameness and hemorrhage associated with the trauma. Chronic injuries can present with a granulating surface plus or minus complications associated with deeper structure involvement. Alternatively, the integument heals, but the abnormal structure of the wall causes altered function and lameness.

126–128 Hoof-wall avulsion. (126) Hoof-wall avulsion that is still attached dorsally. (127) Resection of the distal portion of the avulsed hoof wall and apposition of the proximal margin of the avulsed wall with a wire suture. (128) Stabilization of the hoof wall with a rim cast.

Differential diagnosis

None.

Diagnosis

The avulsion is obvious on presentation, but the underlying damage may not be (126). The coronary tissues and adjacent skin are assessed for viability. Careful exploration is required to ascertain which deeper structures, if any, are involved. Injury to ligamentous or tendonous structures causes lameness due to instability or loss of motor function. Communication with synovial structures that is not obvious is confirmed by flushing the structure from a distant site. Radiography soon after the injury will demonstrate any defects in the bone caused by the injury, and in chronic avulsions may show advanced pedal osteitis associated with the adjacent inflammation.

Management

Complete avulsions are treated like any other wound that is allowed to heal by secondary intention. They should be cleaned and debrided, dressed with appropriate topical antimicrobials and dressings, and bandaged. Systemic antibiotics are administered until the wound surfaces are granulating, analgesia given as needed, and tetanus prophylaxis provided. If the foot is unstable because of the amount of wall lost, a cast or therapeutic shoe maintains the alignment of the foot with the pastern. Partial hoof-wall avulsions, in which the coronary tissues are all present and viable, are best managed by resecting the wall 1–2 cm distal to the coronary band and reconstructing the band (127). The coronary band can be sutured if the outer layers of the hoof capsule have been removed first. A cast may then be applied over the reconstruction for additional stability (128). If the alignment of the coronary band is correct, a new hoof wall may grow that is grossly indistinguishable from the rest of the wall, although defects may persist at and below the margins of the avulsion where the original coronary defect was closed. Partial avulsions that are deemed unviable are converted to complete avulsions. Following either complete or partial healing of

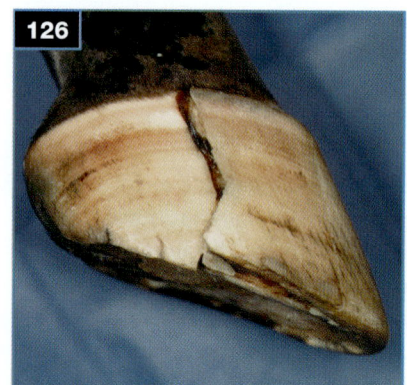
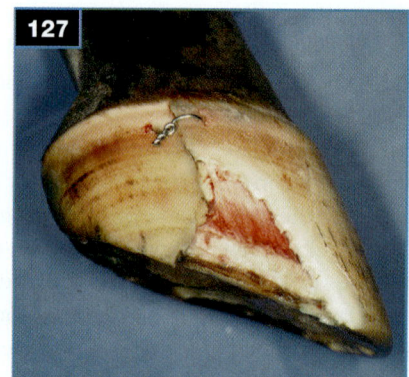
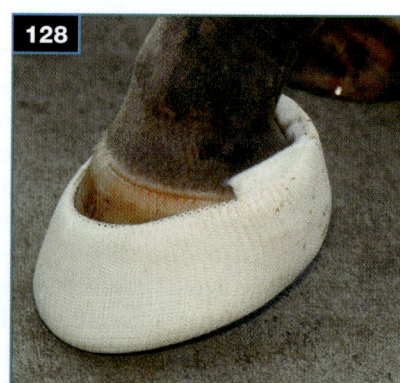

an avulsion, therapeutic shoeing may be necessary to support the side of the foot with the injury, depending on the structural integrity of the new wall. Affected joints and tendons are treated accordingly.

Prognosis
The prognosis depends on the degree of injury to the coronary band and underlying structures. If the coronary band was intact or was successfully repaired, the new wall may closely resemble the original and function normally. If parts of the coronary tissues were lost, the new wall may be surprisingly cosmetic, and functional, with therapeutic shoeing. If the avulsion involves injury to the deeper structures of the foot such as the distal interphalangeal joint or navicular bursa, the prognosis is poorer.

Keratoma
Definition/overview
Keratomas are epithelial tumors of the hoof.

Etiology/pathophysiology
The etiology is unknown, but prior trauma to the hoof has been associated with keratomas in some horses. The tumors originate from the germinal layers of the epithelium of the hoof and occur in the wall or the sole. The tumor develops into an expansile mass, usually deep to the hoof capsule. It may cause pressure lysis of the underlying distal phalanx and/or distortion of the overlying hoof capsule. Histologically, the tumor is characterized by rings of squamous epithelial cells containing abundant keratin. Frequently, the tumors are associated with recurrent secondary infection.

Clinical presentation
The most common presenting symptom is lameness accompanied by distortion of the hoof capsule and recurrent infection.

Differential diagnosis
Other rare hoof tumors; chronic hoof wounds; abscess.

Diagnosis
Most horses with a keratoma are lame. A keratoma may be suspected if the lameness is associated with a distorted hoof capsule and infection, a relatively well-circumscribed round or oval mass of horn is visible on the ground surface of the foot, either in the white line of the distal wall or in the sole, or when a dorsoproximal/palmarodistal oblique radiograph shows a well-demarcated circular or oval area of lysis in the solar margin/parietal surface of the distal phalanx (129). In horses in which a tumor is suspected but cannot be identified on the surface of the hoof capsule, exploration of the capsule is necessary. A definitive diagnosis requires a biopsy and histopathologic evaluation.

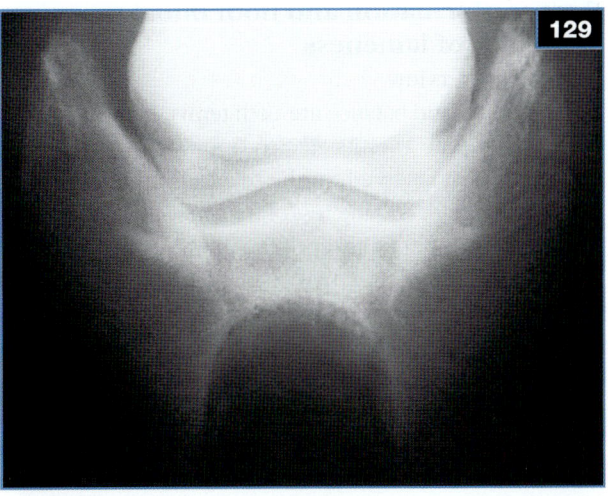

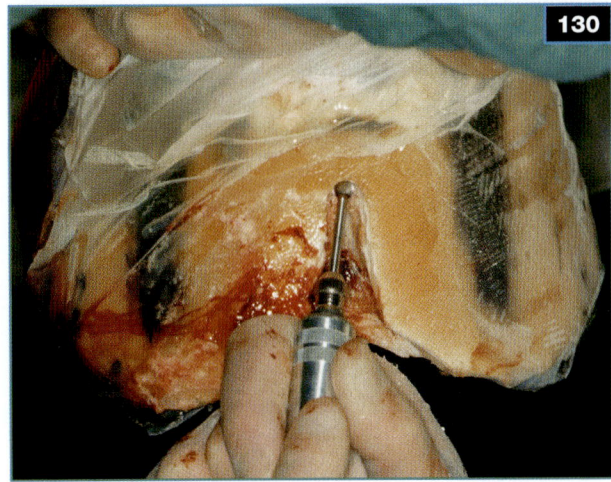

129 Upright radiographic view of of the foot of a horse with a keratoma at the toe, which has eroded a large defect in P3.

130 Surgical removal of a keratoma by resection of the surrounding horn. (Photos courtesy GA Munroe)

Management
Both conservative treatment and surgical excision (130) have been suggested, but the latter is twice as successful. The tumors are excised through a partial hoof-wall resection. The wound is bandaged and the defect heals by secondary intention.

Prognosis
The prognosis for horses with keratomas treated by surgical excision is good. Approximately 80% return to previous athletic performance.

Foot conformation and hoof imbalance as a cause of lameness

Definition/overview

Conformation and balance are both terms that relate to the form of the limb (i.e. its size, proportions, and shape). Balance is best reserved for the relationship between the hoof, the ground, and the rest of the limb. Conformation is used to describe the limb proximal to the hoof (and the rest of the body). Balance is divided into static and dynamic components and is a three-dimensional concept that is traditionally divided into mediolateral and dorsopalmar components. Poor conformation and imbalance refer to changes in the shape of the digit from the normal, near symmetrical form and the way the hoof relates to the ground.

Etiology/pathophysiology

Conformation is dependent on both genetics and development. Balance is also dependent on genetics and development, but also on hoof growth, trimming and shoeing. Poor foot trimming is the most likely cause of imbalance in shod horses. Imbalance occurs in barefooted horses with inadequate care or poor conformation.

The different changes within the foot that are described as imbalance are often interrelated, but some of them are frequently discussed as separate entities.

Contracted heels describes the condition when the heel bulb and heel buttresses are closer together than normal. It is invariably associated with a narrow frog, and frequently with high or underrun heels. The condition is thought to occur secondary to heel pain, reduced weight-bearing by the heels, and subsequent reduced expansion of the heels during the normal cycle of the stride.

Underrun heels occur when the heels are more acutely angled to the ground than normal, and usually occur in horses with excessive length of toe. Typically, the heels are longer than normal and they may be curved dorsally and axially so that the weight-bearing surface of the heels is displaced dorsal to the base of the frog. The foot–pastern axis is usually broken back (see 4-8). While the etiology has not been definitively determined, it appears that some breeds, particularly Thoroughbreds, are genetically predisposed. In other instances, trimming practices that result in excessive length of heel or shoeing that causes excessive weight-bearing on the heels encourage under-run heels. An upright foot with high heels usually accompanies either contracted heels or a flexural deformity of the distal interphalangeal joint. However, in the latter, in contrast to the former, the heels are usually widely spaced. Upright heels are frequently associated with a broken forward foot–pastern axis. When a horse has one upright foot with contracted heels, the contralateral foot often has low/underrun heels.

Sheared heels is a condition in which one heel bulb of the foot is displaced proximally compared to the other, and it is often associated with contracted heels. The exact cause of sheared heels is undetermined, although it is thought to be secondary to inappropriate trimming. Sheared heels may be associated with lameness that is abolished with a palmar digital nerve block.

Imbalance causes lameness by distortion of the hoof capsule and injury to other structures in the limb due to stress redistribution. Dorsopalmar imbalance is divided into broken back and broken forward foot–pastern axis. The former is reported to be associated with navicular disease, distal deep digital flexor tendon strain, heel bruising, hemorrhage in the dorsal white line, and pedal osteitis of the palmar processes. The latter is associated with dorsal sole hemorrhages and pedal osteitis. Mediolateral imbalance (131) is reported to be associated with sheared heels, quarter or heel cracks, sidebone, fracture of the palmar processes, and asymmetrical bruising and pedal osteitis, although for the most part epidemiological evidence to support these observations is lacking.

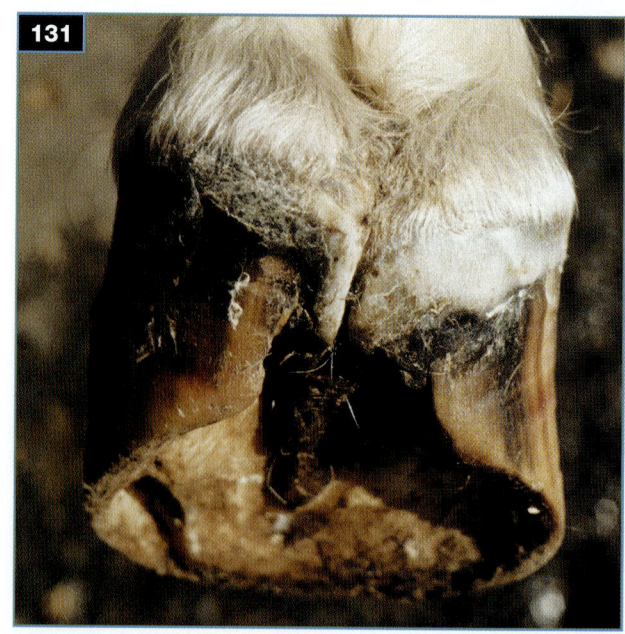

131

131–133 Hoof imbalance. (131) Mediolateral foot imbalance with asymmetry of the heel bulbs and walls of the hoof, sheared and contracted heels, and uneven bearing surface of the wall. (132) Assessing the mediolateral balance of the foot with a shoe in place; note the asymmetry of the walls and bulbs of the heel. (133) Same foot as in 132 with a T square in place demonstrating the asymmetry of the bearing surface (long on the lateral side [left side of picture]). (Photos courtesy GA Munroe)

Musculoskeletal system

Clinical presentation

Horses with hoof imbalance frequently present with lameness, although abnormal shape or movement of the hoof may be an incidental finding in lameness examinations.

Differential diagnosis

Any chronic lameness originating within the foot; healed traumatic hoof wounds.

Diagnosis

Diagnosis of imbalance and poor conformation of the hoof and distal limb is made by careful visual inspection and measurement. Specifically, with the foot on the ground, the length and angles of the wall at the heel and toe and the approximate symmetry of the medial and lateral walls of the hoof, including the presence of underrun and flared wall, are observed. With the foot off the ground, the mediolateral symmetry of the ground surface of the foot is noted as well as its length and width, which are usually approximately equal (132, 133). Horizontal dorsopalmar and lateral radiographs are important to determine the relationship between the hoof capsule and the phalanges. On the former view, the interphalangeal joint spaces should be symmetrical and ideally parallel to the ground. On the lateral radiograph, the solar margin of the distal phalanx should form an angle of 2–10 degrees to the ground, although 3–5 degrees is most common. Gross misalignment of the foot–pastern axis can be detected, but more subtle misalignment is hard to evaluate because it changes as the horse's weight shifts. Regional analgesia may be necessary to localize the lameness to the distal limb and often to the heel region.

Imbalance *per se* rarely causes lameness. Lameness associated with hoof imbalance is usually caused by a subsequent pathologic process in one or more structures other than the hoof capsule. Horses with imbalance may be sound, have lameness related to the imbalance, or lameness unrelated to the imbalance. Frequently, the only way to confirm that the lameness is a sequela to the imbalance is to correct it and observe for improvement in the lameness.

Management

In general, hoof imbalance is treated by therapeutic hoof trimming and shoeing. Improvement may be immediate or take several months. It is extremely beneficial to take serial radiographs to monitor changes in the relationship between the hoof capsule and the phalanges. Conformation cannot be corrected in adult horses. Therefore, therapeutic trimming and shoeing can only compensate for the poor conformation. Frequently compromises are made that enhance the function of one part of the distal limb but may have a negative impact on another.

Specific guidelines for treatment of the different conditions are limited, variably effective, and not well documented. Intentional therapeutic expansion of contracted heels can be very difficult. In those horses in which contracted heels have developed secondary to pain, it is unlikely that treatment will be successful unless the cause of the pain is removed. In horses in which contracted heels are accompanied by a long toe, shortening the toe will encourage the entire foot, including the heels, to expand. In horses in which the long toe is accompanied by underrun heels, rasping the heels back to the base of the frog

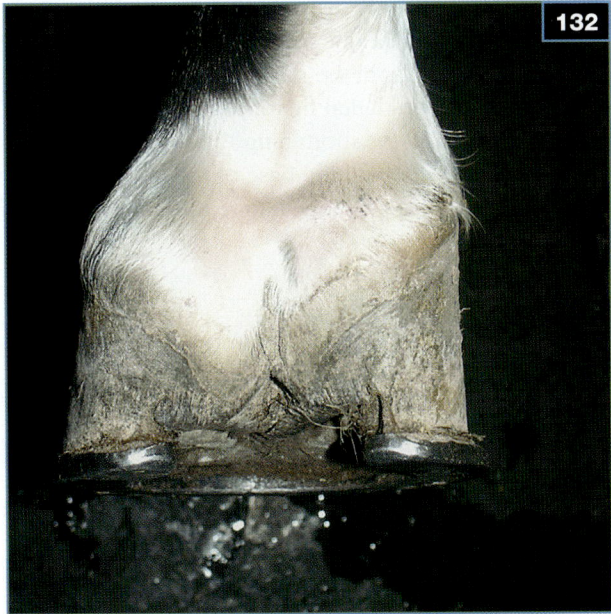

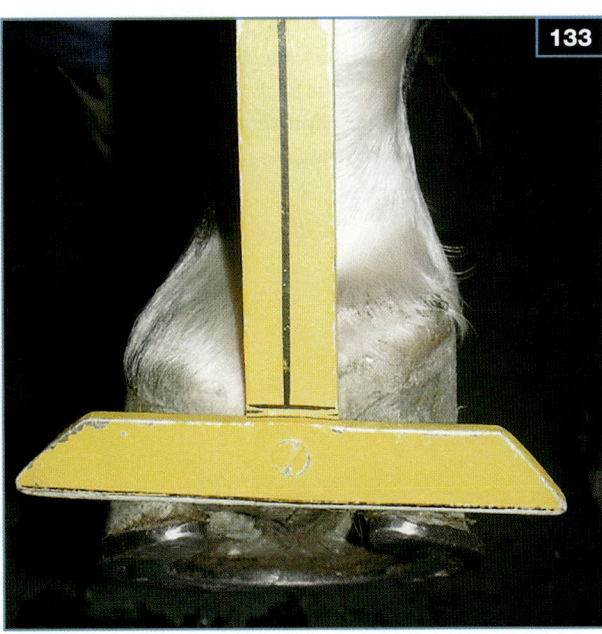

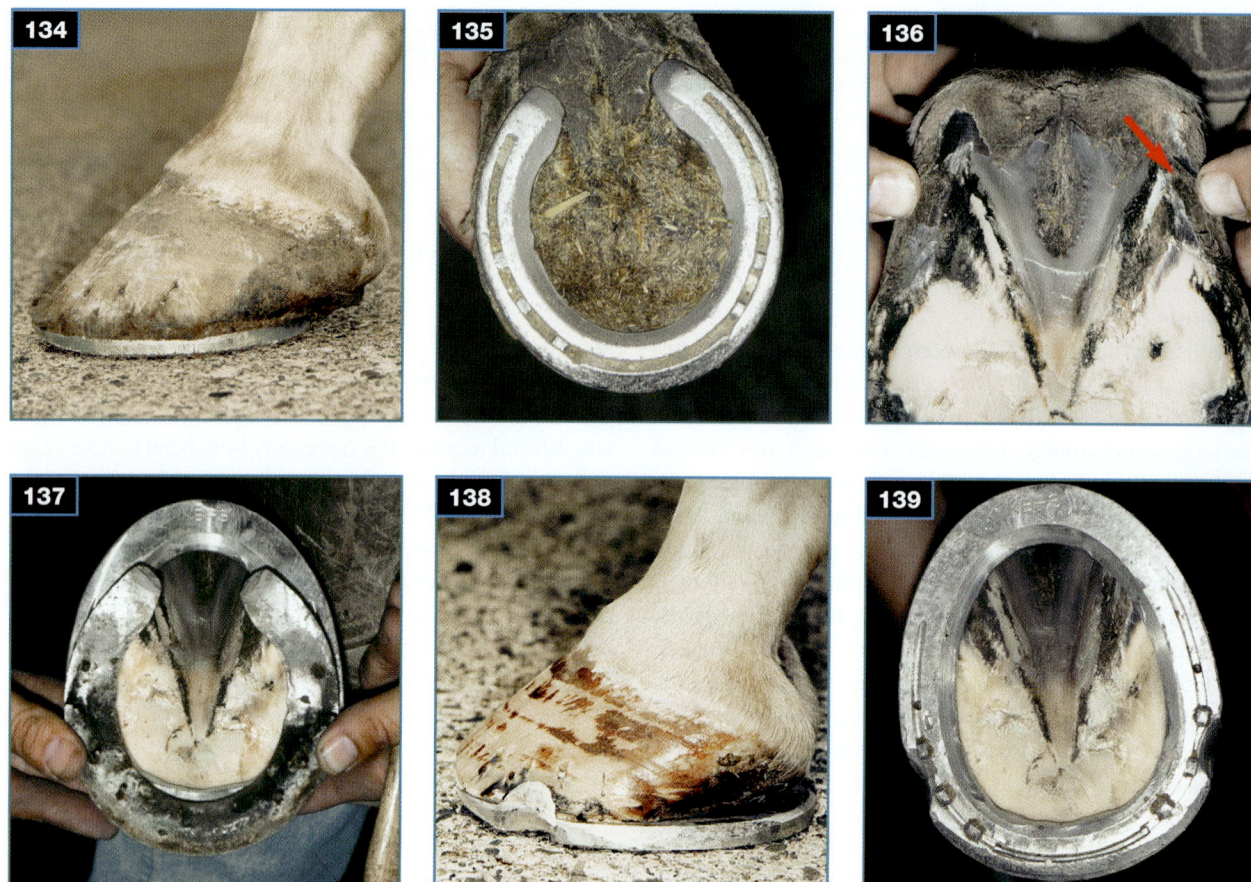

134–139 Hoof imbalance. (134) Lateral view of dorso-palmar imbalance associated with a long toe, low heels, and a broken back foot–pastern axis. (135) Solar view indicating position of the shoe in relation to the ground surface of the foot. (136) The left heel (arrow) has been trimmed back to the base of the frog; note the difference in length between the trimmed and untrimmed heels. (137) The old shoe is superimposed on the new shoe to show the difference in position of break over and coverage of the heels. (138) Lateral view of the foot after shoeing; note the improvement in the hoof pastern angle. (139) Solar view showing the position of the new shoe.

will encourage the heels to grow wider (134–139), but in the author's experience this usually occurs as new hoof from the coronary band, not expansion at the ground surface. Lowering the heels of an upright foot may be counterproductive if the cause of the high heels is not addressed. Lowering the heels of a horse with palmar foot pain may cause a broken forward foot–pastern axis to straighten or a straight one to break back, both of which may increase pain from the navicular bone and bursa or tension in the deep digital flexor tendon. Sheared heels are usually treated by shortening the long heel so that both heels are level with the base of the frog; the foot is then shod with a bar shoe to minimize movement between the heels.

Prognosis

The prognosis for acute imbalance associated with secondary pathology that is readily reversible is good. The prognosis for chronic imbalance, particularly if it is associated with degenerative conditions, is guarded to poor.

Trimming and shoeing as a cause of lameness

Overview

Trimming and shoeing may both cause lameness, although the incidence is unknown. Poor trimming may cause a foot to become unbalanced. Trimming the medial and lateral walls unevenly creates a mediolateral imbalance. Similarly, inappropriate trimming of the heel and/or toe may create a broken foot–pastern axis. Leaving the toe too long creates a dorsopalmar imbalance or broken back foot–pastern axis. Leaving the heel too long may create a broken forward axis. Trimming the sole too thin causes undue pressure on the underlying sensitive structures and predisposes them to bruising.

Attaching steel shoes with nails to horses' feet has some detrimental effects on the biomechanics of the foot, including decreased expansion of the foot, increased maximum deceleration of the foot, increased frequency of vibrations as the foot contacts the ground, and an increase in the maximum ground reaction force. Despite these effects, shoeing is remarkably well tolerated and, indeed, frequently necessary. Both the attachment of shoes and shoe selection can cause lameness to develop.

Attachment of the shoe

Incorrect nail placement can cause lameness. If it directly damages the sensitive tissues immediately underlying the hoof capsule, it will cause immediate lameness (nail prick). The diagnosis can be confirmed by localizing the pain to a specific nail with hoof testers or identifying the incorrect placement on shoe removal. Removal of the nail should resolve the problem. The nail hole is then infused with an antiseptic. More insidiously, a nail that remains within the hoof capsule, but impinges on the sensitive tissues (nail bind), may cause pain secondary to pressure on the sensitive tissues or cause microfracture of the hoof wall internally, with subsequent introduction of infection (140). Lameness does not usually occur for several days following shoeing, but as with direct puncture of the sensitive structures, application of hoof testers should localize the pain. The nail should be removed and, if present, subsequent abscessation treated appropriately.

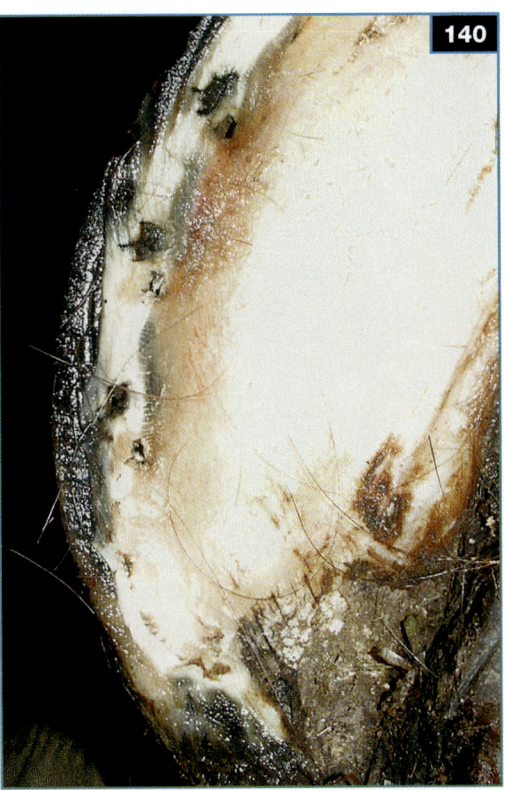

140 A foot in which several of the nails have been placed too close to the sensitive laminae (nail bind). (Photo courtesy GA Munroe)

Shoe selection

Poor shoe choice may also predispose to lameness. A shoe that is too large, either too wide or too long, is more likely to be pulled off, while a shoe that is too small or short is likely to result in pressure at the heels or angle of the sole and predispose to bruising, hoof cracks, and underrun heels. A shoe with a web that is too wide will cause pressure on the sole if the sole is dropped, while a shoe with a web that is too narrow will not protect the adjacent sole. A shoe that is too heavy will cause fatigue, which will in turn predispose the horse to injury.

83

The foot

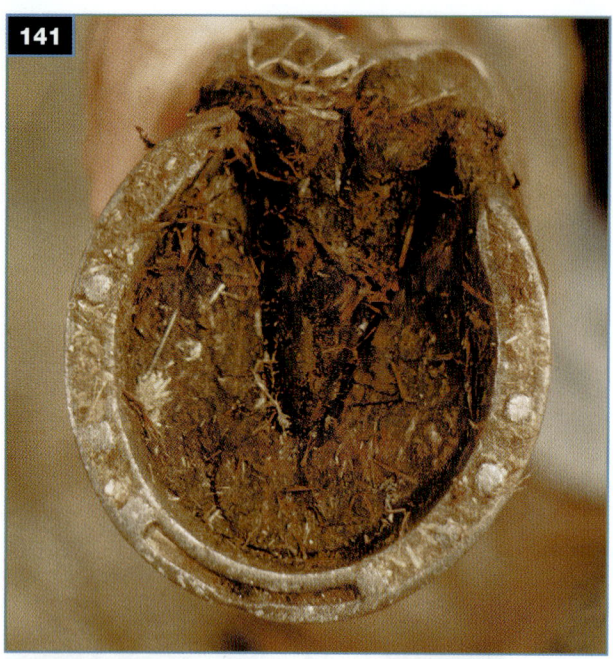

141 This shoe has been placed asymmetrically, leading to foot imbalance and an abnormal landing position. (Photo courtesy GA Munroe)

Fractures of the distal phalanx

Definition/overview
Fractures of the distal phalanx occur in several configurations: fractures of the body and wings of the distal phalanx, fractures of the extensor process, and fractures of the solar margin (142–144). Fractures of the body/wings of the distal phalanx are subdivided into articular and non-articular fractures.

Etiology/pathophysiology
Most distal phalangeal fractures occur following trauma or exercise on hard ground. Occasionally, fractures occur following penetration injuries or weakening of the bone caused by septic osteitis or large cysts. Distal phalanx fractures heal slowly and in some instances only by fibrous union. In either instance some horses will become sound, whereas others develop persistent lameness due to OA of the distal interphalangeal joint.

Clinical presentation
Horses with an acute distal phalanx fracture present with a severe acute lameness. Horses with chronic articular fractures are presented with a chronic lameness of moderate severity.

Differential diagnosis
Abscesses; puncture wounds; navicular bone fracture; acute strain or sprain; separate center of ossification of the extensor process.

Shoe placement
Placement of the shoe should normally be symmetrical about the axis of the frog. When shoe placement is asymmetrical, so that the shoe is placed further laterally than medially, greater stress will be placed on the lateral wall, and vice versa (141). If a shoe is unintentionally rotated, one heel will have greater coverage than the other. The heel with less coverage will be prone to the same problems as if the shoe was too short.

Inappropriate use of traction
Traction devices such as toe grabs or calks are widely used to increase a horse's speed or prevent a horse from slipping. Such devices concentrate stress in the adjacent wall. Additionally, traction devices that elevate one side of the limb more than the other, or elevate the toe or heel, will induce an imbalance in the limb if the horse is standing on a firm surface. Traction devices that prevent a planted foot from rotating as a horse turns place undue torque on a limb and predispose the distal limb to phalangeal fractures. Consequently, it is best to use removable traction devices, use them only when deemed necessary, and use the lowest, broadest devices possible.

Diagnosis
In horses with acute fractures there is heat in the foot, increased digital pulses, and hoof tester pain. If the fracture is articular, flexion of the interphalangeal joints will also be painful. Distal phalanx fractures must be distinguished from several other causes of acute lameness. Radiographs are often not taken initially while other causes are investigated. Dorsopalmar, 45° dorsoproximal/palmarodistal oblique, lateral, and 60° dorsoproximal/palmarodistal oblique projections are routinely performed and, depending on the configuration of the fracture, additional medial or lateral obliques may be required. Repeat radiographs at 7–10 days may identify acute fractures not seen initially. Scintigraphy is effective in demonstrating the location of occult fractures. Regional analgesia is seldom needed.

Chronic fractures of the extensor process may cause distortion of the coronary band. Chronic articular fractures that cause DJD usually demonstrate lameness that is exacerbated with distal limb flexion. Palmar digital perineural analgesia and distal interphalangeal joint analgesia are required to localize the problem, and radiography is required to identify the DJD. Scintigraphy is beneficial to determine the importance of chronic fractures of unknown significance.

Management

Acute fractures of the body of the distal phalanx are usually treated by limiting movement of the hoof capsule in order to reinforce the natural splinting it provides to the distal phalanx. This is achieved optimally by placing a rim cast that incorporates the heel bulbs around the perimeter of the foot. Alternatively, a bar shoe with a continuous rim that extends 1–1.5 cm proximally can be fitted and the space between the rim and hoof wall filled with a synthetic composite. Bar shoes with quarter clips are frequently used, but are not as effective as these other measures. Acute articular fractures in the median plane in adult horses have been successfully treated with internal lag screw fixation. The DJD that occurs with some chronic articular fractures may require treatment with intra-articular steroids and/or a palmar digital neurectomy.

Small fractures of the extensor process are removed arthroscopically. Larger fractures are reduced by internal fixation with a lag screw or removal of the fracture fragment. Solar margin fractures that are not associated with infection are treated with rest and NSAIDs. Fractures associated with infection are treated in the same manner as septic osteitis of the distal phalanx (see p. 87).

Prognosis

The prognosis is good for solar margin fractures and nonarticular fractures of the body of the distal phalanx. The prognosis for articular fractures of the body of the distal phalanx is good in horses less than 3 years old. For older horses with articular fractures treated conservatively, the long-term prognosis is fair for horses not used for racing, but variably guarded to poor, unless treated successfully by internal fixation, for racehorses. The prognosis is good for small extensor process fractures that are removed arthroscopically and fair for removal of larger fracture fragments.

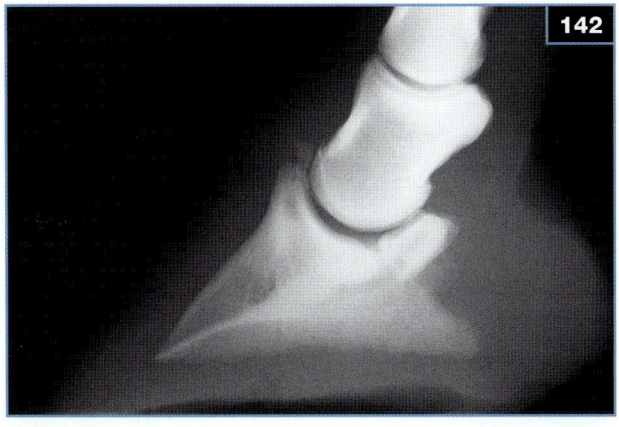

142–144 Distal phalanx fractures. Fracture of the extensor process (142). Mid-sagittal articular fracture (143). Nonarticular fracture of the palmar process (arrow) (144).

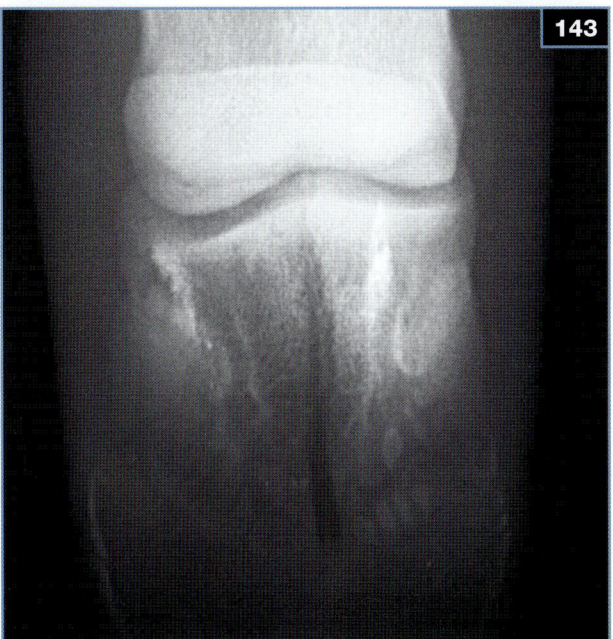

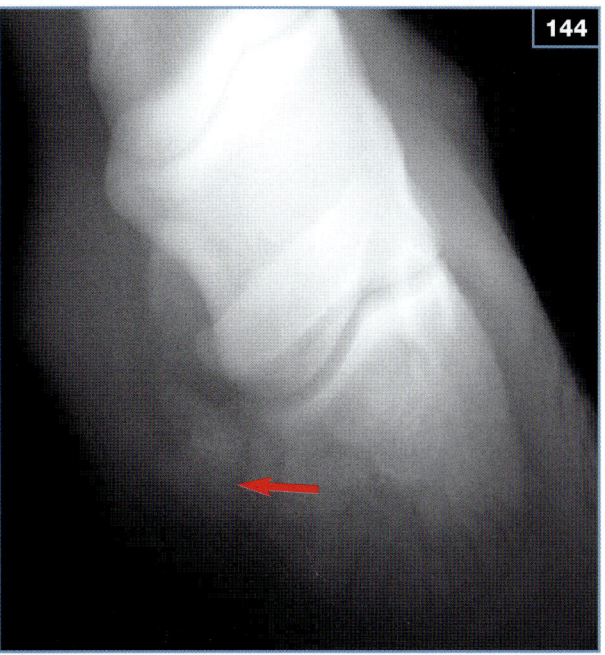

85

Pedal osteitis

Definition/overview

Pedal osteitis is a radiographic description of a pattern of resorption of bone around the solar margin of the distal phalanx.

Etiology/pathophysiology

Bone resorption around the solar margin of the distal phalanx is known to occur following certain inflammatory processes or injuries that induce inflammation (e.g. laminitis and hoof-wall avulsions). It is also seen commonly in horses with flat soles, particularly those horses demonstrating recurrent bruising, and underrun heels. It is therefore a known sequela to some inflammatory diseases in the soft tissues adjacent to the distal phalanx and thought to be a sequela to others. What is not known is whether these radiographic changes can occur following a primary inflammatory response in the bone. Until it is established that this occurs, it is best considered as a radiographic sign rather than a definitive diagnosis, and even then primary pedal osteitis, the definitive diagnosis, will have to be differentiated from secondary pedal osteitis, the clinical sign.

Clinical presentation

Pedal osteitis is most commonly identified in the forelimbs and is frequently bilateral. It is frequently identified in horses with mild to moderate lameness in the forelimbs, but is also a common incidental finding.

Differential diagnosis

Other mild to moderate causes of forelimb lameness; navicular disease; laminitis; bruising; imbalance.

Diagnosis

The classical radiographic image of pedal osteitis shows variable demineralization and an irregular contour of the dorsal margin of the distal phalanx, with vascular channels that fan out as they approach the periphery of the bone. These are best seen on a 45° dorsoproximal/palmarodistal oblique radiographic projection (145). Additional changes, including lipping of the dorsal margin and mineralization on the parietal surface of the distal phalanx, may be seen on lateral radiographic projections. These can also identify pedal osteitis of the palmar processes, seen as scalloping of the solar margin and bony remodeling of the palmar process. This may also be observed on the 45° dorsoproximal/palmarodistal oblique, but is best interpreted in conjunction with the lateral radiographs.

As pedal osteitis is a symptom that appears to reflect either ongoing or past inflammation in the tissues adjacent to the distal phalanx, and is found in sound and lame horses, it is not always possible to determine the clinical significance of the findings. Therefore, it should be interpreted in the light of clinical findings and other

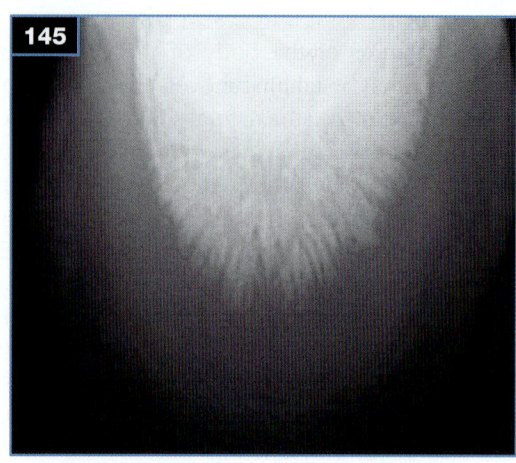

145 Pedal osteitis. Radiograph demonstrating demineralization and irregularity of the solar margin of the distal phalanx and widening of the vascular channels.

diagnostic tests. Particular emphasis should be placed on the thickness and degree of convexity of the sole, as well as the response to hoof tester application. The lameness in most horses in which pedal osteitis is significant will improve with palmar digital regional analgesia. Intra-articular analgesia of the distal interphalangeal joint and navicular bursa analgesia must be interpreted cautiously. If undertaken with appropriate volumes of local anesthetic and the response observed in 5–10 minutes, they are unlikely to improve the lameness, but if larger volumes are used or too long a time is allowed to lapse before the lameness is re-evaluated, a false-positive response is common. Scintigraphic examination may indicate increased radiopharmaceutical uptake in the solar margin area that corroborates the clinical and radiographic findings.

Management

If a primary condition can be identified, it should be treated as such. In those horses in which pedal osteitis is present, but no obvious primary disease can be identified, symptomatic therapy is warranted. Symptomatic therapy usually consists of pain control with nonsteroidal analgesics in conjunction with corrective trimming and shoeing with seated-out wide web shoes and/or pads to diminish concussion on the sole.

Prognosis

The prognosis is related to the primary condition. In horses in which the primary condition is not obvious, but the lameness is chronic and the conformation/balance is poor, the prognosis is guarded.

Septic osteitis of the distal phalanx
Definition/overview
Infection of the distal phalanx.

Etiology/pathophysiology
Septic osteitis of the distal phalynx is usually caused by a puncture wound to the sole or an extension of an abscess. Sequestra of the distal phalanx may develop either as a consequence of a fracture occurring at the same time as the original trauma or secondary to death of the surface of the bone following loss of blood supply. In horses with laminitis, septic osteitis may also occur as a sequela to infection of the lamellae and sole. If a large portion of the distal phalanx is affected, pathologic fractures may occur. Rarely, depending on the location of the infected bone, the infection can spread to adjacent structures.

146, 147 Septic pedal osteitis.
Dorsoproximal/palmarodistal oblique (146) and dorsopalmar (147) radiographs indicating the presence of pedal osteitis (arrow) and a sequestrum (arrow) at the dorsal solar margin of the distal phalanx.

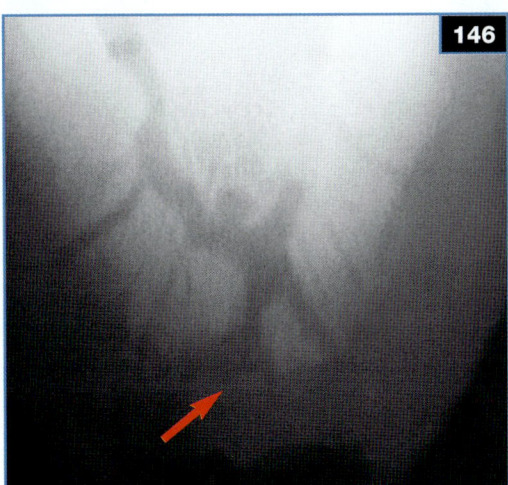

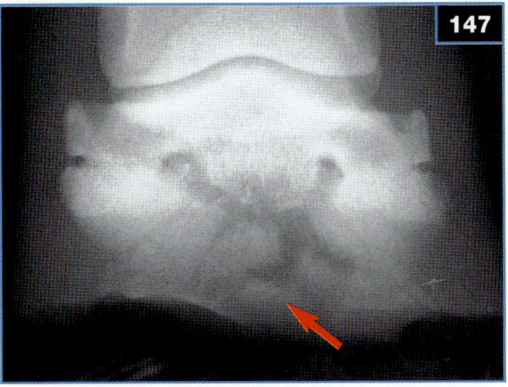

Clinical presentation
Horses with septic osteitis of the distal phalanx usually present with lameness that varies in severity depending on how well the exudate from the affected tissues can drain; severe if drainage is poor and moderate to mild if the drainage is good. A draining wound may be the primary presenting symptom. A history of trauma to the foot or other foot lameness (e.g. abscess) is common.

Differential diagnosis
Severe lameness: abscess; fractured distal phalanx or navicular bone; other deep digital flexor tendon sepsis. Drainage: abscess; other deep digital sepsis.

Diagnosis
The cause of the lameness is usually readily isolated to the foot, either because of the presence of a wound and/or drainage or because of a marked withdrawal response to hoof testers. Standard lateral, dorsopalmar, and dorsoproximal/palmarodistal oblique radiographic projections may need to be supplemented with additional obliques taken at various angles to the median plane to identify septic osteitis of the distal phalanx (146, 147). Usually the radiological symptoms of septic osteitis of the distal phalanx are irregularly marginated areas of lysis around the solar margin of the distal phalanx, although occasionally, radiolucent cavities can present within the substance of the bone. Sequestra are identified as osseous radiodensities surrounded by an area of lysis. Osteitis and sequestra of the planum cutaneum of the distal phalanx may be difficult to detect radiographically because of its concavity. If there is persistent drainage from a wound on the solar surface of the foot, but there is no radiographic evidence of osteitis or sequestration, then surgical exploration of the wound is appropriate.

Management
The treatment of septic osteitis of the distal phalanx with or without sequestration is open surgical drainage and debridement under local or general anesthesia. The wound is bandaged with a topical antimicrobial dressing, and the horse treated with broad-spectrum antibiotics until all exposed surfaces are covered with granulation tissue. NSAIDs are administered as needed and tetanus prophylaxis provided. The wound heals by secondary intention.

Prognosis
The prognosis for returning to work in most cases is good. However, extension of the infection to an adjacent structure, such as the navicular bursa, or pathologic fracture of the bone worsens the prognosis.

Sidebone

Definition/overview
Ossification of the ungual (collateral) cartilages.

Etiology/pathophysiology
The precise etiology of sidebone is unknown, but it is associated with concussion in heavy horses and is more common in older horses. The progressive ossification of the ungual cartilages usually occurs in a distal to proximal direction, although ossification may occur concurrently from a separate proximal center.

Clinical presentation
Sidebone is usually an incidental finding on physical examination or radiography of the foot. Rarely, horses with sidebone present with lameness.

Differential diagnosis
None.

Diagnosis
The ungual cartilages are readily palpated immediately proximal to the coronet in the palmar half of the foot. With marked ossification, the cartilages are not as flexible as normal, although palpation is unreliable at confirming sidebones. Under rare circumstances in which the ossified ungual cartilage is fractured, local heat, swelling, and pain on palpation can be expected. Ossification of the ungual cartilages is readily identified on dorsopalmar and lateral radiographs (148, 149). Separate centers of ossification must be distinguished from fractures. If an ungual cartilage is considered to be the source of the pain causing lameness, the unilateral nature of the pain can be confirmed with a unilateral palmar digital nerve block. Scintigraphy may confirm the identification of ungual cartilages that are causing lameness.

Management
Since most ossified ungual cartilages are asymptomatic, no treatment is required. In horses in which an ungual cartilage can be definitively identified as the cause of acute lameness, NSAIDs and rest are indicated. When the lameness is chronic the horse may be worked with judicious use of NSAIDs. Evaluation of the balance of the horse's feet may indicate that corrective trimming is required for horses with acute or chronic lameness. Lastly, a unilateral neurectomy or surgical excision of the cartilage may be performed in horses with persistent lameness.

Prognosis
The prognosis is good except in the rare circumstances where the lameness is sufficient for the horse to require surgery, in which case it is guarded.

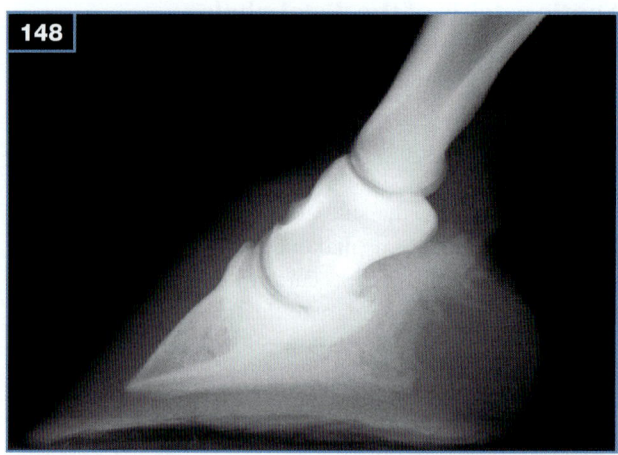
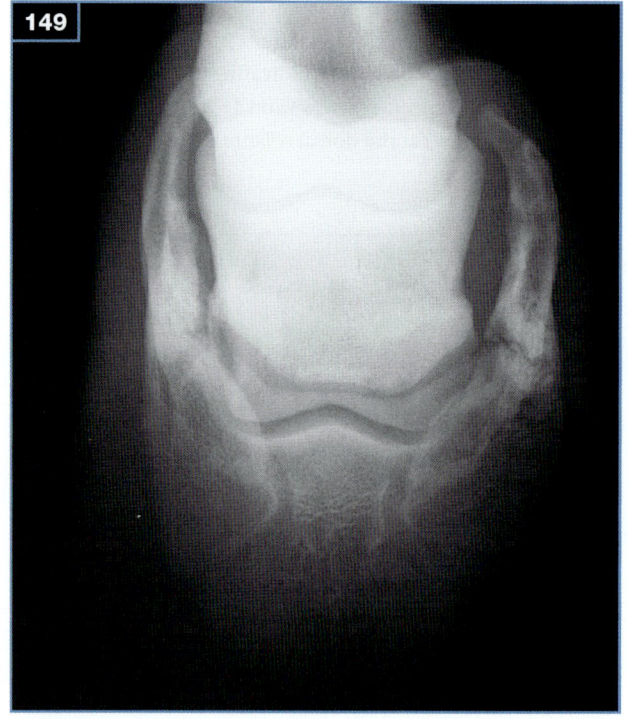

148, 149 Sidebone. Lateral (148) and dorsoproximal/palmarodistal oblique (149) radiographs of bilateral calcification.

Musculoskeletal system

Quittor

Definition/overview
Quittor is defined as septic necrosis of the ungual cartilage.

Etiology/pathophysiology
Quittor usually occurs following direct trauma to the ungual cartilage or from ascending infection from within the foot. The infection is particularly persistent because the ungual cartilage has a poor blood supply. The infection causes a marked unilateral inflammatory response, with swelling and draining sinuses.

Clinical presentation
Quittor is a chronic condition that presents with a unilateral swelling proximal to the coronary band, one or more discharging sinuses, and a varying degree of lameness.

Differential diagnosis
Abscesses that drain at the coronary band (gravel); subcutaneous abscess; puncture wound.

Diagnosis
Diagnosis is based on a history of trauma proximal to the coronary band, lameness, the unilateral location of a swelling, heat and pain on palpation, and one or more draining fistulas (150). If necessary, inserting a probe into a sinus that reaches the ungual cartilage should differentiate quittor from a gravel or subcutaneous abscess. A dorsal palmar and a lateral radiograph with a probe *in situ* will confirm the origin of the sinus in the collateral cartilage or to the palmar process of the distal phalanx.

Management
Necrosis of the ungual cartilage has been treated either conservatively with long-term antibiotics or surgically by excision of the infected tissue. Although treatment with broad-spectrum antibiotics for several weeks may effect a cure, recurrence of the drainage is common. For this reason, in most horses the necrotic cartilage is resected. The surgery is complicated because the ungual cartilage is approximately half inside the hoof capsule and half proximal to the coronary band. Although an elliptical incision over the proximal margin of the ungual cartilage provides access to the necrotic tissue, there is no ventral drainage and treatment through this proximal approach alone is likely to result in recurrence. Consequently, combining the proximal approach with a distal approach 1–2 cm distal to the coronary band by trephination through the hoof capsule provides ventral drainage (151). The proximal incision may be closed by primary intention, while the hoof-wall defect heals by secondary intention (152, 153). Care must be taken to avoid damaging the palmar

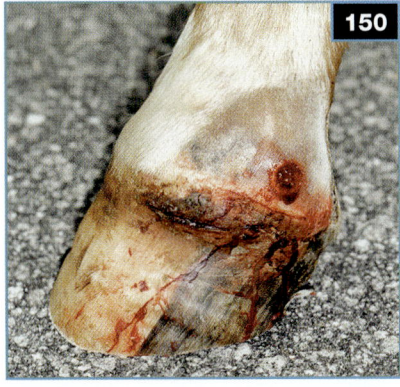
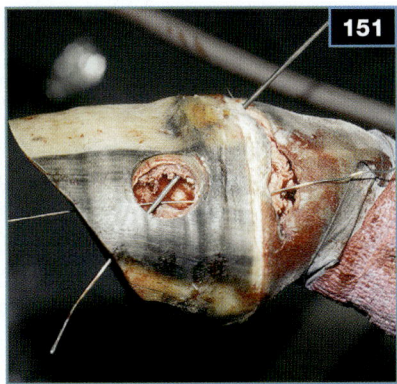
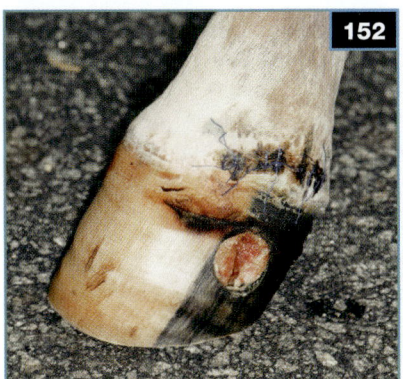
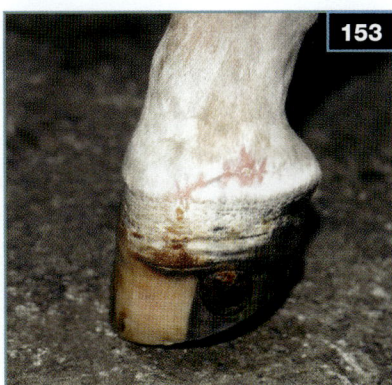

150–153 Quittor.
(150) Lateral swelling and a draining sinus immediately proximal to the coronet, indicative of quittor.
(151) Lateral view of an elliptical incision proximal to the coronet and a trephine hole in the lateral hoof wall to provide drainage; the position of the probe confirms communication between the proximal wound and the white line at the distal aspect of the wall.
(152) The proximal incision has been sutured, but the wound created by the trephine must heal by secondary intention.
(153) Several weeks after the surgery both wounds are completely epithelialized, but the defect in the stratum medium created by the trephine will not be replaced until it grows out past the distal surface of the wall.

reflection of the joint capsule, which lies immediately medial to the ungual cartilage. Postoperatively, the distal limb is bandaged, systemic antibiotics are continued until all surfaces are granulating, analgesia is provided as needed, and tetanus prophylaxis administered.

Prognosis

The prognosis for elimination of the infection is guarded to fair because recurrence is possible regardless of the surgical technique, but if successful, return to normal athletic activity can be expected.

Navicular syndrome

Definition/overview

Navicular syndrome defies a precise definition, but it has been classified as a degenerative disorder of the distal half of the flexor surface of the distal sesamoid or, broadly, as disease affecting the distal sesamoid and all the adjacent structures. Based on the changes observed by diagnostic imaging or pathology, it is best considered a syndrome affecting the distal sesamoid bone, navicular bursa, and the associated insertions of the collateral sesamoidean ligaments of the distal sesamoid bone and origin of the distal sesamoidean impar ligament.

Etiology/pathophysiology

The etiology of navicular syndrome is unknown, but the disease has been correlated with aspects of conformation. It is common in American Quarter horses with small upright feet and in Thoroughbreds with flat soles, under-run heels, and broken back foot–pastern axes. The shape of the distal sesamoid bone itself has been implicated as a risk factor because horses in which the proximal border of the distal sesamoid bone is convex are more likely to have the disease. It has been suggested that the shape of the distal sesamoid bone is inheritable; however, the biomechanical consequences of the shape of the bone are undetermined. Similarly, horses in which the solar margin of the distal phalanx is more acutely angled towards the ground are more likely to have navicular syndrome than those in which the angle is less acute. Biomechanically, it has been demonstrated that pressure on the distal sesamoid bone is negatively associated with the angle the dorsal parietal surface of the distal phalanx makes with the ground (and hence the angle made by the solar margin of the hoof). It also appears that horses with heel pain increase the tension in the deep digital flexor tendon by active muscular contraction, thus prompting the development and/or progression of navicular syndrome. Lastly, the clinical observation that navicular syndrome progresses more rapidly in horses undergoing more strenuous exercise suggests that the effect of conformation is compounded by trauma.

The distal sesamoid bone undergoes natural aging changes in sound horses, including decreased cortical and trabecular bone volume, and degenerative changes in the flexor surface fibrocartilage and opposing deep digital flexor tendon. Exercise increases the thickness of the palmar cortex of the distal sesamoid bone and inhibits the effect of aging on cortical and trabecular bone volume. The pathology of the distal sesamoid bone in navicular syndrome has been studied extensively. The changes reported include defects in the palmar cortex, disruption of the medullary trabeculae, medullary fibrosis, medullary sclerosis, loss of glycosaminoglycans in the fibrocartilage of the flexor surface, and dilation of the vasculature under the flexor surface of the bone (154, 155). Oxytetracycline labeling indicates that the distal sesamoid bone is actively remodeling in horses with navicular syndrome. Additionally in such animals, the subchondral pressure within the distal sesamoid bone is increased. Histologic and molecular studies both suggest that inflammation of the navicular bursa is a feature of horses with navicular syndrome, but its role in the pathogenesis as a primary or secondary event to changes in the distal sesamoid bone and deep digital flexor tendon is unknown. These observations support the hypothesis that navicular syndrome is a degenerative arthrosis-like disease.

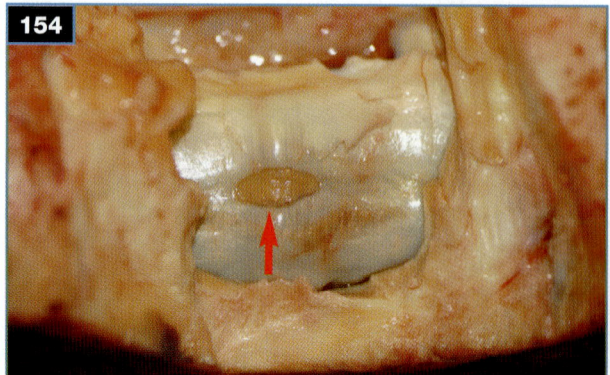

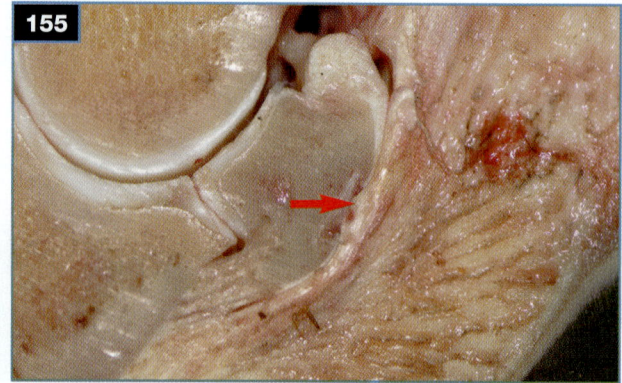

Musculoskeletal system

Clinical presentation

Navicular syndrome is typically a chronic, insidious, bilateral forelimb lameness, although it may occasionally be acute in onset and may only involve one foot. The feet often appear mismatched, one with a lower dorsal hoof-wall angle, the other with higher heels. The disease is frequently associated with broken back foot–pastern axes and underrun heels in Thoroughbred-like horses and upright feet in Quarter horse-like horses. The lameness is characterized by a short-strided gait that is more severe on a hard surface compared with a soft surface, and is exacerbated when the horse is circled towards the side of the more severely affected limb. Flexion of the distal limb joints may exacerbate the lameness. There is a variable response to hoof testers.

Differential diagnosis

Any chronic bilateral forelimb lameness including bruising, pedal osteitis, chronic laminitis, and DJD. Any source of chronic pain originating from the heels including sprain of the distal sesamoidean impar ligament, strain of the deep digital flexor tendon, and sheared heels.

Diagnosis

Diagnosis is based on demonstration of pain originating from the area of the distal sesamoid bone and demonstration of morphologic changes or remodeling within the distal sesamoid bone. Physical examination findings, including conformation, characteristics of the lameness, response to hoof testers and flexion tests, may suggest that a horse has navicular syndrome. Diagnostic analgesia, although readily able to localize pain to the distal limb, may be difficult to interpret in relation to a specific structure or group of structures in the distal limb and must be interpreted carefully in the light of other diagnostic findings. Radiographs are required to demonstrate morphologic changes in the distal sesamoid bone and adjacent structures (**156–159**). Three radiographic projections are

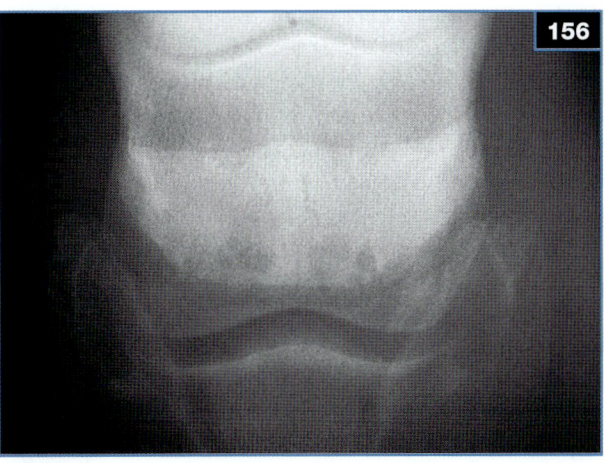

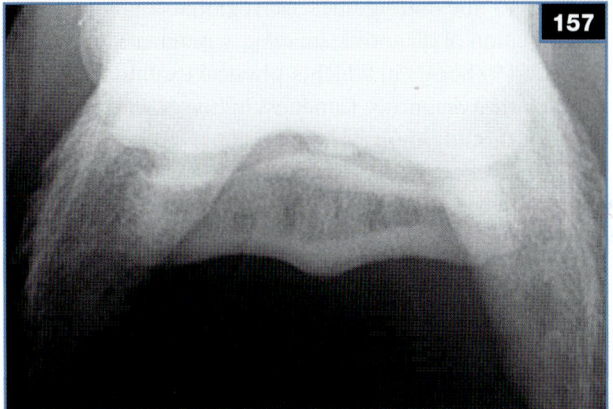

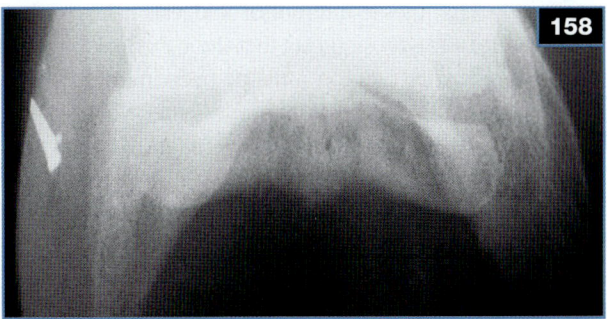

154–159 Navicular syndrome. Erosion on the flexor cortex of the distal sesamoid (arrow) (154). Adhesion between the flexor surface of the distal sesamoid and the deep digital flexor tendon (arrow) (155). Dorsoproximal/palmarodistal (156) and palmaroproximal/palmarodistal oblique radiographs (157) demonstrating an increase in number and size of the distal nutrient foramina/synovial invaginations. Palmaroproximal/palmarodistal oblique radiograph (158) showing loss of the corticomedullary junction, increased radiodensity of the medullary cavity, and erosion of the palmar cortex of the distal sesamoid. Close-up lateral radiograph (159) demonstrating a large enthesiophyte in the collateral sesamoidean ligament of the distal sesamoid (arrow).

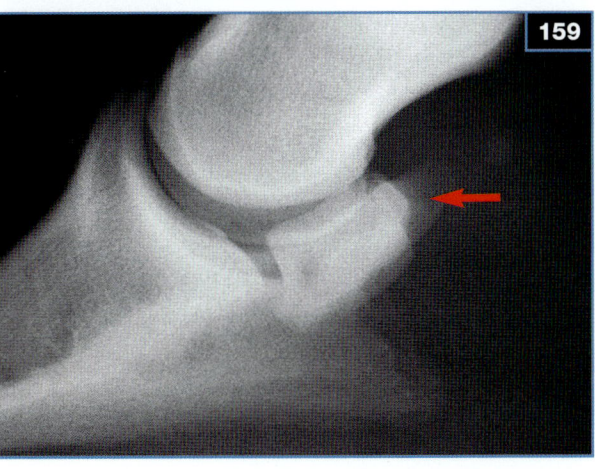

used: a 60° dorsoproximal/palmarodistal oblique, a lateral, and a proximopalmar/distopalmar oblique. The most reliable findings for diagnosing navicular syndrome are defects in the flexor cortex, medullary trabecular disruption (including pseudocyst formation), medullary sclerosis, poor flexor corticomedullary demarcation, and remodeling of the proximal border, including enthesiophyte formation. Synovial invaginations and flattening or thinning of the flexor cortex are more ambiguous. Nuclear scintigraphy is more sensitive than radiography for diagnosing abnormalities within the navicular bone. MRI can detect distension of the navicular bursa and abnormal signals within the bone, as well as differentiate abnormalities of the adjacent deep digital flexor tendon, collateral sesamoidean impar ligaments, distal interphalangeal joint, and phalanges.

Due to the ambiguities of regional analgesia and interpretation of diagnostic imaging, a pragmatic approach is needed in horses in which a physical examination does not provide a diagnosis. Lameness in horses with navicular disease should improve with palmar digital regional analgesia. Assuming the lameness improves, radiography of the foot is indicated. If the radiographs show marked evidence of navicular syndrome, the examination is complete. If the radiographs are ambiguous or do not show evidence of navicular syndrome, either additional diagnostic analgesia or scintigraphy should be performed. A response to distal interphalangeal joint analgesia using 3–5 ml of mepivicaine within 5 minutes strongly suggests that the distal interphalangeal joint is the source of pain. A response in 5 minutes to intrabursal analgesia using 3 ml of mepivicaine strongly suggests that the navicular bursa is the source of pain. Caution must be used in interpreting both of these blocks, because if either too much local anesthetic is used or too much time is allowed to pass before the lameness is re-evaluated, the local anesthetic will diffuse from one synovial structure to the other and around the terminal palmar digital nerve. If these two blocks fail to differentiate between distal interphalangeal joint and navicular bursal pain, then scintigraphy is indicated. Finally, if neither regional analgesia nor scintigraphy can definitively determine the pain in the foot, MRI is indicated. (Note: MRI may supplant scintigraphy in the diagnostic order of events in some practices.)

Management

The treatment of navicular syndrome is more about managing a case rather than curing it and includes therapeutic trimming and shoeing, medical management, and surgery. Trimming is directed at improving dorsopalmar and mediolateral hoof balance. Shoeing modifications include moving back and easing the point of breakover by moving the shoe in a palmar direction; squaring, rolling, or rockering the toe; and elevating the heels. Additionally, egg-bar shoes are frequently effective, probably because they encourage forward rotation of the foot on soft surfaces, which decreases the tension in the deep digital flexor tendon.

Medication with oral phenylbutazone or other NSAIDs on an as-needed basis is standard, although their use in performance horses is highly restricted by competition regulations. The use of isoxsuprine (a vasodilator) may be effective in milder cases. Its use is controversial, because although controlled studies and anecdotal evidence suggest it improves the lameness in some horses, other evidence suggests it is not absorbed and does not improve blood flow to the foot. Injection of corticosteroids and/or sodium hyaluronate into the distal interphalangeal joint or navicular bursa may improve the lameness in mildly to moderately affected horses for 2–4 months.

Prognosis

If therapeutic shoeing and medical management are insufficient to return a horse to its prior performance, the horse may be returned to a lower level of exercise or competition. Alternatively, a palmar digital neurectomy may be performed in horses in which the intractable pain is not associated with pathology that might cause the deep digital flexor tendon to rupture, and the rider is not inexperienced. Palmar digital neurectomies are usually effective for 1–4 years, although the development of neuromas impairs performance in up to 10% of horses. Other surgical techniques such as desmotomy of the collateral ligaments of the distal sesamoid bone and accessory ligament of the DDFT appear to have fallen out of favor.

Musculoskeletal system

Fracture of the distal sesamoid or navicular bone

Definition/overview

The distal sesamoid usually fractures parasagittally, approximately 1–2 cm medial or lateral to the sagittal ridge.

Etiology/pathophysiology

The fracture is caused by trauma such as kicking at a wall or landing hard on an uneven surface. The fractures are slow to heal and usually heal with a fibrous union if untreated. DJD of the distal interphalangeal joint occurs as a sequela.

Clinical presentation

Horses with an acute distal sesamoid bone fracture present with a moderate to severe lameness. Horses with a chronic fracture of the distal sesamoid present with a mild to moderate lameness.

Differential diagnosis

Any disease of the palmar aspect of the foot that causes acute severe lameness or chronic moderate lameness: navicular disease; sheared heels; bruising; puncture wound; abscess; soft-tissue injuries of the foot. The radiographic appearance must be differentiated from a bipartite distal sesamoid bone.

Diagnosis

The history of an acute-onset, moderate to severe lameness, withdrawal response to hoof testers placed across the heels or on the frog, and an absence of swelling or other physical findings is compatible with a distal sesamoid fracture; however, other more common problems are often considered initially. In horses with lameness associated with chronic fractures, regional analgesia, usually a palmar digital nerve block, is needed to localize the pain. Radiography is essential to achieve a definitive diagnosis (160, 161). The most useful projections are 60° dorsoproximal/palmarodistal oblique and the palmaroproximal/palmarodistal oblique views. Superimposition of a paracuneal (collateral) sulcus on the navicular bone in the 60° dorsoproximal/palmarodistal oblique projection can mimic a fracture and must be carefully distinguished by examining the palmaroproximal/palmarodistal oblique projection or by packing the sulcus and repeating the radiograph.

Management

Rest and immobilizing the hoof in a manner similar to that used for distal phalangeal fractures have been used, but fibrous unions and subsequent DJD are common. Internal lag screw fixation of acute distal sesamoid bone fractures has been reported in two uncontrolled studies, with seemingly better results. The technique requires special

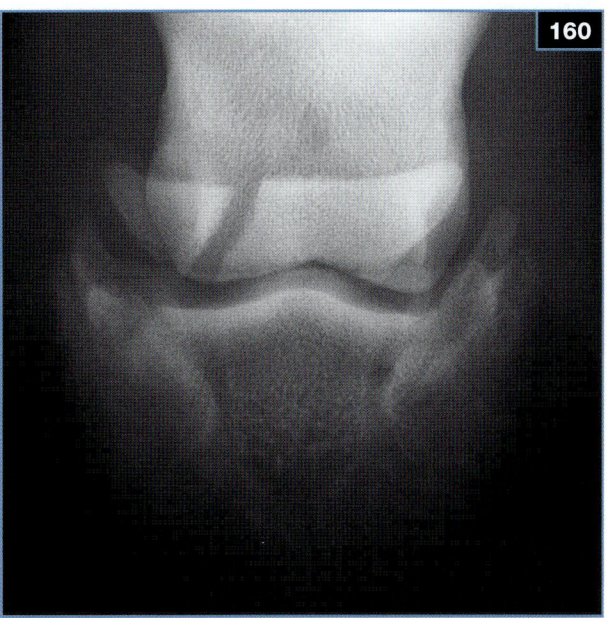

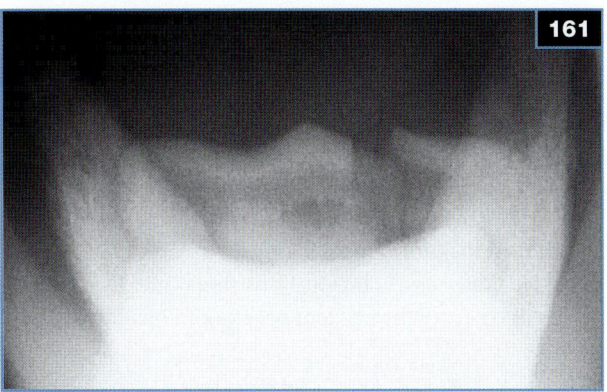

160, 161 Navicular bone fracture. Dorsoproximal/palmarodistal (160) and palmaroproximal/palmarodistal oblique (161) radiographs showing a fracture through the body of the navicular bone.

equipment and expertise. However, this surgery is seldom performed because of the technical challenges and the lack of controlled data supporting superior results. Better results have also been reported following elevation of the heels by 12 degrees for 2 months, which is then gradually reduced three degrees at a time over 4 months. Palmar digital neurectomy is recommended for horses with persistent lameness associated with a fibrous union of the fracture.

Prognosis

Overall, the prognosis for soundness is poor, although the reports of internal fixation or extreme heel elevation offer some hope for successful return to work.

Osteoarthritis

Definition/overview

OA, also referred to as DJD, occurs in both the PIP joint and the DIP joint, and there are similarities between the two.

Etiology/pathophysiology

OA of the interphalangeal joints is usually a sequela to trauma, infection, or, occasionally, subsequent to OCD/subchondral bone cysts. Trauma may be repetitive and low grade associated with constant high athletic performance, which may be exacerbated by poor conformation or foot balance. Alternatively, trauma may result in more acute injuries such as intra-articular fractures, desmitis of collateral ligaments, and direct damage to the articular cartilage. By definition OA is progressive; however, not all arthritis is degenerative, and transient synovitis is not uncommon following either a single episode of trauma or repetitive trauma of short duration.

Clinical presentation

Horses with DJD of the interphalangeal joints often present with a chronic but progressive lameness that is frequently bilateral. The forelimbs are more commonly affected than the hindlimbs. Alternatively, horses with DJD may present acutely as a recognized sequela to known trauma.

Differential diagnosis

Chronic lameness: chronic bruising (pedal osteitis); navicular disease; chronic laminitis; hoof imbalance.

Diagnosis

Physical examination findings, except for the presence of lameness, are usually unremarkable, although in acute and chronic cases involving the DIP joint distension of the dorsal pouch of the joint process can be palpated on the dorsodistal aspect of the pastern immediately above the coronary band (162). Later on in the disease there may be firm swelling abaxially and dorsally associated with OA of the PIP joint and dorsally with OA of the DIP joint following fracture of the extensor process. Regional analgesia is required to localize the disease. Low palmar digital regional analgesia immediately proximal to the ungual cartilages and with low volumes of local anesthetic will result in improvement in the majority of lameness caused by OA of the DIP joint without affecting the PIP joint, while more proximal palmar digital regional analgesia will also improve lameness caused by OA of the PIP joint. Intra-articular analgesia is more specific, although caution must be used in interpreting intra-articular analgesia of the DIP joint because it has been shown to affect branches of the palmar digital nerve to the heels and sole if large volumes of anesthetic are used. Horses with OA of these joints may or may not have radiographic changes. In horses with radiographic changes, the abnormalities include periarticular osteophytes, joint capsule exostoses, loss of joint space, and subchondral bone lysis (163–167). In horses without radiographic evidence of disease, increased radiopharmaceutical uptake during scintigraphy is strongly suggestive, and MRI may identify cartilage loss, small subchondral bone defects, and altered signals in the subchondral bone that are not visible radiographically.

162 This horse has a distended coffin joint (DIP joint) visible as a swelling just above the dorsal coronary band. (Photo courtesy GA Munroe)

163 Dorsopalmar radiograph showing loss of joint space and subsequent collateromotion (rotation in the frontal/dorsal plane) of the distal phalanx in relation to the middle phalanx.

164 Lateral radiograph demonstrating decreased width of the DIP joint and exostoses on the dorsal surface of the middle phalanx.

165–167 Degenerative joint disease of the proximal interphalangeal joint. (165) Lateral radiograph showing mild DJD of the PIP joint, with an osteophyte on the dorso-proximal border of the middle phalanx. Lateral (166) and dorsopalmar (167) radiographs of severe DJD of the PIP joint that demonstrate loss of joint space, severe osteophytes, and exostoses both dorsally and to a lesser extent palmarly and abaxially.

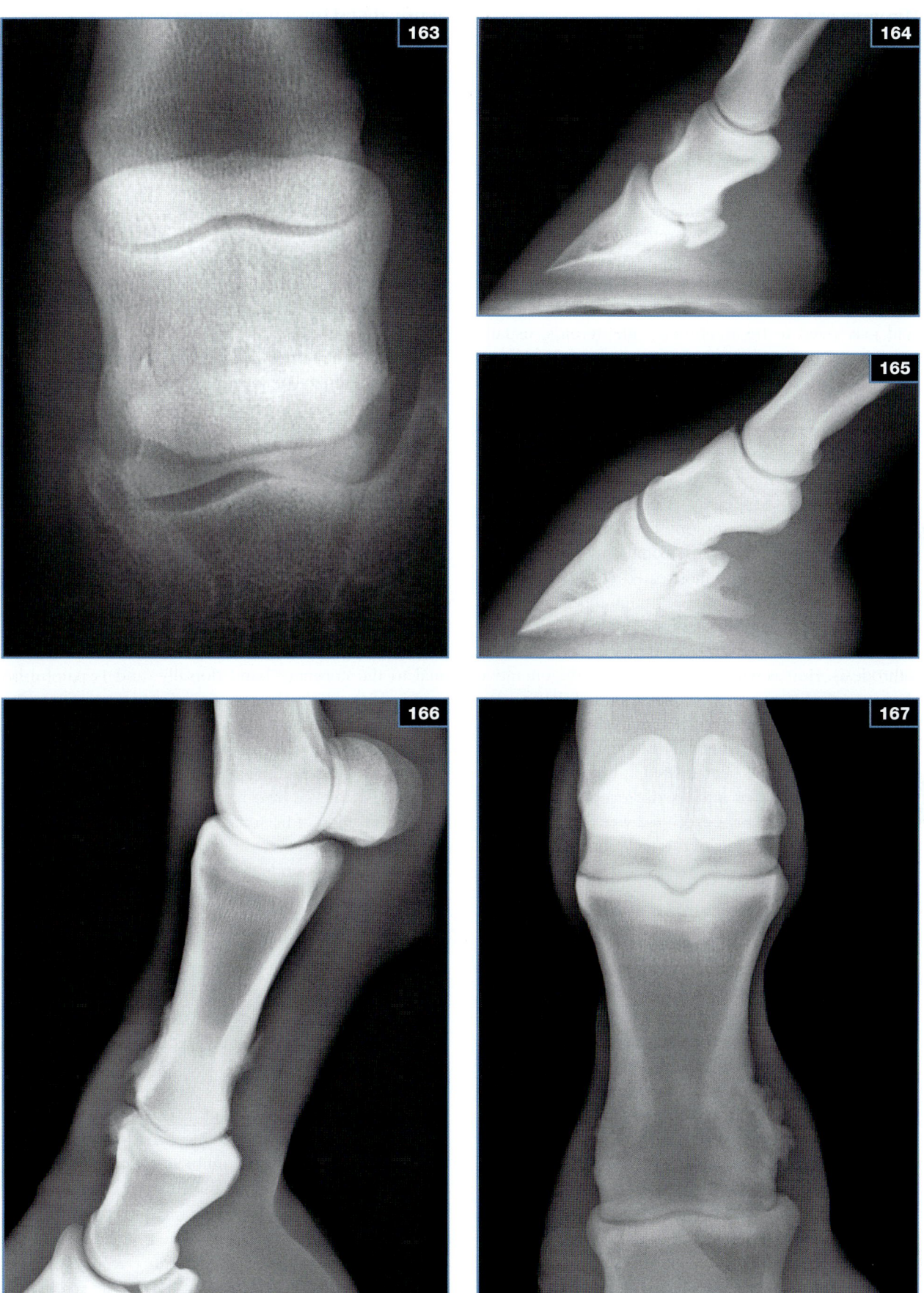

Management

The first line of therapy should be to correct any imbalance that is present. Additionally, shoes that ease breakover and pads that diminish the concussion associated with weight bearing should be used. Medication for OA of the PIP joint and DIP joint depends on the severity of the disease and the type of work expected of the horse. The simplest treatment is to use oral NSAIDs as needed and/or intramuscular polysulfated glycosaminoglycans where competition rules permit and the lameness is mild. Alternatively, injection of the joint with hyaluronic acid may be effective in mildly affected joints. For more advanced disease, intra-articular injections of hyaluronic acid may need to be combined with steroids, usually triamcinolone. The use of intra-articular triamcinolone is not without controversy. In relatively short-term studies it has been demonstrated to be chondroprotective, but clinical experience suggests that repeated injection in the face of continued exercise leads to cartilage destruction. Most clinicians use 6–12 mg, but it is advisable to use the lowest effective dose. Additionally, since the intra-articular administration of triamcinolone has been linked to the development of laminitis, it is commonly held that the combined dose for all joints treated at the same time should be not exceed 18 mg, although this threshold is anecdotal. Advanced disease of the PIP joint that fails to respond to medical therapy should be treated by surgical arthrodesis. Horses with synovitis without degenerative changes of the cartilage or subchondral bone may respond to intra-articular injection of hyaluronic acid and rest, without need for additional treatment. More recently, OA of the DIP joint has been treated by autologous conditioned serum (ACS) or interleukin receptor antagonist protein (IRAP) in the joint every 1–2 weeks on 3–4 occasions. However the results of this technique have not yet been published.

Prognosis

The prognosis for true DJD is guarded. Many joints can be managed medically for months to years, but eventually performance will deteriorate to the point where a horse cannot perform its intended exercise. Successful arthrodesis of the proximal interphalangeal joint is well documented in both fore- and hindlimbs, and will return a horse to athletic performance. The success rate is higher in the hindlimb than in the forelimb.

Septic distal interphalangeal joint

Definition/overview

Infection of the DIP joint.

Etiology/pathophysiology

The DIP joint may become infected from traumatic injuries or joint injection; in foals septic arthritis of the DIP joint may be caused by hematogenous spread of infection. Injuries to the ground surface of the foot that penetrate the DIP joint are also likely to affect the navicular bursa. Joints that become infected following trauma to the coronary band and adjacent pastern may also infect the digital flexor tendon sheath and navicular bursa.

Clinical presentation

Horses with septic DIP joints are usually presented with a severe lameness. There may also be evidence of swelling proximal to the coronary band, particularly dorsally, or a wound.

Differential diagnosis

Abscess; fracture of the distal phalanx or navicular bone; severe strain or sprain; other deep digital sepsis.

Diagnosis

Sepsis should be strongly considered when a horse presents with a severe lameness and diffuse swelling proximal to the coronary band dorsally, and is painful on flexion of the digit. History of a recent injection into the joint, or the presence of a wound in the middle third of the frog or proximal to the coronary band adjacent to the joint capsule, should raise the index of suspicion. Confirmation of sepsis is achieved by centesis (elevated WBC count and the identification of bacteria) or by confirming communication of the joint cavity with an external wound. Exploration of wounds proximal to the coronary band, either digitally or with a sterile probe, may readily demonstrate joint involvement. Infusion of sterile saline into the joint and observing it exiting a wound confirms the communication definitively. Radiography is not usually helpful in the diagnosis of acute joint sepsis, but later on in the course of the disease loss of joint space, subchondral lysis, and periarticular new bone may be present (**168**).

Management

Treatment of a septic DIP joint involves aggressive joint lavage or arthroscopy, systemic broad-spectrum antibiotics, regional infusion of antibiotics, intrasynovial antibiotics, and NSAIDs. Drains can be placed in the DIP joint

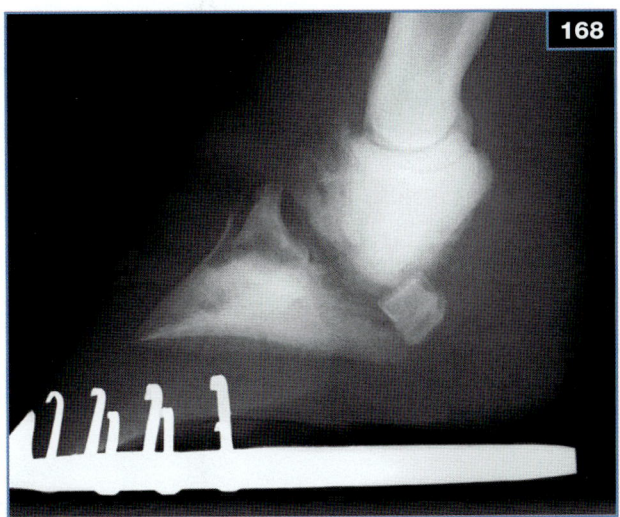

168 Septic distal interphalangeal joint. Lateral radiograph of the DIP joint demonstrating extensive loss of the articular surfaces, exostoses on the dorsal and palmar surfaces of the middle phalanx, a large sequestrum of the extensor process of the distal phalanx, and subluxation of the joint.

to remove harmful products associated with the bacteria and the inflammatory response. Antimicrobials should be continued for at least 2 weeks after closure of any wound communication with the joint and after the DIP joint synovial fluid analysis has returned to normal. In severe chronic cases the joint may be surgically curetted to promote ankylosis with or without cancellous bone grafting. A distal limb cast should be used if arthrodesis is to be encouraged both to stabilize the joint while it fuses and to provide pain relief through stabilization.

Prognosis
For horses in which the infection is controlled before significant degeneration of the articular surface occurs, the prognosis for return to work is fair. For those horses in which there is significant degeneration of the articular surface, the prognosis for survival is guarded and most horses that survive develop DIP joint ankylosis.

Septic navicular bursitis
Definition/overview
Septic synovitis of the navicular bursa.

Etiology/pathophysiology
The cause of a septic navicular bursa is almost invariably a puncture wound to the ground surface of the foot in an area centered on the middle third of the frog. Occasionally, hoof lacerations/avulsions may extend deep enough to involve the navicular bursa. The penetrating foreign body may also directly damage the bone and fibrocartilage of the flexor surface of the navicular bone. The elastic nature of the frog usually seals over any puncture wound and there is often no natural drainage from the wound. Build-up of pressure in the bursa between the deep digital flexor tendon and the navicular bone causes the animal to become severely lame. The close proximity of the DIP joint and digital flexor tendon sheath may lead to these structures becoming infected at the time of the initial injury or, more rarely, secondarily by spread of the infection.

Clinical presentation
The usual presenting symptom is severe lameness in which the horse will not put its heel down during the stride. Depending on the duration of the infection there may be swelling visible/palpable between the heel bulbs and ungual cartilages.

Differential diagnosis
Abscess; fracture of the distal phalanx or navicular bone; severe strain or sprain; other deep digital sepsis.

Diagnosis
A history and/or visible evidence of a puncture wound to the middle third of the frog or adjacent sulci in a severely lame horse that is not putting its heel to the ground is highly suggestive of septic navicular bursitis. Swelling between the heel bulbs and ungual cartilages, pain on flexion of the digit, and a marked withdrawal response following application of hoof testers over the frog add further to the index of suspicion. If a wound is not readily apparent, the foot should be thoroughly explored. Regional analgesia may localize the lameness and greatly facilitates exploration of the frog. Confirmation of bursal sepsis is achieved by centesis revealing an elevated WBC count and/or bacteria. Confirming communication of the bursal cavity with the external wound can be achieved by retrograde flushing (fluid exits from the wound) or radiographic contrast techniques.

97

The foot

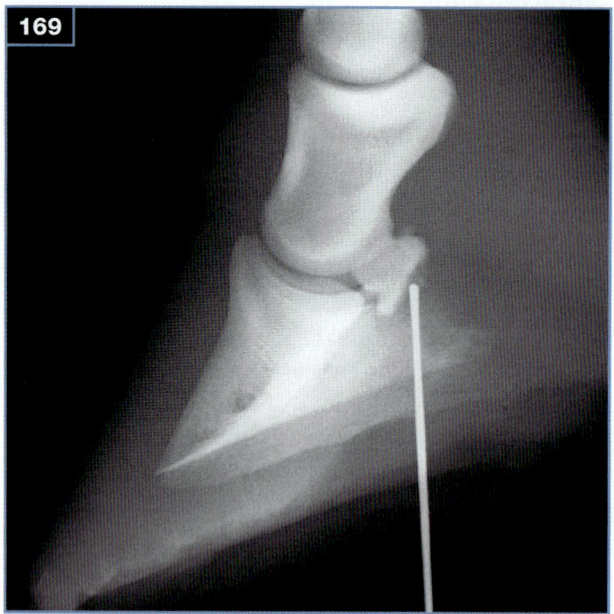

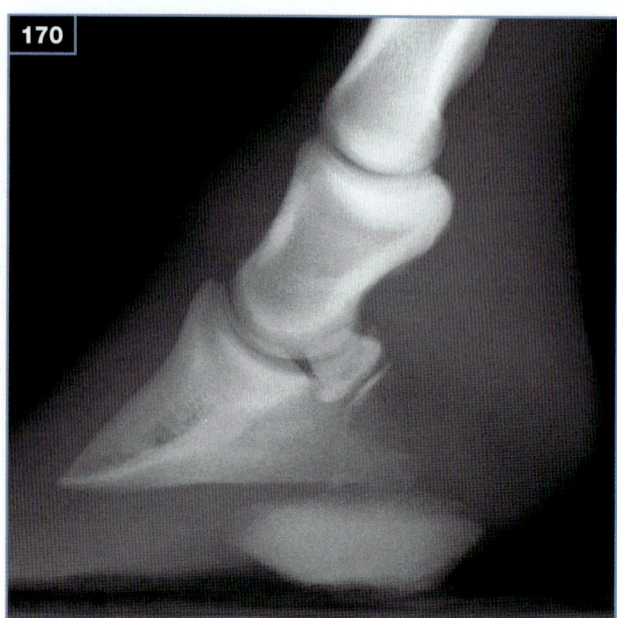

Radiography of the foot in two planes at 90 degrees to each other with either a solid probe (169) or radiographic contrast medium (170) inserted into the wound or bursa is very helpful in reaching a diagnosis. Ultrasound, either through the frog or between the ungual cartilages, can demonstrate increased fluid in the navicular bursa and discontinuities in the flexor surface of the navicular bone. Later in the disease there may be radiographic evidence of lysis of the flexor cortex of the navicular bone (171, 172).

Management

Treatment varies with the duration of infection, presence of damage to the navicular bone, and effect of prior treatment. The hoof capsule surrounding the entry wound on the ground surface of the foot should be removed, the horse placed on systemic antibiotics and NSAIDs, and tetanus prophylaxis provided. Additionally, intravenous or intraosseous regional perfusion of antibiotics, usually gentamicin or amikacin, is strongly recommended. Elevation of the heels by 6–12 degrees greatly decreases stress on the deep digital flexor tendon and increases the comfort of the horse. Horses with punctures to the navicular bursa of less than 2–3 days duration, without radiographic evidence of injury to the navicular bone and with minimal lameness, can be managed more conservatively than those with longer duration, evidence of osseous injury, and marked lameness. Specifically, in the former the overlying hoof capsule should be debrided down to the dermis and if visual evidence of contamination is present in the digital cushion, the debridement may be extended through the digital cushion to the surface of the deep digital flexor tendon. The bursa should be lavaged, with either needles or an arthroscope. The horse is then treated with systemic antibiotics and either intrabursal or intravenous regional perfusion with antibiotics, and carefully monitored. Horses that fail to respond to initial therapy, are more chronic in nature, or have evidence of navicular bone involvement warrant further surgical exploration. The traditional surgical approach, the 'streetnail' procedure, is to fenestrate the deep digital flexor tendon in addition to the hoof capsule and digital cushion in order to permit direct lavage and debridement and ventral drainage (173). Although effective in some horses, this procedure is not benign because adhesions may develop between the surgically created deep digital flexor tendon wound and the navicular bone, and the opportunity for ascending infection is increased. More recently, an endoscopic approach has been developed that offers improved visualization of the navicular

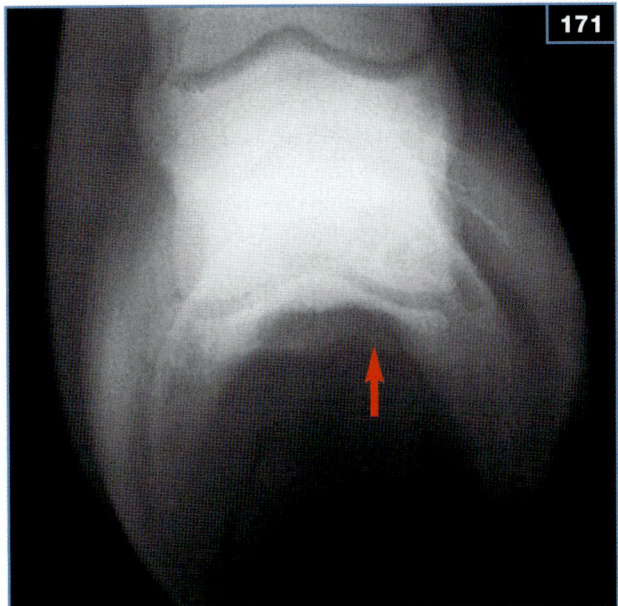

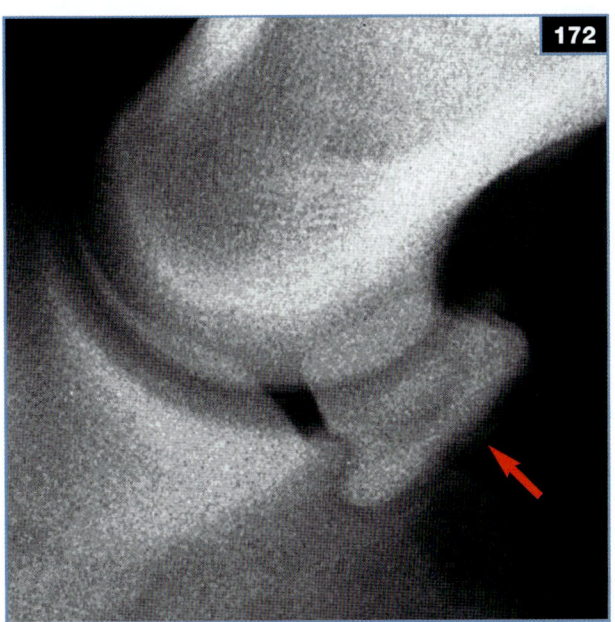

bursa and bone. The original penetrating wound is enlarged to permit introduction of instruments into the bursa to debride the wound and, as such, may offer the additional advantage over the traditional 'streetnail' procedure of a smaller distal wound.

Prognosis

The prognosis for survival and return to work is heavily influenced by the duration before effective treatment and whether there is sepsis of the flexor cortex of the navicular bone. Both have a negative impact, but overall the prognosis for survival is fair and return to performance guarded.

169–172 Septic navicular bursa. Radiographs showing the use of a solid probe (169) and liquid contrast medium (170) to confirm communication between a wound in the ground surface of the foot and the navicular bursa. Palmaroproximal/palmarodistal oblique (171) and close-up lateral (172) radiographs demonstrating erosion of the palmar cortex of the distal sesamoid bone (arrows).

173 Solar view of the foot a few days after a 'streetnail' procedure has been performed.

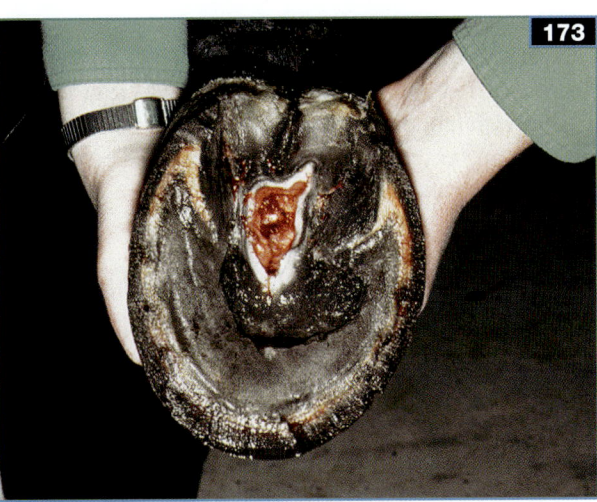

Strains and sprains

Definition/overview

There are numerous ligaments within the foot and two tendons extending into the foot that may sustain sprains or strains following trauma.

Etiology/pathophysiology

Tendons and ligaments sustain strains and sprains in response to abnormal stress. The stress may occur either as a single acute, severe episode or as recurrent trauma of lesser magnitude. The ligaments within the foot can be divided into three groups: the collateral ligaments of the distal interphalangeal joint; the three ligaments that support and maintain the position of the navicular bursa; and the ligaments associated with the attachment of the ungual cartilages to the surrounding structures. The two tendons that extend into the foot are the common digital extensor tendon and the deep digital flexor tendon. Of these structures, the collateral ligaments of the DIP joint, distal sesamoidean impar ligament, and the deep digital flexor tendon have received the most attention. The descriptions of injury to these structures are primarily derived from diagnostic imaging (MRI) because, due to the recent identification of these types of injuries, comparable gross and histopathologic studies are not available. Desmitis has been identified in the DIP joint collateral ligaments and desmitis and dystrophic mineralization in the distal sesamoidean impar ligament. Surface and core lesions have been documented in the distal deep digital flexor tendon, as well as tenopathy of the insertion of the deep digital flexor tendon (174). Involvement of more than one structure is common. For example, injuries of the distal deep digital flexor tendon are commonly associated with injuries of the navicular bone, and injuries of the collateral ligament of the DIP joint may occur in conjunction with injury to the navicular bone, the collateral ligaments of the navicular bone, the deep digital flexor tendon, or the distal sesamoidean impar ligament.

Clinical presentation

Horses with strains and sprains within the foot usually present with moderate acute or chronic lameness. Seldom are there any visible or palpable abnormalities proximal to the coronary band.

Differential diagnosis

Any cause of moderate lameness arising within the foot: navicular disease; bruising; DJD; pedal osteitis; sheared heels.

Diagnosis

As these injuries have only recently been identified on a reliable basis due to improvements in diagnostic imaging, the clinical pictures of the different strains and sprains that may occur are incomplete. There are some generalizations that can be made and some characteristics of individual injuries. Physical examination does not usually identify any visible or palpable abnormalities, although collateral ligament injury may be associated with subtle swelling immediately proximal to the coronary band. The lameness associated with injury to the collateral ligament of the DIP joint is exacerbated by lungeing in a circle. Palmar digital analgesia and intra-articular anesthesia of the DIP joint are likely to partially, but not completely, improve the lameness in most horses with injury of either the distal deep digital flexor tendon or the collateral ligament of the DIP joint.

Usually, primary injuries to the distal deep digital flexor tendon or the collateral ligament of the DIP joint cannot be demonstrated on radiographs except in chronic cases of the latter where well-defined lytic cyst-like lesions have been reported in P3 at the insertion point of the ligament. Nuclear scintigraphic examination may demonstrate increased radiopharmaceutical uptake within a tendon or ligament during the pool phase or at the attachments of ligament or tendon to bone during the bone phase. The definitive diagnosis is based on identifying the injury with either ultrasound or MRI (see 39, 40). Ultrasound is limited to structures that can be visualized either by placing the transducer proximal to the coronary band and directing it distally or by placing it on the frog. Desmitis of the collateral ligament of the DIP joint may be identified on ultrasound by using the proximal approach, although only the proximal third is visible and false-negative results are common. Similarly, ultrasonographic examination may identify lesions in the deep digital flexor tendon in the distal pastern region (175), but again, false-negative results are common. Ultrasound through the frog provides limited visualization of the deep digital flexor tendon and distal sesamoidean impar ligament near the median plane of the limb. Sprains and strains of the ligaments and tendons within the foot are identified using MRI by increased size, symmetry, or altered signal of the affected structure, and this is currently the most effective imaging modality for diagnosing these types of injury.

Management

The aim of treating strains and sprains is to reduce the stresses sustained by the tissues in order to prevent exacerbation of the injury and permit healing. After a period of stall rest, the horse is gradually reintroduced to increasing levels of exercise as the lameness improves. Depending on the severity of the initial injury, this process may last for a period from several weeks to up to a year. In addition to rest, any marked imbalance in the hoof should be addressed, particularly mediolateral imbalance in the case of collateral ligament injury and dorsopalmar imbalance in the case of distal sesamoidean impar ligament or deep digital flexor tendon injury. Recently, some clinicians have been treating some of these injuries by guided injections of stem cells or platelet-rich plasma solutions and/or shockwave therapy, but only anecdotal reports of these techniques and their results are available at present.

Prognosis

The prognosis for return to soundness in horses with primary injuries to the distal deep digital flexor tendon or the collateral ligament of the DIP joint is guarded to poor.

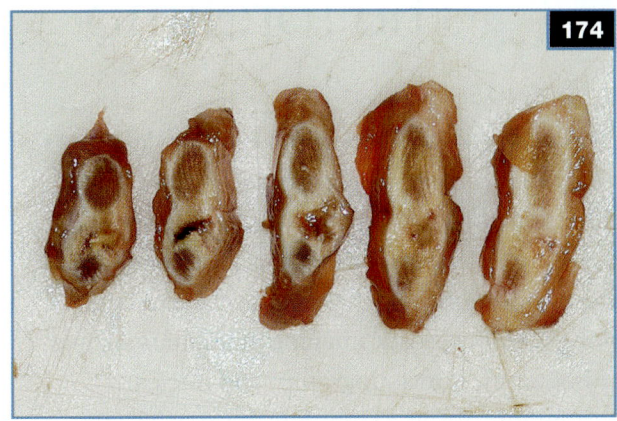

174 Serial sections of the deep digital flexor tendon from the distal pastern demonstrating the linear nature of the tear.

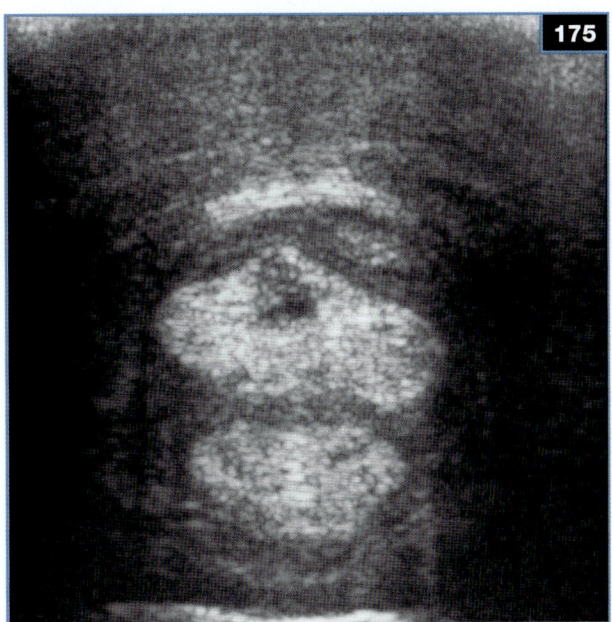

175 Ultrasound of the deep digital flexor tendon proximal to the foot showing a cross-section of a longitudinal tear in the deep digital flexor tendon.

Examination of the horse with forelimb lameness is a common undertaking in equine practice. A full clinical history and detailed examination of the horse are essential for diagnosis and treatment of these conditions. The use of diagnostic analgesia along with diagnostic imaging modalities such as radiography, ultrasonography, and nuclear scintigraphy forms a complete approach to the diagnosis of many conditions. Some conditions are particular to the type of horse encountered (e.g. young racehorses), but many forelimb conditions are seen in all types of horse.

Phalanges

Phalanx fractures

Definition/overview
Fractures of the first phalanx (P1) include incomplete short sagittal (see **52**), complete sagittal, dorsal frontal (incomplete or complete), comminuted, and, more rarely, complete transverse (**176**). Fractures of the second phalanx (P2) include comminuted (**177**), uniaxial and biaxial eminence fractures, avulsion fractures of the palmaroproximal border of P2, and, less commonly, oblique or transverse fractures (**178**).

Etiology/pathophysiology
Although these fractures can occur in all types of horse, fractures of P1 are commonly seen in racing breeds, while horses undergoing sudden turns and stops (e.g. Western riding, polo) can suffer P2 fractures. Injuries at speed and/or from hyperextension of the fetlock can result in P1 fractures. Bending and torsional forces from turning and stopping abruptly result in a 'screwdriver' effect on P1 and P2. Fragmentation of the palmaro/plantaro/proximal aspects of P2 can be due to avulsion secondary to hyperextension or may be an incidental finding.

Clinical presentation
Horses with phalangeal fractures are commonly presented to the clinician as an acute, non-weight-bearing lameness with soft-tissue swelling, although incomplete short sagittal fractures of P1 may be subtle, with pain palpable over the dorsal aspect of P1. Complete fractures of P1 usually exit the lateral cortex and present with a severe lameness, soft-tissue swelling, and crepitation. Dorsal frontal P1 fractures are often seen in the hindlimb. Fetlock effusions are usually present in P1 fractures due to hemorrhage into the joint. Comminuted fractures of P1 and P2 can be highly unstable, with severe lameness and swelling, and they require rapid recognition and external stabilization. Biaxial eminence fractures of P2 can lead to subluxation of the PIP joint and further soft-tissue damage, whereas uniaxial P2 fractures are painful on manipulation, but the PIP joint is stable.

Differential diagnosis
Subluxation/luxation of the fetlock or pastern joint; severe soft-tissue injury (e.g. tendon/sesamoidean ligament damage); synovial sepsis; cellulitis; subsolar abscessation.

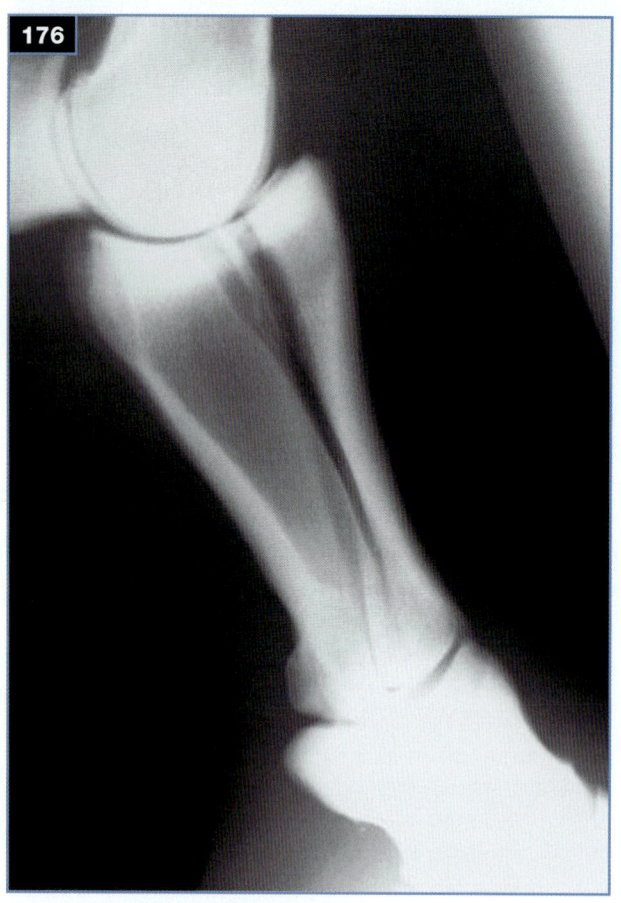

176

176 Preoperative radiograph of an unusual complete and displaced transverse fracture of P1. (Photo courtesy GA Munroe)

Musculoskeletal system

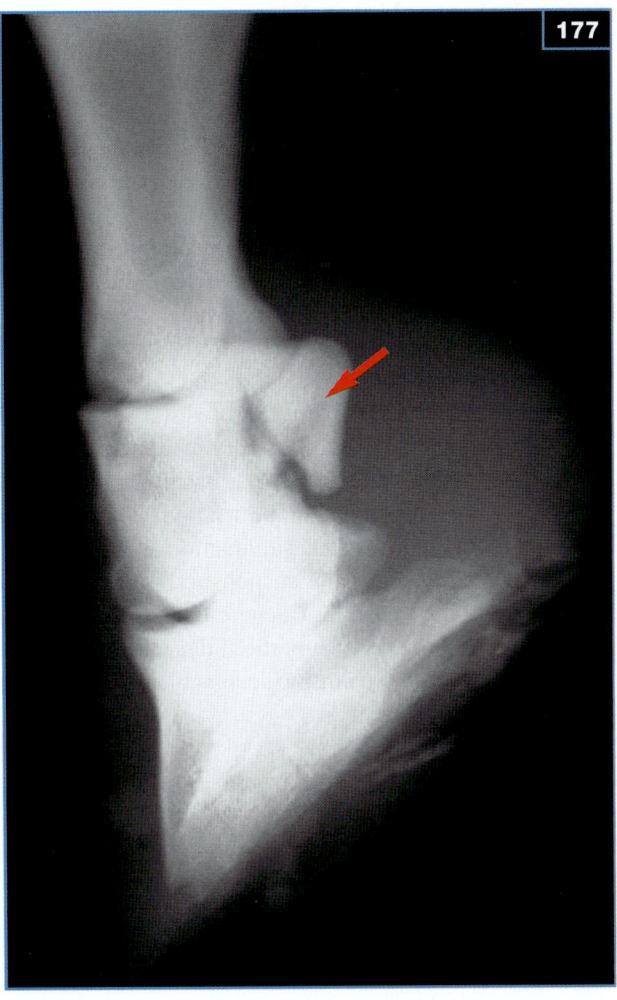

177 Dorsolateral/palmaromedial oblique radiograph of the right forelimb showing a P2 fracture involving the PIP joint. Note the separated palmarolateral eminence of P2 (arrow). (Photo courtesy GA Munroe)

178 Postmortem specimen of a polo pony that sustained a P2 fracture during competition. This view shows the articular surface of the proximal part of P2 and the oblique fracture running across the whole width of the bone. (Photo courtesy GA Munroe)

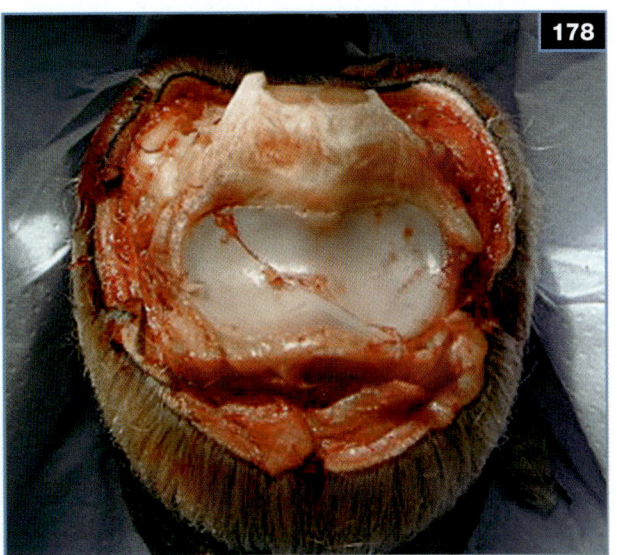

Diagnosis

Diagnosis is suspected from clinical findings, although incomplete fractures may not show obvious clinical signs. Radiography is the imaging modality of choice and it is important to include multiple views for the identification of fracture planes and the number of joints involved. The 125° dorsopalmar/plantar (DP) view is useful for identifying incomplete, short sagittal P1 fractures. Nuclear scintigraphy may be required for the diagnosis of incomplete, nondisplaced fractures.

Management

Phalangeal fractures are treated as an emergency and need to be stabilized externally to prevent further damage to surrounding soft tissues and prevent displacement of nondisplaced fractures. External coaptation to align the dorsal cortices is required. Incomplete, short sagittal P1 fractures may respond favorably to 3 months' box rest or internal fixation. Internal fixation has the advantage of reducing the risk of recurrence and should be employed with fracture lines extending for more than 15 mm from the articular surface (see **53**). Complete fractures of P1 require accurate anatomic reconstruction to reduce the risk of secondary joint disease. Dorsal frontal P1 fractures may respond to rest if they are nondisplaced or undergo internal fixation. Larger fragments require internal fixation. Horses with comminuted P1 fractures are often euthanized. If surgery is attempted, this is as a salvage procedure only. The outcome depends on the presence of an intact strut of bone onto which the fragments can be reconstructed and the degree of concurrent soft-tissue damage. Without an intact strut, a transfixation cast or external skeletal fixation device can be employed.

Comminuted and biaxial eminence fractures of P2 can be repaired by involving arthrodesis of the PIP joint (179). Uniaxial eminence fractures of P2 may be repaired by internal fixation or treated conservatively. Removal of palmar osteochondral fragments of P2 may be required if significant.

Prognosis

The prognosis is good for incomplete short, sagittal fractures of P1 and nondisplaced frontal fractures of P1 managed correctly. The prognosis for complete sagittal P1 fractures is fair for accurate reconstruction, but is reduced if the PIP joint is involved. The prognosis following treatment of comminuted P1 fractures is guarded and euthanasia is often warranted.

Horses can occasionally return to low-level athletic function following PIP arthrodesis for comminuted P2 fractures as long as any secondary complications are avoided. The prognosis for biaxial P2 fractures is markedly reduced with severe concurrent soft tissue injuries. Uniaxial P2 fractures treated conservatively may be at risk of developing OA at a later date.

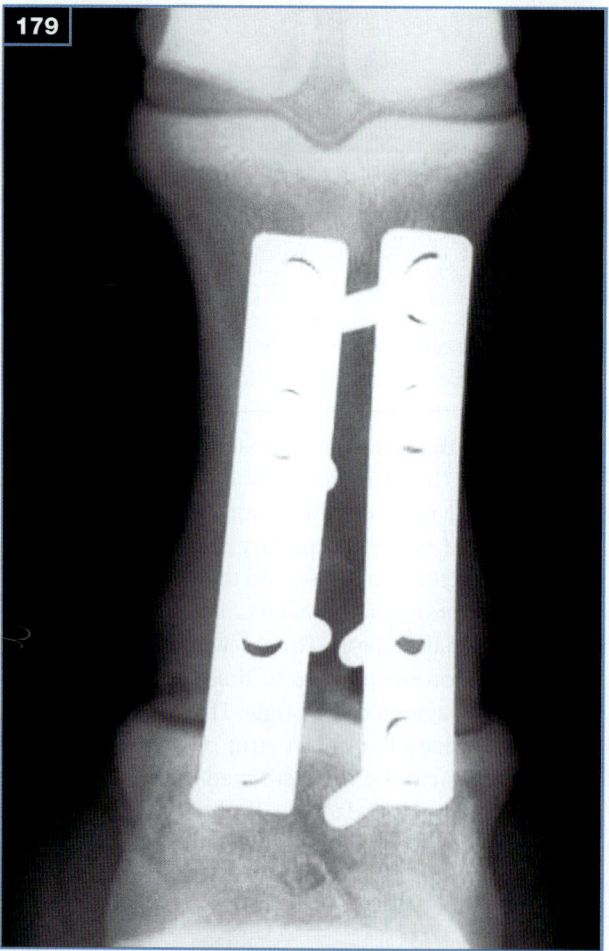

Interphalangeal joint disease
Definition/overview
This section covers conditions affecting the PIP joint, including OA, OCD, and subluxation.

Etiology/pathophysiology
The PIP joint is a high-load/low-motion joint and OA may occur due to 'wear and tear' of the articular surfaces or be secondary to conformational defects, trauma, articular fractures, sequelae to sepsis, or from other conditions disrupting joint integrity (e.g. OCD).

Manifestations of OCD involving the PIP joint include osseous cyst-like lesions (OCLL) of distal P1 or, more unusually, proximal P2 and condylar fragmentation.

Subluxation of the PIP joint is usually traumatic in origin and can occur in either a dorsal or palmar/plantar direction. Dorsally directed subluxation is usually due to severe disruption of the suspensory apparatus (e.g. severe suspensory desmitis). Severe trauma to the distal sesamoidean ligaments or superficial digital flexor tendon branches can result in palmar/plantar subluxation.

Clinical presentation
OA of the PIP joint (or 'high ringbone') may present as a chronic insidious lameness, commonly of aged horses, or, more unusually, as acute-onset lameness. Distal limb flexion tests worsen the lameness, although these are nonspecific. Firm, bony swelling may be palpable over the dorsolateral and/or dorsomedial aspects of the pastern joint. Alterations in conformation may also be present either as a predisposing factor or due to chronicity of the condition.

OCD may present as a low-grade lameness of insidious onset or as acute intermittent lameness in younger horses, usually in the hindlimb. Other clinical signs may be scant, although the young animal may initially be presented for a contralateral ALD.

Subluxation of the PIP joint usually presents as an acute-onset severe lameness. Soft-tissue swelling is often marked and initially localized around the joint. Absence of anatomic incongruity may make the diagnosis more challenging.

Differential diagnosis
Soft-tissue injuries to the pastern; subsolar abscessation; P1/P2 fractures; synovial sepsis.

179 Dorsopalmar radiograph of the horse featured in 177. Two narrow DCPs have been used for a PIP joint arthrodesis following a biaxial P2 fracture. (Photo courtesy GA Munroe)

Musculoskeletal system

Diagnosis

Diagnostic analgesia is required to determine the significance of OA, although intra-articular analgesia may be difficult to achieve. Radiographic signs of DJD (**180**) are usually present to varying degrees, often on the medial aspect of the joint, and can lead to an apparent angular limb deformity if severe.

Diagnostic analgesia and radiography are also important in the diagnosis of OCD. OCLLs are usually present in distal P1 and occasionally in proximal P2 (**181**).

Stress radiography may be required for diagnosis of PIP subluxation. Ultrasonography can be used to examine the collateral ligaments and other soft-tissue structures around the joint following subluxation.

Management

Lameness associated with OA may be improved with the use of NSAIDs along with corrective farriery/shoeing. Intra-articular medication (sodium hyaluronate/corticosteroids) may help if the joint space is accessible. With advanced OA of the PIP joint, surgical arthrodesis is an option. In the hindlimb, tibial neurectomy has also been described for terminally arthritic PIP joints. Osteochondral fragments in the PIP joint can be removed arthroscopically.

Intra-articular medication may resolve clinical signs associated with OCD of the PIP joint. Methylprednisolone acetate has been injected into cyst cavities, leading to resolution in some cases.

Traumatic subluxation of the pastern requires external coaptation. Severe cases may require arthrodesis. Mild cases of dorsal subluxation have been reported in young horses, with no associated soft-tissue disruption, and these often resolve with rest.

Prognosis

The prognosis for OA of the PIP joint is generally guarded to poor, although surgical arthrodesis can result in pain relief if successful. PIP arthrodesis in the hindlimb generally carries a better prognosis than in the forelimb. The outcome of treatment for OCLLs of the PIP joint is generally guarded. Horses treated for subluxation without arthrodesis often re-luxate some time later and the prognosis is generally improved with arthrodesis of the joint.

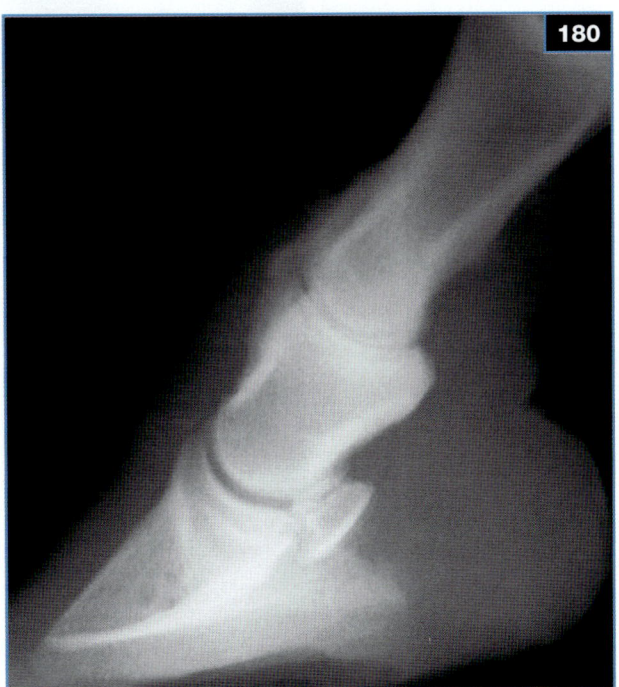

180 Lateromedial radiograph of the PIP joint. Subchondral bone sclerosis, joint narrowing, and marked new bone formation over the dorsal aspect of distal P1, proximal P2, and the proximal interphalangeal joint are present.

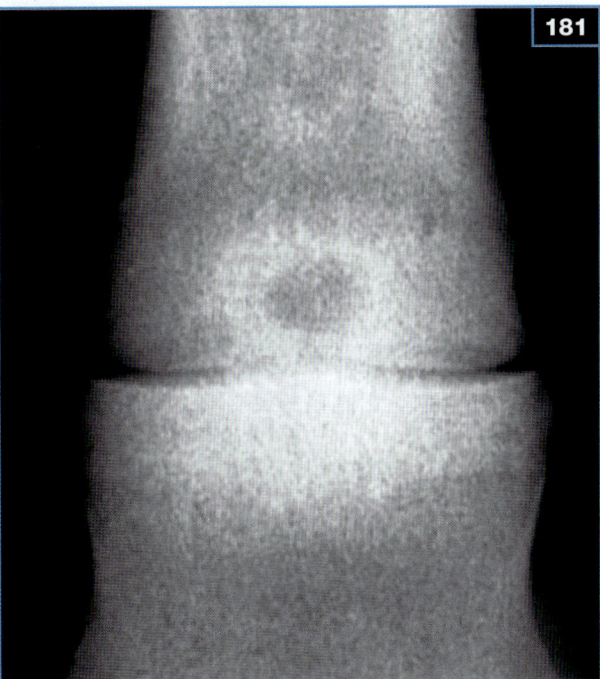

181 Dorsopalmar radiograph of the PIP joint showing an OCLL in the center of distal P1, with connection into the PIP joint. (Photo courtesy GA Munroe)

The forelimb

Sesamoid bones

Proximal sesamoid bone fractures

Definition/overview
Fractures of the proximal sesamoid bones (PSBs) include apical (less than 30% of the height of the bone), mid-body, axial, basilar, abaxial, and comminuted (**182–185**).

Etiology/pathophysiology
Fractures of the PSB may be due to a single traumatic incident at speed, although evidence exists of these bones undergoing stress adaptive remodeling due to exercise. As such, the porosity of the bone reduces, leading to a higher risk of failure.

Clinical presentation
Most PSB fractures result in acute-onset lameness, with swelling and focal pain on palpation over the palmar/plantar fetlock. In cases of biaxial fracture, the fetlock may be dropped due to disruption of the suspensory apparatus. A fetlock effusion is usually present.

Differential diagnosis
P1 fractures; condylar fractures; severe fetlock sprain; fetlock subluxation; sepsis; severe suspensory ligament desmitis; superficial digital flexor tendon (SDFT) tendonitis; digital flexor tendonitis.

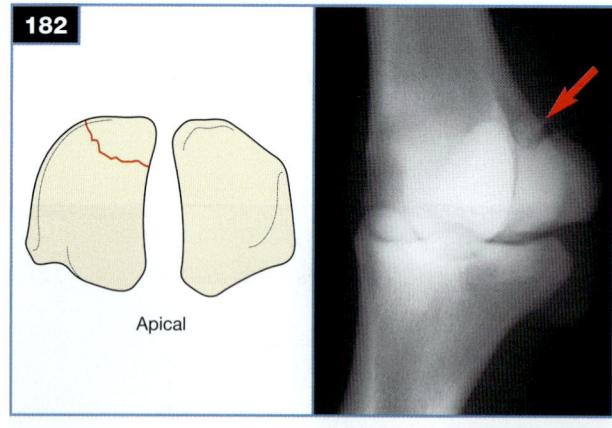

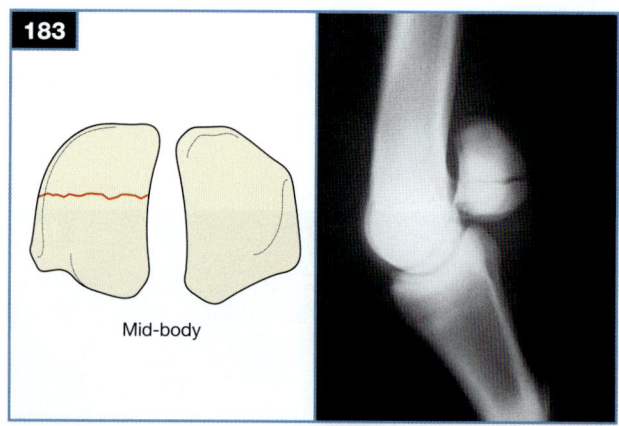

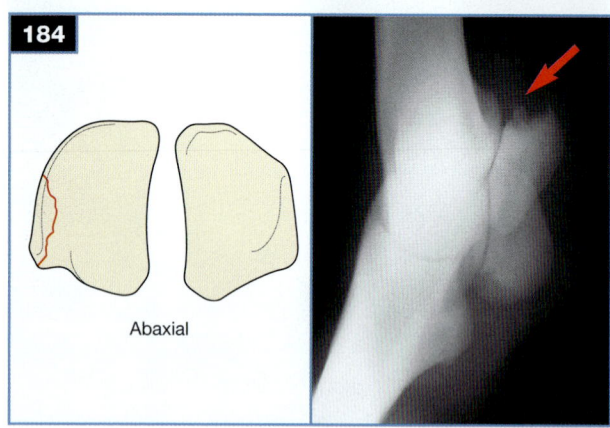

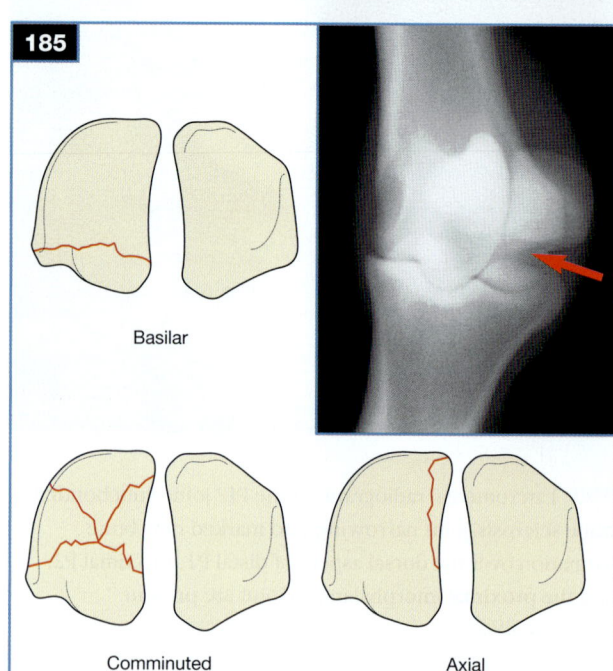

182–185 Classification of fractures of the proximal sesamoid bone with representative radiographs (arrows show fracture location): apical (182); mid-body (183); abaxial (184); basilar (185).

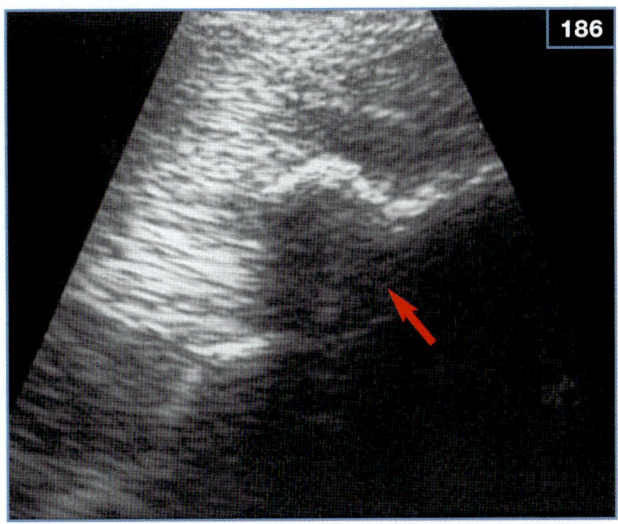

186 Parasagittal ultrasonogram of the medial branch of the suspensory ligament associated with an abaxial proximal sesamoid bone fracture (arrow).

Diagnosis

Clinical examination should alert the clinician to the possibility of a PSB fracture, although in some cases lameness can resolve rapidly. Radiography is important to identify the nature of the fracture(s) and other concomitant damage (e.g. small metacarpal/metatarsal [MC/MT] bone fracture). Multiple views and angles are required for full assessment; for example, the proximal 60° lateral distomedial oblique projection is useful for assessing articular involvement with abaxial fractures. Axial fractures can often be hard to visualize and therefore easily overlooked. Nuclear scintigraphy is sensitive for both complete and incomplete fractures and for evidence of stress remodeling. Ultrasonography (186) is important to evaluate associated structures, such as the suspensory ligament and its branches, the inter-sesamoidean ligament, and the distal sesamoidean ligaments, as damage to any of these will affect long-term prognosis.

Management

Articular apical fractures can be removed by arthroscopy or arthrotomy. Arthroscopy offers the advantage of allowing the clinician to examine the fetlock and assess other joint damage, as well as being minimally invasive. Larger fragments require removal by arthrotomy, and this can be achieved following arthroscopic examination of the joint.

Mid-body fractures are repaired by circumferential wiring or lag screw fixation. Cancellous bone graft is packed into the fracture bed to assist the poor healing associated with PSB fractures.

Basilar fractures are usually articular and have variable involvement of the distal sesamoidean ligaments. Treatment options include rest, removal, or internal fixation. Removal of the fragment can be difficult due to involvement of the distal sesamoidean ligaments. Lag screw fixation is usually not applicable due to the size of the fragment, so circumferential wiring may be attempted. In foals, basilar fractures can be quite large but respond well to 1–2 months box rest.

Abaxial fractures are removed if articular or internally fixated if large enough. Rest is indicated for nondisplaced and/or nonarticular fractures.

Axial fractures are commonly seen in conjunction with lateral condylar fractures of the distal third of MC/MT III. Inter-sesamoidean ligament injuries may be present without fracture and can be difficult to manage. Visualization can be achieved arthroscopically and debridement has been described.

Cases of biaxial PSB fracture (i.e. breakdown injuries) are usually euthanized. If repair is to be attempted, immediate support to immobilize the region is required and fetlock arthrodesis can be performed as a salvage procedure, although this is uncommon.

Prognosis

The prognosis for apical PSB fractures is good following removal provided minimal soft-tissue disruption occurs. Mid-body PSB fractures have an unfavorable prognosis depending on the rate of healing within the fracture bed. Biaxial fractures are usually euthanized. Basilar fractures have an unfavorable prognosis dependent on the size of the fragment; the prognosis worsens with involvement of more than two-thirds of the dorsopalmar/plantar length of the PSB and >3 mm distal displacement of the fragment. The prognosis for axial fractures is guarded to poor, as they are associated with concurrent injuries such as condylar fractures.

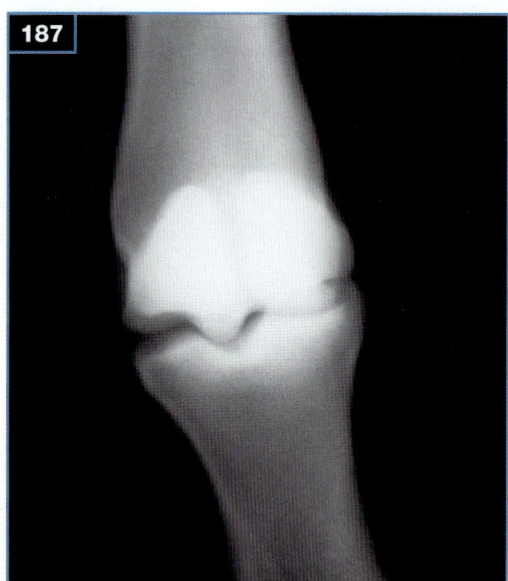

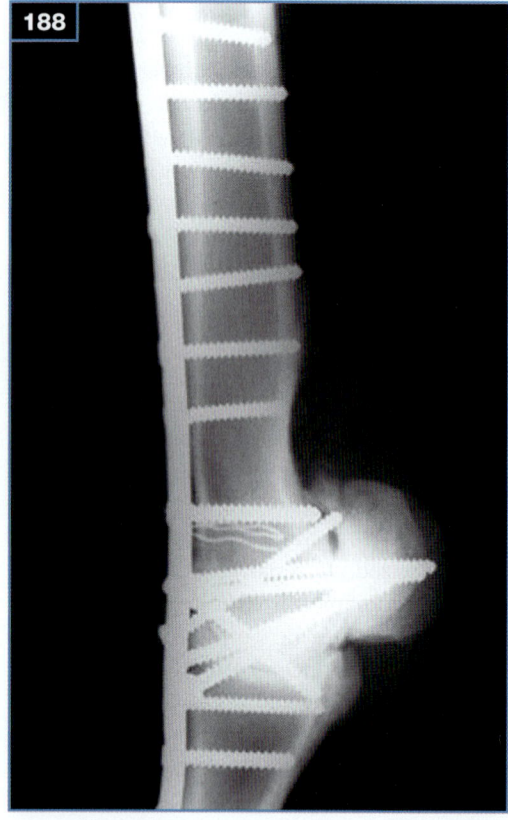

187 Stressed dorsopalmar radiograph showing widening of the joint space on the medial aspect of the metacarpophalangeal joint following medial collateral ligament rupture. (Photo courtesy J Kidd)

188 Intraoperative lateromedial radiograph of a horse undergoing fetlock arthrodesis.

Fetlock joint _____

Fetlock joint subluxation

Definition/overview
Luxation of the metacarpo/metatarsophalangeal joint may be closed or open.

Etiology/pathophysiology
Fetlock joint luxation usually occurs when the horse's foot becomes trapped (e.g. in a cattle grid or due to a fall at speed; for example, a racehorse at gallop). Severe trauma to the region leads to rupture or avulsion of the collateral ligaments of the joint and tearing of the joint capsule and associated structures.

Clinical presentation
The acutely, severely lame horse will usually have anatomic anomalies present, although in closed luxations the joint surfaces may be congruent. Severe soft-tissue swelling develops quickly. Open luxations show obvious derangements. Severe contamination of the joint surfaces will invariably develop in open cases.

Differential diagnosis
Severe joint sprains/soft-tissue damage to the fetlock; intra-articular fractures; sepsis.

Diagnosis
Clinical examination of the limb may indicate severe disruption to the joint, although stress radiography may be required for a definitive diagnosis (**187**). Radiographs are also advisable to check for concurrent injuries such as avulsion fractures. Ultrasonography is indicated to assess damage to the collateral ligaments and other soft-tissue structures associated with the fetlock joint.

Management
Closed luxations can be cast for 6 weeks. With open luxations, early aggressive lavage and debridement are required, followed by casting or fetlock arthrodesis (**188**). The prognosis is guarded, especially in infected open luxations, and euthanasia may be warranted. Long-term sequelae include periarticular fibrosis and OA, most particularly following open luxation.

Prognosis
The prognosis is fair for closed fetlock joint subluxation, but guarded if open and hopeless with severe contamination.

Chronic proliferative synovitis

Definition/overview

Chronic proliferative synovitis or villonodular synovitis of the fetlock refers to the presence of a soft-tissue mass in the dorsal aspect of the joint, commonly affecting the forelimb(s) of the horse.

Etiology/pathophysiology

Chronic repetitive trauma to the dorsal aspect of the fetlock joint from hyperextension leads to hyperplasia of the bilobed synovial pad over the sagittal ridge. This is seen particularly in racehorses. Osteoclastic resorption leads to supracondylar lysis of the underlying bone. Conditions such as the presence of a dorsoproximal P1 fragment may also result in chronic inflammation at the dorsal aspect of the joint. Anecdotal evidence suggests long pasterns may be a predisposing factor.

Clinical presentation

A palpable thickening over the dorsal aspect of the affected fetlock joint is found on clinical examination, with or without a joint effusion (189). Reduction in range of motion of the joint can also be sometimes appreciated and lameness commonly worsens following exercise and fetlock flexion.

Differential diagnosis

Fetlock joint trauma or sprain; fetlock OA; intra-articular fracture or dorsoproximal P1 fragments.

Diagnosis

Radiography may show a crescent-shaped radiolucency on the dorsal aspect of distal third metacarpus due to cortical lysis (190). Dystrophic mineralization may also be present. Contrast arthrography may provide further detail. Ultrasound is sensitive in demonstrating thickening of the synovial pad (>10 mm) and associated joint changes at the dorsal aspect. Radiography should also be performed to examine the joint for other evidence of OA, as changes may also be seen in the palmar aspect of distal third metacarpus.

Management

Medical therapy and changes to the exercise regime may help in some cases. Intra-articular hyaluronan and corticosteroids, with rest initially, followed by an alteration in the training pattern, are often helpful. Surgical excision has been performed arthroscopically.

Prognosis

The prognosis is variable but generally guarded to poor and depends on the presence of DJD. Resolution of the problem can be temporarily achieved, but recurrence is common unless an underlying cause can be found.

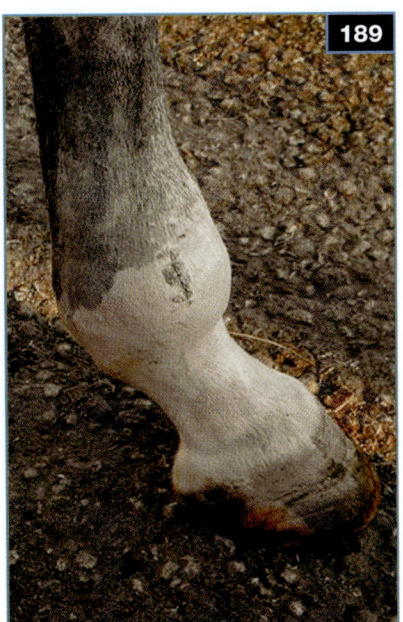

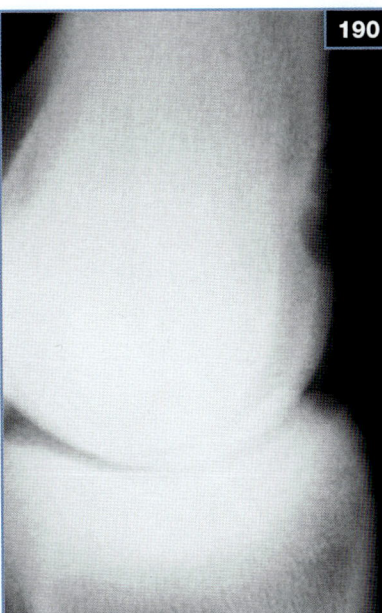

189 Swelling of the dorsal aspect of the metacarphophalangeal joint consistent with chronic proliferative synovitis. (Photo courtesy J Kidd)

190 Lateromedial radiograph of a metacarpophalangeal joint showing a crescent-shaped radiolucency on the dorsal aspect of distal third metacarpus due to cortical lysis. Note also the new bone at the capsular insertion point proximal to the lytic lesion and remodeling of the proximal dorsal aspect of the first phalanx. (Photo courtesy GA Munroe)

Synovitis, osteoarthritis, subchondral bone injury, osteochondrosis, osseous cyst-like lesions, osteochondral fragments of P1

Definition/overview

The fetlock joint is a highly loaded, high-motion joint and acute or repetitive overloading of the joint beyond its physiologic limits can lead to damage to the joint capsule, synovial lining, and subchondral bone as well as the joint surface itself.

Etiology/pathophysiology

Acute joint damage will lead to synovitis developing rapidly. OA (191) is usually a consequence of ongoing damage to an already compromised joint, and it can also be a sequela to other conditions affecting the joint such as OCD, OCLL, intra-articular fractures, or intra-articular sepsis.

Lesions in the subchondral bone of the palmar condylar region of MC III, commonly seen in racehorses, result from sclerosis of the subchondral plate and micro-damage to the articular surface leading to necrosis and collapsing of the articular defect into the subchondral bone (192). This has previously been thought to be a manifestation of OCD, but has now been shown to have a traumatic etiology. Secondary arthritic changes commonly develop.

OCD of the fetlock involves the dorsal sagittal ridge of MC/MT III in young horses, involving flattening or defects of the ridge and osteochondral fragmentation. OCLL in the fetlock usually involves the condyles of distal MC/MT III (193). Dorsoproximal osteochondral fragments of P1 may be incidental findings or associated with hyperextension injuries (194, 195). Although often presented as acute 'chip' fractures, many of these osteochondral fragments are smooth, well-defined bodies, often present in sound horses, that may have developed as separate bodies. It is thought that lameness or poor performance may be associated with the presence of these bodies due to vibration at high speed. Palmaro/plantaroproximal osteochondral fragments of P1 (196) are commonly seen in the hindlimb and can be divided into four types (*Table 3*).

191 Lateromedial radiograph showing severe OA of the fetlock joint. Periarticular osteophytes, remodeling of the palmar aspect of distal MC III, subchondral bone sclerosis, joint space narrowing, and basilar fragmentation are present. Note also the presence of an apical proximal sesamoid fracture (arrow) associated with the pathology.

192 Lateromedial radiograph of the left hind fetlock joint in a 5-year-old Thoroughbred flat racehorse with bilateral hindlimb lameness. Note the flattening of the plantar condyle of the distal 3rd metatarsal bone (arrow), with wedge-shaped subchondral bone sclerosis. (Photo courtesy GA Munroe)

193 Dorsoplantar radiograph showing a discrete circular radiolucency surrounded by a faint rim of sclerosis (arrow) medial to the sagittal ridge on the distal aspect of MT III, consistent with an OCLL. Note the thin communicating channel of the cyst with the articular surface.

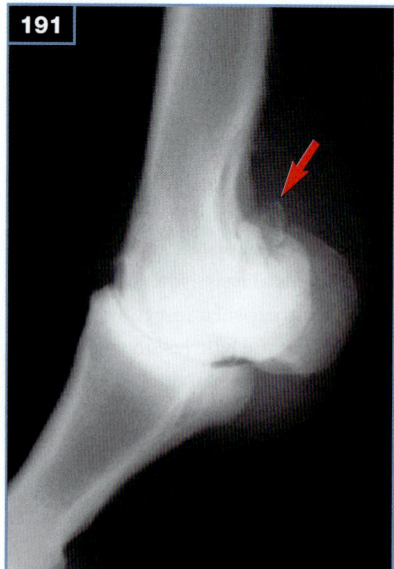

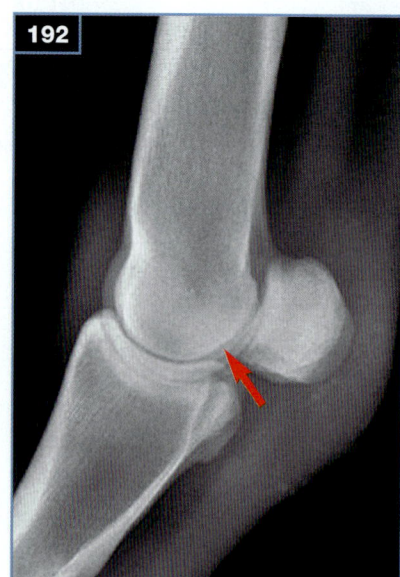

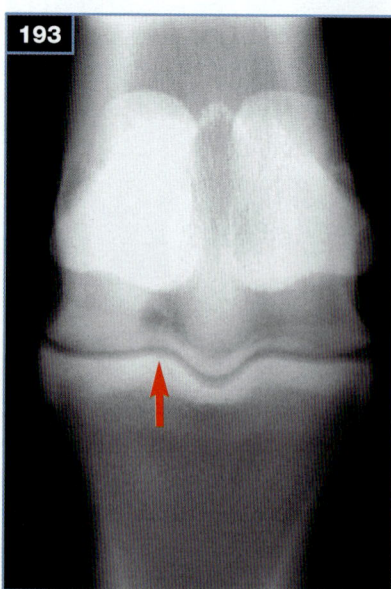

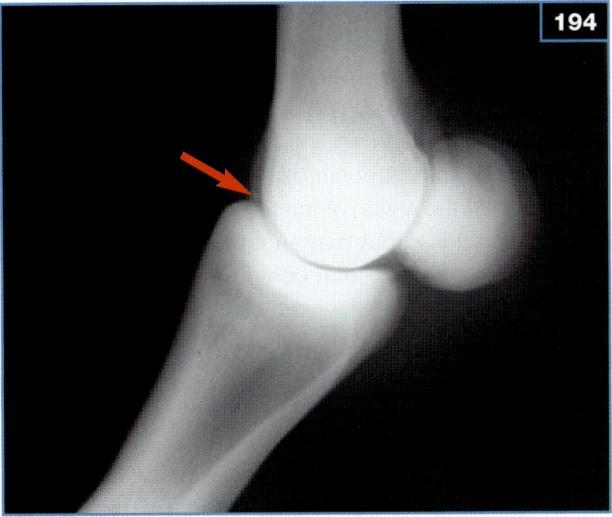

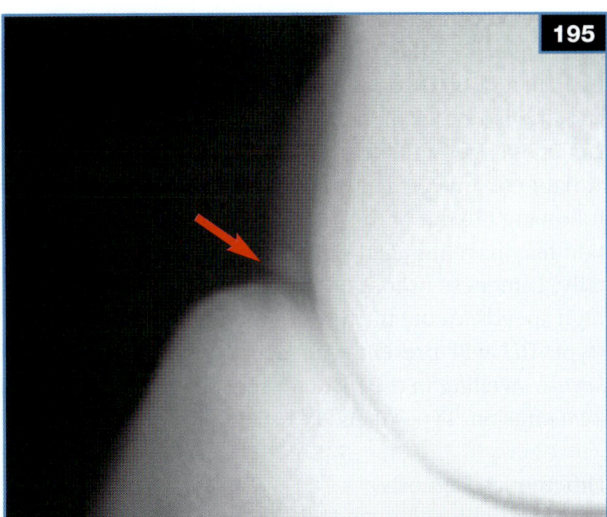

194, 195 Lateromedial radiograph (194) of the fetlock joint showing a discrete radiodense body in the dorsal aspect of the joint (arrow) and magnified image (195) showing location just proximal to the dorsoproximal rim of P1 (arrow).

196 Lateromedial radiograph of the fetlock joint showing a type IV plantaroproximal P1 fragment (arrow). (See *Table 3* for classification.) (Photos courtesy GA Munroe)

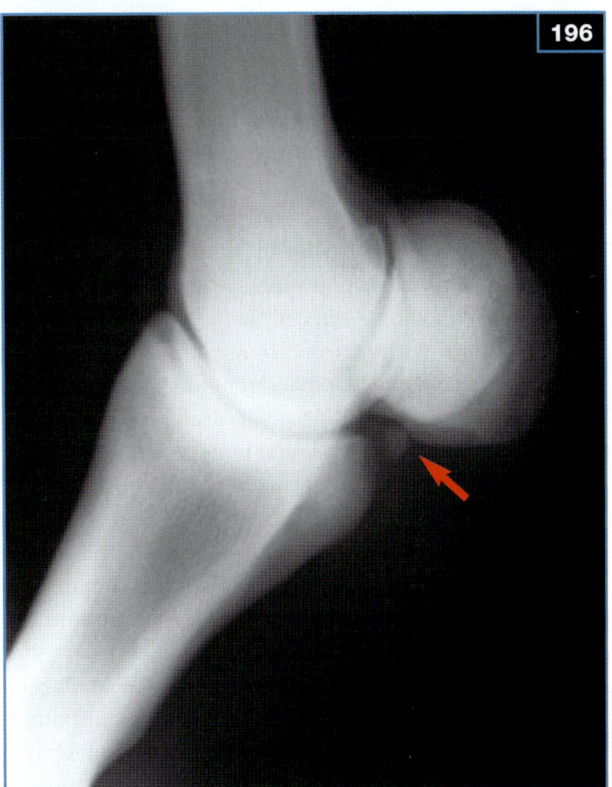

Clinical presentation
Synovitis can present with a mild lameness or loss of performance with mild to moderate joint effusion. Clinical signs worsen following distal limb flexion. OA of the fetlock is usually seen in older performance horses with moderate to severe lameness, minimal joint effusion, and a restriction in range of joint motion due to capsular fibrosis, although it can occur in younger animals following a severe joint injury. Palmar condylar subchondral bone injuries are seen in the young racehorse undergoing intense training, leading to a variable lameness with loss of performance, but in some cases these cases present with severe lameness.

TABLE 3	**Classification of palmaro/plantaroproximal osteochondral fragments of P1**
TYPE	**DESCRIPTION**
I	Axial articular fragment from the proximal palmar/plantar rim of P1, especially on the medial side.
II	Larger, abaxially located fragment, may be partly articular, seen on the lateral aspect of proximal P1 and may represent delayed ossification.
III	Acute fracture of the plantar process of P1.
IV	Usually present in the forelimb at the base of the proximal sesamoid bone, reflecting an old avulsion injury or ossification of the distal sesamoidean ligaments.

OCD in young horses, including foals, usually has variable lameness. An effusion is often present and pain may be detected on flexion of the joint. The remaining limbs should also be examined for the presence of effusions. Lameness associated with OCLL of the fetlock often has a variable severity of lameness or a lameness evident only following flexion of the joint. Osteochondral fragmentation may have minimal signs and may be found incidentally. Lameness or loss of performance may be noted at high speeds. Acute fractures of the plantar process of P1 (type III) will present with acute-onset lameness and severe swelling in the plantar aspect of proximal P1 and joint effusion. Types II and IV usually show minimal signs.

Differential diagnosis
Chronic proliferative synovitis; PSB fracture; sesamoiditis; suspensory branch injury.

Diagnosis
Clinical examination and history may lead to suspicion of fetlock joint disease. Intra-articular analgesia usually leads to some improvement in most fetlock joint conditions, although conditions predominantly affecting the subchondral bone may require perineural analgesia to localize the lameness.

Radiography is an important modality in assessing fetlock-joint conditions. Minimal changes will be evident in acute synovitis. Radiographic signs of OA in the fetlock include periarticular osteophytes, remodeling of the dorsal sagittal ridge of MC/MT III, palmar distal MC III remodeling, palmar condyle subchondral bone sclerosis, irregular basilar fragments, and joint space reduction (see **191**). Intense sclerosis overlying an area of lysis at the distal palmar condylar aspect of MC III may be seen on a lateromedial, flexed lateromedial, or 125° dorsopalmar view with subchondral bone injuries. Fragmentation and OA may be present in severe cases.

OCD of the dorsal sagittal ridge is best evaluated using lateromedial, flexed lateromedial and dorsoproximal/dorsodistal flexed views. The latter view helps to highlight the sagittal ridge. Changes include a defect in, or flattening of, the sagittal ridge of distal MC/MT III, usually in the dorsoproximal aspect, with or without the presence of osteochondral fragmentation. Radiography of the remaining fetlock joints should be undertaken in cases of fetlock OCD.

OCLLs of the distal MC/MT III may be seen on lateromedial, flexed lateromedial and/or dorsopalmar/plantar views. The cyst usually communicates with the joint just dorsal to the transverse ridge and identification of its location is important for potential surgical treatment.

For osteochondral fragments of proximal P1, standard projections including obliques are usually sufficient. To improve visualization of the palmar/plantar aspect of the joint, the X-ray beam should be angled proximodistally by about 20°, with a reduced angle of obliquity (15–20° from dorsal) to minimize superimposition of the distal aspects of the PSBs over the region of interest.

Nuclear scintigraphy may show early evidence of bone remodeling in fetlock-joint conditions, and may be particularly useful in diagnosing early subchondral bone injuries in the palmar condyles with equivocal radiographic changes.

Management
Cases of uncomplicated synovitis or traumatic injury to the fetlock joint respond well to a period of rest and administration of NSAIDs. Intra-articular medication such as sodium hyaluronate and corticosteroids may assist in earlier return to work, but a correct exercise regimen following this is important. Treatment for OA, however, is palliative and a poor response is often seen with intra-articular medication. Correction or improvement of any underlying conditions is also recommended. Treatment of palmar condylar subchondral bone injuries can be difficult and depends on the degree of damage to the joint. Early identification and alteration to training are important in managing these cases. Rest and NSAIDs can be used, but intra-articular medication can be disappointing. Changes to the subchondral bone of the palmar condyle are difficult to assess arthroscopically, but examination of the rest of the joint may give further prognostic information.

Arthroscopic removal of OCD lesions of the dorsal sagittal ridge is recommended to reduce secondary joint disease, although a large defect may be left. However, in cases of mild flattening without osteochondral fragmentation, conservative management is recommended initially.

OCLLs often respond poorly to intra-articular medication and surgery is indicated. A lesion located on, or dorsal to, the transverse ridge may be accessed arthroscopically for curettage. For more palmar located cysts, transosseous drilling may be indicated.

Arthroscopy is warranted for removal of dorsoproximal P1 osteochondral fragments if clinically significant or to reduce the risk of secondary joint disease developing. Type I palmaro/plantaroproximal osteochondral fragments are similarly removed if indicated. Type II fragments are usually left and monitored, although they can be removed if causing lameness. Type III fragments can be repaired by internal fixation or removed (if small). Type IV fragments can be removed, but they are associated with damage to the distal sesamoidean ligaments.

Prognosis

Early, uncomplicated cases of synovitis have a good prognosis. The outcome for OA of the fetlock is generally guarded to poor. Subchondral bone injuries are associated with a guarded prognosis, which becomes poorer with evidence of severe flattening and fragmentation of the palmar condyle and the presence of OA.

OCD of the dorsal sagittal ridge carries a fair prognosis, especially in the hindlimbs, unless extensive. The prognosis and outcome for OCLLs depend on access. Dorsoproximal P1 and type I palmaro/plantaroproximal osteochondral fragments have a good prognosis, although the presence of DJD will significantly worsen this. Type IV fragments tend to have a poor prognosis.

Sesamoiditis

Definition/overview

Sesamoiditis relates to inflammation of the soft tissues around the palmar/plantar aspect of the fetlock and associated bony changes in the PSBs.

Etiology/pathophysiology

Repeated stresses on the palmar/plantar aspect of the fetlock and proximal sesamoid bones lead to tearing of the soft-tissue attachments. A cycle of incomplete healing and further damage can result in an entheseopathy and bony remodeling of the sesamoid bones. Alternatively, an acute single overload injury may result in acute inflammation of the associated soft-tissue structures. The condition is more common in racing breeds.

Clinical presentation

The horse usually presents with a unilateral low-grade chronic lameness, although with acute tearing, a more severe, acute lameness may be present. Pain and swelling are usually evident and, on careful palpation, localized to the PSBs. With chronicity, soft-tissue thickening may be present and larger bony entheseophytes appreciated. Examination of the suspensory ligament may reveal additional soft-tissue involvement in the condition.

Differential diagnosis

Sesamoid bone fracture; injury to the suspensory ligament branches; palmar/plantar annular ligament desmitis/avulsion fracture.

Diagnosis

Regional perineural analgesia is required to localize the lameness. Radiographic assessment of the fetlock joint and PSBs is important. Oblique radiographs highlighting the palmar/plantar aspects of each sesamoid bone yield most information. Bony remodeling and entheseophytosis can lead to changes in the shape and outline of the PSB. Radiolucent lines radiating across the sesamoid bone due to widening of the vascular channels may represent remodeling in the trabecular pattern and need to be differentiated from a fracture (usually distracted) (197). A comparison with the opposite sesamoid bone is required to assess changes in the light of clinical findings, and assessment of other changes in the joint (e.g. OA) is important. Ultrasonography is useful in acute cases with minimal radiographic changes, and for assessment of the suspensory ligament.

Management

Treatment is aimed at reducing the inflammation and preventing recurrence. Cold hosing, rest, and NSAIDs are warranted with a controlled exercise program. Extracorporeal shock-wave therapy has been used successfully in some refractory cases.

Prognosis

Due to the recurrence of lameness, the prognosis for return to full work in cases of sesamoiditis is guarded.

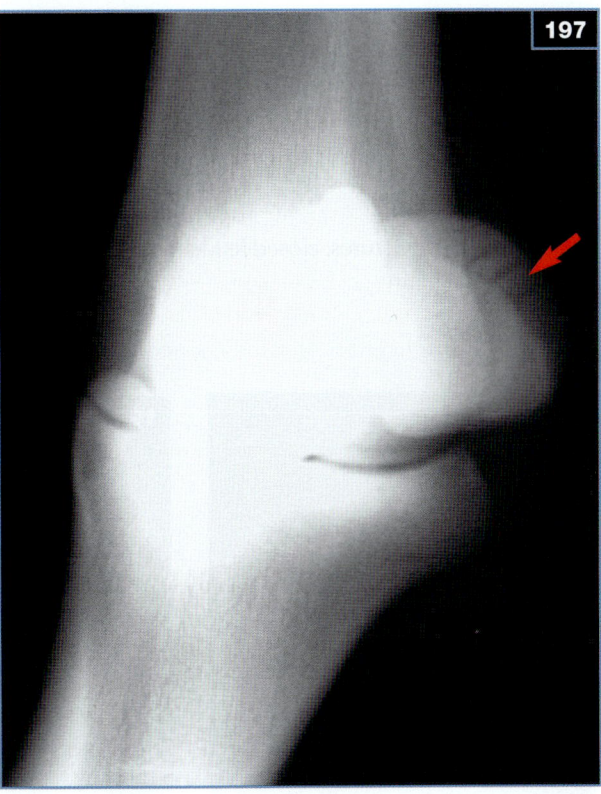

197 Dorsomedial/palmarolateral oblique radiograph of the fetlock showing demineralization of the medial sesamoid bone and radiolucent lines (arrow) radiating through the structure. (Photo courtesy J Kidd)

The forelimb

Metacarpals/metatarsals

Metacarpal/metatarsal III condylar fractures

Definition/overview
MC/MT III condylar fractures are one of the most common types of fracture encountered in racehorses. Lateral and medial condylar fractures can be seen with differing configuration and treatment/prognosis.

Etiology/pathophysiology
The fractures are often encountered as a high-speed injury, although evidence has been shown of pre-existing pathology (sclerosis) in the palmar/plantar aspect of both medial and lateral condyles, suggesting that these fractures are an end point of nonphysiologic stress remodeling of the bone in that region. Both fractures begin at the articular surface of the distal MC/MT III. Lateral condylar fractures commonly exit the lateral cortex approximately 1–3 cm above the physeal scar. They may be nondisplaced or associated with displacement and/or concomitant injuries, such as comminution at the distal palmar condyle or injuries to the PSB(s), including axial sesamoid bone fractures due to avulsion by the inter-sesamoidean ligament. Medial condylar fractures do not exit from the cortex, but continue vertically to either disappear into the diaphysis or spiral in a frontal plane.

Clinical presentation
The horse usually pulls up from exercise very lame, with fetlock swelling and pain evident on clinical examination.

Differential diagnosis
PSB fractures; P1 fractures; closed fetlock subluxation; subchondral bone injury.

Diagnosis
Full radiographic assessment of the affected limb is very important in decision making in these cases. As well as recognition of a fracture, the fracture length, configuration, and degree of displacement all have to be determined (198, 199). Hence the entire length of MC/MT III should be viewed as part of the diagnostic work-up. With lateral condylar fractures, comminution at the distal palmar/plantar condyle may be seen as a 'wedge-shaped' defect at the articular surface with the 125° dorso-palmar/plantar view. The presence of an axial sesamoid fracture, usually on the lateral PSB, also significantly worsens the prognosis. The length and direction of medial condylar fractures as they continue into the diaphysis need to be followed closely, especially at the point the fracture line seems to disappear. Y-shaped fractures, seen mainly in the hindlimb, ascend in a sagittal plane from the medial condyle, do not spiral, and have a high risk of catastrophic failure.

198 Dorsopalmar radiograph showing typical configuration of a lateral condylar fracture exiting the lateral cortex above the physeal scar. (Photo courtesy J Kidd)

199 Dorsopalmar radiograph of a Thoroughbred racehorse with multiple fracture lines in the distal half of MC III, which was treated conservatively. Note the way at least one fracture spirals proximally. (Photo courtesy GA Munroe)

200 Intraoperative dorsopalmar radiograph of a lag screw fixation of a lateral condylar MC III fracture. (Photo courtesy GA Munroe)

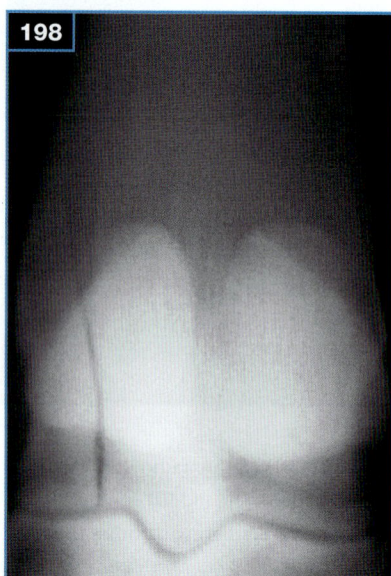

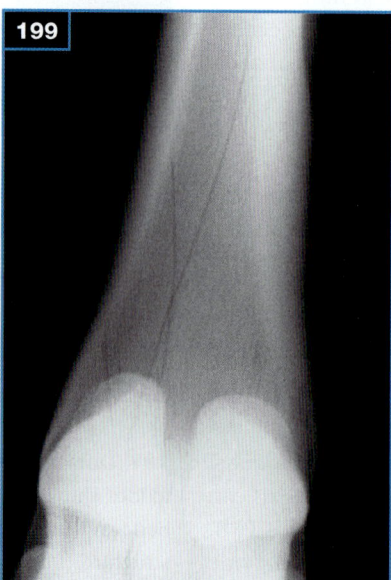

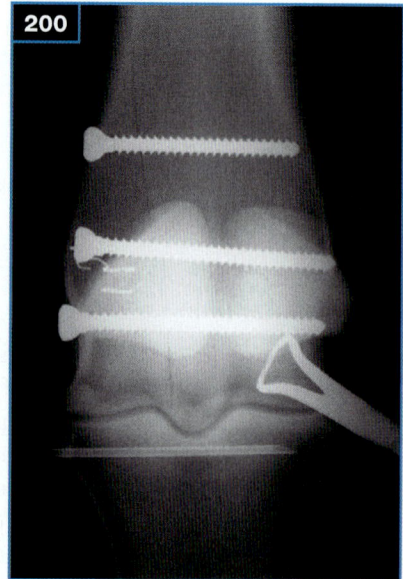

Management
Initial emergency treatment requires external coaptation to protect the region and reduce the risk of nondisplaced fractures becoming displaced. Nondisplaced lateral condylar fractures can be treated conservatively, although internal fixation provides a consistent and predictable time frame for recovery. Displaced lateral condylar fractures are best repaired with internal fixation using the lag screw technique (200). Radiography or fluoroscopy is recommended for intraoperative guidance and arthroscopy can allow direct joint visualization during realignment. Displaced medial condylar fractures are often open and have a degree of comminution, invariably resulting in euthanasia. Repair of nondisplaced medial condylar fractures can be achieved by lag screws or plate fixation, more recently involving minimally invasive techniques.

Prognosis
Nondisplaced lateral condylar fractures, especially of the hindlimbs, carry a good prognosis. Displaced lateral condylar fractures have a fair prognosis for return to racing depending on the accuracy of reconstruction of the articular surface and lack of concurrent injuries. The prognosis for medial condylar fractures varies and is generally significantly worse than for lateral condylar fracture repair.

Metacarpal/metatarsal III fractures
Definition/overview
Fractures of MC/MT III covered in this section include complete diaphyseal and distal physeal fractures.

Etiology/pathophysiology
Most cases of MC/MT III fractures are traumatic in origin. Often a single high-energy impact (e.g. kick) results in a complete transverse fracture, with or without a butterfly fragment. Comminuted fractures are also encountered. Foals trodden on or kicked lead to Salter–Harris type II distal physeal fractures of variable length.

Clinical presentation
There is acute-onset severe lameness with anatomic disruption of the MC/MT III bone. The fracture becomes the pivot point of the forces that should revolve around the fetlock joint. The fracture may present as open or closed and with damage to the vascular supply.

Differential diagnosis
Condylar or P1 fractures (for physeal fractures); septic arthritis or osteomyelitis in foals.

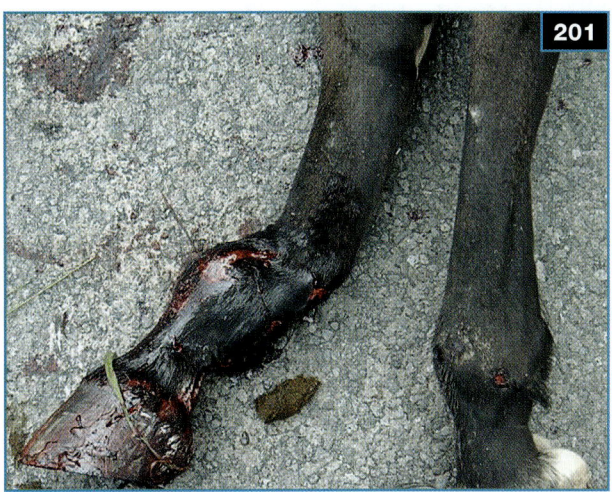

201 This Thoroughbred racehorse was involved in a road traffic accident and has sustained an open comminuted fracture of the distal 3rd metatarsus. It was euthanized immediately. (Photo courtesy GA Munroe)

Diagnosis
Diagnosis is usually made by clinical examination (201), but radiography is important to assess the extent of the fracture and the status of the nutrient foramen. If the fracture line passes through the nutrient foramen in a complete diaphyseal fracture, then the vascularity may be affected.

Management
First aid is important, as further soft-tissue damage and/or conversion of a closed fracture into an open one severely affects prognosis. A Robert Jones bandage with two splints at 90° to each other is recommended. In open, contaminated, or severely comminuted fractures, euthanasia is warranted. Surgical management involves double-plate internal fixation. Newer techniques involve the use of locking compression plates (LCPs). Infection, poor soft-tissue coverage, poor vascularity, and a large metal-to-bone ratio may result in implant failure and therefore the decision to undertake surgical repair has to be justifiable.

Salter–Harris type II fractures can respond to 2–3 weeks' casting (in foals under 6 weeks) followed by bandaging. In older foals, or if the fracture is unstable, internal fixation (avoiding the growth plate) followed by casting is advised.

Prognosis
The outcome is fair if complications can be avoided, but euthanasia is advised in the presence of comminution, contamination, and/or marked trauma to the soft tissues. Closed fractures in young animals carry a favorable prognosis if secondary complications can be avoided.

Sore and bucked shin complex

Definition/overview

The term 'bucked shins' or 'sore shins' relates to bony remodeling and pain over the dorsal cortex of MC III, a condition commonly seen in young horses undergoing intense athletic activities.

Etiology/pathophysiology

Bone is a dynamic tissue and responds to stress (Wolff's law). With cyclic loading, the bony remodeling leads to increased stiffness and reduced porosity, which increases the inertial property of the bone. The porous bone is replaced by secondary osteons and successful remodeling leads to stronger bone adapted to an increased performance. If bone remodeling does not keep up with the increased demand, then a painful periostitis occurs.

Clinical presentation

This problem tends to occur in 2-year-old racehorses recently moved up in their exercise regimen or in older animals returning to the racetrack. The presenting complaint may be of lameness or a lack of performance or dropping off at the end of exercise.

Differential diagnosis

Dorsal cortical stress fractures; traumatic injury.

Diagnosis

Superficial pain may be detected over the dorsal aspect of MC III. Focal soft-tissue swelling may be evident along with periosteal thickening at the region (**202**). Radiography is useful to check for the presence of dorsal cortical fractures, although reduced exposures and various oblique angles may be required to demonstrate periosteal new bone formation. Nuclear scintigraphy will highlight areas of increased bony remodeling.

Management

Management mainly revolves around altering training regimens (i.e. a controlled exercise program involving hand walking until sound, then light exercise for 1–2 months before re-radiography of the area). If the horse is progressing well, it can then be reintroduced to faster work at a level below the initiating cause for 1 month before increasing its level of work again. Extracorporeal shockwave therapy, cryotherapy, and counter-irritants have also been used with variable success.

Prognosis

The prognosis is usually good if the correct management program is followed.

Metacarpal/metatarsal III stress fractures

Definition/overview

These include dorsal cortical stress fractures, longitudinal palmar cortical stress fractures, and transverse distal stress fractures of MC III.

Etiology/pathophysiology

Stress fractures are the end point to the nonphysiologic stress remodeling experienced by high-intensity trained horses. Dorsal cortical fractures are more common in 3–4-year-old racehorses that have had 'bucked or sore shins' as 2-year-olds.

Clinical presentation

Horses are usually presented with lameness that may improve significantly with rest. Other cases may show a reduction in performance, especially towards the end of an intense exercise period.

Differential diagnosis

Bucked shins; local trauma.

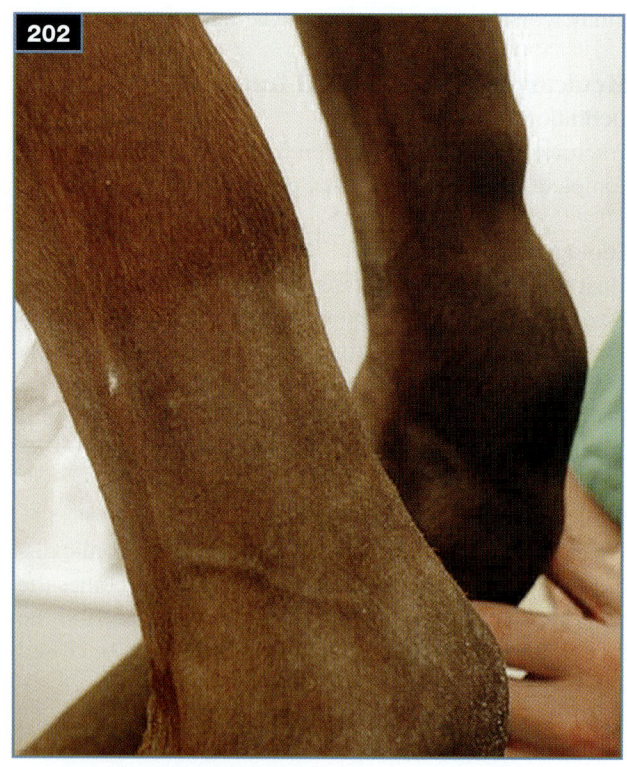

202 Two-year-old Thoroughbred racehorse in dorsal recumbency under general anesthesia about to have arthroscopic surgery of its intercarpal joints. Note the extreme bony swellings on the dorsal aspect of both cannon bones caused by bucked shins. (Photo courtesy GA Munroe)

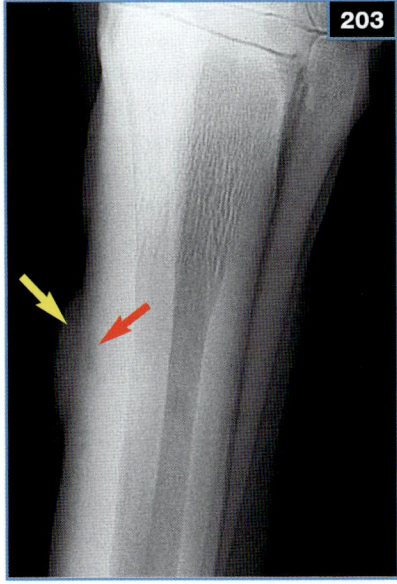
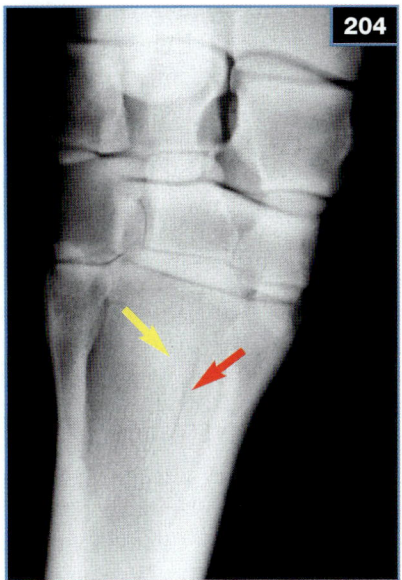
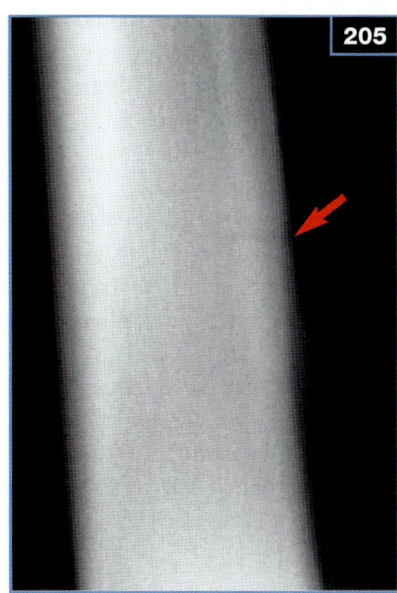

Diagnosis

The clinical history and type of horse may suggest a stress-related problem. Careful clinical examination is required over suspected regions. In cases of dorsal cortical stress fracture, focal pain is detected over the dorsal or dorsolateral aspect of the MC/MT III, with periosteal thickening evident. Cases of palmar cortical stress fracture may be painful on direct pressure over the palmar cortex, adjacent to the suspensory ligament. High suspensory local anesthetic techniques may be required to localize the lameness. A response may be seen on firm palpation or manipulation of the distal MC III with transverse fractures, although this may be inconsistent and difficult to interpret. The lameness may improve on perineural analgesia, but not anesthesia of the fetlock joint. Careful radiographic assessment of the localized area may reveal sclerosis with or without a radiolucent line representing the fracture. With dorsal cortical fractures, a radiolucent line from the dorsolateral cortex may be seen extending approximately two-thirds through the cortex (203). Saucer fractures can be seen if the line also exits in the dorsal cortex. In longitudinal palmar cortical (204) and transverse distal stress fractures (205), proximomedial and horizontal fracture lines may be seen, respectively. Periosteal callus is evident with chronic cases. Nuclear scintigraphy is a more sensitive technique than radiography and may show earlier signs.

Management

Rest and an alteration in training regimen are important in reducing the risk of a catastrophic fracture developing from these stress fractures. Commonly, 1 month of box rest is followed by controlled walking for 2 months. Progress is monitored by clinical re-examination and repeated diagnostic imaging. In clear dorsal cortical fractures, surgical

203 Dorsomedial–palmolateral oblique radiograph of the cannon region of a young Thoroughbred horse showing a dorsolateral 3rd metacarpal stress fracture. Note the obliquely running fracture line in the dorsolateral cortex (red arrow) and the smooth periosteal new bone (yellow arrow).

204 Dorsopalmar radiograph of the corpus and proximal cannon of a horse with a lameness localized to the proximal cannon region by perineural analgesia. Note the longitudinal palmar cortical fracture (red arrow) and surrounding subchondral bone sclerosis (yellow arrow).

205 Horizontal transverse stress fracture in the distal 3rd metacarpus (arrow). (Photos courtesy GA Munroe)

drilling (osteostixis) or screw placement can lead to a local effect on bone remodeling and improve vascularization to the region, aiding recovery. This can be done in the standing horse. Extracorporeal shock-wave therapy has also reportedly led to marked clinical improvement.

Prognosis

The prognosis is usually good, but inadequate time for healing results in a poorer outcome for MC/MT stress fractures. The prognosis with palmar cortical stress fractures worsens in the presence of suspensory desmitis, especially in the hindlimb. Transverse distal stress fractures have a fair prognosis.

Metacarpal/metatarsal II/IV fractures

Definition/overview

MC/MT II/IV or 'splint bone' fractures are relatively common in equine practice.

Etiology/pathophysiology

Many cases, especially MT IV fractues, are a result of direct trauma (e.g. kick, laceration, puncture) (206) and are often open. Distal fractures (207) can result from hyperextension of the fetlock causing stretching of attached fibrous bands and increased loading of the distal aspect of the bone. The fractures often occur at the narrowest point, with distraction of the fragment distally. Acute/chronic overload of the suspensory ligament can lead to overextension of the fetlock and hence these distal fractures are often seen in performance horses (e.g. racehorses) with suspensory desmitis.

Clinical presentation

The horse will commonly present with an acute lameness and moderate swelling, initially centered over the fracture. With direct trauma, an open wound may accompany the fracture. In open proximal splint bone fractures, the presence of joint sepsis may be initially difficult to ascertain in the face of excessive soft-tissue swelling. In chronic infected cases, a discharging sinus or wound that fails to heal may be the initial presenting sign and may indicate bony sequestration. Chronic fractures of the distal aspect of MC/MT II/IV may present as a more subtle problem, only seen at high speed or as a painful swelling close to the suspensory ligament branch.

Differential diagnosis

Exostosis of MC/MT II/IV; suspensory ligament branch injury; osteomyelitis; articular sepsis.

Diagnosis

Clinical evaluation and history may lead to a suspicion of a fracture, although radiography is the key diagnostic tool (208, 209). Evaluation of the carpometacarpal/tarsometatarsal joints and MC/MT III is important to detect concurrent infection/damage (210). It is important to examine the PSBs and suspensory ligament and branches for injuries, therefore ultrasonographic evaluation is also warranted, especially in distal splint bone fractures.

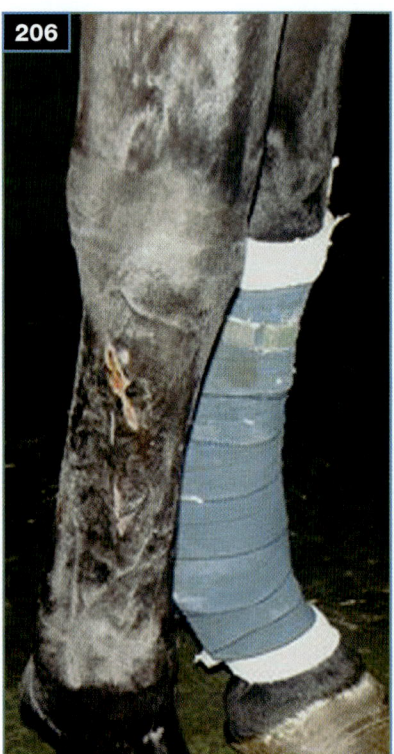

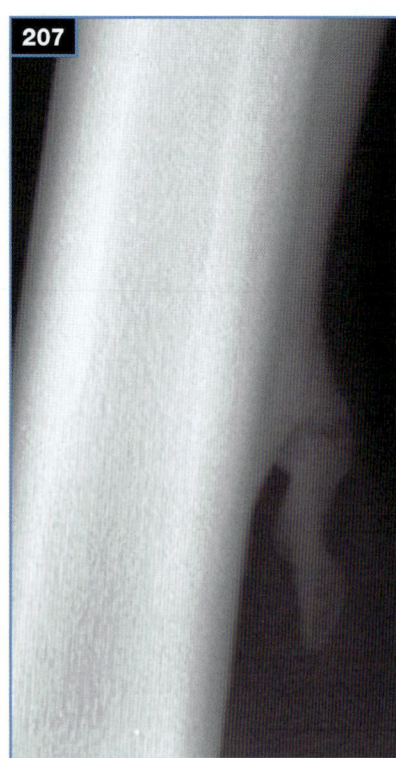

206 Oblique laceration following a kick to the right forelimb lateral splint leading to an MC IV comminuted fracture. (Photo courtesy GA Munroe)

207 Dorsomedial/palmarolateral radiograph showing a chronic fracture of the distal aspect of MC II, with associated bony callus.

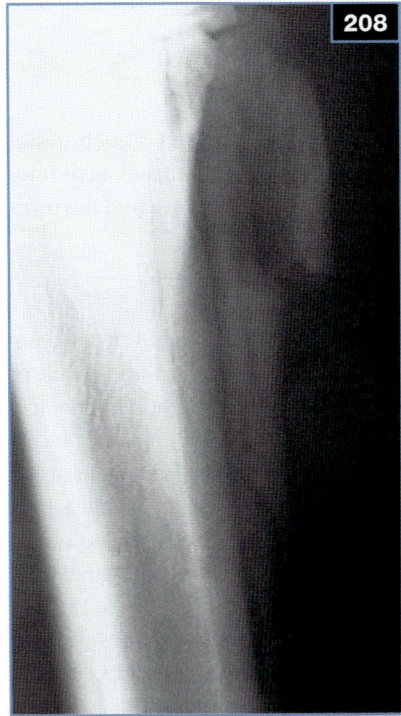

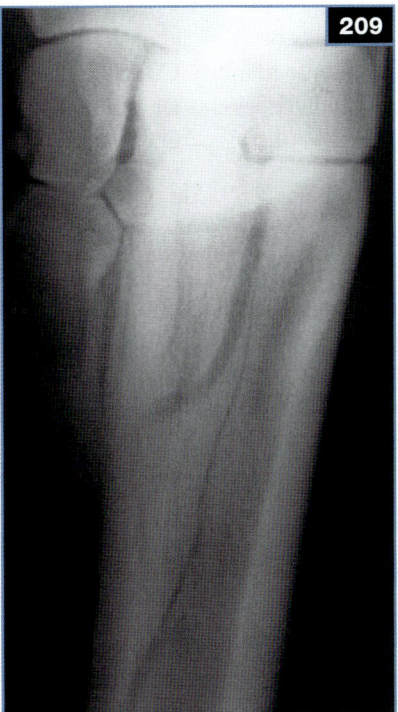

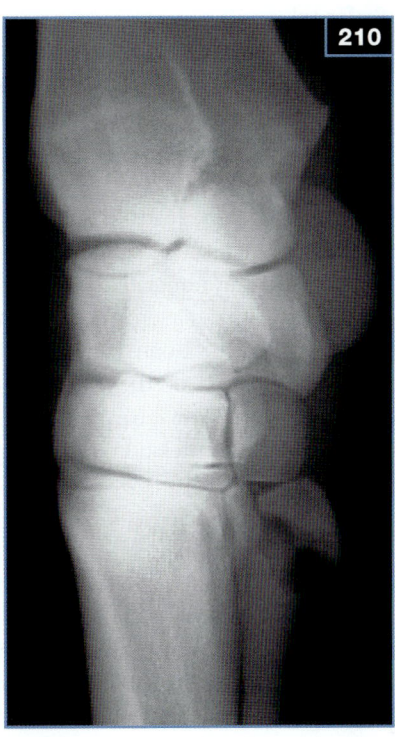

Management

Proximal splint bone fractures can be treated conservatively if minimally displaced and closed. Initial management of open, comminuted fractures may also involve conservative treatment. Surgical intervention is warranted in cases of open, comminuted, displaced fractures and/or if there is involvement of the articular surfaces. Removal of the affected portion distally is recommended and it is possible to remove the whole of MT IV, although careful assessment of other bony structures preoperatively is advised. Internal fixation is recommended if an articular component is present or the affected bone is unstable and unable to be removed. Lavage of the carpometacarpal/tarsometatarsal joints is indicated if sepsis is present.

Distal splint bone fractures can be treated conservatively and healing is monitored by radiography. Concurrent suspensory desmitis is also monitored ultrasonographically. Surgical amputation of the distal splint bone is recommended in cases of nonunion and/or persistent lameness.

Prognosis

Proximal fractures have a fair prognosis, although this worsens with joint involvement and the presence of infection. The prognosis for distal fractures is usually good, but this depends on the presence of concurrent injury to the suspensory ligament and/or the PSBs.

208 Dorsolateral/palmaromedial radiograph of the proximal cannon region of the case shown in 206. Note the comminuted fracture of MC IV, with displacement of part of the proximal fragment to the palmar aspect. (Photo courtesy GA Munroe)

209 Dorsomedial/palmarolateral radiograph of the same case as shown in 206 and 208. Note the nondisplaced fracture of the dorsolateral aspect of the proximal MC III. (Photo courtesy GA Munroe)

210 Dorsolateral/palmaromedial oblique radiograph of the proximal metacarpus showing displaced articular fracture of MC IV. This type of injury will require internal stabilization due to articular involvement of the carpometacarpal joint.

'Splints'

Definition/overview
'Splints' or exostosis of MC/MT II/IV are commonly found in horses and may or may not be associated with lameness.

Etiology/pathophysiology
Trauma to the bone leads to hemorrhage and lifting of the periosteum, with subsequent bone formation. Horses that 'dish' in front may traumatize MC II with the opposing forelimb. Damage to the interosseous ligament because of instability between the bones can lead to splints, especially between MC II and MC III. Young immature animals, especially those with bench carpal conformation (lateral positioning of MC III in relation to the carpus), are particularly predisposed.

Clinical presentation
In the acute phase, trauma will lead to swelling, pain, and lameness. In more chronic cases the soft-tissue swelling and edema may have subsided, leaving a firm, often non-painful fibrous/bony mass associated with the bone. Occasionally, axial impingement on the body of the suspensory ligament can lead to lameness. This may worsen with exercise and improve with rest and the splint becomes transiently 'active'.

Differential diagnosis
Fractures of MC/MT II/IV; soft-tissue trauma.

Diagnosis
Clinical examination is often sufficient to diagnose a splint, but local anesthetic infiltration may be required to assess its clinical relevance, especially in chronic cases. Radiography is important to assess size and potential interference with other structures and to rule out fractures (211). Ultrasonography may be required to assess the locality of the exostosis in relation to important soft-tissue structures such as the suspensory ligament.

Management
In cases of acute trauma or 'active' splints, rest, cold hosing/icing, and NSAIDs may be required. Local infiltration with corticosteroids may reduce soft-tissue inflammation in the short term. Extracorporeal shock-wave therapy has been used in some cases. In severe cases with axial impingement of the suspensory ligament, surgical removal/amputation may be attempted.

Prognosis
The prognosis is good with early treatment and correction of any underlying factors. Chronic cases tend to carry a fair-to-unfavorable prognosis and treatment may be palliative rather than curative.

Carpus

Carpal fractures

Definition/overview
Fractures covered in this section include osteochondral fragmentation (also known as 'chip' fractures), slab fractures, sagittal fractures, comminuted fractures, and fractures of the accessory carpal bone.

Etiology/pathophysiology
Although the clinical signs may be precipitated by an acute incident, osteochondral fragmentation is an end-result of stress adaptation and sclerosis of the subchondral bone. It is commonly seen on the medial aspect of the distal radial and/or proximal third carpal (C3) bones in the middle carpal joint of racehorses. Other locations include the lateral aspect of the distal radial and proximal radial/intermediate carpal bones in the antebrachiocarpal joint, and palmar osteochondral fragments from the accessory carpal bone.

Slab fractures of C3 have been shown to result from nonadaptive remodeling and may be preceded by subchondral lucencies and cartilage damage before a traumatic event causes fracture (commonly through the radial fossa of the bone). Other fractures usually have a traumatic origin.

Accessory carpal bone fractures are seen in horses undertaking jumping activities, with hyperextension causing intense loading on the bone and leading to frontal plane fractures (and occasionally comminuted), or from compression of the accessory carpal bone between the caudal radius and palmar MC III.

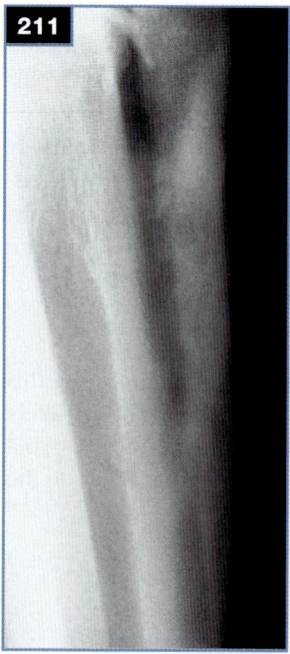

211 Dorsomedial/palmarolateral oblique radiograph of the proximal aspect of the cannon showing ossification of the interosseous space between MC III and MC II. This is a mature reaction and is nonpainful. (Photo courtesy GA Munroe)

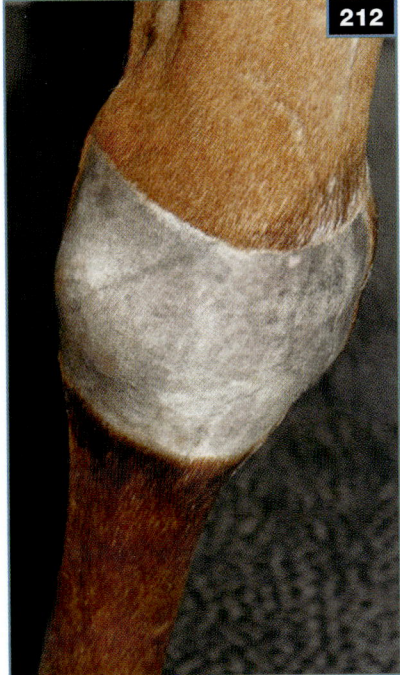

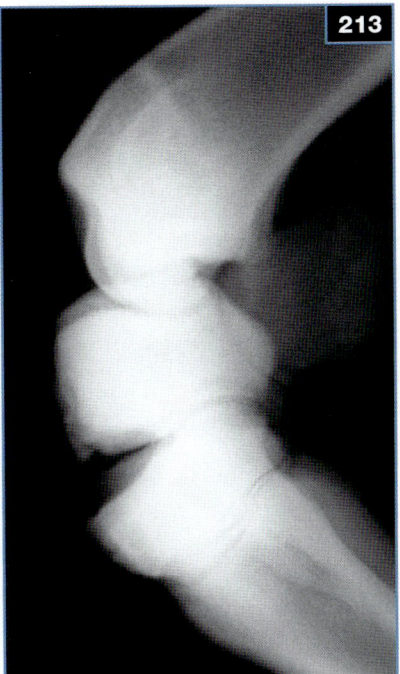

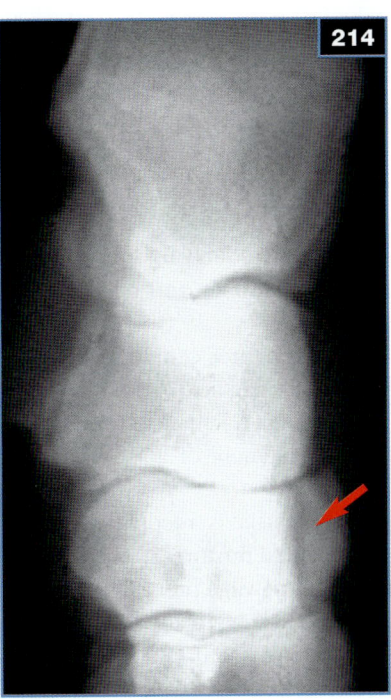

Clinical presentation

The horse usually presents with acute-onset lameness with joint effusion (212), and pain on carpal flexion and direct pressure over the affected bone. Horses with slab fractures are usually more lame, and comminuted fractures or multiple slab fractures affecting more than one row of carpal bones will present with severe lameness, possible carpal collapse, and ALD. Horses with accessory carpal bone fractures are usually severely lame (although on occasion, mildly lame) and tend to stand with a flexed stance. A carpal sheath effusion may be present in these cases.

Differential diagnosis

Intra-articular soft-tissue injuries (e.g. medial palmar inter-carpal ligament (MPICL) damage); extensor tendon sheath tenosynovitis; OA; carpal canal syndrome.

Diagnosis

Full radiographic assessment of the carpus is important with carpal fractures. Small osteochondral fragments will be evident in the joint, usually close to or still attached to the parent bone (213). It is important to check for the possibility of slab fractures in cases of osteochondral fragmentation. Dorsoproximal dorsodistal ('skyline') views (214) are essential for assessing the dorsal aspect of the carpal bones and for the diagnosis of sagittal fractures of C3 (usually involving the radial fossa). Scintigraphy may be more sensitive in incomplete fractures in some cases. If a slab fracture is diagnosed (215), it is important to check all the remaining carpal bones for the possibility of more

212 This horse has a distension of the antebrachiocarpal joint due to chronic osteochondral chip fractures of the distal radius. (Photo courtesy GA Munroe)

213 Flexed lateromedial radiograph of the carpus showing fragmentation of the distal aspect of the radial carpal bone. Note the bony remodeling over the dorsal aspect of the bone.

214 Lateromedial radiograph of the carpus showing a mildly displaced slab fracture of C3 (arrow).

215 Dorsal 55° proximal dorsodistal oblique ('skyline') radiographic view of the proximal row of carpal bones showing a nondisplaced fracture of the intermediate carpal bone (arrow).

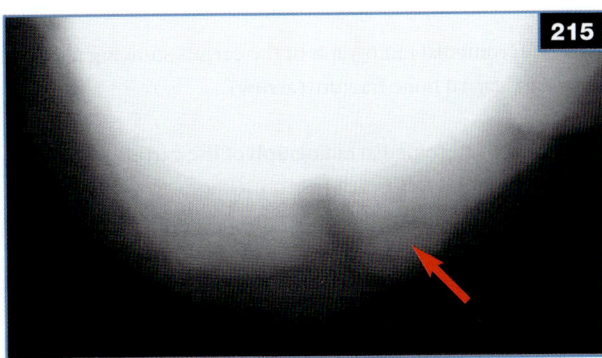

than one fracture. Horses with multiple slab fractures or comminuted fractures need full and accurate assessment of the affected bone(s). Radiography with reduced exposure factors highlights accessory carpal bone fractures (**216**).

Management

Arthroscopic removal of osteochondral fragments is advised to reduce further joint damage and to assess the joint surfaces and intercarpal ligaments (especially MPICL).

Slab fractures can be removed (if less than 8 mm) or repaired by lag screw fixation (**217**), guided arthroscopically. Sagittal fractures of C3 can be treated conservatively or by placement of a screw across the fracture line by arthrotomy.

Euthanasia is recommended with multiple slab or comminuted fractures. Rarely, carpal arthrodesis is undertaken as a salvage procedure.

Conservative treatment is recommended for accessory carpal bone fractures, as large forces act on any internal fixation device, leading to implant failure and loosening. These fractures heal by fibrous union, although any fragmentation in the palmar aspect of the radiocarpal bone may require arthroscopic removal.

Prognosis

The prognosis following osteochondral fragment removal is good, but is related to the degree of cartilage, bone, and/or intercarpal ligament damage as assessed arthroscopically. Slab fractures have a fair to guarded prognosis, but again the outcome depends on the presence of cartilage and bone damage. Sagittal fractures carry a guarded prognosis if treated conservatively, although some heal by fibrous union; however, this is improved with internal fixation. Comminuted carpal fractures have a guarded to poor prognosis and are often accompanied by secondary complications. Fractures of the accessory carpal bone have a good prognosis, although carpal canal syndrome and tenosynovitis may persist.

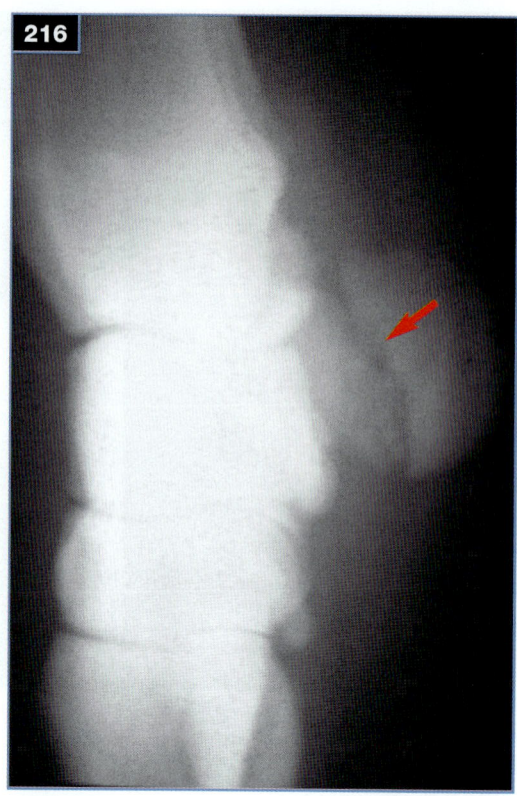

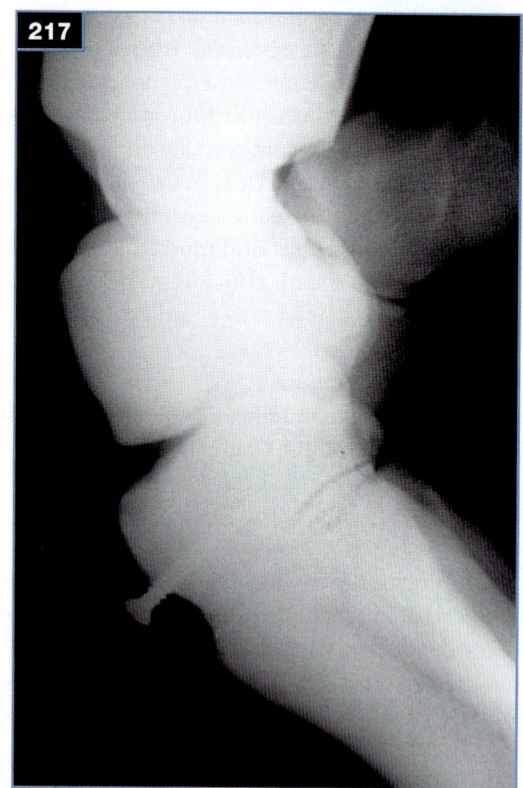

216 Lateromedial radiograph of the carpus showing an accessory carpal bone fracture (arrow).

217 Flexed lateromedial radiograph of the carpus following internal fixation of a C3 slab fracture. (Photo courtesy J Kidd)

218 Carpal sheath distension in the right foreleg. Note the golf-ball-sized swelling proximal lateral to the carpus (arrow). (Photo courtesy GA Munroe)

219 Lateromedial radiograph showing a caudally located osteochondroma (arrow) on the distal radius. (Photo courtesy J Kidd)

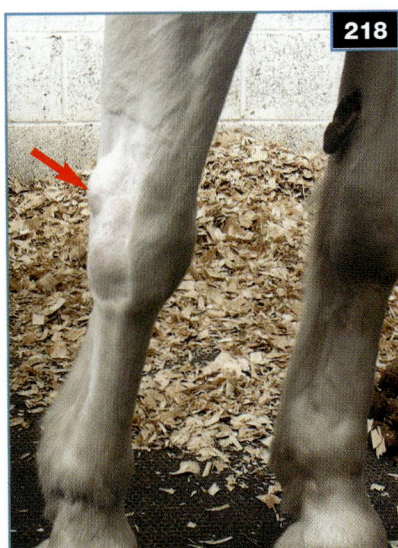

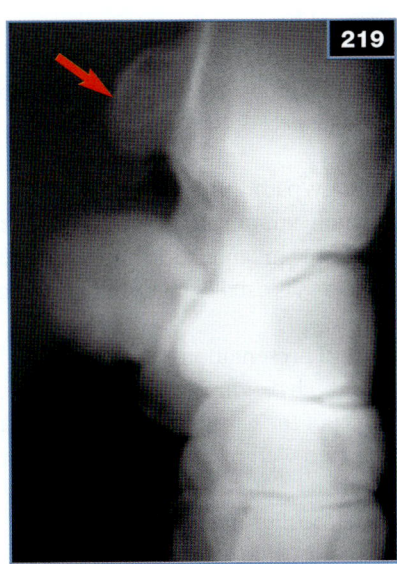

Carpal canal syndrome

Definition/overview
Carpal canal syndrome relates to a number of conditions resulting in a constrictive action on the carpal canal and its contents. These include tenosynovitis of the carpal canal, SDFT or deep digital flexor tendon (DDFT) tendonitis, desmitis of the accessory ligament of the superficial digital flexor tendon (ALSDFT), accessory carpal bone fractures, and osteochondroma.

Etiology/pathophysiology
The carpal canal contains the SDFT and the DDFT as they continue distally to the palmar metacarpus and is bounded dorsally by the palmar carpal ligament, medially by the ALSDFT, laterally by the accessory carpal bone (ACB), and palmarly by the flexor retinaculum and caudal antebrachial fascia. It contains a synovial lining and runs from approximately 7–10 cm proximal to the antebrachiocarpal joint to the proximal metacarpus. Damage to any of these structures can lead to inflammation and pressure on the remaining structures and associated nerve supply, causing pain.

Clinical presentation
Carpal sheath distension is commonly detected in carpal canal syndrome (218). Pain and lameness may be present in acute conditions, although in chronic cases, thickening and filling of the sheath may be palpated with minimal lameness.

Differential diagnosis
Carpal joint diseases; carpal fractures.

Diagnosis
Intrathecal analgesia may be required to localize the syndrome. Synoviocentesis of the carpal canal is required to rule out sepsis. Radiography is important for diagnosing ACB fractures and osteochondroma (219). Ultrasonography is used to examine the ALSDFT, SDFT, DDFT, carpal canal lining, and associated soft-tissue structures surrounding the canal. Comparison with the structures on the contralateral limb is important in detecting true lesions.

Management
Idiopathic tenosynovitis may respond to rest and controlled exercise with intrathecal hyaluronan and/or corticosteroids. Endoscopy of the canal may be required for chronic tenosynovitis. Hemorrhage into the canal from trauma or secondary to fracture may be relieved by drainage, while injection of hyaluronan reduces the risk of adhesions forming. Rest and controlled exercise are advised for ALSDFT desmitis, although the recovery time can be prolonged. Chronic SDFT tendonitis may require desmotomy of the ALSDFT and release of the carpal fascia. Tears in the DDFT within the canal may need to be debrided endoscopically. Removal of an osteochondroma by arthroscopy is recommended, with debridement of any secondarily damaged tissue. Accessory carpal bone fractures respond well to conservative therapy.

Prognosis
The prognosis depends on the cause of the syndrome. Acute tenosynovitis without any underlying complications usually responds well to treatment. Chronicity and presence of adhesions will worsen the outcome. Desmitis and tendonitis within the canal will worsen the prognosis. The prognosis is usually fair to good for accessory carpal bone fractures and osteochondroma.

Carpal hygroma
Definition/overview
Carpal hygroma refers to a subcutaneous swelling over the dorsal aspect of the carpus (220).

Etiology/pathophysiology
Repetitive trauma to the dorsal aspect of the carpus leads to chronic inflammation and a fluid-filled structure forms. Lameness is usually minimal unless it becomes infected.

Clinical presentation
A fluid-filled, nonpainful, fluctuant swelling over the dorsal aspect of the carpus is present. Full carpal flexion may be restricted with marked soft-tissue swelling. If the hygroma is infected, the swelling may be more pronounced, with serous oozing and pain present.

220 This horse has formed a carpal hygroma over the dorsal aspect due to persistent trauma. (Photo courtesy GA Munroe)

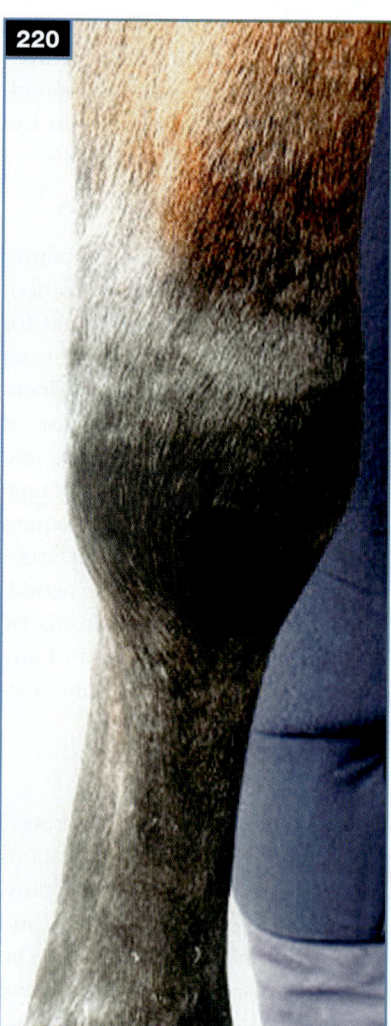

Differential diagnosis
Extensor tenosynovitis; joint distension/herniation.

Diagnosis
Careful clinical palpation and knowledge of anatomy are required to differentiate carpal hygroma from effusions of the extensor tendon or carpal joints. Ultrasonography is useful for examining the hygroma and other nearby structures and looking for the possibility of a foreign body. Radiography can rule out any bony involvement and contrast medium is used to investigate joint or tendon sheath involvement.

Management
Conservative treatment involves rest, local injections of steroids, drainage, and bandaging. Although in some cases these may resolve the swelling, conservative treatment is usually unsuccessful. Surgical treatment requires *en bloc* resection of the tissue, avoiding penetration of the extensor tendon sheaths or joint capsule, followed by a sleeve cast or Robert Jones bandage for 7–10 days.

Prognosis
The prognosis is guarded for complete resolution, as recurrence is common.

Other carpal joint diseases
Definition/overview
Remaining conditions involving the carpal joints include OA, MPICL damage, luxation, and OCLLs.

Etiology/pathophysiology
OA of the carpal joints can have a similar etiology to osteochondral fragmentation, although DJD can exist in the carpus without osteochondral fragments being present. The MPICL prevents dorsal displacement of the middle carpal joint and may be damaged in conjunction with other intercarpal joint disease or exist as an individual entity. Luxation of the carpal joints is usually due to trauma. OCLLs may be seen in the ulnar carpal bone or in C2 along with the presence of C1 and a cyst in the proximal aspect of MC II.

Clinical presentation
Lameness, carpal joint effusion, positive response to carpal flexion, and reduced range of motion are commonly present with OA. Lameness and middle carpal joint effusion are present with MPICL damage, especially when occurring with other middle carpal joint diseases. Horses with luxation of the carpal joint(s) are very lame, usually with an anatomic deviation present. OCLLs are usually incidental.

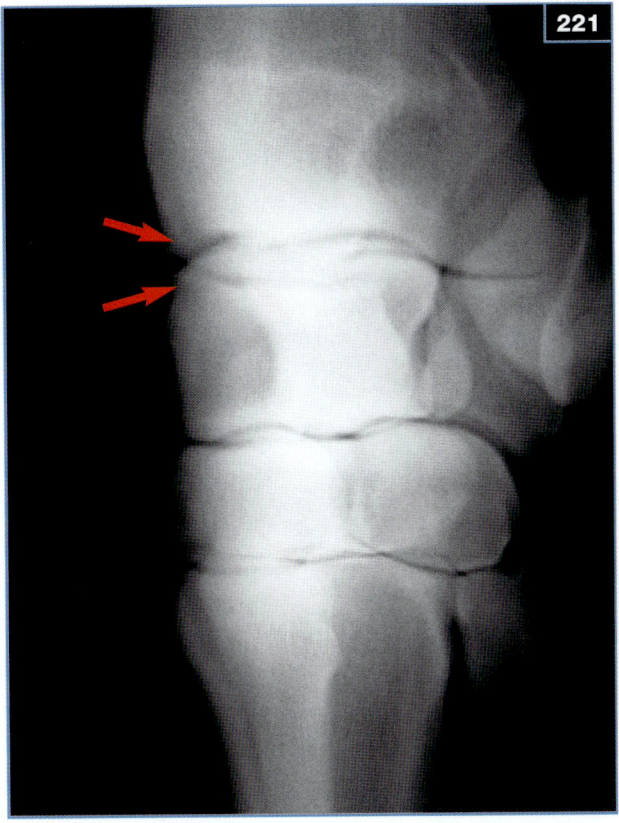

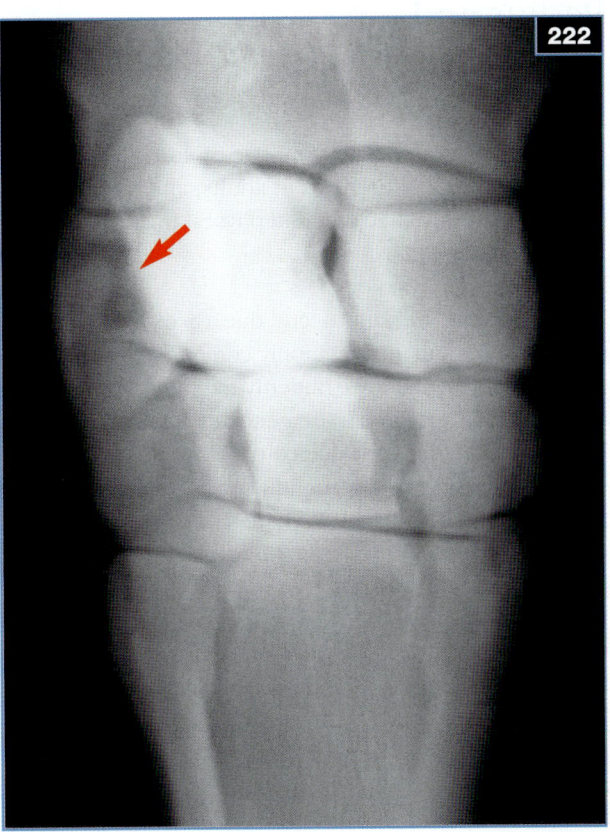

221 Dorsomedial/palmarolateral oblique radiograph of the carpus showing osteophytes present around the antebrachiocarpal joint (arrows).

222 Dorsopalmar radiograph of the carpus showing a radiolucent OCLL in the ulnar carpal bone (arrow).

Differential diagnosis
Carpal fractures; extensor carpi radialis (ECR) or common digital extensor (CDE) tenosynovitis; hygroma; carpal canal syndrome.

Diagnosis
Clinical examination, diagnostic analgesia, and radiography are used to diagnose OA in the carpus. Entheseophytes and osteophytes are usually present on the carpal bones/distal radius (**221**). Nuclear scintigraphy can be more sensitive in young racehorses with early OA. Arthroscopy is important for evaluation of the MPICL, other intercarpal ligaments, and for a general examination of the joint. A diagnosis of luxation is usually obvious from clinical examination, but stress radiography may be required. Radiography is also advisable for examining the carpal bones for the presence of concurrent fractures/avulsion injuries. OCLLs seen radiographically require diagnostic analgesia to determine their significance (**222**).

Management
Palliative treatment can be used for OA, revolving around an alteration to training regimens, NSAIDs, and intra-articular medication. If osteochondral fragments are present, removal by arthroscopy is recommended. In valuable breeding stock with severe OA, partial or pancarpal arthrodesis can be performed. Debridement of the MPICL can be performed arthroscopically and lesions can be graded I–IV. With luxation of the carpus, conservative treatment involves full limb casting for 3 months to allow fibrosis to occur. Alternatively, partial or panarthrodesis can be performed.

Prognosis
The prognosis for OA depends on the number of joints affected, the rate of progression, and the severity of cartilage damage (assessed and graded arthroscopically). The prognosis for MPICL injuries worsens with increasing severity of the lesion and presence of cartilage damage. Luxation of the carpus carries a guarded to poor prognosis, and fibrosis will often lead to restricted movement.

125

Radius and ulna

Radial fractures

Definition/overview
Radial fractures include incomplete or complete spiral or oblique diaphyseal fractures in adults, and transverse or oblique diaphyseal fractures and physeal fractures in foals.

Etiology/pathophysiology
Radial fractures usually occur due to external trauma such as a kick and are commonly comminuted with spiral or oblique configurations. Butterfly fragments may also be present. Fractures in foals are generally less comminuted. Transverse mid-diaphyseal fractures occur due to a cranial blow to the limb, whereas oblique ones result from lateral forces. Salter–Harris type I and type II fractures of the proximal physis can occur with ulnar fractures.

Clinical presentation
Complete diaphyseal fractures present with nonweight-bearing lameness, with instability and crepitus detectable. The horse often stands with the carpus and fetlock flexed, there is severe soft-tissue swelling around the antebrachium, and a wound is commonly present. Horses with incomplete or nondisplaced fractures are lame and may have a wound. Due to the muscular forces acting over the radius, there is a tendency for the limb to abduct. This increases the risk of a closed radial fracture becoming open, severely affecting the prognosis.

Differential diagnosis
Fractures of the humerus, ulna or carpus.

Diagnosis
Clinical examination should lead to a high index of suspicion. Radiography must include multiple views to delineate fracture lines and the presence of comminution (223). In nondisplaced or incomplete fractures, nuclear scintigraphy may be more sensitive if radiography does not yield conclusive results.

Management
In horses weighing less than 250 kg, open reduction and internal fixation may be possible. In adult horses, radial fracture repair is a greater challenge and often results in an unfavorable outcome and therefore euthanasia of the horse is recommended. First aid involves immobilization using caudal and lateral splints with a full-limb Robert Jones bandage. The lateral splint should extend to the mid-scapula to prevent abduction of the limb (224). Incomplete or nondisplaced fractures can respond well to 3–4 months box rest, although some become unstable. Cross-tying the horse to prevent it lying down and getting up is often recommended.

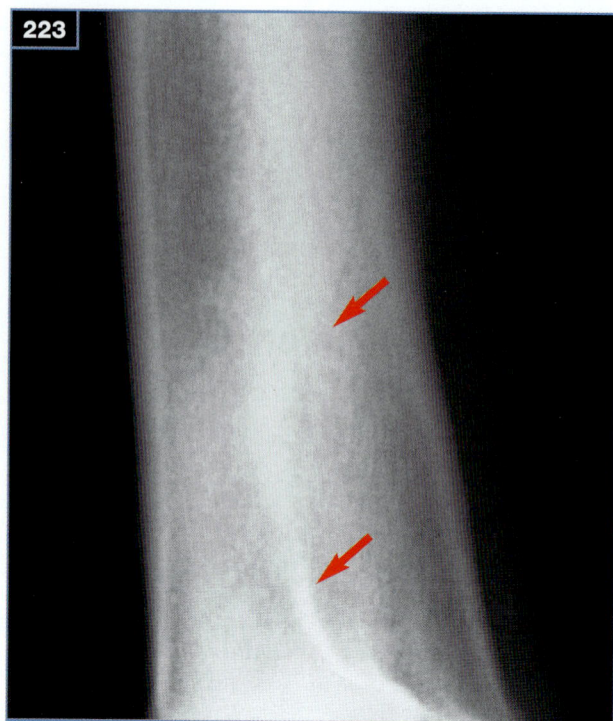

223 Craniomedial/caudolateral oblique radiograph of the mid-radius of a horse with an incomplete Y-shaped radial fracture (arrows). Note the sclerosis accompanying the fracture lines.

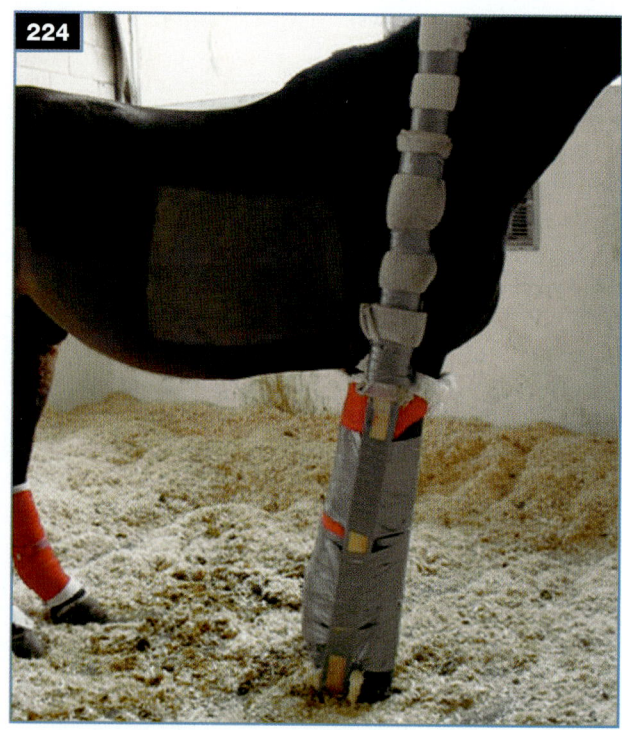

224 Full-limb Robert Jones bandage on a horse with an incomplete radial fracture. Note that the lateral splint extends to the proximal scapula.

For successful surgical reconstruction, the caudal cortex of the radius needs to be intact. Double plate fixation spanning the entire radius is recommended. Complications are common, with infection/implant failure and contralateral limb problems occurring following repair.

Foals less than 6 months of age with simple transverse mid-diaphyseal fractures can be repaired with a single plate, provided the caudal cortex is intact. Other diaphyseal fractures are amenable to double plate fixation. Where Salter–Harris types I and II fractures accompany ulna fractures, the repair of the ulna fracture can be used to engage the radius.

Prognosis
The prognosis is guarded or hopeless in adults, especially if displaced. Nondisplaced fractures carry a fair prognosis if identified early and treated appropriately. The prognosis following radial fracture repair in foals is generally superior to that in adults, although contralateral limb complications can occur.

Ulna fractures
Definition/overview
There are five types of ulna fracture in the horse (225 and *Table 4*).

Etiology/pathophysiology
Usually due to a kick or a fall, but occasionally occuring during fast exercise.

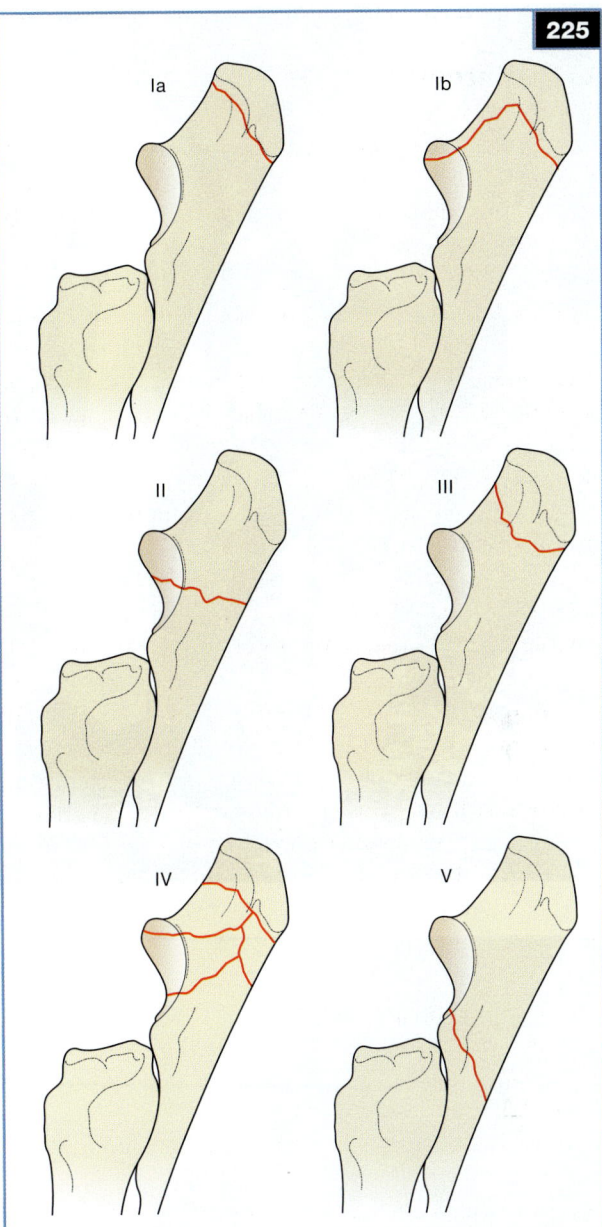

225 Schematic diagram of proximal ulna fracture classification. (See *Table 4* for description.)

TYPE	DESCRIPTION
Ia	Nonarticular fracture involving separation of the proximal ulnar physis, seen in young foals.
Ib	Articular fracture through the proximal ulnar physis and metaphysis, entering the joint near to the anconeal process. Seen in older foals.
II	Simple transverse fracture entering the elbow joint at the mid-point of the trochlear notch.
III	Nonarticular fracture across the olecranon, proximal to the anconeal process.
IV	Comminuted, articular fracture.
V	Distal caudal fracture of the olecranon/ulnar shaft, traversing proximally and cranially to enter the distal aspect of the trochlear notch.

TABLE 4 **Classification of ulna fractures**

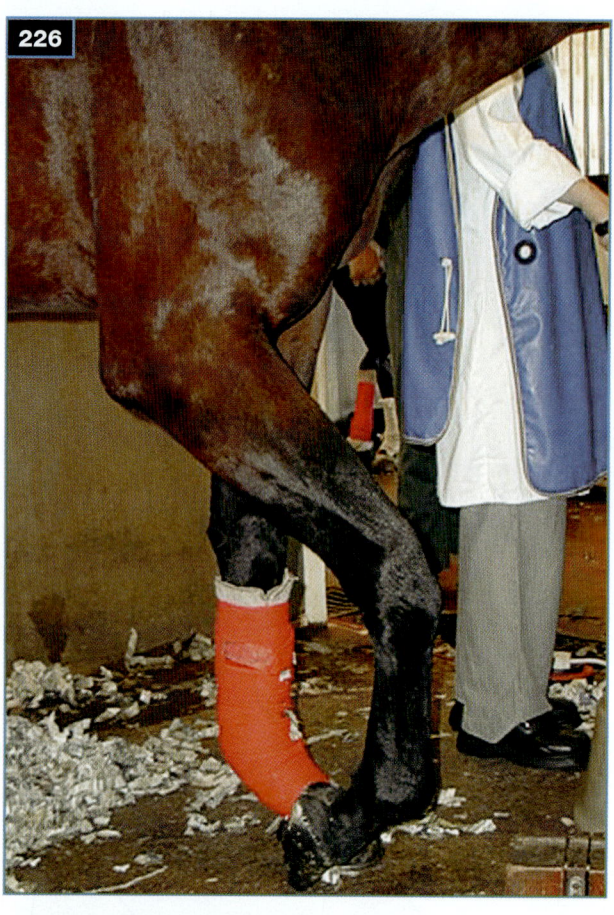

226

226 Ulna fracture in a mature horse. The horse will often stand with its elbow dropped and the carpus in a semi-flexed position due to pain and loss of the stay apparatus.

227 Mediolateral radiograph of the elbow showing a type II articular ulna fracture. (Photo courtesy J Kidd)

228 Mediolateral radiograph of the elbow. A contoured plate has been placed on the caudal aspect of the ulna to stabilize the fracture site. (Photo courtesy J Kidd)

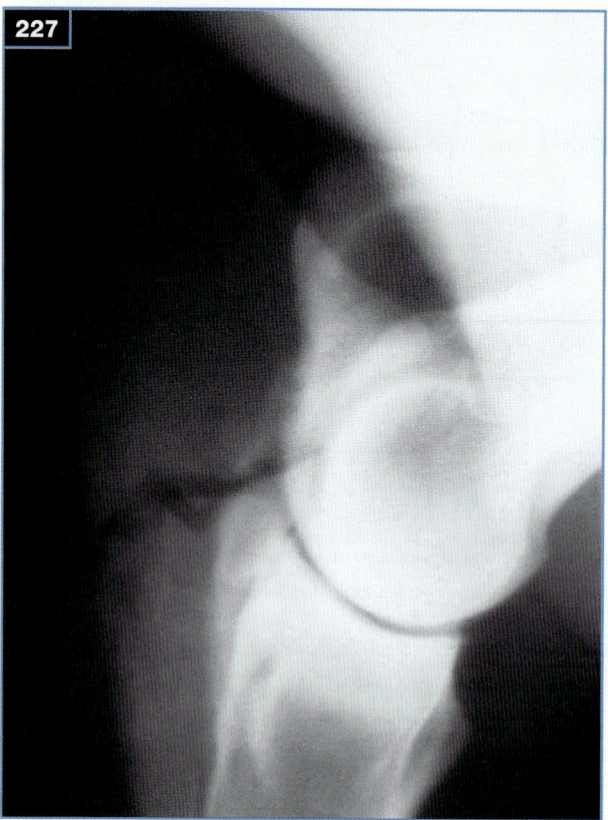

227

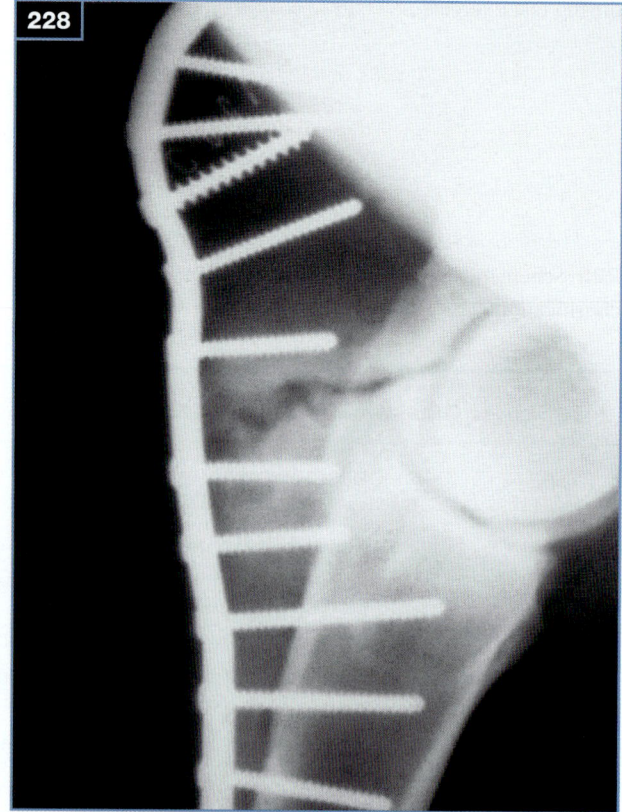

228

Clinical presentation

Due to the loss of the stay apparatus, the elbow drops and the horse will stand with its carpus flexed in a partially nonweight-bearing position (226). Soft-tissue swelling and crepitus can be detected.

Differential diagnosis

Humeral and radial fractures; radial neuropathy.

Diagnosis

Clinical examination and history should point towards the possibility of an ulna fracture. Good radiographs are important for diagnosis and for producing a management plan. A medial-to-lateral projection provides the most information (227).

Management

First aid management involves appropriate treatment of any wounds present. Splinting the carpus into extension can help support the limb. Conservative treatment can be used for types III and V (nondisplaced, nonarticular), but the rate of recovery can be slow and therefore surgical repair can be advantageous. Open reduction and internal fixation are recommended for articular or displaced fractures. The tension band principle is applied by placement of a contoured plate to the caudal ulna or the use of tension band wire fixation (228). Pin and wiring can be used in foals under 6 months old, where plating may affect growth, and in animals weighing less than 250 kg. For successful surgical repair it is important not to place the screws through the concave medial cortex in the proximal fragment, penetrate the joint space, or engage the caudal cortex of the radius in animals up to 18 months old.

Prognosis

The prognosis is usually favorable for internal fixation, especially type II. The prognosis worsens with comminution (leads to DJD) and presence of infection. Type V fractures respond well to conservative treatment given time.

Osteochondroma (supracarpal volar exostosis)

Definition/overview

Osteochondromas are benign, cartilage-capped, osseous projections, commonly involving the distal radius in adult horses.

Etiology/pathophysiology

Osteochondromas may form from aberrant cartilage and undergo endochondral ossification to form multiple cartilaginous exostoses. Due to their location in the carpal canal, an effusion develops and damage to the DDFT can occur.

Clinical presentation

The horse presents with tenosynovitis of the carpal sheath and a variable lameness. Pain may be evident on palpation and from carpal flexion.

Differential diagnosis

See Carpal canal syndrome, p. 123.

Diagnosis

Radiography shows exostosis present, with variable ossification, continuous with the caudal distal radius (see 219). Ultrasonographic assessment of the DDFT is advised.

Management

Intrathecal corticosteroids may lead to a temporary resolution of signs. Removal of the mass is a more definitive treatment and can be undertaken via an open approach or endoscopically. Endoscopic evaluation of the carpal sheath is recommended to check for damage to structures such as the DDFT within the sheath.

Prognosis

The prognosis following removal is good.

Elbow

Hygroma at point of the elbow

Definition/overview
Hygroma of the elbow or 'capped elbow' refers to a non-painful swelling over the point of the elbow.

Etiology/pathophysiology
Hygromas are fluid-filled, acquired subcutaneous bursae caused by repetitive trauma and inflammation. With chronicity, they may become more fibrous than fluid like. Horses with a high action may catch themselves with the shoe of the ipsilateral forelimb. Hygromas can also occur in horses that lie down regularly.

Clinical presentation
The mass is usually nonpainful and not associated with lameness, although it can become infected and therefore be more swollen, painful, and ooze pus.

Differential diagnosis
Ulna fractures; soft-tissue trauma.

Diagnosis
Clinical presentation is usually sufficient for a diagnosis (229). Ultrasonography can be used to delineate the mass, especially when contemplating removal.

Management
Most cases are cosmetic and are not treated, although correction of any underlying cause should be instigated. Drainage and placement of a Penrose drain may resolve some cases. *En-bloc* dissection can be attempted, but wound breakdown is common in this region.

Prognosis
Where surgical resection is undertaken the risk of dehiscence is increased following recovery from general anesthesia, making the prognosis unfavorable in such cases.

Elbow joint diseases

Definition/overview
Elbow joint conditions covered in this section include OA, OCLLs, collateral ligament injury, and elbow luxation.

Etiology/pathophysiology
OA is unusual in the elbow and tends to occur in the older horse. OCLLs are usually found in the medial proximal radius and, less commonly, the distal humerus. Collateral ligament injuries are the result of trauma and, if severe, may lead to joint capsule damage and OA. Luxation of the elbow is seen with severe trauma, often in conjunction with a fracture of the olecranon and/or proximal radius.

Clinical presentation
Horses with OA of the elbow can present with a variable lameness. Joint effusion is usually not palpable. OCLLs may present with severe acute-onset lameness that may vary between examinations. Acute collateral ligament injuries present with swelling around the elbow and resentment to elbow manipulation. Elbow luxation causes a severe lameness, swelling, and anatomic derangements.

Differential diagnosis
Shoulder joint conditions.

Diagnosis
Intra-articular analgesia may localize the lameness associated with conditions of the elbow joint, although only partial improvement may be seen. Radiography is an important diagnostic tool and examination of both elbows is advised. Ultrasonography and occasionally scintigraphy can also be used for diagnosis of collateral ligament injury. Stress radiography of the elbow is required for the diagnosis of elbow luxation.

Management
Palliative treatment is recommended for OA of the elbow. Intra-articular medication may improve the condition. Conservative treatment involving intra-articular hyaluronan and corticosteroids can lead to resolution of clinical signs in some cases of OCLLs. Extra-articular curettage of the cyst leads to improvement in cysts in the medial proximal radius, although results are more disappointing in distal humeral cysts. Mild collateral ligament injuries may improve following controlled exercise for at least 3 months. More severe cases often result in persistent lameness and OA. Surgical repair for elbow luxation often has a poor outcome and euthanasia is advised.

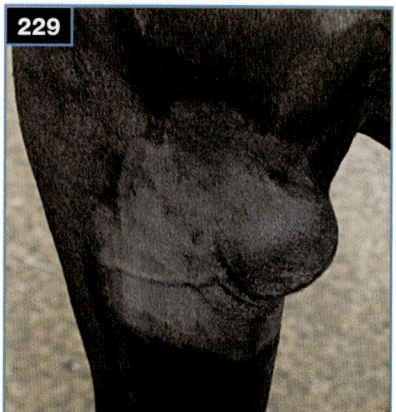

229

229 Chronic subcutaneous bursa in the left foreleg over the point of the elbow. (Photo courtesy GA Munroe)

Musculoskeletal system

Prognosis
The prognosis is guarded for OA of the elbow. A variable outcome is seen with OCD lesions of the elbow, but surgical treatment carries a generally better prognosis than conservative treatment in most cases. A good prognosis is seen for mild collateral ligament injuries, but this is markedly reduced with more severe injuries and capsular tears, leading to DJD of the joint. Luxation carries a poor prognosis.

Humerus and scapula

Humeral fractures
Definition/overview
Fractures of the humerus covered in this section include diaphyseal fractures, fractures of the deltoid tuberosity, and stress fractures.

Etiology/pathophysiology
Trauma can lead to oblique, spiral, or severely comminuted diaphyseal fractures and fractures of the deltoid tuberosity.

Stress fractures of the humerus occur in young Thoroughbreds in intense training on the proximocaudal and/or distal cranial/caudal humerus (230).

Clinical presentation
Diaphyseal fractures present as severe, acute-onset lameness with marked swelling (231), pain, and crepitus. The elbow may be dropped due to loss of the stay apparatus and the horse may rest weight on the toe only. Fractures of the deltoid tuberosity can be acute and painful, although in chronic cases, deep palpation over the deltoid tuberosity may be required to elicit pain. Young Thoroughbreds in training with stress fractures usually develop an acute-onset lameness that can resolve quickly. Pain may be elicited with direct pressure over the regions involved. These fractures may occur soon after returning to exercise after a period of rest.

Differential diagnosis
Ulna fracture; scapula fracture; triceps myopathy; radial neuropathy.

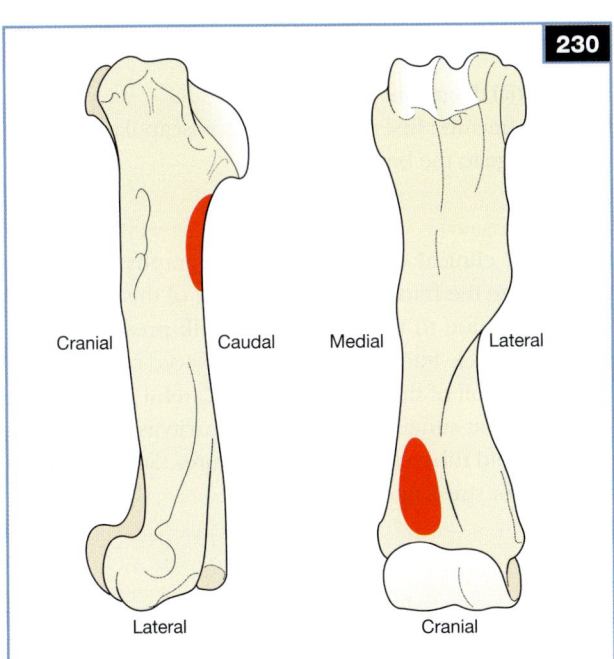

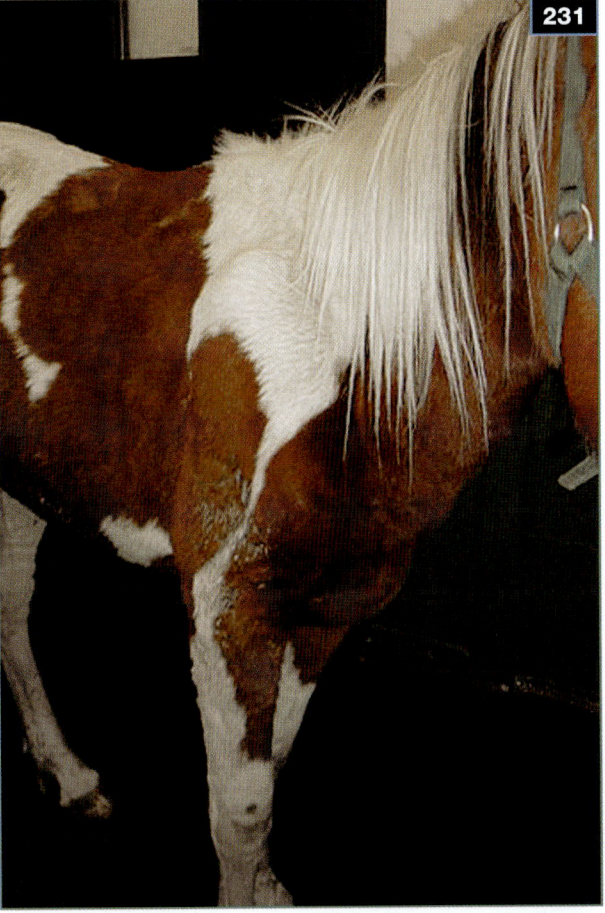

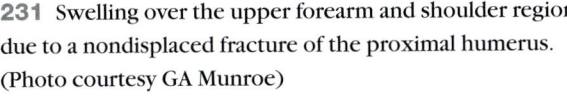

230 Schematic drawing of the equine humerus showing the common locations of stress fractures.

231 Swelling over the upper forearm and shoulder region due to a nondisplaced fracture of the proximal humerus. (Photo courtesy GA Munroe)

131

The forelimb

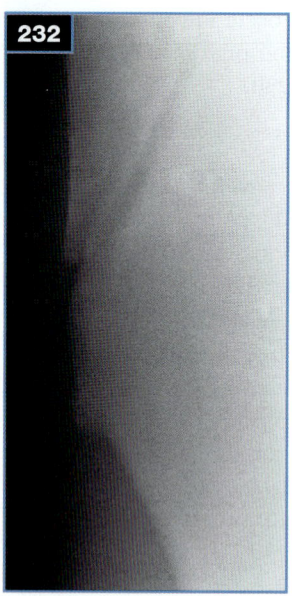

232

232 Lateromedial radiograph of the proximal humerus of the case in 231 showing a nondisplaced fracture starting at the deltoid tuberosity and running proximocaudal towards the shoulder joint. (Photo courtesy GA Munroe)

Scapula fractures

Definition/overview
Included in this section are fractures of the supraglenoid tubercle, fractures of the body of the scapula, and spine and stress fractures.

Etiology/pathophysiology
Apart from stress fractures, fractures of the scapula are usually the result of external trauma such as a fall at speed, collision, or a kick. Supraglenoid tubercle fractures occur through the original physis and may be simple or comminuted. They are more common in animals less than 2 years of age. Scapula body fractures may involve the articular surface and be complete or incomplete. Fractures of the spine of the scapula occur from kicks and can lead to sequestra formation. Stress fractures of the scapula reflect nonadaptive remodeling due to intense training (**233**).

Clinical presentation
Most fractures lead to an acute-onset severe lameness. With chronic fractures of the supraglenoid tubercle, neurogenic atrophy of the supraspinatus and infraspinatus muscles can occur, with suprascapular nerve involvement (**234**). Marked soft-tissue swelling, pain, and crepitus are often present. With fractures of the spine, a discharging tract from a sequestrum may form with time. Stress fractures may result in overt lameness or reduction in performance.

Diagnosis
Diaphyseal fractures usually show severe clinical signs. Deltoid tuberosity fractures may require scintigraphy for localization and radiography for configuration (longitudinal or incomplete oblique) (**232**). Stress fractures of the humerus are sensitive to nuclear scintigraphy. Radiography may reveal new bone on the caudal aspect of the proximal epiphysis or cranial aspect of the distal metaphysis/physis, suggesting previous remodeling has occurred.

Differential diagnosis
Humeral fracture; first rib fracture; suprascapular neuropathy; damage to the brachial plexus.

Diagnosis
Following clinical examination, radiography is used to characterize the fracture (**235**). Imaging of this region can be difficult due to the large tissue bulk present. Supraglenoid tubercle fractures are often displaced craniodistally due to the pull of the biceps brachii. Careful examination of the articular surface on the glenoid cavity is important in supraglenoid tubercle and body fractures. Scintigraphy is sensitive for stress fractures.

Management
Incomplete humeral fractures may respond to prolonged rest. Complete diaphyseal fractures are poor candidates for repair and in the adult require euthanasia. Repairs have been undertaken in horses less than 3 years of age. Nondisplaced deltoid tuberosity fractures respond well to rest. Displaced fractures have been successfully repaired by internal fixation. Removal of infected or open deltoid tuberosity fractures has been achieved by standing surgery. Thoroughbreds in training with stress fractures of the humerus should undergo walking exercise for 3 months before a gradual return to exercise.

Prognosis
The prognosis is hopeless in complete and/or open diaphyseal fractures in adult horses and guarded to poor if reduction and stabilization are attempted, as implant failure is high. Nondisplaced deltoid tuberosity fractures carry a good prognosis and a favorable prognosis in displaced fractures following reduction without complications. Stress fractures carry a good prognosis if correct management is instigated.

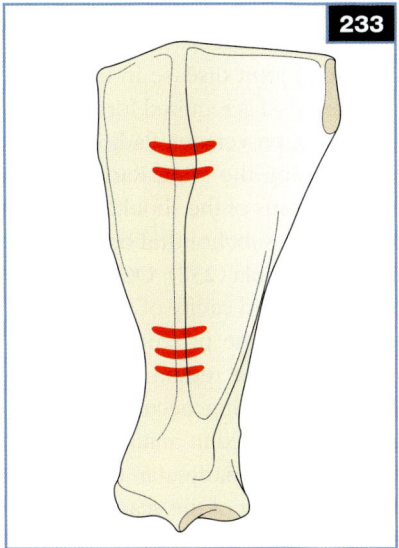

233 Schematic drawing of the equine scapula showing the location of stress fracture sites.

234 Supra- and infraspinatus muscle atrophy in an Arab stallion that was kicked on the point of the right shoulder while covering a mare, and developed a suprascapular nerve paralysis. (Photo courtesy GA Munroe)

235 Craniocaudal radiograph showing a complete nonarticular scapula body fracture (arrows).

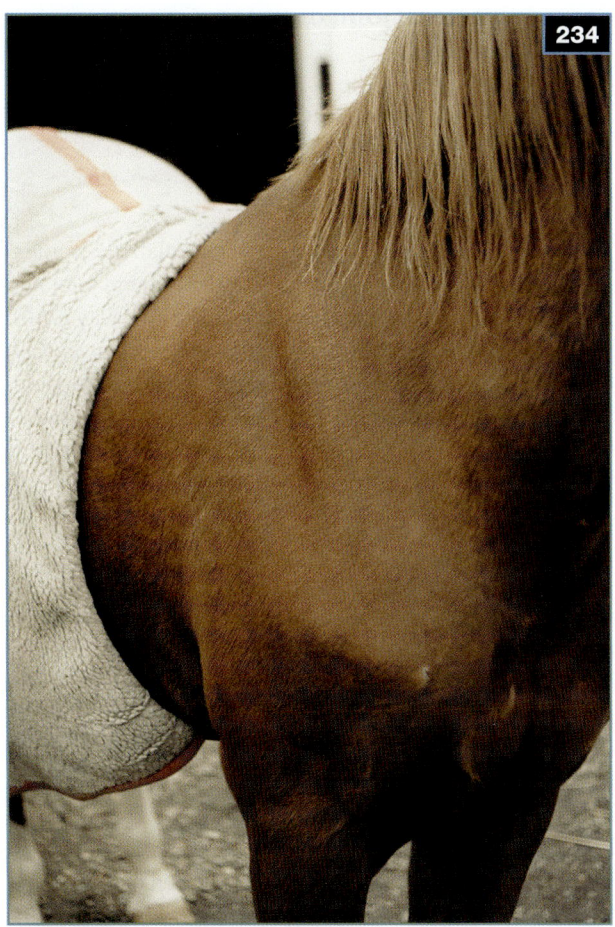

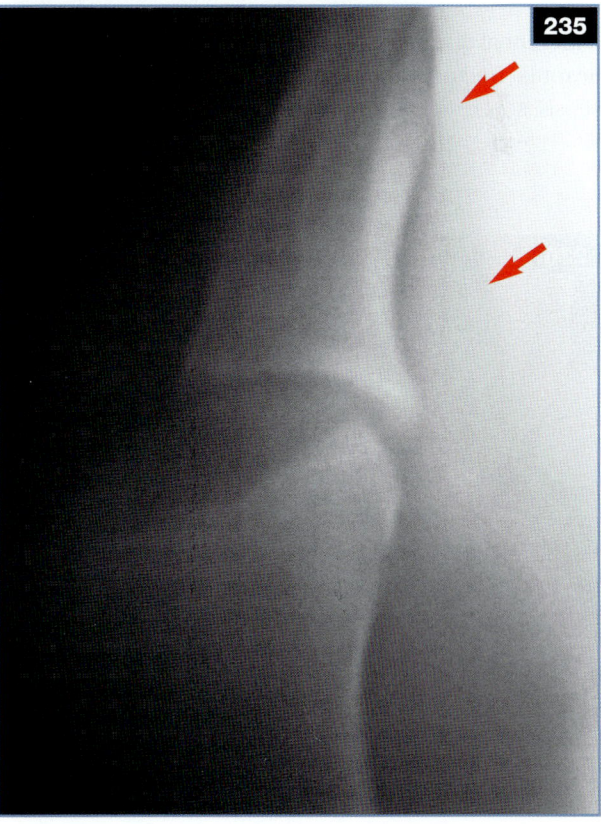

Management
Conservative treatment of supraglenoid tubercle fractures often leads to a poor outcome and DJD rapidly ensues. In acute cases, internal fixation involving lag screws and tension band wiring may be successful, but large distracting forces on the implants may lead to failure. Incomplete, nonarticular fractures of the body of the scapula can respond well to conservative treatment. Complete and/or articular involvement requires euthanasia. Removal of sequestra from fractures of the spine is recommended. Rest and alteration to exercise regimens often resolve problems associated with stress fractures of the scapula.

Prognosis
A poor outcome is associated with conservative treatment of supraglenoid fractures and the prognosis is generally unfavorable if surgery and stabilization are attempted. The prognosis is good for nonarticular body fractures, poor with articular involvement, and good for spinal fractures. The outcome for stress fractures is favorable if diagnosed early and managed correctly.

Scapulohumeral joint diseases

Definition/overview

Conditions involving the scapulohumeral joint include osteochondritis dissecans, OCLLs, OA, dysplasia, and luxation.

Etiology/pathophysiology

Miniature breeds (e.g. Shetland ponies, Falabella ponies) have a predilection for OA of the scapulohumeral joint and this may be related to dysplasia of the glenoid cavity (236). In non-miniature breeds, OA can be secondary to OCD, intra-articular fractures, or trauma to the joint capsule. Scapulohumeral dysplasia has been shown to be due to flattening of the radius of curvature of the glenoid cavity of the scapula. Luxation of the shoulder tends to occur laterally and is seen more often in ponies.

Clinical presentation

Osteochondritis dissecans of the shoulder presents in older foals/yearlings. Moderate/severe lameness may lead to muscle atrophy and flexural deformity of the DIP joint. OCLLs tend to occur in slightly older horses (1–3 year olds) and signs may be precipitated by a traumatic accident. A variable moderate to severe lameness may be present between examinations. OA in miniature breeds can cause a sudden-onset severe lameness. Pain is identified on manipulation of the upper forelimb. Extensive swelling and a reluctance to bear weight are seen with scapulohumeral joint luxation.

Differential diagnosis

Scapula fractures; humeral fractures; bicipital bursitis; sepsis; severe joint sprain.

Diagnosis

History, signalment, and clinical examination may lead to a suspicion of scapulohumeral joint disease in the horse. However, intra-articular analgesia is required for diagnosis and generally leads to some improvement. Radiography is an important tool in examining the joint. Radiographic signs of osteochondritis dissecans of the shoulder include flattening of articular surfaces, subchondral bone lucencies, and remodeling of the scapula (237). OCLLs tend to occur in the middle of the glenoid cavity of the scapula, but occasionally are present in the proximal humerus. Nuclear scintigraphy may show a region of increased uptake with active bony remodeling occurring. Radiographic signs of OA can be advanced in miniature ponies when diagnosed and include periarticular osteophyte formation and marked remodeling of the scapula. Occasionally, fragmentation may be present and the glenoid cavity should be examined for evidence of flattening and dysplasia. Radiographs should be taken in cases of luxation to check for concurrent fractures.

Management

Debridement of the lesion is recommended for osteochondritis dissecans of the scapulohumeral joint, although success is reduced with large lesions and the presence of secondary OA. Intra-articular hyaluranon and corticosteroids may resolve clinical signs associated with an OCLL of the joint. Surgical curettage may be feasible, although this depends on the size and location of the cyst. Palliative treatment including rest and NSAIDs is recommended for OA. Simple, acute luxations can be reduced manually under general anesthesia, with the assumption that periarticular fibrosis will help to stabilize the joint.

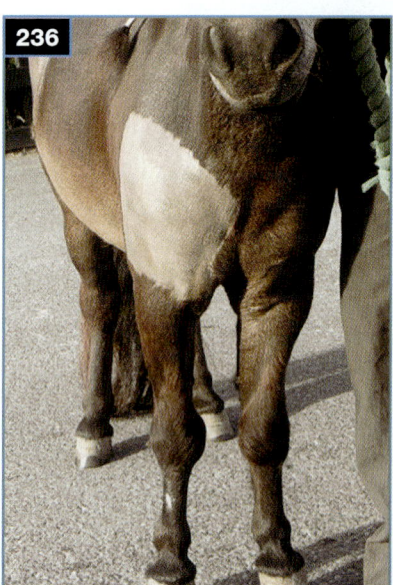

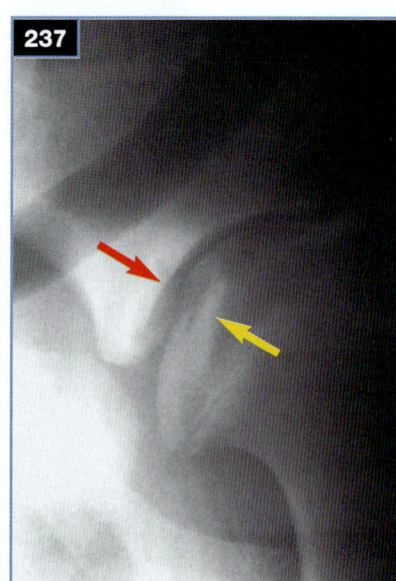

236 An 8-year-old miniature Shetland pony with a chronic right foreleg lameness localized to the scapulohumeral joint by intra-articular analgesia. Note the marked wastage of the muscles of the RF shoulder and forearm brisket.

237 Lateromedial radiograph of the scapulohumeral joint showing OCD lesions on the caudal humeral head (yellow arrow) and the caudal glenoid cavity (red arrow). (Photos courtesy GA Munroe)

Prognosis

The prognosis is poor for conservative treatment of osteochondritis dissecans in the shoulder and although surgical treatment carries a better prognosis, the outcome is usually unfavorable in the long term. Small OCLL lesions have been successfully treated, but the prognosis is guarded for large active ones. OA and dysplasia of the shoulder carry a guarded prognosis. Shoulder luxations have an unfavorable prognosis and often re-luxate. Concurrent intra-articular fractures worsen the prognosis further.

Intertubercular (bicipital) bursitis

Definition/overview

Intertubercular bursitis relates to inflammation of the bursa underlying the origin of the biceps brachii from the supraglenoid tubercle as it passes over the proximal humerus.

Etiology/pathophysiology

Trauma to the region may result in the setting-up of a bursitis. Infection of the bursa can occur due to trauma and may be seen following a puncture wound (e.g. pitchfork injury).

Clinical presentation

Bursitis leads to a mild to moderate lameness that worsens with work and improves with rest. Clinical examination may reveal pain over the upper humerus, with resentment by the horse on retraction of the upper forelimb. Sepsis of the bursa leads to a more severe lameness with pain and swelling over the region (238). A wound or discharging sinus may be present.

Differential diagnosis

Conditions of the scapulohumeral joint; fractures of the scapula and humerus.

Diagnosis

Intrathecal analgesia of the intertubercular bursa leads to an improvement in clinical signs, although in approximately 20% of horses, communication between the bursa and the scapulohumeral joint exists. Synoviocentesis and evaluation are important in the diagnosis of sepsis. Ultrasonography can be used to examine not only the bursa, but also the bilobed bicipital tendon and the surfaces of the humeral tubercles (239). Comparison with the contralateral region is useful for detecting differences. Lesions may also be present in the tendon itself. Radiography, including skyline views of the humeral tubercles, may reveal bony remodeling or mineralization of the tendon of the biceps.

Management

Inflammatory bursitis and tendonitis can be managed by rest and NSAIDs, although recovery is often prolonged. Intrathecal medication including corticosteroids and hyaluronan can also help to resolve signs. Monitoring is undertaken ultrasonographically every 3 months. Infection of the bicipital bursa requires thorough lavage and can be performed endoscopically.

Prognosis

The prognosis is good if bursitis is the sole cause of the lameness, but poorer if there is damage to the bicipital tendon. Cases with chronic bursitis have a worse prognosis.

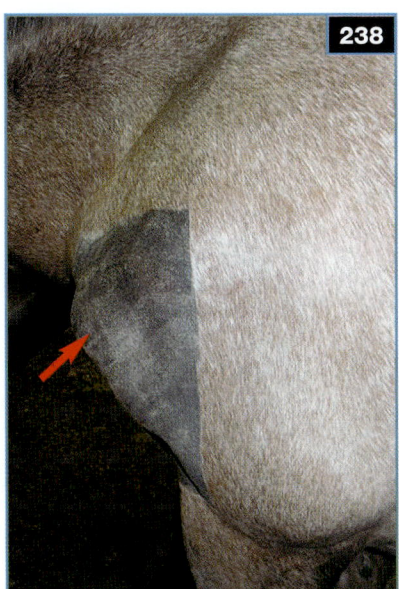

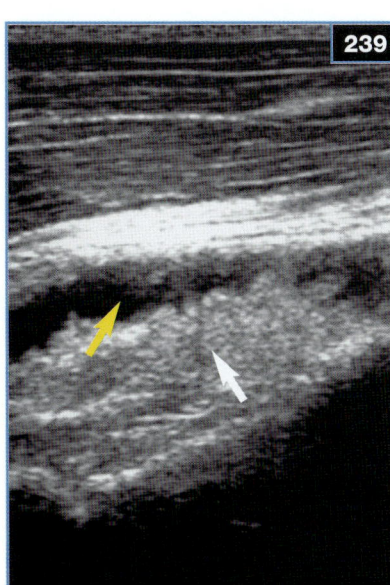

238 An Arab gelding with swelling and pain on palpation over the cranial aspect of the shoulder region following a fall. There is both subcutaneous and bicipital distension (arrow).

239 Longitudinal ultrasound scan over the swelling shown in 238, revealing marked synovial distension (yellow arrow) and marked synovial proliferation (white arrow) within the bicipital bursa. The tendon was unaffected. (Photos courtesy GA Munroe)

The hindlimb is less frequently encountered as a cause of gait abnormality in the horse than the forelimb, although in the last 10 years there has been a considerable increase in hindlimb lameness, particularly in sport and general riding horses. The most common anatomic sites involving lameness are the hock and stifle. Since the conditions seen in the distal hindlimb are similar to those of the forelimb, this chapter discusses hindlimb problems from the hock proximally, including the pelvis.

The hock

Fractures and luxations

Definition/overview

Fractures of the hock include the medial and lateral malleolus of the distal tibia (240), the talus (241, 242) and its trochlear ridges (243), the calcaneus (244), the cuboidal tarsal bones (245), osteochondral fractures of the talus, and incomplete or less commonly complete articular fractures of the dorsoproximolateral aspect of the third metatarsal bone. Luxation or subluxation may occur at the level of the tarsocrural (TC), proximal intertarsal (talocalcaneal–centroquatral) (246, 247) or tarsometatarsal (248) joints with or without a concurrent fracture of the hock. Luxation of the distal intertarsal joint (centrodistal) has not been reported.

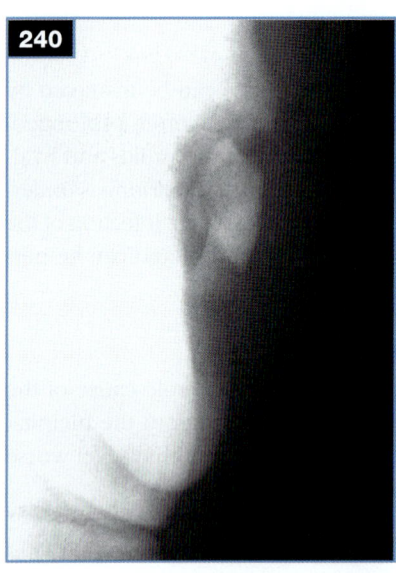

240 Dorsoplantar radiograph of the medial side of the tarsus showing a slightly distally displaced fracture of the medial malleolus of the tibia. (Photo courtesy GA Munroe)

241, 242 Dorsoplantar (241) and plantaromedial/ dorsolateral (242) oblique views of a comminuted fracture of the talus sustained following a kick.

243 A dorsolateral/plantaromedial oblique radiographic view of a tarsus showing a displaced fragment of the medial trochlear ridge of the talus sustained following a kick to the hock. (Photo courtesy GA Munroe)

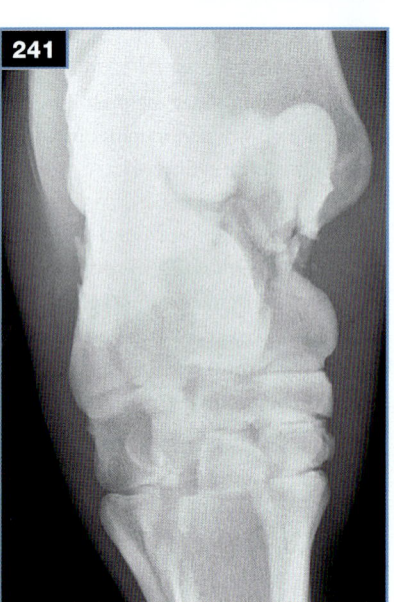

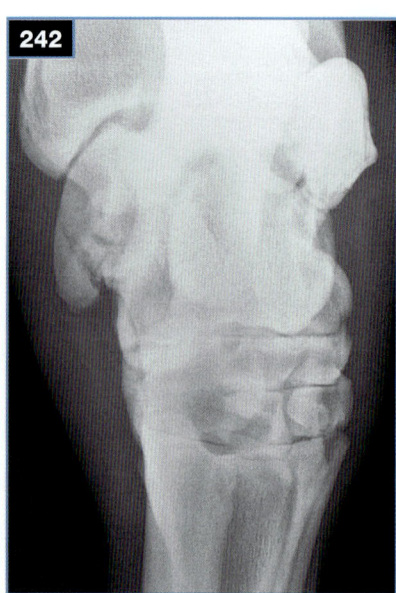

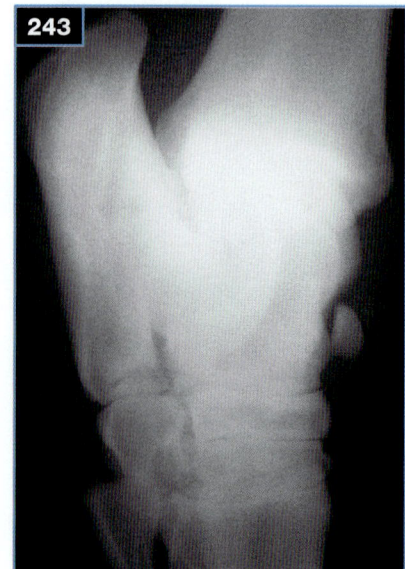

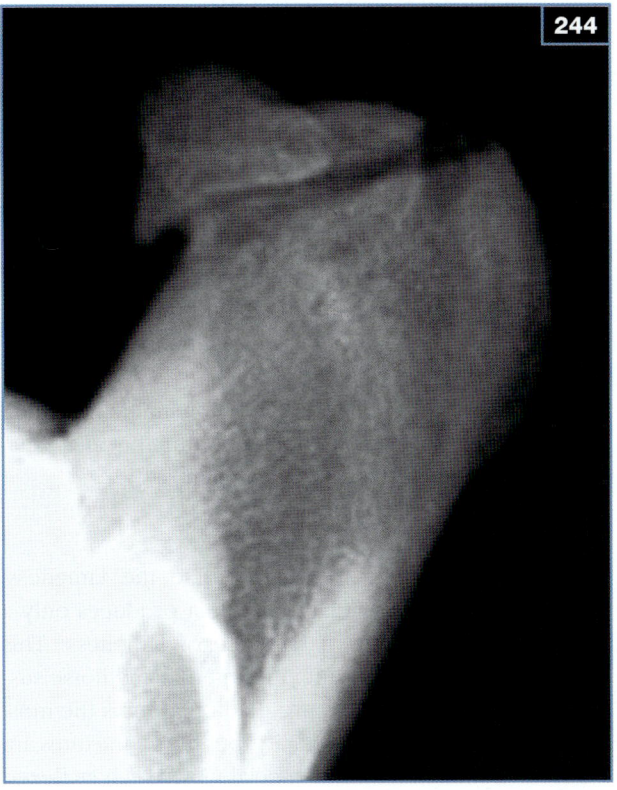

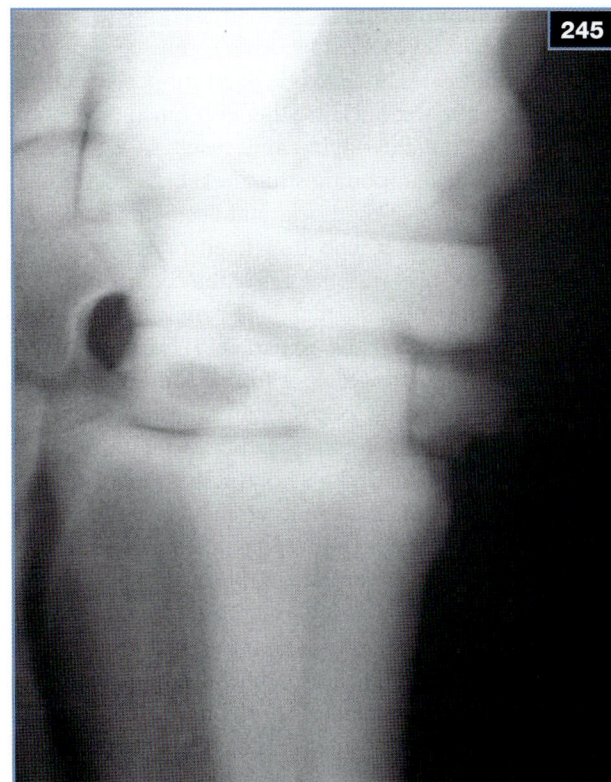

244 Radiograph demonstrating a transverse fracture of the calcaneus in an adult horse following a kick injury. (Photo courtesy MC Schramme)

245 A dorsolateral/plantaromedial radiograph of the tarsus showing a slightly displaced slab fracture of the third tarsal bone sustained after an excessive period of exercise during the convalescent period post tarsal arthrodesis. (Photo courtesy GA Munroe)

246, 247 Dorsoplantar (246) and lateromedial (247) radiographs showing luxation of the proximal intertarsal joint following entanglement of the limb in a horse walker.

248 A stressed dorsoplantar radiograph of the hock demonstrating widening of the tarsometatarsal joint following rupture of the medial collateral ligament and subluxation.

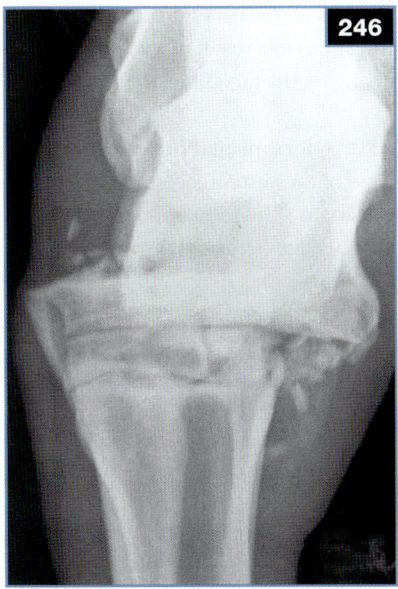

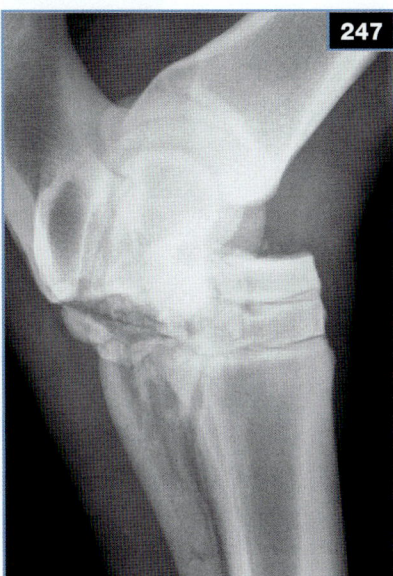

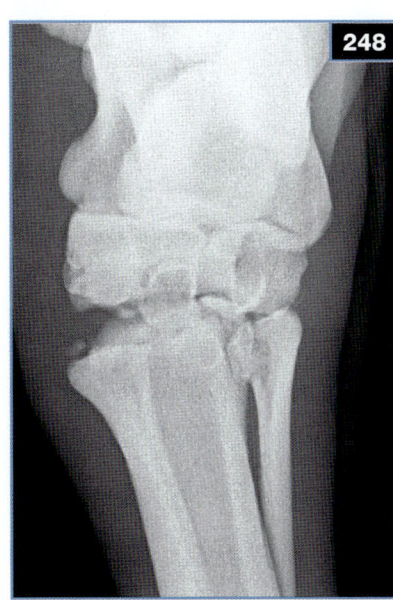

Etiology/pathophysiology

The hock is heavily invested by dense soft-tissue structures that cover the bones and provide good support. Fractures and luxations of the hock are therefore uncommon, are usually of traumatic origin, and result in significant disruption of the supporting structures. External trauma, rotational twisting of the hock, and accidents involving trapping of the distal limb in a fixed object are often described in the history. Fractures of the central and third tarsal bones are uncommon and are mainly seen in racehorses, especially Standardbred trotters. They are occasionally seen secondary to previous fusion of the small tarsal joints. An association has been identified between the presence of wedge-shaped conformation of the third tarsal bone and slab fractures of this bone in mature racehorses. Fractures of the sustentaculum tali may be a sequela to external trauma and may be accompanied by sepsis of the tarsal sheath, which may lead to osteomyelitis.

Clinical presentation

Skin perforation may accompany external trauma. Invariably, horses are lame on the affected limb. The degree of lameness, however, varies from mild to non-weight-bearing according to the extent of damage to the structures within and around the hock. In several cases, mild chronic lameness may precede an acute onset of severe lameness. Lameness caused by fracture of the small tarsal bones may diminish after some rest, but will return when work commences. Horses affected by bilateral fracture of the third tarsal bone may be presented for poor performance rather than hindlimb lameness. Depending on the nature of the injury, palpation may reveal heat, soft-tissue swelling, synovial effusion, crepitation, and pain. Horses suffering from fractures of the calcaneus will have a dropped-hock appearance caused by the loss of function of the gastrocnemius muscle. Luxation of the tarsal joints may be presented as abnormal deviation of the limb at the tarsus, and instability may be identified.

Differential diagnosis

Synovial sepsis; OCD; peritarsal cellulitis; other soft-tissue injuries. Spurs or fragments associated with the distal end of the medial trochlear ridge are a common incidental finding, and do not require any treatment.

Diagnosis

Flexion of the tarsus may exacerbate the lameness. Occasionally, intra-articular anesthesia produces only a partial improvement in the degree of lameness. This diagnostic procedure is contraindicated in any horse suspected of sustaining a fracture. Radiography is the most commonly used imaging modality, but not all fractures are immediately diagnosed and special views such as flexed lateromedial, skyline view of the calcaneus, and modified oblique views may be necessary (249, 250). Occasionally, a nondisplaced fracture may not be radiographically apparent until demineralization has occurred. In these cases, repetition of the radiographs is recommended

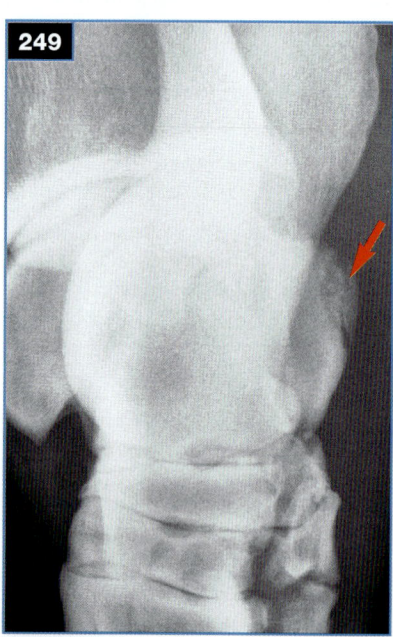

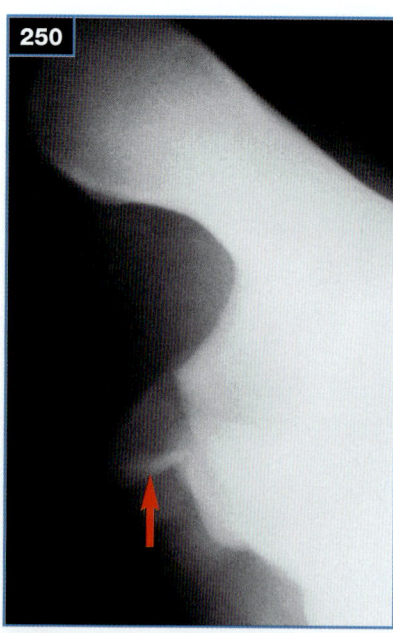

249 A plantarolateral/dorsomedial oblique radiograph of a hock showing a fracture of the sustentaculum tali of the calcaneus as a result of a kick injury involving the tarsal sheath (arrow).

250 A dorsoplantar flexed oblique view of the sustentaculum tali of the calcaneus showing a fracture of the medial edge (left side) (arrow) following a kick to the inside of the hock. (Photo courtesy GA Munroe)

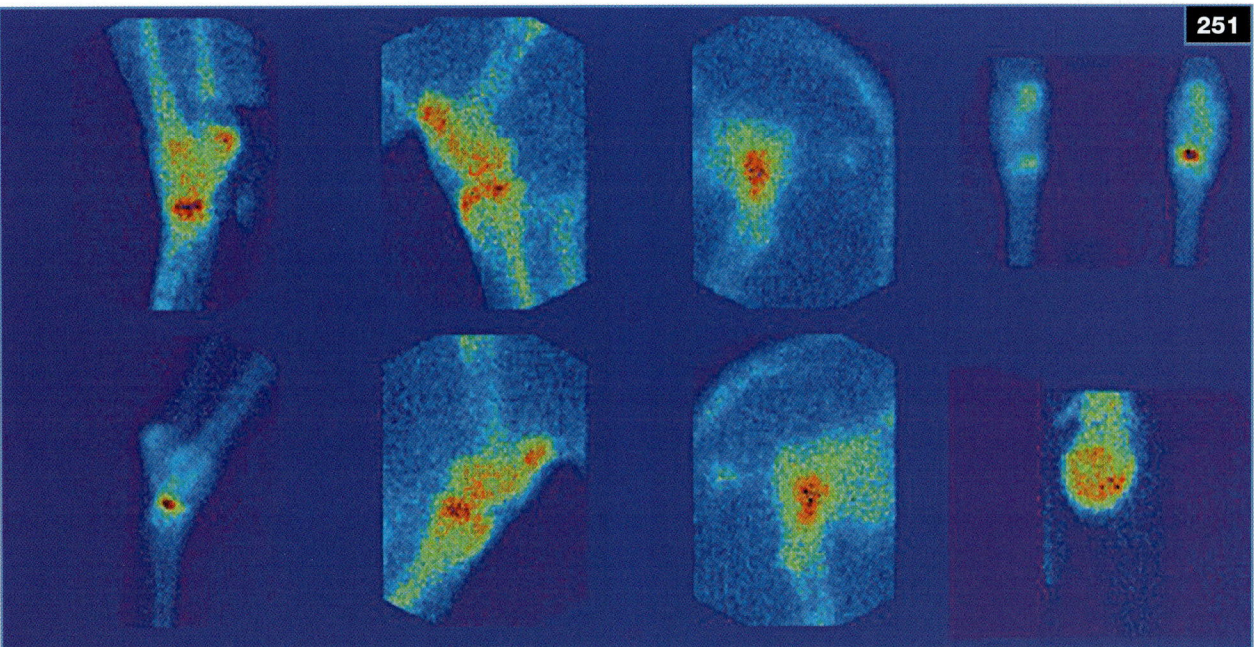

251 A bone scan of the left and right hindlimbs of a horse that presented with acute-onset right hind lameness after jumping a fence. The lameness was localized to the tarsus by regional analgesia, but no radiographic changes were evident. The lower left and upper right scans clearly reveal a focal 'hot spot' over the medial distal row of tarsal bones. Subsequent radiographs some 10 days later confirmed a nondisplaced slab fracture of the third tarsal bone. (Photo courtesy GA Munroe)

within 7–10 days from injury. Stress radiographs may be helpful to diagnose subluxations. Gamma scintigraphy can be beneficial in horses with mild or bilateral hindlimb lameness and in cases where fractures are not demonstrated radiographically (**251**). Ultrasonography is useful to help diagnose concurrent soft-tissue damage. In cases of inconclusive findings it is recommended that the affected limb is compared with the contralateral limb.

Management
Fractures of the lateral malleolus are best treated surgically by removal of small fragments (less than 1 cm). Repair of the larger fragments through an arthrotomy should be considered as it would offer a quicker recovery. Conservative management of minimally displaced small fragments can also be considered.

Arthroscopic removal is the treatment of choice for small fragments off the trochlear ridges. Large fresh fractures may be amenable to internal fixation. Complete sagittal fractures of the talus can be repaired by internal fixation, whereas incomplete fractures can be treated conservatively. Severely comminuted fractures are inoperable and often lead to euthanasia. Small fragments off the calcaneus should be removed or fixed internally. Transverse fractures require internal fixation using a DCP. Open comminuted fractures carry a grave prognosis, and euthanasia is recommended. Chip fractures of the sustentaculum tali require removal via tenoscopy of the tarsal sheath. Some of these are associated with wounds, with possible tarsal sheath sepsis and/or focal osteomyelitis requiring more extensive resection either by tenoscopy or open approaches and long-term antibiotic treatment. In large chips where a significant portion of the flexor surface is fractured, the fragment should be stabilized using screws. Slab fractures of the small tarsal bones can be treated either by box rest or internal fixation, with similar success rates. In cases where the fragments are too small or osteoarthritic changes are evident, surgical drilling to facilitate arthrodesis of the joints is an alternative option. Attempts can be made to reduce luxations, but this, especially with TC luxation, can be extremely difficult to achieve. If reduction is successful, the limb should be placed in a full limb cast for 4–8 weeks.

Prognosis
The prognosis varies depending on the pathology and the involvement of bones, joints, and supporting soft tissues from good (small fragments, especially if they can be removed) to hopeless where there is severe comminution and/or soft-tissue trauma.

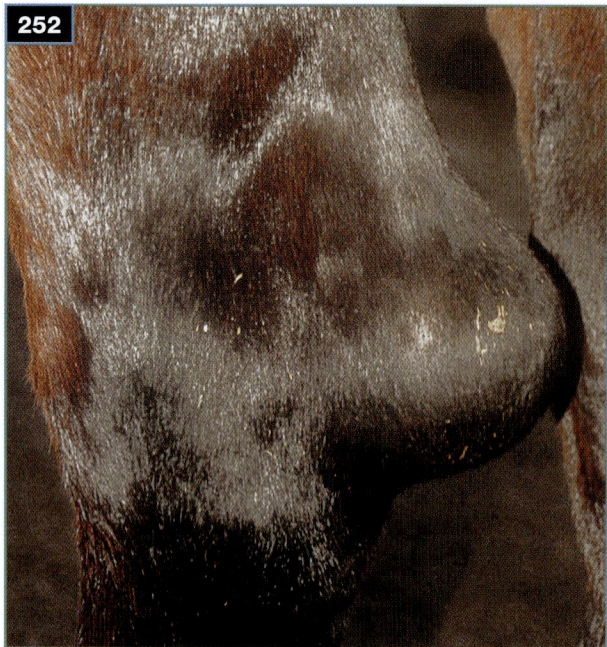

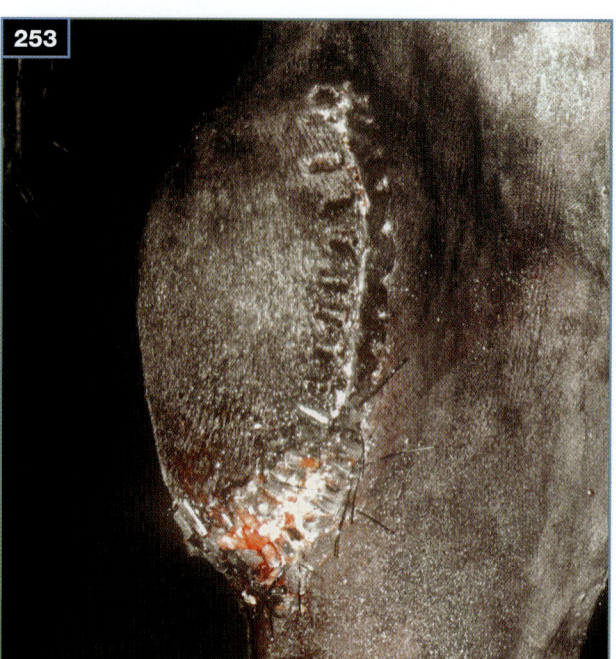

Hygroma of the tuber calcis (capped hock)

Definition/overview

The condition involves a subcutaneous bursa at the point of the tuber calcis, which is naturally present in a proportion of horses, but is more commonly acquired. It is defined as a bursitis, as inflammatory processes take place within the bursa.

Etiology/pathophysiology

Frequently the condition is chronic and characterized by slow development of the bursa as a result of repetitive trauma to the region, until it becomes cosmetically unacceptable to the owner. Excessive fluid is accumulated within the bursa and the wall becomes thickened. The cavity may become filled with fibrous bands and subdivided into smaller cavities by septa. Most commonly, it is a nonseptic condition; however, if the bursa becomes infected, it may enlarge, form an abscess, and rupture.

Clinical presentation

The horse is rarely lame, unless the condition becomes septic or it interferes mechanically with the gait. A local fluctuant swelling is present over the point of the tuber calcis (252), the size and thickness of which are dependent on the stage of the condition. Some pain may be evident in acute cases, but in chronic cases the swelling is nonpainful on palpation.

Differential diagnosis

Gastrocnemius tendonitis and associated bursitis; sprain of the long plantar ligament (curb); tarsal sheath distension (thoroughpin); luxation of the SDFT.

252, 253 Pre- and postoperative photographs of a show horse with hygroma of the tuber calcis. Note the tension-relieving sutures placed in the skin to prevent postoperative dehiscence.

Diagnosis

The clinical presentation of a swelling over the point of the tuber calcis without lameness is very consistent. Ultrasonography is useful to demonstrate the hygroma and its content, and to differentiate it from other conditions. Radiography is usually not required.

Management

Prevention of further trauma and deterioration by using hock boots is recommended. Local injection with corticosteroids and applying a pressure bandage has been used with variable results. Drainage of fluids and implantation of a Penrose drain can be attempted as well, although there is an increased risk of contamination and infection with prolonged use of a drain. Surgery should be avoided due to the very high incidence of wound breakdown, and is only indicated in show horses. It is important to use a pressure-relieving suture pattern (253) and keep the horse cross-tied for 14 days. As the procedure is likely to create a large dead space, the use of a suction drain for a few days and a pressure bandage are recommended.

Prognosis

The prognosis is good for athleticism and guarded for cosmesis.

Tarsus

Intertarsal synovitis/osteoarthritis (bone spavin)

Definition/overview

Osteoarthritis of the tarsometatarsal (TMT) and distal intertarsal (centrodistal) (DIT) joints and, less frequently, the proximal intertarsal (talocalcaneal–centroquatral) (PIT) joint is the most common cause of lameness involving the hindlimbs of mature horses. These are low-motion joints, believed to act primarily as shock absorbers with limited horizontal movement. Although it is usually seen in mature animals, bone spavin can occur in young Thoroughbreds, Warmbloods, Standardbreds, and Western performance horses. 'Juvenile spavin' is the term used for the condition in horses less than 2 years old. Incidence of the condition appears to have little relation to the type of horse or to the type or amount of work it has undertaken.

Etiology/pathophysiology

Many factors may play a role in the development and progression of bone spavin. Normal 'use trauma' as well as abnormal conformation such as 'cow' or 'sickle hock' is believed to provoke formation of the condition. Excessive compression and rotational forces of the tarsal bones during jumps or stops and excessive tension of the ligaments over the dorsal aspect of the hock are all thought to be prominent in the development of bone spavin. Other factors include incomplete ossification and the subsequent collapse of the third and central tarsal bones (254), septic arthritis, fractures of the cuboidal tarsal bones, and OCD. In Icelandic horses the disease appears to have a hereditary component. In the majority of cases there is no correlation between the clinical signs, the degree of lameness, and the severity of radiographic changes.

Clinical presentation

The onset of signs is often gradual. Horses may present with a variety of clinical signs ranging from subtle change in performance without obvious lameness, to moderate or severe lameness. Occasionally, the first sign is identified by a farrier when the horse resists being shod behind. Mild cases may warm out of the lameness and improve after a short time, whereas severe cases tend to worsen with exercise. Generally, hard work usually worsens the lameness within several days, and rest may improve it. Affected horses are presented with a range of gait abnormalities, none of which are specific for bone spavin. These may include reduction in the height of the foot flight arc and shortening of the cranial phase of the stride, toe dragging, axial swing of the foot during protraction and landing on the lateral wall, and asymmetric movement of the tuber coxae. These signs may be accentuated with the worse limb on the inside or, occasionally, the outside when the horse is worked in a circle. Flexion of the affected limb (spavin test) for 60 seconds usually results in exacerbation in the degree of lameness; however, due to the stay apparatus of the hindlimb, it is not specific to the hock.

254 Lateromedial radiograph of the hock in a young foal demonstrating collapse of the central and third tarsal bones.

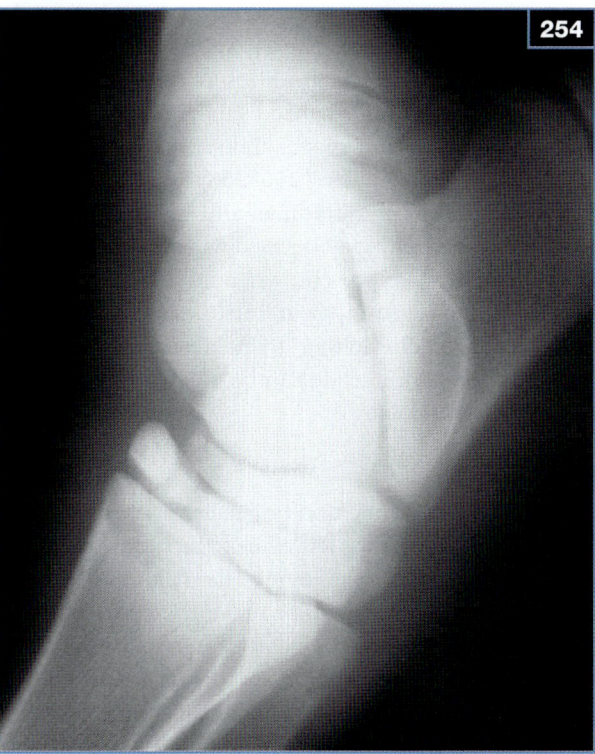

254

The hindlimb

Thickening of the periarticular soft tissue resulting in enlargement on the medial aspect of the hock is an unusual finding that may occur in more chronic cases (255). Muscle wastage, especially of the gluteals, may be identified.

Differential diagnosis
Occult spavin; OCD; proximal suspensory ligament desmitis; stifle problems; talocalcaneal OA; cunean tendon bursitis.

Diagnosis
Intra-articular analgesia of the small tarsal joints is important to confirm the source of pain. Since <40% of horses have a physical communication between the TMT and DIT joints, some clinicians recommend injecting both joints either separately or in combination. Many clinicians, however, inject the TMT joint first and assess the response before attempting the more difficult DIT joint block. Recently, published work has proved that local anesthetics do freely communicate between the lower two joints. The response to these blocks should be assessed within 10 minutes from injection, and improvement in the degree of lameness of >50% is considered positive. Failure to alleviate lameness using these blocks does not rule out the condition. Assessing the effect of local analgesia on the response to flexion test may be misleading and is therefore not recommended. Radiography is always used in the diagnostic process, using four views for each hindlimb. It is important to center the beam accurately in order to evaluate the small tarsal joints. Signs of the disease are usually first evident on the dorsomedial or the dorsolateral aspects of the TMT and DIT joints. Radiographic findings include periarticular osteophyte formation, localized subchondral bone lysis, narrowing of the joint space, and sclerosis of the distal and third tarsal bones (256–258). The correlation between radiographic findings and lameness is poor. Nuclear scintigraphy may be used where no radiographic abnormalities are present, when intra-articular blocks are difficult to perform, or in horses presented for performance problems rather than lameness. Increased uptake of the radionuclide can be identified at the level of the intertarsal joints.

Management
Treatment for this condition originally involved working affected animals with the use of analgesics in an attempt to provoke ankylosis of the joints. The majority of horses, however, do not achieve fusion and the lameness persists. Numerous treatments, both medical and surgical, have been described, suggesting that none provide complete cure in all cases. Determining the treatment is dependent on the clinical and radiographic findings, use of the horse,

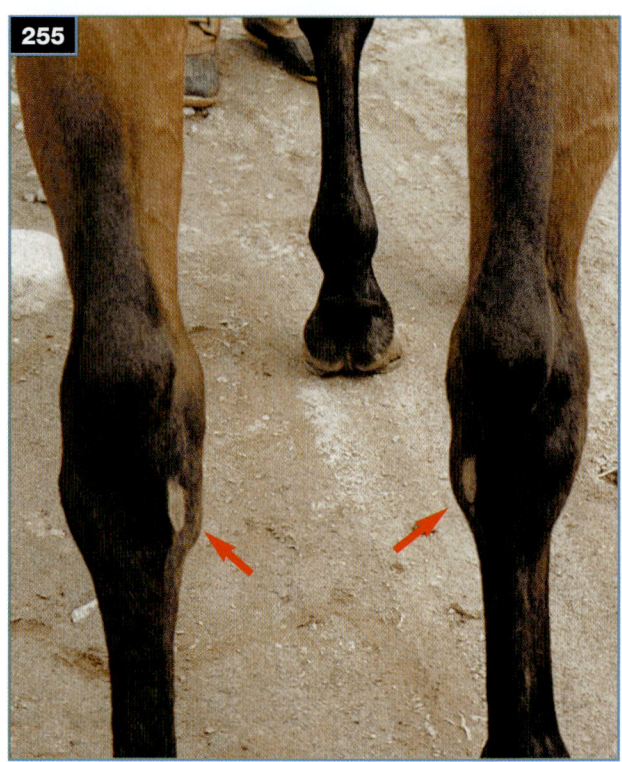

255 This horse was presented with a history of chronic bilateral hindlimb lameness that was diagnosed after radiographs and intra-articular analgesia as bone spavin. Note the distal medial enlargements in both hocks due to soft-tissue filling over the spavin region (arrows). (Photo courtesy GA Munroe)

response to previous treatments, and financial constraints. Horses with little or no radiographic change are best treated with intra-articular medication and a systemic NSAID such as phenylbutazone. Either triamcinolone (4–6 mg/joint) or methylprednisolone acetate (20–40 mg/joint) can be used with or without hyaluronan. This treatment invariably produces an improvement in the lameness and frequently results in soundness; however, many horses suffer recurrent lameness after 2–4 months. Prolonged rest is not beneficial, and these horses should be kept in a box for 3 days and then gradually returned to work. A change in work program either in type or degree can be very useful in decreasing the degree of lameness. Severe radiographic changes or failure to respond to conservative management justifies a more radical intervention. Cutting the cunean tendon is thought to reduce the pressure over the medial aspect of the distal tarsal joints. Although this technique may result in temporary improvement in clinical signs, it is unlikely to restore soundness. Furthermore, since only a few of the clinical cases seen today demonstrate the classically described large prolifera-

142

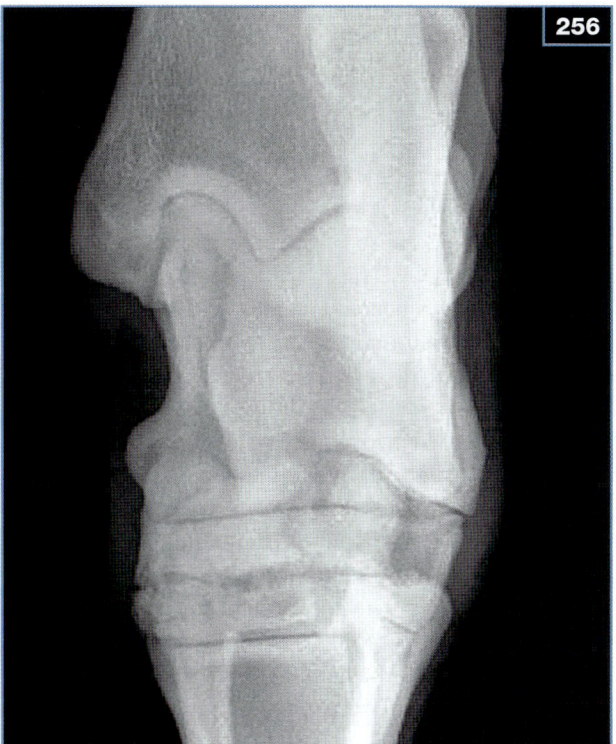

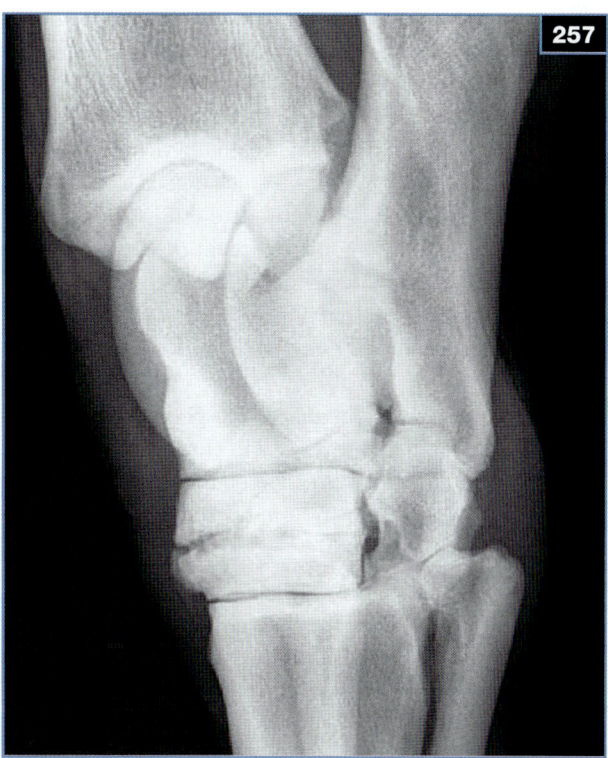

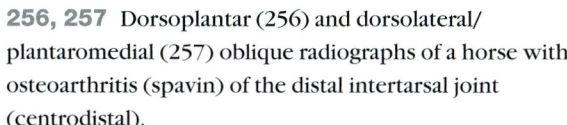

256, 257 Dorsoplantar (256) and dorsolateral/
plantaromedial (257) oblique radiographs of a horse with
osteoarthritis (spavin) of the distal intertarsal joint
(centrodistal).

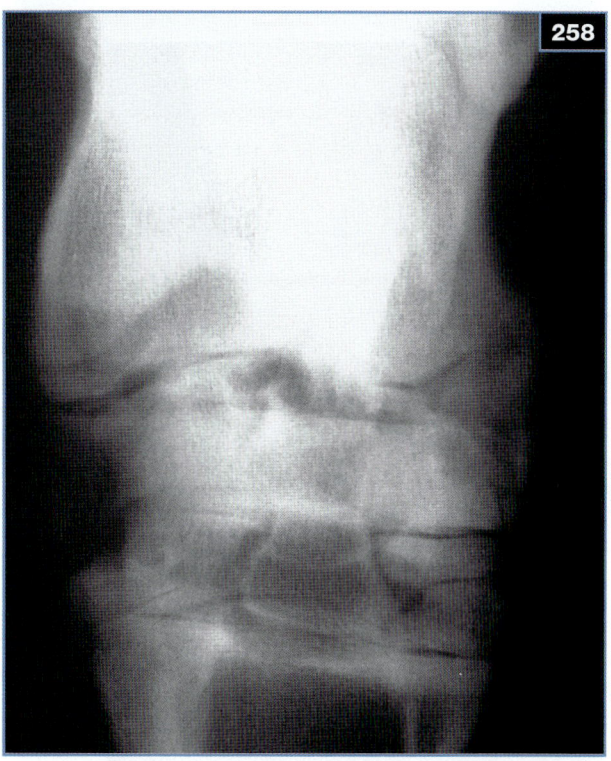

tive exostosis on the medial aspect of the joints, this technique is not unanimously supported. Localized partial
neurectomy of the branches of the tibial nerve and neurectomy of the deep peroneal nerve supplying the small
tarsal joints can be performed and carries a success rate of
65%. The technique, however, requires prolonged anesthetic time and extensive soft-tissue resection, and is only
effective for 1–2 years because of reinnervation. Chemical
arthrodesis can be achieved by injecting a caustic agent,
monoiodoacetic acid (MIA), into the affected joints, usually
under general anesthesia, with a success rate of 40–80%.
More recently, 70% ethanol has been used with more
successful results.

Surgical arthrodesis can be performed in a number of
ways, including simple drilling across the joint (3–6 tracts
with a 4.5 mm drill bit), with or without the addition of
cancellous bone graft after drilling, T-plates, and 4 cm
long, 9 mm diameter Bagby baskets filled with cancellous
bone placed across the joints. The most common technique involves the drilling of three 4.5 mm tracts across
both TMT and DIT joints. The prognosis for soundness

258 A dorsoplantar radiograph of the tarsus showing osteoarthritic changes of both the centrodistal and talocalcaneal
centroquatral joints. Note the marked bone lysis in the upper
joint. (Photo courtesy GA Munroe)

143

with these techniques is 60–75%. Arthrodesis of the small tarsal joints following chondronecrosis induced by intra-articular application of Nd-YAG laser does not appear to be superior to conventional drilling. Extracorporeal shock-wave therapy as a possible treatment has also been reported; however, long-term results are still unavailable. In parts of Europe the biphosphonate drug Tiludronate is licensed for the intravenous treatment of intertarsal OA, but there is little scientific evidence of its effectiveness in this condition at the present time.

Prognosis
The prognosis varies from guarded to poor depending on the joint(s) affected, the severity and chronicity of articular changes, secondary causes of lameness or back pain, the type of work carried out by the horse, and response to treatment.

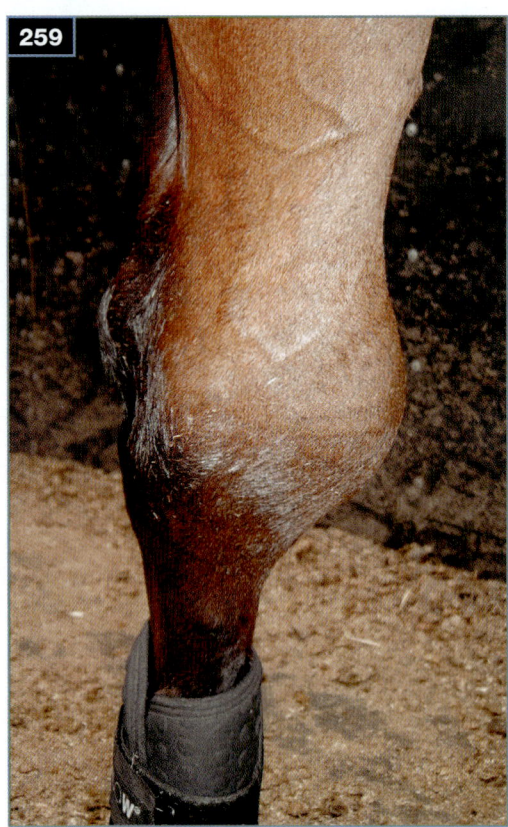

259 Tarsocrural synovitis (bog spavin). Note the large synovial effusion of the joint, especially dorsomedially. (Photo courtesy GA Munroe)

Tarsocrural synovitis (bog spavin)
Definition/overview
Bog spavin is the term describing excessive distension of the TC joint with synovial fluid as a result of acute or chronic synovitis.

Etiology/pathophysiology
The best defined cause of bog spavin includes variable manifestations of OCD (see p. 50). Lesions are recorded in a number of different anatomic sites with different presentations. Other well-defined causes include OA, trauma, sepsis, hemoarthrosis, and intra-articular fractures. Mineral or vitamin deficiencies have also been implicated without clear scientific evidence.

In contrast to the above, other causes of bog spavin, including idiopathic synovitis, cannot be clearly identified and are rarely associated with lameness. It can also be a manifestation of continuous cartilage microtrauma as a result of poor conformational abnormalities, particularly straight hocks. TC joint effusion may also be a result of box rest, particularly in older, well used jumping and dressage horses; however, this should disappear once exercise is initiated. Joint capsule sprain, with or without damage to the collateral ligaments, may also cause TC effusion.

Clinical presentation
The history and clinical signs will vary with the etiology. Excessive effusion of the TC joint is most apparent in the dorsomedial and plantarolateral pouches of the joint (**259**), although the other pouches may be distended as well. In OCD, distension occurs from about 6–24 months of age, is often bilateral, and is associated with variable degrees of lameness related to size and mobility of the lesion, but often mild in nature. There may be a sudden onset, sometimes in association with excessive exercise. In older horses, lameness may be seen in later life due to the onset of OA subsequent to the chronic presence of an undiagnosed OCD lesion. Most horses with idiopathic synovitis are sound, whereas horses with other etiologies such as fractures and sepsis are extremely lame. Local heat, pain, and swelling may be identified, particularly following trauma. Flexion of the hock may induce lameness or exacerbate it in some horses. Mechanical lameness can follow extensive distension of the TC joints.

Differential diagnosis
OCD; joint sepsis; nondisplaced fracture; soft-tissue injury; OA; nutritional deficiencies; systemic problem.

Diagnosis
All cases that are lame need careful assessment, including intra-articular anesthesia. Arthrocentesis in chronic cases is commonly unremarkable. In acute cases, hemarthrosis or

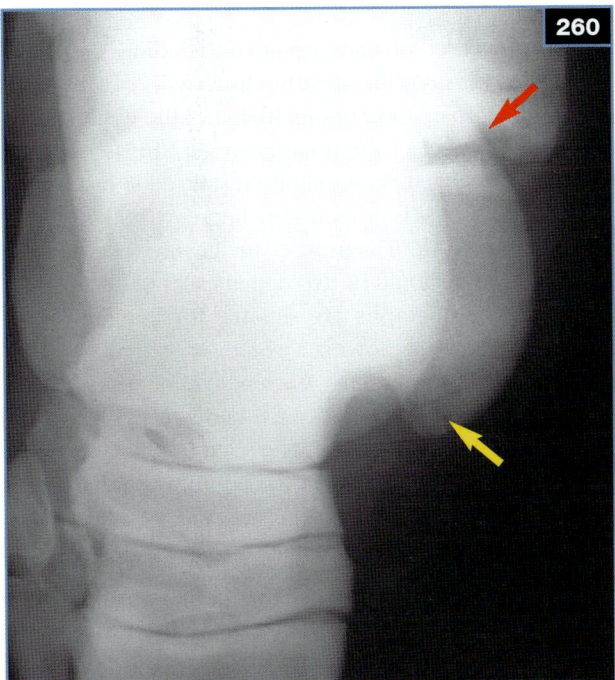
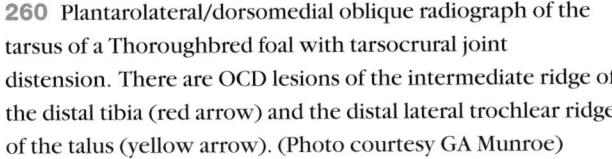

260 Plantarolateral/dorsomedial oblique radiograph of the tarsus of a Thoroughbred foal with tarsocrural joint distension. There are OCD lesions of the intermediate ridge of the distal tibia (red arrow) and the distal lateral trochlear ridge of the talus (yellow arrow). (Photo courtesy GA Munroe)

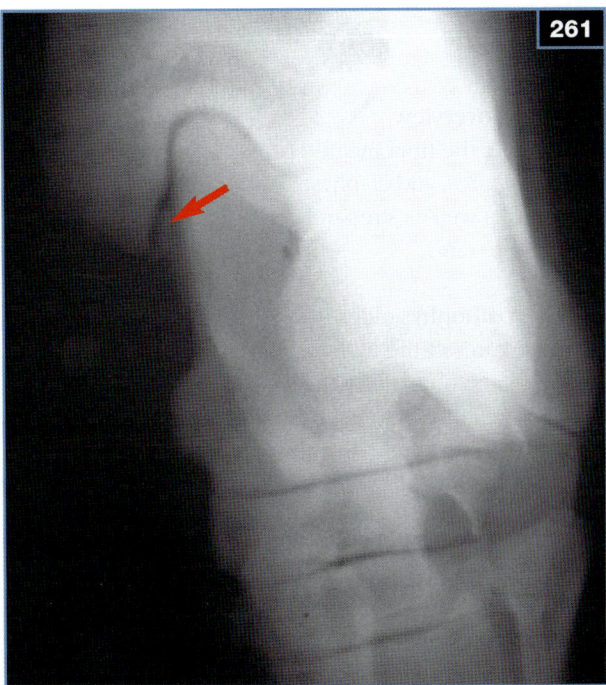

261 Dorsoplantar radiograph of a yearling crossbred horse that presented with moderate tarsocrural joint distension and mild lameness. The lameness was localized to the joint by intra-articular analgesia and this radiograph reveals a medial malleolar OCD lesion just visible as a small defect and separate osseous fragment on the articular margin of the malleolus (arrow). (Photo courtesy GA Munroe)

increased WBC count and total protein may be present. Radiography should include four standard views. In OCD the most common lesion is fragmentation of the intermediate ridge of the distal tibia (260), although these lesions can be seen incidentally in older horses. Less common, but of greater clinical significance, are lesions involving the distal lateral trochlear ridge of the talus (260). The medial ridge is rarely affected. These are variable sized, lytic lesions, which cause a greater degree of lameness. Much less common are small bony fragments axially on the medial and lateral malleoli of the tibia (261). If standard views fail to demonstrate any bony abnormality, it is recommended to include a flexed lateromedial, a dorsal 15° lateral plantaromedial oblique (for medial malleolar lesions), and skyline views. In the absence of radiological abnormalities, more advanced imaging modalities (e.g. scintigraphy, CT, and MRI) or arthroscopic examination may reveal a cause.

Management

No treatment is required if a cause is not identified and the horse is sound. Treatment may be attempted if the owner finds the condition cosmetically disturbing. Drainage of synovial fluid via arthrocentesis, intra-articular medication with steroids and/or hyaluronan, pressure bandaging of the hock, and restricted exercise may prove successful. Recurrence is expected in about 50% of horses. Lame horses that improve on intra-articular analgesia of the TC joint are good candidates for arthroscopic exploration. Some clinically significant OCD lesions will respond to conservative treatment such as rest, systemic NSAIDs, and intra-articular medications such as sodium hyaluronate and corticosteroids. Those cases that do not respond, or where there are large lesions or increased lameness, are candidates for arthroscopic examination of the joint and surgical removal of loose fragments and damaged cartilage.

Prognosis

The prognosis varies with the etiology of the condition, but in OCD is determined by the size and position of the lesions, whether they are bilateral, the use of the animal, and whether secondary OA occurs. The prognosis is guarded for conservative treatment of all clinically significant lesions. With surgical treatment the prognosis is good for distal intermediate ridge and malleolar lesions, and guarded for trochlear ridge lesions.

Tibia

Fractures

Definition/overview

Fractures of the tibia include proximal physeal fractures, fissure fractures, and diaphyseal displaced or nondisplaced fractures, as well as stress-related fractures. Distal physeal fractures are rare.

Etiology/pathophysiology

Stress fractures of the tibia result from an accumulation of stress and microfracture at the level of the caudal or caudolateral cortex of the tibia. These fractures usually occur in 2-year-old Thoroughbreds in training, and are most commonly unilateral. Physeal and diaphyseal fractures are usually of traumatic origin, either following a kick or as a result of a fall. Proximal physeal fractures are most common in foals, usually following a kick or after being stepped on by the mare. These fractures originate medially, separating the proximal epiphysis from the metaphysis and propagating laterally across the physis to about two-thirds the width of the bone where the fracture orientation becomes vertical, commonly forming a Salter–Harris type II fracture. Some of these fractures will be initially minimally displaced, but progressive displacement usually occurs. Most diaphyseal fractures are displaced, spiral in configuration and/or comminuted, and occur at all ages.

Clinical presentation

Horses affected with stress fractures are commonly presented with acute lameness that improves greatly, but only temporarily, after a few days of rest. Severe non-weight-bearing lameness may indicate an incomplete fissure fracture or a complete displaced or nondisplaced fracture. Abduction of the affected limb at the level of the tibia occurs if the fracture is displaced and/or comminuted. A wound may be present at the injured site and also medially if the sharp edges of the fractured bone have penetrated the skin.

Differential diagnosis

Pelvic stress fractures; stress-related injury of the distal aspect of the third metatarsal bone; fracture of any other bone; septic arthritis.

Diagnosis

Diagnosis is based on clinical signs and findings on palpation. Some horses with stress fractures will respond with pain on deep palpation or percussion of the easily palpable medial aspect of the tibia; however, this is not very reliable. Stress fractures should be suspected in racehorses when the lameness is pronounced, improves with rest, and recurs after work. Diagnostic analgesia is commonly impractical and should be avoided in cases of acute lameness. Plain radiographs are suitable for imaging of all displaced fractures; however, some stress fractures and nondisplaced or fissure fractures may initially be radiographically silent and only become evident after 10–14 days. In these horses, bone scintigraphy is the most suitable imaging modality to help with diagnosis. Increased radiopharmaceutical uptake can be seen on the affected cortex, usually in a single area, but occasionally at multiple sites or bilaterally (262, 263).

Management/prognosis

Horses diagnosed with stress fractures should be box rested for 1 month, and then have controlled walking exercise combined with box rest for an additional 2 months before resuming training. The prognosis for a return to racing is good; however, introduction of training too early predisposes to recurrence. Good management prior to referral of horses with complete fracture is crucial, as the lack of soft tissue on the medial aspect of the tibia increases the risk of converting a closed to an open fracture if adequate immobilization is not achieved immediately.

Incomplete fissure or nondisplaced diaphyseal fractures should be treated conservatively with box rest and cross-tying. As this does not fully prevent the horse from lying down, some authors recommend using a sling during the first 10 days. Any displaced fracture, regardless of the degree of displacement, should be internally fixated using DCPs. This procedure is, however, only recommended for horses weighing <325 kg, and immediate humane destruction is recommended for heavier horses as the prognosis in these cases is hopeless (264). Generally, the prognosis in adult horses is unfavorable.

Proximal physeal fractures in foals can be managed conservatively if minimal displacement is present; however, displacement, evident by valgus deformity, usually occurs and internal fixation by a variety of techniques should be recommended. These foals have an excellent prognosis for life and fair for soundness.

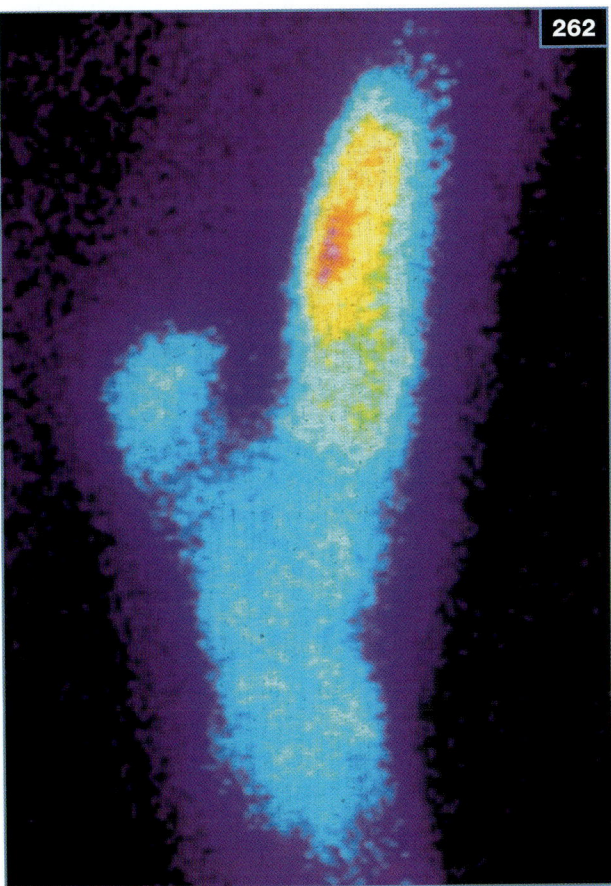

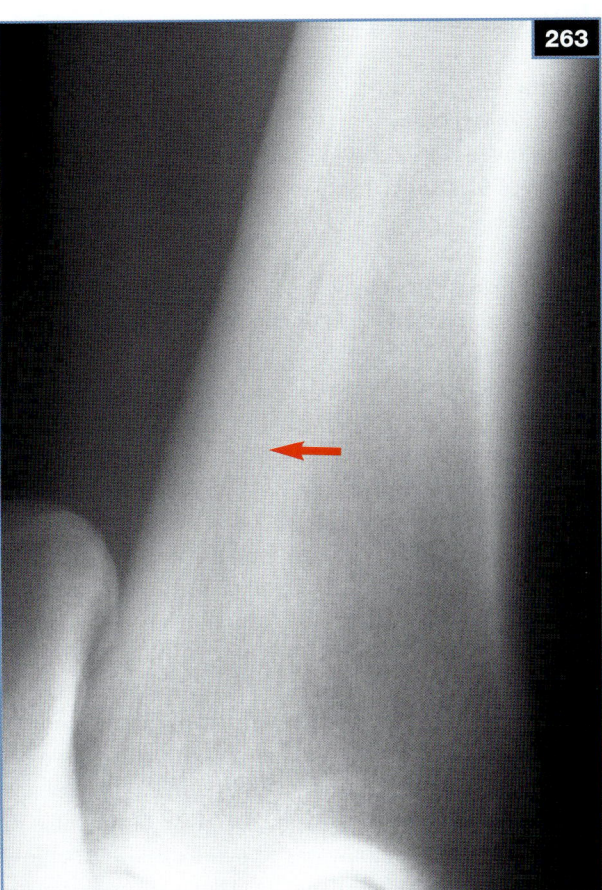

262, 263 Gamma scintigraphy (262) and plain radiograph (263) of a stress fracture at the level of the distal third of the tibia in a racehorse. Note the increased sclerosis evident on the radiograph (arrow).

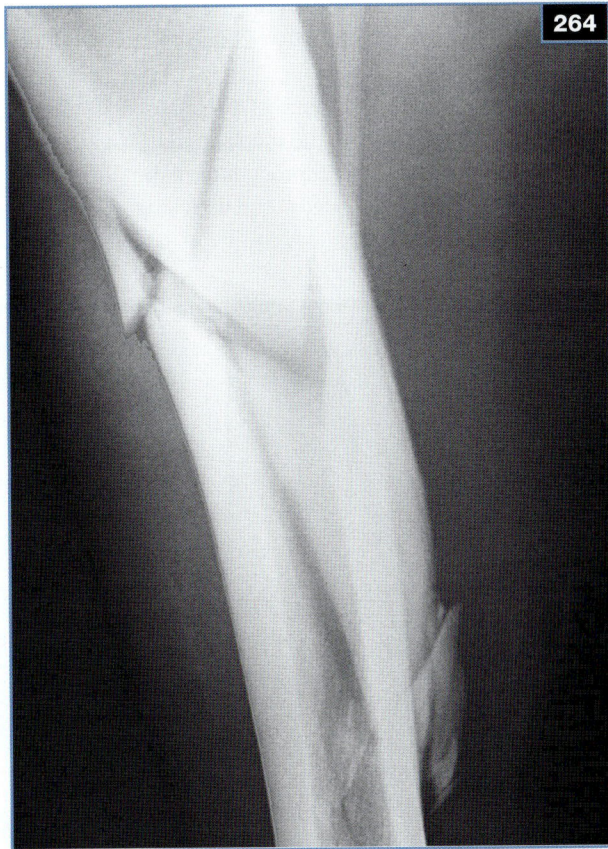

264 Radiograph of a comminuted mid-shaft tibial fracture sustained during recovery from unrelated surgery.

The hindlimb

Patella/stifle joint

Patella

Definition/overview
Conditions associated with the patella include upward fixation of the patella, fractures, fragmentation of the apex, and luxation.

Etiology/pathophysiology
The medial patellar ligament locks the patella and its medial cartilaginous extension above the medial trochlear ridge of the femur as part of the stay apparatus of the hindlimb. Upward fixation of the patella is caused by failure to unlock this mechanism, and is more common in young horses and ponies. It is thought that straight hindlimb conformation predisposes horses to the condition. Other factors include poor body and muscle condition and weak thigh musculature. Upward fixation of the patella can also occur secondarily to coxofemoral luxation, trauma to the stifle region, or sudden box rest of older and/or fit horses. In certain pony breeds the condition is considered hereditary. Acute and permanent fixation is usually unilateral, whereas intermittent fixation can be bilateral as well.

External injury such as a kick or hitting a fixed object while jumping is the most common cause of fractures of the patella. The proximity of the patella to the trochlear ridges of the femur while the stifle is flexed is suggested to predispose the patella to fracture if an external blow is sustained. The medial pole of the patella is most commonly affected, but a variety of other fracture configurations can occur.

Fragmentation of the apex of the patella is closely correlated to desmotomy of the medial patellar ligament. It is suggested that the surgical procedure places the patella in a different position and leads to maltracking.

Lateral luxation of the patella is considered to be inherited and occurs most commonly in miniature breed foals, but it has been reported in other breeds as well. The luxation is usually accompanied by hypoplasia of the lateral trochlear ridge, but it can occur with normal conformation. Medial luxation has to overcome the much larger medial trochlear ridge and is usually induced by trauma to the region.

Clinical presentation
Generally, the degree of lameness varies between mild and severe depending on the condition affecting the patella. Hindlimb flexion commonly exacerbates the degree of lameness, and some horses may resent this manipulation. Upward fixation of the patella causes typical gait abnormalities, and the signs are usually evident during rest or at the start of movement (265). The affected hindlimb is extended caudally and dragged while walking; this may be temporarily relieved after a few strides or remain for a prolonged duration. The release after an intermittent locking

265 This Dale pony has an upwardly fixated patella in the right hindleg, which extends the hock and stifle, causing it to stand with the distal limb joints flexed. (Photo courtesy GA Munroe)

266, 267 Lateromedial (266) and cranioproximal/craniodistal oblique (skyline) (267) radiographs of the stifle demonstrating a sagittal fracture of the medial pole of the patella. Note that the fracture is more difficult to identify on the lateromedial view.

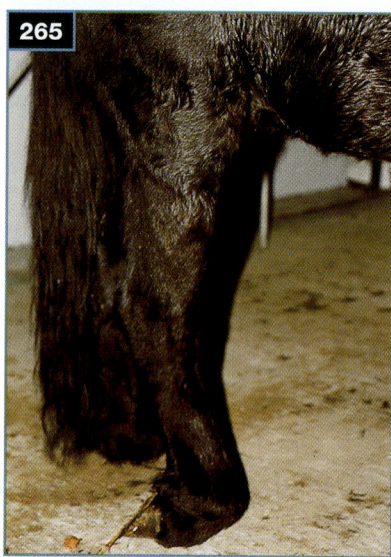

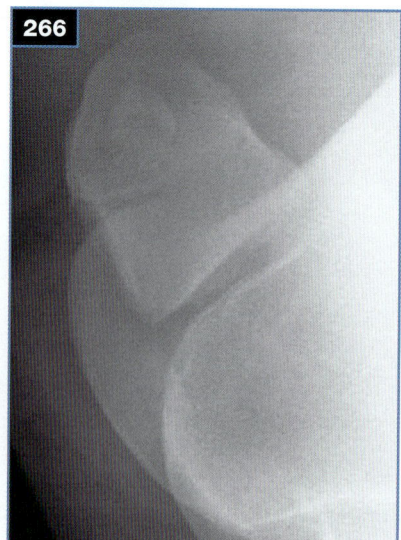

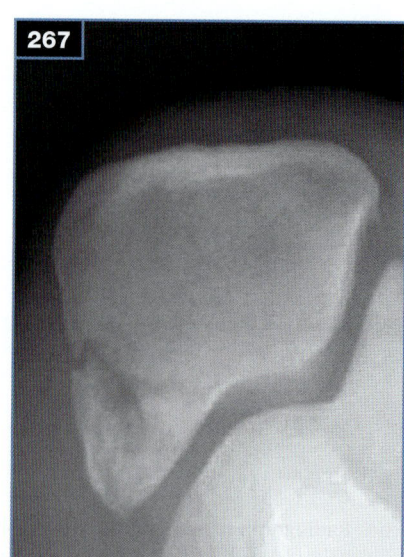

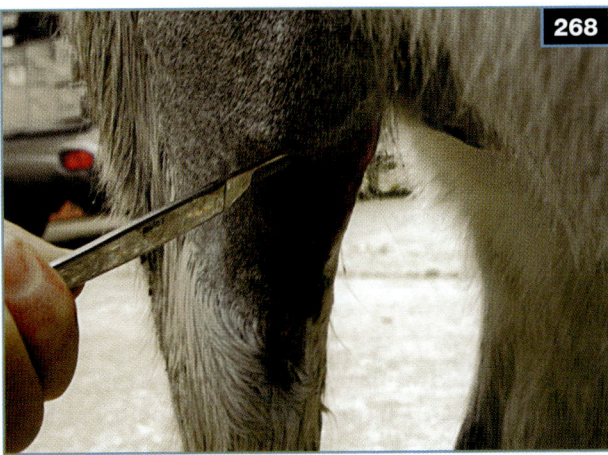

268 Desmotomy of the medial patellar ligament in a standing sedated miniature pony with upward fixation of the patella.

269 Magnified lateral view radiograph of the distal patella of a horse that developed distal patellar fragmentation (arrow) post medial patellar desmotomy. (Photo courtesy GA Munroe)

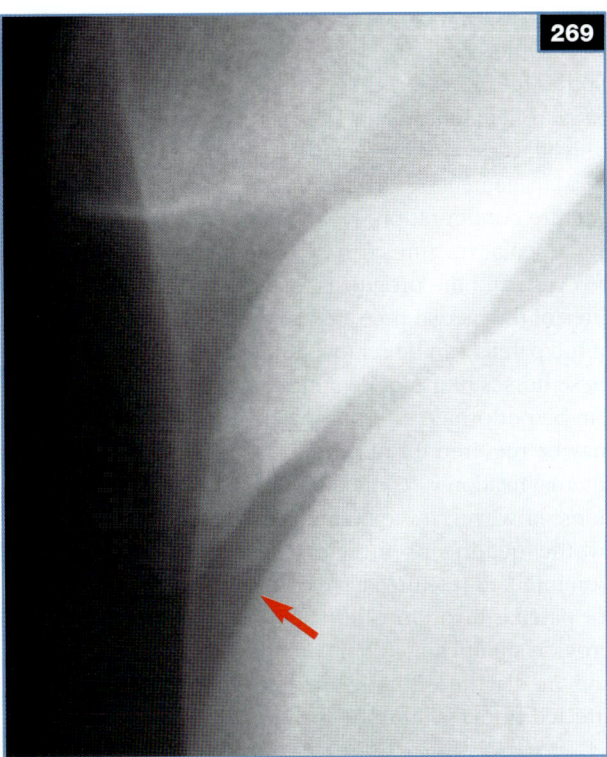

involves a snap followed by rapid hyperflexion of the stifle and hock. The condition can also be manifested as 'delayed release' or 'catching' of the patella, with a sudden jerk observed during flexion of the stifle as the horse moves.

Foals affected with luxation of the patella are unable to extend the stifle and stand in a characteristic crouching position (see pp. 48, 49). Less severe luxation may be manifested as a stiff gait and refusal to flex the affected limb.

Effusion of the femoropatellar joint is common with fractures, fragmentation of the apex of the patella, and all chronic conditions that may promote OA. Horses that develop fragmentation of the apex of the patella after desmotomy of the medial patellar ligament may have excessive fibrous tissue at the surgical site and resent flexion of the affected limb.

Differential diagnosis
Stringhalt; fibrous or ossifying myopathy; OCD; septic arthritis; meniscal and/or cruciate ligament tear; desmitis of the patellar ligaments; fracture of any other bony component of the stifle; low-grade hindlimb ataxia.

Diagnosis
Diagnosis is based on clinical signs, palpation, and imaging findings, including lateral/medial, caudal/cranial, and caudocranial oblique radiographs of the stifle region. Careful palpation of foals with patellar luxation reveals the

position of the patella, the possibility for relocation, and if the luxation is intermittent or permanent. It is extremely important to include a cranioproximal/craniodistal (skyline) view of the patella if a fracture is suspected (**266, 267**), as this may be the only view demonstrating the fracture line. Ultrasonography is useful for demonstrating excessive scar tissue after desmotomy.

Management/prognosis
Upward fixation of the patella should be initially treated conservatively, mainly aiming at reconditioning of the horse and building up muscle mass through exercise and improved nutrition. Many young animals 'grow out' of the condition. Failure of conservative management, or severe clinical signs on presentation, warrant surgical intervention in the form of medial patellar ligament desmotomy, which is easily performed with the horse standing sedated (**268**). Postoperatively, it is recommended to rest the horse in a box for 2 months, providing gentle walking in hand during the second month. After surgery, in the absence of degenerative changes in the joint, horses are expected to return to normal use, although some may develop a slightly restricted gait. Some cases have been reported to develop distal patellar fragmentation and severe lameness post surgery, especially if they are returned to work too quickly (**269**). Splitting the ligament percutaneously under ultrasonographic guidance, either standing or under general anesthesia, has recently been described and appears as

149

effective as desmotomy and without any serious complications. Other clinicians, particularly in parts of Europe and North America, use counter-irritant agents injected into the patellar ligaments as an alternative technique, although with little scientific evidence of its effectiveness.

Management of a fractured patella is determined by the fracture configuration. Horses with small nondisplaced, nonarticular fractures can be treated conservatively with box rest, and the prognosis for soundness is good. Fractures of the medial pole are best removed, and up to 30% of the patella can be removed safely, with the majority of these horses returning to athletic activity. This procedure can be performed arthroscopically; however, arthrotomy may be required for removal of large fragments of bone. Internal fixation is required for all other fracture configurations; however, the extreme pull exerted on the patella by the quadriceps muscle may promote breakdown. Comminuted fractures have a poor prognosis. Treatment for patellar luxation is difficult and commonly does not provide significant athletic prospect. Both lateral release and medial imbrication are important. Breeding from affected animals should be avoided.

Stifle joint injuries
Definition/overview
Injuries of the stifle include fractures of the patella (see above) and desmitis of the patellar ligaments, fractures of the tibial tuberosity and trochlear ridges of the femur, as well as soft-tissue injuries such as meniscal tears or damage to the cruciate, meniscal, or collateral ligaments. Fractures of the intercondylar eminence of the tibia can occur as well, and any penetrating injury into the synovial compartments can result in septic arthritis. Trauma to the articular cartilage is frequently encountered, and the stifle is a common site for OCD and subchondral bone cysts (see pp. 50 and 58).

Etiology/pathophysiology
Fractures of the patella, tibial tuberosity, trochlear ridges, and femoral condyles are most common in horses engaged in jumping/hunting activity after hitting a hard object while jumping. They can also occur following a kick injury or a foreign body penetration. Fractures of the lateral trochlear ridge and, less commonly, the medial trochlear ridge may occur either alone or concurrently with patellar fractures. Fractures of the tibial tuberosity vary in size and may be displaced by the pull of the patellar ligaments. Occasionally, these fractures are intra-articular. Injuries to the articular cartilage may be identified arthroscopically on the femoral condyles and the axial part of the tibial plateau. In about 25% of horses these are considered to be the cause of lameness; however, they may accompany other primary femorotibial joint pathologies.

270 Extensive synovial effusion of the femoropatellar joint in a 2-year-old Thoroughbred with stifle OCD.

271 An oblique radiograph of the stifle demonstrating an osteochondral fragment in the femoropatellar joint capsule (arrow) and entheseopathy of the origin of the middle patellar ligament following a kick injury.

It is suggested that injuries of the meniscus and associated ligaments are caused by a combination of crushing forces with rotation of the tibia and flexion or extension of the stifle. Cruciate injuries are possibly the result of sudden turning of the horse while the stifle is flexed. The medial collateral ligament is more commonly affected than the lateral one. Usually it is in an adult horse and in combination with other soft-tissue injuries.

Fracture of the intercondylar eminence of the tibia is thought to be a sequela to lateral impingement of the medial condyle on the eminence rather than avulsion. Desmitis of the patellar ligaments, usually the middle one, is rare and occurs most commonly in jumping horses. This condition may also occur in horses with intermittent upper fixation of the patella or as a sequela to desmotomy of the middle patellar ligament. Blunt trauma to the region can induce a variety of injuries.

Clinical presentation
Invariably, all affected horses are lame, but the degree of lameness varies from subtle to severe depending on the type, severity, and duration of the injury. Effusion of any of the stifle joint compartments may be palpable (**270**), and signs of local inflammation may be present as well. Commonly, upper limb flexion tests exacerbate the degree of lameness, with some horses resenting flexing of the affected limb. Intra-articular analgesia will greatly improve the degree of lameness in injuries involving any of the joint components; however, occasionally only partial improvement is noted. Evidence of external injury or wounds may be present. Horses with desmitis of the patellar ligaments are lame, have subtle effusion of the femoropatellar joint, and may partially respond to intra-articular analgesia. The majority of horses with injury of the medial collateral ligament will have obvious instability and severe lameness, but only minimal swelling will be visible. They rarely respond to intra-articular analgesia of the stifle joints.

Differential diagnosis
OCD; septic arthritis; rupture of the origin of the long digital extensor tendon and peroneus tertius; femoral fractures.

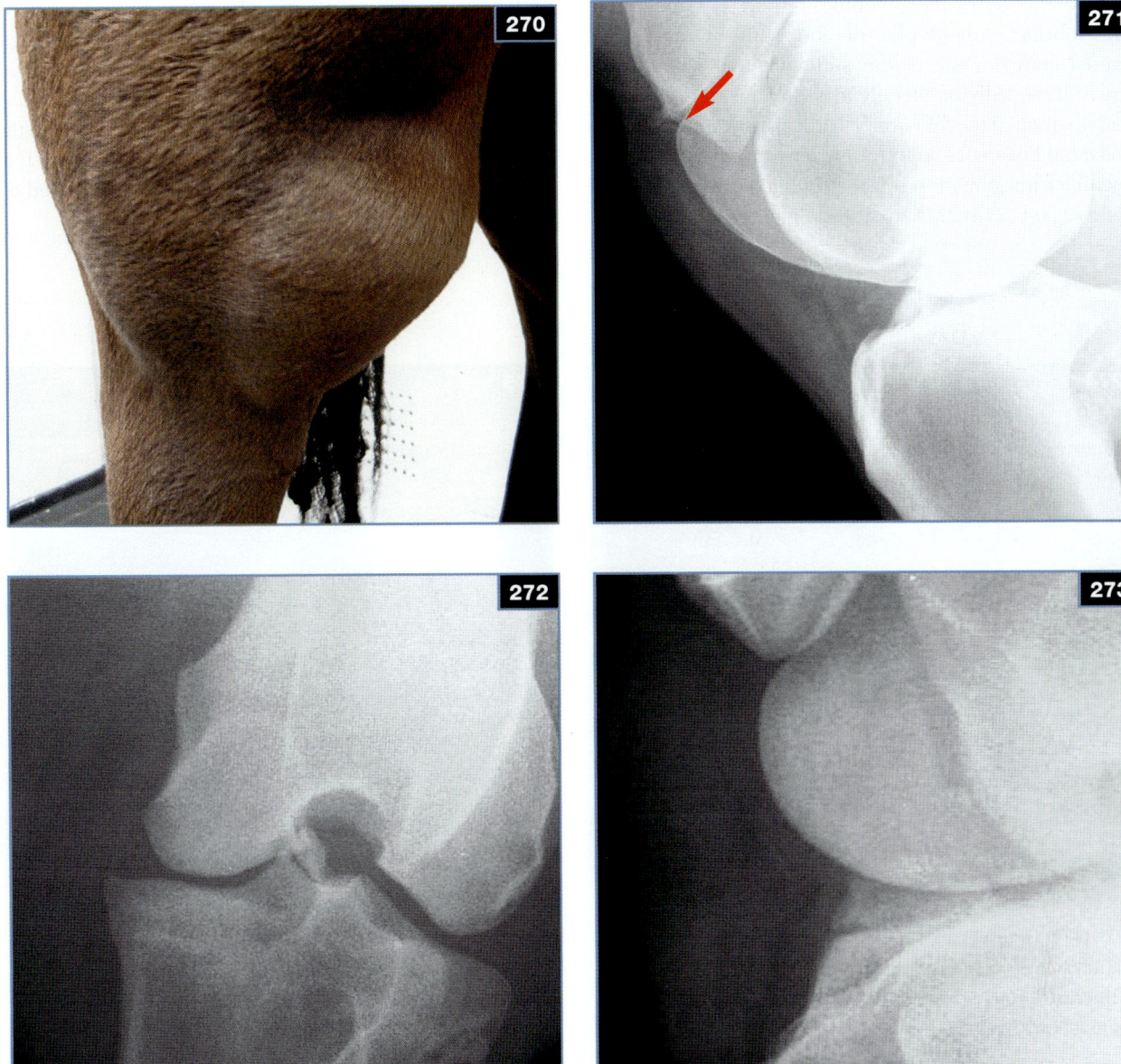

Diagnosis

The reciprocal apparatus coordinates the movement of the whole limb and therefore it is impossible to localize gait abnormalities to the stifle. Clinical findings at the level of the stifle may point to this region as the potential site of pain, but careful examination of the rest of the limb is still mandatory. Due to the unpredictable communication between the different synovial compartments of the stifle joint, it is important to anesthetize all three to localize the pain. If the lameness is severe, local analgesia should be avoided. Radiography and ultrasonography may identify the injury (271–273). Additional views such as a skyline view of the patella, flexed lateromedial, and oblique views

272, 273 Caudocranial (272) and flexed lateromedial (273) radiographs showing a fracture of the medial intercondylar eminence of the tibia sustained spontaneously during exercise.

at different angles are sometimes required in addition to the routine radiographs of the stifle. Obtaining a caudal/cranial view of the stifle while it is manually stressed medially or laterally may demonstrate an abnormal opening of the femorotibial articulation, indicating lost collateral ligament support. Ultrasonography is extremely useful for imaging most soft-tissue conditions affecting the stifle region (274–277), apart from injuries to the cruciate

and meniscal ligaments, which cannot be adequately visualized. It is also very helpful in examining the cartilage of the trochlear ridges of the distal femur. Scintigraphy is indicated in acutely lame horses when a fracture is suspected but the location is not identified. Diagnostic arthroscopy is indicated if no abnormalities are detected on any imaging modality and the lameness is localized to the stifle (278).

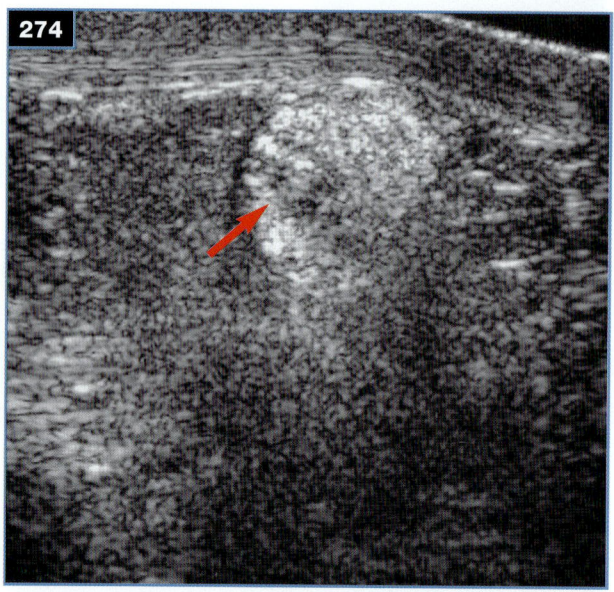

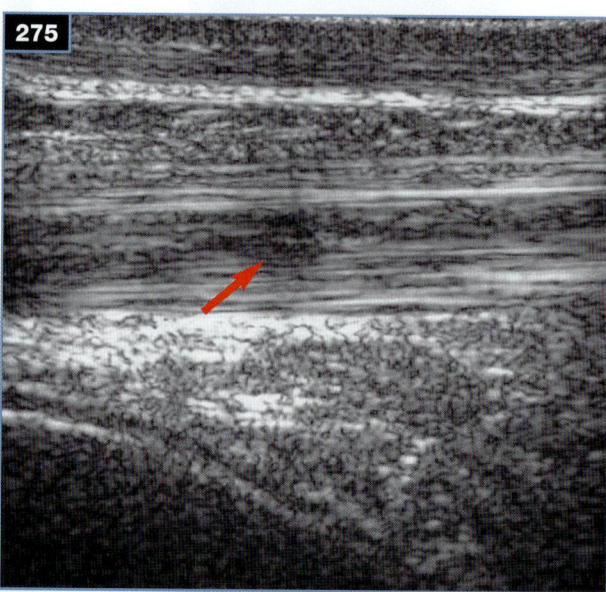

274, 275 Transverse (274) and longitudinal (275) ultrasonographic images demonstrating heterogenicity and disruption of fiber pattern indicative of desmitis of the middle patellar ligament (arrows).

276, 277 Longitudinal ultrasonographic scan of the medial aspect of the stifle demonstrating disruption of the medial meniscus, indicative of a tear (276). Note the normal ultrasonographic appearance of the contralateral meniscus (277).

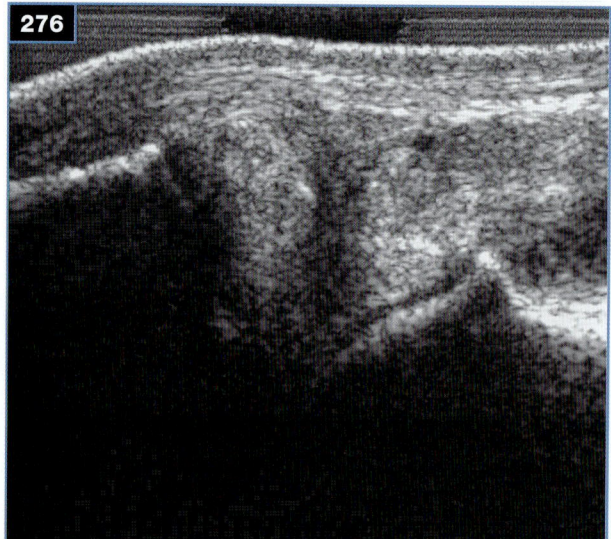

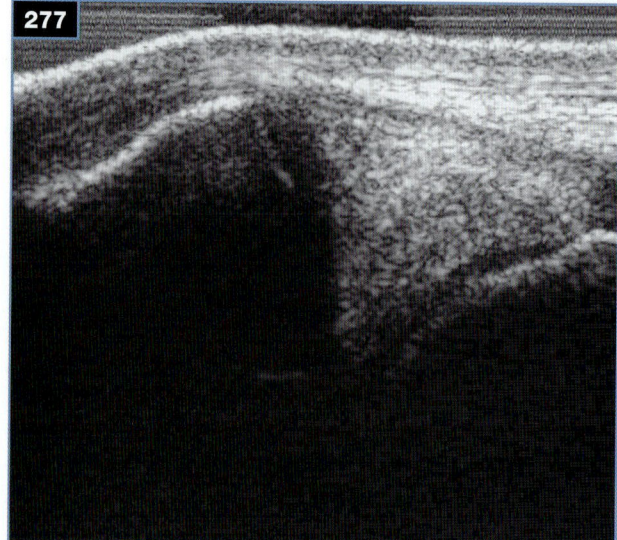

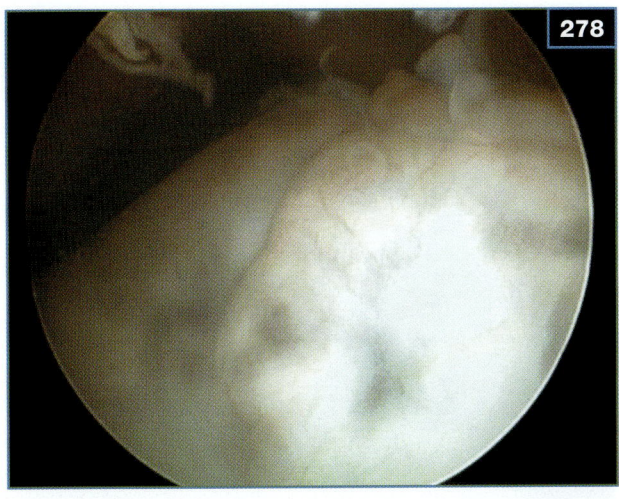

278 Arthroscopic view of the horse in 270 demonstrating OCD of the lateral trochlear ridge of the femur.

Management/prognosis

Treatment for tibial tuberosity fractures is determined by the size of the fragment, the degree of displacement, and involvement of the joint. Horses with minimally or non-displaced fragments may be treated conservatively with box rest. It is advisable to cross-tie these horses to minimize the risk of proximal displacement of the fractured fragment by the pull of the quadriceps muscles via the patellar ligament. Small, displaced fragments are best removed, and large fragments creating loss of function of the patellar ligaments should be fixed internally using a DCP and screws. Generally, the prognosis for horses with tibial tuberosity fractures is good.

Intra-articular fractures should be assessed arthroscopically, small osteochondral fragments should be removed, and the fracture bed debrided. Large fragments should be stabilized internally and this commonly requires an open approach. Arthroscopic evaluation and debridement are the preferred procedures for articular cartilage fragments, torn menisci and their supporting ligaments, and the cruciate ligaments. Surgical repair of a torn cruciate ligament in the horse is technically impossible. The prognosis for soundness is guarded in horses with articular cartilage fragments or meniscal tears, and poor in horses with moderate to severe cruciate ligament injuries.

Horses with desmitis of the patellar ligaments or damaged collateral ligaments should be treated with rest and controlled exercise, and the progress monitored ultrasonographically. Some cases have been treated with shockwave therapy. The prognosis for collateral ligament injury is poor, and some horses with desmitis of the patellar ligament may not return to their previous level of exercise.

Osteochondrosis of the femoropatellar joint

Definition/Overview

The femoropatellar joint is one of the most common sites for OCD in the horse, particularly in the Warmblood and Thoroughbred (see 261). The disease usually presents in actively growing large individuals as foals and weanlings, but may remain clinically silent until the animal starts active work. It may predispose to the early onset of OA of this joint.

Clinical presentation

The condition usually presents before 2 years of age and is particularly seen between 4 and 14 months in excessively growing individuals. In some animals the disease remains asymptomatic in their early life, but presents later either as their work program increases between three and six years of age or where excessive wear and tear leads to OA of the joint. There is usually obvious femoropatellar joint distension, often bilateral, but possibly asymmetrical in degree. The degree of lameness can vary from a mild bilateral stiffness of the hindlimb gait to a marked unilateral lameness, especially where there are large lesions of the lateral trochlear ridge and possible lateral patella instability. The lameness often improves with rest but returns with increased exercise.

Differential diagnosis

Traumatic lesions of the stifle joints and patella; subchondral bone cysts of the medial femoral condyle; sepsis of the femoropatellar joint; in older animals other causes of OA and inflammation of the femoropatellar joint.

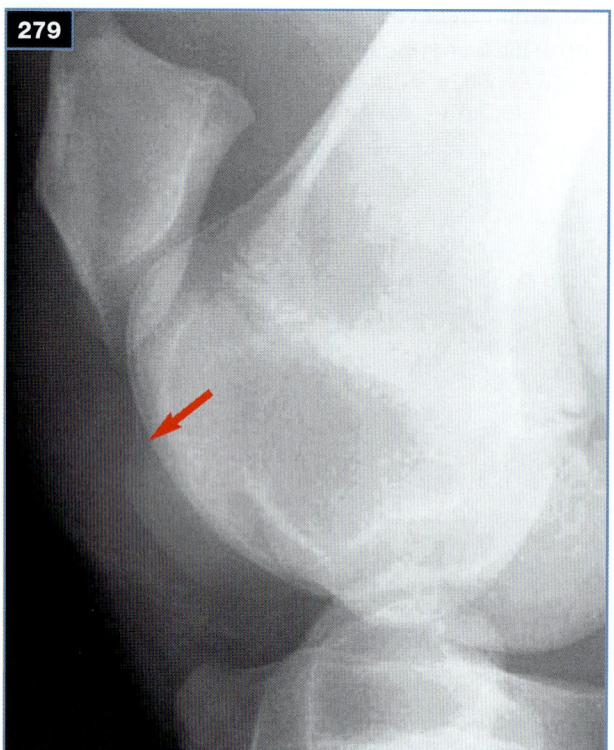

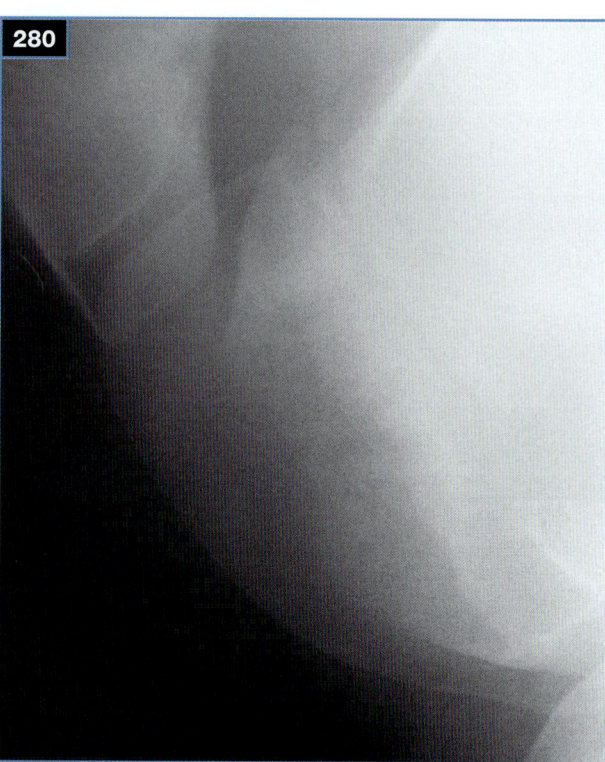

279 Lateral radiograph of the stifle of the horse in 270 demonstrating OCD of the lateral trochlear ridge of the femur (arrow).

280 Lateral radiograph demonstrating a severe OCD lesion of the lateral trochlear ridge of the femur. (Photo courtesy GA Munroe)

Diagnosis

Clinical history and presenting signs are highly suspicious, but confirmation requires radiographs of the stifle, preferably of both limbs. Lateral medial and caudal 60° lateral craniomedial oblique views are the most useful. The most common site for lesions is the lateral trochlear ridge of the femur, although occasionally lesions restricted to the articular surface of the patella are seen. Rarely, the medial trochlear ridge and the trochlear groove are involved. Significant radiographic lesions include: marked flattening of the mid- to upper-third of the lateral ridge; irregularity of the contour of the ridge; one or more subchondral lucent defects in the ridge +/− surrounding sclerosis; osseous density fragments within the ridge defects or free in the joint distally; irregularity of the articular surface of the patella towards the apex +/− surrounding sclerosis; evidence of osteophytic development in older horses with secondary OA (**279**, **280**). Ultrasonography of the femoropatellar joint will identify joint distension and localize trochlear ridge cartilage lesions. Arthroscopy of the joint allows identification of all lesions and assessment of the extent of cartilage damage.

Management

In early or mild cases, conservative treatment with rest, systemic NSAIDs, and possibly intra-articular medications may be adequate to return the animal to soundness in the short term. Some of these animals may develop problems later in life due to the onset of early joint disease and OA. Surgical intervention using arthroscopy is recommended for cases that are significantly lame, have not responded to conservative treatment, and have large lesions, and where an athletic career is envisaged. Horses with OA are treated conservatively in most cases.

Prognosis

This depends on the extent and severity of the lesions, at what age they are detected, and whether affecting one or both limbs. The prognosis is generally guarded to fair for return to athletic soundness for lesions requiring surgical intervention and guarded to poor where OA is evident. Large lesions where instability of the patella is evident have a poor prognosis.

Calcinosis circumscripta

Definition/overview
This is an uncommon condition, more often seen in young horses. The lesions involved in this condition are usually in the subcutaneous tissue close to joints or tendon sheaths. Although most commonly seen in the stifle region, calcinosis circumscripta has also been described in the hock, carpus, neck, and shoulder.

Etiology/pathophysiology
In the stifle, calcinosis circumscripta occurs on the lateral aspect close to the fibula. The cause is unknown. Histologically, the lesion demonstrates dystrophic mineralization of subcutaneous tissue, with evidence of inflammation, hence it is suggested that trauma may be the initiating factor. Tumoral calcinosis is a metastasic condition associated with calcification of multiple periarticular sites.

281–283 Caudocranial (281) and lateromedial (282) radiographs of a horse with calcinosis circumscripta located on the lateral aspect of the stifle. (283) Calcinosis circumscripta lesion removed surgically. (Photos courtesy MC Schramme)

Clinical presentation
The horse is generally presented because of the presence of an unsightly mass. Owners commonly describe the mass as having been slowly increasing in size. The lesion palpates as a firm and well-circumscribed mass closely attached to the underlying tissues, with no involvement of the skin. Occasionally, horses may have a gait abnormality. Tumoral calcinosis is commonly present at multiple sites.

Differential diagnosis
Tumoral calcinosis; osteochondromatosis; mast cell tumor.

Diagnosis
Clinical findings are not specific enough for accurate diagnosis. Radiography reveals localized soft-tissue swelling and amorphous to well-circumscribed accumulations of granular mineral opacity (281, 282).

Management
Most horses are best not treated at all. Surgical excision is indicated only if the lesion causes clinical complications or if the owners insist on removal for cosmetic reasons (283). In these horses, delicate excision is required to avoid penetrating the adjacent femorotibial joint capsule. Recurrence has not been reported.

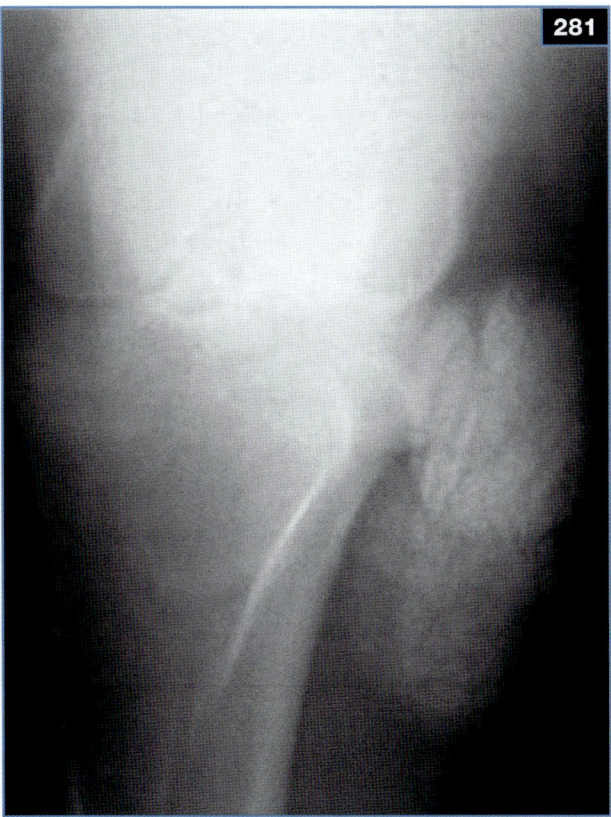

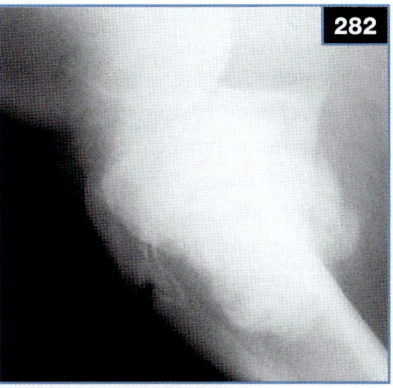

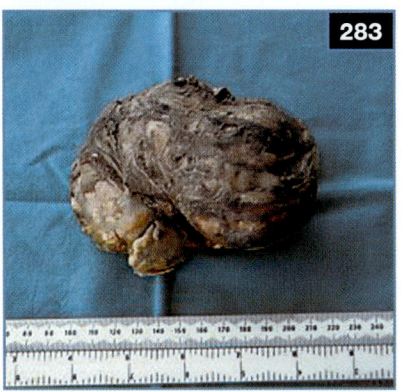

155

Femur

Fractures

Definition/overview
Femoral fractures may occur at any level of the bone. Possible fracture locations include the head, neck, and greater trochanter, as well as fractures at the level of the mid-diaphysis or the distal aspect of the femur.

Etiology/pathophysiology
Femoral fractures are most commonly seen in very young horses, but can be found at any age. Fractures of the femoral head and neck occur almost exclusively in foals, usually after flipping over backwards or severely abducting the hindlimbs. Similarly, other types of femoral fractures occur most commonly after an external trauma such as a kick, a severe fall, or in young foals as a result of being trodden on by their dam. Femoral fractures in adult horses may also result from bad induction or recovery from general anesthesia. Diaphyseal fractures are commonly comminuted, spiral, or oblique in shape, and distal physeal fractures are usually Salter–Harris type II with the metaphyseal component caudally. The extensive musculature surrounding the bone protects femoral fractures from becoming open, and muscle contraction promotes significant overriding of the fracture ends.

Clinical presentation
Affected animals are non-weight-bearing lame, and crepitation and rotational instability are evident while manipulating the limb. The hemorrhage and swelling in the muscle may, however, keep the fracture ends separated, making it difficult to elicit crepitation. Young foals with a proximal physeal fracture can frequently bear some weight on the affected limb. External rotation of the limb, caused by the continuous pull of the gluteal muscles, is common. Swelling and severe edema are present in all diaphyseal and distal physeal fractures, but may be mild in minimally displaced distal physeal fractures and not readily apparent in acute proximal fractures. Overriding of the fracture ends shortens the distance between the greater trochanter and the patella, resulting in an appearance of upward fixation of the patella and, generally, a shorter limb with a higher hock compared with the contralateral limb. Furthermore, the patella itself often feels loose and can be manipulated sideways. Occasionally, a major blood vessel, usually the femoral artery, may be severed by the sharp fracture ends, resulting in clinical signs of acute blood loss or fatal hemorrhage.

Differential diagnosis
Coxofemoral luxation; upward fixation of the patella; fractures of the patella or tibia; pelvis fractures; muscle tear (284).

Diagnosis
Presentation, clinical signs, and findings on palpation and manipulation of the limb are highly suggestive of a fracture, and auscultation with a stethoscope over the femoral region may facilitate crepitus recognition. Proximal physeal fractures are the most difficult to diagnose clinically. Rectal palpation of larger animals may reveal the crepitation while the limb is manipulated. Soft-tissue swelling may be identified on the medial aspect of the thigh. For all fracture types, radiography is required for definitive diagnosis and determination of severity (285, 286). Due to the musculature overlying the bone in an adult horse, diagnostic images can usually be obtained only for the distal aspect of the femur in a standing position, although with the right equipment, oblique views of the coxofemoral joint can be obtained as well. All other cases require general anesthesia, although in small foals heavy sedation may suffice. If a displaced fracture is suspected, induction and recovery are likely to be difficult and general anesthesia is therefore contraindicated. In these cases, ultrasonography may allow tracing of the surface of the fractured bone to confirm the displacement. Scintigraphy is the best imaging modality for diagnosing fractures of the greater or third trochanters; however, these may also be confirmed ultrasonographically.

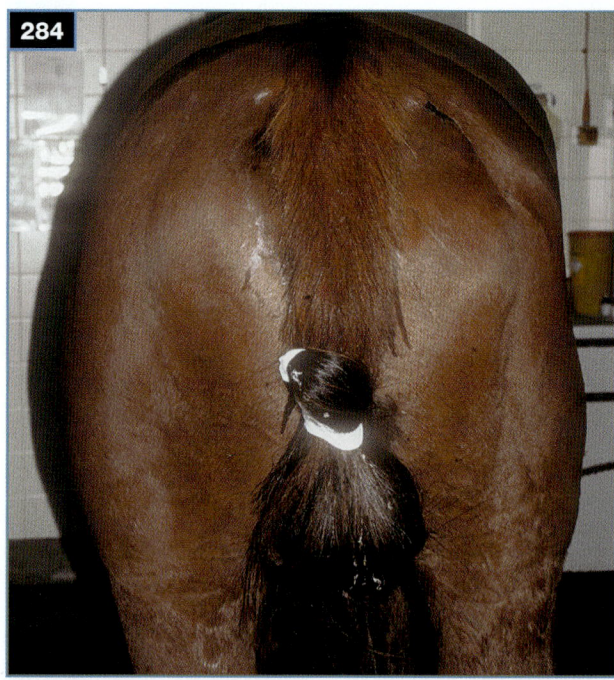

284 Caudal view of a horse with swelling of the musculature of the left hindlimb as a result of hematoma following acute muscle tear. (Photo courtesy RK Smith)

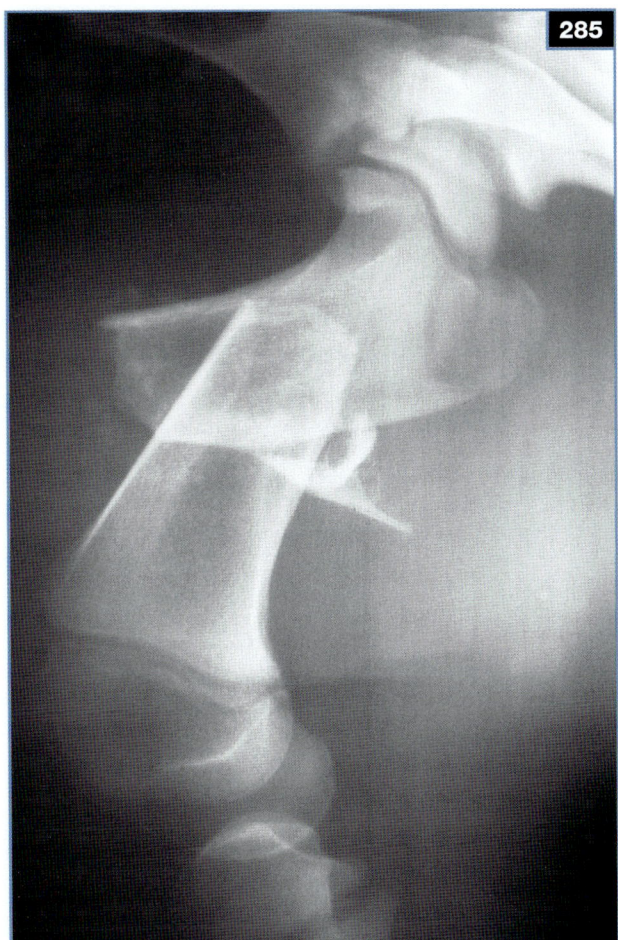 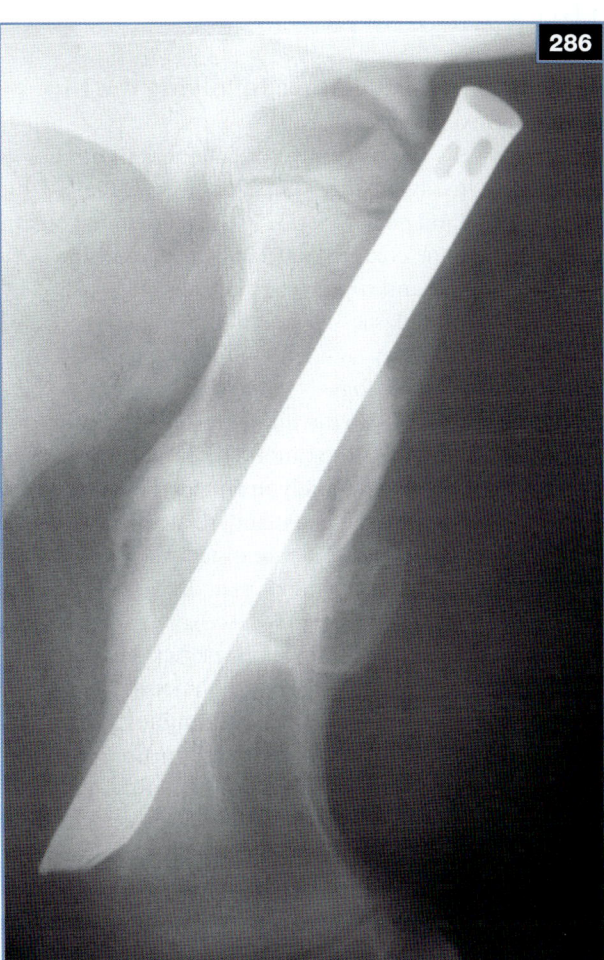

285, 286 Preoperative (285) and postoperative (286) radiographs of a mid-shaft fracture of the femur in a foal.

Management

Treatment depends on a variety of factors such as location, type and severity of the fracture, degree of soft-tissue damage, temperament of the horse, and financial constraints. The most important factor to consider is the size of the affected animal, and euthanasia is warranted for horses heavier than 200 kg with a displaced fracture. Successful repair of diaphyseal or proximal physeal fractures has been achieved only in foals and small ponies, and distal physeal fractures have been successfully treated in yearlings. Internal fixation of diaphyseal fracture requires double plating, and full fracture healing is expected in 50% of cases. Distal physeal fractures can be more difficult to repair due to the smaller distal part of the bone restricting screw placement. In these cases a single special plate may be used. Conservative management of a minimally displaced distal physeal fracture may result in a satisfactory result; however, although a similar approach to the treatment of diaphyseal fracture may lead to healing, complications such as limb shortening, rotational deformity, and contralateral varus deformity are common. A variety of surgical techniques and implants can be use to repair proximal physeal fractures, but the prognosis is guarded as significant complications such as OA of the coxofemoral joint, unstable fixation, and necrosis of the femoral head are common. Conservative management of these fractures is best avoided as it is unlikely to result in a comfortable horse. Box rest is the treatment of choice for a fractured greater or third trochanter.

157

Hip joint and pelvis

Injuries and joint disease involving the hip

Definition/overview

The hip joint is rarely a cause of lameness in the horse. Conditions involving this joint include fractures of the femoral head and neck (see p. 156), fracture involving the coxofemoral joint, coxofemoral joint subluxation and luxation, partial tear and rupture of the round ligament, OA, OCD, and hip dysplasia.

Etiology/pathophysiology

Fractures and damage to the round ligament are the result of trauma to the region, commonly after a fall. The coxofemoral joint is predominantly maintained in position by the round (accessory) ligament and, to a lesser extent, by other smaller ligaments. The rare instances of round ligament rupture/partial tear without joint dislocation result in instability and/or subluxation of the coxofemoral joint and rapid development of OA. Luxation results from damage to the supporting ligaments, unstable fracture of the ilial shaft, or articular fracture of the acetabulum following a fall, violent overextension, or severe abduction or adduction of the limb. The femur most commonly displaces in a craniodorsal direction. Luxation can also occur after application of a full-limb cast and, occasionally, it is manifested as a complication of upward fixation of the patella or it accompanies this condition. Hip dysplasia occurs rarely, but is well recognized and possibly hereditary in Norwegian Dole ponies. This syndrome is usually bilateral, involving malformation of the acetabulum and the head and neck of the femur, which leads to instability, subluxation, and OA, which may also be a sequela to any of the other conditions affecting the coxofemoral joint. OCD occurs very rarely in the coxofemoral joint.

Clinical presentation

Commonly, the horse is presented with an acute lameness following trauma. Horses that have dislocated the hip joint or have just ruptured the round ligament without luxation are severely lame. The affected limb is rotated with the stifle and toe pointed out and the hock turned medially (**287**). When assessed from the back, the hock of the dislocated limb appears to be higher in comparison to that of the contralateral limb, and as a result of this limb shortening the cranial phase of the stride is significantly shorter. The excessive motion of the femur may lead to crepitation and pain when the limb is manipulated. If the round ligament is only partially torn, clinical signs are less

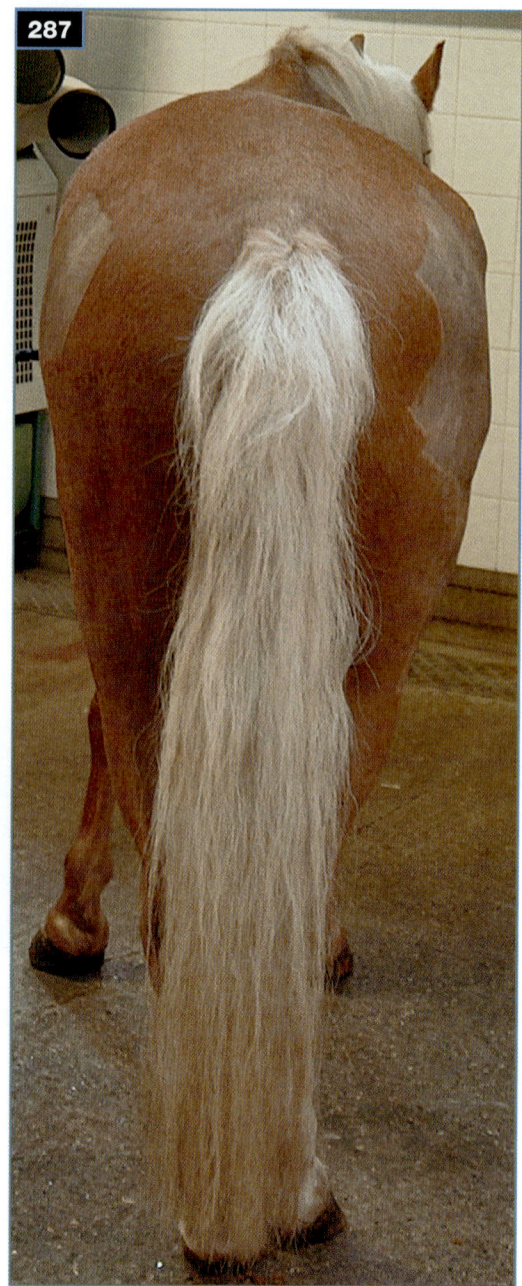

287 Luxation of the right coxofemoral joint in a pony following upward fixation of the patella. Note the pelvic asymmetry and outward rotation of the right hind toe.

288 Ventrodorsal radiograph of the hip region of the pony in 287 demonstrating luxation of the coxofemoral joint.

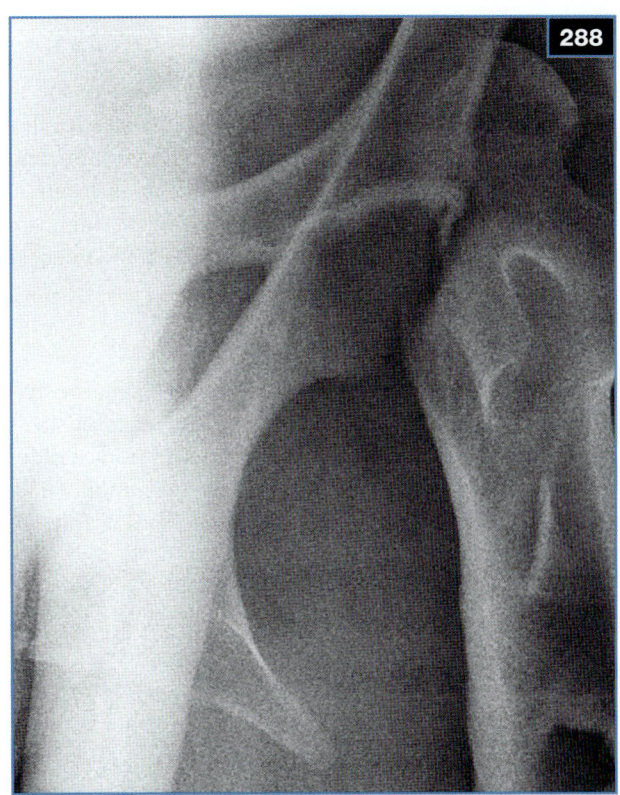

distinct and the horse, other than being lame, may resent abduction of the limb. Chronic cases develop significant gluteal atrophy. OA has no distinct clinical signs other than lameness with or without muscle atrophy.

Differential diagnosis
Upward fixation of the patella; fracture of the pelvis; trochanteric bursitis.

Diagnosis
A history of trauma, severe lameness, and clinical findings, mainly of outward rotation of the whole limb, may be suggestive of hip luxation or rupture of the round ligament. In these cases, radiographs of the coxofemoral joint can be taken in a standing position and luxation of the joint or fractures can be identified (**288**). If luxation is ruled out and in other chronic cases, where OA has developed, intra-articular analgesia of the coxofemoral joint should be performed to localize the joint as the source of pain. This procedure can be challenging, although easier under ultrasonographic guidance, and will usually only improve the lameness rather than completely abolish it. Ultrasound examination of the articular regions of the acetabulum and femoral head is possible and helpful where X-ray machines of suitable power are not available. Nuclear scintigraphy can be performed if a fracture is suspected or if the results of the intra-articular block are equivocal. Scintigraphic findings, however, have to be cautiously interpreted because of possible differences in muscle mass. Definitive diagnosis of OA requires high-quality radiographs obtained under general anesthesia in dorsal decumbency. Diagnostic arthroscopy can be performed, but for horses weighing >300 kg, special long instruments are required.

Management
Closed reduction of a coxofemoral luxation can be achieved under general anesthesia in acute cases only. In chronic cases the acetabulum fills in with granulation tissue preventing relocation of the femoral head back into position. The joint may dislocate again either during recovery or within a few days. Various surgical procedures for open reduction can be attempted, but the prognosis for athletic function is poor. There is no effective treatment for rupture of the round ligament apart from arthroscopic debridement and medication of the joint with corticosteroids, which is also suitable for horses with OA. The prognosis in these cases is guarded.

Fractures of the pelvis
Definition/overview
Any of the bony components of the pelvis are prone to fracture. This includes the ilial wing, tuber coxae, ilial shaft, pubis, obturator foramen, acetabulum, sacrum, and ischium. While previously considered to be an uncommon injury, stress fractures, mainly at the wing of the ilium, are now known to be a common cause of hindlimb lameness in the racing Thoroughbred.

Etiology/pathophysiology
Complete fractures of the pelvis occur as a result of external trauma, falls on the side, or as an end stage of stress fractures in horses in training or racing. In horses older than 6 years the wing of the ilium is most commonly fractured, and in younger animals the other types of fracture occur at similar rates.

Clinical presentation
Affected horses are presented with a variable degree of lameness, depending on the location of the fracture and its duration. Fractures of the ilial shaft or acetabulum commonly produce a non-weight-bearing lameness, although horses with other types of pelvic fracture may be less lame. The lameness is commonly evident at the walk. Fractures of the sacrum or pubis commonly result in bilateral hindlimb lameness, and horses with fractures of the acetabulum have an extremely short limb protraction at the walk. Pelvic asymmetry is common with fractures of the tuber coxae and complete fractures of the ilial wing or shaft (289). Fractures of the tuber ischii usually show asymmetrical positioning and swelling. Other clinical signs may include soft-tissue swelling, muscle spasm, pain and crepitation on palpation and manipulation, subcutaneous hematoma, and, occasionally, penetration of the skin by the sharp edges of the fractured bone (290). While complete fractures of the ilial wing in a racehorse may be present on one side only, signs of subclinical stress fractures in the same site on the contralateral limb are commonly reported. Mares with fractures of the pubis or ischium may have vaginal or vulvar swelling from edema and hemorrhage. Fatal hemorrhage can occur if a major artery is severed by the sharp edges of the fractured displaced bone.

Differential diagnosis
Fracture of the femur; separation of the femoral head; coxofemoral luxation; exertional rhabdomyolysis.

289 Caudal view of a horse with a fracture of the pelvis. Note the distinct pelvic asymmetry.

290 Caudal view of a Thoroughbred racehorse that presented with right hindlimb lameness after a fall. There is an asymmetry of the tubera ischii, with the right side (arrow) not as clearly visible as the left. This horse was confirmed to have a fracture of the right tuber ischii following ultrasonography and radiography of the caudal pelvis. (Photo courtesy GA Munroe)

291 Ventrodorsal radiograph of a pony that had spontaneously fractured its pelvis while in a field.

Diagnosis
Diagnosis is based on history, clinical signs, findings on external and rectal palpation, and imaging. Radiography of the pelvis is easily performed in a foal, but is considerably more difficult in the adult horse. Views of the coxofemoral joint region and ischium can be obtained in the standing sedated horse using powerful machines (291). Most fractures can only be imaged with the horse under general anesthesia. Due to the risk of further damage or displacement during recovery, this is contraindicated. Bone scintigraphy is extremely useful. Ultrasonographic examination is easy, quick, and relatively cheap compared with the other imaging modalities. This modality is useful for fractures of the tuber coxae as well as the ilial wing and shaft (292); however, minimally displaced or incomplete fractures as well as poor callus formation may not be identified with ultrasonography.

Management
Surgical fixation of pelvic fractures in the adult horse is impossible, and the only option is box rest for 2–3 months. Removal of bony fragments that have formed a sequestrum may be indicated. The outcome in terms of functional anatomy depends on the site and initial displacement of the fracture and the extent of further distraction of the fragments by the subsequent muscle contracture.

Prognosis
Horses with fractures of the tuber coxae and ilial wings have a good prognosis for athletic activity, but involvement of the ilial shaft significantly worsens the prognosis. Fractures of the acetabulum carry the worst prognosis for returning to athletic activity.

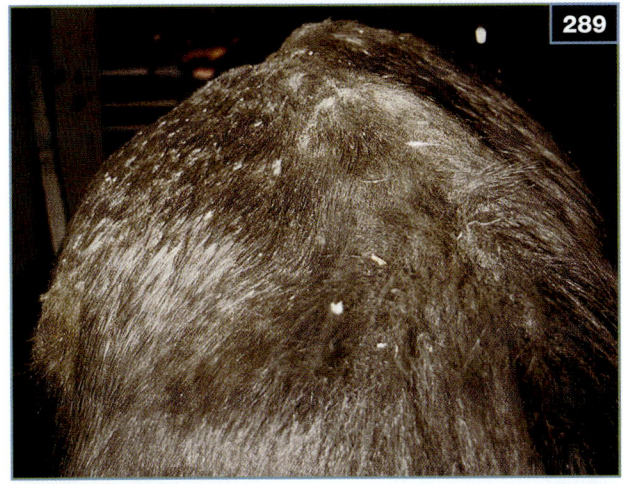

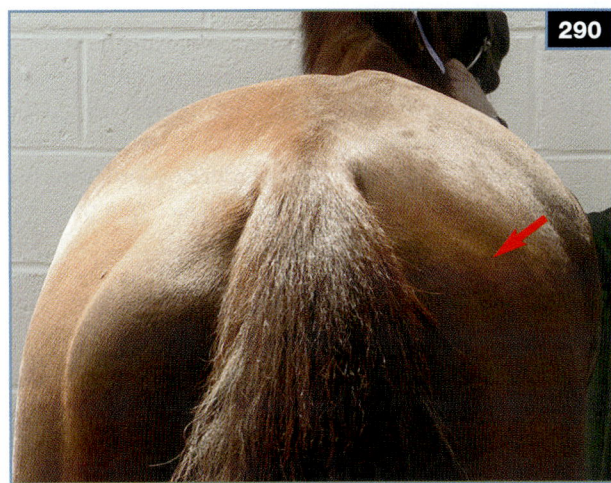

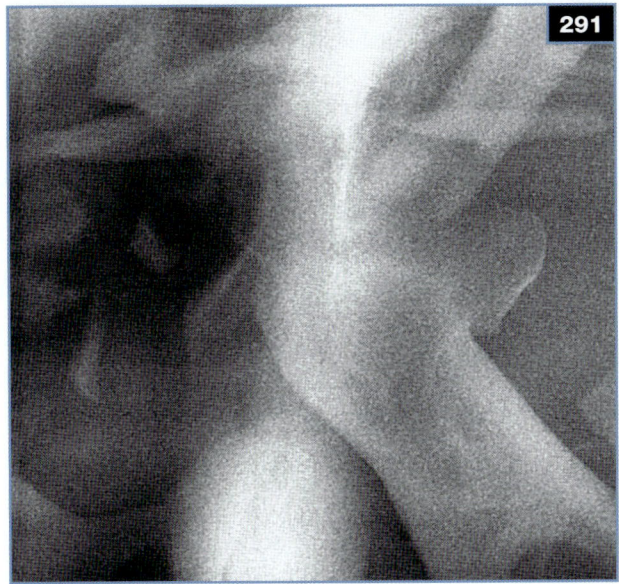

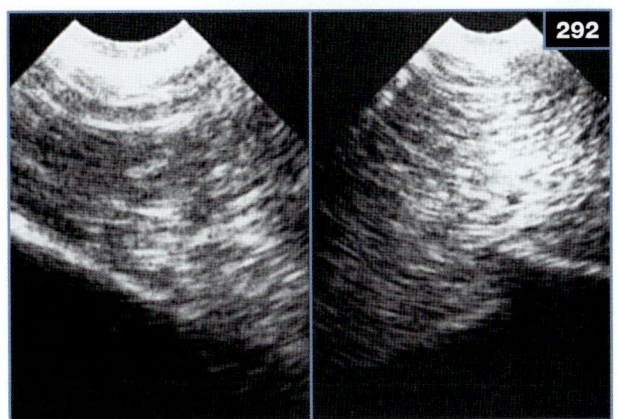

292 Ultrasound scan of the ilial wings. Note the disruption of the echogenic line of the bone indicative of a fracture on the right image compared with the normal appearance of the ilial wing on the left.

Generalized orthopedic diseases

Immune-mediated polysynovitis

Definition/overview
This condition is relatively uncommon, and most reported cases are in foals.

Etiology/pathophysiology
Immune-mediated polysynovitis is caused by deposition of immune complexes in the synovium and complement activation as a sequela to a primary inflammatory focus such as pneumonia, infected umbilicus, or a peripheral abscess. *Rhodococcus equi* is the most commonly reported primary infective agent, but the condition has been reported following equine virus herpes-4 and streptococcal infections. Frequently, more than one joint is involved.

Clinical presentation
Affected animals are presented with an effusion of one or more joints, gait stiffness, and low-grade lameness. If the primary infection source is still active, the animal will have the relevant clinical signs.

Differential diagnosis
Infectious arthritis; idiopathic arthritis; Lyme disease.

Diagnosis
Clinical presentation of multiple joint effusion but minimal lameness is suggestive of the condition. Analysis of synovial fluid collected aseptically from affected joints reveals a WBC count of <20 × 10^9/l, with a mixture of healthy neutrophils and mononuclear cells.

161

Management

The primary cause should be identified and treated accordingly. The condition is self-limiting and recovery is expected within a few weeks. The animal should be restricted to a box and treatment with systemic chondroprotective drugs may be considered. Corticosteroid therapy may be contraindicated in the face of a bacterial infection.

Lyme disease (borreliosis)

Definition/overview

Confirmed clinical cases are rare, but in certain parts of the world such as the north east of the USA and parts of the UK cases are seen regularly. The disease has a significant zoonotic risk in humans bitten by infected ticks in endemic areas.

Etiology/pathophysiology

The causative agent of Lyme disease is a spirochete, *Borrelia burgdorferi*, which is transmitted to the horse through a bite of an infected tick of the *Ixodes* family. These ticks have a 2-year, three-stage life cycle and they can become infected during any stage by feeding on mammalian hosts, commonly the white-footed mouse in the USA and possibly deer in the UK. The stage of the life cycle infecting the horse is unknown. Not all ticks are infected with the spirochete and infection varies by tick species and geographic region. The infective agent is capable of nonspecifically activating various cells of the immune system, leading to the production of proinflammatory mediators, which tend to localize in joints and result in chronic arthritis.

Clinical presentation

Lameness and stiffness in one or more limbs as well as low-grade fever are the most common clinical signs. The lameness is often caused by arthritis, which can involve more than one joint and may become chronic. Other clinical signs include chronic weight loss, swollen joints, muscle tenderness, and anterior uveitis. Neurologic signs may be seen if the bacteria have penetrated the central nervous system (CNS).

Differential diagnosis

OA; OCD; polysaccharide storage myopathy; chronic intermittent rhabdomyolysis; equine protozoal myelitis; immune-mediated polysynovitis.

Diagnosis

Diagnosis of the disease in horses is difficult, and presumptive diagnosis is commonly based on history, clinical signs, housing in an endemic area, and ruling out of other causes. ELISA titers and positive Western blot testing are reported to be beneficial in some cases. Serologic tests, however, do not distinguish between active infection and subclinical exposure. Tests that directly identify the spirochete are being developed.

Management

Treatment most commonly involves administration of tetracycline (6.6 mg/kg i/v q24h) or doxycycline (10 mg/kg p/o q12h). Administration of ceftiofur (2–4 mg/kg i/m q12h) has been reported as well. The duration of treatment may be as long as 30 days, but the rationale for this is empirical. A supportive treatment is occasionally indicated, and may include chondroprotective agents and/or NSAIDs. Clinical signs in suspected cases have been reported to resolve within 1 week of treatment. Aids in prevention of the disease include daily grooming, application of tick repellents containing permethrin, and pasture management and care. An equine-approved vaccination is not yet commercially available.

Musculoskeletal nutritional deficiencies

Definition/overview

Nutrition has a major role in the proper development and function of the musculoskeletal system. Imbalanced nutrition affects horses of all ages and disciplines, starting from the embryo, through the foal and growing horse stage, to the adult. Conditions that may occur as a result of these deficiencies include nutritional secondary hyperparathyroidism, OCD and/or any of the DODs, exertional rhabdomyolysis, and white muscle disease.

Etiology/pathophysiology

Nutrients suggested to affect the musculoskeletal system when deficient include: electrolytes such as sodium, potassium, calcium, and magnesium; minerals such as calcium and phosphorus; trace minerals (copper, zinc, and selenium); vitamins (A, D, and E); protein; and digestible energy. Not only is the actual digested level of these nutrients important, but also the relative amounts of any of these nutrients and the interrelations between them. A malnourished mare may deliver an abnormal or impaired foal, and a nursing foal may develop musculoskeletal abnormalities following inadequate production of milk by the mare or production of milk with improper amounts of minerals or other nutrients.

DODs are thought to be caused in part by abnormal cross-linkage of cartilage matrix and impaired replacement of cartilage by bone as a result of copper deficiency. Copper is an essential component of lysyl oxidase, which is important in the cross-linking of collagen and elastin. Diets high in calcium and phosphorus in young, growing foals have been shown to interfere with copper and zinc absorption, adversely affecting cartilage maturation, and experimental zinc-responsive osteodystrophy has been reported; however, the deficiency has not been confirmed in horses on natural feeds. Electrolyte depletion, mainly of sodium, potassium, magnesium, and calcium, appears to predispose susceptible horses to exertional rhabdomyolysis, as these electrolytes play a key role in muscle fiber contraction. Depletion occurs due to loss in sweat during overstrenuous exercise or as a result of dietary deficiency.

Horses that are fed on a diet high in phosphorus and/or low in calcium, with a phosphorus/calcium ratio of 3:1 or more, may develop nutritional secondary hyperparathyroidism. Feeding excessive amounts of wheat bran may be associated with the condition due to its high content of phosphorus. Grains with a high phosphorus/calcium ratio may result in excessive absorption of phosphorus and reduced absorption of calcium. Various pastures contain high contents of oxalate, which binds calcium and predisposes to the condition. This imbalance leads to hyperphosphatemia, which stimulates parathyroid hormone (PTH) secretion and inhibits the synthesis of the active form of vitamin D in the kidney. As a result of this, osteoclastic activity is increased, resulting in excessive bone resorption and bone loss.

Nutritional myodegeneration (white muscle disease) is due to inadequate selenium intake by a dam during pregnancy or lactation, hence this condition is most common in foals up to 60 days of age, but can also occur in older animals. Although selenium and vitamin E appear to have a synergistic effect in preventing this condition, it appears that selenium deficiency has a more important role.

It is suggested that inadequate levels of protein in a mare's diet can cause hypothyroidism in the fetus, which may persist postnatally and affect normal development. This deficiency may lead to incomplete ossification of the carpal/tarsal cuboidal bones, thus causing ALDs.

Clinical presentation
Clinical signs vary with the condition. Foals and young horses with DODs may be lame and have synovial effusion, swelling at the level of the physeal growth plates, or limb deformities. ALDs may be present at birth, but commonly occur within the first few weeks. Horses affected by nutritional secondary hyperparathyroidism may show symmetrical enlargement of facial bones, upper respiratory noise, and lameness, and young horses may develop physitis and limb deformities. Bone resorption around the lamina dura of the molars and premolars may result in pain and masticatory problems, and in severe cases teeth may become loosened. Exertional rhabdomyolysis results in a stiff and stilted gait in affected horses and occasionally these animals are unable to walk. The hindquarters and back muscles may be firm and painful on palpation, and the horse may sweat excessively and have a high respiratory rate due to the pain. The skeletal muscle form of white muscle disease is mainly characterized by muscular weakness and stiffness, and affected animals may be unable to

stand. Muscles of the limbs are swollen and may be firm and painful on palpation. Muscle fasciculations and a stiff and stilted gait can occur in horses with hypocalcemia and/or hypomagnesemia, both of which are very uncommon. Hypothyroidism in the fetus may cause delayed prenatal and postnatal development, resulting in permanent stunting. Delayed ossification of the cuboidal bones of the carpus and hock is also suggested to be related to this condition.

Differential diagnosis
Septic polyarthritis; neuromuscular disease; polysaccharide storage myopathy; aortoiliac thrombosis; colic.

Diagnosis
Commonly, the only way to diagnose and correct nutritional deficiencies is to evaluate the ration and water ingested. If a problem develops in a nursing foal, it is recommended to ascertain that the mare is producing enough milk and that the composition of the milk, especially with regard to minerals, is correct. In horses with nutritional secondary hyperparathyroidism, clinical laboratory findings may include mild hypocalcemia and hyperphosphatemia; however, these values may be within the reference ranges. Fractional urinary clearance of calcium may be normal or low and that of phosphorus may be normal or high. Serum PTH level is increased. With an acute severe electrolyte deficiency (e.g. after an endurance exercise), serum levels of electrolytes may be below normal ranges; however, in chronic deficiencies, serum concentrations may not reflect total body electrolyte imbalances. In these cases renal fractional excretion should be determined by sampling urine and blood concurrently to determine creatinine and electrolyte concentrations. Measuring of muscle enzyme levels in the serum of horses with exertional rhabdomyolysis is useful; however, the degree of elevation does not necessarily reflect the severity of clinical signs. Horses suspected of having the chronic form of exertional rhabdomyolysis can be subjected to a submaximal exercise test and muscle biopsy. Some clinicians perform nuclear scintigraphy to demonstrate increased uptake of the radiopharmaceutical in the affected muscle.

Management
There is some evidence that supplementing the mare's diet during the last trimester with copper may result in significantly fewer cases of OCD. However, although supplementing the mare's diet to improve milk composition may succeed, if correct balance of mineral is not achieved, weaning of the foal is recommended. Food analysis may prove valid as part of the management of impaired endochondral ossification. Treatment for nutritional secondary hyperparathyroidism requires correction of the ration by

163

increasing calcium and reducing phosphorus intake to the level required, and restricting access to plants containing oxalates. Unless fractures are present, lameness usually disappears within 6 weeks. The objective of treating horses with the acute form of exertional rhabdomyolysis is to reduce anxiety and pain, and because severe rhabdomyolysis may lead to renal compromise, correcting fluid imbalance and inducing diuresis are essential. Horses affected with the chronic form of this condition are better off exercising daily than being rested, and their diet should be assessed and adjusted accordingly to include balanced minerals and vitamins, high quality hay (other than alfalfa), and a minimum of carbohydrates. Limb deformities should be treated according to the location of the deformity, its severity, and the age of the animal.

Fluoride toxicosis

Definition/overview
This condition is a rare event in horses, and refers to skeletal abnormality caused by chronic fluorine intake above the critical levels. Although both acute and chronic forms have been reported, chronic fluoride toxicosis appears to be more common.

Etiology/pathophysiology
Common sources of fluoride include contaminated forage from nearby industrial plants, drinking water containing excessive amounts of fluoride, feed supplements with high fluoride concentration, and vegetation grown on soils rich in fluoride. Fluoride accumulates in the bone and teeth throughout the horse's life and it is therefore a cumulative poison. It is almost fully absorbed from the GI tract, and approximately half is rapidly excreted in the urine; the rest accumulates in calcified developing tissues (i.e. bones and teeth) and therefore young growing animals are more susceptible. Excessive amounts of fluoride affect teeth during development by causing ameloblastic and odontoblastic damage, which results in defective mineralization. The pathophysiology of bone damage is not clear, but the results include abnormal osteogenesis, production of abnormal bone, accelerated remodeling, and, occasionally, accelerated bone resorption.

Clinical presentation
Affected horses may have exostosis formation, especially on the third MC/MT bones, but also on the mandible, ribs, and in sites of tendon insertion and periarticular tissues. They may also have a stiff gait and intermittent lameness and a dry and roughened coat. Poor growth and weight loss can occur as well, and abnormal bones are susceptible to fractures. Teeth may appear mottled and brown discolored, and with hypoplastic enamel. Some teeth may be missing.

Differential diagnosis
Hypertrophic osteopathy; nutritional secondary hyperthyroidism; osteomyelitis; OA; septic arthritis.

Diagnosis
This is based mainly on clinical signs and history of possible exposure. Fluoride in urine and bone can be determined, and analysis of water and feed is advisable. Radiographs may reveal abnormal bone appearance such as thickening and increased density of the bones.

Management
A reduction of the toxic effects of fluoride can be attempted by using substances such as aluminum sulfate, aluminum chloride, and calcium carbonate, but dietary restriction of fluoride-containing substances and removing the affected animal from the source of fluoride are the main options for treatment.

Prognosis
The prognosis appears to be poor if intermittent lameness is present. The teeth never recover from the discoloration.

Hypertrophic osteopathy

Definition/overview

Hypertrophic osteopathy is a noncontagious condition usually demonstrated clinically by bilateral symmetric proliferation of vascular connective tissue and subperiosteal bone of the distal extremities. The condition is also referred to as Marie's disease, hypertrophic osteodystrophy, and hypertrophic pulmonary osteoperiostitis.

Etiology/pathophysiology

The pathophysiology of this condition is not clearly understood, but theories include humoral, neural, and hypoxic mechanisms. Hypertrophic osteopathy has been associated with thoracic pathology such as lung abscessation, tuberculosis, neoplasia, pulmonary infarction, and rib fractures, but it has also been diagnosed in animals with abdominal metastases, and in one report it was twice related to pregnancy.

Clinical presentation

Horses are commonly presented for investigation of the enlarged bones, but signs related to the primary lesion such as cough, nasal discharge, or chronic weight loss may precede and be the reason for investigation. The clinical presentation is variable, but commonly the condition involves progressive deterioration over a prolonged period of time. The distal limbs may be symmetrically or asymmetrically swollen and warm, and there may be some restriction and pain on palpation and manipulation. Affected animals may have a stiff gait and commonly are reluctant to move.

Differential diagnosis

Fluorosis; nutritional secondary hyperthyroidism; and for the primary underlying disease intrathoracic or intra-abdominal mass (neoplasia, abscess).

Diagnosis

Diagnosis is based on clinical signs and radiographic findings. Radiography commonly reveals a palisade pattern of periosteal new bone formation parallel to the cortices of the long bones (293). Although the new bone may be close to the joint margins, the articular surfaces are rarely involved. Bone scintigraphy may show an increased uptake in the distal limb, even before radiographic changes. Hematology and biochemistry may reveal abnormalities related to the underlying cause. Efforts should be made to identify the primary condition. This should include upper airway endoscopy, broncheoalveolar lavage, thoracic radiography and ultrasonography, rectal palpation, abdominal centesis and ultrasonography. More invasive diagnostic procedures may include lung biopsy, pleuroscopy, and laparoscopy.

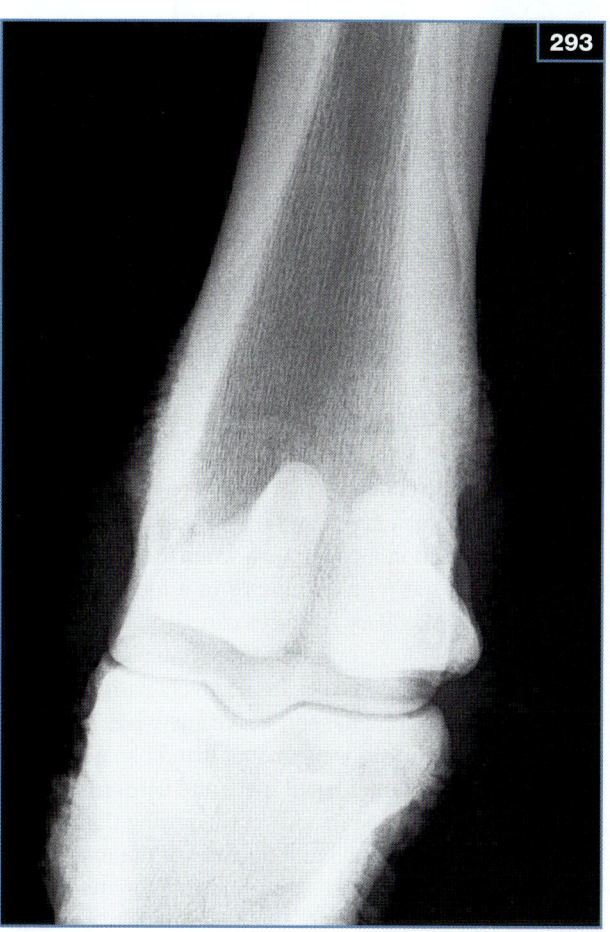

293 Dorsopalmar radiograph of a horse with hypertrophic osteopathy. Note the new bone formation at the level of the third metacarpal bone and proximal phalanx.

Management

The primary lesion should be treated if possible, and the bone lesions may subside following resolution of the primary problem. If no underlying disease is identified, symptomatic treatment, mainly with NSAIDs, is worthy of consideration. In a small proportion of horses the condition may resolve either spontaneously or following treatment of the primary cause.

Prognosis

If the primary lesion is not identified or treated, the prognosis is poor and, because of the debilitating nature of the condition, euthanasia is commonly necessary.

Mandible/maxilla

Fractures

Definition/overview

Fractures of the rostral skull are not uncommon, with the mandible being the most frequently fractured bone of the head. Many rostral skull injuries initially appear dramatic, with profuse hemorrhage and distortion of the bones of the skull, but most carry a good prognosis for full recovery.

Etiology/pathophysiology

Mandibular fractures may result from kicks by companion horses or from self-induced trauma when the horse tries to free itself after trapping its muzzle in a feeder, gate, or similar device. Maxillary fractures can also be caused by other horses, collisions, or self-induced trauma (**294**).

The mandible and maxilla are relatively narrow bones, with thin cortices and little soft-tissue covering. The most common site of fracture is the rostral mandible, where the bone narrows at the interdental space and flares rostrally to accommodate the incisor roots, predisposing this area to becoming trapped. Mandibular fractures at the interdental space are often bilateral. Many fractures of the rostral mandible and premaxilla are open and heavily contaminated, but the high vascularity of the region and relative fracture stability aid rapid healing in most cases, despite a high complication rate. The horizontal and vertical rami of the mandible and the maxilla are fractured less frequently due to protection by the overlying large masseter muscles. Neurologic deficits are unusual with rostral skull fractures.

Clinical presentation

Clinical signs of mandibular fractures vary with severity of injury and whether both mandibles are affected. Horses with small fractures of the incisive portion of the mandible may be able to prehend and masticate normally and show few or no signs, while fractures located more caudally may cause ptyalism, dysphagia, and, in chronic cases, marked halitosis as food becomes impacted into the fracture site. Maxillary fractures are commonly concurrent with nasal and/or frontal bone fractures (see p. 171). If the fragments are severely depressed, there will be involvement of the paranasal sinuses and associated structures and the most prominent clinical sign will be cavitation of the dorsal skull. There may be considerable subcutaneous emphysema as air exits the nasal cavities or sinuses. Visible depression of the dorsal surface of the skull indicates fracture of the maxillary, nasal, or frontal bones. Palpation of the rostral skull may reveal abnormal movement of the rostral mandibular region if there are bilateral fractures, or malalignment of the incisors (**295**). Examination of the oral cavity is important, but it should be performed initially without the use of a gag, which may further displace a fracture. Displaced incisors or laceration of the rostral gingiva should raise the suspicion of a fracture of the rostral mandible or premaxilla (**294**).

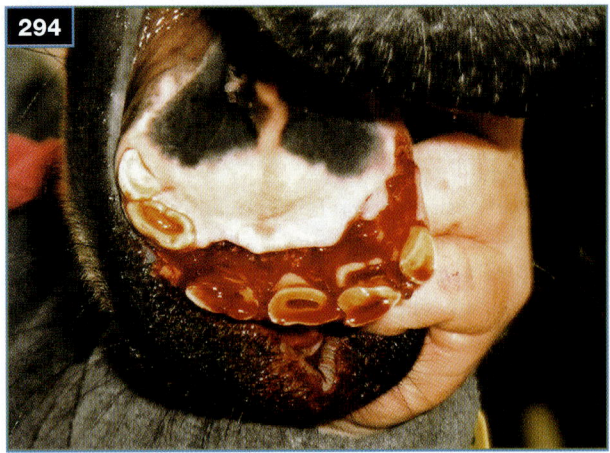

294 This wound had an associated fracture of the rostral maxilla, which was successfully treated by stabilization through a cerclage wire placed from the incisors to the first cheek teeth. (Photo courtesy N Collins)

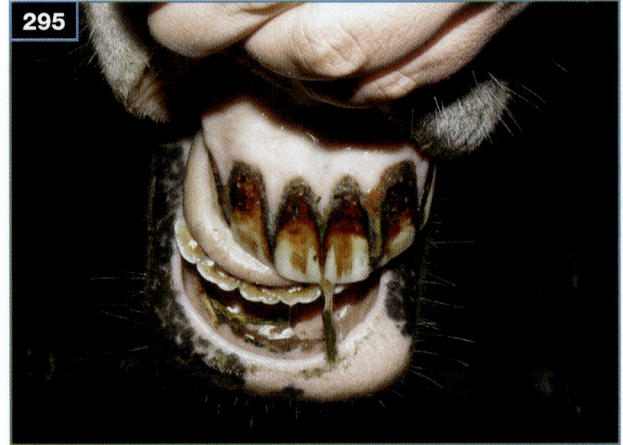

295 Malalignment of the incisors of a horse with a fractured caudal horizontal ramus of the mandible. (Photo courtesy GA Munroe)

Musculoskeletal system

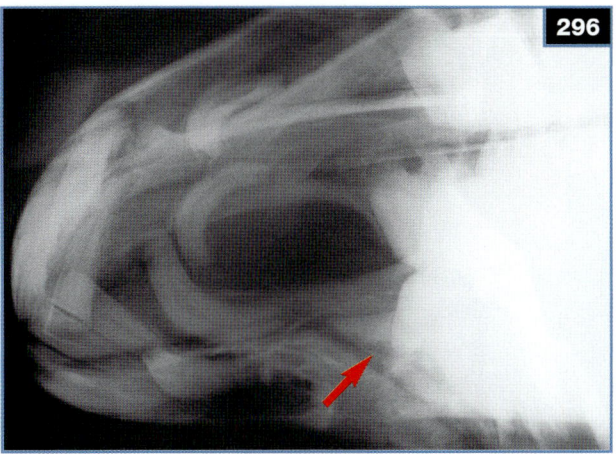

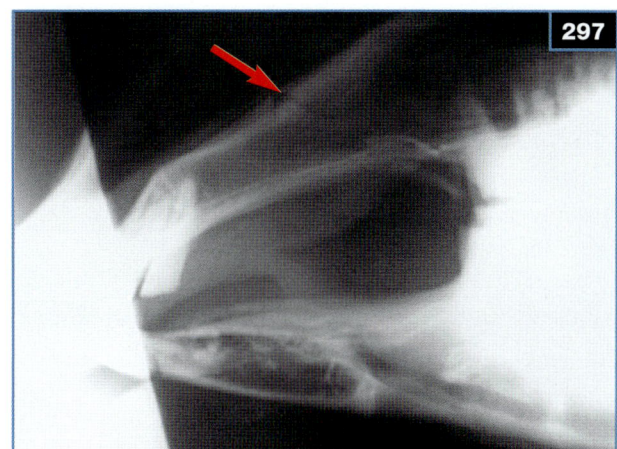

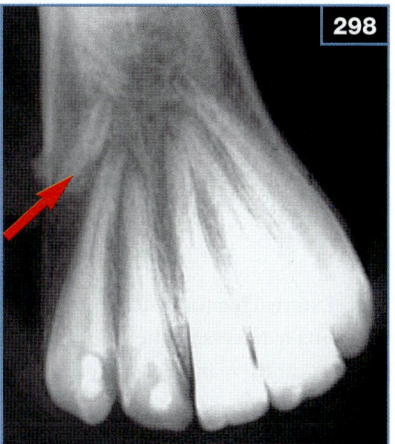

296 Lateral rostral skull radiograph of an oblique fracture of the interdental space of the mandible (arrow). (Photo courtesy GA Munroe)

297 Lateral rostral skull radiograph of an oblique fracture of the premaxilla (arrow). (Photo courtesy GA Munroe)

298 Intraoral occlusal view of the rostral mandible following a fracture of the incisive region and removal of a lateral incisor. Note the remaining small apical tooth fragment (arrow).

Differential diagnosis

Other causes of dysphagia include esophageal obstruction, retropharangeal masses, severe dental disease, botulism, and other neurologic conditions. Soft-tissue trauma of the oral cavity, such as tongue laceration, may result in dysphagia and halitosis. Dental disease is a more common cause of focal ventral mandibular swelling than trauma.

Diagnosis

Although neurologic deficits are less likely following mandibular or maxillary fractures than with caudal skull fractures, assessment of cranial nerve function should be performed early in the investigation of all skull trauma. Radiography is used to confirm a diagnosis of mandibular or maxillary fracture. Laterolateral (**296**, **297**) and dorsoventral views should be obtained under sedation. For rostral fractures, a cassette or nonscreen film can be inserted into the oral cavity to allow evaluation of the affected incisor region without superimposition of the other incisor arcade (intraoral occlusal view) (**298**). For more caudal fractures, the beam is centered on the area of suspected pathology and the temporomandibular joints and hyoid apparatus should also be assessed radiographically (**299**). Maxillary fractures can appear quite complex on radiographs and direct palpation may allow better assessment.

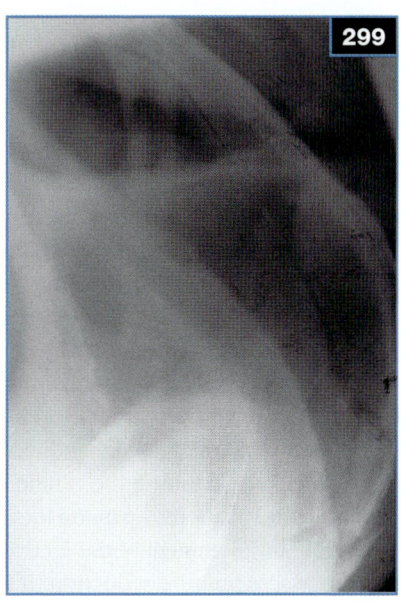

299 Lateral caudal skull radiograph showing a vertical fracture of the vertical ramus of the mandible. (Photo courtesy GA Munroe)

167

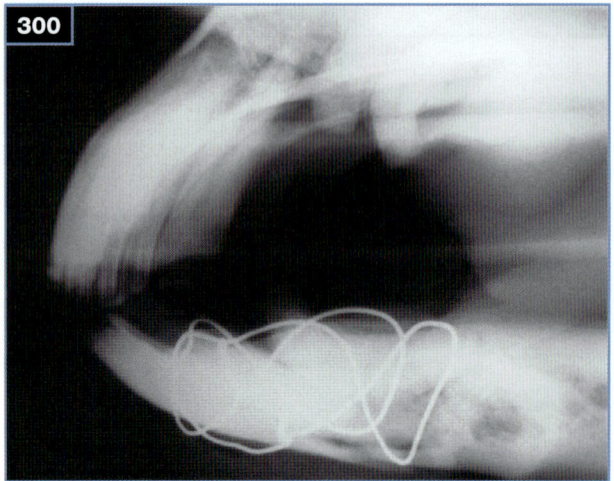

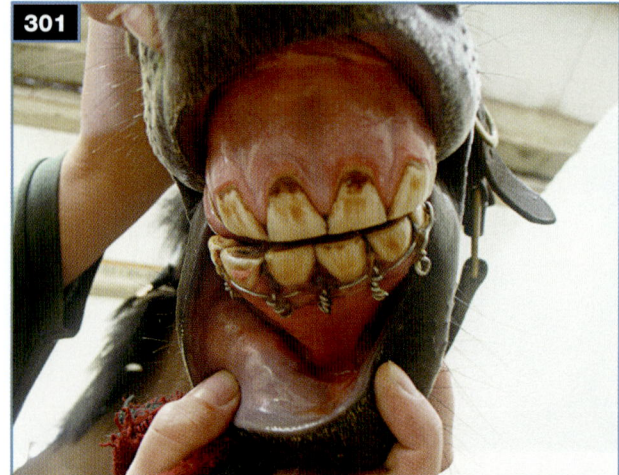

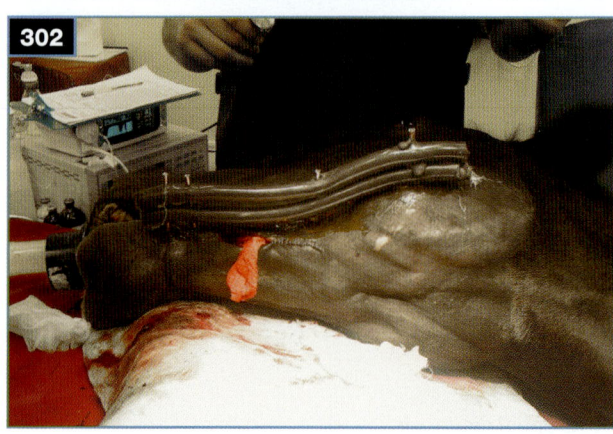

300, 301 Lateral radiograph (300) of the rostral skull of a horse where several cerclage wires (301) have been used to repair a mandibular fracture.

302 External fixator system of intramedullary pins horizontally traversing the rostral and caudal mandible either side of a caudal mandibular fracture and held together by small rubber tubes filled with thermoplastic material. (Photo courtesy GA Munroe)

Management

Minor injuries may heal spontaneously, although they will benefit from wound lavage and debridement. The speed of healing of head injuries is high when compared with injuries involving the distal limbs. More extensive injuries will require fixation. Most fractures involving the incisive portion of the mandible or maxilla can be held in reduction using cerclage wires placed between the remaining intact incisor teeth and the rostral mandible (300, 301). If all the incisor teeth are involved, the canine teeth, if present, can be used to aid fixation by passing the cerclage wires tightly around them. Alignment of the incisor occlusal surfaces is used to assess fracture reduction. It may not be obvious whether involved teeth are viable; however, these can be left at the time of repair and removed later if this proves necessary.

Bilateral fractures involving the mandibular interdental space are treated using tension-band wires, U-shaped frames held by wires around the teeth, or frames using pins through the mandible (302). Unilateral fractures of the interdental space are usually stablized by the contralateral mandible. After fixation, the horse should not be allowed to graze until healing is complete. Internal fixation using bone plates is unusual, but is indicated for those fractures of the caudal mandible that are causing problems with mastication. Caudal cheek teeth involved in the fracture may require removal, but if possible this should be delayed until callus has formed, as the force required to remove these teeth may further destablize an acute fracture.

Fractures of the caudal maxilla, nasal, or frontal bones will inevitably involve the nasal passages and/or paranasal sinuses (see pp. 171–173). Larger fracture fragments require stabilization by cerclage wire fixation to surrounding stable bone. The sinuses and nasal passages should be lavaged for several days to remove blood and contamination and prevent sinusitis. If the periosteum can be salvaged and sutured over the fracture site(s), this will aid healing.

Temporomandibular and temporohyoid articulation

Temporomandibular joint disease

Definition/overview
Disease of the temporomandibular joints (TMJs) is uncommon, with occasional case reports of OA, septic arthritis, and luxation. Recently, diagnostic imaging techniques have proved useful in detecting TMJ abnormalities, and the disease detection rate is increasing.

Etiology/pathophysiology
The TMJ forms the articulation between the vertical ramus of the mandible and the zygomatic process of the temporal bone. It is divided into two compartments by a fibrous disk and is supported by its joint capsule and biconcave shape more than the poorly developed lateral and caudal ligaments. OA of the TMJ is seen in horses with chronic and severe dental abnormalities, but it is unclear whether disease of the joint caused the dental changes or vice versa. In these horses, lateral movement of the mandibles is impeded.

Pain or dysfunction of one or both TMJs interferes with the normal movements of the mandibles, which are vital for prehension and mastication of food. Over time the abnormal dental wear will lead inexorably to pronounced tooth abnormalities that will further interfere with feeding. The masseter muscle atrophy seen with TMJ disease may be due to reduced movement of the mandibles or from damage to the mandibular branch of the trigeminal nerve medial to the temporal condyle. As a result of ingesting poorly masticated food, secondary choke or impactions may occur.

Clinical presentation
Disease of the TMJs is often diagnosed only at an advanced stage. Affected horses show marked problems when feeding (slow feeding, quidding, food pouching in cheeks), masseter muscle atrophy, and weight loss despite a good appetite. Examination of chronic cases will reveal severe dental abnormalities (most commonly 'shear mouth') and oral ulceration. When the mandibles are passively manipulated there will be a reduced range of movement and possibly resentment by the horse. Where there is infection of the TMJ there may be pain on direct palpation of the temporomandibular region. Luxation of the joint is caused by trauma and there may be concomitant signs (wounds, fractures, draining tract). Some clinicians believe that disease of these joints may cause head shaking in some horses.

Differential diagnosis
It is possible to overlook a TMJ abnormality as affected horses have obvious dental abnormalities that may be thought to account for the clinical signs. Dysphagia can be caused by esophageal obstruction (choke), retropharyngeal masses, mandibular or maxillary fractures, guttural pouch disorders, equine protozoal encephalitis (EPM), botulism, and other neurologic conditions.

Diagnosis
Good-quality radiographs will confirm luxation or show bone proliferation and focal bone lysis associated with OA, although in advanced OA the joint space will be obscured by proliferative new bone. Oblique views are required to avoid superimposition of both joints. Septic arthritis, as elsewhere, appears more aggressive radiographically than OA, with joint space widening and a mixed pattern of periarticular lysis and sclerosis. Arthrosonography can depict the intra-articular disk, joint capsule, and articular cartilage. The joint can be injected with local anesthetic to confirm it as the source of pain, preferably under ultrasound guidance.

Management
Sepsis of the TMJ may be treated successfully with a combination of antibiotic medication, local debridement, and flushing. Mandibular condylectomy has also been described as a treatment. Well-established temporomandibular OA carries a very poor prognosis for recovery. Replacement of a luxated TMJ has been performed and may be successful if the injury is recent.

Disease of the temporohyoid articulation

Definition/overview
The temporohyoid articulation is a short cartilaginous region between the proximal extremity of the stylohyoid bone and the petrous temporal bone, which lies immediately ventrolateral to the middle ear region (303). Functionally, it is slightly flexible and thus dampens the movements of the hyoid apparatus during tongue motion.

Etiology/pathophysiology
Disease of the middle ear can result in ossification of the cartilaginous temporohyoid articulation, but cases may present without any history of ear disease.

Extension of infection from the middle ear to the temporohyoid articulation is thought to reduce the flexibility of this region, and normal tongue movements may then result in fracture of the mid-portion of the affected stylohyoid bone without any history of trauma. Due to the proximity of the facial and vestibulocochlear nerves (CNs VII and VIII) neurologic signs are common and fracture of the stylohyoid bone has been associated with acute onset of CN VII and VIII deficits.

Clinical presentation
Affected horses may present with a range of signs indicating neurologic dysfunction, including head tilt, facial nerve paralysis, keratitis, and ataxia. Head shaking or aural discharge may also be observed.

Differential diagnosis
The condition must be differentiated from other causes of cranial nerve disease.

Diagnosis
Osseous enlargement of the proximal aspect of the stylohyoid bone or sclerosis of the tympanic bulla may be diagnosed radiographically, but endoscopy of the guttural pouch has proved more consistently successful (304). Both CT and MRI have been used for definitive diagnosis of temporohyoid osteopathy, including one case without endoscopic evidence of bony abnormalities. Unfortunately, these imaging modalities are currently not widely available.

Management
Although it can be difficult to prove the presence of ear infection at the time of presentation, antimicrobial therapy should nevertheless be initiated as a precaution. A few horses have been treated with partial stylohyoidectomy (where a portion of the middle of the bone is removed as it passes through the guttural pouch) as a prophylactic measure to prevent later fracture. However, as many horses improve using a conservative approach it is unclear whether surgery is necessary.

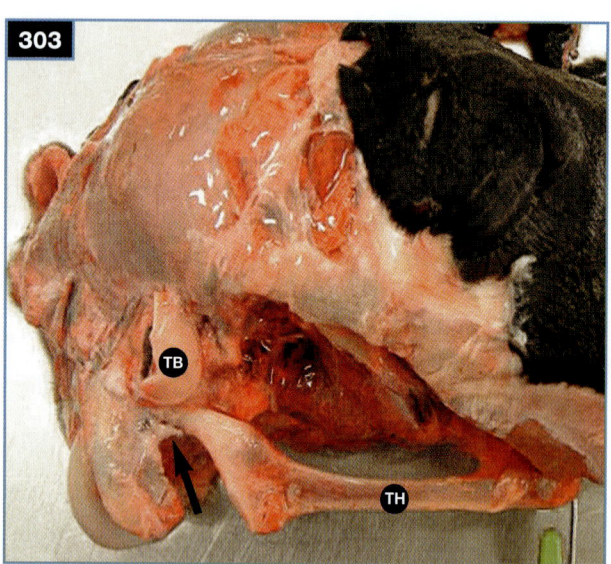

303 Dissection to show the tympanohyoid articulation (arrow) in a neonatal foal. TH = tympanohyoid bone; TB = tympanic bulla.

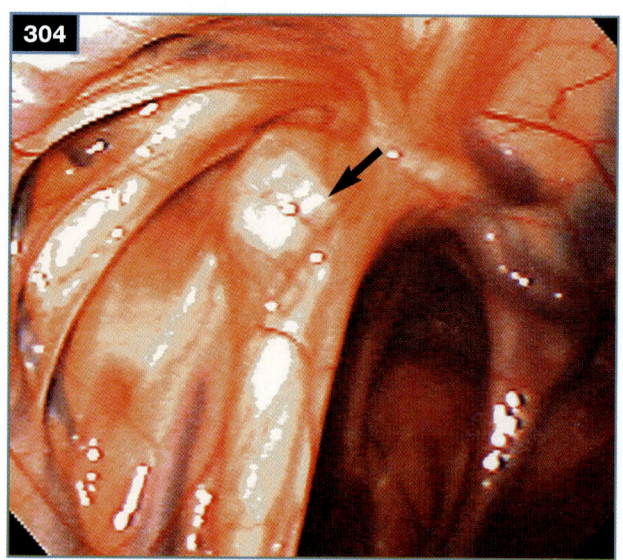

304 Endoscopic view of the guttural pouch of a horse with tympanohyoid osteopathy showing enlargement of the proximal region of the stylohyoid bone (arrow). Radiographs also revealed marked thickening of the tympanic bulla.

Cranium and face

Fractures

Definition/overview

Fractures of the cranium, although rare, may have serious consequences due to neurologic trauma. Two types of cranial fracture occur: basilar skull fractures and dorsal or dorsolateral cranial fractures. In contrast, facial fractures (of the nasal and frontal bones) are not uncommon and may appear dramatic due to profuse hemorrhage and facial distortion, but they are not life threatening. Fractures of the cranium or of the facial region can be either closed or open.

Etiology/pathophysiology

Basilar skull fractures are caused almost invariably by a backward fall, while dorsal cranial fractures are usually a consequence of a head-on collision. Facial fractures usually involve the nasal and/or frontal bones and occasionally also the maxillary or lacrimal bones. They occur by direct trauma either through falling forwards, kicks, or rearing and striking a solid object.

The clinical signs of cranial fractures are caused by associated brain damage and may increase in severity as pressure from edema and subarachnoid hemorrhage grows. The raised intracranial pressure causes cerebral anoxia. Concurrent injuries may include avulsion of the ligamentum nuchae origin, tearing of the rectus capitis muscles, or fracture of the basisphenoid or basihyoid bones.

The frontal and nasal bones overlie the paranasal sinuses and nasal passages. If the fracture is sufficiently displaced, there may be interference with normal breathing. Untreated displaced facial fractures can lead to permanent facial deformity, sequestrum formation, or chronic sinusitis.

Clinical presentation

Horses with a cranial fracture may be so severely affected that they are unable to rise. In other cases, a progression in CNS signs (e.g. ataxia, depression, head tilt, cranial nerve deficits, and nystagmus) and alterations in cardiac and respiratory function may be seen. Irregular breathing, with periods of apnea, is indicative of a poor prognosis. There may also be visible signs of trauma in the region of the poll or the dorsal cranium. Where a cranial fracture has exposed the CNS, cerebrospinal fluid may be seen leaking from an ear canal. Epistaxis is common.

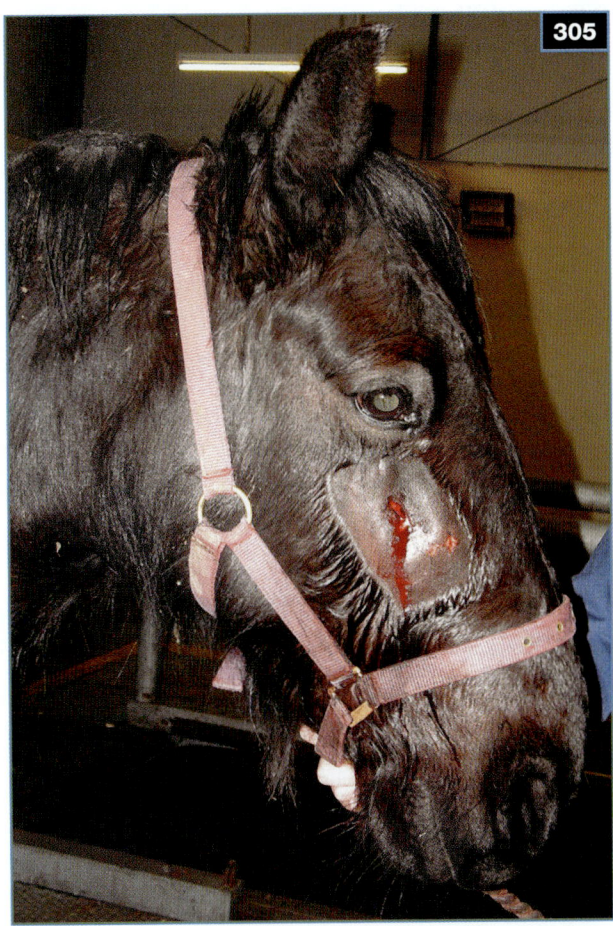

305 This horse sustained a wound to the right side of the skull. Note the depression centered over the maxillary region. Radiographs revealed a slightly displaced fracture of the facial crest.

Horses with facial or cranial fractures are usually presented as emergencies. Facial fractures may have obvious signs of external trauma (**305**); in severe cases there may be open communication with the nasal passages or paranasal sinuses. There will be overlying swelling due to edema and trapped air, and epistaxis and facial asymmetry are common. A wound may be present, but a fracture should not be ruled out where the skin has remained intact. Palpation, if tolerated by the horse, may reveal crepitus. Distortion and partial blockage of the upper airways may cause respiratory stridor.

Differential diagnosis

In most cases of acute-onset neurologic signs, a history of recent trauma involving the head is highly suggestive of a fracture. The neurologic signs are similar to those seen in acute-onset vestibular disease and inflammatory disease of the CNS.

Facial swelling and epistaxis after a fall or other trauma may be due to soft-tissue trauma only. Clinical and radiographic examinations are required to identify horses with facial fractures.

Diagnosis

Several radiographic views may be needed to detect and assess fractures of the cranium. Other radiographic signs suggestive of basilar skull fractures include soft-tissue (blood) opacity within the guttural pouches, ventral deviation of the dorsal pharyngeal wall, and irregular bone opacities ventral to the skull base. In some cases the diagnosis cannot be confirmed radiographically and must be based on the history and clinical signs alone. Diagnosis of fractures of the paranasal and nasal regions is based on the history of trauma, clinical examination, and radiography (306), although radiographs may not clearly demonstrate nondisplaced fractures. These latter fractures can sometimes be confirmed ultrasonographically.

Management

If examined immediately after a fall or collision, the horse should be rapidly assessed for significant concomitant injuries. First aid should be administered as appropriate, and this may include sedation, dexamethasone, and/or NSAID medication. Mannitol given intravenously is effective at reducing intracranial swelling, and furosemide may also be useful. Careful consideration should be given to the possible deleterious effects on the brain of administering large volumes of other fluids. An emergency tracheostomy may be required. If the horse is severely ataxic, it should initially be nursed where it is rather than attempting to transport it. However, the longer a horse remains recumbent after a cranial injury, the worse the prognosis. If the progression of signs indicates rising intracranial pressure, usually in horses with a closed fracture of the cranium, this can be relieved through decompression, performed either through the creation of burr holes in the cranium or via a craniotomy, which also allows the removal of hematomata by careful suction. Although such procedures are currently rare, they are likely to become more common with increasing use of imaging methods such as CT, which allow clinicians to identify and localize intracranial fluid pockets. Open fractures are treated by debridement of contused tissue and blood clots, irrigation, and replacement of displaced bone fragments.

Many small, nondisplaced facial fractures will heal spontaneously, although there is a risk of complications (see above). Where cosmetic appearance is important, and with larger displaced fragments, surgical correction is indicated. Any wound and involved region of upper airway should be lavaged and debrided. Fragments can be wired together once elevated into position after local lavage, debridement, and flushing of the wound and involved sinuses. The periosteum should be preserved where possible and sutured over the defect. Flaps of periosteum and skin have been used to treat large defects.

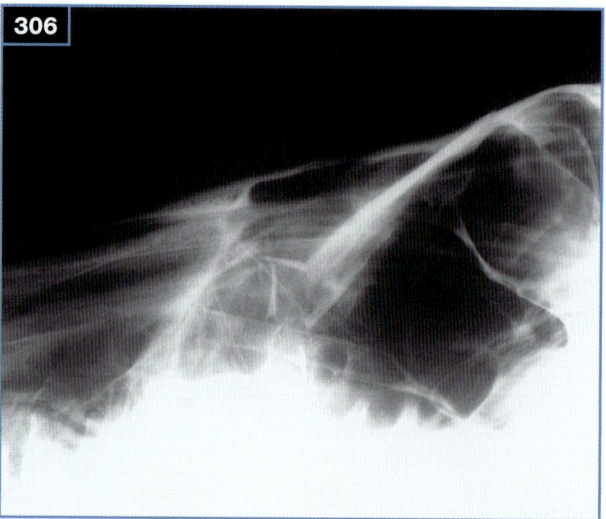

306

306 Lateral radiograph of the maxilla of a horse that sustained a blow to the head and which clearly shows a ventrally displaced fracture of the frontal bone into the paranasal sinuses. (Photo courtesy GA Munroe)

Musculoskeletal system

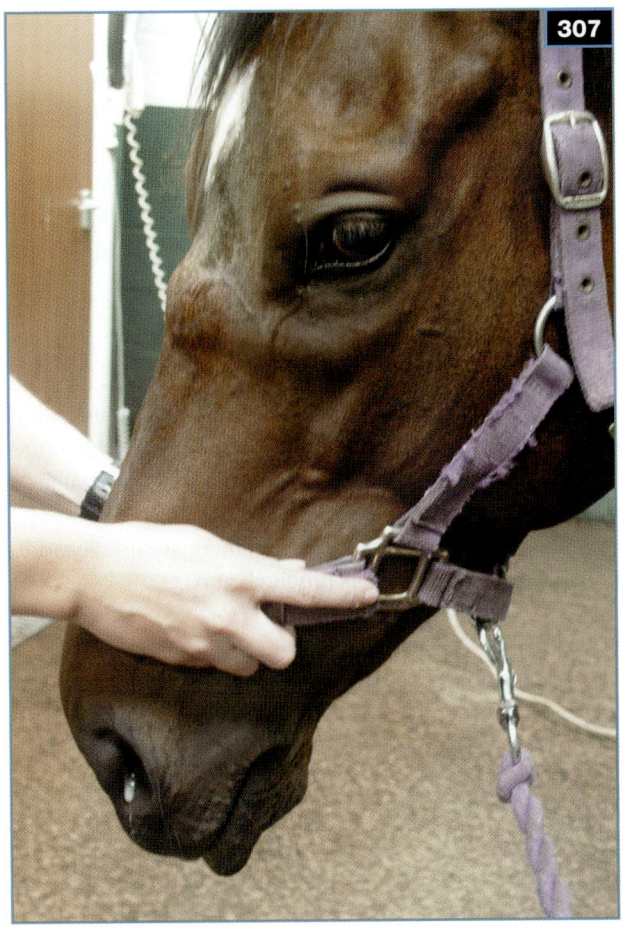

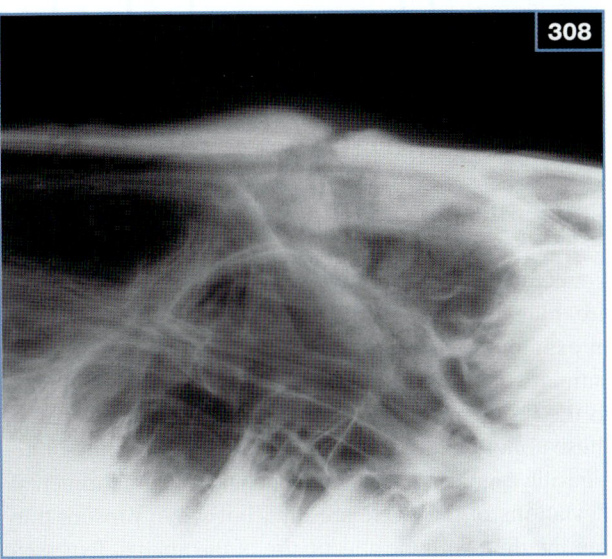

307 Extensive new reaction along the suture lines of adjacent bones of the head, both in the midline and underneath the left eye. (Photo courtesy GA Munroe)

308 On lateral head radiographs there is marked bone proliferation adjacent to the suture. (Photo courtesy GA Munroe)

Nasofrontal suture periosteitis
Definition/overview
Nasofrontal suture periosteitis is a bony swelling, usually idiopathic but commonly thought to be trauma-related, which appears in the dorsal midline at the joint between the frontal and nasal bones (307, 308). It is normally non-painful and its only significance is as a cosmetic blemish; however, it may have the radiographic appearance of a healing fracture.

The axial skeleton

Thoracolumbar/sacral region

Congenital abnormalities

Definition/overview

Congenital, osseous abnormalities of the vertebral column are quite common, with a reported incidence of 20–36% of examined Thoroughbreds having deviations from the standard vertebral formula (C7, T18, L6, S5, Cd15–21) in the thoracolumbar or lumbosacral region, but few of these abnormalities lead to deviations of the spine or are clinically significant. Severe congenital, or developmental, deviations of the spine are rare, but when present they can interfere with the athletic use of the animal. Excessive curvature of the thoracolumbar spine can be ventral (lordosis), dorsal (kyphosis), or lateral (scoliosis) (309).

Etiology/pathophysiology

There are multiple articulating bony surfaces that maintain the thoracolumbar vertebral column in normal alignment (310). Severe curvatures are usually due to an anomaly in one or several vertebrae. Mild lordosis is common in older animals due to muscle atrophy. The age at which the vertebral column deviation becomes apparent depends on the extent of the vertebral anomaly.

Clinical presentation

Affected animals are usually free of pain despite obvious vertebral column deviation (311, 312). Neurologic gait abnormalities are not usually seen, although stride length may be restricted.

Differential diagnosis

Gradually progressive developmental curvatures must be distinguished from mild curvatures of the vertebral column caused by asymmetric muscle contraction. The latter are usually painful to palpation and will respond to analgesic medication. Fractures of the thoracic or lumbar vertebrae may cause lordosis or kyphosis, but there are usually additional clinical signs such as hindlimb ataxia.

Diagnosis

Diagnosis is made by examination and inspection. Radiography is not required for diagnosis, but may be helpful in elucidating the cause of the abnormal curvature.

Management

There are no reports of attempted correction of congenital anomalies of the spine. Owners may wish to breed from mildly affected animals. The inheritance of these anomalies is unknown.

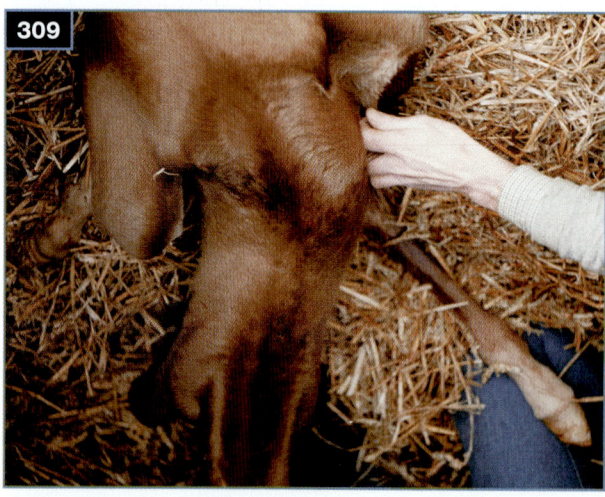

309 Neonatal Thoroughbred foal born with congenital axial and appendicular abnormalities including a lateral scoliosis most evident at the level of the withers.
(Photo courtesy GA Munroe)

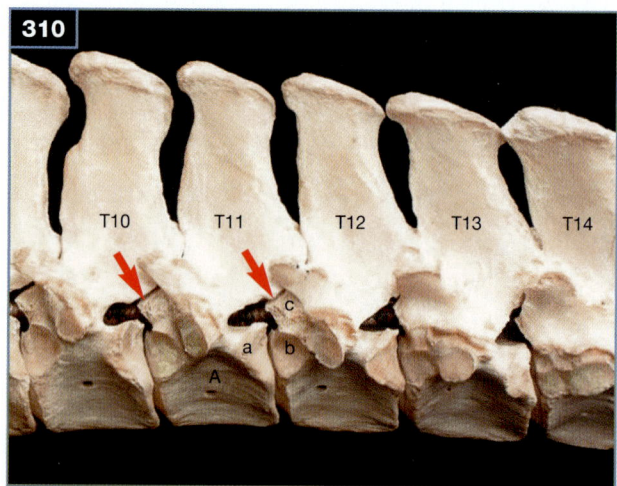

310 Mid-thoracic vertebrae (T10–T14) from a normal mature horse. Note the narrow spaces between the tips of the processes, which point cranially. A = vertebral body of T11, a = caudal costal facet, b = cranial costal facet, c = mamillary process. Arrows = dorsal intervertebral joint space.

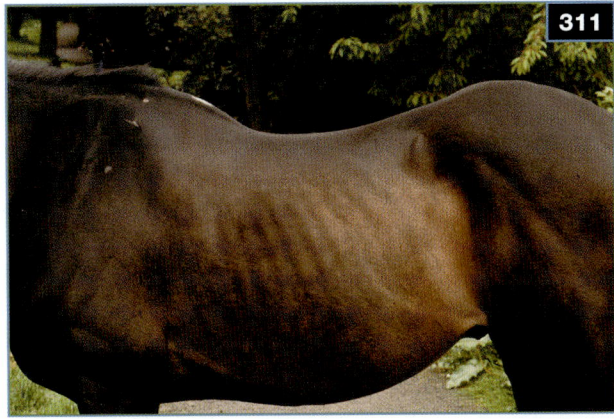

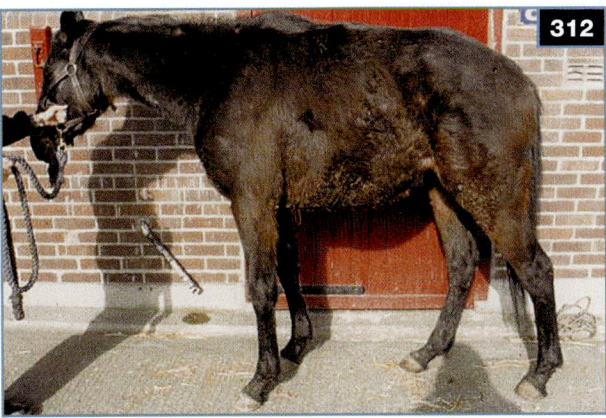

311 A late middle-aged Thoroughbred with lordosis of the back. The horse had no clinical signs of back pain. (Photo courtesy GA Munroe)

312 A 3-year-old Thoroughbred filly with kyphosis.

Soft-tissue lesions

Definition/overview
The soft-tissues of the thoracolumbar and sacral regions include the muscles (epaxial and hypaxial), the ligaments interconnecting the vertebrae, and those attaching the vertebral column to the hindlimbs at the sacroiliac joint. Lesions of the soft tissues may be primary or secondary to osseous pathology. Specific conditions are often poorly defined, and some conditions are diagnosed by inference from known human back disease rather than from evidence of the same conditions in equine athletes. For instance, while intervertebral disk protrusion is a common cause of back pain in humans and dogs, it is a very rare event in the horse, though commonly diagnosed in error.

Etiology/pathophysiology
Acute soft-tissue injuries occur either as a result of repeated low-grade trauma or in a single acute incident such as a fall. When the cervical and thoracolumbar regions of the vertebral column are maximally flexed, for example, the supraspinous ligament is placed under considerable strain. This can occur during a fall or, to a lesser degree, if a horse is continually ridden with a forced and excessive low head carriage. Exertional rhabdomyolysis can affect many muscle groups simultaneously, including those of the back. Disease of the vertebrae may result in secondary strain of muscles and ligaments. Ill-fitting saddles may cause direct soft-tissue trauma at specific sites, particularly the dorsal supraspinous ligament at the caudal aspect of the withers, with the predilection site the tip of the 10th thoracic dorsal spinous process (DSP) (**313**). The supraspinous bursa lying between the supraspinous ligament and the tips of the cranial thoracic DSPs at the withers may become infected following a wound at this site ('fistulous withers') or as a consequence of chronic infection by bacteria such as *Brucella abortus*.

A sufficiently excessive force exerted on a muscle or ligament may cause rupture or detachment from an origin or insertion; however, most injuries are less severe. Ligaments respond to injury by an increase in diameter and the slow repair phase is characterized by irregular alignment of collagen fibers. New bone may form at a ligament origin or insertion site (**314**). Chronic pain probably arises from damage to, and continued tearing of, poorly healed insertion sites (enthesiopathy).

313 Lateral scintigraphic image of the withers of a horse with back pain, with cranial to the left. Note the focal marked increased uptake at the tip of DSP T10 (arrow).

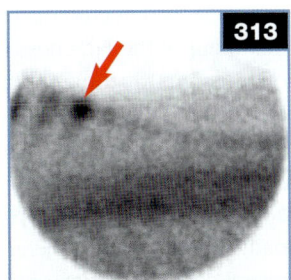

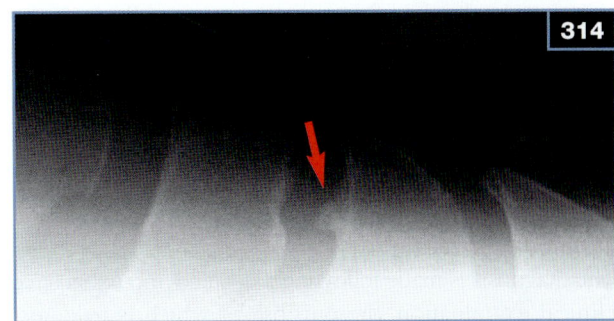

314 Radiograph of several DSP tips in the cranial thoracic region. There is a spur of bone (arrow) on the cranial aspect of DSP T11 without narrowing of the interspinous space.

175

Clinical presentation

Clinical signs of thoracolumbar discomfort ('back pain') in the horse are notoriously varied and can often be attributed to pain elsewhere or equitation problems. Horses with back pain due to soft-tissue lesions may have concomitant uni- or bilateral hindlimb lameness (raising the question which of the two conditions came first), shortened stride length affecting the hindlimbs, poor performance, and deterioration in temperament or other behavioral signs such as bucking when ridden. Often, veterinary attention is only sought at a late stage in the condition, by which time localized swelling and pain on application of pressure are no longer evident. There may be palpable focal enlargement of the supraspinous ligament; the other ligaments can only be examined by ultrasound. Clinical signs in horses confirmed as having pain in the sacroiliac joint region are varied and include poor or asymmetric muscling, either reduced or increased movement of the thoracolumbar spine, and gait abnormalities, which usually worsen when ridden.

Differential diagnosis

Disease of the vertebral bodies shows many of the same presenting signs as soft-tissue lesions and differentiation is often difficult. In conditions such as impingement of the DSPs (see below), the source of pain may arise in part from the interspinous ligaments that occupy the spaces between and attach to the processes. Other causes of poor performance, such as lameness, should be ruled out before it can be assumed that thoracolumbar pain is the cause. If lameness is detected during the examination, successful treatment of the lameness will often result in amelioration of the signs of thoarcolumbar pain. Occasionally, pain associated with impending ovulation can cause signs resembling back pain or mild colic. Caudal aortic or iliac artery thrombosis causes exercise-associated hindlimb lameness of varying degree that may be attributed to back pain. Changes in temperament may be associated with a recent change in rider, or in type of work, rather than back pain. It is important to note that some horses habitually flex their back when first mounted but rapidly return to normal as they start to work. This 'dipping', termed 'cold back' is unlikely to be an indication of back pain. The saddle should be assessed for adequacy of fit. As dental pain can result in some of the signs described above, a full oral examination using a gag must also be performed.

Diagnosis

The diagnosis is made following a detailed and exhaustive clinical examination, the purpose of which is to detect other conditions that may be the cause of the reported clinical signs. Unless a lesion is immediately obvious, it is wise to follow the same diagnostic protocol for all horses presenting with a possible back lesion. The initial clinical examination is aimed at answering the question: Does this horse have thoracolumbar pain? The horse should be observed moving in-hand and when lunged. If the signs are evident only during riding, the horse should be observed with the regular rider, although if the history includes unseating the rider, there are clear safety considerations. In addition to direct palpation of the soft-tissue structures of the back, the hypaxial muscles should be palpated per rectum. CK and AST levels should be measured following a period of strenuous exercise to detect exertional rhabdomyolysis. A full orthopedic examination should be performed.

A useful diagnostic test is to place the horse on a course of phenylbutazone and monitor the response, if any, when ridden. No improvement while under medication suggests that the problems are not due to pain. In such cases, the author has found it invaluable to have access to an experienced trainer or behavior specialist to whom the horse (and rider) can be referred for advice on equitation.

If it has been established that the horse does have 'back pain', then diagnostic imaging is used to localize the pain. Radiography of the bony structures of the thoracolumbar spine may detect bony lesions. Scintigraphic examination using technetium labeled with a bone-seeking pharmaceutical (^{99m}Tc-MDP) is also useful; in all horses with suspected back pain the entire thoracolumbar and sacral spine, pelvis, and both hindlimbs should be imaged. A desmopathy detected radiographically is more likely to be clinically significant if the ligament insertion/origin site also appears as a 'hot spot' on scintigraphy. The supraspinous and interspinous ligaments as well as part of the ligaments supporting the sacroiliac joint can be examined using ultrasound. Increases in diameter of a ligament, when compared either with the contralateral ligament or with normal horses, are regarded as suggestive of injury. Hypo- and hyperechoic regions within the supraspinous ligament have been interpreted as indicators of desmopathy and occur most frequently between T15 and L3. However, noninflammatory metaplasia can occur in this ligament and will also appear hypoechoic on ultrasound imaging (315). Ideally, local anesthesia should be used to confirm a suspected soft-tissue lesion as the source of pain, but this is not always possible. On occasion, when faced with a horse with definite clinical signs of back pain but no evidence of bone abnormalities or pathology in the accessible soft tissues, it must be recognized that there are soft-tissue structures that cannot be examined using current technology, but that may be the source of pain, and a nonspecific diagnosis of soft-tissue pain is made.

Infrared thermographic imaging has been advocated as a means not only of detecting soft-tissue lesions in the thoracolumbar region, but also of detecting sympathetic dysfunction of the nerve roots that innervate the dermatomes of this region. However, as yet there have been no published reports of controlled trials using the technique.

Management
If the damaged ligament or muscle can be accurately located, then targeted treatment is possible. Steroids and irritants have been injected directly into ligaments and reported to be of use. Ultrasound can be used to monitor healing (reduction in diameter, return of fibers to normal alignment). With any significant lesion of a ligament or insertion, prolonged rest is essential. Physiotherapy techniques, including extracorporeal shock-wave therapy, are also regularly used in treating soft-tissue injuries in the back (see pp. 31 and 32).

Many treatments have been devised to treat (often tenuous) diagnoses of thoracolumbar pain in horses. Unfortunately, the literature offers mostly anecdotal reports and opinions, rather than evidence, of their success. Chiropractic manipulation aims to restore apparent malalignments of vertebrae, which are said to cause soft-tissue inflammation and neurologic dysfunction.

Injections of corticosteroids, sometimes combined with sarapin, are frequently administered into interspinous spaces. Mesotherapy involves injections of small quantities of a combination of steroid, local anesthetic, and a myorelaxant subcutaneously into the dermatomes corresponding to the proposed sites of pathology over the thoracolumbar region and is popular in continental Europe. Acupuncture may provide analgesia for some thoracolumbar conditions.

Fractures
Definition/overview
The incidence of complete fractures of the thoracic, lumbar, or sacral vertebrae is low. A survey of 443 horses with a history of thoracolumbar pain included five (1.13%) with vertebral body fractures and eight (1.81%) with fractured DSPs. The vertebral lamina at the base of the DSP appears to be a predilection site for incomplete stress fractures and subsequent remodeling in flat-racing Thoroughbreds, and this may be responsible for poor performance or other signs of back pain. In foals, vertebral end-plate fractures or separations may occasionally be seen following trauma during or soon after parturition (316).

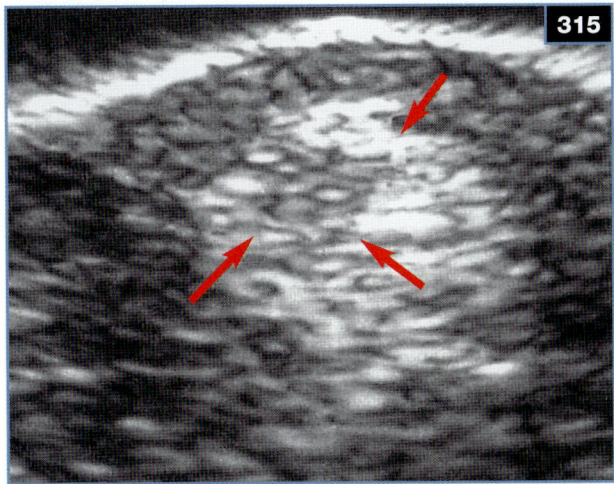

315 Cross-sectional ultrasound view of the supraspinous ligament between DSPs L3 and L4. There is a zone of reduced echogenicity indicated by the arrows.

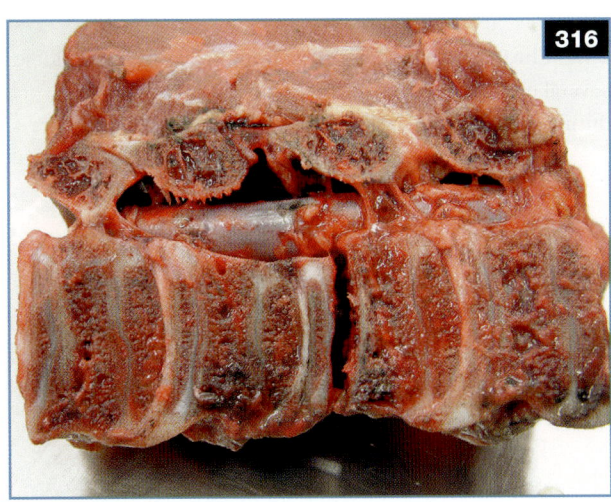

316 Sagittal section through several thoracic vertebrae of a neonatal foal that was unable to rise following parturition. There is separation at one of the vertebral cranial physes.

The axial skeleton

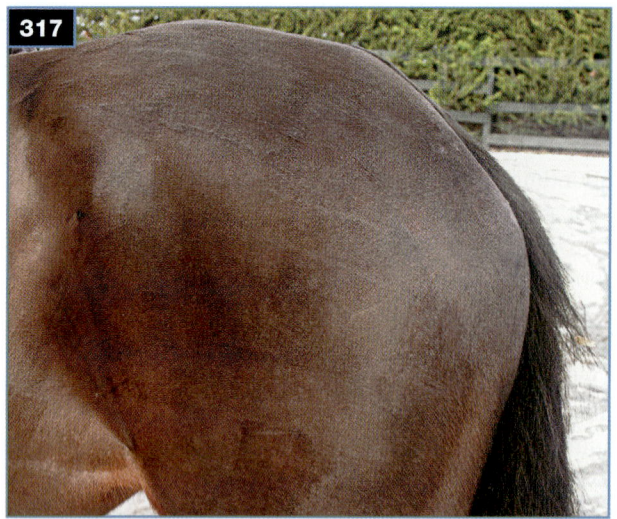

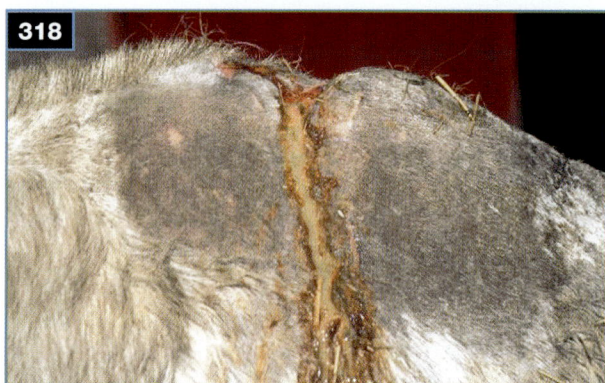

Etiology/pathophysiology

Most vertebral fractures are caused by falls or other severe trauma. The author has experience of a horse that fractured a lumbar vertebra due to muscle spasm caused by tetanus. The most common cause for fractured DSPs at the withers (T2–T9) is a backward fall when rearing. If a horse collides forcefully with a solid object while moving backwards or is hit from behind, a fracture of the (fused) sacral vertebrae may occur (317).

Fractures of the DSPs can become infected if associated with an open wound (318). Due to the poor drainage from the withers region, chronic sepsis of the spinous processes and adjoining soft tissues may result. Closed fractures of the DSPs heal well. Fractures of the vertebral bodies may result in acute and severe neurologic signs due to spinal cord compression. Hindlimb paresis or paralysis with normal forelimb function is suggestive of a lesion caudal to T2. Sacral fractures can cause cauda equina syndrome by pressure on the caudal spinal cord. Stress fractures of the vertebral laminae probably result from repeated mechanical overload. The fractures are incomplete and remodeling occurs as a response.

317 This horse was hit from behind by a vehicle and sustained a fracture of the sacrum. The fracture has healed, but left an obvious angulation in the line of the sacrum halfway between the tail head and the tuber sacrale. (Photo courtesy GA Munroe)

318 Chronic purulent discharge from the withers of a horse several months after it sustained a wound to the withers during a fall.

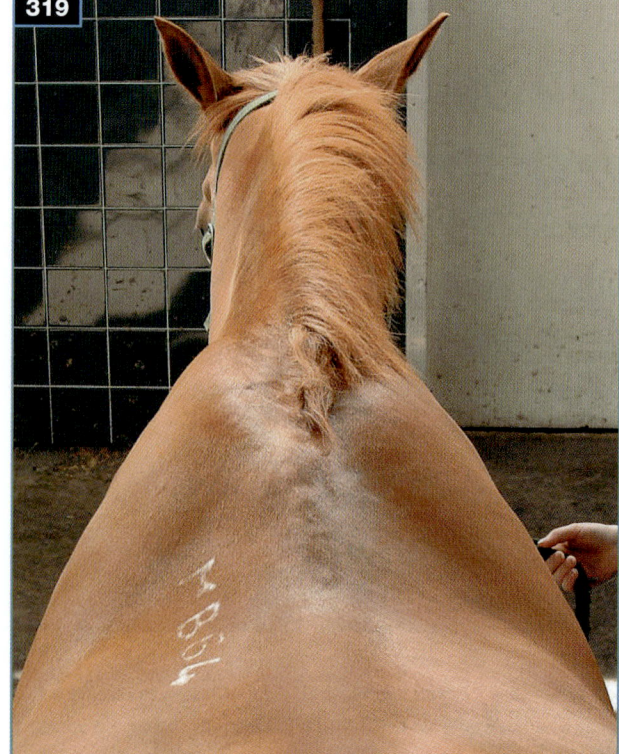

319 View from above of a horse that had fallen backwards earlier that day. Note the swelling over the proximal aspect of the left scapula. Radiography confirmed fractures of the DSPs of T4–T7.

Clinical presentation

The clinical appearance of a horse with a fracture of the axial skeleton will vary depending on the location of the fracture (the vertebra affected and the site within the vertebra) and the degree, if any, of vertebral displacement. At one end of the spectrum, stress fractures of the vertebral lamina may go unrecognized or the horse may show only vague and low-grade signs of back pain or poor performance. In contrast, a severely displaced fracture caudal to T2 will result in hindlimb paralysis, while a complete but minimally displaced fracture may still allow the horse to move without overt discomfort, but showing hindlimb paresis, ataxia, and usually epaxial muscle atrophy.

Swelling will be apparent only in cases with fractured DSPs (319). In cases of open fractures of the withers, there is likely to be considerable purulent discharge from the withers (318). Pain may be apparent on direct palpation of the affected area, and horses with significant vertebral column pain usually resist stimulation of reflex movements of the back.

Differential diagnosis

Horses with lumbar or sacral fractures without neurologic signs can resemble animals with pelvic fractures. If the presenting signs are vague vertebral column discomfort and poor performance, then the other causes of such signs must be considered (see above). Discharge at the withers secondary to an infected fracture(s) should be differentiated from an infected supraspinous bursa ('fistulous withers').

Diagnosis

The diagnostic approach is the same as that outlined above for soft-tissue lesions, unless there are obvious clinical signs such as ataxia, marked swelling, or discharge. If vertebral displacement is present, a deviation of the DSP(s) may be palpable. The DSPs can be assessed ultrasonographically and radiographically in the standing horse (320–322). Good-quality radiographs of the vertebral bodies require high-output X-ray machines, in particular if the caudal thoracic and lumbar regions are being examined. Scintigraphy is very sensitive at detecting the high osseous metabolic rates associated with fractures and would therefore be the imaging modality of choice to confirm a diagnosis of suspected fracture, in particular stress fractures.

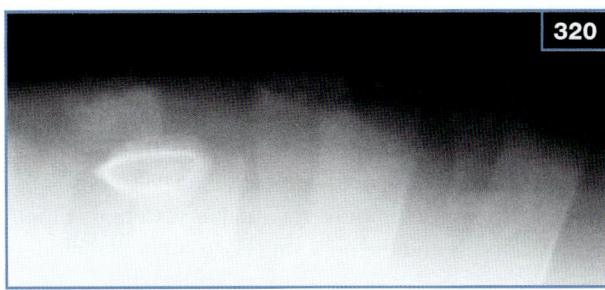

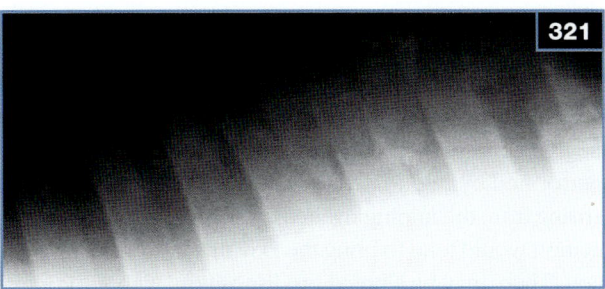

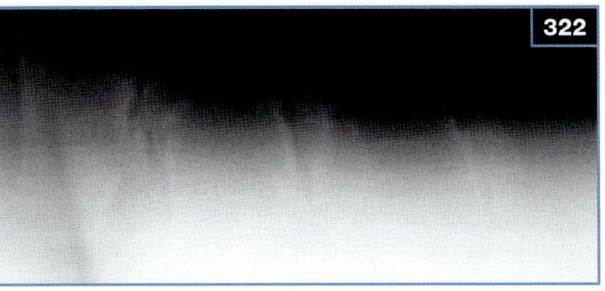

320, 321 Lateral radiographs of the withers region revealing several fractured and distally displaced thoracic dorsal spinous processes. (Photo courtesy GA Munroe)

322 Lateral radiograph of a single dorsal spinous process fracture of T11. (Photo courtesy GA Munroe)

Management

Although surgical management of a sacral fracture has been reported, surgery of most vertebral fractures is currently not feasible. The exception is fractures of the dorsal spinous processes; although removal of DSP fragments is possible, they self-resolve in most cases of closed fractures, albeit often with a cosmetic blemish. Infected fractures at the withers require extensive and often repeated debridement and there is a significant recurrence rate. For other fractures, euthanasia is indicated if there is significant and progressive hindlimb ataxia or paresis. Cases presenting with low-grade signs only should be managed with a period of at least 3 months rest, although no data are available to indicate what rate of return to function can be expected.

The axial skeleton

Impingement of dorsal spinous processes
Definition/overview
Also known as 'kissing spines' and 'overriding dorsal spinous processes', impingement of DSPs is one of the most common conditions known to cause thoracolumbar pain in horses. The spaces between the DSPs in the mid-thoracic or, less commonly, the lumbar vertebral column narrow dorsally and the opposing bone surfaces remodel.

Etiology/pathophysiology
The cause of this condition is unclear, particularly as it occurs in many functionally normal horses (ranging from 30–90% of examined horses in various surveys). It may be that differences in thoracolumbar conformation affect the degree of impingement, and the level and type of work performed by the horse may affect the likelihood of pain arising from the impinging areas. A slightly lordotic conformation would tend to bring the DSP tips into closer apposition. There may be a breed predisposition, with Thoroughbreds or part-Thoroughbreds (which have more narrow interspinous spaces than other breeds) reported to have a moderately higher incidence. Horses that jump are also reported to be at higher risk. Impinging DSPs have been reported in horses that have not been ridden, although it is not known whether these horses suffered back pain.

The incidence is highest in the saddle region (T12–T18) and between two and six DSPs may be involved (323). As the apices of the DSPs approach each other, the dorsal third to half of each affected process increases its rate of remodeling, demonstrated radiographically initially by sclerosis of the subperiosteal bone, followed by development of cyst-like zones of bone resorption. Where DSPs are in contact, pseudarthroses and small bursae may form (324). In horses with painful 'kissing spines', the source of the pain is unclear. Local anesthetic infiltrated diffusely into the narrowed spaces will alleviate the pain transiently, which implies that the soft tissues are a significant source of pain.

Clinical presentation
This is a chronic condition and horses are usually presented for veterinary examination only after signs have been present for a considerable period, and sometimes only after a range of 'alternative' therapies have been tried. Rarely, the onset of signs follows known trauma such as a fall. Clinical signs are nonspecific and can include back stiffness, poor hindlimb impulsion, reduction in jumping ability, and other forms of poor performance. Affected horses usually resent flexion or extension of the back when manipulated. Clinical signs tend to be more severe when more than one or two DSPs are affected, and when the impingement affects the mid-portion or ventral part of the DSP.

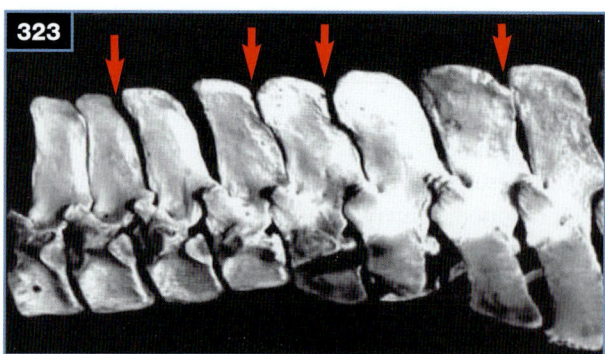

323 Postmortem specimen of the thoracolumbar region (T14–L3) of a horse euthanized due to chronic and severe back pain. Note the multiple sites of impinging DSPs (arrows).

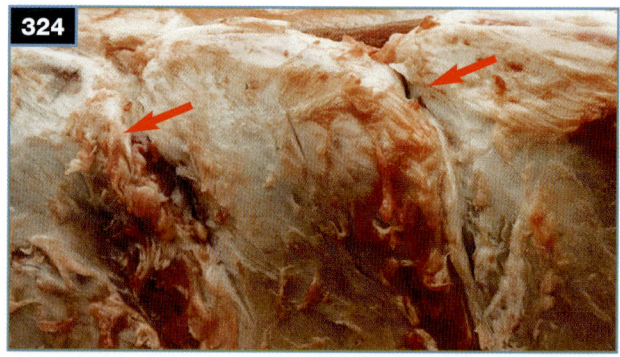

324 Postmortem specimen of three adjacent DSPs that are overlapping; the arrows show the formation of pseudarthroses. (Photo courtesy L Jeffcott)

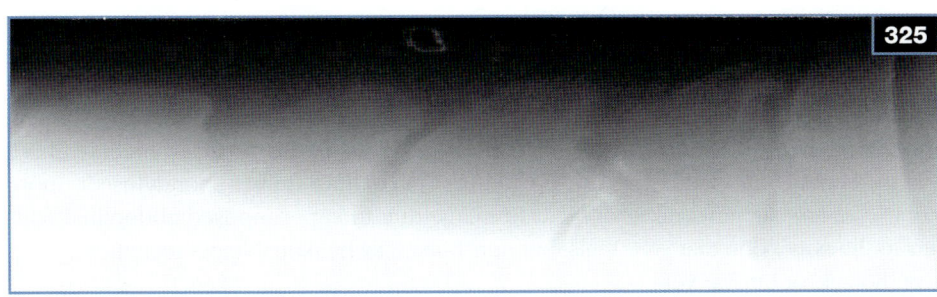

325 Lateral radiograph of the DSPs of the thoracic spine showing multiple overlapping processes with new bone reaction and spur formation. (Photo courtesy GA Munroe)

Differential diagnosis
Soft-tissue lesions of the back and other bone pathology can result in similar clinical signs.

Diagnosis
Palpation and ultrasound examination can detect narrowing of the interspinous spaces, but radiography is required to demonstrate the full extent of secondary changes (**325**). However, as many normal horses have similar changes, further examination is required to confirm that the impingement is causing pain. Local anesthetic is infiltrated into the affected interspinous processes (**326**) and the horse is re-evaluated. If the signs are most evident when ridden, then the horse's response to the rider should be assessed before and after injection. Scintigraphic examination may demonstrate local increased metabolic activity; it is considered that 'hot' impinging DSPs are more likely to be clinically significant than those with normal metabolism.

Management
It is recognized that a proportion of affected horses will recover spontaneously or after several months rest. Physiotherapy and either systemic or local anti-inflammatory and/or counter-irritant medication have all been used with some success. If these conservative treatments are unsuccessful, the involved DSP tips can be removed (**327**), either under general anesthesia or standing sedation, with a reported 72% of horses returning to full work after resection of between one and six processes.

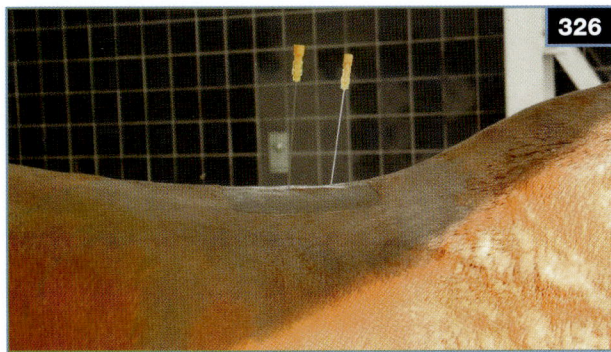

326 Two needles in place prior to injection of local anesthetic into two interspinous process spaces. Correct placement of the needles should be confirmed by radiography.

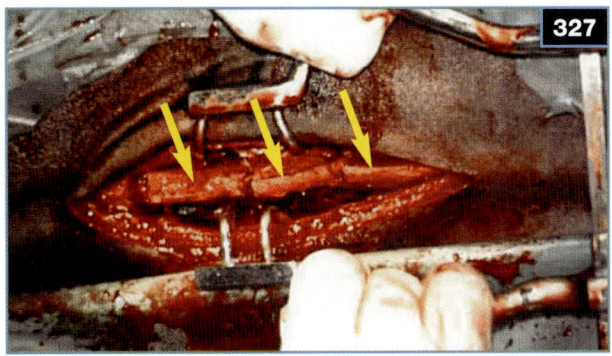

327 Intraoperative view of surgery to remove several thoracic DSP tips. The skin incision has exposed several DSP tips (arrows). (Photos courtesy GA Munroe)

Spondylosis

Definition/overview

Spondylosis ('spondylosis deformans'; 'ventral spondylosis'; 'vertebral spondylosis') in humans is defined as a degenerative disease of the intervertebral disks and vertebrae and proliferation of bone on the ventral and ventrolateral surfaces of the cervical, thoracic, or lumbar vertebral column. In horses, the term refers to the new bone that is produced on the ventral surface of thoracic or lumbar vertebrae. There is no evidence that the intervertebral disks are also affected.

Etiology/pathophysiology

The formation of bone at the sites of soft-tissue attachments on the ventral surface of the vertebrae may represent a form of enthesiophytosis, with wear and tear of the connective tissues leading to new bone formation. This is supported by the fact that the condition is seen more commonly in older horses.

While in humans the disease may cause pain by pressure from proliferating bone on nerve roots, equine vertebral anatomy and function differ considerably from those of humans, with much narrower intervertebral disks and less movement between the vertebrae. These differences may explain why spondylosis in horses is often asymptomatic. The bone proliferation occurs in regions occupied by the ventral longitudinal ligament and the outer annular fibers of the intervertebral disk, ventral to the disk spaces, but it may extend to form a solid plate of bone on the ventral surface of the thoracolumbar vertebral column. Lesions are most common in the region T9 to T15, the vertebrae that are also most commonly affected by impingement of DSPs. In the majority of horses the bone proliferation appears to cause no pain. Occasionally, the plate of proliferative bone can fracture and this has been associated with clinical signs.

Clinical presentation

This condition has frequently been encountered as an incidental finding when the dorsal thorax has been radiographed for reasons other than suspected thoracolumbar pain. The clinical signs are those seen in other chronic back pain conditions and may include back stiffness, poor hindlimb impulsion, poor jumping ability, and reluctance to flex and extend the thoracolumbar vertebral column.

Differential diagnosis

Other osseous or soft-tissue pathology of the thoracolumbar vertebral column can cause some or all of the clinical signs described.

Diagnosis

It is not possible to distinguish spondylosis from other causes of chronic thoracolumbar pain on clinical examination alone. Radiography will confirm the presence of new bone on the ventral aspect of the thoracic vertebrae (328). Caudal thoracic (>T16) and lumbar spondylosis is more difficult to image due to superimposed abdominal contents, but new bone may be palpable per rectum.

Management

As no specific treatment is available, recommendations are limited to long-term rest and the administration of systemic anti-inflammatory medication if warranted by the signs of pain. Due to the difficulty of confirming the diagnosis, there is a lack of meaningful data on which a prognosis can be based.

Osteoarthritis

Definition/overview

OA of the thoracolumbar vertebral column occurs at the thoracic and lumbar dorsal intervertebral joints.

Etiology/pathophysiology

The dorsal intervertebral joints are formed by the cranial and caudal facets of the articular processes in the thoracolumbar vertebral column. The incidence of OA in these joints is unknown and reports differ on the clinical significance of the condition. The lesions are more common in the caudal thoracic and lumbar regions and may occur concurrently with impingement of the DSPs. OA-like changes also occur at the lumbar intertransverse joints, but these are currently not thought to cause pain.

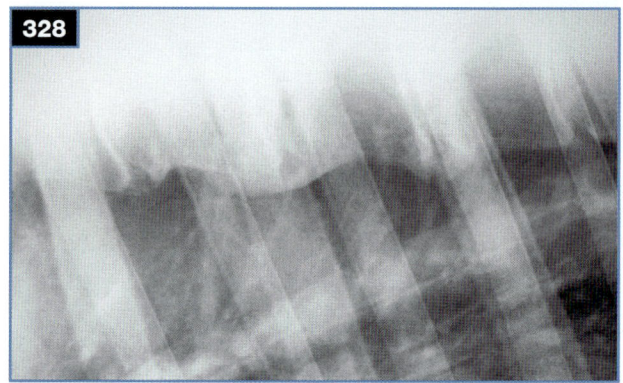

328 Radiograph of the caudal thoracic vertebral column, showing marked smooth new bone formation on the ventral surface of the vertebral bodies (spondylosis).

329 Left ventral right dorsal oblique radiograph of an Irish Sport horse with back pain. Bone scintigraphy localized the problem to the intervertebral articular facet in the caudal thoracic region. The view shows the articular facet between T14 and T17. There is evidence of osteoarthritis, especially in the facet joints of T16 and T17 (arrows).
(Photo courtesy GA Munroe)

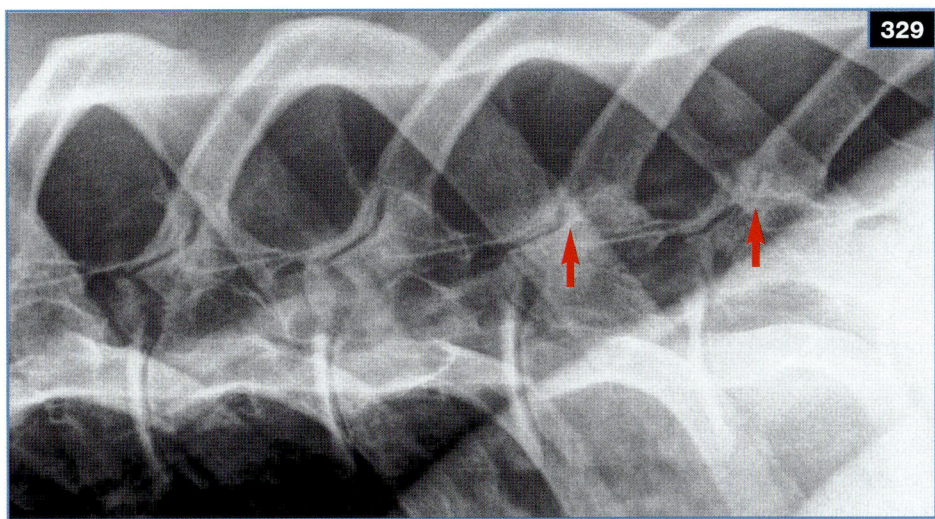

In a postmortem survey of young Thoroughbred race-horses, the majority had evidence of stress fractures of the vertebral lamina adjacent to the dorsal intervertebral joints and there was a positive correlation with the presence of OA, suggesting that laminar stress fractures may be common and may lead to dorsal intervertebral joint OA.

Clinical presentation
The onset of clinical signs is insidious and can range from overt vertebral column pain (resentment at being saddled or ridden; bucking when ridden) to poor performance. There are no clinical signs that can be used to differentiate this condition from other chronic back problems.

Differential diagnosis
As with all chronic back problems, other conditions must be ruled out. If the recommended systematic examination protocol is followed for all examinations for potential back problems, this will rule out hindlimb lameness and behavioral or equitation problems, and confirm that the animal has back pain. Other conditions that can cause back pain are impingement of the DSPs, spondylosis, nondisplaced fractures, and ligamentous or muscular pathology.

Diagnosis
The conventional imaging modalities of radiography, ultrasonography, and scintigraphy are all useful for confirming a diagnosis of dorsal intervertebral joint OA. Achieving adequate radiographic images requires a machine capable of an output of over 100 kV and 200–300 mAs, used in combination with a rare-earth screen/film system. The normal joint space appears as a radio-lucent oblique line sloping from cranial to caudal at an angle of approximately 45° to the vertebral bodies. The lesions have been graded into eight categories based on radiographic appearance. On high-quality radiographs, sclerosis of the articular facets, subchondral lucencies, and periarticular bone proliferation obscuring the joint space can be detected (**329**). Scintigraphy demonstrates increased bone activity in some of these lesions. The clinical impression is that radiographic findings are more likely to be causing pain when the same regions show an increased metabolic rate on scintigraphy. Experienced operators can image dorsal periarticular new bone ultra-sonographically, and this technique can also be employed to guide a needle for periarticular injections.

Management
Affected horses can be treated systemically using NSAIDs, but long-term treatment is not possible in many competitive horse for regulatory reasons and is frequently only transiently useful. Corticosteroids can be injected directly into the muscles adjacent to the dorsal intervertebral joints (multifidus), ideally under ultrasonographic control (e.g. methylprednisolone, with a maximum total dose of 80 mg). The use of acupuncture in horses with back pain has been reported. Mesotherapy is a treatment popular in continental Europe. It entails the intradermal injection of a short-acting corticosteroid combined with a muscle relaxing agent into dermatomes corresponding with the vertebral lesions.

The prognosis for a horse with back pain due to dorsal intervertebral joint OA depends on the severity of the lesions, the number of joints affected, the presence of concurrent lesions such as DSP impingement, as well as the type of work being performed and the ability of the horse and rider. Poor thoracolumbar flexibility and pain caused by multiple affected joints, particularly if accompanied by further lesions elsewhere in the vertebral column, are bad prognostic signs.

Sacroiliac/coccygeal region

Sacroiliac joint and ligament injuries

Definition/overview

The sacroiliac joints function to transmit forces from the hindlimbs to the vertebral column via the pelvis. They are diarthrodial joints with a very low range of gliding movement. The joint has a fibrous capsule and is strengthened by well-developed ventral, dorsal, and interosseous ligaments. Pain from the sacroiliac joint or region is a fairly common diagnosis in horses with hindlimb lameness, but it may be difficult to confirm.

Etiology/pathophysiology

Degenerative changes of the sacroiliac joints have been found in a high proportion of horses in postmortem surveys. The true incidence of clinically significant sacroiliac pathology is unknown. Acute damage to the soft tissues in the sacroiliac region may be caused by trauma such as a fall, but more commonly the presentation is of an insidious onset and the cause is not known. The pathophysiology is unknown.

Clinical presentation

Horses with sacroiliac region pain are more likely to have been used for dressage and show jumping than racing. Clinical signs in horses with confirmed sacroiliac joint region pain are varied and include poor or asymmetric muscling, either reduced or increased movement of the thoracolumbar spine, and gait abnormalities, which usually become worse when ridden. Asymmetric tubera sacrale are frequently encountered as an incidental finding and, contrary to previous reports, are unusual in horses with confirmed sacroiliac region pain (330).

Differential diagnosis

Hindlimb lameness; pain in the thoracolumbar vertebral column; stress fractures of the ilial wing adjacent to the sacroiliac joint.

Diagnosis

Most cases are presented when the condition is chronic and pain is unlikely to be seen on deep palpation over the sacroiliac joints. Radiography of these joints requires general anesthesia and is therefore seldom performed. Ultrasound images of the dorsal part of the dorsal sacroiliac ligament can be obtained by imaging from a dorsoventral direction, either side of the sacral spinous processes (331). The ventral ligament can be imaged via a rectal approach. Scintigraphic images of the sacroiliac region can be obtained with the detector camera placed above the cranial pelvis. In this view, the joint is covered by the wing of the ilium and lies approximately halfway between the tuber sacrale and the tuber coxae. In one study, normal horses showed symmetry of the tubera sacrale and ilial wings while most horses with confirmed sacroiliac region pain showed asymmetry of these regions. Techniques for injecting the sacroiliac joint region with local anesthetic agent to confirm a diagnosis of pain in this region have been described. The author uses a medial approach by placing a spinal needle obliquely from the cranial aspect of the contralateral tuber sacrale, aiming at the ipsilateral greater trochanter of the femur; the same approach is used to deliver anti-inflammatory medications. There are anecdotal reports of severe hindlimb paresis leading to recumbency or profuse hemorrhage following sacroiliac injections, caused by the proximity of the sciatic nerve and prominent gluteal vasculature. Direct injection into the joint itself is not possible in the living horse.

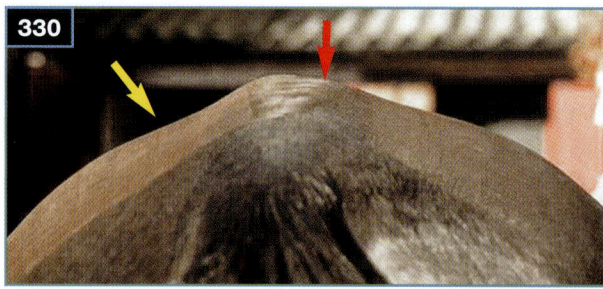

330 Dorsal pelvis of a mature horse. Note that although the right tuber sacrale (red arrow) is lower than the left, there is pronounced gluteal muscle wastage on the left (yellow arrow). This horse had a chronic left hindlimb lameness.

331 Ultrasonography of the dorsal sacroiliac ligaments can be carried out easily in the standing horse. (Photo courtesy GA Munroe)

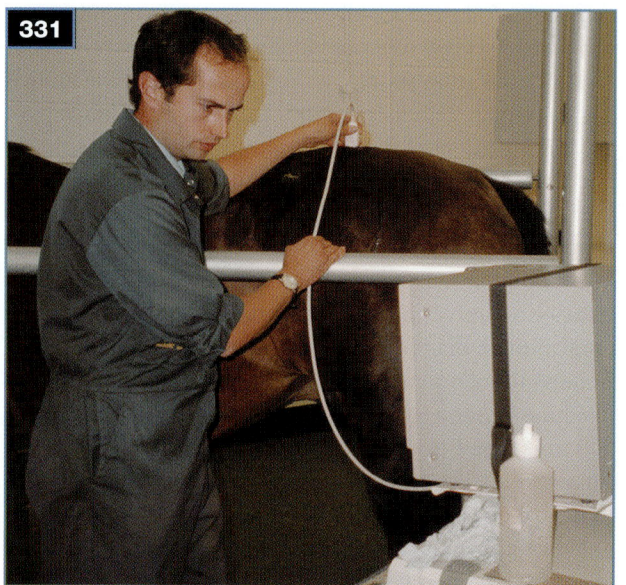

Musculoskeletal system

Management

Rest, continued work, and local and systemic medication have all been advocated for sacroiliac joint disease, but no well-founded reports exist on which to base recommendations. It is generally thought that poor muscling may make the problem worse, and that therefore complete (stall) rest is contraindicated.

Coccygeal vertebrae trauma

Definition/overview

Injuries of the tail occur rarely in the horse compared with cattle because the tail is generally not used to restrain this species.

Etiology/pathophysiology

Tail injuries are most frequently caused by inappropriate bandaging. Rarely, trauma may result from the tail being caught in a door or from another animal.

If the first three coccygeal vertebrae are involved, neuropraxia may result in tail motor weakness and, therefore, fecal and urine (mares) staining. A tight tail bandage left in place for 2–3 days will result in ischemia of the distal tail.

Clinical presentation

Some injuries may go unnoticed until swelling of the tail or excessive fecal contamination becomes apparent. Coccygeal fractures or luxations will result in local swelling, abnormal movement, and pain on manipulation. Ischemic damage is characterized by necrosis (blackening) of the skin.

Differential diagnosis

Other conditions such as polyneuritis equi, EPM, and equine herpesvirus myeloencephalopathy can cause tail paresis, but there will be concurrent signs such as bladder and anal atony. Sacral trauma can also cause tail weakness.

Diagnosis

Radiography of the tail will confirm coccygeal fractures, luxations, and osteomyelitis (332).

Management

The extent of ischemic damage following bandaging injury will take time to become evident. If there are no signs of healing after 2–3 weeks, amputation is indicated. Fractured or luxated coccygeal vertebrae can be stabilized with an intramedullary pin if cosmesis is important, but amputation will achieve swift pain relief.

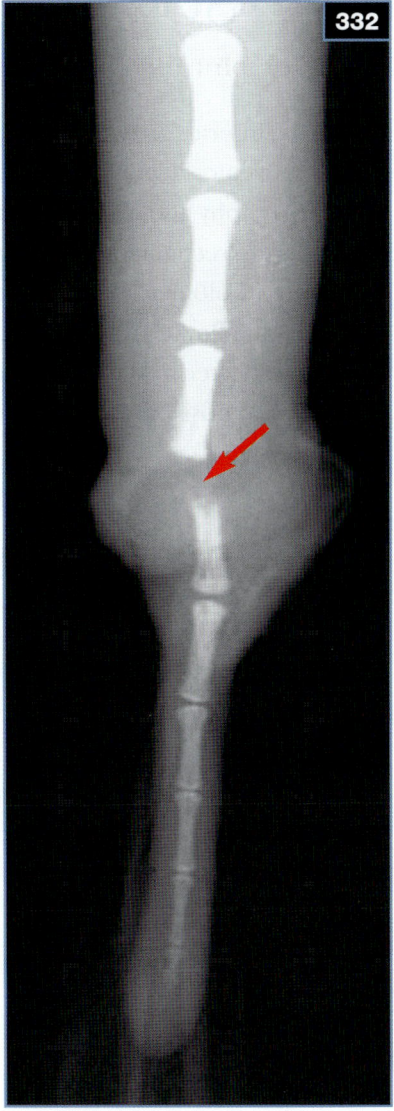

332 Radiograph of the caudal coccygeal vertebrae of a pony 1 month after a tail bandage was inadvertently left in place for 2 days. Note the subluxation of one intervertebral joint, with lysis of one vertebral end-plate (arrow). The distal third of the tail was subsequently amputated and the animal recovered uneventfully.

8 Soft-tissue injuries

Soft-tissue injuries are extremely common in the equine musculoskeletal system. The advent of ultrasonography and, more recently, of MRI has enabled us to recognize an increasing variety of complex pathologies. The treatment of these injuries is still limited, but new technologies are being investigated and their application to clinical cases is a real possibility in the future.

Types of injury

Horses are particularly prone to tendon injuries because of their weight, the extreme anatomic simplification of their distal limb, and the speed at which they can work, all of which can lead to enormous loading upon their tendon structures. These injuries are one of the most significant causes of losses in the equine industry.

Injuries to the superficial digital flexor tendon are the most common and affect a large number of race and sports horses. Suspensory ligament injuries have been found to occur nearly as commonly and affect horses of all types and breeds.

Ultrasonography has uncovered a much wider range of tendon and ligament injuries (e.g. distal sesamoidean ligament, biceps and common calcanean tendons, proximal suspensory ligament desmitis, branch injuries of the SDFT). Similarly, articular and nonarticular ligaments have been identified as a cause of severe lameness (e.g. collateral ligament injuries of the tarsocrural joint and cruciate ligament injuries of the stifle joint).

Tenosynovitis (inflammation of a tendon sheath) is also a commonly recognized form of injury in all types of horse and pony and it can lead to severe lameness in some cases. The complexity of the underlying pathology of these cases is becoming increasingly understood. The prognosis is guarded to poor and an early, accurate diagnosis is paramount to improve the chances for recovery.

Most of these soft-tissue injuries appear to have a similar pathophysiology based on repeat, cyclic and overuse trauma or, less commonly, direct trauma to the limb. This is described in more detail in the superficial digital flexor tendonitis section (see p.188).

Diagnostic techniques

Localization of the site of pain, in some cases by regional or intrasynovial anesthesia, is important as some of these injuries are subtle and difficult to detect using observation and palpation alone. Furthermore, there is often significant regional edema, making precise location of a lesion difficult.

Ancillary diagnostic techniques
Radiography provides very poor detail of soft tissues and ultrasonography has become the technique of choice for most of these injuries. Although used in the past, tenography, consisting of injecting air or positive contrast medium into tendon sheaths (333) or around tendons, has been largely replaced by ultrasonography.

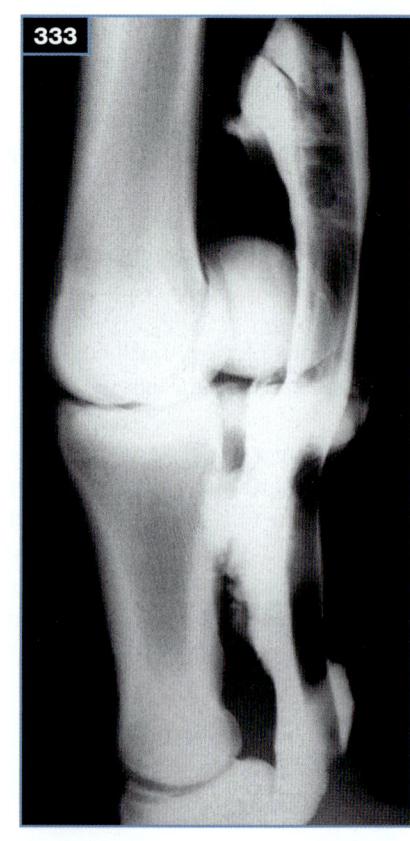

333 Tenography of the digital sheath of a horse. 10 ml of iodinated contrast medium was injected intrathecally into the digital sheath before this lateromedial radiograph was obtained. The outline of the flexor tendons and sheath wall is visible, but there is no detail of the tendon structure and superimposition of the structures makes fine evaluation difficult.

Ultrasonography

Ultrasonography can be used to examine all soft-tissue structures and the insertions of tendons and ligaments, and to assess joints, bone surfaces, and periarticular structures. High-definition equipment is necessary to evaluate structures accurately. Many portable and larger ultrasound scanners are equipped with transducers working at 7.5 MHz or higher, and these are adequate. The choice of probe will vary depending on the location, size, and depth of the structures to be assessed, but linear transducers (334, 335) tend to be most practical in the distal limb. Curved array transducers (336) and lower-frequency systems will be necessary for some applications over areas covered by large muscle masses (e.g. ilial wing fractures) or to approach structures that lie at an angle to the skin (e.g. intra-articular ligaments). The ideal system is one that provides a range of transducers from 4 to 12 or 16 MHz and is based on both linear and curved array transducers. The hair should be clipped as finely as possible (using a #40 clipper blade or finer) over the whole area of interest. It is not necessary to shave the area as this will often lead to swelling and pain. It is possible to scan a horse without clipping, but the hair coat traps air and debris and attenuates the sound beam significantly, causing major losses of information and artifacts. The use of ethanol or surgical spirit helps to improve sound transmission through the hair, but most probes will be damaged by the solvent effect of alcohol. Ultrasonography requires some experience and a thorough knowledge of the normal anatomy to allow an accurate interpretation of the findings. Comparison with the contralateral limb is always useful and will assist the operator in differentiating between normal variations in ultrasonographic appearance and significant lesions.

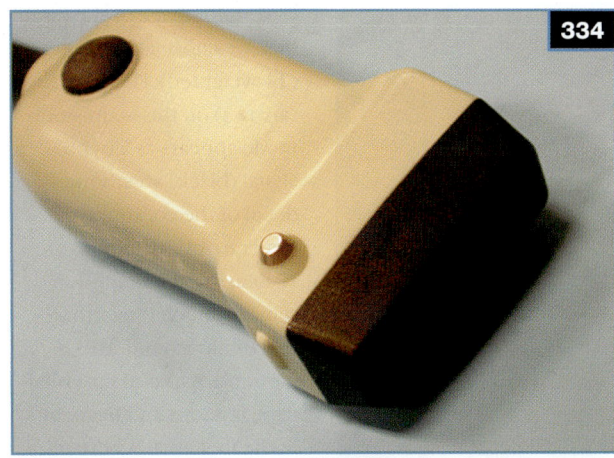

334

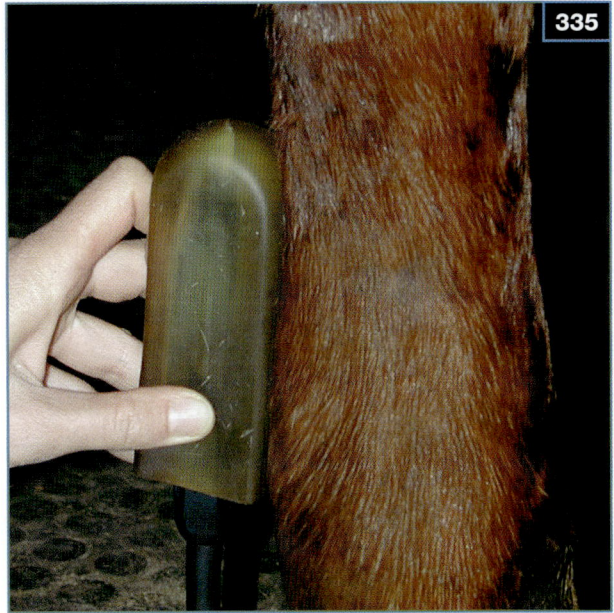

335

334 Pediatric 'T-probe' linear array ultrasound transducer. This is the probe of choice for most musculoskeletal applications in horses.

335 Linear array ultrasound transducers are designed as rectal probes that may also be used for abdominal applications and are therefore more versatile. Unfortunately, these are often of low definition and may be impractical in some anatomic areas because of obstruction by the cable.

336 Curved array ultrasound transducer. Based on the same technology as in 335, the components are placed along a curved line of varying lengths and radii, giving out a pie-shaped image. This type of probe provides a wider field of view in deeper tissues, while reducing the contact area between the skin and the probe. This is particularly useful in uneven areas or when the structures to be visualized are not parallel to the skin surface, as the probe may be tilted in relation to the skin.

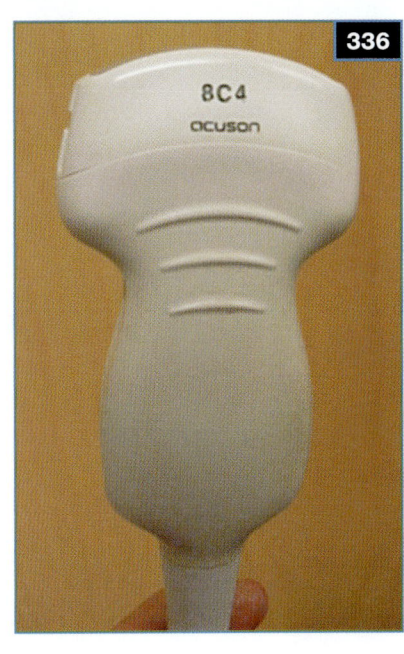

336

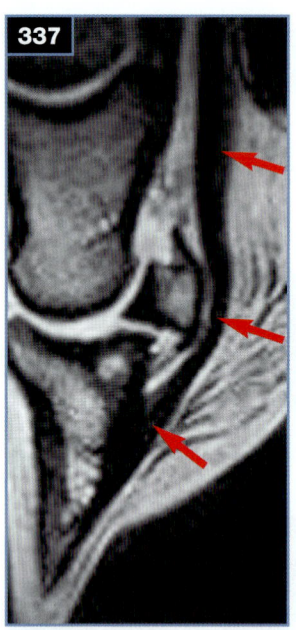

337 MRI image of the distal limb of a normal horse (T1-weighted). The DDFT (arrows) on this acquisition mode appears as a hypo-signal (black) area. Some detail of the contours and structure of the tendon are visible, but the definition remains much lower than that of ultrasound. MRI is particularly useful for visualizing tendons and ligaments in the foot area, where ultrasonography is generally impractical.

Other techniques

MRI has proved to be a very accurate means of detecting and assessing soft-tissue lesions in the musculoskeletal system in man, in small animals, and, more recently, in the horse. In equine orthopedics it has proved very useful for imaging soft-tissue structures that may not be adequately visualized with ultrasonography, in particular in the palmar foot (337). The cost of the examination and the need for general anesthesia in some high-field units (although low-field units have been developed to be used in the standing horse) still limit the practicality of this powerful diagnostic tool. High-definition CT may also provide valuable information about soft-tissue structures, particularly in the foot, but the limitations remain the same as for MRI.

Conditions affecting the tendons and ligaments

Superficial digital flexor tendonitis

Definition/overview

Tendonitis is a common condition affecting all breeds, but particularly racehorses, eventers, and other horses engaged in high-speed pursuits. Progressive, exercise-induced degeneration of the collagen matrix leads to acute, partial rupture of the tendon ('tendonopathy'). After injury, healing is slow and characterized by a high rate of recurrence. Tendonitis is a major source of economic loss in the equine industry. Alternative names include 'bowed tendon', 'tendon strain', and 'tendon break-down'.

Etiology/pathophysiology

The etiology is still incompletely understood. The main cause is probably a mechanical failure of tendon tissue due to overstretching of the fibers beyond the tolerance of the tissue. Although naturally very elastic, the SDFT is stretched to near its physiologic limits during fast exercise as the fetlock drops to near ground level (338). Cyclic strain involves fast stretching–release cycles at fast paces, which appear to weaken the tendon. In most cases, subclinical microtears occur during training or fast exercise. They accumulate quicker than they can heal, progressively mechanically weakening the tendon. An acute, severe episode, involving rupture of a major proportion of the fibers, then occurs with a normal level of exercise. Predisposing factors include heat damage in the tendon core during exercise, hormone-induced biochemical changes in females, intensity of training (number of strides or cycles per hour), and age (age-induced matrix degeneration). There are major biomechanical influences from the hoof

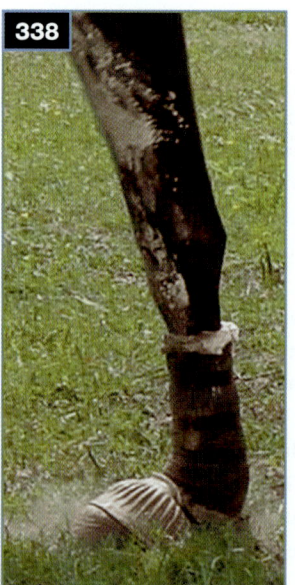

338 View of the distal limb of a racehorse at full gallop. The fetlock drops at maximum weight bearing during the stance phase of the stride because of stretching of the flexor tendons and interosseous ligament. The SDFT, being most palmar, is stretched to a greater degree, nearing its physiological limits (yield point).

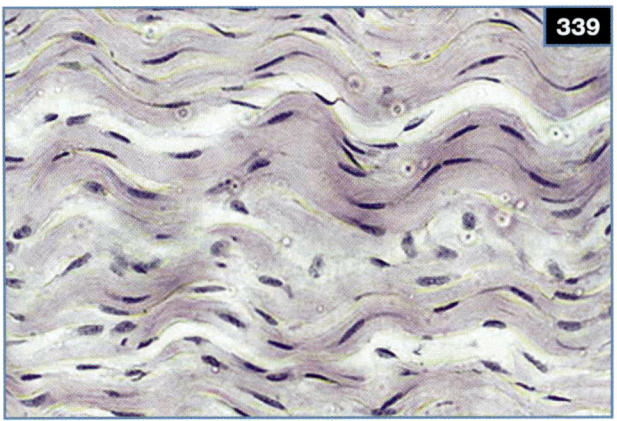

339 Histologic longitudinal section (hematoxillin stain) of the SDFT of a young horse (x100) showing the parallel organization of the collagen fibers and their zig-zag ('crimp') pattern. The dark nuclei of the tenocytes (tendon fibroblast-like cells) are interspersed between fibrils.

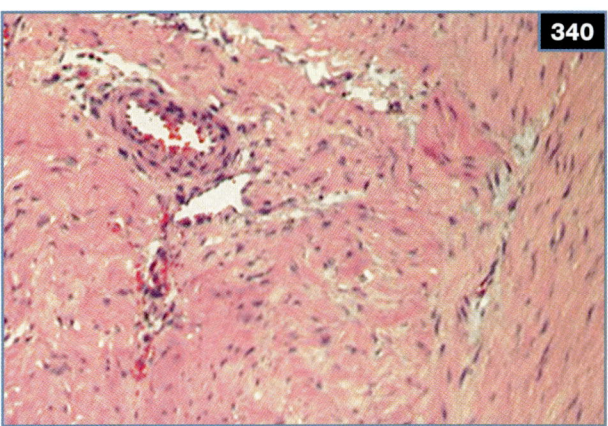

340 Histologic longitudinal section (H&E stain) of the SDFT of a horse presenting with an old tendonitis lesion. There is near complete loss of the longitudinal, parallel arrangement of the collagen and an increase and lack of differentiation of the fibroblastic cells. This image is typical of mature scar tissue.

shape (especially long toe/low heels conformations), ground surface quality (especially soft, deep soil and uneven surfaces), and method of training (duration and length of high-speed training).

Direct trauma, especially from limb interference (over-reach injuries) or hitting jumps, may also cause localized lesions, which tend to be peripheral (palmar or abaxial). There is an associated paratendonitis.

Repeat cyclic trauma leads to alterations of the collagen matrix. Normally, the tendon consists mainly of longitudinally arranged type I collagen fibers (339) and following injury there is an increasing proportion of poorly arranged collagen (especially type III). This leads to decreased elasticity and reduced resistance to cyclic strain. Stretching of the tendon at fast speed, although within theoretically normal tolerance levels, then causes sudden rupture or strain of a large proportion of collagen fibers. Hemorrhage subsequently occurs from endotenon capillary vessels. Platelets degranulate, inducing an acute inflammation with release of collagenases and an influx of inflammatory cells, which cause further damage to the tendon (spread of the lesion may last several days). Healing occurs through fibroplasia and scar tissue formation, which gradually replaces the torn tissue (340). This strong but inelastic matrix may gradually undergo maturation and remodeling with a relative increase of more longitudinally arranged type I fibers. The replacement tissue only matures slowly (over 18 months) and remains less elastic and resistant to cyclic strain than normal tendon. Recurrence with worsening of the lesion is therefore very common (40–80% of cases in racehorses in various studies).

Clinical presentation

The injury is usually associated with a sudden-onset lameness, which occurs during or immediately after exercise. The lameness is variable, but is often severe, especially a few hours after the injury or on the following day. Some horses only show a mild lameness. Heat and swelling over the palmar aspect of the metacarpus (less commonly the plantar metatarsus) develop over the first 24 hours. Pain is usually marked on palpation, but this gradually recedes over 4–10 days, leaving a firm, bow-shaped swelling over the 'tendon' area ('bowed tendon') (341). There may be associated distension of the carpal and/or digital sheath(s).

341 Typical swelling ('bowed tendon') over the mid-metacarpal region of a horse suffering from subacute tendonitis of the SDFT.

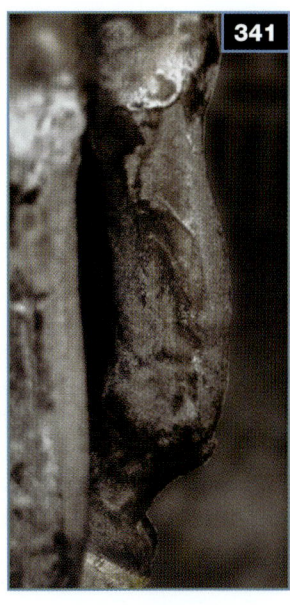

189

Lameness usually recedes after 7–20 days. The severity of the swelling and lameness does not correlate well with the severity of the tear. Early return to exercise may cause a more severe strain.

Differential diagnosis

Subcutaneous or paratendonous trauma (paratendonitis); swelling from inflammation or infection elsewhere in the limb; tenosynovitis of the digital sheath; inferior check ligament desmitis; suspensory ligament desmitis.

Diagnosis

Clinical examination

A diagnosis may be suspected on the basis of lameness associated with swelling, heat, and pain over the palmar metacarpal or plantar metatarsal area. These signs are not pathognomonic and there is little correlation between clinical presentation, palpation, and severity of the lesions as based on ultrasonographic appearance.

Ultrasonography

This is the diagnostic method of choice. It should not be carried out before 7–10 days, as the lesions may initially continue to increase in size. High-definition ultrasound systems using 7.5–12 MHz linear array transducers should be used. A systematic approach must be used and comparison with the opposite limb is valuable. The palmar aspect of the distal limb is clipped from above the accessory carpal bone to the bulbs of the heels and laterally as far as the cannon bone or phalanges. The palmar metacarpus (or plantar metatarsus) is divided into three equal areas (342): proximal third of the metacarpus (zones IA at the level of the carpometacarpal joint and IB); middle third (zones IIA and IIB); and distal third to the proximal edge of the sesamoid bones (zones IIIA and IIIB). A zone IIIC corresponds to the area palmar to the sesamoid bones. The palmar or plantar pastern area is divided into three zones (PI to III). The limb is first assessed from the palmar aspect in transverse planes, then in longitudinal sections (using both sagittal and parasagittal planes). Some ultrasonographers use an alternative system in which they measure the position of lesions in the soft-tissue structures in centimeters from the accessory carpal bone.

The whole area should be assessed, including the suspensory ligament. This is evaluated from the palmar aspect to the middle of the metacarpus or metatarsus, then each branch of the suspensory ligament is assessed abaxially from its corresponding side (lateral for the lateral branch, etc.) in both transverse and longitudinal planes. The origin of the suspensory ligament in the hindlimb is difficult to assess. This is more easily achieved with a curved array transducer from a plantaromedial approach.

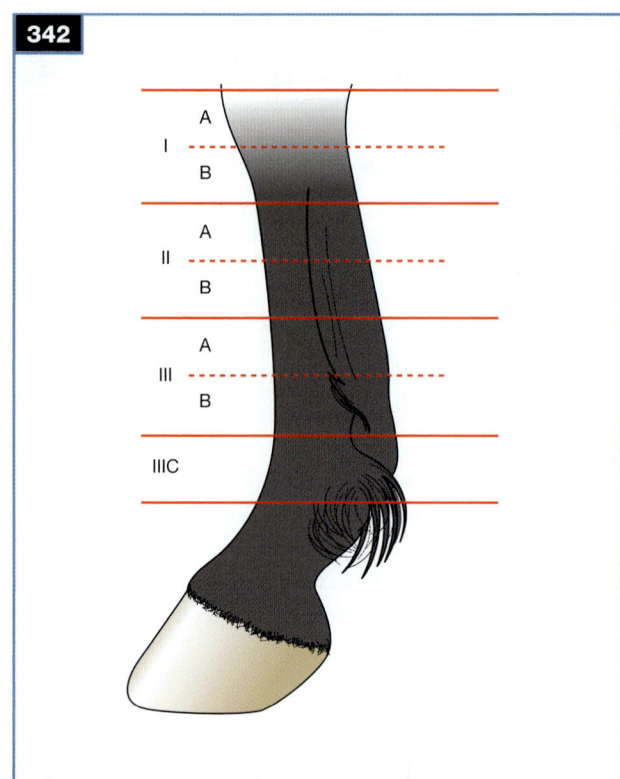

342 Definition of zones I to III and subdivision into zones A and B for each area of the palmar metacarpus.

Typical lesions appear as discrete, well-defined hypo- (dark grey) or anechogenic (black) areas. These are most often located near the center of the tendon (343), but they may occur at the periphery (344). The size of the defect should be measured and its ratio to the whole cross-sectional area of the tendon calculated (most scanners have software that make this possible). Longitudinal scans should always be performed because they will show the extent of the lesion and loss of the normal fiber pattern. The latter gives an insight into the normal fascicular organization of type I collagen-rich tendon (345). Associated swelling of the tendon due to edema, hemorrhage, and cell infiltration causes an increased cross-sectional surface area. Some lesions may be more diffuse and less defined (346). Severe tendon sprains are characterized by a marked, diffuse decrease in echogenicity and significant enlargement (2–3-fold). In completely ruptured tendons the fibrous tissue is replaced by amorphous,

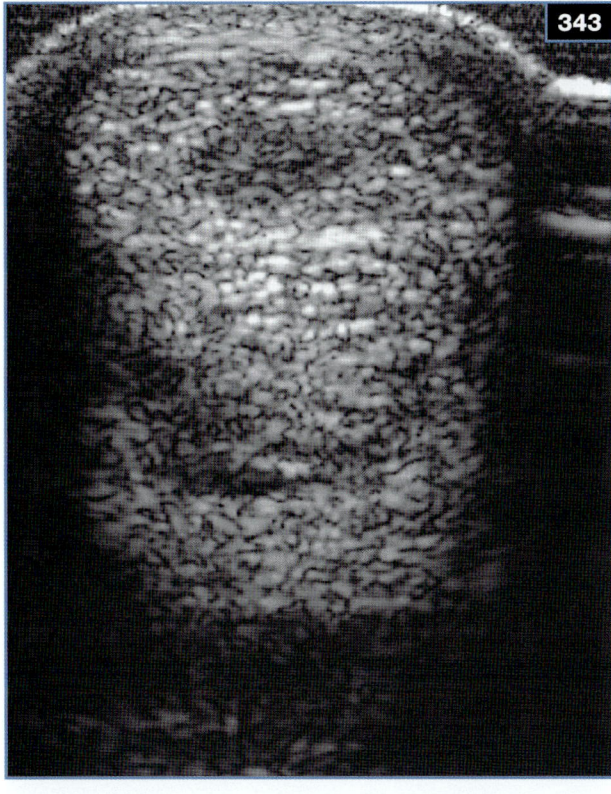

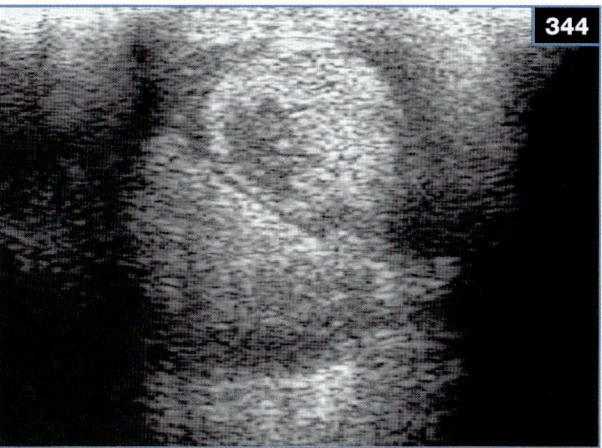

343 A subacute, hypoechogenic central core lesion on a cross-sectional (transverse) ultrasonographic scan of the palmar aspect of the metacarpus. This is the most common site for lesions to occur.

344 A subacute, peripheral hypoechogenic lesion on a cross-sectional (transverse) ultrasonographic scan of the palmar aspect of the metacarpus. This location is less common.

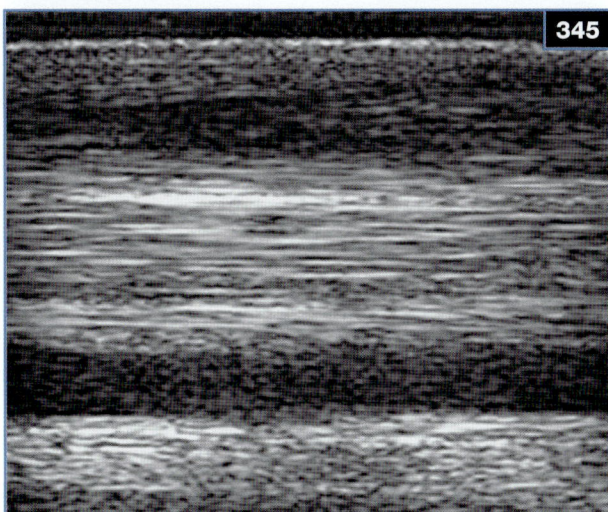

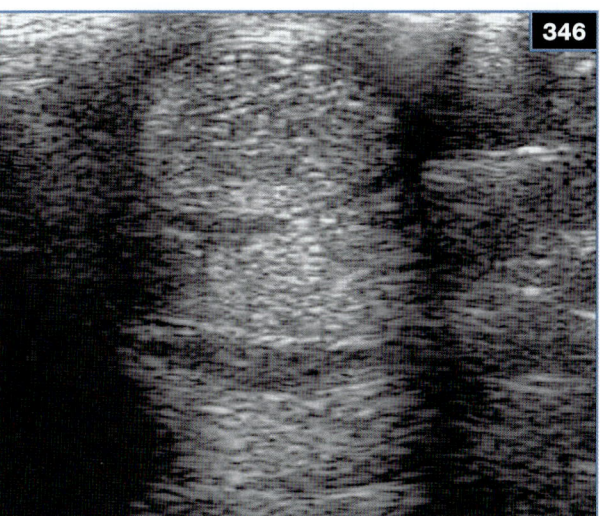

345 Longitudinal, sagittal ultrasonographic section of the SDFT of a horse with subacute tendonitis. There is loss of the normal fiber alignment within the SDFT, which also appears significantly enlarged and hypoechogenic. The underlying DDFT shows a normal echostructure.

346 Diffuse lesion characterized by enlargement of the SDFT and generalized, heterogeneous decrease of echogenicity.

hypoechogenic tissue containing anechogenic foci (hematoma formation). This tissue is gradually replaced by homogeneous, hypoechogenic granulation tissue (347). No normal tendon tissue is visible. The frayed ruptured ends are hypoechogenic and heterogeneous. With time, the echogenicity of the lesion tends to increase because of decreased infiltration and increased collagen deposition. Scar tissue is iso- to hyperechogenic to normal tendon tissue, but lacks a normal fibrillar pattern on longitudinal scans (348). Mineralization may be present in chronic cases, causing hyperechogenic interfaces casting an acoustic shadow.

Lesions most often occur in the metacarpal, unsheathed area. They may also occur, though much less commonly, within either the carpal flexor tendon sheath (349, 350) or the digital sheath (351), where they are probably more often traumatic than spontaneous.

Finally, injuries to the distal branches near their insertion on the middle phalanx are increasingly recognized. The branch will appear enlarged, hypoechogenic, and heterogeneous (352). The lesion may be defined, but often affects the whole cross-section of the branch. One or both branches may be affected. There is usually associated digital sheath effusion.

The initial examination will confirm the diagnosis and determine the localization, size, extent, and severity of the lesion. The latter is based on increased cross-sectional area of the tendon and decrease of echogenicity, cross-sectional surface area (relative to that of the tendon), and proximodistal length of the lesion. Diffuse lesions carry a worse prognosis than central core lesions.

Ultrasonography should be used regularly (every 8–12 s) to monitor the progress and quality of healing, looking for increases in echogenicity (fibrous tissue formation) and fiber alignment on longitudinal scans. Adequate healing is characterized by isoechogenicity of the damaged portion with normal tendon tissue and near-longitudinal alignment of the replacement fibers.

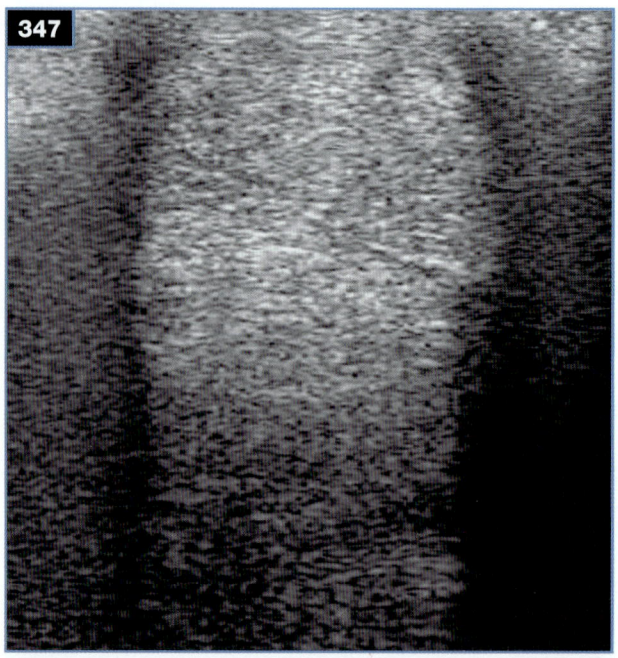

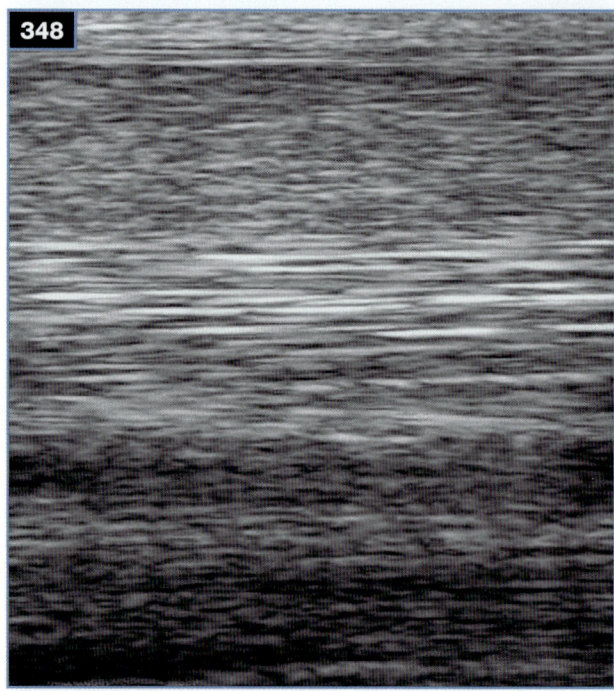

347, 348 Transverse (347) and longitudinal (348) ultrasonographic scans of the SDFT of a horse with chronic tendonitis. The tendon appears normally echogenic on the transverse scan (347), although it is enlarged and heterogeneous, with a mottled appearance. The sagittal scan (348) confirms a lack of longitudinal rearrangement of the fibers. This is typical of poorly remodeled scar tissue.

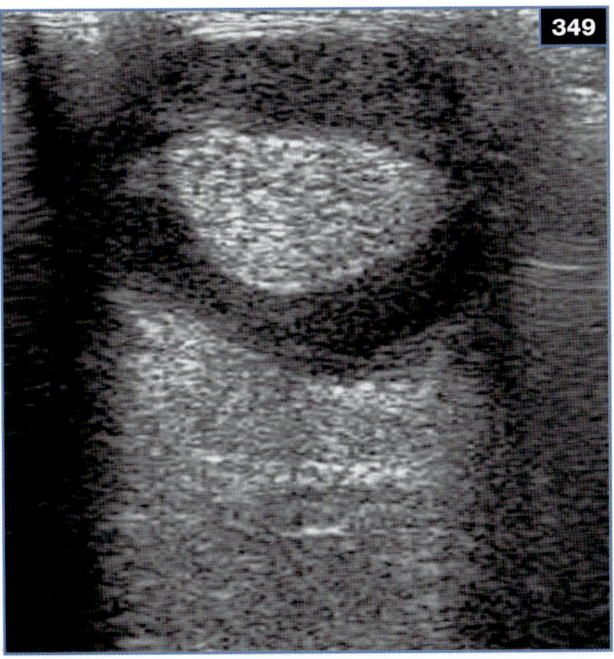

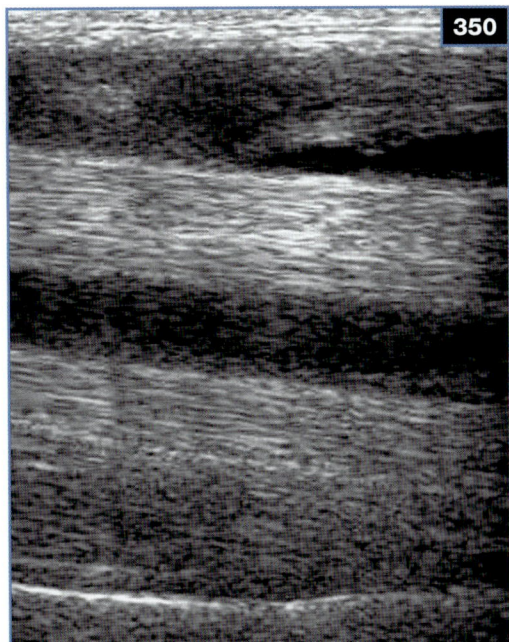

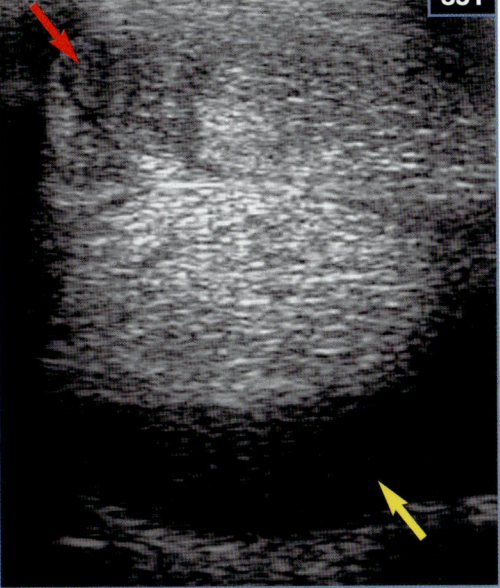

349, 350 Transverse (349) and longitudinal (350) ultrasonographic scans of the SDFT of a horse with complete rupture. The tendon appears completely anechogenic and decreased in size. The tendon tissue has been replaced by a homogeneous, slightly granular structure, typical of granulation tissue. On the longitudinal scan (350), the frayed proximal end of the distal stump presents as a mixed echogenicity and is slightly enlarged, while the rupture segment becomes very thin within the carpal flexor sheath. Note the presence of anechogenic fluid and thickened synovial membrane within the digital sheath (tenosynovitis).

351 Transverse ultrasonograph of the SDFT in the distal metacarpal area, within the digital flexor tendon sheath. The SDFT is enlarged and there is an irregular, peripheral hypoechogenic lesion in the lateral part of the tendon (red arrow). The sheath is distended and a hypoechogenic halo around the tendons suggests synovial inflammation (tenosynovitis) (yellow arrow).

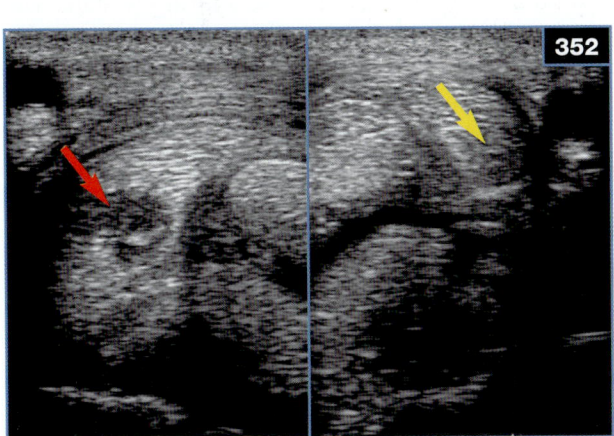

352 Transverse ultrasonograph of the SDFT in the proximal digital (pastern) area. The left image shows an enlarged lateral SDFT branch. It contains a well-defined hypoechogenic lesion (red arrow), although the remainder of this branch also appears heterogeneous. The right image shows the normal medial branch (yellow arrow). The latter is smaller, but is surrounded by hypoechogenic material representing inflamed synovial tissue.

Management

Tendonitis is divided into three phases: an acute (inflammatory) phase lasting 7–10 days; a subacute or repair phase lasting 2–4 months; and a remodeling phase (4–12 months).

Acute phase

Aggressive anti-inflammatory treatment is paramount to reduce deleterious mediators and enzyme release. The animals should be box rested to limit mechanical strain. Steroidal anti-inflammatory drugs may interfere with fibroplasias and probably delay the early repair phenomena. Systemic NSAIDs are used for analgesia as they have little effect on local inflammation. Cold water or ice (for 20 minutes 3–6 times daily) is probably the most efficient local anti-inflammatory treatment: cold induces vasoconstriction, thus decreasing hemorrhage and edema, and reducing the temperature partially inhibits enzyme activity. Topical NSAIDs may also be used. Counter pressure is provided through support bandages, and massage may be helpful.

Subacute phase

As soon as local signs of inflammation have receded (edema and local heat), controlled exercise should be instituted in the form of in-hand walking or use of walkers, treadmills, or underwater treadmills, according to a graduated program (see below) over 6–8 s. The horses may be ridden at a walk 4 s post injury.

Physiotherapy techniques may be used at this stage, although there is little scientific evidence to determine their impact on the recovery rate or rate of recurrence of the injury. Laser, shock wave, and therapeutic ultrasound treatments have been advocated and may help to reduce pain and edema. Their effect on the healing quality is unclear and probably limited. It has been shown that controlled exercise is superior to box or field rest or other treatments alone at this stage.

Recovery phase

If ultrasonography shows adequate repair, the horse may be turned out to pasture or preferably given light exercise (ridden or in a horse walker). Gradual return to training should not be reinstituted for at least 4–6 months and then under ultrasonographic guidance. The use of ultrasound treatment has been said to help reduce adhesions and fibrosis in chronic cases.

A number of biological treatments are currently under evaluation or advocated for clinical use, although there is little consensus on their effectiveness. Intralesional or peritendinous injections of polysulfated glycosaminoglycans and hyaluronic acid have been disappointing. Intralesional injection of growth factors has been described. Among these, only insulin-like growth factor-1 (IGF-1) has been shown to provide some gain *in vivo* in terms of speed of repair, but this may be mainly through increased scar tissue production. Intralesional, autologous platelet-rich plasma is being evaluated clinically, but there are still limited data that show a dramatic positive effect.

Sternebral bone marrow as a source of growth factors and/or stem cells is increasingly being used around the world despite a lack of published evidence regarding its benefits and concerns about potential adverse effects (i.e. large volume required, presence of fat and bone material, small or even negligible percentage of stem cells). To improve the specificity of the treatment, autologous pluripotential stem cells may be isolated from bone marrow or adipose tissue aspirates and grown *in vitro* before being re-injected into the lesion. The results of clinical trials are still awaited in the scientific literature, but presented results show lowered recurrence rates in sport horses and in National Hunt (jumping) racehorses.

Surgical treatments have been suggested, including chemical or physical cautery ('firing'), proximal check ligament (accessory ligament of the SDFT) desmotomy, and percutaneous longitudinal tenotomy ('splitting'). Cautery and blistering have not been shown to produce any advantages and may be deleterious as they promote intertendonous adhesions and paratenon fibrosis. These methods also raise concerns regarding the animal's welfare. The other two techniques are carried out in the subacute phase and appear to increase the speed of recovery, although the repair quality and rate of recurrence may not be improved. These should therefore be used in severe or recurrent cases or in cases where speed of recovery is required. There has been some concern that accessory ligament desmotomy may predispose to contralateral SDFT tendonitis or to suspensory ligament injury in either limb. There is currently no strong evidence that surgical treatments significantly improve the long-term outcome.

Summary: controlled exercise program

- Walking for 30 minutes daily for 4 weeks (in-hand or in walker or treadmill).
- Then walking (in-hand, walker, or under saddle) 45 minutes daily for 4 weeks.
- Follow-up ultrasonographic examination at 8 weeks, then every 8 weeks or prior to changes in exercise level.
- Add 5 minutes trotting to above for following 4 weeks, then 10 minutes trot over the following 4 weeks.
- Gradually add slow canter (15–20 minutes daily) over 4–12 weeks depending on severity of injury and sonographic appearance.
- At that stage (4–6 months), either turn out to pasture for 3–6 months or, preferably, continue controlled exercise as follows: canter one mile daily for 4 weeks, two miles daily for a further 4 weeks.
- Introduce breezes gradually.

No cantering or galloping should be allowed before 6 months after injury as re-injury is likely unless the injury is mild. The protocol should be altered depending on the severity of the injury (increase exercise regimen earlier if the lesion is mild and sonographic appearance indicates adequate repair; delay if severe and sonographic appearance shows poor healing). Return to racing/competing should be envisaged at 9–12 months, depending on the severity of the injury and ultrasonographic evolution at follow-up examinations.

Prevention

Prevention in the future may be through improved training techniques, adequate care of training surfaces, proper farriery, and identification of early degenerative changes in the tendon. It has been suggested that early training before 2.5 years of age may help to increase tendon resistance to strains, but this remains to be confirmed.

Prognosis

The prognosis for soundness is always good, even with severe tears. Tendons always heal. The prognosis for return to the same level of activity and performance is, however, moderate to guarded, depending on the severity of the lesion. Up to 50% of affected racehorses never return to racing, while recurrence occurs in up to 80% of cases. In other athletic activities the prognosis is probably better, but the risk of recurrence remains high. Recent studies suggest that the prognosis for return to athletic activity does not depend on the severity of the initial injury, but rather on the evolution of the ultrasonographic appearance regardless of the initial severity.

Suspensory ligament desmitis
Definition/overview

Suspensory ligament desmitis is actually a form of tendonitis, similar to SDFT tendonitis, and the suspensory ligament (interosseous III muscle) is the second most common site for tendon and ligament injuries in the horse. It is encountered in all breeds, but is most common in the forelimbs of racehorses and in both fore- and hindlimbs in Standardbreds. It is, however, increasingly recognized in the hindlimbs of sports horses. The condition differs depending on the site of the lesion and it is therefore divided into proximal desmitis, desmopathy of the body, and desmopathy of the branches.

Etiology/pathophysiology

The etiology is similar to that of SDFT tendonitis, but it is unclear under what circumstances the suspensory ligament is affected rather than the SDFT. Branch injuries may be occasionally associated with a single excessive or asymmetrical weight-bearing event. Some branch injuries are associated with sesamoid bone injuries (see p. 106). Horses with straight hock and low fetlock conformation may be predisposed to some suspensory ligament injuries, particularly proximally. In some cases, lesions result from mechanical interference with prominent metacarpal or metatarsal bones (periostitis due to 'splints' or fractures), although it is possible in many cases that the periostitis is secondary to ligament strain. Avulsion fractures of the proximal palmar metacarpal or plantar metatarsal cortex are an allied but separate condition. Fatigue stress fractures of the palmar cortex of MC/MT III are unrelated.

The pathophysiology is similar to that of SDFT tendonitis. In the hindlimb, proximal desmitis is suggested to be associated with a compartment syndrome, the ligament and peripheral neurovascular structures being encased in a tight sheath formed by the MC/MT bones and fascia. This could explain the poorer prognosis and lack of healing at this site.

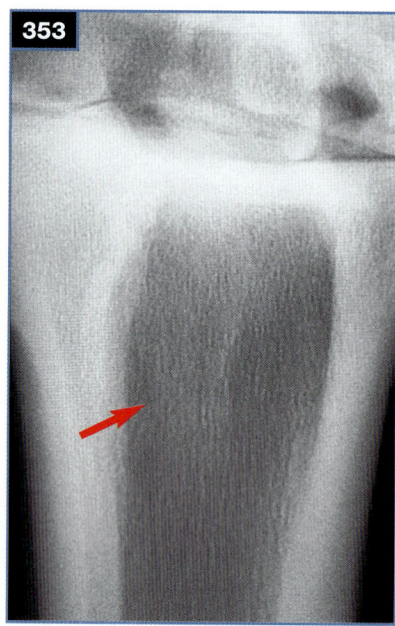 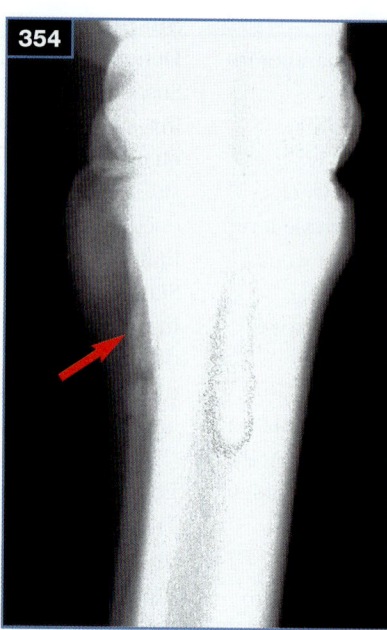

353 Dorsopalmar radiograph of the proximal metacarpus of a horse presenting with proximal suspensory ligament desmitis. There is a slight increase of opacity and loss of trabecular pattern lateral to the palmar sagittal ridge of the proximal metacarpus, suggesting early sclerosis (arrow).

354 Lateromedial radiograph of the proximal metacarpus of a horse with chronic proximal suspensory disease of the forelimb. Note the multiple bony fragments palmar to the proximal third metacarpus due to avulsion fractures of the palmar cortex (arrow). (Photo courtesy GA Munroe)

Proximal suspensory desmitis

Clinical presentation

Lameness varies from mild to severe, often worsening with exercise. In some cases, especially in the forelimb, there may be acute-onset lameness, but many cases, especially in the hindlimb, are chronic and insidious in onset. Lameness may be increased on the circle, especially on the outside limb or when ridden. There may merely be signs of exercise intolerance or poor performance. There are often no specific local signs, but occasionally a nonspecific diffuse swelling of the palmar/plantar cannon region is palpable. In some cases, digital pressure on the proximal suspensory ligament may lead to resentment.

Differential diagnosis

Lesions within the other ligaments and tendons in that region; other causes of inflammation in the metacarpal or metatarsal area; any other causes of lameness and notably, in the hindlimb, bone spavin.

Diagnosis

Diagnosis may be challenging as there are no pathognomonic signs and the ultrasonographic appearance varies.

Clinical examination

A systematic, routine lameness investigation is warranted. Many cases are positive to fetlock flexion and, in the hindlimb, to hock flexion. The use of diagnostic analgesia is essential. The lameness is not altered by distal metacarpal or metatarsal analgesia (lower six-point nerve block), although proximal diffusion of the anesthetic solution may improve the gait. The lameness may or may not respond to proximal metacarpal or metatarsal analgesia (higher six-point nerve block), but it should be abolished by instillation of local anesthetic around the origin of the ligament or by antebrachial (ulnar +/- musculocutaneous and median nerve blocks) or crural regional analgesia (tibial +/- fibular nerve blocks). Some clinicians use a deep lateral plantar nerve regional block in the hindlimb. False-positive and false-negative responses are observed. The lameness may also respond to analgesia of the carpometacarpal or tarsometatarsal joints.

Radiography

There may be sclerosis with loss of the trabecular pattern and thickening of the cortex of the palmaro- or plantaroproximal third metacarpal or metatarsal bone (**353**). Cortical fissures or avulsed fragments may be visible near the origin of the ligament (**354**).

Ultrasonography

Lesions occur within the proximal 2 cm of the ligament. They may be extremely subtle. Comparison with the contralateral limb is warranted. Expected signs include any of the following:

✦ Enlargement of the ligament, characterized by decreased space between it and the check ligament (accessory ligament of the DDFT) or increased width (**355**).
✦ Poor definition of the ligament margins (**356**).
✦ One or several, diffuse or well-defined hypoechogenic areas (**357**, **358**).

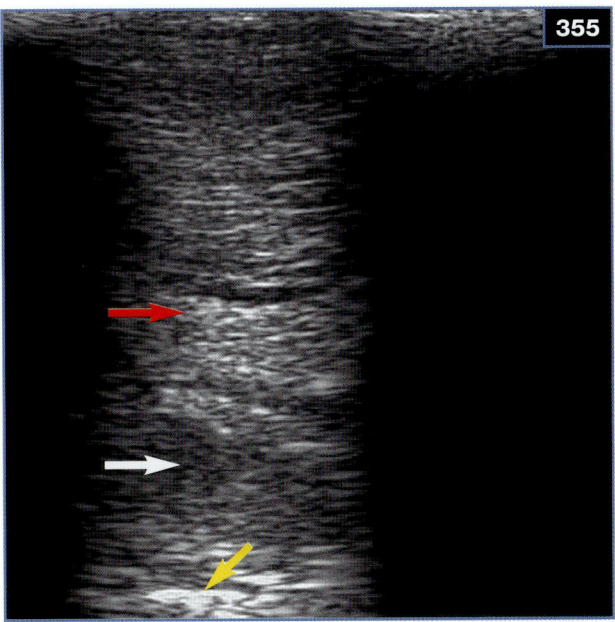

355 Proximal suspensory desmitis in the forelimb of a horse. The ligament appears enlarged and fills up the entire space between the accessory ligament of the DDFT (inferior check ligament) (red arrow) and the third metacarpal bone (yellow arrow). There is also a large, diffuse, hypoechogenic lesion throughout the middle portion of the ligament origin (white arrow).

356 Proximal suspensory desmitis in the hindlimb. The ligament is enlarged and pushes the blood vessels plantarly (red arrow). The plantar borders of the ligament are not clearly defined and merge with the surrounding connective tissue and the tarsal check ligament (yellow arrow).

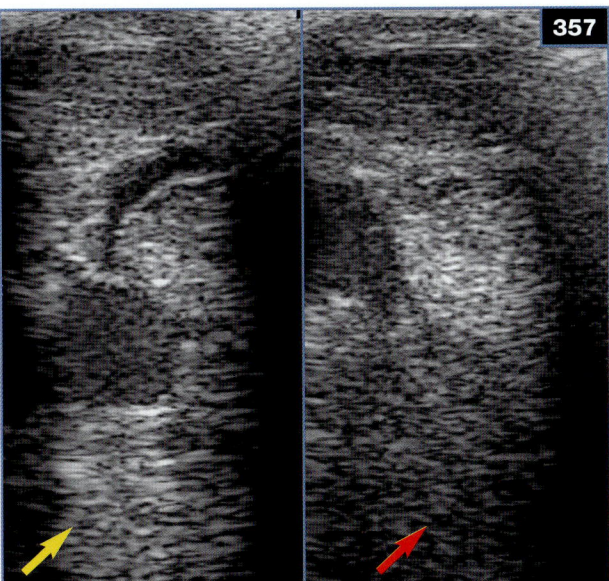

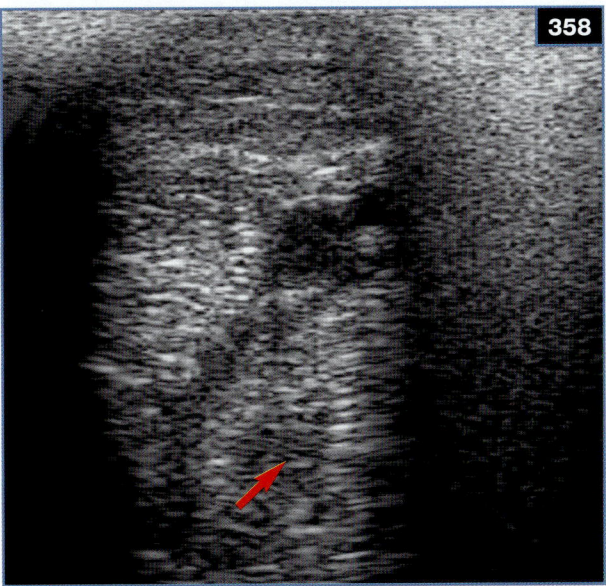

357 Proximal suspensory desmitis in the right hindlimb of a horse. The right image shows a diffusely hypoechogenic ligament (red arrow). The blood vessels, tarsal check ligament and flexor tendons are displaced plantarly and the peri-ligamentous connective tissues are obliterated. The left image shows the normal contralateral (left hindlimb) ligament (yellow arrow).

358 There is a diffuse hypoechogenic area in the center part of the origin of the suspensory ligament (arrow) in the hindlimb of this horse.

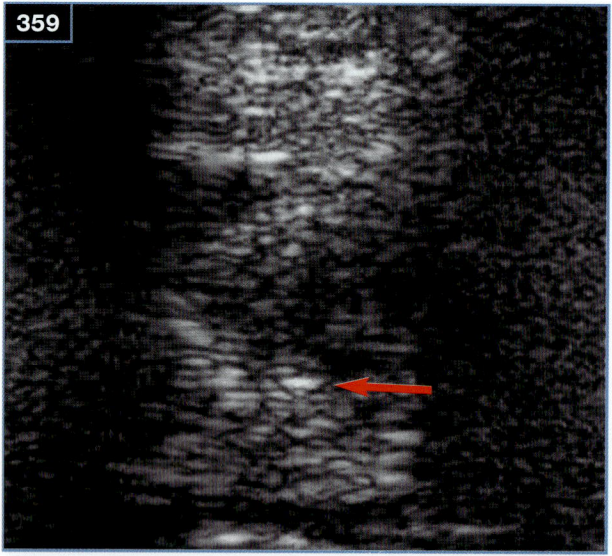

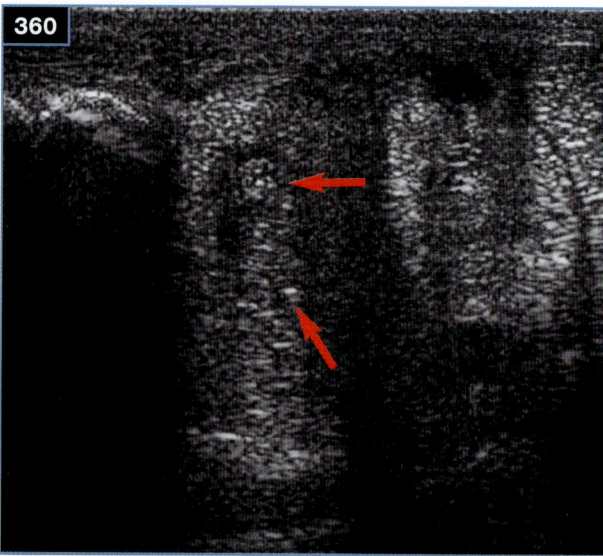

359, 360 Transverse ultrasound scans of the proximal part of the suspensory ligament as seen from the palmar (359) and medial (360) aspect of the limb. This double approach is used to rule out artifacts. Hyperechogenic foci are visible within the ligament which otherwise contains a poorly delineated, heterogeneous, and hypoechogenic lesion.

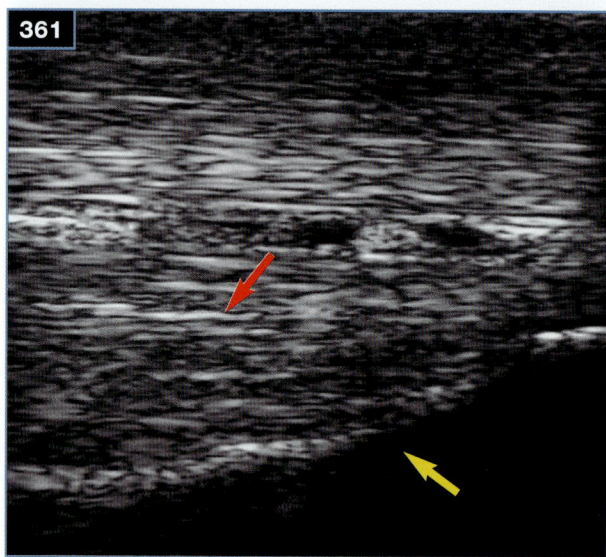

361 Longitudinal ultrasonographic view of the origin of the suspensory ligament in a forelimb. The ligament shows a poorly defined, diffusely heterogeneous echogenicity, partial loss of the fiber pattern, and enlargement leading to obliteration of the connective tissue space between its palmar border and the inferior check ligament (red arrow). The palmar contour of the third metacarpal bone is within normal limits (yellow arrow).

362 Longitudinal ultrasonographic view of the origin of the suspensory ligament in a forelimb. The palmar outline of the third metacarpal bone is irregular and there are two interruptions in the continuity of the cortical line, suggesting new bone production, and possibly the presence of an 'avulsion fragment or fracture' (yellow arrow). This horse also has a decreased echogenicity and loss of the fiber pattern in the suspensory ligament (red arrow).

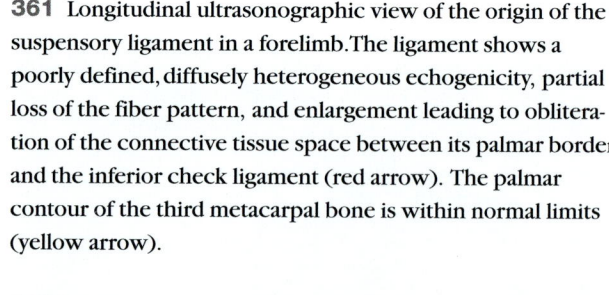

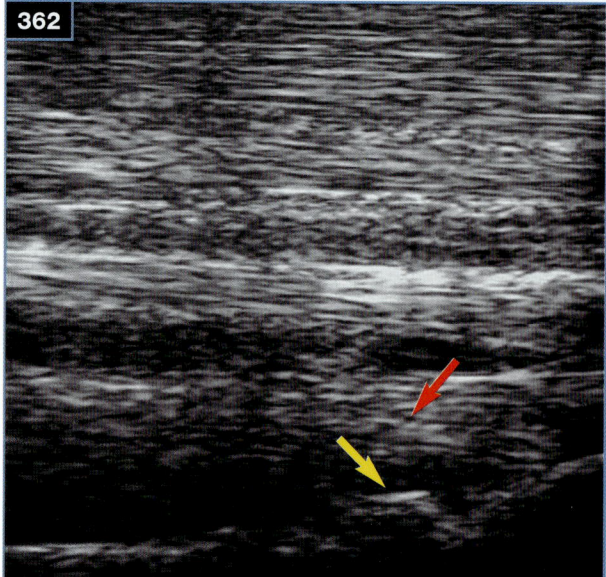

- Hyperechogenic areas in chronic cases, particularly in the hindlimbs (359, 360).
- Irregularity of the palmar (plantar) surface of the third metacarpal (metatarsal) bone (361, 362).

Scintigraphy

Bone scintigraphy shows increased uptake over the origin of the ligament (363) and it can be useful to rule out intertarsal joint disease.

Management

Forelimb proximal suspensory desmopathy

Conservative treatment is undertaken as for SDFT tendonitis. It is based on initial rest with in-hand walking for 5–10 minutes 2–4 times daily for 4 weeks, then gradually increasing to 20 minutes in-hand walking or in a mechanical walker over 4 weeks. Follow-up ultrasonography should be performed at 8 weeks. Some acute injuries in the forelimb will allow a gradual return to work between three and 6 months post injury. Full work should not be resumed before complete resolution of the lesion on ultrasonography. In chronic cases the lesion may persist; if this is the case, return to work is based on the absence of evolution of the lesion on ultrasonography for a period of 3 months. Surgical options or intraligamentous injections of corticosteroids, hyaluronate, or glycosaminoglycans have not been shown to improve the outcome.

Hindlimb proximal suspensory desmopathy

These injuries are often recognized at a later, chronic stage. The same treatment is applied over a duration of at least 6 months. Lameness often persists (in 80% of cases).

Shock-wave therapy has been shown to improve the clinical signs (lameness) in 50% of cases, but not the ultrasonographic appearance of the lesion, particularly in the hindlimbs. The mode of action is thought to be analgesia through destruction of nerve endings. Other forms of physiotherapy have generally not been effective in this condition.

Surgically based treatments are increasingly used, including fasciotomy to relieve the compartment syndrome combined with specific neurectomy of the deep lateral plantar metatarsal nerve. This is, however, a palliative treatment and the lesions persist or may worsen if work is reinstituted too soon. It should therefore be associated with a period of rest with controlled exercise. Percutaneous fasciotomy has been advocated in the US and, in the past, tibial neurectomy was suggested as useful in chronic cases. Many cases have very poor foot conformation and will benefit from corrective foot trimming and shoeing. Intratendinous bone marrow or isolated stem cell injections are currently under evaluation.

Prognosis

The prognosis for return to the same level of performance is good in the forelimb (90%), but it is guarded to poor in the hindlimbs (22% in one study), where lameness often persists. Chronic injuries respond less well to treatment. Recurrence is common, especially where there are signs of bone remodeling.

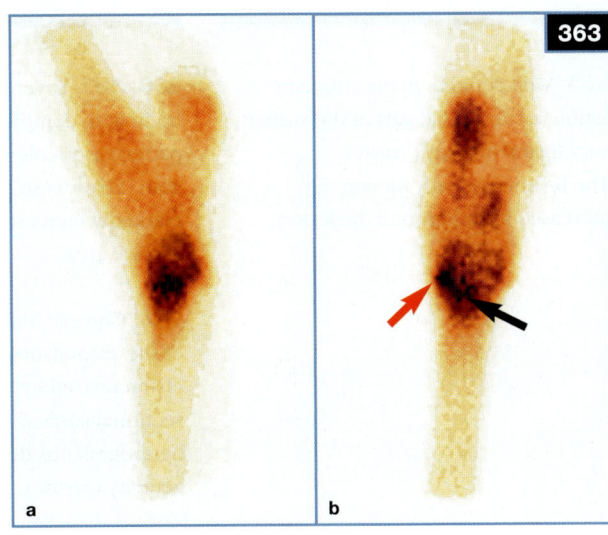

363 Lateral (a) and dorsoplantar (b) ^{99}Tc-MDP scintigraphy of the hock and proximal cannon region of a horse that was suffering from bilateral proximal suspensory desmitis. Note the increased uptake of isotope (hot spot) in the middle of the proximal third metatarsus (black arrow). The focal hot spot laterally is the head of the fourth metatarsus and is normal (red arrow). (Photo courtesy A Font)

Desmitis of the suspensory ligament body
Clinical presentation

The degree of lameness is variable. The condition tends to be unilateral and affects the forelimbs most commonly, except in Standardbred racehorses. Lameness is usually severe at the outset and decreases gradually within 3–6 weeks. There is obvious swelling in the area palmar to the metacarpus and dorsal to the tendons (364). As edema recedes, thickening of the suspensory body becomes obvious on palpation. There may be palpable pain.

Differential diagnosis

Lesions within other parts of the suspensory apparatus and the other ligaments and tendons in that region; consider other causes of inflammation in the metacarpal or metatarsal area.

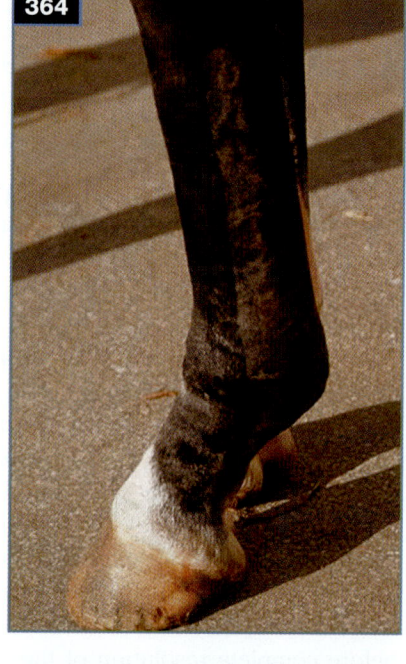

364 Diffuse swelling over the abaxial aspects of the metacarpus due to a subacute suspensory ligament injury.

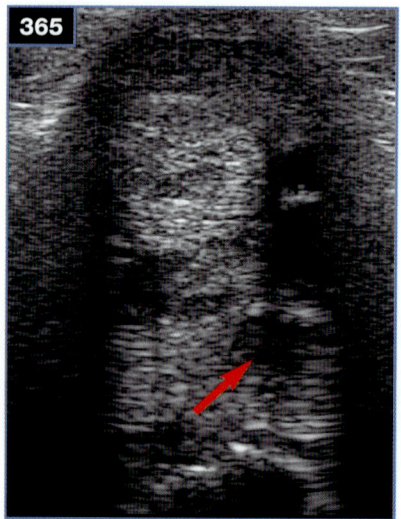
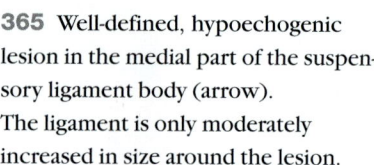
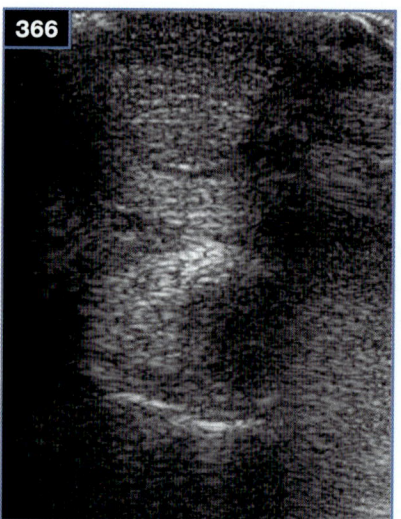
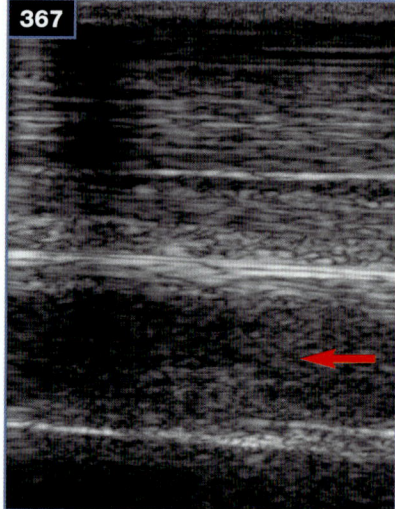
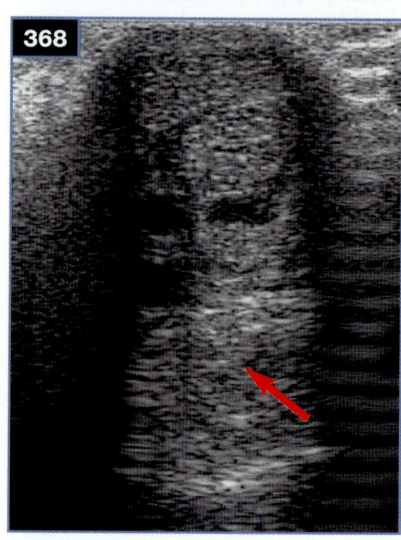

365 Well-defined, hypoechogenic lesion in the medial part of the suspensory ligament body (arrow). The ligament is only moderately increased in size around the lesion.

366, 367 Severe tear in the ligament body with complete loss of fiber pattern as visible on the longitudinal scan (arrow) (367). The ligament is markedly increased in cross-sectional surface area.

368 Chronic, diffuse desmopathy of the suspensory ligament body, characterized by an increased cross-sectional surface area and a diffuse heterogeneous decrease in echogenicity (arrow).

Diagnosis
Clinical examination
Palpation often provides a strong suspicion. Diagnostic analgesia is rarely necessary.

Radiography
It is useful to look for fracture or periostitis of the second or fourth metacarpal or metatarsal ('splint') bones.

Ultrasonography
The lesions are similar to those encountered in the SDFT, with an increased cross-sectional surface area on transverse scans and lesions ranging from discrete anechogenic to diffuse hypoechogenic (365–368). Diffuse lesions are more common. In chronic cases there may often be hyperechoic areas casting acoustic shadow artifacts, compatible with focal mineralization.

Interference with the splint bones is visible as an area of encroachment between the bone surface of the affected splint bone and the ligament. There may be tremendous periligamentous thickening, especially in fractures, but not necessarily associated with desmitis.

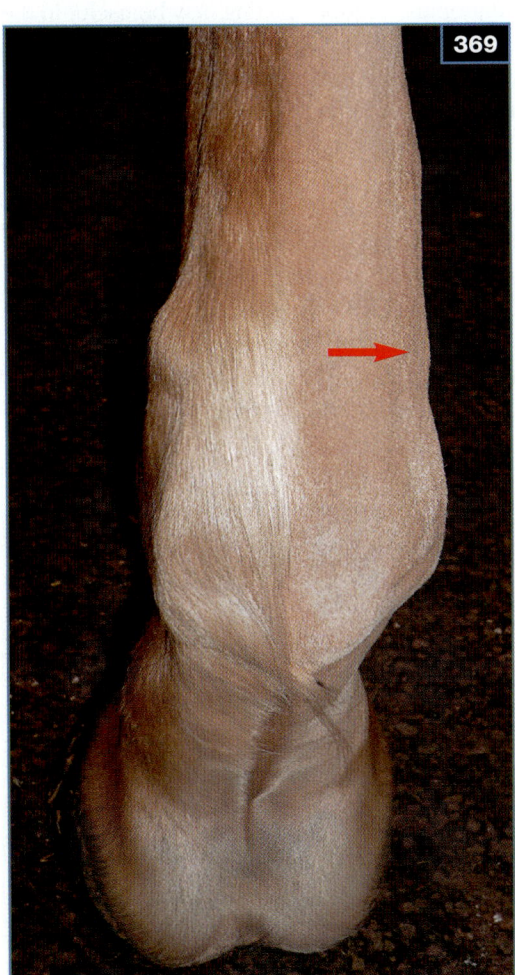

Management
Conservative and medical management is carried out as for SDFT tendonitis. Longitudinal tenotomy ('splitting') may be used. Cautery and blistering are often used, but there is no evidence of any benefit.

Prognosis
The lesions often persist despite clinical improvement and there is often severe intra- and periligamentous fibrosis. Recurrence is extremely common.

Suspensory branch desmitis
Clinical presentation
This is probably the most common injury of the suspensory ligament, especially in non-racehorses. Lameness is variable and depends on the severity of the lesion(s), and is worse if the lesion affects both branches and in acute cases. Local signs are usually obvious, with marked thickening +/− palpable pain of the affected branch(es). Biaxial lesions are more common in the forelimb, and lateral lesions in the hindlimb. However, in the acute stage there may be diffuse edema and distension of the fetlock and digital sheath synovial pouches, making diagnosis somewhat confusing.

Differential diagnosis
Lesions within the other ligaments and tendons in that region; other causes of inflammation in the metacarpal or metatarsal area; synovitis of the fetlock joint or digital sheath; fractures and sesamoiditis of the PSBs.

Diagnosis
Clinical examination
There may be painful and positive fetlock flexion. Observation of local swelling and palpation often provide a strong suspicion (369). Diagnostic analgesia is rarely necessary in acute cases. Concurrent injuries of overextension may involve sesamoid, fetlock joint, or digital sheath damage. In severe bilateral cases the fetlock may drop.

369 Swelling over the medial aspect (right-hand side) of the distal metacarpus providing a strong suspicion of a medial suspensory ligament branch injury (arrow). Ultrasonography is paramount to confirm the diagnosis and establish a prognosis.

201

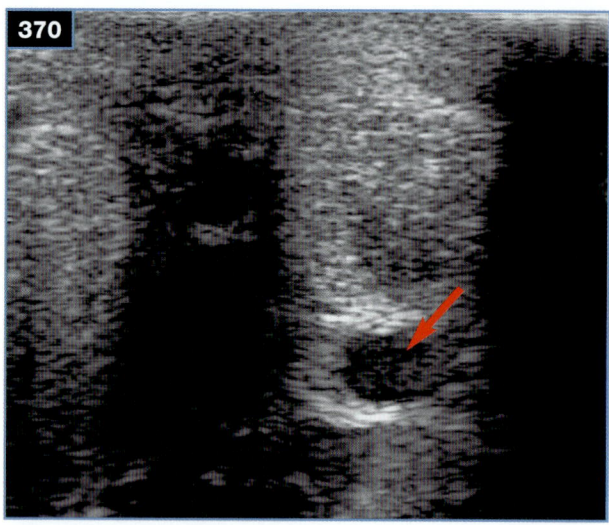

370 Well-defined, hypoechogenic lesion within the medial branch of the suspensory ligament. Note the axial localization of the lesion (in the deep part of the branch) (arrow).

371, 372 Severe, diffuse, hypoechogenic lesion within the medial branch of the suspensory ligament (371) (transverse skyline view) with loss of fiber organization throughout most of the thickness of the branch (372) (longitudinal skyline view).

Radiography

Radiography may be useful to detect distal entheseopathy ('sesamoiditis') or splint bone fractures.

Ultrasonography

The lesions have a similar appearance to those in the SDFT, with increased branch size and well-defined (370) or diffuse (371, 372) hypo- to anechogenic lesions and loss of fiber alignment. The lesions are often axially situated (deep on the image obtained from the abaxial approach) and may or may not extend to the distal insertion on the sesamoid bone. Abaxial, focal lesions may be associated with overreach injuries. The medial branch is most commonly affected. Both branches may be involved and the lesions can extend into the body. Irregularity or bone formation (entheseopathy) at the distal insertion on the sesamoid bone may be present (373, 374). These will produce an irregular bone contour and hyperechogenic areas within the ligament. In chronic or recurrent cases there may be marked ectopic mineralization within the ligament (375, 376).

Management

Conservative and medical management are conducted as for SDFT tendonitis. Tendon splitting may be useful in the subacute stage. These lesions tend to heal slowly. In severe cases, increased fetlock support may be necessary in the early stages of healing. Extracorporeal shock-wave therapy has been used in chronic cases.

Prognosis

Prognosis is related to the severity of the lesion. It is usually fair if one branch is involved, poor if both branches are involved. Sesamoiditis does not appear to affect the prognosis, while intraligamentous mineralization has been associated with a poorer outcome. Re-injury is relatively common and further worsens the prognosis.

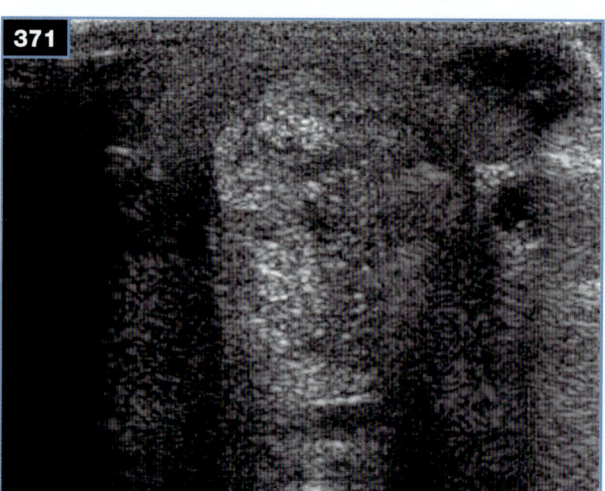

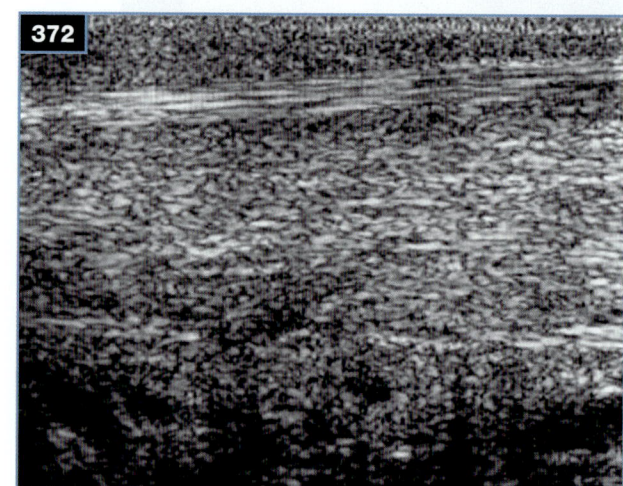

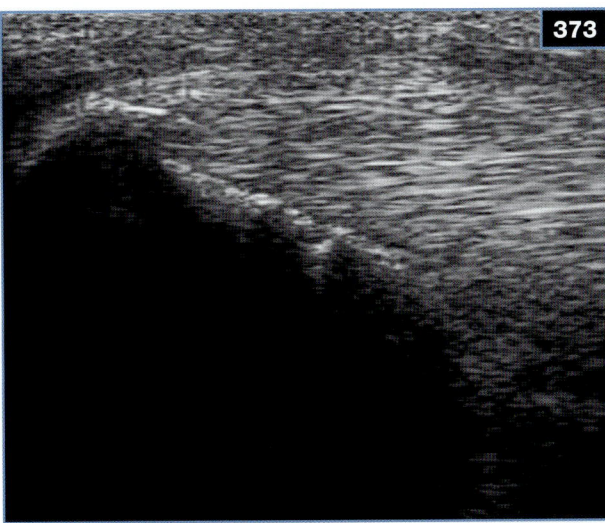 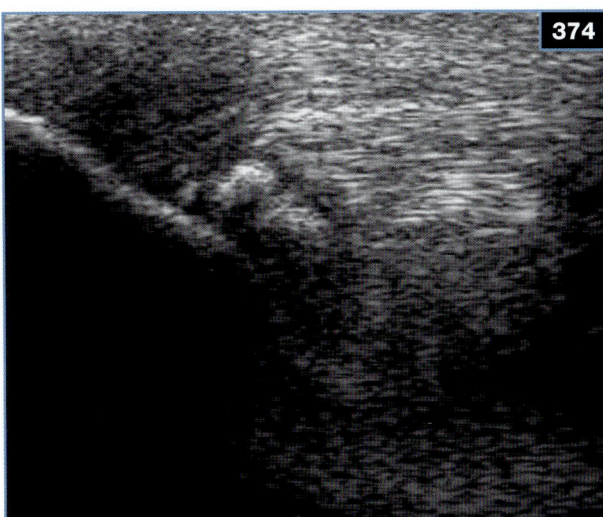

373, 374 Entheseopathy at the insertion of the suspensory ligament branch on the abaxial surface of the PSB, giving an irregular bone contour (373) and/or hyperechogenic spikes protruding into the ligament (374). Note the hypoechogenic, heterogeneous appearance of the area of interface between the ligament and bone (374).

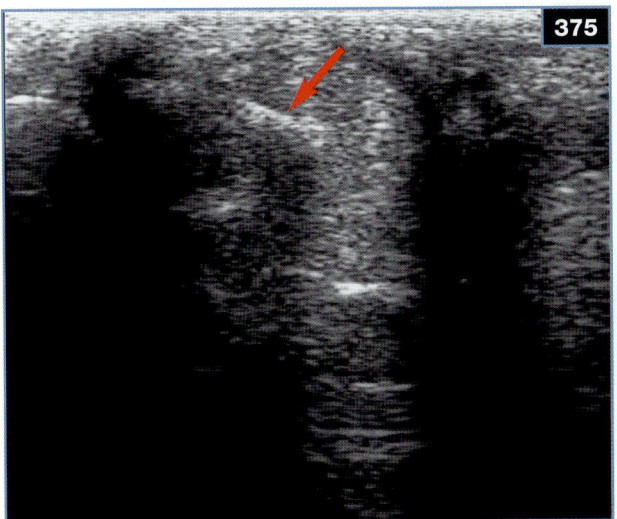 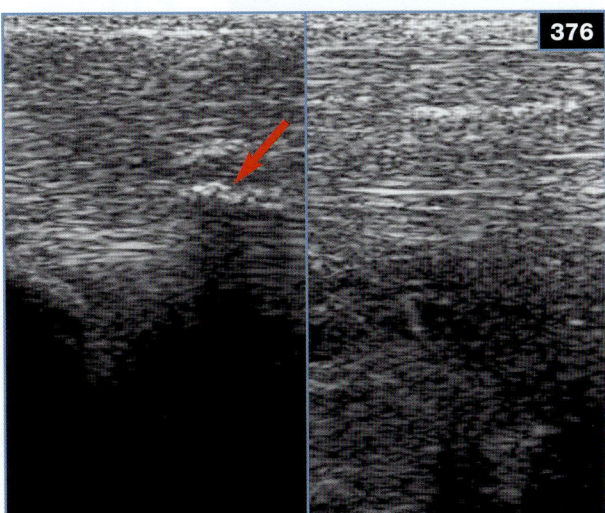

375, 376 Ectopic mineralization within the suspensory ligament branch in transverse (375) and longitudinal (376) scan planes (arrows).

Inferior check ligament (accessory ligament of the deep digital flexor tendon) desmitis

Definition/overview
This condition is similar to SDF tendonitis and is characterized by partial to complete tear of the inferior check ligament. It affects mostly pleasure, draught, and sports horses, and ponies, particularly those over 10 years of age, but all types of horses may be affected. It is most common in the forelimb, but also occurs in the hindlimb (tarsal check ligament).

Etiology/pathophysiology
The etiology is unclear, but probably involves age-related degeneration predisposing to an acute tear. A strain is most likely due to overextension of the DIP joint. It is commonly encountered in ponies kept at grass and in animals used for jumping.

Clinical presentation
Acute lameness occurs during and immediately post exercise. There is usually diffuse swelling in the proximal and middle metacarpal (metatarsal) area, particularly on the medial aspect (377). The condition often evolves chronically, with recurrent bouts of swelling and lameness. Chronic cases show marked thickening of the tendon area. In some cases a flexural deformity of the distal interphalangeal joint occurs with persistent lameness and limb postural changes (378).

Differential diagnosis
Mostly suspensory ligament body desmitis, as swelling occurs in the same area; other causes of diffuse swelling of the palmar metacarpus, including pathology in the distal limb causing edema and congestion of the palmar/plantar veins.

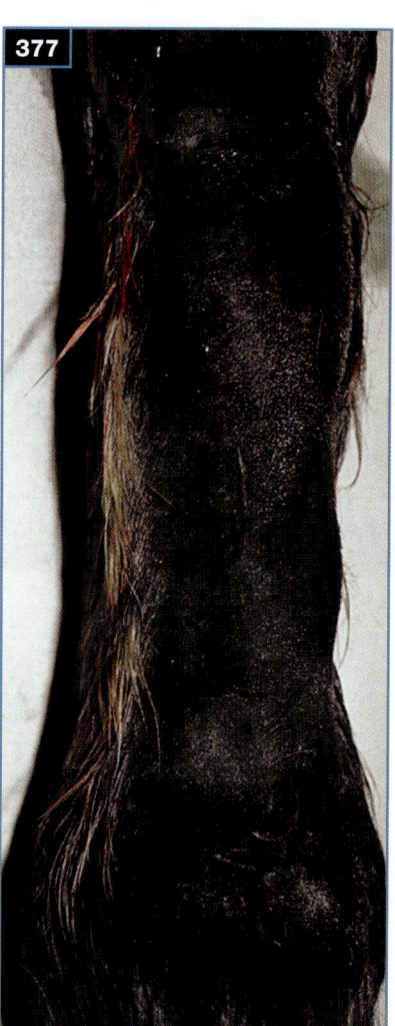
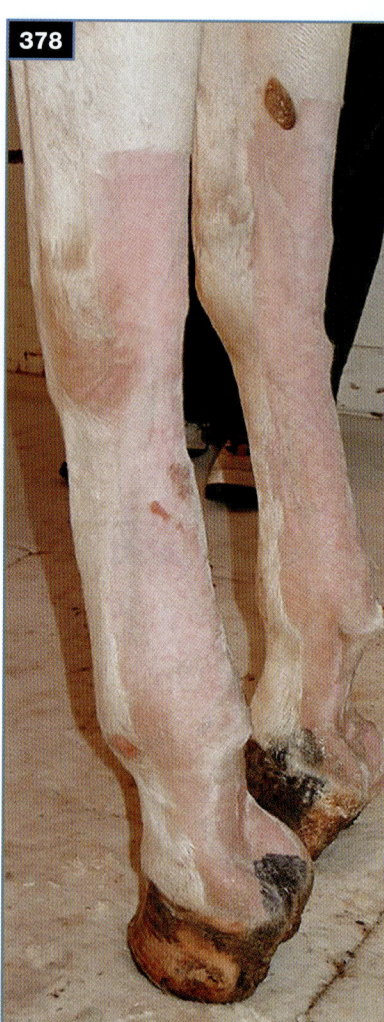

377 Diffuse swelling over the palmar aspect of the metacarpus due to subacute inferior check ligament injury.

378 Chronic inferior check ligament injury associated with severe, acquired loss of extension of the DIP joint ('flexural deformity').

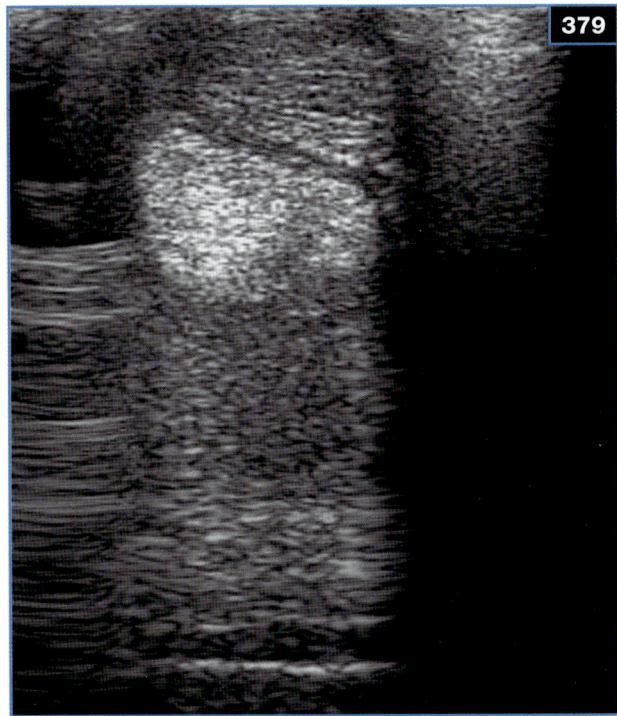

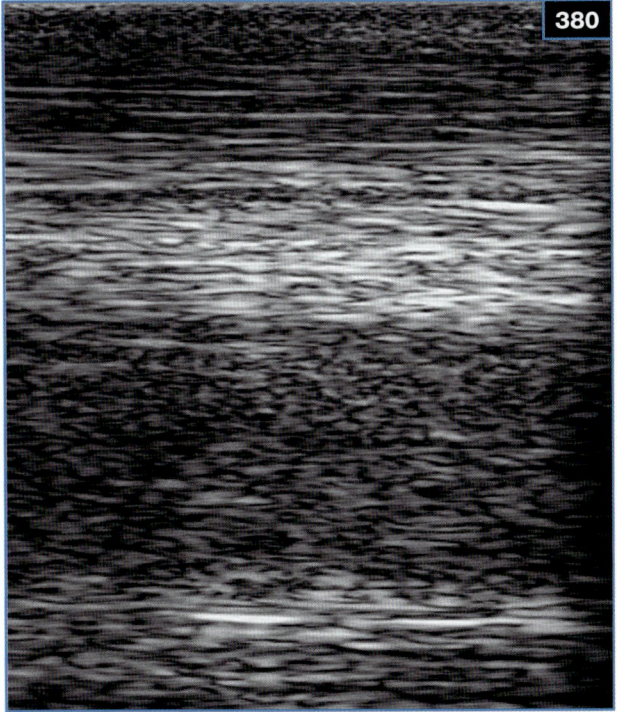

Diagnosis

Clinical examination

Suspicion should be based on swelling over the middle to upper palmar metacarpus area.

Ultrasonography

There is a marked decrease in echogenicity and increased cross-sectional surface area of the inferior check ligament (379, 380). Discrete hypoechogenic to anechogenic lesions may be present, but diffuse, heterogeneous decrease in echogenicity is observed most commonly. The ligament may develop contact with the SDFT, especially medially. Lesions often occur in the middle section of the ligament, but they may extend to the palmar carpal ligament and/or deep digital flexor tendon. There is usually secondary ('sympathetic') effusion within the carpal flexor tendon sheath. With time, the echogenicity increases but the ligament remains markedly thickened. Adhesions with the deep and superficial digital flexor tendons are frequent, especially in chronic cases.

Management

Rest and conservative treatment as for tendonitis are usually effective, and lesions tend to heal more rapidly than in the SDFT. Aggressive physiotherapy with controlled exercise and passive manipulations aimed at decreasing restrictive adhesion formation are useful. In chronic, recurrent cases, surgical resection (desmotomy) of a 5 cm long portion of the check ligament may be effective. Corrective farriery should include keeping the toe short with rolling of the toe of the shoe. The heels should be kept slightly long. Heel wedges have been suggested, but should be avoided as they may cause retraction of the ligament and flexural deformity. If the latter occurs, desmotomy of the check ligament and use of toe-extension shoes are indicated.

Prognosis

Recurrence is common and the desmitis then tends to evolve into a chronic, recurrent form. The prognosis is fair in acute, mild cases, more guarded in recurrent cases. The latter respond well to surgical treatment.

379, 380 Transverse (379) and longitudinal (380) ultrasonographic images showing a subacute, severe tear of the accessory ligament of the DDFT (inferior check ligament). The ligament is extremely enlarged, filling the space between the DDFT and suspensory ligament. Its echogenicity is diffusely decreased and there is complete loss of fibrous organization on the long axis scans.

Distal sesamoidean ligament desmopathy
Definition/overview
This is a rare condition involving strain injury to one or several of the distal sesamoidean ligaments. Short (deep) distal sesamoidean ligament (DDSL) injury is rare, but probably underdiagnosed as it is difficult to confirm. It may be a component of fragmentation or fracture of the base of the PSBs. CT and MRI may be useful to confirm injury in this area. Oblique distal sesamoidean ligament (ODSL) and straight distal sesamoidean ligament (SDSL) tears are rare, but they are occasionally recognized, especially in trotters. They should be considered a part of suspensory apparatus breakdown injuries (including suspensory ligament desmitis and PSB transverse and basilar fractures), although the author has encountered several cases of ODSL injury as a result of overreach injuries.

Etiology/pathophysiology
The etiology is unclear, but this condition is probably due to a single strain injury or trauma with overextension of the fetlock. Surprisingly, these injuries are usually not associated with lesions in the suspensory ligament.

Clinical presentation
The clinical signs are variable. Lameness is usually marked to moderate and there may be obvious distension of the digital sheath. With ODSL, thickening is palpated over the distal abaxial aspect of the affected sesamoid bone. There is pain on passive digital flexion and hyperextension.

Differential diagnosis
Tenosynovitis; deep digital flexor tendonitis; tendonitis of the branches of the SDFT; basilar fracture of a PSB.

Diagnosis
Clinical examination
Lameness localized to the pastern area may be caused by these injuries and in some cases subtle swelling is palpable in the region. Lameness may be abolished with intrathecal anesthesia of the digital sheath.

Radiography
Radiography should be performed in all cases to look for remodeling (entheseopathy) at the base of the PSBs and to rule out associated sesamoid bone pathology (fractures, displacement, lysis). Roughening of the bone or marked new bone production over the palmar sagittal aspect of the distal third of the proximal phalanx diaphysis often indicates entheseous new bone around the insertion of the two ODSLs (381). This is considered to be an incidental finding, not usually associated with desmitis or lameness.

Ultrasonography
This is a difficult anatomic area to scan and may require some experience. Lesions are usually focal and discrete. The DDSLs are difficult to image, but may be seen using a microconvex transducer below the sesamoid bones. MRI and CT may be useful for this purpose. The ligaments appear hypoechogenic and heterogeneous and there is usually evidence of bone remodeling at the sesamoidean and phalangeal insertion areas. ODSL desmitis presents as obvious thickening and decrease in echogenicity, most often near the sesamoidean origin (382, 383). Lesions may be diffuse or discrete and there is usually marked roughening and irregularity of the PSB surface at the ligament origin. SDSL injuries are most often localized in the middle portion of the ligament. A discrete, hypo- to anechogenic core lesion is visualized.

Management
Conservative treatment with rest and controlled exercise as for suspensory ligament desmitis is advocated.

Prognosis
The results are variable and there may be persistent, recurrent lameness. SDSL injuries carry a guarded prognosis, although there have only been few reports and there are insufficient data to make this a general rule.

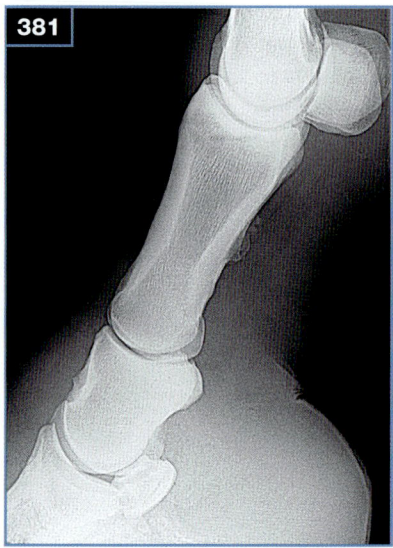

381 Lateromedial radiograph of the distal forelimb of an adult horse showing entheseous new bone over the palmar aspect of the proximal phalanx. This entheseopathy lies within the insertions of the oblique distal sesamoidean ligaments and is considered to be a normal variant. The source of this horse's lameness was elsewhere. (Photo courtesy GA Munroe)

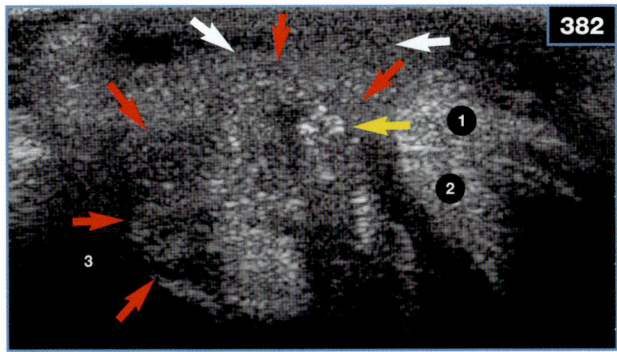

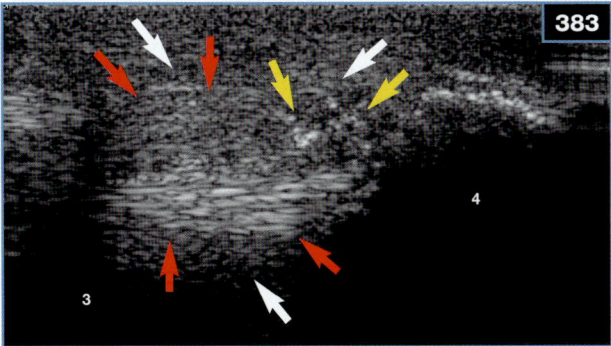

382, 383 Transverse (382) and long-axis (383) ultrasonographic sections of an oblique distal sesamoidean ligament showing a partial tear of its origin on the distopalmaromedial aspect of the PSB. The ligament appears thickened and hypoechogenic and has partially lost its fiber pattern over its superficial half (red arrows). There is significant periligamentous swelling (white arrows) and numerous mineral fragments casting acoustic shadows are visible at the bony origin (yellow arrows). 1 = P1; 2 = SDFT; 3 = DDFT; 4 = sesamoid.

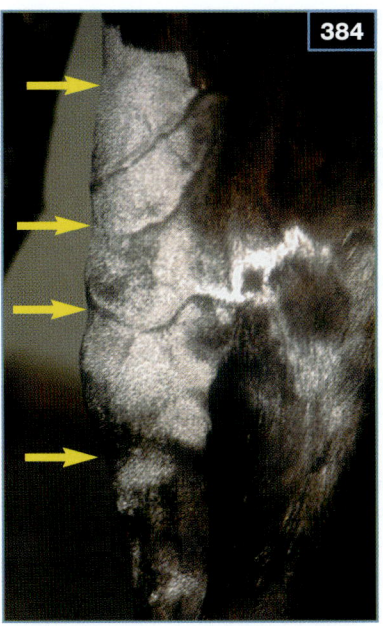

Extensor tendon injuries and tenosynovitis
Definition/overview
Injuries to the ECR, lateral digital extensor (LDE), and CDE tendons in the forelimb, and LDE and long digital extensor tendons in the hindlimb, are common in horses of all breeds and ages through direct trauma to the dorsal aspect of the limb. Tenosynovitis of their sheaths is usually a consequence of trauma, with or without damage to the tendon they surround. Idiopathic tenosynovitis, characterized by nonpainful sheath effusion without evidence of inflammation, is occasionally encountered. Rupture of the CDE tendon is recognized in the foal (see p. 46). Septic tenosynovitis of the extensor sheaths occurs occasionally.

Etiology/pathophysiology
Trauma occurs through kicks or hitting jumps, gates, or wire fences. Wounds and contusions are most common over the dorsal aspect of the distal limb, particularly in the metacarpus/metatarsus, dorsal distal radius, or dorsal tarsal region. In these areas the digital extensor tendons lie directly between the skin and bone and are easily damaged or severed by sharp objects.

Tenosynovitis may be a consequence of direct trauma. The tendon and underlying tissues may also be affected. Hemorrhage in the sheath induces severe inflammation. If severe inflammation, particularly from chronic infection, is left untreated, it may lead to chronic synovial thickening and fibrosis, restrictive adhesion formation, and eventually partial carpal or tarsal joint restriction.

Idiopathic tenosynovitis is of unknown origin. There is increased synovial fluid production, but the synovial membrane is not thickened and no pain is observed.

Clinical presentation
Partial tendon damage usually causes mild to moderate lameness. With complete rupture, the horse is unable to extend the fetlock and digit and tends to buckle over at the fetlock and drag the toe. This gradually improves as the horse learns to compensate by flicking the limb forward. If the LDE tendon is not affected, the horse can regain normal extensor tone within a few days or weeks.

With trauma not involving a wound, there is a painful swelling and thickening due to local hematoma, periosteal contusion, and tendon trauma.

In the carpal or tarsal area (384), the main sign is tendon sheath swelling, characterized by fluid distension arranged longitudinally over the dorsolateral aspect of the

384 Tenosynovitis of the extensor carpi radialis tendon sheath over the dorsal aspect of the carpus. Note the sausage-like appearance of the swelling that follows the longitudinally arranged tendon and is separated into strips by the transverse dorsal carpal retinacula (arrows).

207

Soft-tissue injuries

joint and interrupted over the bones because of restriction by the transverse retinacula. Horses are usually markedly lame, except in idiopathic tenosynovitis, where there is no pain or heat. In chronic, traumatic cases the swelling becomes firm and nonpainful, but carpal or tarsal passive flexion is painful and markedly restricted.

Open skin wounds expose the tendon and/or periosteum. If the tendon is partially severed, the frayed tendon ends are usually visible at the wound edges. If it is totally severed, the cut ends tend to retract for several centimeters proximally and distally, so that the tendon is no longer visible and the periosteum is exposed and often stripped (385). In the tarsal or carpal area there is associated tenosynovitis, which may be open (septic) or inflammatory only.

Differential diagnosis
Trauma to the dorsal metacarpus or metatarsus; unicortical stress fractures of the dorsal metacarpal cortex; contusion and wounds not affecting the tendons; tenosynovitis; synovitis of the carpal joints; hygroma; hematoma or seroma; subcutaneous abscesses and granulomata.

Diagnosis
Clinical examination
There is usually obvious swelling over the affected area. Tenosynovitis of the carpal or tarsal sheath of the CDE or LDE tendon is easily differentiated from other swellings unless there is diffuse edema or fibrosis.

Radiography
Radiographs of the affected area should be obtained to rule out concurrent fractures or new bone formation. The latter may be secondary to the tendon or sheath inflammation and is common in chronic cases (386). Conversely, new bone production may occur secondarily to trauma not affecting the tendon. If extensive, it may occasionally interfere with the extensor tendons and cause secondary tendonitis.

Ultrasonography
This is the method of choice and will confirm tendon involvement with loss of fibrillar pattern, diffusely decreased echogenicity, and increased cross-sectional area (387). In cases of complete rupture, the tendon stumps will be visible several centimeters apart (388). Their frayed ends appear enlarged, hypoechogenic, and markedly thickened. The space between the severed ends is hypoechogenic and amorphous due to hematoma formation. It may contain fluid organized in geometric cavities, separated by thin strands of echogenic tissue. With time, granulation tissue develops and there is a gradual increase in echogenicity as fibrosis takes place.

Tenosynovitis may occur with or without overt tendon lesions. The changes observed resemble those of digital sheath tenosynovitis, with a thickened synovial membrane, anechogenic fluid distension, and mass formation (389-391).

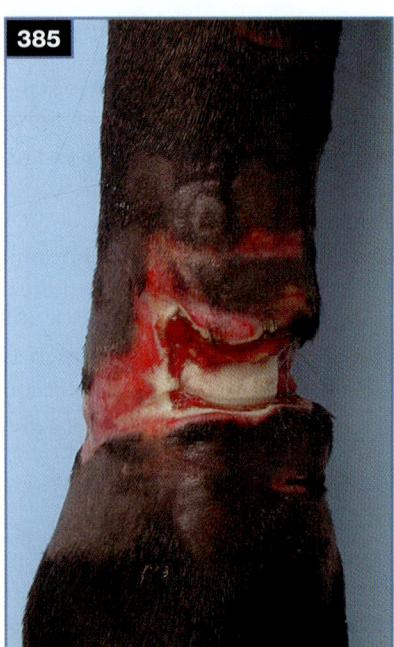

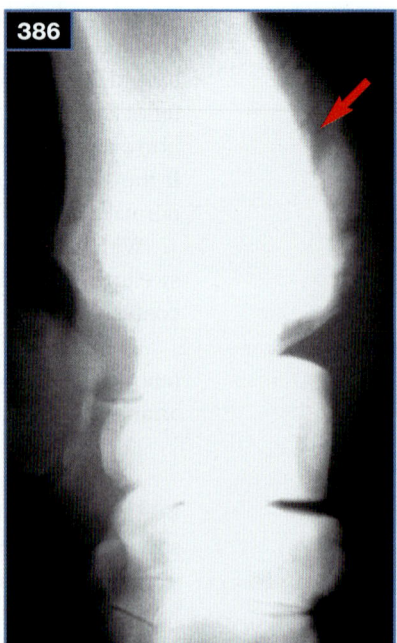

385 Deep wound over the dorsal aspect of the metatarsus, involving complete transection of the long and lateral digital extensor tendons. The severed ends have retracted proximally and distally and the periosteum is completely stripped, leaving the underlying bone exposed.

386 Lateromedial radiograph of the carpus and distal radius of a horse with persistent tenosynovitis of the extensor carpi radialis tendon sheath subsequent to chronic trauma. Note the extensive roughened new bone on the cranial distal aspect of the radius (arrow). (Photo courtesy GA Munroe)

208

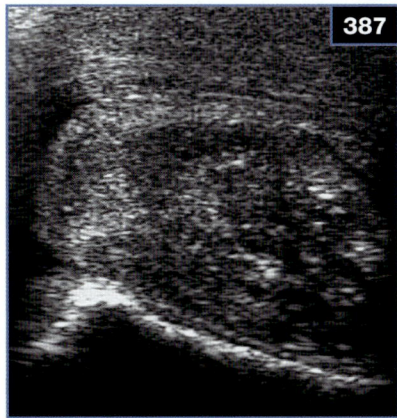

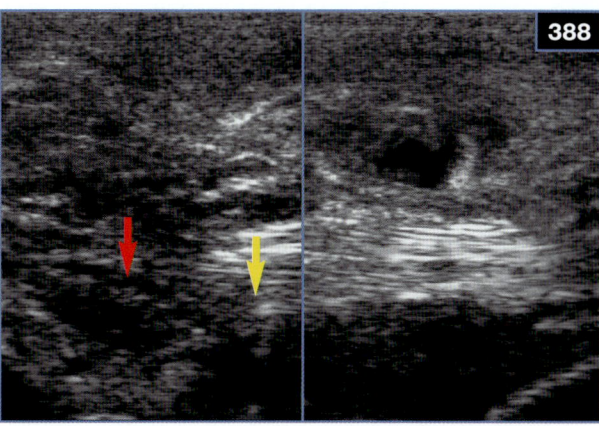

387 Transverse ultrasonographic image over the craniolateral aspect of the distal radius showing an enlarged, heterogeneous, and hypoechogenic extensor carpi radialis tendon.

388 Spontaneous rupture of the extensor carpi radialis tendon. The frayed stumps are separated by hypoechogenic material that fills the sheath, forming an amorphous soft mass (fibrin, granulation tissue) (red arrow). The tendon is enlarged and its echogenicity is decreased (yellow arrow).

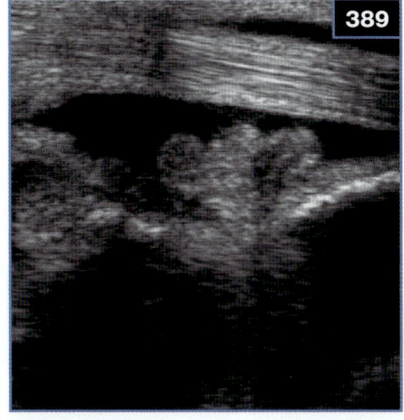

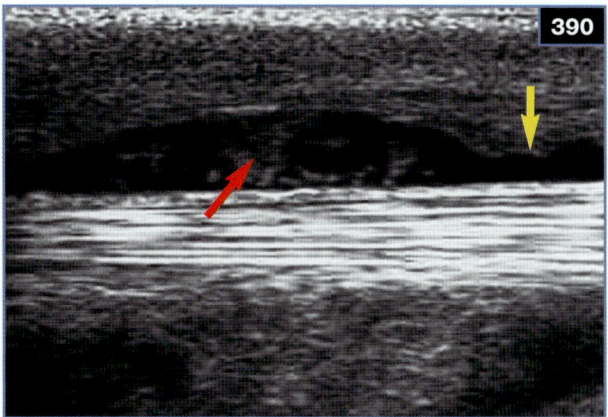

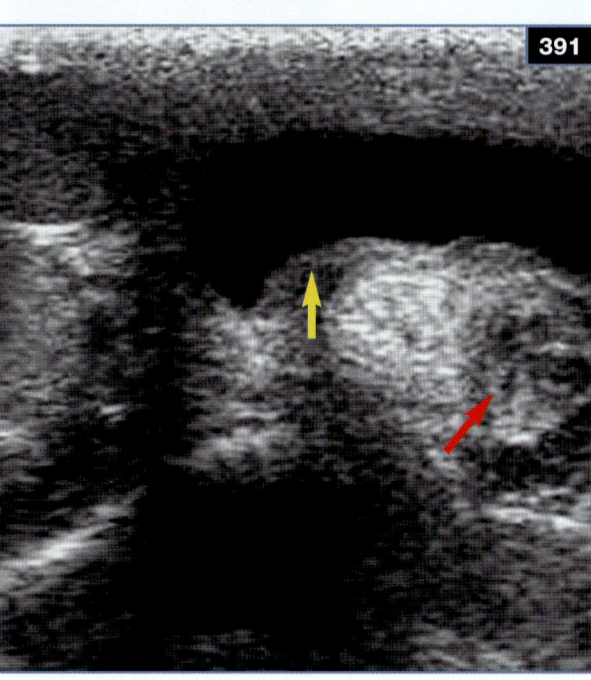

389 Chronic extensor carpi radialis tendonitis (longitudinal scan over the radiocarpal joint). The sheath is distended by anechogenic material. The cauliflower-shaped echogenic image deep to the sheath represents the normal radiocarpal joint capsule, which is folded in extension and highlighted by the overlying fluid.

390 Acute tenosynovitis of the extensor carpi radialis tendon secondary to direct trauma over the dorsal aspect of the carpus (longitudinal scan over the dorsal carpus). The sheath is distended by anechogenic fluid containing strands of echogenic material (fibrin due to hemorrhage) (red arrow). The synovial membrane is moderately thickened (yellow arrow).

391 Chronic tenosynovitis of the long digital extensor tendon tarsal sheath (transverse scan over the dorsal aspect of the tarsus). Note the medial lesion within the tendon (red arrow) and the thickened visceral synovial membrane forming a halo around the tendon (yellow arrow).

Septic tenosynovitis is characterized ultrasonographically by severe synovial changes, heterogeneous lesions that may extend into the tendon, and distension of the sheath cavity by heterogeneous material representing exudate, fibrin, and debris (392, 393).

Management

Conservative treatment of traumatic tendonitis or tenosynovitis based on box rest, systemic and topical anti-inflammatory drugs, and regular in-hand exercise is often effective. Initially, the limb should be hosed for 15–20 minutes with cold water 2–4 times daily. The duration of rest varies with the severity of the lesion, but healing is usually fairly rapid and most horses can return to work within 2–12 weeks. Wounds should be treated as appropriate and the limbs kept bandaged. Casts or splints may be applied over a dressing to limit movement of the wound edges and tendon stumps.

In the case of complete rupture, complete box rest is necessary. The limb should be supported with splints placed over the dorsal and/or palmar or plantar aspect of the limb from elbow or mid-crus to the foot and over a padded bandage. An aluminum or resin splint system that encloses the foot or is attached to the toe of the shoe prevents the digit and carpus or hock from flexing and will thus provide best results. The splint is left on the limb for 3–4 weeks, after which a thick bandage is applied to the limb for a further 2–6 weeks depending on the clinical appearance of the wound. Passive manipulation and physiotherapy may be useful to aid regaining of full joint motion.

Aseptic tendon sheath injuries are treated with box rest, daily in-hand exercise, cold hosing or application of ice packs, and systemic and topical anti-inflammatory drugs. Intrathecal injection of hyaluronic acid may be useful in acute or subacute cases. Short-acting steroidal drugs may be used in cases that fail to respond to conservative treatment alone.

Chronic, adhesive tenosynovitis may be a therapeutic challenge. Complete surgical stripping of the sheath synovium is generally successful in these cases. Tendon resection has been performed for salvage in severe, unresponsive cases, but may not yield a full return to function.

Prognosis

The prognosis is good to fair for most extensor tendon injuries. Severed extensor tendons tend to heal through fibrosis and scar tissue formation, but most horses appear to adapt and regain full function with time.

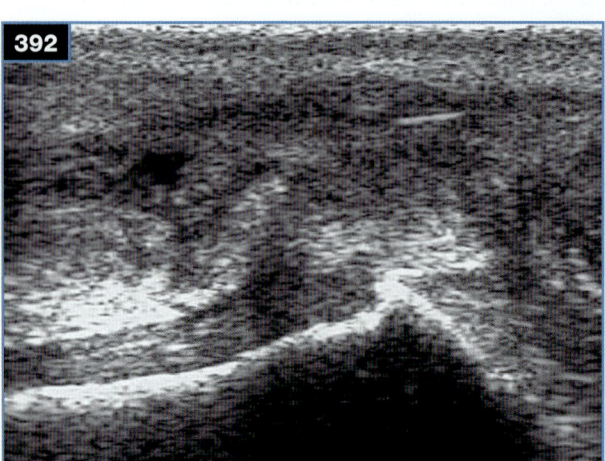

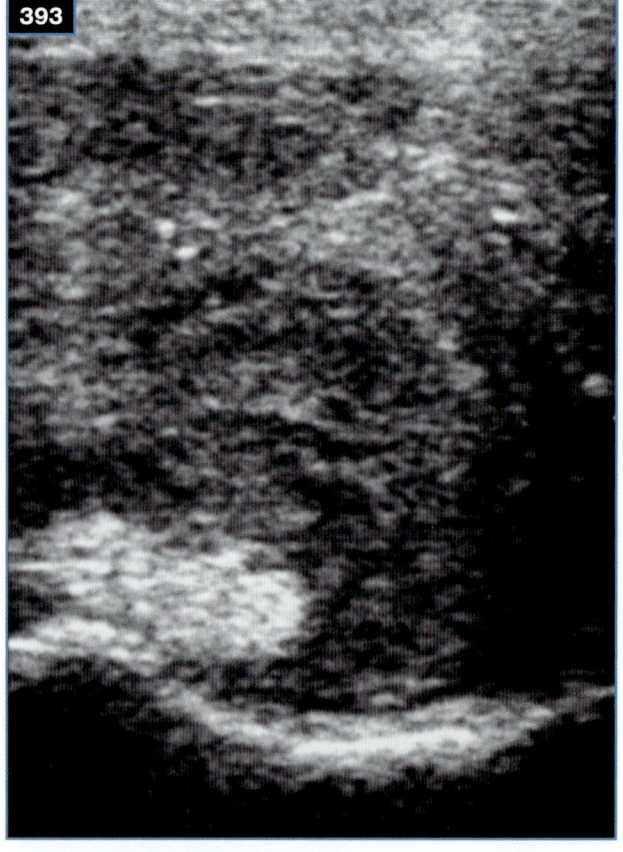

392 Wound over the craniomedial distal forearm extending into the medial aspect of the extensor carpi radialis tendon sheath. The partially frayed, hypoechogenic tendon is visible on the left of the image and is surrounded by fluid and heterogeneous material.

393 Severe septic tenosynovitis of the lateral digital extensor tendon over the tarsus. The tendon is enlarged and hypoechogenic and has lost its normal echostructure. The sheath is obliterated by hypoechogenic material (pus and fibrin) so that its boundaries are no longer discernible.

Ruptured extensor tendon in foals
(See p. 46)

Rupture of the extensor carpi radialis tendon
Definition/overview
Spontaneous partial to complete rupture of the ECR tendon is a rare condition affecting adult horses, particularly those used for show jumping.

Etiology/pathophysiology
The cause is unknown, but may involve repeated trauma to the dorsal carpus, repeat strain injuries, or sudden trauma on a tense tendon during carpal flexion.

Clinical presentation
The tear or rupture occurs in the carpal region, within the carpal sheath of the ECR tendon. Partial tears cause mild to moderate lameness with tenosynovitis and sheath distension. Complete rupture is characterized by sudden-onset lameness with marked sheath distension over the cranial aspect of the distal antebrachium and dorsal carpus. Typically, there is an exaggerated, stringhalt-like flexion of the carpus during the stride, supposedly from a lack of counter resistance to the flexor muscle action.

Diagnosis
Ultrasonography will show tenosynovitis and characterize the partial or complete tendon rupture.

Management
Conservative treatment with support bandaging and splints or a tube cast from elbow to fetlock may be effective, although the gait abnormality and sheath distension usually persist. Tenoscopic debridement of the sheath and frayed tendon ends has been reported to benefit some horses, particularly those with partial tears. Repair of the ruptured tendon is not effective in most cases.

Prognosis
The prognosis for soundness is fair, but it is poor for return to athletic activities. Partial tears may heal adequately after tenoscopic debridement.

Digital flexor tendon sheath tenosynovitis
Definition/overview
Inflammation of the synovial tissues of the digital flexor tendon sheath, usually but not necessarily associated with distension of the sheath (tendinous windgalls).

Etiology/pathophysiology
There may be many causes. Idiopathic tenosynovitis relates to fluid distension of the sheath without lameness or overt signs of inflammation. The cause is unclear, but may relate to a previous inflammatory episode or to a discrepancy between synovial fluid production and elimination.

Primary traumatic tenosynovitis is due to direct trauma to the area of the sheath. There is, reportedly, contusion of the synovial tissues and intrathecal hemorrhage, which induces an acute inflammation. The trauma may be spontaneous and of unknown cause, but these cases are likely to be due to tearing of the synovial membrane through overextension or overuse.

Secondary traumatic tenosynovitis relates to inflammation caused by a lesion of a structure within the sheath or sheath wall. Causes include tendonitis, flexor tendon and manica flexoria tears, fractures of the bones associated with the sheath (phalanges, PSBs), and problems of the annular ligaments.

Sympathetic tenosynovitis is used for noninflammatory, transitory synovial fluid distension due to inflammation elsewhere in the distal limb.

Inflammatory conditions lead to hyperemia and edema within the synovial membrane, which thickens. If the inflammation persists, synovial cells will proliferate, leading to permanent thickening of the membrane and eventual fibrosis in chronic cases. Fibrous adhesions may also develop between the parietal and visceral sheath layers. These anomalies can severely compromise the function of the sheath, causing partial to total restriction of the lower limb.

Clinical presentation

Idiopathic tenosynovitis is characterized by moderate to marked fluid distension of the sheath, often bilaterally. The proximal pouch protrudes laterally and medially to the tendons and proximally to the annular ligament of the fetlock (394). A more distal swelling is palpable in the sagittal plane in the mid-pastern area; however, there is no obvious thickening of the sheath tissues and no heat or pain is noticeable. There is no associated lameness, although flexion of the fetlock may occasionally elicit pain. It is more common in the hindlimbs and in larger animals.

In other forms of tenosynovitis the swelling is similar, but there is variable heat and pain on palpation of the area of the sheath. Pain is typically elicited by deep palpation of the palmar aspect of the pastern and distal limb flexion. Lameness is usually severe and characterized by decreased digital flexion, reduced foot flight arc, and, occasionally, reduced weight-bearing.

In chronic cases the swelling is more diffuse and firm, and pain may not be as obvious on palpation. There is decreased flexion of the fetlock and digit and passive flexion is painful.

Differential diagnosis

Edema of the digit due to inflammation of the foot or pastern, annular ligament syndrome, or fractures of P1, P2 or the PSBs; septic tenosynovitis, suspensory ligament branch injuries and fetlock joint effusion may have a similar presentation.

Diagnosis
Clinical examination

Pain on deep palpation of the palmar or plantar pastern and over the proximal pouch of the sheath area is suggestive of tenosynovitis. The lameness may be partially or totally abolished with an abaxial sesamoid or distal metacarpal or metatarsal nerve block (4- or 6-point). Intrathecal injection of 5–10 ml of local anesthetic solution usually eliminates the lameness, but this is not always specific for the sheath.

Ultrasonography

In idiopathic tenosynovitis the sheath is distended by anechogenic fluid, but the synovial membranes are not thickened. Intrasynovial structures such as vinculae, mesotenons, and the manica flexoria are visible, but they remain thin (less than 1 or 2 mm in thickness) (395).

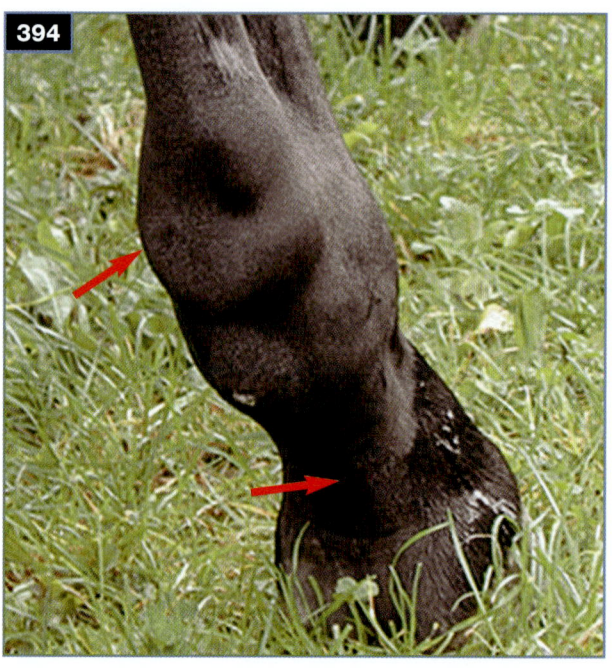

394 Swelling of the digital sheath (tendinous 'windgalls') is obvious proximal to the palmar annular ligament of the metacarpophalangeal joint (top arrow) and over the palmar mid-pastern (bottom arrow).

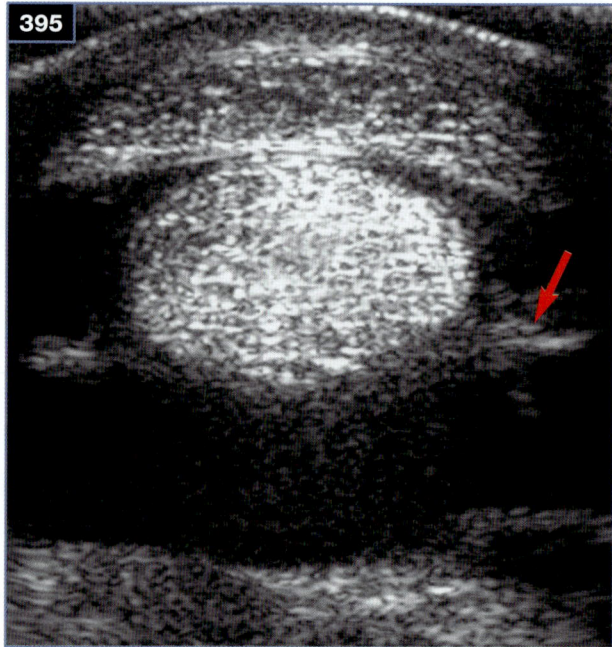

395 Transverse ultrasound scan over the distal metacarpus of a horse with idiopathic distension of the digital tendon sheath. The sheath is distended by anechogenic fluid. The flexor tendons are well delineated, but no thickened synovial membrane is visible. The proximal vinculae of the DDFT are visible within the proximal recesses of the sheath (arrow).

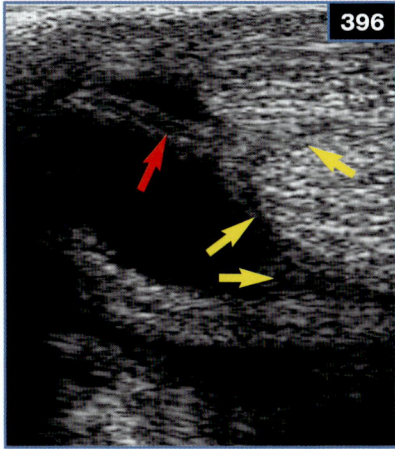

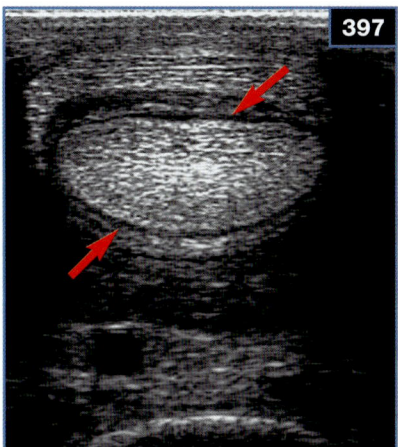

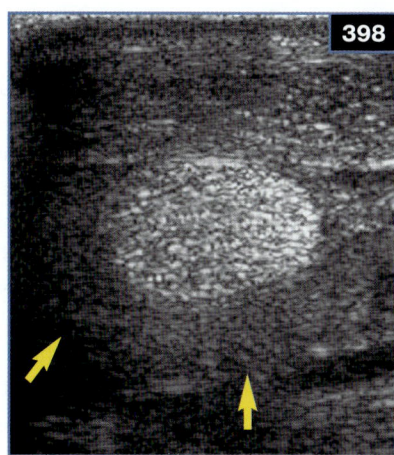

In acute tenosynovitis there is accumulation of anechogenic fluid, although bleeding will produce strands of hypoechogenic material (fibrin strands and pannus) and the fluid may appear echogenic. The synovium is diffusely thickened and hypoechogenic, producing a 2–4 mm thick halo around the tendons (396).

Chronic tenosynovitis presents as partial to complete obliteration of the sheath by a thickened, echogenic synovium (397, 398). Dynamic examination (i.e. while flexing and extending the limb) may show that the tendons and parietal sheath are adhered.

Other lesions include focal or localized hypoechogenic lesions in one or both tendons, erosions of the proximal scutum, and bone production at the insertions of the annular ligaments and/or synovial membrane on the bones. There may also be thickening of the peripheral tissues, including annular ligaments and subcutaneous tissue. Partial tears of the manica flexoria may be seen as a focal, hypoechogenic thickening near the attachment of the manica. In complete tears the redundant manica may be seen to float in one of the proximal recesses of the sheath or, most often, to curl up into a soft-tissue mass lateral to the SDFT.

Management
Idiopathic distension is usually not treated, but some cases, especially if treated early, may respond to rest and pressure bandages. Intrathecal steroid injections may provide temporary resolution of the distension, but in most cases the swelling recurs within a few weeks or months. Aspiration of the fluid is contraindicated as it only provides temporary resolution and may cause bleeding and inflammation in the sheath.

Acute tenosynovitis is best treated by rest with controlled exercise, systemic NSAIDs, cold hosing, and/or application of ice. Intrathecal sodium hyaluronate and/or short-acting steroid injections may be helpful in nonresponsive cases. If superficial lesions are present on the

396 Subacute, traumatic tenosynovitis. The vinculae are thickened (red arrow) and there is a halo of hypoechogenic tissue around the tendons (yellow arrows). The sheath is distended by anechogenic fluid.

397, 398 Chronic, traumatic tenosynovitis. There is a halo of echogenic synovial tissue around the tendons, separating the DDFT from the SDFT and its manica flexoria (red arrows) (397). In extreme cases (398), thickened synovium can totally obliterate the sheath (yellow arrows), enclosing the tendons and vinculae in solid tissue and thus causing restriction of movement in the affected part of the limb.

tendons or scutums, tenoscopy has improved some cases. Physiotherapy is useful to decrease fibrosis, resolve inflammation and distension, and encourage healing.

Chronic tenosynovitis is difficult to treat. Conservative management and physiotherapy may improve some cases. Intrathecal hyaluronate is not indicated. Steroids may be helpful in some cases, but disappointing in others. Tenoscopic surgery to debride adhesions and superficial lesions, and performing a partial synovectomy is helpful in some cases. Annular ligament desmotomy is helpful in some cases.

Prognosis
The prognosis is good for idiopathic distension, although the blemish often persists. Acute cases without lesions to the tendons or scutums carry a fair prognosis, but aggressive anti-inflammatory treatment is warranted. If the tendons are involved, the lesions often persist because of fibrocartilaginous metaplasia and necrosis. Recurrent lameness is usual and the prognosis is therefore considered guarded, especially for lesions of the DDFT. In chronic cases the prognosis is guarded to poor.

213

Palmar/plantar annular ligament syndrome
Definition/overview
The palmar/plantar annular ligament (PAL), or palmar/plantar flexor retinaculum, is a local thickening of the fascia forming a thin, transverse ligamentous band that restrains the digital flexor tendons on the palmar/plantar aspect of the fetlock during flexion. It extends from the periosteum on the abaxial aspect of the PSBs and lies superficial to the digital sheath. It measures between 1 and 2 mm in thickness. The PAL syndrome is characterized by thickening of the ligament, which allegedly induces compression of the tendons and digital sheath, with associated pain and inflammation (tenosynovitis). There is considerable controversy on this point as ultrasonography has revealed that the ligament is rarely affected. The typical notched appearance often associated with the syndrome is actually due to the proximal sheath pouch bulging proximal to the ligament due to synovial distension, regardless of whether the ligament is affected or not (399).

Etiology/pathophysiology
A true PAL syndrome is characterized by thickening of the PAL, most often as a result of direct trauma to the palmar aspect of the fetlock. It may also be due to spontaneous injury, possibly as a result of overextension of the digit. The condition is relatively rare.

Apparent thickening of the tissues palmar to the SDFT is most often due to thickening and fibrosis of the subcutaneous tissues. In tenosynovitis the visceral and parietal sheath layers may also be thickened as a result of chronic inflammation and synovial hyperplasia.

It is questionable whether these conditions actually involve a compressive syndrome, as histology does not show any local necrosis and no major nerves traverse the sheath, unlike in the carpal canal. PAL syndrome is often a part of digital tenosynovitis.

Clinical presentation
Typically, the sign most commonly reported is 'constriction' of the palmar aspect of the fetlock, causing the sheath to bulge proximal and palmar to the ligament. This is not due to PAL thickening, but solely to sheath distension or synovial thickening. PAL thickening may cause diffuse thickening over the whole palmar (or plantar) aspect of the fetlock region, but in most cases there are no specific morphologic signs. There may be local pain on palpation in acute cases. Clearly, most signs are related to the associated tenosynovitis.

Differential diagnosis
Tenosynovitis, cellulitis, edema, and congestion of the palmar veins should be considered.

Diagnosis
Clinical examination
Careful palpation may reveal some thickening and pain over the affected area.

Radiography
Radiography is useful to eliminate other causes of swelling in the palmar fetlock (e.g. fractures of the sesamoid bones). There may be entheseous new bone on the palmar abaxial aspects of the PSBs.

Ultrasonography
This is the diagnostic technique of choice. It will usually demonstrate the presence of tenosynovitis. The PAL is visible as a thin band of tissue with a transversely oriented fiber pattern that covers the palmar aspect of the SDFT. It should measure <2 mm in thickness in an average 500 kg horse (400). The ligament may be thickened in association with tenosynovitis or as a result of chronic trauma (401, 402). Entheseopathy is visible as local thickening on the abaxial aspect of the PAL and irregular bony insertion (403). Ultrasonography shows that the large majority of suspected PAL syndrome cases are due to synovial membrane thickening (404). It is likely that thickening impairs the tendon movement through lack of mobility rather than through compression. Subcutaneous tissue thickening is visible between the echogenic epidermal layer and the PAL (405, 406). In acute cases, a hematoma may be visible at this level.

399 Notched appearance over the palmar fetlock (arrows), sometimes wrongly attributed to annular ligament thickening but actually due to distension of the proximal recesses of the digital sheath proximal to the non-elastic, palmar annular ligament of the fetlock.

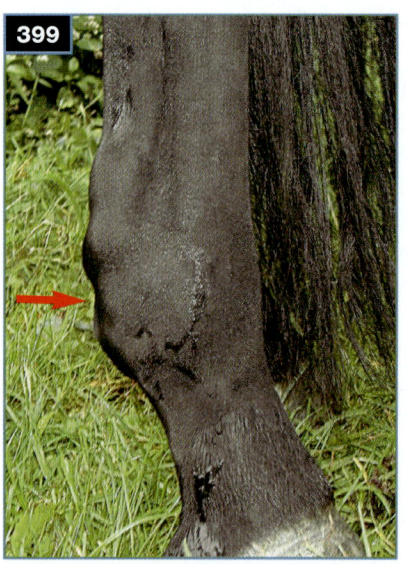

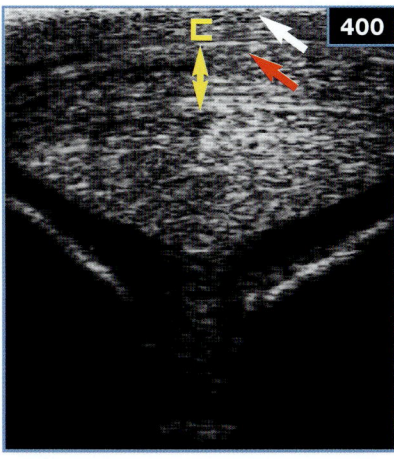 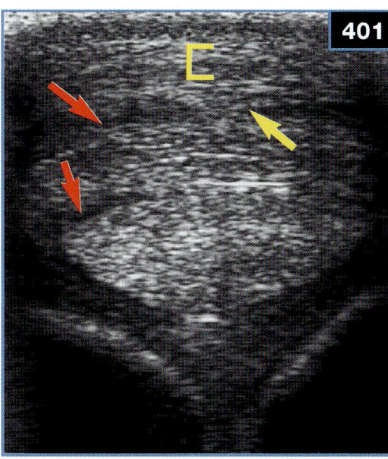 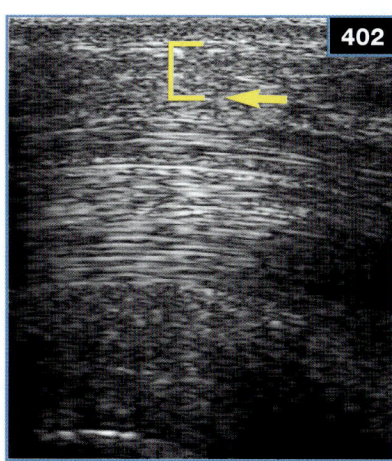

400 Transverse ultrasound scan over the palmar aspect of the fetlock. The normal palmar annular ligament is a thin, fibrous band (yellow bracket) with fibrillar organization, lying directly over the palmar aspect of the SDFT (yellow arrow). Note the barely visible synovial tissue between the tendon and the ligament (red arrow) and the thin subcutaneous tissue (white arrow).

401, 402 Palmar annular ligament desmopathy: (401) transverse and (402) sagittal. Note the thickening and increased echogenicity of the PAL (yellow bracket), associated with mild synovial thickening (red arrows). The yellow arrow shows the mesotenon of the SDFT, outlined by the synovitis.

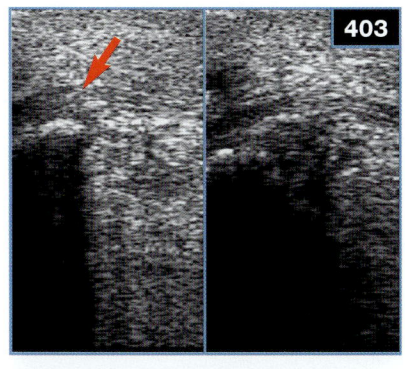 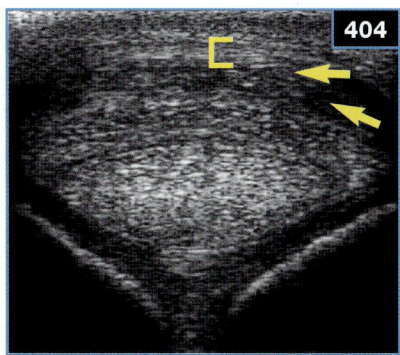

403 Entheseopathy of the lateral insertion of the annular ligament (left image). Note the thickening in comparison with the medial insertion (right), irregular bony contour at the insertion (entheseophytes), hypoechogenicity of the ligament, and loss of fiber pattern (desmopathy) (arrow).

404 Thickening of the synovial membrane due to septic tenosynovitis. The annular ligament is normal (yellow bracket), but the inflamed, space-occupying synovial tissue causes stenosis of the fetlock canal (arrows).

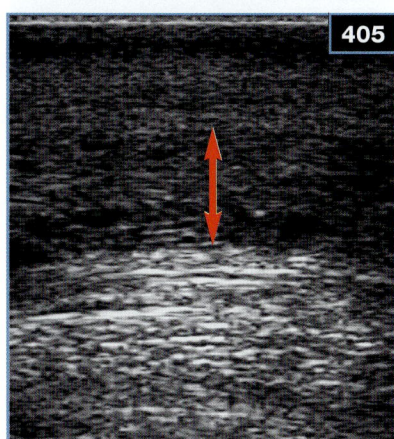 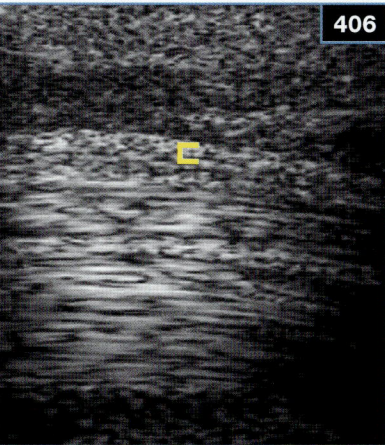

405, 406 Subcutaneous tissue thickening palmar to the annular ligament is unlikely to cause a stenosing syndrome. (405) Transverse ultrasound scan showing a normal annular ligament and synovial sheath. Hypoechogenic thickening of the subcutaneous tissues is probably due to focal contusion/hematoma formation (red arrow). (406) Longitudinal scan of the same area; the annular ligament is indicated by the yellow bracket.

215

Management

If a hematoma or subcutaneous thickening is noted, rest, local anti-inflammatory treatment (e.g. cold-hosing, ice packs) and bandaging until the symptoms resolve are usually all that is necessary. Tenosynovitis should be approached as described earlier (see p. 211). In most cases, thickening of the PAL responds well to conservative management and treatment of the associated tenosynovitis.

In chronic cases it is likely that fibrosis and thickening of all the tissues affect the function and cause reduced flexion and pain. In these cases, transection of the PAL (PAL desmotomy) may provide some relief. The surgery is best performed tenoscopically, as this will allow accurate assessment of the sheath integrity and, if indicated, a partial synovectomy to be performed. The ligament is severed using a retrograde, curved tenotomy knife ('hook blade'), arthroscopic electrosurgical hook blades, or a coblation hook probe. Postoperatively, the horse should be treated as for tenosynovitis, with early passive manipulations of the fetlock to reduce adhesions. Open surgery through a larger skin incision has been used extensively and often successfully, but is associated with a higher risk of wound breakdown and fibrosis.

Prognosis

The prognosis is good in acute and subacute cases with conservative management, guarded in chronic tenosynovitis, and fair with chronic PAL syndrome treated by desmotomy.

Deep digital flexor tendonitis

Definition/overview

Spontaneous traumatic injury to the DDFT nearly always occurs in the digital sheath or within the foot. The two syndromes are differentiated clinically, the first condition being associated with digital tenosynovitis, the second with 'palmar heel pain and navicular syndrome'. Tendonitis of the DDFT has also been described in the distal antebrachium as a result of protruding osteochondromas (see Carpal canal syndrome, p. 123), in the tarsal sheath (see Thoroughpin, p. 218), and occasionally in association with desmitis of the ALDDFT (see p. 204).

Etiology/pathophysiology

DDFT tendonitis is usually a spontaneous strain injury and is due to repeated trauma (cyclic injury) or overextension injury. Direct trauma and puncture of the tendon through the palmar fetlock or pastern area without contamination of the sheath can occur. Injuries are diffuse or focal lesions that tend to extend through the tendon in a reticulated pattern. Healing is often delayed and occurs through fibrosis and fibrocartilaginous metaplasia. Mineralization may occur within the metaplastic foci. Tenosynovitis is usually severe, particularly if the lesion communicates with the sheath lumen.

DDFT tendonitis in the foot is of unknown origin, but is probably related to mechanical imbalance in the foot and abnormal compressive and shearing forces over the palmar aspect of the distal sesamoid (navicular) bone. It may be associated with podotrochlear bursitis and can lead to erosions of the palmar navicular fibrocartilage (distal scutum) and adhesion formation.

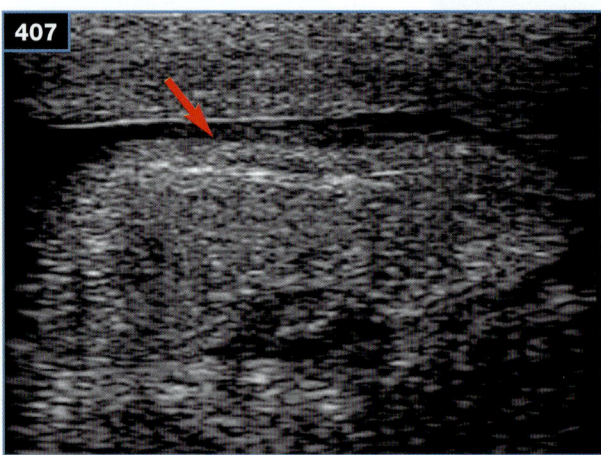

407 Transverse ultrasound scan of the palmar aspect of the pastern at the level of the PIP joint. The lateral part of the DDFT is enlarged and irregular in shape (left side). There is associated thickening of the synovial membrane of the digital sheath (arrow).

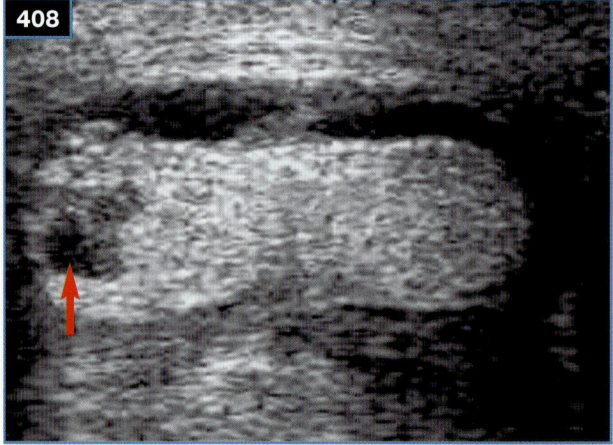

408 Irregular, longitudinal lesion within the lateral part of the DDFT in the pastern region (arrow). The lesion extends to the periphery and synovial sheath cavity, which appears distended. There is, however, no obvious synovial thickening.

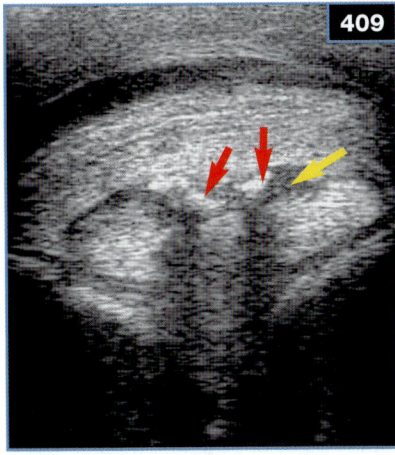
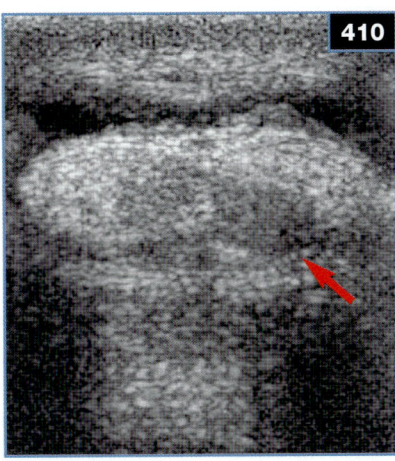
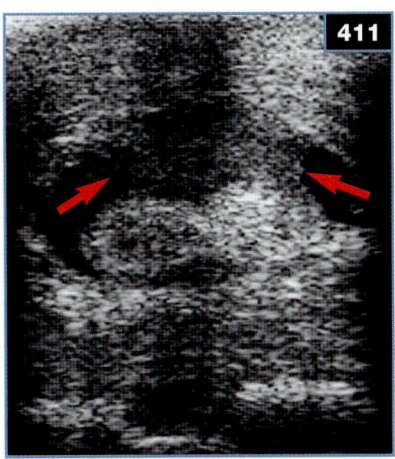

Clinical presentation
Deep digital flexor tendonitis in the digital sheath is always associated with a distension and inflammation of the sheath and is more common in the hindlimb. Lameness varies from mild to moderately severe and is usually unilateral and acute in onset, although sometimes the sheath distension may have been long-standing. Accurate palpation of structures is difficult, but pain is often elicited by distal flexion and/or direct pressure on the tendon. Distal flexion increases the lameness. Intrathecal analgesia of the digital sheath will improve the lameness.

Deep digital tendon injuries in the pastern region can occur as a strain or following direct injury by blunt trauma or puncture wounds. Tendonitis is not common, but is most often seen in mature sport horses as an acute-onset, unilateral moderate to severe lameness in the forelimb. There may be palpable thickening and pain, but minimal digital flexor tendon sheath filling.

Differential diagnosis
Other causes of tenosynovitis need to be considered.

Diagnosis
Ultrasonography
Four types of lesions of the DDFT have been identified in the digital sheath region on ultrasonography: enlargement and change in the shape of the tendon (407); focal hypoechoic lesions within the tendon or on its border (407, 408); mineralization within the DDFT (409); and marginal tears (410). The latter may require surgical exploration to identify the lesion definitively. In addition, there may be adhesion formation in more chronic cases (411) and digital sheath synovitis changes. The lesions are often reticular in pattern and may combine several of the above characteristics. Chronic injuries often lead to dystrophic mineralization.

409 Longitudinal tears of the DDFT in the fetlock region (yellow arrow) associated with mineralization within the lesion (red arrows), visible as hyperechogenic surfaces casting acoustic shadows.

410 Transverse ultrasound scan of the palmar aspect of the pastern at the level of the PIP joint. The medial part of the DDFT (right side) is slightly enlarged. There is a hypoechogenic lesion opening at the dorsomedial aspect, suggesting a superficial tear (arrow).

411 A large adhesion is present on the palmar aspect of the DDFT in the pastern region (arrows). There is mild distension of the digital sheath. The synovial membrane is thickened and irregular, indicating chronic synovitis.

Management
Many cases are treated conservatively as described in the DDFT sheath section (see p. 204). Surgical treatment with tenoscopy to debride the tears has been recommended, but healing often remains slow and the results are often disappointing.

Prognosis
The prognosis is guarded to poor due to poor healing of lesions and persistence or recurrence of lameness. Some horses will make an eventual recovery over a considerable length of time.

Tenosynovitis of the tarsal sheath (thoroughpin)

Definition/overview

The tarsal sheath is the synovial sheath of the lateral digital flexor tendon (LDF). This large tendon runs over the medial aspect of the hock and sustentaculum tali of the calcaneus to join up with the medial digital flexor tendon (MDF) in the proximal metatarsus to form the DDFT. Thoroughpin refers to distension of the sheath, whatever the cause.

Etiology/pathophysiology

The causes are the same as in the digital sheath. Idiopathic distension is by far the most common cause. It is therefore paramount that other causes of lameness are ruled out. Other common causes include spontaneous injury to the tendon (tendonitis) or other sheath components (tears of the mesotenon), probably as a result of overextension of the digit while the hock is flexed, and direct trauma (e.g. kick injuries, interference with the opposite limb). LDF tendon tendonitis is rare, but causes a similar syndrome to DDFT tendonitis. In most cases, superficial tears on the tendon surface are associated with severe tenosynovitis.

Direct trauma to the medial hock tends to cause damage to the prominent sustentaculum tali, with frequent fragmentation of its plantar edge. This also leads to tenosynovitis. If a wound is present, septic tenosynovitis is common.

412 Severe tarsal sheath distension visible as a fluid-filled pouch medially, between the tibia and common calcanean tendon.

Chronic or recurrent sheath inflammation leads to adhesion formation. These are often restrictive and tend to tear repeatedly because of the large range of movement of the tendon over the sustentaculum tali, leading to repeated hemorrhage, chronic inflammation, and marked pain. In severe cases the fibrocartilage covering the sustentaculum tali is eroded and leads to contact lesions on the overlying tendon.

Clinical presentation

Typically, distension of the sheath causes swelling of the proximal pouch in the distal crus, particularly laterally and medially between the tibia and common calcanean tendon (412). A lesser swelling is visible or palpable medial to the DDFT in the proximal third of the metatarsus. There should be no confusion with distension of the calcaneal bursa or plantar pouch of the tarsocrural joint. In idiopathic distension, there is no associated lameness. There may, however, be pain on limb flexion. Tenosynovitis causes a moderate to severe lameness, with restricted hock flexion and decreased foot flight arc.

Differential diagnosis

Other swellings on the caudal distal crus, sympathetic effusion, and tarsal check ligament desmitis may have a similar presentation.

Diagnosis

Clinical examination

The swelling must be differentiated from joint or bursal swelling. Intrathecal injection of local anesthetic solution (5–8 ml) is useful to confirm that pain is due to sheath involvement.

Radiography

Four standard projections of the tarsus and a flexed caudoproximal plantarodistal ('skyline') view of the calcaneus should be obtained. These will confirm sustentaculum tali fragmentation and/or erosion (413). Lytic osteitis may be present in association with wounds.

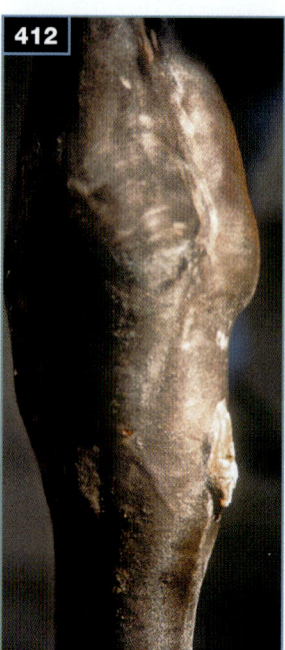
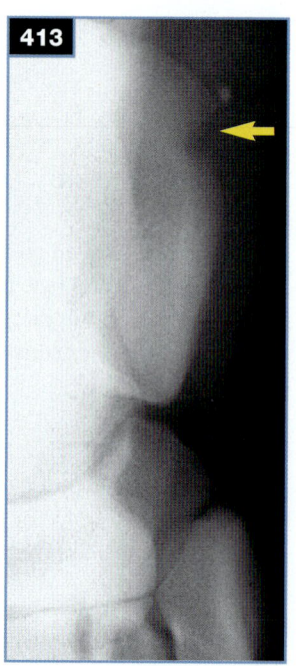

413 Dorso 45° medial/plantarolateral radiograph of the tarsus of a horse that had sustained a kick injury to the medial aspect of the hock. There is a small defect and fragmentation of the edge of the sustentaculum tali of the calcaneus (arrow).

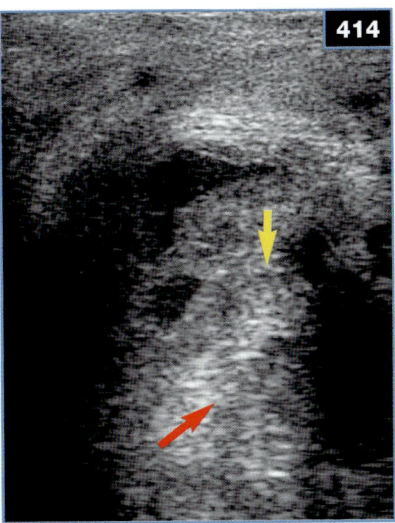 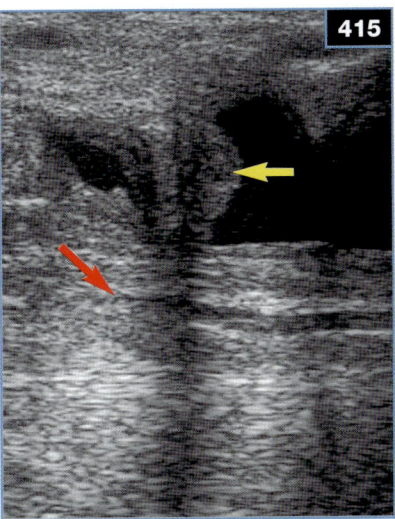 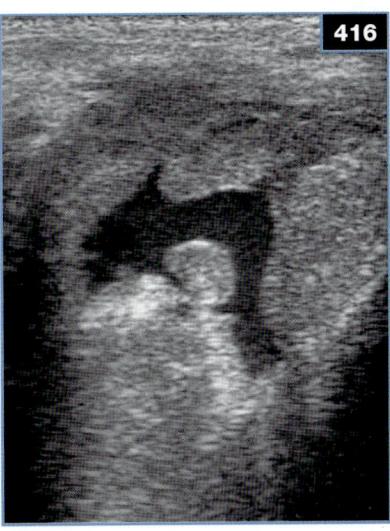

414, 415 Transverse (414) and longitudinal (415) ultrasound scans over the plantaromedial aspect of the proximal hock. The LDF tendon is deformed and frayed (red arrows) and there is a large, fibrous adhesion (yellow arrows) forming a restrictive link to the thickened parietal sheath.

416 Chronic tarsal sheath tenosynovitis. There are several echogenic synovial tissue masses protruding into the sheath cavity.

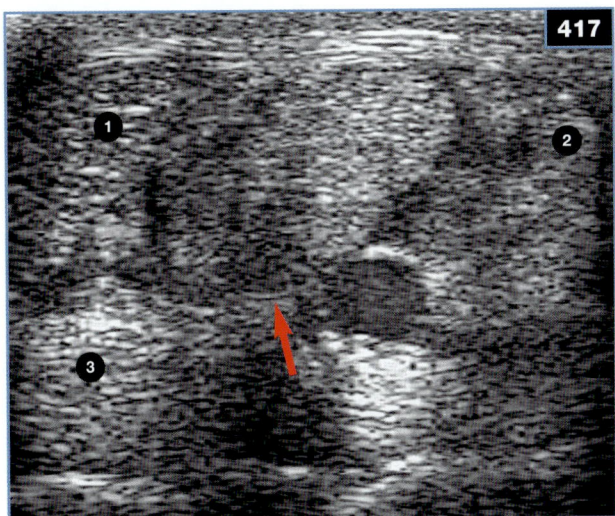

417 Transverse ultrasound scan over the plantaromedial aspect of the distal tarsus. The LDF tendon contains a large, irregular, hypoechogenic lesion at its dorsolateral border (arrow). This was a longitudinal tear forming a deep cleft on the surface of the tendon. 1 = SDFT; 2 = medial digital flexor tendon; 3 = LPL.

418 Longitudinal ultrasound scan over the sustentaculum tali. There is a large, irregular defect at the surface of the latter (yellow arrows). The overlying LDF tendon is hypoechogenic and has lost its normal fiber pattern (red arrow). There is a tremendous amount of synovial thickening in this chronically inflamed tarsal tendon sheath (white arrow).

Ultrasonography

The ultrasonographic signs are as described for the digital sheath. Adhesions are often large and fibrous (414, 415). Chronic tenosynovitis often leads to the production of large synovial masses that obliterate the proximal pouch (416). LDF tendon lesions are variable, but are often diffuse and longitudinally arranged, forming large clefts in the tendon (417). Erosion of the fibrocartilage may be obvious (418). Fragmentation of the edge of the sustentaculum tali is often associated with thickening and decreased echogenicity of the plantar retinaculum.

219

Soft-tissue injuries

Management

The approach is similar to that described for digital tenosynovitis. Chronic cases are often nonresponsive to conservative management. Surgical treatment is recommended in these cases. Tenoscopic examination, debridement of erosive lesions, and partial synovectomy is often surprisingly effective and a complete recovery may be expected in a significant proportion of horses. In horses that do not respond to this approach, particularly as a complication of septic tenosynovitis, aggressive debridement, synovectomy, and resection of the tarsal portion of the LDF tendon has been described as a salvage procedure.

Prognosis

The prognosis is good to fair in acute cases, except in the presence of severe tendon tears. In chronic cases the prognosis remains fair with tenoscopic surgery, although severe tendon lesions are usually associated with a guarded prognosis.

Luxation of the superficial flexor tendon from the tuber calcis

Definition/overview

The SDFT normally attaches to the tuber calcis of the calcaneus via two abaxial fibrous branches; these prevent the SDFT slipping sideways, but allow it to glide over the bone. Rupture of the medial or, less commonly, the lateral branch will cause the tendon to slip in the opposite direction during hock flexion. The condition is usually unilateral, but bilateral injuries have been described.

Etiology/pathophysiology

Probably traumatic either by direct injury or during excessive exercise. Horses with a straight hock and/or fetlock overextension are predisposed. The luxation may be complete or partial (subluxation) and most commonly occurs laterally.

Clinical presentation

Rupture of the branch is acute, causing sudden-onset lameness. Typically, the horse is severely distressed as the tendon slips on and off the calcaneus. The tendon comes off the tuber calcis during hock flexion and returns to its normal position during limb extension. There is associated distension of the calcaneal bursa. The tendon eventually remains in a permanently dislocated position in most cases (419).

Differential diagnosis

Traumatic or septic bursitis of the calcaneal bursa, capped hock (acquired subcutaneous bursa), septic osteitis of the calcaneus, and tendonitis of the deep tarsal tendons should be considered.

Diagnosis

Clinical examination

The tendon may be seen to flick on and off the tuber calcis under the skin. The instability is easily palpated during passive hock flexion. The luxation is most commonly lateral.

Ultrasonography

Ultrasonography will confirm the luxation, calcaneal bursitis, and rupture of the medial (or lateral) calcaneal branch of the SDFT.

Management

Surgical repair is difficult and a variety of techniques have been described. Early treatment and aggressive, vigorous postoperative care can lead to success in some cases. In acute cases, box rest, bandaging, and application of a cast or splint preventing limb flexion may be effective. In most cases, complete luxation will allow the tendon to become stabilized in its dislocated position. Although a mechanical lameness may remain, particularly with lateral luxation, the horses are pain free and may be able to return to their previous level of performance.

Prognosis

The prognosis is guarded for luxation both laterally and medially.

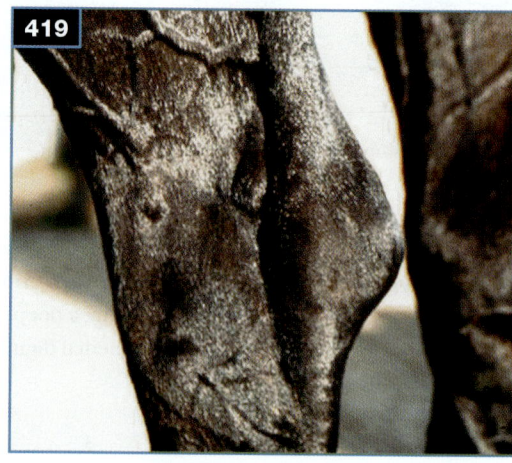

419 Permanent lateral luxation of the SDFT off the tuber calcis. The tendon is visible under the skin, following a straight path over the lateral aspect of the calcaneus.

Rupture of the peroneus tertius tendon

Definition/overview

The peroneus tertius tendon is a fibrous structure lacking muscle fibers that runs from the lateral femoral epicondyle to the dorsal proximal aspect of the metatarsus. It is a major component of the reciprocal apparatus as it forces the tarsus to flex passively when the stifle flexes. Rupture is usually strain induced and spontaneous, although the tendon may be severed in wounds to the cranial aspect of the crus.

Etiology/pathophysiology

This condition is a consequence of a sudden strain injury, the tendon being stretched to rupture through overextension of the hock while the stifle is still flexed. This may occur when the distal limb is caught over a fence, door, or jump or following recovery from anesthesia when the limb is cast or bandaged. Rarely, there may be avulsion of the origin of the tendon on the lateral femoral epicondyle.

Clinical presentation

Typically, the horse can stand normally. Lameness is variable, but there is characteristic overextension of the hock at the end of the stance phase, causing the distal limb to slightly lag behind. There may be swelling and edema in the acute phase over the cranial aspect of the crus.

Diagnosis

Clinical examination

Diagnosis is based on the pathognomonic loss of reciprocal flexion between the stifle and hock. Thus, the hock can be passively extended while the stifle is flexed (420). This also causes a dimpling of the common calcanean tendon ('Achilles tendon'), which is no longer kept taut by the opposing extensor system.

Ultrasonography

Ultrasonography helps to determine the level of the rupture, but is not necessary for the diagnosis. It is, however, useful for monitoring the healing process.

Management

The horse should be box rested for 2–3 months and work gradually resumed over 2–3 months. Surgical repair is unnecessary and conservative management nearly always provides full functional recovery.

Prognosis

The prognosis is good in most cases. Chronic cases may take longer to heal because of scarring and functional lengthening of the peroneus tertius, but gradual fibrosis usually provides eventual recovery.

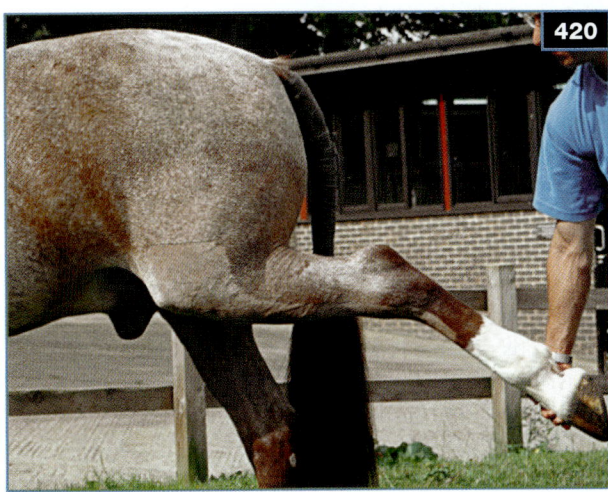

420 Rupture of the peroneus tertius tendon. The hock is extended by pulling the limb backward while the stifle remains flexed. Note the slight dimpling of the common calcaneal tendon due to loss of reciprocal tension from the peroneus tertius tendon. (Photo courtesy R Smith)

Injuries to the common calcanean ('Achilles') tendon

Definition/overview

The common calcanean tendon ('Achilles' tendon) comprises the two tendons of insertion of the gastrocnemius muscle on the tuber calcis of the calcaneus and also the SDFT and the deep tarsal tendon, two ligamentous branches that arise from the fascial reinforcement of the tendon and receive fibers from the biceps femoris, semitendinosus, and semimembranosus muscles. They insert on the tuber calcis, dorsal to the gastrocnemius tendons. Strain injuries are rare, but have been described in the gastrocnemius and in the deep tarsal tendons. The former may be injured at its origin on the femur, but the tendons of insertion are most commonly affected near the calcaneus. Rupture is always traumatic and usually associated with a sharp wound to the caudal aspect of the crus. This structure is part of the reciprocal apparatus and is essential for the animal to bear weight on the limb. It locks the hock into extension when the stifle is extended, either actively during locomotion or passively through locking of the patella on the medial femoral trochlear ridge.

221

Etiology/pathophysiology

Tendonitis is probably due to repeated strain or to a single event causing hyperflexion of the hock while the stifle is extended, although this remains unclear. Spontaneous rupture has not been described, but wounds to the caudal aspect of the crus occur occasionally and may cause partial to complete laceration of the various components of the common calcanean tendon.

Clinical presentation

Tendonitis of the deep calcanean (tarsal) tendons is only occasionally encountered. It is characterized by moderate hindlimb lameness with or without focal enlargement of the distal part of the common calcanean tendon and distension of the calcaneal and gastrocnemius bursae. Tendonitis of the gastrocnemius tendon is also rare and usually affects the distal-most part of the tendon. Focal swelling may be visible and there is usually associated bursal distension. This produces a diffuse enlargement of the area proximal to the point of the hock (421). Lameness is variable and a specific gait abnormality, characterized by lateral rotation of the tuber calcis during the stance phase of the stride, shortened caudal phase, and reduced foot flight arc, has been described. Lesions in the tendon of origin do not give rise to specific signs and the diagnosis can be a real challenge.

Partial laceration usually involves an obvious wound. Lameness is usually severe, but close inspection and ultra-sonography are often necessary to confirm the partial rupture. Laceration of the SDFT disrupts the stay apparatus and causes the hock to partially collapse during weight bearing. Lameness is therefore severe and characterized by a partial flexion of the hock during the stance phase. Complete laceration of the common calcanean tendon is associated with a total inability to bear weight on the limb.

Differential diagnosis

For tendonitis of the deep tarsal or gastrocnemius tendon: bursitis of the calcaneal and/or gastrocnemius bursae ('deep capped hock'); acquired subcutaneous bursa ('capped hock').

Diagnosis

Clinical examination

A suspicion of tendonitis is made through lameness associated with focal swelling over the distal common calcanean tendon area. This is, however, not always evident and regional perineural analgesia may be necessary to confirm the site of pain.

Tendonitis of the origin of the gastrocnemius is difficult to confirm clinically. Anesthesia of the stifle joints is normally negative. Radiography may show new bone remodeling over the caudal distal femoral metaphysis. Scintigraphy is a useful tool for detecting entheseopathy.

Rupture of the SDFT proximal to the hock gives a characteristic dropping of the hock during the stance phase, but this may be difficult to observe because of the associated severe lameness. Complete rupture is confirmed through the pathognomonic ability to flex the hock passively without flexing the stifle.

Ultrasonography

Ultrasonography is necessary to confirm the presence of tendonitis. Deep calcaneal (tarsal) tendonitis is characterized by marked enlargement and decreased echogenicity of the deep tarsal tendons (422, 423). These are difficult to image for an inexperienced operator and care should be taken not to confuse focal edema or gastrocnemius bursitis with this condition. Gastrocnemius tendonitis lesions resemble those observed in the digital flexor tendons and there is usually associated synovial thickening and distension of the gastrocnemius bursa.

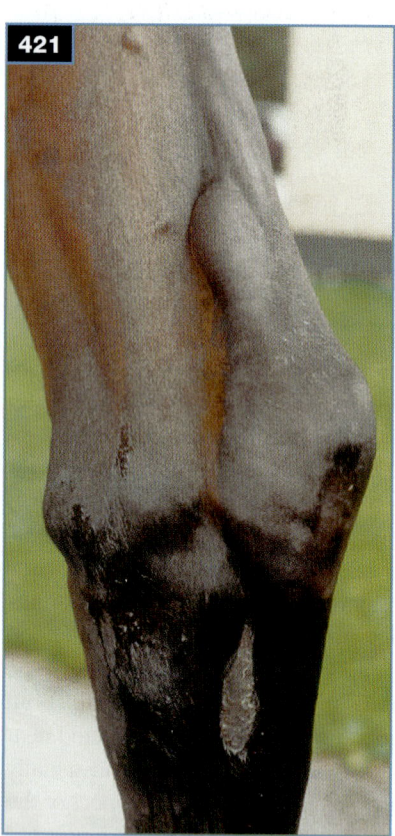

421 This picture of the medial hock shows swelling of the calcaneal bursa just dorsomedial to the common calcaneal tendon. This was associated with injury to the gastrocnemius tendon. (Photo courtesy SJ Dyson)

Musculoskeletal system

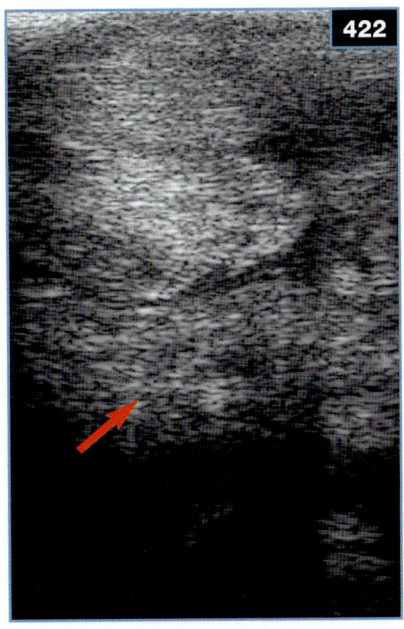

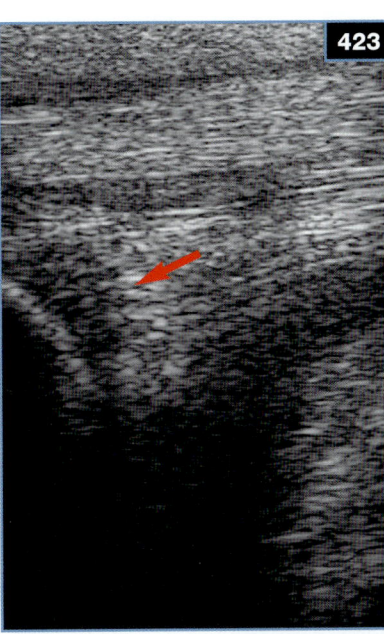

422, 423 Transverse (422) and sagittal (423) ultrasound scans of the common calcanean tendon (arrows) showing severe increase in size and a heterogeneously decreased echogenicity of the deep part of the tendon. These images are typical of deep tarsal tendonitis.

424 Partial tear of the SDFT (yellow arrow) in the distal crus. There is severe calcaneal bursitis (red arrow) due to subacute infection. This was associated with a wound over the common calcanean tendon.

Tendonitis at the femoral origin may be difficult to diagnose, as the tendon is very short and muscle fibers may resemble a lesion. A hematoma may be obvious in acute cases, characterized by focal enlargement and a discrete anechogenic structure, usually organized into several loculated cavities. In chronic cases, entheseopathy with marked bone remodeling may be seen.

Ultrasonography is useful to confirm partial or complete rupture of the SDFT (424). It is not necessary for complete common calcanean tendon rupture as the clinical signs are pathognomonic.

Management
Tendonitis is best treated conservatively with box rest with controlled exercise. It may take a fairly long time (up to 12 months) before the horse with gastrocnemius tendonitis can resume full work.

SDFT rupture is treated with complete box rest, and some limb support (full-limb cast or splints) is advised for up to 3 months. Fibrosis may allow partial to complete functional repair.

Complete common calcaneal tendon rupture should be treated by surgical repair and application of a full-limb cast for 12 weeks, followed by bandage and splint support for a further 6–12 weeks. The repair often fails during recovery.

Prognosis
The prognosis is good for deep tarsal tendonitis, although too few cases have been reported for an accurate prognosis to be established. The prognosis for distal gastrocnemius tendonitis varies from good to guarded depending on the severity of the lesion. It appears to be fair for proximal tendonitis, although very few cases have been reported. Rupture of the SDFT carries a guarded prognosis, but functional recovery is possible in some horses. The prognosis is generally very poor for complete common calcanean tendon rupture. The prognosis is good to fair for tears of the tendon of origin of the gastrocnemius muscle.

223

Curb

Definition/overview

Curb refers to swelling over the distal plantar aspect of the hock, giving it a convex appearance when viewed laterally (425). It was initially considered to be due to injury to the long plantar tarsal ligament, which arises from the plantaroproximal aspect of the calcaneus and runs distally to the head of the fourth metatarsal bone. Ultrasonography has, however, shown that other soft-tissue structures are more commonly affected.

Etiology/pathophysiology

Thickening of any of the soft tissues covering the plantar aspect of the tarsus may be involved. These include the skin and subcutaneous tissues, the fascia, the SDFT, and the long plantar ligament (LPL) of the tarsus. In most cases subcutaneous tissue is involved. The deformity is due to thickening, probably as a result of direct trauma and contusion; for example, when a horse kicks at its stable door or manger. SDFT injuries may arise in this region and give a similar appearance, particularly as there is usually associated peritendinous tissue swelling and thickening. These injuries are most likely a consequence of direct trauma. Plantar ligament desmitis is encountered in a small proportion of cases with a curb-like swelling in horses of all breeds, with a predisposition in those with a sickle hock conformation. A curb-like appearance is observed in young foals with dorsal collapse of cuboidal bones, causing a sagittal deformity (see p. 42).

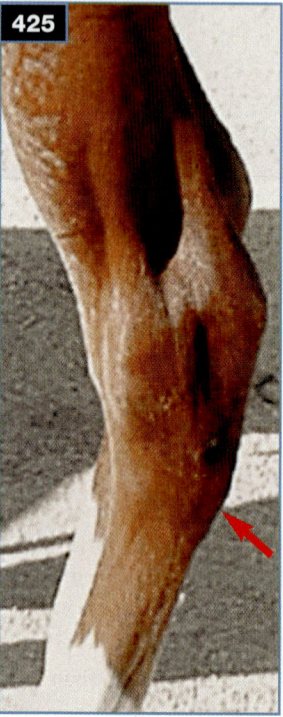

425 Curb deformity due to trauma to the plantar aspect of the tarsus, giving a bowed appearance to this region (arrow).

Clinical presentation

There is a typical deformity over the distal plantar aspect of the hock (425). The swelling may be soft initially, but it is often firm in chronic cases. Lameness may be marked, particularly in cases with SDFT tendonitis, but presents in a more low-grade, recurrent form in plantar ligament desmitis. Many horses do not appear to be lame, although it has been incriminated as a cause of loss of performance in racehorses.

Differential diagnosis

Swelling involving distension of the calcaneal bursa, fracture and osteitis of the calcaneus, and tarsal bone collapse should be considered.

Diagnosis

Clinical examination

The typical deformity is fairly pathognomonic, but ultrasonography is warranted to confirm the diagnosis. Radiography is advisable to rule out other causes.

Ultrasonography

Subcutaneous and peritendinous tissue thickening is obvious (426). SDFT lesions are typically focal hypoechogenic and associated with marked tendon enlargement (427). Plantar ligament injuries lead to ligament thickening (428), although it may be necessary to compare with the opposite limb for confirmation. Although desmitis with thickening without changes in echogenicity has been described as a cause of loss of performance in racehorses, the author has usually observed diffuse or focal hypoechogenic lesions within the ligament. There may be associated bone remodeling, particularly at the distal insertion on the fourth metatarsal bone.

Management

Conservative treatment is preferred in all forms of curb. Box rest, in-hand exercise, and local hosing and anti-inflammatory treatments are used as for other types of tendon/ligament injuries.

Prognosis

The prognosis is good for most cases of curb, although the swelling may persist. SDFT injuries carry a good to poor prognosis, depending on the severity of the lesion.

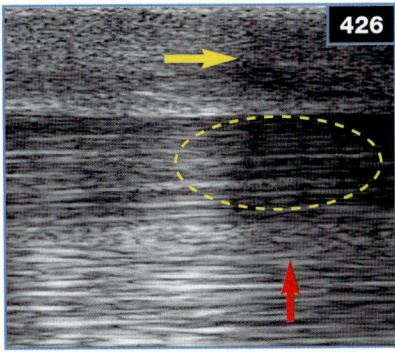 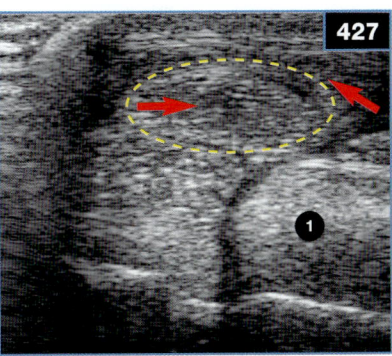 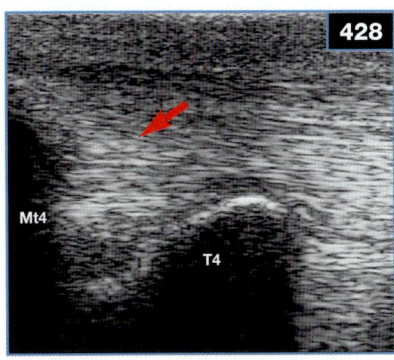

426 Longitudinal ultrasound scan over the plantar aspect of the calcaneus. The SDFT (circled) and LPL (red arrow) are normal, but there is marked thickening of the subcutaneous tissues (yellow arrow), probably as a result of repeated, mild trauma.

427 Transverse ultrasound scan over the plantar aspect of the calcaneus of a horse presenting with curb. The SDFT (circled) is enlarged, with a focal, central, and hypoechogenic lesion (left arrow), as well as a peritendinous, hypoechogenic lesion suggesting paratenon thickening (right arrow). The LPL is normal. 1 = DDFT.

428 Longitudinal ultrasound scan over the plantarolateral aspect of the distal tarsus. The long branch of the LPL (arrow) runs distally from the calcaneus, over the plantar aspect of the fourth tarsal bone (T4), to insert over the proximal aspect of the head of the fourth metatarsal bone (Mt4). There is mild, hypoechogenic thickening of the LPL and overlying subcutaneous tissue. This is a very rare cause of curb-like deformity.

Cunean tendonitis/bursitis

Definition/overview

The cunean tendon is the medial branch of the distal cranial tibial tendon. It arises from the latter over the dorsal aspect of the tarsus and runs obliquely and medially to attach on the head of the second metatarsal bone. A small, subtendinous bursa is present between the surface of the second and central tarsal bones and the cunean tendon. Cunean tendonitis and bursitis have been described as a cause of lameness and poor performance, especially in racing Standardbreds. This condition is the subject of controversy, as most authors believe that the pain is actually due to DJD of the distal tarsal joints ('bone spavin'). Anesthesia of the bursa or of the tarsometatarsal and DIT joints appears to provide similar results in many cases of spavin.

This author has observed one case of cunean tendonitis, confirmed on ultrasonography (**429**). This was most likely due to direct trauma and was associated with marked focal edema.

429 Longitudinal ultrasound scan over the medial aspect of a tarsus with cunean tendonitis. The tendon (red arrow) is enlarged, hypoechogenic, and heterogeneous. The underlying bursa is distended with anechogenic fluid (yellow arrow).

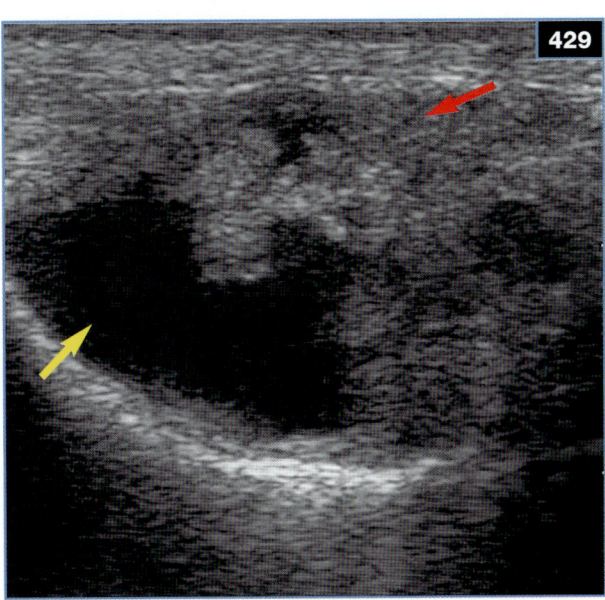

Conditions affecting the skeletal muscles

Hyperkalemic periodic paralysis

Definition/overview
Hyperkalemic periodic paralysis (HYPP) is a genetic disease observed in certain Quarter horses. It causes attacks of paralysis, which can be induced by ingestion of potassium.

Etiology/pathophysiology
HYPP is inherited in the Quarter horse, Appaloosa, and American Paint horse and associated crossbreds as an autosomal dominant trait. It is linked to the lineage of a single Quarter horse stallion named 'Impressive'. The defect disrupts a sodium channel protein, causing altered sodium/potassium exchange through the muscle membrane.

Abnormal sodium influx and leakage of potassium increase muscle fiber excitability, initially causing spontaneous twitching and myotonia, eventually followed by flaccid paralysis. The blood potassium concentration consequently increases.

Clinical presentation
Affected horses exhibit unpredictable attacks of varying severity, from muscle tremor to paralytic recumbency and, rarely, death from cardiac or respiratory arrest. Homozygous animals appear to be more severely affected than heterozygous carriers. The severity varies between individuals and tends to decrease with age. The most common presentation is characterized by bouts of muscle fasciculations, manifested by localized to generalized trembling and weakness. The crises last from a few minutes to several hours. They may be triggered by stress or exercise, but are often spontaneous. In more severe presentations, myotonia leads to hindlimb paresis or involuntary recumbency. Other signs include prolapse of the third eyelid, laryngeal paralysis, facial tremors, and stiff jaws. Affected horses usually recover spontaneously from each bout.

Differential diagnosis
Other causes of hyperkalemia, hypocalcemia, exertional rhabdomyolysis, colic, tetanus, and viral myeloencephalopathies should be considered.

Diagnosis
History and clinical examination are critical. Blood biochemistry demonstrates no abnormality between clinical episodes. Blood samples taken during the crises may reveal hyperkalemia ($\geq$ 6 mmol/l). Electromyography may show increased muscle fiber contractility during or between crises. Inducing hyperkalemia can be useful to confirm suspicion in asymptomatic animals, but this may be risky for the animals (i.e. risk of death, particularly if any concurrent heart or renal disease is present). This should be avoided during clinical episodes.

DNA testing can confirm the gene mutation. The American Quarter Horse Association accepts tests performed in certain licensed laboratories including: Veterinary Genetics Lab at University of California at Davis; Shelterwood Laboratory at Carthage, Texas; Vita-Tech Canada Inc., Markham, Ontario; NSW Agriculture in Australia; Veterinary Diagnostics Center, Fairfield, Ohio; Stormont Labs, Woodland, California; Gene Check, Inc., Ft. Collins, Colorado; and Maxxam Laboratory at Guelph, Ontario.

Management
In mild episodes, light exercise is useful. Injection of epinephrine (3 ml of 0.1% solution i/m per 500 kg) may be helpful. In severe episodes, the hyperkalemia should be reduced by providing intravenous fluids without potassium (e.g. 5% dextrose with or without 1–2 mEq/kg sodium bicarbonate). Calcium gluconate (23% solution, 0.2–0.4 ml/kg diluted in 1 liter of 5% dextrose given i/v over 10 minutes) may help to decrease muscle hyperexcitability. Insulin (0.1 IU/kg i/v with 0.5–1.0 g/kg dextrose) may be administered to improve influx of K^+ into cells, but this requires regular monitoring of blood glucose concentration.

Prevention
With dietary management, it is essential to decrease the potassium intake; therefore, alfalfa, molasses, and bran intake should be decreased or stopped. Equal amounts of hay and grain should be given 2–3 three times daily. Fasting or sudden changes in the diet should be avoided. Regular exercise (e.g. daily pasture exercise and avoid sudden changes in exercise levels) should be provided. Acetazolamide (2 mg/kg p/o q12–8h) may be administered as a preventive therapy.

Prognosis
The prognosis is generally fair. Mild episodes are usually self-resolving. Severe episodes require emergency treatment, but death is rare. The disease may be efficiently controlled by proper management. Affected horses should not be bred.

Postanesthetic myoneuropathy

Definition/overview

This is a myopathy that occurs during the anesthetic recovery period and causes rapid, progressive degeneration of the muscle fibers. Two syndromes are recognized: localized myoneuropathy affecting one muscle or muscle group, and generalized myopathy causing diffuse myodegeneration. It is generally accepted that there may be a peripheral neurologic component, but postanesthetic neuropathy primarily involves the muscles, hence the use of the term 'myoneuropathy'.

Etiology/pathophysiology

Postanesthetic myoneuropathy occurs after general anesthesia. Intrinsic predisposing factors include the weight of the animal, its muscular development, intensive training, and nervous temperament. Extrinsic factors relate to the anesthetic. The risk increases with the duration of anesthesia, arterial blood pressure ≤ 70 mmHg, use of positive pressure ventilation, hard or poorly supporting table padding, and poor positioning. There may be a congenital predisposition of certain individuals to generalized myopathy, probably through hypersensitivity.

This condition is thought to be similar to compartment syndrome in humans. Prolonged pressure applied to muscle masses causes a decreased perfusion and blood stasis in the muscles. Hypotension worsens the situation, leading to hypoxia and ischemia. This induces an anaerobic metabolism, with accumulation of lactate, decreased pH, and edema. The inelastic fascia surrounding the muscle masses causes the compartment pressure to increase. Electrolyte imbalances are associated with muscle hyperexcitability and sustained myotonic contractions. These phenomena lead to fiber necrosis. During recovery, reperfusion brings oxygen to the damaged cells, causing free radical accumulation. Halothane may also lead to the formation of toxic radicals. These induce further muscle degeneration. The release of lactate, electrolytes, cell debris, and particularly myoglobin from the lysed cells induces cardiovascular disturbances and renal toxicity that can lead to renal failure.

Clinical presentation

The signs become apparent during the recovery from anesthesia or soon afterwards. Recovery is prolonged, with difficulty or an inability to stand up, depending on the affected muscles. Muscles are swollen, hard to touch, and feel abnormally warm (430). There is localized to generalized sweating and pain when pressure is applied to the affected muscle masses. Two forms are encountered:

+ *Localized form.* A distinct muscle mass is affected, particularly the triceps, biceps and quadriceps femoris, masseter, longissimus dorsi, gluteals, and hindlimb adductor muscles. The affected muscle mass is hard, hot, and painful with localized sweating (431).

430 Postanesthetic myopathy affecting the left shoulder mass. Note the swollen supraspinous muscle on the left side (arrow) compared with the right side.

431 Same horse as in 430. There is focal swelling and patchy sweating.

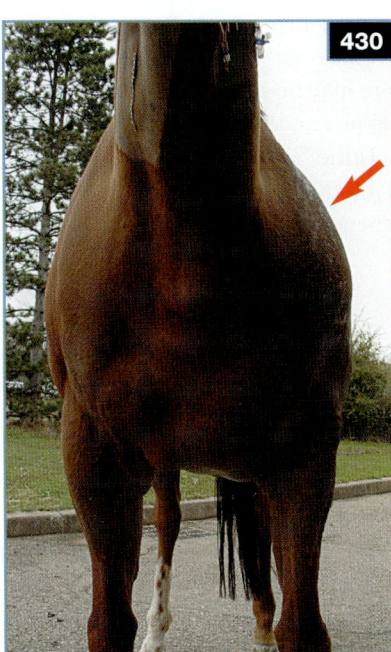
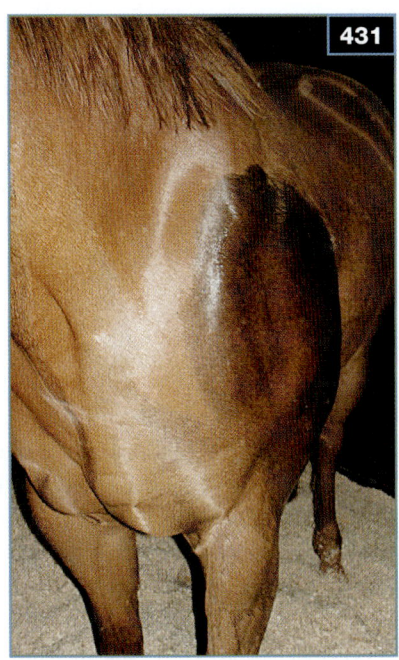

432 Localized, postanesthetic myopathy-induced lameness due to loss of the shoulder muscle mass and triceps functions. The horse is unable to extend its shoulder and elbow.

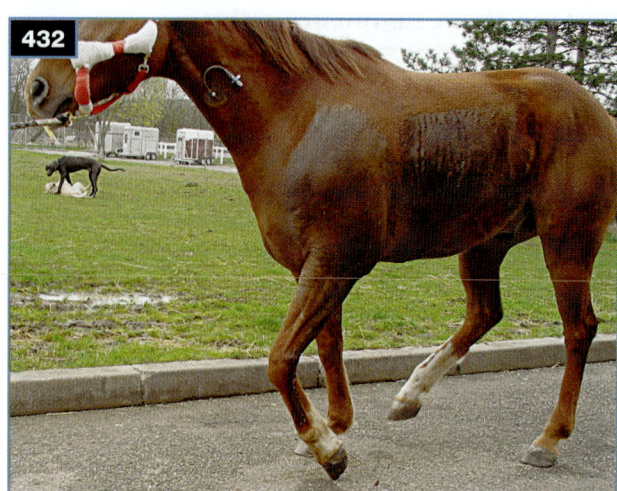

There may be mild to severe lameness in the affected limb(s) (**432**) or complete paresis. If the horse is recumbent, the condition may worsen significantly. In more severe cases the urine may appear orange to dark chocolate brown due to myoglobinuria. The signs usually resolve after a few hours to several days, but muscle atrophy and/or fibrosis may appear in 2–3 weeks and remain.

✦ *Generalized form*. This occurs spontaneously or as a result of prolonged recumbency (e.g. as a complication of localized myoneuropathy). Affected animals are recumbent and show an inability to stand up. Most muscle masses are affected, as noted above, with increased heart and respiratory rates, myoglobinuria to anuria, profuse sweating, distress, and possible cardiovascular shock and death.

Differential diagnosis
Neuropathies, other causes of lameness occurring during recovery (e.g. fractures, muscle tears, sprains), and other causes of prolonged recumbency (e.g. cord or brain disorders) should be considered.

Diagnosis
History and clinical examination are imporant. Blood biochemistry shows increased muscular enzyme concentrations (CK, AST, and LDH) with a peak at around 4–8 hours after the end of anesthesia (CK is often increased 100- or 1,000-fold), hyperkalemia, hypocalcemia, and acidosis with early hyperlactacidemia. There may be signs of renal failure (increased urea and creatinine concentrations) and other vascular imbalances. Urine analysis reveals myoglobinuria and presence of blood. Muscle biopsy is useful to confirm fibrosis or degeneration in subacute or chronic stages.

Management
Medical treatment
Palliative and supportive therapies to limit muscle damage from recumbency include provision of adequate padding, maintenance in sternal recumbency, and regular turning over. A hoist and harness may be used if the horse's temperament allows. Analgesia can be provided by opioids (e.g. morphine 0.1–0.2 mg/kg i/v, percutaneous fentanyl patches), NSAIDs at standard rates, or alpha-agonists (e.g. detomidine, romifidine) combined with acepromazine (0.03–0.05 mg/kg i/m).

Sodium bicarbonate may be added to intravenous fluids if there is an acidosis or urine pH < 7.5.

Myorelaxants can be given. Sodium dantrolene (15–25 mg/kg by slow i/v injection 4 times daily) has been advocated for the treatment of clinical myopathy.

Reperfusion injury can be prevented by giving DMSO (1 g/kg i/v) or dexamethasone (in the acute phase).

Surgical treatment
Fasciotomy is used in man and could perhaps be useful in the acute stage to limit compartment syndrome, but postoperative management is extremely difficult (risk of infection, poor wound healing) and the technique is not usually recommended.

Prevention
✦ Adequate preoperative examination (cardiovascular state) and avoid stress and exertion prior to induction.
✦ Use of adequate padding, with even support of all the dependent muscle masses (air mattresses help prevent muscle compression). The limbs should be kept horizontal, the proximal limbs supported, and compression of muscles with ropes and heavy items avoided.
✦ Avoid hypotension (adequate monitoring, decrease anesthetic depth, treat hypotension *ad hoc*). Improve recovery (analgesia, sedation, calm conditions).

Prognosis
The prognosis is variable depending on the severity and extent of the rhabdomyolysis, but also the animal's temperament. It is generally fair if the horse is able to stand up. Recovery may take a few hours to several days. Prolonged recumbency leads to a poor prognosis.

Exertional rhabdomyolysis

Definition/overview
Exertional rhabdomyolysis is a common syndrome affecting horses of all breeds and characterized by sudden-onset lameness during exercise. It may be a single event or recurrent. Synonyms include 'Monday morning disease', 'tying-up', 'myositis', 'azoturia', and 'paralytic myoglobinuria'. It is recognized as a complex syndrome with four groups of conditions and several possible etiologies.

Etiology/pathophysiology
Two syndromes are described:

+ *Acute or sporadic exertional rhabdomyolysis.* This is a single episode occurring in an otherwise healthy animal with no previous history of rhabdomyolysis. Etiologies and predisposing factors have been suggested, but the actual cause is unclear and probably multifactorial. An association with selenium and vitamin E deficiency, hypothyroidism, and variations in female sex hormone levels has not been shown in studies. Viral infections (e.g. EHV-1 and influenza) may be predisposing factors. Dietary imbalances such as excess energy (grain) can be a major predisposing factor. It can be induced by excessively intense exercise, inadequate training, dehydration, or electrolyte imbalances.

+ *Chronic exertional rhabdomyolysis.* Recurrent episodes occur at the onset of exercise or during low-level work, but may also be induced by stress. The etiology is poorly understood, but it is probably linked to genetic factors, most likely due to an inherent metabolic disturbance affecting muscle cell function. The condition may be triggered by specific environmental stimuli (e.g. weather). It includes three subgroups:
  ◇ EQUINE POLYSACCHARIDE STORAGE MYOPATHY (PSSM). Affects mostly Quarter horses and draught horses, but is described in most breeds. Affects mostly females and is transmitted as an autosomal, recessive trait. It has been associated with an excess storage of polysaccharides in a poorly bioavailable form within the muscle cell.
  ◇ RECURRENT EXERTIONAL RHABDOMYOLISIS. Affects mostly Thoroughbreds, but also Standardbreds and Arabians, particularly mares and young animals, especially nervous individuals. Transmitted as a dominant autosomal trait. The condition is induced by heavy exercise, stress, lameness, and excessive grain feeding. It is due to a defect in calcium exchanges within muscle cells leading to defective excitation/contraction coupling.

◇ MITOCHONDRIAL MYOPATHY. Anecdotal condition described in one Arabian mare. Altered metabolism and/or severe electrolyte imbalances lead to excessive production of lactate and activation of proteolytic enzymes within muscle cells. These lead to cell necrosis and release of cell contents, including enzymes, myoglobin, and lactate.

Clinical presentation
Exertional rhabdomyolysis usually affects the hindlimbs bilaterally. Signs often occur within 15–30 minutes of the start of light exercise. There is sudden-onset stiffness to severe lameness characterized by a reluctance to move and a stiff gait (decreased limb flexion). The affected muscles (mostly thigh, gluteal, and epiaxial muscles and, less commonly, forelimb and neck muscles) are hard, painful, and hot to touch. There is often excessive sweating, distress, and, in severe forms, marked dehydration, congestion of mucous membranes, tachycardia, tachypnea, and hyperthermia. The signs worsen when the horse is forced to move. Rarely, the condition may lead to prolonged recumbency and death. In low-grade cases, poor performance and stiffness may be the only signs.

Differential diagnosis
Cramps, other causes of sudden-onset lameness (e.g. fractures, severe sprains), laminitis, colic, and severe neurologic disorders should be considered. A fatal glycogen storage disorder in Quarter horse foals distinct from PSSM has recently been identified (glycogen branching enzyme deficiency).

Diagnosis
History and clinical examination are important in order to determine whether recurrent disease is present. Blood biochemistry demonstrates markedly increased muscle enzyme concentrations (CK, AST, LDH). A dynamic evaluation with serial blood sampling to establish a time–concentration curve is useful to interpret the results. Affected horses show myoglobinemia, metabolic acidosis, hyperproteinemia, and elevations in the hematocrit. Electrolyte imbalance and renal function should be assessed for signs of renal toxicity. Urine analysis demonstrates myoglobinuria. An exercise tolerance test is useful, especially in recurrent or mild forms. A blood sample is obtained in the resting animal. It is then worked at a fast pace (on the lunge or exercise under the saddle) for 20–40 minutes and resampled at T0 plus 4, 24, and 48 hours. Normal horses should have a mild increase in muscle enzymes and return to normal by 24 hours. In predisposed horses, a marked increase in enzyme levels and a slower return to normal should be expected. Nuclear scintigraphy may help identify some forms of muscle damage.

229

Muscle biopsy is useful, particularly in chronic or recurrent forms (e.g. PSSM) or in case of complications (e.g. myonecrosis, fibrosis).

Management

Nursing should involve keeping the horse in a quiet environment, with complete box rest on thick bedding. It should be fed only hay with water provided *ad libitum*. Massages and cold showers over affected muscles may be useful.

Restoration of hydration through rational fluid therapy is important and should include lactated Ringer's or Hartmann's solution intravenously and/or oral fluids, depending on severity. Electrolyte imbalances should be assessed and corrected as necessary. Potassium chloride and bicarbonate are often useful, but they require strict monitoring.

NSAIDs are used mostly for pain relief: phenylbutazone (4.4 mg/kg i/v q12h) and flunixin meglumine (1.1 mg/kg i/v q12h) are advocated. Other NSAIDs also used include ketoprofen, vedaprofen, and carprofen. Opiates can be used to control severe pain: morphine (0.1–0.2 mg/kg i/v); fentanyl (percutaneous patches).

Acepromazine (0.03–0.05 mg/kg i/m or i/v q8h) has been suggested as a vasodilator, but it is mostly useful as a mild tranquilizer.

Myorelaxants such as dantrolene sodium (10 mg/kg p/o q24h) have been suggested as a useful treatment, but there is limited evidence of their effectiveness. Dantrolene sodium is hepatotoxic and therefore hepatic function should be monitored regularly.

After a few days free exercise in a small paddock, in-hand walking (5–10 minutes) can be reinstituted. A gradual return to exercise should only be resumed once enzyme levels are normal.

Prevention

✦ **Exercise regimen.** Provide regular, daily exercise (work or pasture); avoid complete rest for a full day. Avoid sudden changes in exercise regimen. Ensure adequate warm-up and cool-down periods before and after exercise, respectively; increase pace or level of exercise gradually. Avoid stress by standardizing daily routines and providing a good quiet environment.

✦ **Feeding practice.** Decrease energy (grain) intake. Provide good-quality hay and can use fat and good-quality protein diets, especially in cases of PSSM. Supplements containing selenium and vitamin E have been suggested, but remain controversial. Assess mineral imbalances in diet and correct as necessary.

✦ **Medical preventive treatments.** Acepromazine (0.01–0.02 mg/kg i/m 30 minutes before work) may be useful before exercise, especially when reintroducing work; dantrolene (2 mg/kg p/o q24h. for 3–5 days, then every other day) may also be used, although efficacy remains controversial.

Prognosis

The prognosis is variable, depending on severity, and there may be a number of sequelae (e.g. muscle atrophy and fibrosis if there is widespread necrosis). In most cases, prevention is fairly effective if the horse has only suffered one or a few episode(s). Recurrence is the rule in chronic forms. Preventive measures may help to keep the horse in activity, but are not always effective.

Fibrotic and ossifying myopathy
Definition/overview

This is a rare condition characterized by a severe muscle tear and subsequent formation of fibrous scar tissue (fibrotic myopathy) that may become mineralized (ossifying myopathy). It is encountered in Quarter horses and barrel racers and, rarely, in other breeds. It primarily affects the semitendinosus muscle and, less commonly, the semimembranosus, biceps femoris, and adductor muscles.

Etiology/pathophysiology

Fibrotic and ossifying myopathy are due to spontaneous trauma (muscle strain), probably through repeated overstretching of the muscle in association with rapid pivoting actions around the hind feet and sudden stop and slide actions. It may also be due to external trauma from ropes, kicks, falls, or secondary to a wound, intramuscular injection, or surgical trauma. There may initially be a hematoma, but chronic strain on the healing wound leads to muscle atrophy and the formation of exuberant fibrous tissue within the muscle, most commonly at the muscle/tendon junction. Recurrent inflammation may lead to osseous or fibocartilaginous metaplasia with associated mineralization (ossifying myopathy). A congenital form has been described in yearlings, supposedly through perinatal trauma.

Clinical presentation

In the acute form there may be an acute lameness with focal swelling over the caudal aspect of the thigh. In most cases the condition is encountered in the chronic stage. There is a typical mechanical lameness characterized by a 'slapping' action of the affected hindlimb. The stance and caudal phases of the stride are normal, but in the cranial phase (as the foot goes forward) the stride is suddenly interrupted, the foot being suddenly brought down and backward to slap the ground at the heels. This is due to restriction of the cranial phase by a functional shortening (or lack of stretching) of the caudal thigh muscles. The condition is usually unilateral, although occasionally bilateral, especially if secondary to external trauma to the caudal aspect of both thighs (e.g. in transport).

Differential diagnosis

Stringhalt, shivering, and wobbler's syndrome may have a similar presentation.

Diagnosis

Diagnosis is usually based on history, clinical examination, and observation of the typical gait. The anomaly may be less visible at the trot or canter. A mass or hard 'knot' may be palpable in the affected muscle. There is usually no improvement with the use of analgesic drugs. Ultrasonography is the diagnostic method of choice as it will confirm the presence of an echogenic or hyperechogenic lesion at the muscle/tendon junction (433,434). Mineralization may be visualized and the extent of the lesion (i.e. which muscle(s) are involved) can be determined. This is particularly useful if surgery is to be considered.

Management

In the acute stage the muscle tear may be treated conservatively with rest, NSAIDs, and local application of cold and massages. In the chronic, established stages, surgical treatment is the only option. Myotomy and myotenectomy (combined resection of a portion of muscle and tendon) have been described, but both procedures are associated with a high risk of complications (wound breakdown, recurrence, worsening). Myotenectomy is safer, but it may not provide complete resolution of the gait abnormality. More recently, tenotomy of the tendon of insertion of the semitendinosus muscle on the tibial tuberosity under general anesthesia has been recommended. This may require that a second incision is made over the common calcanean tendon in order to release the aponeurotic insertion of the semitendinosus muscle.

Prognosis

The prognosis for complete resolution is guarded. No improvement can be expected without surgery.

433, 434 Fibrotic and ossifying myopathy. Transverse (433) and longitudinal (434) ultrasound scans of the distocaudal thigh region showing loss of the normal echostructure of the semitendinosus muscle, which appears echogenic and amorphous (yellow arrows) because of diffuse fibrosis, and contains hyperechogenic areas casting acoustic shadowing (red arrows) characteristic of ectopic mineralization.

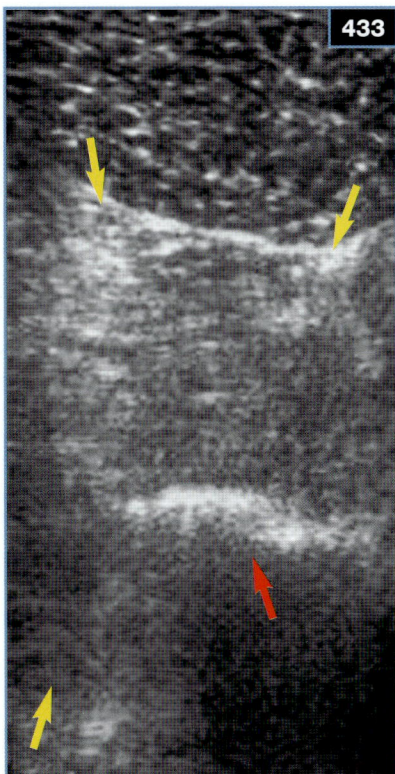
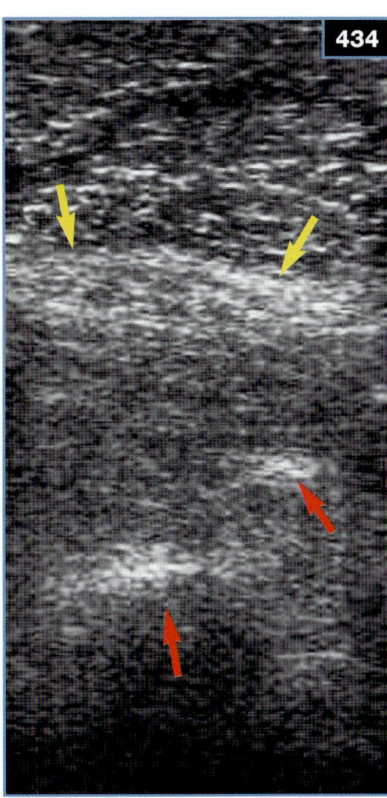

Clostridial myonecrosis

Definition/overview

Clostridial myonecrosis is an acute to peracute condition, characterized by rapid muscle necrosis due to infection by *Clostridium* spp. and associated with severe systemic disturbances (toxic shock). It is also referred to as 'clostridial myositis', 'malignant edema', 'gangrene', or 'clostridial cellulitis'.

Etiology/pathophysiology

The condition can be caused by contamination of a wound, necrotic area, or hematoma by Gram-positive anaerobes, including *C. perfringens*, *C. septicum*, and *C. chauvoei*. Often, several species are involved. It may be secondary to open or puncture wounds, but also to intramuscular or perivascular injections, especially of irritant substances (e.g. NSAIDs, thiopentone), which presumably cause local necrosis and activate dormant spores in the muscle. Contamination via the hematogenous route may also explain abscesses without apparent wound. The disease evolves as a poorly delineated cellulitis with severe, rapidly developing myonecrosis, abscess formation, and accumulation of gas. Severe systemic disturbances occur as a result of the release of exotoxins causing fever, septic shock, and death.

Clinical presentation

In peracute cases the animals present with sudden onset hyperthermia (40–41°C), recumbency, and signs of septic shock (increased cardiac and respiratory rates, congested mucous membranes, increased CRT). There may be localized edema and emphysema in the affected region (especially the neck, breast, or rump area) (435), and stiffness to severe lameness. The disease may evolve to coma and death.

In less severe cases there is hyperthermia, anorexia, and tachycardia. Localized signs may become more obvious, with painful, localized muscle swelling, crepitus, local heat, focal edema, and emphysema. The skin may eventually become cold and tense and exudate may ooze through a wound or fistula. The animal is usually very stiff and reluctant to move, depending on the affected muscle masses.

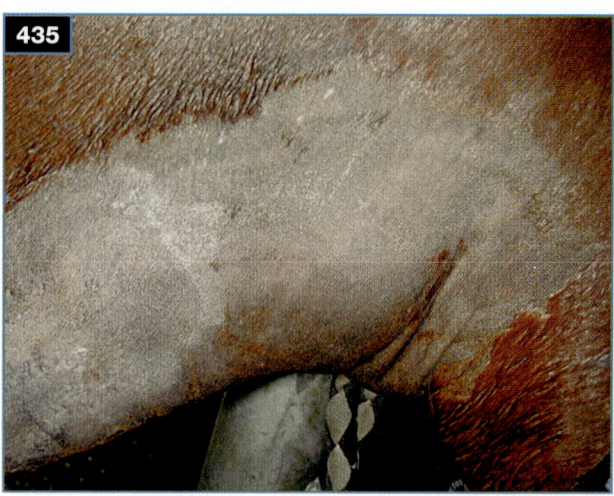

435 Clostridial abscess following a thrombophlebitis. The infection invaded the surrounding muscles and fascia.

Differential diagnosis

Colic; other causes of septic shock; exertional myopathy.

Diagnosis

Clinical examination will demonstrate suspicion of sepsis associated with local signs of myonecrosis and crepitus, especially with a history of a wound or intramuscular injection. Other causes of severe fever or septic shock should be ruled out. Blood tests usually reveal a mild to marked increase in muscle enzymes. Hypovolemia with increased hematocrit and protein concentration is indicative of toxic shock. In the subacute stage, hyperfibrinogenemia and neutropenia will become more obvious. Renal function should be evaluated.

Ultrasonography will reveal the myonecrosis and the presence of exudate (436) and, potentially, of gas (437). There is usually very marked edema in and around the affected muscle(s). An ultrasound-guided, fine-needle aspirate may help to confirm the presence of bacteria. The sample should be submitted for bacteriological examination, and immunofluorescence tests are available to confirm the clostridial infection.

Management

Aggressive fluid therapy (using lactated Ringer's or Hartmann's solutions) is warranted as a supportive measure. The animal should be given NSAIDs (e.g. flunixin meglumine 1.1 mg/kg i/v). Opioids may be used to control pain.

The intravenous administration of antibiotics (e.g. sodium penicillin, 22,000–40,000 IU/kg i/v q2–6h) is important. Combination with metronidazole (15–25 mg/kg p/o q6h) has been suggested, but poor tissue levels may limit its use. If the species can be isolated, specific antitoxin sera may be used.

Local treatment consisting of surgical exposure, debridement, and drainage of the necrotic area is essential. The wound may be left open or a drain can be left in place. Daily lavage of the wound with sterile saline is carried out to remove debris and improve drainage. The wound is left to heal by second intention.

Prevention

Careful antisepsis is warranted for any injection.

Prognosis

The prognosis is often guarded to poor, particularly in acute cases, where death is the most common outcome. Early, aggressive treatment can improve the prognosis and up to a 73% survival rate has been reported in one study.

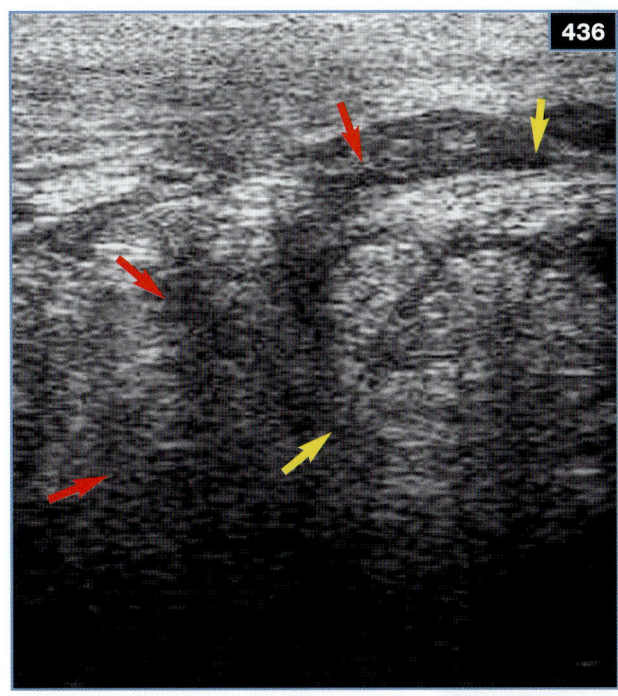
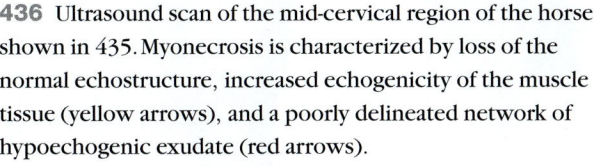

436 Ultrasound scan of the mid-cervical region of the horse shown in 435. Myonecrosis is characterized by loss of the normal echostructure, increased echogenicity of the muscle tissue (yellow arrows), and a poorly delineated network of hypoechogenic exudate (red arrows).

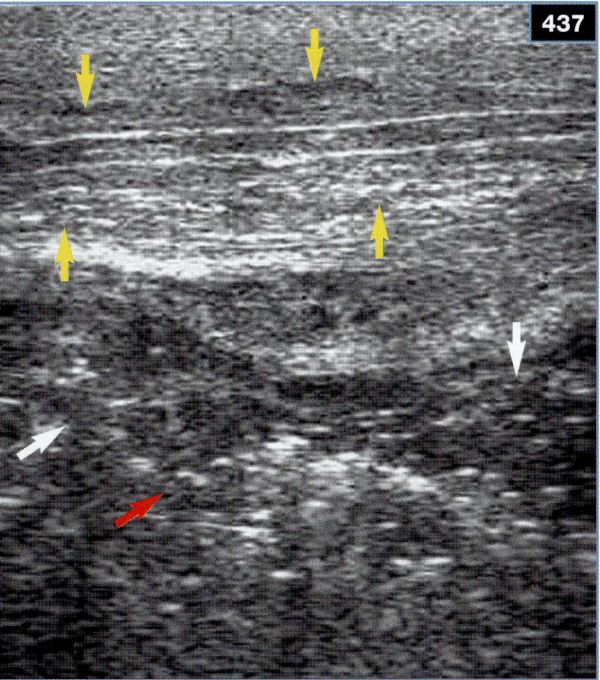

437 Ultrasound scan of the cranial cervical region of the horse shown in 435. There is extensive subcutaneous edema as shown by dissecting, hypoechogenic lines along the fascial planes (yellow arrows). Diffuse heterogeneous and hypoechogenic material within the muscle tissue represents exudate from the cellulitis (white arrows). The exudate contains numerous gas bubbles casting acoustic shadows and comet-tail artifacts (red arrow).

233

Corynebacterium pseudotuberculosis abscesses

Definition/overview

This is a condition characterized by spontaneously occurring intramuscular abscesses and muscle necrosis due to infection by *C. pseudotuberculosis*. It may be associated with ulcerative lymphangitis affecting one or several limbs. The condition is a rare cause of lameness, but it is rarely life threatening.

Etiology/pathophysiology

The abscesses are caused by hematogenous or lymphatic spread of *C. pseudotuberculosis*. There may be a predisposition for horses infested by *Habronema* spp. or other migrating parasite larvae to develop myonecrosis. A localized abscess forms within a muscle mass, most frequently in the pectoral region, but also in the limbs, inguinal region, ventral abdomen, and thorax. A miliary, subcutaneous form (multiple small abscesses in the subcutis) has also been described.

Clinical presentation

As for any other deep abscesses, there is usually local heat, pain, and swelling and there may be associated stiffness or lameness in one or more limbs depending on the location. Multiple small nodules and lymphangitis may be present (438–440). Systemic signs of infection (e.g. fever, anorexia) are rare.

Differential diagnosis

Larva migrans; abscesses of other origin, including brucellosis; tumors; reaction to injections or insect stings or snake bites.

Diagnosis

Diagnosis is based on clinical signs suggestive of a local abscess, with or without a fistula being present. Blood analysis may or may not show neutrophilia. Serology through a synergistic hemolysis inhibition test is useful for intra-abdominal or thoracic abscesses, but has proved unreliable for muscular abscesses. Ultrasonography can confirm the presence and extent of an abscess. It will also permit ultrasound-guided fine-needle aspirate for bacteriological analysis. Bacteriology provides a definitive diagnosis and allows for antibacterial sensitivity testing.

Management

NSAIDs are used for their analgesic properties. Systemic antibacterials (sodium penicillin i/v or procaine penicillin i/m are usually effective, but the antibacterial is best chosen according to sensitivity testing) are useful but not always necessary, except with multiple sites affected or concurrent lymphangitis.

Surgical treatment to expose, drain, and lavage the abscess is warranted. The incision may be carried out under ultrasonographic guidance and it is left to heal by second intention.

Prognosis

The prognosis is generally fair. Healing after drainage may be prolonged and there may be recurrence or delayed healing, but the condition is rarely life threatening and most often leaves no significant untoward effects.

438–440 *C. pseudotuberculosis* causing diffuse lymphangitis-like cellulitis and multiple muscle masses in the neck (438) and limbs (439, 440).

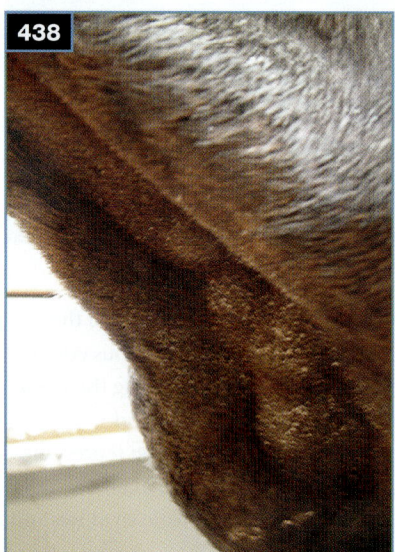
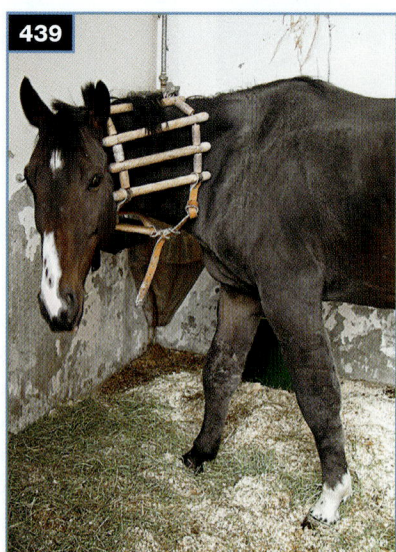
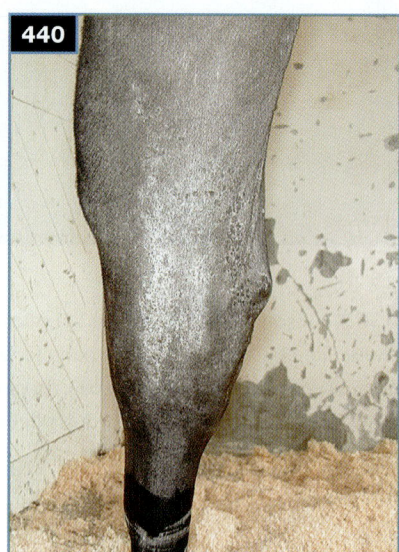

Musculoskeletal system

Hypocalcemia
Definition/overview
Hypocalcemia *per se* relates to a decreased blood calcium concentration causing a stiff gait, weakness, and multiple muscle fasciculation (spasms). This is associated either with lactation in the mare ('eclampsia' or 'lactation tetany') or with exertion, transport, stress ('stress' or 'transport tetany'), or severe metabolic disorders such as colic. It may be difficult to differentiate hypocalcemia from the 'exhausted horse syndrome' (see p. 236).

Etiology/pathophysiology
The recruiting of calcium in the milk of the mare at the peak of lactation (around 60–100 days post partum) predisposes to hypocalcemia, especially in case of stress of exertion, although this is relatively rare. It is most commonly encountered in horses undergoing severe stress and exertion, as in transport, especially in hot weather conditions. Poor dietary intake of calcium is probably a major predisposing factor. Intoxication by the cantharid beetle (found especially in alfalfa hay) may cause hypocalcemia.

Hypocalcemia leads to hyperexcitability of the muscle fibers, making them more sensitive to stimulation. Muscle tremor and 'cramps' occur, affecting skeletal muscles but also, in severe cases, the diaphragm ('flutter') and the heart muscle.

Clinical presentation
Increased muscular tone leads to generalized stiffness, hypometria, and muscle fasciculations and cramps, notably in the facial muscles (trismus, temporal, and masseter twitching), neck and trunk muscles, and occasionally in large proximal limb muscle masses. Muscular hyperactivity leads to hyperthermia and profuse sweating that can cause severe dehydration. If untreated, the disease may progress to diaphragmatic flutter, cardiac dysrhythmia, and, in severe cases, ataxia, recumbency, convulsions, and eventually death within 24–48 hours.

Differential diagnosis
Severe exertional rhabdomyolysis; tetanus; other causes of severe electrolyte imbalances; exhausted horse syndrome.

Diagnosis
The clinical signs are relatively typical. They are tetanus-like, but a medical history of vaccination and lack of a wound helps to orient the clinician towards a diagnosis of hypocalcemia. On blood analysis the serum ionized-calcium concentration should be ≥10 mmol/l. Signs become obvious below 8 mmol/l and severe below 5 mmol/l. Unfortunately, ionized-calcium analysis is not always available and total calcium levels are unreliable because the ionized fraction within the total level is affected by protein levels and acid–base balance. Other electrolytes (P, K, Cl, Na, and Mg) should also be assessed. There may be signs of dehydration and metabolic alkalosis.

Management
The treatment of choice consists of the intravenous administration of calcium gluconate solution (500 ml of 20% solution [for a 500 kg horse] diluted in 2 liters of 0.9% NaCl solution and given over 10–20 minutes). This dose may be repeated as required to effect.

Prevention
Analysis of the mineral intake in the feed and correction of Ca/P imbalances are paramount. Excess phosphates in the diet will prevent absorption of the calcium, thus worsening the situation. Predisposed horses and lactating mares should be protected from unnecessary stress or exertion.

Prognosis
The prognosis is usually good with prompt treatment, but severe forms may not respond to treatment.

Exhausted horse syndrome

Definition/overview

Exhausted horse syndrome is very similar to hypocalcemia. The condition relates to a syndrome of muscle hypercontractility induced by severe electrolyte and acid–base imbalance in horses after a period of hard, sustained exercise. It is most commonly encountered in endurance horses competing over long distances, and especially in hot weather.

Etiology/pathophysiology

The muscle fasciculations and 'cramps' are due to heavy losses of fluid and ions, including sodium, potassium, chloride, and calcium, through sweating. Fluid losses cause hypovolemia and hemoconcentration. Poor oxygenation of the muscles promotes an anaerobic metabolism, with subsequent lactate accumulation and consumption of the stored glycogen.

Clinical presentation

The disturbances provoke a myositis-like syndrome with a similar presentation to hypocalcemia or exertional rhabdomyolysis, although the serum calcium concentration is often normal and no myoglobinuria is noted.

Differential diagnosis

Hypocalcemia, exertional rhabdomyolysis, and various causes of colic should be considered.

Diagnosis

Clinical signs are similar to those of hypocalcemia, with fasciculations affecting the large skeletal muscle masses and generalized stiffness. Characteristically, the muscles are painful on palpation. There may be more or less obvious signs of systemic disturbances including dehydration, mucous membrane congestion, increased CRT, increased heart rate, and often hyperthermia. The animals may be dull or depressed and appear weak. On blood analysis the serum activity of muscle enzymes is often within normal limits or only slightly increased. The hematocrit and protein concentration are increased and an ionogram reveals hyponatremia, hypokalemia, and mild hypocalcemia (ionized fraction). There is usually metabolic alkalosis.

Management

Oral or, in severe cases, intravenous fluid therapy using balanced, polyionic solutions is warranted and is the treatment of choice to re-establish normal circulation. A more specific correction of electrolyte imbalance may be undertaken with care, including potassium (10 mEq/l). If present, hypocalcemia is treated as described above. Glucose should be added to the fluids (10 g/l). It may be useful to cool down the animal using cold showering. The animal should be kept in a cool, dark, and calm environment.

Prevention

It is paramount to provide water regularly during strenuous exercise and to use adequate electrolyte supplements in the water (prior to, during, and after a race, for instance).

Prognosis

The prognosis is usually good with adequate care, but severe cardiovascular shock may lead to organ failure and eventually to death.

Diaphragmatic flutter

Definition/overview

Diaphragmatic flutter is caused by a synchronous contraction of the cardiac and diaphragmatic muscles. The condition may be observed in exerted animals as a consequence of severe imbalances (see hypocalcemia and exhausted horse syndrome above).

Etiology/pathophysiology

Supposedly, severe metabolic and electrolyte imbalance leads to phrenic nerve hyperexcitability. This consequently responds to stimulation by atrial depolarization waves as they course alongside the heart. The diaphragm is therefore submitted to violent contractions at each heartbeat.

Clinical presentation

Brisk, sudden, and painful contraction of the diaphragm is visible at the costal arch and flank. This typical sign may occur in isolation or, more commonly, in association with other disturbances as described in hypocalcemia and exhausted horse syndrome.

Differential diagnosis
Hypocalcemia and exhausted horse syndrome may produce similar signs.

Diagnosis
Typical rhythmic contractions of the flanks synchronously with the heartbeats are seen on clinical examination.

Management
The condition disappears if the underlying anomalies are treated and corrected.

Prevention
(See Prevention of hypocalcemia and exhausted horse syndrome, above.) It has been suggested that food rich in calcium (e.g. alfalfa hay) should be avoided in predisposed animals and in endurance horses.

Prognosis
The prognosis is good if the primary problem can be addressed.

Nutritional myodegeneration
Definition/overview
Nutritional myodegeneration (white muscle disease) is a disease characterized by skeletal and cardiac muscle degeneration. It affects primarily foals of less than 1 year of age, although a rare occurrence in adults has been reported. It is caused by a dietary deficiency of selenium and vitamin E, but there are probably other factors involved in horses.

Etiology/pathophysiology
Nutritional myodegeneration is rare in Equidae. It is most commonly encountered in foals from birth to 1 year of age, apparently as a consequence of selenium-deficient diets during gestation in the dams. Selenium-poor soil and pastures (< 0.05 ppm), or succinoxidase inhibitors in grass or hay, which interfere with vitamin E, may be involved. These substances are important for the integrity of muscle cell membranes. Supposedly, a deficiency will promote degeneration, especially as a result of anaerobic metabolism in muscle cells. Increased intake of unsaturated fats in the milk or diet and strenuous exercise appear to be predisposing factors for the development of nutritional myodegeneration.

Clinical presentation
The presentation varies with age. In neonates, generalized weakness and difficulty to rise can progress to recumbency. There may be associated dysphagia, with resultant inhalation pneumonia.

In older foals (several months of age) the disease follows a period of brisk exercise and may lead to subacute or acute signs. In the milder, subacute form, the animals present with a stilted gait and stiff neck carriage. They may become recumbent after a few hours. The muscle masses are swollen and painful and subcutaneous edema may be observed over the rump, neck, and ventral abdominal/thoracic wall. Myoglobinuria is generally observed. In a more acute form, the foals show a sudden onset of recumbency shortly after exercise. Death occurs within 4–5 hours due to heart failure and/or pulmonary edema.

In adult horses the condition has been reported to cause colic, muscle stiffness and soreness, and edema of the head and neck. Myoglobinuria is also observed. The disease may be lethal due to cardiac failure.

Differential diagnosis
In foals, any cause of sudden onset of recumbency such as septicemia, colic, and tetanus should be considered. In adults, exertional rhabdomyolysis is an important differential diagnosis.

Diagnosis
A strong suspicion is based on the clinical signs and the observation of myoglobinuria. Confirmation of the disease is obtained through blood analysis and the measurement of serum vitamin E and selenium concentrations. Measurement of erythrocyte glutathione peroxidase activity may be more accurate. In acute cases, AST, LDH, and CK show a similar increase to that observed in rhabdomyolysis. Postmortem examination reveals the skeletal muscles as typically pale, with or without white streaks. Subcutaneous edema and brown fatty tissue are observed.

Management/prevention
The specific treatment involves injection of selenium and vitamin E (50 µg selenium and 100 mg vitamin E/kg i/m or slow i/v q24h), but this is rarely effective in very acute cases. Supportive therapy with intravenous fluids and NSAIDs is warranted. Oral selenium and vitamin E supplementation may be efficacious in more chronic cases. A daily dietary intake of 10 µg/kg selenium and 2–5 mg/kg vitamin E is recommended for prevention. Mares should be given oral supplements through the last term of gestation and during lactation. In endurance horses, high doses have been recommended, but the optimal dose rates have not been well defined. Selenite is not an adequate form of selenium as it is poorly bioavailable.

Prognosis
The prognosis is poor in acute forms, but fair if treated adequately in subacute and chronic cases.

Muscular injuries

Definition/overview
Muscle injuries are common but poorly understood causes of lameness and poor performance.

Etiology/pathophysiology
Injuries most commonly occur in equine athletes such as racehorses, showjumpers, eventers, and Western horses. Varying degrees of muscle damage may lead to pain and strain or even tearing of the tissue.

Clinical presentation
Acute muscle damage and subsequent hemorrhage/inflammation may lead to lameness and palpable swelling/heat/pain in affected muscles if superficial. Deeper muscle injuries will not be palpable.

In the forelimb the most commonly affected sites are the biceps brachii, the brachiocephalicus and pectoral muscles, and the superficial digital flexor muscle/tendon junction. In the hindlimb the semimembranosus and semitendinosus, adductor, gluteal, quadriceps, and gastrocnemius muscles are most commonly involved. Muscle spasm and pain are common in the thoracolumbar region (441) secondary to a hindlimb lameness or primary spinal or sacroiliac injury.

Diagnosis
History and clinical examination are important, especially palpation of affected muscles for pain, swelling, and spasm in acute cases and atrophy/fibrosis in chronic cases. Visual appraisal is useful. Full lameness examination is paramount. Muscle-stimulating machines may identify specific muscle injuries. Thermography, nuclear scintigraphy, and ultrasonography can all help locate the site of injury and, in the latter, determine the extent of damage (442, 443). Serum muscle enzymes are rarely useful in such cases.

Management
The type of treatment depends on the specific injury and the stage at which it is diagnosed. Acute injuries may benefit from cold therapies and NSAID therapy. Many of the treatments involve physiotherapy techniques and machines (e.g. laser, therapeutic ultrasound, TENS, electromagnetic therapy, massage, stretching, and manipulation). These are combined with box rest and a controlled graduated exercise program once the acute stages are over. Resolution of the primary problem is essential before any secondary muscle injury can be treated.

Prognosis
This depends on the extent, severity, and chronicity of the specific muscle injury. It varies from good to more guarded in chronic injuries secondary to other problems.

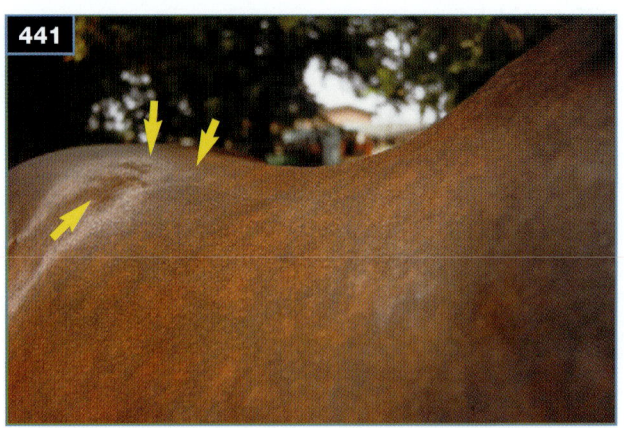

441 Focal swelling due to a spasm (clonic contraction) of the longissimus dorsi. This was found to be secondary to chronic hindlimb lameness from distal intertarsal OA.

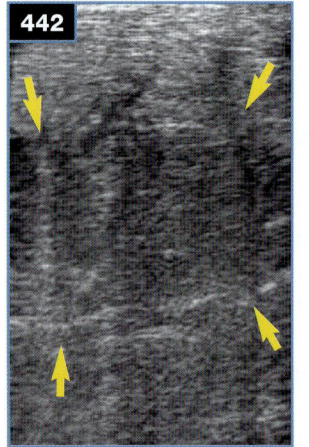 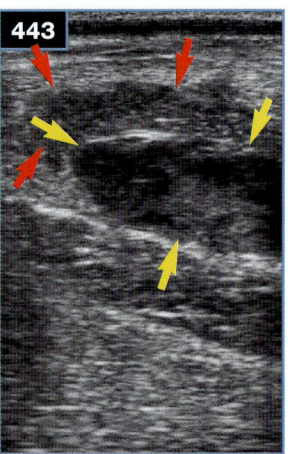

442 Ultrasound scan of the ascending pectoral muscle on the craniomedial aspect of the forelimb, showing an area of diffuse decrease in echogenicity and loss of normal muscle architecture (arrows). This is indicative of a partial tear and granulation tissue reaction within the torn portion of muscle.

443 Longitudinal ultrasound scan of the distal part of the triceps muscle in the caudal upper forelimb area of a horse presenting with acute, sudden-onset lameness and pain on flexion of the elbow. There is a large, anechogenic hematoma at the musculotendinous junction (junction between the muscle belly and aponeurosis) (yellow arrows). The distal part of the muscle appears hypoechogenic and heterogeneous because of fiber retraction, cell infiltration, and necrosis (red arrows). This appearance is typical of a complete muscle tear.

Myotonia

Definition/overview

Myotonia is a rare, nonprogressive condition, probably with a genetic component, characterized by sustained, prolonged muscle contractions and stiffness, more obvious after a period of rest. The condition usually occurs in foals less than 1 year of age.

Etiology/pathophysiology

The etiology is unknown, but probably involves mutation of a gene encoding for a sarcolemmal chloride channel, although it has not been identified. This leads to abnormal neuromuscular conduction and muscle hyperexcitability. Sustained, exaggerated clonic contractions (myoclonia) result from normal stimuli.

Clinical presentation

The foals are lame or very stiff, especially immediately after a period of rest. There may be obvious, symmetrical muscular hypertrophy. Percussion, dimpling, and prolonged muscle contractions are typically observed, either spontaneously or elicited by manipulation of the limbs. Worsening of the signs with time is not usually noted.

Differential diagnosis

Wobbler's syndrome, nutritional myodegeneration, and hypocalcemia should be considered.

Diagnosis

Clinical examination

Dimpling and spasmic contractions on percussion of muscle masses is typical. The main differential diagnosis is myotonic dystrophy, but histologic examination will usually help to differentiate between the two conditions.

Blood analysis

Usually, no significant abnormalities are observed.

Electromyography

Myotonic discharges and high-frequency bursts are noted in certain muscles during needle insertion, movement, or percussion.

Muscle biopsy

Histologic examination reveals few or no abnormalities of muscle morphology.

Management

No treatment is available.

Prognosis

The prognosis is poor for sports activities, but good for survival.

Equine myotonic dystrophy

Definition/overview

Equine myotonic dystrophy is a rare condition, probably with a genetic component, characterized by sustained spasms and muscle contractions as in myotonia, particularly in the gluteal and hindlimb region. It has mostly been described in young Quarter horses and in one horse of Anglo-Arab lineage.

Etiology/pathophysiology

A genetic cause is thought to be involved, but the etiology and pathogenesis are unclear. It is similar to an inherited form of myotonic dystrophy in man.

Clinical presentation

The condition usually affects foals over 4 months of age or young horses. Marked muscular hypertrophy of the hindquarters is usually described. Prolonged muscle contractions (myotonia) are elicited by manipulation of the limbs and they occur spontaneously during locomotion. There may be generalized muscle weakness, stumbling, and multiple tendon contractures. Generalized muscle atrophy, functional kyphosis or scoliosis of the dorsal spine, pendulous abdomen, colic, and testicular atrophy have been described.

Differential diagnosis

Wobbler's syndrome and myotonia may have a similar presentation.

Diagnosis

The clinical examination is as for myotonia, but often with more severe signs. A characteristic is dimpling that occurs following percussion. This condition may worsen with time. Blood analysis is unremarkable. Electromyography is as for myotonia. Histologic examination of a muscle biopsy, unlike in myotonia, demonstrates moderate to severe dystrophic changes in muscle morphology, notably fiber size, type I muscle fiber hypertrophy, increased perimyseal and endomyseal connective tissue, muscle necrosis, and inflammatory cell infiltration.

Management

No successful treatment is available.

Prevention

Affected animals should not be bred.

Prognosis

The condition may be progressive, so euthanasia may be necessary in some cases.

Atypical myopathy (myoglobinuria)

Definition/overview

Equine atypical myopathy (AM) was first identified in 1984 in the UK. It affects horses grazing most of the day in the autumn and/or spring and is frequently fatal. It has been sporadically reported from countries all over Europe, including in recent years the Benelux countries and Spain, and also possibly the USA.

Etiology/pathophysiology

The etiology and pathophysiology are still incompletely understood, but recent epidemiologic studies have determined horse and pasture factors that are associated with AM. Sex, breed, and type of animal are not factors, but age (<3 years or >20 years old), poor to normal condition, lack of work, autumn and spring grazing, adverse weather (strong winds and rain), minimum daily temperatures (0–8°C), certain pastures (permanent pastures that are bare and with humid areas, streams, or rivers within them, had previous cases of AM, areas with dead leaf accumulation), hay fed at pasture, and mechanical harrowing of the pasture are all considered possible predisposing factors. Postmortem examination of AM cases may reveal few macroscopic lesions, although some respiratory and postural muscles (e.g. masseter, brachiocephalic, biceps, infra- and supraspinatus, gluteal) may have pale areas within them. Histopathology performed on frozen muscle samples reveals specific features of accumulation of neutral lipid in type 1 muscle fibers that have undergone a specific type of necrosis and degeneration. These histopathologic findings suggest that the causal agent of AM may induce a dysfunction of oxidative mitochondrial metabolism in the muscle fibers.

Clinical presentation

Clinical signs are acute in onset and include weakness and stiffness, especially of the hindquarters, depression and lethargy, lateral recumbency, myoglobinuria, respiratory difficulties with tachypnea and dyspnea, trembling and sweating, very little sign of pain, hypothermia, and unexplained death at pasture. Less frequent signs include colic, icteric mucous membranes, sometimes with bleeding, dysphagia, head edema, and dysuria with a distended bladder on rectal examination.

Differential diagnosis

Other causes of acute myopathies and myoglobinuria; respiratory difficulty; colic; sudden death; recumbency.

Diagnosis

Diagnosis is based on clinical signs along with laboratory and histopathologic postmortem findings. There is evidence of severe muscle damage with very elevated serum CK, AST, and LDH levels. Serum electrolyte levels are often unaffected and hematology results are inconsistent, but hypocalcemia, hyperglycemia, and high levels of serum triacylglycerols are common.

Management

The possibility of bacterial or fungal toxins as causal agents is reflected in the suggested treatment regimens. The aim is to limit the acute rhabdomyolysis process. Unfortunately, even with very intensive therapy the response is poor. Treatments proposed include oral metronidazole for clostridial infection; broad-spectrum antibiotics; intravenous balanced electrolyte, calcium borogluconate and 5% glucose solutions; insulin and heparin to control the hyperlipidemia and hyperglycemia; vitamin B2; antioxidants such as selenium and vitamins C and E; dantrolene sodium by slow i/v injection; NSAIDs for analgesia; and oxygen administration.

Management is very important and the movement of affected horses should be minimized, although if they are still standing, they should be moved to a stable to allow better care to be available. Affected animals should be kept warm, their bladder emptied regularly, be regularly turned if recumbent, and fed concentrates if still able to eat. This can be maintained unless there is evidence of severe dyspnea (lowered PaO_2), when euthanasia should be considered. Pasture companions of affected cases should be checked regularly and moved to stables, especially the youngest. They should be fed concentrates and kept away from affected pastures in the spring and autumn.

Prognosis

The mortality rate varies from 65–85%, with death occurring within 3–72 hours (mean 26 hours). The few survivors either progress rapidly to full recovery or suffer considerable muscle wastage with prolonged convalescence. An absence of expiratory dyspnea is thought to be a major prognostic factor for survival.

Reproductive system

1   Female reproductive tract
    Graham Munroe, Madeleine Campbell, Zoë Munroe, and Matthew Hanks

2   Male reproductive tract
    Theresa Burns, Tracey Chenier, and Graham Munroe

3   Equine castration
    Luis Lamas and Graham Munroe

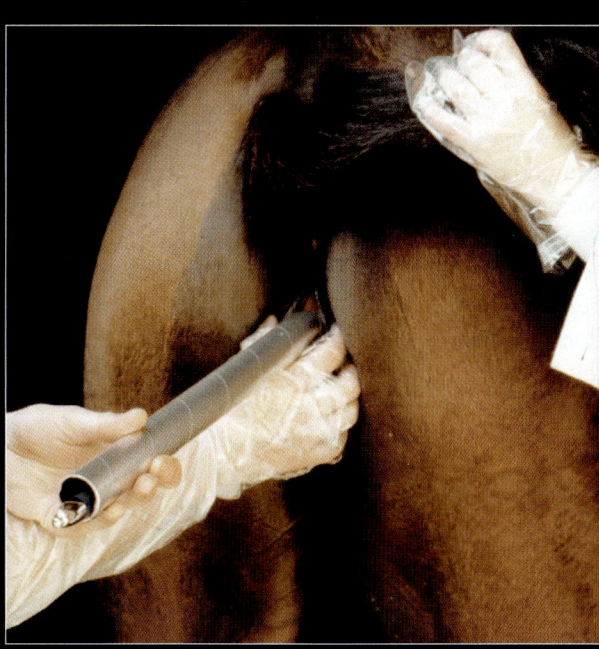

Normal reproductive system

Reproductive seasonality

Mares, like other domestic animals, have an estrous cycle that is a coordinated series of anatomic, endocrine, and behavioral changes that eventually lead to ovulation. Mares are seasonally polyestrus breeders, meaning that they have multiple estrous cycles during a 'breeding season'. Most mares are 'long day' or spring/summer/early autumn breeders, although about 20% of mares continue to ovulate throughout the winter months. The majority of mares enter a period when they stop cycling, known as anestrus, during the winter months. Photoperiod or day length is the most important factor influencing this seasonality and ovarian activity, but the transition between cyclicity, non-cyclicity, and back again is gradual. The effect of the day length is mediated by the hormone melatonin, produced by the pineal gland. Short winter days lead to high melatonin secretion and suppressed gonadotropin-releasing hormone (GnRH) levels from the hypothalamus. With increased day length the periods of high melatonin production decrease, leading to increased pulses of GnRH, which stimulate follicle-stimulating hormone (FSH) and luteinizing hormone (LH) production.

In terms of increased ovarian activity, mares seem to respond best to a photoperiod of around 15–16 hours (i.e. summer). The period from the first spring ovulation to the last in the autumn is the ovulatory phase of the cycle. The periods between the anestrus and the ovulatory phases, which occur in the early spring or late autumn, are called the transition phases. These are associated with periods of no, irregular, or prolonged estrous behavior.

The estrous cycle

During the winter months, in the majority of mares there is a period of anestrus, characterized by small firm ovaries with minimal follicular activity. The uterus is atonic and thin walled, with a pale, dry, and partially relaxed cervix. The mare is neither receptive towards nor rejects the stallion. Levels of LH are low and levels of FSH fluctuate randomly. Plasma progesterone levels are <1 ng/ml, due to the absence of any corpora lutea.

As day length increases, there is an increase in ovarian activity and the mare enters the 'spring transitional' stage of her annual cycle. In the spring the ovaries develop numerous follicles of varying sizes that grow, regress, and do not ovulate. These can be palpated per rectum as the 'small bunches of grapes' ovaries noted in the literature. Initially, the uterus and cervix remain pale and thin walled, but as activity increases there is greater edema of the tract.

Eventually, a follicle progresses through to maturity and ovulates, thereby initiating the ovulatory phase. Plasma FSH levels rise early in the transitional period, causing follicular development, but steadily fall approximately 15–20 days prior to the first ovulation. Plasma luteinizing concentrations are initially low, meaning ovulation will not occur, but they increase slowly until a few days immediately prior to the first true estrus, with a peak around ovulation. Developing follicles in the ovary produce estrogen, but in the transitional mare their levels are not high enough to trigger rises in GnRH and LH, which will lead to the first ovulation. Eventually, a follicle does develop sufficiently to trigger these changes and the mare will show estrous behavior and ovulate. Once the first ovulation has occurred, the mare usually continues to ovulate regularly throughout the remainder of the ovulatory season. The sometimes prolonged transitional phase before a mare starts to ovulate regularly each spring can cause problems for breeders who are keen to breed early foals. This is particularly acute in the northern hemisphere Thoroughbred industry because of the imposed breeding season, which starts in February, at which time only approximately 30% of mares are naturally cycling. This contrasts with the physiologic breeding season for the mare, which starts around March to April in the northern hemisphere (August to mid-September in the southern hemisphere) and runs through to the early autumn. Unnecessary, repeated breeding during this transitional phase can be minimized by careful management and this will avoid contaminating mares and over-using stallions.

During the ovulatory phase the mare develops a cyclic pattern individual to herself and notorious for its inconsistency as compared with other domestic species (e.g. ovulation without estrous behavior, estrus without ovulation, split estrus). The durations of the various components of the cycle are shown below. They show great variability, especially in the transition periods in spring and autumn:

✦ **Estrous cycle**: time period from one ovulation to another; 19–24 days, average 21 days.
✦ **Estrus**: time when the mare shows 'heat', is receptive to the stallion, and stands to be mated; 4–9 days, average 6 days.
✦ **Diestrus**: time between estrus periods when the mare is not receptive to the stallion; 12–16 days, average 14 days.

Ovulation is generally considered to occur approximately 24 hours before the end of estrus, often during the evening or night.

Hormonal changes in the estrous cycle
Early luteal phase
Ovulation and subsequent luteinization result in the formation of a corpus luteum/corpora lutea (CL) and a rapid rise in plasma progesterone. The corpus hemorrhagicum is palpable per rectum for the first 2–3 days after ovulation and the CL can be detected by ultrasonographic scanning for the entire luteal phase. A combination of rising progesterone and low estrogen results in non-receptive behavior and characteristic changes to the genital tract (cervix and uterus become firm or are said to have 'tone').

Mid luteal phase
High progesterone concentration (8–10 ng/ml) leads to a negative feedback on GnRH, causing a decrease in its pulsatile secretion from the hypothalamus. This decrease in GnRH results in inhibition of LH release, but still stimulates release of FSH from the pituitary. FSH release causes waves of follicles to develop. The mare is still non-receptive.

Late luteal phase
Prostaglandin F$_2$ alpha (PGF$_2\alpha$) is released from the endometrium and causes regression of the CL (luteolysis) and so a decline in serum progesterone. Falling progesterone removes the negative feedback on GnRH release. The increased pulse frequency of GnRH increases LH release. Rising LH levels cause follicular growth, maturation, and ovulation. The dominant follicle produces estrogen and inhibin. The latter inhibits the growth of non-dominant follicles. The uterine tone begins to decrease.

Follicular phase
The combination of falling progesterone and rising estrogen results in estrus behavior and increasing receptivity. There are corresponding changes to the genital tract (uterus becomes 'flaccid' and soft with edema, the cervix relaxes and softens, and there are increased secretions). There is gradual growth of the primary follicle/s evident on rectal palpation and ultrasound. Estrogen level reaches a threshold, which results in a positive feedback on LH release, causing a surge in LH, which is responsible for ovulation. Ovulation occurs at the hilar or ovulation fossa.

Identifying the stage of the estrous cycle
Accurate and early recognition of the stage of the estrous cycle in the mare is a central part of modern stud-farm management. A number of techniques are used, often in combination.

Visual inspection and observation of behavioral changes
Often practiced by individual mare owners or where teaser animals are not available.

Teasing
The mare is exposed to a teaser, which is usually a pony or non-valuable stallion, and her behavior assessed for evidence of receptivity. There are many different teasing methods (444).

The signs of estrus when teased by a stallion are: quiet and calm; ears forward; nuzzling; posturing; moving towards the teaser; squatting and frequent squirts of urine; raising tail; eversion of vulval lips and clitoris (winking).

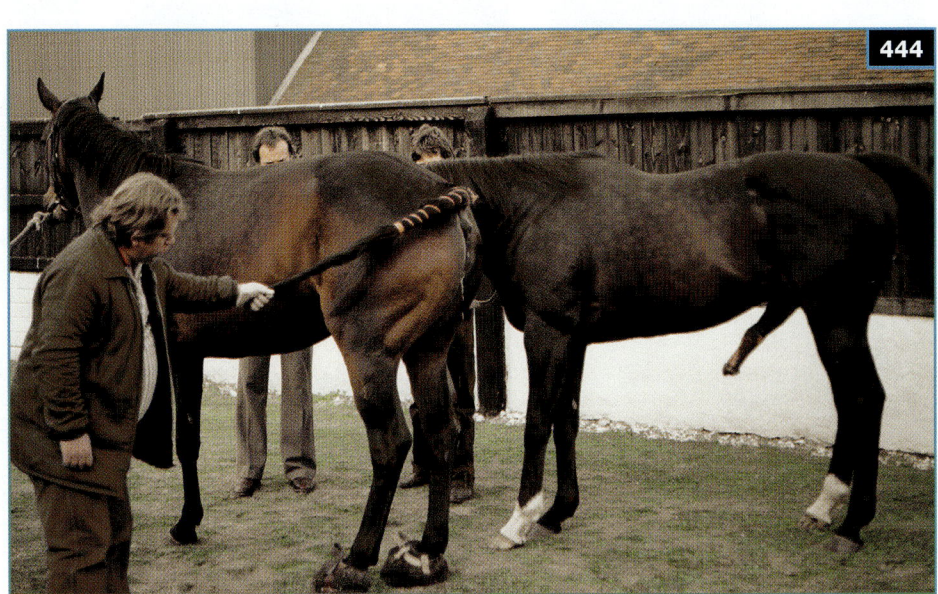

444 Teasing of a Thoroughbred mare by a stallion prior to natural covering. Note the restrained mare with a nose twitch and padded boots on the hind feet. The stallion is presented to the mare from the side to minimize the chances of being kicked.

Female reproductive tract

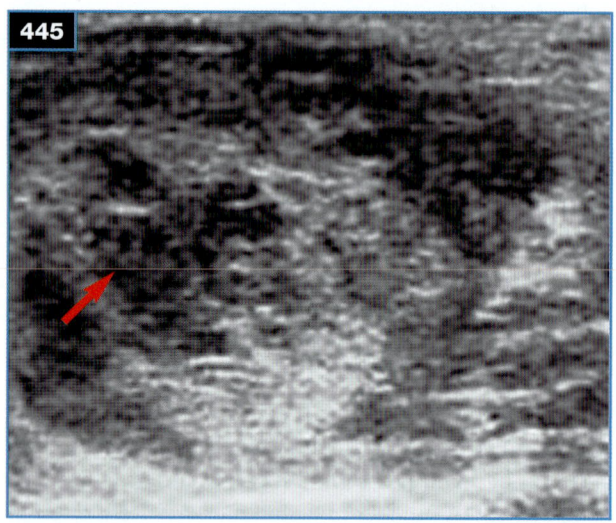

445 Ultrasonographic image of an ovary showing an early developing corpus luteum (arrow). (Photo courtesy T Chenier)

446 Ultrasonographic image of the ovary of a mare revealing a mature corpus luteum with a central cystic structure (arrow). (Photo courtesy T Chenier)

447 Transverse transrectal ultrasonographic image of a uterine horn showing marked endometrial edema during estrus. (Photo courtesy T Chenier)

448 Transverse transrectal ultrasonographic image of a uterine horn showing marked endometrial edema and intraluminal fluid. (Photo courtesy T Chenier)

The expression of teasing behavior can be variable and some mares may need to be 'broken down' by the stallion, which involves the stallion stimulating the mare by nuzzling etc. Maiden mares and mares with a foal at foot will often tease poorly due to fear and uncertainty.

Teasing is a major management method for identifying mares in heat. It is important to note that teasing is a poor predictor of ovulation, but is very useful in differentiating estrus from diestrus. Inadequate teasing can affect reproductive performance on broodmare farms.

Rectal palpation

Rectal palpation is commonly used to determine the stage of the cycle in the mare. Cervical and uterine tone and follicular size and firmness are assessed. Uterine tone is prominent and the cervix is closed (cigar like) when there are high levels of circulating progesterone. Uterine tone is soft and the cervix open and relaxed when there are high levels of circulating estrogen and low levels of progesterone. The ovary will be enlarged with follicular development.

Transrectal ultrasonographic examination

Ultrasound can provide the following information:
- Presence or absence of CL (445, 446).
- Follicle size, shape, and echogenicity.
- Presence of endometrial edema (447).
- Pathology such as uterine fluid (448), endometrial cysts.

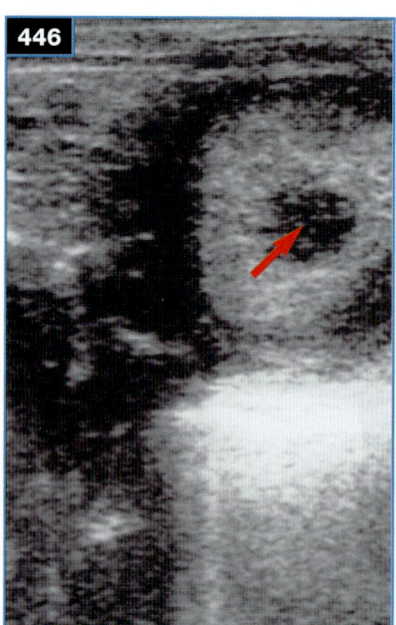

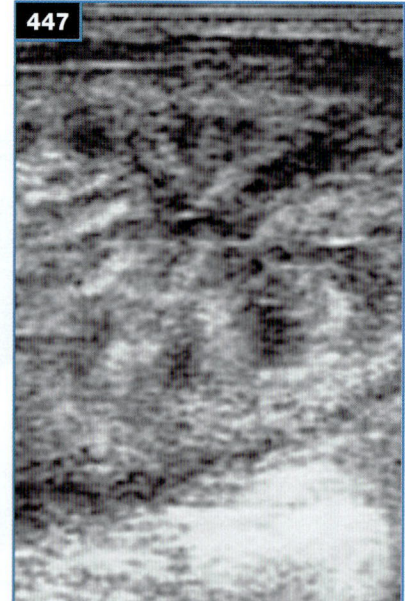

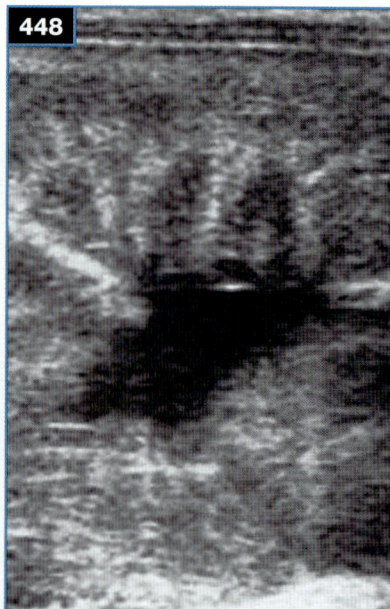

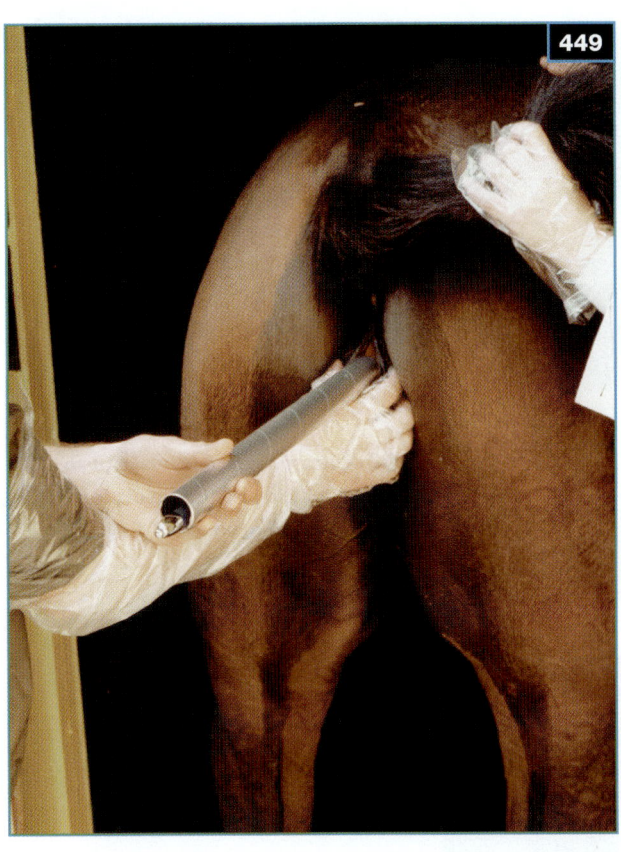

449

449 Introduction of a sterile disposable vaginal speculum to allow visualization of the vagina and cervix and collection of uterine swabs.

A follicle of around 20–30 mm in diameter usually accompanies early estrus. There may also be uterine edema present. Progressive enlargement of the follicle to 40 mm or greater is associated with impending ovulation.

Vaginoscopy
A speculum is passed into the vagina and a visual inspection of the anterior vagina and external os of the cervix is made (449). During estrus the cervix becomes increasingly hyperemic, edematous, and relaxed (pink to red, moist, swollen, and lying on the vaginal floor). In diestrus the cervix becomes paler, dry, tightly closed, and elevated off the vaginal floor.

Endocrinology
Serum progesterone concentration: >1 ng/ml in diestrus; <1 ng/ml in estrus.

Records
Records can be used to predict when a mare is likely to return to estrus following her last known estrus. A mare can be expected to tease at about 14–16 days after the last day of her last estrus (of course this will NOT apply if she is pregnant). Records allow the clinician to pick the best time to concentrate on teasing and palpating a particular mare.

The difficulty of ovulation prediction in the mare
The mare has a relatively long estrus period (5–7 days) and ovulation normally occurs at around 24 hours before the end of the estrus period. No single method exists to predict reliably the precise moment of ovulation; however, the following criteria are of use:

+ *Size of ovulating follicle.* Follicles grow at 3–5 mm/ day during estrus and very few follicles ovulate within 24 hours when <33 mm in diameter. The size of the follicle at ovulation is NOT determined by the size of the mare. Small ponies will ovulate with the same size follicles as large draft breeds.
+ *Change in consistency of ovulating follicle.* Consistency changes from a tense, tight sphere to a soft, fluctuant structure occur in 85–90% of pre-ovulatory follicles.

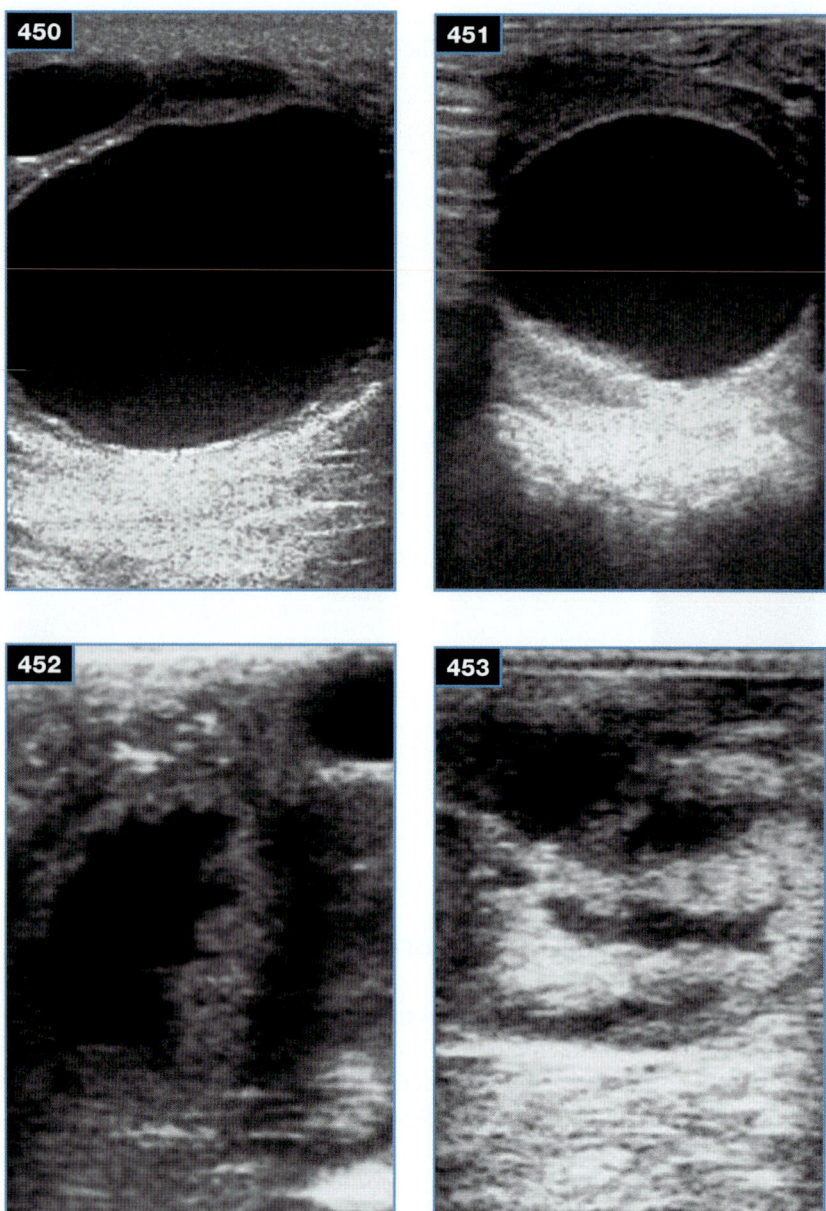

450 Ultrasonographic image of an ovary of a mare in estrus showing a large developing follicle. (Photo courtesy T Chenier)

451 Ultrasonographic image of an ovarian follicle just prior to ovulation. (Photo courtesy T Chenier)

452 Ultrasonographic image of an ovarian follicle during ovulation. (Photo courtesy T Chenier)

453 Ultrasonographic image of an ovarian follicle just after ovulation has occurred. (Photo courtesy T Chenier)

+ ***Change in shape of ovulating follicle.*** A change in shape (detected on ultrasound examination) from a round shape to a pear or conical shape indicates impending ovulation. However, this may not be seen in all follicles and occurs in 85–90% of pre-ovulatory follicles (450–453).
+ ***Change in endometrial edema.*** Edema (detected on ultrasound examination) is maximal at around 1–2 days prior to ovulation and starts to decline in prominence around 24 hours prior to ovulation.

It is important to collate all information in order to help make an estimation of when the mare will ovulate and therefore when to breed her. Fertility is highest when mares are bred within a window from 48 hours prior to ovulation to 6 hours post ovulation (although it is possible to achieve conception up to 20 hours post ovulation).

Examination of the female reproductive tract

A breeding soundness examination (BSE) is performed in the mare to determine a mare's suitability as a broodmare and to identify causes of infertility. Certain parts of the examination are routinely performed during the breeding season as part of the monitoring of the appropriate breeding time in normal mares. Some indications for a BSE are listed below:

✦ Age: >12 years of age.
✦ Examination before undertaking expensive artificial insemination (AI) (especially frozen semen)/embryo transfer program (donors and recipients).
✦ Repeat breeder.
✦ Repeated early embryonic death.
✦ Problem foaling.
✦ History of endometritis/metritis.
✦ Prepurchase examination of a breeding mare.

History

It is essential to collect and record a full history of the mare in general and specifically her reproductive performance. Details of the type of work the horse has previously undertaken, or is undertaking if still performing, should be noted along with any drugs used or injuries incurred. Any history of abnormal estrous cycles while in training can be significant to future breeding abilities. The age of a mare may influence her breeding efficiency (i.e. young mares may be sexually immature or abnormally cycling). Older mares may have declining fertility from 12 years of age onwards due to previous reproductive injuries or wear and tear. A detailed reproductive history should include the number of foals bred (live or dead); the incidence of dystocia, retained fetal membranes, abortions, early embryonic death; breeding history with note of previous fertility or infertility, twins, and history of endometritis; sexual behavior, especially the mare's estrous cycle; treatment history including drugs used and surgery performed; and laboratory results.

Knowledge of the fertility of the sires previously used, as well as the current stallion, plus the method to be used for insemination are important factors to assess.

The general physical condition of the mare should be appraised as poor condition or obesity can affect fertility. Systemic illness such as Cushing's disease may affect the ability to conceive, while other conditions such as chronic laminitis, chronic lower respiratory tract disease or ventral hernias may affect the mare's ability to carry a foal to term safely. Poor diet and other management factors (e.g. stress) can significantly affect fertility rates.

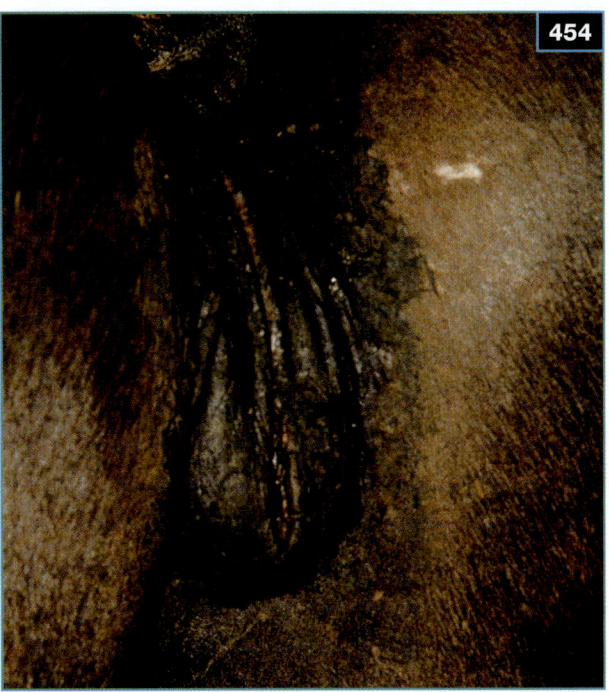

454 Assessment of the vulval conformation of the mare is an essential part of the breeding soundness examination. This aged Thoroughbred mare has a sloping upper part of the vulva, with cranial migration of the anus. The vulval lips are well apposed and have good tone.

Reproductive examination
External genitalia

There are three main anatomic barriers that maintain the integrity of the caudal reproductive tract: the vulva including its labia, constrictor muscles, and perineal body; the vestibular sphincter including the constrictor muscles of the vestibule; and the cervix. These barriers block the aspiration of air and contaminants into the reproductive tract. During estrus the cervix is relaxed and during coitus the vestibular sphincter temporarily relaxes to allow entry of the stallion's penis. Other mechanisms (e.g. uterine contractions and immune-mediated reactions) are thus also important in protecting the reproductive tract against infection.

It is very important to assess the vulval/perineal conformation and to observe any vulval discharge (454). Anatomic alignment of the perineal and pelvic conformation is important for breeding soundness and should be assessed from the back and side. Placing a finger horizontally on the posterior tip of the bony pelvic brim adjacent to the vulval lips allows the clinician to assess where the dorsal vulval commissure is in relation to the bony pelvic brim and also the angle of the vulval commissure. The integrity of the vulval lips needs to be assessed and any injuries noted. Defective vulval conformation (VC) is related to a sunken anus and atrophy of the perineal body. It is more common in older, pluriparous mares that have had repeated foalings and in mares in poor body condition. The vulva is best evaluated during estrus, when it is most relaxed:

✦ *VC good.* Vulval lips are vertical. Lips are closely apposed, making a good seal. Dorsal commissure is either below the bony brim or up to 2.5 cm above.
✦ *VC fair.* Vulval lips inclined up to 30° off the vertical. Lips are apposed, making a good or reasonable seal.
✦ *VC poor.* Vulval lips are inclined more than 30° off the vertical. Poor or ineffective seal. More than half of the vulval commissure is above the bony brim, with a sunken anus.

Poor conformation will commonly lead to pneumovagina, urovagina, accumulation of intrauterine fluid, and endometritis. Foamy, frothy exudate may be detected in the vaginal cavity.

The lips of the vulva should be parted to determine the integrity of the vestibulovaginal sphincter (no air should enter the cranial vagina) and assess the color and moisture of the lining of the vestibule. The integrity of the perineal body is assessed by placing one finger in the rectum and the thumb in the vestibule. At least 3 cm of muscular tissue should be present between the two digits.

Clitoral swab for contagious equine metritis culture

The clitoral sinuses can harbor contagious equine metritis (CEM) (caused by *Taylorella equigenitalis*) and other venereally transmissible organisms such as *Pseudomonas aeruginosa* and *Klebsiella pneumoniae*. It is important to swab the clitoral sinuses and fossa as part of any BSE. Special small fine cotton swabs are required for the sinuses and the specimens should be placed immediately into specific bacterial transport media before dispatch for specialist culture, including microaerophilic. Some countries use a code of practice for CEM and other bacterial venereal diseases, and in some countries the former is a notifiable disease.

Vaginal examination

A vaginal speculum or flexible endoscope can be used to inspect the vaginal mucosa and external part of the cervix. The speculum should be sterile and either disposable or easily re-sterilized. A good focal light source such as a pen torch or transilluminator is essential. Suitable restraint of the mare and protection of involved personnel are important and the tail should be either held out of the way or bandaged. The perineal region should be washed with warm water and dried with a paper towel before the lubricated speculum is introduced. Vaginoscopy can be used to evaluate the presence or absence of pathology and to assess the stage of the estrous cycle. Pathology that may be noticed includes:

✦ Urine pooling.
✦ Uterine or vaginal discharge.
✦ Vaginal tears, hematoma, adhesions, and varicosities.
✦ Persistent hymen.
✦ Cervical tears, trauma, or adhesions.
✦ Rectovestibular/vaginal fistula.

A manual vaginal examination can also be carried out and can give additional information on the vagina and the nature and integrity of the cervix. The perineum should be washed and a gloved lubricated hand introduced gently upwards. It is possible to dilate the cervix manually, sometimes enough to allow palpation of the uterine lumen. Care should always be taken to ensure that the mare is not pregnant before dilating the cervix or introducing any instrument through it, as to do so in a pregnant mare will cause abortion. An endometrial biopsy punch and fiberoptic instrument can also be introduced in a similar way.

Rectal examination

This is a routine procedure in equine stud-farm veterinary work and is used to palpate the cervix, uterus, and ovaries both pre-insemination and during pregnancy. It also facilitates transrectal ultrasonographic examination of the tract, which has become so important in the last 20 years. There are significant risks involved in the procedure, both to the mare (rectal tears) and to the people carrying out the technique. Adequate restraint is therefore essential and the use of stocks preferable. Nervous animals may require sedation or the application of a lip twitch. A careful systematic technique, using copious obstetric lubricant, is important. The nature of the cervix and uterine tone should be assessed. The size, shape, and position of the uterus are important components of manual pregnancy diagnosis and BSE. Careful palpation of the ovaries for follicles and corpus hemorrhagicum are central to stud-farm management. All results, often combined with those of ultrasonographic examination, require careful recording.

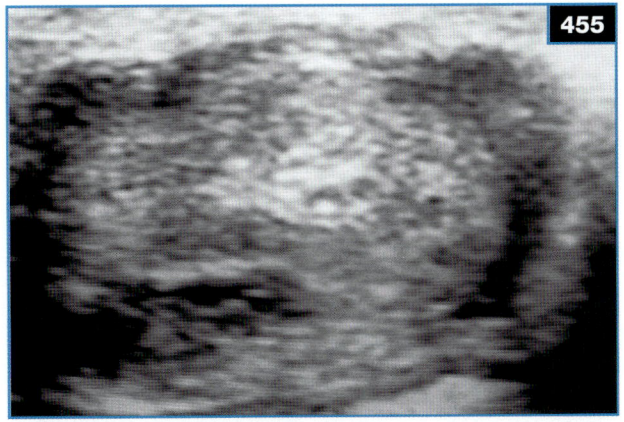

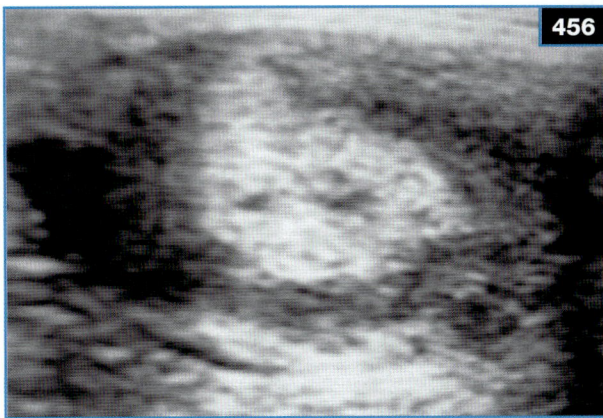

455, 456 Transrectal ultrasonographic images of the ovary of a cycling Thoroughbred mare showing (455) an early and (456) a later developing corpus luteum.

Ultrasonographic examination

This technique, introduced over 20 years ago, has revolutionized the veterinary input into equine stud medicine. Ultrasound waves of the type commonly used are not hazardous and ultrasonographic examination of the reproductive tract increases the quality and accuracy of information. Transrectal ultrasonography is usually carried out with a 5 or 7.5 MHz linear array probe and allows visualization of ovarian structures (size, CL, follicles, neoplasm) (455, 456); uterine size, free fluid or air, edema/folds, cysts, neoplasia, pregnancy from day 11 or 12; and cervical and vaginal abnormalities. A careful systematic examination of the entire tract is essential and careful recording, including using image-capture software or photographs, is essential.

Transabdominal ultrasonography to evaluate fetal viability and placental health is best performed using a linear array transducer of 2.5–3 MHz.

Uterine swab for culture

This is very useful for evaluating the breeding mare, but in recent years the significance of bacterial cultures from this source has undergone some discussion. Cultures from the uterus are possible using a number of different techniques via either a speculum or manual vaginal examination. Use of a sterile double-guarded swab passed directly into the uterine lumen is the best way of avoiding commensal contamination. It is important that the perineum of the mare is washed and dried and an aseptic vaginal examination carried out either manually or by vaginoscopy. The collection of samples for cytologic examination can be carried out at the same time. Cultures are best taken in early estrus since the cervix is relaxing, there are increased secretions from the uterus, and there is less risk of false results or introducing an infection. Swabs, however, can be taken at any time. As the swab is dry, it should either be plated out immediately or be transported in a suitable transport medium. The swabs are plated on blood agar and a selective Gram-negative medium (McConkey) and incubated at 37°C (98.6°F) both aerobically and microaerophilically.

In general, pure cultures and heavy growths are more likely to be significant than light mixed growths, which are often contaminants. The interpretation of culture results is helped by correlating them with the cytologic and/or ultrasound findings. For example, if the culture is positive (moderate to light growth) but the cytology results are negative for inflammatory cells (particularly neutrophils), the culture is likely to be a contaminant. Where cytologic findings are persistently positive with negative cultures, the cause of the inflammatory response should be explored further. The following bacterial organisms, if cultured in significant numbers, should be considered as potentially pathogenic: beta-hemolytic streptococci; hemolytic *Escherichia coli*; *Pseudomonas* spp.; *Klebsiella* spp. (certain capsule types); *Candida* spp.; certain *Staphylococcus* spp.

Uterine cytology

Uterine cytology is a simple but effective method of detecting signs of uterine inflammation, and complements uterine bacteriologic sampling. The presence of neutrophils in uterine cytologic specimens indicates an active inflammatory process. The sample should be collected in early to mid estrus using the same basic technique as for uterine culture. Cytologic samples can be obtained in two different ways:

✦ Using a small-volume uterine flush: 60 ml of sterile isotonic saline is flushed into the uterus and then aspirated. This is then centrifuged and placed onto a slide.
✦ Using a double-guarded swab, which is then 'rolled' onto a slide. The swab can also be used for endometrial culture if the slide is sterile.

The collected smears are stained using, for example, Diff-Quik® and examined for the presence of endometrial epithelial cells and polymorphonuclear neutrophils. It is also possible to have an indication as to whether the mare is anovulatory, transitional, or cycling. The stage of the cycle and the time since parturition should also be kept in mind when interpreting endometrial cytology. For example, the presence of PMNs <5 days post partum is part of the normal cytologic picture at this time.

Endometrial biopsy

This procedure is useful for the diagnosis of endometrial pathology and prognosis for future fertility, but is not necessary in every mare. It is useful for an aged mare, mares with a history of pregnancy loss or chronic endometritis, and in mares being assessed as potential embryo-transfer recipients. Histologic assessment can detect varying degrees of inflammation and fibrosis and evaluate glandular changes. It is a well established and safe procedure. The biopsy is collected using a custom-made 70 cm alligator biopsy punch with a basket size of 20 × 4 × 3 mm. A single biopsy taken from the base of one horn is generally considered to be representative of the entire uterus. Samples can be obtained at any time in the estrous cycle, but the pathologist should be informed of the stage of the cycle and other relevant findings. The collected tissue is placed into fixative (formalin or Bouin's solution) and tissue sections are examined for:

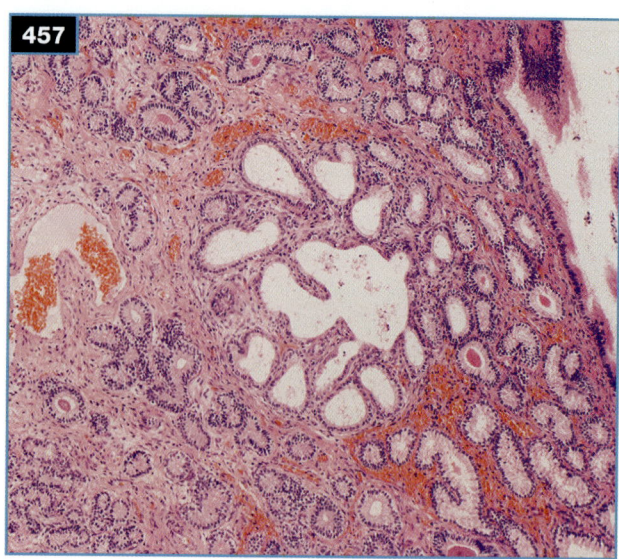

457 Histopathology of an endometrial biopsy specimen from a Thoroughbred mare showing an endometrial gland nest as often seen in older mares with chronic endometrial pathology.

✦ Inflammation or endometritis.
✦ Periglandular fibrosis.
✦ Cystic glandular distension and lymphatic stasis (**457**).
✦ Classification is based on the severity and distribution of the lesions and is associated with the expected ability of the mare to conceive and carry a foal to term:
  ◇ Category I: slight and/or widely scattered pathology; 80–90%.
  ◇ Category IIA: endometrial changes that reduce breeding efficiency but are moderate or reversible. Inflammation is detected; 50–80%.
  ◇ Category IIB: as for IIA but fibrosis is also present; 30–50%.
  ◇ Category III: irreversible and severe changes of fibrosis, cellular infiltration, and lymphatic stasis; 10%.

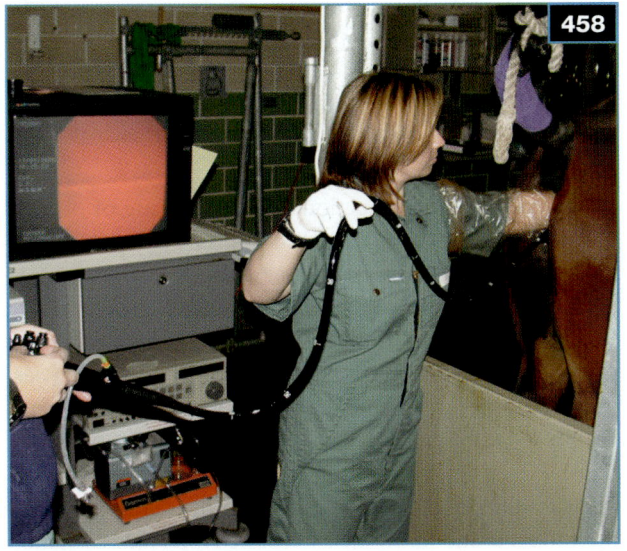

458 Examination of a mare by video hysteroscopy. (Photo courtesy T Chenier)

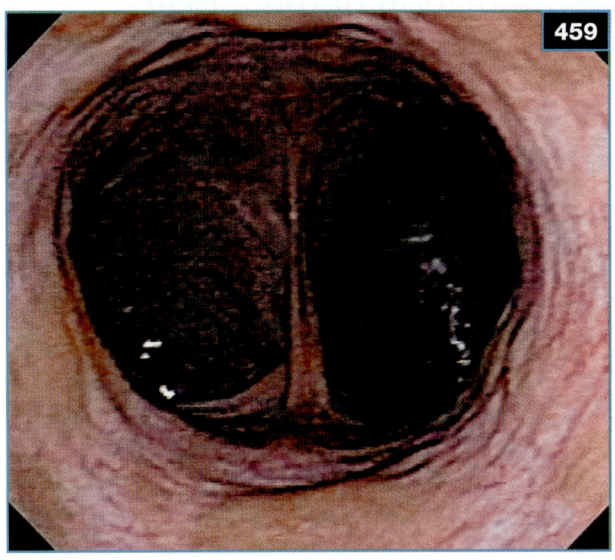

459 Hysteroscopic view of the uterine body and separation into two horns of a normal mare. (Photo courtesy T Chenier)

Fiberoptic examination of the uterus

Hysteroscopy or uteroscopy provides visual information on the endometrium and is carried out using a suitable fiberoptic or video endoscope (**458**). The endoscope needs to be capable of sufficient insufflation and washing to allow the technique to be carried out effectively. It is introduced into the uterus using the same technique as for endometrial biopsy and the uterus is insufflated with about 1–2 liters of air or saline (**459**). This technique is useful in assessing and detecting endometrial cysts, polyps, intraluminal adhesions, and hemorrhagic foci as well as guiding specific site endometrial biopsies. A complete examination of the reproductive tract should be carried out before the endoscopy, as the latter does cause some endometrial damage. Fiberoptic examination is best carried out in diestrus due to difficulties in insufflating the uterus during estrus, when the cervix is relaxed.

Blood endocrine assays

Blood samples for the measurement of hormone concentrations are a routine part of broodmare management. Progesterone assays can determine the presence or absence of luteal tissue within the ovary. They are particularly useful for assessing non-cycling and pregnant mares and for confirming ovulation. Testosterone and inhibin blood levels can be assayed and they may be raised in ovarian granulosa (thecal) cell tumors (GCTs) (see p. 302). Estrone sulfate levels in the mare's blood increase from day 35 of pregnancy and are predominately secreted by the fetus and fetal membranes. They are therefore often used as an indicator of fetal viability (see p. 260).

Karotyping

Karyotype examinations can be performed on animals suspected of having a chromosomal abnormality. Heparinized blood samples are used to harvest lymphocytes, on which chromosomal analysis is carried out. Candidates are mares that have never cycled or have infantile reproductive tracts.

Manipulation of the female reproductive cycle

Advancing the onset of spring transition

The transition of the mare from winter anestrus into the normal cyclicity of the breeding season usually occurs in the early spring. This can present problems to the owner of the mare if it belongs to one of the breeds (i.e. Thoroughbred) that has an artificial birthday for all foals of January 1st (northern hemisphere) or August 1st (southern hemisphere). Breeders will therefore strive for early-in-the-year foals. Early seasonal cyclic abnormality wastes time, increases the workload of the stallion, especially later in the breeding season, and increases veterinary involvement and expenditure. Breeders therefore request techniques that can advance the earliest date of mating in barren and maiden mares.

Artificial lighting

Day length is an important stimulus for the estrous cycle of the mare and the provision of artificial lighting is the best method of advancing the date of the first ovulation. Several methods have been described to offer the mare artificial lighting conditions. Twenty-four hours of lighting is actually detrimental.

A 16-hour light period (16 hours light: 8 hours dark) starting in early December (northern hemisphere) (early June in southern hemisphere) advances the first ovulation by around 60–80 days. A 150W clear bulb per 16m² is required.

Adding 2–3 hours of light at the end of the natural daylight (as dusk falls) is also effective, but the mares have to be kept outside to receive as much natural light as possible.

Another method reported is the 'flash' or 'pulse' system, which delivers 1 hour of light 9.5 hours after the onset of darkness. This system is not widely used commercially. (*Note:* If the lighting system fails for more than 2–3 days, then the mare will go back to where she was before the light treatment.)

Mare management

All barren and maiden mares should be examined early in the year per rectum for an active CL and, if necessary, blood samples taken for plasma progesterone levels to confirm the presence of any active luteal tissue. Those mares with progesterone levels <1 ng/ml should be placed on progesterone withdrawal therapy or GnRH. Those mares with luteal tissue are cycling and can either be induced into estrus by exogenous prostaglandin therapy or be monitored for the onset of natural estrus.

Hormonal methods

Hormonal treatment regimens added to the end of the artificial lighting period can further advance the first ovulation date.

Progesterone

Daily intramuscular injections of 150–200 mg of progesterone in oil +/- 10 mg estradiol 17β for 10 days, or 0.044 mg/kg of the oral progestagen altrenogest daily for 10–15 days usually stops prolonged spring estrous behavior in 1–5 days. Silastic intravaginal progesterone-releasing devices have also been used with success. Following cessation of the treatment the onset of estrous behavior occurs within 1–5 days and ovulation should occur within 7–10 days. Some clinicians combine this regimen with a prostaglandin injection on the last day to ensure that any luteinized tissue in the ovary will be lysed and ovulation will occur. This additional step is unnecessary if the ovary is monitored ultrasonographically and no luteal tissue is noted.

Dopamine antagonists

Drugs of this class (e.g. sulpiride and domperidone) have been used to hasten the onset of the first ovulation in experimental studies, but they are not widely used in general equine stud practice.

Synthetic GnRH

Administration of GnRH to mares results in release of endogenous LH and FSH and is the most successful method of inducing ovulation early in the transition period. In the literature, GnRH has been administered by mini-pumps, implants, and injections. Mini-pumps produce the best results. In the period January to March (northern hemisphere) (July to September, southern hemisphere), injections given three times daily, followed by human chorionic gonadatropin (hCG) administration induces estrus in mares within 12 days. The pregnancy rates following these estrus periods are around 50%.

In the UK, buserelin (2.5–3 ml i/m q8–12h for up to 10–14 days) has been used and the mare scanned for ovarian activity (follicles >25 mm) on day 10. If there is no activity, then the treatment can be repeated. When a follicle >30–35 mm is present, the mare can then be teased, covered, and treated with hCG. Mares can, however, slip back into an anovulatory state after an ovulation with GnRH. In some countries, GnRH is available as an implant (Ovuplant), which is implanted into the mare every 48 hours until she ovulates (2–3 implants). The implants are more successful if a larger follicle (30 mm) is already present. Human goserelin acetate implants (Zoladex, 1.8 mg) are used by some clinicians with some success.

Synchronization of estrus during the breeding season

The reasons for synchronizing estrus during the breeding season include enabling mares to breed on predetermined days (useful for both natural and AI matings), minimizing the time spent on the stud farm, and helping with embryo-transfer programs. The basic approach involves either extending or terminating the luteal phase of the cycle.

Progestagens

These drugs extend the luteal phase and produce two important effects on the cycling mare: 1) they inhibit behavioral estrus (mares will stop exhibiting estrous behavior after 2–3 days of treatment); and 2) they diminish LH levels and block final maturation of follicles and therefore ovulation. This is not 100% effective in the mare.

On average a mare will show signs of estrus for 5 days (3–6 days), and will ovulate 10 days (8–15 days), after cessation of progestagen treatment due to a rebound of LH levels that allows final follicle maturation and ovulation.

Important points to remember are:

+ Progestagens do not interfere with the release of PGF_2 from the endometrium. Therefore, progestagen treatment should continue for 14–15 days.
+ Some mares may ovulate while on progestagens. The new CL formed will therefore be present when the exogenous progestagens are stopped. These mares will not return to estrus until the new CL regresses. To avoid this, PGF_2 can be given at the end of the progestagen treatment period. If PGF_2 is given, the treatment period can be shortened to 8–12 days without any effect on the synchrony of the mares.
+ Some mares develop large follicles towards the end of the progestagen treatment period. These follicles may ovulate rapidly after cessation of the treatment (2–4 days). Mares that ovulate at this time may not show estrus and therefore the opportunity to breed from them may be missed. Scanning mares on the last day of treatment to identify those mares with follicles >35 mm in diameter may identify mares that could ovulate early after synchrony.
+ Synchrony of mares may be improved by administering hCG to mares that have follicles >30 mm in diameter (see below).

Prostaglandin F$_2$ alpha

$PGF_2\alpha$ causes lysis of the CL, resulting in a decline in serum progesterone. A CL will only regress in response to exogenous $PGF_2\alpha$ more than 5 days after ovulation, so it is usual to inject mares on the 6th day after ovulation.

The estrus response starts at about 3–4 days after injection, with ovulation occurring about 5–12 days after injection. Administration of $PGF_2\alpha$ to mares on day 12–14 may not shorten the time to the next ovulation. Mares with follicles >35 mm at the time of $PGF_2\alpha$ administration may ovulate very quickly, or the follicles may slowly regress. Large follicles that slowly regress must then be followed by the development of a new dominant follicle, which takes several days, and these mares often do not ovulate less than 12 days after $PGF_2\alpha$ administration.

$PGF_2\alpha$ can also be given to aid synchrony of mares, as described below.

Synchronization of ovulation

Combination of progestagens and estrogens

Estrogen has a suppressive effect on FSH release. The combination of progestagens and estrogen appears to have a greater negative feedback on LH than progestagen alone. 150 mg progesterone in oil i/m and 10 mg estradiol-17β in oil i/m daily for 10 days, with $PGF_2\alpha$ given on the 10th day, can result in a tight synchrony of estrus and ovulation. Ninety percent of mares treated in this way ovulate between 10 and 12 days after the last treatment. Unfortunately, estradiol-17β and progesterone in oil may not be currently available commercially in some countries. Other estrogens are available (estradiol cypionate and estradiol benzoate), but they have different durations of activity and therefore cannot be recommended for use with the above regimen.

Induction of ovulation during estrus

Human chorionic gonadatropin

HCG has an LH-like effect, helping to mature and ovulate a dominant follicle. hCG is given when the estrous mare has a follicle of 30–35 mm or more. The average dose rate is 2,500 IU (1,500–3,000 IU). Under these circumstances, 90% of mares ovulate within 48 hours of injection. There have been reports of mares that are repeatedly treated with hCG producing antibodies to injectable hCG, causing the mare to fail to respond to the drug.

GnRH implant/injections

Ovuplant is a commercially available biodegradable, silastic implant containing GnRH. Injected into the mare's neck or vulval tissue when the estrous mare has a follicle >30 mm, it gives a response similar to hCG, but with no risk of stimulating an antibody response. The treatment is expensive compared with hCG. GnRH is marketed in an injectable form called Receptal. This does not hasten ovulation unless given twice daily during estrus when a follicle >35 mm is present.

Control of cyclicity in the post-partum mare

Foal heat is the first heat after parturition and generally begins 5–12 days after foaling. As a general rule, ovulation usually occurs 10–11 days after foaling, but this interval shortens later in the breeding season. Studies have shown that pregnancy rates are higher if a mare ovulates >10 days after foaling compared with a mare that ovulates <10 days after foaling. Owners may wish to try and cover a foaling mare on the foal heat to gain time in the race against the January 1st or August 1st deadline. It therefore makes good sense to monitor mares individually 7 days after foaling by vaginal speculum examination, rectal palpation, and ultrasound to select those capable of being bred on the foal heat. The criteria used to help decide this include:

+ Normal foaling.
+ No retained placenta or history of metritis or endometritis.
+ No cervical, vaginal, or vulval damage.
+ Normal uterine involution.
+ Ovulation a minimum of 8 days after foaling and preferably >10 days.
+ There is some evidence that the use of post-mating intra-uterine antibiotics, i/v oxytocin +/- uterine lavage will increase pregnancy rates at the foal heat.

PGF$_2\alpha$ administration

PGF$_2\alpha$ can be used to shorten the first luteal phase in mares that are not ideal for mating on or around day 10. It can be given to mares 5 or 6 days after ovulation when the exact dates are known, or on or around day 20 post foaling to bring them back into estrus 3–4 days post injection.

Delaying the first post-partum ovulation

Progesterone and estradiol in combination, or altrenogest, can be used from day 1 post partum to delay the time to first ovulation. This will delay the first ovulation to beyond day 10 and has been reported to increase pregnancy rates.

Breeding management

Mares can be inseminated either naturally by a stallion or artificially using either fresh or preserved semen.

Natural mating

Mating can occur free with the mare and stallion in a yard or at grass, and this is a system still used at some stud farms, particularly in ponies. There is often minimum input by the stud staff or veterinarian. A supervised mating system is used for the majority of stud farms using natural mating and is the only system permissible in the Thoroughbred if the resulting progeny are to be registered (460). The requirements are:

+ A good teaser stallion(s) is essential to this system and allows the detection of suitable mares to cover.
+ A tease system suited to the farm's management system and the individual mare.
+ An experienced observer and recorder.

Once the mare is considered to be in the breeding season:

+ Mares should be teased three times per week or preferably every other day during the breeding season. This not only determines when mares are to be bred, but is a good method for detecting early pregnancy loss.
+ Those that tease positive are traditionally bred on day 2 or 3 of estrus and then every other day until the end of estrus. In modern systems the goal is to cover the mare as close to ovulation as possible using the minimum number of attempts. This decreases the amount of contamination in the mare's reproductive tract and minimizes use of the stallion, helping to maintain stallion semen reserves and libido.
+ Mares should be bred prior to ovulation when the mare has a dominant follicle (>30 mm) present. If it is necessary to limit the number of matings, the ovaries should be palpated daily and mating should take place just prior to ovulation.
+ If ovulation has occurred, then acceptable conception rates may still be achieved by breeding 12 hours after ovulation. However, it has been shown that there is a greater incidence of early embryonic loss associated with postovulation matings due to the fertilization of an aged ovum.

460 A natural covering of the Thoroughbred mare shown in 444.

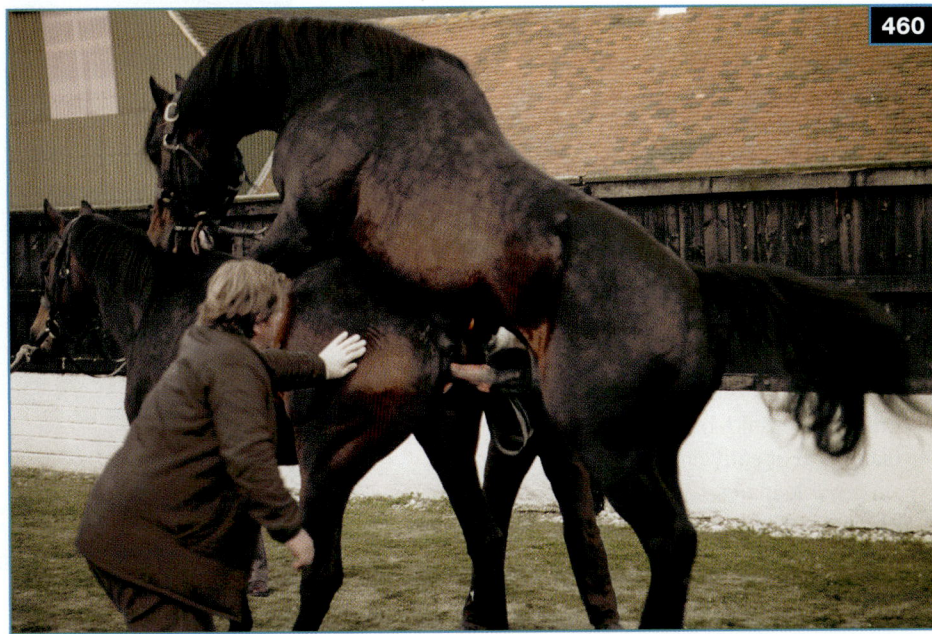

It is important to restrain the mare adequately for mating. A head collar and chain over the nose, a bridle, or a chifney, and/or a twitch can be used to keep the mare still. Some farms place hobbles on the hindlimbs of the mare or tie up a forelimb. The mare's tail should be wrapped in a bandage or plastic bag. The perineal region should be washed three times with mild soap and water before being rinsed and dried with paper towels. On some stud farms the stallion's penis is washed with warm water prior to and, occasionally, post breeding. More controversially, some stud farms use warm water and a mild soap to clean the penis, particularly at the start of the season or where the penis is excessively dirty. Many clinicians believe this is contraindicated.

One person should handle the stallion, one the mare, and a third, if available, should be there to assist the stallion and check for ejaculation by palpating the urethral pulsations in the stallion. A good active and fertile stallion can naturally cover 40–60 mares in one season, although in recent times the tendency has been to ask Thoroughbred stallions to cover well over 100.

Minimal-contamination breeding techniques
Overview
During natural mating ejaculation occurs into the body of the uterus, leading to contamination of the lumen and inflammation of the cervix, vestibule, vagina, and vulva. Techniques applied at mating are aimed at reducing the pathogen challenge to, and any inflammatory reaction from, the intrauterine environment in the pericoital period. These techniques help to improve fertility rates in older multiparous mares, those with a history of endometritis,

and in mares mated at the foaling heat or to stallions infected with *Pseudomonas aeruginosa* or *Klebsiella pneumoniae* (not in the UK under the Horserace Betting Levy Board Code of Practice). It should be considered sound 'good practice' in any mating situation for minimizing the possibility of infection and maximizing fertility.

Technique
+ Only one covering per estrous cycle should be performed, ideally 24 hours prior to ovulation. If required, LH or a deslorelin implant can be administered 24 hours prior to covering in order to induce ovulation.
+ Attend to general hygiene: bandage the tail; wash the vulva and perineum of the mare (some clinicians also wash the penis of the stallion) with clean water, preferably from a spray bottle or from a disposable plastic liner in a bucket (plastic bin liner) to avoid cross-contamination; dry with a sterile paper towel. Do not use chemicals or strong soaps/detergents, as these can be spermicidal. Instil about 100–200 ml of warmed semen extender with antibiotic into the uterus prior to covering. Mating should be fully supervised.
+ Assess the presence of any intrauterine fluid 3–12 hours after mating using ultrasound examination. If a significant quantity of fluid is present after 4 hours, the uterus should be lavaged using 1–2 liters of lactated Ringer's solution warmed to body temperature (37°C [98.6°F]) via an equine uterine lavage catheter or soft tube. Lavage and siphoning should be repeated a maximum of 3–4 times or until

255

Female reproductive tract

the flushing solution emerges clear of debris. Antibiotic solution may be infused after the last flushing, the choice of antiobiotic being either based on the results of culture and sensitivity testing of an endometrial swab prior to mating or a broad-spectrum, water soluble combination. (*Note:* If oxytocin is to be administered intravenously, wait 30 minutes until myometrial activity has subsided before instilling antibiotic.) Oxytocin administered intramuscularly or intravenously 4–8 hours after mating has proved beneficial to conception rates in some mares with a history of chronic endometritis. It also stimulates the drainage of any residual intrauterine fluid, but it may increase the likelihood of early embryonic death in some susceptible mares.

✦ The mare should be re-examined by ultrasound 24 hours later and the oxytocin injection repeated, if required. Only rarely is a second flushing necessary.

Artificial insemination of the mare

AI is regularly used in many types of horse and pony to achieve a pregnancy. Some breeds, however, will not register progeny bred by this technique. Three types of insemination are used in the horse:
✦ Fresh +/- extender.
✦ Chilled extended.
✦ Frozen extended.

The technique and technology of semen collection, extension, preservation, monitoring, and transport are covered in Part 2, Male Reproductive Tract (p. 336).
The advantages of AI are:
✦ An increased conception rate in some stallions and mares with fresh or chilled semen.
✦ Mares can be bred by stallions that would otherwise be geographically inaccessible.
✦ Mares and foals are not subject to transport stress.
✦ Mares can remain in training.
✦ Mare owners save on transport costs.
✦ Reduced contamination of mares and less risk of disease transmission.
✦ Increased flexibility in timing of mating, thus maximizing the use of a stallion during and beyond his reproductive years.
✦ Control/prevention of venereal diseases.
✦ Frozen semen additional benefits include: semen can be kept indefinitely; mare can be bred at any time, including when the stallion is unavailable; worldwide availability of semen; single shipping of semen per season.

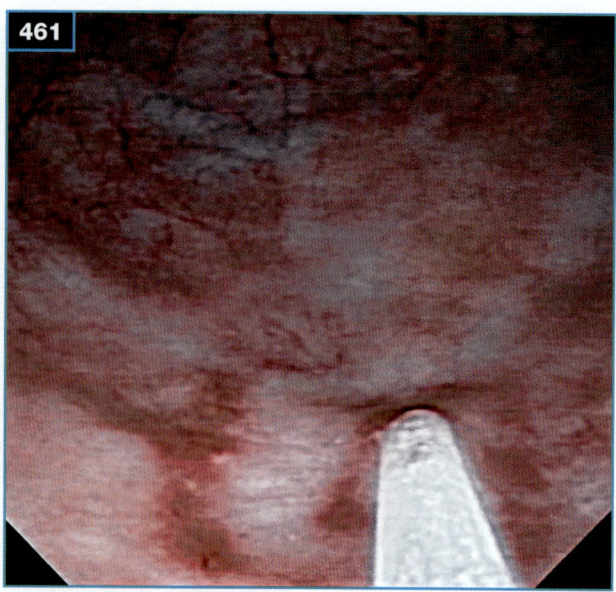

461 Hysteroscopic artificial insemination of a mare. (Photo courtesy T Chenier)

The disadvantages of AI are:
✦ Veterinary input and expenses are greater, especially when using frozen semen.
✦ Mare owners must tease mares, arrange semen shipment, and communicate with veterinarian and stud farm.
✦ Repeat inseminations lead to increased semen collection and shipping costs.
✦ Conception rates using frozen semen are less than that with fresh semen or natural covering. With good management, conception rates are > 75% for fresh semen and > 60% for both cooled and frozen semen.
✦ Various international quarantine requirements for collection and import restrictions.
✦ High semen processing costs and specialized equipment and laboratory facilities required, especially for the production of frozen semen.
✦ There is a huge variation between and within stallions in the ability of their semen to withstand freezing and thawing techniques.

The cost of some AI programs may mean that a full BSE is indicated to avoid insemination in a mare that does not have a uterus capable of facilitating conception and pregnancy. Suggested protocols for insemination of mares with different inseminates are listed below. There is considerable variation among clinicians in their approach to this, particularly when using frozen semen, and the information should be viewed in this light (**461**).

Fresh or chilled semen

✦ Ultrasound scan the mare until she has a >30 mm follicle. Plan to inseminate the mare on the day before ovulation. Some veterinarians use hCG or synthetic GnRH to induce ovulation.

✦ Order semen and plan to have the mare inseminated within 24 hours (48 hours maximum) of collection.

✦ Check motility of semen BEFORE inseminating.

✦ Inseminate using a syringe without latex.

✦ Optimum time for insemination is between 24 hours prior to ovulation and up to 6–12 hours after ovulation.

✦ Check the next day for ovulation and uterine fluid.

✦ Check the mare for pregnancy at 17–18 days post ovulation so that she can be rebred at next estrus if not pregnant.

Frozen semen

✦ Optimum time for insemination is between 12 hours prior to ovulation and up to 6 hours after ovulation.

✦ Ultrasound scan the mare. If in estrus and with uterine edema and a follicle of 30–40 mm, give 2,500 IU Chorulon (hCG) i/v at 22.00 hours or 24.00 hours. Scan the next morning and then at midnight, then at 08.00 hours, 12.00 hours, 16.00 hours, 20.00 hours (i.e. every four hours). Most mares will ovulate between 08.00 hours and 16.00 hours.

✦ Mares with uterine fluid (>15 mm) on the day before insemination should be given oxytocin (2 ml i/v) and allowed to exercise.

✦ If the mare has a follicle of 40–44 mm and is in estrus, scan before giving Chorulon at midnight. Scan at 08.00 hours, 16.00 hours, 24.00 hours, 08.00 hours, 12.00 hours, 16.00 hours, and 20.00 hours.

✦ If the mare is in estrus at the first scan with a follicle >45 mm, do not give Chorulon. Start scanning at 18.00 hours, 24.00 hours, 06.00 hours, 12.00 hours (at least every 6 hours).

✦ On the morning after AI, if the mare has >15 mm of fluid, flush with lactated Ringer's solution until the recovered flush is clear. Give 2 ml oxytocin i/v. Repeat oxytocin injections twice over the day. If the mare has <15 mm of fluid, then treat with oxytocin, as above, only.

✦ Re-examine the mare by ultrasound 8–12 hours after insemination and if ovulation still has not occurred, re-inseminate.

✦ This system is quite intensive in monitoring terms, but it is effective for most mares and can be modified to individual mares depending on their estrous cycle and rate of follicle development.

Frozen semen insemination procedure (462–464)

✦ The semen is usually supplied in 0.5–5 ml straws, which should be stored, handled, and thawed strictly according to the supplier's instructions. Each straw or packet is individually labeled.

✦ Only one straw at a time should be thawed, usually in a temperature-controlled water bath.

✦ Take great care to avoid semen contact with disinfectants, detergents, or tap water and avoid temperature fluctuations.

462–464 The straws containing the frozen semen should be stored in liquid nitrogen and carefully labeled to avoid incorrect insemination (462). They are thawed in a temperature-controlled water bath (463) before insemination. (464) Insemination of a mare with frozen semen using an insemination pipette.

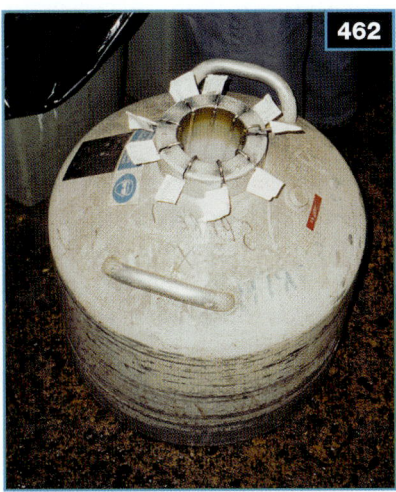

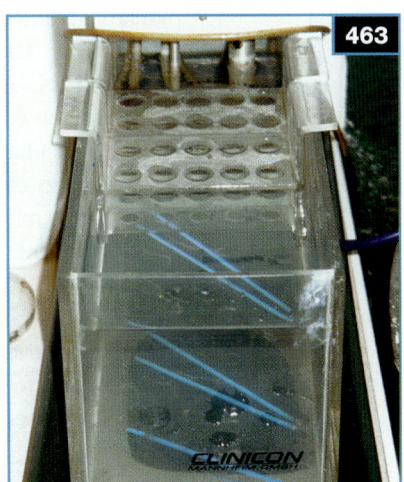

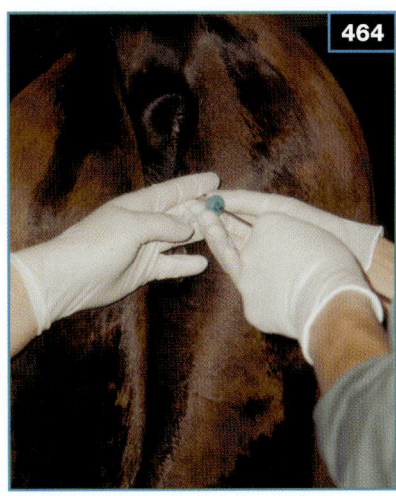

- ✦ Once thawed the semen should be inseminated immediately in its entirety.
- ✦ Transfer the semen from the straw into an insemination pipette or load into an insemination gun.
- ✦ Using a sterile procedure, gloved hands, and a nonspermicidal lubricant (KY jelly) as required, carefully introduce the pipette through the cervix, pushing it gently forward until it reaches the mid to cranial body of the uterus, where the semen should be discharged. Gradually withdraw the pipette.
- ✦ Once thawed, semen should never be refrozen. Many veterinarians examine a small drop of inseminated semen post insemination for motility. In general, it is recommended that there is a minimum of 30% progressively motile sperm after thawing, and dosages of 150–350 x 10^6 of these motile sperm have been reported to result in acceptable conception rates.
- ✦ Insemination of thawed frozen semen has been associated with a severe inflammatory reaction in some mares and this may require postinsemination uterine lavage and systemic oxytocin treatment.

Preparation of the mare for any AI:

- ✦ Empty the rectum.
- ✦ Tail wrapped in plastic sleeve and held to one side.
- ✦ Wash perineal region thoroughly with mild soap/water, rinse, and dry.
- ✦ Use a clean plastic rectal sleeve and sterile hand glove.
- ✦ Use a nonspermicidal lubricant.
- ✦ With fresh or chilled semen the material is drawn into a nontoxic syringe and a sterile insemination pipette passed into the uterus, where the semen is deposited well into the uterine body.

Embryo transfer

Overview

Donor mares are mated and the resulting fertilized ova harvested and either stored using cryopreservation, implanted into a recipient mare directly, or sent to a central embryo-transfer facility where suitable recipient mares are kept. The procedure allows mares with various breeding problems to reproduce and also increases the number of foals that a genetically superior mare can produce in its lifetime. Recent advances in superovulation techniques and more widespread acceptance by breed societies are now resulting in increased use of this technique in mares, but the procedure can be time-consuming and expensive and is therefore used most often in valuable mares.

Uses

Surrogate mares are useful for mares that have difficulty in maintaining a pregnancy themselves, are subfertile, or that persistently have twin ovulations. Genetically superior mares can breed earlier and produce more foals in their lifetime or per year than by natural means. Performance horses need only be out of competition for a couple of weeks a year instead of for the duration of a pregnancy. Cryopreservation of embryos means that pregnancy can be delayed if required, although success rates may be lower using frozen embryos. The technique of oocyte transfer has been developed in recent years in order to help obtain pregnancies from problem, older mares where embryo transfer has very poor success rates. This involves the transfer of a donor's oocyte into the oviduct of a recipient. In-vitro fertilization and cloning techniques are currently being researched.

Technique

Synchronization of estrus between the donor and recipient mares is essential to success, ideally with the recipient mare ovulating 1–3 days after the donor. The success of inducing superovulation in the mare has improved using new combinations of injections of hCG and equine pituitary gonadotropin and this can produce 7–10 ova with 50% viability. The donor mare is mated at the normal time during estrus, usually by AI, and embryos are collected between days 6 and 9 post ovulation (days 7 and 8 have the greatest chance of recovering a viable embryo) via a Bivona foley catheter inserted into the uterus through the cervix. An 80 ml inflatable cuff on the catheter maintains its position in the uterus and seals the cervix. Depending on uterine size, 1–2 liters of a specialist, warmed, flushing solution containing antibiotics (often purchased ready made) is introduced into the uterus via the catheter using gravity feed and then immediately drained into a sterile container through a 75 μm embryo filter (**465**).

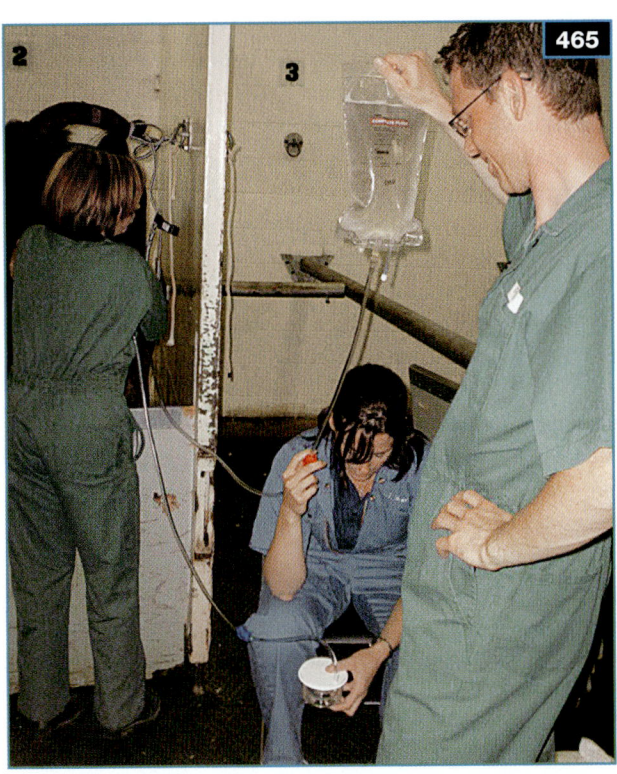

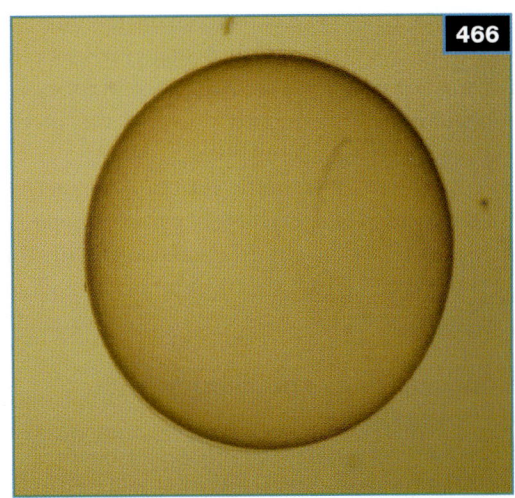

465 Collection of embryos from a donor mare via uterine lavage. (Photo courtesy T Chenier)

466 View of a 7–8 day embryo under high-power magnification. (Photo courtesy T Chenier)

This process is repeated 3–4 times to flush out all the embryos, often assisted by rectal massage of the uterus. The embryos are recovered from the filter by rinsing with flushing solution into a gridded search dish. Embryos are identified using a dissecting microscope (7–10x) and then washed with flushing solution and put into a special holding medium before being graded microscopically for quality, viability, and freedom from abnormalities (466). Embryos can remain viable for up to 24 hours at 5°C (41°F) within a holding medium in a passive cooling device, but where possible the interval between identification and transfer should be minimized, preferably to less than 60 minutes. If no embryos are found, it is possible to place a further two liters of flushing solution into the mare's uterus and, before re-collection, administer oxytocin. Embryo recovery rates can vary and several factors have been identified: days 7–9 collection is more efficient than day 6; older mares have lower collection rates due to poorer fertilization rates and high embryonic loss before day 6; semen quality of the stallion; single ovulating mares only have 50% recovery per cycle.

Recipient mares should be healthy, free from any reproductive problems of their own, cycling normally, and preferably young (3–8 years old). Nonsurgical transfer of the embryo into the uterus of the recipient mare is now the most commonly used technique for transfer, and can have similar success rates (up to 75%) to the more complex surgical implantation techniques. The recipient mare is sedated and premedicated with flunixin meglumine. The mare is maintained on an oral progestagen from the day of transfer for approximately 50 days. A number of different commercial instruments are available for transfer of the embryo. Whichever instrument is used, it must be sterile or covered by a sterile sheath and it must be inserted through the cervix with minimal manipulation.

Prognosis

There are a number of factors that affect the success of embryo transfer. For the recipient mare the factors with the largest effect are uterine tone just prior to transfer and the previous fertility of the mare. The stage of the recipient post ovulation (days 5–9) has no effect. Larger and normal embryos collected on days 7 and 8 have the highest success rate (up to 75%). Chilling embryos before transfer has no effect on pregnancy rates, but freezing embryos does decrease success rates. Day 6 embryos seem to be the best for freezing. The shorter the time between collection and implantation, the more favorable the prognosis. The incidence of embryonic death post transfer between days 12 and 50 can be up to 15–20% and is increased by recipient mares >7 days post ovulation and by poor quality embryos.

259

The pregnant mare

Maternal recognition of pregnancy

The first maternal recognition of pregnancy is thought to occur at about 48 hours post fertilization with the production of a protein called 'early pregnancy factor' (EPF). This protein has been detected in horses, humans, sheep, and mice. It may prove useful in the future for detecting early pregnancy. The embryo enters the uterus at around day 6 post ovulation. At this stage the embryo is either a late stage morula or an early-stage blastocyst. Maternal recognition of pregnancy prevents the production of $PGF_2\alpha$. It is thought to involve:

+ Movement of the embryo around the uterus allowing the embryo to contact every part of the endometrium.
+ Secretion by the embryo of anti-luteolysins/luteotropic substances, which are taken up by the endometrium. The exact nature of these is not fully known.

Endocrinology and maintenance of pregnancy (467)

Progesterone

This hormone is essential for the maintenance of pregnancy. The primary CL is present following the ovulation that led to the pregnancy. The primary CL persists because of the inhibition of $PGF_2\alpha$ secretion described above. After days 35–40 of pregnancy, additional follicles on both ovaries lead to secondary CL that form following ovulation of the developing secondary follicles or luteinization of follicles without ovulation. Secondary CL secrete progesterone. Primary and secondary CL persist until after day 160 and have virtually disappeared by day 210 of pregnancy. The fetoplacental unit begins to secrete progesterone from day 60 and by day 100 is producing enough progestins to maintain pregnancy. Pregnancy in the mare, therefore, is maintained predominately by the placenta. Progesterone assays can be used for pregnancy diagnosis, but it is important to realize that elevated progesterone levels are an indication of luteal tissue and not of pregnancy. However, if blood taken from a mare 18–22 days after the last ovulation still shows elevated progesterone levels, it suggests that an active CL is still present and therefore the mare may be pregnant. False positives do occur, and a high progesterone level at 18–22 days post ovulation may also be due to:

+ Diestrus ovulation.
+ Embryonic loss after maternal recognition of pregnancy (see above).
+ Failure of luteolysis.
+ Pyometra.

Equine chorionic gonadatropin (eCG)

Cells from the embryo attach to the endometrium at about day 35, forming small 'islands' of tissue called 'endometrial cups'. Endometrial cups produce eCG and in the mare this has mainly LH-like effects. It causes resurgence of the primary CL and luteinization of the secondary CL. It is also involved in the maternal immunotolerance of foreign antigens produced by the fetus. eCG is used as the basis for a pregnancy test in mares from days 40–42. The test can have false positives, with the pregnancy having been lost but the endometrial cups being retained.

Estrogen

Maternal serum estrogen levels rise from about day 35 of pregnancy. It is interesting to note that the rise in estrogen concentration at around day 35 does not occur without a functional CL. eCG from endometrial cups apparently stimulates luteal steroidogenesis, resulting in increased estrogen synthesis and secretion from CL tissue. After day 45, additional estrogens are produced by the fetoplacental unit and released into the maternal circulation. Estrogen levels peak at around days 210–250 and then slowly decline. Estrogens are thought to play a role in the development of the vascular supply and endometrial hypertrophy during pregnancy. Assays of estrone sulfate (produced by the fetoplacental unit) can also be used as an indicator of pregnancy and fetal viability, since it is only produced in the presence of a viable fetus. Estrone sulfate assays can be used from days 60–70 onwards.

467 Summary of hormonal events in the pregnant mare. P = progesterone; E = estrogen; eCG = equine chorionic gonadotropin; FG = fetal gonad weight. (Adapted from McKinnon AO, Voss JL (1993) (eds) *Equine Reproduction*. Lea and Febiger, Philadelphia, pp. 27–175.)

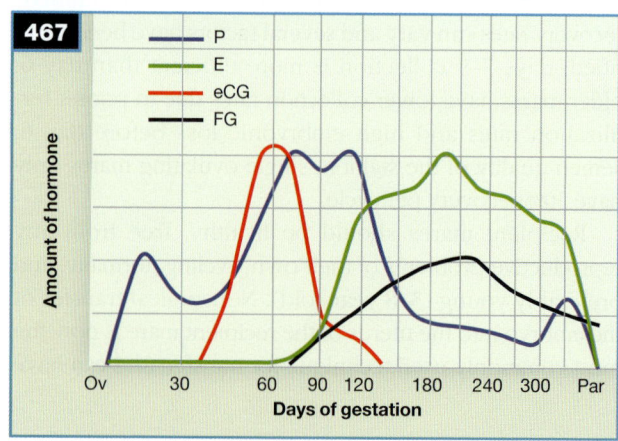

TABLE 5 Main findings on rectal examination of a pregnant mare

GESTATION	UTERINE TONE	UTERINE SWELLING	CERVICAL FINDINGS
16–19 days	Good, firm/turgid	Mild swelling	Closed tight
20–24 days	Good, firm/turgid	Ventral bulge at uterine bifurcation	Narrow and elongated
30 days	Good, firm/turgid	Increasing pregnant horn ventral enlargement	Closed tight
30–50 days	Decreases in pregnant horn. Still good in nonpregnant horn	Continuing increase in size of bulge. Towards end of period starts to include mid uterine horn and uterine body	Closed
50–70 days	Decreases in pregnant horn. Still good in nonpregnant horn	Fluid-filled swelling pregnant horn, body, and some distension nonpregnant horn	Closed
70 + days		Uterus increases in size and moves ventrally. Ovaries start to move closer together. Ballottement of the fetus is possible later in pregnancy (>120 days). Palpation and sizing of fetus may allow ageing by comparison with breed standards	Closed

Pregnancy diagnosis in the mare

This is an important part of stud-farm and individual mare management. There are various techniques available, all of which have advantages and disadvantages, and are best used at various stages of the pregnancy. Establishing that a mare has a normal pregnancy is essential, as early embryonic death is common in the mare and leads to a wasted breeding season. Diagnosis of a twin pregnancy, particularly early enough to allow positive action, is a vital function of the equine stud-farm veterinarian.

Absence of estrus behavior

Lack of detection of estrus 16–22 days post ovulation and following insemination is an indirect test for pregnancy. Unfortunately, not all mares that fail to exhibit estrus behavior are pregnant. Other reasons include: early embryonic death; retained CL; silent or poorly shown estrus; variability in the estrous-cycle timing; lactational anestrus; and teasing at the incorrect time in relation to the true date of the last ovulation. In addition, some pregnant mares show estrus behavior.

Rectal examination

This is a frequently used and effective method, but it does carry risks to mare and veterinarian, depends for its accuracy on the skill of the palpator, and is not applicable to small mares. Palpation per rectum for pregnancy alone is used as early as 16–19 days on intensively managed studs, but in the last 20 years it has usually been combined with ultrasonographic examination. The main findings on rectal examination are shown in *Table 5*.

Vaginal examination

Vaginal examination either directly, via a vaginoscope, or rectally can be used as part of a pregnancy diagnostic examination (*Table 5*).

Ultrasonographic examination

This technique has become established as the most important technique for the diagnosis and assessment of pregnancy in the mare. It is used at the same time as a rectal examination and therefore has that technique's inherent risks. It is able to detect pregnancy very early on (even as early as day 10 in experimental situations with some ultrasound machines) and also to investigate problems of the reproductive tract. Ultrasound examination at days 12–16 is used most effectively to manage mares that present with twin embryos. The timing of the first pregnancy scan can vary considerably depending on the management and breed of the mare. Early-pregnancy ultrasound examination requires careful, systematic use of a linear array 5 or 7.5 MHz transducer. The main characteristics of the conceptus are described below:

261

✦ Days 10–16. At day 10, small spherical vesicles are found most frequently in the uterine body, although they can be found from the tip of a uterine horn to just cranial to the internal os of the cervix. Great care should be taken to examine the entire uterus. At day 16, the spherical vesicles are usually found at the caudal portion of one of the uterine horns. During these early days of pregnancy, the rapidly growing vesicle will have bright echogenic poles that are not associated with the embryonic disk. The vesicle grows from about 2–3 mm (day 10) to about 15–16 mm (day 16) (468, 469).

✦ Days 17–22. The vesicle has a growth plateau between days 17 and 26. After day 17 the vesicle is often irregular/triangular or slightly elongated in shape. This is thought to be due to increased tone and thickness of the uterine wall. The embryo is first visualized within the vesicle between days 20 and 25, usually in a ventral position. The heart beat is usually detected after day 22 and is used to determine embryonic well-being.

✦ Days 23–55. At day 24 the allantois can be seen. As the allantois expands, the yolk sac contracts and so the embryo is lifted dorsally in the vesicle by day 40 (470). After day 40, the yolk sac reduces dramatically and the umbilical cord is formed, which allows the embryo to drop down to the ventral portion of the vesicle by day 50. With knowledge of the approximate age of gestation and the growth characteristics given above, it should be possible to determine twins without too much difficulty when using a 5 MHz ultrasound transducer. For example, twin vesicle walls, when in contact with one another, generally appear vertical, compared with the usually horizontal membranes of allantois and yolk sac of a 3-day-old vesicle.

✦ After day 60 it can be difficult to obtain a complete view of the embryo. This is due to the uterus moving over the pelvic brim and into the abdomen. The presence of twins at this stage can be very difficult to rule out. The age of the fetus can be calculated by measuring parts of the fetus and comparing these with reference measurements. The sex of a foal can often be determined at around 60–75 days. The primitive equine genitalia, the genital tubercle, develops on the body surface of the fetus, between the hindlimbs, after 60 days and is identifiable via transrectal ultrasonography as a highly echogenic, bilobed structure resembling an equal sign (=). Over the next 5 days the tubercle migrates caudally in the female to a position under the tail, whilst in the male it moves cranially onto the abdominal wall behind the umbilicus. Diagnosis requires a scanner of 5–7.5 MHz frequency with good resolution at 12 cm depth. Considerable experience and practice are needed to become accurate in this technique. Abnormalities of the fetus and pregnancy can also be identified (e.g. lack of fetal heart beat, cloudy echogenicity or reduction of fetal fluids, and, rarely, morphologic abnormalities).

✦ Day 180 onwards. Transabdominal ultrasonographic examination is possible. Assessment of fetal membranes and fluids, as well as the fetus, is also possible (471).

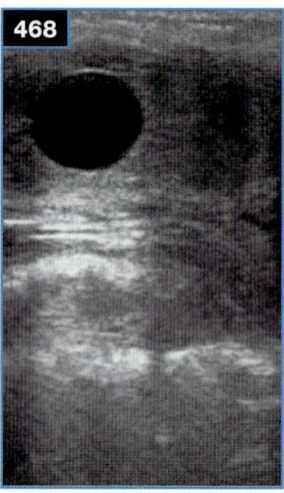
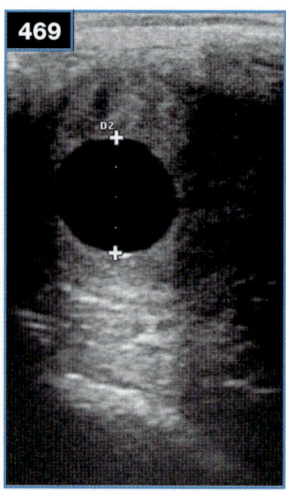

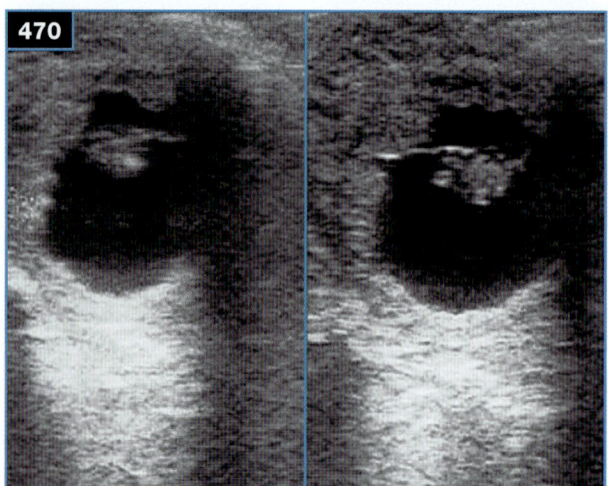

468 Transverse transrectal ultrasonographic image of a single 13-day-old conceptus. (Photo courtesy T Chenier)

469 Transverse transrectal ultrasonographic image of a single 15-day-old conceptus. (Photo courtesy T Chenier)

470 Transverse transrectal ultrasonographic images of a single 34-day-old conceptus. (Photo courtesy T Chenier)

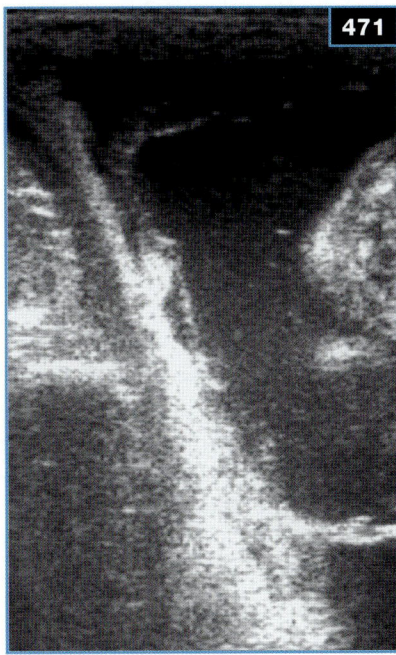

471 Transrectal ultrasonographic image of a single pregnancy in late gestation. Note the large fluid-filled uterus with normal placental lining and, to the right, the fetus. (Photo courtesy T Chenier)

Hormonal tests

Indirect testing of pregnancy can be undertaken by measuring a variety of hormones in the mare's blood or milk. Unfortunately, they can be unreliable if used on their own.

Progesterone

Progesterone levels can be measured in blood or milk, and in the stud farm or practice laboratory situation they are often determined using an ELISA kit. Pregnant mares 17–24 days post ovulation should have progesterone levels >2 ng/ml and often as high as 4–10 ng/ml, but considerable individual variation exists. Retained CL or early embryonic death will also lead to elevated (false-positive) levels. Concentrations continue to rise after day 21 and remain elevated up until days 150–200 before declining, sometimes to <2 ng/ml.

Equine chorionic gonadotropin

Following the invasion of the fetal trophoblast cells into the maternal endometrium and the formation of the endometrial cups, detectable levels of eCG are produced at around days 35–38 post ovulation. Maternal rejection starts at day 60 and the cup cells cease to function at around day 120. Blood concentrations of eCG, often measured by ELISA tests, are useful between days 45 and 90 and in some mares up to day 120. False negatives will be given if samples are taken outside these time limits or with mule fetuses. False positives can occur with embryonic death after day 35.

Estrogen

ELISA tests are available for determining the concentration of estrogen in urine, blood, or feces in pregnant mares after day 60 and up until full term. Peak conjugated estrone sulfate concentrations increase until days 180–240 days of pregnancy (peak days 150–160) and slowly decline thereafter. Estrogen levels are a good indicator of fetal viability, as the fetus and placenta both contribute to their production.

Techniques for assessing fetoplacental health

The continued assessment of the pregnancy in an individual mare and the health of the fetus and its placenta is a normal part of good stud-farm management. The level of assessment required for each individual pregnancy is determined by whether it is categorized as of low or high risk. Maternal conditions or situations that can lead to high-risk pregnancies/foals and, therefore, increased assessment of the fetoplacental unit are:

✦ History of abnormal pregnancy previously or during this gestation.
✦ Premature mammary development and lactation.
✦ History of previous production of premature, dysmature, or septic foals.
✦ History of dystocia or premature placental separation.
✦ History of abnormal pregnancies.
✦ Vaginal discharge in pregnancy.
✦ Excessive abdominal enlargement.
✦ Severe maternal illness including injury, lameness, and infections.
✦ Severe maternal malnutrition.
✦ Twin pregnancy.
✦ Excessively prolonged gestation.
✦ Maternal transport and stress, especially last four weeks of pregnancy.
✦ Severe or prolonged abdominal pain.
✦ Maternal drug treatments, general anesthesia, and/or surgery.
✦ Induction of parturition.

There are a variety of different techniques that can be used, often in combination, to assess the viability of a pregnancy.

Rectal palpation

This is a simple, but fairly unreliable technique, that can determine fetal activity, position, and placental fluids.

Vaginal examination

Vaginal examination has limited risks to mare and pregnancy and allows information to be gathered on the cervix, vagina, and vestibule. The degree of cervical softening can be assessed and samples taken for culture of any abnormal discharge. (*Note*: Take care not to breach the cervix in a pregnant mare, as this can result in abortion.)

Blood hormonal analysis

Serial blood samples assayed for maternal plasma progestin levels can detect trends that may be associated with a compromised fetus. Circulating estrogen levels are an important indicator of fetal viability.

Fetal and placental ultrasonography

Ultrasonography can be performed per rectum and/or, in later pregnancy, transabdominally. It is particularly useful for:

+ Detecting and sexing single or twin pregnancies.
+ Assessing the thickness of the combined uteroplacental unit and the appearance and volume of allantoic and amniotic fluids.
+ Assessing the position of the fetus within the uterus.
+ Measurement of fetal size and gestational age.
+ Assessment of the cardiovascular system including fetal heart rate.

A biophysical profile is built up using a scoring system derived from the following measurements:

+ Combined thickness of uterus and placenta (CTUP): the normal CTUP is <7 mm before day 300 of gestation.
+ Fetal activity: the fetus is rarely inactive for more than 5 minutes. Excessive movement may indicate fetal stress.
+ Heart rate: an inactive fetus with a heart rate <50 or >100 bpm is considered abnormal. When measuring heart rate it is important to remember that an increase of 25–40 bpm is normal following fetal activity.
+ Maximum depth of fetal fluid pool: a depth of around 22 cm is considered normal. It is important to assess the echogenicity of the fluid.
+ Aortic diameter: has been shown to correlate to fetal weight.
+ Uteroplacental contact: any areas of detachment with fluid/exudate visible behind the placenta.

Each variable can be given a value of 2 for normal and 0 for abnormal. A total value of 8 or less is suggestive of an unfavorable outcome. A maximal score, however, is not an assurance of normality, as problems can develop during delivery including premature placental separation, dystocia, and failure of the chorioallantois to rupture. Biophysical profiling of the prenatal equine fetus is an area that requires further research if accurate conclusions are to be made from the findings.

Fetal electrocardiography

This is a technique that has been used for over 25 years and can, if carefully carried out, document the fetal heart rate and the presence of a twin pregnancy. A normal electrocardiograph is used and both a mare and fetal trace obtained. Abnormalities of the fetal heart rate may precede fetal death. It should always be used in association with other assessment techniques because there can be difficulties in obtaining and interpreting the traces (472, 473).

Amniocentesis

Amniotic and allantoic fluid can be obtained by this technique. Research initially suggested that analysis of these fluids may help in determining the maturity of the fetus, but it has no significant advantages over less invasive procedures. It is carried out most safely under ultrasound guidance, but there are potential risks of abortion.

Changes in mammary secretions

The electrolyte levels in the secretions produced by the mammary gland undergo characteristic changes during the last week of gestation (474). Potassium and calcium concentrations rise, while sodium concentrations fall. These changes relate to fetal maturation, but caution should be used in interpreting milk electrolyte levels in maiden and pony mares and also in late-pregnancy mares that are ill, where maternal and fetal preparation for parturition may not be synchronous.

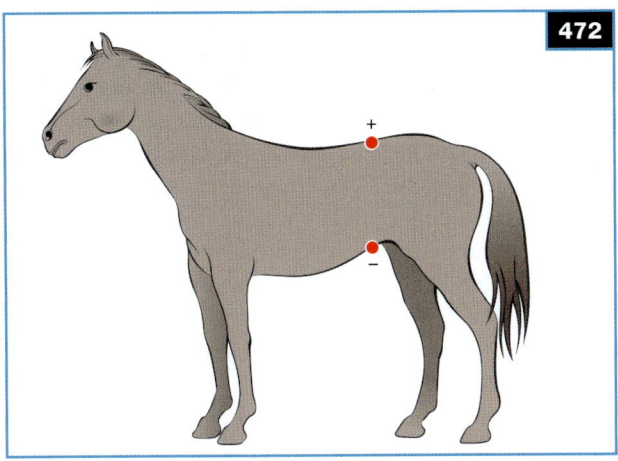

472 Diagram showing the sites of attachment of the leads to the mare for a fetal ECG.

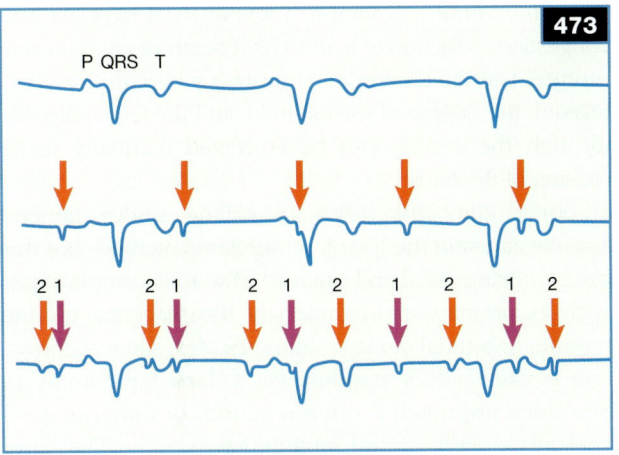

473 Typical ECG traces of (top) a nonpregnant mare, (center) a single pregnancy, and (bottom) a twin pregnancy. Arrows indicate the fetal heartbeat.

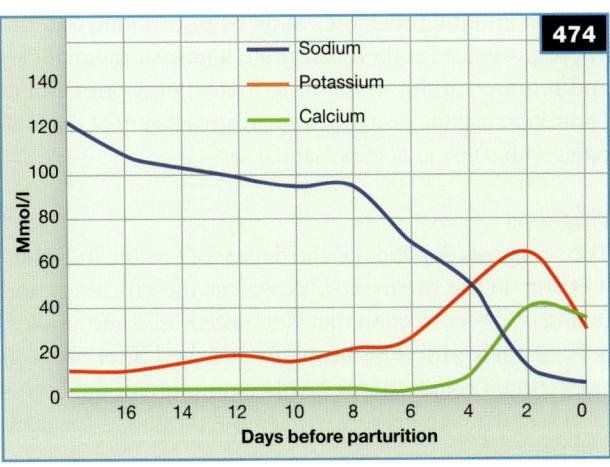

474 Mammary electrolyte secretions in the mare.

Management of high-risk mares

Mares with high-risk pregnancies should be given treatment according to the maternal disease present. Mares with placentitis can be given systemic antibiotics based on culture and sensitivity. Studies have shown that potentiated sulfonamides, procaine penicillin, crystalline penicillin, and gentamicin can all, when administered systemically, cross the placenta and reach therapeutic levels in the fetal fluids. However, the spectrum of action of procaine penicillin and crystalline penicillin is limited and although gentamicin may achieve adequate concentrations to be effective against *E. coli* and *Klebsiella* spp., it does not cross the placenta well enough to be effective against *Streptococcus equi*. For these reasons the broad-spectrum potentiated sulfonamides are the most commonly used antibiotics in cases of placentitis. A swab of the vulvar discharge should be taken to identify organisms and determine antibiotic sensitivity.

There is no evidence that NSAIDs are able to prevent abortion by the inhibition of cyclo-oxygenase-induced prostaglandin release, but they may be useful in mares suffering from any form of endotoxemia. Exogenous progesterone has been shown to stop cloprostenol-induced abortion in experimental models and it has been used in some high-risk pregnancies either as progesterone in oil i/m or altrenogest p/o at standard doses. Clenbuterol, a beta-agonist tocolytic agent used regularly in human medicine, may not be effective in the equine. Any decrease in nutrition requires an immediate response, as this can lead to premature parturition. With a placentitis, the fetus may or may not be infected, even if the placenta appears grossly infected. A weak foal that develops sepsis during the first 12 hours of life has probably acquired a bacterial infection *in utero* and should be treated accordingly.

Identification of the high-risk pregnancy is paramount if the pregnancy is to be given the chance of continuing to term. An assessment of the likely risk category of the live foal born from a high-risk pregnancy will greatly improve the survival of that foal.

Female reproductive tract

Complications of pregnancy

Uterine torsion

Definition/overview

Uterine torsion is an uncommon condition that usually occurs in late gestation, but rarely at parturition. The etiology is unknown. The condition usually presents as abdominal pain, often low grade and intermittent, and the diagnosis is confirmed by rectal palpation. Treatment using a rolling method under general anesthesia has been suggested, but most cases are treated surgically.

Etiology/pathophysiology

Usually occurs in the last trimester of pregnancy (>7 months), but only occasionally in association with parturition. The cause is unknown, but severe trauma, violent rolling (e.g. with a GI tract problem) or sudden fetal movements may be involved. The cervix is rarely involved. Older mares are more susceptible.

Clinical presentation

Most gravid mares with uterine torsion present with abdominal pain that is mild and intermittent, but it may become more severe depending on the degree of torsion, subsequent tension on the broad ligaments, and/or pressure on the uterine wall. Secondary GI complications and uterine rupture due to necrosis will exacerbate the clinical signs and worsen the prognosis. Rarely, torsion at parturition can lead to dystocia.

Differential diagnosis

Abortion or premature parturition; GI tract colic; fetal hypermotility; uterine dorsoretroflexion; hydrops amnion/allantois; uterine rupture (see p. 288); ventral abdominal wall rupture; prepubic tendon rupture; and two other conditions described briefly below:

+ Fetal hypermotility is the term used for violent or excessive foal movements in late pregnancy. The cause is unknown. If the condition persists, it is treated with smooth muscle spasmolytics.
+ Uterine dorsoretroflexion is when the fetus impacts in the pelvic canal during the last trimester. The cause is unknown. The condition is palpable per rectum/vagina. Treatment is with smooth muscle relaxants, reduced feed intake, and regular walking exercise.

Diagnosis

Rectal palpation, particularly of the broad ligaments, is essential to confirm the diagnosis. The tension and position of the ligaments vary in respect to the direction of the torsion. In the more common clockwise (from behind) torsion the left broad ligament courses across the dorsal aspect of the uterus from left to right, and the right broad ligament disappears ventrally. The fetus is usually displaced cranially. The amount of torsion can vary from mild to severe (90°–720°). The greater the rotation, the more effect there will be on the uterine circulation, the placenta, and the fetus.

Vaginal examination, visually or digitally, is often unhelpful because the cervix and cranial vagina are rarely involved. If the cervix is involved, it is not palpable or visible.

Management

Early intervention is vital to prevent local hypoxia and congestion, which may lead to fetal death or even uterine rupture. Uterine torsion at parturition where the cervix is relaxed, the degree of torsion mild, and the fetus palpable through the cervix, can be corrected manually using rocking of the fetus.

Some clinicians advocate rolling under general anesthesia using the 'plank in the flank' method, but this can be unsuccessful and can lead to serious complications such as premature separation of the placenta, uterine rupture, or arterial damage. In most cases, surgical correction is used, either standing via a flank laparotomy (a two-sided approach is often required) or under general anesthesia via a ventral midline laparotomy. The latter technique has the advantage of allowing better visualization of the uterus, ligaments, blood supply, and GI tract and identifying any damage and its subsequent repair, as well as the option of a Cesarean section. In a simple torsion with no complications the uterus is returned to a normal position and the pregnancy allowed to continue to term. These pregnancies then constitute high-risk pregnancies and require careful monitoring thereafter. Correction at parturition usually results in immediate delivery of the foal, often with some judicious manual assistance.

Prognosis

The prognosis depends on the degree of torsion and when it occurs in the pregnancy, as well as the efficiency and timing of the correction that is required. In some studies, 50% of foals and 70% of mares survived after surgical correction. Complications involving rupture of the uterus or vessel damage gravely worsen the prognosis for mare and foal.

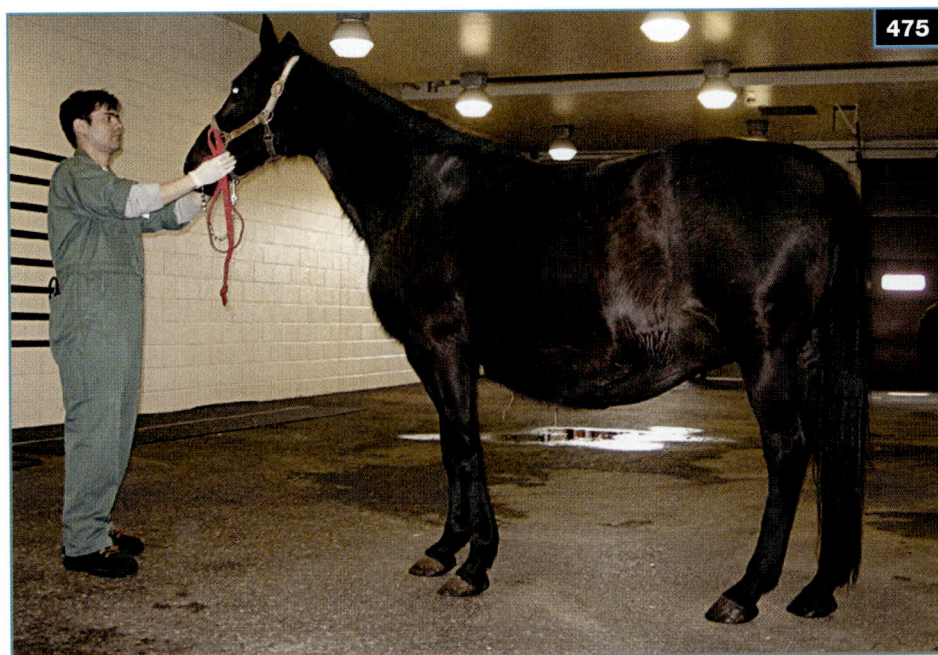

Hydrops amnion/allantois

Definition/overview

This is a sporadically occurring condition of late pregnancy in mares, which involves an abnormality of the fetal membranes (either amnion, allantois, or both together). Fetal abnormalities commonly accompany this condition. Rapid accumulation of placental fluids leads to sudden-onset abdominal enlargement in the last trimester of pregnancy. Circulatory problems, uterine rupture, and rupture of the abdominal wall can all occur secondarily and severely affect the prognosis. Rectal palpation and ultrasonography confirm the diagnosis and the mare should be either induced or aborted.

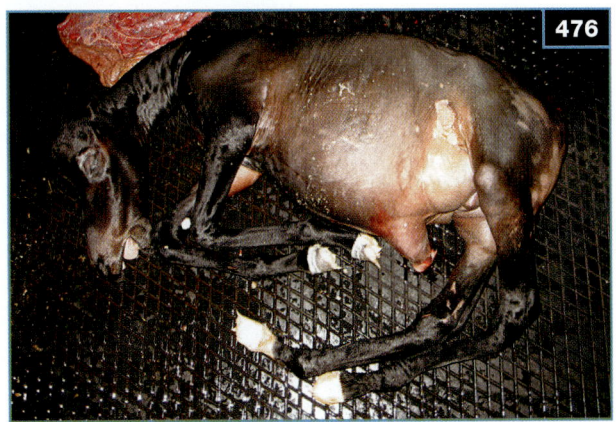

Etiology/pathophysiology

Hydrops is more common in multiparous mares. Hydrops allantois is the more common and is usually due to placental abnormalities, which lead to excessive accumulation of fluid in the allantoic cavity with or without fetal abnormalities such as wry neck, hydrocephalus, and ventral herniation. Hydrops of the amniotic cavity is extremely rare and is due to placental abnormalities, either inflammatory or vascular, and/or fetal abnormalities leading to an inability of the fetus to swallow normally.

Clinical presentation

Hydrops usually occurs in the pregnant mare in the last trimester of pregnancy, with a rapid accumulation of fluid in the uterus leading to visible abdominal enlargement over a few days to weeks (475). In some severe or chronic cases the mare may have problems standing after recumbency, signs of breathing difficulties, low-grade abdominal pain, and, in extreme cases, rupture of the ventral abdominal wall or prepubic tendon. Secondary ventral peripheral edema or inguinal herniation may occur, and uterine rupture has occasionally been reported.

Diagnosis

Clinical signs and rectal palpation can confirm these conditions, but transabdominal or transrectal ultrasonography may help differentiate hydrops amnion from hydrops allantois and detect abnormalities of the placenta and/or fetus. On rectal palpation the uterus is massively enlarged, filling much of the caudal abdominal cavity and making it difficult to detect the fetus. If the foal is identified as being abnormal (476), treatment should be directed more towards saving the mare.

Management

Both conditions are treated either by inducing parturition in late term mares or by aborting the mare. Induction of parturition is most easily achieved in the last 30 days of pregnancy by administering oxytocin (see Induction of parturition, p. 282). Abortion can be induced by manual dilation of the cervix over a 15–30 minute period or by placing dinoprostone (6 mg vaginal tablets) within the cervix for a few hours, after which the allantochorionic membranes can be manually ruptured through the cervical os. Whether abortion or induction is used, assistance with delivery of the foal is usually required because of uterine inertia. It is important to control the drainage of fluid from the uterus in order to minimize fluid imbalance and/or circulatory shock in the mare, which can be fatal. A sterile nasogastric tube can be useful for siphoning out the fluid and regulating the flow. Intravenous polyionic fluids or hypertonic saline may be useful during drainage to help maintain blood pressure.

After parturition or abortion, retention of placental membranes is common and should be treated as soon as possible. Use of an oxytocin drip may stimulate contractions and prevent uterine pooling of blood within the splanchnic circulation. Uterine involution and subsequent fertility are unaffected.

Prognosis

Severe or chronic cases carry a guarded to poor prognosis for the mare, especially if abortion or parturition is not induced quickly and circulatory and/or ventral abdominal wall problems ensue. There are reports of normal foals being born from mares with this condition, but most are abnormal and nonviable.

Rupture of the ventral abdominal muscles
Definition/overview

Rupture of the prepubic tendon and/or abdominus muscles can occur in late-term pregnant broodmares, particularly in older, multiparous animals with previous damage or abnormal pregnancies. Initially, it often presents with a plaque of ventral edema and mild abdominal pain before dropping of the abdomen is noted. Ultrasonography of the abdominal wall can be diagnostic (477–482). Treatment may include abdominal supports, induction of and/or assistance at parturition, surgical repair post parturition, retirement from breeding (except by embryo transfer), and euthanasia. The prognosis is guarded to poor.

Etiology/pathophysiology

Progressive rupturing of the prepubic tendon and/or the rectus/transverses abdominus muscles can occur either singly or in combination in late-pregnant mares. The exact etiology is unclear, but appears to be related to increasing strain on these structures from the weight of the developing pregnancy, leading to weakening and eventual rupture of the supporting tissues. Previous damage, poor fitness, twin and hydrops pregnancies, multiparity, increasing age, and draft breeds may all be predisposing factors.

Clinical presentation

The condition usually occurs in the last trimester of pregnancy and will often present initially as a ventral abdominal edematous plaque of up to 15 cm thickness. There may be abdominal pain, difficulty in moving, and, slightly later, dropping of the abdomen or even asymmetrical bulging. If the prepubic tendon completely ruptures, the mammary gland appears to move cranially and the tuber ischii become more elevated.

Differential diagnosis

Other abdominal hernias or ruptures including post surgery and traumatic; mammary gland/ventral abdominal wall edema.

Diagnosis

History and clinical presentation are very helpful, but confirmation of the damage is best achieved using transabdominal ultrasonography. Rectal examination may identify the prepubic damage in the midline cranial to the pubis.

Management

Abdominal supports have been used in these cases in late pregnancy, but they can be difficult to manage long term (483). In severe or progressive cases, induction of parturition is often considered, but fetal readiness for birth should be checked before this is undertaken. If the mare does reach parturition, this should be closely monitored. Additional assistance is often required due to loss of abdominal pressure. Cesarean section may be used in some cases. Surgical repair of the prepubic tendon ruptures is not possible and in other types of rupture is rarely undertaken due to economic considerations and poor success rates, particularly in severe cases. It is usually carried out after foaling, when all the edema and reaction have subsided, using a mesh implant. Euthanasia may be the only humane course in severe cases. High-value mares can be retired and embryo transfer used to maintain their genetic value. Foals born to these mares are always high risk, particularly due to problems with colostral quality, and they should be treated appropriately.

Prognosis

The prognosis is guarded to poor depending on the degree and extent of the damage, and the stage of pregnancy. In older or more severely affected mares, retirement from breeding, or at worse euthanasia, may be necessary.

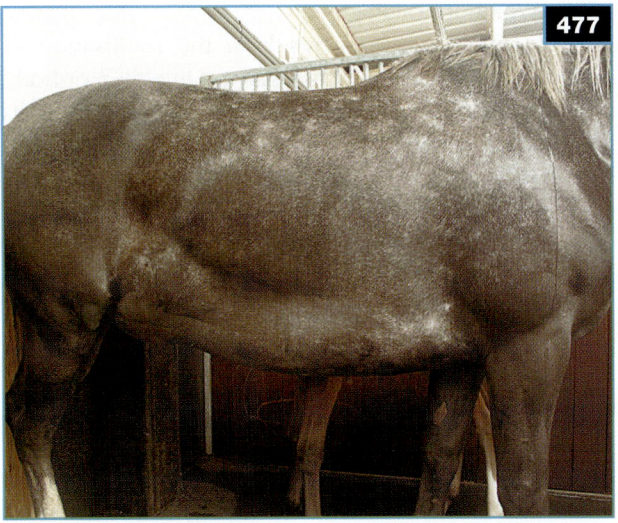

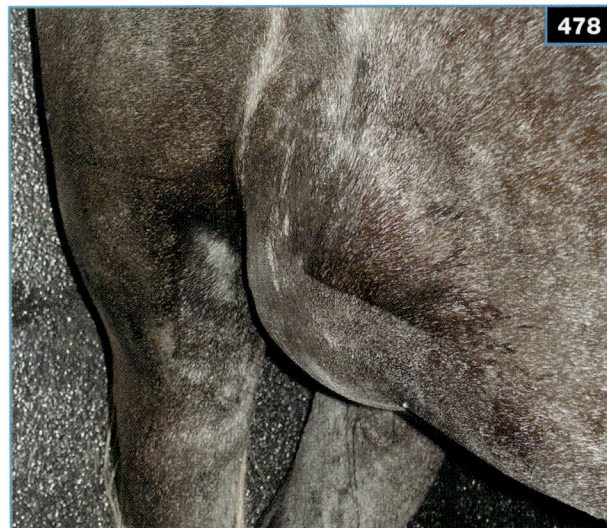

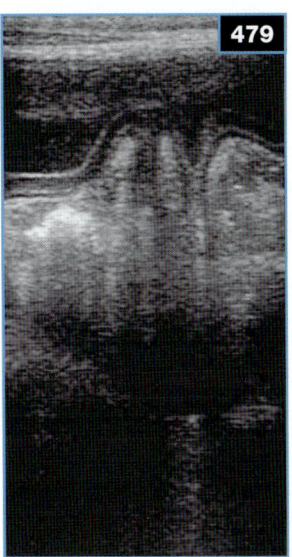

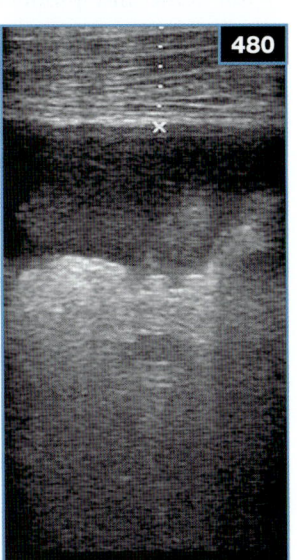

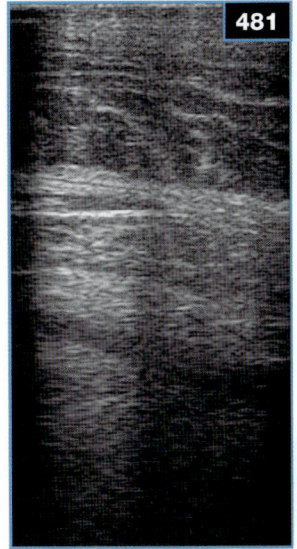

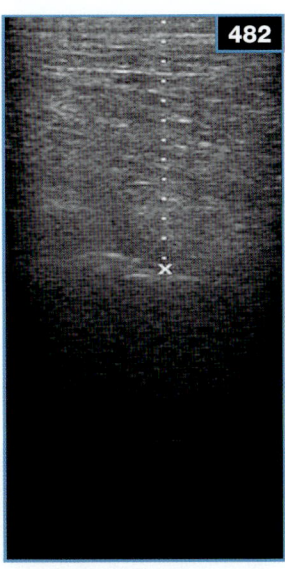

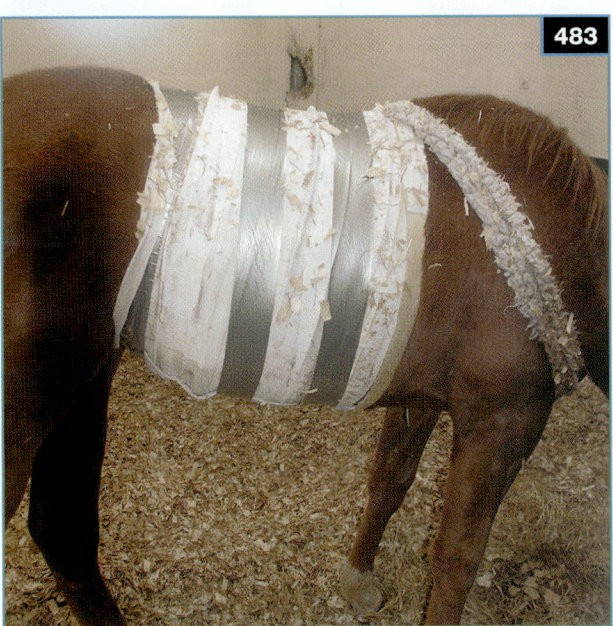

477 Large Danish Warmblood mare on the day of a normal foaling. In the weeks prior to foaling there had been increasing ventral edema and stiffness in the mare.

478 Immediately post foaling, an additional swelling had occurred on the lower right side of the abdomen.

479–482 Ultrasonograms from: directly over the right-sided swelling showing complete loss of the abdominal wall at the right side due to rupture (479); the left side showing normal wall thickness (480); over the ventral midline revealing extensive subcutaneous edema over a thickened abdominal wall (481); and over the prepubic tendon just cranial to the pubis, showing thickening and disruption of the fiber pattern of the tendon (482).

483 Use of an abdominal support bandage in a mare after foaling that had early signs of ventral rupture of the abdominal wall prior to parturition.

269

Twinning

Definition/overview

Multiple ovulations may be synchronous or more than 24 hours apart and the resultant embryos may implant in the same or both uterine horns. Twin pregnancies are not usually sustainable and the mare spontaneously aborts approximately 75% of unilateral and 15% of bilateral twins (**484**), accounting for 20–30% of abortions in the Thoroughbred prior to the advent of routine reproductive ultrasonography. Incidence is breed related, heavy horses exhibiting a proportionally higher incidence, and it is rarely encountered in ponies. Some individuals are predisposed to multiple ovulations for their entire breeding lifetime and multiparous mares generally have a higher incidence. Identical twinning, due to splitting of a single fertilized ovum, is extremely rare in the horse. Diagnosis of twinning is by manual palpation of the embryos/fetuses or by ultrasound scan. Evaluation of every mare at pregnancy examination for twin pregnancy is a core part of modern stud-farm management. Treatment is by manual rupture of one fetus or hormonal induction of abortion of both fetuses. Due to the risks of twin pregnancy to mare and foals, any identified cases should not be allowed to continue beyond mid term.

Etiology/pathophysiology

Multiple ovulations may result in the fertilization of multiple ova at mating, which may fix in either, or both, uterine horns. It has been found that where both twins fix in the same uterine horn at day 16, 83% will undergo so-called 'natural reduction' and scan pregnant with only one embryo at 40 days post ovulation. Of those that have one twin in each horn at 16 days, none will undergo natural reduction and all will scan positive for twins, with one embryo in each uterine horn at 40 days. Twin pregnancies are unsustainable, particularly if unilateral, because of placental insufficiency, and they usually result in the death of one or both fetuses and early abortion. They are very rarely carried to term, and if so, one or both foals are usually born dead or else are severely dysmature. Mummification of one fetus and the pregnancy continuing to full term and producing a normal foal has been recorded.

Clinical presentation

Two or more ovulated follicles are palpable on a routine postovulation rectal examination or ultrasound scan, or two conceptuses at a later stage. Early abortion may occur, or birth of two dysmature or dead foals at term, if the pregnancy is allowed to continue. Abortion is usually later (7 months) for bilateral twins.

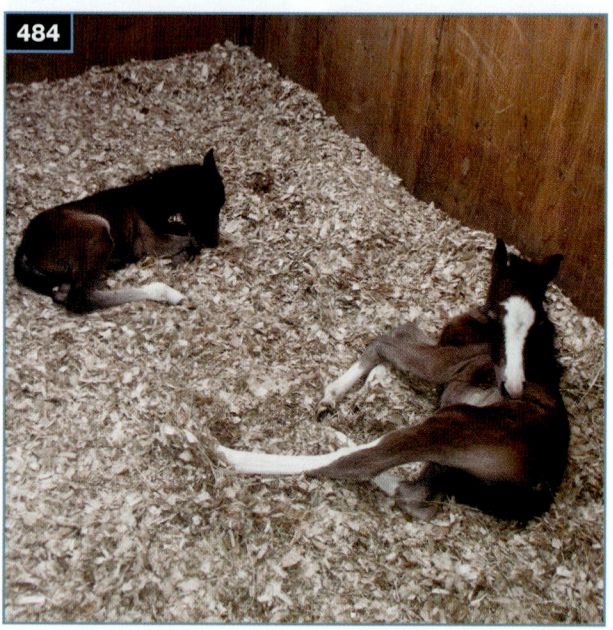

484 A remarkably uncommon situation in which twin foals have been born live to a pony mare and survived. Both were dysmature at birth. Note the disparity in the size of the two foals.

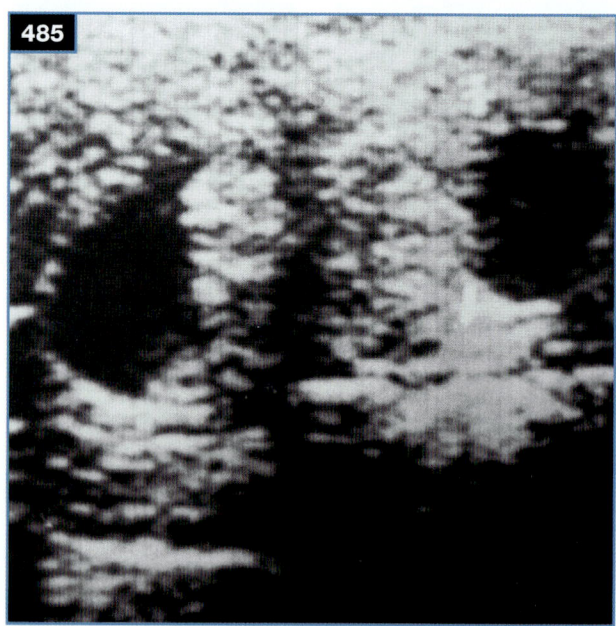

485 Ultrasonographic image showing twin 17-day-old conceptuses, one in each uterine horn.

Diagnosis

A thorough examination of the entire reproductive tract using ultrasound scanning at 14–15 days post ovulation is the best time to identify the still mobile embryos and multiple CL (**485**). High-quality equipment should be used and if twinning is suspected, the examination repeated in 24–48 hours to confirm the presence of twin embryos rather than endometrial cysts, which can confuse the picture (embryos will grow and change shape rapidly, move around at this stage, and are thinner walled). Asynchronous ovulations may also result in difference in size of the embryos, allowing the more immature embryo to be missed if only one examination is carried out. Manual palpation per rectum of the ovaries and uterus during a routine postmating examination may identify two conceptuses, but any findings should be confirmed by ultrasound examination. Identification of multiple follicles and ovulations is not a reason for delaying mating. Because not all the ova may be fertilized, there is a high incidence of early embryonic death in the mare and not all of the embryos may continue to develop.

Management

Termination of one or both pregnancies is the treatment of choice. While the embryos are still mobile (up to 16 days) one embryo (usually the smaller) can be manipulated into a position, usually at the tip of a horn, where it can be manually crushed either against the ultrasound probe or wall of the pelvis, or within the hand. Sedation may be required to facilitate this procedure (using an α_2 agonist such as detomidine) and care is required to prevent injury to the mare. Serial scanning after crushing is essential to check for success and the continuing health of the remaining conceptus. After 20 days and up to 30 days, bicornuate twins can still be crushed as above (it is less successful), but the unicornuate are now fixed by uterine tone. Separation is usually not possible, and further serial scanning is useful to monitor their progress because considerable natural reduction (approximately 50%) occurs in these cases. It is not advisable to attempt the crushing of a blastocyst while it is situated in the uterine body; undue force will be required, which could damage the uterus.

Flushing out of the embryos using uterine lavage is possible before they implant.

After 30 days and up to 60 days (ideally 45–50 days), selective reduction of one embryo/fetus by ultrasound-guided needle puncture and drainage of allantoic fluid through the anterior vagina has been carried out, but success is limited in retaining a viable single normal foal. In even older pregnancies (up to 120 days), one fetus can be injected transabdominally directly into the heart with potassium chloride to induce fetal death and its subsequent abortion. In all cases, repeat examination should be made 3–4 days after twin reduction in order to ensure that the procedure has been successful. In those cases where successful resolution has not been achieved by 34 days, or where removal of both fetuses is required, abortion should be induced using multiple doses of prostaglandin prior to endometrial cup formation, at around 35 days post ovulation.

Prognosis

Manual rupture of one of bilateral twins or unilateral twin embryos during the mobile phase (16–18 days post ovulation) can be very efficient (up to 95% successful). If unilateral twins cannot be separated, skilled clinicians can still attain 50% success in destroying one and maintaining the other. The key to successful treatment of all twin pregnancies is early diagnosis, preferably in the mobility phase. Many of the treatments later on usually result in resorption/abortion of the remaining conceptus and return to estrus in the mare. Natural mechanisms for twin reduction do occur. Approximately 70% of unicornuate twins undergo natural reduction to a single pregnancy before 30 days of gestation. In bicornuate twins, however, almost none undergo natural reduction. If allowed to proceed, twin pregnancies may result in abortion, dystocia, retained placenta, delayed uterine involution, reduced subsequent fertility in the mare, and usually dead or severely dysmature foals. Some mares and breeds (Thoroughbred) are predisposed to multiple ovulation/twinning for their entire reproductive lives. Barren and maiden mares appear more likely than lactating mares to have multiple ovulations.

Placentitis

Definition/overview

Placentitis is a common cause of sporadic abortion and late-pregnancy vaginal discharge in the mare (486). An ascending infection via the cervix can spread, or hematogenous infection may lead to a generalized placentitis, premature placental separation, fetal death, or poor growth and abnormal maturation of the fetus. Abortion, stillbirth, or mummification can also occur. Infection of the fetus may lead to organ damage and death or abnormalities of growth or maturation. Bacterial, viral, and fungal causes have been identified. In late-term pregnancy a live foal may be delivered, which should be classified as high risk, particularly of septicemia.

Etiology/pathophysiology

Possible routes of infection are ascending from a vaginal infection or externally from contact with infected fomites; hematogenous spread; or infection introduced at the time of breeding or iatrogenically from manual reproductive examination. Bacterial causes of infection include: *Streptococcus* spp. (most common isolate), *Staphylococcus* spp., *Escherichia coli*, *Pseudomonas* spp., *Klebsiella* spp., *Salmonella abortus equi*, *Corynebacterium pseudotuberculosis*, *Leptospira pomona* (hematogenous), and *Nocardia* spp. Viral causes of placentitis include: EHV-1 (most commonly) or EHV-4; equine viral arteritis (EVA) virus. Fungal cases are rare and most are caused by *Aspergillus* spp., usually via ascending infection from the cervix. Infection of the placenta results in chorionic villi inflammation/necrosis, interference with chorion/endometrial interdigitation, and placental insufficiency, and usually leads to premature placental separation and either premature delivery or fetal death. Infection can spread from the placenta directly to the foal, resulting in fetal death from septicemia. Infected fetal membranes and fluids, as well as uterine secretions from aborted mares, can be a source of infection in the viral causes of placentitis. Latent infections are possible with EHV-1, which can be activated by stress. Placentitis affecting only a limited area of placenta, or a severe placentitis occurring close to full term, may not cause abortion, but may result in delivery of a live foal, which may be weak, poorly grown, dysmature, or septicemic. In some cases the placentitis may cause sufficient early maturity of the fetal adrenal cortex to occur, which allows the foal to survive despite its early gestational age. Older, multiparous mares with poor perineal conformation may have an increased risk of placentitis.

Clinical presentation

Usually, there are transient systemic signs such as pyrexia, depression, anorexia, peripheral edema, and respiratory signs for 3–7 days in viral placentitis (EHV and EVA infection [see p. 278]). Systemic signs are unusual in bacterial and fungal placentitis. Vaginal/vulval discharge is common in bacterial and fungal placentitis. Abortion or premature delivery may occur immediately or be delayed, but is usually sporadic. Occasional abortion outbreaks occur in viral-induced placentitis. Premature lactation is commonly a sign of placentitis and/or placental/fetal compromise. Postpartum purulent or fetid vaginal discharge within 12 hours of parturition should be investigated and the foal monitored as high risk.

Differential diagnosis

Other causes of abortion. Other causes of vaginal discharge: vulval trauma; premature placental separation; urine staining from urogenital disorder; vaginal varicose veins (old, multiparous mares).

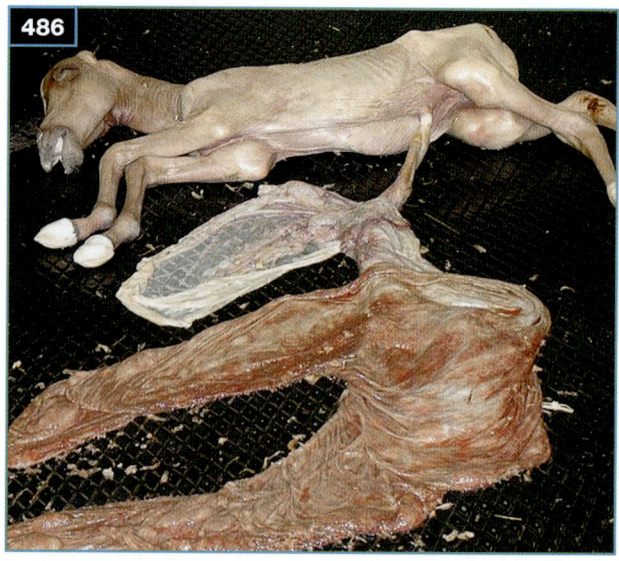

486 Aborted, poorly grown fetus subsequent to a placentitis. (Photo courtesy T Chenier)

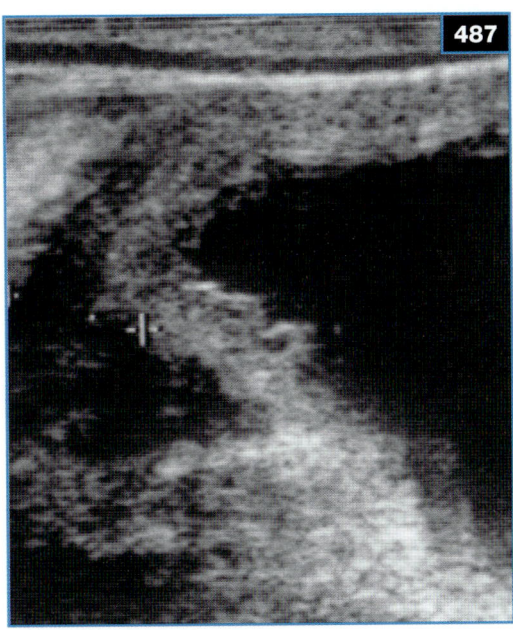

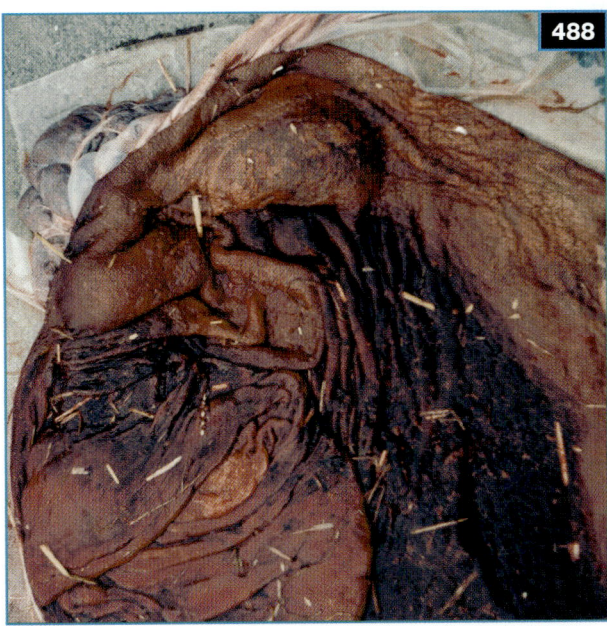

487 Transabdominal ultrasonographic view of an abnormally thickened placenta in a mare with placentitis. (Photo courtesy T Chenier)

488 Part of the placenta of a Thoroughbred mare that had foaled following a late-pregnancy vaginal discharge. There are areas of placental thickening and brown discoloration due to a focal placentitis of bacterial origin.

Diagnosis

Any vaginal discharge should be sampled for culture and/or histopathology. Transrectal and/or transabdominal ultrasonographic evaluation should include assessment of the state of health of the foal and an assessment of the combined thickness of the uteroplacental unit lateral to the cervical star, an increase in which may indicate inflammation or separation (487).

Following abortion or parturition, the placenta and aborted foal should be examined carefully grossly for any diagnostic lesions (488). Culture and histopathologic examination of stained tissue samples and smears from affected areas of the placenta/foal and/or swabs taken from the uterus post abortion may help identify the pathogen (some bacteria are difficult to isolate [e.g. *Leptospira* spp.]). ELISA or agglutination tests are available for identification of some pathogens.

Management

There is often little that can be done to avoid abortion, which is usually inevitable by the time clinical signs are manifested. Broad-spectrum antibiotics, anti-inflammatories, and tocolytic drugs (e.g. clenbuterol or progesterone supplementation) to try to suppress uterine motility may help when the condition is diagnosed early (e.g. in an outbreak).

Where a live foal is delivered, any prematurity or abnormal vaginal discharge in the mare around delivery should immediately class the foal as 'high risk' of being infected and appropriate neonatal monitoring and therapy should be instigated to avoid septicemia.

Strict stud hygiene, immediate isolation of aborted mares and fetuses, and use of vaccination for EHV-1 and EVA, where available, are essential measures to minimize the risk of infection or to control an outbreak. Surgical correction of poor perineal conformation may reduce the incidence of placentitis in some mares.

Prognosis

Abortion is a common sequela to placentitis. Prolonged infection in the mare is uncommon, depending on the causal organism, once abortion has occurred and following treatment. Latent infections can occur in EHV-1 infection, which can be instigated by stress at a later date. The prognosis for a live foal is guarded to poor depending on the causal agent and degree of placental compromise.

Fetal mummification

Definition/overview

If intrauterine fetal death occurs and the cervix remains closed, the fetus is retained and may become 'mummified'. In the case of twins, the live fetus can continue normally to term, when the mummified fetus is delivered at the same time as the normal foal. In single cases, which are rare, the mare may spontaneously abort the dead fetus at any time or enter an extended period of anestrus.

Etiology/pathophysiology

Bacterial or mycotic placentitis may cause fetal death and, where the mare is treated with antimicrobials and proges-terone, this may result in the cervix remaining closed and retention of the dead fetus. If the fetal sac remains sterile, its fluid contents are resorbed, the fetus dehydrates, and it becomes mummified. The most common scenario is in cases of twinning when one of the fetuses spontaneously dies and subsequently mummifies, while the pregnancy is maintained by the remaining live fetus. The mummified fetus may macerate *in utero* over time, or as a result of an ascending infection via the cervix, leading to a vulval discharge.

Clinical presentation

Spontaneous abortion of a mummified fetus can occur at any time in the pregnancy, but most commonly in the second trimester (489). There is prolonged anestrus or variable cyclicity after a positive pregnancy diagnosis. The mummified fetus is delivered at term as a single pregnancy or alongside a normal foaling. Prolonged pregnancy can occur beyond the expected term. In some cases the mum-mified fetus is trapped in the uterus or cervix after parturi-tion and the mare starts to cycle normally. If the fetus undergoes intrauterine maceration, a brown discharge may be seen at the vulva. There are rarely any systemic signs.

Differential diagnosis

Other causes of spontaneous abortion.

Diagnosis

Diagnosis is based on clinical signs. Rectal palpation reveals the uterus contracted around a dry, contorted fetus with no surrounding fluids. Transrectal or transabdominal ultrasonography reveals a highly echogenic contracted fetal mass in the uterus.

Management

In the late-term mare, delivery can be induced following prostaglandin treatment and cervical dilation, often manually. The uterus should be flushed with sterile saline to aid lubrication of the delivery and repeated, possibly post delivery, in order to remove debris and contamination from the uterus. If infection is suspected in the case of maceration, antibiotics should be given depending on culture and sensitivity results. Cesarean section may be required to remove a large mummified fetus.

Prognosis

Undiagnosed fetal mummification may result in the loss of a breeding season, but there are no long-term effects on the breeding potential of the mare provided no infection is involved.

Early embryonic death

Definition/overview

Early embryonic death (EED) is defined as occurring before 40 days of pregnancy and it can result from many factors. Figures for the level of early embryonic loss are affected by the timing of the pregnancy diagnosis. EEDs of between 7% and 16% have been suggested when pregnancy is diagnosed by rectal examination, but this rises to 24% with earlier ultrasonographic pregnancy diagnosis. The highest losses occur in the first 10–14 days, with progressively less over time. Many causes have been proposed.

Etiology/pathophysiology

Genetic factors include: embryonic, chromosomal, and developmental defects; inbreeding; ageing of sperm or oocyte at conception; individual mare or stallion genetic makeup or defects. Management effects include: stresses such as hyperthermia, travel, and water deprivation; poor nutrition prior to conception and in early pregnancy; concurrent systemic illness or severe or prolonged colic; toxicosis, including drug therapy in early pregnancy. Individual mare factors include: age of the mare (with older mares often having over double the rate of loss, mainly due to subfertility); breeding at first postpartum estrus.

Uterine disease can lead to a hostile environment for the embryo (e.g. delayed uterine involution; endometritis and retained intrauterine fluid; chronic endometrial disease such as atrophy, fibrosis, and endometrial cysts).

Endocrine causes such as inadequate endogenous progesterone production by the CL to maintain pregnancy have been suggested, but are often difficult to prove.

Other causes include oviduct obstruction, twinning, and abnormalities of the embryo location.

Clinical presentation

Mares return to estrus following positive pregnancy diagnosis either ultrasonographically (14–25 days) or by manual rectal palpation (21–40 days). They fail to conceive (if EED <14 days) despite normal cyclic activity. Variable other signs occur relating to the cause.

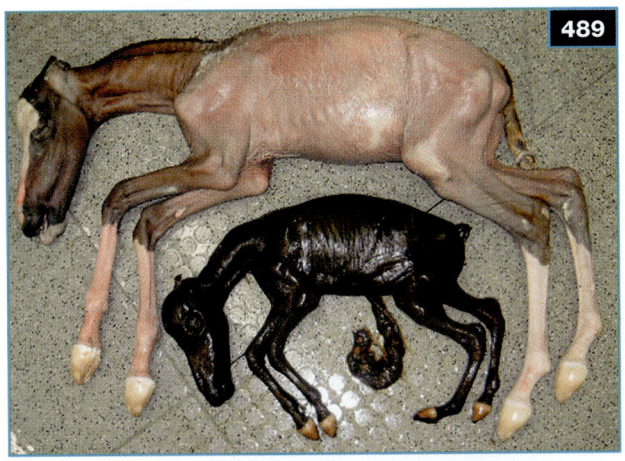

489 Twin abortion in the last trimester of pregnancy showing clear disparity in fetal size. The smaller fetus has already died *in utero* and has undergone early mummification. (Photo courtesy CA Cooke)

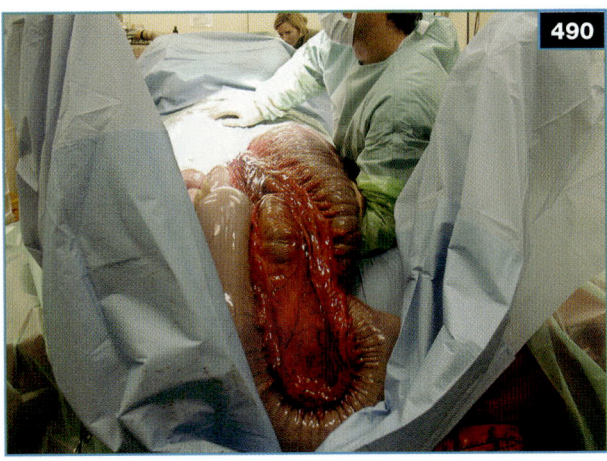

490 Surgical intervention in a broodmare 7 days post foaling that revealed a 360 degree large colon torsion. Note the enlarged and discolored left dorsal and ventral colon, with a hemorrhagic mesentery.

Differential diagnosis

Twinning; embryonic defects; endogenous prostaglandin release following stress; concurrent systemic disease; poor nutrition; oviduct obstruction; reduced oocyte viability with ageing mare.

Diagnosis

Serial ultrasound examinations demonstrate loss of the conceptus. A number of ultrasonographic abnormalities of the abnormal embryo have been identified. Pregnancy diagnosis is possible from 10–12 days by transrectal ultrasonography, but is more regularly performed between 14 and 16 days. An embryo/fetus with a visible heartbeat should be detectable from 25 days onwards in the normal pregnancy. Rectal detection of a pregnancy is variably possible from 18 days onwards.

Management

In mares suspected of early embryonic death, it is generally better to return the mare to estrus and the reproductive tract to the optimal condition for mating as quickly as possible by inducing luteolysis with prostaglandin injections where necessary, treating any obvious causes, and performing intrauterine irrigation to remove any debris. In mares prone to EED, exogenous progesterone supplementation until after the establishment of the endometrial cups has been used with

some limited success. GnRH has also been used at about day 10–12 post ovulation to support the function of the CL. In the majority of cases, early detection of EED by regular examination is the best way to minimize delays in re-mating and thereby increase end-of-year pregnancy rates.

Prognosis

The prognosis is good to guarded depending on the cause.

Gastrointestinal complications of late pregnancy and parturition

Definition/overview

This rare group of conditions is mainly seen in the postpartum mare and includes rupture of the cecum or right ventral colon and contusion of the small intestine/small colon/rectum and attaching mesentery, with possible secondary rupture. Colonic torsion is particularly common in postpartum mares in the first 4 weeks (490).

Etiology/pathophysiology

The cecum and large colon may be traumatized during parturition, particularly if they are filled with ingesta and/or gas. Fetal limbs may directly damage loops of bowel, or prolonged or abnormal straining may damage or rupture bowel trapped in the pelvic canal between the fetus and bony walls. Spontaneous rupture can occur in the cecum

275

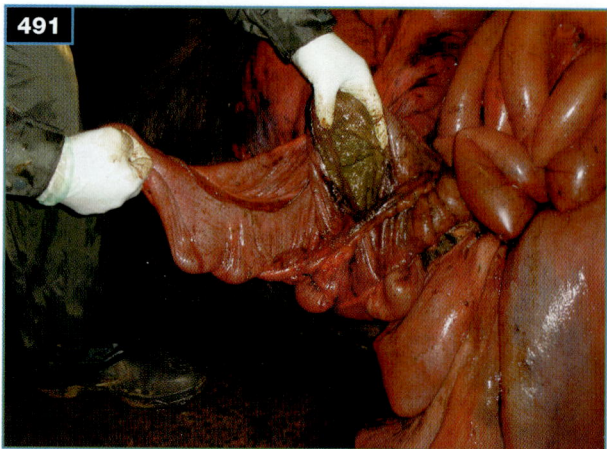

491 Postmortem view of a broodmare that was euthanized after a postfoaling peritonitis. Note the rupture in the cecum.

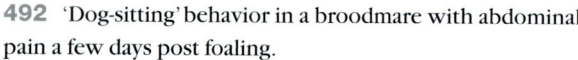

492 'Dog-sitting' behavior in a broodmare with abdominal pain a few days post foaling.

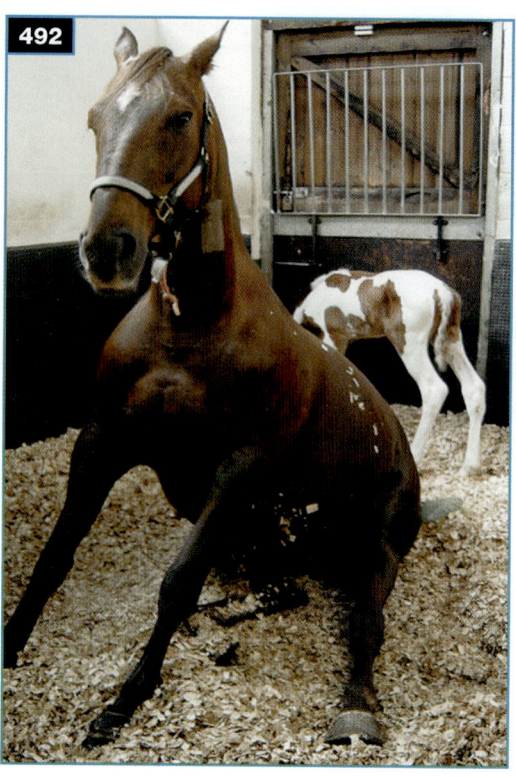

with marked increases of abdominal pressure (491). Ruptures commonly occur within 15 cm of the ileocecal valve, ventrally in the cecum and caudally in the right ventral colon. Contusions of the small intestine, small colon, or even rectum, plus their mesentery, can also occur at parturition. Severe damage can lead to rupture of the bowel or damage to the mesentery, with incarceration or vascular occlusion and segmental ischemic necrosis.

Clinical presentation

The presenting signs will relate to the degree of damage to the bowel and when this occurred (492). Mares that rupture the cecum or large colon early in parturition may present with difficulty in foaling due to weak straining. Delivery of the foal manually usually occurs without complication, but the mare does not recover from the foaling as normal and rapidly develops signs of septic peritonitis and endotoxic shock. Death can occur in 4–6 hours. Where the bowel is damaged but not ruptured, a slower, less marked clinical picture evolves with low-grade abdominal pain, sometimes several days after parturition. The delivery may or may not have been complicated. The colic is accompanied by fever and depression, with poor milk production and abdominal guarding if peritonitis becomes established. Bowel damage can lead to progressive leakage of bacteria and bacterial toxins and result in endotoxic shock, septicemia, and death.

Diagnosis

Peritoneal fluid collection and analysis are essential for diagnosis of peritonitis (neutrophilia and leukocytosis) and bowel rupture (food material). Rectal palpation reveals variable findings from nothing to impacted small colon, painful foci in the abdomen, or roughened, inflamed serosal surfaces. Transabdominal ultrasonography or laparoscopy may be helpful in further differentiation of the diagnosis.

Management

In many cases of rupture the opportunity for treatment is minimal and euthanasia is indicated. Surgical intervention by midline ventral laparotomy may establish the site and severity of damage, but inaccessibility of some lesions, particularly in the small colon and rectum, and the extent of mesenteric damage make many lesions inoperable. Resection of damaged bowel and mesentery followed by anastomosis is particularly challenging in the small colon or cranial rectum. Peritoneal lavage and antibiotics, followed by high levels of systemic antibiotics and intensive care, are essential for mare survival.

Prognosis

The prognosis is poor to grave depending on the degree, site and extent of damage to the bowel, and the amount of peritoneal contamination.

276

Abortion

Abortion in the mare is defined as expulsion of the fetus and its membranes before 300 days of gestation (493). Expulsion after 300 days is usually termed a stillbirth. The overall incidence of abortion varies widely according to surveys, but has been quoted as between 5% and 15%. The causes of abortion can be divided initially into non-infectious, infectious, and unknown. There is some dispute in the literature as to the incidence of these different etiologies. Noninfectious causes are usually the most common (up to 70%), with infectious causes varying between 15% and 45%. Up to 50% of abortions may be undiagnosed. The majority of abortions are sporadic, but in some cases infectious causes can lead to disastrous epidemics for a stud farm. It is essential to establish the individual etiology of each abortion case by a rapid and thorough examination of the aborted fetus and fetal membranes, using a competent diagnostic laboratory. A thorough stepwise investigation must be performed. Until proven otherwise, every aborted mare should be treated as potentially infectious, as in the case of abortion caused by EHV-1. Management of an abortion should follow the guidelines outlined in the country or region's disease-control program (e.g. the Horserace Betting Levy Board's Code of Practice in the UK).

In general:

+ Aborted mares and the aborted material should be immediately isolated from other mares.
+ All in-contact mares should be examined and held in isolation until the cause of the abortion is ascertained.
+ A full history of the mare, its management, and vaccination record should be taken with a view to establishing any causative factor.
+ A postmortem examination should be carried out on the fetus and placental membranes or arrangements should be made to send the material to a diagnostic laboratory.

The clinical signs of abortion vary with different causes, but in some cases the mare may be found to be non-pregnant at the end of the gestational period after being diagnosed pregnant in early pregnancy, yet no abortion has been detected. Premonitory signs are uncommon, but in placentitis cases in late gestation, lactation may be detected. Mares are rarely observed aborting, but if they are, they may show some signs of parturition. Dystocia is extremely rare. Following the abortion there are rarely any complications because the complete fetoplacental unit is usually delivered. Occasionally, part of or the entire placenta is retained.

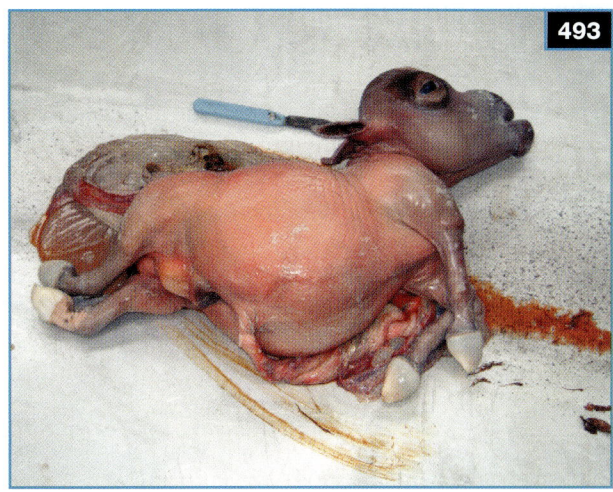

493 Fresh aborted fetus with multiple abnormalities, including the mandible, and small size. (Photo courtesy CA Cooke)

Additional objectives should be to return the mare to health as soon as possible and re-establish normal reproductive function.

Prophylaxis may not be possible with some causes of abortion, but with others it can be very effective. The reduction in the incidence of twins by the routine use of early-pregnancy ultrasonography has considerably decreased twinning as a cause. The identification of endometrial disease can help predict the chances of abortion and may help focus specific treatment pre-conception. Vaccination of pregnant mares for EHV-1 and EVA is helpful under certain circumstances. Bacterial endometritis should be identified and treated, with correction of any condition leading to increased contamination of the reproductive tract.

Infectious causes of abortion
Equine herpesvirus type 1
Definition/overview

In many parts of the world this is the single most important infectious cause of abortion. It may be sporadic or more extensive (termed 'storms'). This virus also causes various respiratory and neurologic disorders (see pp. 451 and 765).

Etiology/pathophysiology

The virus is transmitted by aerosol via the respiratory route and usually spreads slowly between in-contact horses. Abortion material, membranes, and fluids are also very infectious.

Clinical presentation

The timing of abortion is usually around 9 months (>5 months to term), 4–14 weeks post infection, and without premonitory signs. The foal is usually aborted wrapped in its membranes. In some cases the foal may be born alive, but it invariably dies within 24 hours.

Diagnosis

Diagnosis is based on history, fetal and placental pathologic changes, and virus isolation. The aborted material can have quite specific lesions such as excessive serosal fluids, small (1 mm) white areas of necrosis in the liver, an enlarged spleen, and pneumonic lung lesions, pleuritis, and exudate in the airways. The chorion may be edematous, with the chorionic side out (due to rapid expulsion of the fetus). Histologically, there will be foci of necrosis in the liver, lungs, and spleen and intranuclear inclusion bodies within hepatocytes and other cell types. It has been suggested that abortion can be mediated by the production of a vasculitis involving the endometrium and/or the chorion, with antibody–antigen complexes having been found within affected blood vessels.

Management

There is no treatment for the aborting mare or aborted fetus. The mare will develop natural immunity following recovery from the abortion; however, this lasts only 4–6 months and therefore repeat abortions can occur in consecutive pregnancies.

Vaccination of the pregnant mare with a killed vaccine at 5, 7, and 9 months of gestation can substantially decrease the incidence of abortion in groups of mares and in epidemic storms. Other preventive control measures include quarantine of all mares that enter a stud farm until considered suitable to expose to other stock on the farm, batching of pregnant mares of similar gestational age, minimizing the mixing of stock, and isolation of pregnant mares from young stock.

Equine herpesvirus type 4

Abortion can be caused by EHV-4, but these cases are less common and appear to be sporadic rather than abortion storms.

Equine viral arteritis
Definition/overview

EVA occurs worldwide and is the subject of government controls in various countries. It occurs sporadically in the UK (notifiable disease), but is common elsewhere in the world, including the US.

Etiology/pathophysiology

EVA virus is spread to the mare from aerosol contact with the respiratory form of the disease, venereally from a carrier stallion, or via insemination with infected semen. The products of an abortion are also infectious. The disease leads to a vasculitis in a variety of tissues. The incubation period is reasonably rapid (3–8 days). In groups of animals the morbidity rate can be quite high, but the mortality rate is low.

Clinical presentation

There is considerable variation in the range and severity of the clinical signs: pyrexia, depression, and anorexia; nasal discharge; edema of the limbs and ventral abdomen; conjunctival swelling; skin plaques; and abortion.

Diagnosis

Diagnosis of the disease can be difficult, especially prior to abortion. Virus isolation from the aborted fetus, nasal discharges of the mare, and semen from the breeding stallion are helpful. Paired serology testing can be used to confirm exposure of the mare to the virus and indirectly identify carrier stallions. False positives will occur post vaccination.

Management

Treatment is supportive and most animals recover. Prevention includes the use of vaccination and careful management practices. The use of infected carrier stallions should be avoided if possible. Serologic testing of blood samples while horses are in stud-farm quarantine will establish the status of mares prior to breeding with known disease-free stallions or their semen. In an outbreak, all in-contact mares and stallions should be tested and isolated for 3 weeks post recovery. All infected materials should be destroyed and disinfection of all equipment and living areas carried out. A modified live virus vaccine is available under license in the UK, Ireland, France, Germany, and certain states in the US, but with different national restrictions on use. Blood testing for seronegativity prior to vaccination is essential.

Bacterial abortion
Definition/overview
A large number of bacterial species can cause abortions in mares and some clinicians consider this the most important cause of abortion.

Etiology/pathophysiology
Bacteria can be introduced at breeding, ascend through the cervix (most common), or spread hematogenously. Cervical incompetence and/or pneumovagina can predispose the mare to an ascending bacterial infection and abortion. A placentitis develops and the chorionic surface becomes brown and edematous, with possibly an overlying exudate. The bacterial infection may spread to the fetus itself and infect and damage a range of organs. Abortion occurs following fetal death either from septicemia or by progressive placentitis and subsequent placental insufficiency. The most likely etiological agents for bacterial abortion are *Streptococcus* spp. (which are the most common), *E. coli*, *Pseudomonas* spp., *Klebsiella* spp., and *Staphylococcus* spp. Hematogenously spread organisms include *Salmonella* spp., *Streptococcus zooepidemicus*, and *Leptospira* spp. A form of noncervical placentitis, which affects the body of the chorion and the base of the horns and is associated with a nocardioform organism, has been reported in the US, particularly Kentucky.

Clinical presentation
Vaginal discharge and premature lactation may precede bacterial or fungal abortion and these mares should be considered high risk and have detailed fetoplacental assessments carried out. The appearance of the placenta following a bacterial abortion can vary from minimal changes in acute cases to a thickened, edematous placenta, either generally or in localized areas. The chorionic surface is often brown and covered in exudate.

Diagnosis
Bacterial organisms may be cultured or seen on stained cytology smears from samples taken from the aborted fetus/placenta and mare's uterus. Leptospiral abortion is difficult to diagnose as bacterial isolation is often difficult and postmortem findings in the fetus are variable. Immunofluorescence and special staining techniques may allow demonstration of the organism in tissues, and rising antibody titers in the mare are supportive.

Management
Treatment of bacterial placentitis is very difficult and abortion is usually inevitable once the infection becomes established. Prevention of ascending infections and endometritis is essential and is covered in detail elsewhere (p. 313). A vaccine is available for *Salmonella abortus equi* abortion in some parts of the world and other nonequine vaccines have been used in leptospiral abortion. Careful management and hygiene practices are important to avoid exposure to bacterial organisms before and after abortions.

Fungal abortion
This is a rare cause of late abortion (generally >10 months) or stillbirth and is usually an ascending infection through a damaged cervix. The gross appearance of the placenta and fetus is similar to a bacterial abortion, but there may be a mucoid exudate and yellow leathery areas of the placenta. There may or may not be a vaginal discharge. In some cases the foal may be born alive but congenitally infected. Microscopically, fungal hyphae are abundant on smears and histopathology of the placenta, and inflammatory foci are present in the fetal liver. The organism can be cultured in some cases from the uterus. *Aspergillus* spp. are the most frequently encountered fungi involved.

Noninfectious causes of abortion
Twinning
Twinning was once the single most common cause of abortion (see 489). It now accounts for only 6% of abortions following the widespread use of ultrasonography of the reproductive tract in early pregnancy and early recognition and management of the condition.

Umbilical cord problems
Torsion of the cord, or strangulation of the fetus by the cord, leading to fetal asphyxia.

Body pregnancy
Unknown cause.

Villous atrophy
Endometrial scarring or lymphatic cysts can give rise to a reduced ability of the placenta to associate closely to the endometrial surface, thereby reducing nutrition to the foal. These conditions are most commonly seen in the older mare with a history of endometritis.

Fetal anomalies
Genetic or developmental abnormalities of the fetus, which are incompatible with life, may lead to abortion after 6 months of gestation.

Maternal disease
Maternal disease includes any condition, disease, or environmental circumstance that causes stress in the pregnant mare (e.g. maternal injury, pyrexia, endotoxemia, malnutrition, toxic plants, medications, and transport); uterine abnormality; and premature placental separation.

Female reproductive tract

Management of the foaling case

There is a wide natural variation in the duration of pregnancy in the mare (range 320–400 days), but for most mares it is between 330 and 340 days. This variation may in part be due to embryonic diapause, when the embryo stops growing for a variable period of time. The fetus needs to be fully mature before it is delivered at parturition and a number of physiologic changes need to occur in the mare concurrently. This readiness for birth is associated with a variety of changes in the fetus including increased fetal cortisol release, more fetal activity, and digestive and respiratory tract maturation.

Changes in the mare immediately prior to foaling

Endocrinology

There are high levels of fetoplacental-derived estrogen until immediately after parturition. Progesterone rises during the last 20 days to a peak approximately 5 days prior to foaling, while pregnanes, although still high, are gradually decreasing. Both show a sudden drop to baseline levels following parturition. The change in ratio of progesterone and estrogens stimulates uterine muscular ability prior to parturition. Placental relaxin hormone increases in late pregnancy and during parturition, leading to pelvic ligament and cervical relaxation. Prostaglandin levels produced by the fetoplacental unit slowly increase in the last trimester of pregnancy, and more rapidly in the last few weeks. Two peaks are reached during parturition, leading to cervical relaxation and the onset of coordinated uterine contractions. There is a large release of oxytocin as the fetus enters the birth canal and the second stage of parturition starts. Following birth of the foal, the oxytocin levels drop, but smaller pulses are produced in the third stage of parturition when the placenta is expelled. Prolactin produced by the anterior pituitary increases in late pregnancy and leads to the onset of lactation.

Physical signs

Relaxation of the tail head and pelvic ligaments usually becomes evident in the last 2 weeks of pregnancy and progresses towards parturition. The anus, and especially the vulva, progressively soften and relax in the same period. The mammary gland starts to develop slowly about 6–4 weeks prior to parturition, becoming more noticeable in the last 2 weeks. This time frame is mare and age variable. Final development is usually within 24–48 hours before foaling. The mammary gland secretions change in the last month from yellow and serous-like to colostrum, which is thick and pale yellow. Premature lactation and leakage of milk is a sign of a high-risk pregnancy and should indicate further investigation. A waxy material may accumulate on the ends of the teats and is part of the initial colostrum production. It often occurs about 24–48 hours prior to foaling, but this timing and the amount produced are variable. Electrolyte concentrations and the comparative concentrations of the various electrolytes in the milk prior to foaling can be used to determine foaling dates and fetal readiness for parturition: calcium >10 mmol/l (40 mg/dl), sodium <30 mmol/l (30 mEq/l), and potassium >35 mmol/l (35 mEq/l) are indicators of fetal maturity and imminent parturition. Various commercial kits are available to help assess these levels.

Normal parturition

Normal parturition is divided into 3 stages:

✦ *First stage* (494). Signs include lying down; rolling; pawing and other signs of abdominal pain; decreased appetite; sweating; frequent urination and defecation, and occasionally a 'Flehmen' reaction. These signs are associated with uterine contractions and relaxation of the cervix, lasting from 30 minutes to 6 hours, with an average duration of about 1 hour. Mares have control over this stage and are able to interrupt it if they feel disturbed. Fetal movements and the mare rolling and getting up and down help the full-term fetus move from a dorsopubic (i.e. upside down) to a dorsosacral position with its poll/neck and forelimbs flexed. With progression of this stage the foal rotates the front of its body 180° and then extends its neck and forelimbs. Stage one finishes with the rupture of the chorioallantois and the release of the brownish allantoic fluid ('breaking of waters').

✦ *Second stage* (495–498). This is a rapid and very active event. The time between chorioallantoic rupture and the appearance of amnion can be as little as 10 minutes, with the foal delivered within 20–30 minutes (range 10–60 minutes). The foal takes an active part in its delivery and if it has any abnormality, this can substantially affect the process. Signs of second stage parturition include rigorous abdominal contractions of up to 1 minute in length, often with the mare recumbent; rest periods of several minutes during which she may reposition herself; presentation of the whitish amnion at the vulval lips; rupture of the amnion and release of the yellowish amniotic fluid; presentation of the foal's forelimbs (one slightly behind the other with the head resting on the carpi); further contractions until the foal is expelled to hip level, when the mare often takes a rest; and final expulsion of the foal, sometimes associated with the mare standing. The umbilical cord usually separates when the foal moves or the mare stands and it is still regarded as preferable to allow this to happen naturally. The mare and foal should be left quietly at this stage to recover from their exertions and to start the bonding process.

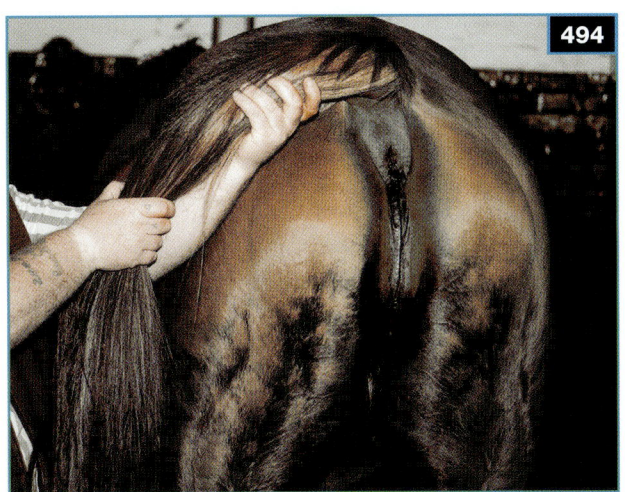

494–498 Thoroughbred mare in first-stage parturition and about to foal (494). Note the elongated and relaxed vulva, raised tail head, and relaxed pelvic ligaments. (495) Second-stage parturition has been initiated and the foal is presented with the head resting on the extended forelimbs. Note the broken amnion wrapped around the limbs of the foal. (496) The foal has been completely expelled and the umbilical cord can be seen still attached to the placenta in the mare. (497) The mare has now stood up and the cord has been broken. The umbilical stump is being treated with an antiseptic spray. (498) The foal has just stood and is being licked by the mare, part of the bonding process.

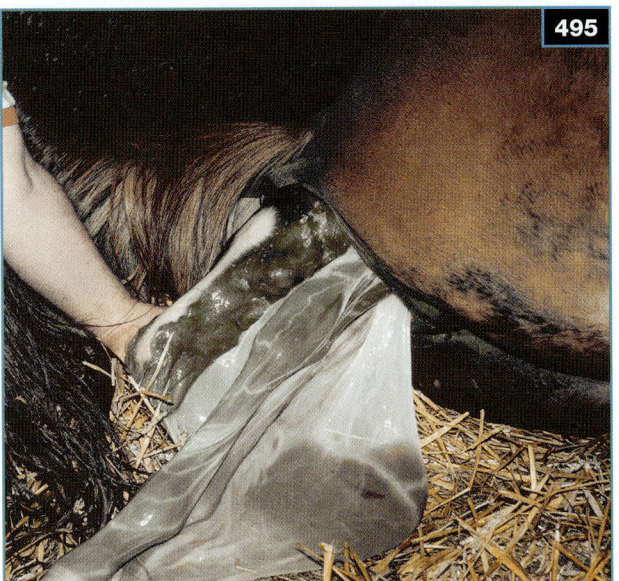

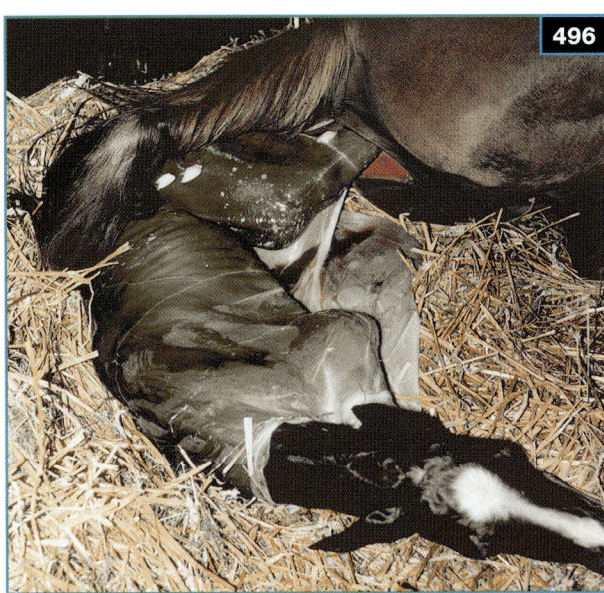

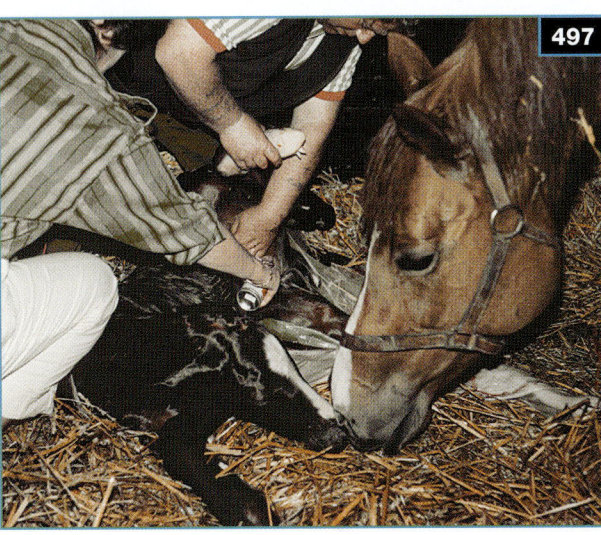

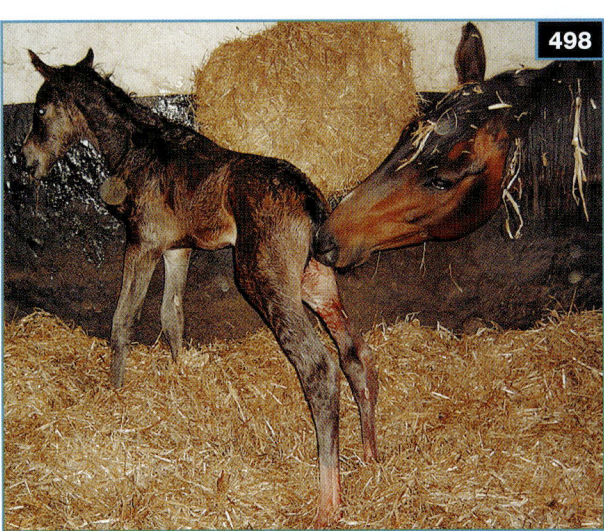

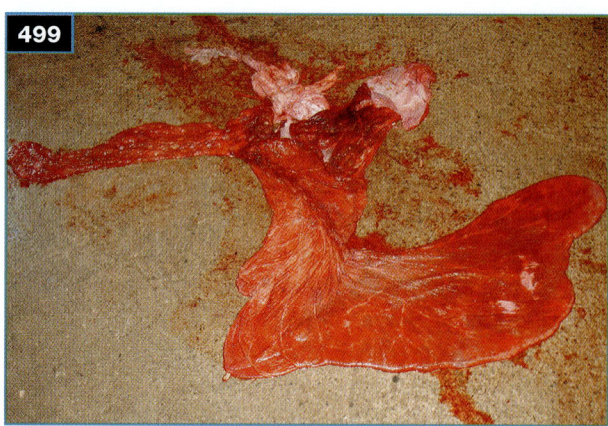

499 This is a normal expulsed placenta showing the allantochorion of the pregnant horn in the foreground and the nonpregnant horn towards the left.

✦ ***Third stage***. This is associated with the passage of the placental membranes and the onset of uterine involution, and usually occurs within 1–4 hours of the foal being born. It is important to differentiate the abdominal pain of this stage from that which can occur in some postpartum complications. The placenta often hangs from the vulval lips, but it should be tied up if it drags on the ground. Once it is expelled it should be examined for completeness and abnormalities (499).

Induction of parturition

Induction of parturition should never be undertaken without first assessing the viability and maturity of the fetus and the stage of gestation of the mare. Failure to ensure that the mare and fetus are ready for birth can result in serious problems for both, including premature placental separation, dystocia, retained placenta, foal prematurity or dysmaturity, failure of passive transfer (FPT), and neonatal maladjustment syndrome. Indications for induced deliveries include high-risk pregnancies, history of difficult foalings or abnormal foals, and injuries to the mare such as prepubic tendon rupture or pelvic injuries. Mares should not be induced purely for the convenience of the owner or attending personnel.

Several criteria need to be met prior to making a decision to induce parturition:
✦ Greater than 330 days' pregnancy.
✦ Sacrosciatic ligaments and vulva should have some evidence of relaxation.
✦ Some cervical relaxation.
✦ Fetus in normal presentation, position, and posture.
✦ Mammary secretion and analysis consistent with fetal readiness for birth. There should be colostrum in the udder.
✦ Milk electrolytes should be used to try and predict fetal readiness for birth. There is an increase in calcium (>10 mmol/l [40 mg/dl]) and potassium (>35 mmol/l [35 mEq/l]) and a decrease in sodium (<30 mmol/l [30 mEq/l]) immediately before induction.

There are several methods of induction described in the literature, each having varying advantages and disadvantages:
✦ ***Oxytocin***. This is the method of choice in any mare over 300 days' gestation. It can be given as a single i/v bolus (up to 20 IU), as an i/v drip (60 IU in 500 ml saline over 15–60 minutes), or 2.5–10 IU i/v every 15–30 minutes. Parturition usually starts within 30 minutes after i/v administration. The abdominal contractions and the whole foaling can be quite vigorous.
✦ ***Corticosteroids***. High doses of dexamethasone i/m every day for >4 days will cause the mare to foal, but there are significant risks to the foal and mare with this technique and it is generally not recommended.
✦ ***Prostaglandin $F_2\alpha$***. Various forms of $PGF_2\alpha$, including fluprostenol and cloprostenol, have been used. It is ineffective if the mare is not ready to foal. The foaling can be rapid, with vigorous contractions, and there are reports of cervical rupture and poor fetal viability following its use.

Preparation for the delivery is paramount, with some practitioners having oxygen and plasma ready to give the foal immediately after birth. All induced foalings should be attended by a veterinary surgeon.

Dystocia

The incidence of dystocia is very low compared with food-animal species, but it does vary from breed to breed and is more common in the young, primiparous mare. Thoroughbreds are thought to have an incidence of 4–5% compared with 8–12% for draft breeds and Shetlands. Long fetal limbs and neck are usually the cause of the problem and true fetal oversize is rare in the horse. Dystocia is one of the few true emergencies in equine clinical practice. A very short period of time can be the difference between a live and a dead foal, as well as serious injury to the mare due to a combination of powerful abdominal contractions and early separation of the placenta. Most clinicians use the criterion that clinical examination of a foaling case is justified if the mare has been in the second stage of parturition for more than 15 minutes without any clear progress in the birth. In some cases, intervention may be unnecessary, but a proper clinical assessment will allow problems to be identified and action taken promptly.

General telephone advice to owner

✦ Keep the mare walking. In the event of a malposture, this will minimize straining and so reduce the likelihood of the foal being impacted into the pelvic canal.
✦ Place a clean tail bandage on the mare.
✦ If it seems as though the mare has premature placental separation, instruct the attendant to rupture the membranes and deliver the foal as soon as possible.
✦ Foals that are stuck at the shoulders or hips should be pulled carefully while rotating the foal slightly. This aligns the widest part of the foal to the widest part of the pelvis and can reduce the circumference of soft-tissue areas such as the abdomen.
✦ If the foal is upside down, then allow the mare to get up and down before trying again to deliver the foal.
✦ Posterior presentations should have traction applied immediately to deliver the foal as soon as possible.
✦ Lacerations can be repaired after the foaling is over.
✦ Have plenty of clean warm water and help available.

Preparation of mare prior to examination

Postparturient uterine infection after assisted foaling is common and serious and every care should be taken with cleanliness and hygiene to minimize contamination.

Restraint

Stand the mare in a clean, dry foaling box ideally, or a set of stocks. A twitch can be a useful way to quickly restrain the mare for examination. Sedate the mare if difficult to examine: low-dose detomidine with or without butorphanol is commonly used. Romifidine can also be used, but it is recommended to always use it in conjunction with butorphanol to minimize the possibility of 'defensive

movements such as kicking'. All α2 agonists cause uterine myometrial contraction to some degree, but the advantages of sedation appear to outweigh the disadvantages. In some cases, general anesthesia may be necessary to allow the required manipulations.

Preparation

Wrap the tail in a bandage and have it held to one side by an assistant. Clean the perineum with dilute warm povidone–iodine solution before examination. Preferably use clean rectal examination gloves or arms cleaned with dilute povidone–iodine. Fresh, clean obstetric lubricant should be used. Most mares tolerate examination very well, but initially stand to one side while examining to gauge the mare's response.

Other medications/procedures for use in the field

Clenbuterol (empirical dose of 12–15 ml i/v for a 500 kg horse), though not licensed for horses in some countries, is mainly used when a mare has to be transported to a hospital facility. It helps reduce straining and possible pelvic impaction of the foal. Multiple doses of oxytocin (10–15 IU i/m q8h) should be given for 2 days post partum to ensure that involution of the uterus has not been affected by the administration of clenbuterol. If this dose produces colic, a smaller dose is given.

Epidural anesthesia

Give 4–7 ml lidocaine or mepivicaine (2%) via an 18G 1.25 cm needle. The injection is placed in a surgically prepared area between the 1st and 2nd coccygeal spaces after a subcutaneous bleb of local anesthetic (**500**). This procedure takes time and is not as easy to do as in cattle.

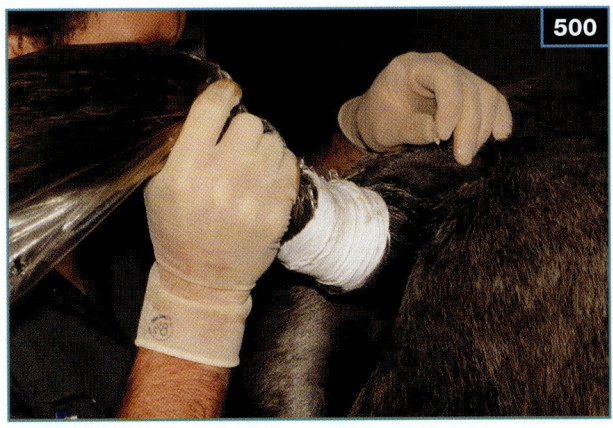

500 Epidural analgesia of the mare is a useful aid in dealing with dystocia cases. A needle is being placed between the first and second coccygeal spaces after aseptic preparation and subcutaneous local anesthesia.

Epidural anesthesia is used if the contractions are too strong to examine or manipulate the foal and/or pulling the mare's tongue out or passing a stomach tube into the trachea has not worked. It does not prevent myometrial contraction.

General anesthesia

General anesthesia is indicated if difficult and prolonged manipulation is required. The mare's hindquarters should be raised. If it is suspected that the mare will require a Cesarean section, then refer the mare rather than trying a general anesthetic first.

Initial veterinary examination

The clinician should ascertain any relevant history such as length of gestation, length of second stage of parturition, past problems with pregnancy or parturition, prior interventions, and other medical problems. A careful and thorough obstetric examination needs to be carried out to establish the cause of the problem. The presentation, position, posture, and health of the foal should be carefully assessed, plus the state of the mare's reproductive tract (i.e. forelimbs/hindlimbs; alive/dead; malposture/deformity; room for manipulation/delivery; one/two foals).

The normal presentation is anterior longitudinal, the normal position dorsosacral, and the normal posture extended head resting on carpi of extended forelimbs. Once all this information is established, a plan can be formulated as to how to rectify the problem.

Foaling technique

After the initial assessment there are four broad courses of action:

+ Deliver the foal after a simple and speedy manipulation.
+ Deliver the foal alive or dead after a relatively prolonged manipulation, using sedation, epidural anesthesia, or general anesthesia. An early decision to undertake this option is essential before the mare and the clinician/helpers become exhausted, the mare's birth canal swells, and the foal dies.
+ Cesarean section. This is the best option in cases of gross deformity or complicated malpostures.
+ If the foal is already dead, perform a 'quick partial fetotomy' (2–3 cuts) to correct a postural abnormality by sectioning the foal into smaller sections that can then be delivered. Full fetotomies are performed, but these nearly always damage the relatively short cervix of the mare and therefore seriously compromise the mare's future breeding prospects. Specialized equipment, including a fetotome, hooks, and an introducer, and technical skills are necessary to minimize damage to the mare.

Summary

+ Apply limb and head ropes as soon as possible before the birth canal gets dry and swollen.
+ Use plenty of clean lubricant.
+ Apply traction in rotation so that the foal presents the least possible circumference.
+ A maximum of 2–3 people should apply traction at any one time.
+ Consider general anesthetic if a malposture is not easily correctable in a standing position. Some malpostures can be delivered safely (e.g. hindlimb up alongside the chest).
+ Consider referral for Cesarean section early if a prolonged manual delivery is anticipated.

Some specific causes of dystocia and recommended action

+ *Incomplete elbow extension*. Should be easily correctable, but will require the trunk to be repelled and the limbs extended.
+ *'Dog sitting'*. Presentation is very difficult to correct standing. Consider general anesthetic or refer for Cesarean section.
+ *Partial dog sitter (one hindlimb back and one limb forward)*. May be deliverable as presented, but may damage cervix.
+ *Retroflexion ventrally of head or head back or flexed*. The foal will require repelling after a head rope has been attached to the head. Traction on head and forelimbs should then allow delivery.
+ *Complete carpal flexion*. May be uni- or bilateral. The affected limb(s) will be in the pelvic canal. The fetal body must be repelled and the hoof cupped in the palm of the hand and then drawn forward into the pelvic canal.
+ *Partial carpal flexion (contracted tendons)*. This is the most common congenital deformity, can be very difficult to deliver vaginally, and a Cesarean section may be indicated. If the foal is dead, then a careful fetotomy incision through the carpus will allow vaginal delivery.
+ *Shoulder flexion*. Unilateral or bilateral. Corrected in two stages: the shoulder flexion is converted to carpal flexion by bringing the radius forward, and then the carpal flexion is corrected.
+ *Posterior longitudinal presentation*. A rare occurrence. Compression of the umbilical cord necessitates rapid delivery if a live foal is to be obtained. Check foal for signs of 'dummy foal' syndrome.
+ *Transverse presentation*. Dorsal or ventral; refer for Cesarean section.

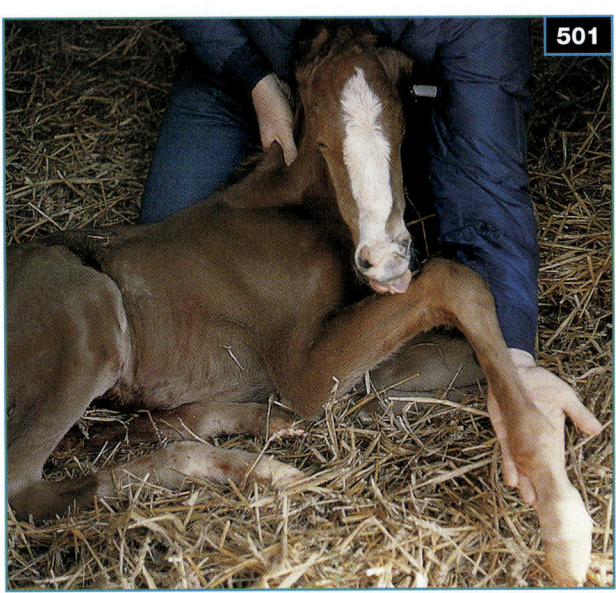

501 A newborn Thoroughbred foal showing contracted foal syndrome, including bilateral carpal flexural deformities and wrynose. The foal presented as a dystocia in the mare because of a partial carpal flexion deformity.

Other causes of dystocia and recommended action

+ *Congenital defects* of the foal often lead to dystocia, but they are relatively rare. Foals with limb deformities such as flexural problems, especially if they are associated with arthrogryposis or contracted foal syndrome (**501**), are the most common. Other syndromes include hydrocephalus, schistosomus reflexus, and fetal monsters. Some of these cases may require Cesarean section for delivery.

+ *Length of gestation*: variable, average 340 days. Mares can have a gestation of greater then 12 months and produce a normal healthy foal. Foals born more than 1 month before term are likely to be weak and require special attention. Overdue foals rarely become too large to foal normally.

+ *Failure to get down*. Mares that do not or cannot get down during the first stage of parturition are more likely to have a malpostured foal.

+ *Pelvic deformities*. Even quite pronounced deformities do not generally impair foaling; however, it is recommended that these mares be watched closely in case a Cesarean section is indicated.

+ *Maiden mares*. Relative oversize is rare, but in maiden mares, pelvic ligament relaxation may be poor, which prolongs parturition. It is debatable if help is required, but careful traction may minimize foal rib damage.

+ *Perineal melanomas*. Can make life painful for the mare. Use of low-dose sedation or epidural anesthesia should improve the situation.

Cesarean section
Indications
Cesarean section is indicated when delivery of the foal is not possible per vagina (e.g. grossly oversized foal; severe fetal malposition that cannot be easily rectified such as 'dog sitter'; transverse presentation; and severe congenital deformities). Problems of the mare that may lead to a decision for a Cesarean section include: previous pelvic injuries; tumors of the vaginal canal or perineum such as melanoma; previous perineal injuries that have not been treated correctly or have scarred excessively; ruptured prepubic tendon injuries; ventral abdominal hernias; uterine torsion. In order to obtain a live foal, surgery needs to be carried out as soon as possible and usually within 1 hour of the start of the second stage of parturition. The procedure requires a general anesthetic, a sterile operating environment, and a trained surgical team, which may not be readily available in some areas and which certainly leads to significant costs to owners. Postoperatively, the mare will have lowered, but still acceptable, fertility rates.

Surgical technique and complications
A variety of techniques have been used in the past, including approaches used under standing sedation. In general, most surgeons perform this operation under general anesthesia, in dorsal recumbency, and via a midline ventral laparotomy extending from slightly caudal to the umbilicus and cranially for 50–60 cm. Occasionally, a paramedian approach is used if there has been previous midline surgery or injury. The most common surgical complication is severe postoperative uterine hemorrhage

from the uterine incision. The incidence of this can be decreased considerably by careful positioning of the initial incision, clamping and ligating the larger vessels, applying a specific hemostatic suture if considered necessary, and the use of oxytocin in the latter part of the operation and postoperatively. Mares require very careful monitoring after the operation in order to identify and deal with other complications (e.g. retained placenta; abdominal incision problems such as local infections and breakdown; laminitis/metritis, particularly in draft breeds; shock; peritonitis; and, in the longer term, adhesions). Usually the mare is not bred until the next breeding season and free exercise is usually limited for the first 3 months postoperatively. Many foals are delivered dead at Cesarean section and any that are alive are high risk and need appropriate intensive care (502). Mare and foal should be reunited as soon as possible because bonding between the two can be a problem.

502 This foal has just been born by Cesarean section and is receiving nasal oxygen and nursing care. (Photo courtesy T Chenier)

The postpartum period

Mares usually recover within an hour of foaling, returning to normal behavior (i.e. looking after their foal, eating, drinking, defecating, and urinating). During this time pulse and respiratory rates return to normal and mucous membranes resume their normal pink color.

Under the changing hormonal balance in the postpartum mare, uterine contractability increases and fluid, bacterial contamination, and cellular debris are expelled from the uterus. Immune reactions are stimulated in the uterus and assist in dealing with any postpartum bacterial contamination. Uterine involution occurs within 6–15 days post partum, with a rapid decrease in uterine size back to normal by 30 days. Mares that have had a difficult parturition, especially those where manipulations were required or whose postpartum management and exercise were compromised, may require additional time and/or treatment to allow resolution of any infection or inflammation and complete involution to occur.

Foal heat

Shortly after foaling the ovaries of the mare start to become active and follicles develop and ovulate between five and 15 days post partum. This is associated with estrus signs or 'foal heat', usually 6–12 days post partum. The length of the foal heat and the period from foaling to beginning of the foal heat decrease in the summer months. Some mares will not show behavioral estrus during the foal heat due to the presence of the foal and the mother's protective instincts. A decision on whether to breed the mare on the foal heat should be made on an individual basis. It depends on the degree of uterine involution as determined during a full reproductive examination, the history of the foaling and the immediate period thereafter, the time of year (particularly in the Thoroughbred), the type of mating used (i.e. natural covering or AI [not frozen semen]), the age of the mare (lesser fertility in older mares on foal-heat breeding), and the time since foaling before breeding (a minimum of 10 days post partum is used by many clinicians). Some clinicians delay the first covering until after the foal heat, but 'short cycle' the mare by injection of prostaglandin 6–7 days following foal-heat ovulation. This induced estrous period is associated with an increased fertility compared with foal-heat breeding.

Postpartum complications

Complications should be suspected and investigated urgently if abdominal pain continues or worsens, if pulse or respiratory rate rises, if the mucous membranes become pale or injected, or if the mare sweats and/or shows no interest in the foal or food.

Postpartum pain

Pain related to uterine contractions in the immediate postpartum period is most common in primiparous mares and tends to be intermittent. There is usually a moderate increase in heart rate, with some sweating. This usually subsides within 1–2 hours. Administration of analgesics is indicated in the worst cases. Rectal palpation of the uterus and the rest of the abdomen should be carried out to help differentiate other more serious causes of abdominal pain such as large colon torsion, which occurs most commonly in recently postpartum mares.

Conditions associated with foaling

Uterine artery rupture

Definition/overview

A well-recognized but uncommon condition that can occur in the late pregnant mare, but more usually in parturient or immediately postparturient mares. It is more common in older, multiparous broodmares, with the ruptured arteries bleeding into the mesometrium or peritoneal cavity. It can present with mild to moderate abdominal pain or, in severe cases, shock and death. Treatment is symptomatic.

Etiology/pathophysiology

The etiology of uterine artery rupture is unknown, but rupture (typically 2–3 cm long and longitudinal) can occur in any of the following arteries: middle uterine, utero ovarian, and external iliac (503). It is more common in multiparous mares >12 years old. Some clinicians believe this may contribute to progressive weakening of the arteries and predisposition to rupture. There may be a predilection to right-sided rupture. Hemorrhage from the damaged vessels initially accumulates in the mesometrium (broad ligament), where it may form a hematoma, which helps stop further bleeding. If the hemorrhage continues and/or the mesometrium ruptures, unlimited extravasation of blood into the peritoneal cavity will lead to hemorrhagic shock. In severe cases, exsanguination and death can occur within minutes to a few hours.

Clinical presentation

Mares are usually affected during or just after parturition, but occasionally late gestational or 24–48 hour postparturient cases occur. Mild or restricted bleeding cases tend to demonstrate mild to severe abdominal pain (depending on the degree of hemorrhage) with signs including Flehmen response, sweating, and anxiety. Severe or unrestricted cases have signs of blood loss shock, including pale mucous membranes, thin, thready, and rapid pulse, delayed CRT, collapse or inability to stand after foaling or recumbency, shaking, and sweating.

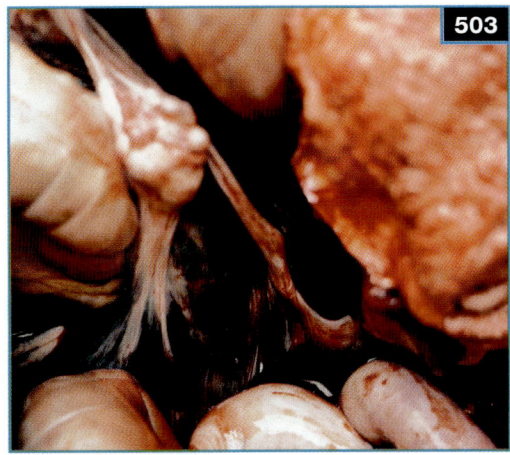

503 Postmortem view of the ovary and broad ligament of a mare that died because of a uterine artery rupture that bled from the ligament into the peritoneum.

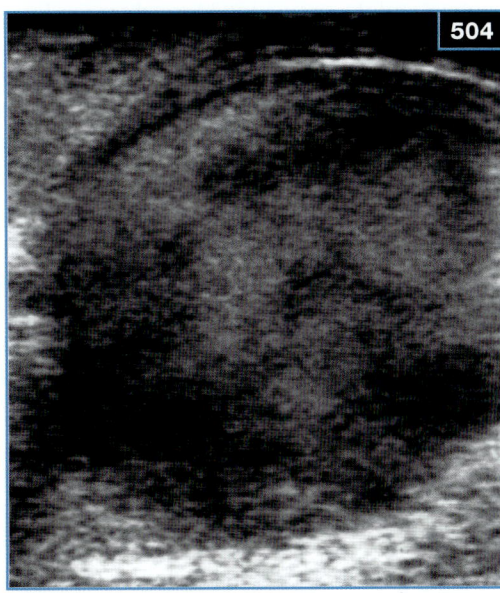

504 A transrectal ultrasonographic view of a hematoma within the broad ligament 24 hours post partum. (Photo courtesy T Chenier)

Diagnosis

In cases that hemorrhage rapidly into the peritoneum, further diagnostic tests, including rectal palpation, are often futile or dangerous because of the behavior of the mare. Mares that present with milder clinical signs, especially abdominal pain, should be examined per rectum very carefully for the presence of a mesometrial hematoma, which can vary in size from an egg to a melon. Palpable pain in the area in the early stages is common. Ultrasonographic examination per rectum (504) is also a

287

possibility and will confirm the condition. Transabdominal ultrasound and abdominocentesis will reveal free blood in the abdominal cavity if the hematoma is torn, and raised protein levels if it is not. Assessment of the hematology parameters of the mare is of variable use. In the peracute case the hematocrit often does not change significantly and will often not change in less severe cases for 12–24 hours.

Management

There is no one reliable treatment and a combination of therapies is often used. It is recommended to keep the mare quiet and minimize any stress in order to keep the blood pressure low. The foal should be kept in a safe place, but in view of the mare. Some clinicians recommend this for several weeks post partum to help prevent hemorrhage recurring. Intravenous formalin solution (50 ml 10% formalin in 1 liter of saline) has been used controversially by some clinicians to decrease the hemorrhage. The use of sedatives in such cases is controversial, as although most of these drugs lower blood pressure, which may help clotting and decrease blood loss, they can lead to severe cardiovascular collapse and death. Fluid therapy has been used in some cases with variable results, but the stress of setting it up may well exacerbate the problem. Two to four liters of warmed hypertonic saline (7%) or Hetastarch given quickly, followed by 10–20 liters of warmed poly-ionic crystalloid solution, will restore some circulatory volume, while other clinicians have used whole fresh blood or plasma to improve blood pressure and help replace clotting factors. Nasal insufflation of oxygen at 5–10 liters/minute has also been used to increase tissue oxygenation. Corticosteroids have been used and, after the initial crisis, broad-spectrum antibiotics, antioxidant drugs, and anti-inflammatory medications such as flunixin meglumine should be administered.

Prognosis

In general, where the bleeding is restricted to the mesometrium and a broad ligament hematoma forms, the mare will survive. The hematoma organizes and fibroses with time and can often be palpated rectally for many years afterwards. The mare can be bred as soon as the hematoma is fully fibrosed, which can be ascertained by ultrasound examination per rectum. Usually this has occurred by the second estrus post partum. It is unknown whether these mares have an increased tendency to further hemorrhages in subsequent pregnancies. Intra-abdominal hemorrhage usually leads to death.

Uterine rupture

Definition/overview

Uterine rupture is an uncommon condition, usually secondary to other problems occurring at parturition. Tears may be partial or full thickness and are often ventral. Partial tears are often not detected and may heal spontaneously with uterine involution. Full-thickness tears can be associated with abdominal pain, severe peritoneal hemorrhage and/or contamination, or even a preparturient peritoneal fetus. Death can occur due to severe peritonitis and/or intestinal complications. Surgical repair via a ventral midline laparotomy and intra- and postoperative peritoneal lavage are essential in treating full-thickness tears.

Etiology/pathophysiology

Spontaneous rupture uncommonly occurs during normal parturition, but more usually it occurs secondary to other conditions such as hydrops, uterine torsion, obstetric manipulations during a dystocia, or, rarely, excessive fetal movement, especially of the hindlimbs. Tears not associated with dystocia tend to occur towards the tip of the gravid horn. Late-pregnancy ruptures may lead to part, or all, of the fetus assuming an intraperitoneal position. The majority of tears occur on the ventral aspect of the uterus and they can be partial or full thickness. The latter can lead to peritonitis and death. A tear of the uterus may involve a large blood vessel and, occasionally, visceral herniation may complicate the condition.

Clinical presentation

Partial-thickness lacerations are often not detected unless the uterus is examined in detail post partum. Uterine rupture is not usually associated with severe hemorrhage into the abdomen, but if this does occur, the mare may present with hemorrhagic shock and rapid death. If the foal becomes partially or entirely intraperitoneal, the mare may develop late pregnancy abdominal pain and possibly intestinal complications related to adhesions and peritonitis. Full-thickness ruptures post partum can heal spontaneously and may not be detected, whereas other cases develop peritonitis due to contamination from the uterus. These present with abdominal pain and guarding, fever, depression, and signs of endotoxemia and septic shock. Occasionally, ruptures (partial or full thickness) are not recognized until uterine lavage is carried out post partum: fluid pumped into the uterus is not retrieved because it flows into the abdominal cavity.

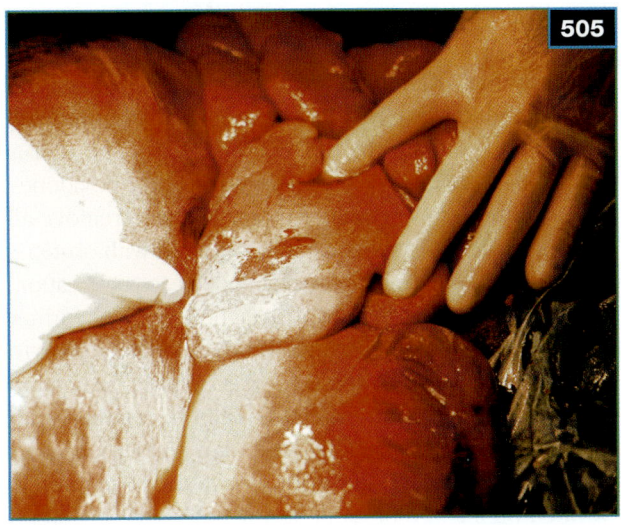

505 View at laparotomy showing a small tear in the uterus of a recently parturient mare. Note the inflamed serosa of the uterus subsequent to generalized septic peritonitis.

Diagnosis

Examination of the uterus manually per vagina, rectal palpation, and transrectal ultrasonography post partum can confirm the presence of most full-thickness ruptures, but partial ruptures are harder to detect. Palpation should be carried out carefully in order to minimize extension of the laceration. All mares that have had a dystocia should be checked post partum for lacerations. Transabdominal ultrasonography is useful in late pregnancy cases to document the position and health of the fetus and detect possible ruptures. Peritoneal fluid analysis will reflect the depth and extent of the laceration and should confirm peritoneal hemorrhage and/or peritonitis. Laparoscopy can be used to confirm the tear and possibly to repair smaller ones.

Management

Secondary intention healing of partial-thickness tears usually occurs as the uterus involutes and no specific treatment is required other than oxytocin to encourage uterine clearance and shrinkage. Uterine lavage should not be carried out as this may exacerbate the problem. Occasionally, partial-thickness tears, which only have the serosa left intact, present and are treated similarly to full-thickness tears with peritonitis. Tears presenting with peritonitis need to be treated by surgical repair with concurrent peritoneal lavage. This is usually achieved via a ventral midline laparotomy with postoperative lavage continuing for several days afterwards (**505**). All mares diagnosed with uterine ruptures (partial or complete) require broad-spectrum systemic antibiotics, anti-endotoxic NSAIDs, and oxytocin (10–20 IU q2h). Mares with peritonitis will require intensive treatment with intravenous fluid therapy and prophylactic treatment for laminitis.

Prognosis

The prognosis is guarded to grave depending on the extent and depth of the rupture, how soon the tear is detected and treated, the degree of hemorrhage and contamination into the peritoneal cavity, and the complications of peritonitis, adhesions, and secondary bowel damage. Partial-thickness tears do heal, but the mare should not be mated for at least 60 days, and then preferably by AI. Mares with full-thickness tears should not be bred from that breeding season.

Uterine prolapse
Definition/overview

Uterine prolapse is an uncommon condition seen in the parturient mare where there has been dystocia, obstetric manipulation or extraction, or excessive straining post partum. Complete uterine prolapse is easily diagnosed and is a true life-threatening emergency, while prolapse or invagination of the tip of the uterine horn is often noted only at the first routine postpartum examination. Treatment involves replacement under sedation and epidural anesthesia.

Etiology/pathophysiology

Uterine prolapse can occur following dystocia, particularly if it is prolonged and/or excessively forceful or quick extraction is carried out. It can also occur following late-gestation abortion and secondary to any condition leading to postpartum straining (e.g. retained placenta, vulval/vaginal lacerations). The uterus is often damaged to some degree and needs to be carefully assessed for tears before replacing. Uterine artery rupture can also lead to fatal hemorrhage.

289

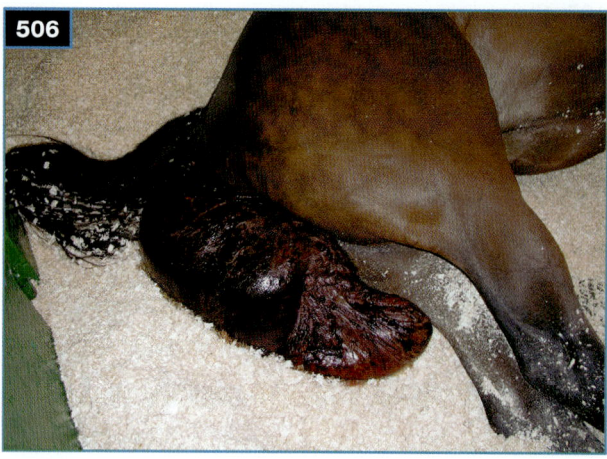

506 A uterine prolapse post partum in a mare that was subsequently euthanized. (Photo courtesy T Chenier)

Clinical presentation

The recently foaled mare (several hours to, rarely, days) presents with varying amounts of everted uterus at the vulval lips (506). The uterus will appear either bright or dark red, depending on the amount of hemorrhage present, with varying degrees of damage and friability, and the placenta may still be attached. There may be rapid development of shock and endotoxemia. Rupture of the ovarian and/or uterine arteries often leads to abdominal pain and rapid death. Any concurrent damage and/or infection will have a negative effect on the mare's future fertility. Rarely, bladder eversion, uterine rupture, and intestinal herniation can occur and seriously alter the prognosis. Invagination of the tip of the uterine horn may present as abdominal pain due to traction on the ovary or it may be subclinical and only detected on subsequent routine fertility examinations.

Diagnosis

Diagnosis is made on clinical signs and rectal/vaginal palpation.

Management

Complete prolapses are emergency cases and require immediate attention. The uterus should be protected as much as possible to prevent further damage. Often the mare is distressed and in pain, which may lead to further self-damage to the uterus. The mare should be restrained and kept quiet, preferably in a standing position, with the use of sedatives/analgesics only if these are essential (drug-induced hypovolemia may cause the mare to collapse). Systemic antibiotics (including oral metronidazole) and NSAIDs (flunixin meglumine) are preferably given prior to attempts to replace the uterus in order to help prevent metritis and counteract endotoxemia. The uterus should be placed on a clean plastic sheet or tray and elevated, preferably to the level of the vulva. This improves the uterine circulation, thereby decreasing edema, and decreases the likelihood of blood-vessel rupture and damage to the endometrium. The uterus should be thoroughly cleaned with warm dilute povidone–iodine solution followed by isotonic saline to remove all debris and identify any damage. Lubrication with obstetric lubricant may assist replacement and decrease desiccation. If the placenta can be easily detached without further damage to the uterus, this should be undertaken prior to replacement. Areas of damage may require protection during replacement and lacerations can be repaired with absorbable sutures. Generally, the uterus is replaced under sedation and epidural anesthesia, with the hindquarters elevated on a slope or bank, but in some cases, general anesthesia and elevation of the mare's hindquarters will be necessary. The prolapse is replaced carefully starting with the vagina, then the cervix, and finally the uterus itself. It is important not to use finger pressure, but to keep the hands flat in order to avoid punctures or lacerations to the friable uterus. Covering the uterus with a plastic bag helps to decrease the incidence of damage. When the uterus returns back into its abdominal position it is essential that it is completely reduced, particularly at the tips of the horns, otherwise re-prolapse and/or damage to the tips may occur. This can be achieved by filling the uterus with warm clean water or, preferably, saline if the clinician's arms are not long enough to reach the tips of the uterus. Irrigation of the uterus and removal of the fluid will also further reduce contamination and the risk of septic metritis. Once reduction is complete (check per rectum) small doses of oxytocin (10–20 IU q2h) will improve uterine involution. Intrauterine antibiotic/saline solutions are used by some clinicians. If the placenta is still retained, specific therapy should be instituted. Some clinicians advocate suturing the vulva to prevent re-prolapse, although it is more likely it prevents a pneumovagina. Recurrence is unlikely unless the uterus is not completely reduced or there is persistent straining for other reasons. Any bowel involvement will usually require surgical treatment via an exploratory laparotomy.

Prolapsed bladders can be replaced after drainage of the urine via catheter or needle.

Initial emergency treatment is followed up by continuing small doses of oxytocin, based on the degree of involution, and fluid therapy, broad-spectrum antibiotics, and anti-endotoxic therapy, depending on the clinical signs of the mare. Uterine lavage is continued until the recovered fluid is clear.

Prognosis

The prognosis varies from guarded to grave depending on the degree of prolapse, the damage to the uterus, secondary problems such as ruptures or vessel damage, and secondary complications such as shock and metritis. Death can occur sometimes even prior to examination. Metritis following replacement is common, and requires early aggressive treatment. The incidence of prolapse is not increased in subsequent pregnancies.

Bladder eversion or prolapse

Definition/overview
These are rare conditions in the horse. They are more common in larger mares, particularly the draft breeds.

Etiology/pathophysiology
Bladder eversion or prolapse usually occurs subsequent to postpartum straining due to reproductive tract injuries, dystocia, retained placenta, or rectal impaction. In prolapse the bladder is forced through a tear in the ventral vaginal wall. In eversion the bladder is everted through the urethral opening.

Clinical presentation
Clinical signs in bladder prolapse are of a bladder with its serosal surface exposed, usually at the vulval lips, while in an eversion the mucosal surface is presented with the ureteral openings visible.

Management
Treatment is usually undertaken with epidural anesthesia in the standing sedated animal. Treatment of prolapse involves emptying and cleaning the bladder before replacing it back into the abdomen via the tear, which is subsequently repaired surgically. In cases of eversion the bladder is emptied, any defects repaired, and the bladder lubricated before careful replacement back through the urethral opening. In some cases, swelling and edema of the bladder require that it is pressure wrapped in a dextrose solution-soaked, cool, soft cloth to reduce the fluid content of the bladder wall prior to replacement. Occasionally, a loop of bowel becomes trapped behind the bladder, preventing replacement. This can be identified on ultrasonographic examination. The urethra may require surgical enlargement and subsequent repair if it is too narrow to allow replacement. Following replacement the cause of any initial straining must be treated, bladder straining prevented by epidural anesthesia, and/or nasotracheal intubation and broad-spectrum antibiotics and NSAIDs administered.

Prognosis
The prognosis depends on the degree of damage to the bladder, the ease of replacement, the need for surgical repair of the urethral opening, and the primary cause of the straining. There is an increased incidence of urinary incontinence after bladder eversion or prolapse.

Rectal prolapse

Definition/overview
This problem is associated with conditions that cause abdominal straining and can include dystocia, retained placenta, and damage to the reproductive tract post foaling (507). (See also p. 588.)

Premature placental separation

Definition/overview
This emergency at parturition occurs when the allanto-chorion separates from the endometrium before the foal breaks through it and enters the pelvic canal. Instead of the normal rupturing of the allantochorion at the cervical star, the mare attempts to push the placenta and foal through the vagina as one unit. The presentation of the allanto-chorion requires immediate intervention and rupturing, with rapid delivery of the foal. Many of the delivered foals are subsequently abnormal and require treatment.

Etiology/pathophysiology
This uncommon complication of late pregnancy/parturition is usually secondary to other problems, particularly of the placenta. It is most commonly seen in ascending infection placentitis, where separation may initially occur at the cervical star. It is a recorded complication of induction of parturition and is also seen with late gestational stress, excessive nutrition, or fescue toxicosis.

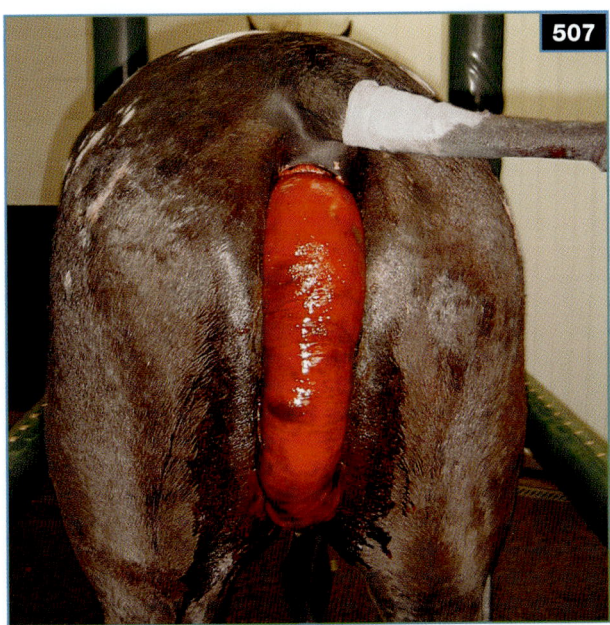

507 A type 4 rectal prolapse in a recently foaled broodmare. The prolapse contained small intestine and damaged mesentery and was not amenable to repair.

Clinical presentation

Signs of an ascending placentitis including a late gestational vaginal discharge may be noted. Occasional cases exhibit vaginal bleeding for a few days prior to parturition. At parturition the red, velvety surface of the allantochorion is presented at the vulval lips at the start of second-stage labor ('red bag delivery') instead of the whitish amniotic sac that normally covers the fetus. As the allantochorion has not broken, there will be no release of the placental fluids ('breaking of waters').

Management

The fetus loses its blood supply as soon as the allantochorion separates and therefore this condition requires emergency action. The allantochorion should be opened quickly either by manual tearing or, if it is thickened, with a sharp object, preferably at the cervical star. The foal should then be delivered as soon as possible and oxygen supplied per nasum if available. These foals constitute a high risk and many are premature, dysmature, maladjusted, and/or septicemic. Appropriate prophylactic treatment and management should be instigated as soon as possible.

Prognosis

The prognosis for the foal born following premature placental separation can vary from guarded to grave depending on the cause and degree of placental damage prior to parturition and the rapidity of response to the abnormal delivery. Following this condition, many foals are born with considerable problems and require extensive and costly treatment to survive.

Retained fetal membranes (placenta)

Definition/overview

Retained fetal membranes is a common complication of the postpartum mare. In normal circumstances the placenta is passed from the uterus within 1–3 hours of birth (third stage of parturition), although there is considerable variation in normality and some mares will retain it for up to 24–48 hours without short- or long-term complications. Retention of fetal membranes has a multifactorial etiology, probably causing abnormalities of uterine motility and/or maturational processes within the microcotyledons. In some mares, especially the larger heavy types, serious complications related to the metritis–laminitis–septicemia complex have been recorded. Treatment is aimed at encouraging release of the fetal membranes and prevention of secondary complications. The prognosis is fair in cases treated early and aggressively, but poor in advanced chronic cases.

Etiology/pathophysiology

Causes of retained fetal membranes include any factor or condition that affects uterine motility, although it does occur following what appear clinically to be normal deliveries:

+ Dystocia, especially after extensive manipulations or embryotomy.
+ Induced parturition.
+ Premature delivery.
+ Abortion.
+ Cesarean section.
+ Deficiencies and imbalances in selenium and calcium/phosphorus.
+ Uterine inertia/fatigue (e.g. post hydrops or twin pregnancy, inadequate exercise or obesity, general anesthetic).
+ Placentitis.
+ Abnormalities in oxytocin release.

The incidence of retained fetal membranes in one survey was suggested to be 2–10% of all parturitions, with a higher incidence in draft or cold-blooded mares, older multiparous mares, and mares that had previously suffered from the condition. Retention of fetal membranes usually involves the tips of the uterine horns, more often in the nongravid horn than the gravid horn. The exact mechanism that causes interference with the normal separation process is at present unknown.

Complications that follow placental retention are more common in larger, heavy mares and are associated with bacterial proliferation in the uterus and a build-up of autolytic enzymes. In addition to endometritis and metritis in the uterus, this bacterial and enzyme mix may be absorbed systemically and lead to a bacteremia/septicemia and endotoxemia, with a high incidence of severe, acute laminitis. Retained fetal membranes may also predispose to uterine prolapse (p. 289).

Clinical presentation

The retained fetal membranes are often observed hanging from the vulval lips, with the amnion most visible outside. By definition, any mare with the fetal membranes still visible after 3–5 hours post partum has a retention, but there is considerable variation across breeds and types. If the mare is still in the third stage of parturition (experiencing uterine contractions), then she will show signs of abdominal discomfort and may well pass the fetal membranes fairly quickly. If they are truly retained, then no discomfort is usually apparent. The mare should receive a full physical examination to detect any of the common complications of retention of the fetal membranes.

Diagnosis

Clinical signs are diagnostic. If the mare develops any of the complications, then bacterial samples for culture and sensitivity from the uterus and blood should be taken, along with blood samples for a full hematology and biochemistry analysis. Subsequently, lateral foot radiographs may be useful in the management of any laminitis. All fetal membranes should be examined once they have been passed to check that they are intact and that there are no abnormalities that may affect the neonate.

Management

The approach to retained fetal membranes varies considerably depending on the duration of membrane retention and the presence/absence of metritis with septicemia. If the retained fetal membranes are trailing down the hindlimbs of the mare, and especially below the level of the hocks, they should be tied up so that they do not interfere with the limbs. The tying of an additional weight to the retained fetal membranes is not recommended as it may predispose to uterine prolapse or tearing of the membranes, but it is used by some clinicians.

Accelerating the release of the fetal membranes is best achieved in the first 24 hours post partum by the use of oxytocin administered slowly (over 15 minutes) in intravenous fluids (50 IU in 500 ml saline, may be repeated after 2 hours), or intramuscular injections (10–20 IU) repeated every 15–60 minutes. Intravenous bolus doses, single or multiple, every 1–2 hours have also been used, but they tend to cause the mare more abdominal pain and are often less successful. In the latter part of the postpartum period, doses of oxytocin may need to be increased slightly to achieve uterine contraction. If oxytocin therapy is unsuccessful, or as an alternative, uterine lavage with 10–12 liters of warm saline/water +/- mild antiseptic solutions (<0.5%

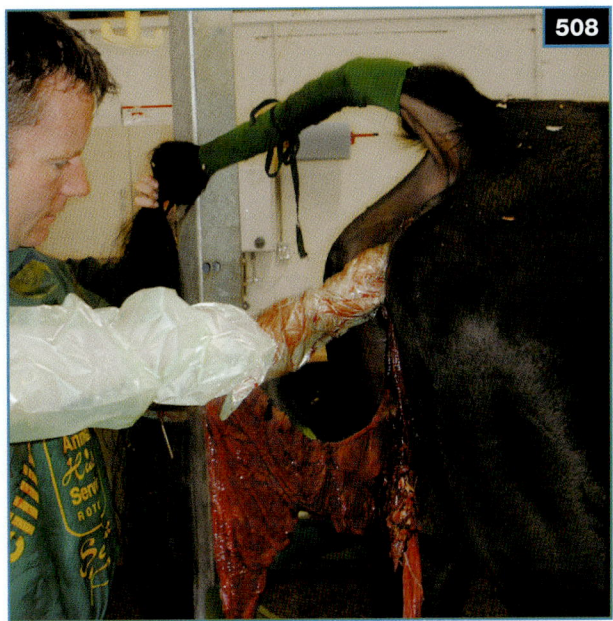

508 A retained placenta being gently retrieved from the uterus after treatment with oxytocin.

povidone–iodine) is used regularly by clinicians to fill the allantochorion, stretch the uterus (possibly releasing endogenous oxytocin), detach the microvilli of the placenta, and encourage passage within 30 minutes. A sterile nasogastric tube is passed beyond the torn distal fragments and into the chorioallantoic sac. The membranes are held tightly around the tube as the fluid is placed in the sac and then the opening is tied off with tape (**508**).

Manual removal of the placenta is generally not advised as it leads to uterine hemorrhage, increased damage and fibrosis of the endometrium, and increased uptake of endotoxins and bacteria. Aggressive removal can predispose to uterine horn-tip invagination and prolapse and/or small parts of the placenta remaining in the uterus. Some clinicians feel that gentle traction and twisting of the placenta is helpful during uterine lavage in order to encourage separation.

Prevention of secondary complications and their aggressive treatment are important. Broad-spectrum antibiotics are indicated unless specific culture and sensitivity results are available. Anaerobic organisms can be involved and are often treated with metronidazole or penicillin. NSAIDs, especially flunixin meglumine, are particularly useful for their anti-endotoxic effects. If the mare becomes endotoxic, intravenous fluids are essential to maintain the cardiovascular system and major organ function.

Female reproductive tract

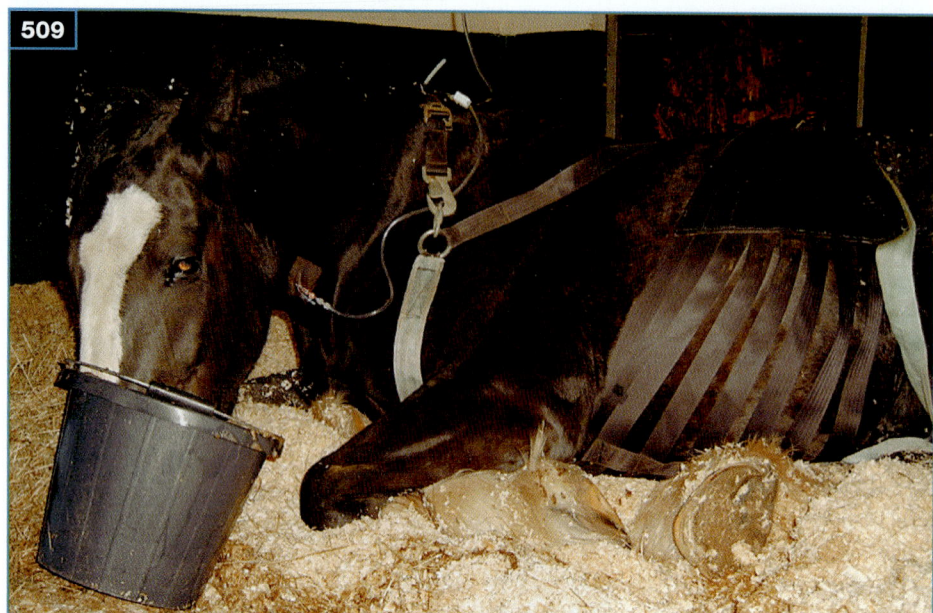

509 A Shire mare that has developed metritis–laminitis–septicemia complex after a retained placenta. The mare is reluctant to stand and is on a deep shavings bed, partially supported in slings.

It is important to check electrolyte levels and supplement if necessary. Tetanus prophylaxis should be checked and boosted if required. The feet of the mare should be supported by placing them on sand, peat, or a small shavings deep bed, or by the use of frog supports (**509**). Aggressive laminitis therapy may be necessary if laminitis occurs (see pp. 69–71).

After release the fetal membranes should be laid out carefully to check for their entirety. If any part is missing, attempts should be made to determine whether it is still present in the uterus, using either sterile intrauterine digital palpation or endoscopy. There is a risk of septic metritis developing if the membranes are retained for >8 hours.

After passage of the fetal membranes, uterine lavage should be performed to completely distend all parts of the uterus including the horn. This will encourage removal of bacteria, fluid, debris, and enzymes and should be repeated every 12–24 hours until the reflux is clean. The use of intrauterine antibiotics is controversial. The mare should receive a complete examination of the uterus at the subsequent foal-heat estrous period, including culture and cytology. The mare should not be bred at the foal heat.

Prognosis
In some mares, retention of the fetal membranes seems to have little effect on their uterine or general health, but in others it can lead to devastating complications and even death. All cases require careful consideration and early treatment if thought necessary. Cases that are ignored or develop serious complications carry a guarded to poor prognosis. Fertility rates are not affected in mares that are treated effectively and quickly.

Cervical injuries
Definition/overview
Most cervical injuries occur at parturition and they vary according to the type and depth of damage. Mucosal defects, adhesions, partial- and full-thickness lacerations, and cervical incompetence can all occur to a variable extent and anatomic position in the cervix. Damage may not be noted until the mare fails to conceive or maintain a pregnancy. Careful digital palpation of the cervix in diestrus, plus vaginoscopy, will detail the type of injury and its extent. Treatment depends on the type and age of injury and its extent and anatomic site, but often involves surgical repair.

Etiology/pathophysiology
The vast majority of cervical injuries occur as a result of trauma during parturition. Attempts by the mare or by outside parties to deliver the foal before adequate dilation of the cervix and/or lubrication, as well as dystocia resolved with the use of fetotomy and/or obstetric manipulation, are common causes of injuries. The least serious injuries are mucosal defects, which can heal by epithelialization, but if this is delayed, substantial fibrous adhesions can form. With time, organization and scarring of the tissue can lead to cervical canal distortion or obstruction. Adhesions have also been recorded where the reproductive tract, usually the uterus, has been infused with irritant or caustic solutions such as iodine-based compounds, which damage the lining mucosa. In some cases the muscular layers of the cervix can be damaged, whereas the mucosal layers are not, or they may heal very quickly. These injuries can lead to cervical incompetence. In the worst injuries the mucosal and all muscular layers are damaged, leading to a

cervical laceration, which is usually wedge shaped in the cervical body (base at the external os). Injuries that affect the function of the cervix may lead to infertility by obstructing the lumen or, more usually, by preventing adequate closure. Transluminal adhesions can be associated with chronic endometritis and pyometra either as cause or effect. Congenital abnormalities and neoplasia of the cervix are rare.

Clinical presentation
Damage to the cervix may be noted at the time of parturition or shortly afterwards. On many occasions it is not identified until the mare is presented for failure to conceive, chronic endometritis, or a failure to maintain a pregnancy beyond 4–5 months.

Diagnosis
Direct observation of the external os of the cervix is useful, but defects, tears, and adhesions are easily missed if this is used alone. Careful digital palpation with a clean, gloved, lubricated hand is the most useful diagnostic aid. Some clinicians use their first finger and thumb. The problems are best identified during diestrus when the cervix is firm and closed, but after a traumatic foaling it is often advisable to examine the cervix within 3–5 days. Mucosal defects are often missed as they heal quickly, unless they are large or deep. The position and extent of any adhesions or defects must be recorded. With incompetence it is possible to pass several fingers through the cervix at diestrus. In more severe cases, before embarking on treatment, it is prudent to assess the rest of the reproductive tract for normal function.

Management
Areas of damaged mucosa should be cleansed at least daily with clean warm saline before an antiseptic emollient cream is applied liberally to minimize infection and adhesions. Most lesions epithelialize by the first postpartum estrus, except those that are very large. Freshly formed adhesions can be manually broken down, followed by twice daily manipulation of the cervix and application of an antibiotic/corticosteroid ointment for 7–10 days. This prevents their re-formation and encourages healing of the exposed areas of submucosa. More chronic adhesions, especially those that have caused physical deformation, require surgical resection and these have a high tendency to recur.

Partial-thickness tears or small full-thickness tears can heal spontaneously by second intention, but a check on the integrity of the cervix should be made at the diestrus period after the second postpartum estrus, and mares should be monitored carefully for signs of incipient placentitis throughout any ensuing pregnancy. Full-thickness tears of greater than half the length of the cervix

are best repaired surgically, no earlier than 4–6 weeks post partum, when, hopefully, all inflammation has subsided and a healthy granulation tissue reaction is present. This is carried out under standing sedation with epidural anesthesia and long-handled instruments. A three-layer closure is invariably used. Postoperatively, 3–5 days of systemic antibiotics and daily application of an antibiotic/corticosteroid ointment help decrease the incidence of excessive scarring and adhesions, which are common sequelae. Mares should be checked 30 days postoperatively for integrity of the repair, as breakdowns are common. The mare should not be mated for 30 days by AI or 90 days by natural service. Some clinicians supplement pregnant mares after surgery with progesterone to promote cervical closure.

Cervical incompetence is difficult to treat, but converting the defect into a laceration, by surgical resection of the overlying mucosa, and then repairing it with a similar three-layer closure can be successful. Mares with severe damage to the cervix, which is not amenable to repair, have been treated by cervical cerclage after early diagnosis of pregnancy.

Prognosis
The prognosis for mucosal damage treated early is good. Adhesions of the cervix can recur if treated as chronic lesions, and these carry a guarded prognosis. Partial-thickness or small lacerations can heal spontaneously and carry a fair to guarded prognosis. Surgical repair of full-thickness lacerations is difficult and expensive, with partial breakdown, scarring, and adhesions possible complications. Fertility following successful repair is fair, but recurrence of the lesion at the next foaling is quite common. Abortion and premature parturition associated with posterior-pole placentitis is a common sequela. Repeat surgery is possible, but more guarded in prognosis.

Metritis–laminitis–septicemia complex
Definition/overview
Retained fetal membranes or any other significant infection of the uterus following foaling can lead to absorption of bacterial toxins and septicemia in the mare. Laminitis caused by circulating toxins resulting in vascular changes is a common sequela. There is a high incidence in heavy horse breeds (509). The progression of symptoms can be alarming and death can occur in severe cases. Postfoaling metritis should be classed as a medical emergency.

Etiology/pathophysiology
Gross contamination and damage to the endometrium during dystocia or retained fetal membranes can lead to bacterial infection of the endometrium and myometrium or even the serosal layers of the uterus. Large volumes of

295

Female reproductive tract

abnormal uterine fluid can accumulate without visible vaginal discharge. The endometrium becomes thin and friable, allowing bacteria and toxins to be absorbed into the mare's systemic circulation, causing septicemia and/or toxemia. These toxins cause peripheral vascular changes that may result in laminitis. The most common causal organisms are Gram-negative bacteria, particularly *Escherichia coli*.

Clinical presentation
Twelve hours to 10 days after foaling, dystocia, or retained placenta, the mare presents with a sudden onset of pyrexia, depression, dullness, vaginal discharge (often discolored, reddish brown, and fetid), abdominal pain, decreased milk production, and increased heart and rates. Acute laminitis (p. 69) may develop within 1–5 days (i.e. digital pulse, coronary band heat, bilateral or quadrilateral limb lameness). In undiagnosed cases, severe septicemia and endotoxemia ensue, with injected mucous-membranes, cardiovascular collapse, shock, and death.

Differential diagnosis
Colic; large bowel torsion; uterine rupture; uterine artery rupture.

Diagnosis
Diagnosis is based on history and clinical signs. Rectal palpation may reveal an enlarged, atonic uterus, which can be doughy, thickened and painful, and contain large quantities of fetid fluid. Ultrasound examination of the uterus confirms the enlargement, with prominent endometrial folds and echodense intrauterine fluid +/- retained placenta. Bacteriological culture and sensitivity of intrauterine fluid samples help direct antibiotic treatment, and blood samples for hematology often show a neutropenia and toxic cells. Palpation of the feet and lateral radiographic views are helpful in diagnosing laminitis.

Management
Immediate, vigorous, uterine lavage with 1–3 liters of warmed sterile saline 0.5% solution of povidone–iodine, using a sterile nasogastric tube and funnel, is required until the egress fluid is clear in order to remove as much debris and toxins as possible. An antibiotic solution effective against Gram-negative bacteria is instilled into the uterus. The procedure is repeated several times every few hours until there is no evidence of uterine debris in the flushings. Thereafter, it is repeated on a daily basis until the initial flush is clear and free of debris. The response to treatment can be monitored by the use of serial ultrasonographic examinations.

Supportive care for the mare includes broad-spectrum systemic antibiotics (including metronidazole), NSAIDs (e.g. flunixin meglumine), intravenous fluid therapy if dehydration or cardiovascular collapse is evident, oxytocin injections to aid uterine clearance of fluids or retained fetal membranes, and early implementation of acute laminitis treatment either prophylactically or therapeutically (p. 71).

Prognosis
Early recognition and treatment determine the prognosis. The condition can be life-threatening if not treated aggressively and early. The onset of laminitis is a poor prognostic sign.

Perineal lacerations
Definition/overview
Perineal lacerations are common injuries, particularly in the primiparous mare, usually associated with fetal oversize and malpresentation where one or both forelimbs is/are presented dorsally over the head and neck. Three types of perineal lacerations occur: 1st degree, 2nd degree, and 3rd degree (510-514). Careful visual examination along with rectal and vaginal palpation will confirm the degree of damage. Treatment varies with the degree of damage. Careful attention to detail in the pre- intra-, and postoperative periods is essential to achieve a good surgical success and return to breeding soundness.

Etiology/pathophysiology
Perineal lacerations occur at foaling and are more common in primiparous mares partly due to the increased likelihood of hymen remnants, especially dorsally, and the increased presence of the vestibulovaginal sphincter. Fetal oversize and malpresentation are also more common in these mares. A particular problem is where forelimbs are presented through the pelvic canal dorsally over the head and neck. The increased prominence of the hymen and/or vestibulovaginal sphincter increases the chance of these forelimbs catching on the dorsal vaginal mucosa during parturition and, with continued expulsion, being pushed through the dorsal vaginal wall and, in severe cases, into the rectum. If the dorsal vaginal wall is penetrated, but not the rectum, continued expulsion leads to damage to the ventral perineal body and dorsal vulva. If the rectum is penetrated, but the foot/feet are withdrawn back into the vagina before further expulsion, then a rectovaginal fistula is created (p. 299). If the rectum is penetrated and the foot/feet are not withdrawn and there is continued expulsion, then the entire caudal perineal body, ventral anus, and dorsal vulva are destroyed (3rd degree perineal laceration). Rarely, the damage occurs to the lateral vaginal wall, caudal rectum, and anal sphincter.

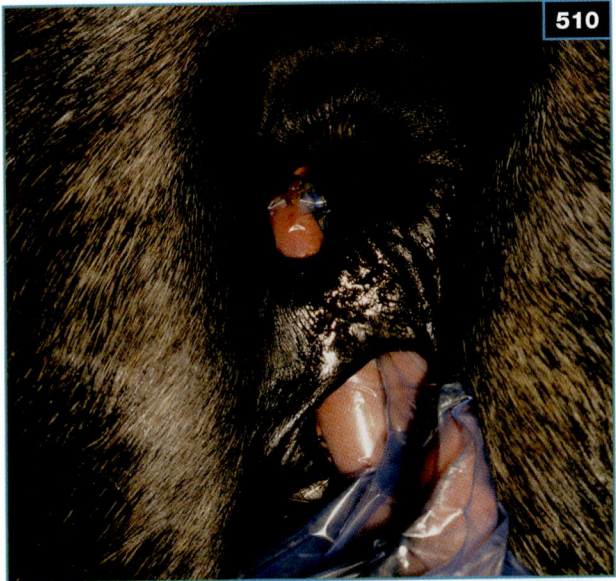

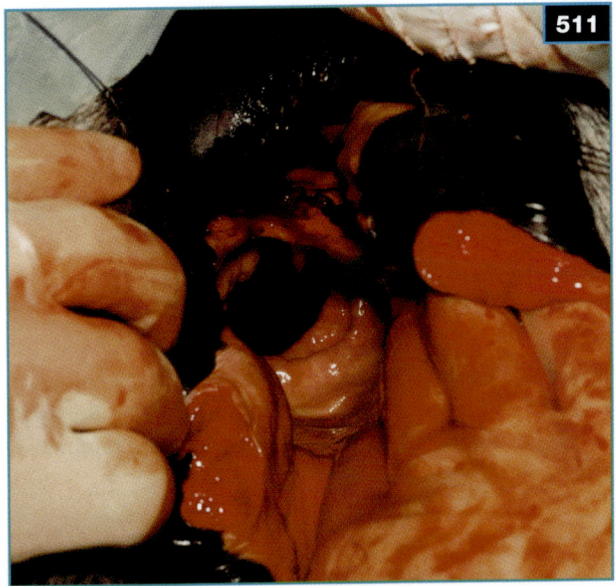

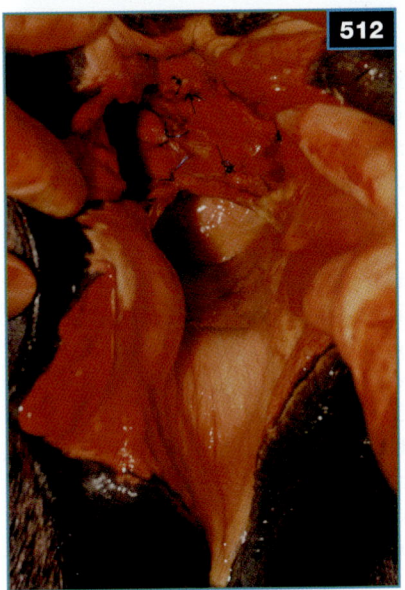

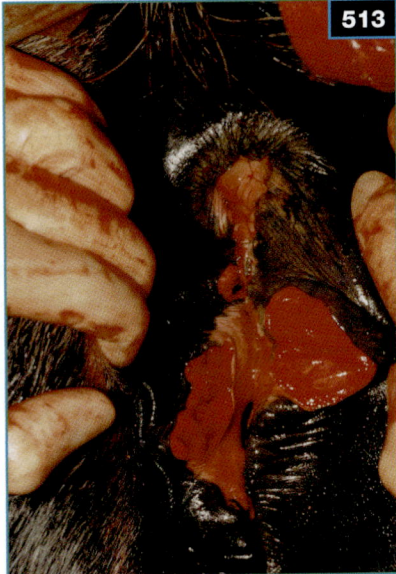

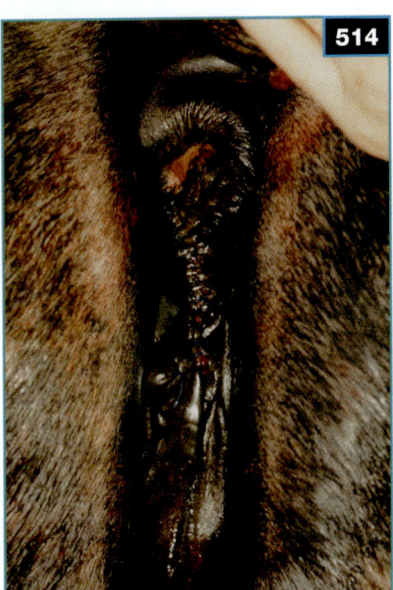

510–514 A Thoroughbred mare is presented with a history of sustaining a third-degree perineal tear 8 weeks previously. It has partially healed at the level of the vulva (510). (511) After suitable preparation the tear is about to be repaired. The part of the vulva that has healed has been sharply severed, revealing the 3rd degree tear. The gloved hand is in the vagina and the black hole leads into the rectum.

(512) The rectal (upper) and vaginal (lower) shelves are being created following careful dissection and the insertion of simple interrupted vertical mattress sutures in the deep layers of each structure. (513) The repair of the shelves is almost complete and the perineal body is about to be constructed. (514) The completed one-stage repair is finished with careful closure of the skin of the perineal body and anal ring.

Clinical presentation

+ 1st degree lacerations involve only the mucosa of the vestibule and dorsal vulval commissure and are the least severe injury.
+ 2nd degree lacerations affect the mucosa and submucosa of the vestibule, the dorsal vulval skin, and some of the perineal muscle.
+ 3rd degree lacerations are the most severe and all layers of the dorsal vestibule, perineal body, caudal rectum, and ventral anus are destroyed.

All of this damage is retroperitoneal, but in rare cases damage can occur more cranially and involve the peritoneal cavity, with the possibility of severe contamination and peritonitis.

Differential diagnosis

Rectovaginal/vestibular fistula; other caudal reproductive tract lacerations.

Diagnosis

Clinical signs and a careful examination visually and by rectal and vaginal palpation will confirm the extent of the damage. In cases that are not repaired immediately, particularly with 3rd degree lacerations, it is important to assess the entire reproductive tract, especially the uterus, for damage and endometritis. The latter is particularly common due to fecal contamination of the caudal tract. Endometrial cytology, culture, and biopsy may be useful in assessing this possibility.

Management

Careful observation at foaling may allow early detection of problems involving the forefeet and the vaginal mucosa and allow immediate cranial repulsion of the foal and redirection of the limbs. This will limit the severity of any injury. If the foal is presented with its limb(s) penetrating into the rectum and possibly protruding from the anus, repulsion may be possible, thereby at least saving the perineal body and ventral anus from damage but leaving a rectovaginal/vestibular fistula.

Second-degree perineal lacerations often heal spontaneously with the assistance of daily cleansing and possibly application of antiseptic creams. Surgical repair is rarely required, but can be performed within 4–6 hours of foaling or after a delay of 2–4 days in order to allow the immediate swelling and inflammation to subside. Many clinicians use a Caslick's vulvoplasty (p. 307) type procedure. Re-breeding is usually delayed until the wound is fully healed (4–6 weeks).

First-degree perineal lacerations can heal spontaneously, but if the perineal body is damaged significantly, the normal anatomy of the vestibule and vulva may become disrupted. This can lead to anal and dorsal vulvar/vestibular sinking, pneumovagina, and ascending vaginal infection (p. 306). Surgical repair is preferred and should be undertaken after all the inflammation and swelling have subsided. Many of these mares will benefit from postfoaling systemic antibiotics and NSAID therapy, tetanus prophylaxis, and daily wound cleaning and application of antiseptic creams to encourage resolution of any infection and inflammation prior to repair. Once healthy granulation tissue is present, careful minimal sharp debridement and anatomic layer repair (especially the perineal muscles) will ensure a return to normal function of the vulvar and vestibular seals.

Third-degree lacerations, if presented immediately after foaling (4–6 hours), can be treated by emergency surgical repair. Many cases are, however, so badly traumatized and contaminated that this is unlikely to be successful or lead to only a partial, poor quality repair. Most cases benefit from a delayed surgical repair. Initial treatment is similar to that for 2nd degree lacerations, but will be required for much longer (2–4 weeks). Manual removal of feces every 6–8 hours may also be required in some mares for varying periods depending on the extent and severity of the injury. The removal of all dead and extensively damaged tissue by careful sharp debridement at an early stage will speed up the process of secondary intention healing, although it is important not to be too aggressive. Granulation, epithelialization, and healing of the damaged areas take between 4 and 8 weeks depending on the severity of the injury. Surgical repair is undertaken once all the inflammation has resolved and is essential if return to breeding is required (see **510–514**).

With mares with a foal at foot the surgery is often delayed until after weaning. Pre- and postoperative measures to improve the success of the surgical repair are essential and must be carried out with great care:
+ Preoperatively. Decrease fecal volume and loosen their consistency to ease defecation and decrease rectal impaction (i.e. give a laxative diet: decrease concentrates; lush green grass; pelleted grass rations; laxatives including magnesium sulfate; bran mashes). Withhold all food 24 hours prior to surgery to reduce surgical contamination by feces.
+ Perioperatively. Medications 24 hours prior to surgery until 5–7 days post surgery should include broad-spectrum antibiotics and NSAIDs. Tetanus prophylaxis.

The surgical repair is undertaken in stocks under standing sedation, preferably with xylazine epidural anesthesia +/- lidocaine infiltration. There are many variations in the surgical procedure, which can be undertaken in one or two stages, but the basic principles of all of them should include: the use of strong absorbable monofilament suture material; minimal tension on the suture lines by careful and extensive dissection of tissue planes allowing apposition without tension; creation of a thick shelf between the rectum and vestibule; and placement of all sutures with good bites of tissue to decrease breakdown of suture lines. The exact surgical procedures are detailed in the standard surgical texts. In one-stage repairs the vagina, perineal body, and rectum are all repaired at the same time. In a two-stage repair the rectovaginal shelf is constructed initially, but the perineal body is rebuilt at a later stage.

The preoperative diet and perioperative medications are continued postoperatively and the external wounds on the perineum are gently cleansed and antiseptic ointment applied daily. The laxative diet is continued for 4 weeks. Monitoring for normal fecal passage is vital and any straining to pass feces must be dealt with urgently. External sutures are removed 10–14 days postoperatively. Endometrial cytology and culture can be performed at the second estrus period after the operation, which allows adequate time for healing and one estrus cycle to help natural resolution of the preoperative contamination.

The mare can be re-bred by AI 4 weeks post surgery or 3 months post surgery for natural covering. Complications of the surgical procedure include total or partial wound breakdown, infection, urine pooling, and constipation.

Prognosis

The prognosis for return to breeding soundness is: good for 1st degree tears; fair for 2nd degree lacerations with surgical repair, but guarded if this is not undertaken; poor for 3rd degree lacerations if not treated surgically, and guarded to fair with surgical repair as long as very careful attention to detail is paid. 1st and 2nd degree tears can occur at subsequent foalings, but it is unusual for 3rd degree tears to do so if they are repaired correctly.

Rectovaginal/vestibular fistulae

Definition/overview

Less common than perineal lacerations (p. 296), but similar etiology with a higher incidence in primiparous mares. Presents as a communicating hole between the rectal and vaginal cavities, with an intact anus, perineal body, and skin. A rectovaginal fistula occurs in the vagina cranial to the vestibular fold, whereas a rectovestibular fistula is caudal to the fold. The latter tends to damage more of the perineal body, leaving, on some occasions, only the perineal skin intact. The size of the fistula can vary from millimeters (where there has been poor healing of a 3rd degree perineal tear and subsequent fistulation) to, on average, 5–10 cm. Some of the largest are the diameter of a foal's head.

Management

The management and treatment of rectovaginal/vestibular fistulae are similar to 3rd degree perineal lacerations, with a suitable delay to allow traumatic inflammation and tissue damage to subside and resolve. Cleaning of the fistula is not possible, but fecal contamination of the vagina, which is quite common, should be removed daily.

Some small fistulae can seal spontaneously with wound granulation and contraction. Delays of a minimum of 4–6 weeks to allow reduction in inflammation, second intention healing, granulation, wound contracture, and tissue fibrosis to occur prior to surgical treatment are based on a similar premise to that for 3rd degree lacerations. The pre- and postoperative preparation and care are similar and just as important.

Several different methods of surgical repair have been described. The intact anal sphincter and perineal body can be excised, essentially converting the fistula into a 3rd degree laceration, and this is repaired by one of the methods described for this injury. This technique is particularly useful where the perineal body is substantially damaged and it has the advantage of a good exposure and the opportunity to reconstruct a strong shelf between the rectum and the vagina. The second repair method involves splitting the perineum transversely between the anus and the dorsal vulva, and continuing this to and beyond the fistula for 3–5 cm. Two holes are thus created, one dorsally into the rectum and the other ventrally into the vagina. These fistulae are then closed with everting suture patterns and the dissection dead space and perineum are sutured closed. Other methods include fistula repair following a transrectal or transvaginal approach, which have the disadvantage of a more limited exposure.

The mare can be re-bred by AI or natural covering as for 3rd degree tears. Complications include total or partial wound breakdown in the rectal and/or vaginal layers and, quite commonly, some perineal dehiscence with secondary intention healing. Infected wounds in the perineum can be treated by drainage and lavage and often resolve. Postoperative constipation and straining are a continual concern and best resolved with careful dietary management.

Prognosis

Small fistulae may heal spontaneously and carry a fair prognosis. Where surgical repairs are necessary, the prognosis depends on the extent and severity of the injury, but it is guarded to fair for return to breeding soundness. Fistulae rarely recur at subsequent foalings.

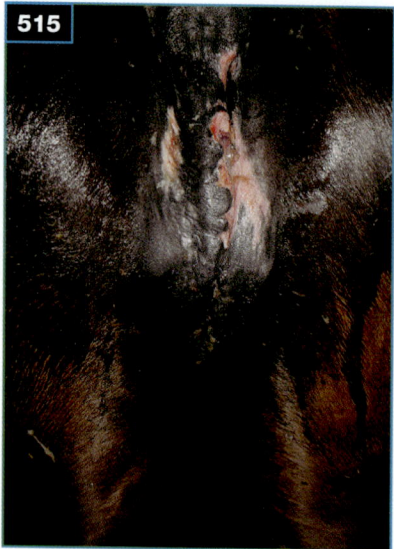

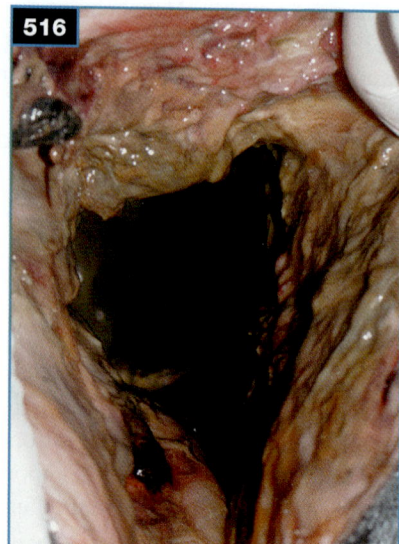

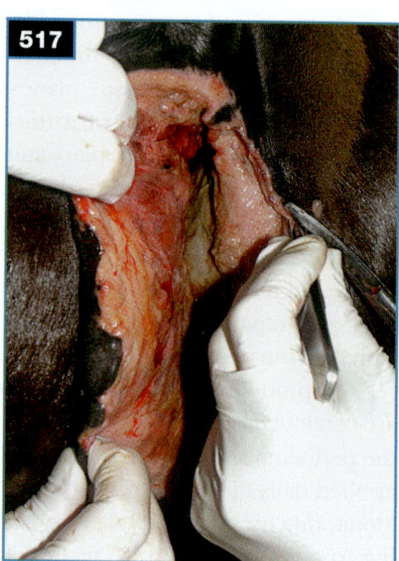

Postfoaling perineal bruising and vulvar hematoma

Definition/overview

Hematomas in the vaginal wall and vulval lips are common, especially in primiparous mares, where large foals have been delivered, and in cases of dystocia, particularly where large amounts of manipulation have been necessary. Considerable edema may accompany the bleeding. In severe cases there may be caudal vaginal or vulval lacerations (515–517). Complications of these cases, if treated correctly, can include severe vaginitis, fibrosis, and abscessation.

Treatment should include fecal softeners to ease the passage of feces through a swollen and painful perineum/pelvic canal, broad-spectrum antibiotics, tetanus prophylaxis, NSAIDs, and emollient creams. Most of the swelling and hematoma resolves uneventfully, but occasionally hematomas in the vulva and vagina may require drainage 7–10 days after foaling.

Delayed uterine involution

Definition/overview

Post partum the uterus usually contracts markedly within the first few days, expelling a brown discharge from the vulva for 3–7 days and contracting to its pregravid state within 35 days. In delayed involution the uterus fails to involute in the normal time frame, remaining flaccid, voluminous, and fluid-filled. Recognition of delayed involution can be a critical factor in deciding whether to mate a mare on the foaling heat.

Etiology/pathophysiology

Delayed uterine involution most commonly follows abortion, dystocia, retained fetal membranes, placentitis, uterine infection or hemorrhage, or lack of exercise.

515–517 A Thoroughbred mare that suffered perineal, vulval, and vaginal bruising and trauma, following major dystocia (515). After retraction of the damaged vulval lips it is clear that there is damage to the vestibule and vagina, while the cervix is still dilated and there is a view directly into the damaged uterus (516). The vulval and vaginal damage is being lightly debrided with sharp scissors after thorough washing with antiseptic solution (517).

Clinical presentation

Often there are no clinical signs, but occasionally there is an increase in vulval discharge. In unusual cases the mare may be dull, have a poor appetite, and show abdominal discomfort.

Diagnosis

The vagina tilts downwards on vaginal examination with or without urine pooling and vaginitis. The uterus is flaccid and voluminous on rectal examination. Hyperechoic intra-uterine fluid is seen on ultrasound examination.

Management/treatment

The intrauterine fluid should be removed by lavage using large volumes of dilute saline/povidone–iodine solution. Oxytocin (30 IU in 500 ml sterile saline) should be administered over the course of 15 minutes to stimulate uterine contractions and involution. Parenteral antibiotics and anti-endotoxic therapy should be administered. Paddock exercise is helpful. There is no evidence that prophylactic oxytocin or uterine lavage in the early postpartum period promotes involution or prevents failure of involution.

Prognosis

Good if treatment is implemented promptly.

Disorders and diseases of the ovary and oviduct

Chromosomal abnormalities of the mare

Definition/overview

Chromosomal abnormalities are uncommon, with the most reported type being the 63XO or gonadal dysgenesis syndrome. This presents as an infertile mare, often with cycling abnormalities and normal external genitalia, but with hypoplastic uterus and ovaries. Definitive diagnosis requires karyotyping on a blood sample. No treatment is available.

Etiology/pathophysiology

Chromosomal abnormalities are usually associated with abnormalities of the sex chromosomes and often lead to ovarian/uterine hypoplasia and infertility. The most commonly reported abnormality is 63XO (gonadal dysgenesis syndrome) – equivalent to Turner's syndrome in humans. Other chromosomal abnormalities include mosaic or chimeric karyotypes (63XO/64XX), 64 XY, 65 XXX, and 65 XXY. These occur during embryogenesis (mitosis) or gamete formation (meiosis) and are caused by chromosomal segregation errors. All breeds can be affected.

Clinical presentation

Often seen in a mare of breeding age which is infertile. The mare may present with persistent anestrus or irregular periods of behavioral estrus, and she can be receptive or passive to mating. Some affected mares may be smaller than normal. The external genitalia are female, with a normal or slightly small vulva.

Differential diagnosis

Other causes of infertility. Ovarian and endometrial atrophy (young [prepubertal] or very old mares); hermaphrodites; postexogenous hormonal administration to athletic animals.

Diagnosis

Affected mares have an underdeveloped uterus and very small, smooth, and firm ovaries (ovarian hypoplasia) on rectal palpation. If a cervix is present, it is usually flaccid and pale on vaginoscopy. There is endometrial hypoplasia on uterine biopsy, but care is required with this procedure in these mares as the uterine wall can be very thin and easily punctured. Definitive diagnosis requires karyotyping (chromosomal analysis) on a blood sample taken into citrate dextrose or heparin (**518, 519**). Rapid transport to a specialized laboratory is essential.

Management

None for reproductive function, but these animals can be used as athletes.

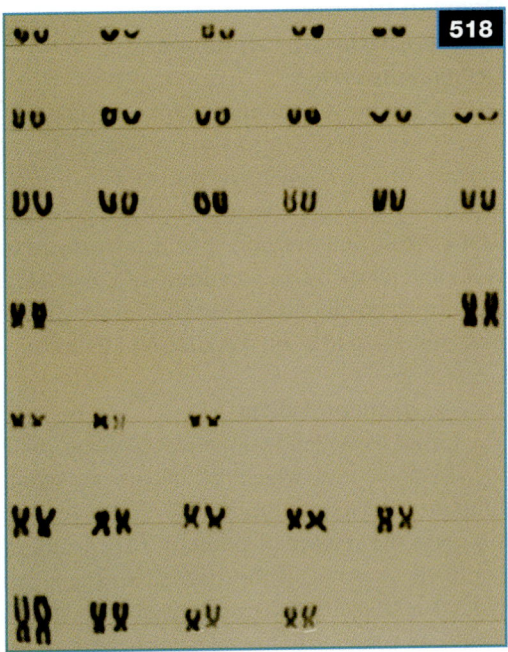

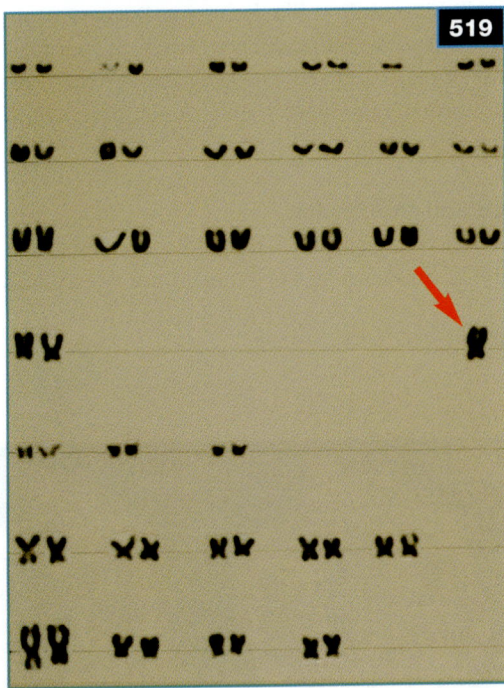

518 Karyotype of a normal mare (64XX).

519 Karyotype of a 63XO mare with a chromosomal abnormality. Note the single X chromosome (arrowed).

Ovarian tumors
Granulosa (thecal) cell tumor
Definition/overview
GCT is the most common ovarian neoplasm. GCTs are usually benign, slow growing, unilateral, and varying in size (6–40 cm diameter). The tumor destroys normal ovarian tissue in the affected ovary and produces diagnostically significant hormones, which cause atrophy of the contralateral ovary and a variety of clinical signs. Treatment by removal of the affected ovary carries a fair prognosis for return to normal cycling and fertility.

Etiology/pathophysiology
The tumor tissue gradually replaces the normal tissues of the affected ovary, which can become quite large in size. Inhibin, released by the neoplastic tissue, is thought to suppress the release of pituitary FSH, leading to almost complete atrophy of the normal ovarian tissue of the contralateral ovary and cyclic inactivity. Occasionally, the ovary can continue to function normally, but conception is rare. Neoplastic thecal cells may produce testosterone, leading to stallion-like behavior. Progesterone levels are low due to ovarian inactivity. Rarely, the neoplastic ovarian tissue causes raised estrogen levels, which may lead to abnormal mammary gland development and signs of nymphomania.

Clinical presentation
A variety of signs are exhibited according to the nature of the hormones released by the tumor. Masculinization may occur, with the mare showing stallion-like behavior of aggressiveness and interest in cycling mares or, in the chronic case, developing a more masculine muscle distribution and even clitoral enlargement. The estrous cycle is often affected, with the mare exhibiting anestrus characteristics, constant estrus (nymphomania), or irregular cycling. On rare occasions the unaffected ovary may continue to function and the mare cycles normally. Tumors have occasionally been diagnosed in pregnant mares.

The affected ovary is usually grossly enlarged on rectal palpation, with no ovulation fossa, and it may be cystic (520). The contralateral ovary is usually firm and small and often shows no signs of activity.

Differential diagnosis
Ovarian hematoma; cystadenoma; teratoma; other ovarian neoplasia, lymphoma/lymphosarcoma.

Diagnosis
Diagnosis is made on the basis of the history, clinical signs, and palpation per rectum of one grossly enlarged, noncycling ovary and a small, firm, variably cycling contralateral ovary, combined with ultrasonography results. Ultrasonography reveals the structure of the affected ovary to be multicystic in the majority of cases (521), but sometimes a single large fluid-filled cysts or a dense homogeneous mass is detected. Occasionally, one or more hematomas may be present within the tumor, leading to a distinctive appearance. The contralateral ovary is usually small and fibrous, often showing no cyclic activity.

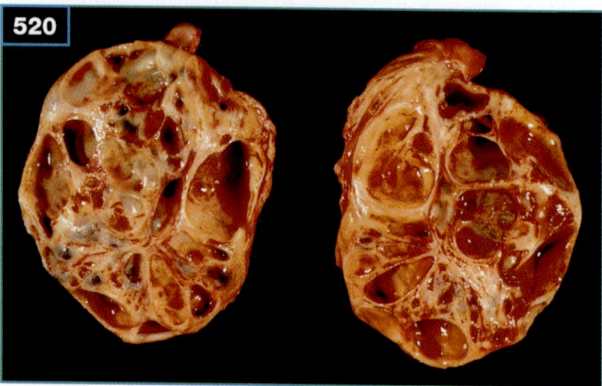

520 Postmortem specimen showing the cut section of a granulosa cell tumor of the ovary. Note the multiple honey-combed structures.

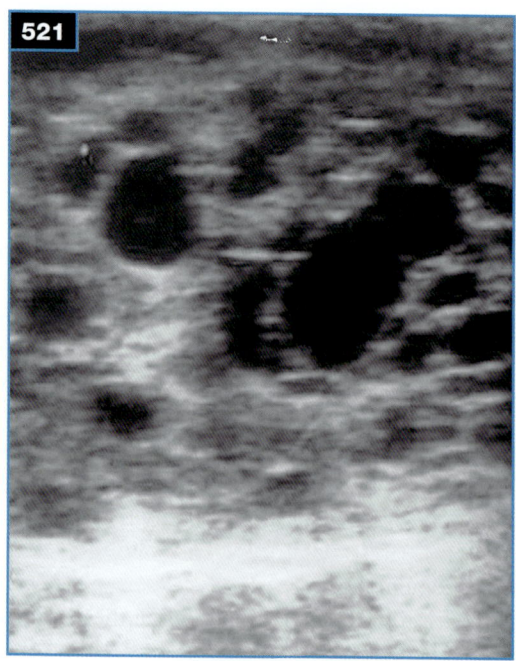

521 Transrectal ultrasonographic view of an ovary with a multicystic granulosa cell tumor. (Photo courtesy T Chenier)

A hormone assay supports clinical findings prior to surgery. The vast majority of mares will have raised serum inhibin levels (>0.7 ng/ml). Testosterone levels are elevated in 50–60% of cases (>50–100 pg/ml) and progesterone levels are invariably low (<1 ng/ml). Occasionally, estrogen levels are raised.

Laparoscopy/laparotomy followed by histopathology of the ovary after its removal will confirm the diagnosis.

Management

Treatment is by surgical removal of the affected ovary via a flank or ventral midline laparotomy (**522**), colpotomy, or laparoscopy. Laparoscopy is the method of choice except when the ovary is very enlarged, when laparotomy may be necessary.

Prognosis

The prognosis for return to fertility is good, cyclic activity usually resuming within 9 months of surgery or the next breeding season if surgery is performed late in the year. Metastasis is rare.

Mares that develop GCTs during pregnancy often continue their pregnancy as normal, but they will have abnormal cyclic activity post partum.

Other ovarian tumors

Definition/overview

Other tumors of the ovary include teratoma, adenoma, cystadenoma, adenocarcinoma, and dysgerminoma. They are nonsecretory, unilateral, and usually not malignant except in the case of dysgerminoma and adenocarcinoma. Teratoma is the second most common ovarian tumor after GCT, but the others are rare.

Etiology/pathophysiology

Adenomas are epithelial and usually unilateral, arising most commonly at the ovulatory fossa or oviductal fimbriae. They are nonsecretory, usually benign, can grow extremely large, are unilobular or multilobular, and the contralateral ovary is usually normal. When they become cystic they are referred to as cystadenomas (**523**). Rarely, noncystic adenomas metastasize, in which case they are termed adenocarcinomas.

Teratomas are solid or cystic tumors arising from germ cells, which are benign and nonsecretory. They contain abnormally placed embryonic structures (e.g. hair, skin, nerves and blood vessels, and even teeth and bone).

The extremely rare dysgerminoma consists of homogeneous primordial germ-like cells, and it is often lobulated or polycystic. The tumor tissue is nonsecretory, but can metastasize rapidly to the thoracic and abdominal cavities. Hypertrophic osteopathy (see p.165) has been associated with dysgerminoma.

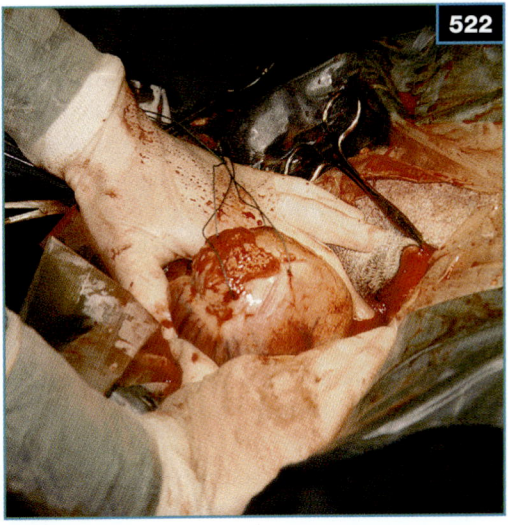

522 Ovarian tumor being removed at laparotomy using a stapling device. Note the enlarged ovary.

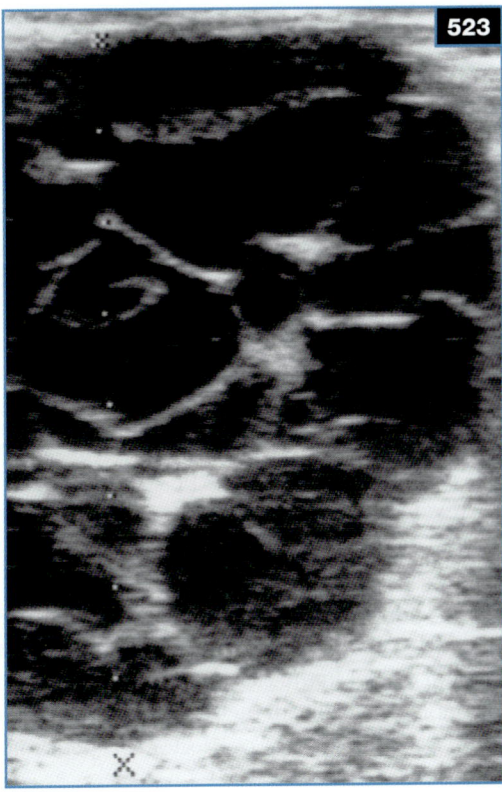

523 Transrectal ultrasonographic view of a left ovary with a cystadenoma. (Photo courtesy T Chenier)

303

Clinical presentation

Most of these tumors are nonsecretory and therefore mares exhibit no hormonal/cyclic aberrations and the contralateral ovary is normal. If the tumor becomes very large, it can cause abdominal pain by traction on the ovarian ligament or even rupture of the ligament leading to intra-abdominal hemorrhage. Fertility is not usually affected unless the tumor becomes so large that it displaces or impinges on the reproductive tract, altering its conformation.

Abdominal metastasis may lead to recurring abdominal pain, colic, weight loss, and/or ascites. In the case of dysgerminoma, the mare may show signs of hypertrophic osteopathy (see p. 165).

A unilateral, enlarged, often cystic and irregularly shaped, abnormal ovary is evident on rectal palpation.

Differential diagnosis

Ovarian hematoma; GCT, other ovarian neoplasia, lymphoma/lymphosarcoma.

Diagnosis

Diagnosis is based on clinical signs and the identification of a unilateral, enlarged, often cystic, abnormal ovary on rectal palpation and ultrasonography. The ultrasonographic appearance varies according to the tissue components of the tumor (523). In the case of dysgerminoma, serum testosterone levels may be very high (up to 2,500 pg/ml), with low progesterone levels. Diagnosis is confirmed on laparoscopy/laparotomy and histopathology of the ovary following removal.

Management

Treatment is by surgical removal of the affected ovary via laparotomy, colpotomy, or laparoscopy. Laparoscopy is the method of choice except when the ovary is very enlarged.

Prognosis

The prognosis following surgery is good for most of these tumors because they are usually hormonally inactive and benign, except in the case of dysgerminomas and adenocarcinomas, which can metastasize rapidly. The prognosis for these is poor unless ovariectomy is performed prior to metastasis.

Ovarian hematoma

Definition/overview

Ovarian hematoma is a unilateral ovarian enlargement due to hematoma formation.

Etiology/pathophysiology

Ovarian hematoma was a common diagnosis prior to the routine use of ultrasonography and was thought to be a result of excessive hemorrhage into the postovulation follicle. It is now considered to be an uncommon event. Ovarian hematomas are thought to be anovulatory follicles that have a blood-filled lumen (i.e. anovulatory hemorrhagic follicles [AHF]).

Clinical presentation

The contralateral ovary, behavioral cycle, and endocrine patterns are normal. Ovarian hematoma is often an incidental finding on rectal palpation.

Differential diagnosis

GCT; other ovarian neoplasia; anovulatory follicle; ovarian abscess; transitional ovary.

Diagnosis

Ultrasonography of the ovary may reveal a mass similar to a GCT, but ovarian hematomas are usually more uniformly echogenic and have an ovulation fossa present and a characteristic homogeneous appearance to their contents. The ultrasonographic appearance of an AHF normally changes more rapidly (i.e. within days) compared with that of a GCT. Hormone assay levels will be normal for AHFs.

Management

Treatment is not necessary as the ovarian structure will be absorbed.

Prognosis

The prognosis is good as there is no long-term effect on the mare unless the structure becomes extremely large (524).

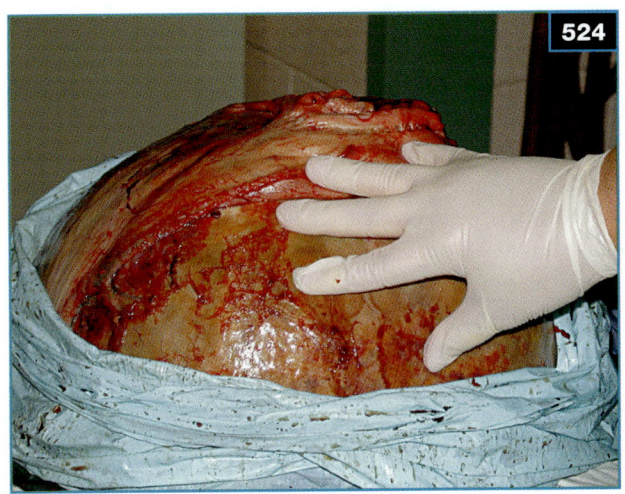

524 An enormously enlarged ovary, due to a hematoma, being removed surgically via laparotomy. (Photo courtesy T Chenier)

Oviduct disease
Definition/overview
Lesions of the oviducts (Fallopian tubes) are rare in the mare, often only being recognized at postmortem examination.

Etiology/pathophysiology
Direct spread of a uterine infection (endometritis) or spread from a body cavity may lead to salpingitis, or it may result from hematogenous spread of an infection from another body system. The resulting inflammation may reduce the patency of the oviduct and lead to delayed sperm or ovum passage, thereby affecting fertility. In extreme cases the lumen of the oviduct or the uterotubal sphincter can be completely occluded. Adhesions between the infundibulum and an ovary or the uterus are a common postmortem finding, but their significance in relation to fertility is unknown. Very rarely, tumors of the oviduct may occlude the lumen, and ovarian cysts or tumors may block the entrance to the oviduct or physically impinge on it. Parafimbrial cysts and fimbrial adhesions may affect the ability of the fimbria to receive the oocyte and pass it to the oviduct. Occlusions can also occur with collagen-type material, at present of unknown origin, particularly in older mares.

Clinical presentation
Oviduct disease can cause reduced fertility and endometritis. Older mares are more likely to be affected (mean age 18 years old).

Diagnosis
A full reproductive tract and fertility examination should be carried out and other more common causes of mare infertility explored before oviduct problems are considered. Patency of the oviducts can be tested using a fluorescent microsphere or starch-grain test, via laparoscopy or ultrasound-guided transvaginal deposition, both of which are difficult and awkward to carry out. The normal transit time from ovary to cervix is between 4 and 7 days. Hysteroscopy of the uterus and evaluation of the uterotubal junction may reveal cysts, adhesions, fibrosis, or other uterine abnormalities, which may cause obstruction. The oviducts can be palpated per rectum, visualized on ultrasound examination, viewed directly via laparoscopy, or examined directly at exploratory laparotomy.

Management
Endometritis should be treated appropriately (p. 314) after swabbing for bacterial culture and sensitivity testing. Hematogenous infections are treated using systemic antibiotics. Adhesions can be broken down surgically and prostaglandin E_2 has been applied to the oviducts via laparoscopy to encourage contractions and improve patency. Hysteroscopic-guided laser surgery of the uterotubal junction has been used in the treatment of abnormalities of this area. Exploratory laparotomy allows the ducts to be lavaged and fimbrial adhesions and cysts removed.

Prognosis
Diseases of the oviduct are not easily diagnosed or treated and therefore the prognosis for these conditions is always guarded.

305

Diseases of the vulva, vagina, and cervix

Pneumovagina and increased contamination of the caudal reproductive tract

Definition/overview

Loss of normal perineal and vulval conformation through a multifactorial mix of conditions such as trauma and the loss of perineal fat as a mare ages compromises the anatomic protective barriers of the normal caudal reproductive tract. This allows the creation of a pneumovagina, which increases the bacterial contamination of the vagina, cervix, and uterus and leads to inflammation and infertility. Careful assessment of the perineal and vulval conformation and structure can be carried out by visual and digital examination. The ascending infection can be confirmed on a vaginoscopic examination with intrauterine bacterial swabbing and cytology. Vulval and perineal body surgery is required in many cases to resolve the problem permanently. Specific endometrial treatment is often not required further after the vulval/perineal problem is resolved.

Etiology/pathophysiology

Mares with good perineal and vulval conformation have a vertical vulva with 80% below the level of the pelvic floor. In some mares a greater percentage of the labia appears to be situated dorsal to the pelvic floor, which compromises vulval function. A proportion of these mares develop a condition where the anus and rectum appear to be pulled cranially towards the caudal abdomen, which leads to the dorsal vulva becoming more horizontal and sloping. Finally, the vulva and its labia/constrictor muscles can be damaged by repeated foalings, leading to stretching and lacerations, as well as repeated vulval surgery. Damage may also occur to the perineal body and vestibular sphincter with or without vulval damage, which further compromises the functional barriers. Other factors include poor inherited conformation, ageing with loss of muscle tone in the body generally and specifically in the caudal reproductive tract, pendulous abdominal conformation, and poor body condition. With the poor function of the caudal tract barriers, air and bacteria/debris can enter the tract, especially at estrus, and create a pneumovagina. The pneumovagina desiccates and inflames the mucosa, which, along with increased bacterial contamination, leads to a vaginitis/cervicitis that can ascend into the uterus and cause an endometritis.

525 Transrectal transverse ultrasonogram of the right uterine horn showing air within the lumen (note bright white hyperechoic foci). This mare had abnormalities of the vulva and vestibule leading to aspiration of air into the proximal reproductive tract. (Photo courtesy T Chenier)

Clinical presentation

The mare may be presented for a BSE, a routine reproductive examination, or following a history of repeated unsuccessful attempts to breed. Abnormal vulval conformation, structure, and/or tone may be noted on visual and digital examination. The angle and length of the vulva have been used to create a Caslick score (length of vulva in cm × angle of declination of vulva), which helps determine the necessity for a Caslick's vulvoplasty operation. Values <150 and preferably <100 are associated with normal anatomy and better fertility rates. The score increases naturally with age. The relative length or percentage of the vulva above the ischium is also a major determinant of the need for surgical treatment. The vulval lips should be parted manually and any aspiration of air into the vagina noted, as this confirms that the vestibulovaginal seal is also compromised. There may also be a history of aspiration of air during normal exercise (vaginal wind sucking).

Differential diagnosis

Other causes of infertility and endometritis.

Diagnosis

History and clinical examination of the external genitalia are usually enough to achieve a provisional diagnosis. The perineal and pelvic conformation will need careful consideration. The vulva is ideally evaluated during estrus. The integrity of the perineal body is best assessed by placement of one finger into the rectum and the thumb in the vestibule (there should be at least 3 cm of muscular tissue between the two). Calculation of the Caslick index will help define if this procedure is necessary. On vaginoscopic examination, there may be air in the vagina and a vaginitis/cervicitis with congestion and mucus/discharge (sometimes frothy and foamy due to air). Samples can be taken to confirm the presence of an endometritis (swabs for bacterial culture/cytology). Rectal palpation and ultrasound examination may reveal an air-filled vagina/uterus (525) and cranial migration of the uterus into the abdomen.

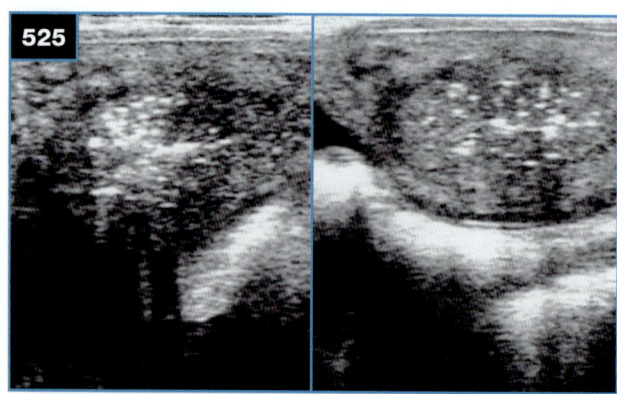

525

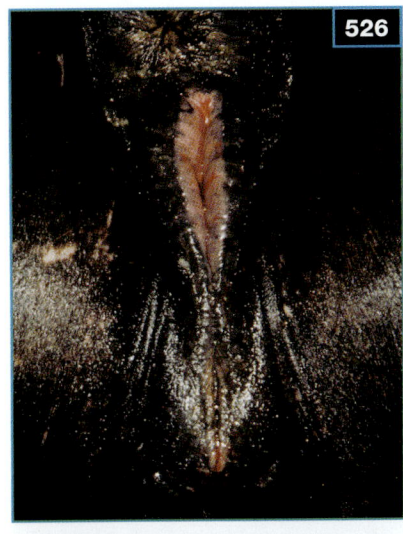

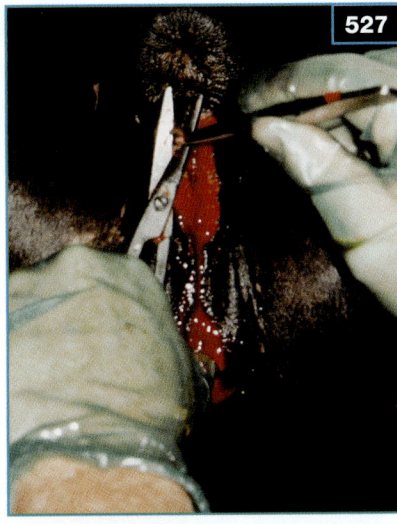

526–529 A Caslick's operation. Local anesthetic has been infiltrated under the edges of the vulval lips down to the level of the pelvic floor (526). Using sharp scissors, a thin slice of mucosa is removed just inside the vulval lips (527). The two edges are now ready to be sutured together (528). The operation is finished with the edges carefully brought together by simple interrupted nylon sutures (529).

530 A Caslick's operation undertaken post foaling that has subsequently broken down.

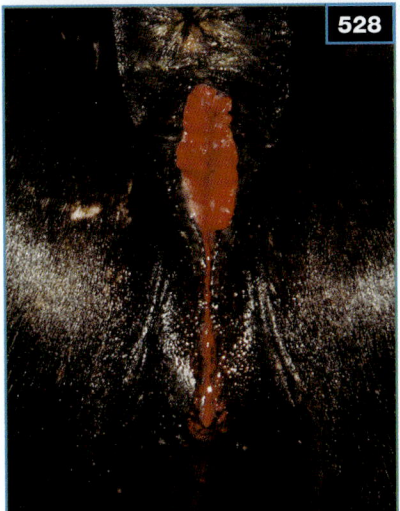

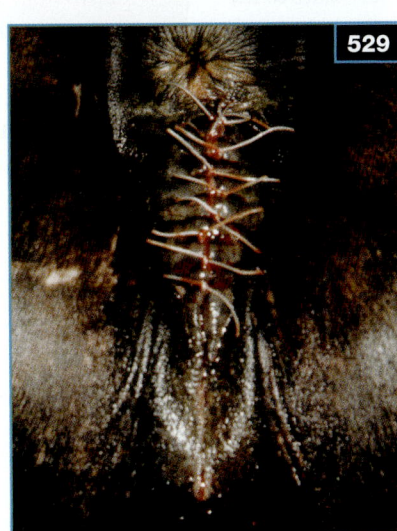

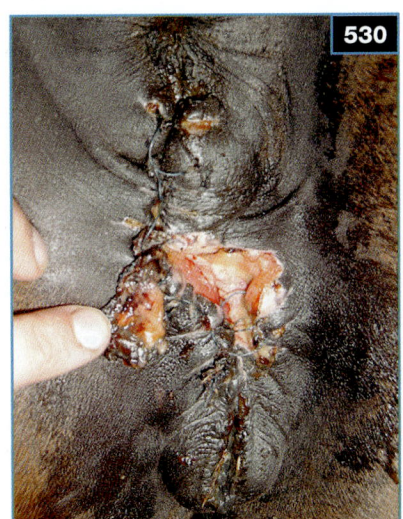

Management

Caslick's vulvoplasty operation is the most important treatment for vulval insufficiency and pneumovagina (526–529). A thin piece of mucosa is removed from either side of the vulval lips and then the two edges are sutured together down to the level of the pelvic brim. The repair must ensure that the dorsal commissure is closed and kept closed. Once the procedure is carried out the mare requires a Caslick's operation for the rest of her reproductive life (530). The Caslick will require opening for breeding and foaling, and rapid repair thereafter to prevent reinfection. Endometritis/cervicitis/vaginitis secondary to the pneumovagina often resolve spontaneously after the Caslick's operation due to the natural defense mechanisms. In older or heavily contaminated mares, specific endometritis therapy may be necessary.

Where a Caslick's operation is ineffective, and especially if there is vestibular insufficiency, it may be necessary to undertake additional surgical procedures. Where there is cranial migration of the anus and rectum, Pouret's procedure may be used to realign the vulval labia. Where there is vestibular and perineal insufficiency, perineal reconstruction is indicated. Both are more technical procedures than the Caslick's operation and are best carried out in stocks under epidural anesthesia.

Prognosis

The prognosis varies with the degree of vulval and/or vestibular insufficiency and subsequent pneumovagina, but is guarded in most cases. The condition is usually progressive during the breeding life of the mare and constant opening and repair of the vulval lips is time-consuming and ultimately contributes to progression of the problem. Perineal and vestibular insufficiency are more difficult to treat and carry a slightly worse prognosis.

307

Female reproductive tract

Urovagina
Definition/overview
Conformational defects of the vestibule and vagina may result in urine pooling in the anterior vagina. Vaginitis, cervicitis, and/or endometritis may ensue, leading to infertility, particularly if the condition becomes chronic. Conformation may improve spontaneously, resulting in resolution, or surgery may be required.

Etiology/pathophysiology
Age, weight loss, foaling/mating injuries, relaxation of the reproductive tract during estrus, Caslick's vulvoplasties that have been extended too far ventrally below the level of the pelvic brim, or a large pendulous multiparous uterus may result in changes in conformation of the vulva/vagina/vestibule, which result in urine pooling in the anterior vagina. Urine pooling may be a temporary state in the first postpartum estrus while the uterus is still involuting.

Clinical presentation
The clinical signs are vulval discharge, failure to conceive, and an abnormal vulval conformation.

Differential diagnosis
Other causes of infertility/subfertility; bacterial endometritis; bacterial vaginitis; CEM; pneumovagina.

Diagnosis
Urine/vaginitis is visible on vaginoscopy at estrus. Urine pooling is evident on manual examination. Ultrasonography may identify fluid in the uterus (urine or endometritis) and/or poor uterine involution.

Management
Many acute cases resolve spontaneously as the uterus involutes fully and the vagina resumes normal conformation. Sexual rest and improvement in the physical condition of the mare also help in some cases. Caslick's vulvoplasties that have been extended too far ventrally should be corrected to allow the normal efflux of urine. Vaginitis/cervicitis/endometritis should be treated appropriately with antibiotics and/or flushing. Some cases of urovagina cause a problem for fertility only while the cervix is open during estrus and the urine refluxes into the uterus. These may be treated medically, with repeated manual scooping out of urine from the vagina, lavaging of the uterus, and use of intrauterine antibiotics while the mare is in estrus and the cervix open.

In more severe, chronic cases a urethral extension procedure, where a mucosal tube is created surgically from the urethral opening to direct urine caudally, may be required.

Perineal body transection (Pouret's operation) may help in mares with poor vulval conformation (**531**).

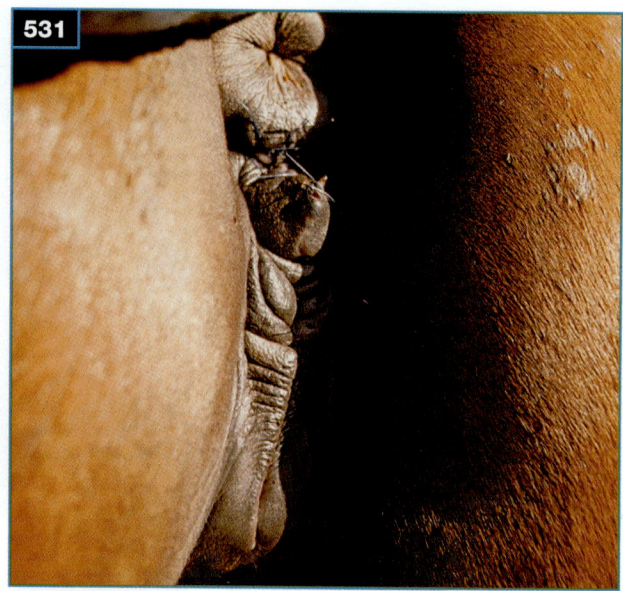

531 This mare has just had a Pouret operation carried out. Note the way the dorsal commissures of the vulval lips are vertical and there is a shelf effect above them before reaching the anus.

Prognosis
The prognosis is good in young mares with the temporary state, and fair for older mares following surgery.

Persistent hymen
Definition/overview
Maiden mares often have a remnant of the hymen present, which varies in size and completeness. Very occasionally it forms a complete membrane, which can bulge between the lips of the vulva.

Etiology/pathophysiology
Some remnant of the hymen is normal in maiden mares and is found just cranial to the urethral orifice at the junction between the vestibule and vagina. It can consist of a loose fold of thin tissue forming a low ridge of less than 2 cm height ventrally on the floor of the caudal vagina. More unusually, there can be strands of tissue more dorsally crossing the vagina, or a complete membrane. The latter condition stops the flow of endometrial gland products down the reproductive tract, and these accumulate behind the membrane causing it to bulge out between the vulval lips.

Clinical presentation

Persistent hymen may present as minor hemorrhage from the vulval lips after the first covering of maiden mares. The condition may prevent the passage of a vaginal speculum and/or hand at the first reproductive examination of the maiden mare. Cases where there is considerable build-up of fluid behind the complete hymen occur in postpuberty mares that are cycling and these may present with a bulging, rounded, bluish-white tissue between the vulval lips, often noted when the mare is moving at grass.

Diagnosis

Diagnosis is by vaginal examination via speculum or manually. Rectal palpation and ultrasonography of the entire reproductive tract will confirm that there is a tract cranial to the membrane and that this is not a severe congenital deformity. There may be fluid accumulated cranial to the hymen in the vagina and, occasionally, in the uterus.

Management

Simple manual vaginal palpation will break down fine strands or folds. In more complete folds it may be necessary to sedate the mare and cut the center with scissors before placing the clinician's fingers through the new hole and breaking the fold down manually. Subsequently, the accumulated uterine fluid drains away.

Prognosis

The prognosis is good for future fertility as long as no congenital defects of the tract are present.

Varicose veins of the vagina

Definition/overview

Prominent and varicosed veins are a common occurrence in the dorsal vaginal wall, at the level of the remnants of the hymen, just cranial to the urethral orifice. They are more common in older mares, especially in late pregnancy, and can cause intermittent vaginal bleeding.

Etiology/pathophysiology

The cause of the varicosity of the veins is unknown, but they increase in incidence with age and multiparity and, once present, persist. They rarely hemorrhage all the time and usually bleeding is associated with partial rupture of the vessels in late pregnancy or, occasionally, estrus. The hemorrhage, which is usually slight, invariably stops spontaneously after parturition.

Clinical presentation

Varicose veins may be detected as an incidental finding at a reproductive examination. They usually present as intermittent slight fresh hemorrhage from the vulval lips in older, late-pregnant mares or, less commonly, during estrus, particularly after breeding. Once the veins are established the bleeding may occur every year in late pregnancy or, in severe cases, at every mating. An increase in incidence and/or severity should be investigated further.

Differential diagnosis

Placental abnormalities; trauma to the reproductive tract, especially post breeding or examination; urinary tract hemorrhage.

Diagnosis

Vaginal speculum examination will detect the enlarged (1–3 mm), thin-walled, bluish veins, usually dorsally at the level of the hymen (532). Severe cases may involve the ventral and lateral walls. Hemorrhage may be seen from the vessels. It is important to rule out other sources of bleeding from the reproductive or urinary tract, including the placenta. Rectal palpation, transrectal or transabdominal ultrasonography, and endoscopy of the tracts may be considered in certain cases.

Management

In incidental cases or where the hemorrhage is intermittent and/or slight, no treatment is necessary. If the hemorrhage is more severe or persistent, the vessels may be cauterized using lasers or diathermy. Some clinicians have tried local injections of 5% formalin solution under endoscopic guidance with some success. Occasionally, large vessels can be ligated with absorbable suture material.

Prognosis

The prognosis varies with the severity of the varicose veins and whether treatment is necessary, but is generally fair to good.

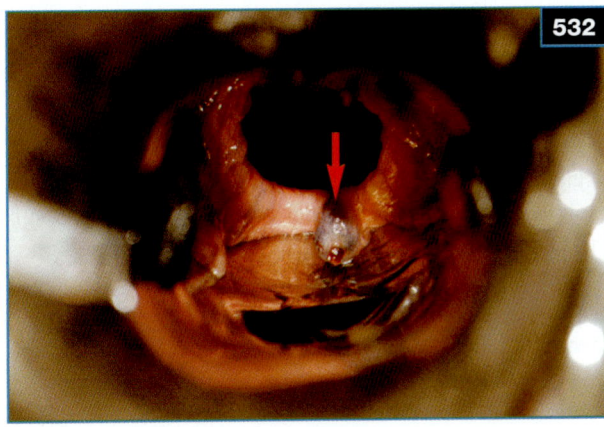

532 A view down a vaginal speculum of a case of vaginal varicosity showing the bluish enlarged vessel in the fold of tissue in the ventral vagina (arrow).

309

Cranial vaginal lacerations

Definition/overview

Cranial vaginal lacerations can occur during parturition, but more commonly they are related to accidents occurring at breeding. Many of the lacerations occur dorsally and are easily missed. Spontaneous healing is very quick in most cases, but occasionally complications, including eventration of bowel or bladder and/or peritonitis following contamination, occur. Surgical repair of lacerations is rarely indicated.

Etiology/pathophysiology

Lacerations during parturition tend to occur in the caudal part of the vagina or cranial vestibule (see Perineal lacerations, p. 296). Cranial vaginal lacerations are usually associated with intromission of the stallion's penis during breeding. Some stallions are more likely to cause these injuries and some clinicians consider them to be related to a discrepancy between the size of the stallion's penis and the mare's vagina. It is more likely to be related to a particular stallion's copulatory behavior.

Clinical presentation

In many cases the laceration in the mare is not detected at breeding and, by the time the mare is examined vaginally again, it has healed. In some cases, fresh blood is noted on the vulval lips and/or the stallion's penis immediately after breeding. Breeding lacerations usually occur in the cranial dorsolateral vaginal wall. Some are small (<5 cm) and only partial thickness, with limited hemorrhage and rapid healing. Any contamination of the ejaculate with blood may affect its fertility. Full-thickness lacerations at this point are peritoneal and contamination by semen and penile/vaginal debris and bacterial flora can lead to peritonitis. If the laceration is noted early, the mare should be monitored for signs of peritonitis for at least 3–4 days and treatment instituted as soon as possible. Severe vaginal lacerations or ruptures, particularly if they are ventral, can lead to bowel or urinary bladder eventration.

Diagnosis

Vaginal speculum examination may lead to air being aspirated into the abdominal cavity if the tear is full thickness and peritoneal, and the vagina then becomes dilated. The tear is often identified in the cranial region just dorsal to the cervix. Alternatively, the vagina can be manually palpated. If peritonitis is suspected, peritoneal centesis and ultrasonography of the abdomen may help confirm this suspicion.

Management

Partial-thickness and small lacerations are often undiagnosed or left untreated and heal spontaneously without incident. Very few lacerations appear to develop into peritonitis. It has been known for mares to conceive from a breeding where a laceration has occurred, suggesting that ejaculation through the tear is rare. Careful monitoring for complications for at least 96 hours, plus prophylactic use of broad-spectrum antibiotics, is usually all that is required for dorsal lacerations. Ventral lacerations, which are rare, have an increased chance of eventration. The chance can be reduced by cross tying (to discourage lying down), plus systemic medications to decrease abdominal straining. If the bowel or bladder eventrates, it should be protected and washed with sterile antibiotic solutions before replacement in the vagina and vulval suturing. An epidural anesthetic will stop straining and allow referral to an equine hospital for surgical replacement and/or bowel resection. If this is unavailable, euthanasia should be considered.

Surgical repair of lacerations with absorbable sutures in the standing sedated mare under epidural anesthesia can be performed in acute lacerations, although this is rare. Some clinicians carry out a Caslick's vulvoplasty operation when there is a cranial vaginal tear in order to reduce the possibility of air aspiration and contamination into the abdominal cavity.

Prognosis

With small or partial cranial lacerations the prognosis is fair. For larger cranial lacerations it is guarded, and for any case with eventration it is poor. Lacerations that occur during foaling can interfere with foaling and may necessitate a Cesarean section if eventration occurs.

Coital exanthema

Definition/overview

Coital exanthema is a sporadically occurring, usually venereally transmitted, EHV infection of both sexes. Initial blisters, usually on the vulval lips, penis, or prepuce, rupture to form ulcers. If they do not become secondarily infected, these heal within 7–10 days. Preventive applications of antiseptic creams and the cessation of mating until healing occurs are all that is required for treatment.

Etiology/pathophysiology

Coital exanthema is a disease of the external genitalia of the mare and stallion caused by EHV-3. It is usually venereally transmitted, although other speculated transmitters include grooming and veterinary equipment. The initial lesions appear on the mare or stallion 5–10 days after an infected mating or contact with a contaminated fomite. Initially, blistering of the skin with vesicle formation occurs

(1–3 mm diameter), with rapid progression to pustules, which rupture, leaving shallow ulcers. Rarely, lesions occur on the lips and nasal mucosa, but the presence of respiratory disease is controversial. It is not known whether latent infections can occur with this specific herpesvirus.

Clinical presentation

The clinical lesions usually occur after a mating, but occasionally they develop spontaneously in mares after minor vulval injuries, damage, or surgery. In the mare, lesions occur mainly on the vulval lips and perineal skin, occasionally on the anus, and rarely in the vestibule. In the stallion, both the penis and prepuce are affected, particularly in the area of the preputial fold. Stallions may show pain on intromission and be unwilling to breed. In both sexes, early in the disease process, there may be swelling and pain in the affected areas. In the stallion there may be pain on urination, especially if the urethral process has lesions. Spontaneous healing occurs quite rapidly in 7–10 days in both sexes provided no secondary bacterial infection of the lesions occurs. The discharge from and the severity of the lesions will increase if bacteria become established. After healing, the site of the lesions may be marked by permanent focal areas of lack of pigmentation (see p. 895).

Diagnosis

Diagnosis is based on clinical signs. Scrapes and biopsies of fresh lesions will show intranuclear inclusion bodies on histopathology.

Management

To help prevent secondary bacterial infections the affected areas of skin should be treated symptomatically with antiseptic creams. If there are other injuries to vulval tissue, these need to be specifically treated. Mating for the stallion and mare should cease until all the lesions have healed. Mares can usually be mated on the next estrous period.

Prognosis

There is no effect on fertility, except in the short term because of delays in breeding or reluctance to breed. Once the lesions are healed they present no further problems, since it is considered that the affected animal is now immune, although it is not known if this herpesvirus can be latent. No vaccine is available for prevention.

Dourine

Definition/overview

Dourine is a venereally transmitted, protozoal disease present in certain parts of the world and subject to international controls. Carrier animals are an important factor in the spread of the disease, along with a very long potential incubation period and slow onset of clinical signs. Clinical signs include fever, characteristic skin lesions, weight loss, and discharges from and swelling of the external genitalia of the mare and stallion. The organism is identifiable from discharges, blood, and fine-needle aspirates of skin lesions. Cases are rarely treated and many countries have a slaughter eradication policy.

Etiology/pathophysiology

Dourine is caused by a protozoal organism, *Trypanosoma equiperdum*, which is transmitted venereally. It is present in the Middle East, certain areas of Africa, Central and South America, and parts of Asia. The condition is subject to national and international control measures to stop the spread of the disease, which is complicated by the existence of clinically unaffected carriers. Epidemics have been reported where carrier or early infected animals are introduced. The course of the disease is slow, but it is progressive and leads to a high mortality rate.

Clinical presentation

The disease is very slow in onset, with an incubation period of up to 26 weeks. Clinical signs include a chronic mild fever, urticarial-like plaques of edema particularly on the flank skin, muscle wasting and weight loss, and, in the later stages, neurologic signs, collapse, and death. In the stallion, early on there is a mucoid or purulent urethral and/or preputial discharge. Later there is scrotal and preputial edema, which may extend cranially towards the ventral abdomen and chest. In the mare, in the early stages, there is a mucoid or purulent vaginal discharge. Later there is perineal and vulval edema, which may extend cranially towards the mammary gland and ventral abdomen.

Diagnosis

Diagnosis is based on history, clinical presentation, and identification of the organism from discharges, fine-needle aspirates from skin lesions, blood, and CSF. Control of the spread of the disease internationally depends on serologic testing to detect previous disease exposure and possible carrier status.

Management

It is possible to treat this condition, but in most countries there are control and eradication measures in force, including slaughter policies, and these need to be checked before any action is taken.

Prognosis

The prognosis is poor to grave, with most affected animals being humanely killed.

Tumors of the female reproductive tract excluding the ovary

Definition/overview

Tumors of the uterus are very rare and the only significant occurrence is leiomyoma. Tumors of the vestibule and vulval area are more common and include polyps, squamous cell carcinoma (SCC), melanoma in gray animals, and, rarely, hamartoma. All occur mainly in older mares. Biopsy for histopathologic diagnosis is essential for differential diagnosis. Many tumors can be surgically removed, with a fair to guarded prognosis for survival and fertility.

Etiology/pathophysiology

Leiomyomas have an unknown cause. Polyps/papillomas are thought to be caused by an unidentified papillomavirus unrelated to the cutaneous form. Both leiomyomas and polyps are benign.

SCC is more common in mares with unpigmented perineal skin. They can be malignant, spreading mainly to the local lymph nodes, but this seldom occurs. More usually there is local spread, especially in the ulcerative form.

Melanoma is very common in older gray animals, especially in the perineum. Most are slow growing and benign, and usually only cause problems due to their space occupation. Rarely, they may become highly malignant.

Vascular hamartomas occur mainly in the vagina, and muscular hamartomas in the perineal muscles. Hamartomas are abnormal accumulations of a normal cell type in a normal or abnormal location. They are benign.

Clinical presentation

Leiomyomas are usually single, occasionally multiple, nodules in the wall of the uterus, varying in diameter from two to 15 cm. They rarely cause any recognizable clinical signs, except for slight bleeding if ulceration occurs, and they are therefore found incidentally on rectal or ultrasonographic examination of the uterus.

Polyps/papillomas are seen protruding from between the vulval lips. Usually, they have a pedunculated neck and little surrounding reaction on the vestibule or vulval lips. They can enlarge slowly to a considerable size and may ulcerate and become secondarily infected.

SCCs come in two types: the proliferative type occurring on the vulval lips, vestibule wall, and clitoral region (**533**); and the ulcerative type, found more likely on the perineum or vulval lips. Secondary infection is common, leading to further tissue damage, increased odor, and serosanguineous discharge. Metastasis to other organs (lungs, vertebral bodies) beyond the local lymph nodes is rare, but may lead to other clinical signs and generalized weight loss and illness.

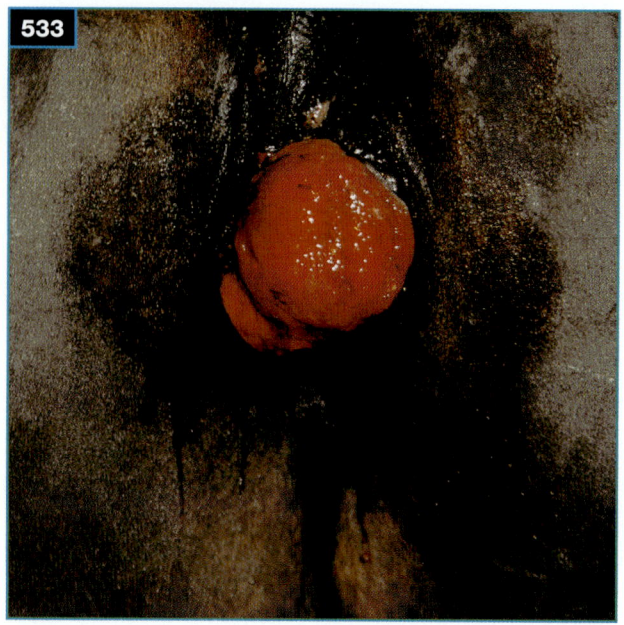

533 A squamous cell carcinoma of the clitoris and ventral vulval lips.

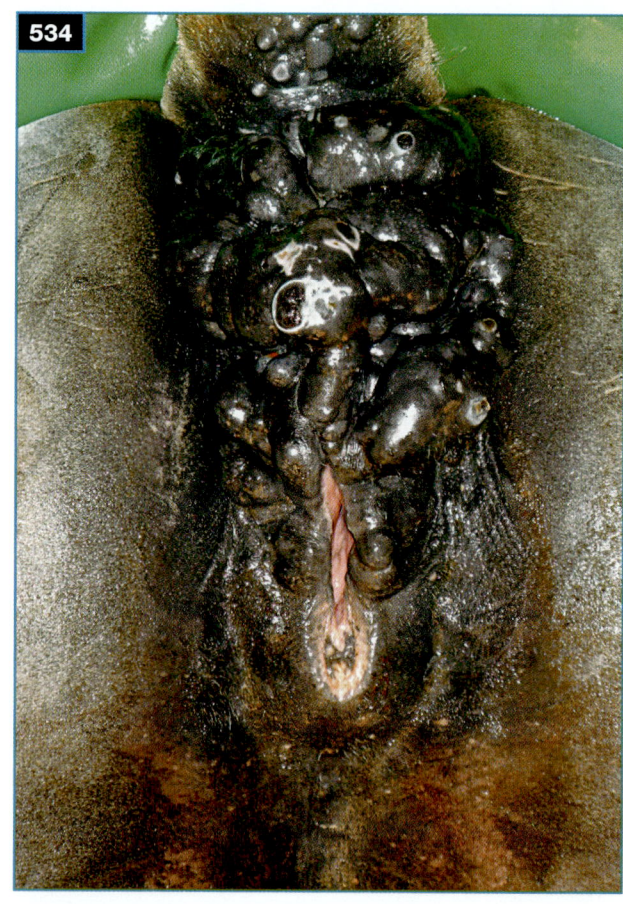

534 Massive infiltration of the perineum, tail head, and dorsal vulva by a melanoma.

Melanomas usually present as typical black lesions of varying size in the perineal skin (534), which may ulcerate with trauma or rapid growth and lead to a thick, black, hemorrhagic discharge. Some mares have either a single large tumor or large numbers of small tumors, which can adversely affect intromission and parturition. Depigmentation may suggest malignancy.

Hamartomas present as large growing masses in the perineum or adjacent muscles, leading to distortion of the normal anatomy.

Diagnosis

Leiomyomas may be detected on rectal palpation as firm spherical masses in the uterine wall. On ultrasonography these are hyperechoic, solid, and spherical. The histopathologic appearance on biopsy is distinctive. Papillomas/polyps have a distinctive appearance on vulval/vaginal examination and can be differentiated from leiomyomas on biopsy. SCCs are typical in gross appearance and on biopsy. The draining local lymph nodes in the inguinal/iliac region should be palpated. Melanomas are also typical in gross appearance and multiple lesions in the perineum and elsewhere around the body are common. Excisional biopsy may confirm the diagnosis and malignancy. Hamartomas on biopsy reveal normal tissue types.

Management

Pedunculated leiomyomas can be removed by a snare passed via an endoscope, or with a CO_2:YAG laser. Papillomas/polyps are easily removed by ligating or surgically severing the pedunculated neck. SCCs that are small, localized, and not extensively ulcerated can be surgically excised, especially on the vulval labia or vestibule. Other treatments include cryotherapy, topical 5-fluorouracil daily for 3 weeks, BCG local infiltration, and radiotherapy. Melanomas are rarely treated, but ulcerated or especially large lesions can be surgically excised. Intralesional cisplatin has been used in large lesions not amenable to surgery. Oral cimetidine therapy can decrease the size of the tumors if used over several months. Repeat therapy can be used if the tumors begin to enlarge again. No treatment is required for hamartomas and surgical resection is difficult because of their poorly defined borders.

Prognosis

Leiomyomas can be difficult to remove completely and fertility may be affected. Papillomas/polyps are easily removed and have a good prognosis for return to fertility.

SCCs have a variable prognosis depending on the type and extent of the lesion (worse in ulcerative types, large lesions, local lymph node spread). Melanomas generally carry a good prognosis, but large or multiple lesions may cause difficulties in defecation and urination as well as affecting mating and parturition. Hamartomas carry a good prognosis unless they enlarge enough to interfere with normal defecation, urination, or breeding.

Diseases and disorders of the uterus

Endometritis

Inflammation of the endometrium (endometritis) is one of the most common causes of subfertility in the mare. Endometritis is categorized into persistent mating-induced endometritis (PMIE), infectious endometritis, chronic degenerative endometritis, and sexually transmitted diseases.

The tubular reproductive tract, especially the uterus, is subjected to a variety of insults during the life of a broodmare including mating, pregnancy, and parturition. These insults include trauma to tissues and contamination with bacteria, fungi, semen, feces, urine, and other liquids/debris. There are cellular (neutrophil phagocytosis), immunologic (production and secretion of immunoglobulins and opsonins), and physical mechanisms that the tract can employ to help defend, restore normal function, and heal in the face of these insults. If any of these mechanisms do not function properly, the uterus will not be able to protect itself and infections will occur and persist. With age and increasing number of pregnancies, physical and immunologic changes in the tract render the mare more susceptible to infection and less able to resolve it. Failure of mechanical clearance of fluid, debris, and inflammatory substances from the lumen of the uterus is thought to be one of the major predisposing factors associated with the development of endometritis.

The multifactorial nature of endometritis has been divided into three categories:
1. Persistent mating-induced endometritis (PMIE).
2. Chronic uterine infection (CUI).
3. Sexually transmitted diseases: *Taylorella equigenitalis* (CEM) [notifiable], *Pseudomonas aeruginosa*, *Klebsiella pneumoniae* capsular types 1, 2, and 5.

Category 3 can occur at any age, but the others are more common in the older multiparous mare.

Persistent mating-induced endometritis

Definition/overview

A mild transient endometritis can be considered a normal event in mares following breeding, foaling, examination, or treatment with foreign substances. It is essential for fertility that the mare resolves this inflammation quickly. In normal mares this happens within 12 hours post breeding. In mares affected by PMIE the uterus is unable to evacuate the uterine contents post breeding within this normal time frame. This leads to prolonged uterine inflammation and poor fertility, with a high incidence of early embryonic death. It is not clear whether the defect in the clearance mechanism of these mares is a muscular problem or a problem in the neuroendocrine events that control muscle contraction. In some (normally pluriparous) mares with a pendulous uterus the muscular contraction of the uterus may be functioning normally, but the fluid is unable to move against gravity and so pools in the uterus. The persistent accumulation in the uterine lumen of inflammatory products and debris leads to further inflammation, edema, and damage, increasing the likelihood of infections and further endometrial damage and fibrosis.

Clinical presentation

Multiparous mares, often in their teens and with poor vulval/perineal conformation and pneumovagina, are particularly predisposed to this condition. Mares of any age with cervical pathology, either stenosis or incompetence, can also be affected. In many mares there are no signs before mating, but subsequently there is fluid accumulation in the uterine lumen within 12–36 hours. There is early pregnancy loss with repeated return to estrus and bacteria and neutrophils evident on endometrial culture and cytology. These mares have difficulty in conceiving unless they are identified and treated.

Diagnosis

Postbreeding examination within 12–36 hours will usually show intraluminal uterine fluid accumulation on ultrasonography and occasionally, in severe cases, intramural edema (535, 536). Many practitioners rely on ultrasound imaging of intrauterine fluid for diagnosis, and they may take endometrial swabs to confirm the presence of neutrophils and bacteria.

Management

Treatment includes the use of an ecbolic drug, intrauterine antibiotics, and uterine lavage, alone or in combination, depending on the perceived severity of the PMIE.

Uterine lavage with 1–3 liters of warmed saline or lactated Ringer's solution between 4 and 8 hours post breeding plus oxytocin (10–20 IU i/v or i/m) should hasten the removal of postcoital debris, contamination, and fluid without affecting the semen and before the mare mounts

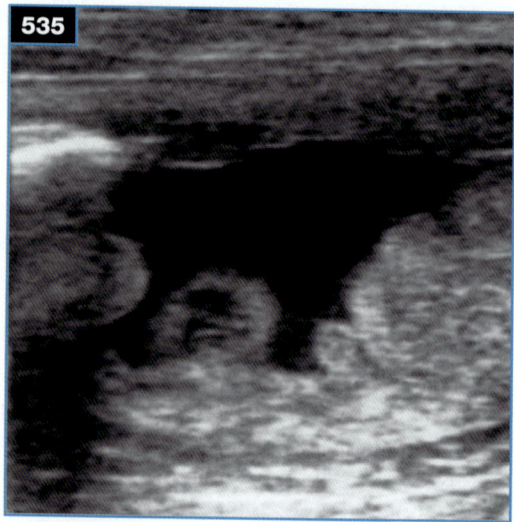

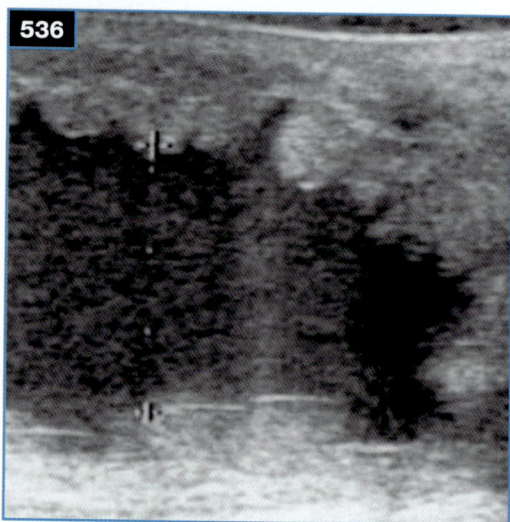

535, 536 Transverse transrectal ultrasonograms of a uterine horn containing (535) anechoic and (536) echogenic, more cellular, luminal fluid. Note the uterine wall edema. (Photo courtesy T Chenier)

a major inflammatory response. Broad-spectrum water-soluble antibiotics (e.g. 1 g ceftiofur in 20 ml of sterile saline) are often infused into the uterus following or instead of lavage. The procedure can be repeated 24 hours after breeding if there is still evidence of fluid accumulation in the uterus. Mares with particularly severe edema in the uterine wall and lymphatic lacunae can have additional treatment with 250 μg cloprostenol, which induces further uterine contractions. However, cloprostenol should not be used after ovulation as it is now recognized that it may induce luteolysis as soon as the day after ovulation.

314

Recently, the use of a single dose of dexamethasone at the time of breeding has been advocated as a means of down-regulating the immune response in mares known to be prone to PMIE. As with any corticosteroid, there is an associated risk of laminitis. Specific infections and physical defects (e.g. perineal defects) need to be identified and treated. If the endometritis becomes chronic and established, particularly if there is active on-going inflammation, severe edema/lacunae, or persistent luminal fluid, sexual rest for two to three estrous cycles is warranted.

Prognosis

Generally, the prognosis deteriorates with age and continuing degeneration of the reproductive tract. It becomes increasingly difficult to establish a pregnancy in these mares despite extensive treatment.

Chronic uterine infection

Definition/overview

CUI can occur in PMIE mares that are repeatedly bred in one breeding season, particularly if they are not treated appropriately. Mares can become susceptible to endometritis where there is a breakdown in their normal uterine defense mechanisms that allows normal microbiological flora to populate the uterus and cause a persistent uterine inflammation. Repeated and untreated severe endometritis will lead to severe and chronic inflammatory changes in the uterus, leading to fibrosis and degeneration.

The most commonly isolated causative organisms of endometritis are: β-hemolytic streptococci (*Strep. zooepidemicus*), *Staphylococcus aureus*, *Escherichia coli*, *Pseudomonas* spp., *Klebsiella* spp., yeasts and fungi (e.g. *Candida* spp., *Aspergillus* spp., *Mucor* spp., *Allescheria boydii*), and *Bacteroides fragilis* (anaerobic).

The infection can be introduced by: pneumovagina and/or incompetent cervix; parturition; copulation, especially if repeated; and veterinary gynecological procedures.

Some specific bacterial infections, and fungal and yeast infections, may be induced by the repeated use of intrauterine antibiotic and/or antiseptic therapy.

Clinical presentation

Mares with chronic infectious endometritis have reproductive histories including repeated breeding, poor fertility, PMIE, conformational abnormalities of the vulva, and repeated intrauterine therapies. They usually present with a vulval discharge of varying nature and amount.

Diagnosis

A reproductive examination usually produces a positive endometrial culture result and neutrophils should be seen on uterine cytology. On ultrasonography there is uterine intraluminal fluid. Endometrial biopsy often reveals chronic endometritis with focal or diffuse cellular inflammation (537).

Management

Initially, until antibiotic sensitivity test results are available, 3–5 days of broad-spectrum, water-soluble antibiotic intrauterine infusion therapy should be given (e.g. ceftiofur sodium, 1 g in 20 ml sterile water for injection q24h). Infusion should be made under minimum-contamination conditions. The perineum and vulva should be hygienically prepared, a sterile plastic insemination pipette inserted along the index finger through the cervix into the uterus using a gloved hand, and the sterile antibiotic infusion delivered into the uterus via a sterile syringe.

537 Histopathology of an endometrial biopsy from a mare with chronic infiltrative endometritis that subsequently responded to sexual rest and intrauterine therapy. Note the diffuse cellular inflammatory reaction (arrows).

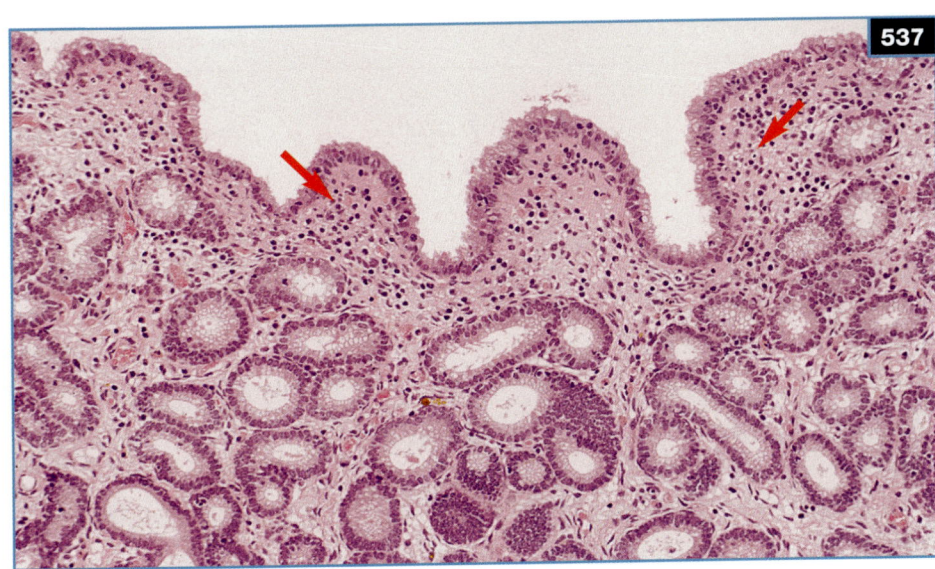

There are few, if any, efficacy studies performed to determine the best treatment for endometritis. In addition, there are few products licensed for intrauterine use or have licensed claims to treat endometritis in the mare. However, some basic principles should be followed whenever treating endometritis in the mare:

✦ Based on the causative agent/s cultured and their sensitivity pattern, select the best therapy (*Table 6*). This may involve systemic and/or intrauterine antibiotics.

✦ ALL intrauterine agents (including Hartmann's solution) cause some degree of intrauterine inflammation. Some antibiotics (e.g. gentamicin and amikacin) will require buffering with sodium bicarbonate solution before being used in the uterus. Infusion volumes of 50–200 ml (larger volumes in older pluriparous mares) into the uterus are adequate.

✦ Try and do no harm! Some therapies such as chlorohexidine gluconate and undiluted iodine solutions produce severe irritation to the endometrium and have been associated with uterine adhesions. Counter-irritant therapy has been used in the uterus of the mare successfully, but it requires very careful use.

✦ Short cycle the mare with PGF_2 to bring the mare back into estrus. Estrogens have been shown to have a positive influence on uterine immune mechanisms.

✦ Administer 20 IU oxytocin i/v and/or remove uterine contents by lavage with sterile saline (Hartmann's or lactated Ringer's solution is best).

TABLE 6 **Drugs and their doses used in the treatment of uterine infections**

DRUG	DOSE	COMMENT
Amikacin sulfate	1–2 g	Gram-negative organisms.
Ampicillin	1–3 g	Not good against anaerobes.
Carbenicillin	2–6 g	Broad spectrum including *Pseudomonas* spp.
Ceftiofur	1 g	Very broad spectrum.
Gentamicin sulfate	0.5–2 g	Gram-negative organisms. Requires buffering.
Neomycin sulfate	3–4 g	Gram-negative organisms. Often used with penicillins.
Oxytetracyclines	1–5 g	
Penicillin (Na or K salt)	5,000,000 IU	Gram-positive organisms, especially streptococci.
Penicillin G	3-6,000,000 IU	Gram-positive organisms, especially streptococci.
Ticarcillin	1–6 g	Broad spectrum, but poor against Klebsiella spp.
Combinations		
Neomycin + penicillin G	2 g/3,000,000 IU	
Gentamicin sulfate + penicillin G	0.5–2 g/3–6,000,000 IU	
Oral		
Enrofloxacin	8 mg/kg	Accumulates and concentrates in endometrium.
Antimycotics		
Nystatin	250,000–1,000,000 IU	Dissolve in 0.9% saline solution.
Clotrimazole	300–600 mg	Daily or every 2–3 days for 12 days.
Vinegar	2% solution	20 ml wine vinegar in 1 liter saline.
Povidone–iodine	1–2% solution	Individual mares may be very sensitive to povidone–iodine, causing uterine pathology. Use with caution!
Irritants		
Saline	Infuse 1 liter at a time	Infuse until recovery becomes clear.
EDTA-Tris	1.2 g + 6.05 g Tris per liter of water	Tritrate to pH 8 with glacial acetic acid. Infuse antibiotic 3 hours later.
Hydrogen peroxide	1:4 dilution with saline	

Adapted from Perkins NR (1999) Equine reproductive pharmacology. *Vet Clin North Am: Equine Pract* **15**(3):687–704.

- 30 minutes later, infuse the uterus with appropriate antibiotics (generally use systemic dose). For streptococcal infections, ceftiofur sodium (1 g in 20 ml sterile water for injection) is now commonly used. Repeat the treatment for 3–5 days.
- It is important to correct any predisposing conformational abnormalities (e.g. Caslick's vulvoplasty) or repair any damage to the external barriers.
- Autologous plasma infusions into the uterus have been used in mares with chronic endometritis both during treatment and 12–36 hours post breeding.
- Minimal-contamination techniques at breeding have been recommended in mares with chronic endometritis (p. 255).
- Always maintain good hygiene during examinations, treatments, and breeding and use AI if possible.
- Sexual rest, for up to 45 days, is particularly useful in severely affected cases.
- Fungal and yeast infections in the uterus will require prolonged intrauterine treatment with antimycotic drugs based on culture and sensitivity results. Some cases have been treated effectively with a saline and vinegar mixture or povidone–iodine and saline solution. Recently, the addition of DMSO to lavaging fluids has been advocated as a way of breaking down the 'biofilm' layer of mucus that can coat the endometrium in cases of fungal endometritis.

Indwelling uterine infusers can facilitate the treatment of mares with CUI. The infuser is held in position in the uterus by an intrauterine device and at the vulva by sutures. It can be left in position for up to a month.

Systemic treatment with antibiotics is rarely indicated because in most cases the infecting organism is in the uterine lumen rather than the endometrium. Oral ketaconazole (2 g p/o q24h for 10 days) concurrently with povidone–iodine flushing, has improved the chance of successful resolution of fungal endometritis in some cases.

'Follow-up' examination including smears/swabs should be made 3–4 weeks after the end of any course of treatment.

Prognosis
Chronic infectious endometritis carries a guarded prognosis, with common recurrence of infections and with increasing difficulty in treating them successfully. Fungal and yeast infections can be very hard to treat. With increasing age and chronicity of infection, degenerative changes in the endometrium worsen the prognosis further.

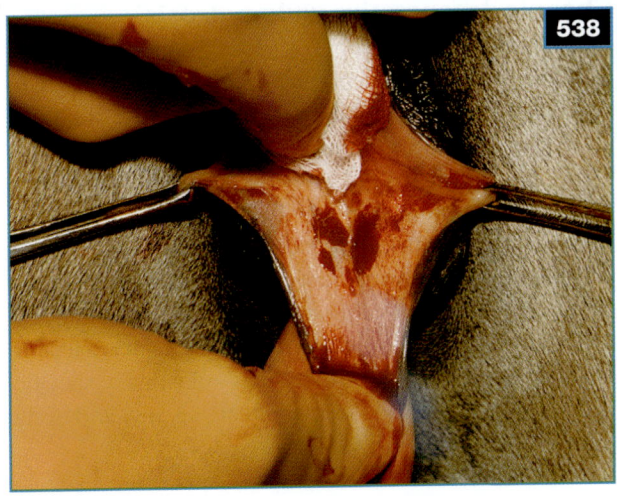

538 Removal of the clitoris as part of the treatment of a *Pseudomonas aeruginosa* infection of the caudal reproductive tract of a mare.

Sexually transmitted endometritis
Definition/overview
Diseases transmitted through breeding horses (venereally transmitted) can be caused by a variety of organisms, some of which are notifiable to government authorities in some countries. The main diseases transmitted venereally include EVA (p. 278), coital exanthema (p. 310), dourine (p. 311) and CEM (p. 248). In addition to CEM, endometritis can be caused by *Pseudomonas aeruginosa* and *Klebsiella pneumoniae* capsular types 1, 2, and 5 and transmitted venereally, either directly from the stallion's penis or from infected semen. These two organisms can be involved in PMIE and chronic infectious endometritis, and clinical signs will be as previously described. If these organisms are cultured, they should be typed if possible and antibiotic sensitivity testing carried out. Treatment, particularly with *P. aeruginosa* infection, can be prolonged and difficult.

K. pneumoniae infection can be treated with 2 g gentamicin in 50 ml sterile water buffered with an equal amount of 7.5% sodium bicarbonate. *P. aeruginosa* is treated with 3.2 g ticarcillin in sterile water. For severe, nonresponsive clitoral infections, which are nonresponsive to clitoral washing with 2% chlorhexidine and packing with nitrofurazone/silver sulfathiazine creams, clitorectomy should be considered (**538**).

The success of treatment for venereal infections should be monitored by collecting three sets of swabs at 2-day intervals, starting 7 days after treatment.

Female reproductive tract

Chronic degenerative endometrosis

Definition/overview

Chronic degenerative endometrosis is a term used to describe a wide range of histopathologic changes found in the endometrium of older mares in particular.

Etiology/pathophysiology

Chronic degenerative endometrosis is degenerative and progressive in nature and generally there is no evidence of active inflammation, although there are infiltrates of lymphocytes, plasma cells, and macrophages. It is a feature of older mares, although the onset is individually specific, and is a sign of uterine 'wear and tear', ageing, and cyclic hormonal effects.

Clinical presentation

The degenerative changes are seen in older mares that have difficulty in conceiving and repeatedly return to estrus, suffer early embryonic loss or pregnancy failure, or carry foals to term that are dysmature. Older maiden mares that have had a successful athletic career may also demonstrate these changes on biopsy outside of the degree expected for their age, and this may explain their poor fertility.

Diagnosis

The major histopathologic changes seen on endometrial biopsy are: fibrosis, which can be diffuse and stromal, periglandular or perivascular; lymphatic stasis; uterine sacculation; transluminal adhesions; glandular nests; and glandular or lymphatic cysts (539).

Management

Evidence-based effective treatments for this group of conditions have not been described, but most therapies are aimed at inducing a superficial endometrial inflammation and tissue loss. It is postulated that as the tissue regenerates itself, it will be in a better histopathologic state than before. Some of the therapies have the potential to cause irreversible damage to the uterus and elsewhere in the tract and so should be used carefully. Mechanical uterine curettage and uterine lavage with caustic substances have been used with variable success. All can lead to intrauterine, cervical, and vaginal adhesions. These therapies should only be used after all other conventional therapies have been tried. After treatment, follow-up uterine biopsies are required to assess any response. All affected mares require breeding and postbreeding techniques to minimize contamination and optimize conception chances.

Prognosis

The prognosis is guarded to poor depending on the degree of histologic changes and the response to therapy.

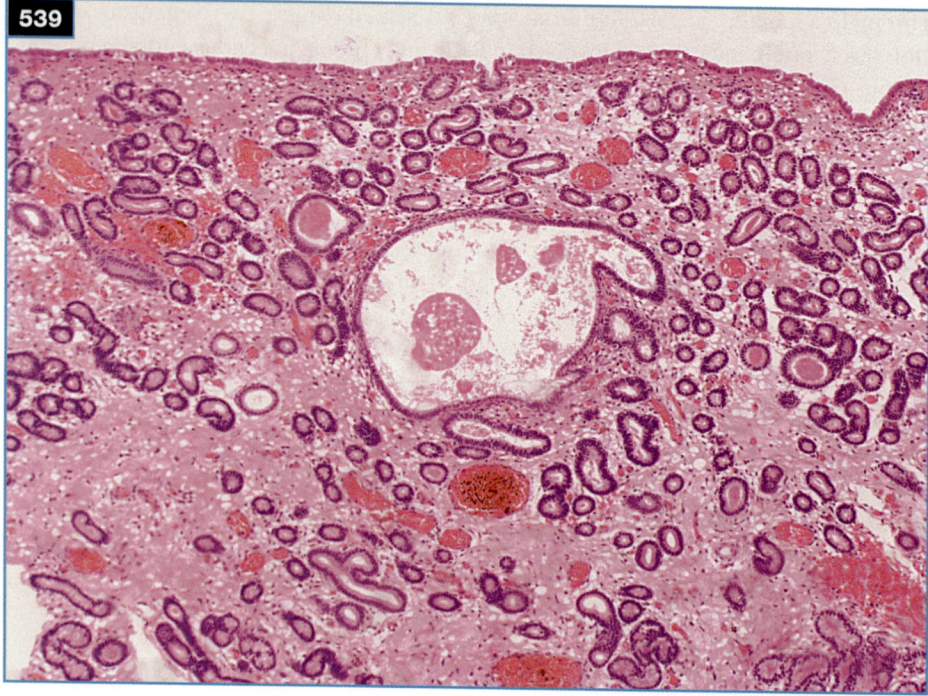

539 Histopathology of an endometrial biopsy from a mare with chronic endometrial degeneration showing a glandular cyst.

Endometrial cysts

Definition/overview

The endometrium of the mare is rich in blood vessels and lymphatics. Dilation and coalescence of these lymphatic ducts can produce a thin-walled, fluid-filled structure within the endometrium called an endometrial or uterine cyst. These are variable in size, can be uni- or multilocular, and can project into the uterine lumen if they become large enough. Their clinical/breeding significance is debatable. They are inconvenient in that they may confuse visual/manual pregnancy diagnosis, but are likely to affect fertility only if they inhibit movement of the embryo around the uterus before day 16, happen to occur at the point at which the embryo initially fixes at the base of one uterine horn, or are so widespread that they limit placental nutrition.

Etiology/pathophysiology

Fibrosis of the endometrium due to age or trauma, or both, can cause a blockage in the lymphatic ducts, which causes lymphatic fluid to 'back up' in the afferent ducts. Dilation and coalescence of these ducts produces one or more fluid-filled cysts.

Clinical presentation

The significance of endometrial cysts is unclear. They are commonly found as an incidental finding on ultrasonographic examination of the uterus per rectum during a pre-breeding examination or during an early pregnancy check, when they may even be mistaken for an early conceptus. This can cause confusion with twin conceptuses. Whether large numbers of endometrial cysts or a single large endometrial cyst can lead to embryonic death or even abortion, due to interference in the development of normal chorionic villi, is still a subject of controversy. It is also possible that they can interfere with the maternal recognition of pregnancy by inhibiting normal movement of the embryonic vesicle between days 6 and 16 of pregnancy, thereby failing to inhibit luteolysis.

It is useful to identify cysts at pre-breeding checks in order to document their presence prior to breeding. Cysts do not increase in size, move, or develop an embryo within them.

Diagnosis

Cysts appear as fluid-filled (hypoechoic) structures on ultrasound examination (540, 541). Most are less than 10 mm in diameter and occur in small numbers (1–3). They can also sometimes be seen on hysteroscopy and large cysts (up to 10 cm) are palpable per rectum.

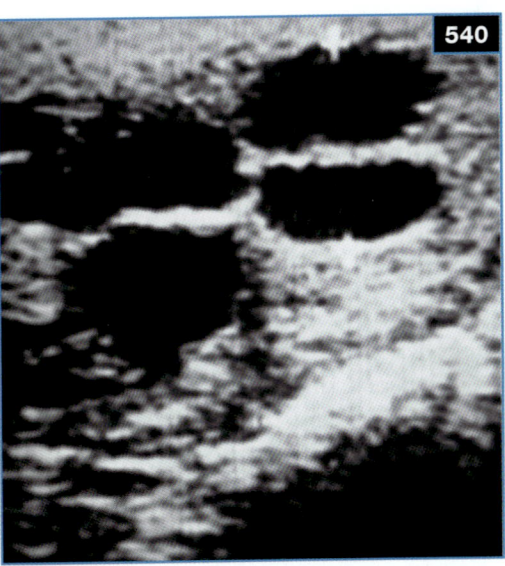

540 Multiple endometrial cysts seen in a 16-year-old Thoroughbred mare on transrectal ultrasonography.

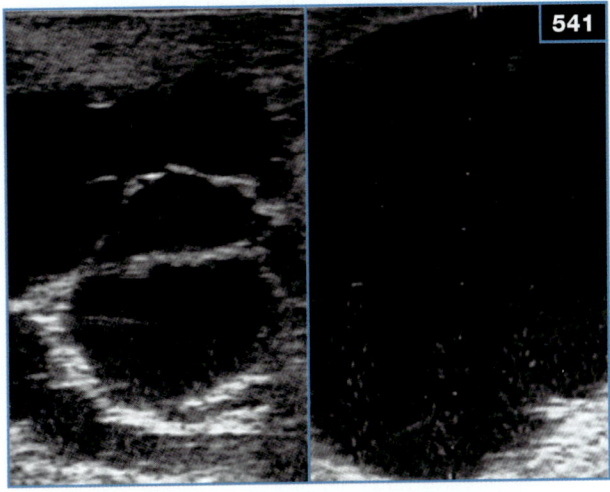

541 Very large and multiple endometrial cysts seen in an aged mare on transrectal ultrasonography. (Photo courtesy T Chenier)

Management

There is disagreement as to whether cysts require treatment. Generally, small cysts in low numbers should not be treated. Large single cysts have been drained under endoscopic guidance, but they have a high tendency to recur. Ablation via diathermy or, preferably, CO_2:YAG laser has decreased recurrence and, with the latter procedure, results in less endometrial scarring and fewer adhesions.

Pyometra

Definition/overview

Pyometra is an accumulation of exudate within the uterus, often of considerable volume. It is a sequela to infection, but the etiopathogenesis is still unclear. Many mares fail to cycle and have an enlarged 'doughy' uterus on rectal palpation. There are usually no systemic signs. It is very difficult to treat and there is a poor prognosis for future fertility.

Etiology/pathophysiology

Pyometra is an uncommon sequela to infection of the tubular genital tract, where large amounts of debris, inflammatory products, and uterine secretions accumulate in the uterus. Often, there is a retained functional CL and this leads to many mares not cycling. Some cases have cervical and/or uterine adhesions that some clinicians feel prevent evacuation of the tract. Some cases, however, do not have adhesions or they are a consequence of the problem rather than the cause. Older mares, often with poor uterine defense mechanisms, are more prone to this condition. The true etiopathogenesis is unknown. Pyometra is more frequently reported in North America in association with chronic *Pseudomonas aeruginosa* infections.

Clinical presentation

Many cases have no or irregular estrous cycle behavior, although the occasional affected mare cycles regularly. There are usually no systemic disease signs and sometimes no vaginal discharge, although in those mares that do continue cycling (and may short cycle) the owner often reports a very thick, purulent vaginal discharge when the mare is in estrus. The mare may be presented for pregnancy diagnosis.

Differential diagnosis

Endometritis; metritis; pregnancy; mummified fetus.

Diagnosis

Rectal palpation reveals an enlarged uterus with a 'doughy' feel. The uterus can contain up to 60 liters of material and mimic a pregnancy. Ultrasonography, transrectally or transabdominally, will confirm the presence of a large uterus without a fetus but containing large amounts of floccular fluid (542). Hematology and biochemistry results are usually unremarkable. Bacterial culture of the uterine fluid may reveal pathogenic bacteria/fungi, but in some cases it is sterile. Cervical adhesions are often detectable per vagina. After drainage of the uterine fluid, endometrial biopsy is vital in order to establish a long-term prognosis for fertility. Many cases have irreparable endometrial damage and some have considerable endometrial atrophy, increasing the risks associated with biopsy collection.

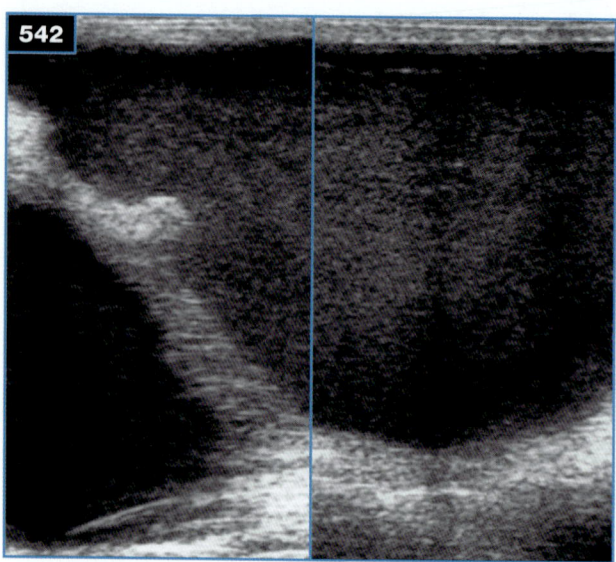

542 Transrectal ultrasonogram of a mare with pyometra. Note the very enlarged uterus filled with large quantities of cellular fluid. (Photo courtesy T Chenier)

Management

Drainage should be established from the uterus by passage of a sterile, wide-bore tube. Passage through the cervix may be affected by adhesions, which will require treatment. Uterine lavage and drainage over a prolonged period may be required, along with specific antimicrobial intrauterine therapy. Ovariohysterectomy has been carried out in some affected mares, but the procedure is difficult, with a high risk of complications in this condition.

Prognosis

For future breeding the prognosis is poor, especially if cervical or uterine adhesions are present or there is recurrence of fluid accumulation. If there are severe, deep, chronic inflammatory changes or end-stage endometrial atrophy, the prognosis is hopeless. Mares that still cycle and naturally expel the exudate may respond to treatment.

Tumors

See Tumors of the female reproductive tract excluding the ovary (p. 312).

Miscellaneous conditions ———————

Hermaphroditism

Definition/overview

Hermaphroditism forms part of the group of intersex conditions and can be divided into true hermaphrodites and pseudohermaphrodites. True hermaphrodites have ovarian and testicular structures. Pseudohermaphrodites have one or the other (i.e. a male pseudohermaphrodite has testes and a female pseudohermaphrodite has ovaries). The reproductive tract in these cases often has elements of the male and female. All pseudohermaphrodites are sterile.

Etiology/pathophysiology

Hermaphroditism is a congenital condition of unknown etiology.

Clinical presentation

Male pseudohermaphrodite

This is the most common type of hermaphroditism. Affected animals present physically with a small vulva, an enlarged clitoris, and a blind-ended, short vagina (543). The urethra usually enters into the vaginal structure and urine is voided from here. Small hypoplastic testicles are normally abdominal (544), although occasionally testicles and a deformed penis-like structure are present in the inguinal regional. The tubular reproductive organs are absent or very small. The animal is a female genetically (XX), but exhibits either stallion behavior or persistent estrous behavior. Testicular feminization is an inherited type of male pseudohermaphroditism where there is a female appearance with a male genotype (XY).

Female pseudohermaphrodite

The external genitalia in this form are either male or, more commonly, small and neither male nor female. The internal reproductive organs are vestigial, with the presence of ovaries. The animal is a genetic male (XY). A specific form of this condition is the XY sex reversal syndrome, where the external physical appearance is of a female with a poorly developed internal reproductive tract and infantile ovaries, but the animal is genetically male.

Diagnosis

Diagnosis is based on a full reproductive examination, including rectal palpation, and ultrasonography, chromosomal analysis, and laparoscopy.

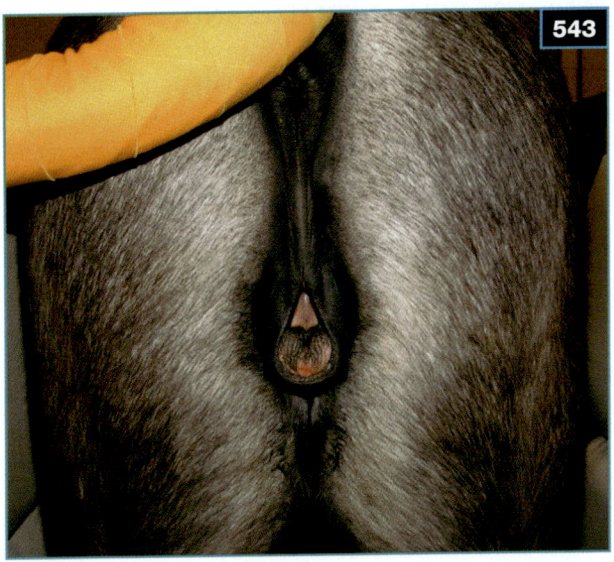

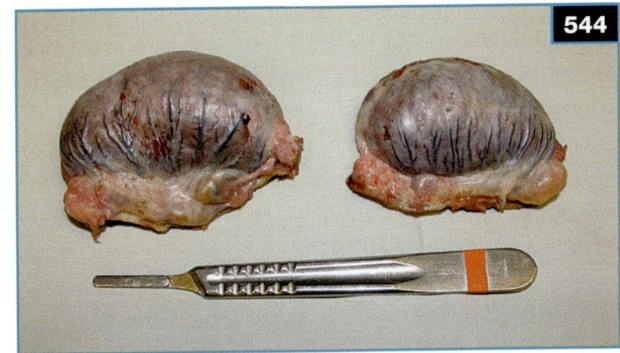

543, 544 The external genitalia (543) and removed gonads (544) of a true hermaphrodite. Note the enlarged clitoris and small vulval opening and removed ovotestes from the abdomen. (Photo courtesy T Chenier)

Management

Surgical removal of any gonadal tissue (usually intra-abdominal) is necessary if the animals are to be used for athletic purposes because extreme reproductive behavior may affect this use. Laparoscopy may be useful in detecting and removing the gonadal tissue.

Prognosis

The prognosis is guarded to poor for athletic use unless surgical removal of the gonadal tissue is carried out. These animals are infertile.

ESTROUS CYCLE ANOMALIES AND ABNORMALITIES
Prolonged or persistent diestrus
Definition/overview
This common cyclic abnormality is the result of the retention of a CL beyond its normal life span. The mare may remain in diestrus for several months and this condition must be differentiated from early pregnancy. A full reproductive examination is useful in the differential diagnosis. The condition is treated very effectively by intramuscular prostaglandin injections, and the mare will return to a normal estrous cycle with usually a good prognosis for a return to fertility.

Etiology/pathophysiology
Prolonged or persistent diestrus is associated with any abnormality that prolongs the life span of a CL outwith pregnancy. In an individual mare the cause is not always clear, but those proposed include: inadequate release of prostaglandins to induce luteolysis; diestrus ovulation leading to an immature CL nonresponsive to luteolysis; maternal recognition of early pregnancy with prolongation of primary CL followed by embryonic death before day 37 (pseudopregnancy type I); chronic endometrial infection; and/or damage leading to decreased prostaglandin release. The retained CL can persist for several months.

Clinical presentation
Mares fail to demonstrate normal estrous cycles and estrous behavior in the breeding season. This may occur at any time of the season and can last for 2–3 months.

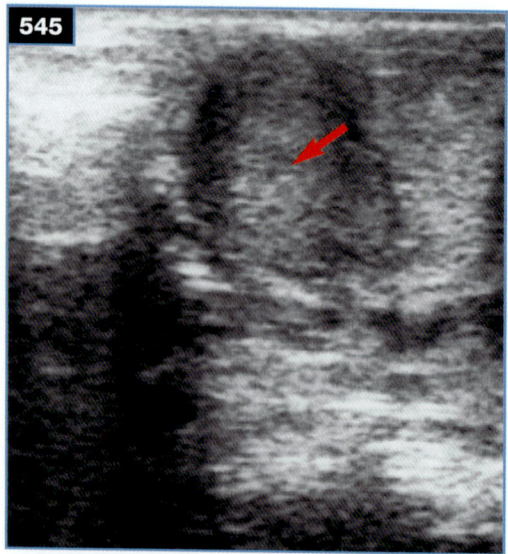

545 Transrectal ultrasonogram of the ovary of a mare in persistent diestrus revealing a mature corpus luteum (arrow). (Photo courtesy T Chenier)

Diagnosis
It is important to differentiate this condition from early pregnancy or causes of anestrus. Rectal palpation reveals a nonpregnant uterus, which is firm and under progesterone stimulation. The ovaries are active with follicular development. Ultrasonography confirms no pregnancy, ovarian activity, and the presence of at least one CL (**545**). Vaginal examination confirms a closed diestrus cervix. Sequential blood samples reveal persistent high levels of progesterone.

Management
Intramuscular prostaglandin or its analogs are the treatment of choice. A mature CL over 5 days old will be lysed and the mare should come into estrus depending on the stage of follicular development present in the ovary. If the ovary contains a larger follicle (>35 mm in diameter), ovulation may occur rapidly (within 48 hours) with a short estrous behavioral period. Where smaller follicles are present, estrus will usually begin within 2–5 days and ovulation towards the end of the estrous period. There is some controversy as to whether the mare should be mated on this first estrus or whether it should be short cycled with another prostaglandin injection and bred on the subsequent cycle.

Prognosis
The prognosis for return to fertility is good except where chronic uterine damage is present.

Behavioral anestrus
Definition/overview
Behavioral anestrus is defined as a lack of behavioral estrus by the mare despite physiologic changes of estrus within the reproductive tract ('silent heat'). It is possibly a behavioral or a psychologic abnormality. It is common in maiden mares or mares with a foal at foot. Diagnosis relies on confirming physiologic estrus without behavioral signs. Management relies either on AI or on careful and persistent teasing to encourage mares to relax and exhibit behavioral signs.

Etiology/pathophysiology
Normally the physiologic reproductive tract and endocrine changes of estrus are coordinated with behavioral estrus, allowing the mare to be receptive to the stallion at the time of ovulation. In this behavioral/psychologic abnormality, mares do not exhibit behavioral estrus despite normal physiologic estrus changes. Performance mares previously administered anabolic steroids may also exhibit problems of reproductive behavior when entering a breeding career, although this is a separate iatrogenic condition.

Clinical presentation

This condition is most commonly seen in maiden mares, particularly those that have had prolonged athletic careers, mares with foals at foot, which are very protective, and nervous mares of any age. It is a particular problem where there is no access to a teaser or stallion, or where little time or effort is placed upon the teasing process. The affected mare may show no signs of behavioral estrus or it can be aggressive towards the teasing stallion.

Diagnosis

Repeated reproductive examinations of the mare, including rectal and ultrasonographic examinations of the ovaries and reproductive tract plus vaginoscopic examinations of the cervix, should be able to identify physiologic estrus changes. Serial plasma progesterone samples (every 4–5 days) should identify when the mare enters estrus (plasma progesterone <1 ng/ml) except early in the year when winter anestrus may still be present. A careful and imaginative approach to teasing with, if necessary, restraint of the mare, plus acute observation by the teasing personnel, may sometimes allow recognition of some estrous behavioral changes.

Management

AI can be used where this is permitted, but accurate timing is not helped by the lack of estrous behavior and reliance has to be placed on serial reproductive examinations. Careful and persistent teasing can help relax mares and many will show estrous behavior eventually. Care is required to protect the stallion and personnel present at covering and some clinicians use low doses of sedation in such cases as an additional aid.

Prognosis

The prognosis is fair with persistent and effective teasing.

Postpartum or lactational anestrus
Definition/overview

This is an uncommon condition less related to lactation than to early foaling dates (decreased photoperiod), poor body condition or nutrition, and stress. Originally it was thought that there was a persistence of the CL after a normal foaling heat, but now it is generally considered to be a true anestrus and ovarian shutdown. Mares either demonstrate a normal foal heat and then do not cycle for between 1 and 3 months or, occasionally, do not cycle at all post partum. Rectal palpation, ultrasonography of the reproductive tract, and serial plasma progesterone samples help differentiate this condition from other cyclic abnormalities. Improving the mare's condition and nutrition plus decreasing stress will help some mares, while intramuscular prostaglandin is effective in a persistent CL.

Etiology/pathophysiology

This problem probably has a number of causes related to photoperiod early in the year, poor body condition and nutrition, and stress conditions. The relationship to lactation *per se* is questionable. It may be related to persistence of the CL (prolonged diestrus) after a normal foal heat or, more rarely, complete ovarian shut down and anestrus after parturition.

Clinical presentation

Most commonly there is a normal foal heat, both behaviorally and physiologically, and then the mare does not return to normal cyclic behavior at the normal interval. Rarely, the mare goes straight into anestrus post partum. It appears to be more common in mares that foal in the early months of the breeding season (February/March in the northern hemisphere) and in older mares in medium to poor body condition. It may be 1–3 months before mares return to normal cyclic activity.

Diagnosis

A full reproductive examination should be undertaken, including rectal palpation and ultrasonographic evaluation of the ovaries and uterus, plus plasma progesterone samples. Those cases with persistence of the CL will have raised progesterone levels and clinical signs as already noted (p. 243). Those mares that enter true anestrus will have plasma progesterone concentrations <1 ng/ml and small inactive ovaries, plus a flaccid uterus and partially open cervix. Any nutritional and/or medical condition leading to poor condition and health requires detailed investigation.

Management

Mares with persistent CL will respond to intramuscular prostaglandin and return quickly to a normal estrous cycle. If the mare is in true anestrus, the treatment is not effective. The mare's environment and nutrition should be improved and any stress factors removed if possible. Similar regimens of management and drug therapy to that undertaken in the treatment of transitional estrus/anestrus have been used with variable success in this condition. In addition, GnRH given via a continuous infusion pump delivering 2.5–5.0 µg/hour has led to cyclic activity within 10–14 days. The GnRH analog buserelin (10 µg q12h) also seems to be effective in some cases. Oral domperidone (a dopamine antagonist) given daily can also induce follicle activity. Prevention using extra light exposure (14½ hours) for early-foaling mares from early December to February/March (northern hemisphere) has been effective.

Prognosis

The prognosis is guarded in true anestrus cases, particularly where conditions are stressing the mare and/or she is in poor body condition. Some mares (particularly older animals) that have difficulty maintaining body condition when lactating repeatedly enter lactational anestrus when they have a foal at foot, and for this reason often only produce a foal every other year.

Diestral ovulation

Definition/overview

It is quite common for mares that are cycling normally to ovulate in diestrus when a CL is already present and functioning. The mare shows no estrous behavior and this ovulation is only detected if the mare is examined regularly by rectal palpation and ultrasonography. This situation appears to be a normal variation in the estrous cycle of the mare and some clinicians feel it may be related to the mid-diestral peak of FSH that occurs in the mare. It usually has no effect on the estrous cycle, but if the ovulation and subsequent luteinization of this follicle occurs 1–4 days prior to prostaglandin release on day 15–16 of the cycle, the immature CL is unaffected and can be retained, leading to prolonged diestrus.

Failure of follicles to ovulate

Definition/overview

This is a separate condition from that seen in the transitional period of mares in the spring and autumn months, as it occurs in the normal breeding season, often in certain mares as a recurrent problem. The cause is unknown. Mares with enlarging follicles that fail to ovulate remain in estrus for prolonged periods until regression or luteinization occurs. Repeated rectal palpation and reproductive ultrasonography will help determine the presence of an anovulatory follicle. Spontaneous resolution of the problem will lead to normal cyclic behavior in most cases, but recurrence is quite common in some specific mares.

Etiology/pathophysiology

The failure of follicles to ovulate can be part of the syndrome of the transitional period seen in the spring and autumn months (p. 242). The follicles enlarge and persist for up to 2 months. Eventually, in the spring, one of the follicles ovulates and the mare starts to cycle normally. In the autumn transitional period the declining gonadotropin levels allow the enlarged follicles to persist throughout the period.

Occasionally, in the normal breeding season, a dominant enlarged follicle does not ovulate and in some mares this can be a persistent problem over a number of estrous cycles. Various names have been used to describe these follicles including anovulatory, hemorrhagic, or persistent. It has been reported to be more common in

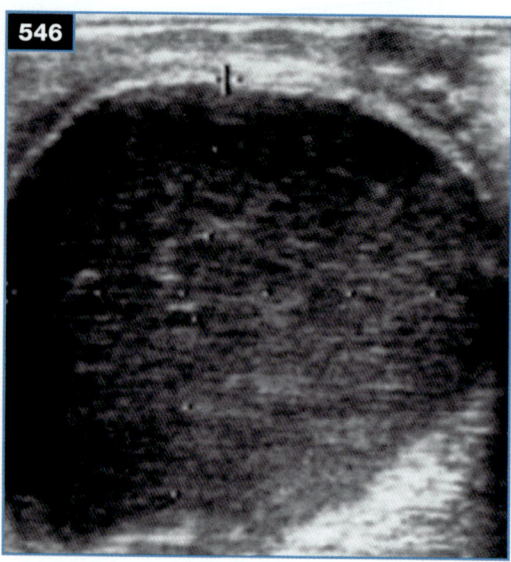

546 Transrectal ultrasonogram of the ovary of a mare that is failing to ovulate. Note the very enlarged anovulatory follicle containing echogenic material. (Photo courtesy T Chenier)

pony mares (5% incidence). The cause is unknown, but it is probably endocrine-related, either from the pituitary gland or, more likely, the follicle itself.

Clinical presentation

Mares with anovulatory follicles may remain in estrus for prolonged periods of up to 15 days. Eventually, the follicle may luteinize and the mare will stop estrous behavior. The luteinized follicle may have a normal life span or be prolonged, leading to persistent diestrus. Mares with anovulatory follicles may accept the stallion, but as no ovulation occurs they do not conceive.

Differential diagnosis

Ovarian tumor, especially GCT; transitional ovaries; ovarian abscess.

Diagnosis

Repeated rectal palpation and ultrasonography of the ovaries are essential to identify and follow-up mares with anovulatory follicles. Affected follicles may develop gradually into very large structures (>10 cm in diameter), but they do not ovulate (**546**). They have a variety of ultrasonographic appearances within the follicle including free-floating focal echogenicities, bands of tissue, hemorrhagic structures, and outer rims that become more echodense with luteinization. The ovary becomes enlarged on rectal palpation, with a large follicle that does not progress to normal maturational changes towards ovulation, but feels firmer and within the ovarian structure. The contralateral ovary is normal and the mare will continue to cycle unless the anovulatory hemorrhagic follicle luteinizes sufficiently to produce enough progesterone to inhibit the return to estrus. Anovulatory follicles will usually regress over a period of 1–2 months, with the ovary returning to a normal size.

Management
Many of these mares will not respond to treatmen, but will (eventually) spontaneously resolve the problem. If the follicle luteinizes, it may respond to exogenous prostaglandins. Recurrence at subsequent estrus periods can occur. Occasional cases will ovulate if diagnosed in the early stages of becoming an anovulatory hemorrhagic follicle and are treated with exogenous hCG or GnRH. Matings on spontaneous or induced ovulations in these cases are rarely successful as the oocyte ovulated is often degenerate and nonviable.

Prognosis
The prognosis is good for return to normal cyclic behavior and ovulation over time, but short-term delays to the breeding program are an inevitable consequence. Recurrence is quite common in some mares. Further delays are possible if the follicle luteinizes and this CL persists, although these usually respond well to exogenous prostaglandins.

Mastitis
Definition/overview
Mastitis is an uncommon condition, usually seen in the lactating or postweaning broodmare. A variety of bacteria are involved, but *Streptococcus* spp. are the most common. The mammary gland is swollen, hot, and painful on palpation in the acute case, but becomes more fibrotic and harder in the chronic form. The mammary gland secretion changes nature and on cytology shows increased neutrophils and, occasionally, bacteria. Bacterial culture and sensitivity testing are essential to direct the correct systemic and local antibiotic therapy. Stripping of the gland, hot compresses, and NSAIDs will all improve the well-being of the mare. Chronic cases are difficult to treat and carry a more guarded prognosis.

Etiology/pathophysiology
Mastitis is usually seen in lactating mares or after weaning and is therefore most common in the summer and autumn months. A variety of bacteria can be involved, but *Streptococcus* spp., especially *S. equi zooepidemicus,* are commonly isolated along with a range of Gram-negative organisms and *Staphylococcus* spp.

Clinical presentation
The udder is usually hot, painful to palpation, and swollen. There may be secondary ventral edema, mammary vein enlargement, and hindlimb stiffness. There may be no other signs or systemic reaction, although occasionally mares may show pyrexia and inappetence. Abnormal secretions are usually retrieved from the gland. Mammary abscesses may form in the gland, either as solitary structures or more widespread, multiple foci. The gland may become hard and fibrotic on palpation in chronic cases.

Differential diagnosis
Mammary gland edema, abscessation, trauma, and neoplasia.

Diagnosis
Clinical signs and the examination of mammary secretions are usually diagnostic. The milk may vary from sanguineous and watery to purulent, with large numbers of neutrophils and possibly bacteria on cytologic examination. Bacteriological culture and sensitivity testing on samples are essential to direct therapy. Mammary gland ultrasonography will help identify the site and morphology of any structure within the gland, and aid direct aspiration of any contents.

Management
Drainage of the mammary gland by stripping from the teats will relieve pressure and make the mare more comfortable. Some clinicians accompany this with hot fermentations to the gland. Systemic antibiotics based on laboratory results may be accompanied by intramammary versions, although the latter have to be placed in each separate gland and can lead to damage to the teat openings. Antibiotic therapy can finish 2–3 days after clinical resolution of the infection. NSAIDs are important to decrease the inflammation, pain, and pyrexia and help the mare feel and eat better. Abscesses may be drained and flushed, often under general anesthesia. Chronic mastitis is difficult to treat due to the extensive fibrosis and sequestration of infection. Mastectomy may be necessary in some of these cases.

Prognosis
Many acute cases respond very favorably and quickly with little long-term damage to the gland. Chronic mastitis carries a guarded to poor prognosis.

2 Male reproductive tract

It is essential that the veterinary clinician possesses a thorough knowledge of the normal anatomy and physiology of the breeding stallion in order to monitor the health and reproductive status of their patients, as well as helping to detect variations from normal when disease conditions arise. The breeding stallion is like a high-maintenance piece of delicate machinery. While breeders may expect him to 'perform' without hesitation and achieve excellent pregnancy rates, this may be far from the case. Stallions are frequently affected by psychologic and behavioral problems, which significantly affect their performance and usefulness. Medical and surgical conditions affecting reproductive ability may be completely unrelated to the reproductive system. A wide array of disease conditions affect the reproductive system, many of which can be career-ending for the breeding stallion if not appropriately managed.

Anatomy and physiology

Neuroendocrine control of stallion reproduction involves the hypothalamus, pituitary gland, pineal gland, vomeronasal organ, and testes. The importance of the pineal gland, and the resulting influence of season, is less obvious in stallions than in mares, because the stallion continues to produce sperm throughout the year, regardless of season. Testicular size, semen production, libido, and hormone concentrations vary by season in the stallion, with maximal values obtained in the spring and summer months, and the lowest in the winter.

GnRH is released in a pulsatile manner by the hypothalamus in response to both neural and hormonal control. Visual, tactile, auditory, and olfactory inputs are important regulators of stallion reproductive physiology. Exposure of stallions to mares increases GnRH and LH concentrations in the pituitary. The Flehmen response, or lip curl, exhibited by stallions investigating mares, directs air across the openings of the vomeronasal glands, which in turn convey olfactory information from pheromones to the hypothalamus. Although its function is poorly understood, the vomeronasal organ and Flehmen response are important components of the social interactions of horses with one another.

GnRH is transported via the hypothalamic–pituitary portal vessels to the anterior pituitary where it controls production and release of the two gonadotropic homones, LH and FSH. These act on the cells of the testis, regulating spermatogenesis and steroidogenesis. FSH regulates production by Sertoli cells of a variety of compounds important in sperm production, including androgen-binding protein, estrogen, growth factors, inhibin, and activin. The latter two protein hormones appear to feed back to the anterior pituitary to regulate FSH release. Sertoli cells function to regulate seminiferous tubular fluid, maintain the blood–testis barrier, and support the developing germ cells. LH regulates the Leydig cells of the testis, stimulating the production of the steroid hormones testosterone, dihydrotestosterone, and estrogen. Testosterone attains high local concentrations within the testis, which are essential for normal spermatogenesis. The steroid hormones also regulate accessory gland function and maintain libido by systemic actions via the bloodstream. Testosterone and estrogen feed back on the hypothalamus and anterior pituitary gland to regulate LH release.

Testicular descent

The testicles normally descend into a scrotal position between the last 30 days of gestation and the first 10 days post partum. In some colts the testes may descend into the inguinal region and remain there for some time before fully descending into the scrotum. The hormonal and physical events leading to testicular descent are poorly understood, and many theories have been proposed. Androgen production by the developing fetal gonads probably plays an important role, as may do müllerian inhibiting factor and epidermal growth factor. Traction of the gubernaculum, which attaches the caudal pole of the testes to the inguinal region, is believed to draw the developing epididymides into the inguinal ring, aided by intra-abdominal pressure, elongation of the vaginal process, and expansion of the inguinal ring.

Scrotum

The scrotum of the stallion is located high in the inguinal region and is much less pendulous than in the ruminant species. The scrotum consists of two distinct pouches that contain, protect, and thermoregulate the testes, epididymides, spermatic cords, and cremaster muscles. The testes are located in the scrotum in order to maintain testicular temperature at several degrees below core body temperature, a necessity for normal spermatogenesis. The wall of the scrotum consists of four layers: skin; tunica dartos; scrotal fascia; and parietal vaginal tunic.

The scrotal skin is thin, generally hairless, and slightly oily. It contains numerous sebaceous and sweat glands, which assist in testis thermoregulation. The tunica dartos layer lines both scrotal pouches and extends into the median septum, seen externally as the median raphae of the scrotum. The degree of contraction or relaxation of this layer allows alterations in the size, shape, and position of the scrotum in relation to the body wall, thereby aiding testis thermoregulation. The scrotal fascia is a loose connective tissue layer between the tunica dartos and the parietal vaginal tunic that allows the testes and associated parietal tunic layer to move freely within the scrotum. The parietal vaginal tunic, which forms during testicular descent, is an evagination of the parietal peritoneum through the inguinal rings. This layer forms a sac that lines the scrotum and is closely apposed to the visceral vaginal tunic, which is the outer layer of the testis. The vaginal cavity is the space between the parietal and visceral layers of the vaginal tunic. Normally it contains a very small amount of viscous fluid, allowing some free movement of the testis within it. The vaginal cavity is a potential space within which considerable fluid may accumulate as a result of a variety of causes.

The scrotum of the normal stallion should appear slightly pendulous, globular, and generally symmetrical. Normal variations may be observed in the positioning of the testes if one is relatively anterior to, or ventral to, the other. The skin should have no evidence of trauma, scarring, or skin lesions. Scrotal skin lesions can cause significant alterations in testis temperature and affect fertility. Palpation of the scrotum of a normal stallion reveals a thin and pliable covering, which slides loosely and easily over the testicles and epididymides within.

Testicles

The testicles of a normal stallion are palpable as two oval structures lying horizontally within the scrotal pouches. Normal orientation of the testicle is ascertained by palpation of the tail of the epididymis and the ligament of the tail of the epididymis (or caudal ligament of the epididymis) at the caudal pole of the testicle (547). The ligament is palpable as a fibrous nodule attaching the tail of the epididymis to the caudal pole of the testicle. It can be relatively large in newborn colts and, on palpation, may be mistaken for a testicle within the scrotum. On occasion, examination of a normal stallion may identify rotation of up to 180° of one or both testicles. Testicle rotation is often transient and a subsequent examination may find the testicle in normal orientation. Rotation must be differentiated from true testicular or spermatic cord torsion, in which stallions demonstrate signs of colic and palpation reveals a painful and swollen testicle.

The testis is encapsulated by the tunica albuginea, a layer of tough collagenous tissue and smooth muscle that is fused to the visceral layer of the vaginal tunic. The tunica albuginea sends supportive trabeculae into the testicular parenchyma, dividing the testis into lobules. The testicle of the stallion does not contain an axially oriented mediastinum testis as is seen in the bull and other species. In the stallion it is located at the cranial pole of the testis, where the excurrent ducts leaving the testis cross the tunica albuginea and enter the head of the epididymis. This results in a mediastinum testis that is less prominent grossly on cut section and almost indefinable ultrasonographically.

Epididymides and excurrent duct system

Each epididymis is a highly convoluted but unbranched duct approximately 70 meters long and having a grossly distinct head, body, and tail. In the stallion the head of the epididymis is a flattened structure that lies dorsomedially along the cranial border of the testis. The body, or corpus, lies along the dorsolateral aspect of each testis and continues as the tail, or cauda, which is a large, prominent structure attached to the caudal pole of the testis. The deferent duct, the excretory duct for sperm, attaches to the tail of the corresponding epididymis, runs along the medial aspect of the testis, and ascends via the spermatic cord through the vaginal ring into the pelvis. Each deferent duct widens into its corresponding ampullary gland and eventually terminates at the colliculus seminalis of the pelvic urethra. The colliculus seminalis is a rounded prominence

547 Gross appearance of the testis and epididymis of the stallion. The body of the epididymis runs along the dorsolateral border of the testis with the head (red arrow) at the cranial pole and the tail (yellow arrow) at the caudal pole.

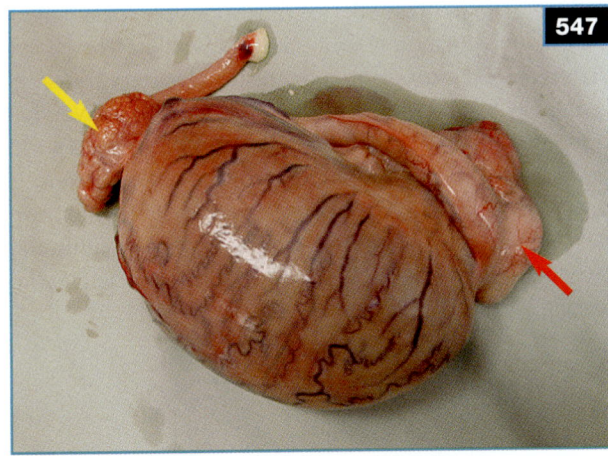

327

situated on the dorsomedial wall of the urethra about 5 cm caudal to the urethral opening from the bladder. This is the site at which the ducts of the accessory sex glands empty into the urethra. Whereas the deferent ducts are not externally palpable in stallions, all portions of the epididymis are usually palpable through the scrotal wall. The head of the epididymis may be difficult to ascertain because of its flattened nature and because the cremaster muscle lies on top of it.

The histologic structure of the epididymis changes as it continues through its different regions, with epithelial height being greatest proximally and smooth muscle components greatest distally. As sperm are transported from the excurrent ducts into the head, along the body, and into the tail, they undergo a number of morphologic and physiologic changes that ultimately render them motile and fertile. Specific maturational changes include: the capacity for progressive motility; shedding of the cytoplasmic droplet; plasma and acrosomal membrane alterations; DNA stabilization; and metabolic changes.

The tail of the epididymis generally serves to store the matured sperm.

Spermatic cord and vascular supply to the testis

Each spermatic cord is enveloped in the parietal layer of the vaginal tunic, which extends distally from the internal inguinal ring. Each spermatic cord contains the corresponding deferent duct, testicular artery, testicular veins, lymphatic vessels, and nerves. The cremaster muscle is situated in the caudolateral borders of each spermatic cord.

The testicular artery descends through the inguinal ring into the cranial border of the spermatic cord in a tortuous manner and divides near the testis into several branches to supply the testis and epididymis. These small branches, embedded in the tunica albuginea, enter the parenchyma via the trabeculae and septa of the testis. A corresponding network of veins leaves the testis and surrounds the testicular artery in a tortuous manner, forming the pampiniform plexus. This countercurrent arrangement of artery and veins, as in other species, is responsible for much of the thermoregulation of the testis in the stallion. The cooler venous blood surrounding the testicular artery transfers heat away from the testicular arterial blood to the venous side, much like a countercurrent heat exchanger. Blood temperature within the branches of the testicular vein is lowered to less than core body temperature by evaporative heat loss through the skin. As a result, blood within the testicular artery is several degrees cooler on reaching the testicle.

Penis and prepuce

The penis of the stallion is musculocavernous in type and can be divided anatomically into a root, a body, and a glans penis. The penis is supported at its root by the paired suspensory ligaments of the penis and the ischiocavernosus muscles. The penile root arises at the ischial arch in the form of two crura, which fuse distally to form the single and dorsal corpus cavernosum penis, and it is enclosed by a thick tunica albuginea. The cavernous spaces making up the erectile tissue of the penis are the corpus cavernosum, corpus spongiosum, and corpus spongiosum glandis. Engorgement of these spaces with blood from branches of the internal and external pudendal arteries and the obturator arteries is responsible for erection. The cavernous spaces within the penis are continuous with the veins responsible for drainage. The corpus spongiosum originates at the pelvis as the bulb of the penis and distally surrounds the penile urethra within a groove on the ventral side of the penis. It continues distally over the free end of the penis to form the glans penis (corpus spongiosum glandis). This is responsible for the distinct bell shape of the stallion's penis that is seen during full erection. The urethral process is distinctly visible at the center of the glans penis and is surrounded by an invagination known as the fossa glandis.

Ventral to the urethra and along the entire length of the penis is the bulbospongiosus muscle. Arising from the urethralis muscle, its smooth rhythmic contractions assist in moving the penile urethral contents (semen and urine) distally. Rhythmic pulsations of the bulbospongiosus muscle are distinctly felt during ejaculation if a hand is placed on the ventral aspect of the penis during collection/natural service. The paired retractor penis muscles also run ventrally along the length of the penis and attach at the glans penis. These smooth muscles function to return the penis to the sheath following detumescence.

The prepuce is formed by a double fold of skin and resembles scrotal skin in that it is essentially hairless and well supplied with sebaceous and sweat glands. It functions to contain and protect the nonerect penis. The external part of the prepuce, or sheath, begins at the scrotum and has a distinct raphe, which is continuous with the scrotal raphe. This external layer extends some distance cranially before reflecting dorsocaudad to the abdominal wall to form the preputial orifice. The internal layer of the prepuce extends caudad from the orifice to line the internal side of the sheath, then reflects craniad toward the orifice again before reflecting caudad to form the internal preputial fold and preputial ring. It is this additional internal fold that allows the marked lengthening (approximately by 50%) of the stallion's penis during erection. During erection, the preputial orifice is visible at the base of the penis just in front of the scrotum, and the preputial ring is visible approximately mid shaft in the penis. Located distal to the preputial ring during erection is the internal layer of the internal preputial fold.

The penis and prepuce of a breeding stallion are best examined following teasing with an in-estrus mare, when the stallion can be observed to drop the penis and attain a full erection. Removal of smegma accumulations may be required for a complete examination of the skin surfaces.

Accessory sex glands

The accessory glands found in the stallion are the prostate gland, seminal vesicles, bulbourethral glands, and ampullae. Their secretions produce the seminal plasma that makes up the majority of the ejaculate volume.

Prostate gland

The prostate gland of the stallion consists of a central isthmus and two lateral lobes that extend along the caudolateral borders of each vesicular gland. Although not always palpable per rectum, the prostate is lobulated or nodular and firm, distinguishing it from the smooth, thin-walled vesicular glands lying next to it. Each prostatic lobe measures 5–9 cm long, 2–6 cm wide, and 1–2 cm thick. Multiple ductules from the prostate enter the lumen of the urethra lateral to the colliculus seminalis. Prostatic secretions appear to contribute to the sperm-rich fraction of the ejaculate. The prostate gland is easily identified ultrasonographically, with its two symmetric, homogeneously echogenic lobes distinctly seen (548). Hypoechoic dilations within the gland parenchyma of each lobe are usually evident. These hypoechogenic spaces are smaller within the isthmus of the gland, and the size of these spaces varies with the frequency of ejaculation and degree of sexual stimulation.

Vesicular glands

The vesicular glands are paired, pyriform, thin walled structures lying laterally to the ampullae, predominantly within the genital fold. Sexual stimulation results in dilation and elongation of the vesicular glands, up to 12–20 cm long and 5 cm in diameter. The distal ends of the glands converge, passing under the prostate as they parallel the ampullae towards their termination at the urethra. The excurrent ducts of the vesicular glands open lateral to the excurrent ducts of the ampullae at the colliculus seminalis of the urethra. Secretions of the vesicular glands make up the gel fraction of the ejaculate. Season influences the output of the vesicular glands, with gel fraction volume being highest during the physiologic breeding season. Individual stallions may produce larger amounts of gel fraction than others. Ultrasonographically, the vesicular glands appear in longitudinal section as flattened oval to triangular sacs, depending on the degree of sexual activity and time since last ejaculation (549). The size and echogenicity of fluid within the glands is extremely variable both within and between stallions. A thin echogenic wall surrounds a fairly uniformly anechogenic lumen. Increased echogenicity of vesicular gland fluid is associated with the highly viscous gel fraction produced by some stallions.

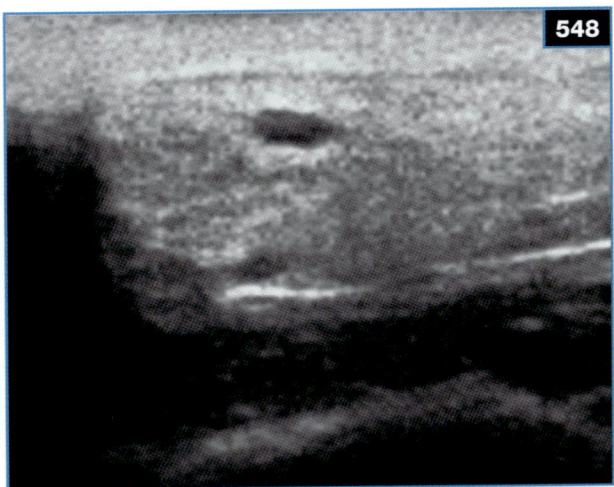

548 Ultrasound image of the prostate of a normal stallion.

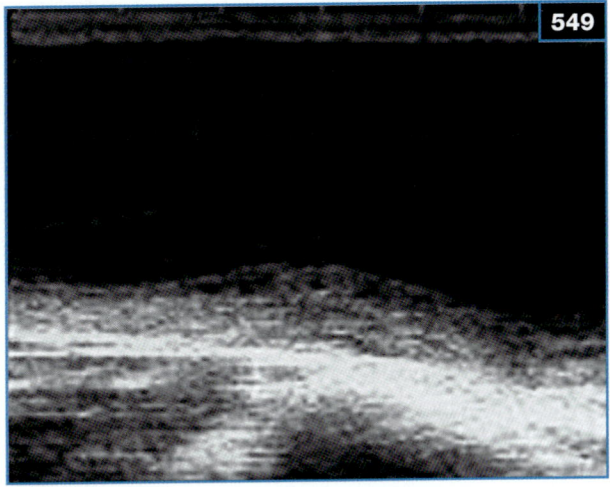

549 Ultrasound image of the vesicular gland of a stallion following teasing. Significant hypoechoic accumulations of fluid are evident within the gland lumen. Vesicular glands vary considerably in their normal ultrasonographic appearance.

329

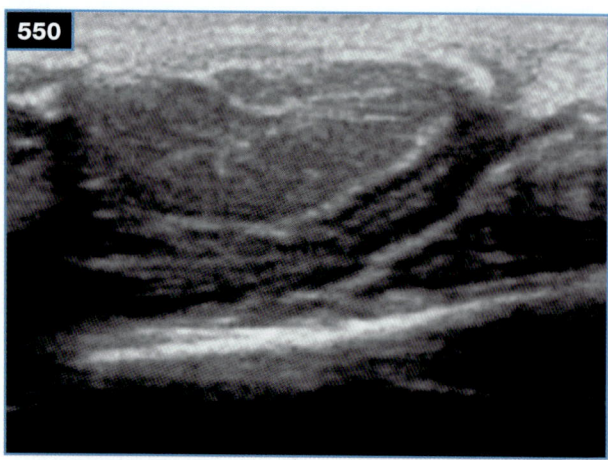

550

550 Ultrasound image of one of the paired bulbourethral glands. They can be visualized by moving the probe slightly to the left or right of the midline pelvic urethra.

Bulbourethral glands

The bulbourethral glands attach to the dorsal surface of the pelvic urethra, about 8 cm caudal to the prostate gland. They are not usually palpable per rectum because they are embedded in the urethralis and bulboglandularis muscles. Similar to the prostate gland, multiple ductules from the bulbourethral glands enter the medial aspect of the urethra distal to the prostatic ductules. Bulbourethral gland secretions make up the majority of the pre-sperm or first fraction of the ejaculate and likely function to cleanse the urethra before ejaculation. Ultrasonographically, the bulbourethral glands appear as oval structures with multiple small hypoechogenic spaces throughout the parenchyma. A thin hyperechogenic line representing the gland wall is surrounded by the hypoechogenic bulboglandularis muscle, which surrounds the gland (550).

Ampullary glands

The ampullary glands are the enlarged distal portions of the deferent ducts. Palpable along the midline of the pelvic floor over the neck of the bladder, they converge caudally, passing beneath the prostate gland, but lie dorsal to the pelvic urethra. At their distal ends they continue through the wall of the urethra, opening into the colliculus seminalis alongside the excretory ducts of the seminal vesicles.

Each ampulla is identified ultrasonographically by the hypoechogenic central lumen surrounded by a uniformly echogenic wall and a hyperechogenic outer muscular layer. Hypoechogenic areas may be seen within the walls and probably represent the glandular areas. In many stallions the uterus masculinus, a remnant of the müllerian duct system, is visible ultrasonographically as one or two cystic structures located between the ampullae.

Breeding soundness examination of the stallion

Handling a stallion for examination

A confident, experienced horse person should handle stallions for examination and breeding or semen collection. The handler should be aware of normal stallion breeding behavior, including vocalization, prancing, and arching of the neck, and not attempt to discourage or correct these. The handler should work with the stallion away from the breeding area first in order to become familiar with the stallion's behavior and establish respect. The stallion should respond to both voice and lead corrections and halt, back up, and turn when asked. Excessive corrections, beatings, or discipline must be avoided as they can establish long-term behavioral difficulties in stallions. Similarly, the stallion must not be allowed to rush to the mare or phantom, as this habit becomes difficult to break. A good fitting, preferably leather halter is essential. A long leather lead rope, preferably with a good quality chain and clasp, is used to provide additional control. Depending on the stallion's experience and behavior, the chain can be placed over the nose and through the halter rings, or through the mouth. Once the handler is comfortable with the stallion, the examiner can approach. Palpation of the external genitalia is probably best performed following semen collection when the stallion is more relaxed, willing to stand quietly, and more likely to tolerate the examination. The handler should always stand on the same side as the examiner, and clear communication between handler and examiner is essential. It can be helpful to stand the stallion against one wall to limit his movement during the examination. The examiner approaches slowly but confidently from the left side at an angle to the shoulder, and moves alongside the stallion until reaching the left flank. It is helpful to run the left hand or arm over the stallion's neck and back as one moves toward the stallion's flank, so the stallion is aware of the examiner's location. The examiner should never surprise the stallion with movements or grasping of genitalia, as the most likely response will be a forceful kick with the hindlimbs. Many stallions squeal and kick out behind when the scrotum or penis is palpated or washed. With training, most stallions become accustomed to routine examination without difficulty.

Introduction

Guidelines for evaluation of breeding soundness in stallions are published by the Society for Theriogenology (www.therio.org). The primary purpose of the BSE is to select stallions that are expected to achieve pregnancy rates of at least 70% when bred to 40 mares by natural service or 120 mares by artificial insemination. A second purpose of the BSE is to diagnose causes of reduced fertility and develop management guidelines to optimize pregnancy rates. The BSE includes accurate animal identification; a complete physical examination; evaluation of libido; bacterial culture of the urethra and semen; evaluation of semen for pH, total sperm numbers, sperm motility, morphology, and longevity; and examination of the external reproductive organs. Additional tests that may be warranted during the BSE include examination of the internal reproductive organs, endoscopy of the urethra, and measurement of motility after semen cooling or freezing. Results must be recorded clearly and permanently.

After the BSE, stallions are classified as satisfactory, questionable, or unsatisfactory. Classification guidelines are listed in *Table 7*. Results of the BSE are not a guarantee of fertility or infertility and must not be represented as such. Occasionally, stallions with apparently adequate results may achieve poor pregnancy rates. In such cases, additional diagnostics, including evaluation of breeding management, and additional sperm staining and function assays, are required to diagnose the problem. In contrast, stallions classified as questionable may achieve adequate pregnancy rates, especially when bred to a limited number of mares. It is important to remember that the BSE predicts fertility based on findings from a single day. Semen quality is expected to change over time depending on factors such as season, stress, and breeding management. In stallions classified as questionable, it is common practice to repeat all or part of the BSE after 60 days in order to assess changes in semen quality. Stallions to be used in cooled transported or frozen-semen programs require testing not included in the standard BSE in order to ensure adequate numbers of sperm remain viable after processing.

Protocol for a breeding soundness examination

Identification and history

The age, breed, and occupation of the stallion are noted. A permanent veterinary record identifying the stallion is created using markings, tattoos, microchips, and/or photographs. Historical information on general management including exercise, nutrition, hoof care, parasite control, disease, and lameness is noted. The owner/trainer should be questioned as to whether the stallion has received any medications, supplements, or performance-modifying substances. Specific information on breeding history includes the number of mares bred per season, overall seasonal conception rate, average number of estrous cycles mares are bred to achieve pregnancy, non-return rates, and numbers of matings or inseminations per estrus. It can be useful to chart this information on a monthly basis to uncover seasonal trends. Additionally, obtaining a description of the stallion's breeding routine from the owner can provide insight into management.

TABLE 7 Classification criteria for stallion breeding soundness evaluation (Society for Theriogenology)

SATISFACTORY CLASSIFICATION

- Good libido.
- Penis anatomically normal and free from inflammatory lesions.
- Bacterial culture does not result in pure growth of a single organism.
- Bacterial numbers decline from pre- to postejaculatory samples.
- Bacterial culture under correct conditions is negative for *Taylorella equigenitalus* (CEM).
- EIA (Coggins) test is negative.
- Two scrotal testes are present.
- Testicles and epididymides are of normal size, shape, and texture.
- Total scrotal width is >8 cm.
- At daily sperm output, the second of two ejaculates collected 1 hour apart contains a minimum of 1 billion progressively motile morphologically normal (PMMN) sperm.

QUESTIONABLE CLASSIFICATION

- At or below standard on two or more of the criteria above.

UNSATISFACTORY CLASSIFICATION

- Uni- or bilateral cryptorchidism.
- EIA (Coggins) test positive.
- Carrier of known genetic disease (e.g. combined immunodeficiency disease of Arabian horses).

Physical examination

The purpose of the physical examination is to ensure that the stallion has the desire and ability to breed. Any condition that may impact on breeding ability should be noted. Lameness, debilitation, respiratory impairment, neurologic disease, and blindness are all important problems that can negatively affect breeding ability. Arthritis in the hindlimbs or spine will impair the stallion's ability or desire to mount and thrust during breeding. Chronic painful conditions often decrease semen quality, probably via stress-related endogenous corticosteroid secretion. Known heritable defects such as parrot mouth and aniridia must also be recorded. Congenitally unilateral or bilateral cryptorchid stallions are classified as unsatisfactory breeding prospects under the Society of Fertility and Theriogenology (USA) (SFT) guidelines due to the hereditary nature of the condition. An owner wishing to use a unilaterally cryptorchid stallion for breeding purposes may be advised to have the retained testicle surgically removed in order to prevent future neoplasia in this testicle, although in some countries, such as the UK, this would be considered unethical.

Testing for infectious diseases

Serum samples are collected and accurately identified for testing for venereally transmitted diseases such as equine infectious anemia (EIA) and EVA. When serum antibodies are found for EVA, semen samples are submitted for viral isolation to detect carrier stallions that are shedding virus in semen. Bacterial culture swabs of the penile shaft, prepuce, urethra, and urethral fossa are submitted to test for *Pseudomonas aeruginosa*, *Klebsiella pneumoniae*, and CEM.

Evaluation of libido

The stallion is exposed to a restrained estrus mare and should show strong interest and achieve an erection within 1–5 minutes (**551**). Determination of adequate libido is subjective and based on many factors such as season of the year, temperament, age, and previous handling and breeding experience. For details on normal and abnormal libido see Observation of libido and breeding behavior (p. 335) and Poor libido (p. 340).

Examination of the external genitalia

The penis and prepuce are most easily examined during teasing and washing for breeding. The skin of the penis and prepuce should be intact and free from erosions, crusts, or masses (**552**). The urethral process should be free from growths. The scrotal contents are most easily examined after semen collection. Structures on either side of the scrotum should be of similar size and consistency. Asymmetry creates suspicion of disease. The scrotal skin should be free from erosions, crusts, and masses. The testicle should be uniformly firm and freely moveable in the scrotum. The head and body of the epididymis are palpable on the cranial and dorsolateral aspect of each testicle. The tail of the epididymis is clearly palpable at the caudal pole of the testicle. The epididymis feels less firm than the testicle. The ligament of the epididymis is palpable running dorsocranially from the tail. If the tail and ligament are difficult to locate, testicular torsion should be suspected. The spermatic cord is palpated running dorsally from the testicle to the external inguinal ring.

Total scrotal width is measured using calipers or ultrasound (**553**); larger widths are associated with increased sperm output. The average for light horse stallions is 9–12 cm. Stallions with total scrotal width <8 cm generally will not produce enough sperm to meet the BSE standard. Each testis of a postpubertal stallion weighs between 150 and 300 g and measures approximately 50–80 mm wide, 60–70 mm high, and 80–140 mm long. Testicular size varies among stallions depending on breed, season, age, and reproductive status. Testis parenchymal weight correlates highly with daily sperm production and therefore is a useful predictor of breeding potential; however, because parenchymal weight cannot be measured in the live stallion, estimates must be used. Measurement of scrotal circumference is difficult in the stallion because the testes are held close to the body wall. Caliper measurements should be used judiciously based on their inherent potential sources of error including caliper sensitivity,

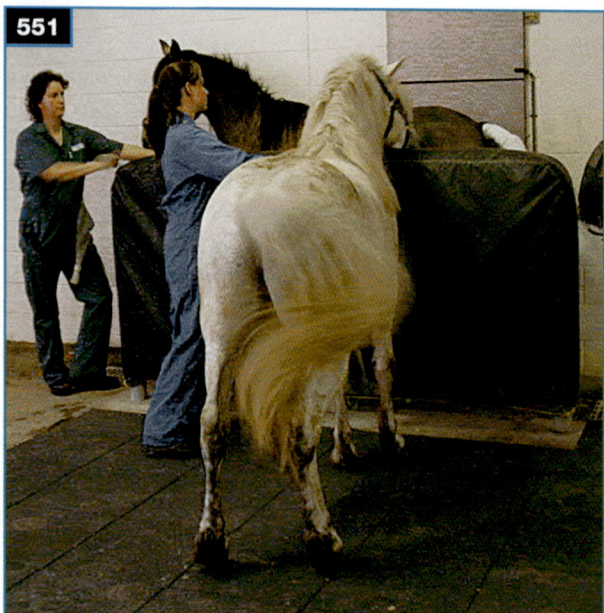

551 A maiden stallion being introduced to an estrus mare over a padded board, and encouraged to tease prior to training to the phantom for semen collection.

552 Lesions on the penis of a 16-year-old Thoroughbred stallion with squamous cell carcinoma. The disease had already spread to inguinal lymph nodes at the time of presentation.

553 Taking the total scrotal width of a stallion. The testes are pushed ventrally into the scrotum with one hand, while the calipers are placed over the widest part of the scrotum with the other hand.

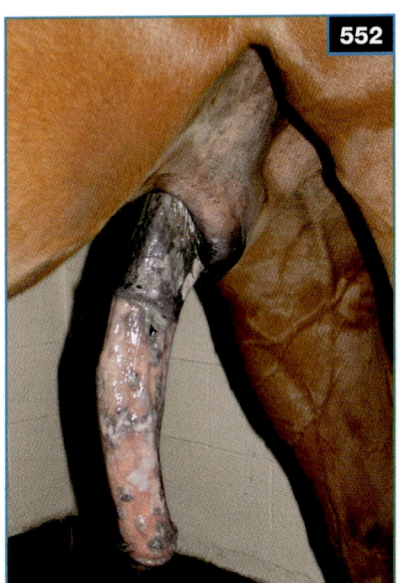

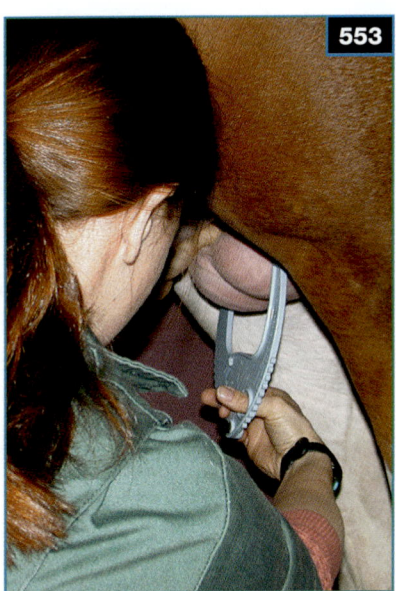

operator technique, and testis location within the scrotum. To measure the total scrotal width, the examiner stands close to the stallion's left flank and reaches under the abdomen to grasp both testicles within the scrotum with the left hand. The calipers are held in the right hand and the measurement is taken across the widest part of the scrotum while the left hand pushes both testicles firmly downward into the scrotum.

The testes should also be measured individually using either calipers or ultrasound for length, width, and height. Ultrasonographic measurements may be more accurate, although proper placement of the probe across the testis to ensure that a cross-sectional image is obtained is critical. Deviation toward an oblique image dramatically affects measurements obtained with this method. The ultrasound probe is placed longitudinally across one testicle, while the examiner's left hand pushes the opposite testicle dorsally out of the way. Once the length has been measured, the probe can be turned to a cross-sectional axis in order to measure the width. Turning the probe once again at the pole of the testicle obtains the height measurement. Testicular volume can then be calculated from the individual measurements and used to predict daily sperm production. As a testis approximates the shape of an ellipsoid, the following formula is used to convert length, width, and height measurements into testicular volume:

Testis volume = $4/3 \pi$ (length/2) (width/2) (height/2) or = $0.5236 \times H \times L \times W$ in cm

Predicted daily sperm production = $[0.024 \times (\text{vol L} + \text{vol R})] - 0.76$

Predicted daily sperm production can be compared with actual daily sperm production as estimated by semen collection during the routine BSE. A stallion whose actual daily sperm production is below that predicted for his testicular size should be further evaluated for disease conditions of the testes, epididymides, and accessory glands.

Examination of the internal genitalia

The internal genitalia are examined by rectal palpation and ultrasonography. Examination is easiest after semen collection. To reduce the risk of rectal tearing or other injury, appropriate patient selection and restraint are critical. The isthmus of the prostate is a firm 3×4 cm structure approximately 10 cm cranial to the anal sphincter. The seminal vesicles are thin-walled structures located craniolateral to the prostate on either side of the ventral midline. In normal stallions they may be difficult to appreciate except during sexual arousal. They are symmetrical and approximately 2 cm wide and 5 cm long. The ampullae are tubular structures located cranial to the prostate and medial to the seminal vesicles, on the pelvic floor. They are approximately 1 cm wide by 12–25 cm long. The internal inguinal rings can be palpated along the abdominal wall cranioventral to the pelvic brim and lateral to the midline. Bending and straightening the index finger while sliding the hand along the appropriate area of the abdominal wall will cause the finger to enter the ring. The ring can then be evaluated for hernia and adhesions.

Bacterial culture

After washing and drying the penis, the glans is stimulated to initiate the flow of pre-seminal fluid. The fluid is allowed to wash the urethral lumen before the urethra is swabbed with a bacterial culture swab; a second swab is taken immediately after semen collection. In addition, an aliquot for bacterial culture is removed from the semen immediately post collection in a manner that minimizes the risk of contamination. In normal stallions, bacteria cultured from samples are inconsistent and bacterial numbers decline after ejaculation. Pure cultures or increased numbers of bacteria on the postejaculation sample are indicative of reproductive tract infection. In countries with CEM, microaerophilic culture should be performed.

Semen collection (see also p. 336)

Prior to a BSE, semen should be collected from the stallion twice daily for 7 days in order to deplete epididymal reserves and reach daily sperm output. During a BSE, semen is collected twice, with 1 hour between collections. Normally, the volume and pH of both collections are similar, but the second collection contains half the total sperm number. During semen collection, a hand should be placed on the ventral shaft of the penis so that the strength of the ejaculatory pulses can be evaluated. Deviations from normal mounting, intromission, and ejaculation are recorded. It is essential that the ejaculate is collected and handled carefully, avoiding exposure to heat (above body temperature), direct light, and contact with spermatotoxins.

Semen evaluation

Initial motility: Total and progressive motility of raw semen should be evaluated within 5 minutes of semen collection. Most normal stallions have progressive motility of >40%. Higher progressive motility is generally associated with higher conception rates, although this is not always the case. In stallions at daily sperm output, a significant change in motility between collections often indicates a semen-handling problem such as cold shock, heat damage, or water contamination.

pH: pH should be evaluated within 10 minutes of collection using commercial pH paper with an appropriate range. Normal pH is 7.2–7.8. Elevated pH may indicate urine or soap contamination or inflammation.

Sperm concentration: During a BSE the sperm concentration in the second semen sample is expected to be approximately half that of the first sample. If the concentration of sperm is roughly the same as the first collection, consider whether complete ejaculation in both collections has in fact occurred. A sharp drop in sperm concentration on the second collection may be seen in stallions with severe testicular or epididymal dysfunction or disease.

Sperm morphology: During a BSE it is generally most important to determine the percentage of normal sperm in the ejaculate in order to calculate the number of progressively motile, morphologically normal (PMMN) sperm. It is thought that in most cases abnormal sperm do not reach the oocyte. However, certain morphologic abnormalities may not impair motility, simply fertility. In these cases, defective sperm are competing with normal sperm at the moment of fertilization, therefore the proportion of defective sperm may be significant.

Number of progressively motile, morphologically normal sperm: The calculation method is demonstrated in *Table 8.* In stallions classified as satisfactory, the second ejaculate contains more than one billion PMMN sperm.

Longevity of motility: For raw semen, at least 10% progressive motility is anticipated after 6 hours in a 37°C (98.6°F) water bath. Poor longevity is associated with short sperm survival time in the mare's reproductive tract.

Hormonal evaluation

The addition of hormonal evaluation in a standard BSE is the subject of some controversy. In normal stallions, where physical examination and semen analysis are within normal limits, hormonal evaluation is highly unlikely to provide any useful information. Veterinarians managing stallions with large books may elect to monitor hormonal status once or twice yearly. When hormonal testing is done, several samples on consecutive days should be taken to avoid sampling in the trough of the normal pulsatile secretion. Baseline serum samples should be tested for FSH, LH, estrogens, testosterone, and inhibin. In stallions with abnormalities on physical examination or spermiogram, additional tests including a hCG stimulation

---

TABLE 8 Number of progressively motile, morphologically normal sperm

SEMEN PARAMETERS

- Volume — 50 ml
- Concentration — 100 million/ml
- Progressive motility — 70%
- Morphology — 50% normal

EXAMPLE CALCULATION

Volume × concentration × proportion motile × proportion morphologically normal

50 ml × 100 million/ml × 0.70 × 0.50 = 1,750 million or 1.75 billion PMMN sperm

test (see p. 357) or GnRH challenge test, can be conducted. Hormonal changes in stallions with testicular degeneration (TD) occur late in the course of the disease, and may be most useful for prognosis. The typical hormonal profile in TD includes high FSH, low estrogen and inhibin, and normal to low levels of LH and testosterone. Estrogen values below <124 pg/ml suggest irreversible damage to the seminiferous epithelium and a poor prognosis.

Examination for venereal disease

Examination for venereal disease includes visual examination of the external genitalia and bacterial culture of the genital skin, pre- and postejaculatory fluids, and semen. The penile, preputial, and scrotal skin are evaluated for erosions, granulomas, and exudates. The testis and epididymides are palpated to detect hard or soft areas and enlargements. After teasing, cultures of the prepuce, shaft of the penis, and urethral fossa are collected. The penis is washed and dried thoroughly. Although washing the genitalia in disinfectant soap is generally contraindicated, here it is necessary to reduce contamination from skin flora. After washing, the glans penis is massaged and the pre-ejaculatory secretions of the urethral gland are swabbed. If possible, semen for bacterial culture is collected in an open-ended vagina. The ejaculate is fractionated and the first fraction provides fluid from the prostate and ampullae. Immediately after ejaculation, the urethra is swabbed again. To collect fluid samples from the vesicular glands, the stallion is teased, then the enlarged glands are massaged transrectally during urethral endoscopy.

Urethral endoscopy

Urethral endoscopy can be used to evaluate hemospermia and accessory sex gland and urinary tract abnormalities. Endoscopy is performed using a thoroughly disinfected and well rinsed, one-meter flexible endoscope with a maximum diameter of 10 mm. Catheters and forceps that can be passed through the biopsy channel should be available to collect samples. Stallions are sedated and restrained in stocks, and the glans penis and urethral fossa are carefully cleaned prior to insertion of the endoscope.

Ultrasonography of the male genital tract (554)

The scrotal contents and spermatic chords are easily evaluated using a portable ultrasound machine with a 5- or 7-MHz linear probe. The testes are uniformly echogenic, while the epididymes are comparatively hypoechoic and granular. Unilateral conditions can be evaluated by comparison with the contralateral side. Biopsy of abnormal areas is facilitated by ultrasonography. Ultrasonography of a cryptorchid testis and the ampullae and prostate glands is performed transrectally; with a cryptorchid testis it can also be performed parainguinally. Adequate restraint and sedation are required to minimize the risk of rectal tears.

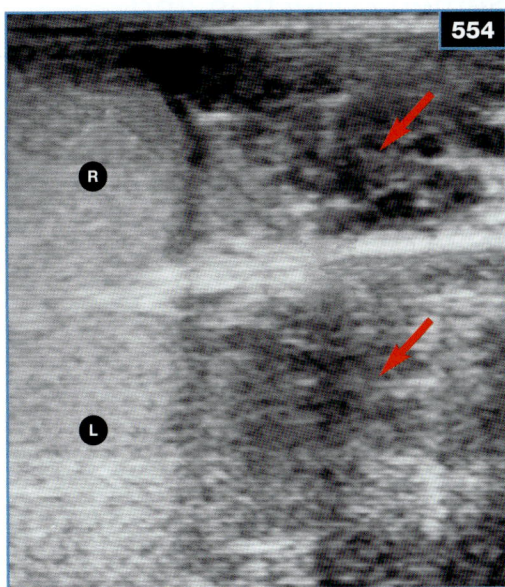

554 Ultrasound appearance of the testis and epididymis of the stallion. Both the right and left testes and epididymal tails (arrows) are imaged.

Observation of libido and breeding behavior

Libido and behavior are observed during the stallion's typical breeding routine (551). Sexually experienced stallions used for breeding in hand will show strong interest in a mare in estrus. Vocalizing and prancing begin soon after the mare is visible. Most stallions will approach the shoulder of the mare and may sniff, then squeal and strike out. If the mare is receptive, the stallion will move towards the mare's hindquarters, nuzzling the flank and perineal region before mounting. The time required to obtain an erection depends on the stallion's previous breeding experience and temperament, but is normally less than 5 minutes. Stallions experienced in collection for AI, either by mounting a phantom or ground collection, also develop an erection rapidly during their usual breeding routine; however, the stimuli are stallion specific. These stallions should exhibit a strong drive to mount the phantom or service the artificial vagina. Experienced pasture-breeding stallions may appear to show little interest in breeding in an in-hand situation or when the mare is not at the peak of estrus. Additionally, they test receptivity carefully by thorough teasing and mounting without an erection. After mounting, intromission of the penis into the vagina or artificial vagina stimulates strong pelvic thrusting. Ejaculation occurs rapidly, and consists of six to eight strong urethral pulsations. After ejaculation, the penis almost immediately becomes flaccid and the stallion relaxes.

Semen collection and evaluation

Semen collection

Collection of semen from a stallion for evaluation or insemination is best accomplished through the use of one of the commercially available models of artificial vaginas. The most common types in use include the Missouri style, the Colorado style, and the Hanover artificial vagina (**555**). The Missouri artificial vagina is light and easily handled; however, the internal temperature cools more quickly than other types. The Colorado artificial vagina holds the temperature well, but it is heavy to use. Commercially available phantom mounts are designed in some cases to have the Colorado device placed inside. This method offers the advantage of requiring one less person (i.e. does not require a semen collector) for the semen collection. However, this type of set-up appears to place the stallion at higher risk of traumatic injuries, particularly to the prepuce and penis. Other methods of obtaining semen include collection of a dismount sample, use of a condom or other collection device in the mare, and pharmacologic ejaculation. The total number of sperm in the ejaculate, however, can only be determined following collection of the entire ejaculate with an artificial vagina. This is an important consideration when a stallion is presented for fertility evaluation. Raw stallion semen is very fragile and poor handling can easily result in poor motility, morphology, and longevity. Rapid changes in temperature and exposure to water, detergents, lubricants, or other chemicals all impact negatively on sperm survival (**556**).

The artificial vagina is designed to hold hot water within a sealed jacket. The warmth and pressure of the artificial vagina on the stallion's penis cause ejaculation. Most stallions ejaculate readily with the temperature set in the range of 43–48°C (109.4–118.4°F). However, the temperature and pressure may be modified to suit a particular stallion's preferences. Care must be taken to ensure that the stallion's penis is fully within the artificial vagina, preventing ejaculated sperm from being exposed to the high temperature of the device and resulting in heat shock. The artificial vagina is fitted with a collection bottle or bag and use of an in-line filter method is recommended. The filter removes most of the gel fraction as well as dirt or smegma. Immediately following collection the semen is moved to an incubator and maintained at 37°C (98.6°F) for the initial evaluation. Semen extender should be prepared immediately before semen collection and kept at 37°C (98.6°F) in the incubator. Semen extenders are commercially available through veterinary supply companies or they can be prepared easily within a laboratory. There are many variations on the market, ranging from simple combinations of sugar and milk solids, to complex buffer solutions. The purpose of the extender is to provide an energy source to support the high metabolic activity of spermatozoa, provide antibiotics to combat bacterial contamination inevitable with collection, and provide protection from cold shock during cooling. The semen from individual stallions varies greatly according to which type of extender it performs best in. Practitioners are encouraged to test several extenders with every stallion to determine which best suits each case. In general, the Kenney style extender containing glucose and nonfat dried skim milk solids is a good initial choice. All slides, coverslips, containers, pipettes, etc. that come in contact with semen should be kept warm.

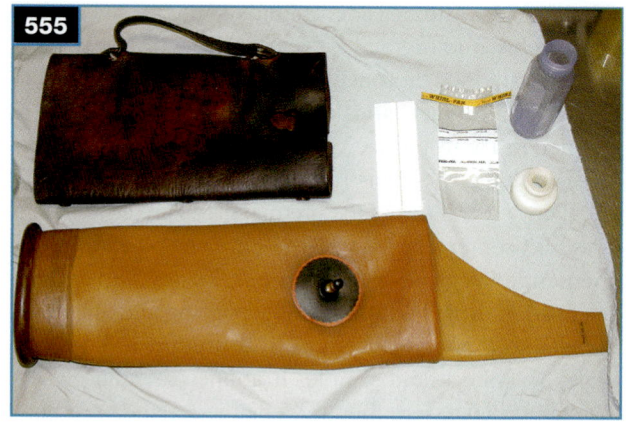

555 The disassembled Missouri artificial vagina, including the rubber liner, leather case with handle, semen filter, collection bag, and bottle.

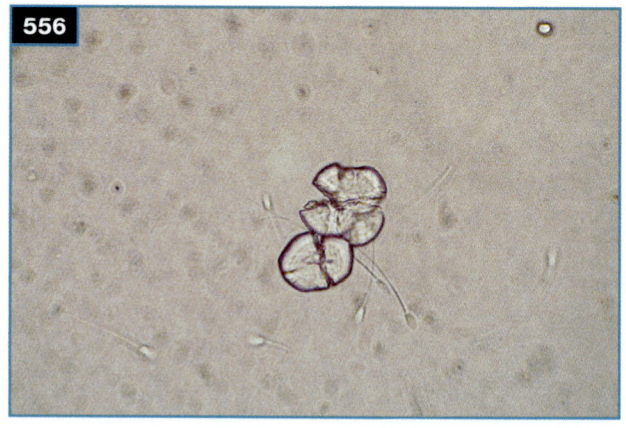

556 These unusual contaminants found within a semen sample were determined to be starch granules and were the result of baby powder applied within the artificial vagina to prevent the rubber sticking together. Contaminants such as powders, soaps, lubricants, and water significantly impact on semen motility and viability.

Semen evaluation

Once collected, semen is commonly evaluated for color and appearance, volume, total and progressive motility, concentration, and morphology. Stallion semen should be white to skim-milk in color and appearance. The ejaculate is divided into sperm-rich (produced by the testes and epidymidides) and gel fractions (produced mainly by the accessory sex glands). The gel fraction should be removed immediately after collection by filtering, decanting, or aspiration.

Semen volume

The volume of both the gel and sperm-rich fractions of the ejaculate should be recorded. Semen volume can be measured using a warmed sterile plastic tube, clean dry baby bottle, or graduated cylinder. Normal semen volume varies greatly depending on breed, age, season, frequency of collection, and amount of time spent teasing the stallion prior to collection. A typical average volume from an adult stallion would be 50–70 ml, with a range of 25–300 ml. The volume varies according to the season: higher in the spring and summer, lower in the autumn and winter. Precopulatory sexual stimulation may increase the gel portion and high frequency of ejaculation will decrease the semen volume. At this time, a small sample of unextended semen is taken for morphology analysis and determination of sperm concentration. The semen volume multiplied by sperm concentration determines the total number of sperm in the ejaculate.

Total and progressive motility

Total and progressive motility can be evaluated prior to dilution with extender by placing a small drop of raw semen on a prewarmed (37°C [98.6°F]) microscope slide with a coverslip. Several fields are evaluated with a magnification of ×200 to ×40 with phase contrast, and the average motility of the fields recorded. Computer-assisted sperm motion analysis (CASA) systems are available that reduce the subjective nature of motility analysis (557); however, their considerable expense makes them of little value in the field situation.

The motility evaluation is repeated with semen extended in a 1:1 ratio. Use of extender prevents agglutination of sperm to one another and to the microscope slide and allows for more accurate determination of motility. Total motility is defined as the percentage of sperm cells moving, in any manner, in the sample. Progressive motility is defined as the percentage of sperm cells moving forward in a progressive manner in the sample. An additional description of sperm velocity or vigor may also be given. One example is a scale of 0 to 4, with 0 being nonmotile, 1 being very sluggish motility, and a score of 4 describing fast or highly vigorous motility. Retrograde or circular motion is abnormal.

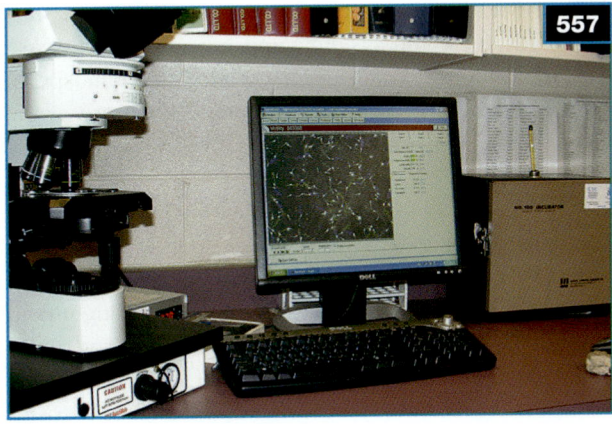

557 Total and progressive motility can be evaluated by computer-assisted sperm motion analysis systems, which reduce the subjective nature of motility analysis.

Sperm concentration

Sperm concentration of the nongel fraction can be determined using a hemocytometer or a densimeter. Densimeters measure the amount of light transmitted through a sample (photometry) and correlate this with the sperm concentration of the sample. Examples of commercially available densimeters include the SpermaCue (Minitube of America) and the ARS System (Animal Reproduction Systems, Chino, CA). Photometric instruments must be calibrated properly and are less accurate at extremely high or low concentrations. Contaminated samples will give spurious results.

The hemocytometer method of determining concentration uses the same counting chamber and Unopette dilution system that is used for WBC counts. Raw semen is drawn into the micropipette of the Unopette and mixed with the diluent. The Unopette is allowed to sit for a few minutes until the sperm become immotile. A coverslip is placed over the hemocytometer chamber and the diluted semen loaded into the chamber by capillary action. Care must be taken to avoid overfilling. With the WBC Unopette system, the sperm visualized in all 25 squares in the center large square are counted. The number of sperm obtained is multiplied by one million to calculate the sperm concentration per milliliter. Both sides of the chamber are counted and the results averaged. The RBC Unopette system can also be used, although the mathematics changes. With the RBC system, the number of sperm in five small squares within the center square (normally the outside four squares and the center square) are counted. The number of sperm counted is multiplied by a factor of ten, which then gives the number of sperm in millions per milliliter. For example, if 12 sperm are counted in five squares, the concentration of sperm is 120 million/ml.

Age, season, frequency of ejaculation, testicular size, sperm reserves, and systemic and reproductive disease can all influence total sperm count. The total sperm number is multiplied by the percentage of progressively motile sperm to give an approximate total live sperm count of an ejaculate.

Sperm morphology

Sperm morphology is determined either by examination of a fixed-stained specimen under oil-immersion bright-field microscopy or by examination of a wet mount using differential interference-contrast microscopy (558, 559). For the stained method, the most commonly used stain is eosin-nigrosin. Other stains that can be used include modified Wright–Giemsa, Indian ink, Spermac, or new methylene blue. A drop of warm semen is gently mixed with a drop of warm stain at one end of a microscope slide. A smear is made using either a second slide or a glass pipette, similar to the method used to make a slide for a differential blood smear. Two hundred sperm should be counted, recording the number of normal as well as abnormal sperm. Sperm with abnormal morphology are categorized as to the type of defect present (i.e. head, midpiece, and tail defects; proximal and distal droplets; and loose heads). Morphological defects can be further classified according to whether they are defects of spermatogenesis (primary), occurring in the efferent duct system (secondary), or caused by incorrect semen collection and/or handling technique (tertiary). Note that in stallions, abaxial attachment of the midpiece to the head is common and such sperm are considered to be morphologically normal. The number of normal sperm should be similar to the percentage of progressively motile sperm, otherwise laboratory error should be suspected.

Some stains (e.g. Indian ink) facilitate estimation of alive:dead ratio because the stain penetrates damaged cell membranes, staining the head of dead sperm.

pH

The pH of the semen should be measured to determine if it is free from urine or purulent material and that a complete ejaculation has occurred. The optimal pH for stallion semen is about 7.7.

Sperm longevity

Sperm longevity should be assessed for all stallions whose semen is being chilled and transported. The semen sample is extended to a concentration of 25–50 million/ml in several different extenders that may vary in the sugar, buffers, and antibiotics used. One sample from each extender is stored at room temperature and another is stored in the transport container. Alternatively, the chilled samples can be stored in the refrigerator by placing the plastic tube containing the sample into a beaker of 35°C (95°F) water to allow slow cooling. The motility of the extended semen in the various extenders is examined at various times: examination intervals suggested might include 12, 24, 36, 48, and 72 hours post collection. The results of this evaluation suggest whether a particular stallion's semen is likely to ship well over prolonged periods of time.

Advanced tests

Advanced tests can be performed that evaluate other aspects of sperm function. Sperm membrane integrity can be evaluated using the hypo-osmotic swelling test or fluorescent probes such as the Fertilight Kit (Molecular

558 A morphologically normal equine sperm with an abaxially attached tail. Abaxial tail attachment is normal in the stallion and can be seen in very high percentages of sperm within an ejaculate. They are not associated with subfertility.

559 An equine sperm demonstrating a proximal droplet (arrow). This is considered a major defect and is associated with reduced fertility if found in high numbers.

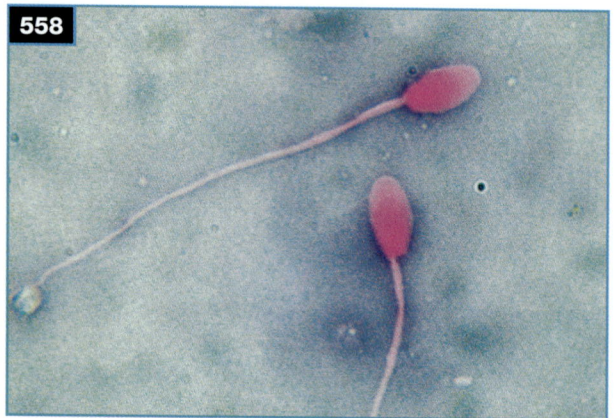

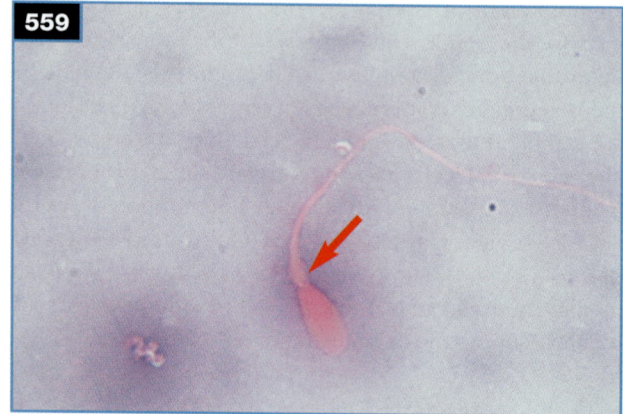

Probes, Eugene, OR). Acrosomal integrity and sperm chromatin structure can also be assessed using fluorescein staining. Fluorescent staining requires specialized microscopic equipment, including flow cytometry, and is therefore generally only available in academic or specialized settings. Scanning electron microscopy can be used to investigate subtle structural abnormalities.

Advanced reproductive techniques

Chilled semen

The transport of chilled extended semen is now commonplace and has greatly influenced the growth of AI. Transport of equine semen across state lines, countries, or continents may require that government permits, certification of disease-free status, or other paperwork is completed. Many commercially available transport packaging systems are now available, ranging from short term (24 hour) cardboard boxes with icepacks to the longer term (48–72 hour) Equitainer. Research has shown that most stallions' semen retains best motility when extended for chilling to a concentration of 25–50 million sperm/ml. Following routine semen collection and analysis, semen is extended and packaged in a leak-proof container such as a Whirl-Pak bag. Clear labeling of the bag and the exterior of the container should include the following information: stallion name; owner; registration number; collection date; motility, concentration, and number of sperm shipped; and mare identification. It is generally accepted that 500 million motile sperm should be included in an insemination dose, although some stallions may demonstrate acceptable fertility with as low as 200 million motile sperm per dose. If semen will not reach the mare for 24–48 hours, the expected decline in motility should be factored in and a higher number of total sperm included in the shipment.

Semen freezing

Cryopreservation allows permanent storage of semen, worldwide distribution of superior genetics, and permits continued breeding while a stallion pursues a performance career or is sidelined by injury or disease. Cryopreserved semen appears to retain its fertilizing ability virtually permanently, provided it is stored properly in liquid nitrogen. The semen from individual stallions varies considerably in response to cryopreservation. While most stallions' frozen semen will result in acceptable fertility rates, the semen from some individuals cannot be frozen successfully. The reasons for individual variation in response to semen cryopreservation are not known. A stallion with poor-quality semen is unlikely to be successful in a cryopreservation program. Perhaps more frustrating is the stallion with

high-quality semen and good post-thaw motility that achieves few or no pregnancies with cryopreserved semen. Per cycle pregnancy rates are generally lower than that expected with natural cover, fresh, or transported breeding programs. Several studies have demonstrated that average per cycle pregnancy rates with frozen equine semen are in the 50% range. Practitioners should discuss the expected results with clients wishing to use frozen semen in their breeding program.

The cryopreservation process involves routine semen collection, centrifugation to remove the seminal plasma, and re-suspension in freezing extender. Depending on the stallion and extender used, semen may or may not be chilled prior to cryopreservation. Freezing extenders contain buffers, antibiotics, sugars, egg yolk, and a cryoprotectant such as glycerol, dimethlyformamide, or DMSO. The extender components protect the sperm membrane from phase transitions and other changes during freezing, and exert osmotic forces to draw water from the sperm cell prior to ice-crystal formation. Several packaging methods are available; however, the 0.5 ml plastic straw is the most widely used. The loaded straws are placed over nitrogen vapor to initiate the freezing process before being plunged into liquid nitrogen. Once frozen the straws are stored in liquid nitrogen until required. It is important to note that while semen is generally referred to as 'frozen', it cannot under any circumstances be kept in a standard freezer. This may be an area of confusion for horse owners. Two types of container are available for frozen semen. A dry-nitrogen shipper is a short-term storage and transport vessel. Liquid nitrogen is used to charge and cool the vessel, but is not kept within the tank. When semen is transported by truck or aircraft, it is imperative that all remaining liquid nitrogen be removed from the dry-shipper. Couriers and airlines will not accept a dry-shipper with liquid nitrogen within it. Models vary in capacity and also in the length of time that the temperature is maintained once charged (from only a few days to 3 weeks). If semen is received in a dry-nitrogen shipper, it is recommended that it be moved immediately to a liquid nitrogen tank. When a dry-nitrogen shipper is opened, a puff of vapor will be seen from the top if the tank is still charged. If there is no vapor, then the tank has lost its charge and the semen has thawed. A liquid nitrogen tank is the best method for storage of frozen semen. These tanks are generally kept on the farm or in the veterinary clinic, and the dry-shipper is used for short-term transport from one liquid tank to another.

Epididymal sperm can be collected from the testicles of a recently deceased stallion and cryopreserved. Testes of a deceased stallion should be removed within 4 hours of death and transported at 4°C (39.2°F) to a laboratory capable of performing the sperm recovery and cryopreservation, within 24 hours.

Ultra-low-dose artifical insemination

Ultra-low-dose AI involves passing a flexible endoscope through the cervix of the mare and depositing an extremely low volume (i.e. 30–150 μl) of semen directly onto the uterotubal papilla. This technique has resulted in pregnancies using concentrations as low as 1,000 motile sperm. Acceptable pregnancy rates (24–29%) have been achieved with insemination of 100,000 motile sperm. This very low dose of sperm allows for careful use of frozen-thawed semen from deceased stallions, and also permits use of sex-sorted sperm. Hysteroscopic insemination has not been found in most cases to improve fertility rates of stallions with oligospermia.

Intracytoplasmic sperm injection

Intracytoplasmic sperm injection (ICSI) involves micro-injection of a single tailless sperm head directly into an oocyte to result in fertilization. The resulting embryo is cultured in the laboratory before being transferred into a recipient mare's oviduct. The technique can be used with epididymal sperm, frozen-thawed sperm, and sex-sorted sperm.

Sperm sexing

Sex-sorting of sperm is performed by flow cytometry and has resulted in the birth of sex-selected foals. The greatest limitation to the procedure with current technology is the low numbers of sperm that can be processed and sorted in a reasonable length of time. This means that either ICSI or ultra-low-dose AI must be used to achieve pregnancies, further increasing cost and limiting the market.

Chromosomal analysis

The normal chromosomal complement in the stallion is 64,XY. Chromosomal analysis may be required to investigate unexplained infertility in a young stallion or to confirm the presence of a chromosomal aberration in an animal with a suspected intersex condition.

Aberrations of the autosomes are rare, as they generally lead to embryonic failure early in development. Sex chromosome abnormalities are the most common finding. Blood samples can be submitted to cytogenetic laboratories for testing. Two tubes containing freshly collected sodium heparin are submitted on ice overnight. The blood sample should be collected aseptically and without contamination of cells from other sources. Live lymphocytes are cultured for 72 hours and the nuclear chromatin collected and stained to perform the karyotype analysis. Specific C- and G-banding techniques are used to identify specific chromosomes. Fluorescent *in-situ* hybridization and PCR techniques are used to probe for translocations, duplication, and deletions, including SRY expression.

Abnormal sexual function in the stallion

Demands placed on many breeding stallions require them to function in an environment that is very different from the natural equine herd. The manner in which stallions are housed and bred, as well as the demands of performance, may cause extreme stress on certain individuals. Prognosis for behavioral problems is good when there is a strong commitment from all the people interacting with the stallion. Calm and consistent handling is the cornerstone of treatment.

Poor libido

Definition/overview

Poor libido occurs when a stallion takes longer than desired by an owner or manager to obtain an erection and ejaculate. It is reported in stallions used for in-hand breeding and artificial semen collection. In pasture mating situations, poor libido as a cause of low pregnancy rate in an otherwise normal stallion has not been reported.

Etiology/pathophysiology

Lack of libido can be caused by a number of physical and psychologic factors. In novice stallions, sexual inexperience may result in slow sexual responses. Endocrinological and physiologic function is usually normal. Genetic selection for placid temperament, stressful housing conditions, and previous punishment for exhibition of sexual arousal all contribute to low libido in young stallions. In experienced stallions a decline in libido can be caused by a negative sexual experience, overuse, use during the nonbreeding season, management changes, orthopedic pain, or systemic disease. Negative sexual experiences include accidents such as kicks or falls, as well as less apparent traumas such as chaffing or burns caused by the artificial vagina or phantom.

Clinical presentation

Young stallions exhibit prolonged sniffing, nuzzling, and Flehmen behavior and are slow to develop an erection and mount. They seem to lack focus and are easily distracted. Experienced stallions may present with declining libido manifested as less vigorous teasing behavior, lack of focus, and more mounts per ejaculation.

Differential diagnosis

Erectile dysfunction; ejaculatory failure.

Diagnosis

The clinician must be familiar with the range of normal stallion behavior. Quiet observation of the breeding routine, including preparation of the mare or breeding mount and artificial vagina, stallion handling and washing, and teasing and mounting behavior, will often reveal the cause of poor libido. For experienced stallions, a detailed history will focus on recent changes in routine, and physical examination will focus on the diagnosis of systemic, neurologic, and orthopedic disease.

Management

The cornerstones of treatment in young stallions are handler education and improved management (e.g. provide light and airy housing, encourage exercise, provide exposure to mares, and eliminate exposure to other stallions). Low-libido stallions usually benefit from being housed in the mare barn. Testosterone levels, libido, and sperm production may increase significantly when a low-libido stallion is no longer housed exclusively with other stallions. Teasing and breeding experiences should be positive and pain free. This is achieved through patient handling techniques with minimal restraint, a safe and distraction-free environment, and exposure to mares in the peak of estrus. Stallions are brought in hand to the breeding area and allowed to tease one or more estrus mares for 30 minutes once or twice daily. Walking and circling the mare and allowing the stallion to tease face to face and mount without an erection may improve arousal. GnRH (50 µg 1 and 2 hours before breeding) increases testosterone levels and may increase libido. *Table 9* gives the indications and dosages for drugs commonly used in stallion reproduction. *Table 10* gives the effects of some medications on reproduction in stallions. In older stallions exhibiting declining libido, appropriate management changes are similar to those for young stallions. Additionally, orthopedic disease should be treated appropriately with anti-inflammatories, shoeing, or joint injections. The breeding process is modified to provide maximum comfort, including ensuring that the phantom or mare is at an ideal height or training the stallion to collect from the ground. The stallion's sexual workload should be minimized by reducing the number of mares bred. A stallion with low libido may only be able to cover three mares per week, compared with high-libido stallions that may breed three or four times per day, 6 days of the week.

Prognosis

In young stallions the prognosis is excellent. In mature stallions the prognosis for improvement is good; however, the breeding schedule may need to be permanently reduced.

TABLE 9 **Pharmacologic agents used to alter sexual function in the stallion**

DRUG	DOSAGE	THERAPEUTIC EFFECT	ADVERSE EFFECTS
Testosterone	50 mg s/c every 2nd day for 7 days	Increase libido	Decrease semen quality; decrease endogenous testosterone production; increase aggression
GnRH	50 µg s/c 2 hours and 1 hour before breeding	Increase libido by increasing endogenous testosterone	Frequent use or overdosage may decrease semen quality
Imipramine	0.5–2.5 mg/kg p/o 2 hours before breeding	Induces masturbation and ejaculation	Mild sedation; dark colored urine
Diazepam	0.05 mg/kg (up to 20 mg max.) slow i/v 5 minutes before breeding	Reduces anxiety	Sedation and ataxia; disinhibition of aggressive behavior
Phenylbutazone	6 mg/kg i/v 1 hour before breeding or 2 mg/kg p/o q12h on an ongoing basis	Relieves pain	GI and renal damage with chronic administration
GnRH vaccine	Not documented	Temporary sterility; dosage, efficacy, and reversibility not evaluated in stallions	Does not eliminate sexual or aggressive behavior in mature stallions; repeated dosing may result in vaccine reactions

TABLE 10 **Performance-altering drugs with potentially negative effects on male fertility**

DRUG	COMMON USE	EFFICACY	ADVERSE EFFECTS
Progestagens (altrenogest)	Decrease sexual behavior	Poor	Temporarily decrease testicular size and semen quality. May cause permanent decreased fertility if used in immature stallions
Phenothiazines (acepromazine, fluphenazine)	Tranquilization, control unruly behavior	Undocumented	Priapism, loss of erectile function
Reserpine	Control unruly behavior	Undocumented	Penile paralysis, loss of erectile function
Anabolic steroids (boldenone undecylenate, nandrolone decanoate)	Improve athletic performance	Undocumented	Severe decline in testicular mass and semen quality

Aggressive behavior

Definition/overview

In many cases of owner-reported aggression, the stallion is exhibiting normal equine behavior; however, the handling of the animal or the available facilities are poor. In other cases, behavior may have escalated to unruliness because of inappropriate management. Stallions can be dangerous and evaluation should be carried out by experienced personnel in a controlled environment.

Etiology/pathophysiology

Aggression in stallions can be caused by a number of physical and psychological factors. Temperament is heritable, and some breeds and lineages are more challenging to handle than others. Psychological causes of aggression are often based on frustration due to inappropriate management conditions. Unruly stallions tend to be handled as little as possible and may spend a large amount of time isolated from equine and human contact, further increasing aggression. Overuse of stallions and semen collection during the nonbreeding season may result in increased aggression.

Clinical presentation

Veterinary evaluation of an aggressive stallion is often precipitated by an injury to a person or horse. Usually, stallions presented for aggression are boisterous and unruly in the breeding environment, and handling and management are poor. Common inappropriate behaviors include excessive biting and striking at the handler, wheeling around, charging towards the mare or phantom, biting the mare during breeding, and kicking out after dismounting. Rarely, a well-managed stallion with good manners will present with a history of unpredictable savage behavior towards people or horses not associated with breeding. These individuals are dangerous and may not be amenable to treatment.

Diagnosis

A complete history of the stallion's management is determined including type of housing, amount of exercise, and daily and breeding routines. A detailed description of the undesirable behavior is obtained from the stallion's manager. The stallion's breeding routine is observed, with careful attention paid to handling techniques and the stallion's attitude and expressions. A complete physical examination including palpation of the external genitalia and lameness examination is performed.

Management

Retraining of aggressive stallions should only be carried out by an experienced team in a safe facility. The stallion should be handled with the least amount of restraint equipment possible, usually a snug-fitting halter with a chain over the nose or a bridle with a snaffle bit, and a dressage whip or 100 cm (39 inches) length of plastic pipe. The whip or pipe is not used for excessive punishment, but can be used to extend the arm length of the handler so that he/she may provide direction while standing at the horse's shoulder. Retraining must begin in an environment that is not sexually stimulating and include teaching the stallion to walk quietly in hand, halt on command, back up, and move the haunches away from the handler. Training should focus on positive reinforcement of appropriate behavior. The goal of the first collection or breeding is improved behavior and a calm and positive experience for the stallion. Use of an extremely docile, estrus mare wearing appropriate protective equipment facilitates success. Behavior can be further shaped during subsequent training sessions. Decreasing social isolation through introduction of a suitable companion horse and through daily grooming, turn out, and exercise decreases aggressive behavior.

Prognosis

With long-term retraining and consistent handling, the prognosis is good. Educating and involving all persons who will have contact with the stallion are very important. In stallions of limited breeding value, castration may be the most appropriate way to prevent human injury and improve the quality of life of the horse. Properly managed stallions that exhibit unpredictable savage behavior towards humans or other horses may warrant euthanasia.

Erectile dysfunction

Definition/overview

Erectile dysfunction is the inability of a stallion to obtain or maintain an erection.

Etiology/pathophysiology

Psychological factors or physical abnormalities of the genital or neurovascular systems can cause erectile dysfunction. Psychological factors are discussed in the section on low libido (p. 340). Conditions preventing retraction of the penis (paraphimosis or priapism) frequently result in erectile dysfunction. Injury during breeding is the most common cause of paraphimosis. Lacerations on breeding phantoms with openings for mounting an artificial vagina, thermometers forgotten in artificial vaginas, and kicks are common causes of trauma. Paraphimosis can also occur secondary to neurologic disease or debilitating illness. Priapism may occur after administration of phenothiazine drugs and reserpine. Occasionally, erectile failure may occur when the partially erect penis folds and becomes trapped within the prepuce.

Clinical presentation

Most stallions present with a history of traumatic injury and chronic paraphimosis. The skin of the penis and prepuce is often thickened and tough, and sensation is impaired. During sexual arousal, the penis fails to become sufficiently turgid for intromission. Most stallions have normal libido, although those that have experienced repeated failed breeding attempts may show poor libido or frustrated behavior.

Diagnosis

Diagnosis is based on history and examination of the external genitalia. In cases where a cause is not evident, breeding behavior is observed and physical and neurologic examinations are performed.

Management

In cases where erectile function is permanently impaired but testicular function is normal, the goal is to develop a protocol for reliable semen collection. Training stallions to ejaculate through manual stimulation and application of hot compresses to the base of the penis is frequently successful. Imipramine (2 mg/kg p/o) followed 2 hours later with xylazine (0.66 mg/kg i/v) induces ejaculation within 20 minutes in approximately 50% of attempts. With either method, exposure to estrus mares in a distraction-free environment will lower the ejaculatory threshold.

Prognosis

Stallions with chronic erectile failure due to physical abnormalities have a poor prognosis for recovery and a fair prognosis for fertility.

Ejaculatory dysfunction

Definition/overview

Any cause of abnormal sexual function will result in a stallion that fails to ejaculate as reliably and quickly as desirable. Stallions whose most significant clinical sign is ejaculatory dysfunction are rare.

Etiology/pathophysiology

Ejaculatory failure is most frequently caused by systemic abnormalities that hinder pelvic thrusting. These include arthritis of the spine and hindlimbs, neurologic disease, and aortoiliac thrombosis. More rarely, abnormalities of the excurrent duct system prevent ejaculation.

Clinical presentation

Presenting complaints include inability to obtain spermatozoa after artificial collection, absence of urethral pulsing or tail flagging at breeding, or a sudden decline in pregnancy rate. Stallions usually show good libido and normal erectile function. Cases caused by musculoskeletal or neurologic disease may adopt atypical mounting positions, tread and readjust the hindfeet, dismount after two or three thrusts, and have a worried or painful expression. Stallions with ampullary blockage show normal libido and pelvic thrusting, but urethral pulsation, tail flagging, and ejaculation do not occur. Occasionally, a stallion will present that appears to ejaculate normally; however, few or no spermatozoa are present in emitted fluids.

Differential diagnosis

Differential diagnoses include severely impaired spermatogenesis, retrograde ejaculation, aplasia of the excurrent duct system, azoospermia.

Diagnosis

Differentiation of causes of ejaculatory dysfunction begins with a complete physical examination to detect arthritis and neurologic disease. Palpation of the external genitalia is performed to detect excurrent duct abnormalities and testicular atrophy. Breeding behavior is observed including the stallion's attitude, number of mounts, position when mounted, vigor of thrusting, and character of urethral pulsations. Emittited fluid is examined for the presence of spermatozoa or spermatazoal precursor cells, and alkaline phosphatase (AP). AP levels >1,000 IU/l indicate testicular and epididymal secretions are present. When retrograde ejaculation is suspected, the bladder is catheterized and high numbers of spermatozoa are found in the urine. In stallions that do not ejaculate after multiple collection attempts, palpation and ultrasonography of the urethra and accessory sex glands are performed. In the normal stallion the ampullae are 1–2 cm in diameter, while in stallions with ampullary blockage they are larger. Endoscopy of the urethra and colliculus seminalis may reveal abnormalities such as inflammation, purulent discharge, or physical obstruction. If no causative abnormalities are detected, treatment is attempted using a trial-and-error approach. In unresolved cases, testicular biopsy to determine spermatogenic activity and cannulation of the ductus deferens to determine patency can be performed surgically.

Management

Treatment depends on the cause of the ejaculatory dysfunction. Stallions with musculoskeletal and neurologic disease are treated with appropriate medications and modification of the breeding routine to facilitate stallion comfort. In stallions with ampullary blockage, oxytocin, transrectal ampullary massage, and collection attempts are repeated 2–3 times daily until ejaculation occurs. Retrograde ejaculation may be treated with behavior modification and imipramine.

Prognosis

Ampullary blockage can be difficult to resolve; however, after resolution, stallions return to previous levels of fertility. Blockage may reoccur after periods of sexual rest. In stallions where neurologic or musculoskeletal disease is impairing ejaculation, function is improved by treatment; however, the prognosis for long-term fertility is guarded. TD and aplasia of the excurrent duct system result in infertility.

Congenital abnormalities of the male reproductive tract

Intersexuality

Definition/overview

Several variations of intersexuality occur in the horse. Female pseudohermaphroditism is uncommon. In these cases the gonads are ovaries, the genotype is female (XX), and the external genitalia are male, although often poorly developed and ambiguous. True hermaphroditism, defined as an individual with both male and female gonads, is extremely rare in the horse. Typically, these animals have poorly developed male external genitalia or, occasionally, poorly developed male and female genitalia, an absent scrotum, and retained abdominal ovotestes.

XY sex reversal is the most common intersex condition encountered in the horse. Wide variations in phenotypic appearance have been reported, ranging from nearly normal females with XY karyotype, of which some are fertile, to intersex mares with male gonads, failed or abnormal müllerian duct development, clitoromegaly and virilization.

In a male pseudohermaphrodite (560, 561) the genetic sex is male (XY-SRY negative) while the phenotype is female with small, inactive ovaries and an underdeveloped tubular tract. The condition may be discovered on karyotyping, when reasons for infertility are sought. Another variation of male pseudohermaphroditism is testicular feminization syndrome. In this syndrome the genotype is male (XY) and the external phenotype is female-like. However, the vagina and uterus are absent and the gonads are abdominally retained testes. The animal typically presents as what is believed to be a filly with stallion-like behavior. The external genitalia are abnormal with an increased distance between the anus and vulva and often an enlarged clitoris. The clitoris may engorge and become penile-like on sexual arousal due to the production of androgens by the testes.

Etiology/pathophysiology

It appears likely that more than one mechanism is responsible for these conditions; however, translocation of the SRY gene from the Y chromosome during spermatogenesis is thought to be responsible in most cases. The SRY gene is the sex-determining region of the Y chromosome that controls much of sexual differentiation by coding for testis-determining factors and Sertoli-cell differentiation in the gonads. Absence of this gene in genetic males results in failure of regression of the müllerian ducts, which form the female tubular tract, since müllerian-inhibiting substance is not secreted by the Sertoli cells. In SRY-positive cases of XY sex reversal, failure of androgen receptor expression on target organs may be responsible for the phenotypic female appearance.

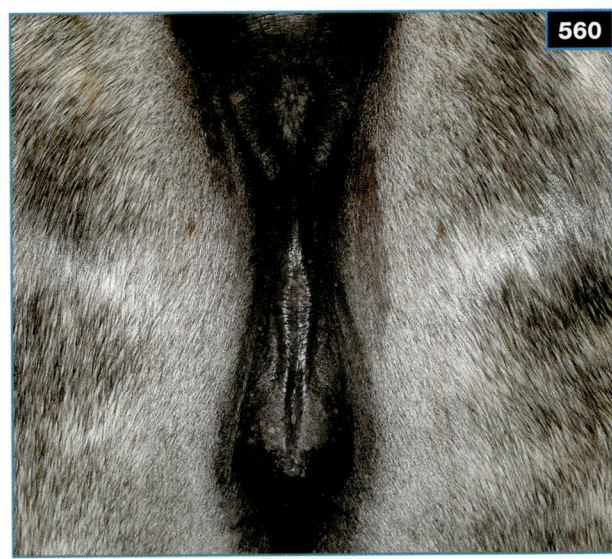

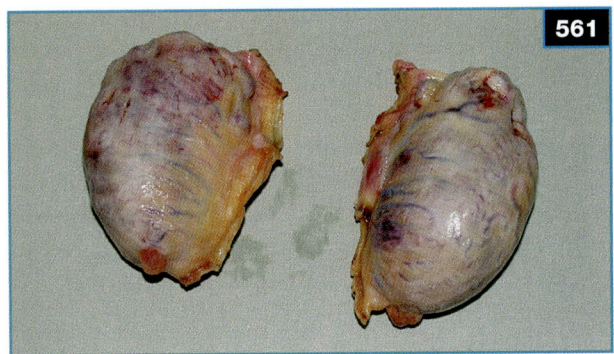

560, 561 View of the external genitalia of a true hermaphrodite (560). The animal presented as a filly with stallion-like behavior. Chromosomal analysis revealed a 64,XY karyotype. Clitoromegaly is often present, but was not seen in this case. A short blind-ending vagina was present. No tubular reproductive structures were identifiable on rectal palpation or ultrasound, but two abdominally retained gonads were found. On histology, these were found to be testes (561).

Diagnosis

Diagnosis of an intersex condition is based on a thorough physical and reproductive examination, as well as cytogenetic analysis.

Management

Surgical removal of retained testes and clitoridectomy should solve behavioral issues and allow the animal to be retained for performance or pleasure purposes.

Prognosis

Affected animals are usually sterile.

345

Cryptorchidism

Definition/overview
Cryptorchidism is failure of normal descent of one or both testes into the scrotal sac. The testis/testes may be located inguinally, abdominally, or subcutaneously outside the scrotum. Testicular descent normally occurs between the last 30 days of gestation and 6 months of age.

Etiology/pathophysiology
The hormonal and physical events leading to testicular descent are not well understood. Elongation of the vaginal process, formed as an outpouching of the peritoneum, occurs due to the pull of the gubernaculum on the tail of the epididymis. Enlargement of the epididymal tail occurs as the fetus grows, resulting in enlargement of the inguinal ring and canal. Traction of the gubernaculum, abdominal pressure, elongation of the vaginal process, and enlargement of the inguinal ring together result in descent of the testis into the scrotum. Fetal gonadal androgen production, müllerian inhibiting substance, and epidermal growth factor probably also play a role in testicular descent. An hereditary component in horses is likely, although the mode of inheritance is disputed. It is possible that more than one genetic mode of inheritance for cryptorchidism exists in the horse. A higher incidence of cryptorchidism occurs in the Standardbred, Quarterhorse, Percheron, Paint Horse, and Welsh Mountain pony than in other breeds.

Clinical presentation
In the case of unilateral cryptorchidism, visual inspection and palpation of the scrotum reveal only one testis. In bilateral cryptorchidism, no testes are palpable within the scrotum, the animal presents with unwanted stallion-like behavior, and it may have been sold as a gelding. Cases of unilateral cryptorchidism with castration of the single scrotal testicle are unfortunately not unusual, and these animals typically present as apparent geldings with stallion-like behavior.

Differential diagnosis
Previous castration of one or both testicles. A true anorchid or monorchid condition can occur, but is very rare.

Diagnosis
Diagnosis is by inspection of the scrotum, and careful palpation together with ultrasonography of the scrotum and inguinal canal. The testis may be retained within the inguinal canal or in the abdomen. Rectal palpation and transrectal/abdominal ultrasonography are useful in locating the retained testis in the abdomen in many cases (562).

Hormonal testing is useful in differentiating bilateral cryptorchidism from previous castration. A serum sample is taken for baseline levels of testosterone and estrogen. If levels are high, testicular tissue is present and no further testing is necessary. If levels are low, a hormonal stimulation test is recommended. Following a serum sample for baseline levels, 5,000–10,000 iu of hCG is administered intravenously. Follow-up samples are recommended 60 minutes, 120 minutes, and 24 hours later. A significant rise (4–5 times) from baseline levels following hCG administration indicates the presence of testicular tissue. An estrogen or estrone sulfate test alone is not recommended for colts less than 3 years of age, or donkeys of any age, as false negatives are common. An hCG stimulation test for both testosterone and estrogen will be more reliable. Due to considerable interlaboratory variation, practitioners should interpret the test using the reference values supplied by their laboratory.

Management
Surgical exploration and removal of the retained testis results in rapid improvement of unwanted stallion-like behavior. The method chosen for surgical removal of the retained testicle depends largely on the location of the testicle and the preference of the surgeon. The most common approaches include the inguinal, parainguinal, and laparoscopic (standing or recumbent) methods:

✦ The *inguinal* approach allows exploration of both the inguinal and abdominal cavities during surgery. With this method, the animal is anesthetized and aseptically prepared. An incision is made either over the scrotal sac or directly over the inguinal ring. The epididymis and/or testicle are located by blunt dissection of the inguinal ring. If the testis in not found, the surgeon places gentle traction on the scrotal ligament (gubernaculum) until the vaginal process is found. The tail of the epididymis is attached to the vaginal process and once found, gentle traction on this structure will expose the testis for removal.

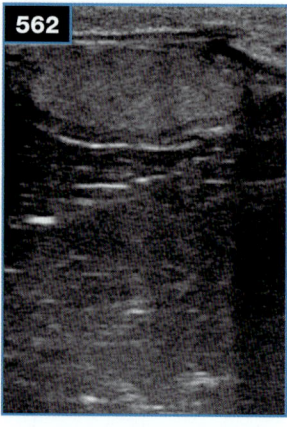

562 Transrectal ultrasound appearance of the retained abdominal testis in a cryptorchid horse.

TABLE 11 Guidelines for total scrotal width by age for light horse stallions

	2–3 YEARS	4–6 YEARS	>7 YEARS
Minimum	81 mm	85 mm	95 mm

TABLE 12 Guidelines for testis length and width for mature light horse stallions

Dimension	Recommended minimum (SD)
Left width	57.8 mm (5.2 mm)
Left length	103.1 mm (8.2 mm)
Right width	55.8 mm (5.8 mm)
Right length	107.5 mm (8 mm)

SD = standard deviation

+ In the *parainguinal* approach, an incision is made several centimeters medial to the inguinal ring. In addition, some surgeons use a pararectal or midline approach in appropriate cases. The surgeon's hand is introduced into the abdomen and the testicle located and removed.
+ If laparoscopic equipment is available, *laparoscopic surgery* may be undertaken. This method has the advantages of reduced patient recovery time, direct visualization of the testicle and any hemorrhage, and closure of the abdominal wall, thereby reducing the chance of postoperative herniation. The procedure can be done on standing, sedated animals or under general anesthesia in dorsal recumbency.

Detailed explanations of surgical methods are available elsewhere, and the reader is referred to surgical textbooks for specific information on these methods.

Prognosis
Exposure of the retained testicle to high temperatures results in increased likelihood of neoplastic transformation. Affected stallions should not be used for breeding purposes due to the hereditary nature of the condition.

Testicular hypoplasia

Definition/overview
Testicular hypoplasia is defined as underdevelopment of one or both testes.

Etiology/pathophysiology
Hypoplasia of the testes is fairly common in the stallion and usually is the result of inherited genetic aberrations or chromosomal defects. The condition may also result from cryptorchidism or exposure to teratogens, toxins, or possibly infections during fetal life. The gonads arise following migration of primordial germ cells from the embryonic yolk sac. Factors that prevent or disrupt this migration, or affect the germinal epithelium following formation of the primitive gonad, lead to testicular hypoplasia.

Clinical presentation
Testicular hypoplasia may be unilateral or bilateral, and ranges from mild to severe. A young stallion with testicular measurements below the minimum recommended for its age may have testicular hypoplasia (*Tables 11* and *12*). Stallions with the condition have small testes, low sperm numbers, poor semen quality, and a history of infertility or subfertility.

Differential diagnosis
The condition must be differentiated from acquired conditions of the testis such as TD. Prepubertal stallions must not be erroneously diagnosed with hypoplastic testicles before growth is complete. Note that it is common during reproductive evaluation of the stallion to observe that one testis (usually the left) is larger than the other.

Diagnosis
Examination of a young, postpubertal stallion with small testes, small epididymides, oligozoospermia or azoospermia, and a history of poor fertility is highly suggestive of testicular hypoplasia. Testicular biopsy may be helpful in confirming the diagnosis (see Testicular degeneration, p. 357).

Management
No effective treatment is known.

Prognosis
Stallions with the condition appear to be predisposed to TD with advancing age. Use of an affected stallion for breeding purposes is discouraged since the condition is likely to be hereditary and often the result of chromosomal aberrations.

Conditions of the penis and prepuce

Phimosis

Definition/overview
Phimosis is the inability of the penis to be exteriorized or protrude from the prepuce.

Etiology/pathophysiology
Normal phimosis occurs in newborn colts whose penis is adhered to the internal prepuce for the first 4–6 weeks of life. Pathologic phimosis occurs most often secondary to swelling and edema following trauma, such as a kick from a mare during breeding (563). Phimosis may also occur with conditions that cause inflammation of the penis, scrotum, and prepuce such as coital exanthema, dourine, and neoplasia. Any animal with significant ventral edema from any cause may have severe edema of the scrotum and prepuce, resulting in prolapse of the internal prepuce and trapping of the penis within the narrowed preputial ring. Once swollen, the effects of gravity worsen the edema and result in more preputial prolapse, swelling, and edema.

Clinical presentation
Careful examination and palpation of the swollen structure reveal that swelling is limited to the prepuce. Digital palpation usually reveals the tip of the penis within the prepuce. If the swelling has been chronic, the skin may be ulcerated, sloughing, or infected.

Differential diagnosis
Swelling and prolapse of the prepuce should be differentiated from involvement of the penis by examination. The cause of the swelling may be unrelated to the penis, prepuce, or scrotum, with the phimosis being secondary.

Management
Edema and swelling are treated by a combination of exercise, hydrotherapy, local massage, anti-inflammatories, and diuretics. Placement of a sling to reduce gravitational effects is helpful in relieving edema (564). Vaseline or other emollient dressings should be applied to help reduce effects on the preputial skin. Diagnosis and treatment of the underlying condition is essential. Rarely, preputial resection (reefing operation) is required to remove permanently diseased tissue.

Prognosis
Phimosis caused by trauma carries a good prognosis. The condition improves quickly following initiation of therapy (565, 566).

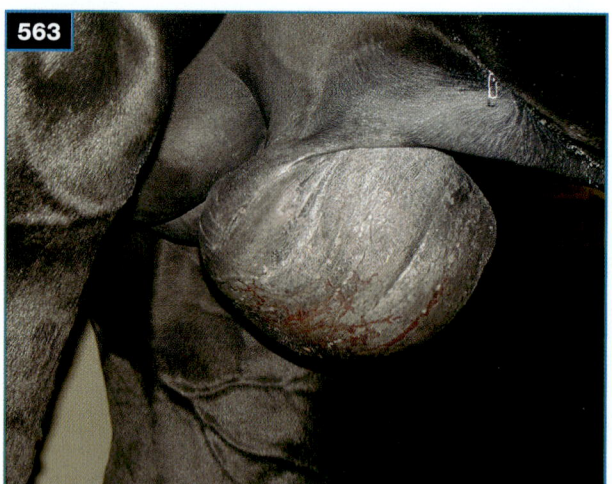

563 Severe preputial swelling and phimosis in a stallion following an accident while mounting a phantom with the artificial vagina affixed inside. The stallion had mounted the phantom aggressively and the prepuce became pinched within the artificial vagina.

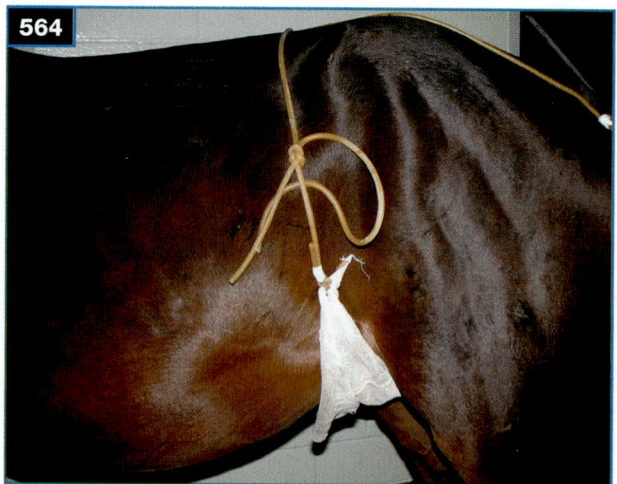

564 Sling applied. The rubber tubing is placed over the back and additional tubing is run between the hindlimbs and tied over the back.

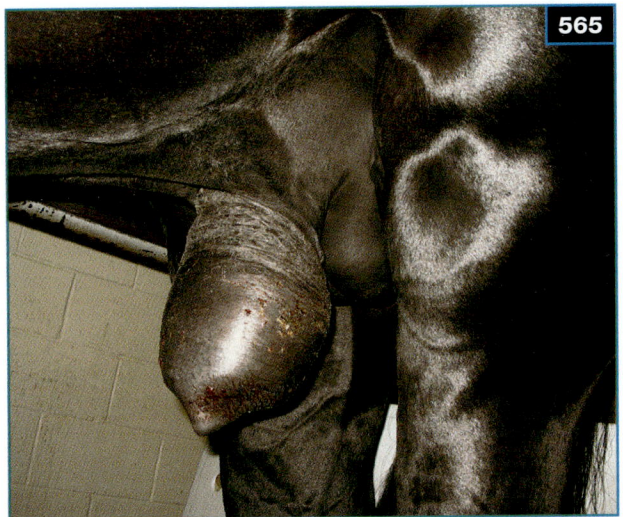

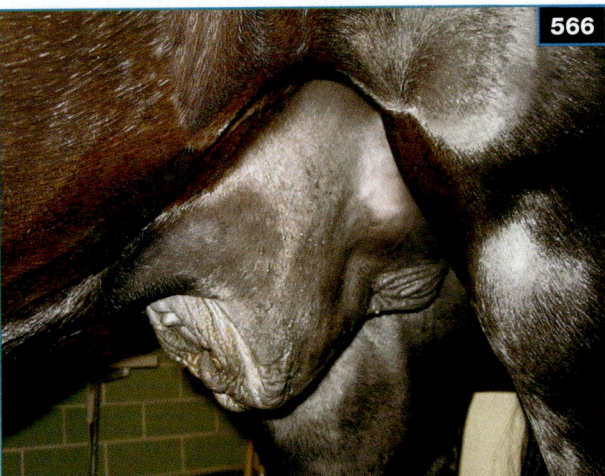

565, 566 Same stallion as in 563, 24 hours after initiation of therapy, which included hydrotherapy, emollients, a support sling, and anti-inflammatories (565). Same stallion 48 hours after initiation of therapy (566).

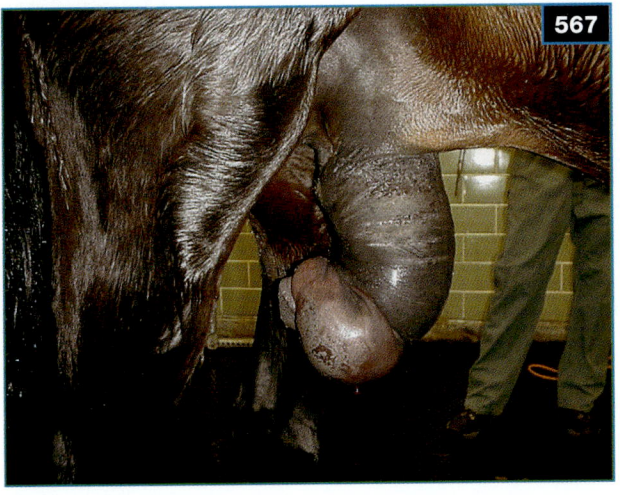

Paraphimosis
Definition/overview
Paraphimosis is the inability of the penis to retract into the prepuce. The effects on penile circulation are rapid and severe. Paraphimosis should be treated as a veterinary emergency.

Etiology/pathophysiology
Paraphimosis may be accompanied by severe preputial edema following trauma. In such cases the rapid swelling of the prepuce prevents the penis from retracting following detumescence. Alternatively, paraphimosis may occur secondary to penile paralysis or priapism (see below). Once prolapsed, a rapid cycle of vascular compromise, edema, and impaired lymphatic drainage ensues. The effects of gravity on the pendulous penis further contribute to this cycle, eventually resulting in necrosis of the skin and gangrene of the penis if left untreated.

Clinical presentation
The animal presents with a prolapsed penis that quickly becomes swollen. In cases of trauma, preputial edema may be also be evident (**567**). Paraphimosis may occur secondary to penile paralysis or priapism following administration of phenothiazine tranquilizers. In these cases, preputial edema is not an initial component of the condition, but may occur over time.

Differential diagnosis
Paraphimosis can be differentiated from simple preputial swelling and prolapse by careful examination of the affected area. A critical evaluation of the history must include previous drug administration.

Diagnosis
Diagnosis is made by identification of the penis outside of the prepuce. This may be more challenging than it appears, particularly when both penis and prepuce are severely swollen and in cases where the penis is only partially prolapsed. Identification of the urethral process is diagnostic.

567 Penile hematoma and paraphimosis in a stallion following a kick from a mare during breeding.

Management

Immediate therapy is required. If the condition is acute, the penis is placed back into the prepuce and retained with an easily fashioned retention device consisting of a cut-off plastic bottle and rubber tubing. The penis is lubricated with vaseline or other emollient dressing and placed within the bottle with the urethral process aligned to the tapered bottle opening, allowing urine to escape via the open bottle cap end. The opposite end of the bottle is lightly padded with tape or foam. The bottle with the penis inside is then gently placed within the preputial cavity and held with the rubber tubing. One set of tubing is passed over the stallion's back and tied, while the other is passed caudally through the hindlimbs and tied dorsally over the back to the first set of tubing. A stallion sling is then placed over the prepuce to ensure proper positioning. The bottle and sling system should be removed twice daily to allow the penis to be inspected and re-lubricated. Alternatively, the penis can be kept within the prepuce using a purse-string suture or clamps placed at the preputial ring. This may require sedation or general anesthesia in the uncooperative animal. If the penis cannot be immediately replaced, it is placed within a sling or similar supportive device to limit the gravitational effects, which will worsen the edema. A combination of manual massage, hydrotherapy, exercise, and anti-inflammatory therapy is indicated. Hydrotherapy should be limited to no more than 20 minutes of cold application per session, repeated every 3–4 hours. Longer application of cold (ice packs, cold hosing) can potentially cause more edema as well as significant damage to the skin and tissues. If gentle massage is not effective in alleviating penile edema enough to allow replacement, pressure wrapping with rubber bandages, beginning at the distal end of the penis, can be used temporarily to reduce edema. In chronic cases the penile skin becomes cracked, oozing, and eventually necrotic and gangrenous. In chronic cases refractory to treatment, partial penile amputation may be required.

Prognosis

The prognosis is dependent on the rapidity with which veterinary treatment is sought and initiated. Preputial and penile dysfunction can occur following successful treatment of prolonged cases due to fibrosis of the skin and damage to the vascular tissues of the penis. Prolonged paraphimosis may also result in nerve damage leading to secondary penile paralysis.

Penile paralysis

Definition/overview

True penile paralysis is an inability to retract the flaccid penis into the prepuce.

Etiology/pathophysiology

Motor innervation of the retractor penis muscle is through the alpha-adrenergic fibers. The most common cause of true penile paralysis in geldings and stallions is the administration of alpha-adrenergic blockers such as the phenothiazine tranquilizers. Other causes of reduced retractor penis muscle tone occur (e.g. spinal disease, myelitis, and exhaustion).

Clinical presentation

The flaccid penis hangs from the preputial cavity. Since lymphatic and venous drainage are disrupted, rapid progression of the condition ensues, with severe penile swelling, skin ulceration, and necrosis.

Differential diagnosis

Paraphimosis; preputial edema; trauma.

Diagnosis

Manual examination reveals a flaccid penis that is often devoid of sensory sensation. Inability to retract the penis during examination is typical.

Management

Initial treatment is as indicated for phimosis and penile and preputial injury and is aimed at reduction of swelling and edema. Placement of the prolapsed, paralyzed penis in a sling apparatus will help to minimize the gravitational effects on circulation. Manual massage may result in sufficient reduction of swelling so that the penis can be replaced in the preputial cavity. Once replaced, the penis may be supported by a sling or a short-term purse-string suture surrounding the preputial opening. If treatment is unsuccessful, phallopexy (penile retraction) or partial phallectomy (penile amputation) is indicated.

Prognosis

The prognosis for return to full breeding capacity is poor.

Priapism

Definition/overview

Priapism is persistent erection, without sexual arousal.

Etiology/pathophysiology

Priapism occurs due to continued filling/engorgement of the corpus cavernosum with blood. Administration of phenothiazine tranquilizers is the primary cause of priapism in stallions and, less commonly, geldings. It is thought that the alpha-adrenergic blocking properties of phenothiazine tranquilizers block the sympathetic nerve pulses that initiate penile detumescence. Once blood flow has been disrupted, a cycle of sludging of blood, edema, thrombosis, and eventually fibrosis occurs. With chronicity, edema and fibrosis further disrupt and occlude blood flow. It has been suggested that exposure of colts to mares following phenothiazine tranquilizer administration increases the risk of priapism.

Clinical presentation

The animal presents following phenothiazine administration with a firm, partially erect penis (568).

Differential diagnosis

The condition must be differentiated from penile paralysis and penile trauma.

Diagnosis

A history of phenothiazine tranquilizer administration is typical and physical findings of a persistent partial erection are diagnostic. Ultrasound imaging of the penis may demonstrate thrombosis.

Management

Early intervention to limit the dependent and gravitational effects, including massage, slings, and emollient dressings, may prevent long-term sequelae if the erection subsides within a few hours. Early administration of benztropine mesylate (8 mg i/v), a ganglionic blocker, has been suggested.

Surgical treatment includes lavage of the corpus cavernosum with heparinized saline to remove sludged blood or intervention to establish vascular shunts between the corpus cavernosum and the corpus spongiosum.

Prognosis

For stallions with priapism that has not resolved quickly, the prognosis is generally poor. Penile amputation may be required.

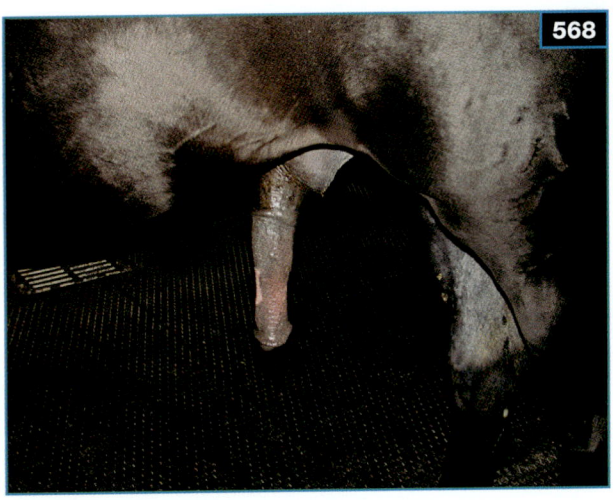

568 Priapism in a stallion. Sustained partial erection following phenothiazine tranquilizer administration.

Penile lacerations/trauma/hematoma

Definition/overview

Trauma to the penis can cause a variable amount of injury, from minor swelling only to significant hematoma of the vascular structures of the penis or open lacerations with severe damage.

Etiology/pathophysiology

Trauma is most commonly caused by a kick from a mare during attempted breeding, when the penis is fully erect and at greatest risk of injury (see 567). Tail hairs from the mare or suture material from a Caslick's stitch may cause laceration of the stallion's penis during breeding. The penis may also suffer trauma during semen collection if the stallion makes forceful thrusts against the phantom before the collector can properly place the artificial vagina. A phantom constructed with the artificial vagina inside predisposes to penile injury during mounting or collection, particularly if the stallion slips and loses footing. Proper construction, maintenance, and use of the phantom are essential for the stallion's safety.

Clinical presentation

In the case of lacerations, blood may be noticed in the semen, dripping from the stallion's penis, or from the mare's vulva after breeding. With blunt force kicks, swelling occurs almost immediately and diagnosis is obvious.

Differential diagnosis

Trauma to the penis must be differentiated from trauma to the prepuce. If the clinical presentation is blood in the ejaculate, a urethral laceration should also be considered a potential cause.

Diagnosis

Thorough examination requires that the stallion's penis is exteriorized, if it is not so already. Determination of the involved structures and severity of injury can then be made.

Management

Penile injuries are emergencies and early treatment is essential for success. Treatment options should be aimed at replacing the penis into the prepuce as soon as possible in order to avoid secondary complications such as paraphimosis. Simple lacerations of the penile skin heal well without suturing if swelling and local infection are controlled. Strict sexual rest is necessary until healing is complete. Deeper lacerations will require general anesthesia and surgical debridement and suturing. Careful evaluation of the extent of the injury is necessary, as deep lacerations may involve the corpus cavernosum and the urethra. Supportive care includes systemic broad-spectrum antibiotics and anti-inflammatory therapy. A significant potential for paraphimosis and/or penile paralysis (see above) exists.

Prognosis

Simple injuries will heal uneventfully with prompt treatment. In more severe cases, recovery is dependent on the severity of the injury and involvement of the corpus cavernosum or urethra. Significant fibrosis can occur following hematoma formation, which may result in penile deviations and incomplete erections.

Smegma accumulation

Definition/overview

Smegma is the foul-smelling accumulation of secretions of the sebaceous and sweat glands of the prepuce. It forms on the penis and, particularly, within the fossa glandis.

Etiology/pathophysiology

Excessive accumulation of smegma may result in irritation and mild balanoposthitis. Significant quantities of the thick, wax-like material may form a 'bean' within the fossa glandis and result in discomfort and difficulty during urination or even ejaculation (569).

Clinical presentation

A foul-smelling odor may be noticed from the stallion's or gelding's sheath or he may experience excessive straining during urination.

Differential diagnosis

Other causes of balanoposthitis, such as excessive force during washing of the penis, use of irritating soaps, or infections such as coital exanthema, should be considered. One of the most common causes of a foul smell from the prepuce is SCC of the penis and/or prepuce.

Diagnosis

Diagnosis is based on observation of the excessive accumulations of the gray to black, thick substance on the penis and prepuce. Examination of the distal penis and exploration of the fossa glandis reveal a 'bean' of smegma, which can be quite large.

Management

Cleaning the penis thoroughly with warm water and cotton before each breeding/collection and periodically throughout the nonbreeding season is recommended. Use of copious amounts of water and limited manual pressure will reduce the irritation caused by washing. Soaps and detergents are not recommended since they may disrupt the normal bacterial flora of the penile and preputial skin, predisposing to growth of pathogenic organisms. If accompanied by balanoposthitis, removal of the irritating smegma is generally an adequate treatment and the irritation resolves spontaneously.

Prognosis

The prognosis is good with good general hygiene.

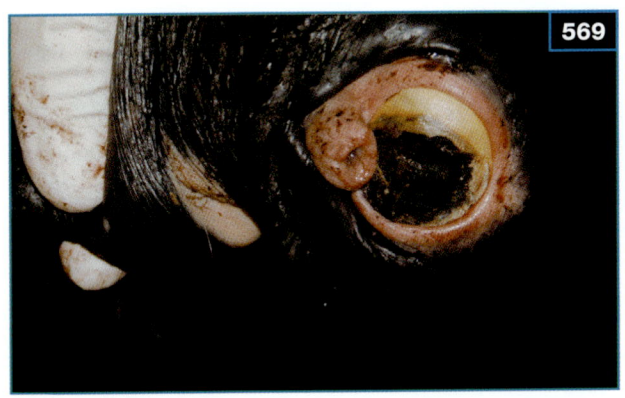

569 Smegma accumulation, also referred to as a 'bean', within the fossa glandis of a gelding that presented with difficulty in passing urine.

Penile deviations

Definition/overview
A penile deviation exists when the erect penis persistently deflects inappropriately, most often laterally or ventrally, making natural breeding difficult.

Etiology/pathophysiology
Deviations are uncommon in the stallion and usually result from fibrosis and adhesions within the vascular structures of the penis following traumatic injury such as penile hematoma. The disruption of normal blood flow to one or more areas of the penis results in incomplete erection, while adhesion formation may result in deviation.

Clinical presentation
A history of penile injury is typical. The stallion may appear normal on physical examination during detumescence. Observation of the stallion during teasing of an estrous mare demonstrates a fully erect penis that deviates to one side or ventrally.

Differential diagnosis
Incomplete erection due to inadequate sexual arousal.

Diagnosis
It is important to perform the examination under optimal conditions with the stallion at the height of sexual arousal and a maximal erection obtained.

Management
If the injury is fairly recent, allowing additional time for healing may result in improvement. Daily manual massage of the erect penis following exposure to an estrous mare and gently directing the penis to its correct position are recommended to help encourage blood flow to the affected areas.

Prognosis
The prognosis is guarded.

Rupture of the penile suspensory ligaments

Definition/overview
The stallion's penis is attached to the ischial symphysis at its base by two short suspensory ligaments, which end continuously with the origin of the gracilis muscle. Rupture of the penile suspensory ligaments is a rare condition, presumably caused by severe trauma, and it results in ventral deviation of the penis.

Etiology/pathophysiology
Severe trauma during breeding results in rupture of the suspensory ligaments. A typical ventral deviation of the penis occurs.

Clinical presentation
Stallions present with severe ventral deviation of the erect penis.

Differential diagnosis
Incomplete erection; ventral deviation due to fibrosis following penile hematoma.

Diagnosis
Diagnosis is based on observation of ventral deviation and ruling out of other causes.

Management
The rarity of the condition makes recommendations for treatment difficult. No reports of surgical correction exist. Affected stallions may respond to pharmacologic ejaculation in order to prolong reproductive usefulness.

Prognosis
The prognosis is guarded.

Conditions of the testes, scrotum, and spermatic cord

Scrotal edema

Definition/overview
Scrotal edema manifests as swelling of the scrotal wall. It may be associated with trauma (**570**), infection, hemorrhage, or other skin conditions such as frostbite.

Etiology/pathophysiology
Damage to the tissues of the scrotal skin or tunica leads to extravasation and accumulation of fluid within the tissue. Uncomplicated scrotal edema may be seen in extremely hot weather; however, the cause is unknown. The insulating effects of scrotal edema will impair proper thermoregulation of the testis and can potentially impact negatively on spermatogenesis.

Clinical presentation
The scrotum may appear to be grossly enlarged and the skin is thickened on palpation. Semen quality is reduced due to effects on thermoregulation, with a reduction in sperm motility and an increase in numbers of morphologically abnormal sperm. Scrotal edema is often seen with scrotal dermatitis. Horses with ventral edema from other causes (e.g. hypoproteinemia) will also have scrotal edema.

Differential diagnosis
Simple scrotal edema must be differentiated from all other causes of scrotal enlargement including intrascrotal hemorrhage, hydrocele, scrotal hernia, neoplasia, and testicular enlargement. Scrotal and ventral edema are classical findings in EVA infection and also in EIA.

Diagnosis
Palpation of the enlarged scrotum reveals thickened skin and difficulty in palpating the underlying testes and epididymides. Scrotal edema is best diagnosed and differentiated from other potential diseases by ultrasonographic examination. A thickened scrotal wall caused by edema of the tissues is characterized by increased thickness of the gray echogenic layer, identifiable as the scrotum and distinct from the testis. Conversely, in cases of intrascrotal hemorrhage or hydrocele, an accumulation of anechoic fluid is typically seen.

Management
Treatment is dependent on the inciting cause. In cases of trauma, systemic anti-inflammatories, diuretics, and cold hydrotherapy are used to combat inflammation and swelling. Care must be taken during hydrotherapy, since excessive cold application can be detrimental to blood flow and tissue and skin health, and also impact on spermatogenesis. Cold therapy should be limited to no more than 15–20 minute sessions every 2 hours. Gentle massage of the scrotum is also effective at improving blood flow and reducing edema of the tissues.

Prognosis
The prognosis is good for complete recovery providing the inciting cause is treated appropriately.

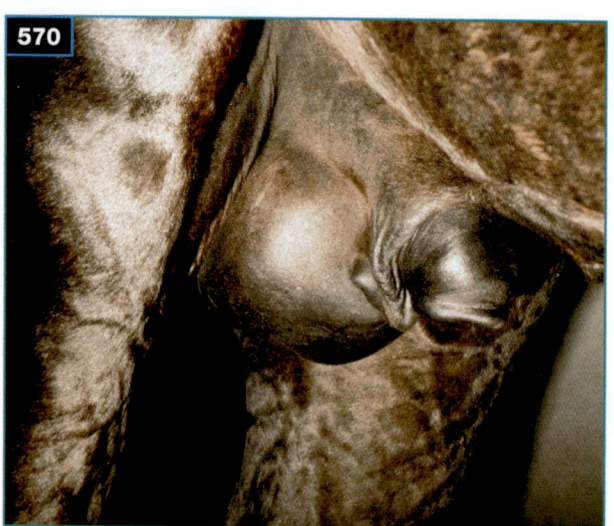

570 Swelling of the scrotal wall, which was associated with trauma from a kick by a mare.

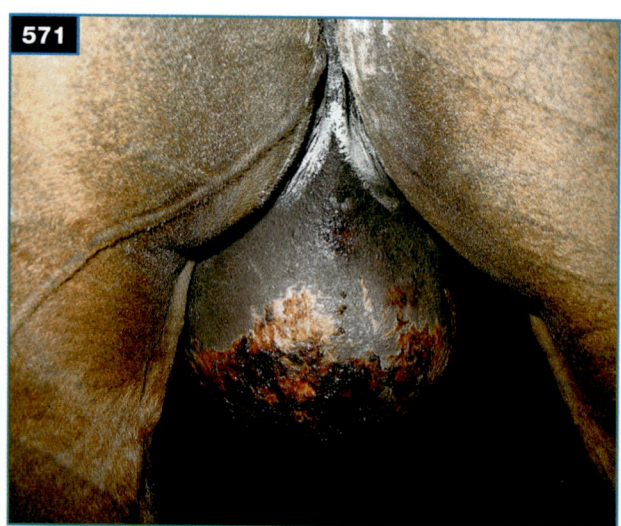

571 Stallion with severe scrotal cellulitis following a kick from a mare.

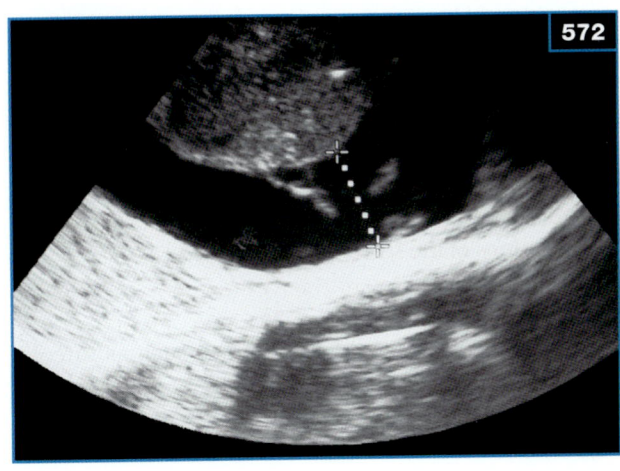

572 Ultrasound examination of the scrotum of a horse that had sustained a kick to this area. Note the presence of hypoechoic fluid (blood) between the parietal and visceral vaginal tunics (hematocele). The testis has not ruptured.

Scrotal and testicular trauma

Definition/overview
Direct trauma to the scrotum can lead to lacerations, edema, intrascrotal hemorrhage, and testis rupture.

Etiology/pathophysiology
Most cases of scrotal and testicular trauma occur during breeding (570, 571) or are due to other severe trauma such as a failed attempt to jump a fence.

Clinical presentation
The amount of swelling depends on the severity of injury. If lacerations are present, the stallion may present with swelling and hemorrhage from the area.

Differential diagnosis
All causes of scrotal swelling including scrotal edema, scrotal hernia, orchitis, testicular torsion, hydrocele, and peritonitis.

Diagnosis
Diagnosis is obvious if there is an accompanying history of a breeding accident or other known trauma. In cases where the origin of the scrotal swelling is unknown, diagnosis is made by thorough examination to rule out all other potential causes of scrotal swelling. Ultrasound examination can be used to determine the severity of injury, the amount of blood accumulation, and whether testis rupture may have occurred (572).

Management
Scrotal trauma should be treated as an emergency since the future reproductive life of the stallion is at stake. Supportive therapy is as for scrotal edema (see above). If ultrasound examination suggests rupture of the testis from the tunica albuginea or significant blood clots are found, surgical exploration is suggested. Lacerations in the tunic should be sutured separately, and fibrinous adhesions and blood clots can be removed at this time. If the affected testis is injured significantly, unilateral castration is recommended as the best option to save the contralateral testis. If the injury is accompanied by laceration, surgical debridement and primary closure should be attempted. Severe swelling is typical following trauma to the scrotum and this significantly complicates wound healing. Systemic antibiotics are recommended, especially when there is significant hematocele, and systemic NSAIDs help control pain and inflammation. The potential for extension of existing scrotal infection to the peritoneal space should not be overlooked.

Prognosis
Effects on spermatogenesis are significant, with an increase in morphologically abnormal sperm occurring within days of injury. Azoospermia may occur about 2–4 weeks post injury. Adhesions may develop between the testis and scrotum, resulting in permanent effects on thermoregulation and spermatogenesis. However, following therapy the affected testis may slowly return to normal size and function 2–5 months following the injury.

Scrotal infection

Definition/overview
Scrotal infection is defined as a bacterial infection of the scrotal sac and/or skin.

Etiology/pathophysiology
Scrotal infection generally follows scrotal trauma, but it can also occur secondary to peritonitis.

Clinical presentation
Stallions with infection of the scrotal sac present with an enlarged, swollen scrotum and pyrexia. History may include trauma or exposure to a mare for breeding. Cases caused by extension of peritonitis into the scrotal sac may present with depression and colic.

Differential diagnosis
All other causes of scrotal enlargement including scrotal edema, scrotal hernia, orchitis, testicular torsion, and hydrocele.

Diagnosis
Diagnosis is obvious when infection is preceded by trauma with or without laceration. Ultrasound examination of the scrotum will demonstrate scrotal edema and pockets of fluid accumulation. Abdominocentesis, a CBC, and fibrinogen estimation should be performed.

Management
Broad-spectrum systemic antibiotics and anti-inflammatories are aimed at controlling the infection and inflammation. Chronic open wounds that do not involve the tunica albuginea should be debrided and lavaged with copious amounts of sterile saline under general anesthesia. Such wounds are best left open to allow drainage.

Prognosis
If the infection can be controlled and it has not extended into the peritoneal cavity or the testis itself, the prognosis is good.

Scrotal dermatitis

Definition/overview
Scrotal dermatitis manifests as injury and inflammation of the scrotal skin.

Etiology/pathophysiology
The scrotal skin is delicate and prone to irritation from foreign substances such as leg paints, fly sprays, alcohol, and soaps. Almost any chemical has the potential to cause contact dermatitis of the scrotal skin. Overly aggressive cold application in cases of scrotal trauma can cause dermatitis. Even slight thickening of the scrotal skin due to dermatitis and its accompanying edema impacts on testis thermoregulation and spermatogenesis. Chronic scrotal dermatitis can cause subfertility and infertility of stallions.

Clinical presentation
The clinical appearance depends on the cause. Slight thickening of the scrotal skin and edema, along with visible lesions of the scrotal skin, are typical.

Differential diagnosis
The presence of other skin conditions such as sarcoid, frostbite, onchocerciasis, habronemiasis, or SCC should be investigated.

Diagnosis
The many potential reasons for dermatitis are best investigated by skin biopsy.

Management
Treatment involves removal of the inciting cause if possible. Onchocerciasis can be treated by administration of ivermectin, which may result in transient worsening of the scrotal edema due to tissue reaction from dying microfilaria. Sarcoids may be surgically excised if they are not extensive.

Prognosis
The prognosis is guarded to poor. Recurrence of sarcoids is common.

Orchitis/epididymitis

Definition/overview
Orchitis/epididymitis is inflammation of the testicle and/or epididymis, causing testicular enlargement.

Etiology/pathophysiology
Orchitis may be bacterial, viral, parasitic, or autoimmune in origin. Bacterial orchitis may be blood borne or caused by ascending or descending infections. Penetrating foreign bodies may cause bacterial orchitis and/or abscessation. Viral causes include EVA, EIA, and influenza. Migration of strongyle larvae has been associated with orchitis. Primary bacterial epididymitis is rare.

Clinical presentation
The affected testicle is painful, hot, and swollen. Orchitis is often accompanied by epididymitis and funiculitis. Signs of systemic illness such as pyrexia, depression, and colic may be seen. A CBC reveals leukocytosis and hyperfibrinogenemia. Semen analysis demonstrates leukocytes within the semen. Chronic epididymitis may be associated with abscessation and the formation of adhesions.

Differential diagnosis

All other causes of scrotal and testicular enlargement should be considered including trauma, torsion, hematocele, neoplasia, and hernia.

Diagnosis

Diagnosis is based on a typical clinical picture and findings on physical examination as described above. Ultrasonography of the affected testicle reveals reduced echogenicity of the testicular parenchyma. Scrotal edema may also be present.

Management

Unilateral castration is recommended if the condition is limited to one testicle. This increases the chances of retaining fertility in the remaining testicle. Systemic antibiotics are chosen according to sensitivity results on culture of the causative organism. Systemic anti-inflammatories and cold hydrotherapy are used to control inflammation and swelling.

Prognosis

If the condition is bilateral, the prognosis for future fertility is poor. In cases of unilateral orchitis, the prognosis for the remaining testicle is guarded to good provided therapy is initiated quickly. Damage to the testis tissues may allow the formation of antisperm antibodies and subsequent formation of sperm granulomas and TD.

Testicular degeneration

Definition/overview

TD refers to the syndrome of progressive decline in fertility of the stallion accompanied by decreasing testicular size and semen quality.

Etiology/pathophysiology

The cause of TD may be idiopathic or known. Examples of conditions that may result in TD are advanced age, neoplasia, testicular trauma, thermal injury, toxins, radiation, administration of androgens or other hormones, nutritional imbalance, vascular lesions, and autoimmune diseases. In idiopathic TD an identifiable cause is not known. Some breeds or family lines within breeds appear to be predisposed to TD. At the cellular level, injury causes degeneration of the seminiferous epithelium of the tubules within the testicle, resulting in disturbances of spermatogenesis. Degeneration may be focal or widespread, unilateral or bilateral.

Clinical presentation

Initially, an increased testicular size and softness may be noted, but with progression of the disease the affected testicle(s) become(s) small and firm, with obvious wrinkling of the tunica albuginea. Semen analysis demonstrates reduced sperm numbers, decreased motility and sperm longevity, and an increase in abnormal morphology. A coincidental drop in fertility is noted.

Differential diagnosis

Testicular hypoplasia; testicular neoplasm.

Diagnosis

The history of a stallion affected by TD typically includes a progressive decline in fertility and a suspicion of poor sperm longevity. Palpation of the scrotum reveals the characteristic wrinkled tunic and small, firm testicles in advanced disease. Ultrasonography of the testicles can be normal or demonstrate increased echogenicity of the testicular parenchyma due to fibrosis and calcification in the tubules. A spermiogram demonstrates low numbers of motile, morphologically normal sperm. In advanced cases, total azoospermia may be present. Round cells (immature spermatids) may be found in the semen sample. Baseline serum samples (use the mean of several daily samples taken at the same time each day) are tested for FSH, LH, estrogens, testosterone, and inhibin. The typical hormonal profile includes high FSH, low estrogen and inhibin, and normal to low levels of LH and testosterone. Estrogen values <124 pg/ml suggest irreversible damage to the seminiferous epithelium. An hCG stimulation test may be useful to determine the ability of the testicle to respond to LH stimulation. Two serum samples are taken 60 and 30 minutes prior to injection of 10,000 iu of hCG and follow-up samples are taken at 30-minute intervals for 3 hours. Stallions with TD typically have lower estrogen and testosterone levels following injection of hCG than normal stallions.

Testicular biopsy will provide a definitive diagnosis. There is mixed evidence regarding the risk of potential for further damage to the already compromised testicle following testicular biopsy. Initial studies in the bovine demonstrated detrimental effects of the open biopsy procedure on spermatogenesis. However, several studies in stallions have demonstrated no gross or histologic evidence of complications to either an open method biopsy or split needle (Biopty gun) method. Testicular biopsy must be performed under strict aseptic conditions.

In cases where it is desirable to biopsy a distinct lesion, ultrasound guidance is used to direct the biopsy. To perform an incisional or open-method biopsy, the patient is placed under general anesthesia. The advantages of incisional biopsy are precise control over the location and size of the biopsy and freedom from artifacts. The disadvantages include potential for adhesions between the skin and testis. This risk is minimized by keeping the incisions as small as possible and by careful suturing.

A needle punch biopsy instrument (e.g. a Tru-Cut needle) may be used to obtain testicular tissue. In most cases general anesthesia will be required, but heavy sedation may be used depending on the stallion's temperament. A very small (0.5 cm) incision is made in the scrotal skin, through which the biopsy needle is introduced. The needle is directed to the center of the testis and the cutting method employed. The advantages of the Tru-Cut method are its ease of use and good correlation of results with the open biopsy method in studies to date. However, the nature of the method carries the potential for significant damage to the testis. In some studies the damage was permanent. In addition, in some studies the amount of tissue obtained was insufficient for histologic evaluation. More recently, a split-needle spring loaded Biopty instrument has been employed for testicular biopsy and has shown good results. This method is less painful and can often be performed on the standing, heavily sedated stallion. The scrotum should be prepared as for aseptic surgery. A bleb of local anesthetic is placed under the scrotal skin in the center of the craniolateral quarter of the testis. A small stab incision is made with a scalpel blade in the scrotal skin. While the testis is held down into the scrotum, the instrument, consisting of a sterile 14 gauge split needle and the spring-loaded Biopty gun, is passed through the incision and placed onto the tunica vaginalis of the testis. The Biopty instrument is fired to obtain the testicular sample. The needle is withdrawn and the skin incision sutured with fine absorbable suture if desired. The advantages of the Biopty technique are the good size of core tissue obtained for histopathology and the relative ease of the procedure. Studies performed to date have not demonstrated any complications on spermatogenesis following the procedure.

Biopsy specimens should be handled very carefully and preferably fixed in Bouin's solution. Histopathology typically reveals a generalized loss of germinal cells, mineralization, vacuolation, and thickening of the basement membrane of the seminiferous tubules. In advanced cases, Sertoli and Leydig cells may also be lost.

Management
Removal of the cause when known may result in partial or complete restoration of fertility, depending on the severity of injury to the seminiferous epithelium. Treatment of idiopathic TD is controversial and has been met with limited success. GnRH injections using subcutaneous pumps are the most widely employed therapy; however, this is time and labor intensive and results are inconclusive.

Prognosis
Most stallions with TD are found to progressively decline in fertility, and some eventually become azoospermic. Breeding management should aim to reduce the number of mares bred per season. Careful monitoring of mares ensures breeding close to ovulation, thus maximizing the chances of conception. Continual monitoring of testicular size and character and monitoring the spermiogram will assist the stallion manager in optimizing the fertility of a stallion with TD.

Torsion of the spermatic cord
Definition/overview
In cases of torsion of the spermatic cord, the cord rotates along the longitudinal axis. The condition may be referred to as testicular torsion.

Etiology/pathophysiology
The orientation of the testis of the stallion in a horizontal fashion within the scrotum is thought to predispose to more frequent spermatic cord torsion compared with many other species. The factors allowing torsion to occur are, however, not understood. The spermatic cord includes the vas deferens, the pampiniform plexus, and muscular and nerve components. Torsion of the cord more than 180° rapidly leads to venous congestion, interference with arterial blood supply, and, as a consequence, detrimental effects on the testis.

Clinical presentation
A 360° torsion of the spermatic cord is usually unilateral and presents with acute severe colic signs, scrotal enlargement, and reluctance to move. A partial rotation of 180° is most often an incidental finding on reproductive evaluation. Such rotations are transient and may recur in the same individual. 180° torsions are not accompanied by pain and have no effect on semen quality.

Differential diagnosis
Inguinal/scrotal hernia; testicular neoplasm; epididymitis/orchitis; trauma; hematocele.

Diagnosis

A 180° torsion is readily diagnosed by palpation of the tail of the epididymis and its associated caudal ligament at the cranial pole of the testicle instead of at its normal location at the caudal pole. In a 360° torsion the tail of the epididymis and caudal ligament are in their usual location; however, the caudal pole of the testis and the tail of the epididymis may be pulled dorsally due to the torsion of the cord. Unilateral scrotal enlargement and pain, accompanied by a thickened, firm, painful spermatic cord, are highly suggestive of cord torsion. Rectal palpation may reveal a thickened, painful spermatic cord within the vaginal ring.

Management

Cord rotation of 180° does not require any treatment. Torsions of more than 180° accompanied by clinical signs of pain and swelling require immediate surgical intervention. The affected testis cannot usually be saved and unilateral castration is recommended. The spermatic cord should be removed proximal to the origin of the torsion.

Prognosis

The prognosis for future fertility of the remaining testis is good provided the condition is recognized and treated rapidly before thermal, ischemic, or immunologic compromise of the unaffected testis occurs.

Varicocele

Definition/overview

A varicocele is an abnormal distension and tortuosity of the veins of the pampiniform plexus within the spermatic cord.

Etiology/pathophysiology

Varicocele is associated with infertility and reduction in semen quality in both men and rams; however, its effect on reproduction in stallions is not known. Effects on fertility are postulated to be the result of inadequate cooling via the pampiniform plexus. Varicoceles are thought to arise from defects in the valves of the spermatic veins or from defects in the fascia surrounding the veins.

Clinical presentation

Varicoceles may be visible by inspection of the neck of the scrotum. Palpation of the spermatic cord reveals a lumpy texture.

Differential diagnosis

Neoplasia of the spermatic cord; cord torsion; funiculitis.

Diagnosis

Ultrasonographic imaging and Doppler examination of the affected cord are diagnostic.

Management

Since there is no clear evidence for a detrimental effect in the stallion, no treatment is currently recommended if semen quality and fertility are good. Unilateral orchidectomy is the only definitive treatment.

Prognosis

The prognosis is good if semen quality and fertility are good.

Funiculitis of the spermatic cord

Definition/overview

Funiculitis is inflammation of the spermatic cord, also known as scirrhous cord.

Etiology/pathophysiology

Funiculitis is most frequently a complication of castration. Other rare causes in intact stallions include trauma, foreign body, neoplasia, orchitis, and strongyle larvae migration.

Clinical presentation

The affected animal presents with swelling of the spermatic cord. If the history includes recent castration, there may be drainage of purulent material from the scrotum and pyrexia. Excessive granulation tissue with chronic infection can result in the formation of a very large cord stump (scirrhous cord). Intact stallions with funiculitis present with a swollen, firm cord and testicular enlargement if funiculitis is an extension of orchitis/epididymitis.

Differential diagnosis

Spermatic cord torsion; spermatic cord neoplasia; varicocele.

Diagnosis

Diagnosis is based on history and clinical signs.

Management

Post-castration funiculitis requires surgical excision, often with the incision left open for drainage. Postoperative antibiotics, anti-inflammatories, walking exercise, and wound cleaning are important. Treatment and prognosis for funiculitis accompanying trauma or orchitis/epididymitis are detailed in the corresponding sections.

Prognosis

The prognosis is good. Recovery may be prolonged in cases where there is considerable surgical dissection and tissue removal.

Hydrocele

Definition/overview

Hydrocele is an accumulation of fluid within the vaginal cavity, between the visceral and parietal layers of the vaginal tunic.

Etiology/pathophysiology

The vaginal tunic secretes a serous fluid to lubricate the vaginal cavity, allowing movement of the testicle within the scrotum for optimal thermoregulation. Normally the fluid is reabsorbed by the lymphatic vessels of the spermatic cord. Any condition causing increased fluid secretion or decreased absorption will result in hydrocele. Causes include inflammatory and noninflammatory conditions (e.g. trauma, neoplasia, orchitis, and extreme hot weather), but the condition is often idiopathic. Since the vaginal cavity communicates with the peritoneal cavity, peritonitis or ascites can also cause hydrocele. Chronic or severe hydrocele can impact on fertility due to the insulating effect of the fluid and the subsequent effect on spermatogenesis.

Clinical presentation

Affected stallions present with unilateral or bilateral painless scrotal enlargement.

Differential diagnosis

All other causes of scrotal enlargement should be considered including cord torsion, trauma, hematocele, scrotal hernia, and neoplasia.

Diagnosis

Palpation of hydrocele is reminiscent of palpating a bag of fluid. The testes and epididymides may not be palpable if there is considerable fluid accumulation. Ultrasound examination reveals anechoic or hypoechoic fluid accumulation between the testis and scrotal skin. An aseptic technique can be used to obtain a sample of the fluid for cytologic analysis and in hydrocele, an amber-colored sterile transudate (low cellularity) fluid is obtained.

Management

In cases of idiopathic hydrocele, drainage of the fluid is not usually effective, as it recurs quickly. Moderate exercise may be helpful. Anti-inflammatory therapy and diuretics are generally of limited value. Most cases of idiopathic hydrocele will resolve spontaneously. Chronic hydrocele can be treated by unilateral orchidectomy of the affected side.

Prognosis

The prognosis is guarded and is dependent on resolution of the inciting cause. Most cases of idiopathic hydrocele will resolve spontaneously.

Scrotal and inguinal hernia

Definition/overview

Scrotal and inguinal hernia involves herniation of intestine and/or mesentery through the inguinal canal, via the inguinal ring, into the vaginal cavity. When the herniation extends into the scrotum, the condition is termed scrotal hernia. If the intestine has penetrated the vaginal tunic, as may occur in the male foal during parturition, the condition is termed a ruptured inguinal/scrotal hernia.

Etiology/pathophysiology

Inguinal hernias commonly occur congenitally in foals as a result of a large inguinal ring, allowing intestine to enter the vaginal sac. The condition may be hereditary and can be unilateral or bilateral (573). Inguinal/scrotal hernias in the adult stallion are generally considered acquired. Affected stallions often have large inguinal rings palpable on rectal examination, which is thought to predispose to the condition. Standardbred, Saddlebred, and Tennessee Walker horses appear to be at greatest risk. Acquired herniation may be the result of increased abdominal pressure during falls, trauma, breeding, or exercise.

Clinical presentation

Foals with congenital scrotal/inguinal hernias present with unilateral or bilateral, soft, nonpainful inguinal or scrotal enlargement at or soon after birth. Palpation of the inguinal region or scrotum reveals crepitation consistent with gas in the herniated intestine. Rarely, these hernias may become incarcerated and present with signs of pain.

Acquired scrotal/inguinal hernias usually present as severe, acute colic due to incarceration of the intestine, often accompanied by scrotal enlargement (574). On rectal examination, distended bowel can be felt entering the inguinal ring.

Differential diagnosis

All other causes of scrotal enlargement should be considered including torsion of the spermatic cord, orchitis, and trauma.

Diagnosis

Ultrasound imaging confirms the diagnosis, as bowel is visualized within the scrotum.

Management

Affected foals should be monitored for evidence of incarceration of herniated bowel. Some hernias will self-correct before 3–6 months of age. Manual reduction of the hernia with the foal in dorsal recumbency, and application of a support wrap (changed every few days) may result in resolution within 2 weeks. If manual reduction is not possible, a ruptured hernia is likely or the hernia becomes incarcerated, and surgical or laparoscopic reduction is required.

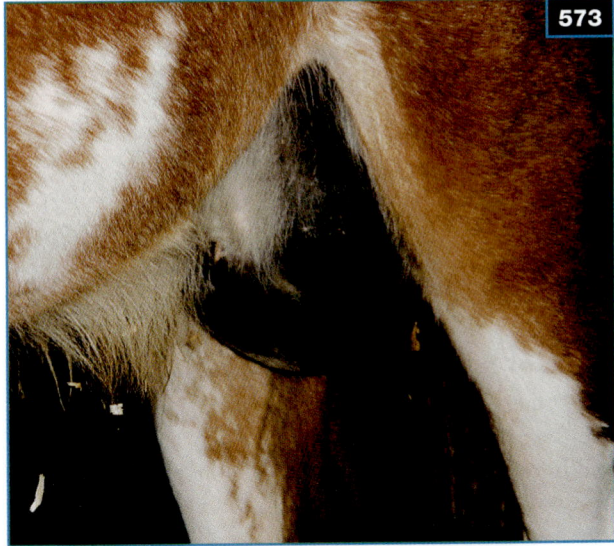

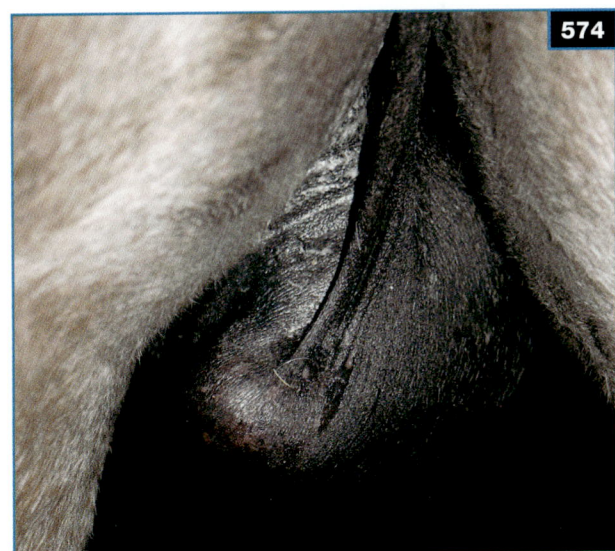

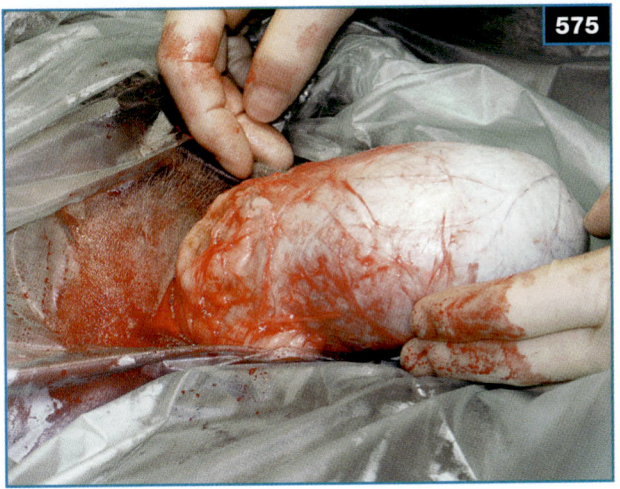

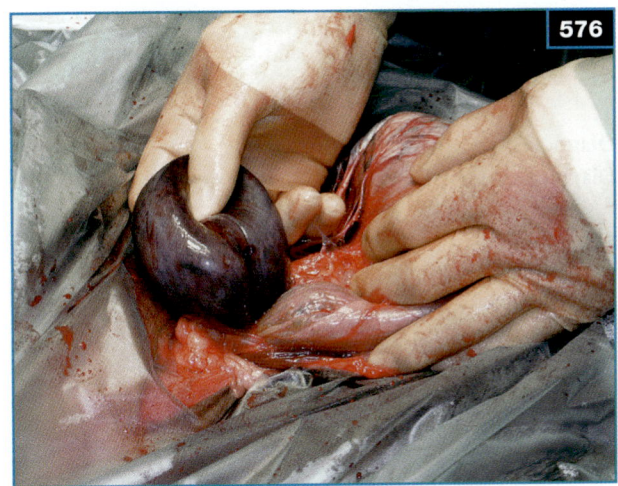

573 Bilateral congenital inguinal/scrotal hernia in a young Clydesdale colt. Scrotal palpation revealed loops of bowel within the scrotal sac, which could be manipulated temporarily back into the abdomen.

574 A 3-year-old Arab colt showing colic and an enlarged, painful right testicle (caudal view).

575, 576 Same colt as in 574. Note the enlarged vaginal sac as it is removed from an inguinal incision (575). An incision through the parietal vaginal tunic revealed a small loop of jejunum that had been trapped and strangulated through the inguinal canal in the vaginal sac. This was manipulated back into the abdomen and resected via a separate midline laparotomy incision (576). The colt was castrated and the superficial inguinal ring closed by interrupted sutures.

Stallions with acquired inguinal/scrotal hernias are treated as emergency surgical colic cases. In affected animals the intestines quickly become severely compromised, requiring resection and anastomosis (575, 576). The testis on the affected side of the hernia is often devitalized due to compression of the spermatic cord by the herniated intestine. Unilateral castration is required in these cases. The inguinal rings are sutured closed to prevent recurrence.

Prognosis

Inguinal hernias may resolve spontaneously in the newborn foal within 4–6 months. Acquired inguinal/scrotal hernias carry a guarded to poor prognosis unless diagnosed and treated rapidly.

Sperm granuloma

Definition/overview

Granulomatous inflammatory reaction results in accumulation of cells into variably sized masses in the epididymis.

Etiology/pathophysiology

Sperm that have escaped the seminiferous tubules, excurrent ducts, or eipididymis are highly antigenic, resulting in a granulomatous reaction around them.

Clinical presentation

The history of an affected stallion may include scrotal trauma, infection, laceration, or orchitis/epididymitis. Palpation of the scrotum reveals single or multiple firm nodules of variable size in the region of the head, body, or tail of the epididymis. Sperm granulomas can cause complete obstruction of the epididymal lumen, resulting in azoospermia.

Differential diagnosis

Neoplasia; epididymal cysts.

Diagnosis

Diagnosis is based on history, clinical signs and biopsy.

Management

There is no known treatment for sperm granulomas. Complete obstructions do not generally change with time.

Prognosis

The prognosis is poor.

Spermiostasis

Definition/overview

Spermiostasis is abnormal sperm accumulation in the efferent ducts, ampullae, and epididymides during sexual rest.

Etiology/pathophysiology

Spermatogenesis continually produces new sperm in an assembly-line fashion. Transit time through the epididymis takes approximately 7.5–11 days. In normal stallions, sperm are stored in the tail of the epididymis for only short periods of time and removed during ejaculation or masturbation. Senescent sperm are also removed in the tail of the epididymis by phagocytosis. Stallions prone to spermiostasis appear to have difficulty with the normal transit and emission of sperm from the epididymis, allowing sperm to accumulate there despite ejaculation. The physiologic reasons behind this condition are not known. Occasionally, spermatozoa may accumulate in the distal ductus deferens and form obstructive plugs, leading to ampullary gland obstruction.

Clinical presentation

Affected stallions appear to ejaculate normally, but have reduced sperm motility.

Differential diagnosis

Other conditions causing alterations to sperm morphology such as TD.

Diagnosis

An ejaculate typical of spermiostasis contains a large number of tailless heads when sperm morphology is examined. These changes to the spermiogram reflect the large number of degenerative, retained sperm in the ejaculate. The stallion may produce extremely large numbers of sperm on some occasions (e.g. 30 billion) and semen of unusually high sperm concentration (>500 million/ml). Sperm and epithelial cell debris may form casts in the ejaculate.

Management

Stallions are best managed by increasing the frequency of breeding or collection to avoid spermiostasis during the breeding season, even if semen is not required. Several ejaculations over a relatively short period of time may be required to return semen quality to acceptable levels in affected stallions. The stallion's frequent collection schedule should be resumed at least 2–3 weeks in advance of the next breeding season to ensure that the semen quality is acceptable prior to the arrival of the first mares of the year.

Prognosis

The prognosis is good.

Oligospermia/azoospermia

Definition/overview

Oligospermia is reduced numbers of sperm in the ejaculate. Azoospermia is complete absence of sperm in the ejaculate. True azoospermia must be differentiated from failure to ejaculate.

Etiology/pathophysiology

Causes include frequent ejaculation, obstruction of the passage of sperm (e.g. ampullary obstruction or sperm granuloma), and decreased spermatogenesis due to disease (e.g. TD).

Clinical presentation

Repeated ejaculations demonstrating below normal levels of sperm for the season of the year confirm oligospermia. In the height of the breeding season (May and June in the northern hemisphere), the total number of sperm in the ejaculate should be >2.0–2.2 billion. In the nonbreeding season (September to January in the northern hemisphere) the total number of sperm should be >1 billion.

Careful observation during breeding or collection will confirm ejaculation has occurred. The tail flag can be visualized, and urethral pulsations can be felt with the hand on the ventral aspect of the base of the penis.

Differential diagnosis
Incomplete or failed ejaculation.

Diagnosis
AP is produced in several locations within the male reproductive tract, with the highest production in the tail of the eipididymis and testicle. Therefore, evaluation of AP levels of the semen of a stallion with no sperm will differentiate between azoospermia and failed ejaculation. The normal AP level in pre-ejaculatory fluid is 10–90 IU/l. AP levels in ejaculatory fluid should be in the range of 1,600–50,000 IU/l. A stallion with apparent azoospermia and AP levels in the pre-ejaculatory range has failed to ejaculate. A stallion with apparent azoospermia and AP levels in the ejaculatory range can be considered truly azoospermic. Stallions with bilateral ampullary obstruction will also have AP levels consistent with the pre-ejaculatory fluid range.

Management
Treatment depends on the cause of the oligospermia or azoospermia. If oligospermia is caused by overuse, careful consideration as to the number of mares that can be bred should resolve the problem. Oligospermia caused by TD is best managed by reduction in the size of the stallion's book. (See Ampullary gland obstruction [p. 364] for a discussion of treatment for this condition.)

Prognosis
The prognosis is guarded depending on the cause.

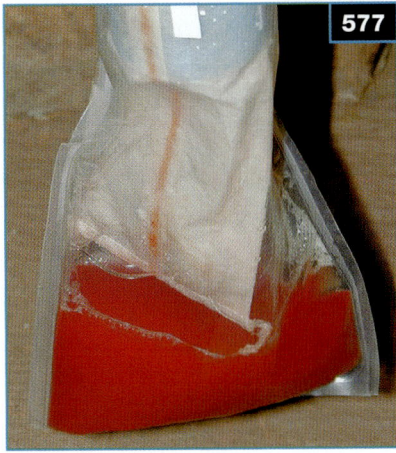

577 Semen collected from a stallion with hemospermia. A urethral laceration was identified by urethroscopy.

Hemospermia
Definition/overview
Hemospermia is the presence of blood in the semen (577).

Etiology/pathophysiology
Blood in the semen may arise from wounds or lesions (habronemiasis or EHV) on the surface of the penis, ulcerations of the penile urethra or urethral process, infections of the accessory glands, urethritis, urolithiasis, varicosities, orchitis/epididymitis, and neoplasia.

Clinical presentation
Blood may be seen dripping from the end of the penis or from the mare's vulva following breeding. Alternatively, a red or brownish discoloration of the semen following collection may be seen. Since hemospermia is associated with reduced fertility, the presenting complaint may include reduced pregnancy rates.

Differential diagnosis
Several conditions as noted above can cause hemospermia. Blood observed following natural cover may originate from the mare, not the stallion. Therefore, the mare should also be examined carefully.

Diagnosis
Since several conditions can be responsible for hemospermia, a thorough examination is imperative. Collection via an artificial vagina and cytologic examination of the semen will confirm the presence of blood versus inflammatory cells, or both, in the ejaculate. Examination should include inspection of the erect penis and urethral process. Urethroscopy using a flexible fiberoptic endoscope can be performed to identify urethral erosions or ulcerations, which are most commonly found at the level of the ischial arch.

Management
Treatment depends on the source of the bleeding. Most surface lesions of the penis heal uneventfully. Infections of the accessory glands are difficult to treat and carry a guarded prognosis. Strict sexual rest is required to allow urethral ulcerations and penile lesions to heal. Generally, 8–12 weeks of rest is recommended. Urethral ulcerations may recur even following prolonged sexual rest. Temporary perineal urethrotomy may assist in healing of these recurrent lesions. Systemic antibiotics and a course of anti-inflammatories are useful adjunctive therapies.

Prognosis
The prognosis is guarded depending on the source of bleeding and extent of the injury/infection.

Urospermia

Definition/overview
Urospermia is the presence of urine in the semen.

Etiology/pathophysiology
The smooth muscles of the bladder neck contract during ejaculation to prevent simultaneous urination. Any condition that affects the nerves and reflex arc responsible for ejaculation can result in urine contamination. Most cases of urospermia are idiopathic. Potential diseases causing this condition include HYPP, cauda equina syndrome, neoplasia, and EHV-1 infection. Urine contamination results in a significant decrease in sperm motility, at least in part due to alterations in pH and osmolality of the seminal fluid. The fertility of affected stallions is therefore decreased.

Clinical presentation
Semen collected for AI may be found to be grossly contaminated with urine on examination for color, odor, observation of urine crystals, and elevation of pH. Stallions may present with infertility or sudden reduction in sperm motility. Urospermia is often sporadic and contamination may not be seen with every semen collection.

Differential diagnosis
Hemospermia and inflammatory products in the semen.

Diagnosis
Examination of the semen for urine components is diagnostic. Creatinine levels >152.52 μmol/l (1.72 mg/dl) and urea nitrogen levels >10.71 mmol/l (30 mg/dl) are highly suggestive of urospermia. Complete physical and neurologic evaluation is suggested due to the potential for systemic illnesses such as EHV-1 infection or space-occupying neoplastic masses to cause this condition.

Management
Treatment of any underlying condition may reduce the frequency of urospermia. In cases of idiopathic urospermia, the stallion is best managed by training him to urinate immediately before semen collection or breeding. Collecting semen into a bottle containing pre-warmed semen extender should minimize the effect of urine on the sperm, but care must be taken to ensure that the extender is kept warm in order to prevent cold-shocking of the sperm. Treatment with alpha-adrenergic agonists such as imipramine hydrochloride (500–800 mg i/v or 100–500 mg p/o per day) or phenylpropanolamine (0.35–0.5 mg/kg p/o q12h for minimum 14 days) before collection may increase bladder neck tone, reducing the chances of urospermia.

Prognosis
The prognosis is guarded since most cases are chronic and intermittent, responding only partially to therapy.

Conditions of the accessory genital glands

Ampullary gland obstruction

Definition/overview
Ampullary gland obstruction is the most common condition of the accessory glands of the stallion. Accumulation of sperm in the ampullae causes partial or complete, unilateral or bilateral obstruction.

Etiology/pathophysiology
The condition is most often observed early in the breeding season or in stallions that are used infrequently for breeding. Prolonged sexual rest can lead to the accumulation of masses of degenerating sperm and gel in the ampullary glands.

Clinical presentation
Complete, bilateral ampullary obstruction presents as azoospermia or, in the case of a stallion breeding naturally, as infertility. Incomplete obstruction presents with semen of very low to zero motility, but high numbers of sperm. Morphologic examination of sperm often reveals a large number of tailless heads.

Differential diagnosis
Incomplete or failed ejaculation; azoospermia of other causes; TD as a cause of poor sperm morphology; poor semen handling as a cause of sperm immotility.

Diagnosis
Diagnosis is based on the clinical presentation and a thorough reproductive evaluation. Rectal examination and ultrasonography demonstrate unilateral or bilateral enlargement and distension of the ampullae. Measurement of AP activity in the ejaculated semen differentiates between true azoospermia and obstruction (see Oligospermia/azoospermia, p. 362).

Management
Treatment involves gentle per rectum massage of the ampullary glands and frequent semen collection in a short period of time to remove the accumulated sperm. Injection of low doses of oxytocin (10–20 IU) prior to massage and collection may assist with resolution of the condition.

Prognosis
The prognosis is excellent. The condition is usually reversible and stallions return to previous levels of fertility.

Accessory genital-gland infections

Definition/overview
The most common accessory genital-gland infection encountered is seminal vesiculitis. Rare cases of prostate infection/abscess have been reported.

Etiology/pathophysiology
The most common causative agents include *Pseudomonas aeruginosa, Klebsiella pneumoniae, Streptococcus* spp., and *Staphylococcus* spp. Infection may occur due to blood-borne infection, ascending infection, or extension of orchitis/epididymitis, or be secondary to urethritis or cystitis.

Clinical presentation
The most common clinical presentation is the finding of polymorphonuclear (PMN) cells and bacteria in the semen. There may be a concurrent history of recent decline in fertility. Infection may or may not be accompanied by gross changes of color to the ejaculate. In acute infections the stallion may present with painful ejaculation or a reluctance to breed, depression, and inappetence. Other systemic signs are uncommon and pyrexia is not a typical finding of accessory-gland infection.

Differential diagnosis
Culture of bacteria from the semen alone does not confirm vesiculitis, as surface colonization of the penis is the most common source of bacteria cultured in semen. Other conditions causing PMN cells in the semen should be considered (e.g. orchitis/epididymitis, cystitis, or urethritis).

Diagnosis
The findings of bacteria and PMN cells in the ejaculate of a stallion should alert the clinician to the possibility of vesiculitis. Rectal examination and ultrasonography may demonstrate enlarged, firm, and painful vesicular gland(s) (**578**). Significant variation, however, exists among different stallions and within stallions across different examinations in the size, degree of dilation, and ultrasonographic character of all of the accessory glands. Therefore, findings of large, dilated glands on rectal examination and ultrasound do not confirm a diagnosis of vesiculitis. Endoscopic examination of the urethra and colliculus seminalis is suggested. In vesiculitis, the gland opening may be inflamed and purulent exudate may be seen draining from it. To confirm the diagnosis, a flexible 5 French polyethylene catheter is passed into the vesicular gland opening via endoscopy and fluid aspirated for cytologic and bacteriological examination.

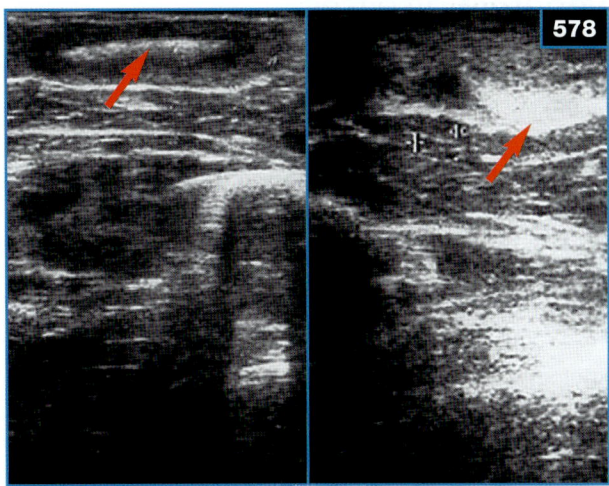

578 Ultrasound images of the vesicular glands of a stallion with bacterial seminal vesiculitis. Hyperechoic secretions are visualized within the vesicular glands (arrows). Ultrasound alone should not be used to diagnose seminal vesiculitis in stallions, as the glands can be variable in appearance.

Management
Vesiculitis is difficult to treat and many infections become recurrent or chronic. A combination of systemic antibiotic therapy chosen based on sensitivity results, systemic anti-inflammatories, and local therapy is most likely to achieve success. Local therapy involves lavaging the vesicular gland via the endoscope and flexible catheter, followed by local instillation of appropriate antibiotics. Following apparent resolution of the infection, periodic semen evaluation and culture are used to monitor for recurrence. Management of a stallion with chronic, low-grade infection can be achieved with the use of appropriate antibiotic-containing semen extenders. Semen should be exposed to the extender with antibiotic for at least 1 hour prior to insemination.

Surgical vesiculectomy has been performed in the stallion, but its effectiveness in controlling chronic vesiculitis is uncertain because of the involvement of other accessory glands.

Prognosis
The prognosis is guarded.

Venereal diseases

Dourine (see also p. 311)

Definition/overview

Dourine is reportable to the World Organization for Animal Health (OIE). North America, Australia, and New Zealand are dourine free. A small number of cases are reported in western Asia, southeastern Europe, southern Africa, and Central America; however, under-reporting is probable and the true prevalence is unknown.

Etiology/pathophysiology

Dourine is a venereal disease caused by the parasite *Trypanasoma equiperdum.*

Clinical presentation

The clinical presentation varies with the breed and the overall health status of the horse. Locally adapted breeds and donkeys may be asymptomatically infected. Clinical disease is characterized by mucopurulent urethral discharge, genital edema, and fever, followed by emaciation, hindlimb incoordination, and penile paralysis. Conjunctivitis and cutaneus plaques may occur. The disease may take weeks to years to progress, but is typically fatal.

Differential diagnosis

Other causes of urethral discharge and penile paralysis.

Diagnosis

T. equiperdum can be identified in urethral exudates and the buffy coat of blood samples; however, false negatives occur, particularly in advanced cases. Complement fixation is the most reliable serologic test, but false positives occur due to cross-reaction with *T. brucei* and *T. evansi.*

Management

Treatment with quinapyramin sulfate may eliminate clinical signs. In most countries, infected animals are euthanized as part of eradication programs.

Prognosis

The prognosis is poor once clinical signs are evident. Euthanasia is warranted to prevent transmission.

Contagious equine metritis (see also p. 248)

Definition/overview

CEM is a highly contagious venereal disease. It has not been detected in Australia or New Zealand, it has been eradicated from North America, and it occurs sporadically in Europe. Control programs are in place to prevent the introduction of CEM to disease-free countries and to eradicate the disease from Europe.

Etiology/pathophysiology

CEM is caused by the bacterium *Taylorella equigenitalis.* Transmission may occur through breeding, AI, or contact with contaminated equipment.

Clinical presentation

Stallions are asymptomatic carriers. Mares bred to carrier stallions develop mucopurulent vaginal discharge, beginning 7–10 days after breeding, and a shortened interestrus interval.

Differential diagnosis

Other venereal infections including *Pseudomonas* and *Klebsiella.*

Diagnosis

Diagnosis is made by isolating the bacteriom from the urethra, urethral fossa, prepuce, or pre-ejaculatory fluid of stallions, or by isolation of the bacterium from the reproductive tract of mares after breeding to a suspect stallion. Swabs must be immediately placed in Ames' medium with charcoal and refrigerated during transport. If transport is delayed, swabs may be frozen. Culture requires a high CO_2 environment and selective media. Serologic testing is not useful in stallions because they do not mount an immune response.

Management

Infection is treated by thoroughly washing the extended penis (teased to penile erection), prepuce, and urethral fossa in 2% chlorhexidine solution, taking care to remove all smegma. This is followed by packing with 0.2% nitrofurazone dressing on 5 consecutive days. (*Note:* Nitrofurazone ointment is no longer available for veterinary use in Europe, and no other effective alternative has been identified.) The US and Canada require quarantine and testing for CEM for all stallions entering these countries.

Prognosis

Infection in stallions is usually eliminated by treatment. Some stallions may develop sensitivity to chlorhexidine, leading to soreness. It is important not to exceed the recommended concentration.

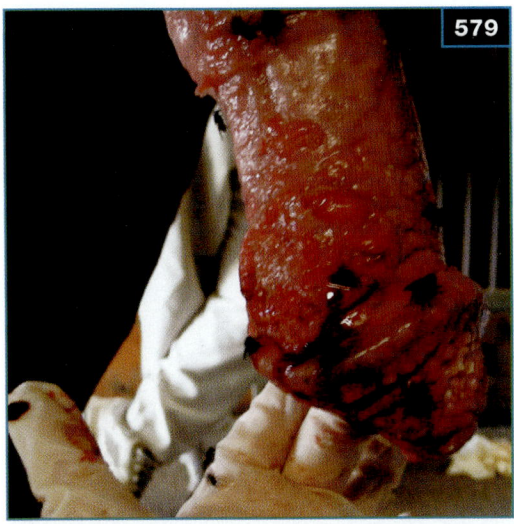

579

Bacterial colonization of the penis

Definition/overview
Iatrogenic bacterial overgrowth can occur on the genital organs of intensively managed breeding stallions or where there is excessive cleaning of the penis in colts and geldings (579).

Etiology/pathophysiology
The external genitalia of the stallion normally harbor a mixed population of commensal bacteria. When the normal bacterial population is disrupted, heavy growth of potentially pathogenic species such as *Pseudomonas aeruginosa* and *Klebisella pneumoniae* can occur. *Pseudomonas* is classified by serotype, phage type, and ability to cause hemolysis. Hemolytic strains are considered infective. Housing stallions on poorly maintained shavings encourages overgrowth of *Klebsiella*. *Klebsiella* is classified by capsular type; types 1, 2, 5, and possibly 7 can be transmitted venereally and are associated with endometritis in the mare. *Klebsiella* does not usually cause accessory-gland infection in the stallion, rather it colonizes itself on the external skin of the penis and prepuce.

Clinical presentation
Mares bred to the stallion have a lower conception rate than expected and may return to heat sooner than 21 days due to endometritis. Uterine culture of multiple mares bred to the stallion results in growth of an identical microorganism.

Differential diagnosis
Other causes of subfertility.

Diagnosis
Culture of the penis, prepuce, and urethral fossa before washing is required. Teasing the stallion to achieve an erection facilitates culture. *Pseudomonas* can be cultured from normal stallions; colonization is diagnosed only when there is a heavy pure growth from culture. After washing and drying the penis, pre- and postejaculatory fluid is cultured and the semen is examined for WBCs to ensure that infection has not ascended to the accessory sex glands.

Management
Prevention is by avoiding the use of antiseptic cleansers when washing the penis. Clean, warm water should be used for routine pre-breeding washing. Both *Pseudomonas* and *Klebsiella* infections can be resistant to treatment. Colonization can be treated by washing the penis in a dilute solution of hydrochloric acid for *Pseudomonas* infections (2.5 ml 38% HCl/l water) or hypochlorite for *Klebsiella* infections (9 ml 5.25% Na hypochlorite/l). Enrofloxacin or other systemic antibiotics are used only if accessory sex glands are infected and following *in-vitro* antibiotic sensitivity testing. Semen extenders or pre-breeding uterine infusions with an appropriate antibiotic will reduce infertility.

In sensitive infections, gentamicin solution (50 mg/ml) or ointment can be massaged into the penile and preputial skin, the urethral fossa, and the diverticulum following sodium hypochlorite washing (5.25%). (**Note:** Gentamicin ointment isno longer available for veterinary use in Europe). In persistent cases, gentamicin-impregnated surgical sponge can be cut to size and inserted into the urethral fossa and diverticulum and left in place for up to 7 days. This can be successful in eliminating infection, but often causes local reaction and soreness.

In *Pseudomonas* infections after washing and removal of smegma, some success has been reported with the use of a 1% silver nitrate solution spray daily for up to 30 days. Periodic treatment with sterile petroleum jelly will help to prevent the penile skin from cracking during treatment.

Thorough disinfection is required to prevent colonization of equipment including buckets and artificial vaginas. Infected stallions should have dedicated equipment to prevent pathogen transmission to other stallions. Periodic repeat cultures should be conducted to monitor these infections. Stallions can be managed in some cases by minimum-contamination breeding techniques and incubating semen in an extender containing the appropriate antibiotic for at least 1 hour prior to insemination.

After antiseptic washing or antibiotic treatment, the penis and prepuce may be treated with a specifically cultured active broth containing a mixture of microflora from normal equine external genitalia to try to encourage rapid recolonization with normal flora and prevent overgrowth with pathogenic bacteria.

Progress should be monitored by follow-up swab samples collected every 2 days from the urethra, urethral fossa and diverticulum, and preputial smegma 7 days after the end of treatment. Three sets of negative swabs can be assumed to indicate successful treatment.

Prognosis

The prognosis is good for treating colonization of the external genitalia, but much worse when infection involves the accessory sex glands, which frequently requires long and repeated treatment programs. Some stallions are never successfully cleared of the infection.

Equine coital exanthema

Definition/overview

This is a self-limiting venereal disease affecting mares (p. 310) and stallions. It has a worldwide distribution.

Etiology/pathophysiology

Equine coital exanthema is a highly contagious disease caused by EHV-3 and spread through coitus or contaminated veterinary equipment.

Clinical presentation

Symptoms develop 4–8 days after infection, with 2 mm diameter red nodules appearing on the penis and preputial skin. These develop into vesicles and then pustules, which rupture, leaving shallow erosions (580). Fertility is not usually impaired, but stallions are reluctant to copulate due to pain. The course of uncomplicated infection is 3–4 weeks. Secondary bacterial infection may occur. Unpigmented scars remain visible after recovery.

Differential diagnosis

Trauma; contact sensitivity; bacterial infection.

Diagnosis

History and clinical signs are suggestive of EHV-3 infection.

Management

Stallions should be rested until the lesions are fully healed. Care must be taken to prevent iatrogenic transmission. Secondary bacterial infections are treated with appropriate topical medications.

Prognosis

The prognosis is excellent.

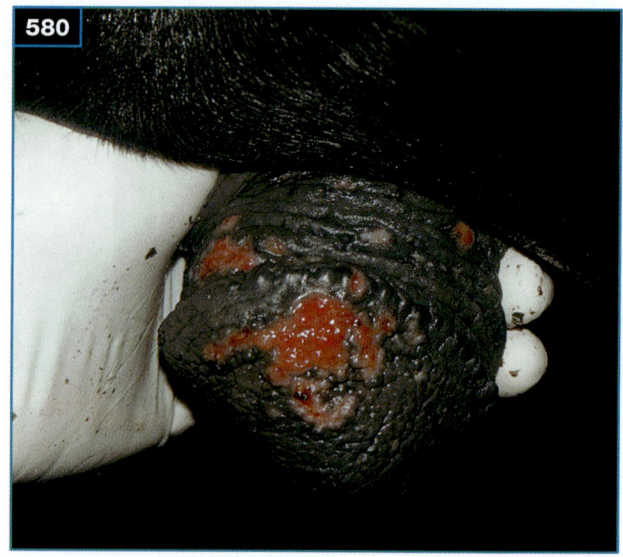

580 Acute coital exanthema ulcerative lesions on the glands of the penis of a stallion.

Equine viral arteritis

Definition/overview

EVA is a viral disease spread by respiratory and venereal routes. Stallions may become permanent carriers. It has a worldwide distribution, but outbreaks are rare. EVA is endemic in Standardbreds in many countries.

Etiology/pathophysiology

The venereal route of transmission is via acutely and chronically infected stallions shedding equine arteritis virus in the sperm-rich fraction of the ejaculate. Acutely infected mares shed virus in body secretions.

Clinical presentation

Asymptomatic infection is common in stallions, geldings, and nonpregnant mares. In symptomatic cases, signs last 1–10 days and include fever, limb and scrotal edema, conjunctivitis and lacrimation, nasal discharge, and skin rash. Scrotal edema may cause a decline in semen quality. In pregnant mares, abortion of partially autolyzed fetuses occurs.

Differential diagnosis

EHV infection.

Diagnosis

In the stallion, diagnosis is made via detection of equine arteritis virus in the semen or by demonstrating seroconversion in a mare after breeding.

Management

There is currently no treatment to eliminate shedding in chronically infected stallions. To prevent infection, stallions should be tested for antibodies to equine arteritis virus before commencing a breeding career. Annual vaccination will prevent infection. Mares being bred to infected stallions should be vaccinated 3 weeks prior to breeding and must be isolated from pregnant mares after vaccination. Currently, a modified live vaccine is available in North America, but only a killed vaccine is available in Europe. Vaccines should be used according to manufacturers' recommendation. Before vaccination of colts, blood must be taken and a pre-vaccination titer documented to allow international transport.

Prognosis

The prognosis is poor in stallions, as infection cannot be eliminated.

Control of equine venereal diseases

Many countries have Codes of Practice for hygienic stud-animal management, and minimal-contamination techniques in AI (e.g. The Horserace Betting Levy Board in the UK, Eire, and France).

Some venereal pathogens are typically not associated with any clinical signs in the stallion (e.g. *Pseudomonas aeruginosa*, *Klebsiella pneumoniae*, *Taylorella equigenitalis*) and postmating endometritis infection in the mare is the first indicator that the stallion is harboring these organisms. All imported stallions and, at the beginning of each breeding season, all resident stallions should be thoroughly screened for venereal infections prior to use, and the first 2–3 mares mated should have clitoral swabs taken post mating.

Following positive isolation or clinical signs of venereal disease, breeding operations should stop immediately. Affected animals should be isolated and screening for infection or carrier status should commence.

Overuse of penile washing or disinfection techniques is to be avoided since this encourages overgrowth of pathogenic species. It has been shown that the normal genital skin flora develop an ecological stability, which can help to prevent the growth of pathogens.

AI using screened semen is an effective control measure for the transmission of venereal diseases (in those countries where registration criteria allow it) provided that the Codes of Practice relating to hygiene are followed precisely.

Skin disease of the external genitalia

Balanitis/balanoposthitis

Definition/overview

Balanitis is inflammation of the penis, while balanoposthitis is inflammation of the penis and prepuce.

Etiology/pathophysiology

The inflammation may be the result of bacterial, viral, or protozoal infections or be caused by chemical irritants such as fly sprays or disinfectants. Overzealous use of soaps and antibacterial solutions can remove the normal bacterial flora, incite inflammation, and result in overgrowth of opportunistic pathogens (**579**). Excessive accumulations of smegma have also been implicated. Bacterial infection may accompany SCC or follow viral infection with equine coital exanthema. Balanoposthitis may also occur in long-standing cases of priapism or paraphimosis, due to prolonged exposure of the penis to adverse environmental conditions and drying of the penile skin. The most common bacteria implicated are *Streptococcus* spp., *Klebsiella pneumoniae*, and *Pseudomonas aeruginosa*. The parasites *Trypanosoma equiperdum* (see p. 366) and *Habronema* can also cause the condition.

Clinical presentation

The stallion or gelding presents with varying degrees of swelling of the penile skin and/or prepuce. Crusting and discharge from the skin surface may occur in severe cases. The stallion may be uncomfortable and resist washing of the penis, collection with an artificial vagina, or natural cover. Balanoposthitis alone is unusual and the clinician should search for underlying predisposing causes.

Differential diagnosis

Neoplasia of the penis; trauma to the penis.

Diagnosis

Swabs of the surface of the penis, the prepuce, urethral fossa, urethra, and of any surface lesions should be submitted for bacterial, viral, and cytologic examination.

Management

Treatment is dependent on the cause of the condition, but sexual rest is indicated until it is fully resolved. Viral infections generally heal uneventfully unless complicated by secondary bacterial infection. Bacterial infections may be treated by local application of antibiotic ointment based on sensitivity results. Systemic anti-inflammatories are useful early in treatment in order to reduce swelling and edema.

Prognosis

This is guarded, depending on the underlying cause.

Habronemiasis

Definition/overview

Habronemiasis is a granulomatous dermatitis caused by hypersensitivity to the larvae of *Habronema* spp.

Etiology/pathophysiology

Adult *Habronema* spp. worms live in the equine stomach and eggs passed in the feces are ingested by fly maggots in the manure. The larvae are transferred to the skin by flies feeding around the mouth, eyes, male genitals, and lacerations. Larvae deposited around the mouth are swallowed and develop into adults in the stomach. Larvae deposited in other regions burrow into the skin, causing a granulomatous dermatitis.

Clinical presentation

Habronemiasis occurs sporadically in a group of horses, but it can occur repeatedly in the same individual. Light-colored horses are most commonly affected. Habronemiasis occurs during warm weather, when fly populations are high. Lesions are pruritic and appear as 1–25 cm reddish open sores, containing characteristic hard yellow granules. In stallions, blood noted in the genital region after mating may be the first detected sign. Proliferative lesions of the urethral process may interfere with urination and ejaculation. Inflammation and swelling of the genital region may disrupt spermatogenesis. Chronic, severe lesions of the prepuce may result in scarring and adhesion, interfering with normal penile erection.

Differential diagnosis

Sarcoid; SCC; granulation tissue.

Diagnosis

Diagnosis is based on history and clinical signs, particularly the presence of yellow granules. Biopsies show eosinophilic inflammation, with areas of necrosis, and in approximately half of cases, degenerating larvae can be detected.

Management

The incidence may be reduced by maintaining a low parasite burden on breeding farms through regular deworming and by limiting exposure of susceptible stallions to flies via appropriate housing, manure management, and use of insecticides. In clinical cases, systemic ivermectin is used to kill larvae, and lesions are debulked and treated with steroid creams.

Prognosis

The prognosis is good with appropriate management.

Tumors of the male reproductive tract

Penis and prepuce

Squamous cell carcinoma

Definition/overview

SCC is the most common neoplasm affecting the skin of the penis and prepuce.

Etiology/pathophysiology

SCC is most common in animals with nonpigmented skin on the penis and prepuce, such as Appaloosas and Pintos. Geldings are more frequently affected than stallions, possibly because they have more smegma accumulation and the penis is less frequently washed. A carcinogenic action of smegma accumulation on the penis has been suggested.

Clinical presentation

Nonhealing erosions or small growths may be noted on the skin during washing for breeding. In nonbreeding stallions or geldings, swelling of the sheath, reluctance to exteriorize the penis, and foul odor may be the first signs noted. The most commonly affected areas are the internal prepuce (581), glans penis (582), and urethral opening. Two presentations are common: a proliferative form, producing cauliflower-like growths that may ulcerate and bleed; and an invasive form that destroys penile architecture and distorts the penis and prepuce. Precancerous skin changes can include discrete areas of depigmentation and thickening of the penile skin (552).

Differential diagnosis

Habronemiasis; other skin tumors such as sarcoid tumors, melanoma, and viral papillomas.

Diagnosis

Diagnosis is made by histopathology of a biopsy. The penis must be fully exteriorized to permit examination of its entirety, including palpation of the base. This may be aided by administration of tranquilizers such as xylazine or acepromazine.

Management

Small SCC lesions can be treated by cryosurgery with liquid nitrogen or carbon dioxide delivered through a cryoprobe or liquid nitrogen spray. Lesions are frozen to a depth of 3 mm, with three freeze–thaw cycles. Small lesions can also be treated by repeated application of 5-flourouracil every 2 weeks. More extensive lesions may be treated by circumferential reefing surgery. In advanced cases, castration followed three weeks later by penile amputation may be necessary (583, 584).

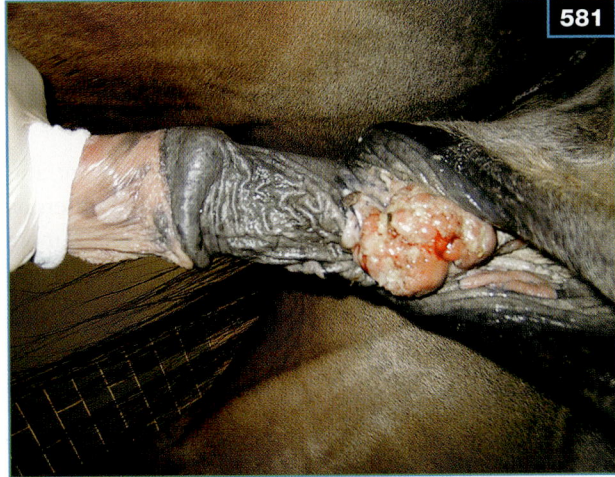

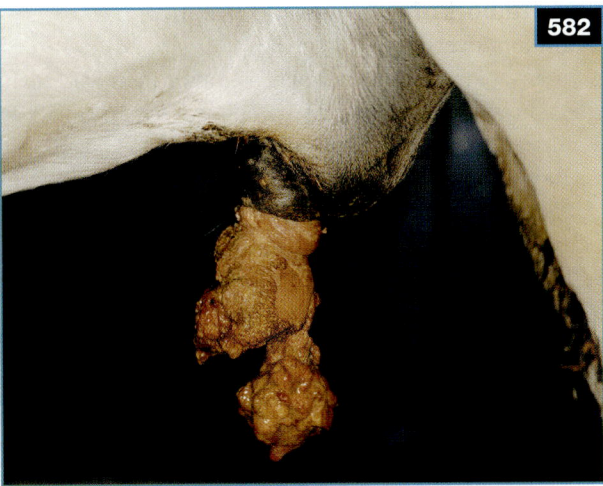

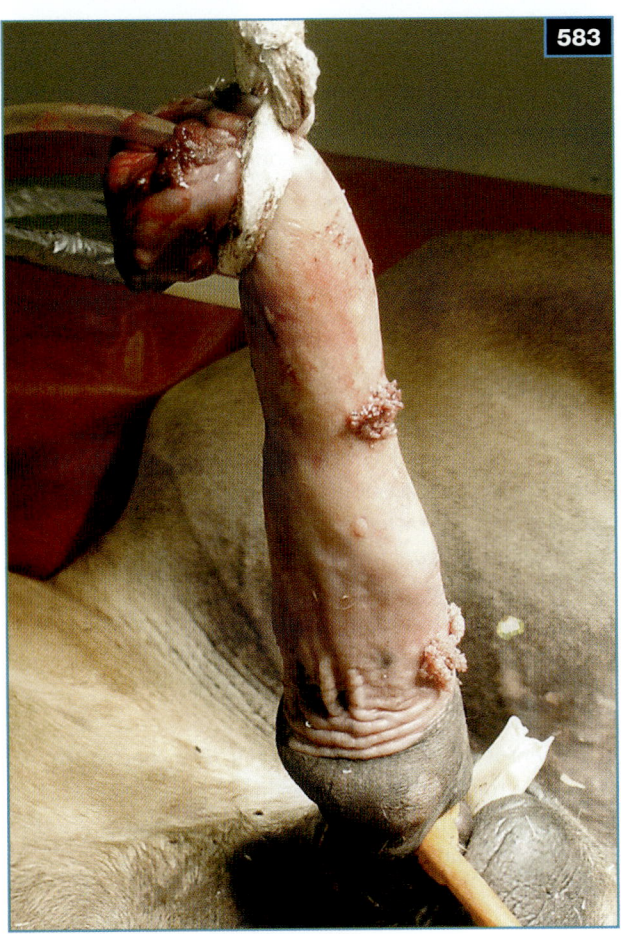

581 Squamous cell carcinoma lesion at the base of the penis of a stallion.

582 A severe erosive and granulating squamous cell carcinoma of the glans and body of the penis of an aged gelding.

583, 584 Immediately preoperative view (583) of the penis of a gelding showing squamous cell carcinoma lesions at two sites on the body and a larger lesion on the glans. The gelding is undergoing a penile amputation (584) and at this stage the urethrotomy incision has just been completed.

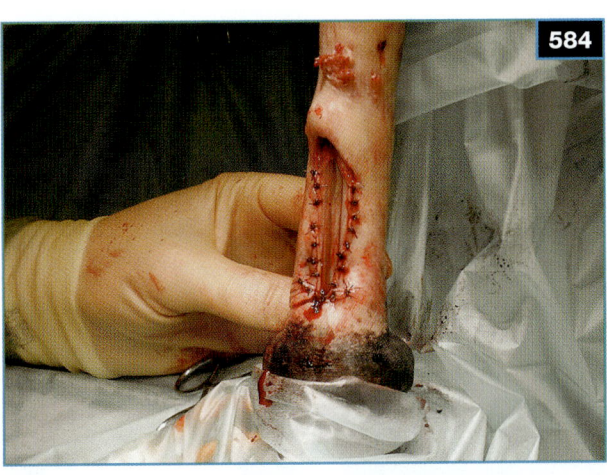

Prognosis
SCC is slow to metastasize. Rectal examination of the superficial inguinal lymph nodes and pelvic lymph nodes for increase in size may indicate metastasis.

Male reproductive tract

Other tumors of the penis and prepuce

Definition/overview

A variety of cutaneous neoplasms, other than SCC, may affect the skin of the penis and prepuce.

+ *Sarcoids* are fibroelastic tumors of the skin and are most common in younger horses. As with other body locations, sarcoids involving the prepuce or penis may be of the fibroblastic nodular (most common), verrucous (warty), mixed, or occult (rare) type. Preputial and penile sarcoids are managed similarly to sarcoids in other locations. Surgical excision is likely the best option, but recurrences are common. Cryotherapy reduces recurrence, but it must be used with caution on penile, preputial, and scrotal skin due to the potential for scarring and fibrosis, which might alter function (penis and underlying urethra) and fertility (scrotum).
+ *Melanomas* may be seen involving the prepuce or penis of older geldings and stallions (585). Examination will find melanomas in other locations such as the perianal or facial regions. Lesions are usually <3 cm, multiple, smooth, round, and hairless. Melanomas are slow to metastasize. Oral cimetidine (2.5 mg/kg q24h) may be helpful in slowing progression.
+ *Viral papillomas* tend to affect young colts or geldings and resolve spontaneously over 4–12 weeks without treatment. Additional lesions are usually found on the muzzle of affected animals.

585 Small melanomas of the base of the penis of an aged gray gelding pony. They were not associated at this stage with any clinical signs.

Testicular tumors

Definition/overview

Testicular tumors of the stallion are uncommon.

Etiology/pathophysiology

Seminomas are the most common testicular tumor and arise from the germinal epithelium of the seminiferous tubule. They are gray and lobulated. Interstitial tumors are rare and arise from the testosterone-producing Leydig cells. They are tan, firm, and nodular. Sertoli-cell tumors are very rare, occurring primarily in retained testes. They are firm and gray-white. Teratomas are rare and occur primarily in retained cryptorchid testes. They may be large and contain various tissues, including bone and hair.

Clinical presentation

Testicular tumors are most common in older stallions. Insidious unilateral scrotal swelling may be noted, but often the abnormal testicle is detected on a routine BSE. In younger stallions, tumors occur primarily in retained cryptorchid testes and are often first noted during castration.

Differential diagnosis

Testicular torsion; abscess; granuloma; trauma.

Diagnosis

Diagnosis is made by palpation and ultrasonographic (high resolution: 7.5 MHz) comparison with the normal testicle. Cryptorchid testes can be examined by rectal palpation and ultrasonography prior to surgery. Tumor type is confirmed by testicular biopsy or, more commonly, by histopathology after castration. Thickening of the spermatic cord, enlargement of the pelvic and abdominal lymph nodes, or histopathologic detection of tumor cells in the cord indicates metastasis.

Management

Treatment is by unilateral castration. The spermatic cord should be transected as far proximal as possible. Ligation may be necessary to control hemorrhage. In cryptorchid stallions, bilateral castration should be performed.

Prognosis

Testicular tumors are usually benign. Return to fertility may be compromised in stallions with long-standing tumors due to old age, hormonal down-regulation, or inflammation of the normal testicle secondary to scrotal edema or unilateral castration.

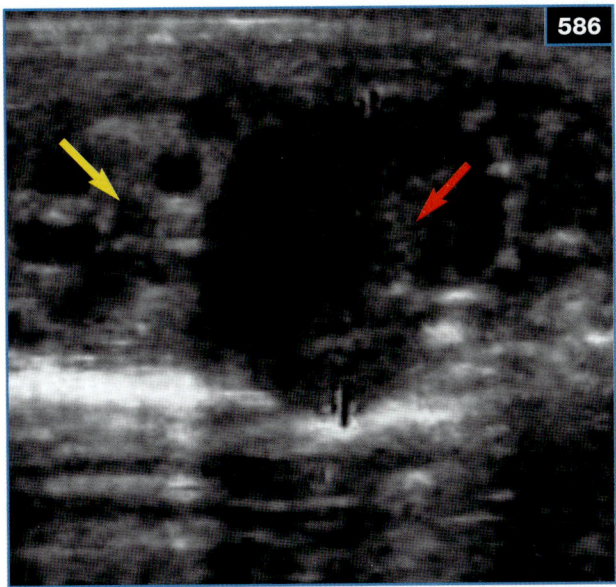

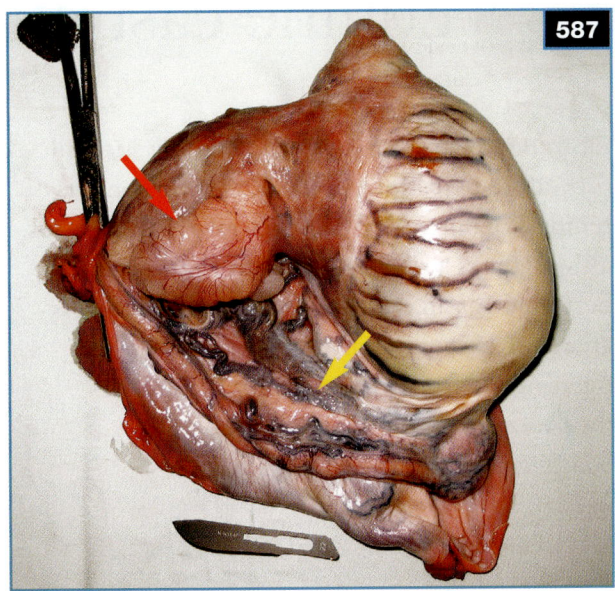

586 Ultrasound image of a hypoechoic, firm mass (red arrow) found in the left spermatic cord (yellow arrow) of a 20-year-old Hanoverian stallion that presented for painful ejaculation.

587 Gross appearance of the testis from the stallion in 586 following unilateral castration. The mass (red arrow) was within the spermatic cord (yellow arrow), with adhesions to the tunic. The histologic diagnosis was a leiomyoma.

Tumors of the spermatic cord
Definition/overview
Reports of spermatic cord tumors are extremely rare in stallions. Fibroma, leiomyoma arising from the wall of cord vessels, and mesothelioma of the tunica albuginea have been reported.

Clinical presentation
The stallion may present for scrotal pain, reluctance to breed, generalized depression, and ejaculatory pain. In some cases no outward signs have been noted.

Differential diagnosis
Thrombosis of spermatic cord vessels; varicocele.

Diagnosis
Palpation of the spermatic cord reveals a mass. Ultrasonographic evaluation may be suggestive of neoplasia (586). Diagnosis can be confirmed histologically by biopsy.

Management
Treatment involves unilateral castration with removal of as much of the spermatic cord as possible on the affected side (587).

Prognosis
The prognosis for life, recovery, and return to fertility is dependent on the type of tumor and whether metastasis has occurred.

Castration is the most common routine surgical procedure performed in the horse and consists of removal of one or, more commonly, both testicles. Although it is a routine procedure and normally performed as an elective surgery, complications are relatively common. A solid knowledge of the urogenital anatomy and preparation for the procedure will greatly reduce the complication rate.

Indications for castration

Most castrations are intended to suppress the development of stallion-like characteristics, and so the age at which the surgery is performed is relevant. Castration in the first 2 months of life is not advisable, as young foals are more vulnerable to stress and infections, but colts over 3 months old can be castrated very successfully, particularly when still suckling. More commonly, colts are castrated several months after weaning or during the first year of life. Competition horses might be kept entire until a later stage to assess their performance and breeding potential. The more a horse is allowed to develop into sexual maturity, the less likely it is that male characteristics will be suppressed.

Other indications for castration include sterilization of a male no longer intended for breeding purposes or as a salvage procedure in cases of severe trauma to the testicles or scrotum. In the latter case, unilateral castration may be performed to maintain breeding soundness.

It is generally accepted that cryptorchids should be castrated, as there is evidence that this condition can have an hereditary predisposition and most breed societies will not allow registration of cryptorchid stallions.

Preoperative considerations

Castration in the vast majority of cases is an elective procedure and as such careful preoperative planning should minimize the potential risks. Castration can be performed at any time of the year, but a dry season when insect numbers are low is preferred.

The environment in which the procedure is to be performed should not compromise the safety of the veterinary surgeon or the patient. If castration is to be performed under general anesthesia, a large open, clean space should be chosen (**588**). For standing castration, padded stocks with a high lateral bar are ideal, but these are not always available and a clean empty stable is adequate when good restraint and assistance are available.

588 Undertaking a routine castration under field conditions using intravenous general anesthesia.

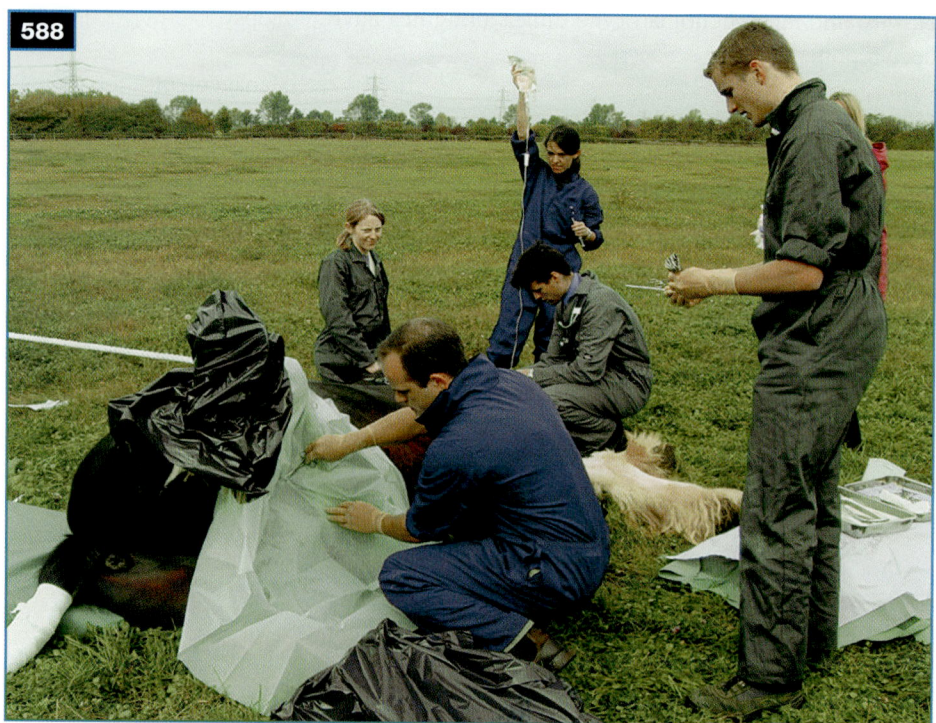

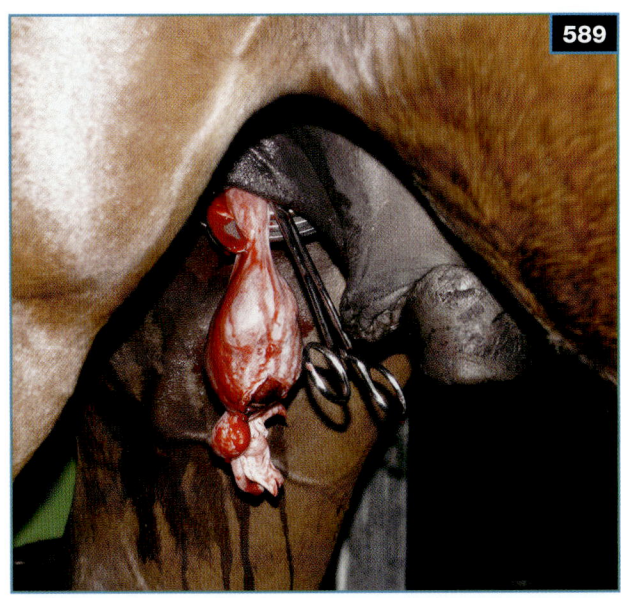

589

589 Standing castration in a 2-year-old colt using sedation and local anesthetic infiltration. The emasculators are just about to be applied. Note the forceps, which are attached to the already-transected ligament of the epididymis.

A careful preoperative examination of the horse should include a physical examination and palpation of the testes to ensure that they are both descended and normal and there is no evidence of herniation. Sedation may help by relaxing the patient and allowing the testes to descend into a scrotal position where they are more easily palpable. Hematologic and blood biochemistry examinations are rarely necessary. If any abnormalities are encountered, a risk evaluation should be carried out and the procedure postponed if necessary.

Preoperative analgesia with an appropriate NSAID is very effective and ideally should be carried out one hour before surgery. Preoperative antibiotics are not normally indicated but if used, minimum inhibitory concentration levels should be achieved by the time of surgery and maintained for 24 hours. Tetanus prophylaxis is vital.

The area should be clipped, if excessive hair is present, and aseptically prepared. Subcutaneous infiltration of local anesthetic solution (5–10 ml of 2% lidocaine) as well as intratesticular infiltration of a similar amount will reduce surgical stimulation and can be done before the final preparation is applied. In field situations, various options of restraint and surgical positioning can be used. If general anesthesia is being given, keeping the limbs open is achieved with ropes held by an assistant and a plastic bag (or rectal glove) can be placed on the higher foot (**588**).

Anesthesia and sedation

Recumbent castration
The chosen surgical technique and the time required for it to be performed influence the choice of anesthetic protocol. For open castration, induction with ketamine following sedation with xylazine and butorphanol allows 15–20 minutes of good general anesthesia; a second half bolus of ketamine and xylazine can be administered, providing approximately another ten minutes of surgical time. The 'triple drip' combination can also be used; the use of guafenesin (5 or 10%) in this mixture, combined with ketamine and xylazine, provides excellent anesthesia and muscle relaxation. Recovery is usually smooth, but the horse should be observed throughout. A head collar and lunge line provide some control over the horse while it stands.

Standing castration
Sedation for standing castration is provided by a combination of an α-2 agonist (e.g. detomidine) and an opioid (e.g. butorphanol). Acepromazine administration should be avoided because of the risk of priapism development. The horse should be restrained by an experienced handler and a skin, ear, or lip twitch may be necessary. Local anesthesia of the scrotum and testis, as described above, will further desensitize the area and facilitate the procedure (**589**).

Surgical techniques

Several surgical techniques can be used to perform castration. The differences between them relate to two aspects of the procedure. The first aspect is the approach, which can be scrotal, parainguinal, or inguinal. The other aspect relates to the layers of tissue incised and whether ligatures are placed around them or not. Laparoscopic-assisted castration can also be performed.

Emasculation is a key step in the procedure, as it provides hemostasis and testicular removal simultaneously. The emasculators should be left in place for at least 2 minutes (590).

The combination of these two aspects leads to various valid permutations in the technique, and the surgeon should be aware of the advantages and disadvantages of each technique and choose the appropriate one for each case.

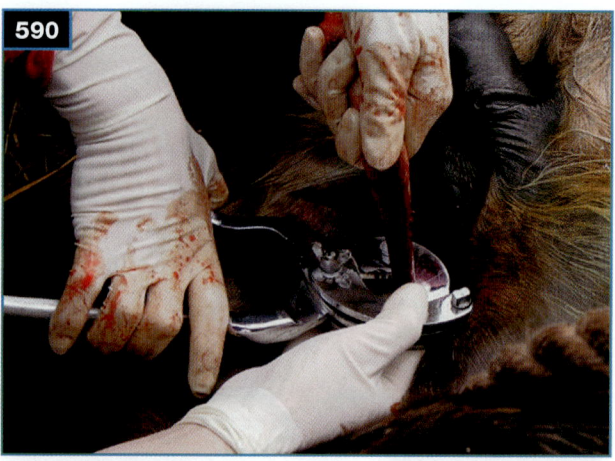

590 Applying emasculators to the dissected spermatic cord of a colt during an open castration. Note that they are applied well clear of the testicle.

Scrotal open castration

Procedure
A scrotal incision from the cranial to the caudal pole of the testicle is performed lateral to the median raffe, with the testicle held tight against the scrotal skin. It is important to ensure that the incision is in the most dependent part of the scrotum. The subcutaneous layers, tunica dartos, and vaginal tunic are incised, exposing the testicle. Some peritoneal fluid might be present in the vaginal sac and blood or a hematoma may also be seen if intratesticular infiltration of local anesthetic was performed. The ligament of the epididymis maintains the testicle's attachment to the vaginal tunic, and this ligament can be transected at this stage, allowing the testicle to prolapse further. The testicular vessels and the ducts deferens can now be emasculated jointly or separately. All layers incised are left open to heal by second intention.

Postoperative care
The patient is stable rested for 12–24 hours and light exercise (small paddock or hand walking) should be encouraged to maintain drainage for a week.

Advantages
This is a fast and technically easy technique that can be performed under standing sedation.

Disadvantages
As no ligatures are placed, there is an increased risk of postoperative hemorrhage and eventration. As wounds are left to heal by second intention, there is an increased risk of infection (acute and chronic) and delay in return to exercise.

Scrotal closed castration

Procedure
This approach differs from the previous one in that the vaginal tunic is not incised. Blunt dissection of the tunica dartos and subcutaneous tissues is usually done with a dry swab. The proper ligament of the testis can prove difficult to break, but this step is essential for correct exteriorization of the testicle. Care should be taken not to cause excessive trauma to the cremaster muscle during dissection, as this may cause unnecessary bleeding (591). Once this dissection has exposed the tubular portions of the testicle (still within the vaginal tunic) a transfixing (4 or 5 metric synthetic absorbable) ligature is placed using the cremaster muscle as an anchor point (592). Once the ligature is placed the whole tubular portion is now emasculated distal to it. The surgeon should ensure that placement of the ligature and the emasculation are performed as proximally as possible. Before removal of the emasculators, grasping an edge of the stump with an Allis tissue forceps will allow retrieval of the stump if hemorrhage is noted. The scrotal wounds are left to heal by second intention.

Advantages
As the vaginal tunic is not entered before it is sutured, contamination of the peritoneal cavity is reduced. The placement of a ligature ensures better hemostasis and reduces the chances of eventration.

Disadvantages
Longer surgery time. As the ligature acts as a foreign body, the risk of postoperative infection is increased. This technique can only be safely performed under general anesthesia.

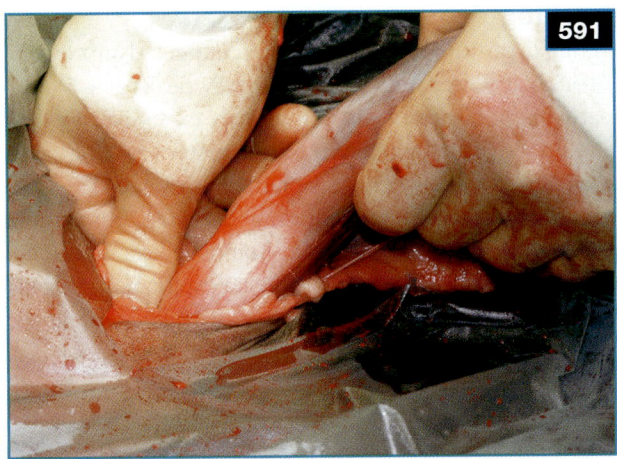

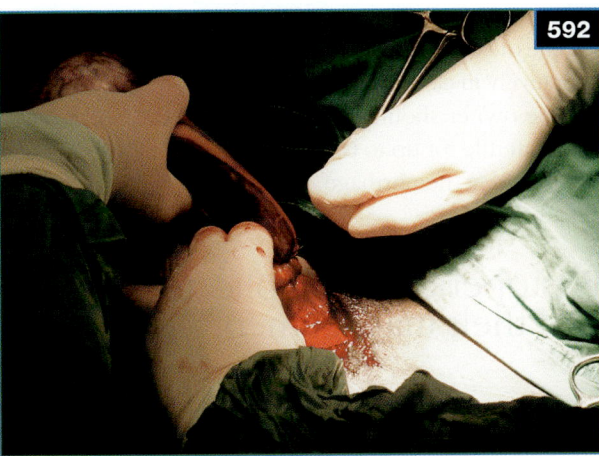

591 Blunt exposure of the vaginal tunic, using fingers and sterile swabs, allows the testicle to be exteriorized sufficiently from the scrotum or inguinal region to allow placement of a ligature and emasculators.

592 Applying a transfixing ligature to the dissected vaginal process during a closed castration under general anesthesia and with strict asepsis.

Scrotal closed castration with primary closure
Procedure
If primary closure of the scrotal skin is to be carried out, the dead space created in the scrotal sac must be closed by suturing the wall of the scrotum to the wall of the median raphe. Intradermal sutures will ensure skin-edge apposition without need for skin sutures. Alternatively, scrotal ablation can be performed to reduce the dead space.

Advantages
Faster healing time and reduced chance of infection.

Disadvantages
As no drainage will occur, strict aseptic technique is required. This might only be achieved in a hospital/clinic environment.

Parainguinal closed castration with primary closure
Procedure
A parainguinal incision is carried out between the scrotum and the thigh over the inguinal canal. The correct site can be identified by pushing the testicle from the scrotum into the inguinal canal and incising over it. Only a small incision is required (5–7 cm). The subcutaneous tissues are then bluntly dissected and the vaginal tunic in the inguinal canal is identified. Blunt dissection around the vaginal tunic is performed and continued in the scrotum to free the vaginal tunic attachments to the subcutaneous tissues. The testicle can then be retrieved through the incision and the procedure continues in the same way as that described for a closed castration. The wound is closed using a subcutaneous layer and an intradermal layer.

Advantages
The same as for a scrotal approach. This approach, however, has been shown to cause minimal complications, and the fast return to work (7–14 days) is appreciated by some owners and trainers.

Disadvantages
The same as for the scrotal approach; however, less swelling occurs with this approach.

Variations
In the closed technique, the vaginal tunic may be opened after the ligature has been placed to allow separate emasculation of the vascular and tubular portions of the cord (open-closed technique). In the closed parainguinal technique, the vaginal tunic can be incised and the testis retrieved through this opening, thus reducing the soft-tissue dissection necessary to retrieve it from the scrotum; however, the inguinal canal must be sutured to prevent hydrocele formation.

Postoperative management
The horse is allowed to recover from sedation or general anesthetic as normal and should be kept under close monitoring for the first 6–12 hours, preferably in a clean stable. Medication with NSAIDs is recommended for 2 or 3 days. If the skin wounds have been left open for drainage, the horse should be walked in hand and/or kept in a small paddock for the first 7 days (preferably on his own). A small amount of swelling and minimal drainage are seen for a few days. If primary closure was performed, exercise should be restricted for 7 days and only minimal swelling around the incision sites is expected.

If no postoperative complications occur, exercise may resume once the skin wounds have closed or 10 days post-operatively in closed castrations.

The owner should be informed that the horse might remain fertile for up to 6 weeks and to monitor for excessive swelling, hemorrhage, and general signs of systemic illness.

Postoperative complications and their management

Hemorrhage

After surgery, a small amount of bleeding is expected and this usually originates from subcutaneous vessels and stops within a few hours. If a stream of blood persists for more than 15 minutes, it should be considered excessive (593).

A decision as to whether to intervene should be made as early as possible in order to minimize blood loss. The horse should be sedated and an attempt made to find the origin of the hemorrhage. Surgical exploration under general anesthesia may be required. In less severe cases, packing of the scrotum with sterile swabs may stop smaller hemorrhages. If the testicular stump is bleeding, it should be re-emasculated and a ligature placed around it. The patient should be given systemic antibiotics for at least 5 days.

Swelling

Minimal postoperative swelling is expected in the first 24–48 hours after surgery and it usually peaks at 4–5 days, particularly in closed castrations. Any excessive swelling should be investigated. In open castrations the most common cause of swelling is premature wound closure or incorrect incision siting causing drainage impairment (594). The castration wound should be examined and opened and palpated by sterile digital exploration. In some cases, increasing exercise will, on its own, reopen the wounds, thus avoiding further manipulation of the surgical sites.

In closed castrations, swellings may be harder to investigate. Ultrasonograhic imaging of the area may help identify the cause of the problem. Bleeding, eventration, and infection can all cause swelling and must be differentiated. In some cases following closed inguinal castration, air gets trapped in the subcutaneous fascial planes during surgery and accumulates in the scrotum; although of no clinical concern, this may be alarming to the owner.

Infection

The reported incidence of postoperative infection after castration varies from 5–20%. Strict aseptic surgery is difficult to achieve in field situations and ascending infection can also occur when the wounds are left open. Although most infections respond well to treatment, they can become very serious if left untreated.

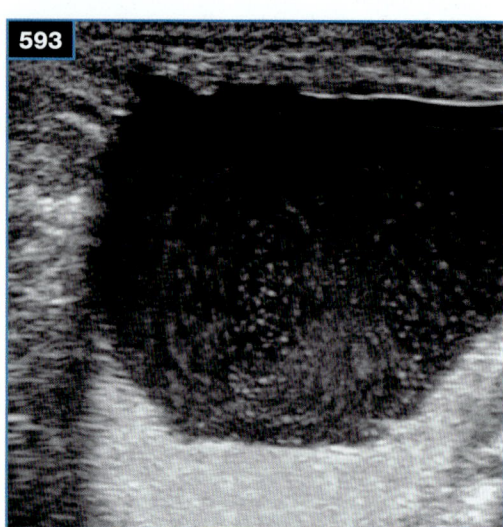

593 Ultrasonographic image of a recently castrated horse with excessive postoperative bleeding, revealing a large collection of blood trapped within the scrotum. The surgical incisions were enlarged and drainage encouraged.

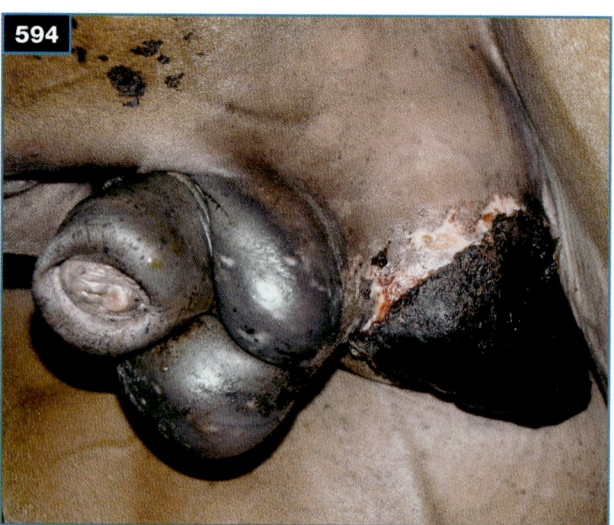

594 This horse had excessive swelling post castration which has led to ischemic necrosis of the scrotum. Note the residual swelling of the end of the prepuce.

Localized infection

The majority of infections are localized to the scrotal and/or inguinal tissues and are mainly caused by impaired drainage allowing bacteria to multiply within the dead space. Most cases are presented with an obvious swelling or a change in discharge appearance and smell (e.g. purulent). Systemic signs may be subtle in the early stages, with depression accompanied by a reduced appetite and pyrexia. Hematological parameters will vary depending on the severity and time elapsed since the beginning of the infection process.

Reopening the surgical wounds is indicated when premature closure has occurred. Antibiotics might be indicated in more severe cases. In surgeries where primary closure was performed, swelling can be more prominent and systemic effects more severe, because drainage is not possible. In the latter cases, treatment with antibiotics might be successful in the early stages, but if pockets of purulent material are present, establishing drainage by opening the scrotum is necessary to achieve a successful outcome.

Peritonitis

Studies have shown that a cellular inflammatory response in the peritoneal cavity occurs after routine castration, mainly due to the presence of erythrocytes in this space following surgery. A more severe response, and indeed a pathogenic one, is expected if infection tracks up the inguinal canal and causes a septic peritonitis. The associated endotoxemia will cause a systemic inflammatory response and related clinical signs. Signs of colic and inappetence may also be present. Analysis of the peritoneal fluid through abdominocentesis will confirm the diagnosis.

Treatment should include establishment of drainage and aggressive broad-spectrum antibiotic therapy as well as preventing the effects of endotoxemia.

Eventration

Eventration after castration means that abdominal viscera have prolapsed through the inguinal ring. This is probably the most serious of the postoperative complications. Eventration of the small intestine is more common than that of the omentum. Prompt and adequate management of the situation should give a moderate to good prognosis. This condition usually occurs in the first few hours after surgery (595).

If eventration has been diagnosed, the patient should be sedated and the prolapsed tissue palpated and anatomically identified. If small intestine has prolapsed, it should be lavaged and kept moist with a wet cloth until, under general anesthesia, the portion of gut is placed into the scrotum and the scrotal wounds sutured closed. The horse

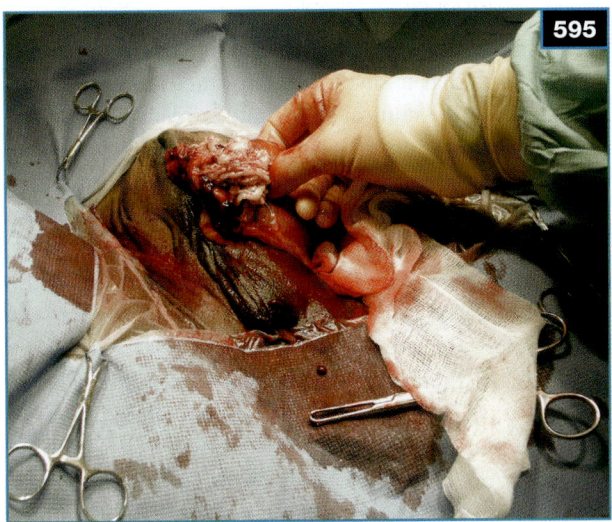

595 This 6-month-old Warmblood was castrated by the open method 24 hours prior to this picture. Investigation under general anesthesia in dorsal recumbency has confirmed eventrated omentum from the left vaginal tunic. This was resected and replaced into the abdomen. The superficial inguinal ring and vaginal tunic were then closed.

should be administered broad-spectrum antibiotics and referred to a surgical facility, as replacement of the small intestine usually requires a celiotomy.

If the tissue that has protruded is omentum, the same procedure can be performed or, if there are financial restraints, some patients will do well after omentectomy performed as proximal as possible using emasculators.

Funiculitis

Funiculitis refers to an infection of the emasculated stump and if the condition is chronic and suppurative, the term scirrhous cord is often used to describe it. 'Champignon' and botryomycosis are also terms used to describe this condition. The most common bacterial isolates from the infected tissue are Gram-positive bacteria (*Staphylococcus* spp. and *Streptococcus* spp.).

It is suggested that the risk of funiculitis is increased if ligatures are placed during the castration; however, this act on its own is unlikely to cause such a problem and a break in sterility during surgery is necessary for infection to occur. Contamination of the end of the emasculators might be the greatest risk factor. Failing to resect the vaginal tunic and external cremaster muscle may also increase the risk of septic funiculitis. In rare cases, the infected tissue may extend proximally into the peritoneum.

Equine castration

The history may reveal that the surgical site healed without complication then, subsequently, a draining tract occurred, or that a small draining tract remained after surgery. The first clinical signs noted are swelling in the area and drainage near the surgical scar. Discomfort in the inguinal area or hindlimb lameness may also be presenting complaints. This condition can remain dormant and clinically silent for several months or even years. Clinical examination reveals a thickened cord palpable within the inguinal region. Ultrasonography will help determine the extent of the infected tissue.

Antibiotic therapy provides temporary improvement, but once discontinued, clinical signs usually return. The treatment of choice for the majority of cases is surgical and involves reopening of the skin around the draining point and careful soft-tissue dissection around the draining tract (596). All infected spermatic cord should be removed by emasculation of the cord proximal to any thickened tissue. No ligatures should be placed and the surgical site is left open to heal by second intention. Systemic antibiotics and NSAIDs are usually required for 5–10 days and drainage is encouraged by regular in-hand walking.

Hydrocele

Hydrocele is a collection of peritoneal fluid in the scrotal region following castration due to persistent communication at the end of the emasculated vaginal tunic. It can occur weeks to months following the surgery and is usually of no clinical consequence. Diagnosis is made by palpation of the swelling, which reveals fluid that can be pushed out of the scrotum and into the abdominal cavity. Ultrasonography may help to rule out the presence of any soft-tissue problems in the area.

Treatment is not normally required except for cosmetic reasons. Surgical treatment requires reopening of the castration site and re-emasculation of the stump. An inguinal approach allows a more proximal emasculation of the tunic and placement of a ligature will further prevent recurrence (597).

Penile damage

Penile damage can occur if the shaft of the penis is confused with one of the testes during surgery and iatrogenic damage occurs. To avoid this, careful pre- and intraoperative palpation should be performed, especially if the surgeon is inexperienced. Treatment depends on the structures damaged. Hemostasis is essential and if the urethra has not been damaged, the wound may be sutured. If extensive damage has been caused, penile amputation or retroversion might need to be performed as a salvage procedure.

Continued masculine behavior

Persistent masculine behavior can be seen in up to 30% of cases following castration. The reasons for this are not fully understood, but are likely to involve innate group behavior between horses. Hormonal influence may also be involved, as androgens are not produced solely by testicular tissue. Cryptorchidism and incomplete castration should be ruled out by hormonal blood tests. The possibility of continued masculine behavior should be discussed with the owners before surgery, especially in older males and those used previously as stallions, as the risk of maintaining masculine behavior is increased.

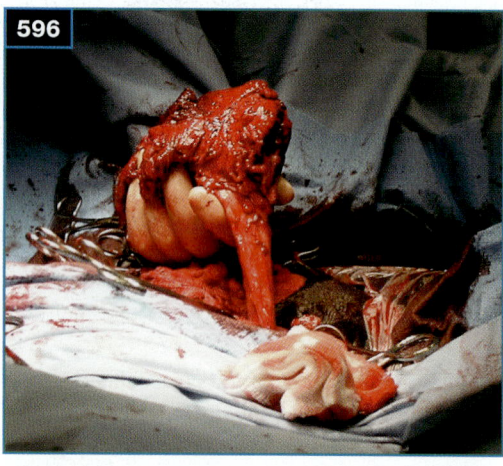

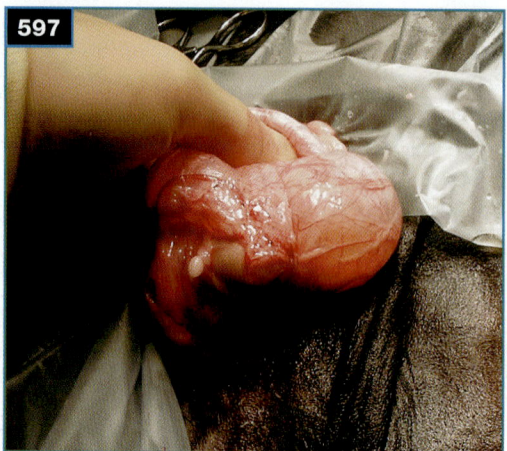

596 This horse had undergone an open castration 4 weeks earlier and presented with a large swelling on the left side of the inguinal region. At surgery, the funiculitis lesion on the end of the vaginal cord is completely exteriorized. Note the normal cord below it.

597 Intraoperative view of a hydrocele found at surgery following swelling in the scrotum of a horse castrated by the open technique several months earlier.

Respiratory system

1 Introduction
Josh Slater

2 Surgical conditions of the upper respiratory tract
Bruce Bladon and Graham Munroe

3 Medical conditions of the upper respiratory tract
Josh Slater

4 Medical conditions of the lower respiratory tract
Joanne Hewson, Luis Arroyo, and Josh Slater

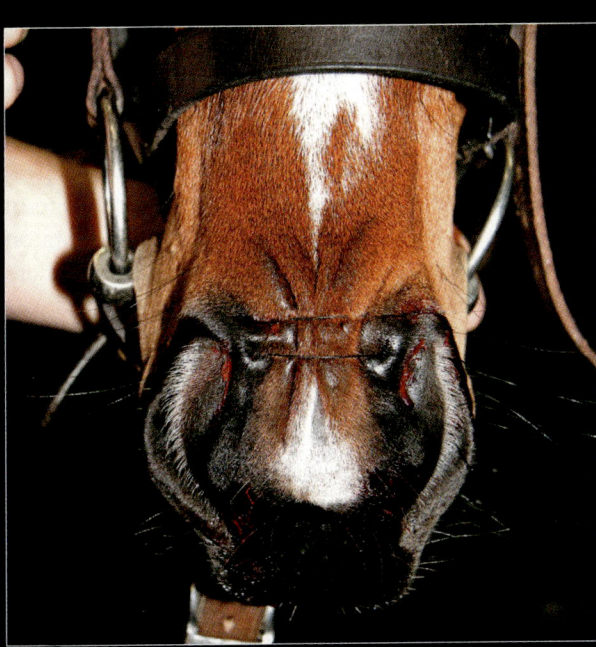

Horses are athletic animals and use only a small proportion of their respiratory capacity at rest. Compared with sedentary animals such as livestock and most small animals, relatively subtle respiratory disease can significantly decrease exercise capacity in equine athletes. Horses therefore usually present for investigation of respiratory disease at a much earlier stage in the disease than other species.

Clinical examination of the respiratory tract

Aims
It is extremely important to remember that:
+ Clinical examination of the respiratory tract at rest can be insensitive in detecting signs, although cases with nasal discharges, epistaxis, or pronounced coughing are obvious exceptions.
+ Respiratory disease detectable at rest, particularly of the lower respiratory tract (LRT), may therefore be of moderate or severe intensity.
+ Horses with significant respiratory disease (sufficient to cause poor performance) may appear normal when examined at rest.
+ Further investigations, especially microbiology, endoscopy, and cytology, are required for accurate diagnosis.
+ Specialist investigations, including respiratory function testing, may be needed to assist diagnosis and assessment of response to treatment.

Nevertheless, by adopting a careful and rigorous approach to clinical examination it is usually possible adequately to assess respiratory function and to diagnose and treat respiratory disease in practice. All regions of the respiratory tract are important for normal respiratory function; therefore, clinical examination must include assessment of each region from the nares to the lungs. The differential diagnoses of respiratory disease are often presented as a list, which is worked through until the correct diagnosis is reached; however, this is unrealistic and not practical. The actual aim of clinical examination should be to reach one of four initial, preliminary diagnoses: infectious upper respiratory tract (URT) disease; noninfectious URT disease; infectious LRT disease; and noninfectious LRT disease.

In most cases, further investigations (e.g. hematology, serology, microbiology, virology, endoscopy, radiography, ultrasonography, thoracocentesis, biopsy, pulmonary function testing) are then required to establish the precise etiology and diagnosis.

Features of different disease classifications
Each of the four groups of diseases has a typical set of presenting signs, although not each individual case will present with every clinical sign on the list.
+ *Infectious URT disease*. Several animals in a group affected; younger animals; pyrexia; depression; mucopurulent or purulent nasal discharge; lymphadenopathy; cough.
+ *Noninfectious URT disease.* Single animal affected; any age; no pyrexia; no depression; mucopurulent or purulent hemorrhagic nasal discharge; variable lymphadenopathy; facial distortion; respiratory noise; possible coughing; possible dysphagia.
+ *Infectious LRT disease.* Individuals or groups; any age; pyrexia; severe depression; mucopurulent or purulent hemorrhagic nasal discharge; often no lymphadenopathy; coughing; tachypnea; dyspnea; may be rapidly fatal.
+ *Noninfectious LRT disease.* Usually individual animals; older horses; no pyrexia; no depression; exercise intolerance/poor performance; mucopurulent or purulent nasal discharge; coughing; tachypnea; dyspnea.

Clinical examination
It is important to follow the same rigorous procedure for all clinical examinations, starting with observation from a distance, followed by close observation, and then hands-on physical examination.

History and signalment
+ Age: young horses are more likely to have infectious or congenital diseases, while older horses more often have noninfectious diseases.
+ Use: athletes with a history of poor performance are likely to have subtle disease on clinical examination at rest.
+ Transport or other stress: pleuropneumonia may be more likely.
+ Mixing with other age groups and through markets/dealer yards: predisposition to URT infections.
+ Single horse affected or several in the group (noninfectious versus infectious diseases).
+ Abnormal respiratory noise at exercise.

◆ Attitude: depression is more common with infectious diseases and the presence of a cough. The equine airway is insensitive compared with other species and coughing is not a sensitive indicator of respiratory disease (it is, of course, a specific indicator of respiratory disease). The character of the cough is not informative; productive coughing in horses is unusual even if there is copious airway discharge.

◆ Nasal discharge: nature and volume. Unilateral or bilateral nature may help to indicate the source of the discharge (i.e. LRT discharges are usually bilateral). Discharge after exercise may indicate an LRT origin. Copious discharge when the head is lowered may indicate a guttural pouch origin.

◆ Vaccination history.

◆ Worming history.

Observation from a distance

The general demeanor should be assessed. Respiratory rate should be evaluated prior to stimulating the horse. Resting rate should be 8–14 breaths per minute. Respiratory effort should be assessed and the respiratory pattern characterized. Normal inspiratory effort is mainly thoracic with some abdominal component. Normal expiratory effort is mostly elastic thoracic recoil with barely detectable abdominal (rectus abdominis) movement.

Close observation

The presence of nostril flare at rest indicates moderate to severe dyspnea. Nasal discharge should be characterized (unilateral/bilateral, serous, mucoid, mucopurulent, purulent, hemorrhagic, epistaxis). Facial symmetry should be assessed, with close attention paid to the maxillary area.

Abnormal noises

There is normally little or no noise during inspiration at rest and light exercise; there may be noise on expiration related to vibration of the false nostril. Fat or unfit horses may make a respiratory noise; this disappears as fitness increases. Breathing and stride patterns are intimately linked. At canter, expiration occurs as the forelimbs strike the ground. Abnormal noises are related to airway obstruction either by dynamic collapse of the airway, physical airway compression, thickening of the airway lining, or an airway mass. Abnormal noise is usually most apparent during exercise because the increased negative pressures cause dynamic collapse of the airway. Abnormal noises are often not present at rest.

Dynamic collapse of the airway causes inspiratory noise, while fixed obstructions cause both inspiratory and expiratory noise. Abnormal noise of nasal origin can be inspiratory and/or expiratory, while abnormal noise of nasopharyngeal or laryngeal origin is usually inspiratory. Abnormal noise of tracheal origin can be inspiratory and/or expiratory.

Physical examination of the respiratory tract

Nares
◆ Assess for patency by feeling for airflow from both nostrils.
◆ Swelling or injury.
◆ Dilation at rest (indicating marked dyspnea) (598).
◆ Discharge.

Nasal cavity
◆ External rostral facial symmetry and swelling.
◆ Percussion (dullness or pain).

Paranasal sinuses
◆ Symmetry and swelling.
◆ Percussion (dullness or pain).
◆ A detailed oral examination (using a gag and some form of light source) is required if sinus disease is suspected.

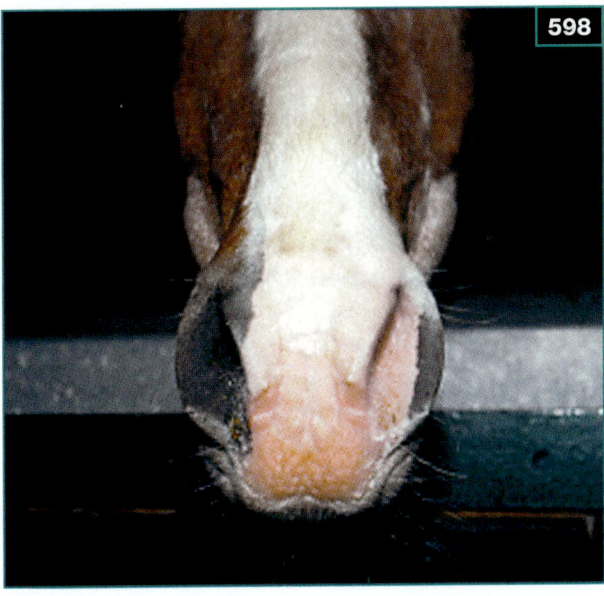

598 Horses with dyspnea may have flared nostrils at rest in addition to tachypnea and dyspnea. Nostril flare occurs with both URT and LRT causes of marked dyspnea.

383

Lymph nodes

+ *Submandibular lymph nodes* are located between the horizontal rami of the mandible and are palpable in normal horses as a group of small, loosely associated lymphoid nodules. These lymph nodes receive drainage from the rostral nasal cavity and nasopharynx and thus become enlarged in most URT infection cases and in some cases of dental disease.
+ *Retropharyngeal lymph nodes* are located immediately dorsal to the esophageal pharynx and immediately ventral to the floor of the medial pouch of the guttural pouch (the nodes are clearly visible through the guttural pouch floor). They are not palpable in normal horses. All lymph flow from the head passes through these nodes; they become enlarged in response to infection, but need to be grossly enlarged before they become palpable.
+ *The parotid lymph node* drains the orbit and ear region, but does sometimes become abscessed in *Streptococcus equi* infection.

Guttural pouches

+ Palpate retropharyngeal area for swelling or pain (not a sensitive indicator of guttural pouch disease).
+ Obvious distension usually indicates tympany, although it may also occur in severe cases of empyema.

Larynx

+ Palpate the dorsal surface of the larynx for symmetry of the left and right dorsal cricoarytenoid muscles and laryngeal cartilages.
+ Slap test: a slap just caudal to the withers induces a brief contralateral adduction of the arytenoid cartilage that can be palpated as a flick of the cricoarytenoid muscle or visualized endoscopically. The reflex requires intact spinal cord ascending white matter pathways (cuneate and gracile pathways in the dorsal funiculus) as well as intact motor pathways in the recurrent laryngeal nerve and functional cricoarytenoid muscles. Recent research has cast doubt on its relevance to the respiratory examination.
+ Induction of cough: squeezing the larynx to induce a cough may provide some indication of laryngeal sensitivity, but this is a highly subjective procedure that has limited clinical value.
+ Auscultation of the larynx may provide some information about the larynx and is worthwhile because laryngeal noise will be audible in the lung field and can confuse thoracic auscultation.

Trachea

Palpation of the trachea can help detect physical deformity, and squeezing the trachea to induce a cough is carried out by some clinicians. This, as for the larynx, is a highly subjective measure of tracheal sensitivity and has limited value.

Auscultation of the trachea is worthwhile because tracheal noise radiates to the lung field and airway discharges pool at the thoracic inlet and provides a valuable estimate of events in the distal airway and lung.

Lung-field auscultation

The auscultation area of the lung field is triangular in shape. Its cranial boundary is the vertical line of the caudal edge of the triceps muscle between the caudal border of the scapula and the olecranon. Its dorsal boundary is a horizontal line from the caudal border of the scapula to the tuber coxae. The caudal border of the lung field slopes cranioventrally from the 16th or 17th intercostal space to the olecranon.

In normal adult horses there is little audible noise in any part of the lung field. Foals and thin adults have much more obvious noise on auscultation. The hilar region, immediately dorsal to the heart base, contains the major divisions of the bronchial tree and there is air movement noise (bronchial sounds) in this region on inspiration, with quiet bronchial sounds on expiration. The peripheral lung field is quiet, with barely perceptible air movement sounds on inspiration or expiration.

The audible area of the lung field may be expanded in horses with severe recurrent airway obstruction or decreased ventrally if there is pleural effusion or pulmonary consolidation.

Auscultation at rest is not a sensitive means of assessing the lung fields because of the slow breathing rate and small tidal volume compared to when being exercised (599). Its sensitivity can be improved by auscultation during and immediately after rebreathing. Abnormal sounds can be accentuated by:

+ Use a large-volume plastic bin liner and fold the free edges over to give better control.
+ Introduce the bag over the horse's muzzle, gather the free bag to form a good seal between the bag and the muzzle, and hold the bag in position under the nose band of the head collar.
+ As the horse rebreathes the air from the bag, its breathing rate and effort increase as carbon dioxide concentration increases.

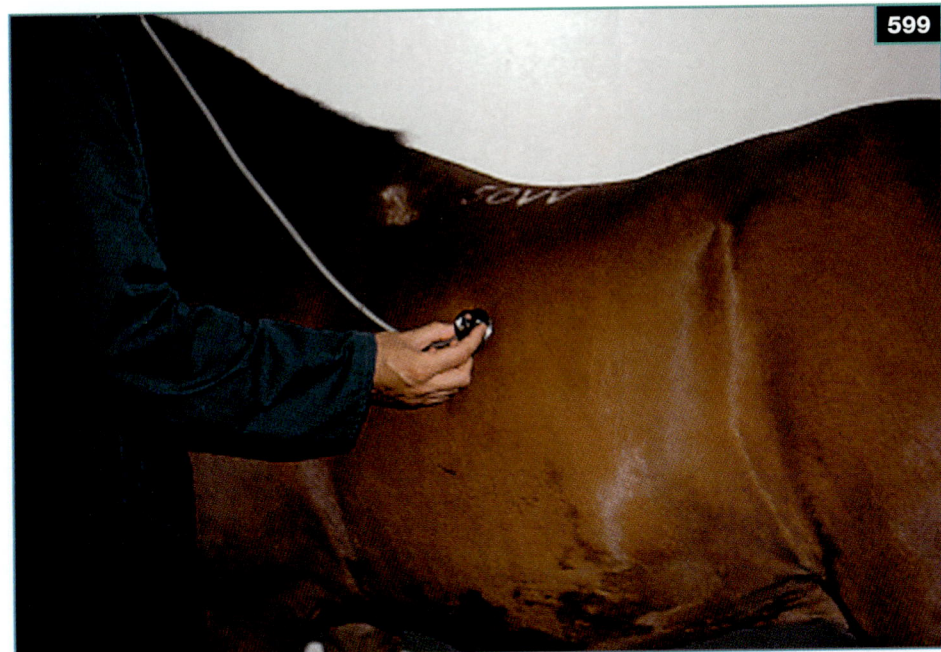

599 Auscultation of the lung field at rest often fails to reveal significant abnormalities because horses have a large respiratory reserve.

+ Keep the bag in place for as long as the horse will tolerate it (the length of time the bag is tolerated for is not an indicator of abnormality); auscultation can be done with the bag in place if desired.
+ The horse will continue to take deep rapid breaths for a minute or two after the bag is removed, accentuating abnormal sounds.

There is a surprisingly small range of abnormal sounds heard in horse lungs:
+ *Wheezes* are musical, sighing sounds generated by air moving through airways narrowed by broncho-constriction and/or discharges. Less marked airway constriction generates bronchial sounds that are harsher and more audible than normal, rather than wheezes.
+ *Crackles* are short, harsh sounds that sound like bubble wrap packaging and are generated by collapsed small airways or alveoli (because of surface tension effects of discharge) snapping open at the end of inspiration and during expiration. Fluid or bubbling sounds are very unusual in horses. Note that, in contrast to humans, crackles are usually not due to emphysema; this is a rare pathology even in horses with severe pulmonary disease.
+ *Friction rubs* are high-pitched, squeaky sounds generated by inflamed pleural surfaces rubbing together, indicating pleuritis or pleuropneumonia.

Lung-field percussion
Percussion is often omitted from the clinical examination, but this is a mistake as valuable information about the presence of pleural effusion and, possibly, the extent of the inflated lung field can be obtained. Percussion can be carried out either by placing the first two fingers of one hand over an intercostal space and tapping these fingers firmly with the tips of the first two fingers of the other hand or, more effectively, by using a plexor and pleximeter.

Working from cranial to caudal, each intercostal space is percussed from dorsal to ventral to identify areas of hyporesonance indicating absence of air-filled lung (i.e. pleural fluid and/or consolidated lung). Percussion is remarkably accurate for identifying pleural fluid lines. Occasionally, hyperresonance may occur in recurrent airway obstruction (RAO) cases due to lung hyperinflation.

Diagnostic tests

Respiratory endoscopy

Respiratory endoscopy is a simple, well-tolerated and extremely informative investigation for both the URT and the LRT. Most endoscopic examinations are facilitated by sedation to reduce coughing, increase patient compliance, and reduce the risk of damage to patient and instrument; however, meaningful assessment of pharyngeal and laryngeal function can only be carried out in unsedated horses because sedation causes relaxation of the nasopharynx, flaccidity of the soft palate, and decreased arytenoid abduction. Endoscopy allows direct examination of most of the tract and can be used to collect lavage and biopsy samples. 1.0–1.5 meters × 8–12 mm fiberoptic endoscopes are standard equipment in equine practices and are suitable for examination of the URT and the proximal trachea, but they are too short for examination beyond the carina. Longer instruments are required for examination of the bronchial tree. Lengths between 1.8 meters and 2.4 meters are needed for collection of bronchoalveolar lavage (BAL) samples.

As for clinical examination, a standard routine should be used for endoscopic examination:

+ Both sides of the nasal cavity: include the ventral and middle meati (to check for discharge from the region of the nasomaxillary openings).
+ Nasopharynx and soft palate.
+ Guttural pouches: entry to the pouches requires an implement (either a closed biopsy forceps [600] or, better, a solid, semi-rigid plastic introducing device inserted via the endoscope's biopsy channel) to lever open the nasopharyngeal ostium of the pouch and allow entry of the endoscope.
+ Larynx: the resting position, movement, and symmetry of the epiglottis, aryepiglottic folds, arytenoids, vestibular folds, vocal folds, and lateral ventricle should be sssessed. Observe during and after swallowing for transient positional abnormalities (e.g. epiglottic entrapment) or sometimes difficult-to-visualize abnormalities (e.g. subepiglottic cysts). Remember that endoscopically-induced dorsal displacement of the soft palate is common and does not necessarily indicate that this abnormality occurs during exercise.
+ Trachea: the proximal trachea is relatively insensitive and can be examined with little coughing. Discharges from the lungs pool at the thoracic inlet.
+ Carina and bronchial tree: the trachea becomes progressively more sensitive along its length and beyond the carina the airway should be desensitized with 1% lidocaine.

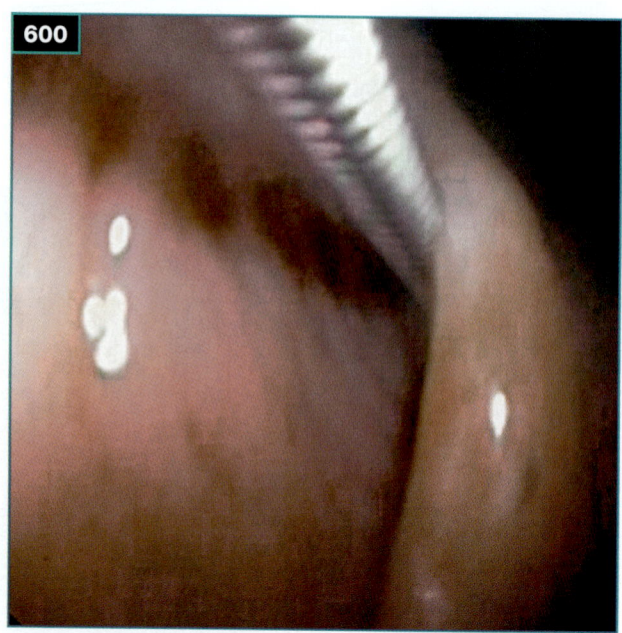

600 Use of a closed biopsy instrument as a guide to assist entry into the guttural pouch. The biopsy instrument is inserted into the pouch and, as the endoscope is rotated, the pouch opening elevates to facilitate entry of the endoscope.

Upper respiratory tract and thoracic radiography

Some regions of the URT are not accessible for endoscopy and radiography can provide valuable diagnostic information about dental disease, sinus disease, the dorsal nasal cavity, and the bone and cartilage skeleton (skull, maxillary and ethmoid turbinates, nasal septum, sinus walls). All views of the head and cranial neck regions of the URT can be obtained with standard general practice X-ray machines. There is considerable superimposition of different structures in the head; therefore, lateral, dorsoventral, and lateral oblique views are required to help interpretation.

Thoracic radiography requires high-powered equipment and is not possible with small portable practice machines. Four overlapping lateral projections are required to image the lung field. Indications for thoracic radiography are chronic unresponsive RAO (pulmonary fibrosis), exercise-induced pulmonary hemorrhage (EIPH) (focal consolidation), pleuropneumonia/bronchopneumonia (pulmonary abscess, pulmonary consolidation), mediastinal masses, and thoracic trauma (pneumothorax). Interpreting thoracic radiographs requires recognition of the four major pulmonary patterns:

- **Bronchial**: increased visibility of the bronchial tree due to chronic airway disease and mineralization of the airway wall.
- **Interstitial**: increased density of the lung interstitium due to inflammation or fibrosis. This is a common, but nonspecific, equine pulmonary radiographic abnormality.
- **Alveolar**: air-filled bronchi (tubular lucencies) silhouetted against fluid-filled alveoli (radio-opaque lung field) producing 'air bronchograms'; associated with pulmonary edema.
- **Vascular**: increased visibility of the pulmonary vasculature, seen in congenital conditions, producing left-to-right shunts (e.g. ventricular septal defect).

These changes indicate pathologic changes and not specific diseases.

Thoracic ultrasonography

This is very useful for identifying pleural fluid or peripheral pulmonary disease (where there is decreased air in the peripheral lung, where lung lesions extend into the pleural space, or where there are adhesions between parietal and visceral pleura). Normal lung is air filled and reflects the ultrasound beam, creating a bright white line at the air interface of the pulmonary surface and not revealing lung detail. Pleural fluid is readily visible and ultrasound can provide valuable information about the nature of the fluid (cellularity and fibrin content) as well as its location within the pleural space and whether there is pocketing. Ultrasound provides a valuable guide for both thoracocentesis and lung biopsy.

Paranasal sinus percutaneous centesis and sinuscopy

The boundaries of the maxillary sinus can generally be defined as follows:
- **Dorsally**: a line drawn from the medial canthus of the eye to the nasoincisive notch.
- **Rostrally**: the rostral limit of the facial crest.
- **Ventrally**: the facial crest.
- **Caudally**: a line drawn from the middle of the orbit to the facial crest.

The boundaries of the frontal sinus are as follows:
- **Caudally**: a line drawn from the temporomandibular joint to the midline.
- **Rostrally**: the midpoint of a line drawn from the medial canthus of the eye to the nasoincisive notch joined to the midline.
- **Laterally**: the medial canthus of the eye.

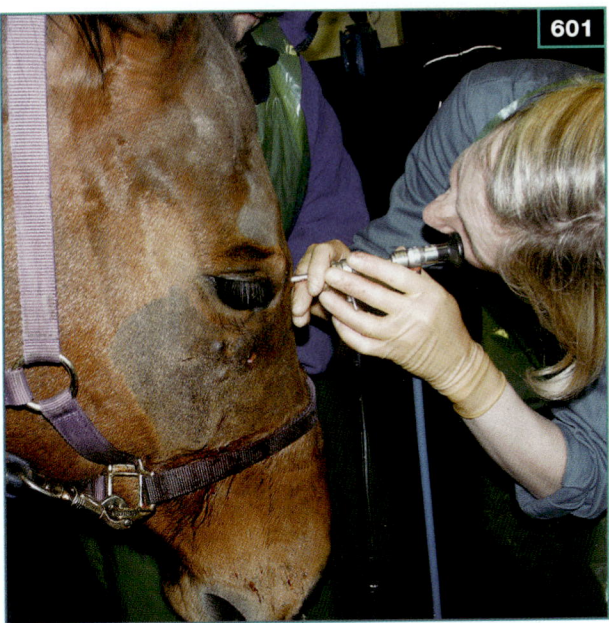

601 Sinuscopy of the frontal sinus carried out under standing sedation. The portal used for this and the one visible beneath the right eye can also be used to collect material from the sinuses (sinocentesis).

Percutaneous sinus centesis

This is a simple means of obtaining a lavage sample from the sinuses in a standing, sedated horse. The entry site for the caudal maxillary sinus is approximately 3–4 cm dorsal to the facial crest and approximately 3–4 cm rostral to the medial canthus. The entry site for the rostral maxillary sinus is approximately 3–4 cm rostral to this. The entry site for the frontal sinus is the midpoint of a line drawn from the medial canthus to the midline. Local anesthetic is infiltrated subcutaneously and a small incision made. A 3–4 mm Steinmann pin in a chuck is used to drill through the bone into the sinus. A catheter can then be introduced and a saline lavage taken.

Sinuscopy

The entry points and preparation for sinuscopy (**601**) are the same as for centesis except that a larger pin size or trephine hole is required to provide access for the endoscope. A trephine hole into the frontal sinus also provides access to the caudal maxillary sinus via the frontomaxillary opening and to the ventral conchal sinus if forceps are used to create an opening into this space.

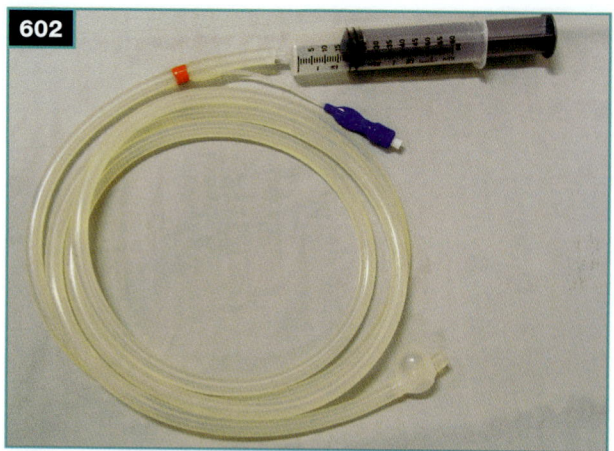

602 Flexible nasotracheal catheter with an inflatable cuff used for performing BAL in horses. The tube is passed blindly into the caudodorsal region of either the right or the left lung for lavage.

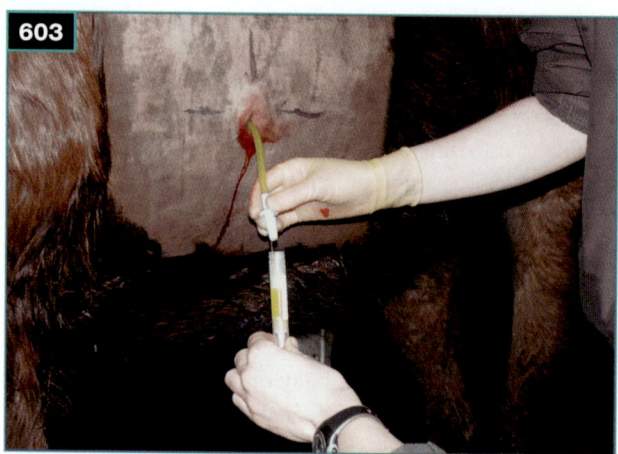

603 A chest drain has been inserted on the left side under aseptic conditions, with local anesthetic infiltration. Note the marks on the skin, which have been made at the point of maximum collection of pleural exudate as determined by previous ultrasonography.

Tracheal and bronchoalveolar lavage

Tracheal lavage (TL) and BAL are essential in all cases of LRT disease. TL and BAL samples are suitable for cytology, bacteriology/virology, and parasitology. As discharges pool in the trachea, TL samples are representative of both lung fields, but generally they provide poor samples for cytology (cells are degenerate) and may not accurately reflect current events in the lung. BAL samples provide an accurate, current reflection of events in the lung, but because only one segment of lung is sampled, they are not representative of the whole lung. BAL samples are thus suitable for generalized lung diseases (e.g. RAO), but they may miss focal abnormalities.

Tracheal lavage

TL is usually performed transendoscopically. There is a small risk of bacterial contamination of transendoscopic samples from the nasal cavity and nasopharynx, but this does not usually invalidate bacteriology results. To avoid this problem, TL can be carried out percutaneously using either a commercial kit or an intravenous catheter. The endoscope is advanced to the mid-cervical trachea or beyond the thoracic inlet and a sterile catheter inserted through the biopsy port. Using a catheter with a sterile plug reduces the risk of bacterial contamination from the head. 20–30 ml of sterile saline is injected into the trachea. This runs either caudally (from a cervically positioned endoscope) or cranially (from a heart-base positioned endoscope) and pools at the thoracic inlet. The catheter is advanced into the saline pool and a sample aspirated.

Bronchoalveolar lavage

BAL requires a 2.4 m endoscope, but samples can be satisfactorily collected 'blind' using a commercial 2.4 m BAL catheter (602). Endoscopic collection is usually carried out by wedging the endoscope in the cranial lung lobe. If a catheter is used, it is wedged and the cuff inflated. 300–500 ml of prewarmed sterile saline should be infused, then 50–250 ml gently aspirated. The fluid should have a frothy appearance because of the presence of surfactant.

Thoracocentesis

Thoracocentesis should be guided by thoracic percussion and ultrasound examination. It can be used to confirm the presence of pleural fluid, obtain samples for cytology and bacteriology, and to drain pleural fluid. The entry site is ventral (about a hand's breadth above the olecranon) at approximately the 8th intercostal space on the left (i.e. caudal to the heart) and the 7th intercostal space on the right, depending on the precise location of the fluid. Ultrasound examination is important because fluid pocketing and adhesions may make drainage difficult. The entry site is the immediate cranial border of the rib at the desired intercostal space (this avoids the intercostal artery, vein, and nerve), taking care to avoid the lateral thoracic vein. The skin is shaved and sterilized and local anesthetic infiltrated subcutaneously and into the intercostal space. A large-bore (30 French) chest drain and a trochar are inserted directly into the pleural space through a stab incision (603). Following entry, the trochar is withdrawn and the drain inserted further; this should provide fluid drainage. If a large volume of fluid is present, the drain can be left in place with a one-way valve to prevent air aspiration.

Lung biopsy

Lung biopsy is rarely undertaken in horses as it has a number of complications including epistaxis, pneumothorax, and sudden death. Biopsy should be reserved for cases where all other investigations have failed to achieve a diagnosis, but a diagnosis is critically required. Biopsy should not be carried out if pulmonary infection is suspected. Biopsy should be ultrasound guided but, as a guide, the entry site is a hand's breadth above the olecranon and just caudal to the heart. Automatic/spring-loaded biopsy needles (e.g. Trucut) should be used and inserted into the lung to a depth of no more than 2–3 cm. Lung biopsy can also be performed under pleuroscopic guidance.

Pulmonary function tests (including blood gas analysis, treadmill, and exercise examinations)

Sophisticated pulmonary function testing is difficult because of the lack of patient compliance. However, by making simultaneous measurements with an esophageal balloon and manometer and a face mask fitted with a pneumotachograph, it is possible to measure pleural pressure changes (an approximate measure of the total work of breathing), pulmonary resistance (a measure of resistance to airflow along the airway – i.e. a measure of broncho-constriction), and dynamic compliance (a measure of the elasticity of the lung). Most pulmonary diseases result in an increase in pleural pressure change, increased resistance, and decreased elastic compliance. These simple estimates of pulmonary function are sometimes useful in assessing severity of disease or response to treatment, but they are not generally required in practice. Blood-gas analysis is simple to perform, but is not abnormal at rest unless moderate to severe pulmonary or cardiovascular disease is present. Arterial blood samples can be collected into a heparinized syringe from the transverse facial artery for immediate analysis. Hypoxia (PaO_2 <80 mmHg) and hypercapnea ($PaCO_2$ >45 mmHg) result from ventilation–perfusion mismatching in the lung. Pulmonary diseases generally cause decreased ventilation, which causes an increase in $PaCO_2$ and a proportional decrease in PaO_2. Treadmill and field exercise testing allow more rigorous assessment of the respiratory (and cardiac, locomotor, and metabolic) systems than examination at rest. The difficulty is standardization so that comparisons with normal horses can be made. For this reason, exercise testing is usually carried out on a treadmill where the exercise test can be controlled and standardized, rather than as track or field tests. Treadmill testing is usually carried out with a treadmill slope of approximately 10% and the running speed increased incrementally from 2–12 ms^{-1} at intervals of one minute until the horse becomes fatigued. Treadmill testing can be combined with simultaneous endoscopy to identify dynamic abnormalities in the nasopharynx including dorsal displacement of the soft palate and dynamic collapse of the larynx and pharynx. A variety of parameters can be measured to follow the response to exercise including heart rate at particular speeds (as fitness increases the speed at which maximum heart rate is reached increases), oxygen uptake (VO_2 max is a measure of fitness and increases with increased exercise capacity), and blood lactate concentration (a measure of aerobic capacity). Recently, overground endoscopy systems have been introduced that allow the URT to be visualized while the horse is performing its normal exercise program.

Thoracoscopy

The thoracic cavity, the mediastinum and its contents, and the lung surface can be assessed using thoracoscopy, which allows direct inspection and can increase the accuracy of diagnosis and prognosis for pleural and some pulmonary diseases. Thoracoscopy can be performed in sedated, standing horses using local analgesia and a rigid endoscope. The right and left hemithorax can both be assessed thoracoscopically, allowing visualization of the dorsocranial thorax and the dorsocaudal thorax. The pleural cavity and lung surfaces can be assessed and the aorta, thoracic duct, azygous vein, and esophagus can also be visualized. The procedure is well tolerated, but some horses may develop a transient pneumothorax.

Nostril

Alar fold disease (redundant/hypertrophy/collapse/stenosis)

Definition/overview
The alar fold forms the ventral aspect of the nasal diverticulum (false nostril) and divides it from the rostral nasal passage. It extends from the alar cartilage caudally to the rostral aspect of the ventral nasal concha. The fleshy fold, which is lined by a mucous membrane, is elevated during exercise and closes off the entrance into the false nostril. Failure of function, or abnormalities, of the alar fold can lead to an abnormal inspiratory noise at exercise. Surgical resection of the fold can be effective.

Etiology/pathophysiology
The cause varies between individuals and many are of unknown etiology, but possibilities include increased size or thickening of the alar folds or abnormal function of the levator nasolabialis muscle (the main elevator of the alar cartilages). Individuals with abnormally narrowed nostrils may also suffer from similar problems. It has been speculated that American Saddlebreds and Standardbreds are more commonly affected because of possible genetic conformation abnormalities of the nostril region.

Clinical presentation
Affected horses present with a loud vibratory noise from the nostril region at exercise, particularly at faster gaits. The noise is usually noted at expiration and inspiration; the former is usually louder, and with no or variable effects on exercise tolerance due to increased airway resistance. In rare cases, noises have been noted at rest. There may or may not be an abnormal nostril or false nostril conformation. Occasionally, the folds are still collapsed into the nostril at the end of work and can be observed.

Differential diagnosis
High blowing is a term used to differentiate a normal situation where the folds vibrate during expiration only and cause no clinical effects. The noise in these circumstances is usually louder at the beginning of work and decreases with increasing exercise. Other differential diagnoses include various causes of abnormal respiratory noise, nostril traumatic damage, and deviation.

Diagnosis
Confirmation that the noise is derived from the alar folds is best achieved by placing a temporary mattress suture through the dorsal nostril and then the false nostril, before taking it over the bridge of the nares, and passing it through the other side in the same manner (604). The suture can be tied on top of a swab in the midline of the dorsal nares. The horse is examined before and after suture placement to assess the difference in noise and performance.

Management
If there is exercise intolerance or the noise is very loud, then bilateral resection of the folds under general anesthesia is indicated. This can be approached through the external nares or after incision through the lateral wall of the nostril. The incision into the fold leads to considerable hemorrhage, which stops with suture placement. Alternatively, the incision can be made with diathermy. Horses are returned to exercise after suture removal at 2 weeks postoperatively.

Prognosis
After surgery the prognosis for noise reduction and return to normal exercise levels is fair, but if there is additional rostral nasal passage narrowing, results may be less effective.

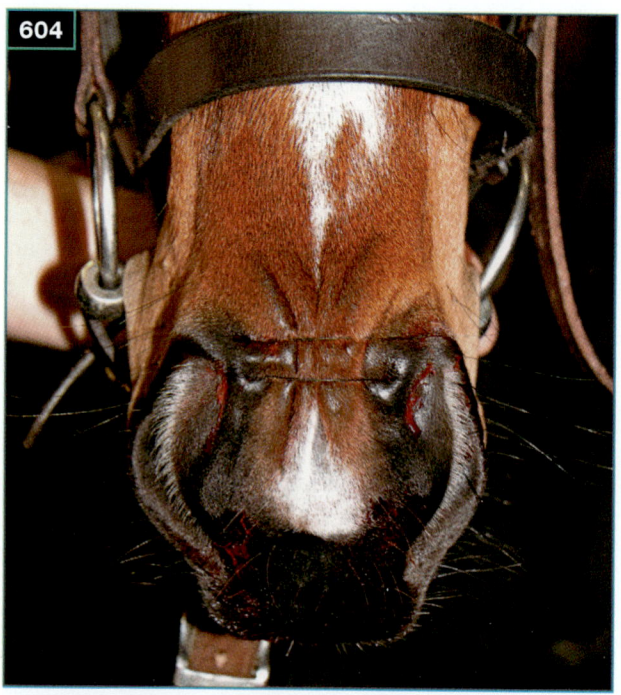

604 Temporary mattress suture placed across the midline as an aid to the diagnosis of alar fold collapse.

Atheroma

Definition/overview

Atheroma is an epidermal inclusion cyst of the false nostril, which presents as a palpable and visible oval-shaped cyst. In rare cases it may have some effect on performance, but it is principally a cosmetic disease. Treatment is removal, either surgically or chemically, with an excellent prognosis.

Etiology/pathophysiology

The epidermal inclusion cyst is formed by keratinizing squamous epithelium with a granular layer, similar to the normal epithelium of the follicular infundibulum, aberrantly located within the dermis of the false nostril. Cysts are congenital, but develop over 1–2 years of life.

Clinical presentation

A visible and palpable soft fluctuant swelling is present on the muzzle, caudal to the nostril (605). It can be up to 5 cm in diameter and can be easily palpated via the false nostril. It is nonpainful, seldom causes any respiratory obstruction, and is of cosmetic significance only.

Differential diagnosis

Possibly skin tumors such as sarcoid, but the clinical presentation is quite typical.

Diagnosis

Diagnosis is based on clinical examination and examination of centesis aspiration of gray, greasy contents.

Management

Atheromas are simply and effectively managed by injection with 10% formalin. In the standing, sedated horse the thick sebaceous contents are aspirated and, following this, a similar volume of formalin–saline is injected, usually about 5 ml. There is swelling for 24 hours and then the cyst gradually regresses over 7 days. Alternatively, a stab incision can be made, under local anesthesia, via the false nostril, into the cyst. The cyst lining is then reamed out using a laryngeal or ventricular 'Hobday' burr. Finally, the cyst can be surgically removed, under local anesthesia and standing sedation, via an approach through the skin overlying the false nostril.

Prognosis

The prognosis is excellent provided all the secretory lining is removed, with recurrence following appropriate management very rare.

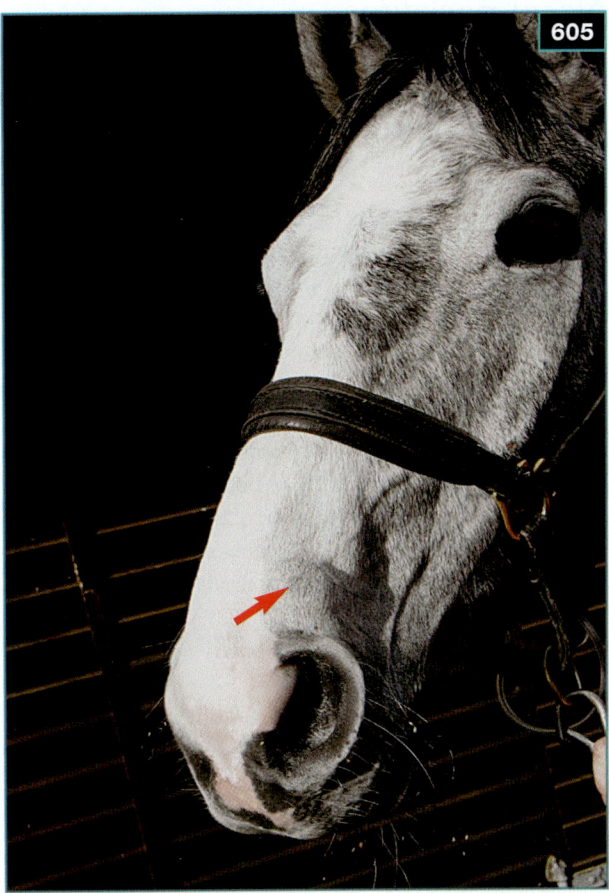

605 A typical epidermal inclusion cyst (atheroma) (arrow) in the false nostril of a young Thoroughbred racehorse.

Nasal passages

Wry nose

Overview (see also p.494)

Wry nose is a complex congenital deformity of the nose, with lateral deviation of the maxilla, nasal bone, incisive bone, and nasal septum to one side, occasionally with a milder mandibular deformity and/or dorsoventral deviation. It is of unknown etiology and is more common in primiparous mares and draft breeds. Some cases may be associated with contracted foal syndrome and may therefore be seen in foals following dystocia. The physical deformity leads to malocclusion and possibly dysphagia. In some cases there are abnormal respiratory noises. Spontaneous improvement has been seen in mild cases and surgical treatment has been undertaken in more severe cases, although this remains controversial and is unlikely to return the animal to normal fast exercise.

Deformity of the nasal septum

Definition/overview

A variety of rare congenital and acquired conditions can cause deviation and/or thickening of the nasal septum. They usually cause abnormal respiratory airflows and noises that are diagnosed on digital palpation, endoscopy, and dorsoventral head radiographs. Some animals are able to cope with these problems without treatment if they perform limited exercise, but surgical removal of the septum may be necessary in some cases.

Etiology/pathophysiology

Multiple conditions have been reported to result in thickening and deviation of the nasal septum. Thickening is seen in hamartoma, congenital cystic degeneration, trauma leading to fracture of the frontal and nasal bones, amyloidosis, severe bacterial or mycotic infection of the septum following URT disease, neoplasia, and wry nose. Deviation is associated with congenital malformations (e.g. wry nose) and expanding masses in the nasal cavity or paranasal sinuses such as neoplasia or cysts.

Clinical presentation

The respiratory obstruction varies with the cause, but it can be severe, leading to nasal passage obstruction, especially at exercise, with an abnormal respiratory noise (marked nasal stertor) and exercise intolerance. Facial swelling and/or asymmetry may also be present.

Differential diagnosis

The most likely cause of reduced airflow in one nostril with marked stertor is conchal swelling. This can be associated with an expansile mass within the paranasal sinuses (e.g. a sinus cyst or severe primary sinusitis) or a large progressive ethmoidal hematoma.

Diagnosis

Digital palpation via the nares may reveal abnormalities of the rostral septum and abnormal airflows may be detected. Endoscopy of the nasal passages may be unrewarding or impossible due to the severity of the swelling and narrowness of the meatus. Dorsoventral head radiographs may reveal bony and septal deformities, but soft swelling can lead to increased density in the entire nasal cavity. CT or MRI of the head may be very helpful in these cases.

Management

Some animals with mild deformities or thickening may be able to cope without treatment during limited exercise. In severe cases or where return to athletic ability is desired, surgical removal of the septum is necessary. This involves the removal of the rostral 75% of the septum under general anesthesia and is associated with considerable intraoperative hemorrhage. Consideration should be given to whether the surgery is justified or whether an alternative salvage procedure such as permanent tracheostomy might be preferable.

Prognosis

The prognosis for a cosmetic outcome is good; however, the prognosis for a functional outcome is more guarded. Significant complications such as excessive granulation tissue at the cut edge of the septum, persistent respiratory noise, collapsed nasal bones, and adhesion formation to the nasal conchae usually limit the horse's resulting airway and an abnormal respiratory noise continues.

Choanal atresia/stenosis

Definition/overview
This is a rare congenital condition involving failure of development, or narrowing, of a hole (the choana) between the nasal passages and the nasopharynx. It can be unilateral or bilateral. Bilateral cases are almost invariably fatal at birth. Unilateral cases will usually survive, but have a poor athletic potential. Occasionally, there is a congenital narrowing or stenosis of the airway at this level that presents, later in life as the animal starts to exercise, as a respiratory noise and/or exercise intolerance.

Etiology/pathophysiology
The nostrils develop caudally by fusion of the palatine processes. The bucconasal membrane separating the nasal cavities from the pharyngeal cavity thins progressively until it is two layers of epithelium (oral and nasal). The membrane perforates before parturition. The precise cause of failure of this membrane to rupture is unknown. In humans, choanal atresia is frequently (47%) associated with other congenital abnormalities including ocular, cardiac, and genitourinary defects.

Clinical presentation
Bilateral cases present with severe respiratory distress at birth. Foals are almost invariably dead by the time veterinary attention is available, but occasional cases learn to mouth breathe and survive.

Unilaterally affected horses usually present with respiratory signs at a young age. The presentation varies, associated with any other abnormalities, but includes respiratory noise, lack of airflow from one nostril, and reduced exercise tolerance.

Differential diagnosis
Bilateral: all causes of respiratory obstruction and distress in the newborn foal can appear similar, most importantly aspiration of fetal fluids and membranes. Unilateral: other causes of respiratory distress in the young horse, including permanent dorsal displacement of the soft palate, and an expansile mass within the paranasal sinuses, including sinus cysts, should be considered.

Diagnosis
Endoscopic examination is definitive (606). This can be difficult to interpret as the endoscope cannot be passed through to the pharynx. Examination via the contralateral nares usually allows orientation and subsequent diagnosis in a unilateral case. Contrast radiography has been used to delineate the deformity. In stenosis cases, one or both of the entrances from the nasal passages to the nasopharynx may appear narrowed.

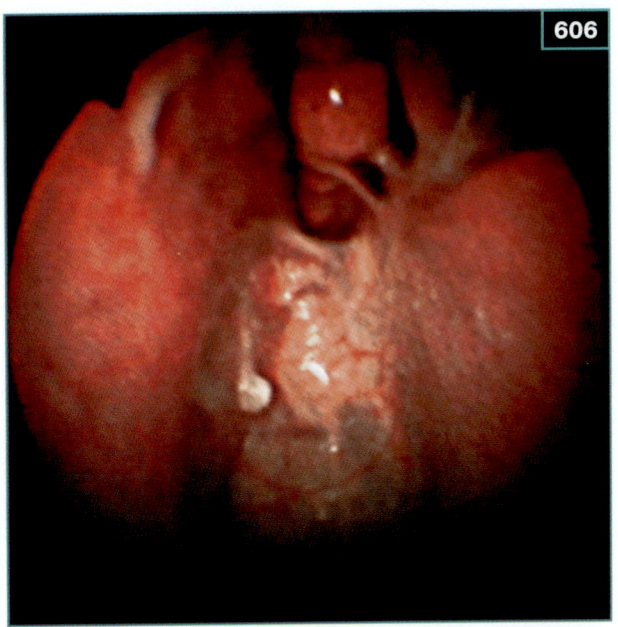

606 Endoscopic view of a unilateral (left side) choanal atresia. The foal presented with respiratory noise, dysphagia and permanent displacement of the soft palate. The left side of the picture is the caudal nasal septum, the upper aspect is the ethmoturbinates, the right side is the caudal ventral turbinate, and the lower aspect is the abnormal membrane covering the upper part of the ventral meatus.

Management
If bilateral, then life support would require orotracheal intubation or a tracheotomy. If the atresia is membranous, then endoscopic laser surgery to ablate the membrane is possible. Many cases are much more substantial, with thickened tissue and bone frequently present; a fron-tonasal bone flap has been used to allow surgical removal of the obstruction. Intranasal surgery using laparoscopic instruments has been reported. An alternative approach is to the caudal aspect of the atresia via a laryngotomy.

Prognosis
Prognosis for survival of unilateral cases is good, but for return to normal exercise tolerance is variable depending on the severity of the lesion. Concurrent congenital abnormalities may seriously affect the long-term prognosis.

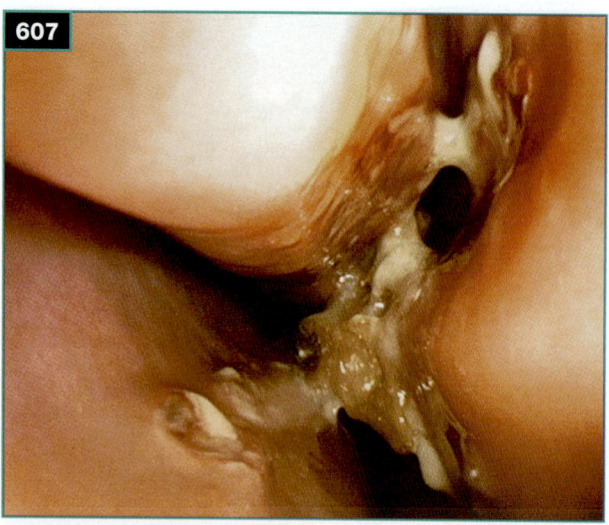

607 Large mycotic plaque in the middle meatus. This horse had a history of intermittent epistaxis.

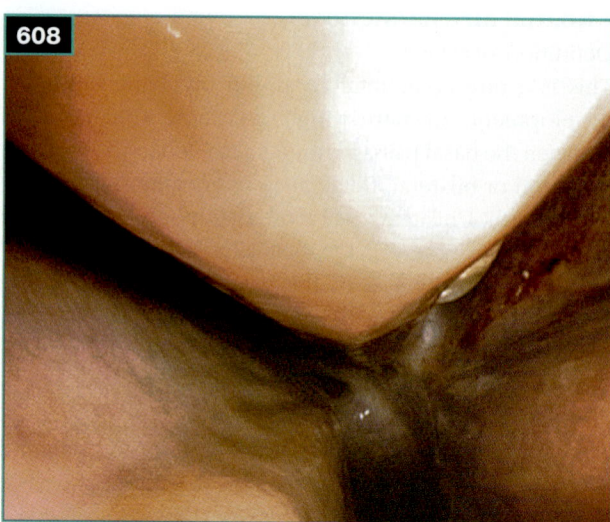

608 The same lesion 48 hours after dislodging the mycotic plaque and irrigating the area with enilconazole.

Fungal rhinitis

Definition/overview

Fungal rhinitis is an infrequent complication of other nasal or sinus disease or treatment. The condition is predisposed (as with most fungal infections) by treatment with antibiotics. The other feature of fungal infections, the erosive nature of the fungal plaque, is also pertinent to this disease. Primary fungal infections of the URT, which are caused by specific fungal species, are rare and tend to occur in certain parts of the world. Such infections include cryptococcosis, rhinosporidiosis, phycomycosis, and coccidioidomycosis.

Etiology/pathophysiology

The most commonly isolated fungus is *Aspergillus fumigatus*, but *Pseudoallescheria boydii* has been cultured. These are mainly secondary invaders of tissue damaged by trauma, sinonasal surgery, nasal or sinus masses such as progressive ethmoidal hematoma, or persistent nasal discharge either from disease of the paranasal sinuses or from the lungs. Primary fungal rhinitis and sinusitis is unusual, particularly in temperate climates, but it has been recorded where animals are stabled with moldy hay and straw. The excessive use of antiseptics or antimicrobials may predispose to fungal infections. The resulting fungal plaques are able to erode into the nasal tissue, leading to bleeding.

Clinical presentation

Fungal rhinitis results in a chronic, unilateral, usually malodorous nasal discharge, often with variable amounts of blood and a mucopurulent or purulent character. The client often ignores the discharge until it becomes bloodstained. If the disease follows surgery, there may be a worsening or persistence of the discharge. There may be submandibular lymph-node enlargement.

Differential diagnosis

Other causes of chronic nasal discharge and epistaxis include progressive ethmoidal hematoma, guttural pouch disease, and other paranasal sinus diseases.

Diagnosis

Endoscopic examination is diagnostic (**607, 608**). One or more mycotic plaques of variable size are usually visible on the ventral or dorsal conchae in the nasal passages. There is often evidence of turbinate damage or deeper bone damage and necrosis. The plaque is often yellowish or greenish-white and covered in thick exudate. Samples should be taken, preferably from the plaques under endoscopy, for cytology and culture and susceptibility testing.

Management

Treatment should consist of removal of the plaque(s), treatment with antifungals, and correction of any predisposing causes. The plaques in the nasal passages are often conveniently debrided, under endoscopic control, using a cleaning brush for the biopsy channel of the endoscope. This often provides just the right amount of friction to remove the plaque. Following removal of the plaque, the area is irrigated with antifungal solution delivered via the endoscope. Further treatment for another 1–2 weeks can be done using a small animal urinary catheter to deliver the solution blindly to approximately the right position in the nasal passages. Antifungal solutions used include enilconazole, miconazole, keto-conazole, and natamycin. The use of nystatin powder can also be useful where lesions are difficult to lavage with solutions, particularly in the paranasal sinuses. Some clinicians use systemic iodides in addition, but these are rarely necessary. The use of antimicrobial or antiseptic solutions and treatments should be withdrawn if possible.

Prognosis

The prognosis is very good. Recurrence or persistence of lesions is rare and is a sign that the fungal infection is a result of an underlying disease. Limiting the use of antibiotics helps to reduce persistence.

609–611 Three sections taken through the head, starting at the rostral end of the facial crest, passing caudally ~2 cm/slice. The nasal cavities are colored light green, the caudal maxillary and frontal sinus compartments are dark green, and the rostral maxillary and ventral conchal sinus compartments are blue. Note the complex curve of the rostral maxillary and ventral conchal sinuses, resulting in very little contact with the side of the face, and the 'bulla' of the rostral maxillary sinus, the bubble-shaped roof (arrows).

Paranasal sinuses

Primary sinusitis

Definition/overview

This is a common condition, particularly of animals with a history of URT disease. The anatomy of the paranasal sinus compartments is very complex (609–611). From a clinical standpoint the sinus compartments can be divided into two: the rostral maxillary/ventral conchal (lateral and medial to the teeth and infraorbital canal) and all the others. The other sinus compartments include the frontal, conchofrontal, and caudal maxillary. The latter all commu-nicate with each other through large openings and drain via a single slit-like opening in the caudal middle meatus of the nasal passages. The rostral maxillary sinus has its own separate drainage ostium in the middle meatus.

Etiology/pathophysiology

A URT infection with viruses or, occasionally, bacteria (*Streptococcus* spp.) leads to increased mucus production and compromised mucociliary clearance, with stagnation of the mucus in the dependent sinuses. Surrounding mucosal inflammation further compromises the relatively small and poorly sited drainage ostia. The mucosal lining can become hyperplastic with chronicity and secondary bacterial infection is common, further increasing the production of fluid (increasingly purulent) and decreasing drainage. A mixed bacterial growth is often isolated. With chronicity, empyema and inspissation of the exudate can occur. In primary sinusitis of the rostral maxillary and ventral conchal sinuses, the drainage is even more restrict-ed and once empyema is established, successful drainage is much harder to achieve. With increasing exudate there may be expansion of the conchal walls of the paranasal sinuses and increasing obstruction of the airway.

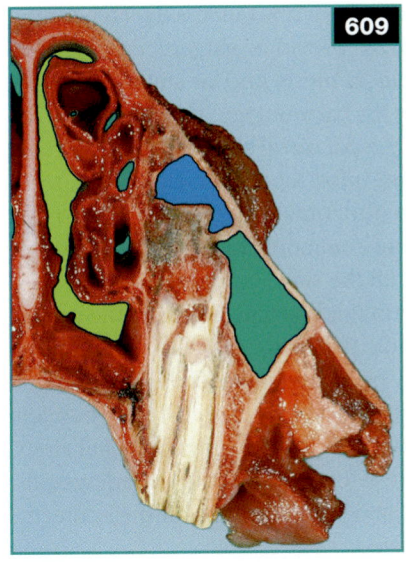
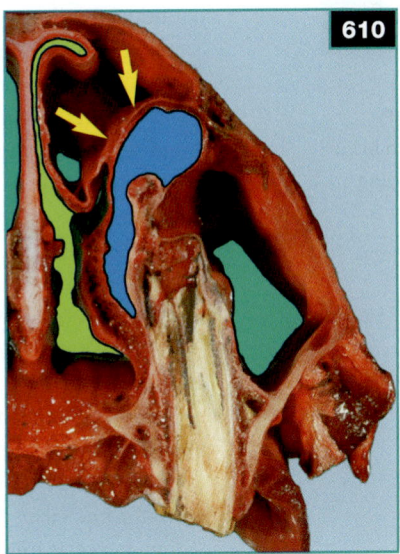
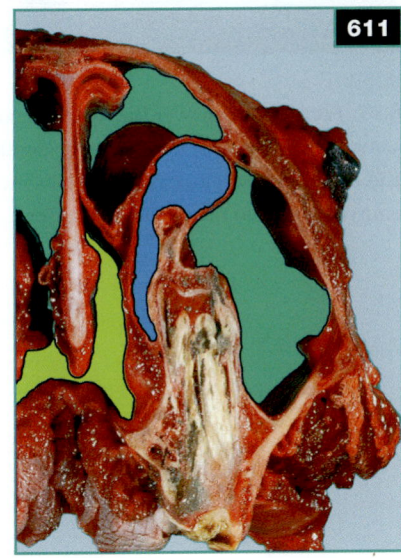

Surgical conditions of the upper respiratory tract

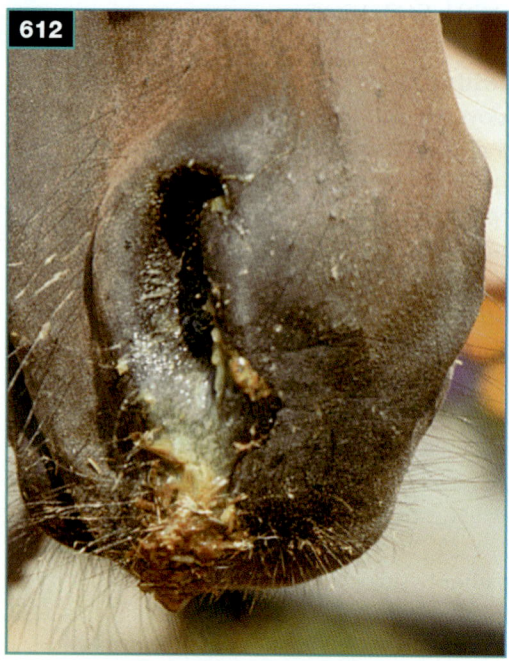

612 Unilateral purulent nasal discharge typical of sinusitis.

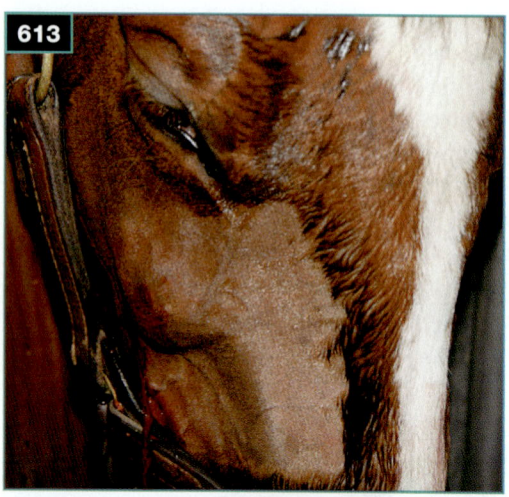

613 Facial swelling over the rostral maxillary sinus. Swelling here is unlikely to be dental in origin and usually reflects an expansile mass, including empyema, within the paranasal sinuses.

Clinical presentation

Primary sinusitis most commonly presents with a unilateral mucopurulent or purulent nasal discharge, often copious in quantity and, in chronic cases, increasingly malodorous (**612**). Bilateral cases do occur, but are uncommon. The discharge may increase after exercise or feeding from the ground. There is often unilateral lymphadenopathy of the submandibular lymph node on the affected side. Less frequently, conchal swelling leads to nasal distortion, resulting in reduced airflow, an abnormal respiratory noise, and, occasionally, exercise intolerance. External facial swelling may also occlude the nasolacrimal duct, resulting in epiphora and/or ocular discharge. The facial swelling is located over the paranasal sinuses caudal to the rostral edge of the facial crest (**613**).

Differential diagnosis

The most important differential diagnosis is secondary sinusitis, particularly that due to dental disease. Other causes of unilateral nasal discharge include guttural pouch disease (particularly empyema), rhinitis (particularly fungal rhinitis), and occasionally mucopurulent tracheal discharges, which are preferentially expelled down one nostril.

Diagnosis

Diagnosis is based on the history, clinical signs, endoscopy, sinoscopy, and radiography. Resonance on percussion over the sinuses may be reduced, but this is an unreliable test. The mouth requires careful examination for any cheek-tooth pathology, most particularly in the caudal four teeth. Endoscopy is less valuable in sinusitis than in many other conditions of the URT, but it should be possible to establish whether there is any conchal swelling and/or discharge from the caudal maxillary sinus drainage angle, visible at the caudal end of the middle meatus, rostral to the ethmoid labyrinth. It is not possible to advance the endoscope into the maxillary sinus unless the architecture has been damaged by previous surgery or extensive mycotic infection. Sinocentesis and/or sinoscopy allow collection of samples for bacteriology, visualization of the lining, and lavage of the paranasal sinuses.

Radiography is the most important diagnostic technique. One or more horizontal free gas/fluid interfaces may be noted or, more commonly in primary sinusitis, so much discharge that all the sinus compartments are filled completely, resulting in fluid opacity replacing the normal gas density of the sinus (**614–616**). On dorsoventral views of the head there may be displacement of the nasal septum by gross distension of the sinus. Occasionally, the purulent material becomes confined to the ventral conchal sinus, where it may be more difficult to identify on radiographs. In chronic cases the lining of the sinuses or their contents may become mineralized.

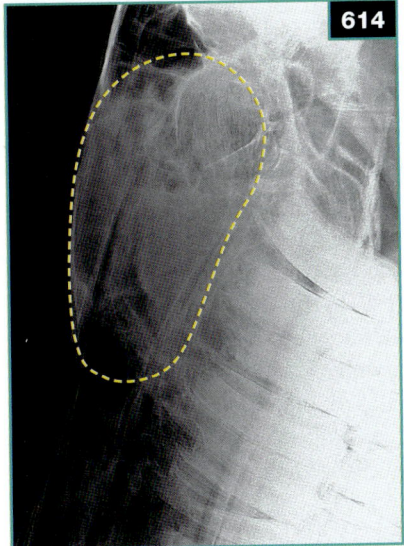

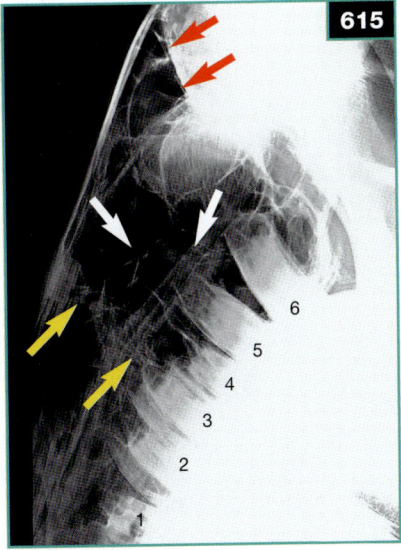

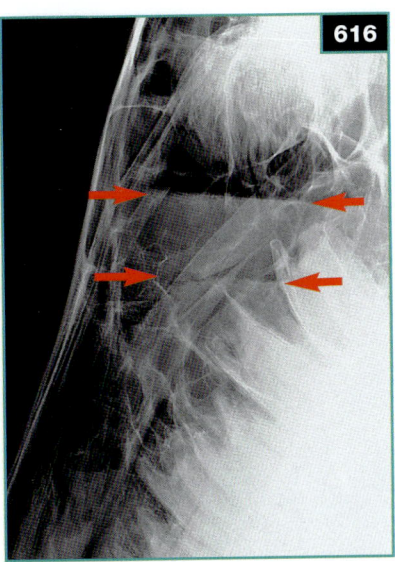

Differentiation from secondary sinusitis is by excluding other possible causes. In a few cases, establishing a diagnosis may be difficult and advanced techniques such as CT and scintigraphy may be helpful.

Management

The management of primary sinusitis depends on its severity. In a simple early case with fluid lines visible in the sinus compartments, treatment with systemic antibiotics for 1–3 weeks is usually curative. Treatment can be guided by culture of nasal discharge or by fluid obtained from the sinus following trephination. Oral treatment with potentiated sulfonamides is often effective. Some clinicians use steam or volatile inhalations. Continued regular light exercise, grazing, and feeding all food off the floor will encourage drainage.

Cases that fail to respond to conservative treatment are often managed by sinus lavage, although inspissated material will not respond to simple flushing alone. A trephine hole is made either in the caudal maxillary sinus, on the flat plate of bone below the eye and above the facial crest, or, alternatively, the frontal sinus can be used. The frontal trephine is located at the medial canthus level, approximately half way from the midline to the medial canthus (617). These portals can also be used for sinuscopic examination of the sinuses. A Foley or other self-retaining catheter is placed, the balloon inflated, and the catheter sutured to the skin. The sinus is then irrigated with copious volumes of fluids, preferably under pressure, including tap water, saline, or dilute (0.05–0.1%) povidone–iodine disinfectant solution q12–24h for 5–7 days. Instillation of an antifungal agent after irrigation is recommended by some clinicians, as fungal sinusitis is a common complication of sinus lavage.

614 Laterolateral radiograph of a 3-year-old Thoroughbred with a history of unilateral nasal discharge. There is increased density of the entire rostral and caudal maxillary paranasal sinuses (dotted line).

615 Laterolateral radiograph of a normal horse's head, showing the rostral edge of the maxillary sinuses (yellow arrows), the caudal edge of the frontal sinus (red arrows), and the 'bulla' of the rostral maxillary sinus (white arrows). The teeth are numbered as cheek teeth from 1 rostral (206) to 6 (211). The fourth cheek tooth (209) is easily identified as the shortest (and hence oldest) tooth.

616 Multiple fluid lines (arrows) within the paranasal sinus compartments.

617 The incision for trephination of the frontal sinus. This horse has had a previous frontonasal flap created on the other side and the scar is clearly visible.

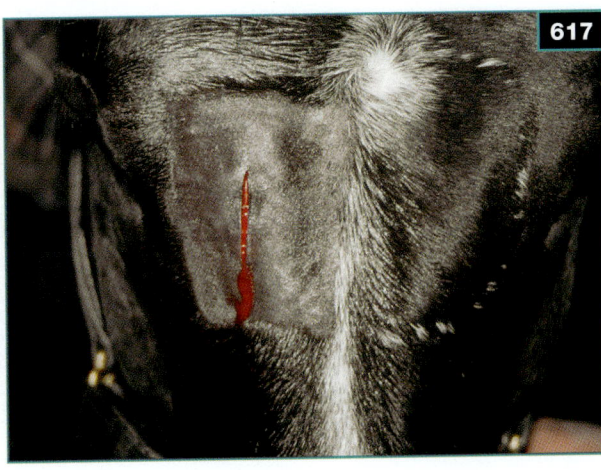

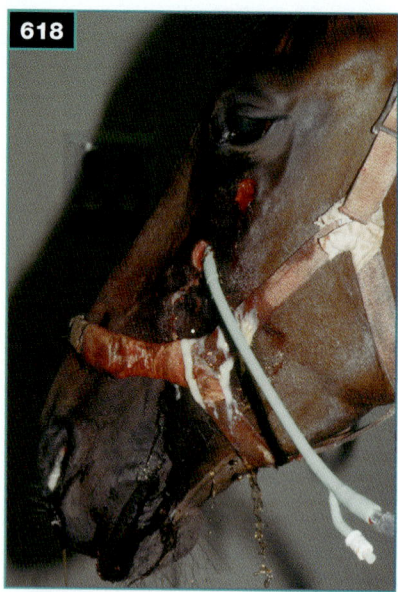

618 Irrigation of the rostral maxillary sinus. Note the trephine in the caudal maxillary sinus and the copious amounts of pus both at the nose and on the head collar, having drained from the trephine.

619 The 'bulla' of the rostral maxillary sinus (arrows), distended by purulent contents, is clearly visible endoscopically from a frontal trephine.

620 Removal of the roof of the rostral maxillary sinus, using arthroscopy rongeurs.

621 Inspissated material removed from the rostral maxillary sinus. This material will not be removed without surgery, no matter how much the sinuses are lavaged.

The most common cause of failure of treatment for primary sinusitis is not inadequate drainage or insufficient lavage, but is ongoing sinusitis of the rostral maxillary and ventral conchal sinus compartment. Trephination of the rostral maxillary sinus is more difficult as the sinus is small, particularly in young horses, and a large amount of the space is occupied by the root of the fourth maxillary cheek tooth. The site for trephination of the rostral maxillary sinus is 1–2 cm caudal and 1–2 cm dorsal to the rostral edge of the facial crest (**618**). The rostral maxillary and ventral conchal sinuses are separated by the infraorbital canal and the maxillary cheek teeth, and communicate by a space over the canal. Trephination and subsequent irrigation can be unsuccessful as the ventral conchal sinus remains poorly lavaged and the formation of inspissated pus is common.

Surgery is indicated in cases of primary sinusitis that have not responded to conservative therapy and sinus lavage. Removal of the inspissated pus from the rostral maxillary sinus can be achieved by removing the 'roof' of the sinus (the bulla) so that the rostral maxillary and ventral conchal sinuses communicate via a large dorsal opening with the caudal maxillary sinus (**619, 620**), and then lavaging vigorously with a high flow of fluid. All the solid inspissated material must be removed (**621**). Fistulation of the maxillary sinuses through to the nasal passages by removal of much of the floor of the conchofrontal sinus and some of the lateral wall of the ventral conchal sinus will improve the drainage of the sinuses and is beneficial in some cases. If extensive surgical manipulation such as extensive mucosal resection and fistulation is required in these cases, general anesthesia and exposing the sinus via a large frontonasal or maxillary bone flap are required. Where fistulation into the nasal passages is not necessary and drainage from the caudal maxillary sinus is adequate, surgery can be completed in the standing sedated horse via a large nasofrontal flap or using one or two trephine holes and endoscopic guidance.

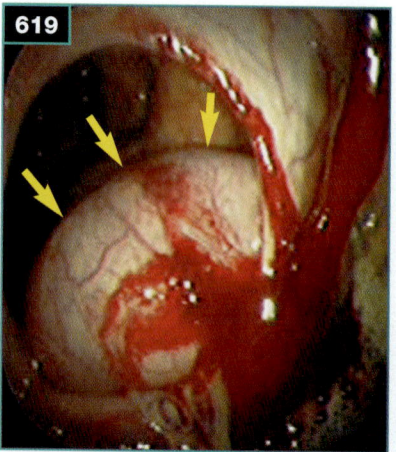

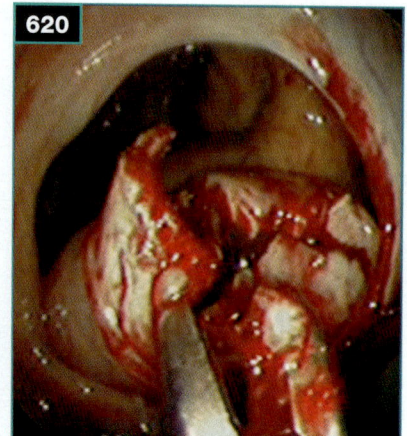

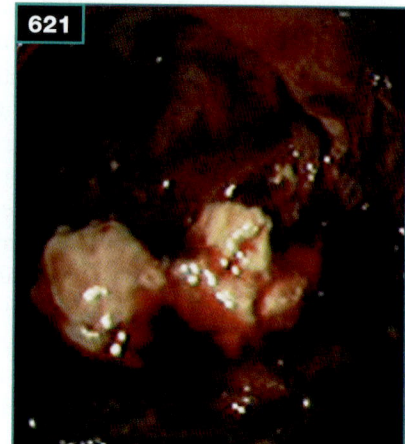

Prognosis

The prognosis for primary sinusitis is good, as many cases respond to conservative treatment or lavage. Those cases requiring surgical intervention carry a more guarded prognosis, and complications such as the development of mycotic sinusitis or the establishment of infection in the trephine holes or bone flap can delay resolution and necessitate repeated surgical procedures.

Secondary sinusitis

Definition/overview

This is a sinusitis secondary to another disease. The most widely described form of secondary sinusitis is dental sinusitis as a sequela to periapical dental infection. Other causes include sinonasal neoplasia, facial fractures or trauma, occlusion of drainage by expansile lesions such as progressive ethmoidal hematoma and sinus cysts, immunosuppression, especially in Cushingoid older ponies, and fungal sinusitis.

Etiology/pathophysiology

The roots of the upper fourth cheek teeth (and occasionally the caudal root of the third tooth) are usually in the rostral maxillary and ventral conchal sinuses, while the fifth and sixth cheek teeth are in the caudal maxillary sinuses. Periapical infections of these teeth can result in sinusitis. The caudal third and the fourth cheek teeth are most commonly involved.

The most common neoplasm of the nasal passages is squamous cell carcinoma (SCC), though many other tumors have been reported from the paranasal sinuses (e.g. lymphosarcoma, adenocarcinoma or ossifying fibroma, or neoplastic-like conditions such as fibrous dysplasia). Any condition that either forms a focus of necrotic or infected tissue within the sinuses or occludes the normal drainage channels can result in secondary sinusitis.

Clinical presentation

The clinical presentation is similar to that of primary sinusitis, although in dental-derived sinusitis the unilateral discharge is invariably purulent and malodorous from the beginning. Tooth-related sinus disease cases often exhibit a fetid halitosis, which is readily detected. Space-occupying lesions within the sinus usually have less nasal discharge, but they may present with facial swelling and/or unilateral epiphora and/or nasal obstruction. Rarely, both primary and secondary sinusitis can extend from the frontal sinus into the CNS to cause a meningoencephalitis or into the eye via the sphenopalatine sinus to result in blindness and exophthalmos.

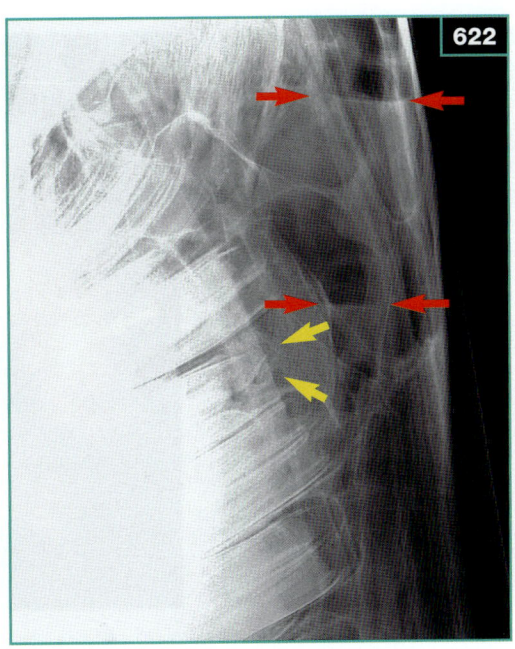

622 Secondary sinusitis caused by periapical infection of tooth 209 in a 3-year-old Thoroughbred. Note the multiple fluid lines (red arrows) and the periapical endosteal sclerosis associated with loss of the clear outline of the lamina dura (yellow arrows).

Differential diagnosis

Primary sinusitis is the principal differential diagnosis, but a specific cause for the secondary sinusitis is essential to make a treatment plan and give an accurate prognosis. In secondary sinusitis a malodorous fetid breath is more common and smaller amounts of fluid are found in the sinuses, with fluid lines on radiographs. Mycotic sinusitis is an important differential diagnosis and can develop as a result of treatment for a primary sinusitis.

Diagnosis

The diagnosis of secondary sinusitis is similar to that of the primary version. Radiographic diagnosis of periapical dental infection (see pp. 486–488) may not be reliable in some cases, particularly so when dealing with the caudal maxillary teeth (**622**) or in younger horses. Specific arcade oblique and/or intraoral radiographic views can be helpful. Lavage of the sinus for several days to help remove as much fluid and pus as possible prior to specific sinus and tooth-root radiographic views may help define specific tooth or sinus problems. Oral examination and radiography should always be combined to increase the

399

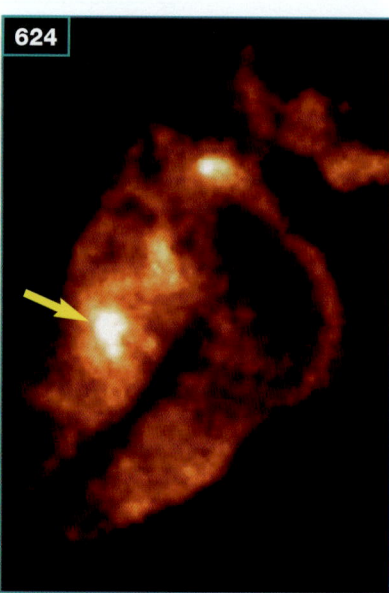

623, 624 Dorsal (623) and lateral (624) scintigrams of a 3-year-old Thoroughbred showing a marked increase in uptake of the radioisotope around the fourth cheek tooth, 209 (arrows).

specificity of a precise diagnosis. Scintigraphy can be used in the diagnosis of periapical dental infection and generally a periapical abscess results in marked uptake of the radioisotope over the root of the tooth (623, 624). Unfortunately, sinusitis also results in a marked increase in uptake of the isotope in the bone around the sinus, particularly for mycotic sinusitis. Recently, CT and MRI have been used in the differential diagnosis of sinus disease.

Tumors and cysts can be visible on sinoscopy, although initial lavage of the discharges for several days may be necessary to ensure adequate visualization (625).

Management

The management of secondary sinusitis depends on the underlying disease. If this can be treated, the underlying sinusitis will usually resolve with conservative management or, at the most, lavage of the sinuses via a trephine hole. Dental disease can be treated by conservative dentistry techniques or by tooth removal. Tooth removal is either by oral extraction, via a buccotomy, or repulsion via a trephine hole or facial flap exposure. Once the infected tooth has been removed (626), the sinusitis usually resolves provided there is no subsequent oro-antral fistula due to the alveolus not healing post removal. Oro-antral fistulae (627) can be frustrating to manage and may require prolonged treatment and multiple surgeries. It is essential to achieve a seal between the sinus and the oral cavities by packing material in the dental socket.

Management of neoplastic secondary sinusitis is generally unrewarding. Tumors can be removed by large frontonasal flaps; however, most are highly invasive and complete removal is very difficult, with aggressive recurrence common.

Prognosis

The prognosis for dental sinusitis is guarded to fair provided tooth removal is successful and oro-antral fistulae do not develop. Lack of resolution of the sinusitis or recurrence indicates continued infection of the sinus by a leaking fistula, persistent diseased tissue such as dental or bone fragments, and/or infection in the alveolus or maxillary bone/turbinates. Secondary fungal and/or anaerobic bacterial infections are quite common in these cases postoperatively. Most fistulae will heal with time; however, the economic aspect of the ongoing treatment can be considerable. Neoplastic sinus disease has a poor prognosis as most tumors in this region are invasive and/or malignant.

625 Postmortem cross-section through the head of a horse with a squamous cell carcinoma of the maxillary sinuses. The invasive nature of the tumor is clearly visible.

626 Radiograph of a recently purchased horse. Prepurchase examination had not established that the horse was missing a tooth. Sinusitis developed shortly after purchase and radiographs revealed a fragment of dental material (arrow) associated with the dental socket. (Photo courtesy M Morley)

627 Postmortem photograph of a severe oro-antral fistula. There is gross food contamination and empyema of the caudal maxillary sinus.

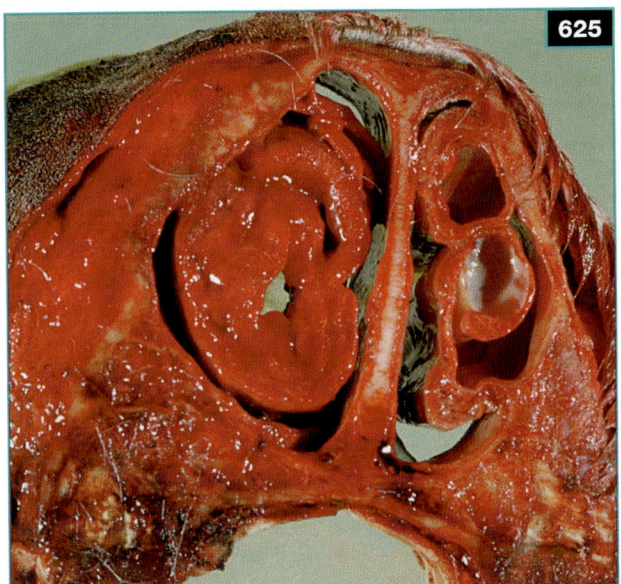

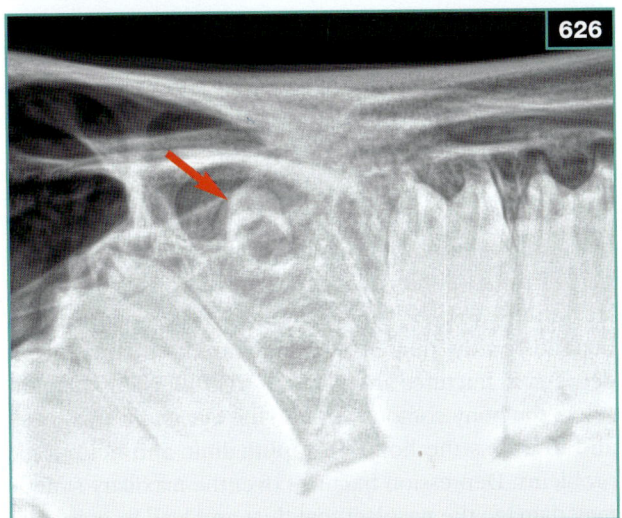

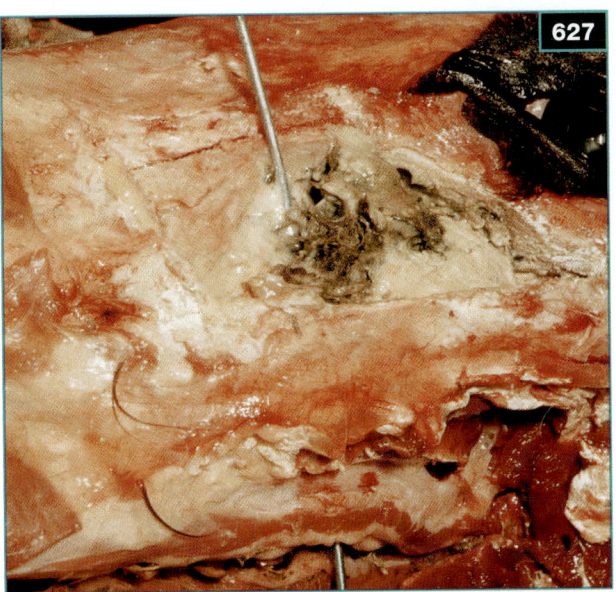

Fungal sinusitis

Definition/Overview

An infrequent condition of the paranasal sinuses, often secondary to another disease process. The disease can be a complication of the treatment of sinusitis and should be anticipated when possible.

Etiology/pathophysiology

As with most fungal infections in temperate climates, the condition is usually secondary. One of the principal causes of mycotic sinusitis is prolonged antibiotic or antiseptic solution treatment, often for sinusitis. Thus it is common for the original primary sinusitis to resolve, but mycotic sinusitis to develop during treatment. This is a confusing presentation as the clinical signs will often not alter, though the disease process changes. Mycotic infections can be secondary to other conditions such as tumors. Primary mycotic sinusitis is recognized, but it is hard to be definitive that this was the original condition. Fungal infections are very erosive and in some advanced cases damage to the nasal conchae or infraorbital canal can develop.

Clinical presentation

The clinical presentation is typical of sinusitis. There is a unilateral nasal discharge and usually unilateral enlargement of the submandibular lymph node. There is usually a chronic history and often a history of previous treatment. Facial swelling is very rare, as is facial ulceration. The discharge is frequently malodorous.

Differential diagnosis

The differential diagnosis includes almost all other causes of sinusitis. Due to the chronic nature of the condition, most horses are investigated for secondary sinusitis.

Diagnosis

Endoscopic examination of the nasal meatus usually reveals no abnormalities or, possibly, scanty discharge from the nasomaxillary sinus drainage angle. Radiography is also frequently unrewarding with limited signs, possibly some fluid lines in the maxillary sinuses, but often no abnormalities. Gamma scintigraphy frequently reveals an intense increase in uptake of the radioisotope. Care must be taken when interpreting the scan as it is possible to misdiagnose the uptake as a periapical tooth abscess. It is important to remember that dental disease is not the only cause of increased uptake of radioisotope in the paranasal sinuses.

Diagnosis requires direct sinus endoscopy (sinoscopy) via a trephine hole in either the caudal maxillary or the frontal sinuses (628). Orientation of the endoscope within the paranasal sinuses can be difficult; the two key features are the sharp-edged frontomaxillary opening and the linear infraorbital canal. Mycotic plaques have a typical diphtheritic appearance and microscopic examination is definitive, with millions of fungal hyphae easily identified.

Management
Removal of the diphtheritic plaques is therapeutic and as much fungal material as possible should be removed at the time of diagnosis. This is achieved with arthroscopy rongeurs through an enlarged or second trephine hole. The sinus is then irrigated with antifungal agents via an indwelling (Foley) catheter. Enilconazole is usually chosen in the UK, where a product licensed for ringworm treatment is available. Irrigation is continued for 2–3 weeks.

Prognosis
The prognosis is good. In the large majority of cases, complete resolution is achieved after a few weeks topical medication, although repeated debridement of lesions may be required.

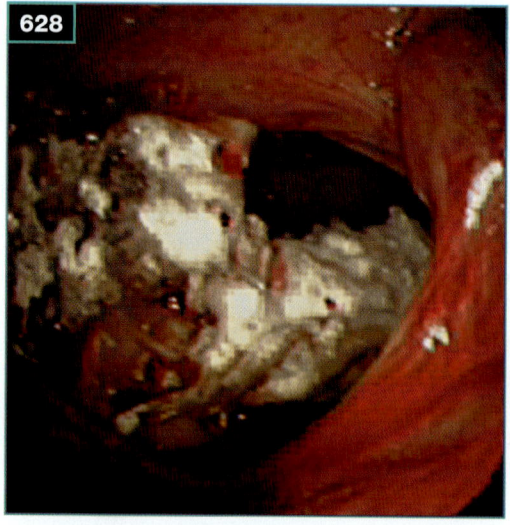

628 Mycotic sinusitis viewed endoscopically by a trephine hole into the frontal sinus.

Facial trauma involving the nasal cavity and paranasal sinuses

Definition/overview
This is a relatively common condition of variable severity. Injuries can be caused by impacts with solid objects during falls or collisions, or by kicks from other horses. Variable degrees of soft- and bony-tissue damage can occur and can secondarily cause injury to the eye, URT, and cranial vault.

Etiology/pathophysiology
The etiology is trauma, but this is not always confirmed in every case. There may or may not be skin lacerations depending on the specific cause. The degree of bony damage can range from superficial trauma to nondisplaced cracks to depression fractures, some of which are comminuted. Large areas of bone overlying the paranasal sinuses and, occasionally, the nasal passages can be damaged in the most severe cases.

Clinical presentation
There is often mild to moderate epistaxis on the affected side, which may last for several days and may become increasingly mucopurulent if secondary infection ensues, most particularly if the paranasal sinuses are involved. Variable soft-tissue swelling over the site of the injury occurs rapidly and may initially disguise the true extent of any bony deformity. Wounds are variably present and can range from small punctures to large flaps of skin or severe lacerations (629). The degree of bony deformation depends on the degree, site, and extent of damage, but depression fractures are common (630). It is important to assess the bony contours around the eye and cranial vault and to assess the horse for ophthalmic and neurologic problems. Depression fractures over the maxillary sinuses may damage the nasolacrimal duct and lead to epiphora. Subcutaneous emphysema can be present if the injuries penetrate into the paranasal sinuses or nasal cavity.

Differential diagnosis
Differential diagnoses include conditions that cause head deformity, including expansile masses or erosive tumors within the paranasal sinuses. It is important to eliminate other causes of epistaxis, particularly guttural pouch mycosis, ethmoidal hematoma, and fungal rhinitis.

Diagnosis
Clinical examination will reveal the extent of any laceration and careful palpation will often reveal the extent and severity of any fractures. A full ophthalmic and neurologic examination should be undertaken. Radiography may be used, including lesion-specific oblique views, but it is often difficult to interpret the results. Some facial fractures can appear very subtle on radiographic images owing to the complicated anatomy and the thin nature of the bone.

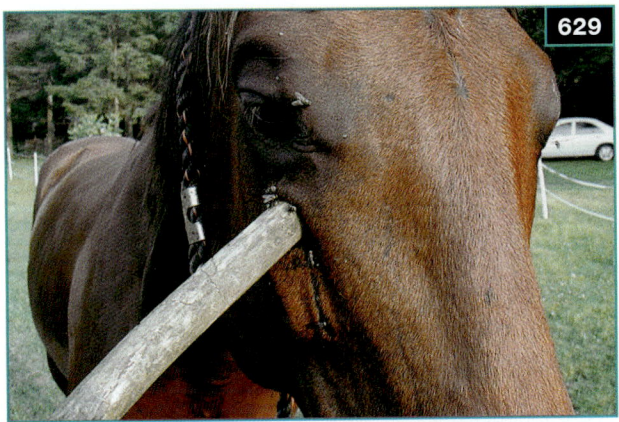

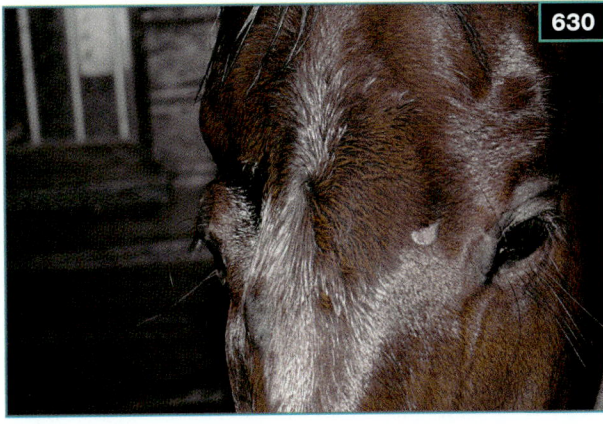

629 Facial injury. This horse was found with a stake in its head. It appeared that the wound was at least 24 hours old. Despite this the horse made a complete recovery following removal of the stake and debridement of the fractured bone fragments. (Photo courtesy B Fraser)

630 Horse with a depression fracture of the frontal bones and the zygomatic arch following a kick injury.

631 Curved 2.7 mm AO plate used to stabilize the depression fracture illustrated in 630.

It is important to assess the paranasal sinuses for the presence of blood, often seen as fluid lines in one or more of the sinuses. Damage to the orbit or cranial vault should also be considered. Ultrasonography of fractures and swellings can also be used and is easier to undertake and to interpret. Subcutaneous emphysema may obscure the image.

Management
Small skin punctures should be cleaned regularly and lavaged with mild antiseptic solutions for a few days. Simple lacerations are repaired in the standing sedated horse primarily, after careful preparation, with skin staples. Immediately following the injury a course of antibiotics and NSAIDs will decrease the swelling and pain, as well as reduce the incidence of secondary sinusitis. If large quantities of blood are present in the sinuses, these can be lavaged for several days via catheters placed in the appropriate sinus. If the facial bones are fractured, management depends on the degree of injury. Non- or minimally displaced fractures can be treated conservatively and usually heal well. More displaced and depressed fractures can also be treated conservatively, but may leave cosmetic defects and, if the nasal bones are involved, the possibility of functional respiratory obstruction. Fragments of bone that have lost all periosteal attachments are probably best removed, which can often be achieved in the standing horse. Larger fractures, especially when there are depressed fragments, are best managed under general anesthesia with the aim of anatomic restoration of the fractured bone. This should be carried out within 48 hours of the injury if possible, before the fracture line starts to stabilize. Depressed fracture fragments can be raised back into position with elevators, bent

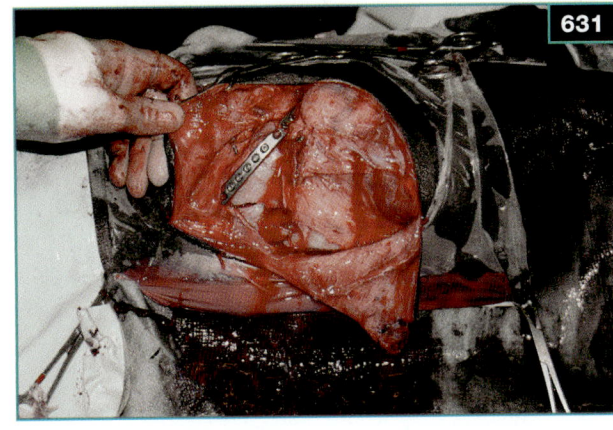

Steinmann pins, or bone hooks, and may be stable when returned into alignment. Occasionally, nylon or wire sutures are required to stabilize the fracture lines. Where there is extensive bone loss, some surgeons have used fluorocarbon polymer or carbon fiber to restore the facial contour. Small bone plates and screws can be used for periorbital fractures in order to restore the orbit, but are seldom necessary on the flat bones of the sinus compartments (631).

Prognosis
Almost all facial wounds and fractures will heal, usually without any functional problems. The cosmetic result varies with the original injury and whether it is treated conservatively or surgically. Most cases have a firm swelling left after healing has finished, although remodeling of the bone contours continues for months after the fracture has healed.

Surgical conditions of the upper respiratory tract

Nasal amyloidosis

Definition/overview

This is a rare disease in the horse, where deposits of amyloid occur in various sites of the URT. There are a variety of clinical signs specifically associated with the deposits in the respiratory tract. Nasal amyloidosis is rarely associated with other primary systemic disease, but other signs such as weight loss may occur if there is a primary disease process. Treatment of the primary disease problem is essential, along with removal of the localized deposits.

Etiology/pathophysiology

Amyloid is a protein substance formed secondary to chronic immunologic stimulation, which in some cases is not identified. The URT is one of the more common sites of deposition and these can occur with or without skin deposits.

Clinical presentation

Amyloid deposits have been recorded in the nostrils, alar folds, nasal septum, and nasal conchae and, more rarely, in the nasopharynx and guttural pouches (632). Presenting clinical signs may include nasal discharge, often containing small amounts of blood, nasal obstruction and subsequent respiratory noise, and exercise intolerance. If a primary disease process is present, a variety of other signs including weight loss may be present.

Differential diagnosis

Other causes of nasal discharge, epistaxis, and soft-tissue formation in the URT should be considered.

Diagnosis

Clinical examination of the nostrils may reveal thickened and raised nodular masses in the mucosa, often with areas of hemorrhage. Endoscopy can be used to examine the rest of the URT for their presence elsewhere. Biopsy and histopathology will confirm the diagnosis. Any generalized signs should be investigated thoroughly before treating the nasal lesions.

Management

The underlying primary disease needs to be identified and treated, but in some cases no cause is identified. Local surgical excision of the nostril lesions can be undertaken and laser ablation of nasal and other URT lesions is possible transendoscopically.

Prognosis

Local URT lesions can recur and carry a guarded prognosis, while the primary problem can have a poor prognosis.

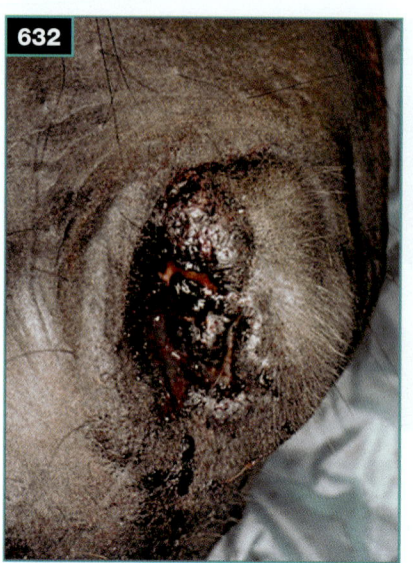

632 A horse that presented with intermittent bilateral epistaxis and which on examination had firm, ulcerated, multiloculated masses in both nostrils. Biopsy confirmed amyloidosis. There were also masses involving both palpebral conjunctivae.

Progressive ethmoidal hematomas

Definition/overview

Ethmoidal hematomas develop from the nasal or sinus surface of the ethmoidal labyrinth and behave as a tumor, being progressive and expansile, but histology does not reveal any neoplastic tissue. Most commonly, affected horses are presented with a low-grade nasal discharge, often containing blood, and are identified by endoscopy. A variety of surgical options are available for their treatment.

Etiology/pathophysiology

The etiology is unknown, but is not neoplastic. The pathophysiology is of repeated submucosal hemorrhage from the surface of the ethmoidal labyrinth and underneath normal respiratory epithelium, and is associated with significant fibrosis. The mass usually consists of a mixture of blood, hemosiderin, and fibrous tissue with macrophages and giant cells. It is unknown why the hemorrhage is repetitive, resulting in progression of the lesion.

Clinical presentation

There is an increasing incidence in older horses and, according to some reports, also females and Arabians and Thoroughbreds. The clinical presentation is of low-grade recurrent unilateral epistaxis or serohemorrhagic non-odorous nasal discharge. The blood in the discharge is often old and not related to exercise. Occasionally, cases are presented with airway obstruction, abnormal respiratory sounds at exercise, and poor performance. Larger masses can cause facial deformity, spread into the pharynx causing dysphagia, or extend down the nasal passages to become visible at the nares. Rare cases have been associated with neurologic signs due to expansion through the cribriform plate and head shaking.

Differential diagnosis

The differential diagnosis includes guttural pouch mycosis, trauma, mycotic rhinitis, polyps, and sinonasal neoplasia.

Diagnosis

Endoscopic examination is the definitive diagnostic tool for the caudal nasal passage lesions that arise from the nasal surface of the ethmoid (633). Ethmoidal hematomas can be smooth-walled or can ulcerate and bleed, and are usually reddish green/yellow in color. Some large lesions can enlarge around the caudal part of the nasal septum and appear on endoscopy of the other nasal passage. Bilateral lesions are frequent and both sides should be evaluated. Paranasal sinus lesions are unlikely to be visible on per-nasum endoscopy unless they invade through the conchae; however, they can be detected on sinoscopy (634).

Standing radiography of the head in a lateral projection can be useful in assessing the location and size of a progressive ethmoidal hematoma, especially in sinus or larger lesions. The appearance is of a soft-tissue mass, usually with quite a defined outline, rostral or dorsal to the ethmoidal labyrinth (635). Dorsoventral views may confirm its presence within or without the paranasal sinuses. Fluid lines may also be present in the sinuses due to secondary sinusitis or hemorrhage. In small lesions or where they are in obscure positions, such as the spheno-palatine sinus, MRI and/or CT may be helpful.

Management

There are a number of possible techniques for treatment of progressive hematoma and the actual technique used will depend on the size, position, and accessibility of the lesion(s) and the available equipment and finance. Surgical resection of ethmoidal hematomas via a large fronto-nasal flap under general anesthesia, is a long-established technique for nasal lesions, but is invariably very hemorrhagic and involves destruction of significant portions of the caudal nasal architecture. Hematomas present within the sinus compartments can also be removed this way.

633 Endoscopic view of an ethmoidal hematoma obscuring part of the view of the ethmoid turbinates. Note the typical appearance and mild hemorrhage from the mass. (Photo courtesy TRC Greet)

634 Progressive ethmoidal hematoma within the frontal sinus, viewed by direct sinus endoscopy.

635 Standing lateral radiograph of the paranasal sinuses in a horse presenting with intermittent unilateral epistaxis and mild mucopurulent nasal discharge. Note the soft-tissue tear-drop-shaped mass situated rostral to the ethmoid within the frontal sinus. Following biopsy via sinoscopy it was confirmed as an ethmoidal hematoma.

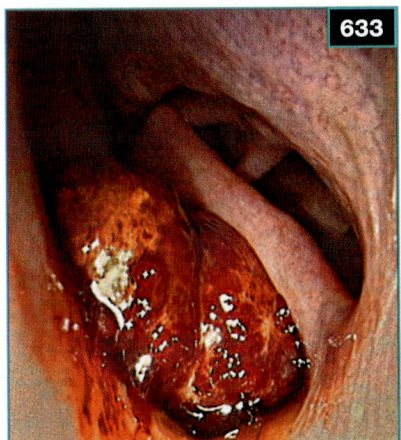

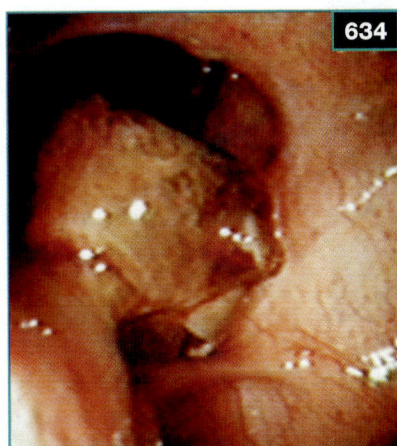

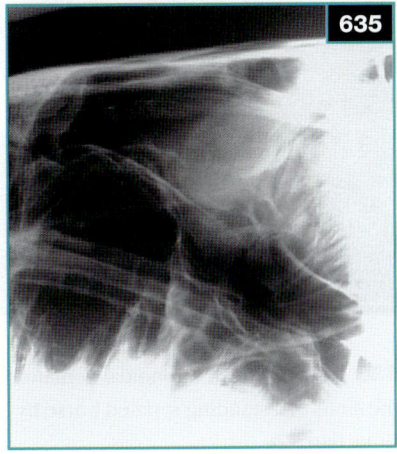

405

A frontonasal flap can be performed in the standing horse and good surgical access is achieved to hematomas in the paranasal sinuses with much less hemorrhage than under general anesthesia (636). Transendoscopic laser ablation of progressive hematomas has been used successfully both with Nd:YAG and diode lasers in the caudal nasal passage and sinuses of the standing sedated horse. Only smaller lesions of <5 cm diameter are recommended for this procedure. Repeated treatments at weekly intervals may be necessary. Other less commonly used techniques include the cryogenic ablation of small hematomas on the nasal side via endoscopy and snare excision via endoscopic guidance.

The most favored technique at present involves injection of the lesion with 10% formalin via an endoscopic catheter, either up the nasal passages or via a sinoscopy approach, in the standing sedated horse. The hematoma is injected with variable amounts of formalin (usually 10–20 ml) until the mass starts to distend and the solution begins to leak from the injection site. The lesion then undergoes necrosis and sloughing over the next 2–3 weeks. Formalin injection is usually repeated every 3–4 weeks until the

mass is ablated. Multiple injections are necessary, usually about 2–5 (up to 18 has been reported). Death was reported in one horse when the hematoma invaded the cribriform plate. Repeated injection is more complicated in horses where the mass is within the paranasal sinuses. Intermittent injection is feasible, but repeated trephination becomes traumatic to the horse. Injection within the sinuses can result in significant chemical sinusitis, though this usually resolves with medical management and lavage.

Prognosis
The prognosis is guarded. Recurrence is common and occurs in approximately 15–50% of cases within a 1–2 year period, due to regrowth, incomplete removal, or the development of new lesions. Follow-up endoscopy every 6 months is recommended to detect early recurrence. Repeated injection with formalin or transendoscopic laser ablation is feasible. Some cases will be lost due to client frustration at repeated veterinary attention and expense, with limited prospect of a permanent cure.

Sinus and nasal neoplasia
Definition/overview
Tumors of the nasal passages and paranasal sinuses are uncommon. Foul smelling nasal discharge, often with blood within it, and nasal obstruction are common clinical signs, but there is considerable variation depending on the site and extent of the mass. Radiographic and endoscopic examination of the head, plus biopsy for histopathology, are essential to determine a clear prognosis for treatment and long-term survival. Surgical removal may be possible via facial flap approaches, but recurrence is common.

Etiology/pathophysiology
Many of the tumors are malignant and/or locally invasive and tend to occur in older animals. Some tumors are benign, but damage areas by local expansion. Lesions may occur in the local tissues of the nasal passages and paranasal sinuses, but invasion of these areas from adjacent structures such as in the mouth and palate can also occur. The most common types of tumor are SCC, adenocarcinoma, fibroma, chondroma, lymphoma, osteoma, osteosarcoma, and hemangiosarcoma. Odontogenic tumors derived from tooth-forming elements are rare and usually occur in young animals.

Clinical presentation
The clinical signs vary with the location and extent of the mass. Early localized cases may be identified incidentally or be presented because of localized secondary infection of the mass. Drainage from the paranasal sinuses may be affected, leading to a secondary sinusitis. Nasal discharge is often foul smelling, bloody, purulent, and usually unilateral unless the mass is so extensive as to invade the

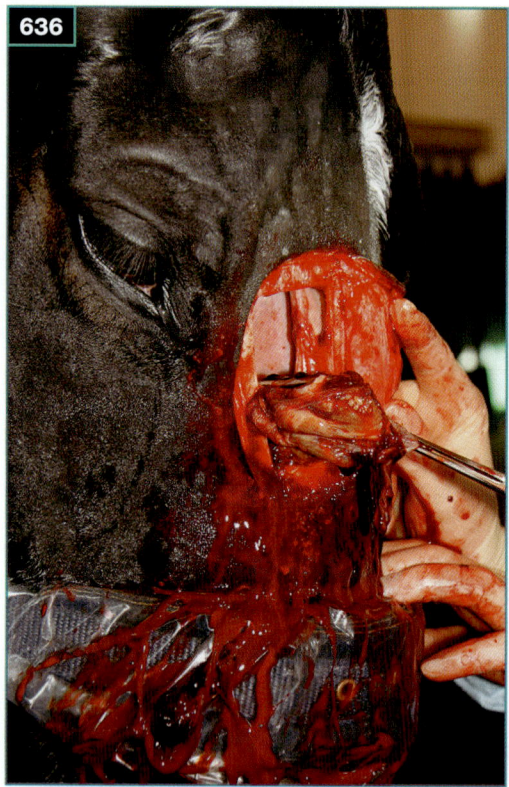

636 Removal of an ethmoidal hematoma from the sinus of a standing sedated horse by a frontal sinus flap.

other side of the head. Expansion of the mass can lead to facial swelling, airway obstruction, and exophthalmos. Those tumors involving the mouth may present with halitosis and occasionally dysphagia. In rare cases the mass may appear at the nares.

Differential diagnosis
Other causes of secondary sinusitis, including maxillary cysts, chronic primary sinus empyema, progressive ethmoidal hematomas, and nasal polyps, should be considered.

Diagnosis
A thorough clinical examination including evaluation of the mouth and palpation of local lymph nodes is essential. Endoscopy of the nasal passages and/or paranasal sinuses may allow biopsy and subsequent histopathologic diagnosis. Radiography of the head may identify poorly demarcated, solid, soft-tissue masses, especially in the sinuses. Tumors of dental origin may be mineralized. Masses involving the orbit can be visualized with transocular ultrasonography. In some cases the extent of the mass may only be visualized on CT/MRI scans.

Management
Frontonasal and/or maxillary bone flap surgery will allow the extent of the tumor to be ascertained, in terms of sinus involvement, and in some specific benign or limited sized cases, excision is possible. Some small nasal tumors can be treated by transendoscopic laser ablation or intralesional formalin injection.

Prognosis
The prognosis is determined by the chronicity, extent, and severity of the lesion. Many cases are extensive before they are diagnosed, making successful treatment unlikely, the chance of recurrence high, and the long-term prognosis poor. Benign lesions that are well circumscribed can be successfully treated by conventional surgical excision, laser ablation, or even intralesional formalin injections.

Nasal polyps
Definition/overview
Nasal polyps are benign pedunculated growths arising from the nasal mucosa, possibly secondary to other inflammatory problems such as periapical dental disease. Polyps may be incidental findings or cause nasal discharge or respiratory obstruction. Diagnosis is made by endoscopic examination and biopsy histopathology. Treatment by direct surgical excision or transendoscopically leads to a good prognosis.

Etiology/pathophysiology
Polyps are benign pedunculated proliferative masses of inflammatory tissue that arise from, and are covered by, nasal mucosa. They may be attached to the nasal septum, conchae, or elsewhere in the nasal passages and are usually single and unilateral. They vary in size from 2–20 cm in diameter. It is unclear as to their origin, but some clinicians believe they may be associated with dental periapical disease.

Clinical presentation
Nasal polyps are more common in older horses and are often insidious in onset, with no or minimal early signs. Occasionally, there may be a unilateral mucopurulent nasal discharge, particularly if sinus drainage is obstructed. If dental disease is present, this will be the overriding clinical presentation. Large polyps can obstruct the airway, leading to abnormal respiratory sounds and occasionally dyspnea. Some large lesions can extend down the nasal passages to appear at the nares.

Differential diagnosis
Other causes of expansile lesions of the nasal passages and paranasal sinuses include progressive ethmoidal hematoma, sinonasal neoplasia, maxillary cysts, and sinusitis-derived swelling of the conchae. By far the most common nasal polyp diagnosed endoscopically is the greater ethmoid bone. This is normal and care should be taken not to consider this a pathologic finding.

Diagnosis
Polyps are invariably detected on endoscopy of the nasal passages and should be biopsied to confirm their identity. Radiography of the dental arcade and oral examination of the teeth should be carried out to ascertain if they are secondary to dental disease.

Management
Nasal polyps can be treated by a variety of surgical techniques depending on their size and position. Surgical excision may be possible via facial bone flap approaches; the hemorrhage in such cases is decreased by the use of electrosurgery. Transendoscopic electrosurgery and laser ablation have also been used and snaring using endoscopic guidance can be effective in pedunculated accessible lesions. Any concurrent dental problems also require treatment.

Prognosis
The prognosis following surgical removal is good, although recurrence can be a problem.

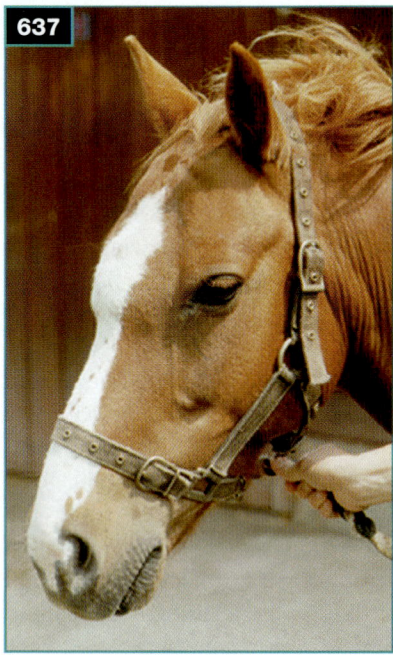

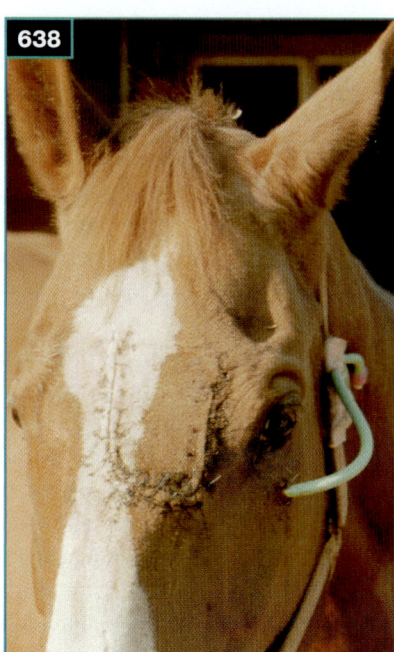

637 Facial swelling over the frontal sinus. Swelling in this area is almost invariably caused by an expansile mass within the sinus compartment, in this case a sinus cyst.

638 The horse in 637 following removal of the sinus cyst, using a frontal flap with a caudal base. A Foley catheter has been placed for postoperative lavage of the sinus.

Paranasal sinus cysts

Definition/overview
Swelling rostral to the rostral edge of the facial crest is frequently caused by dental disease. By contrast, swelling caudal to the rostral edge of the facial crest is almost invariably caused by an expansile mass within the paranasal sinuses. Paranasal sinus cysts are an unusual condition, but are one of the most frequent expansile lesions of this area (637). The cause of the condition is unclear and the precise pathology is debatable. One author has speculated that there is a link between this condition and progressive ethmoidal hematoma.

Etiology/pathophysiology
The etiology and pathophysiology are unknown. Paranasal sinus cysts are fluid-filled structures that are either single- or multiloculated. They have an epithelial lining that produces a yellow, mucoid-like fluid. They usually develop in the maxillary sinus, including the ventral conchal sinus, but can expand into the frontal sinus.

Clinical presentation
Sinus cysts can occur in the first year of life, but they are more common in adult horses. Facial swelling over the maxillary and conchofrontal sinuses is common, frequently associated with unilateral nasal discharge due to obstruction of the drainage ostia and secondary sinusitis. Nasal obstruction of varying degrees due to conchal swelling also occurs in some cases. Sinus cysts can be found during exploratory sinus surgery. The expansile pressure of the lesion is such that the outline of the sinus and nasal turbinates can be distorted. Thinning of the nasal bones may lead to increased resonance on percussion. Exophthalmia occasionally occurs due to pressure behind the orbit. Care should be taken in assessing swellings that do not appear to be quite typical of the outline of the sinus cavity. Occasional cases can appear to be rostral to the facial crest or caudal enough to be involving the cranium.

Differential diagnosis
Other expansile lesions of the paranasal sinuses, including fibrous dysplasia in the young horse, progressive ethmoidal hematoma, squamous cell carcinoma, and primary sinusitis, should be considered.

Diagnosis
Radiology reveals a soft-tissue or fluid density within the sinus. Sometimes, the density has a typical rounded appearance indicative of an encapsulated lesion. Frequently, there is associated fluid accumulation that obscures this outline and the radiological appearance is simply of increased radiodensity within the paranasal sinuses. There may be distortion of the normal sinus outline and structures, soft-tissue mineralization, and nasal septum or vomer bone deviation. Trephination of the sinus usually results in a flow of clear, vivid yellow fluid, which is typical of a sinus cyst. Nasal endoscopy may reveal rounded masses in the middle meatus or, if confined to the sinuses, diffuse narrowing or obstruction of the meatus due to turbinate expansion.

Management

Surgical removal via a large facial bone flap is indicated. Either a maxillary or frontonasal flap can be used depending on the position and extent of the cyst (638). It may be possible to remove the cyst in its entirety as the cyst membrane can separate from the sinus lining quite easily in some cases. If small areas of the cyst are left behind, they do not appear to cause any significant complications.

Prognosis

The prognosis is excellent with surgical ablation. Recurrence is rare. Complete recovery can be anticipated and the cosmetic outcome is usually very good.

Intranasal foreign bodies: overview

This is an uncommon condition and is usually caused by the aspiration of pieces of wood, seeds, and other vegetative material. Clinical signs in acute cases include nasal discomfort with intense and persistent sneezing, facial rubbing, and epistaxis. More chronic cases will have an increasingly purulent and malodorous unilateral nasal discharge. Diagnosis may be possible in rostral nasal passage sites by direct visual examination, but more commonly, endoscopic examination of the entire nasal passages will identify the foreign body. Rarely, the foreign body is radio-opaque and is visible on head radiographs. Treatment by endoscopically-guided retrieval in the standing, sedated horse followed by a short course of systemic antibiotics and NSAIDs is usually effective.

Iatrogenic trauma of the nasal passages

Definition/overview

This is a common complication of nasogastric intubation or nasal endoscopy.

Etiology/pathophysiology

Epistaxis can result from iatrogenic trauma to any of the nasal turbinates, with the ethmoturbinates being the most vulnerable and vascular.

Clinical presentation

Epistaxis, which can be very mild or can be profuse, is observed almost immediately on passage or withdrawal of a stomach tube or endoscope.

Differential diagnosis

There are few differential diagnoses. Probably the most significant is guttural pouch mycosis, though this type of onset is rare.

Diagnosis

Diagnosis is based on a history of passage of an endoscope or nasogastric tube. Further investigation is only warranted if the epistaxis does not stop or recurs without further nasal intubation. Endoscopy is seldom of any value in the face of acute hemorrhage, as visibility is so limited.

Management

No treatment is necessary as the hemorrhage is invariably self-limiting. It is useful to tie the horse up so that blood contamination is limited to one area, preferably one that is less visible to clients. Prevention is far more important than cure. Frequent mistakes include using an inappropriately sized stomach tube and passing the tube into the middle meatus and then into the ethmoidal labyrinth (639).

Prognosis

The prognosis for full recovery is excellent.

639 A parasagittal section of the head of a horse which was euthanized due to progressive ethmoidal hematoma.
The section illustrates how ethmoidal trauma results from endoscopy or intubation via the middle meatus (white dotted line), while the ventral meatus, which is ventral to the nares, opens harmlessly into the nasopharynx (yellow dotted line).

Pharynx and larynx

Nasopharyngeal cicatrix

Definition/overview

This is a rare condition where a web of fibrous tissue traverses the nasopharynx causing constriction and obstruction. Outbreaks have been recorded and there is an association with grazing. The condition is much more frequent in hot climates, and is probably most frequently recognized in Texas, USA.

Etiology/pathophysiology

The cause is unknown. Recent suggestions implicate *Pythium*, a fungus; however, the condition appears to be caused by inflammation rather than the characteristic presentation of pythiosis. Following inflammation, secondary healing can result in a web of scar tissue forming over the floor of the nasopharynx. Almost all cases are associated with deformity of other laryngeal or pharyngeal cartilages such as the arytenoid, epiglottis, or cartilage of the ostium of the guttural pouches.

Clinical presentation

The most common presenting signs are poor performance, abnormal respiratory noise, and dyspnea, although the condition can be subclinical. It is more commonly reported in horses older than five years of age and in females.

Differential diagnosis

Other causes of respiratory noise and poor performance, including dorsal displacement of the soft palate, recurrent laryngeal neuropathy, and arytenoid chondritis, should be considered.

Diagnosis

Endoscopic examination is diagnostic. A web of fibrous tissue is present within the nasopharynx, involving the soft palate alone or the entire circumference of the pharynx and often causing constriction. Other abnormalities are often present including arytenoid chondropathy, epiglottic deformity, and guttural pouch osteum deformity. Careful assessment of the laryngeal cartilages is important, because functional abnormalities are frequently dependent on these rather than the pharyngeal cicatrix.

Management

Treatment may not be necessary if there is no effect on performance. Mild cases often respond to laser ablation of the scar tissue. Cutting of the cicatrices and bougie dilation have also been used in a few cases. Treatment of other associated lesions may be required. Medical treatment with antibiotics and anti-inflammatories is generally ineffective. If there is severe webbing or marked swelling of the arytenoid cartilages, permanent tracheostomy or insertion of a permanent tracheotomy tube is indicated. Prevention in the Texas region has included 'dry lotting' (removal of access to pasture). This is imperative to prevent recurrence in treated cases. Alternatively, the horse can be moved to a more temperate climate.

Prognosis

Recurrence following treatment is very common, especially if the horse returns to the same environment. If the horse can be moved to a different climate, the outlook is fair.

Pharyngeal cysts

Definition/overview

Developmental cysts are uncommon, but they may occur, most commonly in a subepiglottal position (see p. 411) and occasionally on the dorsal pharynx or soft palate. Dorsal pharyngeal cysts may be remnants of the craniopharyngeal duct or Rathke's pouch, while palatal cysts may have a salivary origin. Cysts are usually incidental endoscopic findings, but they can be associated with respiratory noise and, presumably, obstruction in some horses.

Etiology/pathophysiology

The etiology of pharyngeal cysts is unknown, but they are speculated to be of embryologic origin. They are more commonly reported in Thoroughbreds and Standardbreds.

Clinical presentation

Cysts are usually identified during endoscopic examination (640). The significance of the cysts is hard to determine, but clients who learn that their horse has one will seldom be happy until something has been done about it.

Differential diagnosis

Pharyngeal lymphoid hyperplasia and other pharyngeal masses should be considered.

Diagnosis

The endoscopic appearance is usually quite typical and no further diagnosis is necessary. Transendoscopic aspiration is feasible, but the diagnostic value is questionable. The probable loss of volume and hence definition of the cyst would limit further therapy.

Management

If accessible, surgical resection or laser ablation of the cyst could be considered. Intralesional injections of formalin using a procedure similar to that described for progressive ethmoidal hematomas (641) have been used. Usually, up to 5 ml of serous fluid can be withdrawn from the cyst before it is refilled with a similar volume of 10% formalin.

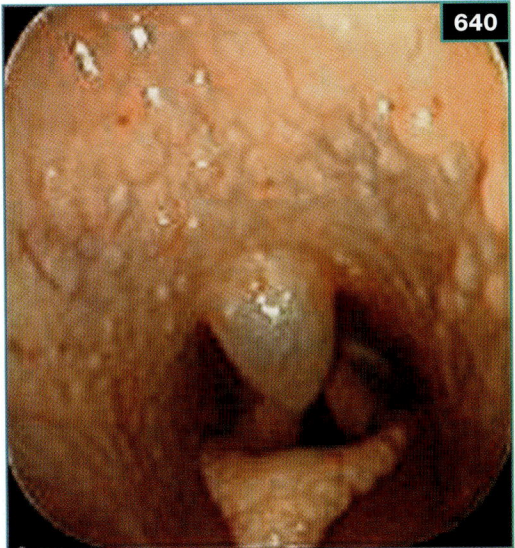

640 Pharyngeal cyst in the dorsal wall of a New Forest pony.

641 Intraoperative endoscopic view of injection of the cyst with 10% formalin.

642 Endoscopic view of the pharynx of a horse with a history of poor performance in National Hunt racing. A subepiglottic cyst is visible in the mucosa between the soft palate and the epiglottis (arrrow). This cyst was intermittently visible, frequently being below the soft palate and only occasionally 'popping up' above it.

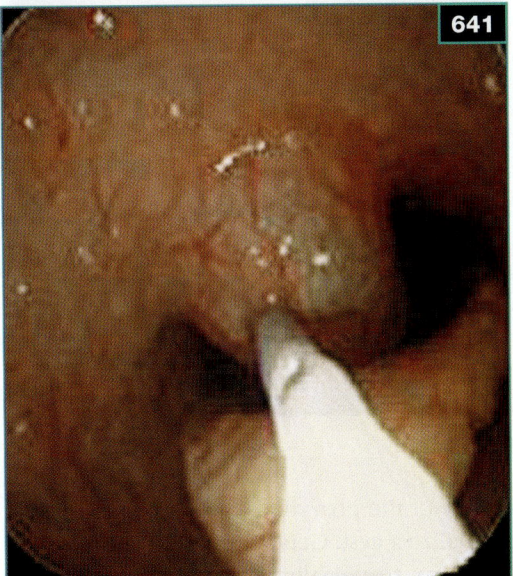

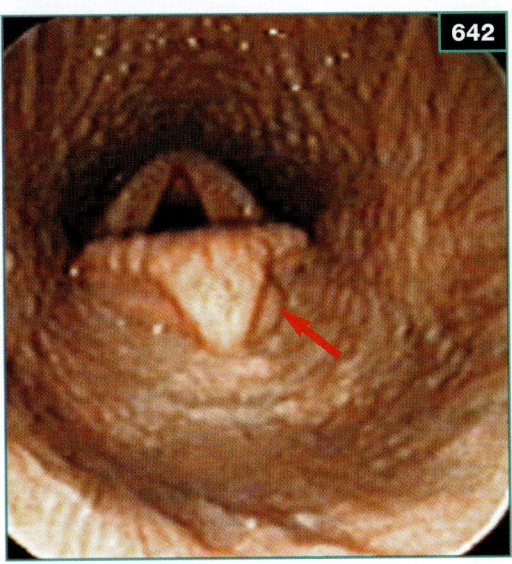

Prognosis

The prognosis is good, as these cysts are seldom clinically significant. Ablation or injection with formalin usually results in a small, scarred area on the pharyngeal wall. Recurrence has not been observed.

Subepiglottic cyst

Definition/overview

This is a congenital condition in which the severity of the cyst varies from a life-threatening respiratory obstruction of the newborn foal to an incidental finding in an adult horse (642). The cysts frequently cause dysphagia. Many of the clinical signs can be attributed to dorsal displacement of the soft palate, which is presumably caused by the space-occupying effect of the cyst.

Etiology/pathophysiology

Subepiglottic cysts are probably caused by failure of the glosso-epiglottic duct to fully atrophy. The cause of this failure is not known. They are recognized in all breeds, but are most commonly reported in Thoroughbreds and Standardbreds. The cysts are smooth-walled, 1–5 cm in diameter, occasionally multilobular, and filled with straw-colored sticky fluid. They form between the base of the tongue and the epiglottis within the loose mucosa in this position.

Clinical presentation

The severity of the clinical signs associated with sub-epiglottic cysts varies enormously. Obviously, the size and location of the cyst affect this, but it is not immediately apparent why some cysts will cause a foal to develop a respiratory obstruction, while other similar sized ones are not noted until adulthood.

411

There are a variety of clinical presentations:
+ Severe respiratory obstruction at birth or shortly afterwards. Emergency management of the airway may be necessary including nasotracheal intubation or emergency tracheotomy.
+ Respiratory noise in a foal usually noticed while the foal is turned out. The noise may be intermittent and have a sudden onset as the cyst precipitates an epiglottic entrapment or dorsal displacement of the soft palate.
+ Dysphagia in the foal or young horse. Typical signs of dysphagia are noted (i.e. coughing, especially during eating, and bilateral nasal discharge of mucoid material containing food). In the suckling foal there will be reflux of milk from the nares. The onset of dysphagia can be relatively sudden despite the congenital nature of the condition.
+ Poor performance, often with respiratory noise and/or choking up at exercise, in the young or adult horse. The author has observed medium sized cysts in horses that have been in race training for several years.

Differential diagnosis

The differential diagnoses vary depending on the clinical presentation. The important differential diagnoses are other causes of permanent dorsal displacement of the soft palate: guttural pouch mycosis; congenital abnormalities including unilateral choanal atresia, subepiglottic infection or foreign body; and primary epiglottic entrapment. Other important causes of dysphagia in the young horse include fourth branchial arch defects, soft palate hypoplasia, and cleft palate.

Diagnosis

Endoscopic examination is the primary diagnostic aid. Many cysts are clearly visible endoscopically. Several deglutition sequences should be observed. Frequently, the cyst will be observed to 'pop' into view above the soft palate and then disappear back underneath it. In many cases the cyst will not be visible and will remain subpalatal throughout the examination. In this situation, malleable 'esophageal' grasping forceps can be very valuable. Following anesthesia of the pharynx by transendoscopic infusion of 50–100 ml of local anesthetic solution (including allowing local anesthetic to flow down the nasal passages), the forceps can be passed into the pharynx via the contralateral nostril. Under endoscopic guidance the forceps can be used to grasp the subepiglottic mucosa and elevate it. This allows a clear view of the free border of the soft palate, as well as assessment of the subepiglottic tissues. Elevation will almost invariably reveal a cyst, if present.

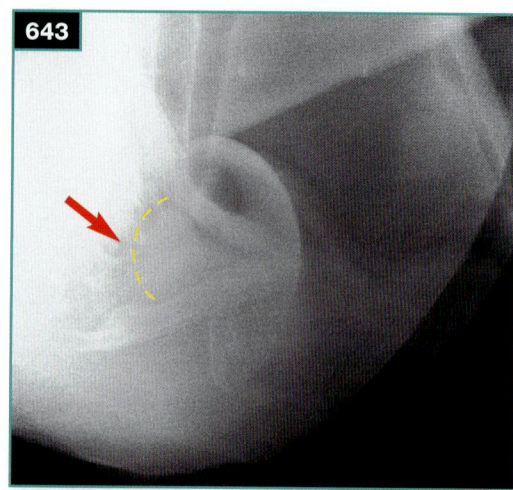

643

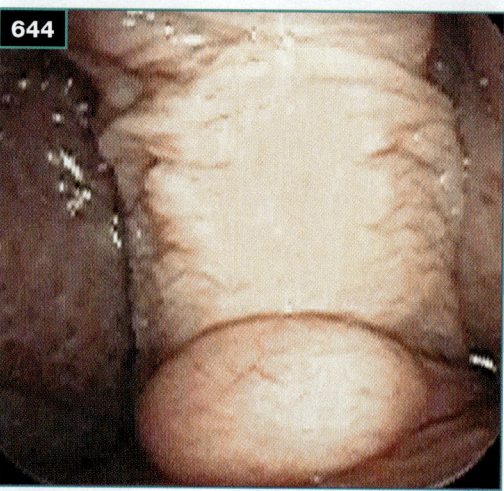

644

Radiography of the pharynx is frequently used in an attempt to visualize a cyst. Generally, a lateral radiograph of the oropharynx (especially if taken with the mouth opened) reveals a triangular-shaped gas radiolucency. Occasionally, a rounded soft-tissue density is observed, which is typical of a subepiglottic cyst (643). In many cases there is no gas between the base of the tongue and the epiglottis. In this case the radiograph is nondiagnostic, as many normal horses have no gas here and the epiglottic cyst is the same density as the surrounding tissues.

Younger horses can be less tractable and endoscopy with grasping forceps may not be well tolerated, even under sedation. In this case the subepiglottic tissues have to be visualized via endoscopy of the mouth. In most cases this requires a general anesthetic. A disposable vaginal speculum is usually passed to separate the tongue and soft palate. A 'scope' can then be passed up the speculum and a good view of the subepiglottic tissues is achieved. The tissue is normally quite loose and floppy, but cysts are quite obvious with a distended rounded outline (644).

Respiratory system

643 Laterolateral radiograph of the pharynx of the horse in 641. The rounded subepiglottic cyst (arrow) is visible ventral to the soft palate. In this horse there is a pocket of air ventral to the epiglottis as well as dorsal to the soft palate, providing excellent contrast, which is often lacking.

644 Intraoral endoscopic examination of the subepiglottic mucosa, with a typical subepiglottic cyst. Despite the inconvenience of a general anesthetic, intraoral endoscopy is often necessary for diagnosis.

645 Intra-operative photograph of a large subepiglottic cyst during surgical removal via ventral laryngotomy.

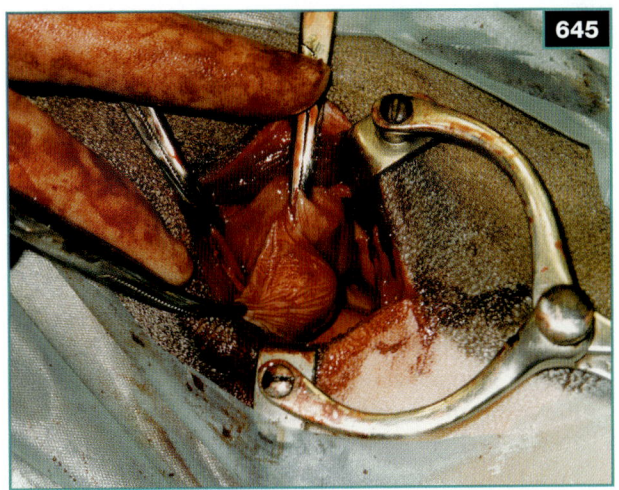
645

Management

Treatment is by surgical removal, although cysts may be an incidental finding in some cases. It has been reported that the cyst can be removed, under general anesthesia, via the mouth using a snare of Gigli wire that is tightened to excise the cyst and overlying mucosa. The author has not been successful with this technique. Alternatively, the cyst can be surgically excised via a laryngotomy (**645**). The mucosal defect is left to heal by secondary intention. Removal by pharyngotomy has been reported, but appears to offer little benefit. An Nd:YAG laser, via an endoscope inserted via the mouth under general anesthesia, can be used to dissect the cyst free.

Prognosis

The prognosis is excellent following complete removal, as recurrence is rare. The outlook for return of normal pharyngeal function in cases of dorsal displacement of the soft palate is also good. Dysphagia and respiratory obstruction are usually prevented immediately.

Pharyngeal lymphoid hyperplasia
Definition/overview

This is an extremely common condition of the young horse (<3 years old), and is considered a normal developmental process rather than a genuine disease. It appears to be a response to exposure of the URT to new antigens. The condition resolves with age. It is unusual for lymphoid hyperplasia to result in airway obstruction except in the most severe cases, although respiratory noise is a frequent finding.

Etiology/pathophysiology

It is a normal response for the pharyngeal lymphoid tissue to hypertrophy in response to exposure to antigenic stimuli such as viruses, bacteria, and other respiratory irritants (e.g. dust and spores), which are increasingly confronted by a young horse while traveling, entering training, and mixing with its peers. The pharyngeal tissues respond by secreting mucus and local immunoglobulins. As the horse and its immune system mature, the hypertrophy resolves and the condition is unusual after 5 years of age.

Clinical presentation

The most common reason for the detection of pharyngeal lymphoid hyperplasia is as an incidental finding during a 'routine' endoscopic examination. The majority of the time there is no interference with the performance or health of the horse, but in extensive and severe cases there may be an abnormal respiratory noise and possible effects on performance due to airflow turbulence and/or reduction. It has been implicated as a possible factor in the occurrence of dorsal displacement of the soft palate.

Differential diagnosis
The differential diagnoses include all the other causes of respiratory noise.

Diagnosis
Endoscopic examination is diagnostic and a grading system has been established (646):

+ *Grade 1:* occasional small white focal spots on the dorsal pharyngeal wall.
+ *Grade 2:* multiple raised nodules on the dorsal and lateral pharyngeal walls.
+ *Grade 3:* large hyperemic nodules over the whole of the dorsal and lateral pharyngeal walls.
+ *Grade 4:* larger edematous follicles coalescing into broad-based edematous plaques or polyps. Rarely, there may be associated petechial hemorrhages.

Grades 3 and 4 may be associated with clinical signs.

Management
No change in management or treatment is usually necessary as the lymphoid hyperplasia is probably not affecting the horse and it will improve with maturity. Treatment has been used in severe cases and has included intensive vaccination programs against the common URT viruses, pharyngeal sprays of antibiotics and anti-inflammatories, and pasture rest. Grade 4 cases have been treated surgically by some clinicians with topical trichloroacetic acid, electrocautery, cryotherapy, and transendoscopic laser. Excessive removal of tissue has led to pharyngeal cicatrix formation.

Prognosis
The prognosis is very good as the condition usually resolves spontaneously with time.

Pharyngeal foreign bodies
Definition/overview
Despite their fibrous diet and their enthusiasm for impaling themselves with all manner of objects, pharyngeal foreign bodies in horses are uncommon. Two types are recognized: oropharyngeal foreign bodies that have been ingested, and nasopharyngeal ones that have been inhaled.

Etiology/pathophysiology
Generally, thorns and twigs can be inhaled or ingested during browsing in hedges or trees, grazing on trimmings, exercising near low trees, or from hay containing abnormal contents. Oral foreign bodies are usually sharp objects and penetration can lead to the establishment of infection in the surrounding tissues including the retropharyngeal region.

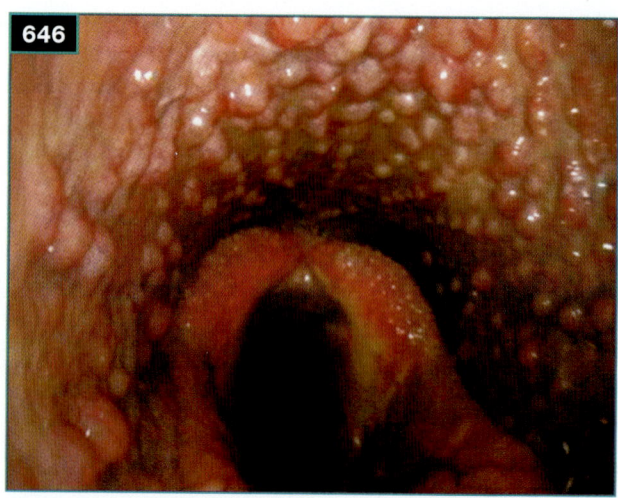

646 Moderate pharyngeal follicular lymphoid hyperplasia (Grade 2) in a 2-year-old Thoroughbred racehorse. This was an incidental finding when the horse was presented for endoscopy and tracheal wash sampling to assess any lower airway inflammation.

Clinical presentation
Nasal foreign bodies can present with marked epistaxis, particularly while the horse is being exercised, due to damage to the nasal turbinates. Coughing can be present in nasopharyngeal cases and horses can be quite distressed, with palpable throat pain and resistance to flexion of the throat region. In longer-standing cases there may be a purulent and foul smelling nasal discharge. Uncommonly, there may be swelling in the retropharyngeal region if secondary deeper infection has occurred.

Oropharyngeal foreign bodies usually present with sudden onset oral phase dysphagia. Coughing and nasal return of food and saliva may be present, but the primary sign is marked dropping of food, visible difficulty or reluctance to swallow, and marked inappetence.

Differential diagnosis
Guttural pouch mycosis and strangles are the most important differential diagnoses of nasopharygneal foreign bodies. Oropharyngeal foreign bodies can be a diagnostic challenge. Many conditions can present with similar signs of dysphagia, including dental disease and pharyngitis.

Diagnosis

Endoscopic examination is often diagnostic for pharyngeal foreign bodies. Careful assessment of the nasal turbinates can reveal a foreign body or damage caused by the passage of the object from rostral to caudal. Objects that become lodged in the retropharyngeal region may require ultrasonography, radiography, or even CT/MRI to locate them. Oropharyngeal foreign bodies can be particularly difficult to diagnose. Endoscopy may reveal swelling of the epiglottis and subepiglottic tissues or permanent dorsal displacement of the soft palate (647). Radiography may reveal subepiglottic swelling and will reveal the foreign body if it is radiodense. Palpation using a suitable mouth gag in the sedated horse may reveal a foreign body if it is not too far caudal. None of these techniques is infallible. In some cases, endoscopic examination of the mouth and palpation of the oropharynx under general anesthesia may be necessary to confirm the diagnosis.

Management

Spontaneous removal of the foreign body may occur from the nasal passages or mouth. If not, pharyngeal foreign bodies can usually be removed without complications once appropriate restraint has been applied; this almost always requires general anesthesia. Oropharyngeal foreign bodies can then be removed by digital manipulation and nasopharyngeal ones by the use of grasping forceps under endoscopic visualization. Significant hemorrhage can result from the removal of either, but packing the defect to control hemorrhage is unwise. Pharyngeal packing can result in respiratory obstruction during recovery from anesthesia, and the hemorrhage, though dramatic, is seldom life threatening. Once removed, treatment with antibiotics and anti-inflammatory agents is appropriate to control postoperative swelling.

Prognosis

The prognosis is good as long as the foreign body is completely removed. Complications include incomplete removal, secondary infections, and swellings/reactions affecting other structures.

Intermittent dorsal displacement of the soft palate

Definition/overview

Dorsal displacement of the soft palate (DDSP) can be intermittent or persistent. Intermittent displacement usually occurs during exercise and is a common cause of dynamic respiratory obstruction, exercise intolerance, and abnormal respiratory noise. It is principally a disease of the racehorse, but eventers and even dressage horses are occasionally affected. It can be difficult to diagnose with certainty, and diagnosis is usually based on history, with clinical and endoscopic examination to rule out other

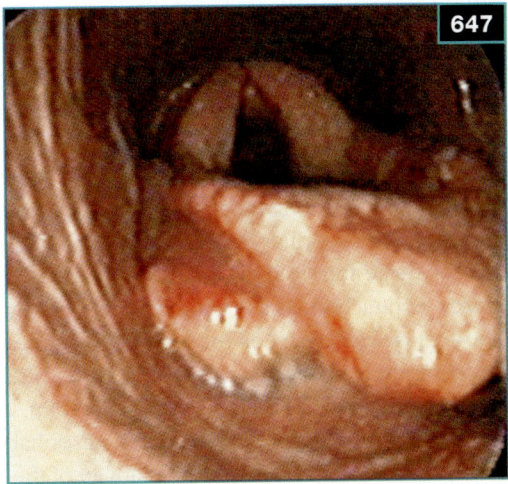

647 Marked subepiglottic swelling and ulceration caused by an oropharyngeal foreign body.
A twig with numerous thorns was removed digitally through the mouth under general anesthesia.

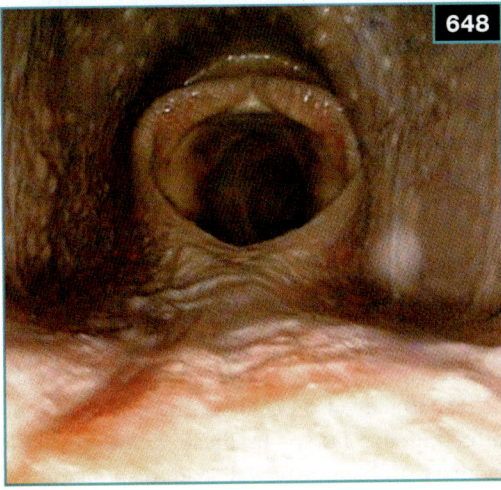

648 A horse showing dorsal displacement of the soft palate at rest. The soft palate is dorsal to the epiglottis, obscuring its normal outline, and the free border of the soft palate is clearly visible.

conditions (648). There are a variety of conservative and surgical treatments for this condition.

Etiology/pathophysiology

In this condition the caudal border of the soft palate displaces from its normal subepiglottic position and can then obstruct the airway at the entrance to the larynx. The cause of DDSP at exercise is unknown and there may be different causes in different horses. During galloping exercise the resting minute volume of a horse increases

415

Surgical conditions of the upper respiratory tract

20-fold and this is achieved by the generation of significant pressure changes in the upper airway by the muscles of ventilation, including the diaphragm. At exercise the pressure during expiration is approximately 15 mmH$_2$O, while during inspiration it is −30 mmH$_2$O. In addition, because of the pressure changes, the airway impedance is nearly doubled during inhalation due to narrowing of the airways. The nasopharynx can only stabilize itself in the face of these intraluminal pressure changes by skeletal muscle contraction, as it is entirely without bony structure. These muscles may act on the hyoid apparatus and larynx, affecting their position and subsequently the shape and tension in the nasopharynx (extrinsic factors). Also, there are skeletal muscles in the palate and nasopharynx themselves that can affect the dynamic stability of the nasopharynx (intrinsic factors). Neuromuscular weakness of the extrinsic and/or intrinsic muscle may lead to the palate being unable to support itself in the face of pressure changes, but as yet it is not apparent what is the cause of the neuromuscular weakness. In many cases it may be due to a lack of individual ability or fitness; however, there are reports of horses that were performing well but then developed DDSP, suggesting other acquired factors are relevant to these cases.

A previous theory of the etiology of DDSP included an association with epiglottic hypoplasia or flaccidity, whereby the abnormal epiglottis was unable to hold the soft palate in the correct subepiglottic position. It has been shown, however, that horses with spontaneous or surgically created retroversion of the epiglottis into the airway at fast exercise, or where the epiglottis has been removed, do not demonstrate DDSP, and indeed the soft palate remains anchored around the base of the larynx.

DDSP may also occur secondarily to other conditions affecting the horse. In these cases, resolution of the primary problem may well lead to spontaneous improvement in the displacement. Primary problems include: general unfitness; cardiovascular disorders; lower airway disease; recurrent laryngeal neuropathy; palatal problems including clefts and injuries, ulceration, and cysts; pharyngeal paralysis; severe abnormalities of the epiglottis such as deformities, entrapment, inflammation, or subepiglottic cysts; pharyngeal discomfort caused by lymphoid hyperplasia, inflammation, infections, swellings, or excess discharges; more controversially, conditions that lead to mouth pain and/or mouth breathing such as dental disease and biting problems; and, finally, neck position, especially in dressage or show animals.

Clinical presentation

The classic presentation is a horse that is performing well, but will suddenly dramatically slow down and at the same time make a vibrant 'gurgling' respiratory noise ('choking up'). Racehorses may not produce this during training, but may suddenly stop or 'go backwards' once under pressure in the last furlong or so of a race when they come under maximal pressure. Once the palate is relocated by the horse, it no longer makes the noise and is able to resume galloping without problem. Billowing of the cheeks has also been noted in some cases due to attempted mouth breathing.

Treadmill endoscopy has revealed a wide variation in the classic presentation. It has been shown that up to 30% of cases of DDSP may not make an audible respiratory noise, which is actually the vibration of the caudal palate edge during expiration. Sound-spectrum analysis reveals a low-frequency noise in almost every case, though it can be below the range of human hearing. Similarly, the noise may not be the classic vibrant noise and may be more harsh, leading to confusion with other respiratory obstructions. Many horses will develop DDSP at the start of exercise and will perform moderately throughout, leading to a suspicion that the horse is of limited ability.

Differential diagnosis

All other causes of dynamic respiratory obstruction, especially recurrent laryngeal neuropathy, which usually has a slightly different presentation and noise, should be considered. Other primary problems that may affect the horse's performance, including limited athletic ability, should also be evaluated.

Diagnosis

Diagnosis is based on history, clinical signs, and endoscopic examination, initially at rest, to rule out some of the primary problems already mentioned. Palpation of the larynx should be undertaken. Intermittent DDSP during resting endoscopy is common in normal horses and should not be overinterpreted, but persistent displacement, either with or without attempts at swallowing, is suspicious and should be investigated further. It is normal to occlude the nostrils of the horse and observe whether pharyngeal collapse or DDSP occurs in response to the lower airway pressure. Definitive diagnosis requires endoscopic examination at exercise either on a treadmill or using overground video endoscopy (649). Comparison between resting and exercising endoscopy does show that findings of DDSP or palatal/pharyngeal flaccidity at rest are not predictive for DDSP at exercise. Sound-spectrum analysis is in its infancy, but does show some promise in the diagnosis of DDSP.

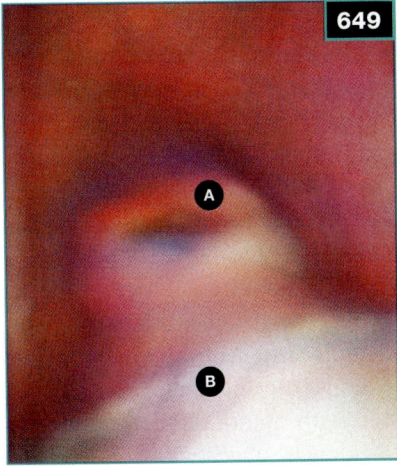

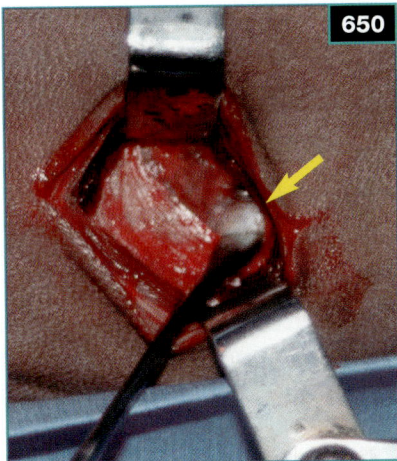

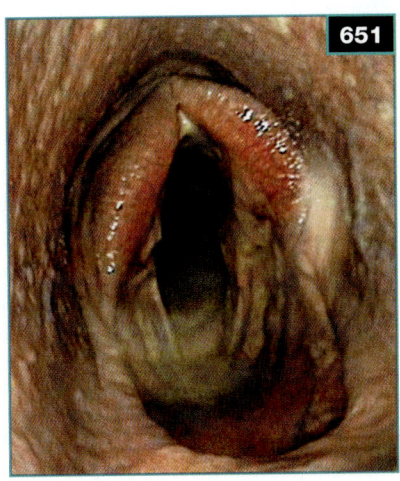

Management

A myriad of procedures have been used to treat DDSP. If any primary or predisposing conditions are diagnosed, these need to be treated. Conservative measures include a period of rest followed by increasing the fitness of the horse. Studies have shown that this approach may be as effective as surgical treatment. A tongue-tie or strap has traditionally been advocated to stop the horse retracting its tongue. This consists of a leather or other material (such as a pair of tights) tied around the tongue and then around the lower jaw. Recent research has failed to show any benefit. Australian or figure-of-eight nosebands have been used to stop the horse opening its mouth during exercise, although with modern concepts of the pathophysiology of this condition they seem unlikely to work. Recently marketed is the 'Cornell Collar', a piece of tack placed around the larynx and designed to produce rostral tension on the larynx relative to the hyoid. Many of these devices are subject to regulations under the rules of racing or competition of the relevant organizations. In the UK the Cornell Collar is banned for racing and a tongue-tie must be declared and inspected prior to the start.

Surgical myotomy of the 'strap' muscles (sternothyrohyoid muscles) was advocated to prevent caudal retraction of the larynx and hence DDSP. The procedure has been carried out under standing sedation or general anesthesia and its main complication was seroma and/or wound infections. Recent research has shown that myotomy results in increased respiratory impedance and that these muscles are important secondary muscles of respiration. The technique has been adapted to tenotomy of the insertion of the sternothyroid muscle on to the thyroid cartilage of the larynx – the 'Llewellyn' procedure (**650**). This can be combined with a laryngotomy, during which some surgeons perform a staphylectomy.

649 Dorsal displacement of the soft palate at exercise, photographed during high-speed treadmill video endoscopy. This frame is taken during exhalation, resulting in the palate billowing up into the nasopharynx as air gets underneath it, resulting in maximum airway obstruction.
A = arytenoids; B = soft palate.

650 The 'Llewellyn' procedure. The tendon of insertion of the sternothyroid muscle (arrow) has been elevated into a laryngotomy incision, prior to transection.

651 A horse with excessive shortening of the soft palate following a staphylectomy. The epiglottis can be positioned dorsal to the soft palate, but almost immediately slips off the free border, resulting in DDSP. The horse was mildly dysphagic, but was still a successful racehorse.

A staphylectomy is a resection of tissue from the free border of the soft palate, performed via a laryngotomy. It has been a widely used surgical technique. It was based on the discredited concept of intermittent DDSP being due to an elongated soft palate. Some surgeons have used physical or chemical cautery to thicken or stiffen the free border of the palate but, more commonly, a variable amount (1–2 cm) of tissue is surgically removed from the free border of the soft palate via a laryngotomy. Intermittent cases of DDSP have developed dysphagia associated with excessive shortening of the soft palate (**651**). Treadmill studies have suggested that horses that have had a staphylectomy do develop DDSP at exercise very easily, but this is associated with less respiratory obstruction than might be the case with nontreated horses, probably because of the reduction of the bulk of tissue available to cause an obstruction. Other procedures that have been

417

included during a laryngotomy include ventriculectomy and cordectomy, and subepiglottic resection.

Following treadmill observation that billowing of the palate preceded DDSP (652), surgical techniques to stiffen the palate were developed. Oral palatopharyngoplasty ('Ahern' procedure) involves removing an ellipse of the oral mucosa of the soft palate and then sewing the edges together, effectively tightening the soft palate (653). This was traditionally combined with subepiglottic resection. The procedure used to be quite popular, but interest has declined; horses appeared to suffer significant postoperative discomfort with reduced appetite, and the results did not appear superior to those of any other technique. Thermal palatoplasty, either photocautery using a laser or actual cautery using red-hot irons, has had considerable interest (654). The technique (particularly actual cautery) is simple to conduct and should produce the goal of stiffening the soft palate. Horses, surprisingly, appear much more comfortable after the procedure than they do following palatopharyngoplasty. They are also able to return to exercise rapidly after only 2 weeks or so rest. The published results do not appear to be better than those of any other surgery.

The most recent procedure advocated for treatment of DDSP is thyrohyoidplasty – the 'tie-forward' procedure (655). In this procedure a permanent suture is placed between the thyroid cartilage on either side and the basihyoid bone. The head is flexed as the sutures are tightened, resulting in rostral displacement of the larynx relative to the basihyoid of 4–5 cm. The basis of this procedure is experimental data showing DDSP at exercise following transection of the thyrohyoid muscle, which is subsequently reversed by a thyrohyoidplasty. Early results suggest significantly higher efficacy for this procedure than other treatments for DDSP. A larger series of results and direct comparison with other procedures still need to be evaluated.

Prognosis

The prognosis for almost all procedures used to treat DDSP is 60%. Various studies of the procedures available show comparable success rates, between 50% and 70%. High-quality controlled clinical trials are lacking and with the many variables associated with racing performance such studies will be necessary to draw firm conclusions on the efficacy of the procedures.

Surprisingly, myectomy of the sternothyrohyoid muscles has been associated with a success rate of 60%, despite experimental evidence that the procedure is detrimental. Similarly, epiglottic augmentation has been shown to be associated with one of the higher success rates, despite recent evidence suggesting no role of the epiglottis in the disease process. Finally, conservative management alone has been associated with a similar success rate to those of the surgical procedures.

652 Billowing of the soft palate observed during high-speed treadmill exercise by video endoscopy. Billowing like this almost invariably precedes DDSP at exercise.

653 Postoperative view of a palatopharyngoplasty. A partial thickness ellipse of palatal tissue has been resected and the incision repaired with simple interrupted silk sutures.

654 The soft palate of a horse following thermal palatoplasty by actual cautery.

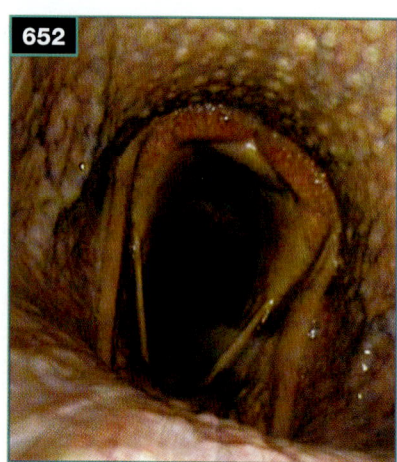

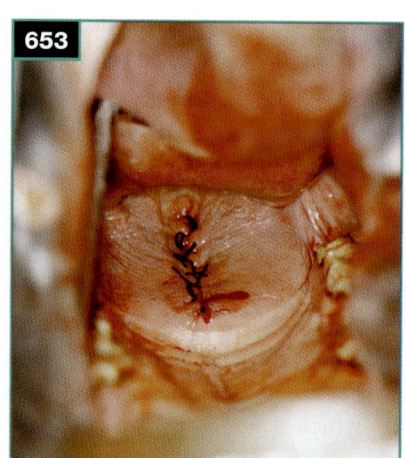

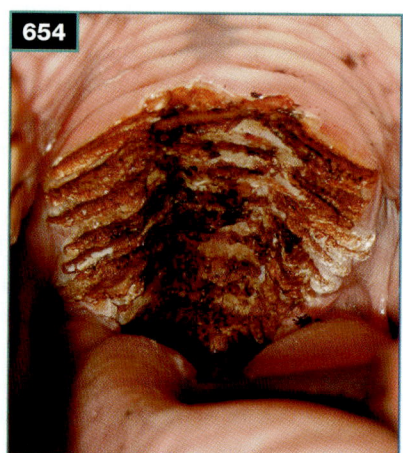

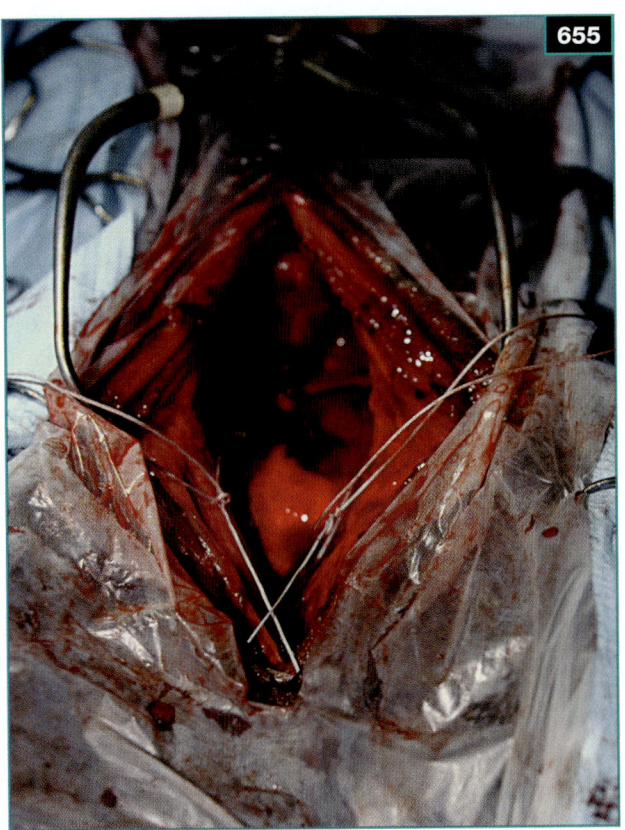

655 The 'tie-forward' procedure. The sutures are placed through the caudal edge of the wing of the thyroid cartilages and around the basihyoid bone. Next the sutures are tightened, with the head flexed to 90°, to displace the larynx 4–5 cm rostrally.

656 Permanent dorsal displacement of the soft palate. Despite numerous deglutition sequences, the soft palate remained displaced. In this case the ulcer on the free border raises suspicion of a lesion ventral to the epiglottis. The horse was managed supportively, including antibiotic and anti-inflammatory therapy, and made a recovery.

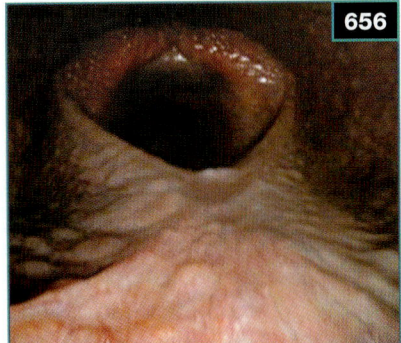

Permanent dorsal displacement of the soft palate

Definition/overview
Permanent DDSP is less common than the intermittent form and is caused by either physical or neurologic abnormalities. Clinical findings can include respiratory obstruction and/or noise, exercise intolerance, dysphagia, and coughing.

Etiology/pathophysiology
There are multiple causes of permanent DDSP. The condition is usually caused by physical obstruction of the subepiglottic space, including subepiglottic cysts, palatal cysts, foreign bodies, and even severe pharyngeal lymphoid hyperplasia. It can also be associated with neurologic abnormalities, in particular pharyngeal paralysis, the most common cause of which is guttural pouch mycosis.

Clinical presentation
Permanent DDSP tends to be associated with marked respiratory stertor at exercise, including at trot or even walk. Performance is usually markedly affected. Most horses are unable to canter due to respiratory obstruction. Pharyngeal-phase dysphagia is another frequent feature, leading to coughing during eating and nasal return of feed material and saliva.

Differential diagnosis
This is a unique clinical finding so there is no specific list of differential diagnoses. Some relevant conditions include cleft palate and palatal hypoplasia in the foal and esophageal obstruction (choke) in the adult horse.

Diagnosis
Diagnosis is usually established by endoscopic examination (656). DDSP is observed and the palate is not replaced in a subepiglottic position despite stimulation of deglutition on several occasions. Care should be taken as some horses will show DDSP as a response to endoscopy; however, patient observation, with the scope withdrawn as far into the nasopharynx and as far away from the larynx as possible, will normally result in replacement of the soft palate in a subepiglottic position in most normal horses. If permanent DDSP is identified, endoscopy of the guttural pouches is indicated. Endoscopy of the oropharynx is also frequently indicated; however, consideration needs to be given to restraint for this procedure in order to prevent trauma to the endoscopic equipment.

The diagnosis can also be confirmed by radiography, including contrast studies. This allows identification of the soft palate dorsal to the epiglottis. It may also allow identification of soft-tissue masses ventral to the epiglottis causing physical DDSP.

Management

Management depends on identification of a specific etiology; for instance, management of guttural pouch mycosis or resection of subepiglottic cysts. In some cases when a specific cause is not identified, and the condition proves to be permanent despite management with anti-inflammatory and antibiotic treatment for a prolonged time, the symptoms can be relieved, but not resolved, by staphylectomy surgery.

Prognosis

The prognosis depends on the cause. Generally, a physical cause that can be treated, such as a subepiglottic cyst, is associated with an excellent prognosis. A neurologic cause is associated with a guarded to poor prognosis. Some pharyngeal function will return in some horses treated successfully for guttural pouch mycosis. Other causes of pharyngeal paralysis have a poor prognosis.

Pharyngeal collapse

Definition/overview

Pharyngeal collapse can be the result of a space-occupying lesion in the peripharyngeal tissues, leading to severe compromise of the airway. The guttural pouch can distend downwards, resulting in dorsal pharyngeal collapse, while distended retropharyngeal lymph nodes can compress the pharynx caudally and laterally.

Dynamic pharyngeal collapse is another cause of airway obstruction that has become apparent since the development of treadmill endoscopy. Dynamic dorsal, ventral, lateral, dorsal and lateral, or complete pharyngeal

collapse has been observed. Ventral pharyngeal collapse has been implicated as a precursor to DDSP. Treadmill studies have shown clinically that almost all cases of DDSP are preceded by billowing of the soft palate up into the airway (ventral pharyngeal collapse).

Etiology/pathophysiology

The nasopharynx is an unsupported muscular tube; it can contract completely, notably during deglutition. As a result, without appropriate muscular tone, the pharynx is unable to resist the changes in airway pressure at exercise. Neuromuscular weakness will result in collapse of the nasopharynx, similar to the pathogenesis of DDSP. Attention has focused on pharyngeal inflammation, including previous evidence of pharyngeal lymphoid hyperplasia and inflammation in the region of the pharyngeal nerves in the guttural pouch, but a causal relationship has not been established. Ventral pharyngeal collapse is quite specifically associated with dysfunction of the tensor veli palatine muscle. Other causes of pharyngeal collapse in the literature include rostral respiratory tract obstructions leading to increased negative pressure in the pharynx (nasal deformities or masses), myopathies causing weakness, and neuropathies. Physical compression from surrounding pathology such as guttural-pouch empyema or lymph-node swelling can lead to pharyngeal collapse. In many cases, no cause is identified.

Clinical presentation

Pharyngeal collapse associated with surrounding swelling will produce dyspnea. The horse may have marked stertor at rest and stand with its head extended. Dynamic pharyngeal collapse presents as a dynamic airway obstruction of the performance horse, with associated signs of exercise intolerance and abnormal respiratory noise. Collapse of the ventral nasopharynx, or billowing of the soft palate, is a specific obstruction noted on treadmill endoscopy.

Differential diagnosis

The presenting signs of dynamic pharyngeal collapse may lead to a tentative diagnosis of DDSP, but they are not specific enough to reliably rule out any of the other airway obstructions of the performance horse. The principal differential diagnoses of permanent pharyngeal collapse are nasal occlusion and severe recurrent obstructive lower airway disease.

Diagnosis

Permanent pharyngeal collapse is readily diagnosed by endoscopy (657). Unless the pharynx is so collapsed as to preclude careful examination, the area of the swelling will provide valuable information as to the location of the swollen tissue. Further examination of the guttural

657 Permanent pharyngeal collapse, secondary to guttural pouch empyema.

pouches is indicated to assess swelling in this area. Oral examination should be undertaken; abnormalities such as fractures of the sixth cheek tooth can result in severe swelling and respiratory obstruction.

Radiography may also be helpful in the diagnosis of permanent pharyngeal collapse; however, this can be frustratingly nonspecific, just showing soft-tissue swelling that has already been appreciated by endoscopy.

Dynamic pharyngeal collapse requires treadmill endoscopy to diagnose. Diagnosis might be suspected if pharyngeal collapse is observed following nasal occlusion during endoscopy at rest, but this is little more than speculative.

Management
Permanent pharyngeal collapse requires treatment of the underlying condition (e.g. drainage of guttural pouch empyema, drainage of retropharyngeal abscesses, or relief of guttural pouch tympany). If this cannot be readily achieved or the horse is in distress, then a tracheotomy should be carried out immediately. Dynamic dorsal or lateral pharyngeal collapse does not have a specific treatment. Generally, treatment with rest and anti-inflammatory medications is provided. Collapse of the ventral nasopharynx can be treated by palatoplasty, either by surgical tension plasty or by thermo- or photocautery. Both techniques are reviewed under DDSP (see p. 418).

Prognosis
Permanent pharyngeal collapse caused by a treatable condition has a good prognosis. Once the swelling has resolved, there appears to be no long-term 'stretching' or other distortion of the pharynx. Dynamic dorsal and lateral pharyngeal collapse is anecdotally presumed to have a good prognosis, with most horses improving with increased maturity and resolution of inflammation. No detailed case studies are available and it has been suggested that this good prognosis may be slightly optimistic. Ventral pharyngeal collapse has a prognosis similar to that of DDSP. There is little evidence that surgical attempts to stiffen the palate are of any benefit, despite appearing logical.

Recurrent laryngeal neuropathy
Definition/overview
Recurrent laryngeal neuropathy is probably the most important cause of upper airway obstruction in the horse. It has been recognized for centuries and remains a major cause of economic loss to the horse industry. Idiopathic recurrent laryngeal neuropathy is associated with the length of the recurrent laryngeal nerve, and hence is more frequent in large horses. The left side of the larynx is almost invariably affected, as the left nerve is longer.

Equine idiopathic recurrent laryngeal neuropathy is a common condition in all large breeds of horses. Microscopically, the disease is present in all horses and clinical signs are frequent in all types of performance horse. The spectrum of the disease varies enormously. Some horses showing asymmetry of the rima glottidis at rest will run on a treadmill (and presumably race) with no further collapse of the arytenoid cartilages, while other horses, which appear mildly afflicted at rest, will develop marked collapse associated with severe respiratory stertor and poor performance at exercise.

Etiology/pathophysiology
Idiopathic equine recurrent laryngeal neuropathy is a distal axonopathy. The precise cause of the axonopathy is not known, but a genetic predisposition seems highly likely. It is postulated that transport of nutrients to the distal axon may be involved. Large-diameter myelinated nerve fibers are preferentially affected. The result is 'die back' of the nerve from the distal (laryngeal) end. This results in neurogenic atrophy of the intrinsic musculature of the larynx. The only significant laryngeal muscle not innervated by the recurrent laryngeal nerve is the cricothyroid muscle.

Pathologic changes are first observed in the principal adductor muscles of the larynx such as the cricoarytenoideus lateralis. These changes are seldom of clinical significance. Neurogenic atrophy occurs next in the cricoarytenoideus dorsalis, the principal abductor of the larynx. These changes are clinically significant.

Clinical presentation
The presentation is usually of an athletic horse with inspiratory respiratory stertor that in some cases is also performing poorly. The abnormal sounds range from a soft musical whistle to a harsher roaring sound. The sound usually gets louder and longer with increased work, but disappears very quickly after the animal stops. At canter and gallop, equine breathing is coupled to locomotion. As the hindlimbs are driving forwards, the colon and other abdominal contents are driven into the diaphragm and the horse will exhale. As the limbs are forced back (during the weight-bearing phase of the stride), the opposite occurs and inspiration results. It is possible for a horse to overcome this, but the metabolic cost of breathing then outweighs any extra ventilation. Therefore, a rider or observer can listen and watch and determine if a horse is making an inspiratory or an expiratory noise. Tradition has it that expiratory noise is normal and often vibrant ('high blowing'), but that inspiration should be silent. Equally, tradition has it that an inspiratory 'whistle' is associated with collapse of the vocal cord and a harsher noise, a 'roar', is associated with collapse of the arytenoid cartilage. Research using sound analysis of treadmill cases has

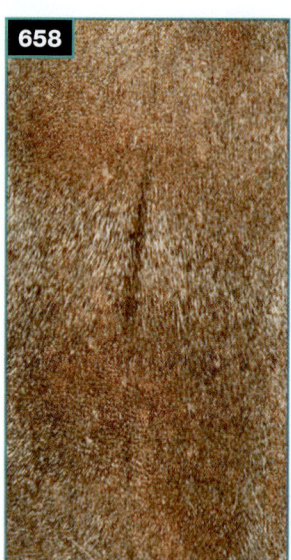

658 A previous laryngotomy scar, not detected until the horse had been anesthetized and the hair clipped in preparation for surgery.

Diagnosis

Listening to the horse during exercise (at a canter and/or gallop), either on the lunge or ridden and on both reins, is recommended prior to undertaking other diagnostic techniques.

Adductor function fails initially and therefore affected horses are often unable to close their glottis. This can be detected as an audible expiration at a time when no respiration would be expected. If the horse is threatened suddenly, or forcibly stimulated to contract the abdominal musculature by any means, an afflicted horse may let air pass through the glottis, resulting in a grunt (the 'grunt to a stick test'). Palpation of the larynx is essential. The skin on the ventral aspect of the larynx should be felt and should be rolled gently between the fingers. A previous laryngotomy scar can be noted as a thickened cord in the skin (**658**). The lateral aspect of the larynx should be felt for the normal anatomic structures of the larynx. The lateral lamina of the thyroid cartilage should be palpable, overlapping the cricoid and forming a complete lateral side to the larynx, with the ventral portion of the ring of the cricoid palpable emerging from underneath and slightly caudal to the thyroid cartilage. Finally, with the operator facing forwards, fingers are slid up underneath the sterno-mandibularis muscle and forwards to palpate the dorsal

revealed that a large number of airway obstructions give similar inspiratory noises.

Severe cases can present with dyspnea and even collapse. Recurrent laryngeal neuropathy following perivascular injection often occurs in association with Horner's syndrome. Recurrent laryngeal neuropathy caused by guttural pouch mycosis is often detected as part of an endoscopic examination for another presenting sign, notably dysphagia or epistaxis.

Differential diagnosis

There are several causes of recurrent laryngeal neuropathy and it is important not to overlook these in the rush to diagnose idiopathic recurrent laryngeal neuropathy. Other causes include infections such as guttural pouch mycosis or equine protozoal myelopathy, trauma (including perivascular injection of irritant substances such as during jugular-vein injection), and toxicoses (including lead and organophosphates).

The differential diagnosis includes most of the upper airway obstructions of the exercising horse including axial deviation of the aryepiglottic folds, pharyngeal collapse, epiglottic retroversion, fourth branchial arch defect (4-BAD) syndrome, or arytenoid chondritis. DDSP has some features of presentation that are similar, but has several that are distinctly different. Notably, DDSP will usually present with a low-frequency expiratory noise, which only occurs at extreme exercise.

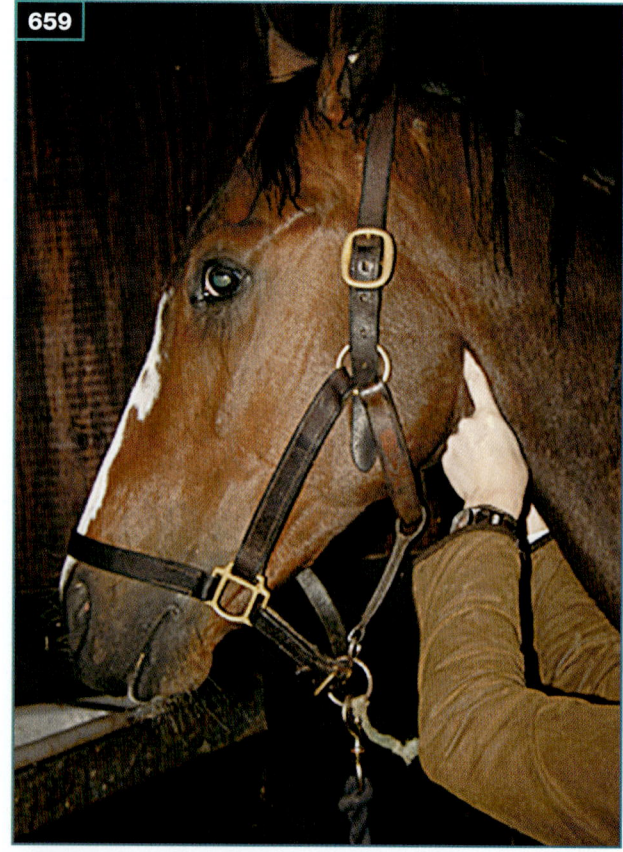

659 Palpation of the muscular process of the arytenoid cartilages. The operator has to face forwards and reach up above the larynx, underneath the vertical ramus of the mandible.

660 Opening of the guttural pouch ostium and contraction of the pharynx during deglutition.

661 Symmetrical complete abduction of the arytenoid cartilages following deglutition in a horse with Grade II.1 recurrent laryngeal neuropathy.

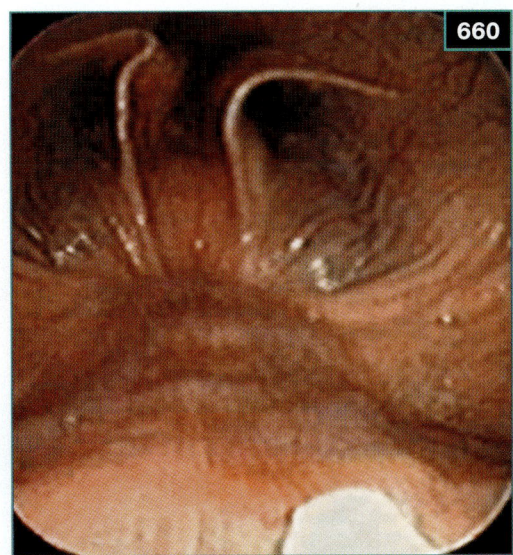

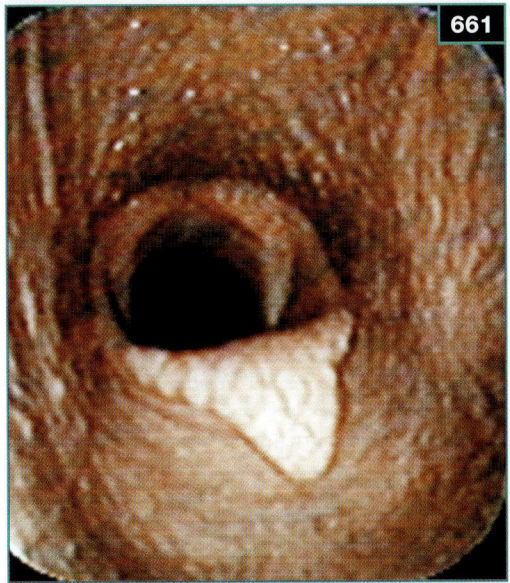

aspect of the larynx (659). Both sides are palpated concurrently so they can be compared. Normally, the muscular process of the arytenoid can be appreciated as a smooth rounding of the dorsal larynx. If there is extensive muscular atrophy, the process can be felt as a sharp promontory on one side. Some clinicians use the slap response in assessing these cases.

Endoscopic examination of the arytenoid cartilage is initially undertaken at rest. The normal movements of the larynx should be observed carefully for a few minutes. Bilaterally symmetrical abduction of the arytenoids occurs during inspiration. Asymmetry of the rima glottidis is obvious in severe cases, but this can be subtle and more difficult to assess in milder degrees of the disease. The larynx should be examined with the endoscope passed up both nostrils to negate the effect of the eccentric positioning of the endoscope in the nasopharynx. Some horses have a degree of asynchronous movement of the arytenoids at rest and it can be difficult to assess the significance of this. The effect of nasal occlusion and deglutition (stimulated by flushing water down the endoscope through the biopsy channel) in inducing abduction of the arytenoids should also be observed (660, 661).

The degree of laryngeal neuropathy can be classified by one of many scoring systems. The one recommended here is the Havemeyer system (*Table 13*) (from the Dorothy Havemeyer workshop on recurrent laryngeal

TABLE 13 **Havemeyer system for classification of laryngeal neuropathy**

ENDOSCOPIC FINDING	HAVEMEYER SCALE	LANE SCALE	US SCALE
Symmetrical at rest; full synchronous movement	Grade I	1	1
Some asynchronous movement; full abduction easily obtained	Grade II.1	2	2a
Some asymmetry at rest; full abduction obtained and maintained	Grade II.2	3– to 3	2b
Asymmetry at rest; full abduction attained but not maintained	Grade III.1	3 to 3+	3
Asymmetry at rest; full abduction not attained	Grade III.2	4– to 4	3
Asymmetry with little arytenoid movement	Grade III.3	4+	3
Total paralysis of the arytenoid	Grade IV	5	4

Surgical conditions of the upper respiratory tract

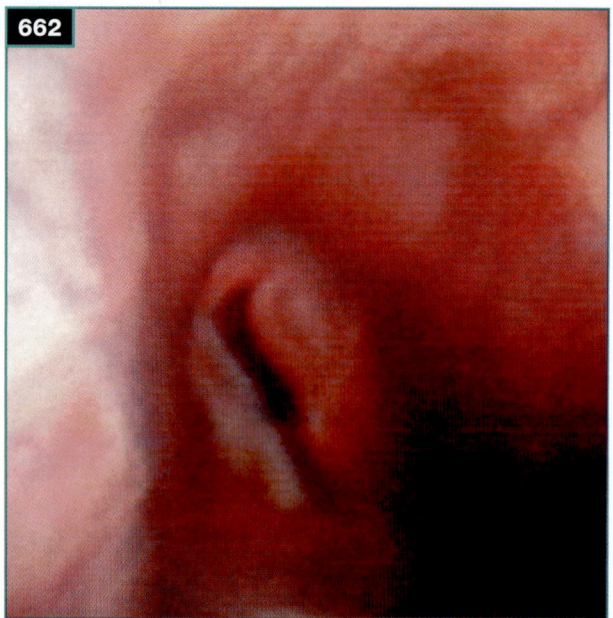

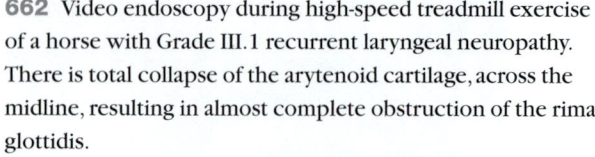

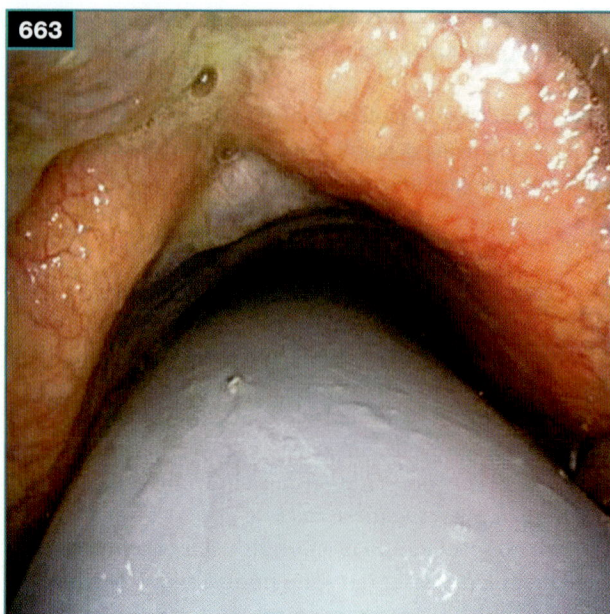

662 Video endoscopy during high-speed treadmill exercise of a horse with Grade III.1 recurrent laryngeal neuropathy. There is total collapse of the arytenoid cartilage, across the midline, resulting in almost complete obstruction of the rima glottidis.

663 Apparent hyperabduction intraoperatively. However, it is very difficult to interpret endoscopy unless the image is vertical. Under general anesthesia, with the endotracheal tube in place, it is difficult to assess how upright the picture is, so removal of the endotracheal tube for further assessment is indicated.

neuropathy), which is based upon the 0–4 system popular in North America. The 0–5 system more widely used in Europe has many advantages over this, but for international concord the Havemeyer system is used throughout. Unfortunately, there is surprisingly poor correlation between the endoscopic appearance and clinical findings.

Treadmill or overground endoscopy is used in certain cases where the diagnosis is more obscure and where complete assessment of laryngeal function is required. It is particularly useful in clarifying the significance of asynchronous movement of the arytenoids (Grades II.2–III.1). At high speeds, collapse of the arytenoid cartilage towards or even across the midline can be observed in a significant number of cases (**662**).

Management

The management of recurrent laryngeal neuropathy depends on the degree of the neuropathy and the athletic potential of the horse. Generally, the maximum demand for air is found in flat-racing horses, followed by National Hunt, then eventing, show-jumping, and dressage horses. A grade of II.1 or lower is usually considered within normal limits, and treatment for recurrent laryngeal neuropathy is only indicated if further diagnostics determine a more serious problem (i.e. marked muscular atrophy or,

preferably, exercise endoscopy evidence). Horses with Grades II.2 and III.1 recurrent laryngeal neuropathy usually have normal exercise tolerance, and treatment for vocal cord collapse may be used if clinical signs are compelling (see Vocal cord collapse, p. 435). Grades III.2 and higher recurrent laryngeal neuropathy are usually significant and result in collapse of the arytenoid cartilage during strenuous exercise. There is a poor correlation between the degree of change observed at rest and the ability of the horse to maintain abduction of the arytenoid cartilage at exercise. Thus, treatment should always be guided by careful assessment of the clinical signs, the degree of muscular atrophy, the character of the respiratory noise at exercise, and, if possible, by endoscopy during exercise.

Grades III.3 and IV recurrent laryngeal neuropathy are usually associated with severe respiratory obstruction at exercise, and surgery is necessary for all but the most sedentary horses. Many surgical procedures have been tried. The Hobday/Williams procedure (ventriculectomy/cordectomy) is reviewed under Vocal cord collapse. Only laryngoplasty (tie-back) and neuromuscular pedicle grafting will be reviewed here (permanent tracheotomy is also appropriate in some cases and is discussed under Airway obstruction, p. 440). Arytenoidectomy is also advocated in some situations (see Arytenoid chondritis, p. 426).

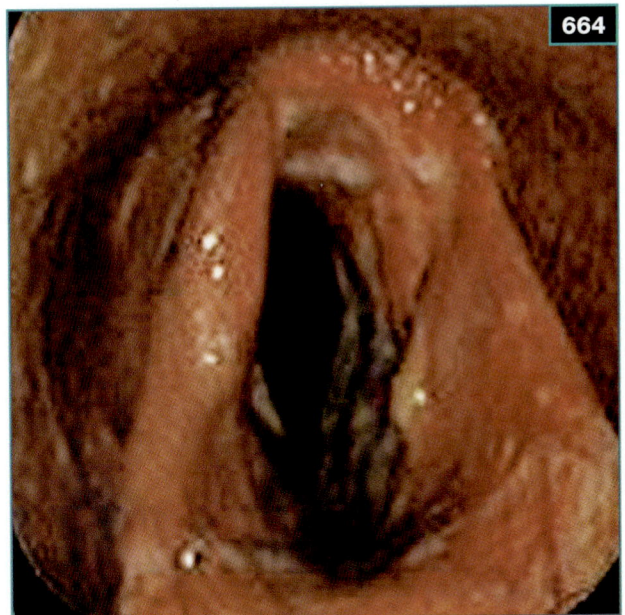

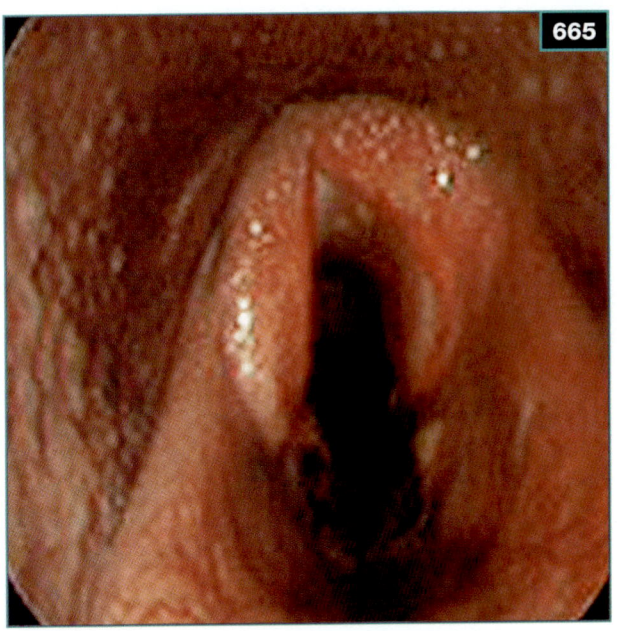

664 Hyperabduction of the arytenoid following tie-back surgery.

665 Endoscopic view of the larynx immediately following tie-back surgery showing a typical degree of left laryngeal abduction.

The laryngoplasty (tie-back) procedure has been used for over 30 years, and despite its many failings, there are few more practical alternatives. The procedure involves the placement of a suture, or sutures, on the outside of the larynx between the cricoid cartilage and the muscular process of the arytenoid. It is intended that the suture mimics the action of the cricoarytenoideus dorsalis muscle in a partially contracted position (663). It is usually combined with a ventriculocordectomy. The complications of tie-back surgery are important. A permanent implant is used and if infection were to localize on the suture, then removal would be the only effective treatment. Infection may be associated with poor surgical technique or, more likely, penetration of the airway during placement of the ligature, particularly at the cricoid. Multifilament materials are much more prone to infection than monofilament materials such as nylon. Postoperative dysphagia is a well-known complication. It has been shown that sham surgery with removal of the ligature results in some dysphagia, thus surgical scarring and neural damage from the dissection will have some effect on deglutition. The fixed abduction of the arytenoid cartilage is the most likely cause of dysphagia (664,665). The degree of dysphagia is very variable and is not directly correlated with the degree of abduction. It is recommended always to feed horses from

the ground following laryngoplasty and to feed dampened food with a more 'sticky' consistency. Fresh grass is one of the most difficult materials to swallow and any horse suffering significant postoperative dysphagia should be prevented from grazing. Following a tie-back, almost all horses will cough occasionally during eating. Occasional horses will develop intermittent pyrexia and occasionally frank pneumonia. Removal of the implant is usually recommended in severe cases and the prognosis is favorable for an improvement in eating, rather than a cure. Due to the degree of scarring, the airway function usually only deteriorates partially, rather than reverting to preoperative levels.

Failure of the tie-back is well recognized. This is usually associated with the ligature cutting through the muscular process of the arytenoid, but it can be caused by failure of the ligature itself or the cricoid implantation. It is quite normal for the tie-back to slacken progressively over the ensuing months and years, even if it does not fail completely. Failed tie-backs can be treated by repeating the procedure, although the degree of abduction obtained is never as much as the first time, or by arytenoidectomy.

The complications of laryngoplasty have led to a search for techniques to re-innervate the larynx. The most

Surgical conditions of the upper respiratory tract

successful technique published was nerve anastomosis. This requires surgical skill and specialist equipment, so has not become popular. A neuromuscular pedicle graft procedure has been described and used by some surgeons, but has not been widely accepted.

Prognosis

The prognosis is guarded. Recurrent laryngeal neuropathy is an incurable, progressive disease. Surgical procedures to alleviate it are available and can be successful, but all have significant complications.

Arytenoid chondritis

Definition/overview

Arytenoid chondritis is an important cause of airway obstruction due to inflammation, thickening, and distortion of the arytenoid cartilage, which leads to exercise intolerance and an abnormal respiratory noise.

Etiology/pathophysiology

A progressive inflammatory process develops within the corniculate process or medial body of the arytenoid cartilage, which, due to its limited blood supply, is difficult to resolve once established. The inflammation leads to distortion of the cartilage, dystrophic mineralization, protruberances of damaged cartilage and/or infected granulation tissue, and fistula formation. The tracts may drain mucopurulent material and there is a decreased abduction of the affected arytenoid. The cause is unknown, but may include trauma to the cartilage and/or infection following mucosal damage. The condition is usually unilateral and is more prevalent in North America than elsewhere.

Clinical presentation

The presentation is similar to other respiratory obstructions with poor performance associated with a stridor-like inspiratory noise. The disease may have an acute onset or be chronic and insidiously progressive. The severity of signs varies with the degree of damage and subsequent obstruction. In severe and bilateral cases, clinical signs may be evident at rest or walk. Coughing occurs in some cases.

Differential diagnosis

Most of the other respiratory obstructions of the racehorse, in particular recurrent laryngeal neuropathy, will present with similar noise and performance limitations.

666 Horse with chondritis of the left arytenoid cartilage following an infected tie-back surgery. The granuloma on the abaxial aspect of the left arytenoid could be missed on a casual examination.

667 A large granuloma (arrow) on the axial and ventral border of the arytenoid cartilage. The horse has had a left ventriculectomy and cordectomy surgery.

668 'Kissing lesion' (yellow arrow) on the right arytenoid cartilage with a discharging granuloma on the left arytenoid cartilage (red arrow).

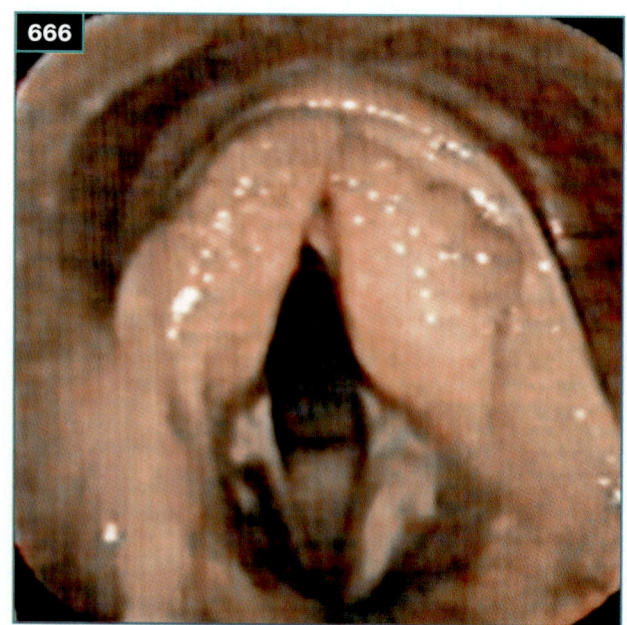
666

Diagnosis

Endoscopic examination is diagnostic, but requires care as the condition is easily misdiagnosed as recurrent laryngeal neuropathy, particularly in a left-sided case of chondritis (666). There will be limited movement of the affected arytenoid cartilage, but further assessment will reveal swelling of the corniculate process, which may be associated with mild rostral displacement of the palatopharyngeal arch. The most reliable diagnostic feature is a small discharging sinus, usually on the axial border of the cartilage, which is often associated with a granuloma (667). A 'kissing lesion', a small reddened or ulcerated area, is commonly identified on the contralateral corniculate process (668). Bilateral cases may have a very narrowed rima glottidis. Palpation over the affected arytenoid may increase the clinical signs of airway obstruction and noise. Lateral radiographs of the larynx may reveal focal mineralization.

Management

Traditional management of arytenoid chondritis is surgical arytenoidectomy, which is also used as a treatment for recurrent laryngeal neuropathy, typically after failure of a laryngoplasty. Partial arytenoidectomy, involving removal of all the arytenoid apart from the muscular process, has been shown to be superior to subtotal arytenoidectomy, where a rim of corniculate cartilage is left *in situ*. The procedure is performed through a laryngotomy and can be associated with a number of complications. A prolonged course of antibiotics and NSAIDs (6 weeks) may cure early cases and can control the swelling and discharge from the arytenoid cartilage for a reasonable period in some more established cases. This is usually associated with a marked improvement in arytenoid motility. Significant axial granulomas and kissing lesions do not usually resolve with this treatment regimen, but they can be removed either by transendoscopic laser surgery or by conventional surgery via a laryngotomy.

Prognosis

Partial arytenoidectomy has a guarded prognosis for return to athletic activity. The procedure is also associated with the complication of dyspnea in the short term, caused by marked postoperative swelling, and dysphagia. Coughing during eating may occur, especially in bilateral cases, and aspiration pneumonia has been recorded. The conservative approach warrants a guarded prognosis, but with this regimen the majority of the more mildly affected cases will be able to perform, though probably at a lower level.

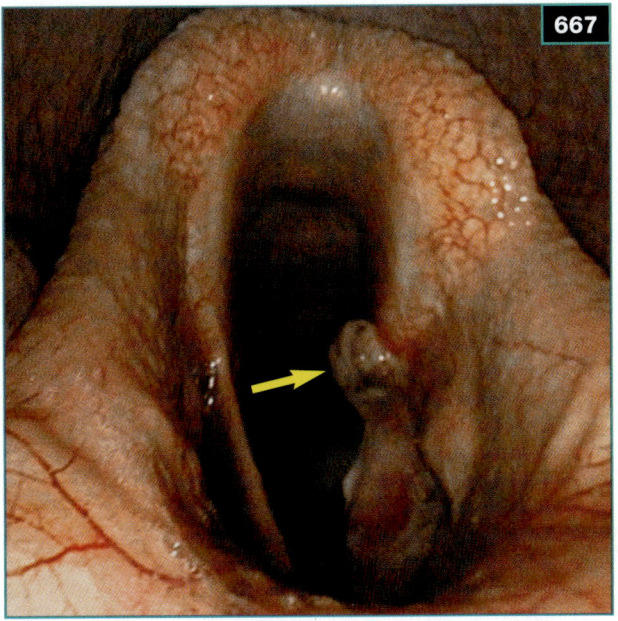

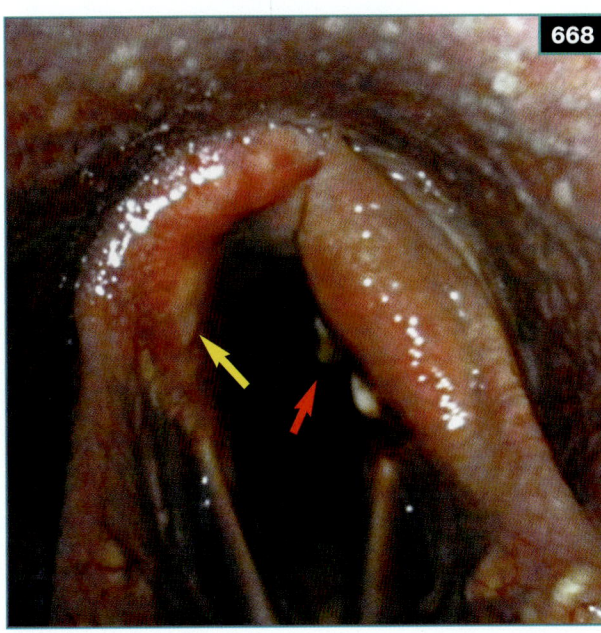

Surgical conditions of the upper respiratory tract

Fourth branchial arch defect syndrome
Definition/overview
Embryologically, the larynx is derived from the fourth and sixth branchial arches. The cricoid and arytenoid cartilage, along with the principal intrinsic muscles, derive from the sixth arch, while the wing of the thyroid cartilage, the crico- and thyropharyngeus muscles (the upper esophageal sphincter), and the cricothyroid muscle (responsible for tension in the vocal fold) derive from the fourth arch. A variety of laryngeal abnormalities caused by hypoplasia or aplasia of the structures that derive from the fourth branchial arch are recognized and are best described collectively as 4-BADs. The literature is confusing and one of the common presentations, rostral displacement of the pharyngeal arch, is sometimes described as a distinct condition. Other terms include cricolaryngeal dysplasia and congenital cricopharyngeal–laryngeal dysplasia. The condition is more common than is generally recognized, is frequently missed, and has a marked impact on a horse's athletic ability.

Etiology/pathophysiology
Studies of large numbers of yearlings and two-year-old Thoroughbred horses before starting training have suggested an incidence of approximately two per 1,000 horses. A genetic link has not been identified, so the likely etiology is embryologic damage or failure during development of the fourth branchial arch. The condition is congenital and is not progressive. There appears to be a predilection to affect the right side of the larynx. This unilateral incidence is not fully understood, so it may be that many left-sided cases are misdiagnosed as recurrent laryngeal neuropathy.

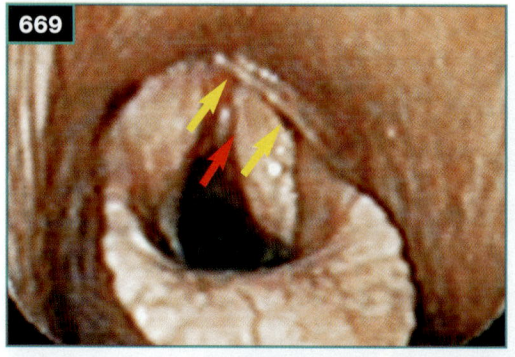

669 A horse with 4-BAD syndrome. The horse presented with chronic intermittent colic and the left wing of the thyroid cartilage was absent on palpation. There is asymmetric abduction of the arytenoid cartilages (red arrow) and unilateral rostral displacement of the palatopharyngeal arch (yellow arrows).

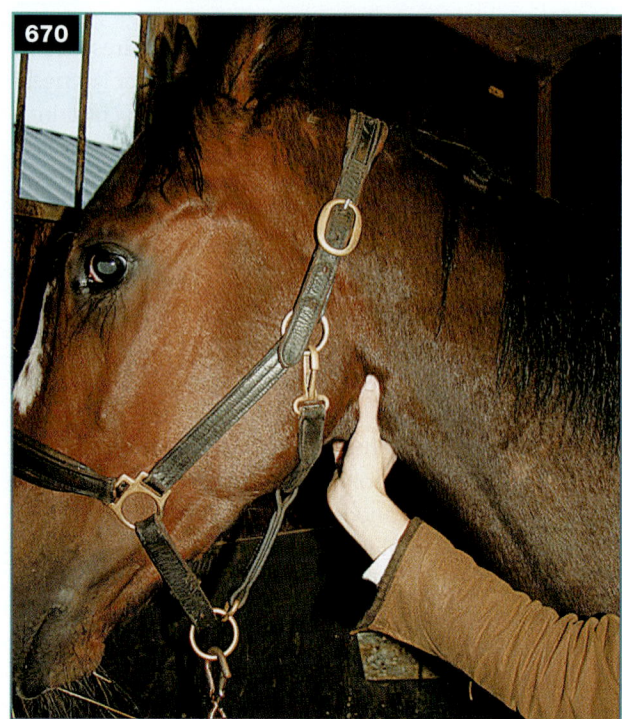

670 Palpation of the larynx. This horse has a 4-BAD and the lateral wing of the thyroid (which should be where the operator's thumb is) is missing.

Clinical presentation
The precise structures that are involved alter the clinical condition. If the wing of the thyroid cartilage is missing, along with the associated cricothyroid muscle, then the presentation may be similar to recurrent laryngeal neuropathy, with collapse of the vocal fold occurring during high-speed exercise. Endoscopic examination at rest will often reveal asymmetry of the rima glottidis, raising suspicion of recurrent laryngeal neuropathy. Great care must be taken to examine the horse carefully if right-sided recurrent laryngeal neuropathy is diagnosed: almost all cases of right recurrent laryngeal neuropathy relate to guttural pouch mycosis, perivascular injection, other trauma, or a 4-BAD. If the crico- and thyropharyngeus muscles are absent, then rostral displacement of the palatopharyngeal arch (RDPPA) will develop. This was previously considered a condition in its own right and is visible endoscopically. With RDPPA, the upper esophageal sphincter will be incompetent, which can result in aspiration of air into the proximal esophagus. Horses with a 4-BAD can therefore present as horses with eructation or even recurrent tympanitic colic (669). Horses with RDPPA can present with dysphagia.

Differential diagnosis

The most important differential diagnosis for the majority of cases of 4-BAD is recurrent laryngeal neuropathy. This is particularly important if surgical correction is considered, as laryngoplasty is frequently impossible in horses with a 4-BAD due to the cartilage abnormalities. Eructation is frequently diagnosed by owners as 'wind sucking' or 'crib biting', but is quite distinct. Thus, a horse may be managed inappropriately for stereotypic behavior.

Diagnosis

Diagnosis of a 4-BAD can be challenging. The most reliable technique is palpation of the larynx, which reveals abnormalities in almost all cases. In a normal horse the wing of the thyroid is palpable as a flat plate protecting the lateral aspect of the larynx. Immediately caudal and ventral to the thyroid, the cricoid is palpable as a complete ring around the larynx, partly obscured by the wing of the thyroid. In 4-BADs, one of the most consistent findings is absence of the wing of the thyroid. In this case the complete cricoid ring can be palpated, feeling similar to a large tracheal ring. In front of the cricoid is a space, palpably similar to the cricotracheal space, but comparison with the contralateral side should prevent any confusion over the precise location of the structures (670).

Endoscopic examination can reveal asymmetry of the arytenoid cartilages, typical of recurrent laryngeal neuropathy, or it can be normal. Rostral displacement of the palatopharyngeal arch is clearly visible endoscopically as a rim of tissue partly obscuring or overlying the dorsal aspect of the arytenoid cartilages. RDPPA can be unilateral or bilateral.

Radiography of the larynx and proximal trachea may reveal air in the proximal esophagus. This finding is usually only present if RDPPA is visible endoscopically. Occasionally, no abnormalities are evident at rest and treadmill endoscopy is necessary to reveal dynamic RDPPA or dynamic vocal-fold collapse.

Management

There is no effective treatment for RDPPA and the abnormality is permanent. Some horses with a 4-BAD have been managed with some success by bilateral ventriculectomy and cordectomy, presumably in cases where dynamic collapse was linked to these structures. Bilateral cordectomy has been associated with the formation of a web of scar tissue across the ventral aspect of the larynx.

Prognosis

The prognosis is poor. 4-BADs are permanent congenital abnormalities and many affected horses are ineffective athletes. A few horses have been salvaged to win some races by ventriculectomy and cordectomy surgery.

Epiglottitis

Definition/overview

Epiglottitis is a rare condition that occurs as a result of infection becoming established within the epiglottic cartilage. As with arytenoid chondritis, the condition appears to be primarily found in racehorses and there is an anecdotal association with all-weather surfaces.

Etiology/pathophysiology

An inflammatory process develops within the elastic cartilage of the epiglottis. It appears that the infection is less likely to become permanently established in the epiglottic cartilage than in the arytenoid.

Clinical presentation

Respiratory noise and poor performance are the usual presenting signs. Occasional cases are presented with dysphagia, though this is unusual.

Differential diagnosis

The principal differential diagnosis following endoscopic examination is pharyngeal foreign bodies, which can be associated with significant epiglottic swelling, epiglottic entrapment, smoothing of the outline of the epiglottis, and general pharyngitis.

Diagnosis

Endoscopic examination is diagnostic. The epiglottis is swollen and the normal crenated outline is lost (671).

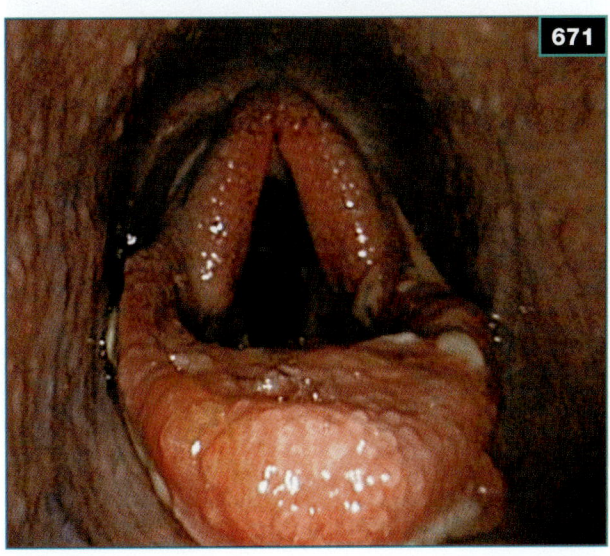

671 Epiglottitis in a young Thoroughbred racehorse.

The epiglottis is often hyperemic and is frequently observed in a more vertical orientation than normal because of the swelling. Occasionally, there may be an abscess on the dorsal surface, which is identified as a rounded swelling. Purulent discharge can be noted from the cartilage occasionally if there is ulceration of the mucosal surface.

Management

A prolonged course of antibiotics, possibly associated with NSAIDs, is indicated. Corticosteroids can be indicated if swelling is severe enough to result in respiratory obstruction at rest.

Prognosis

The prognosis is good. Recurrence of the swelling and discharge are less usual than in arytenoid chondritis. It has been suggested that a proportion of cases progress to develop conditions such as DDSP.

Epiglottic entrapment

Definition/overview

This is a common condition where the cartilage of the epiglottis becomes enveloped by the underlying glosso-epiglottic mucosa and aryepiglottic folds. The cause of the entrapment is often unclear, but careful examination is vital to differentiate any secondary causes. Epiglottic entrapments vary in stability. Some horses have permanent entrapments, while others are more intermittent and can be missed on a single examination. In athletic horses, the incidence at rest, on endoscopic examination, has suggested a range of 0.75–3.3%.

Etiology/pathophysiology

The etiology is often unknown, but inflammation of the aryepiglottic folds and loose subepiglottic tissue may be a factor in some cases. Animals with congenital epiglottic hypoplasia and subepiglottic cysts seem to be predisposed. It is not known how the loose tissue of the glossoepiglottic fold and the aryepiglottic fold becomes caught over the end of the epiglottis. The mucosa rapidly becomes thickened and ulcerated near the tip of the epiglottis (672).

Clinical presentation

The typical presentation is a vibrant respiratory noise, which may be inspiratory and/or expiratory. The severity of airflow obstruction varies with the degree of entrapment and associated swelling and inflammation, plus any secondary DDSP. There may be associated poor performance and other signs of DDSP. Occasional cases can present with dysphagia, including coughing after eating, or head shaking, or be asymptomatic.

Differential diagnosis

DDSP is the primary differential diagnosis, with similar respiratory noise.

Diagnosis

Endoscopic examination is usually diagnostic. Stable epiglottic entrapments are easily diagnosed. Care must be taken to assess the epiglottis carefully. The normal epiglottis should have a crenated edge, with pronounced vasculature. In an entrapment, the epiglottis is present

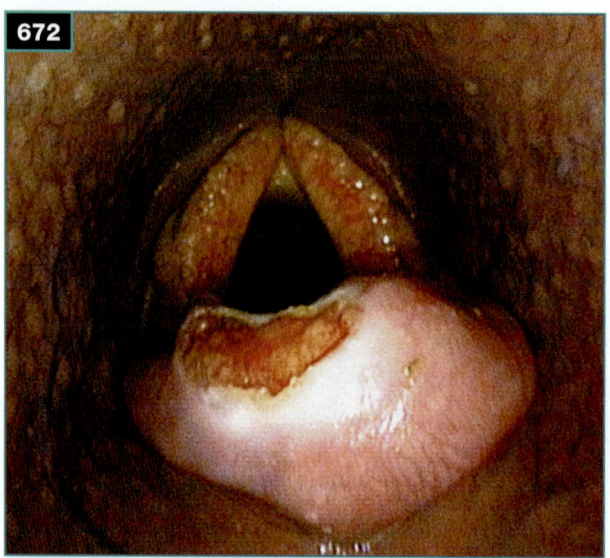

672 Epiglottic entrapment with ulceration of the entrapping glossoepiglottic mucosa.

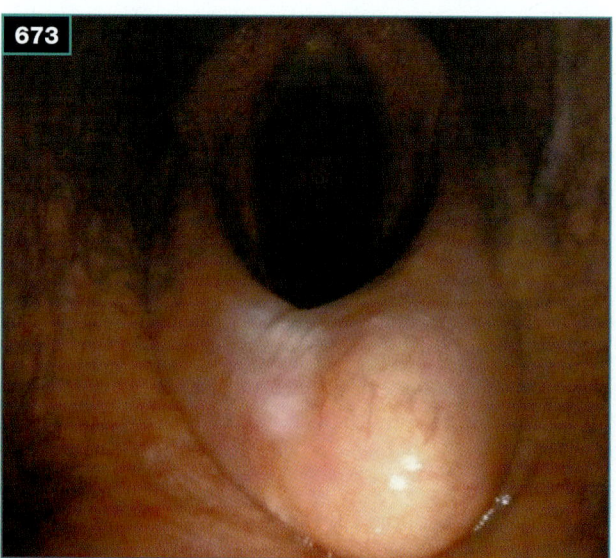

673 A nonulcerated epiglottic entrapment, illustrating the nonvascular smooth edge to the entrapping mucosa.

(unless there is a secondary DDSP), but it has a smooth edge and no vasculature due to the covering mucosa (673). The coverage of the epiglottis is variable. In long-standing cases the caudal edge of the entrapment may become ulcerated and, occasionally, the apex of the epiglottis may erode through the entrapment.

Intermittent entrapments are more of a diagnostic challenge. Almost all entrapments are precipitated by deglutition, not by exercise; therefore, careful assessment of several deglutition sequences is indicated. Treadmill/overground endoscopy is rarely necessary for diagnosis, as most cases can be diagnosed at rest.

Radiography of the pharynx can reveal the blunted outline of an entrapped epiglottis, epiglottic hypoplasia, and subepiglottic cysts (674).

Management

Intermittent cases can be managed successfully by anti-inflammatory medication. Medication is usually administered as a nasal spray using a canine urinary catheter. A combination of DMSO, hydrocortisone, and propylene glycol is often used.

Most cases of epiglottic entrapment are managed surgically. Stable entrapments can be managed in the standing, sedated horse. The pharynx is anesthetized using topical anesthetic delivered by the endoscope. A custom-built hook knife (Sontec Instruments) is then passed via the contralateral nostril and used to hook the entrapping membrane. The knife is then progressively withdrawn until the membrane is transected down the midline. The entrapping membrane is tough and considerable traction is necessary to transect it. Great care is necessary to ensure no trauma to other pharyngeal structures, particularly the soft palate. The entrapped mucosa can also be incised via a transendoscopic laser following topical local anesthesia.

Due to the risks of iatrogenic palatal trauma, and the limitation that standing surgery is only suitable for stable entrapments, many surgeons prefer to perform the procedure under general anesthesia. The same hook knife can be used, passed via the mouth. Accurate placement of the knife can be confirmed by palpation in most horses, provided the surgeon does not have particularly large hands. In smaller horses the procedure can be conducted under oral endoscopic examination (675). In cases where transecting the entrapping membrane does not release the entrapment, resection via a laryngotomy is necessary.

Prognosis

The prognosis is good. Recurrence is recognized in a small percentage of cases managed by simple transection of the membranes. Excision of the glossoepiglottic mucosa can result in chronic coughing due to exuberant granulation

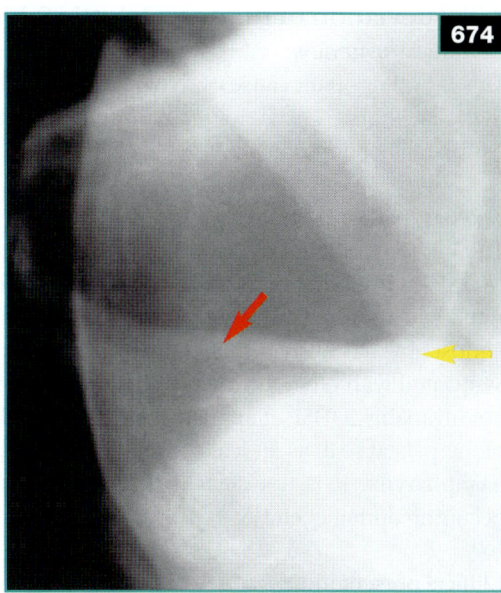

674 Lateral standing radiograph of the pharynx of a horse with an entrapped epiglottis. Note the rounded end of the epiglottis (yellow arrow) and clear soft tissue band running towards the larynx (red arrow), which is the edge of the entrapped membrane.

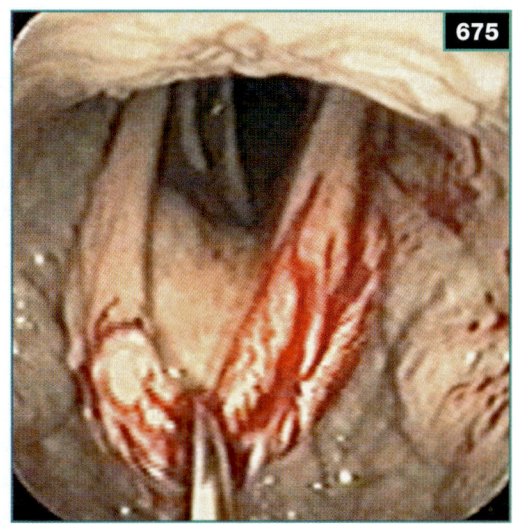

675 Axial transection of the entrapping mucosa using a hook knife passed through the mouth.

tissue formation and low-grade dysphagia in some horses. Iatrogenic trauma to the epiglottis or pharyngeal structures, especially in standing procedures, is a risk. Most cases of epiglottic entrapment make a rapid and uneventful recovery.

Axial deviation of the aryepiglottic folds

Definition/overview

This is an important cause of dynamic airway obstruction in the racehorse. It was not recognized before the advent of treadmill endoscopy.

Etiology/pathophysiology

The etiology of axial deviation of the aryepiglottic folds (ADAF) is not known. The condition has not been replicated by experimental denervation procedures. Treadmill endoscopy has shown that the condition is sometimes associated with other airway obstructions, commonly, but not invariably, DDSP. It appears to be associated with loss of the palatal seal, as air leaks from the oropharynx to the nasopharynx. It is not clear if the same mechanism is occurring during exercise.

Clinical presentation

ADAF usually presents as a typical airway obstruction of the performance or racehorse. The typical history is of poor exercise performance associated with a harsh inspiratory noise. There is no characteristic feature of the inspiratory noise. There is no known breed or gender bias, but there may be a higher incidence in young horses (2–3 years old).

Differential diagnosis

All the causes of inspiratory noise and poor performance in the racehorse should be considered. Many experienced clinicians with access to treadmill endoscopy consider the noise identical to that associated with collapse of the arytenoid cartilage with recurrent laryngeal neuropathy. Care should be taken with a diagnosis of ADAF alone, as most cases are associated with other respiratory obstructions.

Diagnosis

Treadmill or overground endoscopy is required to establish a diagnosis of ADAF (676). There is dynamic collapse, towards the midline, of one or both of the aryepiglottic mucosal folds (more commonly right sided) that extend between the lateral epiglottis and the corniculate process of the arytenoid cartilages. The degree of deviation varies between cases and this determines the degree of clinical signs and possible treatment options. Other concurrent URT endoscopic findings include axial collapse of the vocal cords, left laryngeal hemiplegia, intermittent DDSP, right laryngeal dysfunction, and dorsal pharyngeal collapse.

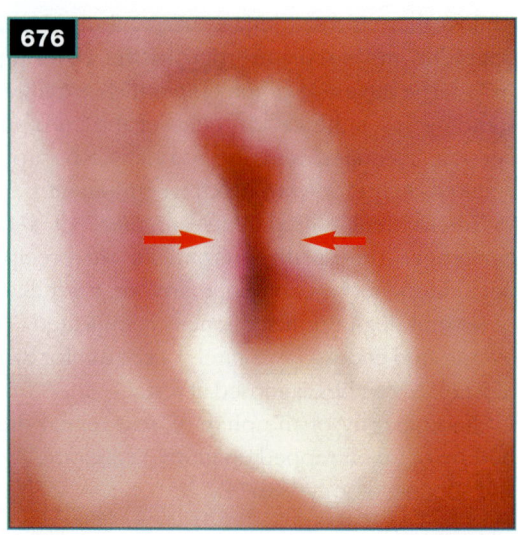

676 Horse showing marked axial deviation of the aryepiglottic folds (arrows) during high-speed treadmill endoscopy.

Management

Surgical resection of the aryepiglottic folds is the treatment of choice for moderate to severe cases or where there are no concurrent abnormalities. This can be performed via a laryngotomy incision *per os*, usually under general anesthesia, or per nasum under standing sedation, and endoscopic guidance using a transendoscopic laser. Postoperatively, the horse is medicated systemically with antibiotics and NSAIDs for 5–7 days. Topical antibiotic and anti-inflammatory pharyngeal sprays may also be used. Coughing and dysphagia do not appear to be serious complications of this procedure, despite being recognized complications of subepiglottic resection for the treatment of epiglottic entrapment.

Prognosis

The prognosis is guarded. The response to surgery is quite good in the short term, but over a longer period (one year or so) the respiratory noise tends to recur. The aryepiglottic folds appear to re-form on endoscopic examination quite rapidly.

Epiglottic flaccidity
Definition/overview
There is controversy as to whether this condition, associated with loss of epiglottic rigidity, exists. Some clinicians believe it may be involved in the etiology of some cases of DDSP and retroversion of the epiglottis. It is still normal in some clinical practices to comment on the stiffness or maturity of the epiglottis when carrying out URT endoscopy in a young horse. There has been no evidence published to link epiglottic flaccidity objectively with DDSP or other airway obstruction.

Etiology/pathophysiology
The proposed etiology is that stiffness of the epiglottis is critical in maintaining the soft palate in a normal, sub-epiglottic position. It has been empirically observed that the epiglottis often appears flaccid in younger (yearling) horses, which has led to the suggestion that the epiglottis may be immature in some of these cases.

Clinical presentation
The clinical presentation is intermittent DDSP.

Differential diagnosis
Differential diagnoses include all other causes of DDSP and many other causes of upper airway obstruction. Epiglottic hypoplasia is a similarly controversial condition and is the principal differential diagnosis.

Diagnosis
The diagnosis is established by endoscopic examination in the nonsedated horse and the observer's opinion of the appearance of the epiglottis (677). This is complicated by the fact that the epiglottis faces the observer, making assessment of length difficult. Assessment of texture may also be difficult. A flaccid epiglottis is generally considered to be one that is flattened against the soft palate throughout its length, with the edges curling upwards. This criterion does not consider the position of the soft palate. It may be that the epiglottis is being flattened by a soft palate that is devoid of tone and is billowing upwards into the airway. This is usually observed as a precursor to DDSP when endoscopic examination is performed during exercise.

The findings of either a flaccid epiglottis or soft palate at rest are of limited diagnostic value. It is reasonably well established that changes at rest are a poor predictor of changes at exercise. Thus, a horse with a flaccid epiglottis at rest may perform perfectly well at exercise.

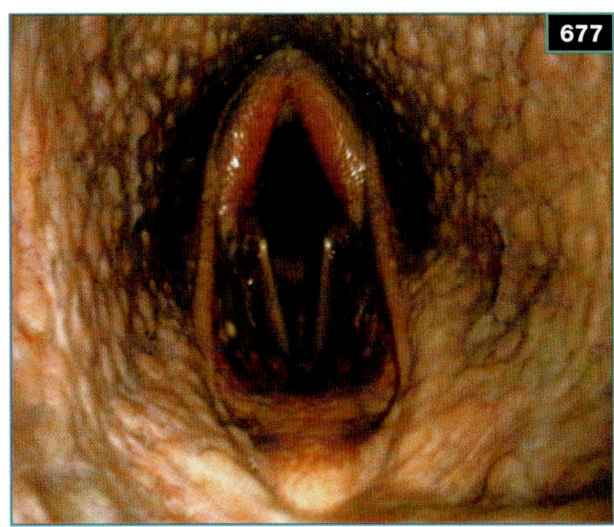

677 Endoscopic view of the larynx of a 2-year-old Thoroughbred. The epiglottis appears flaccid, flattened against the soft palate. However, it is difficult to determine whether it really is flaccid and if it is of any clinical relevance.

Management
The treatment for epiglottic flaccidity is augmentation with polytetrafluoroethylene (Teflon) paste injected into the subepiglottic mucosa via a ventral laryngotomy. This surgery is commonly used as one of a series of procedures for the treatment of DDSP, rather than a specific treatment for epiglottic flaccidity alone. Published results suggest that the surgery is quite successful; however, it is widely accepted to be another surgery for DDSP and associated with a similar success rate to most other procedures.

Prognosis
In published studies, 73% of Thoroughbreds and 53% of Standardbreds showed improved racing performance following epiglottic augmentation surgery. Complications of excessive granulation and abscess formation have been reported in some cases post surgery. The prognosis for epiglottic flaccidity generally is considered to be good, as the endoscopic appearance of the pharynx improves in most horses with increasing maturity.

Epiglottic hypoplasia

Definition/overview

Epiglottic hypoplasia is another controversial condition that is rare. Similar to epiglottic flaccidity, the hypothesis is that the epiglottis is crucial in maintaining the soft palate in a normal subepiglottic position; therefore, a short epiglottis is more likely to be associated with DDSP. Initial studies suggested that the epiglottis was shorter in horses with a history of DDSP, but more recent studies have not verified this finding.

Etiology/pathophysiology

Epiglottic hypoplasia is believed to be a congenital condition.

Clinical presentation

The clinical presentation is intermittent DDSP and/or epiglottic entrapment.

Differential diagnosis

The differential diagnoses include all other causes of DDSP and, in turn, all other causes of upper airway obstruction. Epiglottic flaccidity is the primary differential diagnosis for an epiglottic cause of DDSP.

Diagnosis

The diagnosis is initially made by endoscopic examination, but it should be confirmed by radiography. A lateral radiograph of the pharynx and larynx is taken with a radio-opaque object of known dimensions (preferably spherical to eliminate any parallax errors) taped to the horse in the midline (**678**). A comparison of the actual and measured dimensions of the object gives an accurate measurement of radiographic magnification. The length of the epiglottis can then be measured from the basihyoid to the tip of the epiglottis on the radiograph, and its true length calculated using the magnification factor. An epiglottis that measures less than 5.5 cm in a Thoroughbred (normal 8–9 cm) is considered to be hypoplastic.

Management

There is no effective surgical solution to lengthen the epiglottis. In the majority of cases the length of the epiglottis is an incidental finding unrelated to the DDSP.

Prognosis

Genuine epiglottic hypoplasia has a poor prognosis. Otherwise, the prognosis is as for DDSP, where approximately 60% of horses will improve, regardless of treatment.

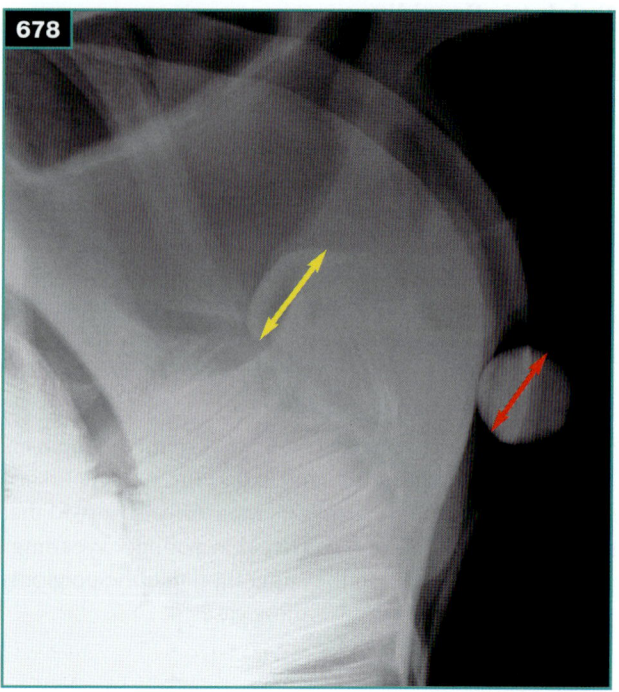

678 Radiograph showing measurement of the epiglottis, (yellow line, 48.3 mm) with measurement of a known diameter radio-opaque sphere (golf ball, red line, 38.4 mm) placed in the midline of the horse to provide a magnification factor. This is the only effective way of measuring an epiglottis; an end-on endoscopic view is not accurate.

Epiglottic retroversion

Definition/overview

Epiglottic retroversion is an interesting condition that was not recognized prior to the advent of high-speed treadmill video endoscopy. The recognition of this condition revealed that the epiglottis probably had nothing to do with DDSP. During epiglottic retroversion the epiglottis is aspirated into the trachea, but the soft palate is observed tightly clasped around the larynx. This observation brought into question the relevance of the two conditions described above (Epiglottic flaccidity and Epiglottic hypoplasia) and altered the focus of research into the cause of DDSP.

Etiology/pathophysiology

Experimental studies have shown that epiglottic retroversion can be induced by nerve blocks of the hypoglossal and glossopharyngeal nerves and by anesthesia of the geniohyoid muscle. It is presumed that the cause of the naturally occurring disease is a neuromuscular weakness of this muscle. As with DDSP, it is not known if this is the limiting factor in a horse's athletic ability or the result of acquired disease.

Clinical presentation

Affected horses are presented with poor performance associated with a vibrant respiratory noise.

Differential diagnosis

Most other dynamic respiratory obstructions of the performance horse should be considered. The most important differential diagnosis is DDSP.

Diagnosis

Diagnosis requires endoscopy at exercise (679). There are no distinctive features of the condition at rest. Without treadmill endoscopy or other endoscopy at exercise, most cases are treated for DDSP.

Management

Epiglottic resection has been attempted and results in severe dysphagia. Permanent tracheotomy can be considered to bypass the larynx. A suture from epiglottis to thyroid cartilage has been described, but limited results are available. Most horses are treated by epiglottic augmentation (see Epiglottic flaccidity).

Prognosis

The prognosis is guarded. Some success has been reported with surgical augmentation, and some return to function may develop with rest.

Vocal-cord collapse

Definition/overview

Collapse of the vocal cord is part of the recurrent laryngeal neuropathy complex recognized on treadmill endoscopy.

Etiology/pathophysiology

The recurrent laryngeal nerve innervates the vocalis muscle of the vocal cord as well as the other principal abductor and adductor muscles of the larynx. The function of this muscle is for vocalization, with the adjacent laryngeal ventricle for resonance. Loss of abduction of the arytenoid cartilage will reduce tension in the vocal cord, and loss of tone in the vocalis muscle will further slacken the cord. It has been shown that the cricothyroid muscle (innervated by the cranial laryngeal nerve) is essential to maintain vocal cord tension, and loss of function of this muscle will also result in vocal-cord collapse.

Clinical presentation

Affected horses have poor performance associated with respiratory noise. The classic musical 'whistle' of a horse with recurrent laryngeal neuropathy is probably associated with collapse of the vocal cord and the passage of air over the open laryngeal ventricle.

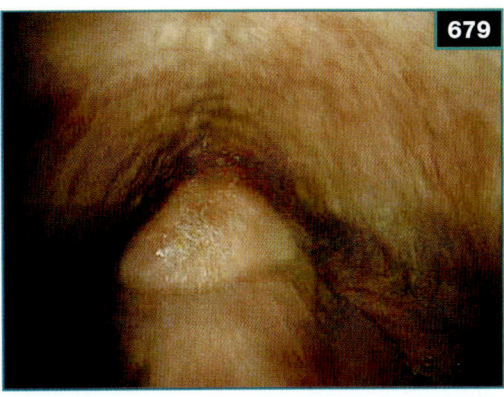

679 High-speed treadmill endoscopy view of epiglottic retroversion. The soft palate is in a normal position, implying that the epiglottis is not pivotal in preventing DDSP. (Photo courtesy S Barakzai)

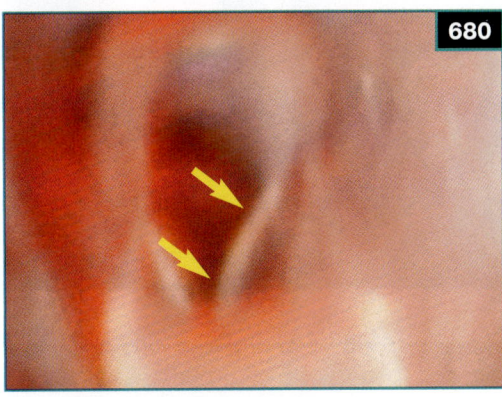

680 Vocal cord collapse (arrows) evident during strenuous exercise on a high-speed treadmill.

Differential diagnosis

Most other dynamic respiratory obstructions of the performance horse should be considered. The most important differential diagnosis is whether the horse has only vocal-cord collapse, or whether it is associated with collapse of the arytenoid cartilage as well.

Diagnosis

Precise diagnosis of vocal-cord collapse requires treadmill endoscopy or another method of endoscopy at exercise (680). Even then the question will remain: 'Would the arytenoid have collapsed if the horse had gone faster?'. Therefore, in the majority of cases diagnosis is based around a musical inspiratory noise associated with a moderate (Grade II.1 to III.1) recurrent laryngeal neuropathy at rest.

Management
Surgical treatment of vocal-cord collapse is very successful using a ventriculocordectomy via a ventral laryngotomy, under general anesthesia or using a laser in the standing horse without the need for a laryngotomy. Resection of both cords is not recommended, as this can result in the exposed tissue healing together, producing a web of scar tissue that obscures the ventral larynx (**681,682**).

Prognosis
The prognosis for resolution of the respiratory noise following cordectomy is very good. The prognosis for improvement in performance is more guarded, as the vocal cord can contribute a large amount of respiratory noise, while collapse of the arytenoid results in the major respiratory obstruction. Even if the procedure appears to be successful, recurrent laryngeal neuropathy is a progressive condition so further respiratory noise and obstruction may develop.

Trachea

Tracheal trauma

Definition/overview
Lacerations of the neck occasionally involve the trachea or the esophagus. Generally, the priority with such a laceration is control of hemorrhage from one of the major vessels of the neck, followed by assessment of any neurologic compromise such as recurrent laryngeal function and damage to the vagosympathetic trunk. There may be open or closed wounds in the trachea.

Etiology/pathophysiology
Tracheal trauma typically occurs as a result of a kick, wire injuries, fence posts, metal objects, or falls.

Clinical presentation
In open lacerations to the trachea there will be an accompanying wound of the neck. There may initially be severe hemorrhage followed by subcutaneous emphysema if the trachea is perforated. With time there may be pyrexia, disseminating cellulitis, increased swelling, tracheal compression, and respiratory obstruction. Attention may be drawn to tracheal trauma by frothing of the blood in the area. Closed injuries to the trachea due to blunt trauma are more difficult to diagnosis. There is no skin wound, but there may be rapid and severe development of subcutaneous emphysema and edema, respiratory stridor caused by obstruction by the wound edges, and possible obstruction of the trachea from external compression by swellings and/or wall injury.

Differential diagnosis
There are no specific differential diagnoses; more relevant is the potential involvement of other structures. The common carotid artery lies dorsolateral to the trachea, with the vagosympathetic trunk deep to it. The esophagus is usually left of, and dorsal to, the trachea. The recurrent laryngeal nerve lies dorsal to the trachea, in the deep tissues of the neck.

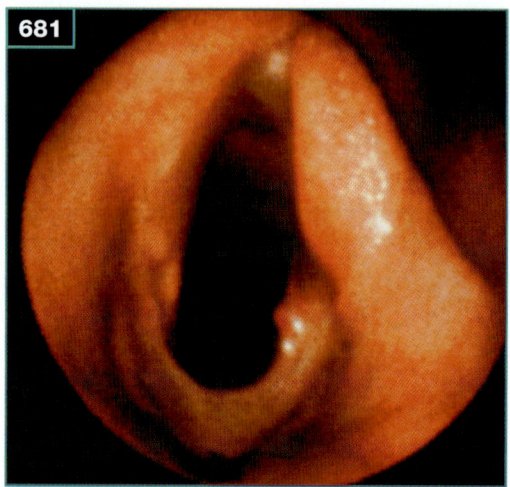

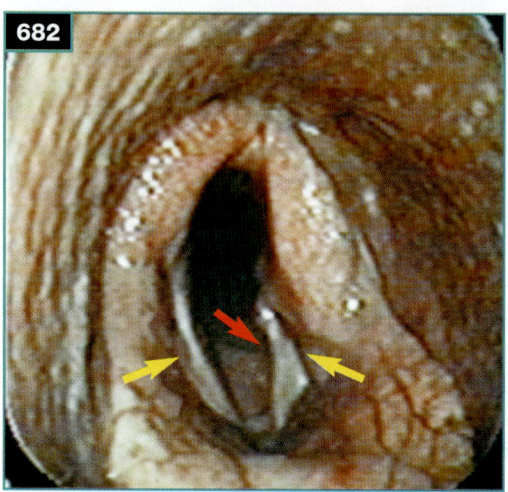

681 'Web' larynx formation, a complication of bilateral vocal cordectomy.

682 Endoscopic view of a horse showing Grade III.3 recurrent laryngeal neuropathy. The horse has also been 'Hobdayed'; the ventricles (yellow arrows) are filled with scar tissue and the left vocal cord (red arrow) has been partially ablated.

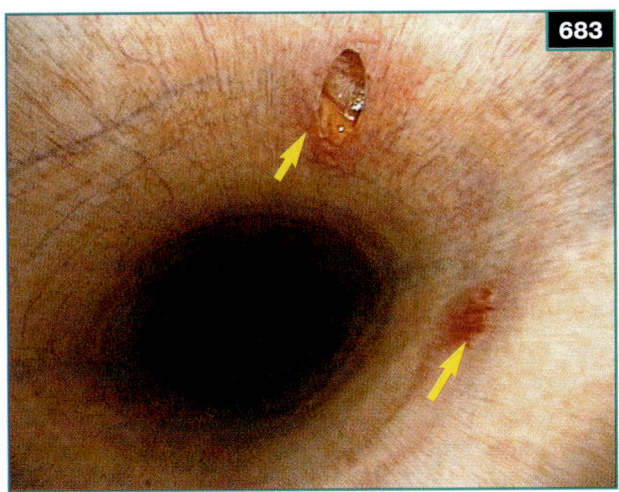

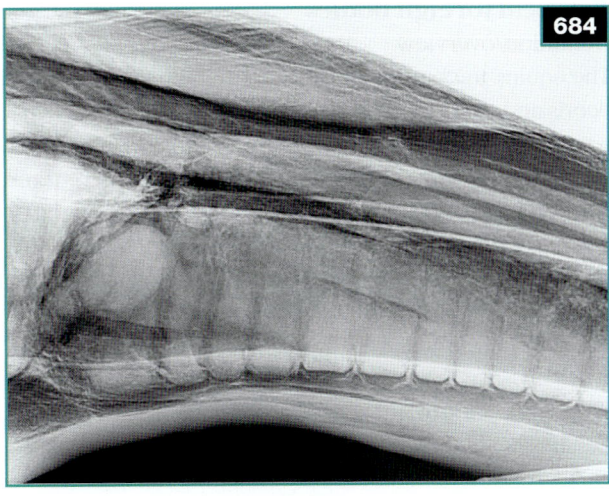

683 Endoscopic view of laceration of the dorsal trachea. The horse presented with subcutaneous emphysema and it was postulated that the blunt trauma that had resulted in laceration of the dorsal trachea had been caused by crushing of the trachea against the cervical vertebrae.

684 Laterolateral radiograph of the upper neck from the same horse as in 683. The emphysema is visually interesting, outlining the esophagus, but does not help isolate the source of the gas.

Diagnosis

Direct examination, sterile palpation of the wound, and endoscopic examination of the trachea will reveal the laceration from the outside and inside, and allow assessment of how much is damaged (**683**). Radiography and ultrasonography will often reveal gas in the soft tissues of the neck in such cases and possibly deformity of the tracheal outline or rings (**684**), while contrast studies help assessment of esophageal integrity.

Management

Any lacerations should be debrided and ventral drainage established. Closure of the wound is usually contraindicated as it can result in severe abscessation, with further compression and damage. Healing by second intention should be encouraged by regular careful wound management and antibiotic/anti-inflammatory medications. In closed wounds, topical pressure and anti-inflammatory measures (i.e. systemic antibiotic and anti-inflammatory medications) are helpful. Suction decompression of the emphysema using wide-bore needles is also surprisingly effective in many cases. If severe respiratory obstruction is present, a temporary tracheotomy distal to the injury may be required. Primary surgical repair of tracheal injuries is possible in some cases.

Prognosis

The prognosis is fair. Generally, if treated appropriately and early, lacerations to the trachea will heal with no long-term problems. Extensive subcutaneous emphysema can track caudally into the thorax or mediastinum, leading to life-threatening complications. Tracheal lacerations can result in disturbance of the airflow and respiratory noise from tracheal stenosis, particularly if there is extensive damage to the tracheal rings.

Tracheal foreign bodies

Definition/overview

The equine trachea has an amazing ability to clear itself of debris and although foreign material is quite common, this is seldom significant. An endoscopic examination immediately after a race will often reveal large chunks of track surface in the trachea and these are almost invariably cleared without complication. The only foreign bodies of significance are those that may get stuck in the trachea, notably twigs and thorns, which are fortunately rare (685).

Etiology/pathophysiology

The foreign body is most commonly inhaled, but ingested material can sometimes enter the trachea. Foreign material with barbs or thorns tends to work its way distally, but stops itself being coughed up. Once wedged in the airway, the foreign body will cause pain and a local reaction. The significance of the foreign body reaction depends on the location of the fragment, but if lodged in the distal trachea or bronchial tree, it may lead to severe necrotizing pneumonia and pleurisy.

Clinical presentation

There is usually a sudden onset of severe or paroxysmal coughing, with subsequent bilateral mucopurulent nasal discharge and possibly LRT disease. Occasionally, epistaxis will also occur in the early stages. In long-term cases there is chronic coughing with malodorous breath.

Differential diagnosis

Other causes of bilateral nasal discharge and coughing should be considered.

Diagnosis

Endoscopic examination is almost invariably diagnostic. If the foreign body is beyond the carina of the trachea, it can usually still be examined by anesthetizing the carina with 20–30 ml of local anesthetic, followed by passing a long (>2 m) scope further along the bronchi, following the purulent discharge.

Management

The challenge of tracheal foreign bodies is communicating to a client that something that can be quite easily visualized can be so difficult to retrieve. Surgical removal is difficult, so most have to be removed by using an endoscopic technique. Most of the proprietary endoscopic tools, such as biopsy forceps and cages, are too flimsy for use in the horse; therefore, a snare is used. Snaring the foreign body can be extremely challenging, involving many hours of patient attempts with the horse under sedation. In certain situations it can be beneficial to pass the endoscope via a distal tracheotomy. This limits the complications associated with a short endoscope and with withdrawing the object through the nostrils. The foreign body may break up on removal and require additional procedures to remove the remaining fragments. Broad-spectrum antibiotics are administered postoperatively and other medications may be needed, determined by the degree of involvement of the LRT.

Prognosis

If the object can be located and removed completely, the prognosis is good. Bronchitis or pneumonia can usually be resolved with appropriate treatment once the foreign body is removed. Inability to retrieve the object is a frequent complication, in which case the prognosis is grave.

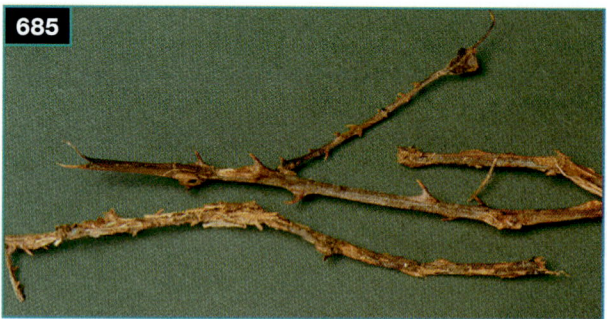

685 Several twigs with thorns removed from the trachea of a horse, under general anesthesia, using an endoscopic snare. (Photo courtesy JG Lane)

Respiratory system

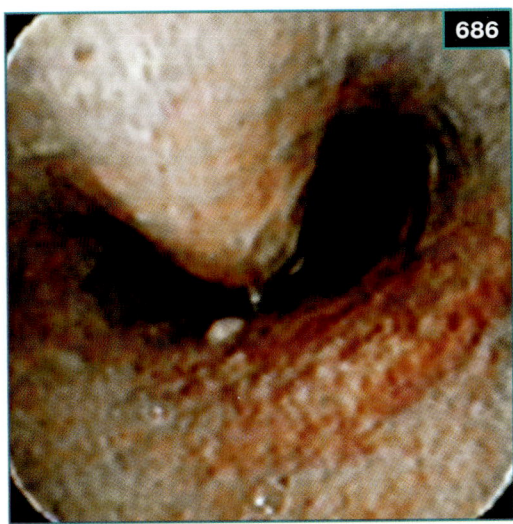

686 Marked collapse of the dorsal tracheal ligament in a pony, concurrent with coughing.

Tracheal collapse

Definition/overview
Tracheal collapse is an uncommon condition seen in a variety of situations. The most important form is an idiopathic dorsoventral collapse, which is frequently intrathoracic. The condition is almost always found in donkeys and small ponies, especially Shetlands and miniature ponies. A lateral collapse (scabbard trachea) of the cervical trachea is also reported in the Thoroughbred. Typically, there is dyspnea and stridor, with diagnosis achieved by external tracheal palpation, endoscopy, and lateral neck and thoracic radiographs. Both conservative and surgical treatments have been successfully used.

Etiology/pathophysiology
Tracheal collapse can develop secondary to conditions such as external compression from enlarged lymph nodes, abscesses, and tumors (mediastinal); trauma around the trachea or to the structure itself; severe expiratory dyspnea as a result of pulmonary disease; and during standing sedation if animals rest their necks on bars at the front of stocks. Dorsoventral tracheal flattening (in the first few tracheal rings) is recorded in the Thoroughbred and its crosses, but is often incidental. Dorsoventral tracheal collapse in ponies is the most common and is caused by a tracheal cartilage ring deformity, although the precise etiology is not known. Some cases in young animals may be developmental, but many are in older animals and

could be degenerative in origin. The condition is usually associated with flattening of the tracheal cartilage rings (reducing dorsoventral distance), with resultant stretching of the dorsal tracheal ligament. Other sorts of deformity may occur concurrently at different sites in these animals and also incidentally in other horses and ponies.

Clinical presentation
In many small ponies and donkeys the condition may be asymptomatic because of limited workload or mild changes. Affected ponies usually present with a history of respiratory distress, including significant respiratory stertor and coughing. The pony or horse may be normal at rest and only show clinical signs during exertion or during hot or humid weather. Exercise-induced pulmonary hemorrhage may occur in severe cases because of increased thoracic pressures. Deformities of the trachea of the Thoroughbred may be asymptomatic, but may present as poor performance with respiratory noise.

Differential diagnosis
For dorsoventral tracheal collapse of the pony the primary differential diagnosis is recurrent airway obstruction.

Diagnosis
Palpation of the trachea in cases of dorsoventral deformity may reveal a sharpened edge to the lateral aspects, especially in the cranial part of the neck, although this may be an incidental finding. Difficulties may be encountered in palpation distally (where the defects are most common) and in thick-skinned, fat, small ponies. With scabbard trachea deformity, palpation will often reveal distinctive ridges on the ventral midline of the deformed trachea in the upper cervical region. Diagnosis is usually achieved by endoscopy (**686**). A markedly wider, flatter, and restricted trachea is usually apparent in the dorsoventral deformity, particularly associated with coughing or deep breathing (inspiratory narrowing cervical lumen, expiratory narrowing intrathoracic lumen). The mucosal lining may be red and inflamed. In scabbard trachea deformity there is slight lateral flattening of the upper tracheal lumen, but often an adequate airway space. Lateral radiographs of the distal cervical and thoracic trachea may be helpful; however, the radiograph must be timed to coincide with the part of the respiratory cycle for the tracheal collapse to occur.

Management
Initially conservative treatment is recommended including restricting exercise, keeping the horse cool in hot weather, and treating concurrent respiratory tract disease. Acute severe cases may benefit from intranasal oxygen and cooling regimens. Systemic corticosteroids will reduce any mucosal swelling in the trachea as well as control any concurrent lung inflammation. This medical therapy may

439

result in only short-term improvement. Surgery to stent the collapsing trachea has been reported using an external stent, such as a plastic syringe case. Surgical management is seldom practical due to the extent of the tracheal collapse and possible intrathoracic location. Scabbard trachea in the Thoroughbred is often incidental and usually not treated, but it can be managed by permanent tracheotomy if permitted by the relevant regulatory authorities and if the horse is destined for an athletic career. Resection and anastomosis of the cervical trachea is reported. The horse must be trained to wear a martingale to avoid raising the head, and a maximum of five tracheal rings can be resected.

Prognosis
The prognosis is guarded to poor as dorsoventral tracheal collapse is generally a progressive condition with no reliable surgical solution. Medical management results in short-term improvement only in some cases; however, many small ponies do very little work and can cope with the problem in the short term. Collapse secondary to other diseases may only partially or temporarily improve even if the underlying condition is resolved. Scabbard trachea is also incurable, but is seldom progressive.

Tracheal stenosis
Definition/overview
This is a rare condition either secondary to tracheal surgery or trauma or as a primary congenital deformity. Occasional cases of stenosis are noted associated with external compression by mediastinal tumors, right-sided aortic arch, or streptococcal mediastinal abscesses.

Etiology/pathophysiology
Congenital stenotic defects are very rare. The usual cause of tracheal stenosis is tracheotomy surgery. When performing a tracheotomy care should be taken not to transect too much of the annular tracheal ligament, with 30% being quite adequate for an emergency airway. With permanent tracheotomy tubing it is preferable not to transect an entire tracheal ring.

Clinical presentation
Mild stenosis may not produce any clinical signs. Poor performance with a harsh respiratory noise is the typical presentation. A history of prior tracheotomy surgery is not always available.

Differential diagnosis
Most upper airway obstructions can be included as differential diagnoses.

Diagnosis
Palpation of the trachea and auscultation should be performed. Endoscopic examination is definitive. Care should be taken to place appropriate significance on tracheal lesions, as they often result in more disruption of the airflow than might be anticipated.

Management
Surgical techniques to ablate the stenotic area are available, including laser surgery, tracheal resection and anastomosis, and external tracheal prosthesis. Recurrence of the stenosis is quite common. A second permanent tracheotomy tube, slightly further caudally in the neck, may be an alternative solution.

Prognosis
The prognosis is guarded for tracheal surgery and good for permanent tracheotomy, albeit with the complications of management of the tube. The prognosis for resolution of the stenosis without surgery is hopeless.

Airway obstruction
Definition/overview
Airway obstruction is encountered occasionally in equine practice.

Etiology/pathophysiology
There are numerous causes, including severe unilateral idiopathic recurrent laryngeal neuropathy, bilateral recurrent laryngeal neuropathy following toxicoses such as lead or organophosphates, acute hepatic failure, pharyngeal swelling following allergic reaction or abscessation (e.g. strangles infection), and, most commonly, after general anesthesia.

Clinical presentation
Horses can present in severe 'air hunger' with the head stretched out, the nostrils flared, and marked thoracic excursion. Generally, upper airway obstruction results in inspiratory dyspnea, while lower airway obstruction results in expiratory dyspnea. Some horses will present with collapse. Noncardiogenic pulmonary edema is a common sequela of upper airway obstruction in the horse, so bloodstained frothy nasal discharge is often involved.

Differential diagnosis
Obstructive lower airway disease is the most important differential diagnosis. Passage of a nasotracheal tube (see below) can be useful to establish if there is an upper or lower airway obstruction.

687 A suitable emergency tracheotomy tube, and the 'pattern' for constructing one. This system works extremely well in emergencies and a suitable container is almost invariably available.

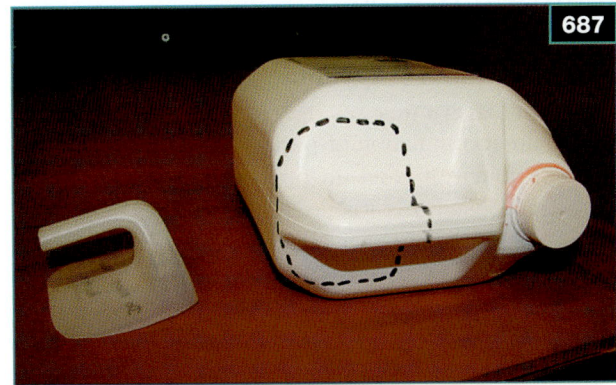

Diagnosis

Endoscopic examination is diagnostic; however, in many cases there is insufficient time for diagnosis, an endoscope is unavailable, or examination may precipitate an episode of collapse.

Management

An airway can be provided by nasal intubation in some cases, but in others this is impossible. Emergency tracheotomy is often necessary with or without the use of local anesthetic infiltration and aseptic skin preparation. A cut-off portion of stomach tube is effective, as is the cut-off hollow handle of a typical 5-liter container (**687**). The tube should then be tied in place around the neck. In some jurisdictions (e.g. the UK) it is still permissible to race a horse with a permanent tracheotomy tube (**688**). This procedure can be used to allow athletic activity from a horse with an inoperable or unsuccessfully treated upper airway condition. A slightly wider tracheotomy is necessary to seat the tube. The tubes can be maintained successfully, with regular removal and cleaning, for many years.

Prognosis

Once an airway is established, the prognosis is dependent on diagnosis and management of the underlying condition. Horses with severe swelling from snake bites or stings have an excellent prognosis. Once the swelling has subsided, the tube is removed. Second-intention healing is almost invariably uneventful over the next few weeks. Horses with surgical conditions of the upper airway can be treated, as appropriate, for the underlying condition. These horses can be managed with temporary or permanent tracheotomy tubes for many months or even years. Finally, horses with expansile conditions of the upper airway such as tumors have a poor prognosis.

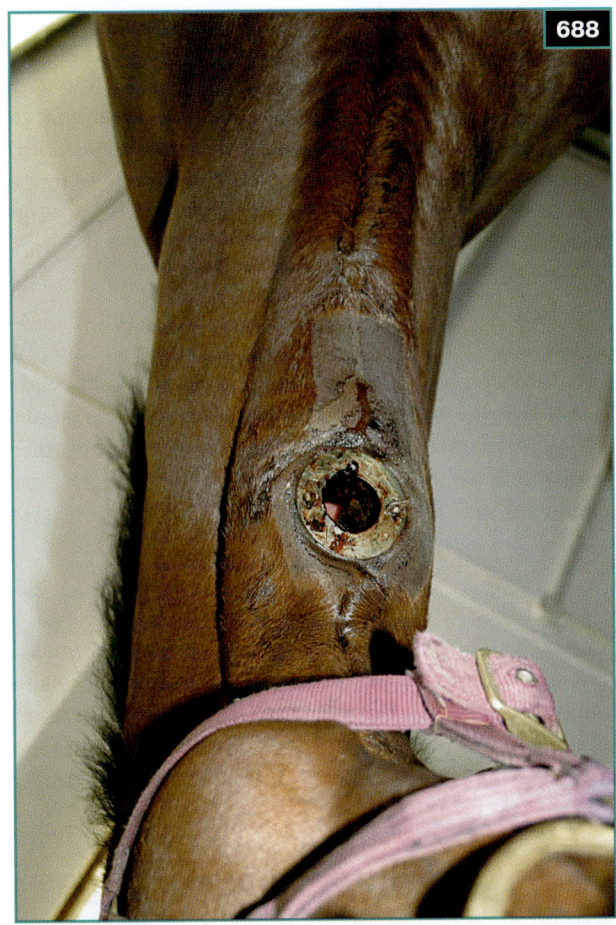

688 Permanent tracheotomy tube in a point-to-point horse with severe recurrent laryngeal neuropathy that did not respond well following 'tie-back' and 'Hobday' surgery.

Surgical conditions of the upper respiratory tract

Guttural pouch

Guttural pouch empyema
Definition/overview
This is an accumulation of purulent material within the guttural pouch. It is an uncommon condition, but is a differential diagnosis for unilateral purulent nasal discharge. The guttural pouch is a commonly recognized site for colonization by *Streptococcus equi equi* (strangles) and any purulent material in this region should be viewed as contagious and probably strangles related, unless proven otherwise.

Etiology/pathophysiology
The etiology is usually a *Streptococcus* spp. upper airway infection that localizes in the guttural pouch either as a primary infection or secondary to a URT viral infection or other guttural pouch disease. The guttural pouch seems to be unable to clear these organisms as effectively as much of the remainder of the upper airway. Thus, horses can become chronic carriers or prolonged shedders of *S. equi*. Sometimes, the infection remains subclinical, but it can be associated with frank empyema of the guttural pouch. This in turn can remain as liquid pus accumulation, or the pus can inspissate. Inspissated pus in the guttural pouch tends to result in the formation of multiple rounded accumulations known as chondroids (689). Once the pus becomes inspissated, the *Streptococcus* infection is often less significant and anaerobic infection may become more relevant.

Clinical presentation
A unilateral, or predominantly unilateral, purulent nasal discharge is almost invariably the presenting sign. Swelling in the parotid region may be noted clinically, as distension of the pouch is frequent. Distension of the pouch into the airway, especially the nasopharynx, can cause dyspnea

and an abnormal respiratory noise. The disease almost invariably has a chronic history, which can vary from unilateral discharge despite treatment through to intermittent unilateral discharge for over a year.

Differential diagnosis
The primary differential diagnosis is sinusitis. Most cases have been treated with a presumptive diagnosis of sinusitis for a period. Discharge from the lower airway, which can be quite purulent, can sometimes appear down one nostril and create the incorrect impression of a URT disease.

Diagnosis
Endoscopy usually provides a definitive diagnosis. Endoscopic examination of the nasopharynx may reveal unilateral dorsal pharyngeal swelling. Purulent discharge from the guttural pouch ostia may be present; however it is normal for horses to aspirate some material from the nasopharynx into the openings of the guttural pouch during swallowing, so identification of material is not diagnostic (690). The opening to the guttural pouch is under the dorsal aspect of the cartilage flap located in the dorsal pharynx, and it is important to pass the endoscope up the ventral meatus in order to facilitate entry into these openings (691–693). Once in the pouch, visibility is often obscured by purulent material. The lining of the pouch may be markedly thickened, limiting identification of normal structures (694). Opening the pouch will often result in a flow of fluid from the ostium, but the ventral aspect of the pouch is almost invariably obscured. The contralateral pouch can be normal (695) or may also be involved.

Radiography of the guttural pouch is diagnostic of fluid or soft-tissue infiltration of the pouch. Chondroids can occasionally be visualized on radiographs, but they are usually associated with some fluid accumulation, which can obscure their outline.

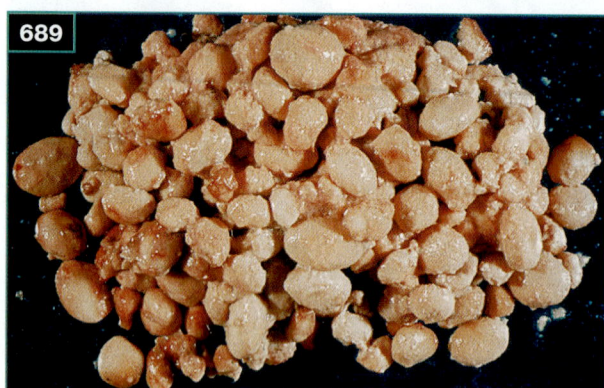

689 Accumulation of chondroids removed surgically from a pony with guttural pouch empyema.

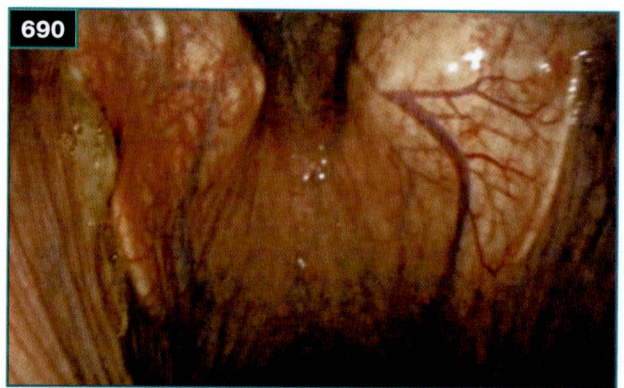

690 Purulent material discharging from the right guttural pouch ostium.

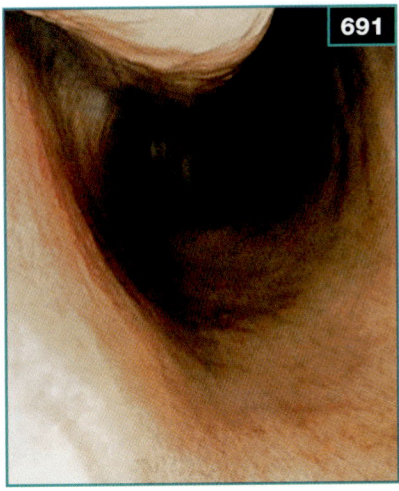

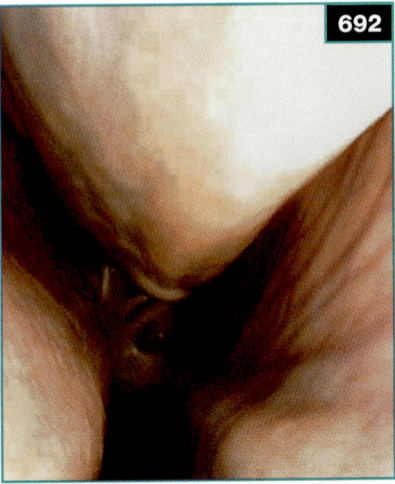

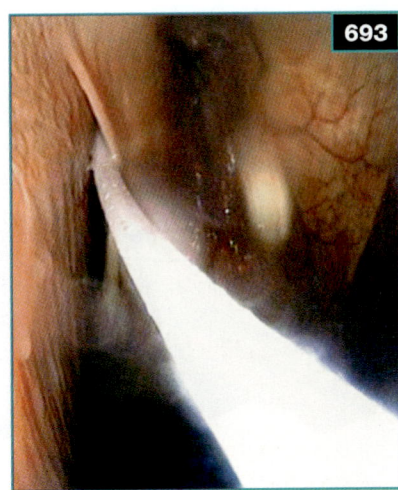

691, 692 The ventral meatus (691), with the U-shaped ventral conchus dorsally, as opposed to the Y-shaped middle meatus (692). An endoscope must be in the ventral meatus to enter the guttural pouch.

693 A length of polyethylene tubing advanced down the biopsy channel of the endoscope, under the dorsal aspect of the cartilage flap and into the guttural pouch.

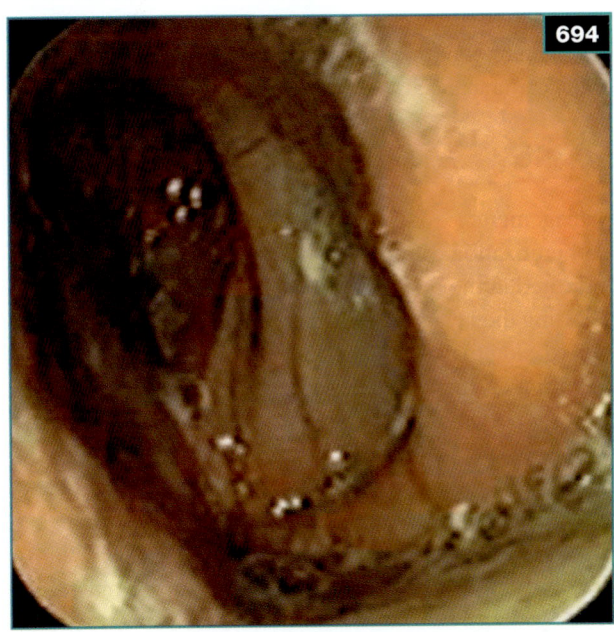

694 Endoscopic view of guttural pouch empyema with liquid purulent material, showing thickening of the lining of the pouch. Culture of the fluid yielded *Streptococcus equi equi*.

695 Normal guttural pouch showing the stylohyoid bone (black arrow), which divides the pouch into medial (right) and lateral compartments. The internal carotid artery (red arrow) is in the medial pouch, along with the neural fold containing the glossopharyngeal and hypoglossal nerves and the cervical sympathetic trunk (yellow arrow). The vagus nerve branches off medially from this fold (white arrow). The external maxillary artery and its numerous branches are in the lateral pouch (green arrow).

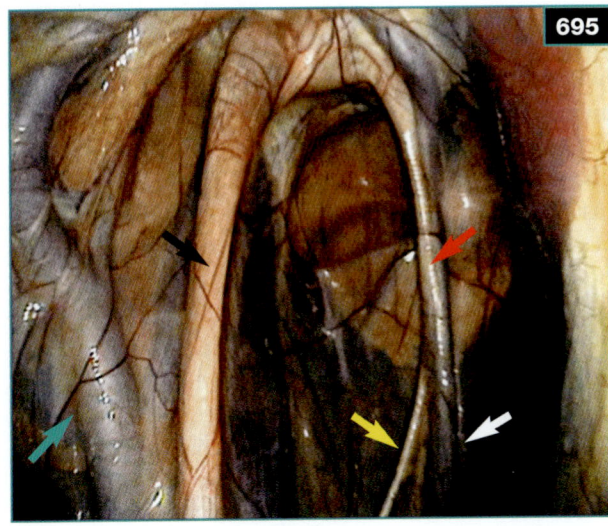

Surgical conditions of the upper respiratory tract

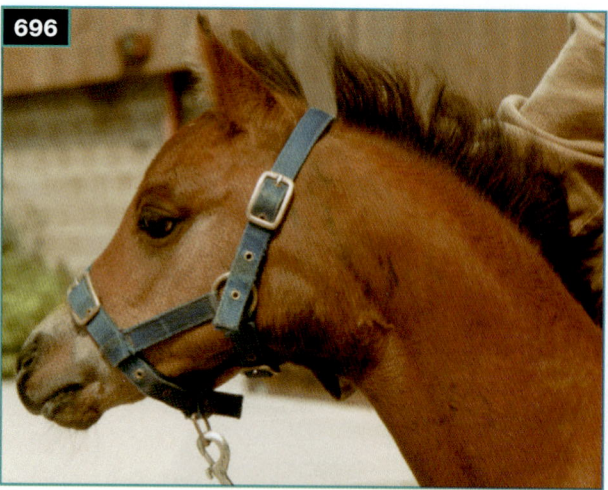

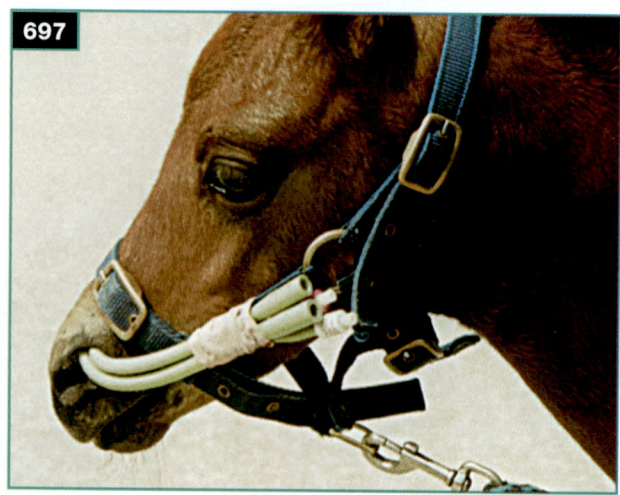

696 Foal showing marked swelling of the parotid and throat latch regions. The swelling was soft, fluctuant, and painless. Radiography confirmed that it was a large gaseous distension of the guttural pouch.

697 The same foal as in 696 (which was bilaterally afflicted) with a Foley catheter present in each guttural pouch, both passed by the same nostril. The catheters were maintained for 3 weeks, which resulted in resolution of the tympany.

Management

Catheterization of the guttural pouch and lavage are indicated in the first instance. Great care must be taken in selecting the lavage agent. Irritant materials such as iodine or peroxide may cause serious neurologic damage due to the number of critical cranial nerves passing through the guttural pouch and are therefore contraindicated. Lavage with antibiotic solutions is also dangerous. Much of the material lavaged from the pouch is ingested and, as with oral penicillin treatment, lavage with crystalline penicillin may lead to complications such as severe diarrhea. Simple warm water is relatively nonirritant and surprisingly effective. Systemic antibiotic treatment is recommended and should be based on the results of culture and sensitivity. Almost always, the antibiotic of choice is penicillin.

Following a period of lavage, further examination is indicated. If the guttural pouch is clear, but thickened and inflamed, withdrawal of the catheter and subsequently of antibiotic treatment should be considered. If there is still purulent material in the pouch, inspissation of the pus and chondroid formation should be considered likely. In this instance, further lavage can be attempted, including with acetylcysteine solution, and the antibiotic treatment should be altered. Once formed, chondroids can be broken down by lavage or removed endoscopically, but this can be difficult and surgical removal may be necessary. Surgical approaches to the guttural pouches are well established, but they do carry significant risks of complications. It is important to remove as much material as possible at surgery, but also to establish good postoperative drainage as complete resolution at surgery is unlikely.

Prognosis

The prognosis for simple empyema is good. Most cases resolve satisfactorily with lavage. The prognosis following chondroid formation is guarded. Complete removal of the chondroids is difficult to achieve, and recurrence has been noted even when surgery was initially successful.

Guttural pouch tympany

Definition/overview

This is an uncommon condition of the foal, although yearlings are occasionally affected. The condition occurs due to a congenital dysfunction of the pharyngeal opening of the pouch associated with a build-up of excessive amounts of air in the guttural pouch. The condition can be unilateral or bilateral.

Etiology/pathophysiology

The etiology is unknown, but guttural pouch tympany is probably a congenital defect. The ostia are usually patent, but are not functioning correctly, allowing a one-way accumulation of air in the pouch.

Clinical presentation

Foals usually present with marked swelling of the parotid region (696). Palpation reveals a tympanic swelling, which is quite painless. Dysphagia or dyspnea may be present if the swelling is extreme.

Differential diagnosis

The clinical presentation is quite characteristic. The most likely confusing differential diagnosis is a retropharyngeal abscess. These can present with identical pharyngeal swelling, but palpation will reveal a firm painful mass.

Diagnosis

Radiography is the most valuable technique to confirm the diagnosis. A lateral radiograph will reveal the extreme distension of the guttural pouch. Endoscopy on initial examination will reveal marked dorsal pharyngeal swelling. Entry to the guttural pouch causes collapse of the pouch and reveals no abnormalities of the internal structures.

Management

The majority of cases can be managed very successfully by chronic catheterization of the guttural pouch. A large-bore (Ch 28) Foley catheter is placed within the affected guttural pouch(es) and left *in situ* for up to 6 weeks. This usually results in sufficient scarring and alteration of the ostium of the guttural pouch to prevent it forming a one-way seal in the future (697). Unilateral cases can be managed by creation of a fistula in the septum between the two pouches. This can be performed endoscopically using a laser. Finally, if long-term catheterization is not successful, then a second ostium can be created in the dorsal pharynx, again using transendoscopic laser surgery.

Prognosis

The prognosis is fair. Most cases resolve with chronic catheterization. Recurrence is rare.

Guttural pouch mycosis

Definition/overview

This is an important but uncommon condition. Clinical signs vary depending on the structures involved in the guttural pouch, but the most common and important sign is severe epistaxis (698).

Etiology/pathophysiology

The etiology is unknown, but fungal infection becomes established in the guttural pouch. The mycotic plaque that forms on the pouch wall is highly erosive and, depending on where the plaque occurs, different structures can be damaged. The internal carotid artery is frequently involved, as the plaque forms on the roof of the medial compartment caudal and medial to the temporohyoid articulation. The pharyngeal branch of the vagus nerve and the recurrent laryngeal nerve are also involved in some cases. Less commonly, the plaque is more lateral, resulting in damage to a branch of the external carotid artery, the external maxillary artery.

Clinical presentation

The most common presentation is severe epistaxis. Usually, horses are discovered after a hemorrhage, but the stable is often heavily contaminated with blood, giving the traditional 'slaughterhouse' image. The next most common presentation is acute-onset, often severe, pharyngeal-phase dysphagia. This includes coughing when eating and discharge of food, mucus, and saliva from both nostrils. The discharge is often stained with dark blood as well. Other cranial neuropathies can include laryngeal hemiplegia, facial paralysis, and Horner's syndrome. Pain in the caudal head/cranial neck region can also occur, leading to head carriage and position changes.

698 Life-threatening epistaxis caused by guttural pouch mycosis.

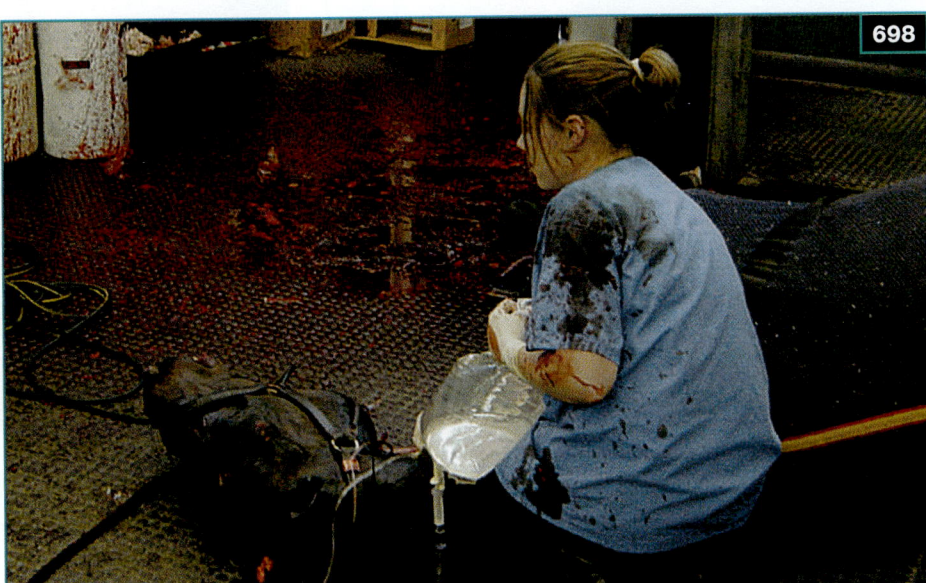

Surgical conditions of the upper respiratory tract

Following the initial bleed, horses will variably continue to discharge dark blood from principally one nostril (699). If untreated, a second severe bleed usually occurs a few hours or days later. The first bout of epistaxis is seldom fatal, but this is highly variable and should not be relied upon.

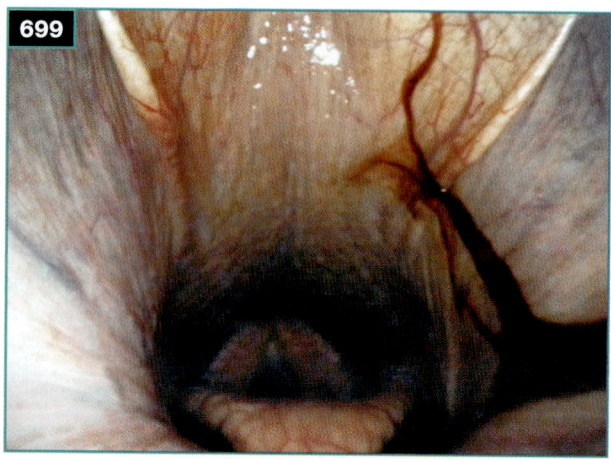

699 Dark blood discharging from the left guttural pouch. The horse had a history of marked epistaxis the previous day. At this stage, preparation for surgery is indicated. The guttural pouch can then be examined immediately prior to induction of anesthesia, in case examination dislodges a blood clot and precipitates another life-threatening hemorrhage.

Differential diagnosis

The principal other cause of severe epistaxis is nasal trauma. Exercise-induced pulmonary hemorrhage can be severe, but obviously always has a history of strenuous exercise immediately beforehand. Dysphagia has multiple causes; however, pharyngeal-phase dysphagia is generally neurogenic in origin. Various poisonings (e.g. lead) can cause neurogenic damage. Masses below the epiglottis can cause permanent DDSP and dysphagia, and if the mass is caused by a foreign body, the onset can be acute.

Diagnosis

Endoscopy is the principal diagnostic aid, but care must be exercised during examination. Examination of the naso-pharynx will usually reveal a large blood clot distending the ostium of the guttural pouch. Horses with blood in the pharynx from other causes will often aspirate some into the guttural pouch ostium during swallowing. Therefore, a small trickle of blood from the ostium is not necessarily significant. A large blood clot is not usually mistaken and is quite obvious during examination. Following this examination, the operator needs to decide whether to examine the pouch itself. This decision is not as easy as might be anticipated. Endoscopic examination may dislodge a blood clot and precipitate a fatal hemorrhage. It is reasonable to admit a horse to a surgical facility following tentative diagnosis of a large blood clot in the guttural pouch. The horse is then prepared for surgery and examined endoscopically in anesthetic induction. Any hemorrhage at this point can be controlled by proceeding with surgery. If the guttural pouch is examined endoscopically, the

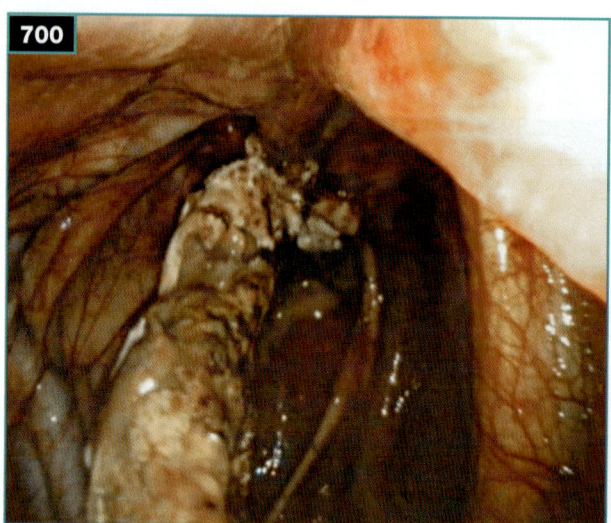

700 Large fungal plaque in the guttural pouch, lying principally over the stylohyoid bone, but extending medially and dorsally across toward the sigmoid flexure of the internal carotid artery and the neural fold.

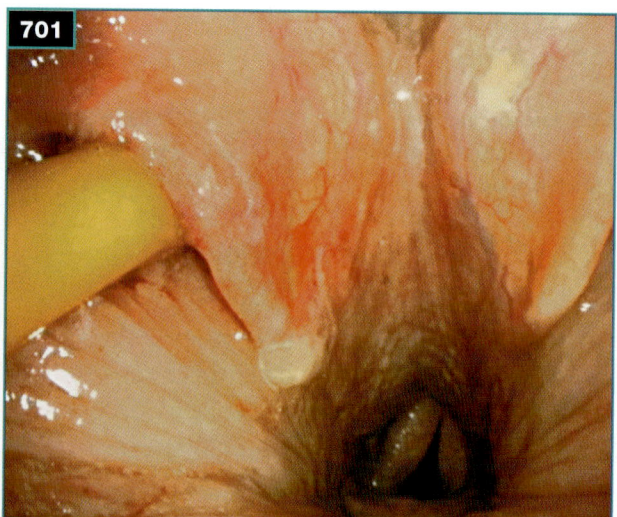

701 Foley catheter implanted into the right guttural pouch. These catheters can usually be maintained for several weeks without complication, and can be easily replaced if dislodged.

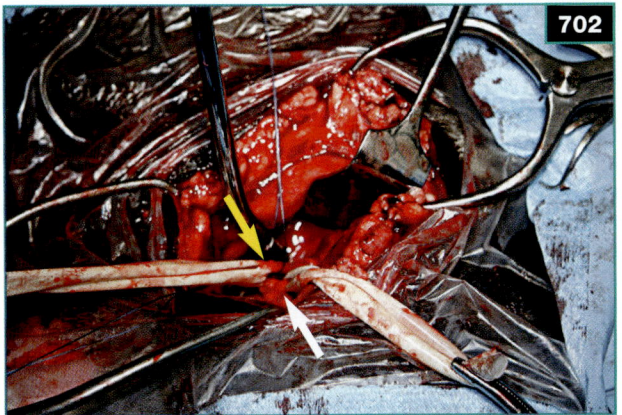

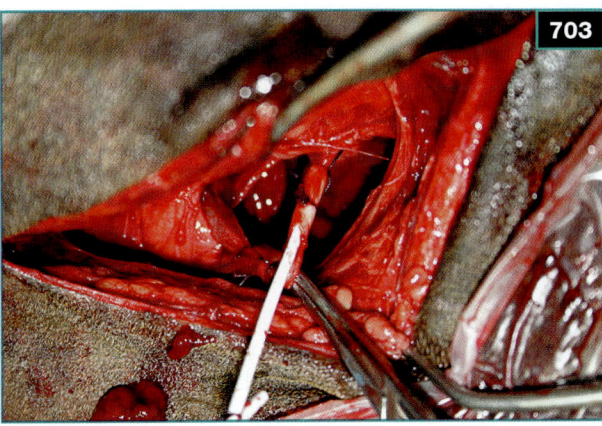

702 The internal carotid artery has been identified and elevated toward the incision (yellow arrow). The occipital artery has also been elevated (white arrow). The arteries are surprisingly elastic and can be elevated quite safely, in order to ensure accurate identification.

703 A 6 Ch Foley catheter has been advanced 15 cm up the internal carotid artery and the balloon inflated. The artery has been double ligated distal and proximal to the arteriotomy.

information gained can be limited, as visibility is frequently obscured by blood. The principal aim of the examination is to localize the fungal plaque (**700**). A dorsomedial location is usually associated with internal carotid hemorrhage, while lateral mycosis is often associated with external maxillary hemorrhage.

In all patients it is important to assess laryngeal motility, as this is frequently affected in horses with mycosis. Guttural pouch mycosis often results in total paralysis of the larynx (Grade IV) and lesser grades of hemiparesis are more likely to be idiopathic recurrent laryngeal neuropathy. Examination of the guttural pouch is always recommended following a diagnosis of right-sided recurrent laryngeal neuropathy.

Dysphagic patients often exhibit permanent DDSP. Repeated attempts at swallowing should be observed, usually by flushing water into the nasopharynx. This should result in active contraction of the pharynx and bilateral opening of the guttural pouch ostium, followed by replacement of the soft palate in a subepiglottic position.

Radiography can also be used in diagnosis. A lateral radiograph of the parotid region may reveal fluid lines in the guttural pouch or more irregular blood clots forming soft-tissue densities.

Management

Medical management can be pursued, but surgery is generally recommended for all hemorrhaging patients as fatal hemorrhage can occur before antifungal treatment has a chance to be successful. In dysphagic patients, medical management is more appropriate, but consideration should be given to prophylactic vascular occlusion even in this situation.

Medical management is topical administration of antifungal agents such as enilconazole. A Foley catheter is implanted in the guttural pouch (**701**). The catheter with a slight bend in the distal 1–2 cm is passed using a wire stiffener down the center of the catheter; alternatively, a Neilson catheter, also with a bent tip, can be used. With an endoscope in the contralateral nostril, the catheter is passed via the ipsilateral nostril with the bend downwards. Once in the pharynx, the catheter is rotated and advanced so the bend is upwards. This usually opens the ostium of the guttural pouch and the catheter is advanced easily and the balloon inflated. The pouch is then irrigated daily with antifungal agents. Some clinicians insufflate antifungal powders (nystatin) into the pouch in order to improve contact of the medication onto the fungal lesion.

Surgical management as a matter of urgency is advised for all hemorrhaging cases. Simple ligation of the internal carotid and occipital arteries has been recommended (**702**), but the collateral circulation in both the internal and external carotid arteries is substantial and proximal and distal vascular occlusion is preferred. Occlusion of the internal carotid proximally (closer to the heart) results in no change in blood pressure and only a 19% reduction in flow in the internal carotid artery in the guttural pouch, while occlusion of the common carotid artery results in an increase in flow.

Currently, two methods of proximal and distal vascular occlusion are favored. The use of embolization coils under fluoroscopic control is a very elegant system, with minimal surgical morbidity. A simpler technique is catheterization of the selected vessels using embolectomy or Foley catheters (**703**). The external carotid artery is harder to occlude distally by catheterization as there are numerous collateral branches. The most important is the palatine artery, which can be exposed in the mouth, caudal to the incisors, immediately adjacent to the maxilla. Simple ligation of the external carotid artery and the palatine artery has been reported to result in unilateral blindness.

Prognosis

The prognosis is excellent if appropriate arterial occlusion is achieved in the absence of neurologic disease. Intra-operative complications are common and warrant a guarded approach initially. The prognosis for the return of neurologic function is guarded. Many horses improve following resolution of the mycosis, but some deficits can remain. This is of particular importance in performance horses that present with recurrent laryngeal neuropathy due to guttural pouch mycosis. The prognosis for improvement in such cases is guarded.

Temporohyoid osteoarthropathy

Definition/overview

This is a rare but apparently increasing condition involving bony proliferation and pain associated with temporohyoid articulation. The disease is highly variable in presentation.

Etiology/pathophysiology

The precise cause of temporohyoid osteoarthropathy is not known. It has been postulated that the condition is a septic arthritis of the temporohyoid joint, following an extension of middle ear disease. However, there is no evidence of underlying middle ear infection in most cases, though some horses do have a history of prior 'strangles' infection. The course of the disease is somewhat unpredictable, but most horses are presented with an acute history. It is suggested that ankylosis of the temporohyoid joint is prevented by the constant movement of the stylohyoid bone via the tongue. This results in continuing inflammation around the joint and hence swelling that can press on nerves adjacent to the joint, particularly the facial and vestibulocochlear nerves. The movement can also result in pathologic fracture of the basisphenoid bone.

Clinical presentation

The clinical presentation is variable and clinical signs can include oral phase dysphagia, head shyness, nondescript pain in the parotid area, difficulty in ridden exercise, altered head carriage (704), and reluctance to flex the neck. A relatively consistent feature has been quite marked pain on squeezing the mandibles together, leading to severe reaction from the horse. The presentation is often acute despite the apparently chronic nature of the disease.

Diagnosis

Endoscopy of the guttural pouch is the most reliable way of establishing a diagnosis. Usually, there is swelling and inflammation associated with the temporohyoid articulation (705). These signs can be difficult to interpret as they are somewhat subjective. Comparison with the contralateral side can be helpful (706). Fracture of the stylohyoid bone can be observed as marked thickening of the bone. Purulent or serous discharge can be noted from the articulation (707). Other diagnostic aids are often used due to the slightly confusing nature of the clinical signs. Diagnosis in the majority of cases is possible using CT, when signs of marked thickening around the temporohyoid joint are usually observed. Radiography may be of benefit when fractures of the stylohyoid bone can be observed and dorsoventral or occasionally oblique views can reveal sclerosis of the petrous temporal bone relative to the contralateral side. Many cases show no radiographic abnormalities. In the majority of cases, scintigraphy reveals an increased uptake of radioisotope in the region of the temporohyoid articulation on dorsal views of the head.

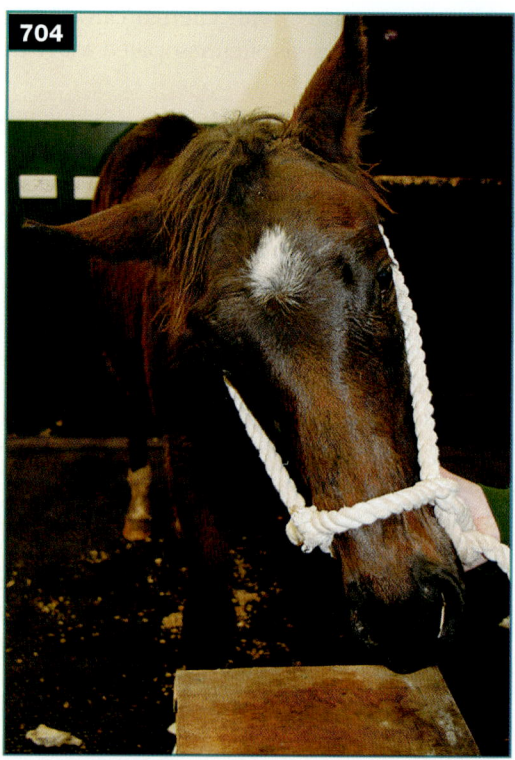

704 Marked head tilt in a yearling. The horse had a history of sudden-onset head tilt and facial neuropathy. Endoscopy revealed marked swelling of the right temporohyoid joint. The head tilt is presumably caused by damage to the vestibulo-cochlear nerve.

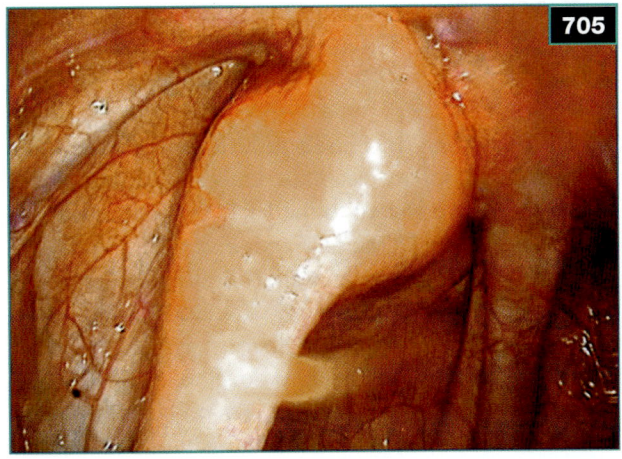

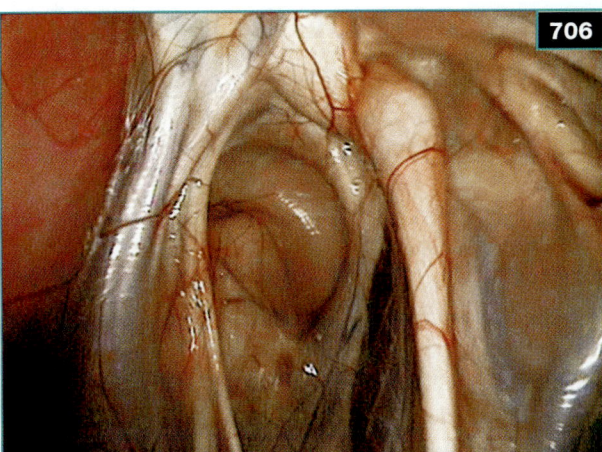

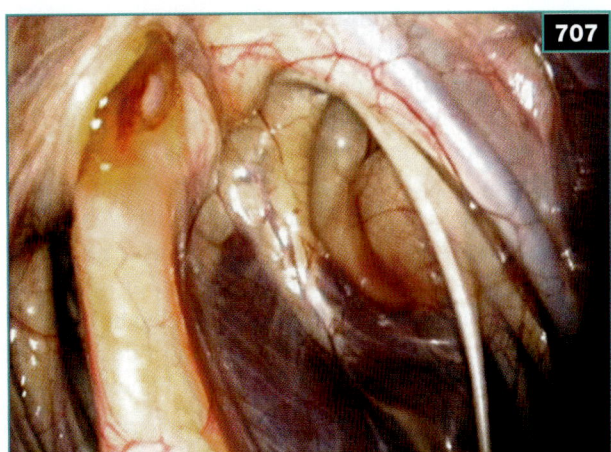

705 Marked thickening and reddening of the mucosa overlying the right temporohyoid joint from the yearling in 704.

706 The contralateral guttural pouch of the horse in 705.

707 Serous discharge from the temporohyoid joint of a horse with dysphagia. This horse responded to a prolonged course of antibiotics and anti-inflammatory agents.

Management

Antibiotic treatment can be sufficient in some cases, but the clinical signs frequently recur. Surgery is recommended in the majority of cases and is designed to reduce the movement, and hence pain, emanating from the temporohyoid articulation. Initially, removal of a section of stylohyoid was used, but now resection of the ceratohyoid is recommended. This is approached by a paramedian incision over the palpable basihyoid bone. The ceratohyoid is dissected out, taking care not to traumatize the hypoglossal nerve (708). The bone is removed in its entirety, leaving cartilage ends behind, hence reducing the prospect of bony reunion.

Prognosis

The prognosis following certaohyoidectomy is good. The majority of horses make a full recovery and are able to resume full exercise. The prognosis is more guarded following stylohyoidotomy as repair of the bone and recurrence of clinical signs can occur.

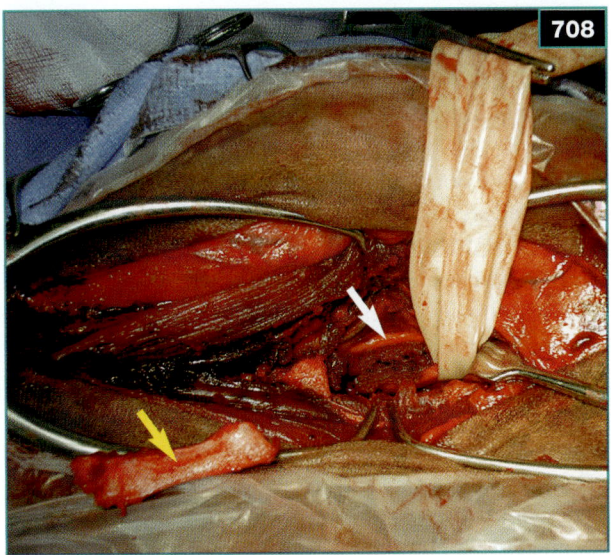

708 Ceratohyoidectomy. The resected ceratohyoid bone (yellow arrow) and the hypoglossal nerve (white arrow) can be seen.

449

Surgical conditions of the upper respiratory tract

Viral diseases

Equine influenza

Definition/overview

Equine influenza is a highly contagious respiratory disease with high morbidity and low mortality caused by Orthomyxoviridae type A influenza viruses. Influenza is usually a self-limiting URT disease, but it may be complicated by secondary bacterial respiratory infections and the virus occasionally causes LRT disease, myocarditis, and postviral fatigue syndromes. Severe or fatal disease is very unusual except in debilitated horses. It affects naïve horses of any age, but disease is typically seen in young horses when first introduced into training yards. Large, economically devastating outbreaks can occur in susceptible groups of horses (e.g. the recent Australian outbreak) or when new viruses with sufficient antigenic differences from vaccine strains enter groups of vaccinated horses. Infection causes pyrexia, depression, nasal discharge, and a persistent harsh, dry cough. Horses usually recover with rest and symptomatic treatment. Vaccination against equine influenza virus is compulsory under the rules of most racing authorities and the Fédération Equestre Internationale.

Etiology/pathophysiology

Equine influenza viruses are type A orthomyxoviruses. They possess two major surface proteins, a neuraminidase (N) and a hemagglutinin (H). Equine influenza viruses possess either H7N7 (formerly known as A/Equine 1 viruses) or H3N8 (formerly known as A/Equine 2). H7N7 viruses have not circulated in the UK for several years and equine influenza currently appears to be caused predominantly by H3N8 viruses worldwide. There are two lineages of H3N8 viruses in circulation, known as European and American lineages. American lineage viruses have been responsible for recent equine influenza outbreaks in the UK and Europe. Influenza viruses undergo 'antigenic drift' whereby amino acid substitutions in antigenic sites of the hemagglutinin molecule create sufficient antigenic differences for vaccine- (or disease-) induced antibodies to fail to neutralize the new virus.

The virus is transmitted from infected horses by aerosol (across distances up to 50 m) or by respiratory droplets, either directly from horse to horse or indirectly via fomites. Virus survival in the environment is short-lived and environmental reservoirs of infection are not important in transmission. After entry into the horse, the virus infects respiratory epithelial cells, causing destruction of ciliated columnar cells, loss of epithelial integrity, exposure of cough receptors, increased mucus production, and decreased mucociliary clearance. Clinically apparent infection is usually restricted to the URT. Limited virus replication does occur in the LRT and, in a small minority of horses (mainly foals or immunocompromised animals), clinically apparent pulmonary disease occurs. Virus-induced impairment of mucociliary clearance can allow secondary bacterial infection to develop, mostly by resident airway microbes (especially *Streptococcus equi* subsp. *zooepidemicus* and members of the genera *Pasteurella*, *Actinobacillus*, and *Haemophilus*). In contrast to the equine herpesviruses, orthomyxovirus replication is restricted to respiratory epithelial cells and the virus does not appear capable of invasion and causing viremia; persistent infections do not occur and latency is not established.

Clinical presentation

There is a sudden onset of signs of acute URT infectious disease, with an incubation period of 1–3 days and duration of less than 3 weeks. The first clinical sign is pyrexia (41.1°C [106°F]) with depression and anorexia. There is serous nasal discharge that becomes mucopurulent, lymphadenopathy (mainly submandibular lymph nodes and occasionally retropharyngeal lymph nodes), and a persistent, dry, harsh, hacking cough. Complications such as secondary bacterial LRT infections (pneumonia and pleuropneumonia), vasculitis, mycocarditis, and chronic postviral fatigue syndromes may be more likely to occur in horses that are exercised and/or kept in unhygienic stable air environments. Clinical disease in vaccinated horses is usually mild and may be difficult to identify. Disease is generally more severe in foals, yearlings, and young adult horses.

Differential diagnosis

All other viral and bacterial causes of infectious URT disease, especially equine herpesviruses, equine viral arteritis (EVA) virus, and *S. equi* subsp. *equi*, should be considered.

Diagnosis

Clinical signs are suggestive, but not diagnostic, of influenza virus infection. Diagnosis requires demonstration of live virus or viral antigens from nasal swab samples or seroconversion to equine influenza virus. Virus isolation is time-consuming, costly, and gives false negatives. Virus antigen detection is more rapid and reliable than virus isolation. This may be performed using an ELISA test for equine influenza virus nucleoprotein or a 'horse side' test using a kit designed to detect human influenza A virus. Serology can be carried out using a hemagglutination inhibition test, but a more sensitive serologic test is single radial hemolysis (SRH). SRH titers provide a measure of protective immunity such that horses with titers >150 mm^2 are generally protected against challenge with homologous virus.

Management

Influenza is usually a self-limiting disease provided clinical cases are properly managed. Affected horses should be rested for 3 weeks and, if stabled, kept in a dust-free environment with good air hygiene. Training and poor air hygiene delay recovery, predispose to secondary infection, and may cause chronic postviral fatigue syndromes. Broad-spectrum antimicrobials are often administered, but are usually unnecessary. NSAIDs may be used to control pyrexia if required. Other treatments may be employed (e.g. clenbuterol [to improve ciliary clearance] and mucolytics), but are not usually required. Strict infection control including suspension of movement on and off infected premises should be employed to prevent spread of infection to adjacent yards. Within the affected yard, barrier precautions should be established to try and prevent spread.

Equine influenza is controlled principally by vaccination. A variety of vaccines are available including inactivated (whole killed virus), subunit, and canary pox recombinant vaccines. These are all delivered by intramuscular injection. In North America, an intranasal modified live virus vaccine is also available. Current recommendations are that vaccines should contain American and European lineages of virus. Vaccination against equine influenza is required by some organizations. The primary vaccination course consists of two injections given 21–92 days apart, with a third dose given 150–215 days later. Annual boosters are given thereafter. Horses may not race until 8 days after any vaccination. Although Jockey Club (UK) rules specify that booster doses be given every 12 months, there is evidence that to provide optimum immunity in young horses in training, an additional 6-month, rather than 12-month, booster after the third vaccination of the primary course may be required before adopting the routine of annual boosters. In the face of a severe epidemic, the third vaccination of the primary course should be given 2–3 months after the second vaccination and subsequent boosters should be given at 6-monthly intervals. Mares may be vaccinated 8–4 weeks before foaling to provide optimum levels of colostral antibody. Foals born to vaccinated mares should not be vaccinated for equine influenza before 4 months of age.

Prognosis
The prognosis for full recovery is good.

Equine herpesvirus infections
Definition/overview
Equine herpesviruses 1 and 4 (EHV-1 and EHV-4) are ubiquitous in horse populations worldwide and have major economic and welfare impacts on all sectors of the horse industry. EHV-1 causes respiratory disease, abortion, paralysis, and ocular disease, while EHV-4 is generally (but not exclusively) associated with respiratory disease only. EHV-1 establishes viremia that disseminates virus to the uterus, CNS, and eye; EHV-4 generally does not cause viremia. Morbidity is high. Mortality is generally low, but may be high in some outbreaks of neurologic disease. Serologically, the prevalence of EHVs in Thoroughbred populations approaches 100%, but estimates of the prevalence of EHV respiratory disease vary from 10–60%. Natural immunity is short-lived. Both viruses establish lifelong latent infections, which reactivate periodically and spread virus to new, susceptible horses. Control is by management precautions and vaccination.

Etiology/pathophysiology
There are nine eqine herpesviruses (EHV-1 to EHV-9); EHVs 1 to 5 are associated principally with horses and EHVs 6 to 8 (also known as asinine herpesviruses 1 to 3) are associated principally with donkeys. The alpha herpesviruses EHV-1 and EHV-4 are respiratory viruses and are regarded as the two most important EHVs that infect horses. EHV-3 causes venereal disease (see pp. 310 and 368). EHV-2 and EHV-5 are gamma herpesviruses with uncertain clinical significance, although EHV-2 has been linked to outbreaks of respiratory disease in young horses and also to keratoconjunctivtis.

EHV-1 has tropism for a range of cells including epithelial, endothelial, lymphoid, and neuronal cells. EHV-4 usually establishes productive infection in epithelial cells only. Following infection of the URT epithelium, EHV-1 infects endothelial and lymphoid cells in the lamina propria and establishes a cell-associated (CD+ T lymphocyte) viremia. During viremia there is a leukopenia, principally a lymphopenia, with a leukocytosis, mainly a lymphocytosis, on recovery. The source of infection is either aerolized virus in respiratory secretions from infected or reactivating horses or uterine fluids from aborted mares. Viremia disseminates virus throughout the body. In the uterine endothelium, CNS, and eye, viral infection of vascular endothelium results in thrombosis and ischemia, causing abortion, paresis/paralysis, and chorioretinal disease. Virus may cross the chorioallantois to reach the fetus, or placental ischemia may be sufficiently extensive for sudden abortion of a virus-negative fetus.

Lifelong latency is established following primary infection in circulating T lymphocytes and also trigeminal ganglion neurons. Latent virus forms a reservoir of virus that, through periodic reactivation from latently infected horses, maintains EHV in the horse population. Reactivation occurs in response to stress (e.g. transport) and can be induced by administration of corticosteroids. Reactivation results in shedding of infectious virus in nasal secretions and, although usually asymptomatic, may result in clinical disease, including abortion and/or neurologic disease, in the reactivating horse.

Clinical presentation

The incubation period following experimental infection with EHV-1 is short (<48 hours), although longer incubation periods of up to 10 days have been suspected in the field. The severity of URT disease varies and is mild or subclinical in horses previously exposed to the virus, but it is more obvious in naïve horses. In naïve horses there is depression and biphasic pyrexia of 10 days' duration. Nasal discharge is initially serous, but becomes mucopurulent. There is some coughing and lymphadenopathy. Viremia persists for up to 20 days and animals usually recover within 21 days of infection. In some horses an ill-defined poor performance syndrome develops. A chronic postviral fatigue syndrome is suspected to develop in some recovered horses, but such disease is poorly defined and difficult to diagnose.

Differential diagnosis

Differential diagnoses for EHV respiratory tract disease include all other causes of infectious URT disease with or without abortion, especially influenza virus and EVA.

Diagnosis

Definitive diagnosis of EHV infection requires laboratory investigations (serology, virus isolation, detection of virus antigen, or DNA) as EHV respiratory disease closely resembles other causes of infectious URT disease. Demonstration of a leukopenia and lymphopenia followed by a leukocytosis and lymphocytosis on recovery is suggestive of a viral infection, but is not diagnostic for EHV infection. Concurrent abortions or neurologic disease should greatly raise the index of suspicion. A rising complement fixation titer (CFT) against EHV-1 or EHV-4 on paired serum samples 10–14 days apart is diagnostic. Elevated virus neutralizing antibody titers are also diagnostic but, because these remain elevated for months after infection, do not necessarily indicate recent infection. Virus antigens can be detected in nasal swab samples by fluorescent antibody or ELISA tests. Virus isolation (demonstration of cytopathic effect on susceptible cell lines) can also be carried out, but this is time-consuming and prone to false-negative results.

Virus DNA can be detected by PCR, which is highly sensitive and specific, but which may also give false-negative results. Confirming the diagnosis in horses that do not shed infectious virus is difficult, but seroconversion provides good evidence of infection; xanthochromia in a CSF sample is suggestive. Latently infected horses can be identified by PCR detection of virus DNA in leukocytes.

Management

Affected horses should be separated from the herd and maintained in strict barrier housing conditions. Horses with uncomplicated URT disease simply require rest and stabling in a clean, dust-free environment. Antibiotics are not generally required, although broad-spectrum antibiotics (e.g. potentiated sulfonamides) are frequently used, unnecessarily, in general practice. Other respiratory medicines (e.g. mucolytics and beta 2 agonists) are also not required. Immunostimulants (e.g. inactivated *Propionibacterium acnes*, mycobacterial cell wall abstracts, or interferon alpha) are used by some practitioners in horses with suspected chronic postviral disease, but such products are not licensed in all countries and are not indicated for acute disease. Very strict hygiene must be maintained around aborted mares because uterine fluids are highly infectious.

Prognosis

The prognosis is good for respiratory disease, although some horses may develop chronic fatigue/poor performance syndromes.

Equine viral arteritis

Definition/overview

EVA causes respiratory disease and abortion and thus shares many clinical features in common with EHV-1 infection. Stallions become carriers, shedding infectious virus in semen, and they are the main reservoir of infection and transmission of virus to susceptible horses. The disease is notifiable in many countries. EVA can be controlled by vaccination.

Etiology/pathophysiology

EVA is caused by a togavirus and has worldwide distribution. The virus is mainly transmitted directly from horse to horse by aerosolized respiratory secretions and also venereally from carrier stallions to mares. Indirect transmission via fomites is also possible. There is initial virus replication in the respiratory tract followed by cell-associated viremia, which disseminates virus to the reproductive tract. Viremia is associated with a leukopenia, principally a lymphopenia, and a leukocytosis, mainly a lymphocytosis, develops on recovery. Virus replication in the walls of small arteries and veins causes vasculitis. In stallions, persistent infection of the accessory sex glands, mainly the ampulla, is established and infectious virus is shed in semen for several years, although semen quality and fertility are not affected. Infection of mares via venereal or respiratory routes at the time of covering causes early embryonic death. Infection of pregnant mares at any time of gestation via the respiratory route causes fetal death. Serologic surveys in the UK have revealed marked breed differences in the incidence of seropositive horses and carrier stallions, presumably reflecting differences in stud management and practice, with Standardbreds having a significantly higher incidence than other breeds.

Clinical presentation
The incubation period seems to be highly variable in the field, possibly up to 21 days. Initial clinical signs are pyrexia, depression, and anorexia. Clinically obvious respiratory disease may develop, but in many mares and stallions disease is mild or subclinical. Respiratory signs, if present, are typical of infectious URT disease and include nasal discharge, lymphadenopathy, and coughing. There may be marked conjunctivitis and lacrimation. In some horses there are clinical signs relating to vasculitis including conjunctival and periorbital edema, scrotal and preputial edema, and edema of the limbs. There are usually no clinical signs relating to early embryonic death. Where abortion occurs, the expelled fetus is generally autolyzed. Carrier stallions are clinically normal and show normal libido and fertility.

Differential diagnosis
All other causes of infectious respiratory disease and abortion, especially EHV-1 infections, should be considered.

Diagnosis
The clinical features of EVA disease are not pathognomonic, although an outbreak of respiratory disease associated with marked conjunctivitis, edema, and infertility or abortion is highly suggestive. Leukopenia with lymphopenia followed by leukocytosis with lymphocytosis on recovery is suggestive of a viral infection, but is not diagnostic of EVA infection. Confirmation of diagnosis requires demonstration of virus, virus antigens, or virus nucleic acids in nasal swab or semen samples. A rising virus neutralizing antibody titer on paired serum samples taken 10–14 days apart is diagnostic.

Management
The disease is notifiable in many countries and suspected or confirmed cases must be reported. Clinical cases should be isolated and maintained with strict barrier conditions. Affected horses require little veterinary attention, as clinical disease is often mild and self-limiting or subclinical.

NSAIDs can be used to control pyrexia and improve welfare. Antibiotics are usually not required and other respiratory medicines (e.g. mucolytics) are not indicated. Prevention and control of EVA in many countries is based on testing and exclusion or restriction of movement of affected horses. For example, in the UK, horses imported from a country where EVA is known or suspected to occur are isolated on arrival for 21 days. Blood samples taken on arrival and 14 days later are tested for antibodies. Mares and stallions are tested for antibodies before breeding. The disease can be controlled by vaccination but, because of the notifiable status, the vaccine can only be used under the supervision of regulatory agencies in many countries. Veterinary certification of vaccination is usually required (to distinguish vaccinated horses from infected and convalescent horses) and it is therefore important that the horse is confirmed seronegative before vaccination.

Prognosis
The prognosis is good for recovery from clinical disease, but EVA causes major economic loss because of breeding failure through early embryonic death and abortion.

Other viral infections
Adenovirus infections are common, based on serology, but cause subclinical disease only. Clinical disease caused by an adenovirus has only been seen in immuno-compromised animals, specifically Arabian foals with severe combined immunodeficiency (SCID). The clinical significance of adenovirus infections in young horses in training is uncertain and there are no data to suggest that infection impacts on training, causes poor performance, or predisposes to other, more serious, respiratory disease.

African horse sickness (AHS) is endemic in southern Africa and causes high morbidity and mortality in susceptible horses. It is a notifiable disease in many countries. AHS is caused by an orbivirus related to bluetongue virus of sheep. The virus requires an insect vector, *Culicoides imicola*, for transmission. The geographical distribution of the vector extends into southern Europe and it is possible that climate change may eventually extend its range further. The severity of clinical signs varies considerably. In the peracute disease form there is sudden death due to pulmonary edema. In the acute disease form there is death from pulmonary edema and myocardial failure. In the subacute disease form there is myocarditis with accompanying signs of heart failure and death in around 50% of cases. The least severe form of the disease ('horse sickness fever') occurs in horses with some immunity to the virus or in resistant species (zebras and donkeys). In this form there is transient URT disease and low mortality. Vaccination can be used to control the disease.

Hendra virus is a zoonotic morbillivirus that has a fruit bat reservoir and can cause fatal pneumonia and encephalitis in horses and humans. The virus was first described in Hendra, Australia, in 1995. Transmission appears to require very close contact with bat uterine secretions or infected horses. In the limited number of equine outbreaks there have been high morbidity and mortality. The disease resembles AHS because of rapid death with acute pulmonary edema. Fatal infections of Australian equine veterinarians have occurred.

Bacterial disease

Strangles

Definition/overview

Strangles is a highly contagious bacterial infection of the URT characterized, in its most severe form ('classical strangles'), by abscessation of the lymph nodes draining the URT and a variety of other, potentially fatal, sequelae including disseminated abscessation and purpura hemorrhagica. An alternative manifestation is a mild, transient URT disease without abscesses referred to as 'atypical strangles'. Strangles affects naïve horses and ponies of all ages and types, although younger animals kept in large open populations are generally most likely to become affected. Some horses develop chronic infections of the guttural pouch and act as carriers, reservoirs of infection, and a source of contagion to other horses.

Etiology/pathophysiology

Strangles is caused by the Lancefield Group C *Streptococcus equi* subsp. *equi*. It is closely related to the other common equine Group C *Streptococcus*, *Streptococcus equi* subsp. *zooepidemicus*, but can be differentiated by sugar fermentation tests and PCR. *S. equi* possesses a variety of virulence determinants, of which the surface M protein (the major immunogenic and antiopsonic protein) and its antiphagocytic hyaluronic acid capsule are best characterized. Most pathogenic isolates are capsulated and possess full-length M proteins; isolates with less capsule or truncated M proteins are less pathogenic, possibly because of reduced resistance to phagocytosis.

Infection is acquired by direct horse-to-horse transmission of infected respiratory-tract secretions or indirectly via infected droplets on water troughs and buckets, feeding utensils, hands, veterinary equipment, and tack. In contrast to the respiratory viruses, aerosol transmission does not appear to be important. Bacterial survival in the environment is short-lived (<1 week if cultures are dessicated or exposed to UV light). Bacteria can survive for a few weeks (possibly up to 2 months) in water troughs or in droplets of water or pus on wood and tack. Bacteria colonize the nasopharynx (and other regions of the URT including the paranasal sinuses and guttural pouches), producing typical clinical signs of URT infectious disease. Bacteria may cross the respiratory epithelium and reach drainage lymph nodes (mainly the submandibular and retropharyngeal lymph nodes) where they persist, despite efficient neutrophil recruitment to the site, and cause abscesses. Occasionally, parotid lymph-node abscesses develop. Retropharyngeal lymph-node abscesses may become very large and compress the airway, causing dyspnea (hence the term 'strangles') before rupturing either externally or internally into the guttural pouch, causing guttural-pouch empyema.

Chondroids (balls of inspissated pus that contain viable bacteria) may develop in chronic cases of guttural-pouch empyema. Persistent (months to years) guttural-pouch infection may develop in a small proportion (<10%) of recovered horses. These animals are often asymptomatically infected and shed bacteria intermittently in respiratory-tract secretions.

In most cases, bacteria do not disseminate beyond the head, but in a small proportion of horses bacteria disseminate widely via the blood and lymph circulations, causing metastatic abscessation ('bastard strangles') in the abdomen (abdominal viscera and peritoneum), thorax (lungs, pleura, and mediastinum), CNS, eye, skeletal and cardiac muscle, and tendon and joint sheaths. *S. equi* antigens in the circulation can trigger purpura hemorrhagica, an immune-mediated vasculitis causing petechial hemorrhages, subcutaneous and visceral edema, and sometimes skin sloughs of the extremities. The milder form of the disease, known as atypical strangles, causes transient URT disease with lymphadenopathy, but no abscessation or other complications. It is not clear why there are two forms of the disease, but bacterial strain differences, horse genetic differences, and previous immune exposure of the horse are probably all factors. Bacteria isolated from atypical cases retain their virulence and are capable of causing more severe disease in other horses.

Clinical presentation

Severe 'classical' disease

The incubation period is variable (1–14 days), even following experimental challenge. Pyrexia (up to 42°C [107.6°F]) is the earliest clinical sign and persists for up to 2 weeks. Affected horses are depressed and anorexic for 1–2 weeks. Nasal discharge (709) becomes increasingly purulent and persists for 2–3 weeks. Lymph-node enlargement is palpable from 2–3 days after infection, but abscesses usually develop 2–3 weeks later (710). Large, unruptured retropharyngeal abscesses can cause moderate to marked airway compression, with ventral deviation of the trachea and occlusion of the nasopharynx (711),

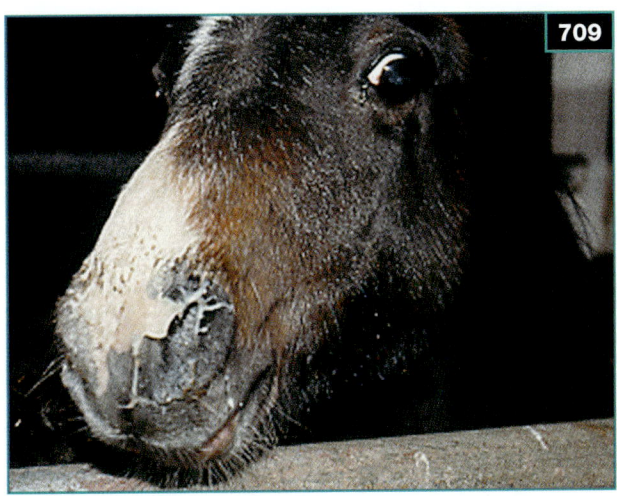

709 *S. equi* infection ('strangles') causes a moderate to profuse bilateral mucopurulent nasal discharge.

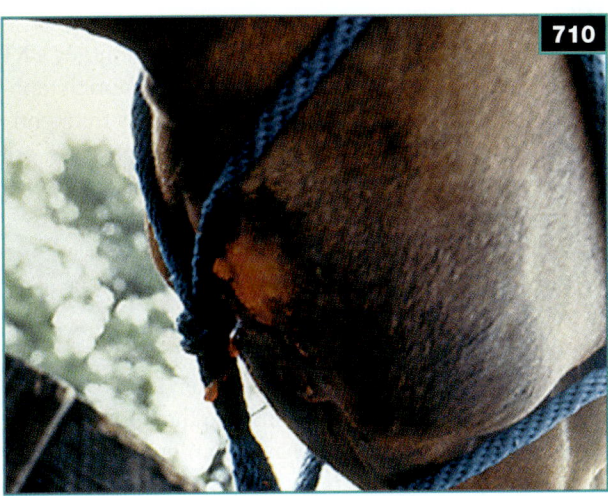

710 This horse with *S. equi* infection has a draining submandibular lymph-node abscess. Abscesses can also develop in the parotid and retropharyngeal lymph nodes. (Photo courtesy DP Lunn)

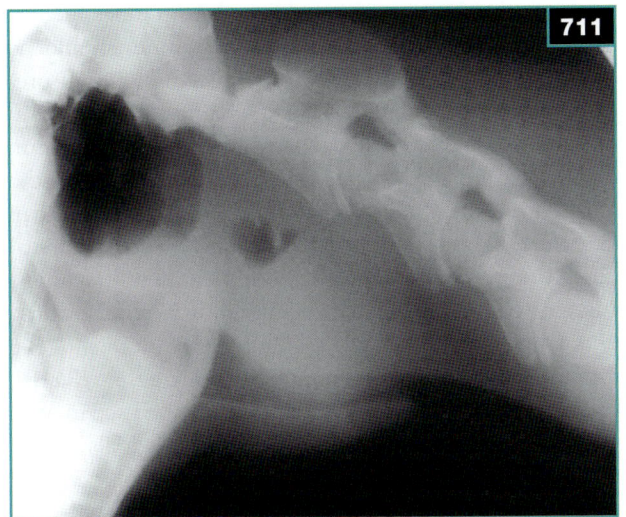

711 *S. equi* infection. Nonruptured retropharyngeal lymph nodes can be become large enough to compress the naso-pharynx and trachea, causing dyspnea. This radiograph shows ventral deviation of the trachea caused by a large nonruptured retropharyngeal lymph-node abscess. (Photo courtesy DP Lunn)

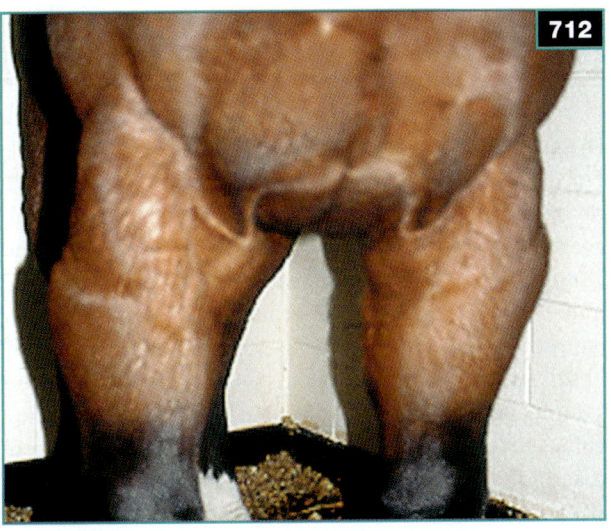

712 Purpura hemorrhagica can be characterized by large plaques of proximal limb and ventral trunk edema. (Photo courtesy DP Lunn)

resulting in inspiratory dyspnea and possibly stertorous inspiratory noise. Guttural-pouch empyema causes inter-mittent, mostly unilateral purulent nasal discharge. There is usually no obvious guttural-pouch swelling externally. The pouch may be painful on percussion or palpation. Metastatic abscessation presents with clinical signs relating to the region where abscesses develop, with more general-ized signs including weight loss, intermittent pyrexia, and anorexia. Purpura hemorrhagica cases show widespread subcutaneous edema (712) with petechial hemorrhages, possibly skin sloughs, and clinical signs relating to visceral injury.

455

Mild 'atypical' disease

This form is transient and self-limiting. It resembles URT viral infectious disease, with pyrexia, depression, lymph-node enlargement, and nasal discharge, and is frequently not recognized as *S. equi* infection if samples are not collected for microbiology. The more serious sequelae associated with 'classical' disease (lymph-node abscesses, guttural-pouch empyema, metastatic abscessation, and purpura hemorrhagica) do not develop.

Carriers

Clinical signs for carriers are variable. In most cases, guttural-pouch carriage is subclinical, although sometimes there is intermittent nasal discharge. Carrier horses usually have some guttural-pouch pathology, although this may be subtle, and obvious empyema is less common. If the paranasal sinuses are the sites of carriage, there may be clinical signs of sinus disease.

Differential diagnosis

Other causes of URT infectious disease including equine influenza virus, EHV-1 and -4, equine rhinovirus, and EVA virus. Abscesses may be caused by other bacteria, particularly *S. equi* subsp. *zooepidemicus.*

Diagnosis

For classical disease, history and clinical findings of an outbreak of URT infectious disease with abscesses are characteristic of *S. equi* infections. However, history and clinical examination findings are not diagnostic for the milder ('atypical') disease because this resembles other types of URT infectious disease. Microbiological culture of nasal swabs (nasopharyngeal swabs provide a better sample, but nasal swabs are usually adequate in acute clinical cases) or pus aspirates confirms *S. equi* infection. A serological test has been recently introduced in the UK with over 90% sensitivity and specificity of exposure to the antigen. It takes 2 weeks for a positive result to occur. The test will also identify carrier animals. Endoscopy confirms guttural-pouch abnormalities and is useful for visualizing retropharyngeal lymph-node abscesses bulging under the floor of the medial compartment of the pouch. Ultrasonography can be used to investigate retropharyngeal abscesses. Radiography is an alternative means of assessing the retropharyngeal region and the guttural pouches and can be useful for identifying pus in the paranasal sinuses. Identifying carriers is not cheap or easy and requires detection of live bacteria or bacterial DNA. A series (at least three) of nasopharyngeal swabs (nasal swabs are not suitable) or nasopharyngeal washes at weekly intervals submitted for culture and PCR (to detect bacterial DNA) is required to identify carriers, because shedding can be intermittent. Alternatively, a single guttural-pouch lavage submitted for culture and PCR provides adequate sensitivity.

Management

The three aims of managing an outbreak of strangles are to prevent spread of infection to new premises, to limit the spread of infection within the infected premises, and to ensure that carriers are identified and treated at the end of the outbreak. Movement of horses on and off the infected premises should be suspended in order to reduce the risk of infection spreading elsewhere. Personnel should be briefed about the risk of indirect transmission and precautions taken with hand washing, clothing, footwear, and tack. Management of clinical cases requires strict isolation and barrier nursing. On suspicion of *S. equi* infection, the yard should be divided into dirty (affected) and clean (unaffected) areas and horses assigned based on clinical signs (initially pyrexia). Antibiotic treatment of clinical cases is controversial, with some clinicians advocating antibiotics should never be used for fear of prolonging the clinical disease, reducing immunity, or increasing the risk of metastatic abscessation. Antibiotics may be used in early cases with pyrexia and depression, especially foals, and to improve welfare and reduce the period of bacterial shedding. In-contact horses can also be treated with antibiotics provided they can be moved to a clean area and are not subsequently exposed, because early treatment will prevent them from mounting a protective immune response. Antibiotics should not be used in horses with developing abscesses; these should be managed by hot fomentation and encouraged to burst. Large retropharyngeal abscesses may need needle drainage under ultrasound guidance. At least 1 month after the end of the outbreak the yard should be screened for carriers. Carriers can be successfully treated by guttural-pouch lavage and antibiotic treatment. Chondroids should be removed endoscopically or surgically if they cannot be retrieved via the nasopharyngeal ostium. The affected pouch should be lavaged daily with approximately two liters of saline via an indwelling Foley catheter. Benzyl penicillin should be instilled into the pouch after each lavage. Lavaging should continue until the pouch is negative on culture. Infusion of antimicrobial gel into the pouch can be effective at elimination of guttural-pouch colonization in *S. equi* carriers (*Table 14*).

Prevention relies on management measures. New arrivals should be kept quarantined until confirmed free from *S. equi* infection by three nasopharyngeal swabs collected at weekly intervals. New cases should be isolated, investigated, and treated promptly. Yards with endemic infection should screen all horses to identify carriers by nasopharyngeal swabs (not nasal swabs) and/or guttural-pouch lavage. A live attenuated intramucosal vaccine has been available in Europe since January 2005, but was withdrawn for technical reasons in 2007. However, it has recently been relaunched. In the USA and Australia, bacterin, M protein, and live attenuated intranasal vaccines are available.

The Horserace Betting Levy Board in the UK has established guidelines on strangles (http://www.hblb.org.uk and follow the links).

Prognosis

The prognosis is variable. For mild disease ('atypical strangles') the prognosis is good. For the more severe disease ('classical strangles') the prognosis depends on whether complications develop. The majority of horses recover once abscesses have resolved, but up to 10% of cases develop complications, which delay recovery or may be fatal.

TABLE 14 Recipe to make 50 ml penicillin gel for guttural-pouch infusion

- Add 2 g of gelatin to 40 ml sterile water.
- Heat or microwave to dissolve the gelatin.
- Cool gelatin to 45–50°C.
- Add 10 ml sterile water to 10,000,000 units sodium penicillin G.
- Combine penicillin solution and cooled gelatin.
- Dispense into syringes and leave overnight at 4°C to set.

From: Verheyen K, Newton JR, Talbot NC *et al*. (2000) Elimination of guttural pouch infection and inflammation in asymptomatic carriers of *Streptococcus equi*. *Equine Vet J* **32**:527–532.

Infectious conditions

Rhodococcus equi pneumonia

Definition/overview

Rhodococcus equi is a primary respiratory pathogen and causes pulmonary disease (suppurative bronchopneumonia and lung abscesses) in foals between one and 6 months old (713, 714). *R. equi* also causes extrapulmonary abscesses, mainly in the abdomen and in bones of affected foals. *R. equi* bronchopneumonia or pleuropneumonia in older foals and adults is rare. The reservoir of infection is the environment, mainly soil, although recently it has been demonstrated that high bacterial numbers are also exhaled in the breath from infected foals, suggesting a direct contagious aspect to this disease. Most foals with milder pulmonary disease recover and progress to useful athletic careers. The prognosis for abdominal and bone abscesses is guarded. There is currently no *R. equi* vaccine.

Etiology/pathophysiology

R. equi is a Gram-positive pleomorphic rod-shaped bacterium. It is a soil-living, environmental organism, which colonizes and cycles through the equine intestinal tract. In the environment, *R. equi* replicates efficiently in hot, dry, dusty conditions and prefers light or sandy soils.

Disease thus occurs in certain geographic locations only. Following ingestion, the organism replicates in the intestinal tract and, especially in foals, large numbers of bacteria are shed in feces. Densely stocked mare and foal paddocks can thus develop an enormous build-up of bacteria. Pulmonary infection occurs from inhalation of bacteria-laden dust. Intestinal tract and abdominal infection occurs either following ingestion of a sufficient infectious dose from soil or secondary to pulmonary disease due to swallowing of bacteria-laden pus. Abscesses can develop at other sites by hematogenous dissemination from the lung or gut. Abscesses develop because *R. equi* establishes intracellular infection and persists within macrophages. The ability to survive within macrophages is conferred by a plasmid encoding a group of 'virulence-associated proteins' (Vap proteins) that act to prevent phagosome–lysosome fusion and hence prevent respiratory-burst killing of infected cells. Virulent strains are all Vap-positive. In the lung, *R. equi* causes suppurative bronchopneumonia, lung abscesses, and mediastinal and tracheobronchial lymph-node abscessation. Lung abscesses may be discrete or diffuse, 'miliary' abscesses. In the abdomen, abscesses develop mainly in the wall of the jejunum, cecum, and colon, and in mesenteric lymph nodes, but they may occur in any of the abdominal viscera. In the skeleton, *R. equi* causes osteomyelitis in long bones and vertebrae.

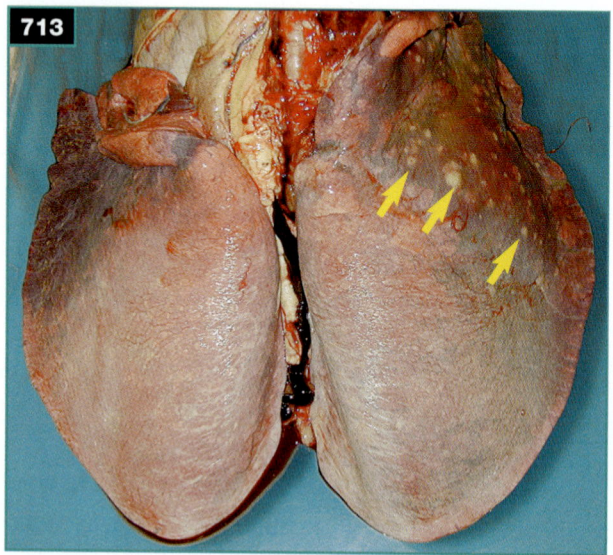

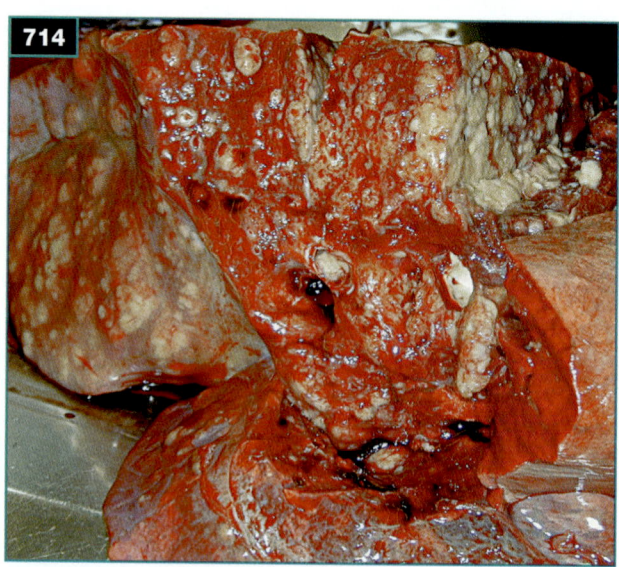

713 Dorsoventral view of the lungs of a foal with *R. equi* infection as seen at necropsy. Multifocal abscesses (arrows) are visible in the lung parenchyma.

714 Cut surface of the lung of the foal in 713 at necropsy, showing multifocal abscesses containing purulent material.

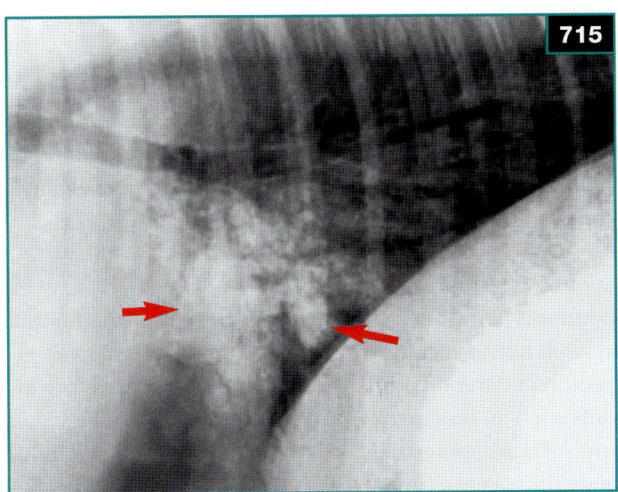

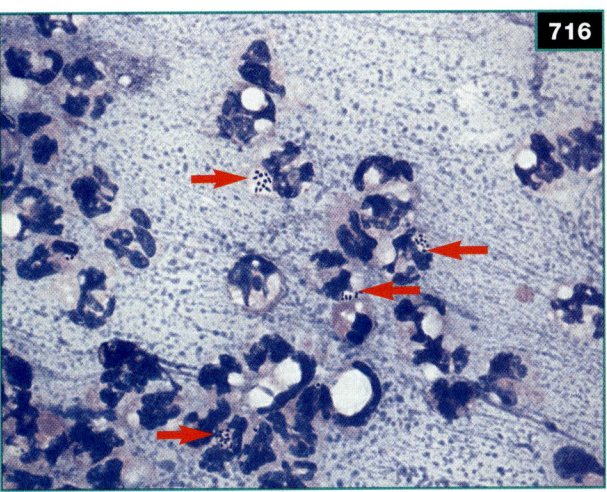

715 Thoracic radiograph of a foal with *R. equi* infection. Multifocal abscesses (arrows) are visible as opacities within the lung field. (Photo courtesy J Prescott)

716 Cytology of tracheal aspirate fluid from a foal with *R. equi* infection. Variably preserved neutrophils are the predominant cell type. Intracellular rod-shaped bacteria are visible (arrows). (Photo courtesy D Bienzle)

Clinical presentation

Clinical signs occur in foals between 1 and 6 months old. Disease in younger and older foals or adults is rare. Clinical signs are usually insidious in onset and slowly progressive, although some foals present with acute-onset pulmonary disease. Microbiological surveys of foals suggest respiratory infection is acquired within the first 2 weeks of life, with clinical signs appearing several weeks later. Careful clinical monitoring, including changes in total leukocyte numbers, detects infected foals earlier in disease progression than reliance on clinical signs alone. Clinical signs include pyrexia, depression, anorexia, coughing, and nasal discharge. Depending on the extent of pulmonary disease, there may be wheezing and crackling on auscultation. Pulmonary consolidation may be detectable by auscultation and percussion if extensive. Abdominal abscesses cause pyrexia, depression, diarrhea, colic, and weight loss. Immune-mediated synovitis, seen predominantly in the tibiotarsal and stifle joints, may present as marked joint effusion, with minimal lameness other than a stiff gait. In contrast, osteomyelitis is extremely painful and causes severe lameness. Affected bones may fracture. Vertebral abscesses may progress to cause neurologic signs.

Differential diagnosis

Other causes of juvenile pneumonia should be considered including other bacterial bronchopneumonias (*Streptococcus zooepidemicus*, *S. pneumoniae*, *Actinobacillus* spp., *Pasteurella* spp., *Klebsiella* spp., and *Bordetella bronchiseptica*), parasitic bronchopneumonia, *Pneumocystis jiroveci* (formerly *P. carinii*) infection, and acute bronchointerstitial pneumonia.

Diagnosis

R. equi is the most common cause of pneumonia in foals between 1 and 6 months old. Affected foals develop leukocytosis and neutrophilia and an increase in plasma fibrinogen. Ultrasonography and radiography can provide an early diagnosis of pulmonary abscesses (**715**). Definitive diagnosis is by demonstration of *R. equi* by cytology (**716**) and bacterial culture of tracheal aspirate samples. PCR assays based on the Vap genes provide increased sensitivity over culture, but may yield positive results in foals without clinical disease. Similarly, serology and fecal culture are unreliable because seroconversion and GI tract colonization in the absence of disease are common.

Management

The intracellular persistence of *R. equi* makes antimicrobial treatment difficult. The standard treatment is long-term (1–2 months) oral combination therapy with erythromycin (estolate 25 mg/kg p/o q6h, phosphate 37.5 mg/kg p/o q12h) and rifampin (5–10 mg/kg p/o q12–24h). These antimicrobials are concentrated in macrophages and thus target the site of bacterial persistence. Treatment is expensive and adverse reactions, including fatal clostridial diarrhea or hyperthermia, may occur. A newer alternative to erythromycin is azithromycin, which allows reduced-frequency dosing (10 mg/kg p/o q24h for 5 days, then q48h) and possibly reduced side-effects. Clarithromycin (7.5 mg/kg p/o q12h), in combination with rifampin, is also widely used. Foals with severe pulmonary signs may require hospitalization, oxygen therapy, inhalation and systemic therapy with bronchodilators, and fluid therapy.

The incidence of *R. equi* infection can be reduced by maintaining young foals (<4 weeks old) on clean grass paddocks and avoiding dusty, overcrowded dirt paddocks with little grass. This reduces the environmental burden and hence the risk of infection of the foal in its first weeks of life. Close surveillance of foals for signs of respiratory disease, including regular hematology screens to identify foals with raised total WBCs, neutrophilia, and raised fibrinogen, allows early separation and treatment of affected foals. In an effort to limit propagation of disease at the farm level, affected foals should be removed from pasture, since they shed high numbers of bacteria in feces. In high-risk facilities, hyperimmune equine plasma can be administered to newborn foals at birth and again at 3–4 weeks of age to reduce the risk of respiratory infection early in life.

Prognosis

The prognosis is poor for foals with severe pulmonary disease, even if treated aggressively. For foals with less severe disease the prognosis is moderate to good. Foals that recover do progress into training and have an effective athletic life. Racing performance in Thoroughbreds does not seem to be affected. The prognosis for foals with extrapulmonary abscesses is generally poor.

Bacterial pneumonia

Definition/overview

Bacterial pneumonia is characterized by inflammation of the lungs that occurs as a result of bacterial colonization of the pulmonary parenchyma. Most cases are secondary to viral respiratory infection, although primary bacterial infections can occur.

Etiology/pathophysiology

Common pathogens isolated from bacterial pneumonia in adult horses include *Streptococcus zooepidemicus*, beta-hemolytic *Streptococcus* spp., and Gram-negative organisms such as *Pasteurella* spp., *Escherichia coli*, *Klebsiella* spp., *Enterobacter* spp., and *Pseudomonas* spp. Gram-negative bacteria can be the sole cause of pneumonia, but they are more commonly isolated in combination with streptococcal pneumonias. *Streptococcus equi* and *Streptococcus pneumoniae* are less common causes of pneumonia. Anaerobic bacteria such as *Bacteroides* spp. and *Clostridium* spp. are mainly found in complicated cases with pleuropneumonia.

Bacterial pneumonia in neonatal foals is usually caused by *Streptococcus* spp., *E. coli*, or *Actinobacillus* spp. In older foals, *Rhodococcus equi* is more common, especially in foals from endemic farms or areas.

The immune defense mechanisms of the upper airways prevent most bacteria from reaching the lungs under normal conditions. In addition, any bacteria penetrating the respiratory system to the level of the lungs are rapidly destroyed and removed by cellular and humoral defenses of the LRT. However, commensal bacteria of the URT may invade the lungs if respiratory immune defenses are damaged or otherwise impaired by viral respiratory infection or stressors such as prolonged transport of an animal.

In response to infection of the lungs, inflammatory cells, especially neutrophils, are recruited to combat infection, but they may also contribute to tissue destruction and loss of organ function. Accumulation of cellular debris, serum exudate, and fibrin within the airways further impairs gas exchange.

Clinical presentation

Common clinical signs include fever, depression, tachypnea, nasal discharge, coughing, and exercise intolerance. Fever can be intermittent.

Differential diagnosis

Viral, fungal, and parasitic pneumonias should be considered. Allergic airway disease (e.g. inflammatory airway disease [IAD], heaves) and primary or secondary pulmonary neoplasia such as lymphosarcoma may also cause similar clinical signs.

Diagnosis

A diagnosis of bacterial pneumonia is made on the basis of history, physical examination, and laboratory and radiographic findings. On auscultation, lung sounds may be harsh with increased bronchial tones, crackles and/or wheezes, or even friction rubs in complicated cases involving the pleura. Thoracic percussion may reveal areas of lung consolidation or abscessation, or fluid accumulation within the pleural cavity (pleuropneumonia).

The WBC count is usually elevated, characterized by a mature neutrophilia with or without band cells. Hyperfibrinogenemia is common, and increased total plasma proteins may be seen in chronic cases as a result of hyperglobulinemia.

Thoracic radiographs are usually confirmatory and are particularly helpful for assessing treatment response and as a prognostic indicator. Thoracic ultrasonography may show areas of consolidated or atelectatic lung, and/or parenchymal abscess(es) depending on their location in the affected lung.

Tracheobronchial aspirates should be obtained and samples submitted for bacterial culture, Gram staining, and cytology examination. Samples could be collected using a bronchoscope (if there are no signs of respiratory distress) or via transtracheal aspiration.

Management

Ideally, therapy should be based on culture and susceptibility results of samples collected from the lower airways. Streptococcal pneumonias respond well to therapy with penicillin, but because mixed bacterial infections are common, broad-spectrum antimicrobials are more desirable. Penicillin/aminoglycoside combinations are commonly used initially. Other antibiotics that offer a moderately broad spectrum of activity against Gram-negative and Gram-positive organisms include second- and third-generation cephalosporins, ampicillin, and/or trimethoprim-sulfa. Additional therapy with metronidazole is often used if an anaerobic infection is suspected.

NSAIDs are indicated to control inflammation and pain. Other treatments of bacterial pneumonia may include moderate intravenous fluid administration to hydrate respiratory secretions in order to facilitate clearance from the respiratory tract. Prolonged rest from strenuous exercise is critical. Treatment failure or relapse may occur if the duration of medical treatment and adequate rest are not enforced.

Prognosis

The prognosis is good if uncomplicated cases are managed promptly with adequate antimicrobial therapy and rest. The prognosis may dramatically change if complications such as pulmonary abscessation and/or extension of the infection into the pleural space occur.

Bacterial pleuritis/pleuropneumonia

Definition/overview

Bacterial colonization of the pulmonary parenchyma can result in pneumonia and/or pulmonary abscess formation. Extension of the infection and inflammatory process to the pleural space results in pleuritis or pleuropneumonia.

Etiology/pathophysiology

The most common organisms associated with pneumonia include *Streptococcus zooepidemicus* or other beta-hemolytic *Streptococcus* spp., which can be complicated with infection by Gram-negative bacteria such as *Pasteurella* spp., *Escherichia coli*, *Enterobacter* spp., *Klebsiella* spp., and *Pseudomonas* spp. Anaerobes such as *Bacteroides* spp. and *Clostridium* spp. may also be involved, but are less common. *Mycoplasma felis* has been identified as an additional cause of pleuritis in horses.

Pleuropneumonia may occur spontaneously, but some common risk factors include recent transportation, viral infection, esophageal obstruction (choke), or general anesthesia.

Bacterial pleuropneumonia results from exudative fluid accumulation in the pleural cavity in response to inflammation and infection. As large amounts of fluid containing bacteria, neutrophils, fibrin, and cellular debris accumulate in the thoracic cavity, layers of fibrin develop over the visceral and parietal pleura. Adherence of visceral and parietal pleura by fibrin leads to loculation of fluid, as well as the development of an inelastic fibrin membrane over the pleural surfaces that may limit lung expansion within the thoracic cavity during respiration.

Clinical presentation

In the acute stage of disease, signs may include fever, depression, increased respiratory rate with a shallow pattern, exercise intolerance, nasal discharge, and intermittent coughing. Other signs may include rapid weight loss, sternal and/or limb edema, and gait stiffness, and horses may stand with abducted elbows due to pleural pain that can be elicited by palpation of the thoracic wall. Signs may be mistaken as colic. In chronic pleuropneumonia, signs may be limited to intermittent fever, weight loss, and exercise intolerance.

Differential diagnoses

Other infectious pneumonias, including viral, fungal, parasitic, or even RAO, should be considered. Primary lung neoplasia is uncommon, but thoracic lymphoma or metastatic tumors such as SCC may be considered as differential diagnoses for the presence of pleural fluid.

Medical conditions of the lower respiratory tract

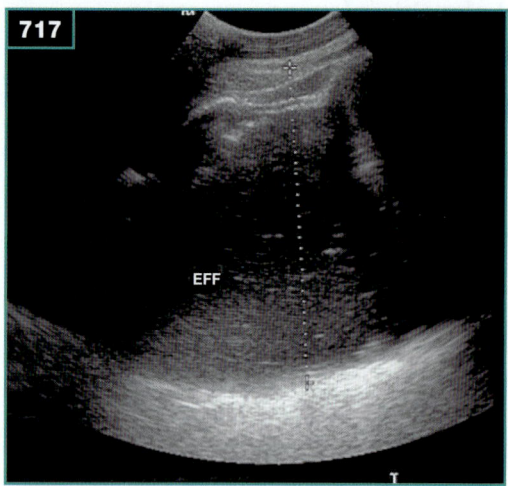

717 Transthoracic ultrasonography of a horse with pleuropneumonia reveals the presence of pleural effusion (labeled EFF) between the parietal and visceral pleura in the left hemithorax. A similar effusion was detected in the right hemithorax.

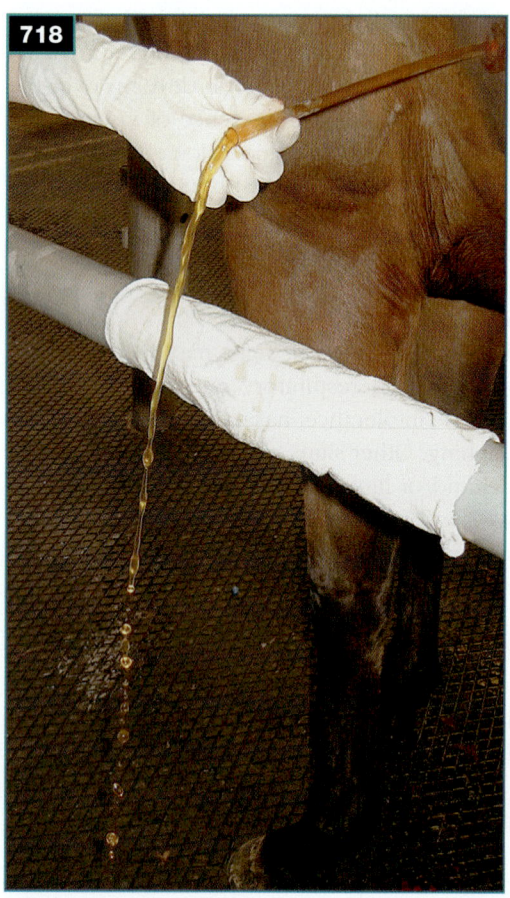

718 Aseptic placement of a chest drain to remove pleural effusion from the left hemithorax.

Diagnosis

History, clinical signs, and physical examination are usually suggestive. Careful auscultation of the thorax may detect even subtle abnormalities in early disease, including crackles or wheezes, decreased lung sounds in the ventral lung field, mucus movement within the trachea, and/or pleural friction rubs. Bilateral chest percussion is essential and helps to determine both the presence and amount of pleural fluid within each hemithorax. A pain response may be elicited during percussion in acute cases.

An inflammatory leukogram (neutrophilia, may include band neutrophils) is common. Hyperfibrinogenemia is also common.

Thoracic ultrasonography is the preferred diagnostic tool for characterization of pleural fluid (**717**). Consolidated or atelectatic lung may also be visible depending on its location. The entire field of both lungs should be assessed to detect any abscesses, loculation of fibrinous fluid, or adhesions; to provide important information regarding prognosis; and to monitor response to treatment over time.

Thoracocentesis is indicated to further characterize the pneumonia, to isolate organism(s) involved, and as a therapeutic measure (**718**). Cytologic examination of pleural fluid should be performed, as well as Gram staining for bacterial organisms. Increased cellularity of pleural fluid ($>10–20 \times 10^9$ cells/l), composed predominantly of neutrophils, is consistent with pleuropneumonia. Extra- and intracellular bacteria may be visible. All fluids should be cultured both aerobically and anaerobically for organism identification and antimicrobial sensitivity testing, although the presence of anaerobes may be difficult to prove due to difficulties culturing these organisms. *Myco-plasma* culture is also useful.

Thoracic radiography may be used to assess roughly the extent of pulmonary involvement in horses with pleuropneumonia (**719**), but it should be performed after thoracic drainage has been accomplished in order to optimize visualization of the lung parenchyma.

Bronchoscopy may be performed in horses that are not showing signs of significant respiratory distress in order to obtain samples of airway exudates from the distal trachea and mainstem bronchi for cytology and culture (**720**).

Management

Broad-spectrum antimicrobial therapy is required. Antimicrobials commonly used are penicillin combined with an aminoglycoside; ceftiofur; or trimethoprim-sufamethoxazole. Metronidazole is sometimes used to provide added efficacy against anaerobes. Bacterial culture and antimicrobial sensitivity testing should be carried out to verify drug selection. In many cases, prolonged antimicrobial treatment is required, necessitating transition to an oral antimicrobial after the initial period of treatment.

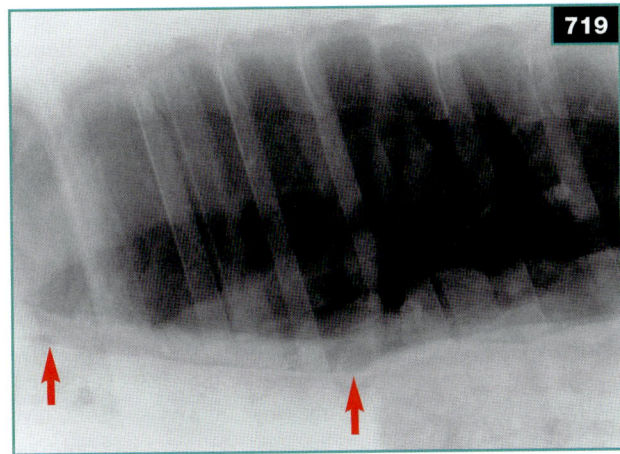

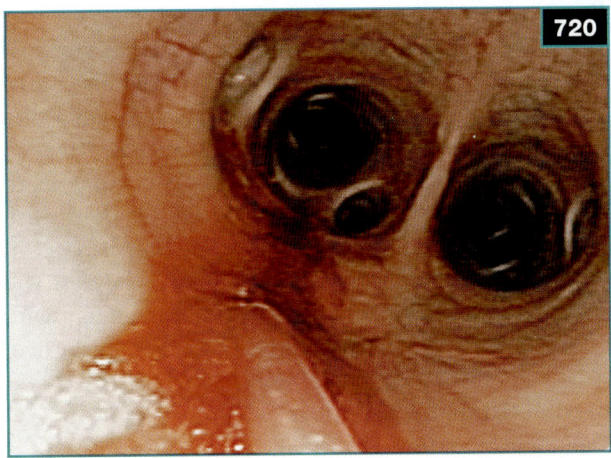

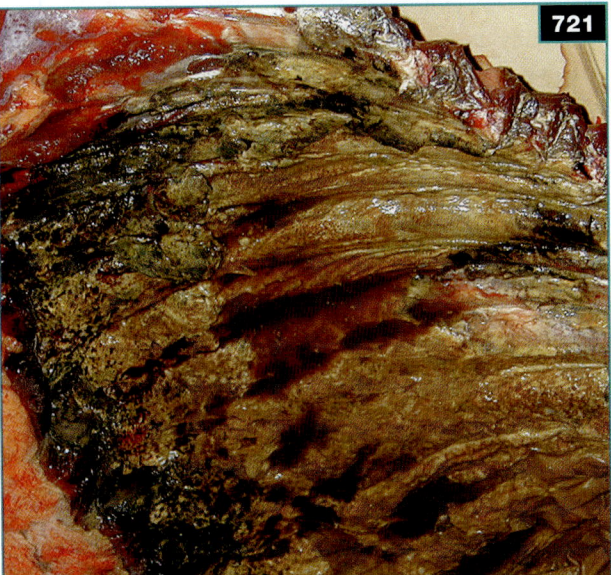

719 Lateral chest radiograph of the horse in 718 prior to thoracic drainage. A fluid line is visible (arrows) and structures in the ventral region of the thorax are obscured due to the presence of the pleural effusion.

720 Bronchoscopic view of the carina in a horse with pleuropneumonia secondary to rupture of a pulmonary abscess. Using bronchoscopy, it was possible to localize the abscess to the right lung by viewing serosanguineous discharge coming from the right mainstem bronchus. Aspiration of this discharge was performed using a catheter passed through the biopsy channel of the bronchoscope, allowing for culture and antimicrobial susceptibility testing.

721 Appearance of the chest wall of a horse with pleuropneumonia as seen at necropsy. A thick layer of fibrin ('fibrin peel') is present covering the parietal pleura.

If any pleural fluid is present, pleural drainage is also indicated to facilitate optimal response to systemic antimicrobial therapy and to alleviate clinical signs associated with pleural fluid accumulation. Drainage can be performed using a cannula, large bore intravenous catheter, indwelling chest tube, or by thoracostomy, depending on the character and volume of the pleural fluid. Thoracocentesis may be a single event or chest tubes may be left in place with a one-way valve to permit ongoing drainage. Intravenous fluid therapy is also indicated if large volumes of pleural fluid are to be removed or if signs of endotoxemia or dehydration are evident. For horses with very cellular or flocculant pleural fluid, pleural lavage can be achieved by infusing a physiologic fluid solution through the chest tube and then allowing free flow drainage by gravity. Alternatively, fluids can be infused through a separate tube placed dorsally in the thorax and allowed to drain through the ventral chest drain. Additional therapy should include NSAIDs (following restoration of hydration) in order to control pain and inflammation. More severe pain may be managed by butorphanol, morphine, or fentanyl.

Prolonged rest and good nutritional support are essential to a satisfactory recovery.

Prognosis
Survival and return to previous athletic function are largely dictated by the severity and duration of the disease. Prognosis for survival is usually good if early diagnosis and aggressive treatment are provided. In contrast, horses with fibrinous loculation and abscess formation, or those with extensive pulmonary necrosis evident on ultrasonography, typically have a poorer prognosis for long-term survival (**721**).

463

Medical conditions of the lower respiratory tract

Pneumocystis jiroveci (formerly *P. carinii*)

This unicellular eukaryote (currently classified as a fungus) is a respiratory tract commensal that causes interstitial pneumonia in immunocompromised foals or foals with other causes of pneumonia, especially *R. equi*, between six and 12 weeks of age. It rarely causes pneumonia in older foals or adult horses. Infection is difficult to diagnose because the organism is unculturable. *P. jiroveci* cysts can be identified with macrophages from BAL samples. The prognosis for affected foals is poor, but treatment with trimethoprim/sulfonamide combinations may be effective.

Mediastinal abscessation

Definition/overview

Mediastinal abscessation is uncommon. Abscessation may develop from translocation of bacteria via the bloodstream into mediastinal lymph nodes from the lymphatic system during pleuropneumonia or through extension of infection from a neck or chest wound.

Etiology/pathophysiology

Streptococcus equi and *Rhodococcus equi* are most frequently associated with mediastinal abscesses in horses, although *Aspergillus* sp. was isolated from a mediastinal granuloma in one horse.

During pleuropneumonia, lymphatic drainage of bacteria to bronchial lymph nodes may lead to mediastinal abscessation. Penetrating wounds to the neck and chest or rupture of the esophagus may also lead to infection of the mediastinum, with subsequent abscess formation as infection localizes.

Clinical presentation

Clinical presentation will vary with the inciting cause. Specific signs of mediastinal abscessation may not be obvious with concurrent pleuropneumonia or severe wounds. When mediastinal abscessation is the primary problem, nonspecific signs of weight loss, inappetence, and intermittent fever are common. Tracheal compression may result in progressive inspiratory impairment. Laryngeal dysfunction may occur from damage to the recurrent laryngeal nerve.

Differential diagnoses

Mediastinal lymphadenopathy, neoplastic mass, or cyst should be considered.

Diagnosis

Clinical signs are nonspecific. Chronic inflammatory hematologic changes include anemia, leukocytosis with neutrophilia, hyperproteinemia, and hyperglobulinemia.

Deviation of the trachea or mainstem bronchi may be observed endoscopically, resulting from external compression of these structures by the abscess. Transthoracic ultrasonography may show pleural effusion, which is frequently present in horses with mediastinal masses. Typically, mediastinal masses cannot be viewed by transthoracic ultrasonography due to interruption of the ultrasound waves by overlying aerated lung. However, ultrasonography at the thoracic inlet may allow visualization of the mediastinal mass and characterization of its contents. Ultrasound guidance is also useful for obtaining centesis samples for cytology and culture. Thoracic radiography is frequently useful in identifying the presence of a mediastinal mass. Thoracocentesis to drain pleural effusion is important prior to chest radiography in order to optimize visualization of thoracic masses. CT may be useful to confirm location and identify associated structures of mediastinal abscesses in foals.

Management

Sporadic reports of successful resolution have included long-term antimicrobial administration. Antimicrobial therapy should target the causative organism through culture and antimicrobial sensitivity testing. Empirical therapy should be based on the suspected etiologic agent and the efficacy of the drug in the treatment of abscesses. Surgical drainage of the abscess improves the response to antibiotic therapy, but is difficult and is generally limited to abscesses at the thoracic inlet.

Prognosis

The prognosis is variable depending on the location of the abscess within the mediastinum. Some horses may respond to long-term antimicrobial therapy, but the overall prognosis is guarded.

Glanders and melioidosis

Definition/overview

Glanders (farcy) is regarded as one of the most serious contagious diseases of Equidae. It is caused by infection with *Burkholderia mallei*. The disease has been eradicated from many parts of the world, but it is endemic in the Middle East, Africa, India, SE Asia, China, and Mongolia. It is absent in the USA and the UK, where it is a notifiable disease. Most countries have strict import regulations (testing and/or quarantine) to control the spread of *B. mallei* infection. Glanders is a respiratory disease that also has skin (farcy) manifestations, and it is a significant zoonosis in endemically infected countries. Disease in horses is usually initially chronic, and affected horses almost always die from acute-onset pneumonia following a long debilitating illness. Disease in donkeys and mules is usually acute, with rapid death from pneumonia. Melioidosis is a similar disease caused by the related bacterium *B. pseudomallei* and occurs in the Far East and northern Australia.

Clinical presentation
Glanders and melioidosis are generally chronic diseases, with initial respiratory disease progressing to a more acute form with skin ulceration and ulceration and abscess formation throughout the respiratory tract. There is an insidious onset and slowly progressive respiratory disease with typical URT infection clinical signs (nasal discharge and lymphadenopathy), but often with nasal mucosal ulceration. This mild and chronic disease may continue for several months, but a more acute disease, possibly triggered by stress or intercurrent illness, develops. In the acute form there is pyrexia, depression, coughing, weight loss, and clinical signs of pneumonia (tachypnea and dyspnea) due to abscessation and ulceration along the URT and in the lungs. Cutaneous ulcerative lesions ('farcy') also develop along the limbs, especially the medial thigh and hock, which discharge a yellow-brown pus containing granules. There is often marked lymphatic cording.

Differential diagnosis
Other causes of URT and LRT infectious disease should be considered.

Diagnosis
The initial clinical signs are nonspecific and horses may appear quite well during the chronic form of the disease. The later, acute form, with LRT signs, nasal ulceration, and skin ulceration over the medial hindlimbs, is more characteristic. Postmortem examination reveals variable sized abscesses containing brown/yellow granular pus throughout the respiratory tract and in other organs including the liver and spleen. Isolation of the organism confirms the diagnosis.

Management
Glanders and melioidosis respond poorly to treatment and the prognosis is poor. An intradermal skin test using bacterial antigen (the mallein test) is used to identify carriers or horses that have been exposed to the organism and have antibody. The disease is a zoonosis and infection-control precautions must be followed when handling tissues that might be infected. Further information is available from various governmental sources.

Obstructive conditions

Heaves
Definition/overview
Heaves is an episodic condition characterized by obstruction of the lower airways in response to inhaled allergens in the environment. It is also referred to as recurrent airway obstruction (RAO), and formerly as chronic obstructive pulmonary disease (COPD).

Etiology/pathophysiology
Obstruction is a consequence of bronchoconstriction and airway septal thickening from inflammatory cell infiltrate and edema, as well as blockage of airway lumen by mucus and inflammatory cells.

Affected animals have airway hyperresponsiveness to inhaled antigens (aeroallergens). Although multiple agents in the environment may act as allergens, molds and dusts in improperly baled hay are most frequently implicated as the cause of heaves exacerbation. It is not currently known whether heaves is a sequela to IAD in some horses. A genetic propensity to develop heaves has also been suggested.

Clinical presentation
A seasonal pattern of heaves exacerbation is often reported. Clinical signs during exacerbation frequently include expiratory dyspnea accompanied by a visible 'heave line' as the external abdominal oblique muscles are used to facilitate expiration. Nasal discharge is serous to mucopurulent, and intermittent to paroxysmal coughing may be observed. Flaring of the nostrils may be seen. Severe cases may have depression, lack of interest in feed due to difficulty breathing, rocking of the animal as it breathes, and a wheeze may be audible at the nares during expiration.

Differential diagnoses
Pulmonary infections (viral or bacterial) and pulmonary neoplasia may have a similar presentation.

Diagnosis
Clinical history may suggest a seasonal pattern of occurrence, corresponding with increased indoor housing during periods of inclement weather such as in the winter months. Lack of improvement in response to antibiotic treatment is also frequently reported.

Thoracic auscultation during use of a rebreathing bag is indicated in all cases except animals demonstrating signs of dyspnea or respiratory distress. Frequently, crackles and wheezes are identified over the lower airways and movement of secretions within the trachea may be audible. Percussion may reveal an expanded caudodorsal margin to the lung field due to hyperinflation of the lungs as a consequence of air-trapping, although this must be differentiated from a gas cap in the cecum when percussing the right side of the abdomen.

Radiographic changes are not specific for heaves and may include an increased interstitial and/or bronchial pattern. Thoracic radiographs may be helpful to exclude bronchopneumonia as a differential diagnosis.

Bronchoscopy is useful to assess airway hyperreactivity, hyperemia, edema, and bronchoconstriction, and to evaluate the presence and nature of any airway secretions (722). BAL is the test of choice to diagnose heaves. BAL may be performed transendoscopically using the biopsy channel of a sterilized bronchoscope for fluid infusion and aspiration, or blindly using a flexible nasotracheal catheter passed into the bronchi. Cytologic assessment of BAL fluid is required to determine the type(s) of leukocyte contributing to the airway inflammation (723). In general, an elevation in the percentage of neutrophils (>25%) in the differential cell count is seen in animals during episodes of clinical exacerbation of heaves, although elevated percentages of mast cells and eosinophils may also be observed.

Management

Clinical cure is not generally possible in horses with heaves, so treatment is aimed at achieving and maintaining remission from clinical signs. This is best done through persistent and aggressive environmental management to reduce exposure to inhaled allergens (*Table 15*). Hay should be good quality with minimal dust and molds present, or preferably changed to haylage, or the animal may benefit from transition to a pelleted complete feed. Continuous pasture turnout is recommended to optimize ventilation. If the animal is to be housed indoors for any period of time, effort should be made to avoid periods of dusty activities such as during cleaning and bedding of stalls, feeding hay, and sweeping. The stall should also not be located near to an arena or hay-storage facility; overhead hay storage is particularly detrimental. Bedding should be wood shavings or peat moss rather than straw or sawdust.

Alleviation of lung inflammation is achieved through therapy with corticosteroids given via oral (e.g. prednisone, prednisolone), parenteral (e.g. isoflupredone, dexamethasone), or inhalation (e.g. beclomethasone, fluticasone) routes of administration (*Table 16*).

During episodes of heaves exacerbation, rescue therapy may be required in animals demonstrating dyspnea or respiratory distress. This is best achieved through bronchodilation with rapid-acting drugs such as beta 2-adrenergics (e.g. salbutamol, clenbuterol), followed by longer-acting bronchodilation (e.g. salmeterol).

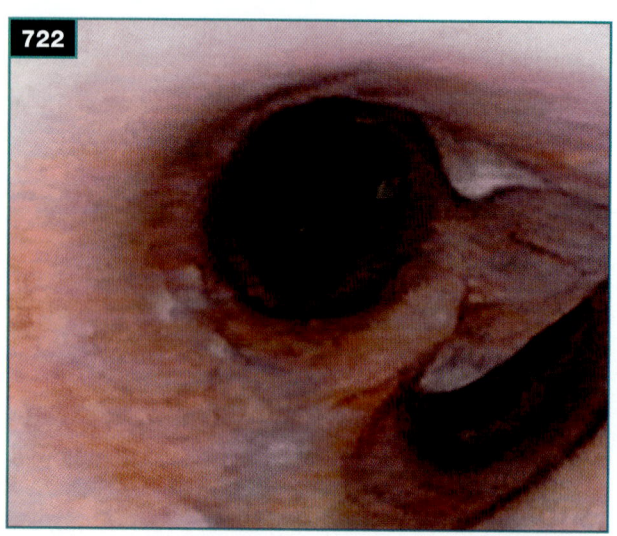

722 Bronchoscopic view of the carina in a horse with heaves during severe exacerbation of clinical signs. The carina is markedly blunted due to edema, and flecks of mucus are visible. Airways are hyperresponsive, resulting in excessive coughing and constriction of the airways in response to passage of the bronchoscope.

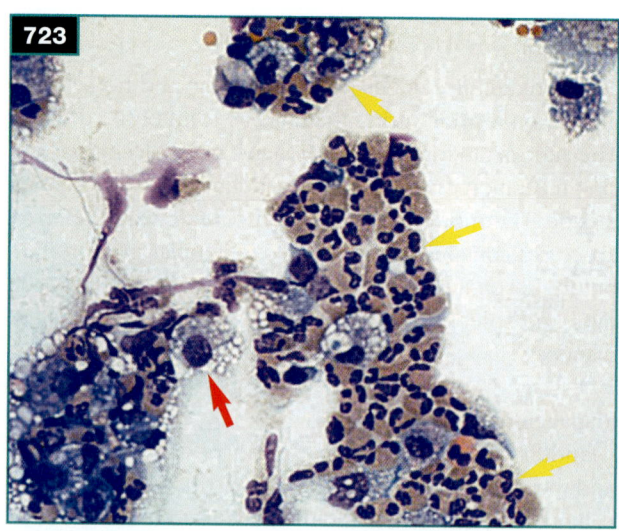

723 Cytology of BAL fluid from a horse with heaves during exacerbation of clinical signs. Well-preserved neutrophils (yellow arrows) are the predominant cell type. Pulmonary alveolar macrophages are also visible (red arrow).

TABLE 15 **Environmental modification options for management of inflammatory airway disease and heaves**

- Feed only good-quality hay using bales that are visibly free from any dusts or molds when the bale is broken open. Do not feed horses using round bales.
- Soak hay by fully immersing it in water for at least 15 minutes prior to feeding. Change the water used to soak the hay daily in order to prevent accumulation of endotoxins and microbes.
- Feed hay on the ground. Do not use a haynet or elevated manger.
- As an alternative to hay, feed 'dust-free' options such as haylage, hay cubes, or complete pelleted rations.
- Concentrates are usually an insignificant source of dust. Adding molasses to concentrates and grains may reduce the respirable dust.
- Optimize ventilation by providing continuous pasture turnout (24 hours/day or as much as possible).
- Ensure appropriate ventilation of the stable.
- For any period that affected horses must be indoors, house them in a stall with ventilation to the outside of the barn (e.g. window).
- Do not stable affected horses next to hay or straw storage or arenas.
- Avoid straw or sawdust as types of bedding. Use shredded paper, large wood shavings, peanut kernels, or peat moss instead. Stalls adjacent to heaves-affected horses should be managed similarly.
- Affected horses should not be indoors during 'dusty' periods such as mucking and bedding of stalls or sweeping.
- Regular cleaning and disinfecting of stables is recommended to prevent the persistence of dust and infectious agents in the environment.

Prognosis

Heaves is generally a lifelong disease in affected horses, with progression in severity of signs and development of chronic airway remodeling occurring in animals with unregulated airway inflammation. The prognosis for achieving and maintaining remission from clinical signs is variable and is highly dependent on the owner's ability to institute aggressive management changes that are successful in reducing exposure to inhaled allergens all year round.

Summer pasture-associated obstructive pulmonary disease

Definition/overview

This is a recurrent disease of adult horses that are kept on pasture. It is most common in the warm and humid months of June to September in the southeastern USA and in the UK. Animals gradually recover during the winter and spring months, but may experience a return of clinical signs the following summer.

Etiology/pathophysiology

The pathophysiology of airway inflammation in this condition is poorly understood, although it is presumed to represent an inflammatory response to environmental allergens that are encountered at pasture. Airway hyperresponsiveness has been linked to increased bronchial smooth-muscle sensitivity to 5-hydroxytryptamine in affected horses.

Clinical presentation

The presentation is similar to heaves. Signs may include nasal discharge, nostril flaring, coughing, tachypnea, labored expiratory effort, expanded lung field on chest percussion, and crackles and wheezes throughout the lung fields on thoracic auscultation.

Differential diagnoses

Heaves and viral or bacterial pneumonia are the most common differential diagnoses.

Diagnosis

Clinical signs and history of seasonality are suggestive. Radiography can be useful. An interstitial pattern is present, with pulmonary overinflation in chronic cases. Increased mucus is evident in the upper airways on bronchoscopy; however, this in itself is not diagnostic. BAL is a useful tool. Cytologic examination of the fluid should be performed. An increased cell count with an increase in nondegenerate neutrophils is diagnostic.

Management

Management factors are critical. Indoor housing during the summer months is important. Drug therapy as described for heaves is an important adjunctive measure (*Table 16*), but response may be limited if environmental modification is not feasible.

Prognosis

Although the prognosis for resolution of the disease is poor, careful environmental and medical management may induce remission of clinical signs in affected animals.

Medical conditions of the lower respiratory tract

TABLE 16 Common drugs used for the treatment of inflammatory airway disease and heaves

DRUG	DOSE	ROUTE*	COMMENTS
Bronchodilators			
Albuterol	0.8–2 µg/kg q3h	Inhalation: MDI	Rapid onset of duration of activity with short duration of effect (0.5–3 hours).
Ipratropium bromide	0.5–1 µg/kg q6h	Inhalation: MDI	Rapid onset of action with moderately long-lasting effect (4–6 hours). No known side-effects.
Salmeterol	63–210 µg q8h	Inhalation: MDI	Rapid onset of action with long-lasting effect (6–8 hours).
Fenoterol	1–2 mg	Inhalation: MDI	Rapid onset of action.
Clenbuterol	0.8–3.2 µg/kg q12h	P/o or inhalation: nebulized	Also increases the rate of mucociliary clearance. Side-effects include sweating, trembling, tachycardia, and excitement.
	0.8 µg/kg q12h	I/v or i/m	
Aminophylline	5–10 mg/kg q8–12h	P/o or i/v	Therapeutic plasma concentrations vary among horses and margin of safety is very narrow. May cause excitement. Dilute i/v dose in 1 liter of saline and administer over 30–60 minutes while monitoring animal for signs of toxicity.
Corticosteroids			
Dexamethasone	0.04–0.1 mg/kg q12h (0.2 mg/kg q12h for p/o)	I/v i/m, or p/o	Increased dosage required for oral administration due to limited bioavailability with oral dosing.
Dexamethasone 21-isonicotinate	0.04–0.06 mg/kg q3d	I/m	Depot form of dexamethasone.
Prednisolone	2.2 mg/kg q24h	P/o	Good GI absorption.
Isoflupredone acetate	10–14 mg q24h	I/m	Repeated administration has induced significant hypokalemia in other species.
Triamcinolone acetonide	0.09 mg/kg once	I/m	Depot drug with prolonged effect after single dose (e.g. 3–5 weeks).
Beclomethasone dipropionate	3500 µg q12h or 500 µg q12h	Inhalation: MDI	Minimal systemic effects due to low dose plus delivery by inhalation. Actual dose depends on delivery system used.
Fluticasone propionate	2000 µg q12h	Inhalation: MDI	Minimal systemic effects due to low dose plus delivery by inhalation.
Cromogens			
Sodium cromoglycate	80–200 mg q12–24h	Inhalation: nebulized	Mast cell stabilizer. Prophylactic use only.
Nedocromil sodium	24 mg q12h	Inhalation: MDI	Mast cell stabilizer. Prophylactic use only.

*Inhaled drugs must be administered using an equine delivery device/mask in combination with a metered dose inhaler (MDI) or nebulization system.

Parasitic conditions

Lungworms
Definition/overview
Dictyocaulus arnfieldi causes parasitic pneumonia in horses. Donkeys and foals are the patent hosts; in horses the infection is usually nonpatent. Infection in donkeys is usually subclinical. Clinical signs are due to the presence of adult worms and late-stage larvae in the bronchi and bronchioles. Clinical signs closely resemble those of RAO. Lungworm infection can be successfully treated with anthelminthics.

Etiology/pathophysiology
D. arnfieldi is a nematode and has a typical lifecycle with a migratory larval phase. Donkeys and foals with patent infections shed eggs containing first-stage (L1) larvae or hatched L1 larvae onto pasture. Within days, these mature to the infective L3 stage. On ingestion, L3 larvae mature into migratory L4 larvae, which enter mesenteric lymphatics, then the circulation via the thoracic duct, and reach the lung hematogenously. L4 larvae migrate into the alveoli and develop into L5 and then adults in the airway (bronchi and especially bronchioles). In donkeys and foals, but not usually in adult horses, patent infection develops.

Adult females lay eggs containing L1 larvae that are coughed into the pharynx and swallowed. Eggs containing L1 larvae may be passed in feces or eggs may hatch in the gut, releasing L1 larvae into the feces.

Clinical presentation

There are usually no (obvious) clinical signs in donkeys. Foals similarly show few, if any, clinical signs. In adults the clinical disease closely resembles heaves. Affected horses are bright, presenting with a history of coughing and decreased exercise capacity. There may be moderate tachypnea and dyspnea at rest and wheezes and crackles are audible on lung auscultation.

Differential diagnosis

Other causes of pulmonary disease, especially heaves and primary eosinophilic pulmonary disease should be considered.

Diagnosis

Clinical examination is not diagnostic, although a heaves-like disease in one or more horses in a group at pasture in the late summer that have been grazing with donkeys should raise suspicion. In donkeys and foals only fecal examination using the modified Baermann technique will reveal larvae. This is not a useful investigation in horses because patent infections are not established. In horses, airway lavage samples will reveal eosinophilia with L5 larvae and/or adult nematodes. Note that airway eosinophilia is not pathognomonic for pulmonary parasitism.

Management

D. arnfieldi can be successfully treated with a variety of anthelminthics including benzimidazoles, ivermectin, and moxidectin. Benzimidazoles are given for 5 consecutive days, whereas single doses of ivermectin and moxidectin are highly effective. Regular anthelminthic treatment of donkeys will control shedding of eggs and L1 larvae and reduce pasture contamination. Picking up droppings and sweeping also help to reduce pasture contamination.

Prognosis

The prognosis is good.

Parascaris equorum
Definition/overview

Parascaris equorum causes parasitic pneumonia in foals and yearlings, typically towards the end of their first summer at pasture. Adult parasites live in the small intestine and clinical signs are caused by larvae migrating through the lung. Solid immunity develops after infection so that disease is uncommon in foals older than 12–18 months. Infection can be treated successfully with anthelminthics. The prognosis is good.

Etiology/pathophysiology

P. equorum is a large ascarid. Adult females can reach 50 cm in length, whereas males are smaller (up to 25 cm). Adults live in the small intestine and lay eggs containing L1 larvae, which are then shed onto pasture in feces and quickly mature (<2 weeks) into the infective L2 larvae inside the egg. The females produce large quantities of eggs and a single infected foal can shed millions of eggs each day. Foals become infected by ingestion of L2 larvae within eggs from the pasture. After ingestion, L2 larvae migrate through the small intestinal wall and reach the liver as L3 larvae via the hepatic portal vein. Larvae migrate through the liver and reach the lungs via the heart and pulmonary artery within 2 weeks of infection. L3 larvae migrate through alveolar capillary walls into the airway, where they are coughed up into the pharynx and swallowed. In the small intestine, larvae develop into L4 larvae and then adult worms, thus completing the life cycle. The prepatent period is between 3 and 4 months.

Clinical presentation

Foals between 6 and 12 months old are most commonly affected, typically towards the end of their first summer at pasture. The disease is sometimes referred to as 'summer colds'. Clinical signs include modest pyrexia, nasal discharge, weight loss, coughing, tachypnea and dyspnea, and crackling and wheezing on auscultation of the lung field. Heavy infections of adult parasites can cause death due to small-intestinal obstruction and rupture.

Differential diagnosis

A variety of causes of pneumonia in foals and yearlings may have a similar presentation.

Diagnosis

An outbreak of pulmonary disease in foals at pasture is highly suggestive of P. equorum infection. Confirmation is by fecal egg counts and demonstration of thick-walled ascarid eggs.

Management

P. equorum can be treated using any of the available anthelminthics including benzimidazoles, ivermectin, and moxidectin. Fecal egg count reduction testing of foals should be done regularly to detect resistance to macrocyclic lactones, in which case early treatment with pyrantel or benzimidazoles may limit development of high burdens in the intestinal tract that predispose to ascarid impactions.

Prognosis

The prognosis is good for most cases, although death from small-intestinal rupture in very heavily infected foals can occur. Solid immunity develops on recovery from infection and infections in foals older than 12 months are unusual.

469

Miscellaneous conditions

Aspiration pneumonia

Definition/overview
Aspiration is a potential cause of serious pneumonia. It may occur in adult horses and foals for a variety of reasons.

Etiology/pathophysiology
There are many potential causes of aspiration. In foals, aspiration of milk may occur because of congenital abnormalities or improper supplemental (bottle or nasogastric tube) feeding. Inadvertent drenching or passing a nasogastric tube into the lungs and depositing fluids, pharmaceutical products, or other substances into the lower airways is a common cause of aspiration in adult horses. Aspiration of saliva and feed material is also a common complication of esophageal obstruction (choke) and may occur during general anesthesia. Dysphagia caused by any reason may also predispose to aspiration.

The quantity and composition of the aspirated fluid/material will largely dictate the clinical signs, progression of disease, and outcome. When large quantities of fluids are aspirated, animals may die acutely. More frequently, they develop pneumonia, which can progress to lung consolidation, pleuropneumonia, gangrenous pneumonia, and/or pulmonary abscessation.

Clinical presentation
Acute clinical signs following aspiration are similar to those of other forms of pneumonia, including tachypnea, cough, anxiety, and increased lung sounds. Shortly after aspiration, a raspy, fluidy sound may be heard during respiration. Ingesta may be observed at the nostrils (724).

Differential diagnoses
Viral or bacterial pneumonia, including pleuropneumonia, should be considered.

Diagnosis
History and physical examination are suggestive, particularly a history of recent esophageal obstruction or nasogastric intubation for fluid administration. Thoracic radiography is a useful tool (725). Ventral consolidation is common due to gravitational flow of aspirated material to this region of the lung. In animals without respiratory distress, bronchoscopy may be useful to visualize fluid or food debris within the trachea as confirmation of aspiration (726). Cytologic examination of tracheal or bronchial aspirates may reveal extra- and intracellular bacteria or foreign material such as mineral oil. The reason for aspiration must be explored. Careful clinical examination may be required to identify possible primary causes and direct subsequent testing.

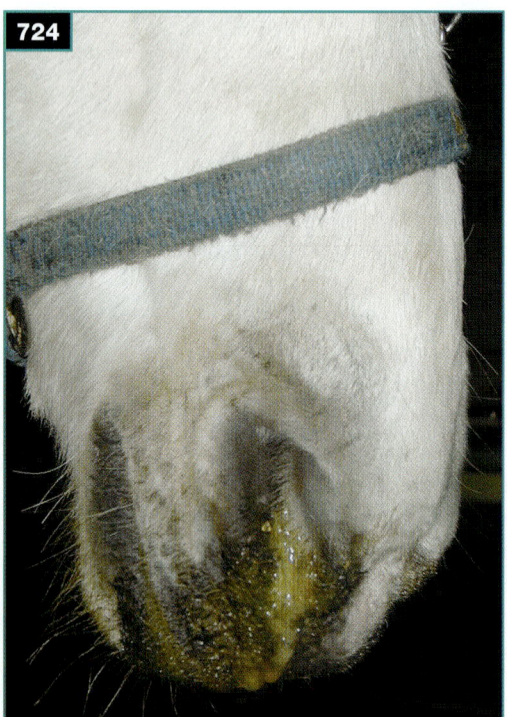

724 Esophageal obstruction in a horse subsequent to improper soaking of beet pulp prior to feeding. Feed material is visible at the nares of the horse.

725 Thoracic radiograph of the horse in 724 showing ventral consolidation due to pneumonia from aspiration of feed material into the lungs.

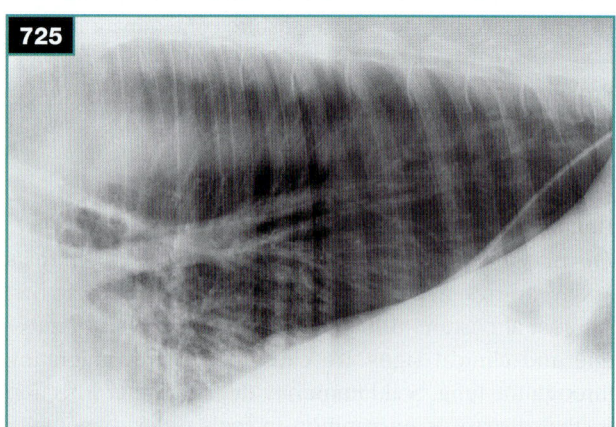

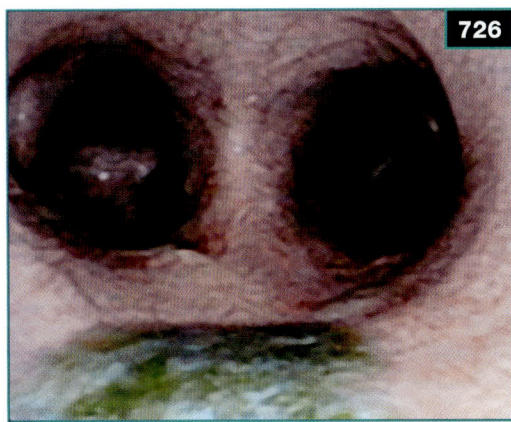

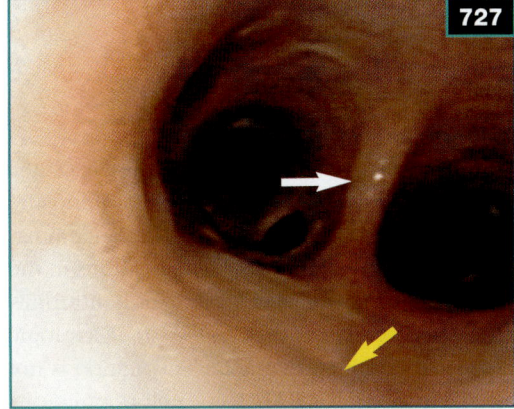

726 Bronchoscopic examination at the carina of the horse in 724 revealed feed material within the trachea down to the level of the tracheal puddle.

727 Bronchoscopic view of the carina in a horse with IAD. Mucus is visible at the tracheal puddle (yellow arrow), and the carina is blunted due to edema (white arrow).

Management

Broad-spectrum antimicrobial administration to target both Gram-positive and Gram-negative as well as anaerobic bacteria is indicated. NSAIDs are also beneficial to control lung inflammation. Specific measures to address the cause of aspiration and prevent further aspiration are required.

Prognosis

The prognosis is variable, depending on the severity of the pneumonia, the inciting cause, and the ability to prevent ongoing aspiration. The volume and nature of the aspirated material or fluid, type(s) of bacteria introduced into the lung, and time of initiation of treatment may influence the outcome.

Inflammatory airway disease

Definition/overview

IAD (otherwise known as nonseptic IAD) is an inflammatory process of the lower airways that causes pulmonary dysfunction and reduced exercise tolerance in affected horses.

Etiology/pathophysiology

Multiple inciting agents have been proposed as causes for the small-airway inflammation in young horses with IAD, including recent viral infection, exposure to environmental irritants (e.g. dusts, noxious gases) or sources of endotoxin, and pulmonary hemorrhage. Some clinicians have speculated on the role of bacteria, particularly in racehorses. An association has been reported between the presence of bacteria in tracheal aspirate samples and IAD; however, a causal relationship has not been proven and there is insufficient evidence to confim an infectious cause of this condition. Currently, the exact pathophysiology of this condition remains unknown. It is most likely multifactorial in nature.

Clinical presentation

Reduced athletic performance and/or prolonged time for recovery from exercise are frequently the only presenting signs. Nasal discharge may be present, ranging from serous to mucopurulent, and coughing may be observed during exercise or at the time of feeding.

Differential diagnoses

Other common causes of reduced performance, particularly musculoskeletal abnormalities, cardiac dysfunction, neurologic disorders, and other respiratory diseases (upper airway obstruction, viral infection, bronchopneumonia, exercise-induced pulmonary hemorrhage, lungworm, neoplasia), should be considered.

Diagnosis

Careful auscultation of the thorax during use of a rebreathing bag may reveal the presence of increased bronchial tones, wheezes, and/or crackles, as well as movement of secretions during tracheal auscultation. Absence of these signs does not, however, preclude a diagnosis of IAD. Often, no abnormalities are detected with even a thorough physical examination.

Radiography is of no diagnostic use to confirm IAD, although radiographs may help to exclude diagnoses of bronchopneumonia or pulmonary abscessation. Bronchoscopy is useful to assess airway hyperreactivity, hyperemia, edema, and bronchoconstriction, and to evaluate the presence and nature of any airway secretions (727).

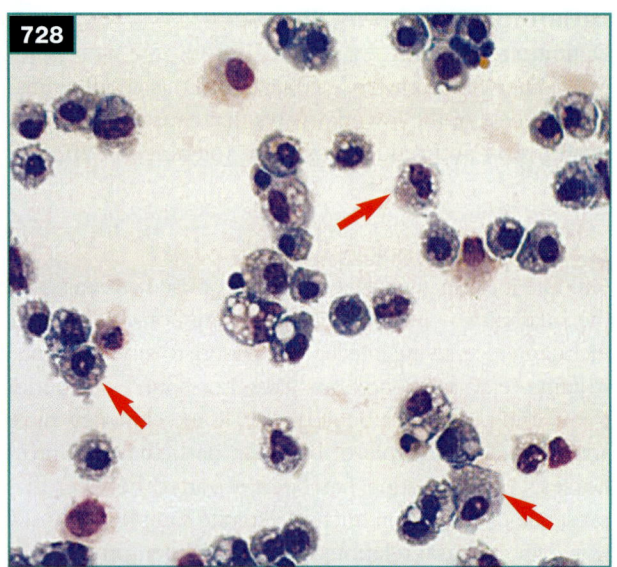

728 Cytology of BAL fluid from a normal horse. The predominant cell type is pulmonary alveolar macrophages (arrows).

729 Cytology of BAL fluid from a horse with IAD. Leukocytes are seen trapped in mucus. Mast cells (red arrows), an eosinophil (yellow arrow), and granules from globular leukocytes (white arrows) are present.

730 Cytology of BAL fluid from a horse with IAD. Multiple eosinophils are present (red arrows). Pulmonary alveolar macrophages containing eosinophilic granules in phagosomes are also visible (yellow arrows).

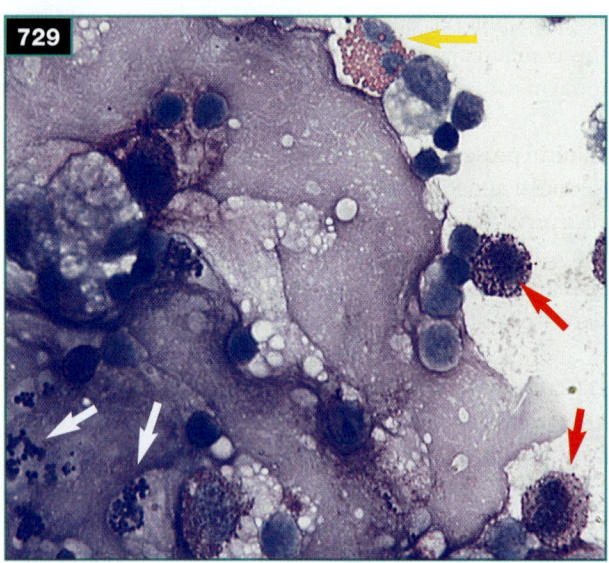

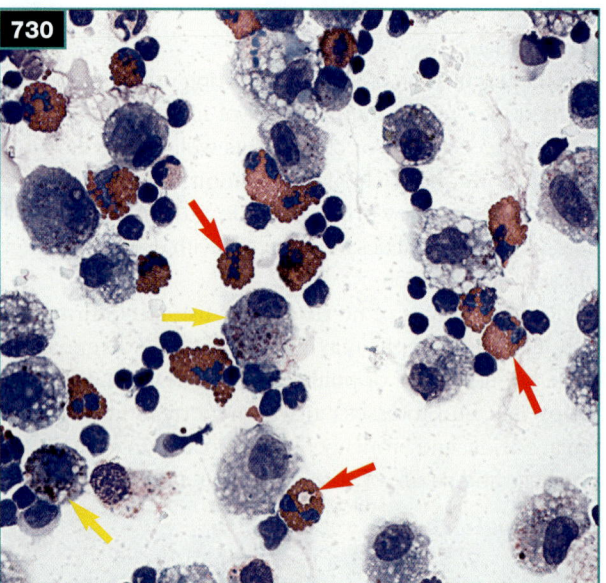

BAL is the test of choice to diagnose IAD. Cytologic assessment of BAL fluid is required to determine the type(s) of leukocyte contributing to the airway inflammation. In general, IAD is characterized by elevations in the percentage of eosinophils, mast cells, and/or neutrophils in the differential cell count (**728–730**). Cytologic assessment of fluid obtained by tracheal aspiration is not an adequate substitution for BAL, since cell populations correlate poorly between samples obtained via tracheal aspirate versus BAL.

Management
The key to recovery from IAD is adequate rest of affected horses and environmental modification to significantly reduce exposure to respirable particles (*Table 15*). Many recommendations regarding medical therapy for IAD are extrapolated from studies in heaves-affected horses. Treatment includes inhalation therapy with mast-cell stabilizers and/or corticosteroids depending on the type(s) of cell identified on the BAL differential count. Oral and parenteral corticosteroids may instead be used to reduce cost, but they require a higher overall dose to be administered to the animal. Bronchodilators may also be useful prior to light exercise, but should be avoided during periods when the animal is housed indoors (*Table 16*). Low-dose interferon-alpha has been shown to improve the outcome in horses with IAD in two recent studies.

Prognosis
Since the pathophysiology of IAD is currently poorly understood, the long-term impact of IAD on athletic performance of affected animals is uncertain. Some animals may respond fully to treatment and return to a normal level of performance, while others will show variable response to treatment and may deteriorate over time.

731 Thoracic radiograph of a horse with granulomatous pneumonia. Multifocal opacities are visible throughout the lung field.

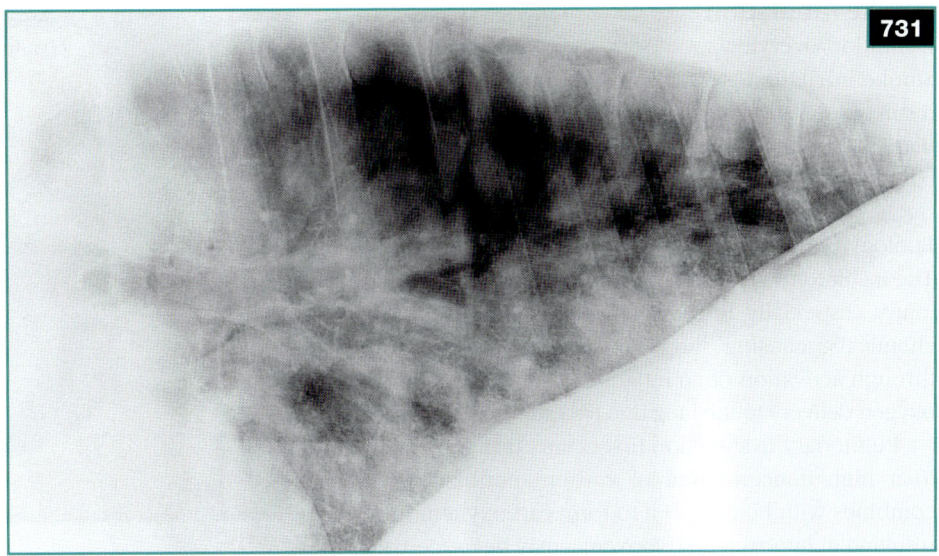

Granulomatous pneumonia

Definition/overview
This is an uncommon, multisystemic granulomatous disease that resembles sarcoidosis in humans. No seasonal, breed, age, or sex predispositions have been identified.

Etiology/pathophysiology
Currently, recognized causes include fungal, bacterial, and/or parasitic agents, silicate pneumoconiosis, and neoplasia. However, in many cases a cause cannot be identified.

The pathophysiology is poorly understood, but is presumed to involve an abnormal host immune response to chronic exposure to an antigen. In humans, the pathologic changes caused by mycobacterial or some fungal infections resemble granulomatous pneumonia, and atypical strains of mycobacteria have been identified in fixed tissues of human patients with sarcoidosis. However, such organisms have not been identified or isolated in affected horses.

Clinical presentation
Chronic signs of weight loss, anorexia, depression, and fever are common, and skin lesions are frequently present. Horses may have progressive respiratory signs including exercise intolerance, tachypnea, cough, nasal discharge, and abnormal lung sounds. Clinical signs do not respond to antibiotic therapy and NSAIDs.

Differential diagnoses
Fungal, parasitic, or bacterial pneumonia and pulmonary neoplasia should be considered.

Diagnosis
For disease caused by silicate pneumoconiosis or coccidioidomycosis, the geographic origin of the horse from an endemic area may be suggestive. Hematologic testing is indicated and evidence of a chronic inflammatory process (anemia, neutrophilia, hyperfibrinogenemia, and increased globulins) is often present. Thoracic radiographs are very important (731). A miliary or nodular interstitial pattern may be present throughout the lung. Tracheal aspirate and BAL cytology are nonspecific. Mild suppurative inflammation may be present. Lung biopsy is required for diagnosis. Sampling of the nodular masses is optimized by ultrasound-guided lung biopsy. Histopathology reveals noncaseating granulomas affiliated with bronchi and bronchioles. Intracellular crystalline material may be observed in silicosis.

Efforts to elucidate a cause should include serum immunodiffusion testing for antibodies against *Coccidioides immitis*, selective histopathologic staining of lung tissue for fungal and mycobacterial agents, and bacterial and fungal culture of tracheal aspirate or BAL fluids.

Management
Adequate target therapy cannot be prescribed since the cause remains unknown. Corticosteroids are widely used in these cases, but there is no information supporting their efficacy.

Prognosis
The prognosis is poor because of the lack of a proven treatment. Affected horses are commonly euthanized because of progressive and severe debilitation associated with the disease.

Smoke inhalation

Definition/overview

Smoke inhalation is a clinical syndrome that occurs as a result of inhalation of harmful gases, vapors, and/or particulate matter contained in smoke, usually originating from barn fires (732).

Etiology/pathophysiology

The insult to the respiratory tract occurs by direct thermal injury (especially in the URT) and inhalation of toxic chemicals, causing lung injury directly or indirectly through activation of an inflammatory response and low oxygen delivery to the lung due to combustion processes.

Pulmonary dysfunction first occurs through exposure to a high concentration of carbon monoxide, which combines with hemoglobin to form carboxyhemoglobin, resulting in hypoxemia. Hypoxemia may be exacerbated if concurrent bronchoconstriction in the lower airways occurs in response to the irritating effects of noxious gases. Pulmonary dysfunction may subsequently progress due to pulmonary edema formation as a consequence of lung inflammation, plus airway obstruction from the accumulation of inflammatory and necrotic cells in the airways. Extensive destruction of airway epithelium also impairs host respiratory immune defenses, predisposing to secondary bronchopneumonia.

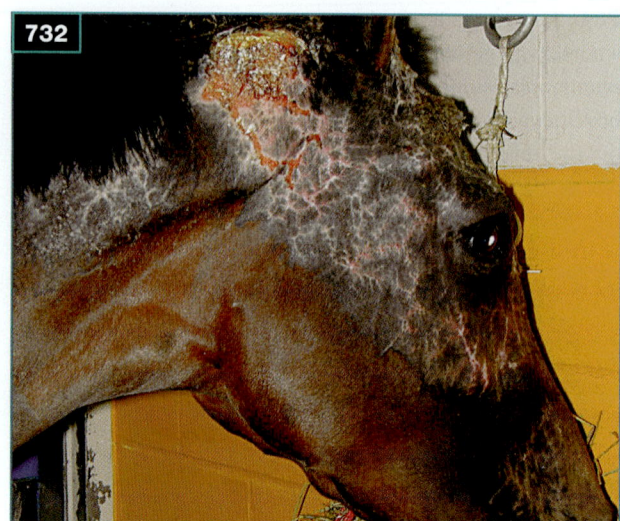

732 External skin burns subsequent to a barn fire. Smoke inhalation resulted in marked damage to the respiratory epithelium, causing respiratory distress in this horse from excessive debris within the trachea and bronchi.

Clinical presentation

Clinical signs will depend on the degree of exposure and the types of gas inhaled. Animals may be mildly affected or clinically normal after smoke inhalation, with severe disease developing 12–24 hours later. Severely affected animals may show signs of hypoxemia, depression, disorientation, and ataxia. Tachypnea, dyspnea, and respiratory stridor may occur. Crackles, wheezes, or decreased air movement may be obvious on initial chest auscultation, but may take up to 12–24 hours after the initial insult to develop. Nasal discharge is common due to edema or inflammatory exudate in the upper airway.

Diagnosis

History and physical examination are usually diagnostic, but the presence of external thermal injuries is confirmatory. Blood-gas analysis should be performed if available. A venous concentration of carboxyhemoglobin above 10% is consistent with carbon monoxide toxicity. In horses without signs of significant respiratory distress, thoracic radiographs, bronchoscopy, and cytologic evaluation of tracheal aspirate or BAL fluid are useful ancillary techniques to confirm the diagnosis and determine the optimal treatment.

Management

Tracheotomy may be required in cases of upper airway obstruction resulting from severe edema and inflammation, or to remove pseudomembranes from the trachea in order to facilitate ventilation of the lung. Humidified oxygen support by nasal insufflation or via a transtracheal catheter is recommended. Bronchodilators may be indicated in cases of severe bronchoconstriction. Diuretics and NSAIDs are usually required to control edema, inflammation, and pain. The use of corticosteroids is controversial and is usually avoided. Some cases may require the use of analgesics such as fentanyl, morphine, or ketamine. Supportive therapy is commonly indicated including intravenous fluids, plasma transfusion, or parenteral nutrition supplementation. High-risk patients or those with confirmed bacterial infections should be treated with appropriate antimicrobials.

Prognosis

The prognosis is variable. Prolonged exposure to gases and extensive or severe thermal injuries carries a poor prognosis. The onset of clinical signs may be delayed, therefore close monitoring is indicated in any animal that has been exposed to smoke.

Pneumothorax

Definition/overview
Pneumothorax is an accumulation of air or gas in the pleural space causing partial or total collapse of the lung. It is uncommon in horses and usually occurs as a result of trauma. Pneumothorax is usually bilateral due to the fenestrations in the mediastinum of horses.

Etiology/pathophysiology
Pneumothorax may result from an open chest wound, rib fracture, blunt trauma to the thorax, rupture of an emphysematous vesicle on the surface of the lung, barotrauma, or spontaneously without evident cause. Horses with pneumonia may develop bronchopleural fistulas, resulting in pneumothorax. Procedures of the thorax (e.g. surgery or lung biopsy) may also result in pneumothorax.

Air may gain entry into the pleural cavity either through a wound in the thoracic wall or by a defect in the lung parenchyma allowing communication between the airways and the pleural space. By definition, simple pneumothorax involves intrapleural pressure that is less than or equal to atmospheric pressure, such that air may enter and exit the chest cavity freely with each breath. In such cases, insufficient negative pressure is generated within the chest cavity to expand the lungs for ventilation. In contrast, respiratory embarrassment from tension pneumothorax escalates more rapidly due to continued influx of air into the chest cavity while no exit of air is possible. In such cases the intrapleural pressure quickly exceeds atmospheric pressure and causes life-threatening compression of the lungs as the chest cavity fills with air.

Clinical presentation
The clinical signs may range from a mild increase in respiratory rate and sweating to tachypnea, dyspnea, and cyanosis. Oral mucous membrane color is often abnormal, but may range widely in appearance from pale to congested, toxic, or cyanotic depending on the degree of pneumothorax and the underlying cause. On chest auscultation, lung sounds are absent in the dorsal lung field and percussion may reveal hyperresonance over the affected area. Subcutaneous emphysema, if present, may obscure these findings.

Differential diagnoses
Diaphragmatic hernia and pleural effusion may produce similar signs.

Diagnosis
History, evidence of trauma to the thoracic cavity, or the presence of subcutaneous emphysema is suggestive. Thoracic radiographs are important. Air within the pleural space compresses the lung ventrally, and is seen as an absence of pulmonary vasculature over the caudodorsal lung field and a sharp lung border in the dorsal and caudal regions (733).

Careful ultrasonographic examination of the middle and dorsal areas of the thorax may reveal air artifact images. These air artifact images, in combination with the inability to identify a sliding motion between the visceral and parietal pleura, are findings consistent with pneumothorax.

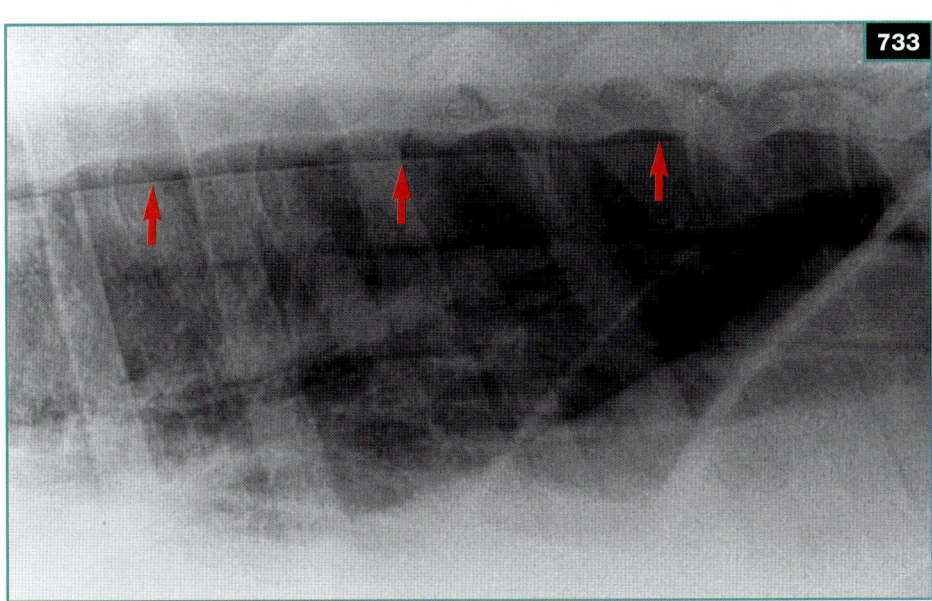

733 Thoracic radiograph of a horse with pneumothorax resulting from an open chest wound. The dorsal margin of the lung is visible as a line below the thoracic vertebrae (arrows).

Management

Treatment of the underlying disease or cause should be addressed. Horses with simple pneumothorax can recover with confinement and rest. In case of hypoxemia, intra-nasal oxygen insufflation can be administered. Removal of the free air from the pleural cavity may be required in more severely affected cases (734). Air suction of the thoracic cavity is performed in the upper mid-thorax between the ribs. The area is surgically prepared and the site desensitized with local anesthetic. A full-thickness skin stab incision is made and a teat cannula or small-bore thoracic tube is inserted into the pleural space. If suction equipment is available, the cannula or tube is attached to the system and suction is applied. Alternatively, a three-way stopcock tube system can be used, with repeated aspiration of air using a large syringe. Once the air is removed from the chest cavity, allowing reinflation of the lung, the cannula/tube should be removed and the incision sutured closed.

Prognosis

The prognosis is commonly dictated by the underlying cause, with cases of pneumothorax secondary to pleuro-pneumonia having a poorer prognosis compared with other causes of pneumothorax.

734 Two indwelling chest drains were placed in the horse in 733 in order to remove air (dorsal drain, red arrow) and pleural effusion (ventral drain, yellow arrow). Negative pressure was applied to the dorsal drain using a suction apparatus. Heimlich valves were attached to both drains for unidirectional movement of gas and fluid, preventing further pneumothorax from the presence of the drains.

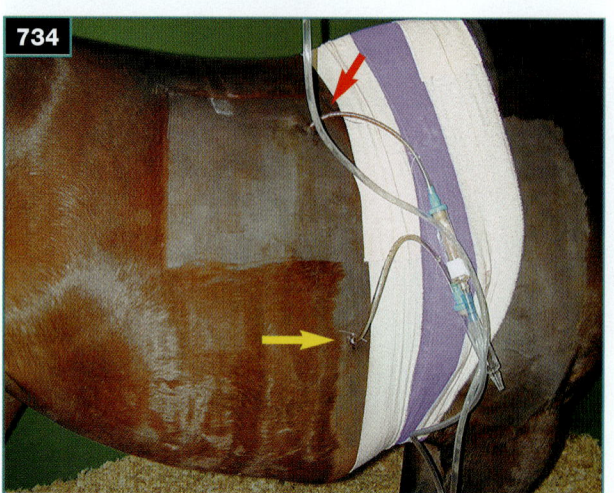

Chylothorax

Definition/overview

The accumulation of chyle in the pleural cavity is infrequently reported in horses. Chylous fluid is generally odorless and of milky and opalescent appearance. Currently, the number of equine cases of chylothorax is limited to a few case reports in foals.

Etiology/pathophysiology

Conditions affecting the thoracic duct (e.g. congenital abnormalities, traumatic rupture, or neoplastic erosion) are the most common causes of chylothorax in humans and have been reported in domestic small-animal species. However, in the majority of cases the cause is unknown. Similarly, in the majority of foals diagnosed with chylothorax the cause could not be determined.

Clinical presentation

Clinical signs reported in foals diagnosed with this condition include tachypnea, dyspnea, cough, lethargy, and pyrexia. Muffled lung sounds on auscultation have also been reported.

Differential diagnoses

Pleuropneumonia, hemothorax, hydrothorax, and diaphragmatic hernia should be considered.

Diagnosis

A fluid line is evident on chest percussion, with lung sounds decreased in the ventral lung fields. Thoracic ultrasonography is useful to detect fluid in the pleural cavity and to guide thoracocentesis. The physical appearance of the fluid is suggestive, but it is important to distinguish between true chyle and pseudochyle. Chyle fluid does not clear on centrifugation and chylomicron globules can be seen under microscopic examination. Special staining with Sudan III or IV, or oil red 0, will confirm the chylomicron globules. Triglyceride levels are usually increased in chyle compared with serum. Cytologic analysis may be variable. Generally, chyle is rich in lymphocytes, but in more chronic cases nondegenerate neutrophils may predominate.

Management

The treatment of chylothorax in small animals is variable and limited information is available in horses. Foals have been successfully managed with supportive care, broad-spectrum antimicrobials, thoracic drainage, and dietary management. Surgical management of chylothorax in small animals has yielded limited success, but has not been reported in horses.

Prognosis

The prognosis for long-term survival is not well known due to the limited number of cases. However, successful medical treatment had been reported in foals.

Hemothorax

Definition/overview

Blood accumulation in the pleural cavity may result from trauma to the pleural or pulmonary vessels or rupture of a large thoracic blood vessel (735). Other causes include hemangiosarcoma, coagulopathy, or iatrogenic hemothorax after thoracotomy or lung biopsy. Unilateral or bilateral hemothorax may be present, largely depending on the cause of the hemorrhage and whether the mediastinum is intact. In some cases of traumatic hemothorax, pneumothorax may also occur.

Clinical presentation

Clinical signs may be variable, depending on the cause. Horses may have signs of tachypnea, distress, pain, and shallow respiration following rib fracture. Animals may die acutely from severe hemorrhage in cases of rupture of a large vessel, or may develop anemia and hypoproteinemia over time if there is more gradual hemorrhage into the thoracic cavity.

Differential diagnoses

Other fluids in the thoracic cavity such as pleuropneumonia or hydrothorax may produce similar signs.

Diagnosis

Clinical examination is nonspecific, but may reveal decreased lung sounds ventrally and muffled heart sounds that radiate over a wide area. Percussion may detect ventral areas of dullness, but this procedure may be painful, especially in cases of thoracic trauma. Thoracic ultrasonography is the method of choice to detect fluid within the chest cavity. Blood within the thorax should appear homogeneous with no flocculation. Thoracocentesis for cytology, packed cell volume (PCV), and total protein concentration is indicated if a clear diagnosis of hemothorax cannot be reached when ultrasonographic findings are combined with history and physical examination. Thoracocentesis is accompanied by a risk of iatrogenic infection. In cases of hemothorax caused by thoracic trauma, the fluid should also be submitted for culture. Thoracic radiographs may be useful for identifying an underlying cause such as rib fracture.

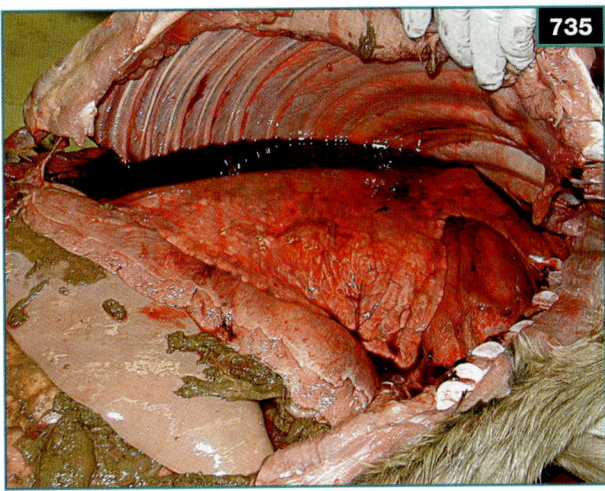

735 Hemothorax in a foal that occurred as a result of rib fracture from external trauma.

Management

The underlying cause should be addressed (i.e. fractured ribs should be stabilized if possible). Drainage of the chest is controversial and should only be performed to alleviate distress in cases with respiratory compromise resulting from excessive fluid accumulation or in the presence of infection. Many cases of hemothorax are treated successfully without drainage. Drainage is generally not recommended if hemothorax is due to clotting disorders. Supportive medical therapy, including intranasal oxygen supplementation, analgesics, intravenous fluids, or whole blood or plasma transfusions, may be necessary. Administration of fluids should be performed gradually to prevent systemic hypertension exacerbating hemorrhage in the acute period of treatment.

Prognosis

The prognosis is variable and depends largely on the underlying problem. Uncomplicated thoracic trauma may respond to medical therapy, but cases that develop secondary pleuritis carry a worse prognosis. Prognosis is also poor in cases of hemothorax secondary to neoplasia or clotting disorders.

Hydrothorax
Definition/overview
Hydrothorax is the accumulation of serous fluid in the pleural cavity, usually secondary to infectious causes such as AHS or noninfections conditions such as multicentric lymphoma, congestive heart failure, or hypoproteinemia.

Clinical presentation
Clinical signs reflect the volume of fluid accumulation and the underlying disease process. Signs may range from mild to severe, including dyspnea and cyanosis.

Differential diagnoses
Pleuropneumonia, hemothorax, and chylothorax may present similarly.

Diagnosis
Physical examination may reveal dyspnea, absent lung sounds ventrally, and dullness on percussion over the lower areas of the thorax. Thoracic ultrasonography is the method of choice to detect fluid within the chest cavity. The fluid should appear clear and homogeneous, with no flocculation. Thoracocentesis for cytology, PCV, and total protein concentration is indicated, but is accompanied by a risk of iatrogenic infection. Thoracic radiographs may be useful to identify an underlying cause such as neoplasia.

Management
The underlying cause should be addressed if possible. Drainage of the chest is controversial, and should only be performed to alleviate distress in cases with respiratory compromise resulting from excessive fluid accumulation.

Prognosis
This condition itself is not fatal, although the underlying disease dictates the prognosis.

Exercise-induced pulmonary hemorrhage
Definition/overview
EIPH refers to the presence of blood in the airways after exercise. Rapid bursts of intense exercise are most commonly associated with EIPH; consequently, affected animals include sprint-racing horses worldwide. The majority of racing horses experience some degree of EIPH during exercise. Other high-performance equine athletes (e.g. barrel-racing, cutting, reining, roping, polo, cross-country or 3-day-eventing, show-jumping, hunter-jumper, steeplechase, and draft horses) may also be affected. EIPH is of great concern to the racing industry due to the financial implications from decreased performance, lost training days, necessity for pre-race medication, and banning of horses from racing in some jurisdictions.

Etiology/pathophysiology
The exact cause of this condition is currently unknown, but a number of theories have been proposed. The most accepted explanation is stress failure of pulmonary capillaries as a result of high transmural pressure generated during exercise. However, this theory fails to explain the caudodorsal location within the lung where hemorrhage is first seen or the pattern of progression that occurs with EIPH. Another explanation, one that explains the site of initiation, nature of the lesion, and pattern of progression of EIPH, is that locomotory forces generated by the forelimb during galloping are responsible for damaging the lung. EIPH is commonly accompanied by airway inflammation, as detected by BAL, and the role of inflammation in the pathogenesis of EIPH is uncertain. Increased upper airway resistance, from nasal, pharyngeal or laryngeal dysfunction, can exacerbate EIPH. It is possible that the cause of EIPH is multifactorial in origin; therefore, multiple variables may need to be taken into account to better explain this condition.

Clinical presentation
The main clinical sign is the presence of blood within the airways; however, the majority of affected horses will not actually demonstrate epistaxis as the blood is often coughed up and swallowed. Horses may be slow to return to a resting respiratory rate after exercise, accompanied by prolonged peripheral vasodilation and sweating. Poor performance may occur, but in many horses EIPH does not appear to interfere with performance capacity.

Differential diagnoses
Other causes of epistaxis include guttural pouch mycosis, ethmoidal hematoma, pneumonia or pleuropneumonia, atrial fibrillation, and hemangiosarcoma. Less common causes of lung bleeding such as lung abscess, neoplasia, or foreign body should also be considered.

Diagnosis
Epistaxis is only seen in a small percentage of horses with EIPH after exercise. EIPH is currently diagnosed by endoscopic visualization of blood in the trachea post exercise (736–738). Endoscopic examination is recommended 90 minutes after exercise in order to increase the probability of detecting hemorrhage from distal airways in mild cases of EIPH.

Hemosiderin in alveolar macrophages (hemosiderophages) can be detected in BAL fluid (739). Although this confirms previous lung hemorrhage, it is not possible to estimate the time or severity of hemorrhage by cytology. Radiography, ultrasonography, and nuclear scintigraphy appear to have limited diagnostic value in the evaluation of EIPH, and their interpretation is difficult.

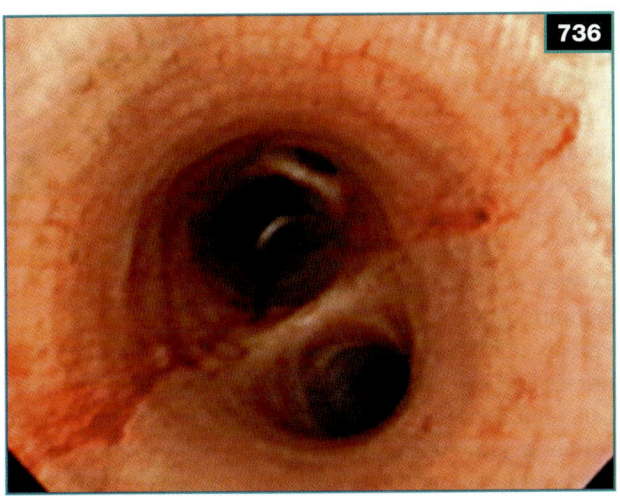

736 Bronchoscopic view of the carina in a horse with mild pulmonary hemorrhage as seen 30 minutes after intense exercise. A small trace of blood is visible from the right mainstem bronchus.

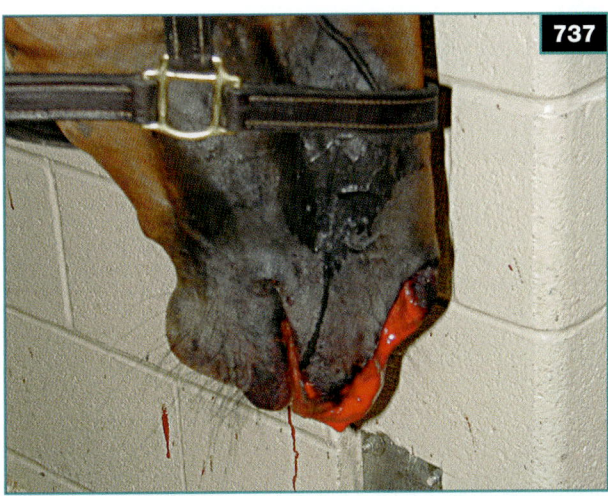

737 Severe pulmonary hemorrhage may appear as bilateral epistaxis following intense exercise. However, the majority of horses with pulmonary hemorrhage do not show blood at the nares because the blood is carried up the trachea by the mucociliary apparatus and is swallowed.

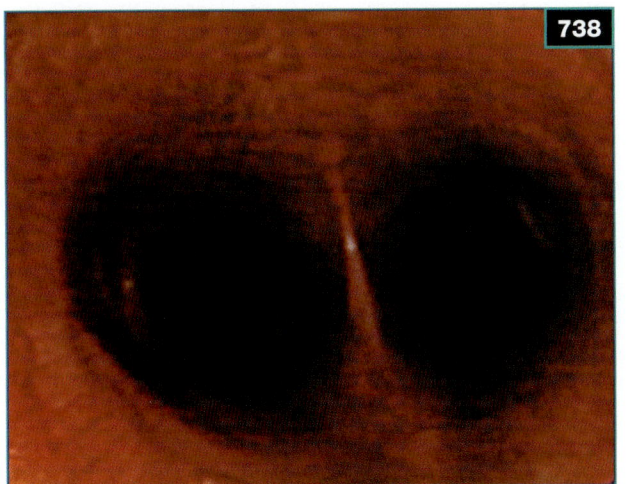

738 Bronchoscopic view of the carina in a horse with severe pulmonary hemorrhage, as seen immediately following a period of intense exercise. Streams of blood are present from both mainstem bronchi, and flecks of blood are seen throughout the rest of the trachea.

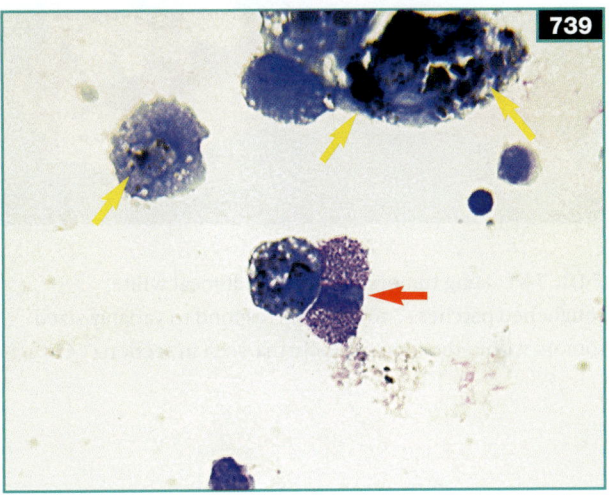

739 Cytology of BAL fluid from a horse with previous pulmonary hemorrhage. Hemosiderin is visible as dark pigment within pulmonary alveolar macrophages (yellow arrows). A mast cell (red arrow) is also present in this sample.

Management

Furosemide is widely used to manage EIPH during exercise, especially in the Thoroughbred racing industry. This medication may reduce the severity of hemorrhage in some horses, but it does not prevent bleeding completely. Currently, several additional treatments are used for EIPH, but their efficacy in treating and/or preventing this condition is unknown. Bronchodilators, broad-spectrum antimicrobials, and corticosteroids may improve general pulmonary health, but their impact on EIPH has not been demonstrated. Commercially available nasal strips have been shown to reduce upper airway inspiratory resistance and reduce the severity of EIPH during intense exercise. An emerging treatment is the use of hyperbaric oxygen therapy in affected horses, although scientific evaluation of the benefits of this treatment is currently lacking.

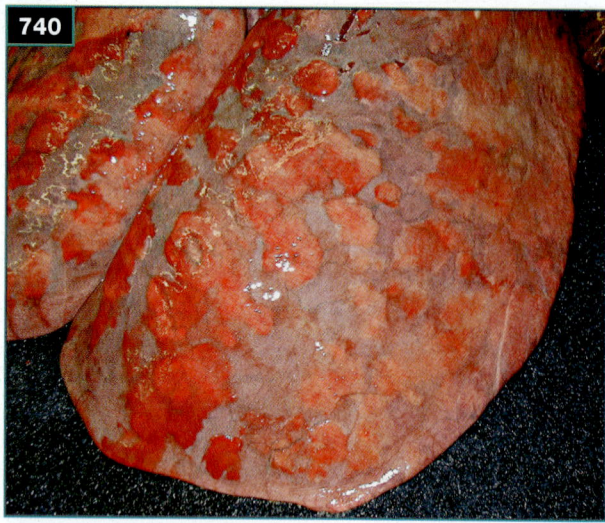

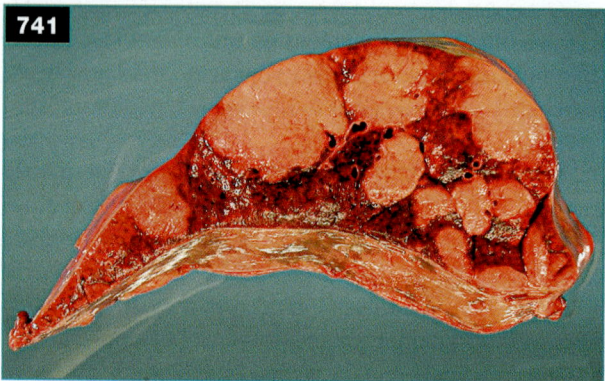

740, 741 Lung tumors. Note the multifocal white, roughened patches (740), that correspond to variably-sized tumors within the lung parenchyma, seen in section (741).

Prognosis
In the majority of horses with mild EIPH, the prognosis for performance is unaffected, but in more severely affected animals, pulmonary hemorrhage may be performance-limiting. A poor understanding of the pathogenesis, progression, and appropriate treatment of this condition makes the prognosis uncertain in such animals.

Lower respiratory tract neoplasia
Definition/overview
Primary pulmonary neoplasias are reported infrequently in horses and include pulmonary lymphosarcoma, granular cell tumor, pulmonary adenocarcinoma, bronchogenic carcinoma, pulmonary carcinoma, bronchogenic SCC, pulmonary chondrosarcoma, and bronchial myxoma (740, 741). Affected animals are generally mature horses (>7 years of age). Similarly, metastatic pulmonary neoplasias are uncommon in horses, but occur more frequently than primary lung tumors. These include hemangiosarcoma, squamous cell carcinoma, adenocarcinoma, fibrosarcoma, hepatoblastoma, chondrosarcoma, and undifferentiated sarcomas or carcinomas among others. Lung metastatic tumors have been reported in animals as young as 3 months of age.

Clinical presentation
Clinical signs are nonspecific, but may include depression, exercise intolerance, weight loss, and fever, which can be intermittent. Other signs such as cough, epistaxis, or dyspnea may occur. Pleural effusion is common, especially in some metastatic tumors.

Diagnosis
Diagnostic screening tests that may help to identify neoplasia include cytologic examination of tracheobronchial aspirates, BAL fluid, or pleural fluid.

Thoracic radiographs usually identify the presence of one or multiple soft-tissue opacities and may suggest the presence of pleural effusion. Ultrasonography will confirm the presence of pleural fluid and may also reveal an irregular lung surface or architecture for masses located at the lung surface. Ultrasound-guided biopsy of thoracic or pulmonary masses may allow antemortem diagnosis of lung tumors by histology, histochemistry, and/or immunohistochemistry.

Prognosis
The prognosis is generally poor, although it may depend on the type of tumor. By the time the tumor is clinically evident and is subsequently diagnosed, lesions are frequently advanced and the animal has developed systemic complications.

4

Gastrointestinal system

1   Upper gastrointestinal tract

Henry Tremaine

2   Lower gastrointestinal tract

Scott Weese, Ludovic Boure, Simon Pearce, and Nathalie Cote

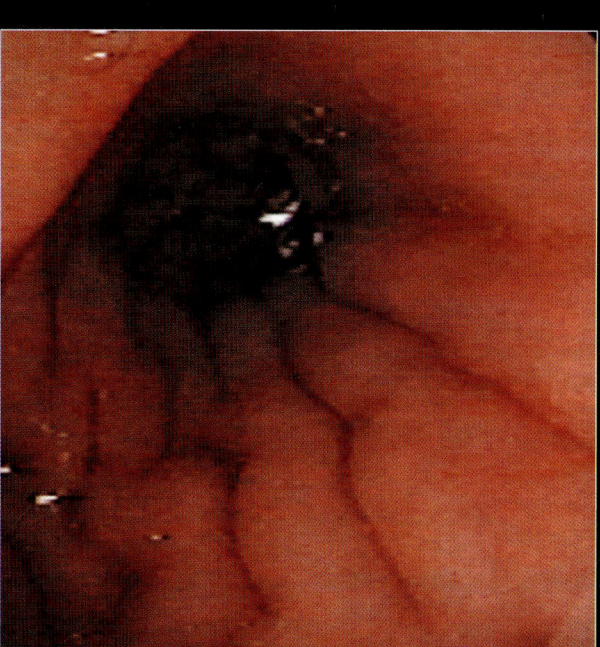

Upper gastrointestinal tract

The equine alimentary tract comprises the oral cavity and its associated structures and the pharynx, esophagus, stomach, small intestine, cecum, colon, and rectum, and presents a challenging field of investigation for the equine clinician. A detailed knowledge of the structure and function of the different components of the tract is a prerequisite for understanding disturbances present in the diseased state. The complicated anatomy, physiology, and pathology requires the use of a variety of techniques to enable the clinician to investigate and treat thoroughly any diseases affecting the GI system. The function of the GI tract can be summarized as the prehension and processing of food and water to provide water and nutrients for normal metabolic activity and, therefore, any disease that affects the alimentary tract is liable to have far-reaching effects on other body systems.

Examination of the oral cavity and teeth

Introduction

An examination of the oral cavity should be performed using a full mouth speculum (gag) to enable a thorough visual and digital examination. Diseases affecting the oral cavity may not result in clinical signs until quite advanced, and a cursory look into the oral cavity can easily result in diseases in their early stages being overlooked. Many horses will require sedation in order to complete this procedure thoroughly and safely; alpha-2 agonists such as romifidine, detomidine, and xylazine, in combination with opiate partial agonists such as butorphanol, at standard doses, are suitable for this. A bright light source is essential and head torches are a convenient way of illuminating the oral cavity for examination. The examination is best conducted in the sedated horse with the horse's head supported on a head-stand or suspended halter. The occlusal surfaces and buccal palatal margins of all teeth should be inspected; subsequently, a dental mirror is used to demonstrate the occlusal surfaces and interproximal spaces. In addition, digital palpation should be performed to detect defects that may be obscured by the tongue, and the teeth should be counted carefully to avoid missing supernumerary teeth. Lesions are identified and `recorded (e.g. on a dental chart) and a treatment plan formulated that may be staged on different occasions for complicated treatments. Dental defects should be recorded using the Triadan system (742) and dental charts are a convenient method of doing this. A more detailed examination of the occlusal surfaces of the caudal cheek teeth can be performed with the assistance of an endoscope.

742 Triadan representation of adult equine teeth.

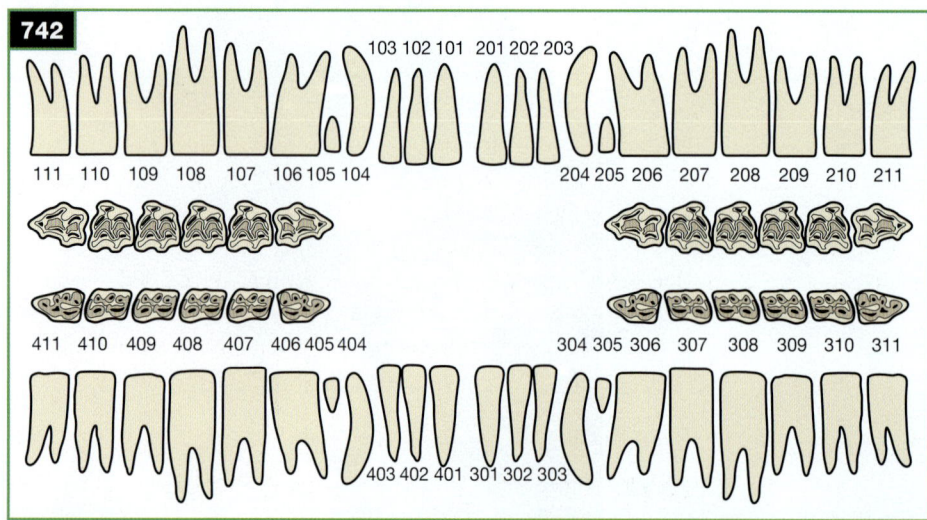

742

103 102 101   201 202 203

111 110 109 108 107 106 105 104   204 205 206 207 208 209 210 211

411 410 409 408 407 406 405 404   304 305 306 307 308 309 310 311

403 402 401 301 302 303

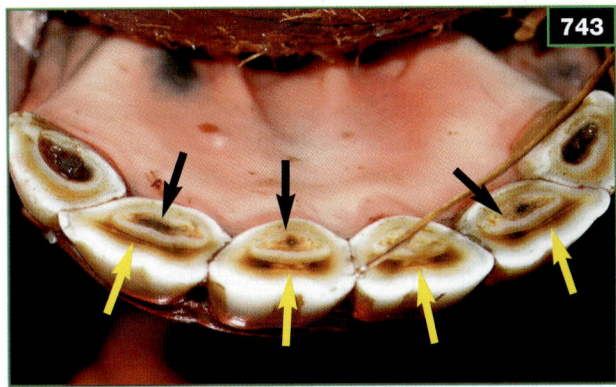

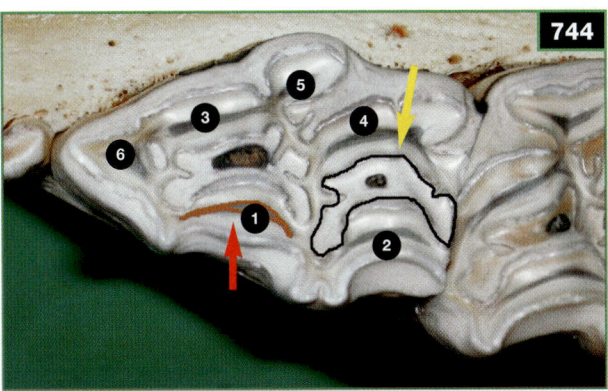

743 Occlusal surface of the incisors in a horse of 7–9 years of age. The ring of infundibular enamel or dental mark is clearly visible (black arrows). On the rostral aspect of this, the brown dental star or secondary dentine lining the pulp is visible on the central and middle incisors (yellow arrows).

744 Occlusal surface of maxillary tooth 106 showing infundibular enamel (yellow arrow, delineated in black) and secondary dentine (red arrow), which corresponds to the pulp horns (labeled 1–6).

The incisors are examined initially without a speculum for contact and evenness of bite. Lateral displacement of the mandible relative to the maxilla (termed 'lateral excursion') will result in the cheek teeth coming into occlusion when the mandible is displaced 1–2 cm to that side. Further displacement of the mandible will result in separation of the incisors and the angled occlusal surfaces of the upper and lower cheek teeth will slide over each other. This is repeated on the contralateral side and the occlusion should be symmetrical. Next, a cheek retractor is placed in the commissure of the lips to displace the cheek, allowing inspection of the buccal aspects of the maxillary teeth and also their degree of occlusion, both at rest and when the mandible is displaced.

Normal dentition and age-related changes

Horses have 24 deciduous teeth, which can be represented by the formula 2 × (Di 3/3, Dc 0/0, Dp 3/3) = 24. The formula for the permanent dentition is represented by 2 × (I 3/3, C 1/1, P 3 or 4/3, M 3/3) = 40 or 42. There are no deciduous molars and the 1st premolar (termed the 'wolf tooth') is variably present. Each tooth is composed of an exposed clinical crown and a larger reserve crown, which is embedded in the bony alveolus. Attrition at the occlusal surface occurs at 2–3 mm/year and continuous eruption of the reserve crown maintains approximately 2 cm of exposed crown.

Incisor teeth

Incisor teeth are simple rooted or brachydont teeth. Each mandible and incisive bone contains three incisors, which are in close apposition to each other, arranged in an approximate semicircle. Once in wear, the occlusal surfaces of opposing incisors meet closely to enable close cropping of grass (743). Inspection of the occlusal surfaces reveals a conical indentation in the enamel and cementum, which when worn appears as a ring of enamel or infundibulum (termed the dental cup), the appearance of which varies with the age of the horse. Progressive attrition reveals the brown-stained secondary dentine laid down by odontoblasts in the pulp cavity. This is called the 'dental star' and it lies labial to the infundibulum.

Canine teeth

The canine teeth are present in male horses and occasionally in female horses. They erupt in the interdental space midway between the corner incisor and the first premolar, with the lower canine being more rostral. The canine teeth are brachydont and sustain no attrition of the occlusal surfaces. Their role is in defense rather than mastication. The reserve crown is sickle shaped and extends caudally towards the apex.

Premolars and molars

The first premolars (wolf teeth) are often rudimentary, with a short reserve crown. They lie variably from the middle of the interdental space to a position in close apposition just rostral to the second premolar. They are present in most horses and historically have been removed, although the medical reasons for this are currently being reviewed. The remaining premolars and the three molars termed 'cheek teeth' differ between the mandibular and maxillary arcades.

The maxillary cheek teeth have occlusal surfaces containing two crescent-shaped infundibula (744). The marginal enamel on the palatal and buccal aspects

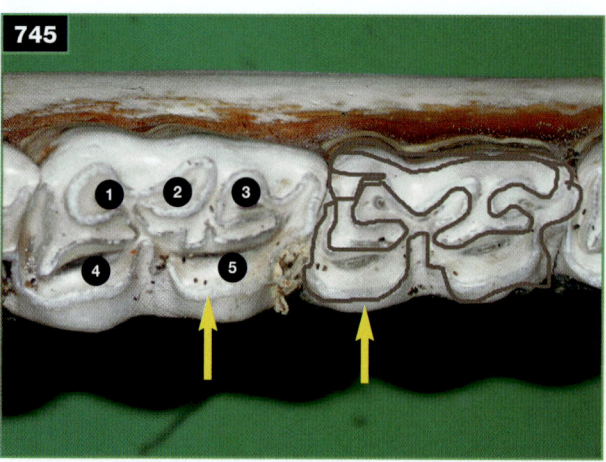

745 Occlusal surface of mandibular teeth 408 and 409 showing continuous enamel (yellow arrows, delineated in black on 408) and secondary dentine, corresponding to pulp horns 1–5 (labeled).

contains undulations forming sharp cingula on the latter aspect and transverse ridges giving the surface a serrated appearance. The maxillary teeth have one large palatal root and two buccal roots. The 1st and 6th cheek teeth typically have an additional pulp cavity at the rostral and caudal aspect, respectively. The apices of the first two maxillary cheek teeth and the rostral root of the 3rd (107s, 108s) typically lie in the maxillary bone. The remaining roots of the 3rd tooth and those of the 4th cheek (109s) tooth lie in an alveolus in close association with the rostral maxillary sinuses. The alveoli surrounding the apices of the 5th and 6th cheek teeth lie in the caudal maxillary sinus on each side.

The mandibular cheek teeth in contrast have no infundibula, but they have infolding of the peripheral enamel, which creates ridges on the occlusal surface once they are in wear (745). Each of the first five teeth in the mandibular arcade has two major roots, with the sixth having an additional pulp cavity and a smaller root. The maxillary arcade is 23–30% wider than the mandibular arcade at any point (anisognathism). The apices of the mandibular cheek teeth lie in the mandible and they are aligned in an approximately straight line, as viewed rostrocaudally.

Composition of equine teeth

Equine teeth are composed of a laminate of three mineralized tissues arranged around the dental pulp, which contains the nervous and vascular supply to the tooth. Equine dental enamel is the hardest substance in the skeleton, comprising 96% inorganic hydroxyapatite crystals. There is no self-reparative process in enamel, but there is very high wear resistance, which makes it vulnerable to cracking. Dentine is the second hardest skeletal tissue; it comprises 70% of the mass of the tooth and is composed of 70% hydroxyapatite and 30% organic tissues, which confers higher elasticity than enamel and increased resistance to cracking. Dentine can be categorized into primary and secondary dentine. Secondary dentine in hypsodont teeth is produced by the odontoblasts lining the pulp cavity throughout the life of the animal in response to attrition at the occlusal surface. It maintains the physical barrier between the oral cavity and the pulp. Equine pulp is incompletely studied, but it consists of a meshwork of connective tissue, reticulin fibers, and vascular and neurologic elements. The vasculature in the pulp passes through wide apical foramina in young horses to fulfill the nutritional requirements of the active odontoblast. The apical foramina are radiologically narrowed in aged horses.

Cement is similar to bone in composition, comprising approximately 65% impure hydroxyappatite crystals. It lines the reserve crowns of the teeth and, in the case of the incisors and maxillary cheek teeth, lines the infundibula. The peripheral cementum grows throughout life, whereas the infundibula cement is devoid of vascularity and can be considered as dead tissue. The cementum's main function is for attachment of the Sharpie's fibers. The cement in the enamel invaginations in the enamel lakes of maxillary teeth is incomplete and may be hypoplastic, resulting in carious defects that may result in apical pulpitis. The periodontal ligament complex consists of a layer of vascular innervated connective tissue comprising the cementum, collagen and the alveolar periosteum. The connective tissue fibers (termed 'Sharpie's fibers') suspend the tooth in the alveolus and provide compressive elasticity and resistance during mastication. Radiographically, the Sharpie's fibers insert into a layer of dense lamellar alveolar bone known as the lamina dura denta.

Dental nomenclature

The Triadan system is now in widespread use for equine dental nomenclature. It avoids the confusion between the notation of the premolars and molars as the cheek teeth 1–6 (starting with the second premolar), as preferred by many authors in Europe, and the classification into premolars and molars as preferred by authors in the USA. Under this system, each tooth has a unique identification number (742).

TABLE 17 Eruption ages of equine teeth

TOOTH	TRIADAN NUMBER	ERUPTION AGE	IN WEAR
Deciduous incisors			
Central	501	3 days	
Middle	502	3 weeks	
Corner	503	3 months	
Deciduous premolars			
1st cheek tooth	506	birth	
2nd cheek tooth	507	birth	
3rd cheek tooth	508	birth	
Permanent incisors			
Central	101 (2, 3, 401)	2.5 years	
Middle	102	3.5 years	
Corner	103	4.5 years	
Canines	104	5 years	
Permanent premolars			
1st premolar (wolf tooth)	105	2–2.5 years	
2nd premolar (1st cheek tooth)	106	3 years	3.5 years
3rd premolar (2nd cheek tooth)	107	4 years	4.5 years
4th premolar (3rd cheek tooth)	108	1 year	1.5 years
1st molar (4th cheek tooth)	109	2 years	2.5 years
2nd molar (5th cheek tooth)	110	3–3.5 years	3.5 years
3rd molar (6th cheek tooth)	111	?????	?????

Age-related changes in the appearance of teeth with eruption and aging (*Table 17*)

As the occlusal surfaces of the teeth are worn during food prehension and mastication, their appearance changes. The cementum and enamel covering the surface are worn as the horse chews. This results in exposure of primary dentine on the occlusal surface and the enamel takes on the appearance of a continuous raised ridge surrounding the dentine and bounded by the peripheral cementum. In the incisors and maxillary cheek teeth the infundibula become raised concentric circles or crescents.

In the incisor the central enamel of the infundibulum (dental mark) is filled with nonregenerative infundibular cement and the invagination (dental cup) becomes filled with organic material, which undergoes oxidation to gain a dark appearance. As the tooth erupts the infundibulum becomes narrower and the amount of organic material becomes reduced, resulting in gradual obliteration of the dental cup (746). Eventually, in aging horses (9–11 years), the infundibular enamel is worn away in the central

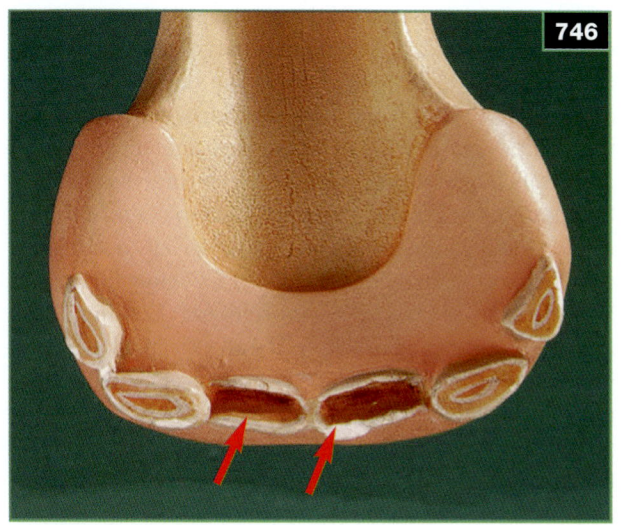

746 Cast of rostral mandible of a 2.5-year-old horse showing erupted permanent central incisors, with a large infundibular cup (arrows).

485

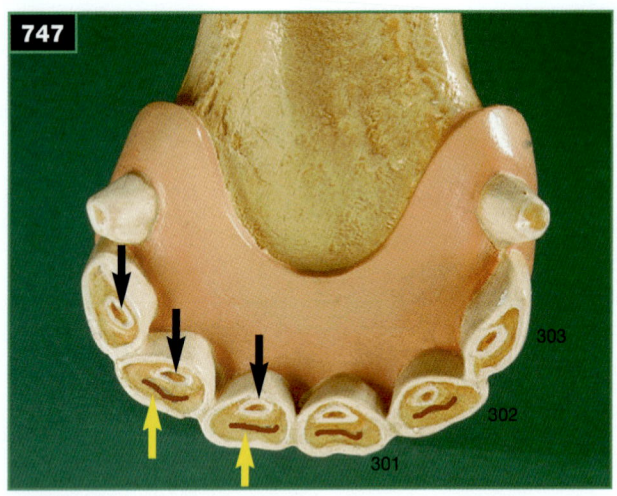

747 Incisors of a 9-year-old horse showing permanent incisors (301, 302, 303), with ovoid infundibular dental marks (black arrows) and rostrally located brown secondary dentine forming the dental stars in the central and middle incisors (yellow arrows).

In horses aged 2–4 years old, the tooth is growing in length at its apical aspect and is also in the process of erupting (or, additionally, displacing deciduous premolars). During this time the tooth exhibits its maximal length and occupies the full depth of the bone in which lies the alveolus. Thus in 2- and 3-year-old horses and ponies the mandibular medulla is full to its depth, with the reserve crowns of the erupting 07s and 08s. In many cases some modeling of the ventral mandible occurs to accommodate this increase in length of the tooth at the time preceding and during eruption. This is observed and palpated as bilaterally symmetrical, bony, nonpainful swellings on the ventral mandible overlying the apices of the 07s and 08s. These are particularly prominent in horses derived from Arab breeds. Similar corresponding swellings resulting from maxillary modeling occur, but are less obvious due to the overlying levator nasolabialis muscle. These are more commonly detected in miniature and native northern European breeds. Radiography can demonstrate significant thinning of the mandibular cortex at these sites. At this age, reserve crowns of the maxillary 08–11s occupy most of the space in the rostral and caudal maxillary sinus. As the tooth erupts with age, the alveolus remodels and the sinus cavity increases in volume. As the teeth erupt, the alveolar bone remodels to gradually fill the interdental spaces and has an increased radio-opacity in aged horses.

Dental imaging

In addition to oral examination, ancillary techniques are sometimes necessary to reveal additional diagnostic information about suspected dental disease. Radiography is the most widely used and, despite certain limitations, enables examination of dental apices and changes to surrounding alveolar bone. Nuclear scintigraphy has been demonstrated to be a useful complement to radiography, especially for the diagnosis of suspected dental apical disease at an early stage.

incisors first, followed by the middle and corner incisors, and the dental mark eventually disappears to leave an occlusal surface consisting entirely of dentine.

As the occlusal surface is worn, the pulp cavity eventually becomes exposed. Odontoblasts lining the pulp chamber produce secondary dentine in the pulp cavity, which maintains the separation of the pulp from the oral cavity. The secondary dentine becomes darkly stained and appears rostral to the 'dental mark' as a 'dental star', which appears at between 8 and 10 years of age, commencing at the central incisors (747). The exact age at which the appearance changes varies between individuals and breeds and it is generally accepted that in contrast to historical belief, these changes are not sufficiently accurate or reliable to be used as definitive means of aging the animal. Knowledge of such changes is useful for checking documentation and can be used to place an individual in an age range based on the appearance of the incisors. Other features such as the timing of the appearance of hooks and Galvayne's groove are unreliable. The angle between the upper and lower incisors becomes more acute with age, and this is reflected in changes in the shape of the occlusal surface from oval in young horses to triangular or trapezoid in geriatric horses and ponies. Some variation has also been described between different breeds of horse.

Eruption of the cheek teeth with age results in some modeling of the maxilla and mandible as the tooth erupts.

TABLE 18 **Examples of exposure factors for the equine head**		
VIEW	KV	MAS
Lateral–lateral	73–81	6.6–10
Lateral 30° dorsolateral oblique or lateral 45° ventrolateral oblique	73–81	6.6–10
Dorsoventral	77–85	10
Intraoral (incisors)	66	6.3

Gastrointestinal system

748 Lateral–lateral projection.

749 Lateral 30° dorsolateral oblique projection.

750 Lateral 45° ventrolateral oblique projection.

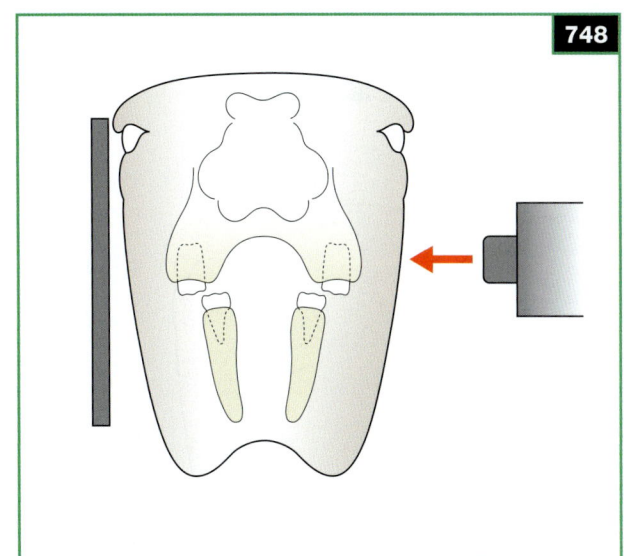

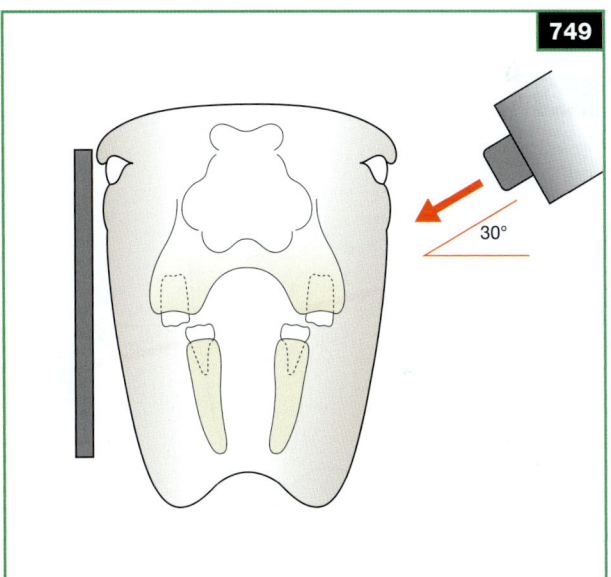

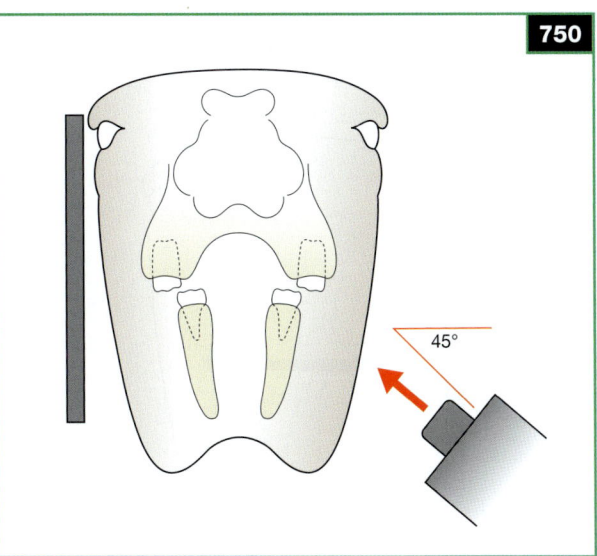

The sharp radiographic contrast between the air in the paranasal sinuses and the nasal cavities, the mandibular bone, and the more radiodense cheek teeth means that diagnostically useful images of the maxillary and mandibular cheek teeth can be obtained without difficulty. Interpretation of equine dental radiographs can be difficult, but it is facilitated by obtaining good-quality radiographs. Most portable machines have sufficient kV output to obtain diagnostic radiographs of the horse's head in the field situation. Examples of exposure factors are shown in *Table 18*, but an exposure technique chart is best compiled for each individual machine and for the film–screen combination used. High-resolution films with a wide gray scale (e.g. mammography films) produce the most detailed images and digital radiography appears to offer increased sensitivity.

Sedation is necessary to reduce head movement and motion blur. A head-stand or stool is useful to support the horse's head with minimal movement. The normal halter should be replaced with a rope halter or one made of radiolucent material. A minimum of two people is usually necessary to position the horse's head and cassette accurately, and adequate radiation protection, including lead gowns and gloves or sleeves, is mandatory. Cassette holders should always be used and these may be mounted on handles or suspended from a stand. The primary beam should always be collimated to prevent exposure of any parts of the assistants, even if they are wearing lead protection.

Standard views include the lateral–lateral projection (**748**) (sometimes referred to as a lateral projection) and the lateral 30° dorsolateral oblique (**749**) and lateral 45° ventrolateral oblique (**750**) projections. The exact angle of obliquity necessary to obtain diagnostic radiographs with the oblique views varies between approximately 30° and 45° for different individuals and breeds. The lateral–lateral view results in superimposition of the contralateral maxillary and mandibular cheek teeth rows, which can result in difficulty in interpreting changes to individual dental apices. This view is useful for demonstrating the presence of exudate in the paranasal sinuses, which are radiographically visible as fluid lines. There is minimal parallax distortion in a rostrocaudal direction on this projection, and it is therefore frequently used with radio-opaque markers such as metal probes.

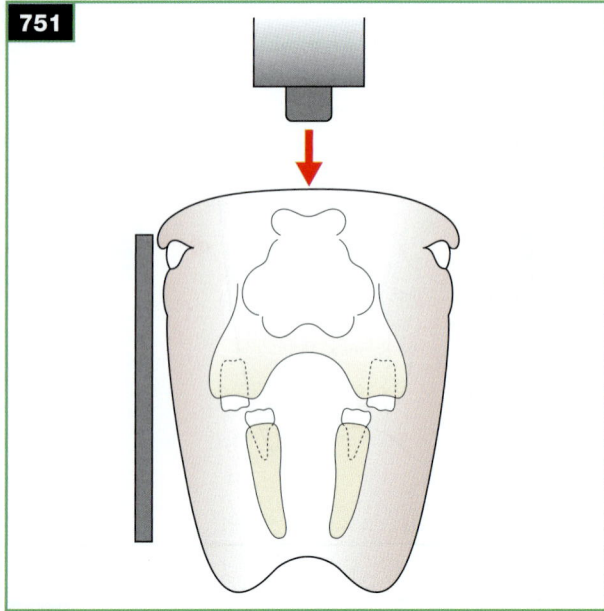

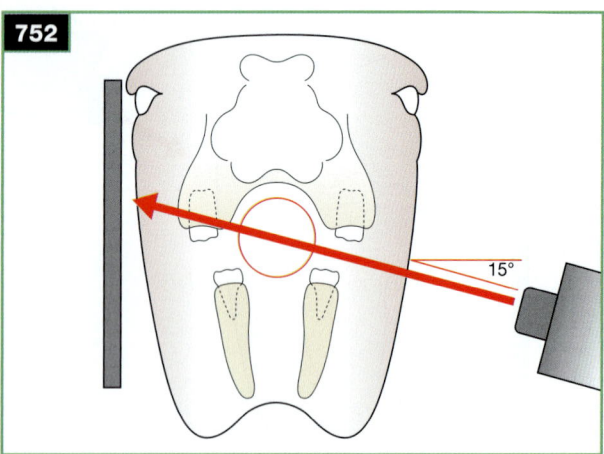

15°

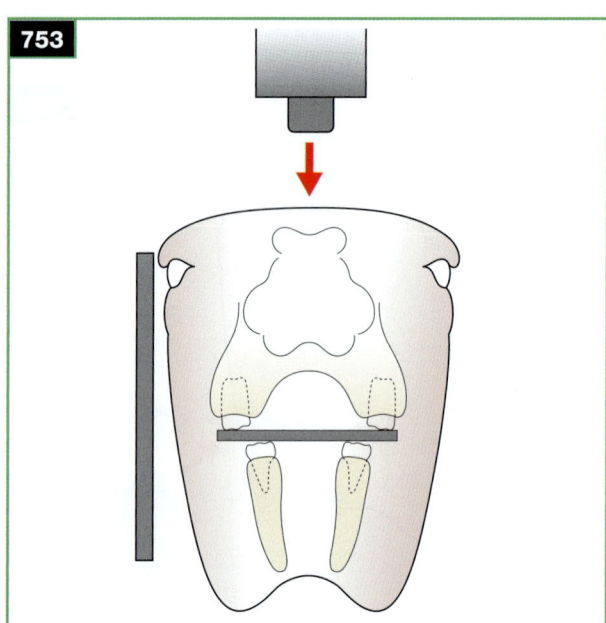

751 Dorsoventral projection.

752 Lateral 15° ventrolateral open-mouthed oblique projection.

753 Dorsoventral intraoral projection.

The lateral 30° dorsolateral oblique projection results in radiographic separation of the contralateral cheek teeth rows and is used to image the apices of the maxillary cheek teeth. The lateral 45° ventrolateral oblique projection is used to image the apices of the mandibular teeth. The latter two projections may be further improved by separating the maxillary and mandibular cheek teeth rows using a Butler's gag or plastic tube gag. Additional views that may be useful include the dorsoventral (DV) (**751**) or ventrodorsal (VD), open-mouthed oblique (OMO) (**752**), and ventrodorsal or dorsoventral intraoral projections (**753**). The dorsoventral projection can be further modified by displacement of the mandible to one side to reduce the superimposition of upper and lower cheek teeth rows. The OMO projection is particularly useful for examining the erupted crowns of the cheek teeth. Lateral 15° ventrolateral projections are used to image the maxillary cheek teeth and lateral 10–15° dorsolateral projections are used for the mandibular cheek teeth. The exact angle depends on the size and breed of horse and the individual teeth that are of most interest. Horses with a steeply angled occlusal surface of the caudal mandibular cheek teeth may require multiple views at different angles to image all the teeth without superimposition.

Routine dental examination and prophylaxis

Routine dental care necessitates a regular dental examination and correction of any dental disorders in order to restore normal occlusion and enable normal mastication. Examination visually and digitally with a full-mouth speculum such as a Hausmann's or Meister-type gag is a prerequisite before performing any procedures (**754**).

A check-list for routine examination is listed below:

✦ Examination of body condition of animal.
✦ Observation while eating forage.
✦ Palpation of temporomandibular joints and temporal muscles.
✦ Palpation of buccal molar arcades through the cheeks.
✦ Palpation of submandibular lymph nodes.
✦ Lateral movement of the mandible to check excursion.
✦ Examination of the incisor tables to check compatibility with documented age.
✦ Application of gag (sedation if required).
✦ Visual examination of all four molar arcades.
✦ Digital palpation of each tooth.
✦ Recording of observations and intended treatments.

- Perform dental treatments on molar arcades.
- Removal of speculum.
- Perform incisor treatments.
- Elevation of cheek to visualize buccal aspect of maxillary arcade.
- Irrigation of the mouth and cleaning of all instruments.

For a full description on the management of equine dental diseases the reader is directed to references specific to this topic. All dental examinations should commence with a thorough examination of the head and structures surrounding the oral cavity. In order to examine the oral cavity thoroughly, a full mouth speculum and a bright light source such as a head lamp should be used. The aim of routine prophylaxis is to restore normal masticatory function to the occlusal surfaces and to remove any focal dental overgrowths resulting from uneven wear, which may be causing soft-tissue trauma or preventing normal masticatory movement. This is done using a combination of manual rasps, of which there are many types, or by using rotating tungsten carbide or industrial diamond burrs, powered by a variety of electrical, cable-driven, or pneumatic motors. The manual rasps are more suitable for smaller overgrowths and are very safe to use in field situations. When using solid carbide blades care must be taken to avoid accidental trauma to the gingivae, which will cause undesirable hemorrhage. The rasps are applied to remove sharp edges from the occlusal surfaces and from the buccal aspects of maxillary teeth and the lingual aspects of the mandibular teeth. Practice is necessary to acquire proficiency for effective rasping, using both hands in an ergonomically comfortable position. The mechanical

tools are more efficient and can be used to more precisely remove dental material. However, if used irresponsibly, they can cause excessive heating of the tooth, removal of excessive occlusal surface, and exposure of vital pulp. Horses should always be sedated when using such tools to enable accurate treatment with precise visual control. Water cooling of some description is advised to cool and lubricate the burr and to remove dental dust. A repeated examination of the whole mouth, including an assessment of the occlusion, should be performed after any treatments to assess progress.

Diseases of the teeth and oral cavity

CONDITIONS ASSOCIATED WITH ERUPTION OF THE TEETH

Diseases associated with the development and eruption of the teeth are most commonly detected in younger horses up to 4 years of age when the teeth are erupting and the deciduous dentition is replaced by the permanent dentition. Anatomic abnormalities that are a consequence of developmental abnormalities may also have secondary consequences in older horses.

Cemental hypoplasia

Definition/overview

Developmental abnormalities in the infundibular cement result in a defect in the cemental layer that can predispose the tooth to diseases affecting the deeper layers.

Etiology/pathophysiology

Cementum is laid down in the incisor and maxillary infundibula prior to eruption by invasion of the invagination in the enamel surface by a layer of cementoblasts. Cement formation occurs with maturation and increasing density of the cementoblasts until eruption, at which point this cementum becomes avascular and ceases to develop. The condition is seen in maxillary cheek teeth, and the 4th cheek tooth (Triadan 109, 209) appears to be most commonly affected. Mandibular teeth with no infundibular cementum may have peripheral cemental hypoplasia, which is less often clinically significant.

Clinical presentation

Cemental hypoplasia can be seen as a deep pocket on the occlusal surface of the maxillary cheek teeth into which food can become packed, with further cemental dissolution. It may represent a benign variation on normal development and has variously been described as infundibular necrosis and cemental caries. It is unclear whether severe cemental hypoplasia of the enamel lakes can predispose to weakness and fracturing of the tooth

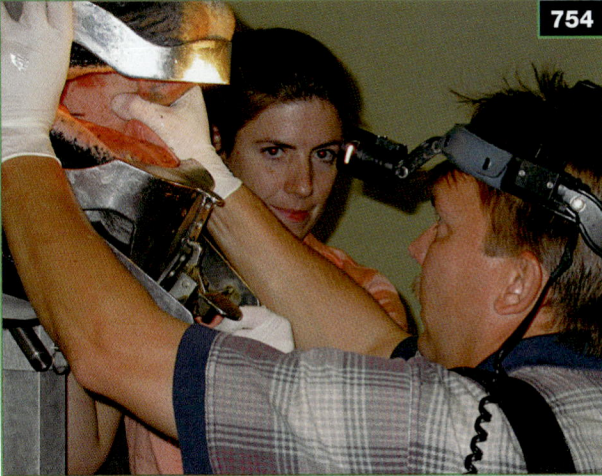

754 A good full-mouth speculum and a powerful light source are prerequisites for a thorough dental examination.

489

through the infundibula. Most parasagittal fractures involving maxillary cheek teeth occur in a plane adjoining buccal pulp cavities, but fractures adjoining infundibula affected by caries also occur.

Differential diagnosis
Caries of the teeth can be the consequence of abnormalities of wear or iatrogenic dental fractures.

Diagnosis
Careful oral examination and the use of dental probes should be adequate for diagnosis.

Management
The presence of cemental hypoplasia may be clinically insignificant. It has been suggested that such cases are likely to predispose to caries. Currently, teeth with advanced caries usually require removal by extraction, repulsion, or buccotomy. It is possible that in the future, viable pulp sealing may be increasingly used to prevent the progression of cemental hypoplasia to caries.

Oligodontia
Definition/overview
Oligodontia is defined as the loss or absence of teeth in an arcade or row.

Etiology/pathophysiology
Oligodontia is common and most acquired cases result from tooth loss following periodontal disease in aged horses or traumatic injury to the developing permanent secondary dentition prior to eruption. Following loss of a tooth, migration of the adjacent teeth occurs, which may result in complete obliteration of the space and shortening of the arcade.

Clinical presentation
The condition may present as a range of secondary dental disorders including dysmastication, overgrowths, and oral dysphagia.

Diagnosis
Diagnosis is based on careful oral examination in conjunction with radiography, if indicated.

Management
Loss of a cheek tooth in a mature horse frequently leads to a palpable space between the remaining teeth and invagination of the empty alveolus with fibrous tissue. Super-eruption of the tooth opposing the absent one can occur in the opposing arcade. More frequent reduction of overgrowths in the super-erupting and adjacent teeth may be required.

Heterotopic polyodontia (dentigerous cysts)
Definition/overview
Dentigerous cysts are congenital abnormalities due to an embryologic disorder leading to anatomically inappropriate dental tissue, often close to the pinna (755).

Etiology/pathophysiology
Heterotopic polyodontia is a well-recognized condition involving the presence of ectopic dental tissue containing rudimentary enamel and other dental elements. The condition can present at any age and is often coincidental with the age of eruption of the teeth (usually less than 3 years). The most common site is at the base of the pinna. The cyst has a stratified squamous epithelium and goblet cells that secrete a seromucinous fluid, which commonly discharges through a duct onto the skin, often halfway up the leading edge of the pinna. The degree of development and organization of the dental elements varies from minimal mineralization of the cyst to partially molarized, rudimentary teeth. The lesion is derived from an embryologic abnormality of the first branchial arch, which becomes displaced into the temporal region.

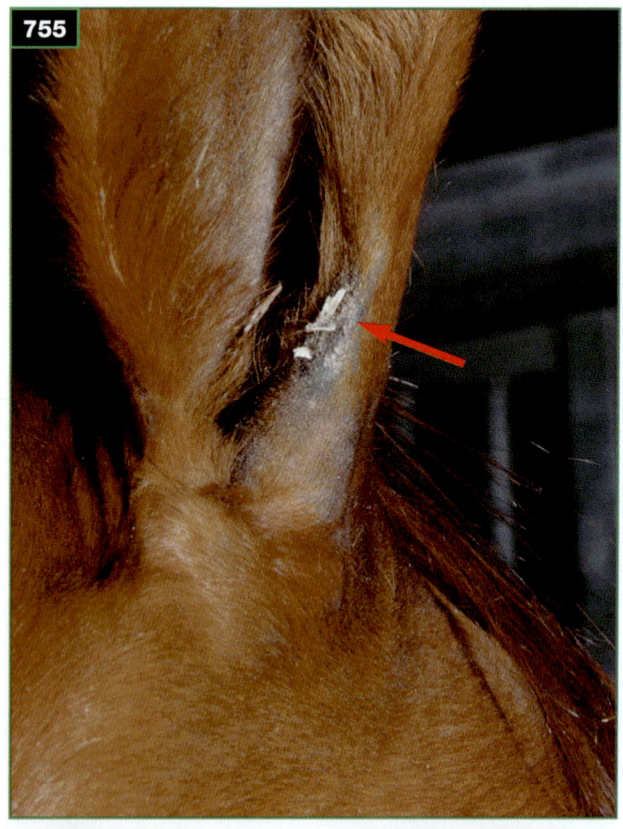

755 The tract discharging from the base of the pinna in this horse (arrow) is typical in cases of dentigerous cyst.

Clinical presentation

Clinically these lesions present as nonpainful swellings over the temporal bone, which characteristically have a duct discharging mucoid or mucopurulent exudates from an orifice at the base or edge of the pinna.

Differential diagnosis

Discharging sinus tracts, sequestra, and skull fractures should be considered.

Diagnosis

The site of the lesion can make radiography awkward, but lesion-orientated oblique projections complement the standard views and ultrasonography can be helpful. It is important to assess the depth of the lesion before embarking on treatment.

Management

In cases where clinical abnormalities are present, careful surgical excision of the lesion, including the entire cystic lining, is recommended. Recurrence is rare following complete removal of the cyst lining.

Rudimentary teeth ('wolf teeth')

Definition/overview

The presence of vestigial brachydont 1st premolars.

Etiology/pathophysiology

The 1st upper premolar (Triadan 105, 205) is commonly present in both male and female horses (756). These vestigial 'wolf teeth' are present in an estimated 20–60% of horses, according to different studies. They are usually in contact with the 106 and 206 and are rarely in occlusion. More occasionally, molarized 105s and 205s are present. Traditional practice has been to remove the wolf teeth under standing chemical restraint and local analgesia. Historically, reduced performance and bit sensitivity has been attributed to discomfort associated with the impingement of the bit over the wolf teeth, with little or no supportive data in most cases, especially where the tooth is a normally situated vestigial wolf tooth. The recent but controversial practice of excessive rasping of the buccorostral aspects of the 106 and 206 to create 'bit seats' is said to be impaired by the presence of wolf teeth, and has been cited as another reason for their removal. Undoubtedly, in some cases, especially where the 105 or 205 is very large, erupting in a rostral or buccal position or when there is clear indication of pain over, for example, an unerupted tooth, the removal of the whole vestigial tooth under standing chemical restraint and local analgesia is indicated. Entrapment of the buccal mucosa between the bit and the wolf tooth or rostrolateral aspect of the 2nd premolar can result in discomfort. Consequently, a lack of responsiveness on the bridle is attributed to their presence.

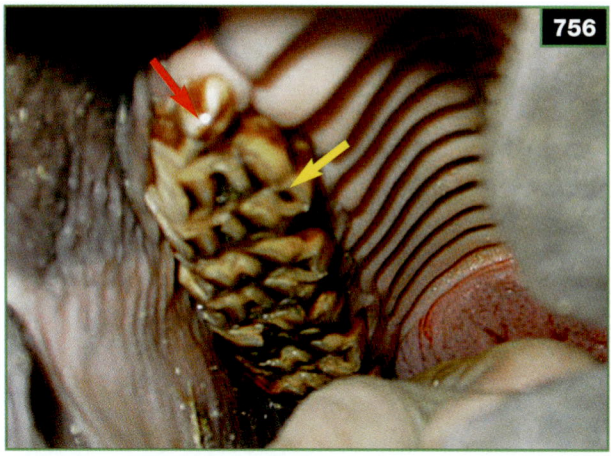

756 A wolf tooth (105) (red arrow) *in situ* rostral to the 1st cheek tooth (106) (yellow arrow) in an adult horse.

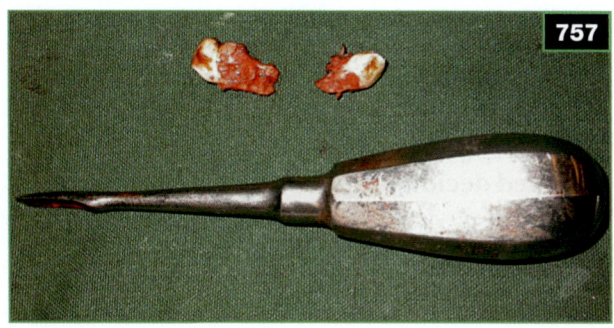

757 These vestigial 1st maxillary premolars (105, 205), or wolf-teeth, have been extracted under sedation and local analgesia.

Clinical presentation/diagnosis

Palpation of the rostral arcade will reveal the presence of erupted or subgingival wolf teeth. Aberrantly placed teeth or very large wolf teeth should be radiographed to assess the size and placement of the apical portion before attempts at extraction.

Management

Wolf tooth removal is easily accomplished in the field. Sedation of the horse is helpful and local analgesia of the tooth using an infraorbital nerve block, local subgingival infiltration of mepivicaine, or topical application of cinchocaine to the gingival mucosa is advised. The gingiva is elevated from all around the tooth using a circular Burgess-type elevator or a small curve-bladed periodontal elevator (757). Very large molarized wolf teeth may require extensive periodontal separation before they are

491

sufficiently loose to extract. Once periodontal elevation is completed the tooth can be extracted using a small pair of incisor or specialized wolf-tooth extractors. Subgingival wolf teeth can be exposed by a small incision in the overlying gingival mucosa. Periodontal attachments can be carefully loosened using an osteotome placed pointing caudally between the rostrally angled tooth and the hard palate. The alveolus can be packed with gel foam or gauze to prevent food impaction, although this is rarely necessary. Failure to loosen the periodontium sufficiently can result in fracture of the tooth. Remaining sharp fragments should be elevated and removed to enable healing of the alveolus. Subgingival apical fragments rarely cause clinical signs and loose fragments may be removed after several days, during which time they usually migrate to a more superficial position. Mandibular lower 1st premolars (Triadan 305, 405) are rare and, if present, can usually be palpated on the ventral mandible rostral to the first cheek tooth. They are commonly small, but vary in size and position and are more likely to be associated with discomfort with the bit. They are a noteworthy observation during prepurchase examinations. The technique for their removal is as previously described.

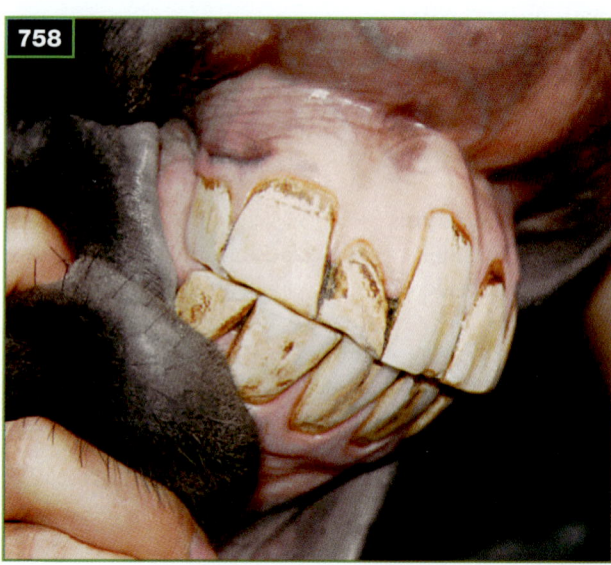

758 Retained deciduous incisors are a common incidental finding. They can be removed easily under sedation.

Retained deciduous teeth

Definition/overview
This condition involves the presence of retained deciduous teeth after eruption of the permanent dentition (**758**).

Etiology/pathophysiology
Retained deciduous incisors are a common presenting finding during routine dental examinations. During normal eruption the permanent incisors emerge on the palatal and labial aspects of their deciduous counterparts, which are shed as their gingival attachments are lost. Occasionally, the permanent dentition erupts, leaving the temporary incisors displaced labially but retaining the gingival attachments. Temporary premolars are commonly retained in young horses due to compression in a rostrocaudal direction along the arcade. This results in failure of the deciduous teeth or 'caps' to be shed even after they have apparently lost their gingival attachments. It is most commonly the deciduous 07s and 08s that are retained, and accumulation of ingesta underneath the shell-like caps can exaggerate the mild periodontitis associated with normal eruption, resulting in painful gingivitis.

Clinical presentation
Although the deciduous teeth may resemble the erupting teeth on the occlusal view, the labial aspect of the tooth appears much smaller, with the gingiva appearing to expose less clinical crown.

Retention of deciduous premolars is a common finding in racing Thoroughbreds and a reluctance to perform is sometimes attributed to deciduous premolar retention. Removal of retained caps is indicated if the division between the temporary and permanent dentition can be palpated on the buccal/palatal aspect of the tooth, indicating that the gingival attachment has receded and that the cap is being retained solely by compression between the adjacent teeth.

Diagnosis
A thorough oral examination should detect this problem.

Management
The remaining periodontal attachments of the temporary incisors are easily parted with a curved elevator after sedation and local analgesia of the horse; the tooth may then be extracted with minimal effort using a small dental extractor, with an excellent cosmetic prognosis. Single-handed cap extracting forceps are available specifically for this purpose. Premature extraction of the molar caps may lead to exposure of the occlusal surface of the permanent dentition before the complete maturation of the cementum, potentially resulting in an increased risk of caries.

Maleruption

Definition/overview
Maleruption is misalignment of the teeth within an arcade as a result of asymmetric or delayed eruption of the teeth.

Etiology/pathophysiology
The eruption of the permanent cheek teeth to replace the primary dentition is a carefully coordinated sequence of events. Disturbances resulting in alteration of the position of the permanent tooth buds or anatomic variations resulting in relative shortening of the maxilla or mandible can result in impaction of the erupting tooth and, consequently, predispose to disease processes. Dental impactions can result in displacement during eruption, with subsequent misalignment of the tooth arcade, or they can predispose to apical compression, with resultant hypoxic ischemia.

Clinical presentation
Maleruption resulting in misalignment is usually obvious on oral examination. Such maleruptions are commonly bilateral and careful inspection for early signs of misalignment should be performed at each dental examination. The consequences of misalignment are malocclusion with the opposing arcade, resulting in the development of focal overgrowths, and the development of diastemata, or gaps, between the adjacent teeth in the row. Diastemata enable food accumulation adjacent to the gingival sulcus and accumulation of destructive bacteria in periodontal pockets. This causes gingivitis, gingival recession, and peripheral cemental caries. This condition appears to be painful, with affected horses often exhibiting signs including slow eating and quidding (oral dysphagia) and, in chronic cases, development of periodontitis.

Diagnosis
Oral examination will reveal the presence of maleruptions. Radiography may be indicated to demonstrate secondary consequences such as deep periodontal disease or caries.

Management
Treatment of the secondary consequence is often indicated, although extraction of individual malerupted teeth may be a component of the management.

DEVELOPMENTAL DISEASES OF THE ROSTRAL SKULL AFFECTING DENTAL ERUPTION

Brachygnathia and prognathia

Definition/overview
Brachygnathia and prognathia involve a relative asymmetric growth rate between the rostral mandible and incisive bone, resulting in an overshot or undershot incisive bone.

Etiology/pathophysiology
Brachygnathia, or parrot mouth (759), is a common disorder in which the incisive bone overgrows the rostral mandible, causing a malocclusion of the incisors. The maxillary incisors lie rostral to the mandibular ones, with no occlusion, or partial occlusion in milder cases. The heritability of this condition is unclear, but certain stallions have been associated with an increased incidence of the condition, although many mares with the condition have successfully bred morphologically normal foals. Prognathia, or 'sow mouth', is a rare condition in which the incisive bone grows at a less rapid rate than the mandible, resulting in 'underbite'.

Clinical presentation
The condition is diagnosed in foals. Grazing may be impaired where there is no occlusion, but most horses compensate sufficiently for a satisfactory weight gain. The cosmetic appearance may be prejudicial to a show career, but the occlusion of the cheek teeth is usually not similarly affected and normal mastication is possible. Severe cases of prognathism may potentially suffer from nostril collapse and abnormal respiratory noises.

Differential diagnosis
Trauma to the rostral mandible and wry nose should be considered.

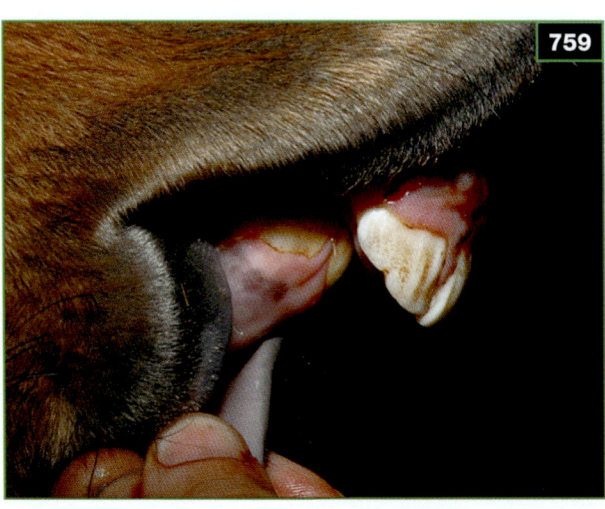

759 Brachygnathia refers to asymmetric growth between the rostral mandible and the incisive bone resulting in this over jet (or bite, depending on the severity) or 'parrot-mouth', which can be surgically corrected in foals up to 6–9 months of age.

Diagnosis

Diagnosis is based on clinical oral examination and radiography.

Management

Correction using tension-band retardation of the growth of the incisive bone in combination with bite plates is advisable in the case of severe defects. Maximum benefit is derived by early correction (from 1 month of age) when growth of the bone is rapid. Careful attention to incisor alignment may be necessary during the animal's life in order to prevent lesions on the mandibular gingiva from impinging on the upper incisors.

Campylorrhinus lateralis (wry nose)

Definition/overview

Wry nose is a complex congenital deformity of the face leading to lateral deviation (760). Although this is a disease affecting the formation of the rostral skull bones, it has important consequences for dental eruption.

Etiology/pathophysiology

Wry nose occurs due to a dysplasia of the incisive, nasal, or vomer bones and maxilla on one side, which results in a lateral deviation of the face and nostrils to the affected side. Deviation is also present in the nasal septum and hard palate, and occasionally the mandible, with dorsoventral deviation also recorded. There is no proven breed predisposition (Arabs and draft breeds may be over-represented) and the heritability of the condition is unproven. It has been suggested that fetal malpositioning may be a contributing factor, as primipares have an increased incidence.

Clinical presentation

The condition is immediately identifiable at birth by clinical examination. Deformity can result in severe airflow obstruction and noise, and difficulty feeding. Careful examination for other congenital abnormalities such as cleft palate and axial/appendicular deformities is required.

Differential diagnosis

Brachygnathia; trauma.

Diagnosis

Clinical appearance and radiography are used for diagnosis.

Management

Mild deformities may resolve spontaneously with growth. Reconstructive surgery with osteotomy of the shortened maxilla and palatine bone after elevation of the soft tissues, followed by realignment and immobilization with external fixators, has been used, but remains controversial. Many neonates are euthanized when the condition is identified.

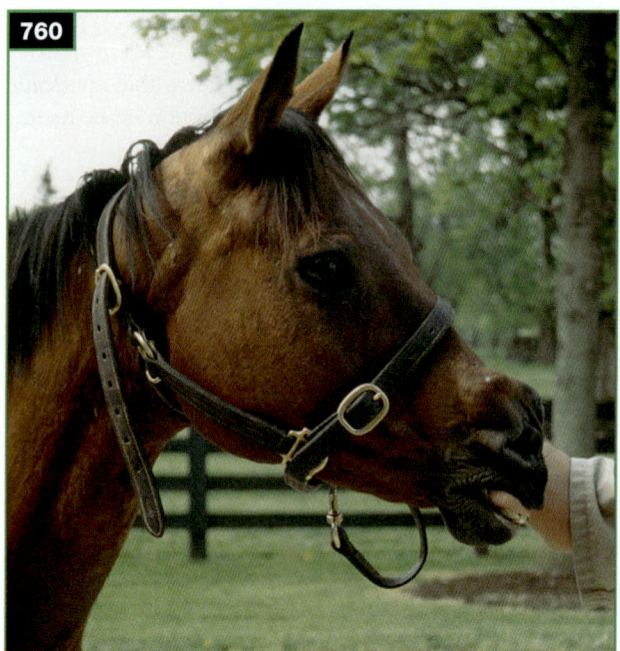

760 A Thoroughbred mare with wry nose, which, unusually, has been reared and used for breeding. Such animals do not appear consistently to produce offspring with the same defect.

ACQUIRED DENTAL DISORDERS
Diastema and periodontitis

Definition/overview

Diastema is defined as an inappropriate space between two teeth of the same type, which is considered to be pathologically significant in Equidae. Periodontitis is inflammation of the periodontal tissues, including the periodontium, and may also include gingivitis.

Etiology/pathophysiology

Primary periodontitis is rare in the horse and plaque accumulation has not been identified as a major factor in this species. Periodontitis usually accompanies the presence of diastema, possibly due to misalignment or age-related loss of mesiodistal compression, which allow the development of periodontal food pockets and bacterial accumulation in the gingival sulcus, resulting in gingivitis and periodontitis.

Clinical presentation

A history including slow eating, spilling of food, difficulty with mastication of long-fibered diets, and even weight loss are suggestive of this syndrome.

Diagnosis

An oral examination, including using a dental mirror, will identify the presence of food trapped in periodontal pockets (761). The condition is common in aged horses, which have reduced areas of periodontal attachment and short reserve crowns, resulting in a physiologic reduction in the mesiodistal compression. In chronic cases, multiple teeth may be digitally loose.

Management

The aim of therapy is:

+ To reduce periodontal food accumulation.
+ To treat alveolar periodontitis.
+ To remove dental overgrowths and transverse ridges that may be preventing normal mastication and contributing to diastema development. Correction of these wear abnormalities will assist normal mastication.
+ To remove grossly loose teeth that have no periodontal attachments and are functionally redundant.

Treatment of widespread diastemata with periodontal pocketing is achieved with variable success and can be disappointing. Periodontal debridement and lavage are achieved by focused lavage of the interdentium, removal of gross food accumulation, and debridement of the periodontal pockets with descaling or air abrasion devices. Widening of the diastemata and packing of the periodontal pockets with acrylic materials have been described anecdotally as preventing recurrence, but controlled data on the efficacy of these techniques are currently lacking.

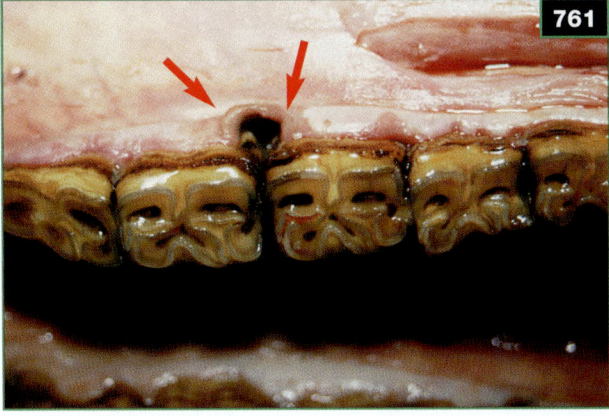

761 Severe periodontal pocketing (arrows) resulting from diastema and periodontal food impaction.

Alveolar periodontitis and gingivitis can be treated with antibiotics and antiseptic mouthwash solutions. This will result in temporary improvement. If the diastema is due to a focal displacement, dental removal can be considered and is effective in relieving the cause of the diastema in some cases. In most cases, removal of overgrowths, the feeding of reduced-fiber food, antibiotic therapy, and widening of valve diastema results in clinical improvement, but recurrence is highly probable and constant management is a more realistic aim than total clinical cure.

Apical infections of the cheek teeth

Definition/overview

Infections of the apical pulp of the tooth manifest as localized pulpitis with ensuing caries. These are acquired disorders, but are probably predisposed by impaction of the dental sac during eruption.

Etiology/pathophysiology

Dental apical infections are one of the most commonly observed endodontic lesions of equine teeth. They are seen in all types of horses and mostly occur at 3–5 years of age for mandibular teeth and 2–7 years of age for maxillary cheek teeth. Mandibular teeth 307, 308, 407, and 408 are most frequently affected in the lower jaw and maxillary teeth 108, 109, 208, and 209 are most commonly involved in the upper jaw. The etiology of dental apical infections is unclear in many cases. It is possible that the mechanisms for apical infection are slightly different in maxillary and mandibular teeth. It has been suggested that infundibular cemental hypoplasia, which has been identified in ultrastructural examination of maxillary teeth, may predispose to apical infection, although this does not appear to be the mechanism in all cases. Mandibular teeth lack infundibula and, despite this, are recorded with apical infections with a similar frequency to maxillary teeth. Incisors, which also have infundibula, are rarely affected by apical infections. Bacterial contamination of the pulp, after penetration of porous dentine on the occlusal surface or by hematogenous spread, may be the initiating event. It has also been suggested that congenital enamel defects predispose to lines of weakness in the tooth, which when exposed to the forces of mastication, result in fissure fractures that can communicate between the occlusal surfaces and adjacent pulp cavities, resulting in apical infection. Pathologic fracture of teeth along such fault lines is commonly observed in maxillary cheek teeth, but rarely in mandibular teeth. Bacterial contamination results in edema and eventual hypoxic necrosis and swelling of the pulp. This leads to vascular occlusion, especially in mature teeth with narrow apical foramina, and eventual pulp necrosis. This is clinically detectable as unilateral swellings on the mandible and maxilla (when rostral maxillary teeth are infected).

Clinical presentation

Maxillary and mandibular unilateral swellings, which can be painful initially, but appear to become less so as the condition becomes more chronic, are observed. Eventually, the apical infections abscessate and discharge through tracts in the thinned mandible or, more rarely, through the maxillary bone, unless aspiration or trephination over the swelling is attempted (762). Caudal (08, 11) maxillary apical infections frequently discharge into the maxillary sinuses, resulting in a sinus empyema, which can involve the rostral maxillary, caudal maxillary, or ventral conchal sinuses, depending on which tooth and dental root are involved and the degree of destruction of the maxillary septum. It is rare to have involvement of more than a single tooth, and the abscess is usually localized over a single dental root, although this may result in necrosis of the adjacent pulp. Cases with dental sinusitis usually present with a malodorous unilateral nasal discharge, submandibular lymphadenopathy, and reduced resonance to percussion over the affected sinuses.

Differential diagnosis

Mandibular fractures; dental cysts; primary maxillary sinusitis; trauma.

Diagnosis

Examination of the occlusal surfaces of both maxillary and mandibular cheek teeth does not usually reveal defects indicative of pulp exposure or gross caries in such cases. The diagnosis can be confirmed by radiography or scintigraphy (763). Multiple radiographic projections, including lateral, lateral 30–45° dorsolateral, and dorsoventral views should be obtained in the standing sedated horse. Radiographic changes associated with dental apical infections include the presence of a radiolucency of the affected apex, which is often surrounded by a region of radiopaque sclerotic bone (especially in chronic cases). More subtle indications of infection of a dental apex include loss of definition and widening of the periodontal space and loss of the lamina dura denta. Occasionally, in the presence of chronic infection, a granular radio-opacity is observed (termed 'coral pattern' or dental rhinitis) in the nasal cavity, resulting from dystrophic mineralization in the nasal conchae. Dorsoventral projections are also useful for imaging periodontal remodeling on the buccal aspects of the maxillary cheek teeth or the lingual aspects of the mandibular teeth. Comparison with the contralateral tooth may facilitate detection of subtle dental apical changes. In chronic cases of mandibular apical infections, with a

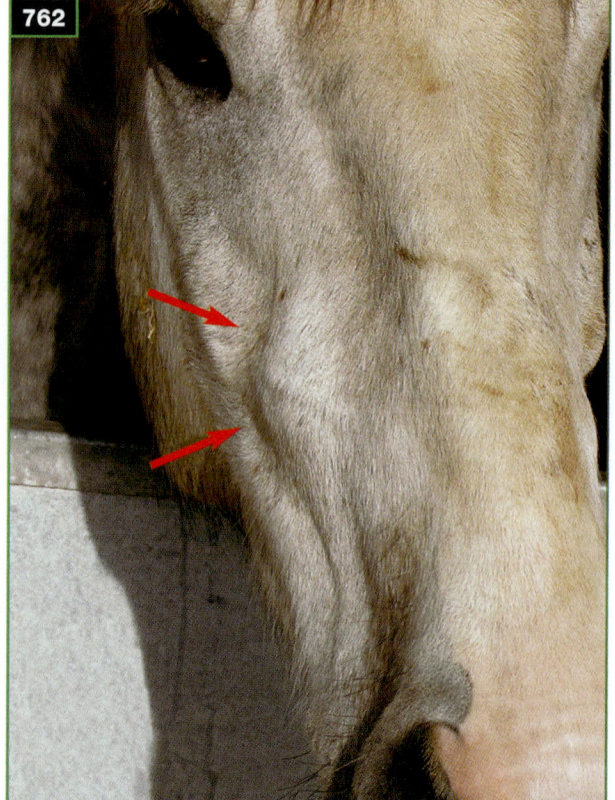

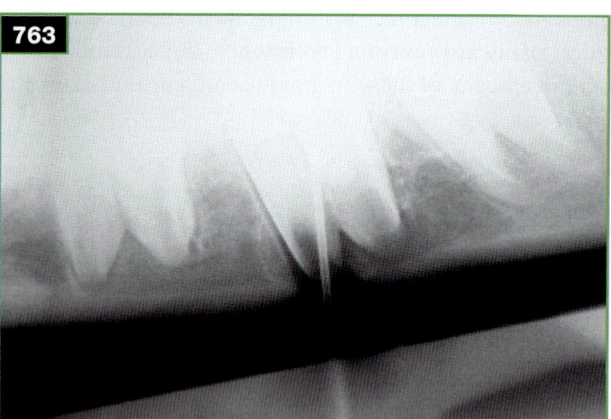

762 This 8-year-old horse displayed focal nonpainful swelling in the right maxillary region (arrows), which is indicative of a rostral maxillary apical infection.

763 Lateral 45° oblique radiograph of the ventral mandible of a 7-year-old horse showing a radio-opaque probe placed in a draining mandibular tract, which is demarcating the infected root of the apex of cheek tooth 208.

discharging tract, additional radiographs should be taken after placing a radio-opaque marker into the tract to identify the tooth and root involved. Apical infections of the caudal maxillary teeth may be associated with sinus empyema, which is seen as fluid lines on erect lateral radiographs (764). Radiographs are neither very sensitive nor specific in detecting early dental apical disease and additional ancillary techniques such as scintigraphy (or CT if available) may be considered if economic factors permit. Scintigraphy has been shown to be sensitive for detecting dental apical infections, due to focal radionuclide uptake over an apical infection; however, the poor specificity of scintigraphy does not enable such lesions to be confidently distinguished from localized primary sinus empyema.

Management

In young horses with wider apical foramina, long-term (2–4 weeks) antibiotic therapy using broad-spectrum antimicrobials (e.g. trimethoprim-sulfadiazine and/or metronidazole administered p/o) can result in clinical remission. In older horses with narrow apical foramina, it appears that despite antibiotic treatment, a nidus of infected necrotic pulp remains in the pulp cavity, resulting in only a transient clinical improvement in response to antibiotics. Apical curettage and drainage has been reported for successful treatment of mandibular apical infections, although case numbers are low and the outcome has been variable. Most commonly, the infected tooth will require removal by repulsion (765), oral extraction (766), or via a lateral alveolar buccotomy. Endodontic root canal filling for cheek teeth with apical infections has also been reported, but with limited success. The use of these techniques is not currently widespread due to technical limitations.

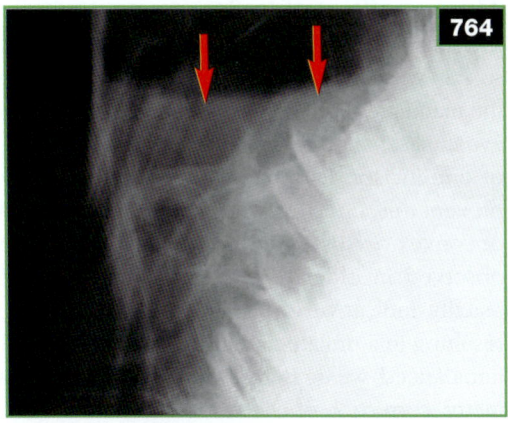

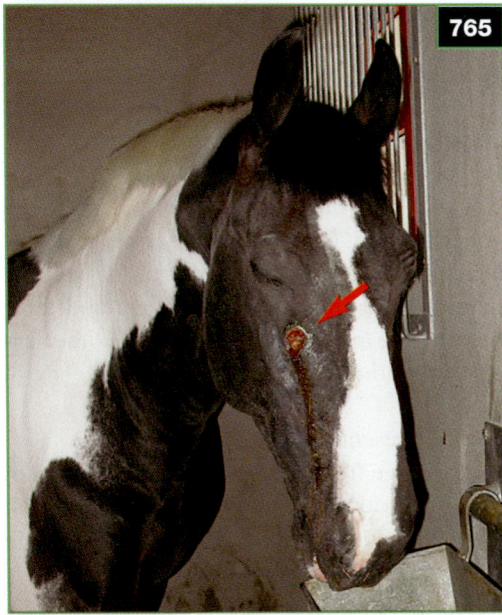

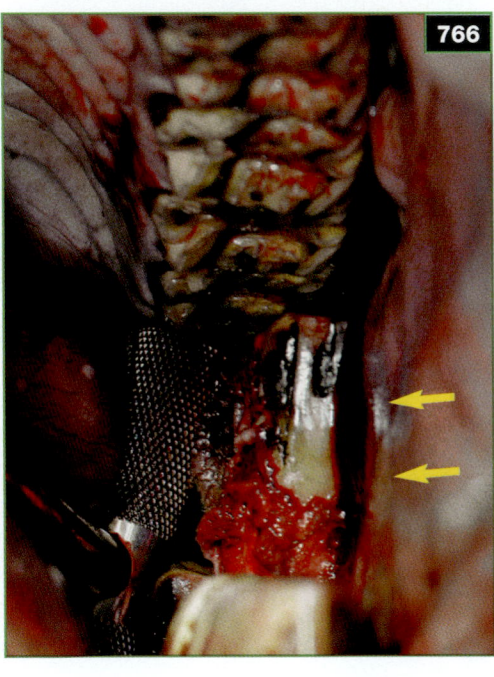

764 A lateral radiograph showing fluid lines (arrows) in the frontal and maxillary sinuses due to the presence of inflammatory exudates.

765 A maxillary cheek tooth in this horse has been repulsed via a trephine hole (arrow), which is being allowed to heal by granulation.

766 A maxillary cheek tooth in the process of being extracted *per os* showing long reserve dental crowns (arrows), with hemorrhagic periodontium.

497

Abnormalities of incisor wear

Incisors are used for cropping forage and they rarely sustain wear abnormalities alone. Full lateral movement of the mandible results in occlusion of the molar arcades and eventual separation of the incisors by about half the width of one incisor. Extreme overgrowths of an incisor may prevent this, but such defects are uncommon. A concave or convex occlusal angle when the incisors are closed is observed in older horses. A slanted occlusal angle is usually indicative of abnormalities of the cheek teeth, resulting in a unilateral masticatory action and leading to imbalanced wear. Before correcting any incisor asymmetry, correction of cheek tooth abnormalities should be performed. Horses with stereotypical behavioral problems, including crib biting, will experience accelerated wear of the incisor tables, giving the appearance of a prematurely aging horse.

Incisor fractures

Etiology/pathophysiology

Fractures involving the incisors are common, especially in young horses (767). Such injuries are usually the result of a kick, or occur as avulsion injuries when a horse is mouthing high-tensile wire fencing and traps the wire between the incisors, causing fracture of the incisor with its alveolus during violent evasive behavior.

Clinical presentation /diagnosis

Hemorrhage from the mouth may often be detected. An oral examination will reveal avulsion of the incisors. Radiography, including intraoral views, will demonstrate the configuration and extent of the fracture.

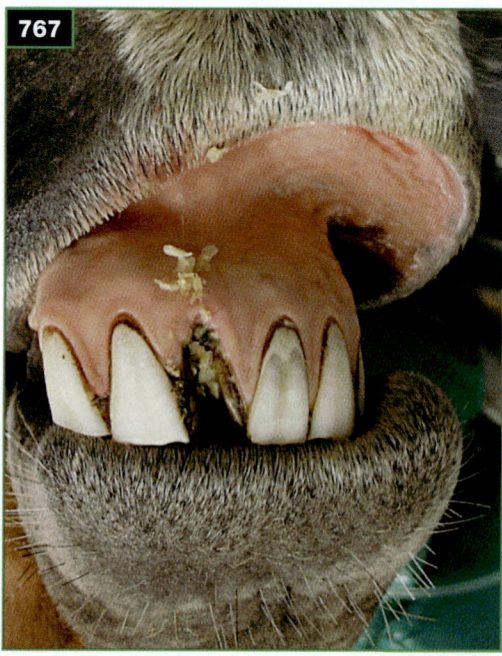

Management

Even in those cases with severe contamination, the incisors can often be salvaged if anatomy is restored by wiring the avulsed incisors to the adjacent teeth and to the incisive bone or rostral mandible. Noneruptted permanent incisors are often able to erupt without complication even when the primary dentition is lost.

Disease of canine teeth

The canine teeth, which have no role in prehension and mastication of food, are rarely involved in dental disease. Fractures of the canines as a result of trauma can lead to pulp exposure and abscessation, which appears to be associated with considerable discomfort. Removal of canine teeth is technically difficult due to the curvature of the apical portion in a caudal direction, necessitating a lateral alveolar buccotomy. Calculus accumulation on the canines is common in older male horses and is facilitated by the fact that the canines are not in constant contact with the cheeks during mastication. Normally, this accumulation is asymptomatic, but in severe cases, gingivitis and eventual gingival recession can occur. Removal of the excess calculus with a dental elevator is easily accomplished in the conscious horse during routine dental examinations.

Focal dental overgrowths, dental points, shear mouth

Definition/overview

During normal mastication in the horse the mandible is lowered and then raised in a dorsal movement, circumducting from buccal to lingual, to bring the mandibular teeth into occlusion in an axial direction so that the occlusal surfaces shear over each other in a grinding action. This is referred to as the 'power stroke' and is driven by the powerful masseter and pterygoid muscle groups. Due to the anisognathism in the equine mouth, only one molar arcade is in occlusion during each masticatory stroke.

The temporomandibular joint is maintained by a tight joint capsule that permits free lateral movement and a degree of rostrocaudal movement.

Etiology/pathophysiology

When the horse lowers its head into the grazing position, the mandible drops and moves rostrally and normal occlusion would be expected at this point. The range of lateral movement appears to be wider when chewing grass or

767 Chronic fractured permanent central incisor, impacted with food material. (Photo courtesy GA Munroe)

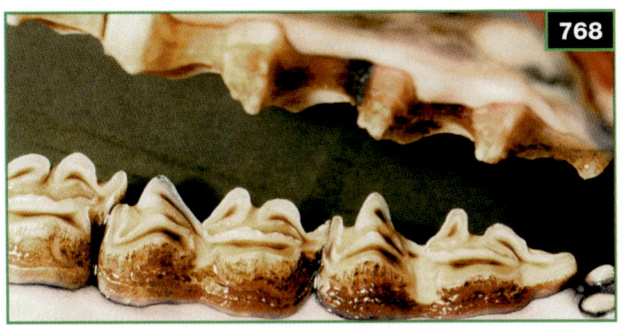

768 Overgrowths on the buccal and lingual aspect of the cheek teeth. (Photo courtesy GA Munroe)

forage than when chewing concentrated processed feeds. The rotary chewing action is reflected in the angled occlusal surface (10–15° to the horizontal) and results in increased wear on the palatal aspect of the maxillary arcade and of the buccal aspect of the mandibular arcade. Factors that limit lateral jaw movement can result in exaggeration of the angle of the occlusal surface due to uneven wear over the tooth. Ultimately, this leads to the development of focal overgrowths (due to reduced attrition) on the lingual mandibular teeth and the buccal maxillary teeth (**768**).

Clinical presentation
These focal overgrowths develop sharp enamel points, which can impinge on soft tissue and cause masticatory pain and ulceration. Overgrowths of cingula (folding of palatal enamel) on the buccal aspect of the maxillary teeth can become particularly prominent.

Diagnosis
Such overgrowths are detected by palpation during thorough routine examinations and are particularly prevalent on the 10s and 11s. Continuing development of these overgrowths can result in occlusal angles approaching 45° (termed 'shear mouth'). These grossly exaggerated overgrowths physically prevent lateral masticatory movement, resulting in a scissor-like action, and further exacerbation of the problem ensues.

Management
Removal of these overgrowths is a fundamental part of routine dental prophylaxis. Correction of severe shear mouth may be a long-term project, necessitating gradual reduction of the overgrowths over a period (e.g. 6 months) in several treatments.

Correction of focal overgrowths is achieved using a variety of instruments including rasps of different handle types fitted with blades made from chipped or solid tungsten carbide. In addition, motorized or air-powered instruments with tungsten carbide or diamond-tipped burrs can be used in sedated horses to reduce quite large overgrowths rapidly. Care is required with these instruments because excessive use can damage the teeth.

Rostral and caudal overgrowths ('hooks, beaks, ramps')

Definition/overview
Prominent overgrowths can develop on the rostral and caudal aspects of the arcade resulting from uneven wear (dysmastication).

Etiology/pathophysiology
Focal dental overgrowths at the rostral and caudal aspects of either the maxillary or mandibular arcades can result from several mechanisms. Anisognathism of the maxillary and mandibular arcades can lead to the development of a rostral overgrowth (hook) on the 106 and 206, or on the 311 or 411, probably due to a relative caudal displacement of the mandible during mastication resulting in incomplete occlusion. It is possible that domesticated horses that are fed with the head raised may be more susceptible to this. The presence of caudal mandibular overgrowths, which may cause trauma to the tongue and other soft tissues, may remain undetected on cursory visual examinations of the mouth. Rostral overgrowths, in addition to interfering with mastication, can be a contributing factor to equitation problems when ridden due to pain caused by entrapment of gingival mucosa between bits and the sharp buccal/rostral overgrowth.

Clinical presentation/diagnosis
Hooks may present as masticatory disorders, oral pain, excessive salivation, and equitation problems. Careful oral examination and palpation will demonstrate the presence of such overgrowths.

Management
Historically, these overgrowths were removed using dental chisels and molar cutters. Such crude instruments are cumbersome, unpredictable, and have a high risk of iatrogenic pulp exposure. Removal of these overgrowths using mechanical grinding instruments enables more precise correction of the overgrowths, with reduced risk of pulp exposure provided that they are used with care in order to avoid overheating the teeth.

Excessive transverse ridges (ETRs)

Definition/overview

This condition consists of the presence of exaggerated ridges in a buccopalatal or buccolingual direction. They are focally prominent and may be associated with reduced masticatory movement and impaction of food into diastemata on the opposite arcade.

Etiology/pathophysiology

Transverse elevations on the occlusal surfaces of the teeth are a normal consequence of mastication and are usually present on the surface of equine teeth in normal wear. The elevations on the mandibular teeth interdigitate with the corresponding depressed areas on the maxillary teeth, and it is plausible that such an arrangement, in combination with the different rates of wear of the dental tissues, enhances the efficiency of mastication. In horses with impaired mastication, exaggeration of these transverse ridges can potentially restrict rostrocaudal mandibular movement and manifest as poor tolerance of the bit and reduced performance in technical disciplines. It appears unlikely that normal transverse ridges significantly restrict movement, since when ridden with the bit in place and the mouth closed with incisors in occlusion, the molar arcades are not in occlusion.

Diagnosis

ETRs are easily detected on oral examination and can be documented by radiography.

Management

Removal of the ETRs to free up movement is attributed with improved performance, but the removal of transverse ridges in horses without clinical signs during routine examinations is not justified.

Step mouth and wave mouth

Definition/overview

Severely uneven mastication can result in severe 'steps' in the occlusal surface of the arcade (step mouth) or undulation of the occlusal surface in a rostral to caudal direction (wave mouth).

Etiology/pathophysiology

Abnormal masticatory movement can also result in one area of the arcade undergoing attrition at an increased rate relative to other parts. The result is an arcade in which the occlusal surface undulates, with areas involving one or more teeth with a longer clinical crown and adjacent areas in which the crown is shorter. The undulations on the maxillary and mandibular arcades complement each other when the arcades come into occlusion. They are common in aged horses that have suffered chronic reduced masticatory movements. Step mouth is the consequence of a local oligodontia or displacements allowing super-eruption of a single tooth, which becomes prominent (>1 cm) to the remainder of the arcade. Locking of the jaw is possible if complete interdigitation occurs and normal mastication is prohibited.

Clinical presentation/diagnosis

Severe step mouth and wave mouth can be the consequence or cause of additional masticatory disorders and can be associated with oral pain. Oral examination will reveal the presence of significant unevenness of the arcade.

Management

Correction of wave mouth is possible until dental eruption ceases (at about 20 years of age). Once normal mastication is restored, the tendency for the condition to recur is reduced. In severe cases, gradual correction is advisable and, in aged horses, preservation of dental tissues is desirable. Step mouth should be corrected gradually with the eventual aim of reducing the prominent tooth to the level of the arcade and bringing the remainder into occlusion. The pulp may extend to within 7 mm of the occlusal surfaces and correction of a large (>1 cm) step mouth should be carried out gradually with repeated treatments. Mechanical burrs offer the safest and most effective method for the correction of step mouth.

Cheek teeth fractures

Etiology/pathophysiology

Dental fractures are sustained as a result of trauma, in the case of rostral mandibular fractures, or iatrogenically. Traumatic fractures of the cheek teeth are most common in the rostral mandibular teeth and the incidence decreases with caudal position in the arcade. Traumatic maxillary fractures are usually iatrogenic, occurring during attempted dental extraction or removal of hooks using obsolete molar cutters. Idiopathic dental fractures occur commonly in the maxillary cheek teeth; the 4th (109, 209) maxillary tooth is most commonly involved. Fractures of these teeth are typically parasagittal and can occur along a plane in the buccal aspect of the tooth, with displacement of a lateral slab of dentine and enamel. In other cases the fracture occurs along a line connecting two adjacent pulp cavities or connecting infundibula. The etiology of these fractures is unclear, although it is possible that pre-existing structural weaknesses are predilection sites for dental fracture when subjected to the forces of mastication, especially if overgrowths are present.

Clinical presentation

Displacement of the slab often results in buccal trauma and ulceration, which causes dysmastication.

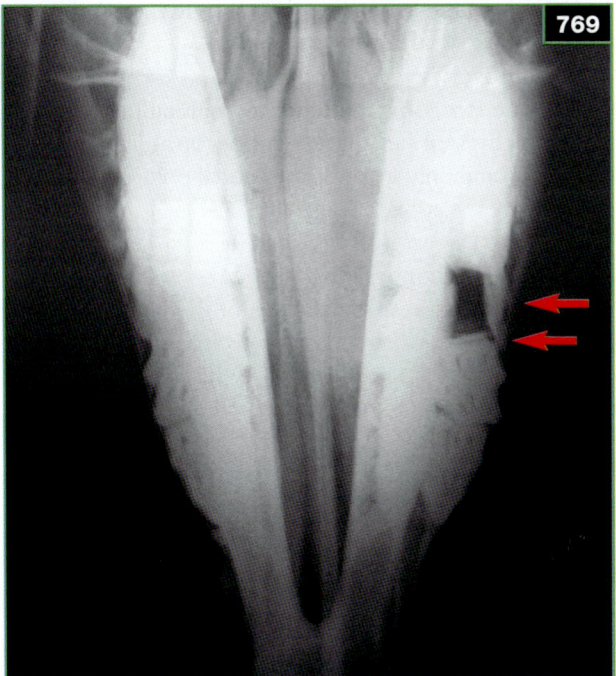

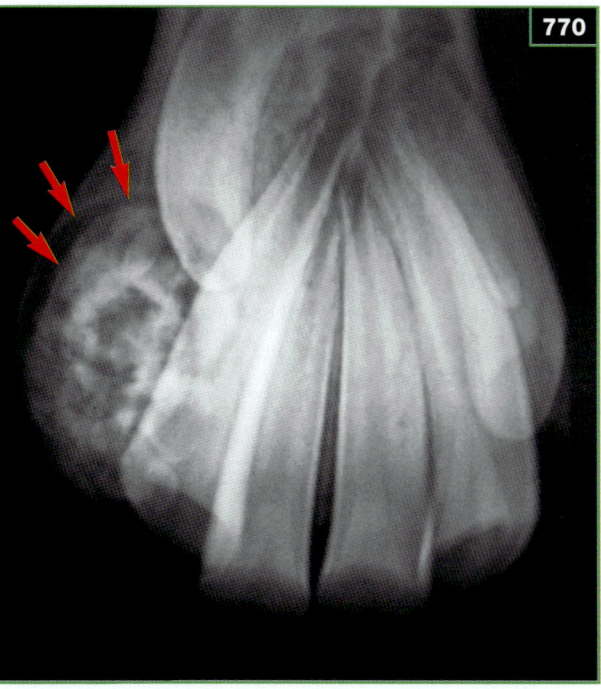

769 Dorsoventral radiograph showing a parasagittal fracture of maxillary tooth 209 (arrows), which was associated with caries and maxillary sinusitis.

770 Well-circumscribed, radio-opaque mass (arrows) on the rostral mandible, typical of an ameloblastoma.

Diagnosis
Diagnosis is based on clinical examination, and supportive evidence can be obtained from radiographs (especially dorsoventral projections) (769).

Management
If the buccal slab does not extend the full length of the reserve crown and does not involve pulp exposure, removal of this slab with correction of overgrowths may enable the remainder of the tooth to be salvaged, especially when the alveolus remains intact. If the plane of the fracture is sagittal and involves pulp exposure, the condition is usually associated with gross caries, necessitating complete dental removal. In cases with dental fractures accompanied by sinusitis, treatment of the sinusitis and removal of any contamination from the oral cavity will be necessary before remission of the clinical signs.

ORAL NEOPLASIA
Definition/overview
Neoplasia affecting the oral cavity may be a consequence of tumors of both dental and nondental origin. Tumors of the oral cavity are relatively rare and although numerous individual case reports are found in the literature, there are few series involving large numbers. Frequently they are detected incidentally during a routine oral or dental examination. They are often at an advanced stage, limiting the options for treatment and rendering the prognosis for complete remission guarded to poor.

Etiology/pathophysiology
Dental tumors may be epithelial in origin and odontogenic such as cementomas, ameloblastomas (770), odontomas, and other calcifying epithelial odontogenic lesions. Mesenchymal odontogenic tumors include myxomas and dentigerous cysts. These tumors are classified according to the inductive effect of the neoplasm on other tissues. Dental tumors, although invariably benign, may be locally invasive and may disrupt adjacent tissues by their expansion.

Dental tumors including ameloblastomas and odontomas, and mandibular tumors of nondental origin including osteomas, ossifying fibromas, and SCCs, can all result in gross changes to the dental apices and reserve crowns,

501

which may be accompanied by swelling of the affected alveolar bone with increased or decreased radio-opacity. The immature cells in ameloblastomas are frequently non-calcified and are usually well circumscribed. SCCs typically lead to destruction of the mandible, resulting in loss of mineral density and eventual periodontal or palato-dontal diseases and loosening of the teeth.

Clinical presentation
Oral and dental tumors present as asymmetric swellings of the maxilla and mandible that may be associated with masticatory disorders. Aggressive lesions may be associated with secondary dental disease and, if intraoral, halitosis. The gross appearance of many lesions is similar and histopathologic examination is usually necessary for a specific diagnosis. The histologic classification of some oral neoplasms, especially those belonging to the fibro-osseous groups, is a specialized science and the classification follows that described for such lesions in human patients. Lesions are defined according to their tissue of origin (i.e. as being derived from dental tissue, bone, or soft tissues) and as having varying degrees of malignancy. Non-neoplastic lesions such as exuberant granulation tissue can be mistaken for tumors by their similar gross appearance.

Differential diagnosis
Apical abscessation; maxillary and mandibular fractures.

Diagnosis
Diagnosis is based on clinical appearance supported by radiography and histopathologic analysis of biopsies.

Management
The treatment options are often limited by the advanced stage of the lesion and the anatomic location, which can preclude surgical access. The low incidence means that reports of comparative treatment of such lesions are lacking in this species. Radical surgery, including hemimandibulectomy or hemimaxillectomy, has been performed successfully in individual cases. Radiotherapy with iridium-192 and cobalt-60 has been used in standing sedated horses. Debulking followed by cobalt-60 therapy has also been used successfully. Chemotherapy using intralesional cisplatin has been described for successful treatment in individual case reports.

NONDENTAL DISEASES OF THE ORAL CAVITY
Cleft palate (palatoschiasis)
Definition/overview
Cleft palate is a congenital defect resulting in an incomplete symphysis. It can affect the upper lip and hard palate, but most commonly involves the caudal portion of the soft palate.

Etiology and pathophysiology
The defect is the result of failure of the lateral palatine processes to fuse, which normally occurs at approximately day 47 of gestation. The heritability has not been definitively established in horses.

Clinical presentation
Primary cleft palate (affecting the upper lip and rostral hard palate) is very rare and presents as a sagittal facial deformity with incomplete aponeurosis of the upper lip. The signs are usually evident during a cursory examination at birth or once the foal commences to suck. Secondary cleft palate presents with nasal reflux during feeding as milk entering the oral cavity passes into the nasal cavity and exits via the nares, bilaterally during sucking. Examination of the hard and soft palate will reveal a defect, which varies from approximately 1 cm to the whole caudal portion of the soft palate. Complications result from the dysphagia and can include failure of passive transfer of gammaglobulins from colostrum, dehydration, hypoglycemia, and aspiration pneumonia.

Diagnosis
Clinical detection of the lesions may be further confirmed by nasal or oral endoscopy. The sagittal defect in the palate is pathognomonic for this defect and any foals with a bilateral nasal discharge when feeding should be carefully examined for this condition. A full investigation should include tracheoscopy and standing thoracic radiography for the presence of food aspiration and pneumonia.

Management
Techniques for the surgical repair of palatal defects have been described, but reports of success are confined to individual cases and the prognosis for the attainment of athletic ability would appear to be guarded. The techniques recommend repair at the earliest opportunity, and repair of lesions confined to the soft palate offers a slightly better prognosis than those involving the hard palate. Repair involves a ventral approach, with mandibular symphectomy to facilitate access and a multilayer repair to reduce palatal tension on the anastomosis. Complications are common and include osteomyelitis of the mandible, while dehiscence of the repair with fistula formation is frequent. Foals of low value are euthanized without treatment in most cases.

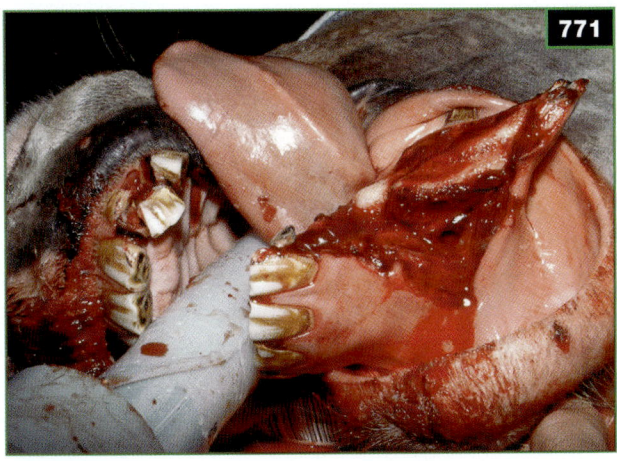

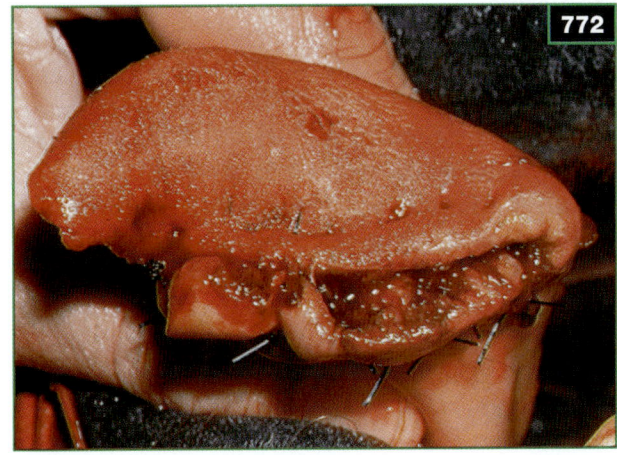

771 A severe laceration of the oral mucosa associated with a mandibular fracture and avulsion of lower incisors.

772 Lacerations of the tongue should be repaired if there is any possibility of viability. They can heal surprisingly well.

Lacerations/wounds and foreign bodies

Definition/overview
Acquired traumatic lesions of the oral cavity can occur for a variety of reasons and may appear dramatic, but they often heal very well.

Etiology/pathophysiology
Ingestion of sharp foreign bodies, entrapment of loose soft-tissue structures or rostral mandible and incisive bone (771), or laceration of the mouth and tongue occur sporadically in horses, resulting in painful lesions that may be complicated by loss of vascularity or the presence of embedded foreign material. Lacerations involving the lips are common in young horses as a result of becoming hooked on sharp objects and rearing to escape.

Clinical presentation
Traumatic wounds to the mouth involving foreign bodies or very sharp dental overgrowths may bleed profusely initially, but they rapidly cease discharging and, in normal circumstances, will heal spontaneously in 3–10 days. The presence of foreign material in the wound will result in delayed healing or the formation of a sinus tract communicating with the foreign body. Eventually, abscessation may occur. Such cases may present with a painful soft-tissue swelling in the oral cavity, particularly in the intermandibular space, which may be palpable externally. Fetid discharges may exude from sinus tracts associated with foreign bodies, and halitosis, hypersalivation, and pain when masticating may be observed. Regional lymph nodes, including the submandibular lymph nodes, may be enlarged. Lacerations to the tongue may be associated with a reluctance to accept the bit or pain when ridden on the bridle.

Differential diagnosis
Painful swellings in the vicinity of the oral cavity must be distinguished from abscesses due to systemic diseases such as those caused by *Streptococcus equi* var. *equi*. Discharging tracts from the gingiva can also be associated with mandibular fractures and, occasionally, sequestra in the interdental spaces as a result of bit trauma. Tongue lacerations are often obscure due to the high mobility of the tongue and the difficulty of examination when it is injured.

Diagnosis
Most lacerations are clearly visible on a thorough oral examination and only minimal further investigation is necessary. Injuries associated with chronically discharging tracts should be assessed radiographically to rule out the presence of sequestra or fractures.

Management
Most oral lacerations heal spontaneously with minimal intervention other than tetanus prophylaxis and broad-spectrum antibiotics. Damage to salivary ducts can be associated with chronic salivary fistulae, many of which granulate eventually. The provision of a semi-liquidized diet can enable animals with severe oral pain to eat. Severe lacerations can be repaired in multiple layers with absorbable sutures to accelerate healing. Some tongue lacerations involving almost full-thickness transection may require surgical debridement and repair under general anesthesia. Any potentially viable tissue should be salvaged wherever possible, and even apparently severe wounds can heal surprisingly well with surgical repair using multiple layers of absorbable sutures, despite the contaminated operating field (772). Loss of the rostral portion of the tongue can adversely affect the ability of the horse to accommodate a normal bitted bridle.

503

Stomatitis

Definition/overview
Stomatitis is defined as inflammation of the soft tissues of the oral cavity.

Etiology/pathophysiology
Stomatitis is an uncommon condition in horses and is usually associated with inflammation secondary to other disease processes. Viral stomatitis may affect the dorsum of the tongue and the lips, and is usually self-limiting in adult horses. This disease is caused by a rhabdovirus and is enzootic in some regions of North America. It tends to be seasonal in nature, occurring in summer, and is believed to have an insect vector. Stomatitis has also been attributed to infection of the lips and gums with *Actinobacillus lignieri*. Migrating *Gasterophilus* larvae in the oral mucosa may also cause a painful stomatitis. Stomatitis may also result from ingestion of caustic chemicals, severe periodontal disease secondary to food impaction in the interdontium, and trauma.

Clinical presentation
Increased salivation may be observed with stomatitis. The presence of raised vesicles on the lips or tongue, gingival reddening or hemorrhage, ulceration of the tongue and lips, and reluctance to masticate can all indicate stomatitis. Rupture of the vesicles in viral vesicular stomatitis results in large painful ulcers. Careful oral examination to identify the primary cause is essential before deciding upon treatment.

Differential diagnosis
Inflammatory disease of the oral cavity may be easily confused with neoplastic conditions such as SCC, and the presence of the primary cause (e.g. dental disease) must be identified.

Diagnosis
Clinical findings can be confirmed by oral endoscopy, radiography to eliminate the presence of dental apical disease, and biopsy of any lesions suspected to be neoplastic. Confirmation of the etiology in vesicular stomatitis is by serologic investigation.

Management
Treatment of any inciting cause (e.g. dental overgrowths, diastemata, or caries) is essential. Debridement of infected or necrotic material from lesions will accelerate the healing process. Diet modification using moistened gruel until vesicular ulcers granulate and epithelialize will aid patient care. Additional treatments such as broad-spectrum antimicrobials, soft diet, and mouthwashes can be useful.

Lampus

Definition/overview
Lampus describes the condition of swollen soft tissues covering the hard palate, resulting in loss of occlusion of the incisors.

Etiology/pathophysiology
Historically, hyperemia and swelling of the gingiva on the ventral aspect of the hard palate was observed in young horses that were in the process of shedding their deciduous incisors and typically were grazing coarse forage. The transient hyperemia and inflammation of the gingival tissues coincidental with dental eruption are now considered to be normal physiologic conditions in a percentage of horses. The condition was historically treated by cauterizing the hard palate to induce cicatrization or by making incisions caudal to the upper incisors, resulting in hemorrhage, which reduced any venous congestion.

Differential diagnosis
In older horses, edema of the hard palate associated with certain abrasive or spikey leaves is very similar in appearance to the juvenile condition.

Management
No pathologic lesions have been identified with this condition and the current view is that there is no justification for any treatment. The swellings almost invariably recede spontaneously and without any negative consequences. Slight edema or loose palatal gingiva may ensue in a few cases. Treatment with NSAIDs may be useful if the condition is judged to be sufficiently painful to impede eating.

Oral photosensitization

Definition/overview
Inflammation of unpigmented tissues can occur as a result of exposure to intense light. Photosensitization may occur secondary to hepatic disease and in association with ingestion of certain plant materials and other chemicals.

Etiology/pathophysiology
Photosensitization can be a consequence of hepatic photosensitization, aberrant pigment formation, or topical contact with photodynamic agents. Photosensitization has been identified after ingestion of plants (including St John's wort, perennial rye grass, and trefoil), chemicals (including rose Bengal acetate, methylene blue, sulfonamides, and tetracyclines), and fungi (including blue-green algae and fungi present on lupins). Photosensitization of hepatic origin has been associated with fireweed, ragwort, fiddle neck, and rattleweed intoxication. The pathogenesis is

similar, irrespective of the source of the photodynamic substances. In hepatic photosensitization the photodynamic agent is phylloerythrin. The photodynamic metabolites are deposited in the skin and activated in contact with light by absorbing energy, which results in free radical release and subsequent cell membrane damage involving various lysozymes and cytokines.

Clinical presentation
Typically, areas of nonpigmented skin and mucocutaneous junctions, including the lips and eyelids, may become inflamed and erythematous after exposure to sunlight. There are signs of swelling and pain at the affected sites. Clinical signs, including raised or erythematous areas of nonpigmented skin with evidence of self-trauma in response to pruritus, can be observed. Vesicles and bullae may eventually form, leading to crusting and necrosis. The clinical signs continue to become more severe as long as the animal is exposed to the triggering light or until the photoactive metabolites are further metabolized to nonactive products. Clinical signs of liver disease including inappetence, jaundice, and weight loss may be detected in more acute or severe cases.

Differential diagnosis
Photosensitization is included in a list of diseases resulting in erythematous skin lesions, especially when these are confined to nonpigmented areas. The lesions can be similar in appearance to those of other immune-mediated skin diseases and hypersensitivities. Grossly, the lesions may resemble SCC or papilloma, but they are generally more widespread. Lesions caused by self-trauma due to the photosensitive pruritus must be distinguished from other hypersensitivity and traumatic lesions. Clinical signs of liver disease are often nonspecific, but persistent jaundice, weight loss, and inappetence must be investigated.

Diagnosis
Biopsy of the skin lesions will demonstrate a type 1 immune-mediated hypersensitivity, without evidence of neoplasia. The reaction may be clearly demarcated histologically into the nonpigmented and pigmented areas. Diagnosis of liver disease is covered elsewhere (see Chapter 5).

Management
Removal of the subject from the source of radiation will prevent continuing worsening of the clinical signs. Management of the primary cause, if possible, is important. Skin lesions will often respond to administration of dexamethasone (0.1–0.2 mg/kg i/v) and can usually be reduced with oral prednisolone (1 mg/kg p/o).

Prognosis
The prognosis depends on the cause of the photosensitization, but is guarded in cases secondary to advanced nonreversible hepatic disease. Specific features of liver disease are described elsewhere (see Chapter 5).

Diseases of the hyoid apparatus
Definition/overview
The hyoid apparatus is the trapeze-like arrangement of bones that suspends the larynx and tongue from the base of the skull. The bones comprise paired ketarohyoid, epihyoid, stylohyoid, and thyrohyoid bones joined by a single basihyoid and the linguohyoid, into which inserts the base of the tongue. Injuries affecting the hyoid apparatus include fracture of the hyoid apparatus and temporohyoid osteopathy, in which periosteal reaction around the temporohyoid articulation can result in enlargement of the hyoid bones and ankylosis of this articulation.

Etiology/pathophysiology
Primary fractures of the hyoid apparatus are extremely rare. They are reported to arise occasionally following severe trauma to the ventral aspect of the head, although the physical protection accorded by the skull and mandibles renders such precise trauma extremely unusual. Pathologic fracture of the stylohyoid bones is suspected in cases with temporohyoid osteopathy in which ankylosis of the articulation has occurred. This obscure disease has been described as a chronic sequela of auditory-tube and guttural-pouch inflammation associated with guttural-pouch mycosis or empyema. The strain put on the stylohyoid during swallowing is suspected to be sufficient to cause fracture of the weakened bone where the articulation is fused.

Clinical presentation
Signs may include nasal discharge and neurologic disease if secondary to guttural-pouch empyema or mycosis. Swelling in the parotid region may be palpated. Slow eating or difficulty with swallowing may be detectable on the affected side. Fracture at the petrous temporal articulation can result in ascending infection, leading to meningitis with progressive neurologic signs. Palpation of the larynx and manipulation of the larynx or tongue are resented when the condition is painful.

Differential diagnosis
Conditions affecting the hyoid apparatus must be differentiated from other causes of dysphagia including botulism, tetanus, equine grass sickness, dental lesions, guttural-pouch mycosis, jaw fractures, and temporomandibular luxations.

505

Diagnosis

Endoscopic examination of the guttural pouch may reveal gross deformity of the stylohyoid bones, particularly at the articulation with the petrous temporal bone. In some cases changes are not endoscopically visible. Lateral radiographs, obliqued in a rostrocaudal direction to separate the radiographic superimposition of the stylohyoid bones, may reveal lysis or proliferative changes to the margins of the stylohyoid bones.

Management

Freeing of the articulation by removal of one section of the stylohyoid bone has been attempted, but the prognosis is guarded in many cases. Fractured stylohyoid bones appear to form a bony union with callus formation, although it is unclear in such cases whether the fracture is associated with the temporohyoid syndrome.

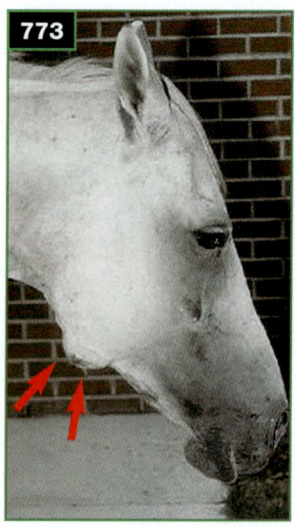

773 A horse with a distended salivary duct (arrows) due to obstruction in the submandibular region.

Diseases of the salivary glands

The salivary glands of the horse consist of paired parotid, sublingual, and submaxillary glands, of which the parotid glands are the largest and produce the greatest volume of saliva. Saliva contains electrolytes, the concentration of which is dependent on flow rate, which is variable, but up to 50 ml/minute has been recorded in ponies. Diseases affecting the salivary glands are rare in horses and most are acquired as a consequence of trauma. A single case of congenital salivary-tract atresia has been reported.

Trauma to the salivary glands and ducts

Definition/overview

Parotid-duct trauma is the most commonly encountered salivary disorder. The parotid salivary gland lobules drain via multiple small ductules, which converge and anastomose to form the parotid duct. The parotid duct passes ventrally on the medial side of the mandible before traversing its lateral border to ascend rostral to the masseter muscle before entering the oral cavity via the parotid papilla at the level of the 3rd cheek tooth.

Etiology/pathophysiology

Trauma to the parotid duct can result from kicks to the mandible, lacerations, and surgical treatments including dental and guttural-pouch surgery.

Clinical presentation

The most common location of parotid-duct damage is on the ventral aspect of the mandible where the duct passes from the medial to the lateral aspects. Small wounds to the duct lead to saliva leakage, with staining of the hair in some cases. This is usually short-lived and resolves spontaneously after a few days as the duct heals by granulation.

If a large volume of saliva is draining continuously, a salivary fistula can develop; if the skin heals but the duct fails to do so, a salivary mucocele follows (773).

Diagnosis

The clinical appearance and production of saliva in response to stimulation of food are normally diagnostic. Retrograde contrast radiography has been attempted.

Differential diagnosis

Sinus tracts due to foreign body penetration; dentigerous cysts; tooth root infections.

Management

Wounds to the parotid gland usually heal by granulation. When surgical debridement is indicated, care should be taken to avoid iatrogenic damage to branches of the salivary duct. The withholding of feed and feeding via a nasogastric tube to reduce salivary stimulation can be attempted, albeit generally with limited success. Fistulae resulting from trauma to the gland also heal by granulation in most instances. Persistent salivary-duct fistulae can be treated surgically, with the intention being to repair the damaged duct. The duct is approached by surgically debriding the fistula and dissecting down to the duct. A thin salivary catheter is then passed caudad towards the gland and rostrad towards the salivary papillae in the oral cavity. The duct is sutured with fine absorbable material (5-0 polydioxanone or polyglactin). The end emerging from the papilla is sutured to the cheek and the tube left *in situ* as a stent for 3 weeks.

A more simple surgical solution is to ligate the salivary duct proximal to the fistula. Unless salivary flow is re-established, partial atrophy of the gland follows. Sclerosis of the duct by catheterization and injecting it with iodine solution has also been suggested to achieve occlusion of the duct. The preferred sclerosing agent is 10% buffered formalin, which is injected and kept in contact for 1–2 minutes. Other agents have been used, but with more serious side-effects including facial edema.

Trauma to the sublingual glands can result in a sublingual salivary mucocele. These lesions, which are located lateral to the frenulum, can easily be treated by marsupialization into the oral cavity.

Salivary gland calculi (sialoliths)

Definition/overview

Salivary calculi are precipitations of mineralized material within the salivary glands or ducts.

Etiology/pathophysiology

Salivary calculi are rare in horses. They are of clinical significance if they become lodged in the salivary papilla at the orifice of the parotid salivary duct. The calculi consist of calcium carbonate and sloughed cells and they can reach several centimeters in size.

Clinical presentation

Distension of the duct proximal to the calculus may be detected by palpation.

Differential diagnosis

Inflammation of the parotid gland, parotid melanoma, retropharyngeal or submandibular lymphadenitis, and guttural-pouch enlargement may have a similar clinical presentation.

Diagnosis

Salivary calculi are often radio-opaque and therefore visible on plain radiographs. Ultrasonography may reveal hyperechoic matter within the parenchyma of the salivary glands or within the ducts.

Management

The calculus can be freed by incising the buccal mucosa via an oral approach in the sedated horse. The sialolith is expressed into the oral cavity and the duct heals by granulation. A more technically difficult approach is to incise the skin and duct over the calculus, after local desensitization, and subsequently meticulously to close the duct with fine sutures, after ensuring that the distal portion is patent. Permanent stenosis of the duct causes chronic distension and mucocele formation.

Sialoadenitis

Definition/overview

Sialoadenitis is inflammation of the salivary glands or ducts.

Etiology/pathophysiology

Transient inflammation of the salivary gland can occur following trauma to the gland or after duct obstruction, but it is uncommon. This phenomenon may be observed in grazing horses in Europe and Australia, particularly in the early growing season, but it appears to be rare in the USA.

Clinical presentation/diagnosis

The glands are bilaterally swollen, but nonpainful, a few days after grazing at pasture. Sialoadenitis may occur sporadically or as a herd outbreak.

Management

Most cases resolve spontaneously when the horse is removed from the pasture, provided that duct patency is unobstructed.

Salivary gland neoplasia

Neoplasia affecting the salivary gland is rare. Adenocarcinomas, acinar cell tumors, and mixed-cell carcinomas have been reported. Enlargement of the parotid gland associated with advanced melanoma is not uncommon in gray horses, and the swelling may be sufficiently large to impinge into the pharynx and restrict airflow in extreme cases. Dissection of the melanoma from the gland tissue is virtually impossible, and radiation therapy has been used to achieve remission in a few cases. Medical treatment using the H2 receptor antagonist cimetidine (2.5–5.0 mg/kg q12h p/o) has been reported to result in remission in a small series of cases, but the efficacy of this treatment appears to be inconclusive.

Ptyalism

Ptyalism or excessive salivation may occur in response to oral pain, periodontal disease, mucosal penetration by a foreign body, and ingestion of the fungus *Rhizoctonia legumincola*. The clinical signs may also be associated secondarily with other diseases including rabies, esophageal obstruction, pharyngeal dysphagia, and stomatitis. Where the ptyalism is caused by a fungal infection, the excess salivation is induced by the toxin slaframine, which is a parasympathomimetic. The toxin may also induce lacrimation, anorexia, and diarrhea. Investigation should be directed at identifying the primary cause and this should include an oral examination, pharyngeal endoscopy, and passage of a nasogastric tube.

507

Diseases of the esophagus

Anatomy of the equine esophagus

The esophagus is located dorsal to the larynx and then rotates slightly to the left of the midline as it descends towards the thorax. It consists of stratified squamous mucosa within a spiraling muscular tube, which contains both striated and smooth muscle in the cranial two-thirds and smooth muscle layers only in the caudal third. There is no serosal layer and the outer adventitial layer is suspended within the mediastinum. The esophagus occupies a position dorsal and slightly to the left of the trachea and is in close association with the carotid arteries within the carotid sheath and the cranial sympathetic trunk and recurrent laryngeal nerves. The cranial esophageal sphincter is about 5 cm long and comprises the esophagus together with the cricopharyngeus and the thyropharyngeus muscles, which occlude it when contracted. During swallowing, the food bolus is voluntarily passed into the pharynx using the tongue and pharyngeal muscles under a complex mechanism involving CNs IX, X, XI, and XII. The larynx is moved ventrally and caudally, the epiglottis is retroverted as the bolus passes into the oropharynx, and the esophageal sphincter muscles relax, allowing the bolus to pass into the esophagus. Thereafter, swallowing is an involuntary reflex controlled by branches of the vagus (CN X) nerve. The esophagus enters the stomach via the cardiac or caudal esophageal sphincter, a tight muscular ring approximately 10 cm long that prevents esophageal reflux under normal circumstances.

Clinical signs of esophageal disease

Eesophageal disease often presents as signs of swallowing difficulties. Dysphagia, nasal discharge, hypersalivation, and sweating are all associated with esophageal obstruction. Aspiration of food spilling from an obstructed esophagus can also result in coughing and signs of aspiration pneumonia. Perforation of the esophagus can lead to a painful mediastinal cellulitis, while esophageal reflux syndrome in foals can cause intermittent signs of esophageal pain associated with food ingestion.

Diagnosis of esophageal diseases

Physical examination

A physical examination should include careful palpation of the neck from the larynx to the thoracic inlet for signs of swelling, pain, edema, cellulitis, crepitus, or firm masses. General physical parameters such as circulatory function, hydration status, hematologic parameters, electrolyte imbalances, and neurologic examination of the CNs should also be included. Cautious passage of a round-ended, well-lubricated nasogastric tube should be attempted. It may be advisable for the horse to be sedated for this procedure. Severe resistance to the passage of the nasogastric tube suggests an esophageal obstruction, and attempts to force the tube through or past the obstruction are contraindicated as they may lead to esophageal wall perforation. The absence of a swallowing reflex may indicate the presence of neurologic dysfunction, which should be considered in the context of other neurologic deficits. A thorough oral examination should be performed to check for any pharyngeal obstructions or causes of oral dysphagia.

Esophagoscopy

Esophagoscopy is essential in order to examine the lumen of the esophagus. It is safe and convenient to perform in the conscious sedated horse. A 2 m endoscope is sufficient to reach the cardia in most horses, although a 3 m endoscope can be useful for gastroscopy as well. Care must be taken when passing the endoscope into the pharynx to avoid retroflexion of the end of the endoscope into the oral cavity, with resultant crushing of the end of the endoscope. This can be avoided by the placement of a Hausmann's gag for esophagoscopy, or by passing a short wide-bore nasogastric tube into the cranial esophagus before introducing the endoscope. The lubricated endoscope is passed all the way down the esophagus into the stomach. The esophageal lumen can then be examined by inflating the esophagus as the endoscope is withdrawn. Constant irrigation will be necessary to identify mucosal lesions. The normal esophagus is collapsed with longitudinal folds, which flatten when it is distended. Good distension is required to avoid missing small focal or longitudinal esophageal perforations. If the esophagus is obstructed with food, the cranial end of the bolus and the type of feed can be identified, but visibility may be poor in the presence of food and saliva in the lumen.

Radiography

Both plain and contrast radiographs should be included in a thorough esophageal investigation. The esophagus is of soft-tissue density and it cannot normally be identified as a discrete structure on plain films. If the horse has previously had a nasogastric tube passed, or if it has a disorder of the cranial esophageal sphincter muscles such as with 4th branchial arch syndrome, a gas density shadow representing air in the lumen can be identified. The presence of granular shadows caused by food stationary in the lumen can be considered an abnormal radiographic finding.

Contrast radiographs are indicated whenever there is a swallowing defect or where there are irregularities or masses associated with the esophageal lumen. Dynamic studies involving fluoroscopic imaging during swallowing are very useful and can demonstrate the presence of duplication cysts or diverticula. External compression of the lumen by masses, generalized cranial megaesophagus, strictures, and vascular ring anomalies may be diagnosed on contrast radiographs or on fluoroscopy. Contrast radiographs can be achieved using gas or barium sulfate, or water-soluble iodinated solution. Barium sulfate mixed into a paste with feed enables voluntary ingestion and swallowing to be imaged. If esophageal wall perforation is suspected, care must be taken with potentially irritant or toxic contrast media. Negative contrast is obtained by inflating the esophagus via a cuffed nasogastric tube placed in the cranial esophagus. Such images are useful for demonstrating foreign bodies, diverticula, and mural perforations, which can become filled with air.

Normal peristalsis can create the impression of irregular lumenal folds and strictures on contrast films. A radiograph taken immediately after distension of the esophagus by injection of contrast medium via a cuffed tube can avoid such artifacts. It should be noted that if evaluation of swallowing reflexes is desired, the study should be attempted without sedation, since most sedatives will affect the swallowing reflexes.

CONGENITAL AND DEVELOPMENTAL DISEASES OF THE ESOPHAGUS

Congenital diseases of the esophagus are rare in horses. Congenital stenosis, persistent right aortic arch, esophageal duplication cysts, intramural duplication cysts, and idiopathic megaesophagus have all been reported.

Congenital persistent right aortic arch
Definition/overview
Congenital persistent right aortic arch is a rare anomaly in which the 4th right aortic arch develops into the functional aorta instead of the normal left vessel.

Etiology/pathophysiology
This is a congenital condition resulting in a fibrous remnant of the ductus arteriosus. The fibrous ductus arteriosus acts to occlude the esophagus between the aortic arch and the left pulmonary artery as the esophagus courses caudally past the heart base into the abdomen.

Clinical signs
Clinical signs are of esophageal dysphagia and obstruction, including salivation, and cervical esophageal distension. The esophagus is usually dilated cranial to the obstruction with diffuse esophagitis.

Differential diagnosis
Esophageal obstruction; 4th branchial arch defects; megaesophagus.

Diagnosis
Diagnosis is based on clinical signs of esophageal dysphagia. This can be confirmed by plain and contrast radiographs showing dilatation of the esophagus proximal

to the ductus arteriosus. In addition, esophagoscopy demonstrates a dilated proximal esophagus with an apparent stricture just cranial to the level of the heart.

Management
Successful surgical correction has been reported in one foal. Euthanasia may be more practical.

Esophageal duplication cysts and intramural duplication cysts
Definition/overview
Esophageal duplication cysts are congenitally replicated segments of the proximal esophagus as a result of bifurcation of the embryonic esophageal tube. Intramural duplication cysts are evaginations within the wall of the esophagus lined by stratified squamous epithelium; they are separated from the main esophagus.

Etiology/pathophysiology
The lesions arise congenitally as elements of the embryonic alimentary endoderm become separated from the main alimentary tube. These lesions result in external compression on the esophageal lumen causing effective obstruction.

Clinical presentation
A palpable swelling may be present in the cervical esophagus, which increases as the cysts enlarge. The swellings can cause impingement of the true esophageal lumen and may result in intermittent esophageal dysphagia and signs of 'choke'.

Differential diagnosis
Esophageal obstruction; thyroid masses; cervical abscessation; parotid salivary gland enlargement; esophageal diverticulum.

Diagnosis
Esophagoscopy may reveal a lumen to be present in the case of duplication cysts; this has been reported in young animals involving both the esophagus and components of the esophagus and trachea. Contrast esophagrams may show accumulation of contrast in the lumen of duplication cysts, which often communicates with the esophageal lumen. Cutaneous ultrasonography is a useful technique for evaluating such lesions noninvasively, and aspiration may demonstrate squamous cells, supporting the diagnosis of an esophageal cyst.

Management
Successful treatment of the cysts has been performed by marsupialization of the cyst. Attempted removal of the cyst *in toto* can be complicated by dehiscence of the esophageal lumen and mediastinitis.

Megaesophagus

Definition/overview

Megaesophagus involves persistent dilatation of the esophagus, resulting in failure of peristalsis and accumulation of ingesta in the esophagus.

Etiology/pathophysiology

Primary megaesophagus is a consequence of motor dysfunction of the esophageal musculature. Congenital esophageal dilatation syndrome involving neural and muscular components has also been described. Secondary megaesophagus can be associated with other conditions such as equine grass sickness, botulism, toxicity with lead, thallium or anticholinesterase, and following sedation with acepromazine and detomidine. Neurologic dysfunction associated with acquired diseases such as EPM and EHV-1 infection can also result in temporary megaesophagus. A transient megaesophagus can be observed after persistent esophageal obstruction or indwelling nasogastric tube placement.

Clinical presentation

Observation while grazing can reveal palpable dilatation of the esophagus on the left hand side of the neck, which may be reducible when the head is raised (774). Such impaction is more obvious when solid food is being ingested and may not be obvious with liquid food. Since the obstruction is incomplete, such animals may learn to compensate and to maintain body condition. Aspiration pneumonia is a secondary complication.

Differential diagnosis

Esophageal obstruction; esophageal diverticula.

Diagnosis

Cases of megaesophagus may present with obstruction at the caudal esophageal sphincter with damming of ingesta cranially, which may be visible on plain and contrast radiographs.

Management

Dietary management will help avoid complete esophageal obstruction and aspiration of food. Metoclopramide and bethanecol have been used to improve muscular tone in the distal esophagus, and to reduce gastroesophageal reflux. Transient secondary cases may gradually improve after conservative treatment, but permanent megaesophagus with persistent dysphagia carries a guarded prognosis.

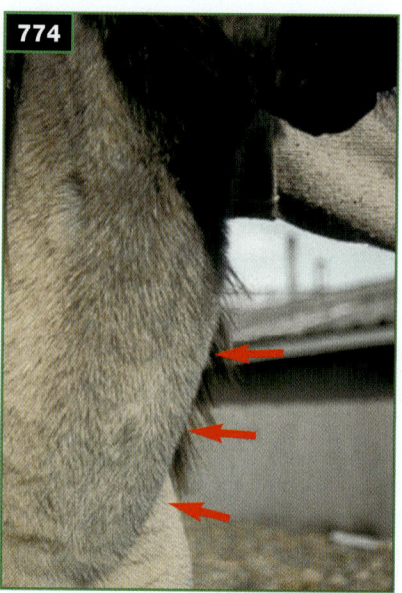

774 Swelling on the left side of the neck (arrows) due to a megaesophagus in which food has accumulated.

Gastroesophageal reflux syndrome

Definition /overview

This is a condition in which gastric contents are refluxed into the caudal esophagus.

Etiology/pathophysiology

Reflux esophagitis is the consequence of repeated episodes of gastric fluid regurgitation into the distal esophagus. The gastric acid results in chemical injury to the mucosa; eventually, mucosal sloughing and ulceration can occur. Reflux esophagitis may occur in combination with gastric ulcer disease, motility disorders including intestinal ileus, or distal esophageal sphincter dysfunction. It is most common in weanlings, but can also occur in adults. Acquired esophagitis can also occur during indwelling nasogastric tube placement, frequent nasogastric tube passage, or after esophageal obstruction.

Clinical presentation

The clinical signs are nonspecific, including signs similar to those of esophageal obstruction. Discomfort when ingesting, including gagging, bruxism, hypersalivation, and anorexia, may all be exhibited. The inflammation can also cause esophageal hypomotility, with secondary obstruction with food if the horse continues to eat.

Differential diagnosis

Colic signs in foals; gastric ulceration; cardiac sphincter stenosis; esophageal obstruction.

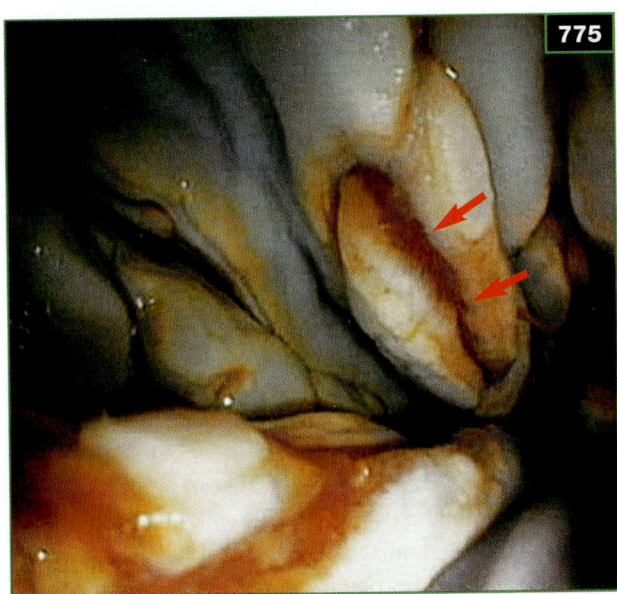

775 Striated ulceration of the mucosa in a young horse with gastroesophageal reflux syndrome.

Diagnosis

Thorough esophagoscopy after clearing obstructions to examine for signs of esophagitis is indicated (**775**). The presence of patchy or linear ulceration is diagnostic for esophagitis. A careful examination for any underlying cause, including gastroscopy, is necessary to prevent chronic recurrence.

Management

Any primary cause such as esophageal obstruction should be removed. Treatment with H2 receptor antagonists (e.g. ranitidine or cimetidine) or omeprazole is beneficial in reducing gastric acid production and ongoing chemical damage of the esophageal mucosa. Alteration in feeding regimens to prompt continuous gastric outflow can also reduce symptoms. NSAIDs may be indicated for their fibrinolytic effects to help reduce the likelihood of fibrous stricture formation at the distal esophageal sphincter, although their use should be carefully restricted in neonates to avoid increasing the possibility of gastric ulceration. Gastric protectants such as sucralfate are of questionable benefit, but they may contribute by physical protection of the ulcerated mucosa. The feeding of semi-liquidized food will help reduce the likelihood of esophageal obstruction at the distal esophageal sphincter.

Stricture of the distal esophageal sphincter as a result of fibrosis is thought to be a consequence of chronic reflux esophagitis and is occasionally diagnosed in young and adult horses.

ACQUIRED ESOPHAGEAL DISORDERS
Esophageal obstruction ('choke')
Definition/overview
Esophageal obstruction is a relatively common problem that occurs from physical obstruction of the esophagus with ingesta.

Etiology/pathophysiology
Physical obstruction of the esophagus with an impacted food bolus is the most commonly diagnosed esophageal disorder in the adult horse. Inadequate soaking of proprietary or preserved foods is cited as the most frequent predisposing cause. The presence of motility disorders within the esophagus has been cited as a cause, but is unproven, although the occurrence of esophageal obstruction in horses at grass suggests an underlying problem. Sugar beet pulp that is inadequately soaked is the most commonly implicated foodstuff in many regions. Absorption of saliva by the food bolus results in swelling and lodgement in the esophagus, commonly at the thoracic inlet where the diameter is narrowest and where the esophagus changes direction. Spasm of the esophageal muscle distal to the bolus can occur, preventing its further passage by peristalsis. Horses commonly continue to eat after esophageal obstruction, leading to a food accumulation, which extends proximally almost as far as the larynx.

Clinical presentation
Nasogastric reflux of food and saliva can be observed from both nostrils and, occasionally, from the mouth. Hypersalivation, dysphagia, and possible abnormal lip movements are associated with esophageal obstruction. Other clinical signs include coughing and retching attempts during swallowing, anxiety, with elevated pulse and respiratory rates, and sweating on the neck. An inability to swallow despite ongoing saliva production can lead to dehydration and electrolyte disturbances including hypochloremia if significant saliva losses are incurred.

Differential diagnosis
Esophageal diverticula, congenital anomalies, cardiac sphincter incompetence, grass sickness, and botulism may present with similar signs.

Diagnosis

Attempts to pass a nasogastric tube will be met with resistance at the proximal end of the obstructing bolus. This should be performed with care, particularly if the obstruction has been present for a while. Esophagoscopy may indicate the type of food and can demonstrate the presence of lumenal defects or a diverticulum, but the view is often obscured by food (776). Radiography may reveal gas, fluid, and food retention.

Management

Many horses tolerate obstruction for 24 hours or more without significant esophageal mucosal damage. Nevertheless, the potential for electrolyte and fluid disturbances, dehydration, inhalation pneumonia, and esophageal ulceration demands a prompt response to the condition.

Spontaneous clearing of the obstruction will occur in many cases if relaxation of the esophageal muscle spasm can be achieved. Assessment of the horse's hydration status and supplementation with intravenous polyionic fluids is desirable and will contribute to spontaneous correction of the obstruction. Smooth-muscle relaxants such as N-butylscopolammonium bromide (Buscopan), acepromazine, diazepam, and alpha-2 agonists (including xylazine, detomidine, and romifidine) are all used, with anecdotal success. In addition to causing muscle relaxation, the alpha-2 agonist reduces anxiety and promotes a lower head carriage, which assists oral drainage. Oxytocin has been reported to encourage muscle relaxation during esophageal obstruction, although the mechanism is unclear. Softening of the bolus by irrigation with warm water through a narrow irrigation tube can be effective.

Great care should be taken to avoid excessive force when advancing the tube, which could perforate the delicate esophageal mucosa. The horse should always be sufficiently sedated so that its head remains lowered throughout the procedure. The water should be infused slowly enough to allow drainage around the tube without excessive overflow into the trachea. It must be assumed that some aspiration will occur during this procedure. As the bolus is softened, it is gradually removed with the egress water, allowing cautious advancement of the tube. Great patience is required to completely remove the obstruction when the bolus is extensive. Cases with chronic or severe obstruction, or where the risk of aspiration is increased, can be more effectively corrected under general anesthesia, when a cuffed endotracheal tube can be placed in the esophagus. The horse is positioned with its head dependent to encourage drainage from the esophagus, allowing a narrower tube to be placed in its lumen for ingress of fluids. This enables ingress and egress of fluids and ingesta via the cuffed tube without the risk of aspiration and over a longer period of time, enabling a gradual and controlled softening and bougienage of the impacted ingesta. A cuffed endotracheal tube should be left *in situ* while the horse recovers in order to prevent any possible aspiration during recovery. Broad-spectrum antimicrobials should be administered if aspiration has occurred.

Esophageal ulceration

Definition/overview

Esophageal ulceration involves full-thickness erosion of the esophageal mucosa.

Etiology/pathophysiology

Esophageal ulceration can occur secondary to esophageal obstruction. Circumferential ulceration is particularly hazardous since the cicatrization of the healing ulcer can lead to a permanent esophageal stricture, which will result in repeated episodes of esophageal obstruction at this site. Ulceration is also observed in the distal esophagus associated with gastroesophageal reflux.

Clinical presentation

Affected horses may present with hypersalivation, recurrent esophageal obstruction, discomfort when swallowing food, and chronic colic.

Differential diagnosis

SCC of the esophagus.

776 Esophagoscopy showing an atypical obstruction with grass.

Diagnosis

Diagnosis is by esophagoscopy, when the red submucosa is visible surrounded by the frayed edges of the eroded stratified squamous epithelium (777). Contrast esophagrams may show some stricture at the site of a circumferential ulcer (778).

Management

Treatment with NSAIDs such as phenylbutazone will delay fibrosis. Repeated endoscopic monitoring of the healing site and feeding of moistened softened food are advisable, before reintroducing a normal diet. Fibrosed strictures can involve all layers or just the muscular and adventitious layers. Full-thickness strictures, which form after deep, circumferential ulcers, can be observed endoscopically and demonstrated on contrast esophagrams. Treatment by resection of the scar and anastomosis has been attempted with limited success due to the re-formation of a stricture at the anastomosis site. Longitudinal esophagotomy, including longitudinal sectioning of the scar with second-intention healing, results in a traction diverticulum, which is less likely to obstruct than the circumferential scar. Partial-thickness strictures that do not involve the mucosa have been successfully treated by esophagomyotomy. The lumen of strictures following circumferential ulceration is at its narrowest 30 days after the ulceration; thereafter it increases and has been reported as largest at 60 days. Esophageal dilators have been used for bougienage dilation, but they have met with very limited success in horses.

Esophageal diverticula

Definition/overview

Esophageal diverticula are pathologic evaginations of the esophageal mucosa resulting from a defect in the muscularis layer.

Etiology/pathophysiology

Esophageal diverticula are usually acquired lesions. Two types have been described. Traction diverticula are the result of fibrosis and adhesion of periesophageal scar tissue following a partial- or full-thickness wound. In addition, they occur following the healing of a ventral esophagotomy by second intention. Pulsion diverticula form when a defect of the esophageal muscularis occurs. The intact esophageal mucosa prolapses through the muscular defect and then increases in size as the diverticulum becomes impacted with food.

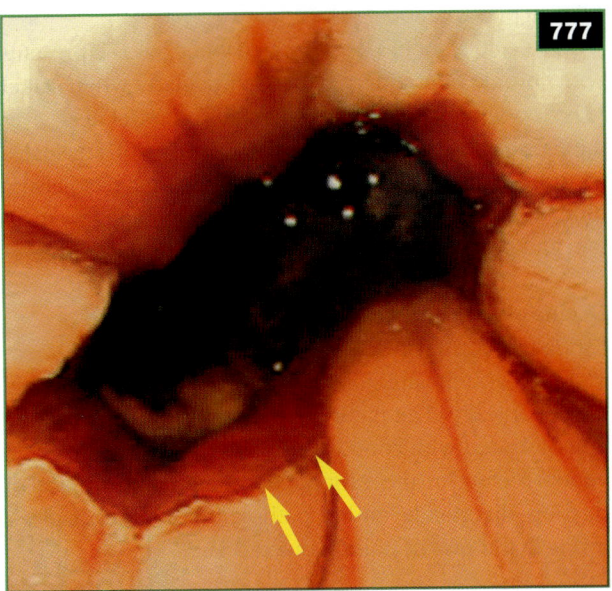

777 Esophagoscopy of a horse's esophagus after chronic obstruction, showing circumferential mucosal ulceration (arrows).

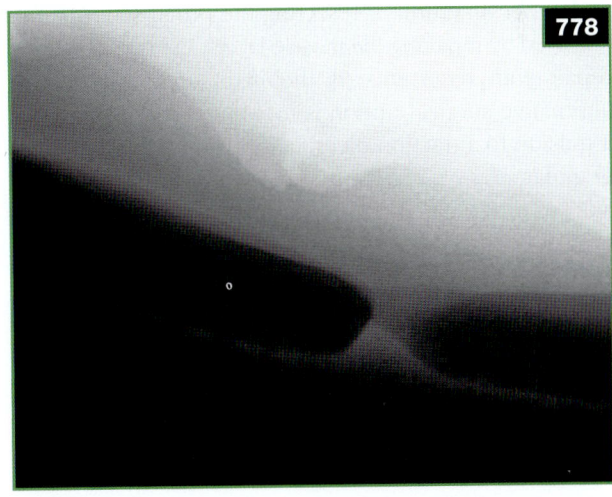

778 Contrast esophagram showing narrowing of the esophageal lumen due to a circumferential esophageal stricture.

513

Clinical presentation

A diverticulum should be suspected when a horse presents with chronic intermittent choke, particularly when out at grass, or when there is a swelling of the cervical neck over the esophagus that does not prevent passage of a nasogastric tube. Care must be taken when passing a nasogastric tube to avoid the end of the tube passing into the diverticulum and perforating the mucosa.

Diagnosis

Esophagoscopy will often reveal flattening of the lumen, and food accumulating in the diverticulum may be visible endoscopically. The nature of a diverticulum can best be demonstrated with contrast esophagrams, which reveal a ventral defect in the esophageal lumen in the case of traction diverticula and a pathognomonic 'hour-glass' image in the case of pulsion diverticula (779).

Management

Traction diverticula rarely cause obstruction and, in most cases, do not require intervention. Pulsion diverticula can be treated by a surgical approach to the esophagus over the diverticulum, longitudinal division of the muscle layer, and either inverting or resecting the prolapsed mucosa, followed by repairing the muscle layers. Breakdown of the repair with recurrence is the main complication. An alternative surgical option is to convert the defect from a pulsion to a traction diverticulum, which is allowed to granulate. Careful feeding of soft food for 4–6 weeks is advised in all cases.

779 Contrast esophagram showing the pathognomonic 'hour-glass' pattern produced by a pulsion diverticulum.

Foreign body penetration and esophageal fistula

Definition/overview

Foreign bodies may cause focal perforation of the esophageal mucosa, with consequences including cellulitis, abscessation, and esophageal dysfunction. Fortunately, such lesions are uncommon in horses because they are relatively fastidious feeders. Failure of complete healing of esophagostomy incisions can result in an esophageocutaneous fistula.

Etiology/pathophysiology

Perforation of the esophageal mucosa by sharp ingested foreign bodies leads to egress of saliva into the interstitium and development of a cellulitis, which eventually abscessates. This results in pain, peristaltic dysfunction, food impaction proximal to the site, and, in some cases, mediastinitis and endotoxic shock.

Clinical presentation

Dysphagia, esophageal obstruction (choke), painful swellings of the neck, hypersalivation, pyrexia, and endotoxic shock.

Differential diagnosis

Primary choke; injection abscesses; diverticula; mediastinitis from other causes.

Diagnosis

Esophagoscopy may reveal the mucosal defect when the esophageal lumen is fully dilated with air, although this can prove to be elusive. Contrast esophagrams may be helpful, although false-negative images are possible.

Management

Some foreign bodies can be retrieved from the esophagus endoscopically, but contrast radiography may be necessary to demonstrate their location. A surgical exploration under general anesthesia may be necessary to remove the foreign body and allow effective drainage of any surrounding septic exudates. The presence of cellulitis or an abscess may cause pain on swallowing and esophageal dysfunction. The abscess may burst into the lumen of the esophagus or subcutaneously to form an esophageal fistula. Periesophageal infections should be cultured to optimize antibiotic administration. If healing of the fistula does not occur after establishing drainage, then surgical resection of the discharging tract followed by closure may be necessary. Antibiotics with a broad-spectrum activity against anaerobic organisms are indicated. Culture and sensitivity testing are recommended wherever possible.

Esophageal rupture

Definition/overview
Esophageal rupture involves traumatic disruption of the esophageal mucosa and other layers.

Etiology/pathophysiology
Rupture of the esophagus can follow prolonged obstruction, over-aggressive nasogastric tube use, or ingestion of foreign bodies (780). Drainage of saliva results in rapid cervical swelling due to the cellulitis, and swallowed air can disperse to form subcutaneous emphysema, which can be demonstrated on radiographs. Extension of cellulitis towards the mediastinum and thoracic cavity can be life-threatening.

Clinical presentation
Cervical swelling, dysphagia, and dyspnea are typically present. Signs of systemic toxemia may be apparent.

Diagnosis
Esophagoscopy and contrast radiographs are critical. Transthoracic ultrasound can be used to demonstrate periesophageal abscesses.

Management
Small, acute defects may be treated by attempted surgical debridement and lavage of the interstitium, combined with inversion and attempted repair of the perforation. An indwelling nasogastric tube allows alimentation, which bypasses the defect. All chronic or heavily contaminated defects are more easily treated by surgical drainage of the affected area and the creation of an esophagostomy caudal to the rupture to allow continued feeding (781). The damaged area is allowed to heal by second intention.

Esophageal neoplasia
Esophageal neoplasia is rare in the horse. Esophageal extension of an SCC originating in the gastric mucosa is the most commonly reported type. The prognosis for such lesions is very guarded and the prognosis for resection is dubious.

Esophageal surgery and esophagostomy
Esophageal surgery in the horse, as with other species, is associated with a high risk of complications and should only be undertaken with careful planning and experience. The absence of a serosal layer results in a high incidence of dehiscence with attempted mucosal repairs and anastomosis. The destructive nature of exudates containing saliva and food means that any leakage results in cellulitis and abscessation. Dissecting mediastinitis can ensue, which can progress to severe depression and endotoxic shock and carries a very poor prognosis. The close proximity of the esophagus to many vital structures leads to a high risk

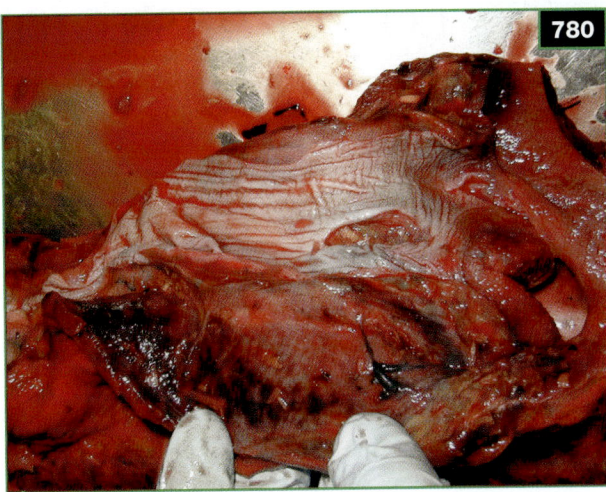

780 Postmortem appearance of an iatrogenic esophageal tear that occurred following nasogastric intubation.

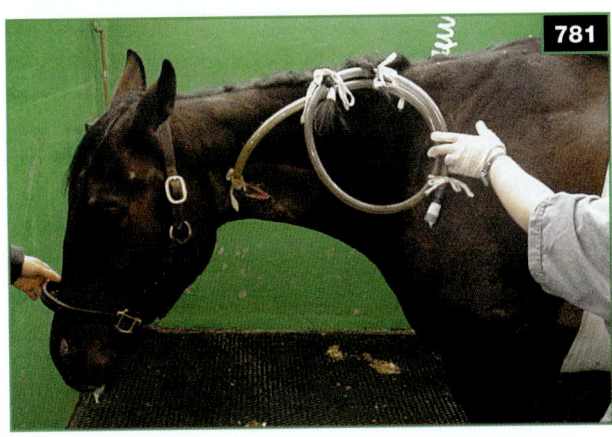

781 Esophagostomy tube.

of iatrogenic damage to other structures including the vagal nerve, sympathetic trunk, and carotid arteries.

Esophagostomy may be indicated to enable passage of a transesophageal feeding tube to allow second-intention healing of proximal esophageal lesions or following pharyngeal surgery. A nasogastric tube is placed into the esophagus before incision of the overlying tissues under local or general anesthesia. Complications include subcutaneous leakage of saliva or gastric reflux, which can lead to a dissecting mediastinitis. After removal of the feeding tube the esophagostomy will close by second intention and a small traction divertuculum can remain.

515

Physical examination

Evaluation of the GI tract (782) should include knowledge of the animal's history, observation of the animal and the surroundings, and a complete physical examination. History should include signalment, occupation of the horse, diet and feeding practices, recent management changes, deworming and dental care schedule, temperament and vices, availability and quality of water, medication received, and duration and occurrence of the problem. Evaluation of the surroundings (e.g. water source, housing condition, and pasture) can provide very useful information. Special attention should be given to assessing the physical appearance of the horse, its body condition, abdominal contour, and skin trauma.

A thorough physical examination should be performed, including evaluation of other body systems such as the cardiovascular, respiratory, neurologic, musculoskeletal, and reproductive systems. This is important, as GI problems can be mistaken for other body system abnormalities and vice versa.

The dentition should be assessed for congenital (e.g. parrot mouth, wry nose) or developmental abnormalities that may be associated with anorexia or have effects on normal eating patterns. The presence of feed material in the oral cavity should be noted. A neurologic examination might be required if there are concerns about the ability of the horse to eat properly. Observation of eating can be useful in some situations.

The neck should be palpated for the presence of masses, crepitus, or pain. While the esophagus usually runs down the left side of the neck, both sides should be examined because it will course down the right side in some horses. Passage of a nasogastric tube will also help in certain esophageal abnormalities.

Qualitative evaluation of intestinal motility can be performed via abdominal auscultation. Transit time can also be a useful assessment of intestinal motility. Passage of mineral oil in the feces following administration via a nasogastric tube should be observed after 8–12 hours.

The consistency, color, and volume of feces should be noted, as should the presence of sand, gravel, or large food particles. An increase in the size of particles in the feces can be indicative of poor mastication or decreased transit time.

Gastrointestinal tract auscultation and percussion

Auscultation is an important component of examination of the GI tract; however, results must be taken in the context of the entire clinical presentation and should not be over-interpreted. Multiple locations should be evaluated. At a minimum, dorsal and ventral quadrants should be ausculted over both abdominal walls. The frequency and character of borborygmi should be noted. Patience is required because of the intermittent nature of borborygmi, particularly sounds associated with cecal contraction. Decreased or absent sounds are indicative of decreased intestinal motility, while increased sounds suggest hypermotility. Sounds of a fluid nature may be present in horses with colic or impending colitis. Simultaneous auscultation and percussion should also be performed to detect 'pings', which indicate underlying gaseous distension.

Palpation per rectum

Evaluation of the intestinal tract per rectum is a useful diagnostic tool that should be performed, if possible, on all horses with colic. The main limitation is that only approximately 40% of the abdomen is palpable in an average horse. Iatrogenic rectal tears can occur, but proper restraint (including chemical restraint) and technique can greatly reduce the risk. The horse should be handled by an experienced person and sedated (i.e. xylazine ± butorphanol) if required. Infusion of lidocaine (60 ml of 2% lidocaine in a 450 kg horse) into the rectum can reduce straining. Ample lubrication should be used. Patience is important and excessive force should never be used. Forcing the arm forward in a straining horse may lead to a rectal tear.

To reach a diagnosis by per-rectum examination it is important to have a good knowledge of the normal anatomy as well as an understanding of displacement and change that can occur in different pathologies.

Normal findings
Left abdomen
The pelvic flexure is located cranially and ventrally to the brim of the pelvis. It is knee-shaped, and bands may be felt if there is some content within. The thin, sharp, caudal edge of the spleen is present against the abdominal wall. The nephrosplenic ligament and posterior pole of the left kidney are palpable dorsomedial to the spleen. The cranial mesenteric artery (CMA) can sometimes be felt caudally and medially to the left kidney, running forward along the aorta.

Right abdomen

The cecum, more particularly its ventral tenial band, is felt running forward and down.

Mid abdomen

The small colon is characterized by the presence of fecal balls, sacculations, and an antimesenteric tenial band. The bladder is found just cranial to the pelvic rim. The small intestine is usually not palpable. In males, the inguinal rings should also be evaluated for any abnormal content such as omentum or small intestinal loops. In mares, the uterus and ovaries should be palpated.

Potential abnormal findings
Stomach

The stomach is not palpable; however, if excessive distension of the stomach is present, the spleen can be displaced caudally.

Small intestine

Small intestinal distension is characterized by the presence of one or more loops of 5–12 cm diameter, smooth-surfaced viscera. It is not always palpable when present, depending on the location of distended intestinal loops. Palpation of the wall of the small intestine should be performed to evaluate the degree of edema.

Cecum

Palpation of distinct contents within the cecum or a tight ventral tenial band running in a vertical plane is indicative of cecal tympany or impaction. In the case of gas distension, the apex of the cecum may be directed dorsally and the ventral tenial band may be in an oblique or transverse position. With some large colon displacements, the cecum may not be found in its normal location.

Large intestine

Large-colon impactions are usually located in the left ventral colon and, less commonly, in the right dorsal colon. As a general rule, feed impaction feels like firm bread dough, which is easily indented by digital pressure, but in which the impressions remain. The free tenial bands of the colon are palpable and run longitudinally. Sacculations are not palpable because of the distension. With impaction of the right dorsal colon, a mass can be felt in small horses in the right quadrant. With gas or fluid distension, the colon can be indented, but the impression does not remain. A gas-distended pelvic flexure is often displaced on the right side or cranially. Edema of the colonic wall is usually indicative of large-colon torsion. Tympany and/or impaction of the left colon with a band running dorsally toward the nephrosplenic space is consistent with left dorsal displacement of the large colon.

Small colon

Small-colon impaction is characterized by palpation of a doughy, sausage-like structure about 10 cm in diameter and usually longer than 30 cm. Other abnormalities that may be palpable on *per-rectum* examination include intraluminal foreign bodies, enteroliths, or intussusception.

Rectum

The absence of feces or presence of mucus-covered feces indicates a decrease in GI transit, which is often secondary to an obstructive disease. If blood is present locally or on the rectal sleeve, the rectum should be palpated carefully for the presence of a rectal tear.

Others

The peritoneal wall should be felt for roughening or a gritty feeling, which will be an indication of peritonitis following bowel rupture.

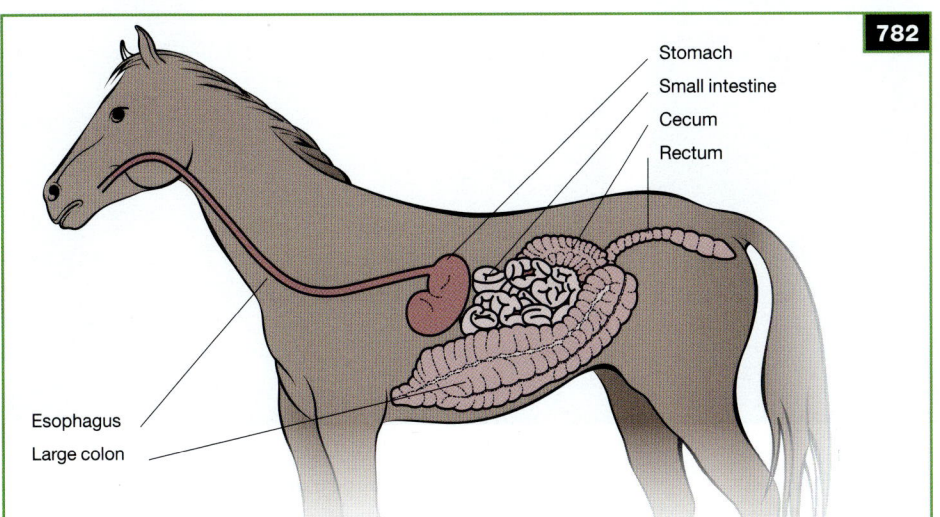

782

Stomach
Small intestine
Cecum
Rectum

Esophagus
Large colon

782 The basic anatomical components of the GI tract and their approximate positioning in the horse . (The small colon is not visible from this viewpoint.)

783 Survey abdominal radiograph in a foal with meconium impaction. Note the radiodense meconium in the cranial abdomen (arrow).

784 Barium enema in a foal with meconium impaction. The contrast dye stops at the level of the impaction.

Diagnostic tests

Nasogastric intubation

Nasogastric intubation is an essential component of colic examination in horses of all sizes, provided an appropriate-sized tube is used. Passage of a nasogastric tube allows for identification and relief of accumulated fluid or gas in the stomach and identification of esophageal obstruction, and provides an administration route for water, electrolyte solutions, mineral oil, or other substances. Creation of a siphon by priming the tube with water is required to confirm the presence of gastric reflux, because there is not always spontaneous reflux, even with severe gastric distension. Adequate manual or chemical restraint should be used to prevent injury to the horse or veterinarian, and the positioning of the tube in the esophagus, not the trachea, should be confirmed before anything is administered.

Radiography

Abdominal radiography has limited applications in adult horses. Identification of sand accumulation or enteroliths is the most common use of abdominal radiography in adults.

Radiography can be very useful in foals and small horses. Survey or contrast radiographs can be taken. Gaseous distension of the stomach, small intestine and large intestine, intestinal obstructions, and the presence of free gas in the abdomen can be identified (783, 784). A combination of lateral and ventrodorsal radiographs is most useful. Contrast radiography is often used for the diagnosis of meconium impactions, but it can also be used to assess intestinal patency and gastric emptying.

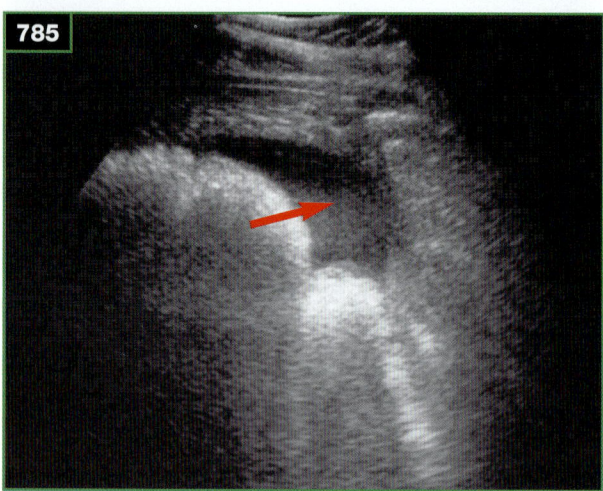

785 A pocket of peritoneal fluid (arrowed) is evident ultrasonographically in a horse with acute colic.

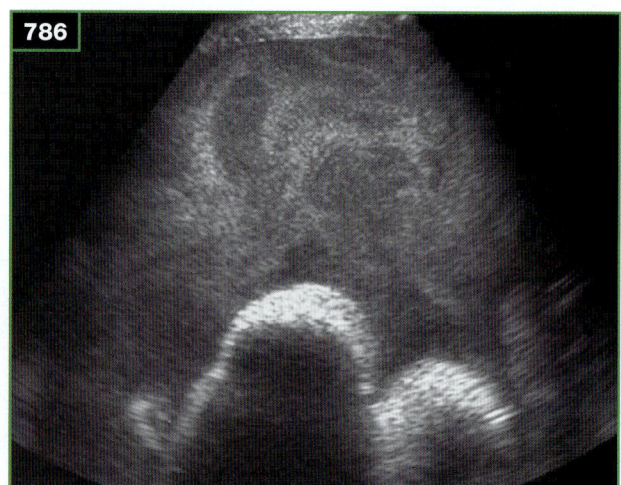

786 Ultrasonographic appearance of hemoperitoneum in a horse with blunt abdominal trauma.

Gastrointestinal system

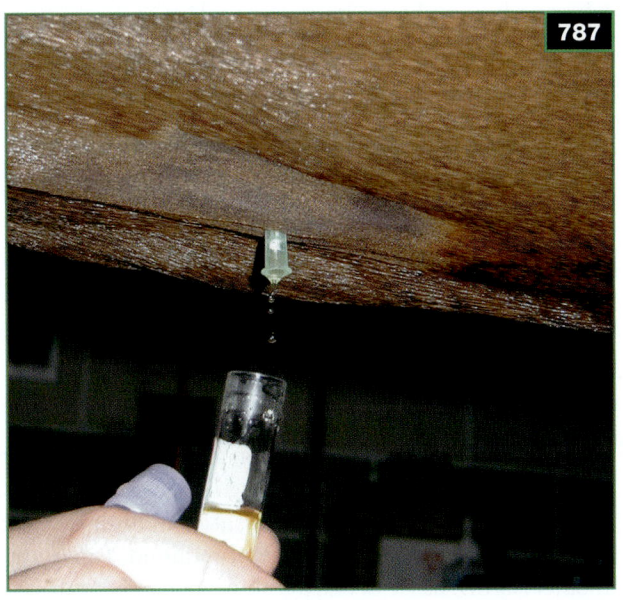

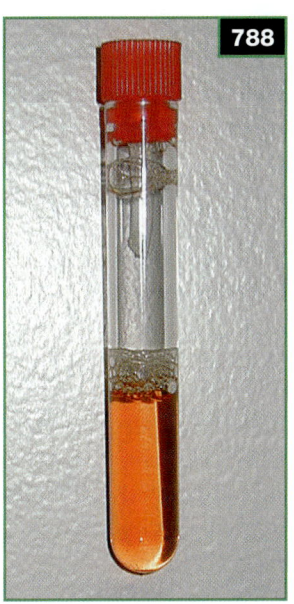

787 Free flowing abdominal fluid during abdominocentesis.

788 Serosanguineous abdominal fluid from a horse with a strangulating small-intestinal lesion.

Ultrasonography

Ultrasonographic examination can be very useful in the diagnosis of GI disease, although its limitations must be recognized. The main limitation, beyond inexperience of the ultrasonographer, is that there is only adequate penetration of 25–30 cm. Intestinal gas can also result in interference. However, using a combination of transabdominal and transrectal approaches, a significant percentage of the abdomen can be examined.

In adult horses, 2.5–3.5-MHz probes are typically used, while the small size of foals allows for the use of 5.0–7.5-MHz probes. Examination of the abdomen should be approached in an organized manner to ensure that all relevant areas are examined. Application of alcohol to the haircoat is usually adequate in horses without excessive coat. If image quality is not adequate, the haircoat should be clipped.

Ultrasonography can be useful for identification of peritoneal effusion (785), distended small intestine, thickened intestinal walls, adhesions, masses, intussusceptions, left dorsal displacement of the large colon, hemoperitoneum (786), and splenic abnormalities, among other lesions.

Abdominocentesis

Abdominocentesis is most often utilized to assist in determining whether colic surgery is indicated; however, it can also be useful in the evaluation of chronic weight loss, chronic diarrhea, chronic inflammatory disease, fever of unknown origin, or evaluation of peritoneal effusion.

Transabdominal ultrasonographic examination is useful for identifying an accumulation of peritoneal fluid and to avoid the spleen. Otherwise, the preferred site is approximately 10 cm caudal to the xiphoid and 5–10 cm to the right of midline. The area should be clipped and surgically prepared. An 18 gauge, 1.5 inch needle is adequate for most horses. A larger needle may be required for very fat animals and those with ventral edema. Occasionally, a change in resistance or 'pop' may be felt when the peritoneum is entered, or fluid may flow spontaneously (787). A small volume (1–2 ml) of air can be aseptically injected into the needle to dislodge any tissue that may be blocking flow. If no fluid is obtained, a second needle can be inserted 3–6 cm from the first. Alternatively, a teat cannula can be used. The area should be infiltrated with 2% lidocaine and a stab incision made through the skin and superficial tissue. Controlled force should be used to enter the peritoneal cavity. Abdominocentesis will not always yield fluid and this is not an abnormal or unexpected finding.

Visual examination of the fluid, plus determination of total protein or specific gravity (SG), can provide adequate information in most cases. Normal peritoneal fluid is clear to slightly yellow in color. Total protein level should be <25 g/l (2.5 g/dl). The fluid may be dark yellow or orange and turbid with peritonitis or compromised intestinal viscera (788). Bloody or red-tinged fluid should be

519

interpreted with caution, as iatrogenic bleeding may discolor a normal sample. A high PCV is suggestive of splenic puncture and determination of total protein content of the supernatant is not reliable. Intestinal contents may be evident as dark, flocculent, foul-smelling fluid. Enterocentesis is possible, particularly when a needle is used. If abdominocentesis fluid is suggestive of rupture of an intestinal viscus, sampling should be repeated at one or more distant sites.

Cytologic examination of peritoneal fluid can be useful in certain circumstances. It is very useful for differentiation of enterocentesis versus intestinal rupture. Intracellular bacteria and degenerate neutrophils should be present if intestinal rupture has occurred. Total nucleated cell count should be $<5 \times 10^9/l$. Bacterial culture should be performed if septic peritonitis or chronic inflammation is suspected.

Carbohydrate absorption tests

Carbohydrate absorption tests are used to assess small-intestinal absorption, mainly in horses with chronic weight loss or hypoproteinemia, or in cases of suspected inflammatory bowel disease. The principle of the test is that monosaccharides (i.e. D-xylose, glucose) are normally readily absorbed in the small intestine. These tests involve oral administration of the carbohydrate, followed by analysis of serial blood samples for the specific carbohydrate. The main advantage of xylose over glucose is that unlike glucose, xylose is not metabolized, so blood levels more closely represent intestinal absorption. However, xylose is more expensive and glucose testing is more readily available.

Both tests should be performed following an 18–24 hour fast. A baseline blood sample is collected, then xylose or glucose (0.5–1.0 g/kg as a 10–20% solution in water) is administered via a nasogastric tube. Sedation should be avoided because of the effects on gastric emptying. Blood samples are then collected every 30 minutes for 3 hours or until an adequate increase in blood carbohydrate level is observed. Blood glucose levels should increase by at least 75%, while blood xylose levels should reach 1.33–1.68 mmol/l (20–25 mg/dl) in most horses. A peak in glucose or xylose typically occurs within 60–90 minutes. A flattened absorption curve suggests impaired small-intestinal absorption; however, delayed gastric emptying can cause the same result. Care should be taken in interpreting results because attenuated absorption curves have been reported in normal horses. 'Normal' test results do not necessarily indicate normal small intestine; segmental disease may not be identified if the remaining small intestine has a normal absorptive capacity.

Use of analgesics in colic

The goal of analgesic therapy in colic is to relieve pain in order to facilitate examination, to benefit animal welfare, to prevent self-induced trauma, to lessen pain-induced ileus, or to allow for safe transportation to a referral facility. A 'standard' regimen for analgesia is not available and analgesic administration should be tailored towards each case (*Table 19*). Overly aggressive analgesic therapy should be avoided so that deterioration of disease is not masked, particularly where early surgical intervention may be required.

Flunixin meglumine is most commonly used. Because flunixin is a potent analgesic that can mask severe pain, the use of lower doses (0.25–0.50 mg/kg i/v) has been recommended by some for initial treatment, with further doses administered up to the full dose, if required. Dipyrone, another NSAID, has lesser analgesic properties but can also be used. N-butylscopolammonium bromide (Buscopan) is an antispasmodic and anticholinergic that may relieve intestinal spasm and is useful in spasmodic colic, but is not indicated in other types of colic.

Alpha-2 adrenergic agonists have a potent analgesic effect; however, they also have adverse effects on GI motility and should be reserved for situations where there is poor response to NSAIDs, where NSAIDs are contraindicated, or where rapid onset of analgesia and sedation is required. Xylazine, alone or in combination with butorphanol, can be very useful, providing short-term (15–30 minutes alone, 30–120 minutes with butorphanol) analgesia and sedation. Detomidine is more potent, but it should be used judiciously because of profound effects on intestinal motility and blood pressure. Chloral hydrate can be useful, in conjunction with analgesics, for its sedative properties. Constant-rate infusion of butorphanol or lidocaine may be useful in severely painful horses, particularly postoperative cases. Lidocaine also has prokinetic properties, which may be useful in some cases, but is contraindicated if an obstructive lesion is present. Morphine is not commonly used because of the potential for hyperexcitability and ileus, but it is useful in some non-responsive cases. Acepromazine has no analgesic effects and causes peripheral vasodilation, which is contraindicated in dehydrated or hypotensive horses, and should be avoided.

TABLE 19 Analgesic drugs used for the treatment of colic

DRUG	DOSE	ROUTE	COMMENT
Flunixin	1.1 mg/kg q8–12h	i/v	Good analgesic effect
Dipyrone	5–22 mg/kg	i/v	Less potent than flunixin
Ketoprofen	2.2 mg/kg	i/v	
Meloxicam	0.6 mg/kg	i/v	COX-1 sparing, may have reduced adverse effects
Phenylbutazone	2.2–4.4 mg/kg	i/v	Not generally recommended for colic. No advantage over other NSAIDs
Buscopan	0.3 mg/kg	i/v	Antispasmodic, only for spasmodic colic
Xylazine	0.25–0.5 mg/kg	i/v or i/m	Short-term sedation/analgesia
Detomidine	10–20 µg/kg	i/v or i/m	Potent analgesic, more likely to cause hypotension and ileus
Butorphanol	0.02–0.1 mg/kg 13 µg/kg/hour	i/v or i/m i/v	Use with α-2 agonist CRI
Lidocaine	1.3 mg/kg loading dose, then 0.05 mg/kg/min	i/v	Also has prokinetic effects. Rarely, neurotoxicity occurs

General disorders of the lower gastrointestinal tract

Ileus

Definition/overview
Ileus is an impairment of aboral transit of ingesta due to abnormal or absent intestinal motility. Ileus can be secondary to an obstructive intestinal disease (obstructive ileus) or can be paralytic (adynamic).

Etiology/pathophysiology
Any intestinal insult can induce an adynamic ileus. Local insults include intestinal distension or impaction, enteritis/colitis, serosal irritation from abdominal surgery, or peritonitis. Electrolyte imbalances (especially hypokalemia or hypocalcemia), certain drugs (alpha-2 agonists or opioid analgesics), endotoxemia, pain, and general anesthesia can also have a deleterious effect on motility. Vascular or obstructive intestinal injuries such as torsion, entrapment, and strangulation will cause an obstructive ileus.

The extrinsic nervous system and local enteric nervous system control GI motility. In the extrinsic nervous system, intestinal motility is stimulated by parasympathetic activity (acetylcholine), while sympathetic stimulation (norepinephrine) has an inhibitory effect. An imbalance between these two components results in ileus.

Clinical presentation
Ileus is often secondary and clinical findings of the primary disease may predominate. In general, adynamic ileus is associated with depression, mild to severe abdominal pain, anorexia, and decreased fecal output. Borborygmi are usually absent or reduced. Heart rate and respiratory rate are often elevated. Signs associated with hypovolemia can also be present due to intestinal sequestration of fluids. Accumulation of fluid in the stomach because of a lack of progressive motility can result in severe pain. In cases of obstructive ileus, the clinical signs are usually more severe and endotoxemia can be present.

Differential diagnosis
Adynamic ileus should be differentiated from obstructive diseases that require surgical intervention.

Diagnosis
Distended small intestinal loops are often palpable per rectum. In cases of ileus involving the large intestine, cecal or large-intestinal distension can be palpated. Passage of a nasogastric tube is a vital diagnostic and therapeutic procedure. The volume of reflux should be recorded. The PCV is often increased and total protein levels may be increased or decreased depending on the degree of intestinal protein loss and hemoconcentration. Leukopenia may be present if ileus is associated with an acute inflammatory response. Sequestration of fluid in the intestines may result in hypokalemia, hypocalcemia, hypochloremia, and hyponatremia. Peritoneal fluid is usually normal. Ultrasonographic examination is very important to characterize intestinal size, wall thickness, and motility.

Management
Supportive therapy, including intravenous fluid therapy, withholding of feed and water, and frequent gastric decompression is critical. This may be achieved by passage

521

TABLE 20 Prokinetic drugs that have been used for the treatment of ileus

DRUG	ACTION	DOSE
Cisapride	Acts on entire GI tract. Oral administration may not be effective if significant gastric reflux is ongoing. Rectal administration is not effective. Should not be used in horses treated with certain drugs such as erythromycin.	0.1–0.6 mg/kg p/o q8h
Erythromycin lactobionate	Improves small- and large-intestinal motility.	1 mg/kg in 1 liter saline given i/v for 1 hour q6h
Metoclopramide	Improves gastric and proximal small-intestinal motility.	0.1 mg/kg/hour CRI
Lidocaine	May act by reducing the release of catecholamines systemically, suppressing the reflex inhibition of gut motility, stimulating smooth muscles directly, or by decreasing the inflammation locally.	1.3 mg/kg i/v bolus over 5 minutes, followed by 0.05 mg/kg/minute in saline CRI
Bethanecol	Stimulates cholinergic (muscarinic) receptors, resulting in increased peristaltic activity in the stomach and intestinal tract.	(1) 2.5 mg s/c 2 and 5 hours postoperatively (2) 0.025–0.1 mg/kg s/c q6–8h (3) 0.3–0.4 mg/kg p/o q6–8h
Neostigmine	Competes with acetylcholine for acetylcholinesterase, resulting in accumulation of acetylcholine and increased intestinal muscle tone.	0.004–0.022 mg/kg i/v

of a nasogastric tube or by the use of an indwelling naso-gastric tube. Fluid rates should be calculated based on the initial fluid deficit, maintenance requirements, and ongoing losses. Electrolyte imbalances should also be corrected because of the negative effect of hypokalemia and hypocalcemia on motility.

Analgesia is often required. Drugs with inhibitory effects on intestinal motility should be avoided if possible, but they are sometimes necessary.

Multiple prokinetic drugs have been used, but none have proven completely satisfactory due to undesirable side-effects or an inconsistent response (*Table 20*).

In cases of large-colon stasis, enhanced motility may result when laxatives are administered by nasogastric tube via the gastrocolic reflex. Suitable laxatives include mineral oil (10 ml/kg), sodium sulfate (0.15–0.5 g/kg), or magnesium sulfate (0.5–1.0 g/kg) in four liters of warm water, or dioctyl sodium succinate (DSS) (10–30 mg/kg of a 10% solution).

If ileus persists or an underlying obstructive cause is suspected, an exploratory laparotomy should be performed to decompress the intestine or correct the primary problem.

Prognosis

In cases of obstructive ileus, the prognosis will depend on the underlying cause. In the case of adynamic ileus, the prognosis is good to fair.

Intestinal stricture

Definition/overview

A stricture is a reduction of the intestinal lumen that typically occurs following local trauma.

Etiology/pathophysiology

Formation of a stricture can be related to an enterotomy or intestinal resection and usually occurs at the surgical site. Stricture can also occur in a site of resolved entrapment, nonperforating duodenal ulceration, and possibly from duodenitis/proximal jejunitis. Proximal duodenal stricture caused by severe gastroduodenal ulceration is classically found in foals more than 2 months of age. Those found at the level of the ileocecal valve may result from tapeworm injury.

Strictures usually result from local ulceration or inflammation, with subsequent formation of fibrous tissue. The deposit of fibrous tissue will eventually remodel and contract, potentially resulting in decreased lumen diameter.

Clinical presentation

Clinical presentation varies with the region affected. If a duodenal stricture is present, poor growth, depression, anorexia, fever, bruxism, reduced gastric emptying, severe gastric ulceration, and intermittent colic may be observed. If the ileum is affected, signs can range from chronic mild intermittent colic to, less commonly, severe peracute colic as with obstructive lesions. Strictures at the level of the pelvic flexure or small colon may be characterized by intermittent colic, recurrent impactions, or intestinal tympany.

Differential diagnosis

Differential diagnoses, of which there are a variety, depend on the degree of intestinal obstruction and the location of the stricture.

Diagnosis

+ *Duodenal stricture.* Laboratory findings can include dehydration, hypochloremia, hyponatremia, and azotemia. Contrast radiography (barium series) will demonstrate a delayed gastric emptying – the barium remains pooled in the stomach for >90 minutes. Nasogastric reflux may be present, but small-intestine distension is not palpable. Endoscopic examination of the gastric and duodenal mucosa may be useful in order to identify a stricture or the underlying cause or secondary problems such as gastric ulceration.
+ *Ileal stricture.* A chronic adaptive small-intestinal distension may occur. The increased diameter of the small intestine may be palpable per rectum or identified ultrasonographically. If total obstruction is present, severe intestinal distension with decreased intestinal motility will be evident.
+ *Stricture of the pelvic flexure or small colon.* An impaction at the level of the pelvic flexure or the small colon is often palpable per rectum. Gaseous distension of the large intestine and, possibly, the small intestine may be present if the obstruction is severe. In some cases, narrowing of the lumen may be felt.

Regardless of the location, exploratory surgery is often required to definitively identify the stricture.

Management

+ *Duodenal stricture.* Surgery is required. If the stricture is distal to the opening of the hepato-pancreatic ampulla, a duodenojejunostomy to bypass the lesion and a jejunojejunostomy to avoid stagnation of intestinal content are needed. Pyloric stenosis can be corrected by performing a side-to-side gastro-duodenostomy.
+ *Ileal stricture.* Surgical treatment is required. An ileocecal bypass is performed with or without resection of the ileum.
+ *Stricture at the level of the pelvic flexure or small colon.* Some strictures, such as a pelvic flexure, may be corrected surgically by a longitudinal incision closed transversally if the stricture is not severe. In the remaining cases, resection and anastomosis of the affected segment are needed.

Prognosis

The prognosis is fair to poor for duodenal stricture, good to fair for other locations.

Cantharidin toxicosis (blister beetle toxicosis)

Definition/overview

Cantharidin is a highly irritating toxin that can cause GI, urogenital, and cardiac damage following ingestion.

Etiology/pathophysiology

Cantharidin is found in a variety of blister beetles, particularly those of the *Epicauta* species. These beetles are found over much of the US, particularly in the southwestern part of the country. Horses are usually exposed via ingestion of alfalfa hay containing dead beetles that were trapped in the hay during harvesting. Simultaneous cutting and crimping of forage may increase the chance of blister beetle contamination. Blister beetles tend to live in clusters, and are usually not evenly distributed between or within bales of hay from the same cutting. The concentration of cantharidin in beetles can be variable. Ingestion of as little as 4–6 g of dried blister beetle may be fatal.

Cantharidin is very irritating to mucous membranes and skin, causing acantholysis and vesicle formation. Sloughing of the GI mucosa may occur following ingestion, particularly in proximal regions. Compromise of the intestinal mucosa may result in fluid loss, protein loss, alteration of electrolyte homeostasis, and absorption of bacterial toxins normally excluded by the mucosal barrier. Dehydration, hypovolemic shock, toxemia, and abdominal pain may rapidly develop. Renal tubular necrosis may also develop. Ulceration of the renal pelvis, ureters, and bladder mucosa is common. Cardiac toxicity is less common, but may occur and is characterized by ventricular myocardial necrosis and pericardial effusion. Hypocalcemia develops for unknown reasons.

Clinical presentation

Clinical signs may be apparent hours to days following cantharidin ingestion. The severity of clinical signs is dose dependent. GI, urinary, cardiac, and systemic signs may be apparent. Abdominal pain, anorexia, depression, sweating, and frequent drinking or soaking the muzzle in water are most commonly observed. Oral mucous membranes are hyperemic, with a prolonged CRT. Oral ulceration is uncommonly observed. Profuse salivation is sometimes present. Body temperature, heart rate, and respiratory rate are usually elevated. If myocardial damage is present, heart rhythm may be abnormal. Pollakiuria and stranguria may be observed, with grossly evident hematuria present later in the disease. Synchronous diaphragmatic flutter, muscle fasciculation, and weakness may be present as a result of hypocalcemia. Sometimes, horses may have a stiff gait suggestive of acute myositis. Sudden death occurs in some cases.

Differential diagnosis

Other causes of GI, urinary, and systemic disease must be considered, depending on the clinical presentation.

Diagnosis

Clinical and laboratory findings are nonspecific. A history of eating alfalfa hay or other alfalfa products supports the suspicion in endemic regions. Identification of blister beetles in hay is highly suggestive; however, a failure to identify blister beetles does not rule out the disease. The PCV is usually elevated. Total protein level is usually normal or elevated initially, but hypoproteinemia may develop over time. Neutrophilia may be present as may hypocalcemia, hyperglycemia, and hypomagnesemia. Serum urea and creatinine levels may be elevated and urinalysis should be performed to differentiate prerenal from renal disease. Hyposthenuria may be present for unknown reasons in some cases. Microscopic hematuria will be evident early in the disease, with gross hematuria occurring later. An elevation in creatine kinase (CK) may be present in severely affected animals and may indicate a poorer prognosis. Esophageal and gastric inflammation or ulceration may be evident endoscopically.

Cantharidin can be identified in urine or intestinal contents in the first few days of disease; however, availability of testing may be limited. Urine (minimum 500 ml) or gastric contents (minimum 200 g) should be submitted.

Management

There is no antidote. Supportive therapy is essential. The hay source should be changed to prevent further intoxication. Removal of recently ingested cantharidin may be attempted via administration of mineral oil (4–6 liters per nasogastric tube) or activated charcoal (1–3 g/kg per nasogastric tube). Intravenous fluid therapy with a balanced electrolyte solution should be commenced. Administration of diuretics (furosemide, 1 mg/kg i/v or i/m q6h) has been recommended to increase cantharidin excretion; however, diuretics should not be administered until the horse has been rehydrated. Analgesics may be required. Supplementation of intravenous fluids with calcium borogluconate may be required and is ideally based on repeated evaluation of serum calcium levels. Magnesium supplementation is less commonly required. Sucralfate (20 mg/kg p/o q6–8h) may be useful if gastritis or gastric ulceration has developed. Administration of broad-spectrum antimicrobials is frequently recommended based on concerns of bacterial translocation from affected intestine; however, there is little evidence to support this concern. Nephrotoxic antimicrobials such as aminoglycosides should be avoided.

All other potentially exposed horses should be treated with mineral oil or activated charcoal.

Prognosis

The prognosis depends on the amount of toxin ingested and the severity of disease at the time of treatment, but is poor overall. Early and aggressive treatment is required. Persistent tachycardia, tachypnea, and elevated CK levels are poor prognostic indicators.

Spasmodic colic
Definition/overview

Spasmodic colic is probably the most common type of colic in adult horses.

Etiology/pathophysiology

The specific etiology is unclear. An association between *Anoplocephala perfoliata* (tapeworm) infestation and spasmodic colic has been reported. Excitement, excessive grain, moldy feed, physical exertion, diet changes, and weather changes have also been proposed as causes. Individual horses may be predisposed to recurrent spasmodic colic for unknown reasons.

Abnormal contractions, or spasms, of the small intestine may result in the development of abdominal pain through stimulation of stretch receptors. Intestinal spasms are transient and do not result in intestinal obstruction.

Clinical presentation

Affected horses usually display signs of mild to moderate abdominal pain, including anorexia, rolling, flank-watching, kicking at the abdomen, pawing, recumbency, and straining to urinate or defecate. Pain is usually intermittent. Heart rate may be normal or elevated consistent with the degree of pain, but rarely exceeds 60 bpm. Borborygmi are usually increased. Feces may be normal or soft. Signs of severe pain are uncommon, but can be observed transiently.

Differential diagnosis

A variety of causes of colic should be considered, particularly tympanic colic and large-colon impaction.

Diagnosis

Physical examination findings are suggestive but not diagnostic. Usually, no abnormalities are palpable per rectum; however, loops of small intestine undergoing spasm may be detected. Gastric reflux is not present. Borborygmi are increased and intestinal hypermotility may be evident ultrasonographically. Peritoneal fluid and hematology are unremarkable. A presumptive diagnosis is often made by clinical presentation and response to therapy.

Management

Many horses with spasmodic colic require no treatment. Analgesics are commonly administered. Administration of an analgesic/spasmolytic drug combination may be useful (*Table 19*). Fluid therapy is rarely necessary, although it may help restore normal intestinal motility. Feeding should be restricted until signs of colic and the effects of analgesics have abated.

Prognosis

The prognosis for full recovery is excellent. Most affected horses respond to a single treatment course. If pain is progressive or poorly responsive to analgesics, the diagnosis should be reconsidered.

Ileocolonic aganglionosis (Overo lethal white syndrome)

Definition/overview

This is an inherited (homozygous recessive), congenital disorder of white-patterned horses characterized by myenteric aganglionosis and fatal functional intestinal obstruction.

Etiology/pathophysiology

Ileocolonic aganglionosis results when a foal inherits two copies of the lethal white gene. Breeding of two horses that are heterozygous for the lethal white gene will result in development of this condition in approximately 25% of foals. Typically, horses carrying the gene responsible for this condition display the Overo color pattern, but this is not always the case. The gene is most common in American Paint horses, but may also be found in other breeds, particularly Quarter horses, Pintos, and Saddlebreds.

This is an autosomal recessive condition, therefore the abnormal gene must be acquired from both parents. This gene codes for endothelin receptor B; however, it is unclear how the alteration in endothelin B receptor produces ileocolonic aganglionosis. There is a complete absence of myenteric ganglia from the terminal ileum to the small colon.

Clinical presentation

Affected foals may be entirely white or have small areas of pigmentation, mainly on the forelock and tail. Irises are white. Foals are normal at birth, but develop signs of colic within the first 4–24 hours of life (**789**). Abdominal pain and distension are progressive as intestinal distension develops. A small volume of feces can occasionally be passed following enema administration.

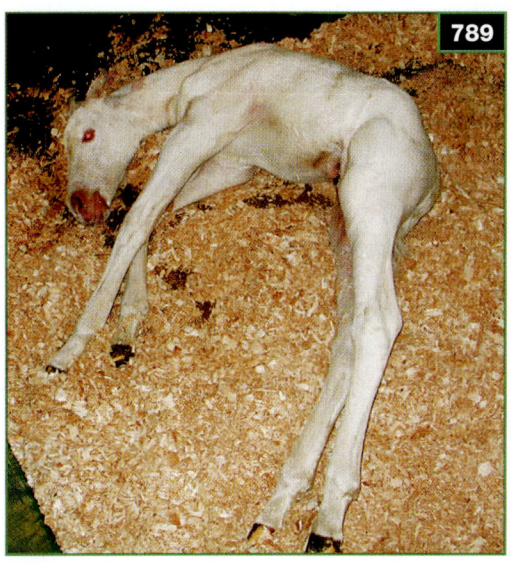

789 Foal with ileocolonic aganglionosis displaying signs of colic.

Differential diagnosis

Many other causes of colic and abdominal distension should be considered, including intestinal accident, meconium impaction, intestinal atresia, severe enteritis with impending diarrhea, and uroperitoneum.

Diagnosis

Progressive abdominal distension and lack of defecation in a white foal of an Overo–Overo mating within the first 48 hours of life is highly suggestive. Abdominal radiographs or ultrasound only demonstrate intestinal distension. Confirmation of the diagnosis is made at necropsy via demonstration of a lack of myenteric ganglia in the small colon or by demonstration that the foal is homozygous for the gene mutation.

Management

No treatment options are available. Breeding stock should be tested for the genetic mutation. A heterozygote should not be bred to another heterozygote.

Prognosis

This is a fatal condition and foals should be euthanized.

Intussusception

Definition/overview

Intussusception is a condition where the intestine telescopes into itself (790, 791). The intussusception consists of an intussusceptum, the leading edge of the orad intestine telescoping into the outer distad segment, the intussuscipiens.

The relative frequency of intussusception varies geographically and anatomically. It is more common in younger horses (<3 years), and may be more common in Standardbreds, Thoroughbreds, and ponies. The most common locations include jejuno-ileal, ileocecal, cecocecal, and cecocolic sites; however, other sites such as the ascending and descending colon have also been reported.

Etiology/pathophysiology

The etiology of intussusception has been hypothesized as a physical consequence of motility waves in a certain structure meeting a structure of different mechanical and functional properties. This may occur at sites of anatomic differences, such as at the jejuno-ileal junction or at the ileocecal valve. The intestine may also become predisposed to intussusception by alteration of the mechanical function or by the presence of intestinal parasites. The tapeworm *Anoplocephala perfoliata* is most often associated with intussusception, but larval cyathostomes have also been implicated. Other potential risk factors include motility-modifying drugs, enteritis, and surgical modification to the intestine.

The consequence of the formation of an intussusception is that the effective intestinal lumen is reduced and the blood supply to the intussusceptum may be compromised. Damage to this blood supply can cause edema and necrosis of the intussusceptum.

Clinical presentation

Two discrete clinical presentations have been reported; acute colic and chronic low-grade colic. The length of the intussusception partially explains the difference in clinical presentation, with short intussusceptions causing a partial intestinal obstruction and a low-grade chronic colic, and longer intussusceptions resulting in marked luminal obstruction with more acute, severe signs of discomfort.

Poor physical condition with varying degrees of intermittent or continual abdominal pain is characteristic of the chronic presentation. Affected horses also are frequently anorexic and depressed. With the acute presentation, signs of acute colic are present. Affected horses may be in great pain, with concurrent elevations in heart rate. Signs of toxemia may be present if there is significant intestinal compromise.

Differential diagnosis

Differential diagnoses may include causes of chronic ill-thrift including heavy parasite burdens, intestinal neoplasia, and inflammatory intestinal infiltrates. Acute colic may be difficult to differentiate from other causes of small-intestinal entrapment/obstruction.

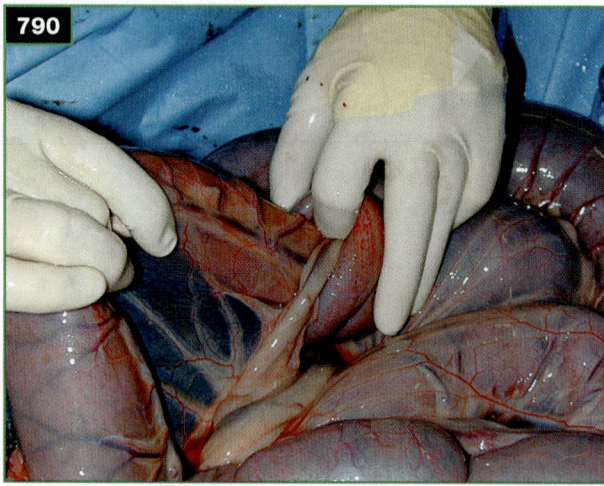

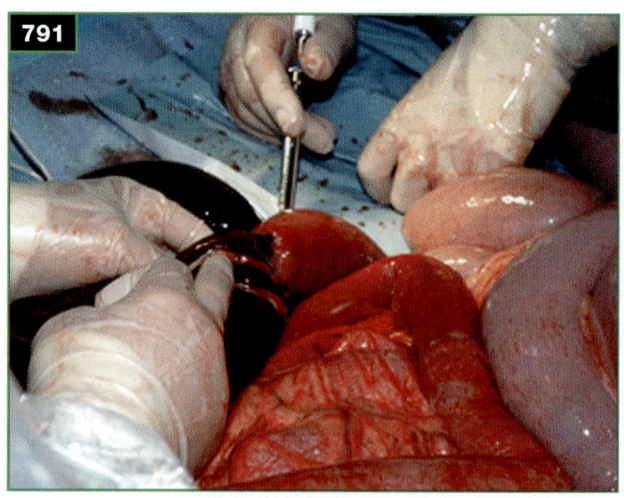

790 Jejuno-jejunal intussusception. The intussusceptum (left side of the picture) is clearly observed to invaginate into the lumen of the intussuscipiens (right side of the picture).

791 Note the hemorrhagic strangulation lesion on the intussusceptum (left side of the picture).

Gastrointestinal system

792 Typical cross-sectional appearance of the ultrasono-graphic image of a small-intestine intussusception. In this image the intussusception wall appears as concentric rings and is frequently described as a bullseye or target lesion.

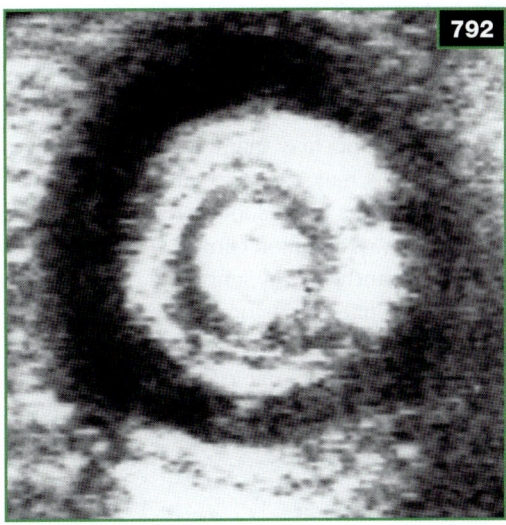
792

Diagnosis

Diagnostic evaluation is frequently consistent with luminal obstruction of varying degrees. Findings may include pal-pation of distended small intestine per rectum and naso-gastric reflux. Abnormalities found on abdominocentesis are inconsistent. Palpating an ileocecal intussusception (right dorsal quadrant) has been a consistent rectal finding in some studies. An ultrasonographic 'target' or 'bullseye' lesion consisting of concentric rings of intestine may be seen (792). A definitive diagnosis is made on exploratory laparotomy.

Management

Surgical correction is required, usually with resection of the affected portion of intestine. The details of the surgical intervention are dependent on the site, chronicity, and ability to reduce the lesion. For reducible intussusceptions, reduction may be used alone. For ileocecal intussusceptions, this may be combined with a jejuno(ileo) cecostomy or a jejuno(ileo) cecal bypass. For cecocecal and cecocolic intussusceptions, reduction may be combined with a partial typhlectomy if the cecum is considered to be of questionable viability, and for jejuno-jejunal anastomoses the affected segment may be resected and the remaining bowel anastomosed.

Irreducible ileocecal anastomosis has been treated by transecting the ileal stump and performing an ileo/jejuno-cecal anastomosis. However, this method may leave a considerable amount of ileum in the cecum, which may obstruct the cecocolic orifice or the newly created ileo/jejuno-cecostomy. Therefore, a technique has been described to resect the ileum within the cecal lumen.

Irreducible cecocolic intussusception also presents a therapeutic challenge, and many cases are euthanized intraoperatively. Surgical options include colostomy to assist correction and, failing that, intraluminal amputation of the intussusceptum. More recently, jejuno or ileal colo-stomy has been described for the treatment of irreducible cecocolic lesions, with favorable results.

Prognosis

The prognosis for reducible intussusceptions is fair and is a reflection of the portion of intestine involved, the chronicity, the amount of damaged tissue, and the surgical procedure required to correct the lesion. For irreducible intussusceptions the prognosis is poorer, the surgical techniques for correction are more technically demanding, and postoperative complications are common.

Foreign bodies

Definition/overview

Ingestion of items that are not normal components of the diet may result in obstruction of and/or damage to the intestinal tract.

Etiology/pathophysiology

Foreign body ingestion may occur as a result of accidental ingestion of foreign material contained in feed or inten-tional ingestion of abnormal items (pica).

Because of their often irregular shape and indigestibil-ity, foreign bodies may lodge along the GI tract. As a consequence of slow intestinal transit, foreign bodies accu-mulate ingesta within and around themselves. The adher-ent ingesta begin to solidify, increasing the size of the mass (enterolith) and precluding breakdown, which contributes to lodging of the mass in the intestine.

As with other causes of bowel obstruction, GI foreign bodies result in gas/fluid distension of the bowel proximal to the obstruction. In proximal obstructions this may lead to gastric distension and reflux; however, gastric reflux may also develop in cases of large-bowel obstruction.

Lodging of a foreign body within a section of bowel may lead to ischemia and pressure necrosis, increasing the likelihood of intestinal rupture at the site of the obstruction. Less commonly, rupture may occur more proximal to the obstruction due to marked distension of the bowel.

Penetrating foreign bodies may lead to abscess or sinus formation. This may also result in adhesion formation between abdominal organs. Leakage from an abscess or sinus tract caused by a penetrating foreign body has the potential to cause severe peritonitis.

Clinical presentation

Ingestion of foreign bodies may occur in horses of any age, but younger horses may be more commonly affected due to their adventurous nature. The clinical signs are usually nonspecific and may manifest over several weeks. The clinical signs may vary according to the location of the foreign body as well as the severity of intestinal obstruction. The most common clinical signs are colic of variable frequency and severity, anorexia, lethargy, weight loss, and abdominal distension. Horses may continue to pass feces depending on the location and completeness of the obstruction. In some cases, acute peritonitis without any preceding signs may occur secondary to intestinal perforation.

Differential diagnosis

Other causes of nonstrangulating obstruction (e.g. phytobezoars, food impaction) are the major differential diagnoses for foreign body impactions.

Diagnosis

Palpation per rectum may be useful for identifying distended bowel, but in most cases it is not possible to palpate the foreign body. Gastroscopy is effective at diagnosing gastric foreign bodies. Nasogastric reflux is characteristic of more proximal obstructions, but is not specific to foreign bodies. Ultrasonographic examination may show distension of the bowel, but it is unusual to be able to visualize the obstruction. A definitive diagnosis is usually made during an exploratory laparotomy.

Management

Some cases may be managed medically by hydrating the bowel using intravenous and oral fluids in conjunction with lubrication of the ingesta with mineral oil (4 liters via a nasogastric tube). The use of DSS (7.5–30 g/450 kg) to break down the obstruction has been used, with anecdotal success in some cases.

If unresponsive to medical therapy, an exploratory laparotomy and enterotomy are indicated to identify and remove the foreign body and any associated damaged bowel (793, 794). In some cases the foreign body may need to be massaged aborally to a location more suitable for enterotomy.

Behavioral reasons for foreign body ingestion should be addressed to minimize the likelihood of recurrence.

Prognosis

Medical treatment may resolve some foreign body obstructions, in which case the prognosis for a full recovery is good. For those cases that require surgery, the prognosis is dependent on the extent of bowel damage and the accessibility of the obstruction. If a large amount of the bowel has been damaged or the vascular supply has been compromised, then the prognosis is guarded. An obstruction causing leakage of ingesta and peritonitis would have a grave prognosis.

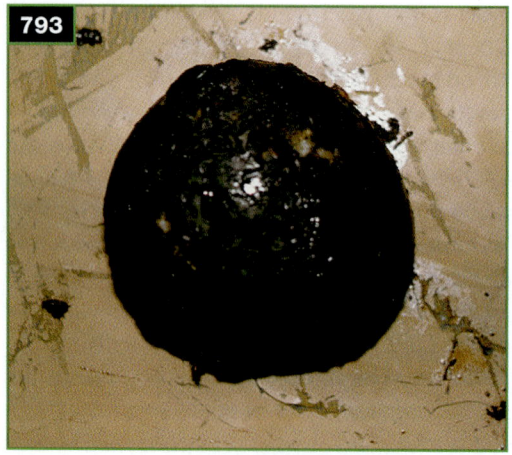

793 Large solitary (round) enterolith. (Photo courtesy GA Munroe)

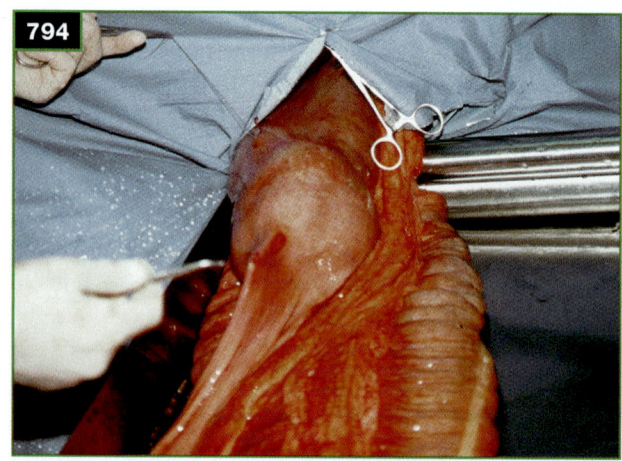

794 Intraoperative view of the right dorsal colon, where two stay sutures have been applied before performing an enterotomy to exteriorize a large round enterolith.

Granulomatous enteritis

Definition/overview

Granulomatous enteritis is a form of inflammatory bowel disease. It is most commonly reported in Standardbred horses and a familial predisposition has been postulated. Young horses (1–5 years old) are most commonly affected.

Etiology/pathophysiology

The etiology is unknown and the pathophysiology is unclear. It is characterized by infiltration of the intestinal wall with macrophages and epithelioid cells. Villus atrophy subsequently develops, resulting in malabsorption and maldigestion. Impaired dietary protein absorption and small intestinal mucosal ulceration may contribute to hypoproteinemia. Lesions are more common and severe in the small intestine, particularly the ileum. The large colon is less frequently affected.

Clinical presentation

The most common presenting complaints are weight loss and anorexia. Edema may develop, consistent with the degree of protein loss. Diarrhea and colic are less commonly observed. Significant small-intestinal fluid loss can be masked by the absorptive capacity of the normal large colon. Attitude is normal initially, but depression and weakness may develop over time.

Differential diagnosis

Other causes of protein loss and weight loss should be considered, including protein-losing nephropathy, lymphocytic–plasmacytic enteritis, eosinophilic entero-colitis, and intestinal lymphosarcoma.

Diagnosis

Hypoproteinemia, consisting mainly of hypoalbuminemia, is common. Anemia is commonly present and may be the result of chronic disease or immune-mediated hemolytic anemia (IMHA). A direct Coombs test, and assessment of serum iron and total iron binding capacity (TIBC) should be performed in anemic horses. The WBC count is usually normal. Urinalysis and abdominocentesis are usually normal, although aseptic peritonitis may be present in some cases. Abdominal ultrasound examination should be performed, but is usually unremarkable.

Carbohydrate absorption testing should be performed. Decreased absorption is usually present, except with early disease or focal lesions. Rectal mucosal biopsy can be diagnostic if disease also involves the rectum. Surgical biopsy of the ileum has the highest diagnostic value. Many cases are only diagnosed definitively at necropsy.

Management

Treatment is often unrewarding, based on the typical poor response to treatment and the severity of disease by the time granulomatous enteritis is diagnosed or suspected. Long-term dexamethasone (40 mg/adult horse i/m q96h for 4 weeks, then 35 mg/adult horse i/m q96h for 4 weeks, with continued tapering of dose) has been reported to be successful in a limited number of horses. Parenteral nutrition may be required initially in severely affected animals. Surgical resection of the affected area is not likely to be practical because a large portion of the intestinal tract is usually involved.

Prognosis

The prognosis is poor. Most horses are euthanized because of poor response to medical treatment and deterioration of condition.

Eosinophilic enterocolitis/multisystemic eosinophilic epitheliotropic disease

Definition/overview

Eosinophilic enterocolitis (EE) is an uncommon form of inflammatory bowel disease. Multisystemic eosinophilic epitheliotropic disease (MEED) involves the intestinal tract and other organs.

Etiology/pathophysiology

The etiology is unknown. No breed or familial pre-dispositions have been reported for EE. Most cases of MEED have been in young (≤ 4 years of age) Standardbred horses.

EE is characterized by eosinophilic infiltration of all layers of the intestine and fibrosis. MEED is characterized by infiltration of the mucosa and submucosa of the intestine with eosinophils, lymphocytes, and macrophages, as well as invasion of other organs. Liver and pancreatic disease is common. Basophilic enterocolitis is thought to be a variant of MEED.

Clinical presentation

The most commonly reported presentation of EE is abdominal pain. Weight loss is uncommon and diarrhea is rare. In horses with MEED, weight loss is almost invariably present and diarrhea is common. Approximately two-thirds of horses with MEED have skin lesions, consisting of exudative dermatitis of the face, limbs, and ventral abdomen. Lingual and buccal ulceration may be present. Ulcerative coronitis and loss of chestnuts may also occur.

Differential diagnosis

A variety of differential diagnoses must be considered, depending on the clinical presentation. Causes of colic, weight loss, hypoproteinemia, and skin lesions may need to be evaluated.

529

Diagnosis

Hematologic abnormalities are uncommon with EE. Carbohydrate absorption tests are typically normal and rectal mucosal biopsy is rarely diagnostic because eosinophilic infiltrates can be present in the rectal mucosa of normal horses. Diagnosis is based on surgical biopsy and histologic examination of affected intestine. Circumferential fibrous bands may be present in the intestinal wall, resulting in intestinal distension.

Hypoproteinemia, mainly from hypoalbuminemia, is common with MEED. WBC numbers are usually normal, but some horses may have a marked eosinophilia. Biochemical changes may be present depending on the involvement of other organ systems. Rectal mucosal biopsy can be diagnostic in many cases by identification of eosinophilic granulomas associated with vasculitis and fibrinoid necrosis of intramural vessels, in contrast to eosinophilic infiltrates that may be present normally.

Management

Horses with EE have a better prognosis than horses with other forms of inflammatory bowel disease; however, the long-term prognosis is still guarded. Oral corticosteroids (prednisolone, 1 mg/kg p/o q12h for 28 days, followed by gradual tapering) may be effective. Intestinal obstruction by fibrous circumferential bands may cause recurrent colic. Some affected horses can be managed by feeding small meals of a pelleted complete ration, while resection of the affected area(s) may be required in others.

Treatment of MEED is usually unrewarding, although one horse treated repeatedly with parenteral dexamethasone was reported to survive for at least 18 months.

Administration of larvicidal anthelmintics has been suggested for both EE and MEED because nematode larvae have been postulated as having a role in the pathogenesis of the diseases.

Prognosis

The prognosis for EE is reasonable. Horses that respond to corticosteroid therapy often do not experience a recurrence of disease. The presence of fibrous circumferential bands worsens the prognosis; however, surgical intervention may be successful. In contrast, the prognosis for horses with MEED is very poor.

Chronic colic
Definition/overview

Chronic colic is an uncommon but frustrating problem that is often difficult to diagnose and manage. Chronic colic has been defined as colic persisting for 3 days or longer; however, this definition also encompasses cases of acute colic that are poorly responsive to initial therapy. Some cases of chronic colic are recurrent and persist for long periods of time.

Etiology/pathophysiology

The causes of chronic colic are varied and often difficult to identify, even with aggressive diagnostic testing. Some cases are extensions of acute colic episodes (e.g. large-colon impaction, cecal impaction, peritonitis, or enteritis). Other causes include colonic displacement, colonic torsion (particularly in pregnant mares), lymphosarcoma, other GI neoplasms, intestinal adhesions, abdominal abscess, ileal obstruction, grass sickness, sand impaction, pyloric stenosis, diaphragmatic hernia, right dorsal colitis (NSAID toxicity), verminous arteritis, pleuritis, urinary tract disease, liver disease, reproductive tract abnormalities, enteroliths, intussusceptions, and gastric ulceration.

The pathophysiology is varied depending on the inciting cause.

TABLE 21 Important historical information in the investigation of recurrent colic

- Age
- Duration of ownership
- Appetite
- Ability to maintain good body condition
- Fecal consistency
- Reproductive status: pregnant, recently bred, recently foaled
- Pain: duration, recurrent/continuous, frequency, intensity, response to analgesics, patterns of onset (e.g. associated with feeding)
- Deworming history: deworming program, recent deworming
- Diet: type, quality, amount, frequency of feeding, recent changes
- Management changes: exercise, turn-out, change in routine, co-mingling with new horses, place in hierarchy with co-mingled horses
- Dental prophylaxis
- Previous medical problems: colic, abdominal surgery, extra-intestinal infection (i.e. S. equi), NSAID therapy
- Water: access, quality, change in source, intake

Clinical presentation

Intermittent or continuous colic of 3 days' duration or longer is the main presenting complaint. Pain may range from mild and intermittent to severe and continuous.

Horses with a poor response to initial treatment of acute colic tend to be in more pain and more systemically compromised than those with recurrent, long-term colic. These horses are more likely to be dehydrated and have signs of cardiovascular compromise. Weight loss and poor body condition may be evident in some cases.

Differential diagnosis

Chronic colic is a vague syndrome encompassing a vast number of GI and extra-intestinal disorders.

Diagnosis

A thorough history is essential (*Table 21*). A complete physical examination is essential to identify both intestinal and extra-intestinal abnormalities. The linea alba should be palpated for a scar from previous laparotomy if the complete medical history is unknown. It is not unusual to find no significant abnormalities during examination of horses with chronic, recurrent colic. In general, a thorough diagnostic testing plan is required, which may include many of the tests described in *Table 22*.

Management

The management of chronic colic varies with the inciting cause. Specific treatments in cases when a cause has been identified are described elsewhere. Management of idiopathic cases is frustrating and often unrewarding. A variety of treatments can be attempted including diet change, change in location, deworming, and anti-ulcer treatment. Deworming with fenbendazole (10 mg/kg q24h for 5 days) is often attempted. Provision of a diet consisting of ready access to good-quality hay or pasture with minimal grain or pelleted ration can be attempted. Alternatively, some horses will respond to elimination of hay from the diet by switching to a complete pelleted feed.

Prognosis

The prognosis is highly variable and depends on the inciting cause. It ranges from very good (i.e. gastric ulceration) to very poor (i.e. GI neoplasia, grass sickness, and intestinal adhesions). Overall, this is a frustrating condition in many cases because an etiology is often not identified.

TABLE 22 Diagnostic options for chronic colic

COMMON INITIAL TESTING

Hematology: complete blood cell count, serum biochemical profile, plasma fibrinogen assay

Urinalysis

Palpation per rectum

Abdominal ultrasonography

Abdominocentesis

Gastroscopy

Salmonella culture of feces

Fecal sand analysis

Abdominal radiography

FURTHER TESTING

Hematology: serum bile acids

Rectal mucosal biopsy

Thoracic radiography

Thoracic ultrasonography

Reproductive tract examination

Cystoscopy

Liver biopsy

Exploratory laparoscopy

Exploratory laparotomy with multiple intestinal biopsies

Grass sickness (equine dysautonomia, mal seco)

Definition/overview

Equine grass sickness (EGS) is a geographically important debilitating and frequently fatal cause of GI disease. EGS has been most widely reported in the UK, but it is also present in several mainland European countries and South America, where it is termed 'mal seco'. There are anecdotal reports of EGS in North America.

Etiology/pathophysiology

There is increasing evidence supporting the role of *Clostridium botulinum* type C. EGS is a seasonal disease, with case occurrence peaking in April and June in the northern hemisphere. Virtually all affected horses are grazing animals, and the risk of disease is highest in horses aged 3–5 years. Previous identification of cases on the farm and recent changes in pasture are risk factors. Clusters of cases are not uncommon. It has been suggested that changes in feed, pasture, weather conditions, and parasite burden may affect the GI microflora and allow for *C. botulinum* growth and toxin production.

531

The pathophysiology is still unclear; however, primary nerve cell damage from *C. botulinum* neurotoxins may be involved.

Clinical presentation

Acute, subacute, and chronic forms are recognized. Clinical signs of the acute form are predominately depression, anorexia, and colic. Affected horses are initially in good body condition. Borborygmi are decreased and progressive abdominal distension develops. Muscle tremors are common and may be severe, particularly over the shoulders, triceps, and flank. Patchy sweating is common. Tachycardia may be severe and higher than expected considering the apparent degree of abdominal pain. Body temperature is normal to slightly elevated. Pytalism is common, as is dehydration, which may be severe. Nasogastric reflux may be present and stomach rupture, with ensuing peritonitis, may occur if gastric decompression is not performed. Dysphagia can be present, but may not be recognized because of the anorexia accompanying severe disease.

The subacute form is similar to the acute form, although of lesser severity. Tachycardia is usually present; however, signs of distress or severe abdominal pain are uncommon. Nasogastric reflux is uncommon. Dry feces are commonly present.

The chronic form may be of insidious onset, characterized by weight loss, depression, a 'tucked-up' or 'wasp-like' abdomen, weakness, and dysphagia. Mastication is typically slow and labored and esophageal spasm may be noted after swallowing. Intermittent diarrhea, bilateral nasal discharge, and chronic rhinitis may be noted.

Differential diagnosis

A variety of other causes of acute colic, chronic colic, chronic weight loss, and dysphagia should be considered, but the most important factor is differentiation of EGS from causes of colic that would require surgical intervention.

Diagnosis

Palpation per rectum is important to identify other causes of colic. Dry, mucus-covered feces are common. Concurrent large-colon impactions may be present with the acute form. Clinical signs, signalment, identification of risk factors such as a recent change in grazing or previous disease on the premises, and exclusion of other differential diagnoses is suggestive of EGS.

Ileal biopsy with histologic identification of changes to enteric nerve plexi provides a definitive diagnosis. Postmortem confirmation of the diagnosis is more common, with demonstration of characteristic neural degeneration of autonomic ganglia, intestinal wall nerve plexi, brain, and spinal cord.

C. botulinum type C can be more commonly identified in the intestinal contents of horses with EGS; however, it can also be found in some normal horses, therefore intestinal culture is not useful diagnostically.

Management

Treatment of the acute and subacute forms is not indicated because affected horses invariably die. Some horses with chronic EGS can recover. Intravenous fluid therapy with a balanced electrolyte solution is required if the horse cannot drink. Provision of adequate nutrition, either by force-feeding, feeding via nasogastric tube, or parenteral feeding, is critical. A high-energy, high-protein diet should be provided. Abdominal pain should be controlled as described previously. Administration of cisapride (0.5–0.8 mg/kg p/o q8h) has been recommended. Long-term treatment (months) is required and horses should be stabled during the treatment period.

Affected horses and herdmates should be removed from the affected pasture, if possible. Reduction in grazing time, particularly of young horses, and supplementation of feeding have been used, but the effect of these measures is unclear.

Vaccination with *C. botulinum* type C toxoid may be a preventive option in the future and this possibility is being evaluated.

Prognosis

Mildly affected horses with the chronic form may recover fully given adequate supportive care. A significant expenditure of time and money is required because of the severity of disease and gradual recovery. Horses that recover may return to normal function, although peak performance may be affected and residual problems with eating dry fibrous food may persist. One study reported that 81% of surviving horses returned to their original competitive work, with the remaining 19% returning to other work. Well over 1 year may be required for return to full competitive work. Mild, recurrent colic may persist in some cases.

Acute and subacute cases are invariably fatal and prompt euthanasia is indicated.

Intestinal adhesions

Definition/overview

When the serosal surfaces of two abdominal organs become adherent, the site of attachment is termed an abdominal adhesion. Clinical problems associated with abdominal adhesions in horses include recurrent abdominal pain with or without intestinal obstruction.

Etiology/pathophysiology

Abdominal adhesions usually form following abdominal surgery, particularly small-intestinal surgery or repeat celiotomy. Peritonitis or prolonged ileus may also induce the formation of abdominal adhesion in horses. Foals under the age of 30 days are reported to be substantially more susceptible to postoperative adhesion formation.

Abdominal adhesions form at a peritoneal injury site as a result of an imbalance between fibrin deposition and fibrinolysis. Inflammation and ischemia increase fibrin deposition and decrease fibrinolysis. Adhesions begin to form within 48 hours of an injury as a fibrin cover appears on the injured serosal bed. Adhesions are well formed by 5–7 days, but are usually not irreversible until after 7 days, when the collagen content increases to a level that cannot be inherently broken down. Permanent fibrous adhesions are usually formed by 7–14 days. Extensive well-defined adhesions are often covered by mesothelium and contain blood vessels and connective tissue fibers, including elastin.

Clinical presentation

The most common clinical sign is recurrent colic. Acute nonstrangulating or strangulating intestinal obstruction can occur in horses with abdominal adhesions. Poor body condition and an inability to consume a high-roughage diet may also be associated with mild restrictive adhesions. Clinical signs associated with postoperative abdominal adhesions are usually observed 1–4 weeks after surgery.

Differential diagnosis

Any clinical condition that may induce acute nonstrangulating or strangulating intestinal obstruction, recurrent colic, and poor body condition should be considered.

Diagnosis

Abdominal adhesions are diagnosed most frequently during exploratory laparotomy (795, 796). Rarely, they can be palpated per rectum as a tight band running from one viscus to either the body wall or another viscus. Ultrasonography may be helpful with the diagnosis of abdominal adhesions. Intestinal adhesions should be suspected in horses with a history of previous celiotomy and appropriate clinical signs. The ventral midline should be palpated for evidence of previous surgery, particularly when the complete health history of the horse is unknown.

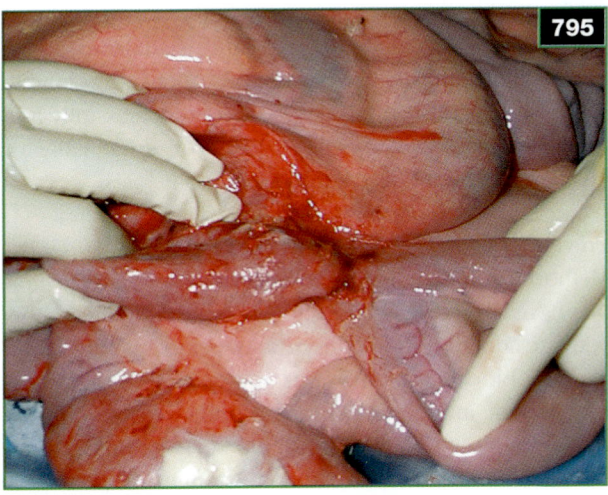

795 Example of fibrinous adhesions that cover injured serosal surfaces.

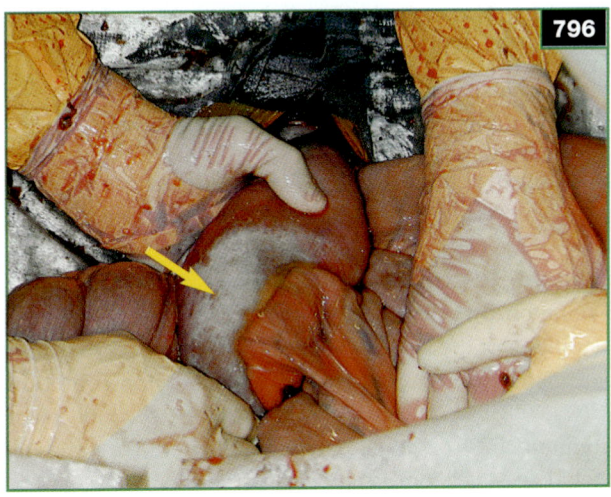

796 Example of a focal mesentery-to-intestine adhesion. Note the ischemic (pale) area on the intestinal surface that most likely induced the formation of this adhesion (arrow).

Management

If the signs of colic resulting from adhesions are mild, medical treatment can be attempted. This includes the use of laxatives, analgesics, and modified diets. Low-residue feeds, such as completely pelleted feeds or alfalfa cubes, may pass through the small intestine more easily and reduce the risk of obstruction. After several weeks on a modified feeding regimen, a normal diet may be reinstituted if the fibrous adhesions have remodeled and become less obstructive. In some cases pelleted feed may be required for the duration of a horse's life.

533

Surgical treatment for bowel obstruction associated with adhesions includes resection and anastomosis or bypass of the affected bowel, with or without adhesiolysis. Laparoscopic adhesiolysis has been used successfully in a small number of equine cases as well as experimentally for the treatment of induced adhesions in pony foals.

Prevention
Methods for preventing postoperative adhesion formation that have been evaluated include perioperative treatments with s/c administration of heparin or verapamil (a calcium channel blocker), intravenous administration of a combination of antimicrobials and flunixin meglumine or dimethylsulfoxide, i/p administration of solutions of high-molecular-weight heparin, omentectomy, and postoperative peritoneal lavage. Results of recent experimental studies evaluating bioresorbable hyaluronate–carboxymethylcellulose membranes for the prevention of experimentally induced abdominal adhesions in adult horses are promising. However, despite all the experimental and clinical studies, no definitive method for adhesion prevention in horses has been developed.

Prognosis
Horses with adhesions causing clinical signs have a reported prognosis of between 0 and 20% for long-term survival.

Gastrointestinal neoplasia
Definition/overview
Neoplasia of the GI tract is a relatively rare occurrence in horses. Lymphosarcoma is the most common condition (797, 798) and gastric SCC is the second most common (799). Other, rarely encountered neoplasias include gastric leiomyosarcoma, gastric leiomyoma, gastric adenocarcinoma, intestinal leiomyosarcoma, intestinal leiomyoma, intestinal adenocarcinoma, intestinal myxosarcoma, disseminated leiomyomatosis, omental fibrosarcoma, and mesothelioma.

Etiology/pathophysiology
The etiology is unknown. The pathophysiology is variable, depending on the type of neoplasm and location. Clinical signs develop as a result of intestinal obstruction, maldigestion/malabsorption, blood loss, peritoneal effusion, and chronic inflammatory response.

Clinical presentation
Clinical presentation will vary with tumor type and location. Weight loss and recurrent colic are the most common abnormalities. Appetite may be decreased, normal, or increased. Neoplasia should be considered in horses with weight loss in the presence of a good or excessive appetite. Weakness, acute colic, depression, or abdominal distension may also be present.

Differential diagnosis
A variety of causes of weight loss and chronic colic must be considered.

Diagnosis
Anemia may be present as a result of chronic disease, bone marrow infiltration, or blood loss. WBC count and morphology are usually normal. Hypoproteinemia is common as a result of maldigestion, protein loss, or chronic inflammation. Elevations in certain enzymes may reflect involvement of other organ systems. Hypercalcemia is less common in horses than in other species, but it can occur.

Specific diagnosis of GI neoplasia may be difficult. Firm masses or abnormal intestine may be palpable per rectum. Esophageal, gastric, and proximal duodenal tumors may be visualized and biopsied endoscopically. Abdominocentesis may yield neoplastic cells, particularly with mesotheliomas. Ultrasonography should be performed to evaluate peritoneal fluid, intestinal distension, and intestinal wall thickness. Rectal mucosal biopsy may be useful with diffuse or distal disease, and can be used to differentiate intestinal neoplasia from inflammatory bowel disease.

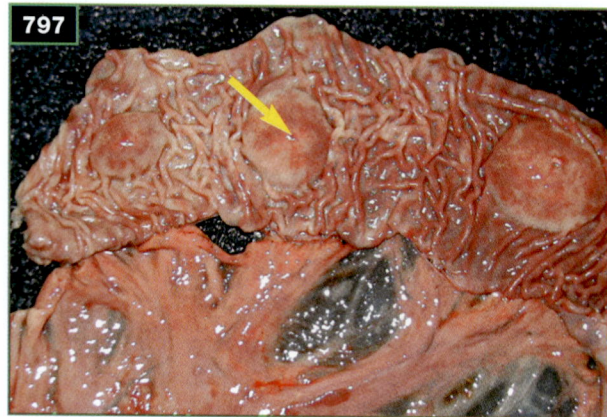

797

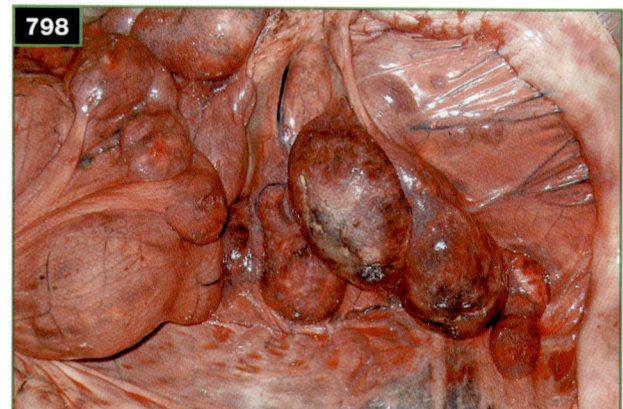

798

Carbohydrate absorption tests can be used to assess small-intestinal absorption, but cannot specifically diagnose neoplasia. Exploratory laparotomy or laparoscopy is preferred. Often, a definitive diagnosis is only made at necropsy.

Management
Treatment of GI neoplasia is usually unrewarding. Focal, benign lesions may be removed surgically. Resection may also be successful with some other tumors provided adequate margins are resected. Prior to surgery, radiographs of the thorax, ultrasonographic examination of the liver, and, potentially, bone-marrow biopsy should be performed to ensure that metastasis has not occurred.

Often, palliative therapy is attempted. Parenteral dexamethasone has been used with variable success in certain neoplasms. There is little information available regarding the use of antineoplasic drugs in the horse. A variety of drugs have been tried on limited numbers of horses, with inconclusive results. Nutritional support is often required in conjunction with medical treatment.

Prognosis
The prognosis is guarded to grave for virtually all GI neoplasms. Rarely is complete surgical excision a possibility. Neoplasms are usually not detected until a relatively advanced stage. Occasionally, small GI tumors may be detected during celiotomy for other reasons.

797 Mucosal surface of the small intestine in a horse with intestinal lymphosarcoma. Note the markedly enlarged Peyer's patches (arrow).

798 Multiple large mesenteric lymph nodes are evident in this horse with intestinal lymphosarcoma.

799 Gastric squamous cell carcinoma in a 19-year-old horse that presented for weight loss.

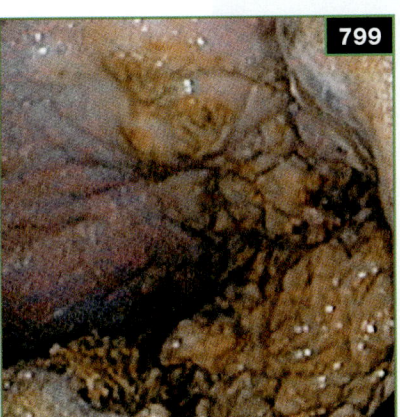
799

Disorders of the stomach

Gastric squamous cell carcinoma
Definition/overview
Gastric SCC is the most common neoplasm of the equine stomach.

Etiology/pathophysiology
The etiology is unknown. Affected horses are usually ≥ 6 years of age.

Gastric SCC originates from the squamous epithelium of the stomach or distal esophagus. Tumor growth rate appears to be variable. Metastasis has been reported to occur in 50–75% of cases, particularly into the thoracic cavity. Tumor spread may be via direct invasion of adjacent tissues or through blood or lymphatic vessels.

Clinical presentation
Signs of SCC are nonspecific and include weight loss, anorexia, chronic colic, pyrexia, weakness, and lethargy. If the esophagus or cardia is involved, dysphagia or ptyalism may be present. Other clinical signs may be present depending on whether the tumor has metastasized.

Differential diagnosis
Other causes of chronic colic, weight loss, and nonspecific disease must be evaluated. Typically, SCC is diagnosed during thorough evaluation of weight loss or chronic colic.

Diagnosis
Nonspecific hematological changes may be present including anemia, leukocytosis, hyperfibrinogenemia, and hypoalbuminemia. Peritoneal fluid is variable, ranging from normal to turbid with an increased total protein and nucleated cell count. Neoplastic cells are uncommonly identified in peritoneal fluid. Gastroscopy is an important diagnostic tool, allowing direct visualization of the tumor (799). Multiple biopsies should be taken to confirm the diagnosis. The stomach can also be visualized ultrasonographically, and ultrasound-guided biopsy can be performed if gastroscopic biopsy is not possible. Ultrasonographic examination of the liver, spleen, and pleura, and thoracic radiography may demonstrate metastatic masses.

Management
There are no viable treatment options.

Prognosis
By the time of diagnosis, the prognosis is grave.

Gastric parasitism: *Habronema* spp. *and Draschia* sp.

Definition/overview

Gastric parasitism caused by *Habronema* and *Draschia* occurs sporadically worldwide and is of varying clinical significance. Gastric habronemiasis is of lesser significance than cutaneous habronemiasis (see p. 909). *Draschia* infection is more likely to produce clinical gastric disease.

Etiology/pathophysiology

The parasitic nematodes *Habronema muscae, H. microstoma,* and *Draschia megastoma* are involved.

Habronema and *Draschia* eggs are passed in the feces of infected animals, and the L1 larvae are ingested by muscid fly larvae. As the fly larvae mature, so do the parasitic larvae. When the adult fly feeds around the mouth of a horse, the infective L3 parasitic larvae migrate from the mouthparts to the skin of the horse and are swallowed or, less commonly, the fly is swallowed whole. Adult worms develop in the glandular portion of the stomach over approximately 2 months. The presence of adult worms in the stomach may induce mild hemorrhagic gastritis. Nodules of adult worms and necrotic debris develop with *Draschia* infection.

Clinical presentation

Infection is usually inapparent. In rare instances, nodule formation may affect gastric outflow via physical obstruction of the pylorus.

Differential diagnosis

Gastric ulceration, gastritis, gastric SCC, and other gastric tumors should be considered in severe cases.

Diagnosis

Due to the typical lack of clinical signs, diagnosis of gastric *Habronema* and *Draschia* infection is often made incidentally. Mild gastritis (*Habronema*) or the presence of nodules (*Draschia*) is most commonly identified during gastroscopy. *Habronema* worms, which are 0.75–2.5 cm in length and slender, may be visible. Endoscopic biopsy of *Draschia* nodules can be diagnostic. Eggs and L1 of both genera are difficult to find on fecal flotation. Direct fecal smears may be more useful, but identification is still difficult. Eggs may be identified in gastric fluid.

Management

Ivermectin (0.2 mg/kg p/o) or moxidectin (0.4 mg/kg p/o) are effective. Measures to control flies would be beneficial.

Prognosis

The prognosis is excellent unless gastric outflow is obstructed. If an outflow obstruction is present, the prognosis is unclear and response to treatment must be observed.

Gastric parasitism: *Gasterophilus* spp. and *Trichostrongylus axei*

Definition/overview

Gastric infection by *Gasterophilus* spp. (bots) or *T. axei* is very common and typically of little significance.

Etiology/pathophysiology

Multiple bot species may be encountered. *G. nasalis, G. hemorrhoidalis,* and *G. intestinalis* are most common and are found worldwide. *G. pecorum* may be involved in Europe, Africa, and Asia. *T. axei* may also cause gastric parasitism.

Most adult *Gasterophilus* flies attach eggs to the hairs of the legs, shoulders, lips, or intermandibular space of horses during the late summer and fall (**800**). Eggs are 1–2 mm in length and creamy-white to orange in appearance. Eggs around the mouth hatch spontaneously, while eggs at other sites may hatch in response to warmth provided by licking. In contrast, *G. pecorum* eggs are deposited in pasture and ingested during grazing. Larvae enter the mouth, penetrate the tongue or buccal mucosa, and reside in these tissues for several weeks before entering the stomach via the pharynx and esophagus. *G. nasalis* larvae tend to attach to the pylorus and duodenum, *G. intestinalis* to the nonglandular mucosa around the cardia, and *G. hemorrhoidalis* to the duodenum and rectum. L3 larvae are then passed in feces and pupate in the soil. There is only one generation per year in temperate areas.

Infective L3 of *T. axei* are ingested on pasture and tunnel into the gastric wall. Gastritis may result, and small erosions can be produced by the congregation of large numbers of parasites in a small area.

800 Numerous bot eggs are visible on the haircoat over the medial aspect of this limb.

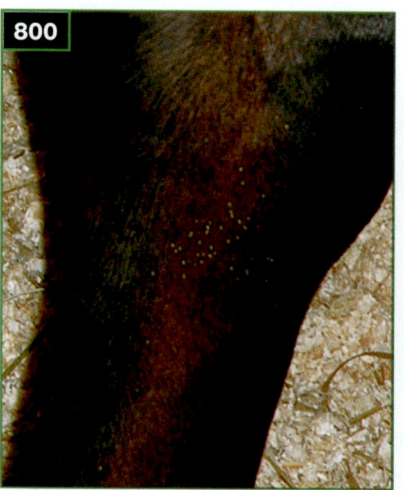

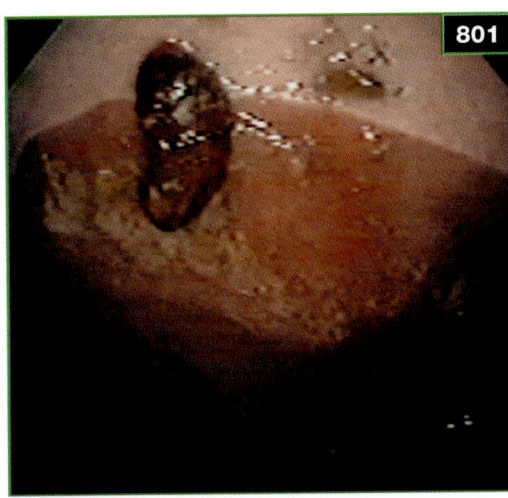

801 A *Gasterophilus intestinalis* (bot) larva is present in the stomach of a normal horse

Clinical presentation

Infection is usually inapparent. Adult bot flies may be of greater significance because of annoyance while they are flying around horses and depositing their eggs.

Diagnosis

Bot infection can be inferred by the finding of eggs deposited on the horse. L3 larvae may be identified in feces. *G. intestinalis* larvae are often identified incidentally during gastroscopy (**801**). With *T. axei* infection, gastritis may be evident endoscopically. The worms are small (<7.0 mm) and may be difficult to identify. *T. axei* eggs may be identified in fecal flotation.

Management

Ivermectin (0.2 mg/kg p/o) and moxidectin (0.4 mg/kg p/o) are effective against bots. Bot infestation is rarely associated with disease; however, annual boticidal therapy is usually recommended. In temperate areas, boticidal therapy should be administered in midwinter once there is no longer ongoing exposure to bot eggs. Physical removal of eggs that have been deposited on the skin can be performed, but based on the limited clinical significance and ease of deworming in the winter, this may not be a particularly useful activity. *T. axei* is susceptible to most anthelmintics.

Prognosis

Excellent.

Gastric ulceration

Definition/overview

Gastric ulceration is a common problem, particularly in performance horses. The prevalence of gastric ulceration in certain groups (e.g. racing horses) can reach 60–90%. Up to 50% of foals may also be affected. While the clinical relevance of ulceration is unclear in some cases, gastric ulcers can produce abnormal clinical signs.

The equine stomach is comprised of two distinct areas: the glandular and the nonglandular (squamous) regions. The glandular mucosa is protected primarily by mucus and bicarbonate secretion and prostaglandin-mediated mucosal blood flow. The nonglandular mucosa has fewer protective mechanisms and is more prone to damage by hydrochloric acid and pepsin. Ulceration of the nonglandular mucosa is most common, particularly close to the margo plicatus, which is the most acidic nonglandular area.

Etiology/pathophysiology

Gastric ulceration is a multifactorial condition that results when the protective mechanisms of the gastric mucosa are overwhelmed. Recognized risk factors include withholding of feed, infrequent feeding, decreased roughage in the diet, 'stress', intense exercise, concurrent disease, and NSAID administration. NSAID administration is associated with ulceration of the glandular mucosa in adults and both the glandular and nonglandular mucosa in foals. There is no evidence that *Helicobacter pylori* plays a role in gastric ulceration in horses.

Clinical presentation

In adult horses, decreased appetite (particularly for concentrates), decreased performance, and weight loss are common complaints. Intermittent, low-grade colic, poor haircoat, and lethargy may also be observed. In foals, anorexia, intermittent colic, bruxism, salivation, and diarrhea are most common. Some foals may have severe ulceration without any clinical signs. Gastric rupture secondary to ulceration is very rare in adults and uncommon in foals, but it can occur without preceding signs of ulceration. In adults and foals, clinical examination is typically unremarkable with the possible exception of decreased body condition and poor haircoat.

Differential diagnosis

A variety of causes of mild colic, partial anorexia, or ill-thrift must be considered. Gastric ulceration can occur concurrently with other diseases, therefore a full clinical evaluation is required.

Diagnosis

Clinical signs may be suggestive, but are not diagnostic. Hematology is typically unremarkable, as anemia and hypoproteinemia are uncommon even with severe ulceration. Fecal occult blood testing is usually negative even with severe gastric bleeding. Gastroscopy provides a definitive diagnosis. With the exception of nursing foals, gastroscopy should be performed after a 12–24 hour fast. Nursing foals should be fasted for approximately 4 hours. A grading system can be used to evaluate gastric ulcers (*Table 23* and *802–805*). If severe ulceration is present, duodenoscopy should be performed concurrently if possible, particularly in foals and weanlings. Sucrose permeability testing, based on evaluation of urine sucrose following intragastric administration of sucrose, may be a useful adjunctive test for the identification of horses with greater than Grade I ulceration, and could be useful if gastroscopy is not an option. Identification of severe gastric ulceration in a foal should prompt an evaluation of gastric emptying because gastric outflow problems can produce severe ulceration. A full colic examination should be performed in horses with abdominal pain. Diagnostic testing should not necessarily cease with identification of gastric ulceration because ulcers could be secondary to another disease.

Management

A combination of drug therapy and management changes is important. A variety of drugs are available for the treatment of gastric ulcers (*Table 24*). Omeprazole is the best evaluated drug and the relative efficacy of other treatments is less clear. H2 antagonists may be useful, but may be more effective at relieving clinical signs than promoting full healing of ulcers. Antacids have not been shown to be beneficial for treating ulcers; however, they may temporarily ameliorate clinical signs during early treatment with H2 antagonists or proton-pump inhibitors.

TABLE 23	**System for gastric ulceration**
GRADE	**DESCRIPTION**
0	Intact mucosa with a completely normal appearance or the presence of mild diffuse hyperemia and hyperkeratosis
1	Small (<2 cm) single ulcer or smaller multifocal ulcers
2	Large (> 2 cm) single ulcer or large multifocal ulcers
3	Extensive ulceration that may involve coalescence of multiple ulcers. Bleeding may be evident

Treatment duration depends on disease severity. In moderate to severe cases, treatment of at least 21–28 days should be given. Ideally, gastroscopy should be repeated prior to cessation of treatment (*806*). Horses with severe or recurrent ulceration that are not taken out of training may benefit from preventive therapy following treatment.

Management changes are also critical. Horses should be fed a hay- or pasture-based diet and should have roughage available at all times. Turnout is preferred. Concentrates should be decreased or withheld. In moderate to severe cases, performance should cease during the treatment period. Possible stressors should be addressed.

Prognosis

The prognosis is excellent if appropriate treatment is provided, though recurrence is likely if long-term management changes are not made. Perforation of gastric ulcers carries a grave prognosis. Routine anti-ulcer prophylaxis of sick or hospitalized horses is controversial. It is debated whether sick horses, particularly foals, respond adequately to anti-ulcer therapy and there is additional concern that raising gastric pH may be a risk factor for the development of infectious colitis, as has been shown in humans.

TABLE 24	**Options for the treatment of gastric ulceration**				
DRUG	**CLASS**	**DOSE**	**ROUTE**	**INTERVAL**	**COMMENT**
Cimetidine	H2 antagonist	25 mg/kg	p/o	q6–8h	
Ranitidine	H2 antagonist	6.6 mg/kg	p/o	q6–8h	Oral administration is preferable
		1.0–1.5 mg/kg	i/v	q8h	
Omeprazole	Proton-pump antagonist	4 mg/kg	p/o	q24h	Best evaluated treatment
		2 mg/kg	p/o	q24h	Preventive therapy
Sucralfate		20–40 mg/kg	p/o	q6–8h	'Bandage effect'. Not recommended as a sole treatment
Misoprostol	PGE analog	2 µg/kg	p/o	q24h	Unknown efficacy; potentially useful with glandular ulceration

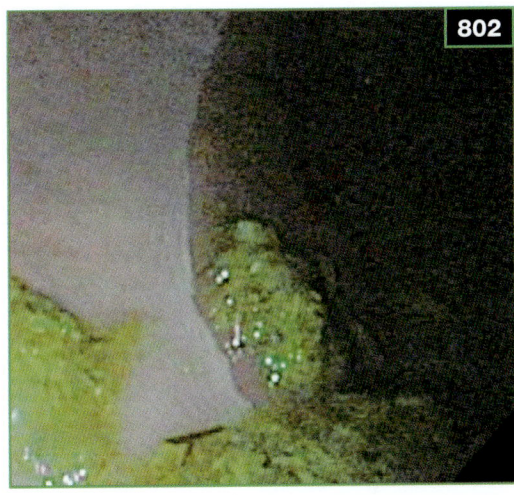

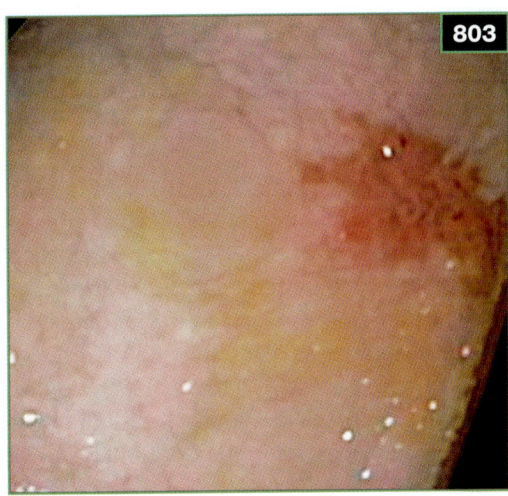

802 Normal stomach (Grade 0). The area of glandular mucosa is to the right of the image and the non-glandular area is to the left.

803 Grade 1 gastric ulceration characterized by a single superficial ulcer.

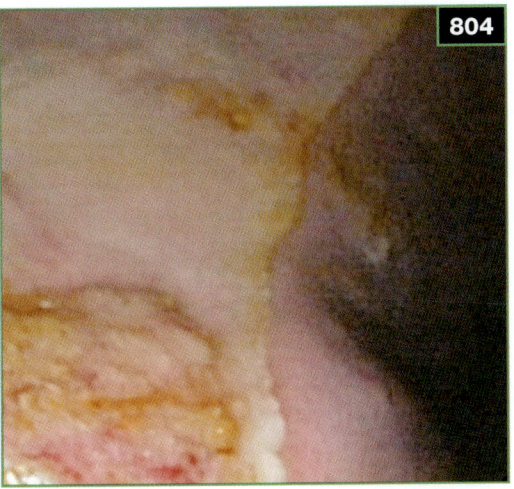

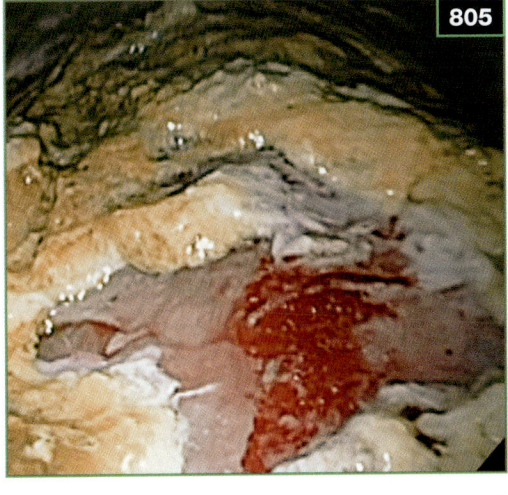

804 Grade 2 gastric ulceration. A large ulcer that is deeper than the ulcer in 803 is evident, as are smaller ulcers in the distance.

805 Grade 3 gastric ulceration. Note the bleeding ulcer.

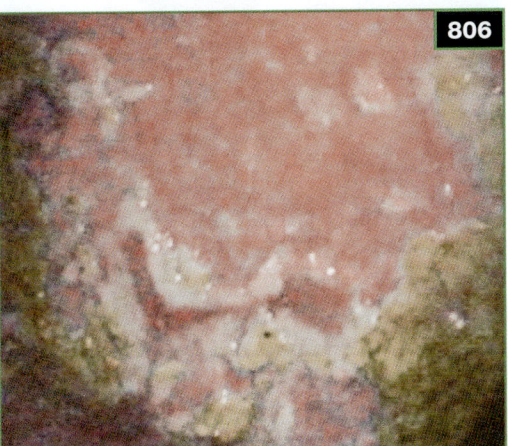

806 Image of the gastric mucosa depicted in 805 following treatment with omeprazole.

Gastric dilation

Definition/overview

Distension of the stomach by gas or fluid can cause signs of colic and potentially result in gastric rupture.

Etiology/pathophysiology

Gastric dilation may be primary or secondary. Primary dilation occurs as a result of excessive gas production following ingestion of highly fermentable feed material or excessive consumption of water following exercise. Secondary dilation occurs as a result of an obstructive small-intestinal lesion, excessive intestinal secretion, or disrupted intestinal motility. The stomach distends with ingested fluid, stomach gas, and reflux of fluid from the small intestine.

If aboral movement of gas does not equal production, then gastric dilation occurs. When the stomach is distended, the conformation of the gastroesophageal junction changes so that the cardiac sphincter is tightly closed and fluid and gas cannot move from the stomach into the esophagus. As dilation increases, signs of colic may develop.

Clinical presentation

Nonspecific signs of colic are most commonly observed. Pain may be severe and heart rate may be markedly elevated (>100 bpm) if the stomach is very distended. Tachypnea may be present because of compression of the thoracic cavity by a large, distended stomach. Other clinical abnormalities may relate to the underlying disease process in horses with secondary gastric dilation.

Differential diagnosis

Other causes of colic should be investigated. Particular attention should be paid to small-intestinal disorders that may result in gastric distension.

Diagnosis

Gastric dilation is identified and relieved by passage of a nasogastric tube as part of a thorough colic evaluation. No abnormalities are typically detectable per rectum unless gastric dilation is secondary to a small-intestinal lesion; however, marked gastric dilation can displace the spleen caudally. Gastric distension may be evident ultrasonographically. A thorough evaluation for small-intestinal lesions is warranted.

Management

Decompression of the stomach and resolution of the primary cause, if present, are the most important components of treatment. If a large volume of gas or fluid reflux is obtained, the nasogastric tube should be left in place or intubation repeated as often as hourly. The nasogastric tube can be removed once gas and fluid reflux are minimal. Surfactants such as DSS are not effective. Surgical intervention may be required if an obstructive small-intestinal lesion is present. If primary gastric dilation is suspected, diet and management should be evaluated.

Prognosis

The prognosis depends on the cause. The prognosis for primary gastric dilation is excellent. The prognosis for secondary dilation depends on the severity of the inciting lesion. The presence of spontaneous gastric reflux is a very poor prognostic indicator because of the typical severity of disease and the potential for complications such as aspiration pneumonia.

Gastric impaction

Definition/overview

Gastric impaction is an uncommon cause of colic.

Etiology/pathophysiology

Dental disorders, gastric ulceration, poor-quality diet, abnormal GI motility (e.g. grass sickness) and gastric outflow obstruction may be associated with gastric impaction, although many cases are idiopathic. Gastric impactions may occur concurrently with large-colon impactions.

Accumulation of excessive amounts of ingesta in the stomach from a variety of causes may result in gastric impaction (807). Impacted ingesta become dessicated, firm, and resistant to rehydration. Gastric distension may result in signs of abdominal pain.

Clinical presentation

Nonspecific signs of colic will be displayed, ranging from mild to severe. Heart rate will be elevated consistent with the degree of pain. Respiratory rate may be elevated if the enlarged stomach compresses the thorax. Signs of toxemia or cardiovascular compromise should not be evident.

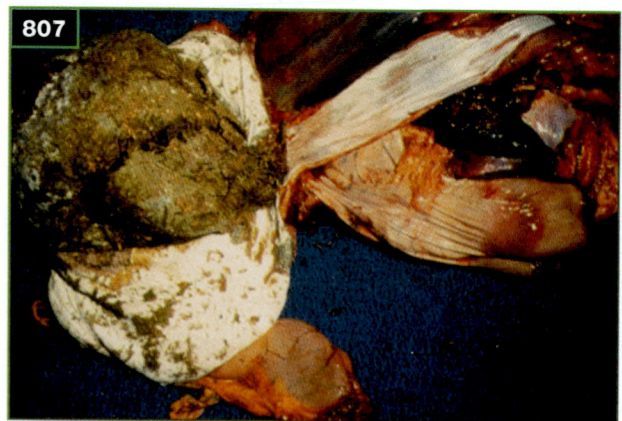

807 Gastric impaction. Note the large mass of dry ingesta in the stomach.

Differential diagnosis
A variety of other causes of acute colic must be considered. Primary gastric impaction should be differentiated from gastric impaction secondary to abnormalities of gastric motility or gastric outflow such as pyloric stenosis and grass sickness.

Diagnosis
Medical diagnosis of gastric impaction is difficult. Difficulty passing a stomach tube through the cardia suggests that gastric distension is present. Recovery of feed material during gastric lavage after 18–24 hours of fasting is suggestive of gastric impaction or delayed gastric emptying. Palpation per rectum is usually unremarkable. Abdominocentesis is normal unless gastric rupture has occurred. Gastroscopy can be useful; however, it is difficult to differentiate an impaction from a full stomach. If feed has been withheld for 18–24 hours and a large volume of feed material is still present, then an impaction is likely. Gastric impactions are often identified at surgery.

Management
If identified during surgery, 2–4 liters of saline can be infused transmurally, followed by manual massage of the stomach. Affected horses should be kept off feed until the impaction has resolved; however, free access to water should be provided. Overhydration using intravenous fluid therapy may be useful, although less so than with large-colon impactions. A nasogastric tube should be left in place or passed frequently. The stomach should be lavaged via repeated administration and drainage of 2–6 liters of warm water. Care should be taken not to use too much pressure when infusing water to lessen the chance of gastric rupture. Gravity flow is preferred over the use of hand pumps. If the horse appears to be in pain, infusion should be stopped. Gastric lavage should be repeated frequently. The use of DSS (250 ml of 8% solution with 4–8 liters of water) has been recommended following gastric lavage on the theory that it facilitates penetration of water into the impaction, but this is unproven. Frequent, repeated dosing of DSS should be avoided because it can be irritating. Mineral oil is less effective because it will likely slide around the impaction rather than soften it. Bethanechol (0.02 mg/kg s/c q6–8h) has been recommended; however, there is a theoretical increased risk of gastric rupture. Gastroscopy should be used to evaluate response to treatment and confirm that the impaction has passed. Risk factors should be identified and addressed.

Prognosis
Gastric impactions can be frustrating because of the time required for some impactions to resolve. However, provided a serious primary problem such as grass sickness or pyloric obstruction is not present, the prognosis is good.

Pyloric stenosis
Definition/overview
Pyloric stenosis is a rare condition that results in delayed gastric outflow.

Etiology/pathophysiology
Pyloric stenosis may be a congenital lesion or occur secondary to severe gastric and duodenal ulceration, particularly in foals, weanlings, and yearlings.

Chronic ulceration of the pylorus can result in fibrosis or hypertrophy. If gastric outflow is inhibited, accumulation of food material and gastric acid will occur.

Clinical presentation
Intermittent colic, lethargy, and chronic weight loss are the most common clinical signs. Salivation, bruxism, and anorexia may also be present. Vital parameters will be normal if signs of colic are not apparent. Diarrhea is sometimes present.

Differential diagnosis
Gastric ulceration and duodenal ulceration are the main differential diagnoses; however, all other causes of weight loss and chronic colic should be considered.

Diagnosis
Hematologic changes, if present, are nonspecific. Palpation per rectum and abdominocentesis are usually normal. Nasogastric reflux may be present depending on the severity of gastric outflow disruption. Gastric ulceration will be evident endoscopically, but it will not be possible to determine whether ulceration is primary or secondary. An attempt should be made to visualize the pylorus and to enter the duodenum. The pylorus may not be visible because of residual fluid in the stomach. Ultrasonographic examination of the abdomen can be used to assess gastric distension, duodenal thickness, and duodenal motility. Food material may be present in the stomach despite fasting. Barium radiography has been used to evaluate gastric emptying and is particularly useful in foals. Other methods to evaluate gastric emptying include nuclear scintigraphy, oral glucose absorption testing, and acetaminophen absorption testing. Definitive diagnosis is made at surgery.

Management
Medical treatment should be attempted initially in case gastric outflow is being affected by inflammation, not stenosis. H2 antagonists or proton-pump inhibitors should be administered as for gastric ulceration. General supportive care, including intravenous fluid therapy, may be required. Dietary change can be instituted initially, depending on the severity of clinical signs. This should consist of frequent feeding of small meals of grass, slurries,

541

or a pelleted ration. If oral feeding is not tolerated, parenteral nutrition should be considered, particularly in foals. Bethanecol (0.025–0.10 mg/kg s/c q6–8h or 0.3–0.4 mg/kg p/o q6–8h) or metoclopramide (0.05–0.25 mg/kg s/c q6–8h or 0.6 mg/kg p/o q4h) can be used in an attempt to increase the rate of gastric emptying. Both drugs can be associated with adverse clinical signs. Medical treatment, particularly nutritional support, may be most useful for improving the horse's condition prior to surgery. Surgical intervention may be required. It has been recommended that if improvement is not evident within 5 days, surgical intervention should be considered. Successful treatment via gastrojejunostomy or gastroduodenostomy has been reported.

Prognosis

If there is not a prompt response to treatment, medical therapy is unlikely to be effective. While successful surgical treatment has been reported, the overall prognosis is guarded to poor.

Gastric rupture

Definition/overview

Gastric rupture (808) is a fatal condition that is usually secondary to distension of the stomach with gas, ingesta, or fluid.

Etiology/pathophysiology

A variety of situations can result in the development of gastric distension, which can proceed to gastric rupture. Primary distension from excessive gas production, grain engorgement, and excessive water consumption after exercise can occur. Distension secondary to obstructive small-intestinal lesions, proximal duodenitis/jejunitis, and ileus is more common. Less commonly, gastric impaction or infarction of an area of the stomach wall may be encountered. Perforation of gastric ulcers is uncommon, but can occur, as can idiopathic rupture. It has been suggested that the use of stiff or nearly frozen stomach tubes may pose a higher risk for iatrogenic gastric rupture. There is no apparent age, breed, or gender predisposition.

The stomach of an average adult horse has a capacity of 20–25 liters under maximal distension. Rupture can occur from the forces of excessive distension and/or ischemic necrosis of the gastric wall because of a pressure-associated decrease in local blood flow. Once the stomach wall has been perforated, severe septic peritonitis will develop rapidly. The majority of tears occur along the greater curvature.

Clinical presentation

Once the stomach ruptures, there may be a short period where the horse appears to improve clinically because the pain associated with gastric distension will have been relieved; however, as septic peritonitis develops, there will be a rapid deterioration. Progressive signs of depression, colic, toxemia, dehydration, cardiovascular compromise, sweating, and shaking will develop. Heart rate will increase and can be severely elevated (>100 bpm). Mucous membranes may be dark red, purple, or blue, and CRT may be markedly prolonged. Borborygmi will be decreased or absent.

Differential diagnosis

Septic peritonitis of other causes, severe enterocolitis, septicemia, and pleuritis should be considered.

Diagnosis

Bloody nasogastric fluid may be obtained following passage of a nasogastric tube. The presence of gastric reflux does not rule out the presence of a gastric rupture. Gastroscopy can be used to identify a defect in the stomach wall; however, visualization may be limited because of difficulties in insufflating the stomach. Gastroscopy could result in progression of a partial tear via gastric insufflation. Hematology may be normal initially; however, neutropenia with a left shift and degenerative changes in neutrophils will develop. Total plasma protein levels will decrease as peritonitis progresses, while the PCV will increase. Excessive flocculent peritoneal fluid will be evident ultrasonographically. Fibrin may be apparent. Abdominocentesis should be performed. The fluid may have a gross appearance of ingesta in some cases. In others, variable elevations in WBC count and degenerative changes in neutrophils may be present. Peritoneal fluid may be normal in some cases, particularly if rupture has occurred very recently or if gastric contents have been sequestered initially by omentum. Definitive diagnosis is obtained at surgery or necropsy.

Management

Once the stomach has ruptured, severe septic peritonitis develops rapidly. There are limited reports of successful surgical repair of seromuscular tears, and one report of successful repair of a tear that involved all but the serosal layer. Once there is gross contamination of the abdomen, there are no viable treatment options.

Prognosis

Gastric rupture with abdominal contamination is invariably fatal.

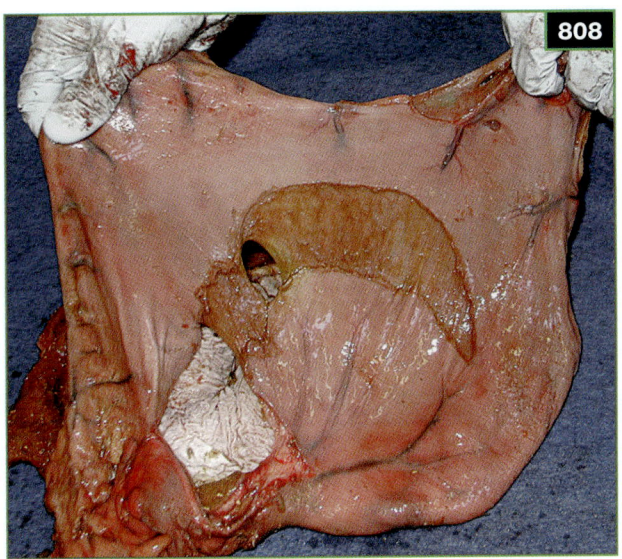

808 Spontaneous gastric rupture in a horse. Note the area of serosal tearing and the large perforation.

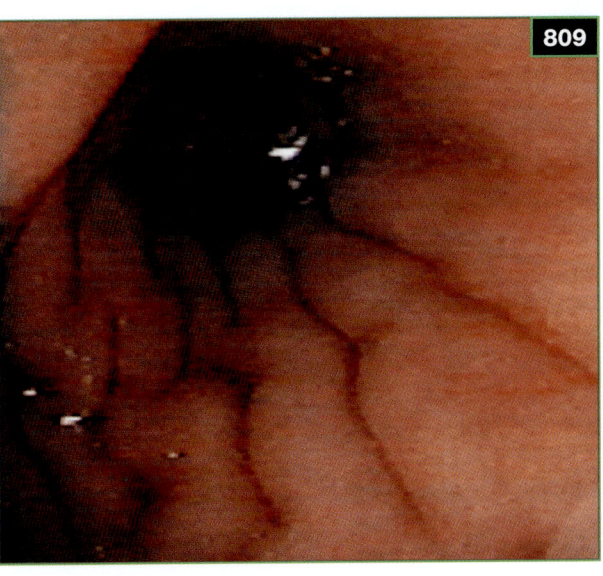

809 Endoscopic view of a normal duodenum.

Disorders of the small intestine

Duodenal ulceration

Definition/overview

Duodenal ulceration is less common than gastric ulceration, but it is more difficult to diagnose and can be more serious. Typically, gastric ulceration is present concurrently. Duodenal ulcers are most common in horses less than 2 years of age, and foals only a few days old may be affected. Perforating ulcers are more common in the first 2 months of life.

Etiology/pathophysiology

The etiology of duodenal ulceration is not well understood. Risk factors for gastric ulceration may apply to duodenal ulceration.

In basic terms, duodenal ulceration develops when protective mechanisms are overwhelmed. The most important protective mechanism in horses is the presence of bicarbonate-rich secretions. Factors affecting protective mechanisms have not been adequately identified. Segmental ulceration, often in the area of the entrance of the bile duct, is most common. In some cases, inflammation associated with ulceration can result in duodenal stricture, which can subsequently affect gastric emptying. Perforation of duodenal ulcers can occur, often with few prodromal signs.

Clinical presentation

Clinical signs from duodenal ulceration are the same as those from gastric ulceration, in part because gastric ulceration is often present concurrently. In foals, bruxism, excessive salivation, rolling on the back, and anorexia may be observed. Diarrhea may also be present. Foals with duodenal ulcers may be more likely to be pyrexic or depressed. In older horses, mild to moderate colic signs may be present. Decreased appetite (particularly for grain), weight loss, and ill-thrift may also occur. If duodenal stricture is present, poor growth, intermittent colic, bruxism, excessive salivation, depression, and fever may be observed.

Differential diagnosis

Gastric ulceration is the main differential diagnosis. A variety of other causes of intermittent colic and diarrhea should be considered.

Diagnosis

Duodenoscopy (809) is the standard for diagnosis and should be performed in all animals with consistent clinical signs, particularly those with severe gastric ulceration or evidence of decreased gastric outflow. Contrast radiography (barium series) is used to identify delayed gastric emptying (>2 hours) and duodenal strictures.

543

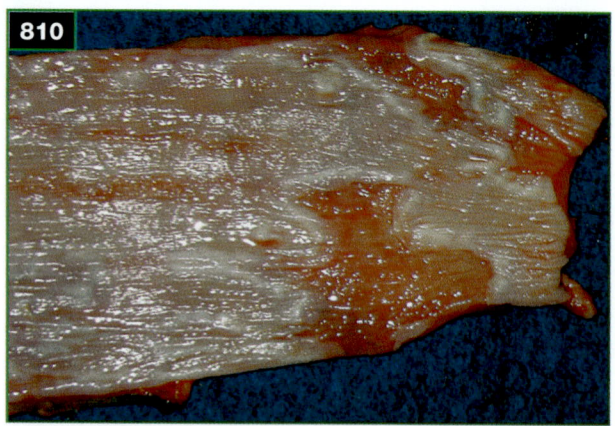

810 Multifocal erosions of the duodenal mucosa.

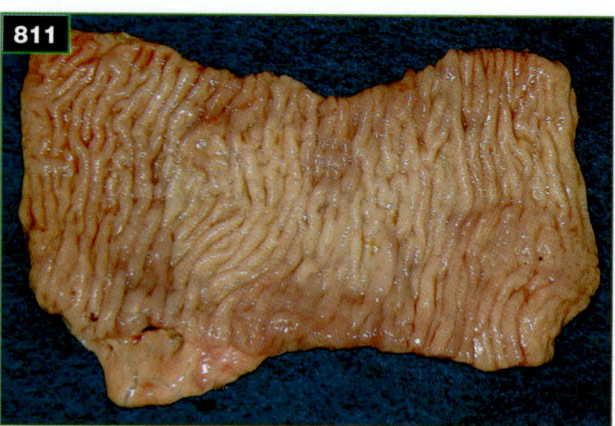

811 Mucosal surface of the ileum of a 6-month-old foal with *Lawsonia intracellularis* infection. Note the thickened, corrugated mucosa.

Management

Suppression of gastric acidity is the main treatment. This can be achieved by a variety of drugs (*Table 24*). Omeprazole appears to be the most effective available drug. Concurrent treatment with sucralfate is likely indicated. The required duration of treatment is unclear, though a minimum of 1 month is usually indicated.

Ensuring proper gastric emptying is important for decreasing secondary gastric ulceration and for delivering administered drugs to the small intestine. If gastric emptying is delayed, bethanecol (0.025–0.10 mg/kg s/c q6–8h or 0.3–0.4 mg/kg p/o q6–8h) or metoclopramide (0.05–0.25 mg/kg s/c q6–8h or 0.6 mg/kg p/o q4h) may be useful.

In addition, management factors that may predispose to ulceration should be addressed. These include reducing stress factors and management changes, limiting stall confinement, and increasing hay feeding or grazing.

Prognosis

The prognosis is variable, depending on the degree of duodenal damage (810). Duodenal stricture carries a guarded prognosis. Peritonitis from a perforating duodenal ulcer carries a grave prognosis.

Lawsonia intracellularis infection (proliferative enteropathy)

Definition/overview

Also known as proliferative enteropathy, *Lawsonia intracellularis* infection has emerged as an important disease in foals.

Etiology/pathophysiology

Lawsonia intracellularis is an obligate intracellular organism that can cause proliferative enteropathy in a number of species, particularly pigs.

Infection with *L. intracellularis* is via the fecal–oral route; however, the source of infection is typically not identified. It has been suggested that young animals may be the reservoir. Following ingestion, the organism invades enterocytes, particularly in the jejunum and ileum and affected cells proliferate, causing hyperplasia (811). The complete pathophysiology is not understood. The large intestine is not affected, therefore fecal consistency may be normal even with severe small-intestinal disease.

Clinical presentation

Foals 4–7 months of age are most commonly affected. The development of disease is often slow and insidious. Clinical abnormalities are often not noted until the disease is quite advanced. The most common presenting complaints are weight loss, depression, edema, diarrhea, and ill-thrift. Colic may be present but is not typical.

Foals are usually in very poor body condition, have ventral and limb edema, a pot-bellied appearance, and poor haircoat. Severe weakness may be present in advanced cases. Often, multiple foals on a farm will be affected.

Differential diagnoses

Depending on the clinical presentation, intestinal parasitism, malnutrition, maldigestion, severe gastric and duodenal ulceration, clostridial diarrhea, salmonellosis, NSAID toxicosis, protein-losing nephropathy, protein-losing enteropathy, hepatic disease, and plant or chemical intoxication should be considered.

Diagnosis

Severe hypoproteinemia (<40 g/l) [4g/dl]), consisting of a marked hypoalbuminemia (<15 g/l [1.5 g/dl], occasionally <10 g/l [1.0 g/dl]) is the most consistent hematological abnormality. The degree of hypoproteinemia is usually more severe than would be expected with the severity and duration of the diarrhea (if present). Leukocytosis, consisting of a neutrophilia, may be present. Mild to moderate hyponatremia, hypokalemia, hypochloremia, and hypocalcemia may be present, particularly in diarrheic foals. Other sources of protein loss such as renal disease and third-space sequestration should be investigated.

Thickened loops of small intestine may be evident on transabdominal ultrasonography; however, these are not always present.

While a presumptive diagnosis is often made based on clinical presentation, severe hypoproteinemia, and exclusion of other causes of disease, specific testing should be performed. Specific testing for *L. intracellularis* involves serologic testing or PCR testing of feces. Coinfection with other enteropathogens such as *Salmonella* spp. and *C. difficile* can occur, therefore testing for multiple pathogens should be performed.

On postmortem examination, much of the small intestine, mainly the jejunum and ileum, is usually remarkably thickened and corrugated. *L. intracellularis* can be detected histologically using silver stains. Confirmation of the diagnosis can be performed on intestinal tissues via immunohistochemistry or PCR.

Management

Antimicrobial therapy is usually administered, although some clinicians suspect that the disease may be self-limiting. Antimicrobials must be able to penetrate intracellularly. Erythromycin (erythromycin estolate 25 mg/kg p/o q6–8h or erythromycin phosphate 37.5 mg/kg p/o q12h), with or without rifampin (10 mg/kg p/o q24h), has been used with anecdotal success. Oxytetracycline and chloramphenicol have also been used with apparent success. The required duration of antimicrobial therapy is unclear and foals are often treated for a minimum of 21–28 days. There are currently no established guidelines indicating when therapy can be ceased.

Fluid therapy may be required in diarrheic foals, but should be used sparingly because of the hypoproteinemia. Oncotic support with plasma or synthetic colloids is often required. The goal of oncotic therapy is not to return total protein levels to normal, rather to provide oncotic support to alleviate any negative consequences of hypoproteinemia. Parenteral nutrition may be required in severely affected foals.

When one affected foal has been identified on a farm, all other foals should be considered at risk. It is important for owners to pay close attention to the body condition of at-risk foals, ideally through physical contact. Regular assessment of total protein may be useful for identifying early disease and allowing early intervention. Testing all at-risk foals via fecal PCR or serology may also be useful.

Prognosis

With appropriate treatment, the prognosis for affected foals is reasonable. Prognosis is worse in foals with severe weight loss and hypoproteinemia. Some foals may be so weak that they become recumbent. These foals carry a poor prognosis, even with aggressive support, including parenteral nutrition. Rapid clinical response to therapy has been observed; however, gross small-intestinal changes and hypoproteinemia require weeks to months to resolve.

Rotavirus enteritis
Definition/overview

Rotavirus is a common cause of diarrhea in foals less than 3–6 months of age. Foals as young as 1–2 days of age can be affected. In some areas, rotavirus may be the most commonly identified cause of diarrhea in young foals. Outbreaks are not uncommon.

Etiology/pathophysiology

A variety of different equine rotavirus serotypes have been identified. Rotavirus is prevalent in the horse population and most horses are likely to be exposed early in life.

Foals are infected via the fecal–oral route. Following ingestion, rotavirus invades villus epithelial cells in the small intestine. Fluid absorption is decreased and secretion can be increased. Lactase-producing cells that reside at the tips of the villi may be damaged, and secondary lactose intolerance may be an important aspect of this disease.

Foals can shed rotavirus and be a source of infection before clinical signs develop, while diarrheic, and for variable lengths of time after resolution of disease. Some foals can shed rotavirus for up to 8 months. While adult horses do not develop clinical disease, they may be a source of infection. Rotavirus can persist in the environment for long periods of time (up to 9 months in some situations); therefore, once on a farm, rotavirus can be difficult to eradicate.

Clinical presentation

Most affected foals are diarrheic, mildly depressed, partially anorexic, and pyrexic. Other signs may precede diarrhea by 24 hours, and depression and anorexia may worsen as dehydration develops. Young foals are usually more severely affected, while older foals may only develop very mild disease. The typical clinical course is 3–5 days in duration, but diarrhea may persist for longer periods in some cases. Signs of toxemia and sepsis should not be present.

Differential diagnosis

Foal heat diarrhea, salmonellosis, clostridial enteritis, and parasitic diarrhea should be considered.

Diagnosis

Identification of rotavirus in feces via ELISA, a latex agglutination test, or electron microscopy is the clinical standard for diagnosis, but interpretation is complicated by the potential for rotavirus shedding by subclinical carriers. For this reason, it is prudent to also test for *Salmonella, Clostridium difficile* and *C. perfringens* to identify coinfection. Diagnostic testing is important for identification of disease for which specific treatments are indicated (e.g. clostridial enteritis) and for determining appropriate infection-control practices.

Management

Specific management depends on the severity of disease and the age of the foal. Very young foals are more likely to require intensive treatment. Fluid therapy is the most important aspect of treatment. Intravenous fluid therapy with a balanced electrolyte solution is required in dehydrated foals. Nutritional support may be required, particularly in young foals. Diagnosis and management of lactose intolerance should be considered and is covered elsewhere (see p. 548).

Rotavirus is not invasive nor does it typically cause significant mucosal damage, therefore the risk of bacterial translocation is low and antimicrobial therapy is not usually indicated. Antimicrobials should be considered in young, severely compromised foals and in any case where sepsis is suspected.

Vaccination of mares during gestation to confer passive immunity to foals has been studied; however, field efficacy has not been demonstrated. Some clinicians report that vaccination may be useful in farms with outbreaks or endemic disease.

Infected foals and their dams should be isolated. Good general farm management including implementation of isolation and quarantine protocols and proper disinfection is very important for prevention of rotavirus diarrhea. Rotavirus can persist in the environment for several months.

Prognosis

The prognosis is very good if adequate supportive care can be provided. Complications are uncommon.

Duodenitis/proximal jejunitis

Definition/overview

Also termed anterior enteritis or proximal enteritis, duodenitis/proximal jejunitis (DPJ) is an inflammatory condition of the small intestine that results in fluid distension of the small intestine, gastric reflux, toxemia, colic, and depression. While DPJ has been reported in most regions of the US, there is anecdotal evidence that the prevalence of disease may be greater in southern states. Most cases occur in the summer months; however, the reason for this is unclear. The vast majority of cases are in horses more than 2 years old.

Etiology/pathophysiology

The etiology is unknown; however, an infectious cause is highly suspected. Recent evidence has implicated *Clostridium difficile*. There is an anecdotal association with high-grain diets and possibly dietary changes, although this has yet to be proven.

Lesions tend to be restricted to the duodenum and proximal jejunum. Inflammation of the affected areas of small intestine results in increased net movement of fluid into the lumen. While intestinal motility may be present, motility may not be coordinated and progressive, and small-intestinal distension develops. Ileus may occur as a result of intestinal distension, electrolyte disturbances, toxemia, or pain. As fluid accumulates in the small intestine, signs of colic develop. Eventually, gastric distension may occur. Gastric distension typically causes the most severe signs of colic, and gastric rupture may occur if the stomach is not decompressed.

Clinical presentation

Acute onset of colic is the most common presentation. Occasionally, depression and fever may be noted before colic signs develop. Colic signs are largely attributable to gastric distension. Horses can be in great pain if the stomach is markedly distended. Large volumes of gastric reflux may be produced. Following decompression of the stomach, horses will often appear more depressed than painful, as opposed to when a strangulating small-intestinal lesion is present. Tachycardia is common, and can be very high (80–120 bpm). Heart rate usually correlates to the degree of gastric distension; however, mild to moderate tachycardia often persists after decompression. Varying degrees of dehydration, fever and toxemia may be present. The appearance of the gastric reflux is variable: a reddish color and a fetid odor may suggest enteritis, but these are not consistent. Laminitis is a common complication, occurring in up to 30% of cases.

Differential diagnosis

The main differential diagnoses early in disease are strangulating and nonstrangulating obstructive small-intestinal lesions. Less commonly, primary ileus can produce the same clinical signs. One of the greatest initial diagnostic challenges in these cases is determining whether a surgical or medical lesion is present.

Diagnosis

Multiple loops of distended small intestine are usually palpable per rectum. Ultrasonographic examination of the abdomen typically displays multiple loops of distended small intestine. In general, intestinal loops are more motile than strangulating lesions; however, this is not always the case. Abdominocentesis can be useful in some cases. Abdominal fluid may have a high total protein (>30 g/l) (3 g/dl) with normal cell count (<5 × 10^9 cells/l), but results are variable. Abdominal fluid changes are typically not as severe as with strangulating lesions.

Surgical exploration is the only definitive diagnostic test and should be considered when there is a reasonable suspicion of a strangulating lesion. Differentiation of DPJ from a strangulating small-intestinal lesion is critical; however, it is not always possible. Certain clinical findings, including fever, depression following gastric decompression, hypermotility of intestinal loops on ultrasonographic examination, and an increased abdominal fluid total protein with a normal cell count, suggest DPJ.

Management

Initial goals should be stabilization of the patient and deciding whether surgical exploration is required. Gastric decompression is critical and should be performed early in the examination of any horse with signs of severe abdominal pain. A nasogastric tube should be left in place or passed frequently because large volumes of reflux can be produced. If more than 5 liters of reflux are obtained, the stomach should be decompressed hourly. As the amount of reflux decreases, the frequency of decompression can be decreased.

Intravenous fluid therapy is almost invariably indicated because of dehydration, toxemia, and an inability to provide oral water: 50–100 liters/day may be required in some cases. Electrolyte abnormalities can be associated with poor intestinal motility, so serum or plasma electrolyte levels should be monitored if possible. Supplementation of the balanced electrolyte solution with potassium chloride or calcium borogluconate may be required. Total potassium supplementation should not exceed 0.5 mEq/kg/hour.

The clinical signs of DPJ are very similar to those of surgical small-intestinal lesions, therefore exploratory laparotomy is not uncommonly performed. The decision on whether surgery is indicated can be difficult and if unsure, it is often wise to err on the side of surgical intervention to ensure that a surgical lesion is not overlooked.

Hypoproteinemia may develop and oncotic support may be required. Plasma may also be beneficial if signs of endotoxemia are present. Synthetic colloids can be used if plasma is not available.

It is unclear whether antimicrobials are required, either for treatment of a primary infection or prevention of bacterial translocation. Penicillin is often used because clostridial organisms may be involved. Broad-spectrum coverage is not unreasonable, but care should be taken when using aminoglycosides because of the potential for nephrotoxicity. Metronidazole (25 mg/kg per rectum q8h) has been used because of the suspected involvement of *C. difficile*, but its efficacy is unclear.

Analgesic (1.1 mg/kg i/v q12h) or 'anti-endotoxin' (0.25–0.30 mg/kg i/v q8h) doses of flunixin meglumine may be useful for controlling pain, attenuating pain-induced ileus, and for purported 'anti-endotoxin' effects. Analgesic doses of NSAIDs should be used judiciously in dehydrated or hypotensive animals. Other anti-endotoxin therapies such as administration of polymyxin B (6000 IU/kg i/v q12h) should be considered in toxemic horses. Prokinetic therapy has not yet been shown to be effective.

Affected animals should be closely monitored for complications such as laminitis or catheter-site thrombophlebitis. Food and water should be withheld until refluxing has ceased. Parenteral nutrition may be required in horses that continue to reflux for several days. Oral medications should be avoided because of unpredictable absorption.

Prognosis

The prognosis is reasonable if aggressive supportive care can be provided. Reported survival rates range from 25 to 94%. Response to treatment is highly variable. Some horses may cease refluxing within 24 hours, while others may continue to reflux for more than 1 week. The typical course of disease is 3–7 days and the prognosis is good for horses that stop refluxing within 72 hours. Complications such as laminitis are not uncommon, and euthanasia is sometimes required for economic reasons if prolonged treatment is required.

Lactose intolerance

Definition/overview

Lactose intolerance is occasionally identified in foals.

Etiology/pathophysiology

Lactose intolerance occurs following damage to the small-intestinal villi. Typically, this is secondary to infectious causes of enterocolitis; however, the initial cause may not be identified in all cases. Primary lactose intolerance has not been reported in foals.

Lactase, the enzyme responsible for converting lactose into glucose and galactose, is normally present in entero-cytes on the tips of villi in the small intestine. Secondary lactose intolerance occurs when lactase-producing cells have been damaged. In foals it is usually associated with infectious enteritis.

Diarrhea and colic are the main presenting signs. Other clinical abnormalities are not common and foals are typically bright and alert. Over time, weight loss, weakness, seizures, and death may occur, although serious problems are rare. Lactose intolerance should be considered in foals that are bright and alert, yet have persistent diarrhea with occasional gaseous distension or signs of colic, and particularly in those foals that have experienced an episode of suspected infectious enteritis. Lactose intolerance may also be present transiently with enteritis of virtually any etiology, but not be readily apparent because of the primary disease.

Differential diagnosis

Clostridial enteritis, salmonellosis, rotaviral enteritis, idiopathic colitis, and other causes of diarrhea, maldigestion, and malabsorption should be considered.

Diagnosis

Other causes of diarrhea (*Salmonella, C. difficile, C. perfringens*, rotavirus) should be ruled out or treated. Lactose intolerance can occur concurrently with infectious enteritis.

Response to supplementation with oral lactase is suggestive but not diagnostic. The oral lactose tolerance test is most widely used to diagnose lactose intolerance (*Table 25*).

Management

The standard approach to management of affected foals is supplementation with oral lactase (1,500–3,000 IU p/o q4–12h). Weaning should be considered in older foals, particularly if oral administration of lactase is problematic. Supportive treatment or treatment of the primary cause should be provided if necessary.

Prognosis

Lactase production should be restored in a few days to a few weeks, depending on the severity of the primary insult. Permanent lactose intolerance has not been reported. The prognosis is excellent if adequate supportive care is provided.

TABLE 25 Protocol for lactose tolerance testing in foals

1. Fast the foal for approximately 4 hours.

2. Obtain a baseline blood glucose level. Stall-side testing with a glucometer can be performed. Red blood cells will consume glucose *in vitro*. If samples must be stored or shipped for >1 hour before testing, plasma or serum should be separated or tubes containing sodium fluoride should be used.

3. Administer 1g/kg lactose, as a 20% solution in water, via bottle or nasogastric tube.

4. Determine blood glucose levels every 30 minutes for 3 hours.

5. An increase in blood glucose of <2 mmol/l indicates maldigestion or malabsorption. The peak value is usually obtained at 60–90 minutes.

6. A glucose absorption test should be performed on all foals with an abnormal lactose tolerance test to differentiate maldigestion from malabsorption.

7. Glucose absorption test is performed as described for the lactose tolerance test, substituting lactose with 1 g/kg glucose. An increase in blood glucose of at least 75% should occur.

Ascarid infection

Definition/overview

Ascarid infestation is common in horses, particularly those housed on crowded pastures with frequent mixing of horses and inadequate parasite-control programs. Ascarid impaction is an uncommon but life-threatening problem that typically occurs after deworming weanlings with large parasite burdens.

Etiology/pathophysiology

Infection occurs following ingestion of infective *Parascaris equorum* larvae that develop within 10 days on pasture from feces of infected horses. Following ingestion, the larvae migrate through the wall of the small intestine, pass through the liver via the portal vein, and eventually reach the pulmonary circulation. Larvae molt in the lung, ascend the trachea, and are swallowed, with final molting and maturation occurring in the small intestine.

Clinical presentation

Ascarids can be present in the small intestine without any obvious clinical signs. Clinical ascarid infestation is usually nonspecific and characterized by a pot-bellied appearance and varying degrees of decreased growth rate, poor hair-coat, and lethargy. Ascarid impaction is a serious condition characterized by acute, often severe, colic. Ascarid impaction should be considered in all cases of colic that develop in foals shortly after deworming. Intestinal rupture may occur, with the associated development of peritonitis.

Differential diagnosis

A variety of other causes of ill-thrift such as malnutrition, poor management, other intestinal parasites, and chronic infection should be considered. Many other causes of colic may produce similar clinical signs to those of ascarid impaction.

Diagnosis

A peripheral eosinophilia may be present during the period of larval migration, but this is not a sensitive indicator of infection. Hypoproteinemia may be present with severe chronic burdens. Fecal flotation should be performed and ascarid eggs are readily identified after the 10–12 week prepatent period. It has been suggested that egg counts of >100/g indicate that treatment is required.

In foals with ascarid impaction, signs of small-intestinal obstruction are present. These include gastric reflux and ultrasonographic identification of distended small intestine. Occasionally, ascarids are identified in gastric reflux or via ultrasound (**812**).

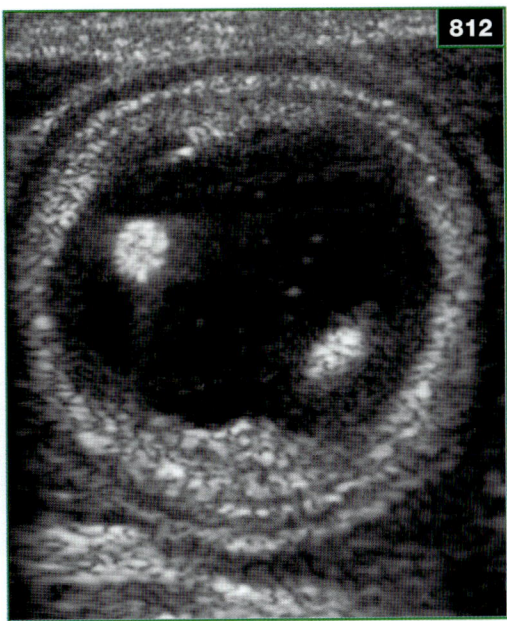

812 Cross-sectional ultrasound image of a foal with ascarid impaction. Note the two cross-sectional images of ascarids within the intestinal lumen.

Management

Routine deworming should be started in foals at 6–8 weeks of age and repeated every 8 weeks for the first year. Broodmares should be dewormed regularly, including during the third trimester, to decrease environmental contamination. Fenbendazole (5–10 mg/kg p/o q24h for 5 days), levamisole (8.8 mg/kg p/o), pyrantel pamoate (6.6 mg/kg p/o), ivermectin (0.2 mg/kg p/o), or moxidectin (0.4 mg/kg) should be effective. Daily administration of pyrantel tartrate (2.6 mg/kg) is also effective. It should be noted that ivermectin resistance has been reported. If a large ascarid burden is suspected, it may be beneficial to deworm initially with slower-acting anthelmintics (e.g. fenbendazole) as opposed to avermectins to reduce the chance of ascarid impaction. Deworming programs for yearlings and adult horses are variable and should be designed for the individual farm based on farm type, horse numbers, horse movement, pasture crowding, and ability to properly manage pastures.

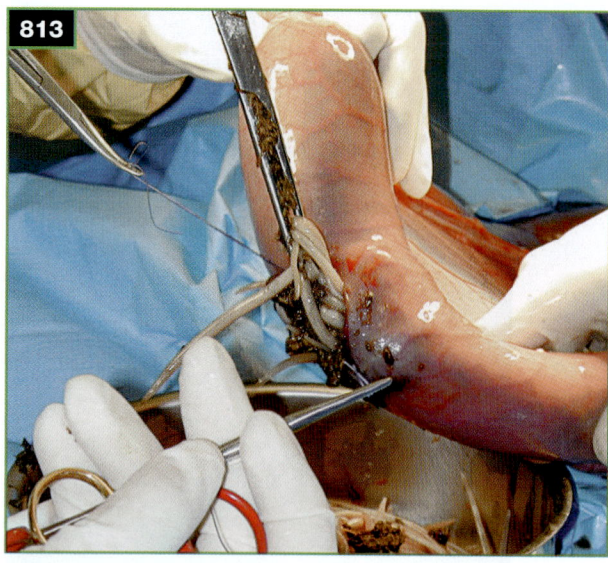

813 Enterotomy to remove ascarids in a foal with an ascarid impaction.

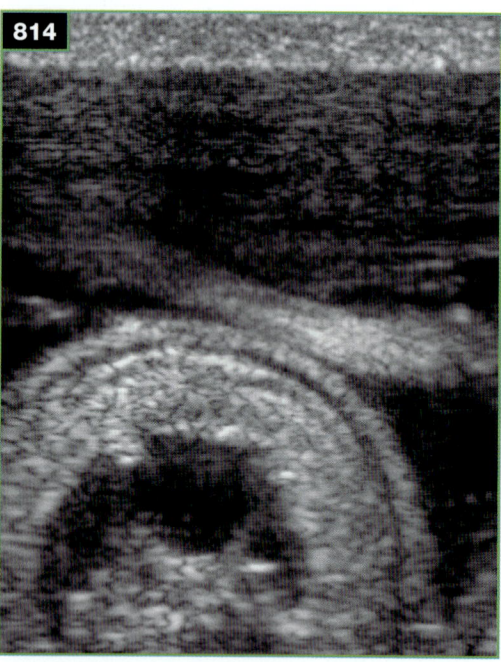

814 Longitudinal image of an ascarid that was free within the abdomen of the foal in 812. Intestinal rupture occurred following ascarid impaction.

Ascarid eggs can remain viable on pasture for years, so prevention of pasture contamination is important. Proper pasture management, including avoidance of overstocking, removal of feces, pasture rotation, and routine deworming of all animals with access to the pasture, is essential. Routine fecal analysis of all horses, or a sample of horses (particularly foals), is useful for evaluating the effectiveness of the deworming program.

Emergency surgery is usually required in foals with ascarid impaction and signs of intestinal obstruction (813).

Prognosis
The prognosis with ascarid infestation is excellent. The prognosis for ascarid impaction is guarded because of the frequent requirement for emergency surgery and the complications that can ensue with small-intestinal surgery in young horses. Intestinal rupture secondary to ascarid impaction is rare, but can occur (814).

Strangulating lipoma
Definition/overview
Strangulating lipomas are the most common cause of small-intestinal strangulation in older horses.

Etiology/pathophysiology
Lipomas are benign fatty masses that can develop in the mesentery of older horses. They are thought to be most common in fat, older horses and ponies, particularly geldings.

A lipoma, in itself, is inconsequential, but over time it may enlarge and develop a pedicle that may wrap around a section of small intestine, resulting in strangulation (815, 816). Once the vasculature is compromised, the affected intestine rapidly loses viability.

Clinical presentation
Acute, severe colic is the most common presentation. Some horses may be in great pain and tachycardic (up to 120 bpm). A nasogastric tube should be passed immediately on any horse in severe abdominal pain, particularly if gross abdominal distension is not noted. Some relief of pain will be achieved via easing of gastric distension; however, tachycardia and signs of colic are usually still apparent and may continue to be severe. Signs of toxemia (hyperemic mucous membranes, prolonged CRT) and cardiovascular compromise are often present. Borborygmi are often absent. Response to analgesics may be poor.

Differential diagnosis
Other causes of small-intestinal distension, including small-intestinal volvulus, epiploic foramen entrapment, proximal enteritis, ileal impaction, and intussusception, should be considered.

Diagnosis

Nasogastric reflux is usually present. Multiple loops of distended small intestine are typically palpable per rectum. Occasionally, small intestine will not be palpable, but will be detected ultrasonographically (817). Round, distended, amotile small intestine is suggestive of intestinal compromise. The PCV and total plasma protein may be elevated initially as a result of dehydration; however, as disease progresses, total plasma protein levels will decrease. Peritoneal fluid changes occur as the intestine becomes compromised. Initially, the protein level and WBC numbers increase, followed shortly by changes in color and turbidity (788).

Management

A nasogastric tube must be passed to relieve gastric reflux. The tube should be left in place if reflux is present. Nothing should be given per os or via a nasogastric tube. Prompt surgical intervention is required. Stabilization via intravenous fluid therapy, gastric decompression, analgesia administration, and antimicrobial prophylaxis are required prior to surgery. The strangulating lipoma should be removed, along with any other lipomas that are identified. Frequently, devitalized intestine is identified and resection is required.

Prognosis

The prognosis is guarded. The length of affected intestine and the degree of compromise are important factors. Intestinal resection is usually required, and complications are not uncommon. Most horses appear to tolerate resection of 60% of their small intestine. Resection of >60% of the small intestine increases the likelihood of malabsorption and resection may not be an option in some cases depending on the length of compromised intestine. Short-term survival rates of 30–72% have been reported. The incidence of postoperative complications, such as prolonged ileus and laminitis, seems to be higher in older horses. Other complications, such as adhesions, anastomosis-site abscessation, dehiscence, or stricture, can occur.

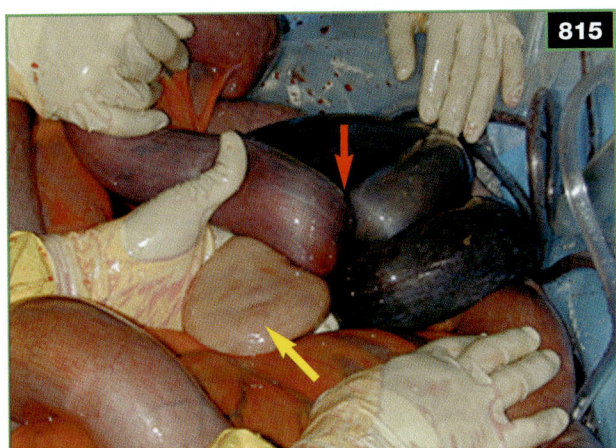

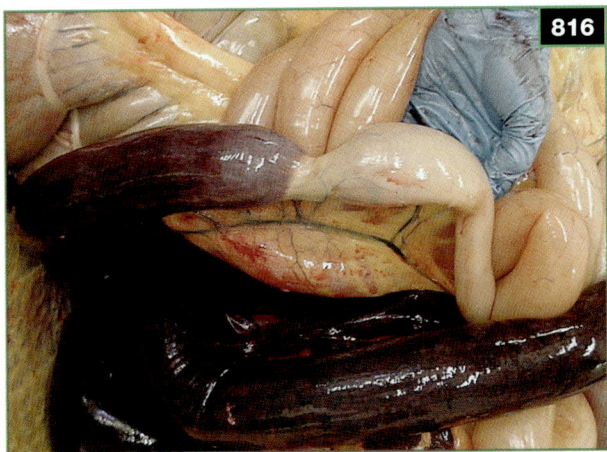

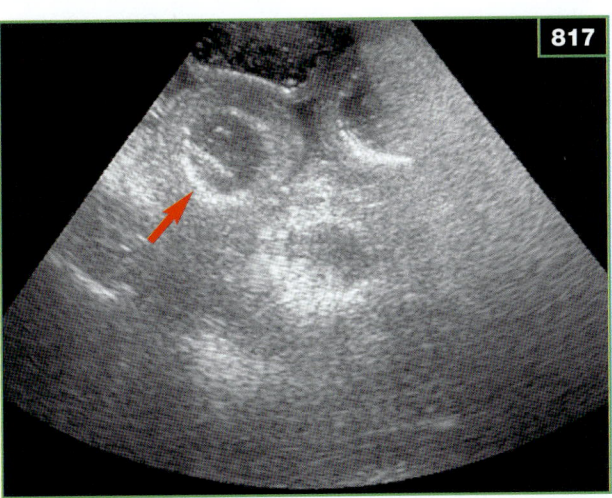

815 Pedunculated lipoma (yellow arrow) causing strangulation of the small intestine (red arrow).

816 After removal of the lipoma depicted in 815, a marked line of demarcation is evident at the site of strangulation.

817 Small-intestinal distension in a horse with strangulating lipoma. Note the extremely thickened intestinal wall (arrow).

Small-intestinal volvulus

Definition/overview

Volvulus of the small intestine involves a rotation of more than 180 degrees around the long axis of the mesentery of the small intestine. It may involve only a segment of intestine (**818**) or the entire small intestine if the rotation is at the base of the mesentery. It most often occurs in horses less than 3 years of age.

Etiology/pathophysiology

The volvulus can be primary or secondary to another lesion such as an anastomosis site, entrapment, or a mesodiverticular band. These lesions probably provide a fixed axis for rotation of the bowel. Abnormal intestinal motility may also predispose to primary volvulus. Volvulus occurs in the mesenteric portion of the small intestine from the jejunum to distal ileum. The duodenum has a short mesenteric attachment that cannot rotate.

Following rotation of the intestine around an axis, the peristalsis of the intestine orad to the lesion causes further mesenteric twisting, bringing both orad and aborad intestine into the volvulus. After the volvulus occurs, increased intestinal movement to relieve obstruction is noted initially, followed by a decrease and eventually absence of motility (ileus). Venous and luminal occlusion will result in fluid accumulation in the affected segment of small intestine and increased intraluminal pressure. The condition is worsened by secretion of more fluid by the intestinal wall. Arterial blood usually continues to enter the affected segment, furthering development of edema. Eventually, the intestine orad to the volvulus becomes distended and gastric distension will eventually develop. Sequestration of fluid in the small intestine may produce dehydration. Necrosis of the intestine creates leakage of protein, RBCs, and bacteria, which can result in peritonitis and endotoxic shock.

Clinical presentation

An acute onset of potentially violent colic is observed. The severity of pain may decrease in some cases concurrent with intestinal necrosis. Moderate abdominal distension can be evident, but is absent in some cases. A marked elevation in heart rate is common and respiratory rate can be concurrently elevated. Body temperature is usually normal. Mucous membranes are pink to cyanotic and the CRT is normal to very prolonged. Spontaneous nasogastric reflux is uncommon.

Differential diagnosis

Other causes of small-intestinal strangulation including pedunculated lipoma, intussusception, epiploic entrapment, and herniation.

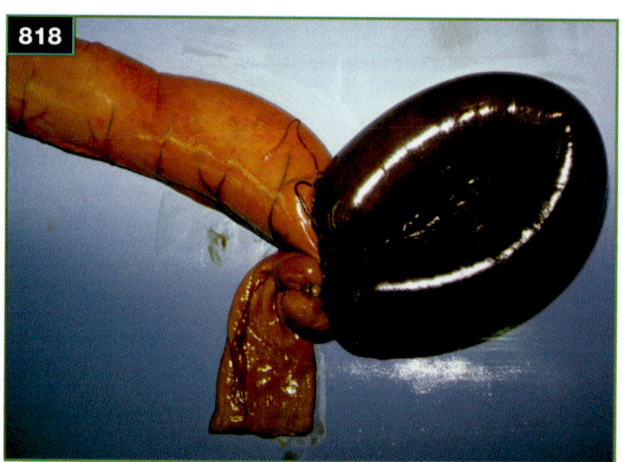

818 Postmortem specimen of a small-intestine volvulus. Note the typical appearance of small-intestine hemorrhagic strangulation. (Photo courtesy S Laverty)

Diagnosis

Small-intestinal distension is usually palpable per rectum. Thickening of the intestinal wall may be appreciated in some cases. Passage of the gastric tube will often yield spontaneous or provoked reflux fluid with alkaline pH, but gastric decompression may not result in any improvement in clinical signs. Hypovolemia with eventual metabolic acidosis develops rapidly. Abdominocentesis usually yields a serosanguineous fluid with an increased nucleated cell count and total protein level. On ultrasonographic examination, distension of small-intestinal loops (>5 cm) with absence of motility can be appreciated. An increase in intestinal-wall thickness may be present.

Management

Surgical intervention is required. Cardiovascular compromise is common and stabilization is required prior to induction of anesthesia. At surgery, the bowel is untwisted and any compromised intestine is resected. Often, so much of the ileum is compromised that it is impossible to carry out an end-to-end anastomosis. In these cases a jejuno-cecal anastomosis (end-to-side or side-to-side) is performed. If >60% of small intestine is involved, euthanasia is usually recommended because of the potential for maldigestion and malabsorption.

Prognosis

The prognosis is generally poor due to the large amount of small intestine that can be involved and the frequency of complications associated with small-intestinal resection. Intestinal adhesions, abscessation of the anastomosis site, and functional obstruction of the anastomosis are common complications.

Muscular hypertrophy of the ileum
Definition/overview
Hypertrophy of the muscular layers of the ileum, with accompanying reduction of the lumen, can result in obstruction of the intestinal lumen (**819**).

Etiology/pathophysiology
Muscular hypertrophy may be primary or secondary. If secondary, it is usually associated with stenosis of the ileum or the ileocecal valve. Causes of the stenosis include ileocecal intussusception, strongyle larvae migration, or mucosal or mural lesions. Muscular hypertrophy occurs as a compensatory mechanism in theses cases. If primary, idiopathic hypertrophy of the ileum may also occur. The etiology of this condition is believed to be an imbalance in the autonomic nervous system and dysfunction at the ileo-cecal valve. There may be an increased risk with a heavy tapeworm burden.

Both the circular and the longitudinal muscular layers of the ileum are affected. The abnormalities can extend to the distal jejunum. In some cases, several segments of the small intestine may be affected. The hypertrophied muscle narrows the lumen, causing a partial obstruction. This obstruction can result in local impaction and distension of the small intestine orad to the lesion.

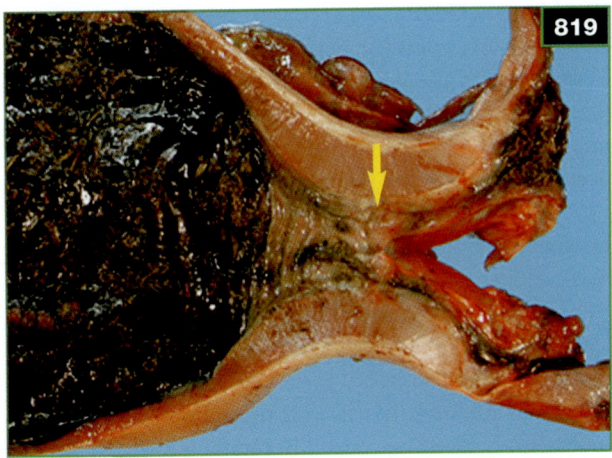

819 A case of severe ileal hypertrophy (arrow). This horse experienced several episodes of medical colic before requiring an exploratory laparotomy. Massive distension of the entire small intestine was found, reflecting the chronic nature of the ileal hypertrophy.

Clinical presentation
The clinical signs will depend of the degree of obstruction. Intermittent colic (especially after eating), anorexia, and chronic weight loss of 1–6 months' duration are common. Partial obstruction may result in mild to moderate intermittent signs of colic, but if the obstruction is total, the horse will be presented with more severe signs. Nasogastric reflux may be present depending on the severity and duration of the luminal obstruction.

Differential diagnosis
A variety of other obstructive or strangulating lesions of the small intestine should be considered. Intestinal lympho-sarcoma may also result in thickened small intestine.

Diagnosis
Distended loops of small intestine may be palpable per rectum. Loops of small intestine with a thickened wall may be palpable in the upper right abdominal quadrant. These findings may also be observed via ultrasound examination, which can provide an objective assessment of wall thickness. In severe cases the intestinal wall can be up to 25 mm thick. If the lesion is obstructive, small-intestinal distension orad to the lesion may be visualized as well. Nasogastric reflux may be present if a complete obstruction has developed. Abdominocentesis usually yields normal fluid. Hematology is unremarkable.

Management
Mild cases, where surgery is not an option, may be treated conservatively with a laxative diet. The potential association with intestinal parasites means that the deworming program should be evaluated. The severity and frequency of clinical signs are used to determine whether surgery is required. Longitudinal myotomies of the serosal and muscular layers at regular intervals may be useful. If the lesion is localized, a single myotomy with transverse closure can be performed. However, the success rate with myotomy is only fair and an incomplete or complete ileocecal or jejunocecal bypass, depending on where the lesion ends, is recommended. An incomplete bypass may result in impaction of the remaining loop, thus obstructing the newly created opening. Furthermore, passage of food in the remaining loop can still cause local pain. A complete jejunocecal anastomosis with formation of an ileal stump alleviates this problem.

Prognosis
If the lesion is localized and does not involve the remainder of the small intestine, the prognosis is fair to good. If anastomosis (with or without resection) is performed, local dehiscence of the anastomosis site, stricture, and adhesions can occur.

Ileal impaction

Definition/overview

Obstruction of the ileum from accumulation of ingesta in the ileum orad to the ileocecal opening is termed an ileal impaction. It most commonly occurs as a primary condition, but it can also be secondary to ileal pathology.

Etiology/pathophysiology

The condition is seen more often in Europe and the southeastern US. The condition in the US is possibly related to feeding coastal Bermuda hay. In Europe the condition is thought to be secondary to local infestation with tapeworms or mesenteric vascular thrombotic disease. In a recent study, feeding coastal Bermuda hay and failure to administer anthelmintic with efficacy against tapeworms was associated with increased risk of ileal impaction. In the US the disease is more commonly seen between June and November.

Coastal Bermuda hay is often dry and fibrous. Feed with a high-fiber content may cause violent peristalsis, resulting in extraction of water from the mass of ingesta, thus creating a drier and firmer mass. Tapeworms may be a risk factor because of the edema and ulceration created at their attachment around the ileocecal orifice, thereby disturbing the motility and lumen diameter.

Clinical presentation

The impaction causes a simple mechanical obstruction, therefore the clinical signs are usually mild early in the condition. As ileal distension progresses, signs of pain increase, but these are not usually as severe as those seen with surgical lesions and they usually subside in 6–10 hours. The abdominal pain then returns as gastric and orad small-intestinal distension increases. Gastric reflux may be present if the condition has been present for a while. Borborygmi are usually decreased. The heart rate is variably elevated, often to approximately 70 bpm. Dehydration with secondary circulatory compromise eventually arises following sequestration of fluid in the intestine and reduced oral intake.

Differential diagnosis

Because ileal impaction results in a simple obstruction, the main differential diagnoses are adynamic ileus and DPJ. In more advanced cases, obstructive small-intestinal conditions must be considered.

Diagnosis

Small-intestinal distension is usually palpable per rectum. In approximately 25% of cases the impaction is palpable on the midline medial to the cecum. Gastric reflux may be present, depending on the chronicity. Abdominocentesis usually yields normal fluid unless intestinal compromise has developed from chronic and/or severe intestinal distension, when the protein level usually increases. A long-standing impaction may result in local necrosis and peritonitis.

Management

Supportive medical therapy consisting mainly of intravenous fluid therapy and analgesics may be successful in early cases. Intermittent gastric decompression may be required and a nasogastric tube should be left in place or passed regularly to detect and relieve gastric distension. Diagnosis may be difficult and impaction may be secondary to another lesion, therefore surgical intervention is common. At surgery, massaging the impaction may break it down without recourse to an enterotomy. Intraluminal infusion of saline may be necessary in some cases. If the condition is secondary to ileal inflammation, hypertrophy, or local dysfunction, an incomplete or complete jejuno-cecostomy may be necessary.

Prognosis

In general, the prognosis is fair to good and is better than with most other small-intestinal disorders. The shorter the duration before surgical intervention the better the prognosis. Postoperative ileus is common.

Meckel's diverticulum

Definition/overview

Meckel's diverticulum is an embryonic remnant of the vitelline duct that results in the formation of a blind sac that communicates with the lumen of the small intestine.

Etiology/pathophysiology

The diverticulum can become impacted with ingesta, resulting in chronic colic. If the impaction is severe, necrosis can occur, followed by peritonitis. Inflammation of the diverticulum may also produce adhesions to other loops of intestine. Wrapping of the diverticulum around adjacent or other loops of small intestine, thus causing strangulation, is possible. Persistent vitello-umbilical bands may act as an axis for small-intestinal volvulus.

Clinical presentation

Clinical signs are most commonly seen in adult horses. Signs are usually nonspecific if luminal obstruction is not present, and may be intermittent and chronic. In these cases, intermittent signs of abdominal discomfort with possible periods of inappetence are reported. Clinical signs are severe if a strangulation or volvulus occurs. Meckel's diverticulum can also be identified as an incidental finding on exploratory laparotomy or necropsy.

Differential diagnosis

A vast array of causes of chronic or acute colic should be considered.

Diagnosis

Small-intestinal distension may be palpable per rectum if total luminal obstruction is present. It may be possible in some cases to palpate the impacted diverticulum as a blind sac with firm contents. Ultrasonographic examination of the abdomen may demonstrate distended small intestine aborally to the diverticulum. If a necrotic diverticulum is present, the peritoneal fluid WBC count and total protein may be elevated. Hematologic changes are nonspecific and variable.

Management

Exploratory laparotomy is indicated in horses with severe signs of small-intestinal obstruction, peritonitis, or chronic signs of colic. A longitudinal resection of the diverticulum with a transverse closure is recommended. A local resection of the ileum may be necessary. In the case of strangulation the affected intestine is resected and an anastomosis performed.

Prognosis

The prognosis is good if rupture and resulting peritonitis are not present or if resection is not needed. In the presence of strangulation or volvulus the prognosis is fair.

Mesodiverticular band

Definition/overview

A mesodiverticular band is a congenital abnormality that results in the formation of a band extending from one side of the mesentery to the antimesenteric surface of the small intestine. It results from the persistence of the paired vitelline vessels as they extend from the aorta to the umbilicus.

Etiology/pathophysiology

A triangular space is created where the mesodiverticular band forms one edge of the triangular hiatus and the adjacent mesentery and jejunum form the others. These structures form a sac where herniation can occur.

Incarceration of the small intestine can result when a loop of small intestine, most commonly the jejunum, passes into the depths of the hernial sac and becomes trapped within it (820). The distension of the entrapped intestine creates pressure on the mesentery, resulting in a rent. Strangulation of a segment of jejunum in the mesenteric rent (821) may provide a fulcrum around which the surrounding intestine may form a volvulus.

Clinical presentation

The clinical signs are consistent with small-intestine strangulation. These signs include mild to severe signs of colic and moderate to severe elevations in heart rate, with eventual gastric reflux. It also can be an incidental finding on exploratory laparotomy or necropsy. There is no age or sex predilection.

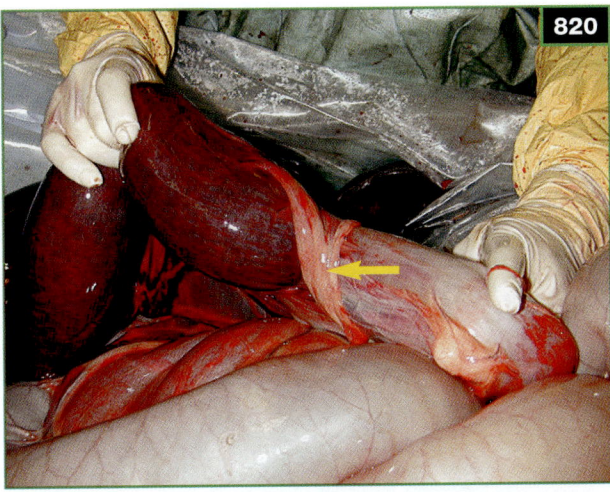

820 A mesodiverticular band that was associated with a small-intestine volvulus (arrow). This picture was taken after correction of the volvulus. Note the hemorrhagic strangulation lesion on the small intestine (left side of the picture).

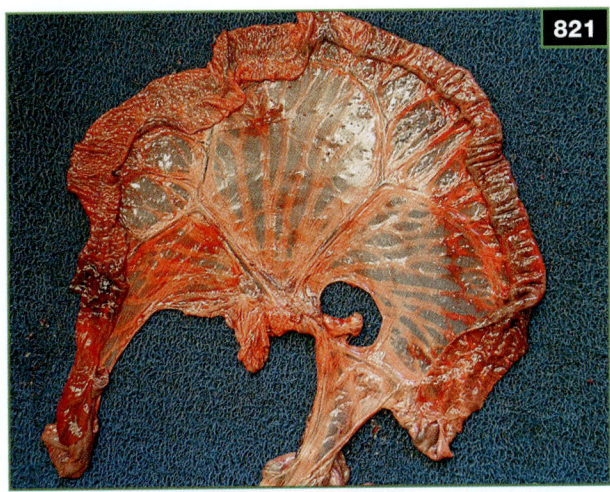

821 Postmortem specimen of a mesenteric rent located close to the root of the jejunal mesentery.

555

Differential diagnosis

Any other obstructive lesion of the small intestine, such as volvulus, strangulated lipoma, or mesenteric rent, can produce similar clinical signs.

Diagnosis

Distended loops of small intestine are typically palpable per rectum. Nasogastric reflux may be present, depending on the duration of obstruction. Ultrasonographic examination of the abdomen may demonstrate distended small-intestinal loops, potentially with intramural edema. If necrosis has occurred, serosanguineous fluid with an increased nucleated cell count and total protein level will be present on abdominocentesis.

Management

Surgical correction is required. At surgery, the incarceration is reduced followed by a resection and anastomosis of the compromised intestine. Often the mesodiverticular band contains a vitelline artery and the potential role of that artery in the blood supply to the jejunum should be evaluated prior to resection.

Prognosis

The prognosis is fair when resection is needed. The prognosis is worse if small-intestinal volvulus is present concurrently.

Epiploic foramen entrapment

Definition/overview

The epiploic foramen is a virtual space on the visceral surface of the liver, where small intestine can become incarcerated (**822**). It is an uncommon condition. Thoroughbreds, Thoroughbred crosses, and male animals appear to be predisposed.

Etiology/pathophysiology

The epiploic foramen lies on the visceral surface of the liver near the portal fissure. It is a narrow opening of approximately 4–10 cm in diameter, limited cranially by the hepatoduodenal ligament and caudally by the junction between the pancreas and the mesoduodenum. The structures bordering the epiploic foramen are the caudate process of the liver, the caudal vena cava dorsally, the right lobe of the pancreas, and the portal vein ventrally. It has been hypothesized that the caudate process of the liver atrophies with age and the potential opening of the epiploic foramen becomes wider, facilitating entrapment of the small intestine. A link between aerophagia and epiploic foramen entrapment has also been reported. In the UK, many cases occur in the winter months when animals are stabled.

The distal jejunum and ileum are the most commonly involved, possibly due to their long mesentery. Entrapment can be from right to left or left to right. In the right-to-left herniation the small intestine passes from the peritoneal cavity through the epiploic foramen and into the omental bursa (left side) (**823**). However, the left-to-right entrapment is more common, where the intestine enters from the visceral side of the liver to lie subsequently between the right liver lobe and the dorsal body wall.

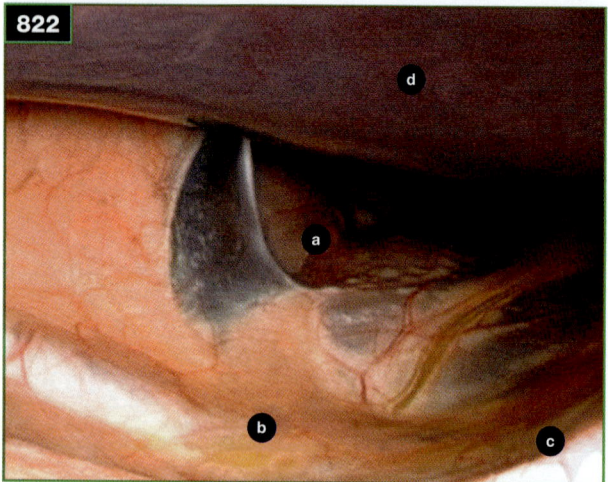

822 Laparoscopic view of the opening of the epiploic foramen (a), the pancreas (b), the duodenum (c), and the liver (d).

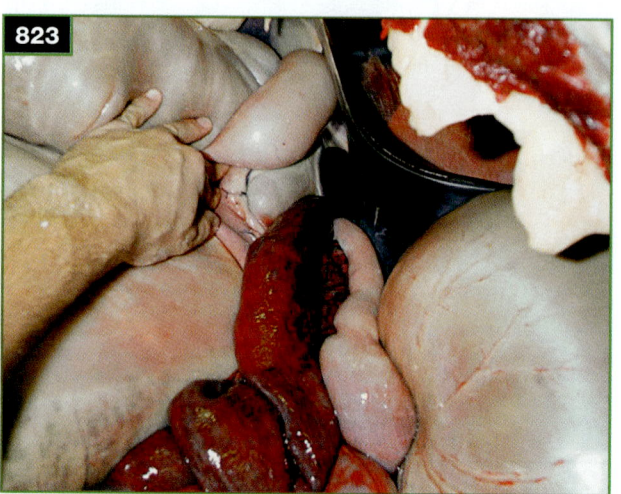

823 Postmortem view of a right-to-left epiploic foramen entrapment. Note the typical appearance of small-intestine hemorrhagic strangulation.

Gastrointestinal system

Clinical presentation

Clinical signs are inconsistent, which may hamper diagnosis. Some horses may display acute violent onset of colic, which subsides and is followed by depression. Other cases may show no signs of abdominal pain and/or gastric reflux. Despite the presence of a necrotic bowel, some horses may have normal vital parameters. Absence of clinical signs of shock may be explained by the fact that the infarcted bowel is in an enclosed area, which may slow down the absorption of endotoxin. Severe hypovolemic shock or even sudden collapse is possible if the portal vein or vena cava ruptures.

Differential diagnosis

Any other small-intestinal obstructive disease such as strangulated lipoma, volvulus, intussusception, and entrapment in a mesenteric rent can cause similar signs.

Diagnosis

Diagnosis may be difficult. The small intestine is incarcerated very cranially in the abdomen, therefore small-intestinal distention may not be palpable per rectum. Nasogastric reflux may not be present until late in the disease because of the typical involvement of distal portions of the small intestine. In most cases an increase in peritoneal fluid protein level is noted. Peritoneal fluid WBC count may also be increased, but this is not consistent. Free blood in the abdomen may be present if rupture of one of the main vessels has occurred. While performing ultrasonographic examination of the abdomen, the right middle body wall region should receive special attention. If amotile and edematous small-intestinal loops are detected in this region, an epiploic entrapment should be suspected. Definitive diagnosis is achieved at surgery.

Management

Surgery is required, and reduction of the entrapped loop is performed. In some cases of severe distension and edema of the affected intestine, resection of one of the branches involved in the entrapment may be necessary successfully to reduce the entrapment. Alternatively, an enterotomy can be performed 1 meter proximal to the obstruction to empty the intestinal contents. In most cases the intestine is nonviable and requires resection. It is possible to rupture the vena cava or portal vein while trying to reduce the entrapment, especially if the condition has resulted in compromise of the vascular wall. This is a fatal complication.

Prognosis

The prognosis is guarded to fair depending on whether resection is necessary or not. Reported long-term outcomes vary from around 35 to 70% and are often poorer than for other small-intestinal surgical conditions. The most common complication postoperatively is ileus.

Inguinal rupture

Definition/overview

Inguinal ruptures result from herniation of intestine through the inguinal canal followed by rupture of the peritoneum or, less commonly, the vaginal tunic, resulting in the presence of intestinal loops in the subcutaneous tissues of the scrotal region. It is often referred to as a direct inguinal hernia.

Etiology/pathophysiology

Inguinal rupture is most commonly seen in foals after parturition secondary to a traumatic rupture of the vaginal tunic or peritoneum, probably caused by compression during parturition. The intestine passes through a rent in the parietal tunic and scrotal fascia. Inguinal rupture may also be caused by a fall or a jump in the adult horse and can be associated with a considerable length of intestinal herniation.

Clinical presentation

Foals are usually presented for depression or mild colic signs and a pendulous swelling extending from the inguinal region to the cranial aspect of the prepuce. If strangulation is present, the colic signs will be more severe. Friction between the swelling and the inner thigh may result in cold, edematous, or necrotic skin locally. Loops of bowel can usually be palpated subcutaneously and in some cases there is evidence of peristalsis underneath the skin. The hernia is usually difficult or impossible to reduce compared with a nonruptured inguinal hernia. Inguinal rupture in the adult can occur in both sexes and produces similar signs.

Differential diagnosis

Nonruptured inguinal hernia, scrotal hematoma, seroma, or hydrocele should be considered.

Diagnosis

Physical examination and hematology are usually in the normal range unless there is intestinal strangulation or concomitant disease. Palpation of intestine outside the inguinal region and the presence of swelling and abrasions are diagnostic. Ultrasonographic examination of the region may reveal loops of small intestine surrounded by subcutaneous accumulation of fluid. Absence of the vaginal tunic enclosing the intestine may be observed. If strangulation is present, the intestinal wall may be thickened and intestinal motility decreased.

557

Management

Surgical treatment is advisable to avoid strangulation, local adhesions of the small intestine, or total rupture. An inguinal approach is selected and the hernia is reduced. If present, the testicle is removed and the vaginal tunic closed. Closure of the vaginal tunic may be impossible in some cases because of edema and trauma. The external inguinal ring is closed subsequently. If the skin has been stretched excessively, part of it is resected or a drain is placed locally to avoid seroma formation. The other testicle should also be removed.

Prognosis

The prognosis is good if there is absence of strangulation or full-thickness trauma at the level of the skin. Complications are usually limited to formation of seroma and local infection. Postoperative ileus is also possible.

Scrotal hernia

Definition/overview

An inguinal hernia results from passage of abdominal contents into the inguinal canal. If the intestine passes through the external inguinal ring and into the scrotum, it is a scrotal hernia (824).

Etiology/pathophysiology

Scrotal hernias can be direct or indirect. In an indirect hernia, the herniated intestine is located inside the vaginal tunic beside the testis. In a direct hernia, the intestine herniates through a rent in the peritoneum and lies subcutaneously. Indirect hernias are more common. The condition may be congenital or acquired.

Congenital hernia in the foal is present at birth and is considered an inherited defect. It is secondary to an abnormal vaginal ring. Acquired hernias in the adult are usually unilateral and may occur secondary to conditions that increase the intra-abdominal pressure such as breeding or trauma. They can also develop post castration for up to a few days.

Clinical presentation

Congenital hernia in the foal

This is usually observed in the first few days of life. Standardbred and draft breeds are predisposed. It may be unilateral or bilateral and is often observed after straining to pass meconium. On palpation of the scrotum, fluid-filled intestinal loops can be detected and borborygmi may be audible locally. Most of the hernia is easily reducible, but re-herniation occurs immediately when pressure is removed. The foal may present with signs of colic if strangulation occurs; however, this is rare.

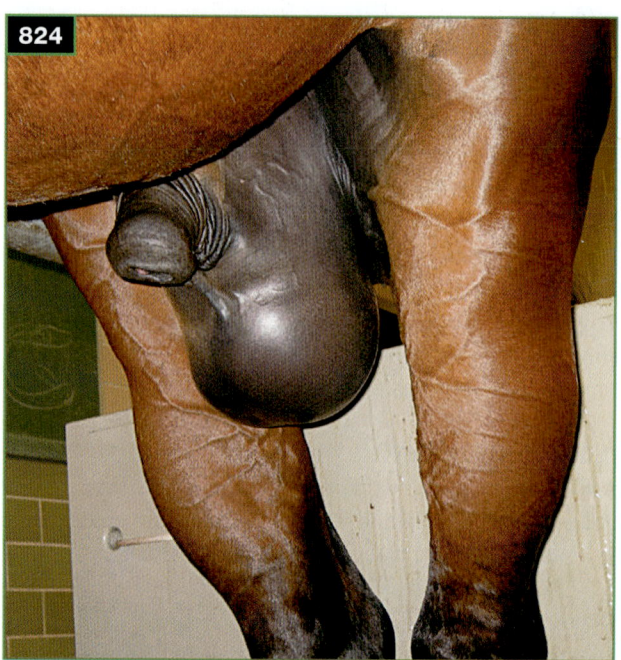

824

Acquired hernia in the adult

Most acquired hernias are unilateral. They are infrequently reducible and more commonly result in acute intestinal strangulation (825). The scrotum and inguinal region may be swollen and cold to the touch. Thickening at the neck of the testicle is usually present. The horse is usually presented for colic because of incarcerated small intestine. Signs of abdominal pain range from mild to severe, with decreased to absent intestinal motility. Reflux may be obtained on passage of a nasogastric tube depending on the duration of the obstruction.

Differential diagnosis

In foals, scrotal distension may also be caused by uroperitoneum, trauma, or abscessation. In adults, testicular torsion is the main differential diagnosis, but orchitis and hydrocele should also be considered.

824 A stallion affected with a severe left scrotal hernia.

825 Intraoperative view of strangulated small intestine in the stallion pictured in 824.

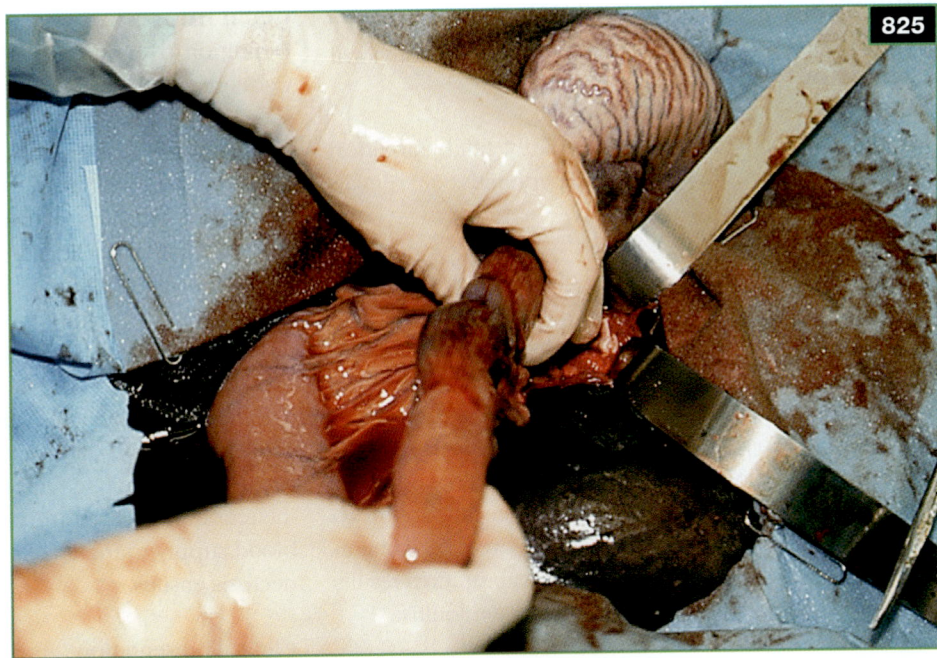

Diagnosis
Congenital hernia in the foal
Diagnosis is made on physical examination. Ultrasonographic examination of the inguinal region demonstrates the presence of normal motile small-intestinal loops in the vaginal tunic. Less frequently, the tip of the cecum or pelvic flexure can be herniated.

Acquired hernia in the adult
Palpation of the scrotum and testicular region will identify an abnormality. A definitive diagnosis is made on per-rectum palpation, when two loops of small intestine are detected passing into the internal inguinal ring. Other distended loops of small intestine may also be palpable within the abdominal cavity. Ultrasonographic examination of the distended scrotum can help differentiate testicular torsion from scrotal hernia, particularly if palpation per rectum is not feasible. Distended loops of small intestine may be evident on transabdominal ultrasonographic examination.

Management
Congenital hernia in the foal
Most resolve spontaneously by 3–4 months of age. Daily manual reduction is recommended. A local bandage following manual reduction can also be applied; however, formation of pressures sores by the bandage is possible. Surgery is indicated if the hernia becomes incarcerated, if it is very large, or if it has not spontaneously resolved by 6 months of age. A bilateral closed castration is recommended.

Acquired hernia in the adult.
Supportive therapy is imperative, as these horses are often systemically compromised. It may be possible to reduce acute herniation by careful per rectum and/or external manipulations; however, reducible hernias occur infrequently. Prior to performing any manipulations, the stallion should be sedated and epidural anesthesia administered to avoid local trauma. The incarcerated loop is grasped gently per rectum and traction is applied. Alternatively, this procedure can be performed under general anesthesia. Rectal tear is a potential complication. In the majority of cases, immediate surgical correction of the condition via an inguinal approach +/– laparotomy is recommended. Intestinal resection is often necessary. The inguinal region is approached initially, the vaginal ring is enlarged, and the intestine is returned into the abdomen. Ideally, a laparotomy is then performed to verify the integrity of the intestine, and the small intestine is decompressed and resected if needed. In some cases the nonviable intestine can be resected in the inguinal region, especially in cases where it would be difficult to reduce back in the abdomen because of the location of the intestinal segment that is involved. A unilateral or bilateral castration is performed to prevent future herniation, followed by closure of the vaginal tunic and the superficial ring.

Prognosis
The prognosis is excellent in foals. In adults, if the condition is diagnosed rapidly and a resection is avoided, the prognosis is good. However, if strangulation has occurred, the prognosis is fair to poor.

559

Disorders of the cecum

Cecal rupture

Definition/overview
Cecal rupture is a rare and invariably fatal condition because of the rapid onset of septic peritonitis.

Etiology/pathophysiology
Rupture may occur due to marked distension or devitalization of the cecal wall. Cecal rupture can occur secondary to cecal tympany, impaction, or infarction. Idiopathic cecal rupture can occur in mares following parturition (see 491), in hospitalized horses treated with NSAIDs, and in the absence of any history of disease. It has also been suggested that severe tapeworm infection may be associated with cecal rupture. It is not uncommon for cecal rupture to occur without any prodromal signs. The gross contamination of the abdomen that occurs with cecal ruptures results in the rapid development of severe septic peritonitis.

Clinical presentation
There may be a short period following cecal rupture when the horse appears to have improved because of the immediate relief of severe distension. Shortly afterwards, progressive signs of depression, colic, toxemia, dehydration, cardiovascular compromise, sweating, and shaking will develop. Heart rate will increase and can be severely elevated. Mucous membranes may be dark red, purple, or blue and CRT may be markedly prolonged. Borborygmi will be decreased or absent.

Differential diagnosis
Septic peritonitis of other causes, severe enterocolitis, septicemia, and pleuritis should be considered.

Diagnosis
Hematology may be normal shortly after rupture; however, neutropenia with a left shift and degenerative changes in neutrophils will develop. Total plasma protein levels will decrease as peritonitis progresses, while PCV will increase. Excessive flocculent peritoneal fluid will be evident ultrasonographically. Fibrin may be apparent. Abdominocentesis should be performed. Dark, foul-smelling peritoneal fluid will often be recovered. A gritty feel to the serosal surface may be detected per rectum. None of these findings can be used to differentiate cecal rupture from rupture of another intestinal viscus. Definitive diagnosis is obtained at surgery or necropsy.

Management
There are no viable treatment options.

Prognosis
Cecal rupture is invariably fatal.

Cecal infarction

Definition/overview
Cecal infarction is an uncommon cause of colic.

Etiology/pathophysiology
Prior to the availability of avermectin anthelmintics, *Strongylus vulgaris* infestation was the most likely cause of cecal infarction. Cyathostominosis may also be associated with cecal infarction. Disseminated intravascular coagulation (DIC) can result in thrombus development in blood vessels, including major vessels in the cecum. Young horses are more commonly affected.

The pathophysiology is dependent on the inciting cause. Extensive collateral circulation is present in the cecum, therefore large thrombi are required to cause cecal infarction. If a large thrombus lodges in certain locations, blood supply to the cecum is compromised and ischemic necrosis ensues.

Clinical presentation
Unless cecal rupture has occurred, most affected horses present initially with mild to moderate abdominal pain. Tachycardia is present consistent with the degree of pain and underlying disease. Signs of concurrent disease, particularly in cases thought to be associated with DIC, may obscure signs of cecal infarction.

Differential diagnosis
A variety of causes of colic must be considered. In addition, cecal infarction must be differentiated from the underlying condition in cases associated with DIC.

Diagnosis
Clinical examination and palpation per rectum are nonspecific. A thickened cecal wall may be evident on ultrasonographic examination, but this is often difficult to interpret. A firm mass may be palpable in the right caudal abdomen; however, this finding is not pathognomonic for cecal infarction. Increases in peritoneal WBC count and protein level will be present. Peritoneal fluid color will be abnormal and will worsen over time. Definitive diagnosis is made during surgery or necropsy.

Management
Surgical resection of all infarcted tissue is required. This may not always be possible, depending on the extent of the infarction. The underlying cause must also be addressed. If parasitism is thought to be the cause, farm management should be evaluated.

Prognosis
The prognosis is good as long as the infarction is not so large as to preclude resection. Prompt intervention is required to avoid the onset of peritonitis.

Cecal torsion

Definition/overview
Cecal torsion is a rare condition.

Etiology/pathophysiology
In most cases the etiology of cecal torsion is unknown. There is a report of cecal torsion in an animal with anatomic abnormalities of the cecocolic fold and in another case with multiple mesenteric defects. Large-colon volvulus may predispose to cecal displacement or volvulus. When this occurs, the axis of rotation involves the dorsal mesenteric attachment of the cecum.

Clinical presentation
Cecal torsion is accompanied by severe, acute pain and metabolic derangements consistent with strangulation of a large organ. Characteristic signs of colic are displayed.

Differential diagnosis
Any form of strangulating intestinal accident would be a differential diagnosis, particularly a large-colon volvulus.

Diagnosis
Physical examination findings are consistent with colic, but not specific for cecal torsion. Cecal tympany may occur with cecal torsion as outflow obstruction develops, in which case distension and tympany of the right flank may be noted. Gaseous distension of the cecum is often palpable per rectum. If cecal tympany does not develop, rectal findings are unrewarding for a specific diagnosis of the condition, and characteristic hematologic or abdominal fluid abnormalities have not been reported. Hematologic and abdominocentesis results will vary with the degree of cecal compromise. Definitive diagnosis is made during exploratory laparotomy.

Management
Surgery is required. A typhlotomy and decompression may be valuable for the immediate postoperative period, particularly if cecal motility is diminished. If the cecum is devitalized at the time of surgery, a partial typhlectomy can be performed; however, inability to remove the entire cecum, and the possibility of devitalized tissue at the anastomosis site, may cause unacceptable morbidity and postoperative mortality in cases with significant ischemic damage to the cecum. In these cases, intraoperative euthanasia is often elected.

Prognosis
The prognosis for cecal torsions is dependent on the viability of the tissues at the time of surgery. With de-rotation early in the course of the disease, the prognosis can be good. Recurrence of cecal torsion has not been reported, and may therefore be expected to be low. If a congenital defect is detected at the time of surgery, recurrence of a similar problem may be encountered.

Cecal impaction

Definition/overview
Cecal impaction is relatively uncommon, but it is the most common cause of cecal disease in horses. Arabian, Morgan, and Appaloosa horses, and horses >15 years of age, may be at higher risk.

Etiology/pathophysiology
A variety of risk factors have been identified or suggested. These include general anesthesia, pain, hospitalization, poor dentition, poor-quality feed, and parasitic infestation. The role of tapeworms in cecal impaction is controversial. Hypertrophy of the cecal base may also be a cause of chronic or recurrent cecal impaction.

The pathophysiology is unclear, but likely involves decreased or abnormal cecal motility. This allows for retention of ingesta in the cecum, particularly at the apex. The blind-ended nature of the cecum may facilitate impaction formation.

Clinical presentation
Affected horses display signs of colic ranging from mild and intermittent to severe and protracted. Pain is usually mild and slowly progressive. Fever should not be present. Heart rate is variably elevated. GI sounds may be normal or decreased, but there is typically a decrease in or absence of borborygmi over the right dorsal paralumbar fossa. Signs of cardiovascular compromise should not be evident.

Differential diagnoses
Colic due to a variety of other causes can present in a similar manner.

Diagnosis
Physical examination and hematology are nonspecific. Palpation per rectum is diagnostic. An impacted cecum typically feels firm and doughy. Sometimes, the impaction is not palpable if it is present at the cecal apex, but the medial cecal band is tight and difficult to move. Cecal impaction can occur concurrently with impaction of the large colon or other abnormalities, so a thorough examination is essential.

Management

Cecal impactions can be frustrating to treat because they tend to take longer to resolve than large-colon impactions. There are no clear guidelines for the management of cecal impactions or when to intervene surgically.

Medical treatment is usually attempted initially and mainly involves feed restriction and fluid therapy. Intravenous fluid therapy is useful and may speed resolution if an adequate volume is used. Oral fluid therapy may also be used. Mineral oil, DSS, or osmotic cathartics (e.g. sodium sulfate) are often used, but their efficacy is unclear. Analgesics should be administered as required. The potential usefulness of prokinetics is currently unclear.

Surgery is typically recommended when there is a poor response to medical therapy or when there is significant cecal distension or abdominal pain. The potential for cecal rupture exists even with apparently small impactions, and some authors recommend early surgical intervention. Typhlotomy is usually performed to remove the impaction.

Prognosis

Most cecal impactions resolve with medical therapy, but some may require prolonged treatment. Cecal rupture is a major concern and can occur without warning. It should be suspected in any horse with cecal impaction that deteriorates suddenly, and carries a grave prognosis. Recurrence of cecal impaction is common in some animals. Presumably this is because of underlying problems in intestinal motility, intestinal-wall damage from the initial impaction, or the continued presence of predisposing factors. Surgical bypass may be indicated in recurrent cases.

Cecal tympany

Definition/overview

Gaseous distension of the cecum, otherwise known as cecal tympany, is a cause of colic.

Etiology/pathophysiology

Primary and secondary cecal tympany may occur. Primary cecal tympany occurs in the absence of an outflow obstruction and arises via excessive gas production in the cecum and/or a reduction in cecal motility. Dietary changes, lush pasture, and high-grain diets may be predisposing factors. Secondary cecal tympany occurs as a result of a cecal outflow obstruction (e.g. large-colon displacement, impaction, or volvulus).

Clinical presentation

Nonspecific signs of colic of varying severity will be evident. Heart rate will be elevated consistent with the degree of pain. Very high heart rates and severe pain can be present with severe tympany or as a result of an underlying process such as a large-colon volvulus. Bloating of the right paralumbar fossa may be evident and an area of resonant tympany is usually present over the right flank. Borborygmi may be decreased on the right side. Abdominal distension may be evident. Signs of toxemia or cardiovascular compromise should not be present with primary cecal tympany. Tachypnea may be present if there is significant abdominal distension and pressure on the thoracic cavity.

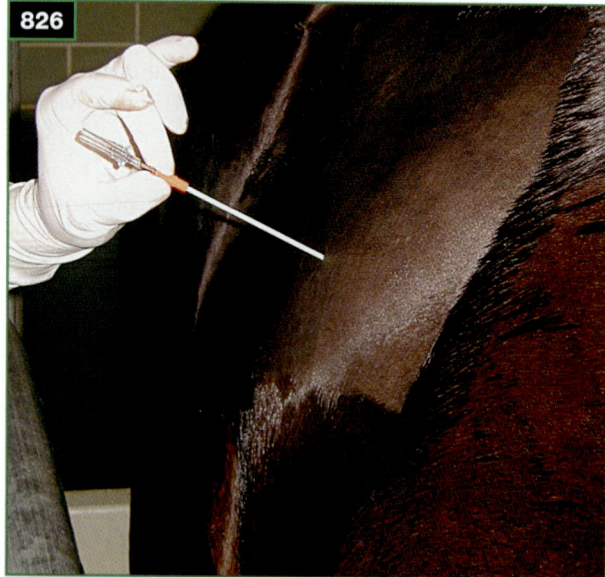

826 Cecal trocarization in a horse with progressive abdominal distension and pain.

TABLE 26 **Protocol for cecal trocarization**
• A tympanic area over the right paralumbar fossa should be clipped, surgically prepared, and blocked with 2% lidocaine.
• Ultrasonographic confirmation that no vital structures are underlying is useful.
• A 14G catheter or trocar set should be used. The catheter or trocar should be inserted perpendicular to the skin surface, until gas escapes. Suction can be used to expedite decompression.
• It might be beneficial to inject 10 ml of sterile saline through the catheter prior to removal to lessen contamination of the body wall as the catheter is removed. Some degree of local peritonitis is expected, and severe peritonitis may develop secondary to laceration of a viscus or leakage from the site of intestinal puncture.
• Broad-spectrum antimicrobial prophylaxis (e.g. sodium/potassium penicillin 20,000 IU/kg i/v q6h and gentamicin 6.6 mg/kg i/v q24h) is indicated.

Differential diagnosis

Other causes of colic, particularly those resulting in gaseous distension of the large colon, should be considered.

Diagnosis

Diagnosis is based on per-rectum detection of a large, gas-distended cecum in the right side of the abdomen. If marked distension is present, the base of the cecum may protrude into the pelvic canal and it is sometimes difficult to differentiate cecum from large colon. Other diagnostic tests are unlikely to differentiate the cecum from the large colon.

Management

The approach to cecal tympany depends on the severity of signs and whether primary or secondary tympany is present. For secondary tympany, the inciting cause must be addressed. Most cases of primary cecal tympany will respond to withholding of feed, walking, and analgesics. Analgesic therapy is described earlier (see p. 547).

Intravenous fluid therapy is indicated in dehydrated horses and may be useful in all cases. If marked cecal distension is present, either with primary or secondary tympany, cecal trocarization may be required (**826** and *Table 26*). Cecal rupture is a concern, mainly with severe and/or chronic distension. Exploratory celiotomy and cecal decompression or typhlotomy may be required. Very rarely will typhlectomy be indicated. This should be reserved for severe, recurrent primary cecal tympany where management changes have had no effect.

Management (particularly diet) should be evaluated. Access to lush pasture should be restricted, high-grain diets should be avoided, and dietary changes should be made gradually.

Prognosis

The prognosis for primary cecal tympany is very good. Recurrence is most often the result of ongoing management issues rather than a primary cecal abnormality. The prognosis for secondary cecal tympany depends on the primary cause.

Tapeworm infection

Definition/overview

Infestation with tapeworms is common worldwide. While typically benign, infestation with *Anoplocephala perfoliata* can be associated with colic, particularly if large numbers are present.

Etiology/pathophysiology

A. perfoliata, *A. magna*, and *Paranoplocephala mamillana* are tapeworms that can be found in horses; however, *A. magna* and *P. mamillana* are not typically considered to be pathogenic. In some areas the prevalence of tapeworm infestation can very high (up to 80%). This is usually in temperate climates as compared with hot and arid areas.

Tapeworms have an indirect life cycle. Horses are infected by ingestion of Oribatid mites, the intermediate host. Adult tapeworms can be found in the intestinal tract 1–2 months following ingestion. *A. perfoliata* is most commonly found around the ileocecal junction.

Mucosal congestion, focal ulceration, and mucosal thickening may develop at the site of *A. perfoliata* attachment. In most cases, no clinical signs result; however, inflammation at the site is thought to predispose to the development of ileocecal intussusceptions (**827**). Studies have also associated *A. perfoliata* infestation with spasmodic colic and ileal impaction, and they may be associated with an increased incidence of colic overall. The risk appears to be proportional to the tapeworm burden, and tapeworm-associated colic appears to be more common in horses 5 years of age or younger.

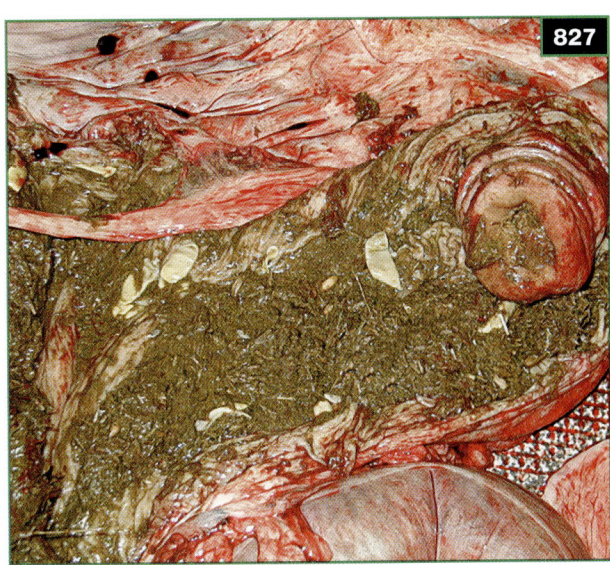

827 Ileocecal intussusception. Note the numerous tapeworms.

Clinical presentation
Most horses that are harboring tapeworms display no clinical abnormalities, and tapeworm infestation itself is not thought to produce signs of ill-thrift, weight loss, or diarrhea. Clinical signs ranging from ill-thrift to severe colic may be observed as a result of intussusception, spasmodic colic, or ileal impaction secondary to tapeworm infestation. These are covered in detail elsewhere.

Differential diagnosis
A variety of causes of colic should be considered in horses with tapeworm-associated colic.

Diagnosis
Fecal flotation is commonly used, but the sensitivity can be poor depending on the testing methodology. Some solutions that are effective for flotation testing of other parasite eggs are not effective. A saturated sucrose solution (450 g in 350 ml water) has been reported to be more effective. *A. perfoliata* eggs are D-shaped with a thick shell. The poor sensitivity of fecal flotation has led to serologic assays being evaluated and these may be available in some areas. Adult tapeworms are uncommonly found in feces and, if present, might suggest a high burden.

Management
Most routinely used anthelmintics are not effective against tapeworms and they are often overlooked in deworming programs. Pyrantel pamoate can be effective when used at a dose of 38 mg/kg p/o, which is twice the nematocidal dose. Daily administration of pyrantel tartrate (2.6 mg/kg) is likely to be effective as well; however, less information is available. Praziquantel (1.0–1.5 mg/kg p/o) is effective against tapeworms, and products containing a combination of ivermectin (0.2 mg/kg) and praziquantel (1.5 mg/kg) are available in many countries. Optimal deworming regimens have not been reported, but it is important to ensure annual deworming of horses 5 years of age or younger. The optimum frequency of deworming of older horses is less clear.

Prognosis
Simple infestation with tapeworms carries an excellent prognosis because of the ease of treatment and limited clinical signs. The prognosis is poorer if a tapeworm-associated intestinal accident has occurred.

Disorders of the large colon _____

Colitis
Definition/overview
Acute colitis is a potentially life-threatening disease characterized by diarrhea and varying degrees of depression, dehydration, toxemia, abdominal distension, and abdominal pain.

Etiology/pathophysiology
A variety of pathogenic organisms may be involved, including *C. difficile*, *C. perfringens*, *Salmonella* spp., and *Neorickettsia risticii* (Potomac horse fever [PHF]). Identification of the etiologic agent can be difficult because of limitations of available tests and incomplete understanding of the GI microflora. In most regions the majority of cases are idiopathic. Severe, peracute idiopathic colitis is sometimes termed colitis X. Outbreaks of colitis can occur, particularly in equine hospitals and on breeding farms.

Salmonellosis
Salmonellosis occurs when the appropriate combination of host (immune status, GI microflora, pain), bacterial (pathogenicity, dose), and environmental (stressors) factors is present. Fecal–oral inoculation or proliferation of small numbers of *Salmonella* organisms already in the GI tract may occur. Large numbers are typically required to cause disease in normal animals. Compromised animals (young, concurrently ill, antimicrobial treated, hospitalized) may be infected with much lower doses. Certain *Salmonella* strains may be able to cause disease with lower numbers (**828**).

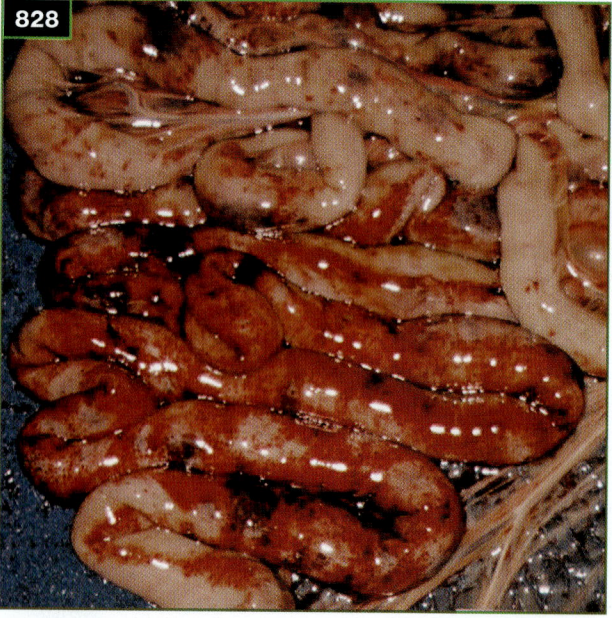

828 Marked hyperemia of the serosal surface of the small intestine of a foal with fatal salmonellosis.

TABLE 27 Toxin production by different *Clostridium perfringens* types

Type	TOXINS					
	alpha	beta	epsilon	iota	beta-2	enterotoxin
A	√				±	±
B	√	√	√		±	±
C	√	√			±	±
D	√		√		±	±
E	√			√	±	±

Clostridium difficile *infection*

C. difficile is a spore-forming bacterium that can be found in a small percentage of normal horses, particularly young horses and those treated with antimicrobials. In some situations, *C. difficile* can proliferate and produce toxins. It is unclear whether *C. difficile* infection (CDI) develops following ingestion of toxigenic strains of *C. difficile* or overgrowth of *C. difficile* residing in low levels in the GI tract; it is likely that both situations occur. Although antimicrobial therapy is a risk factor for the development of CDI, the absence of a history of antimicrobial administration does not rule out CDI.

Clostridium perfringens-*associated diarrhea*

C. perfringens is a Gram-positive spore-forming anaerobic bacterium that can produce a wide variety of toxins (*Table 27*). The clinical relevance of some strains is unclear. *C. perfringens* enterotoxin and beta-2 toxin have been associated with diarrhea in adult horses and foals. Type C strains have been implicated in severe enterocolitis in foals. *C. perfringens* is a normal inhabitant of the GI tract of a large percentage of normal horses and foals. In some situations, *C. perfringens* can overgrow and produce a variety of toxins. Antimicrobial therapy, dietary changes, stress, concurrent disease, and transportation may be predisposing factors.

Potomac horse fever

N. risticii (formerly *Ehrlichia risticii*) is an obligate intracellular bacterium that has an affinity for monocytes. Most cases occur during summer and early fall. There tends to be close proximity to freshwater. A variety of aquatic invertebrates may be involved in the natural transmission of the disease. The mechanism by which *N. risticii* causes diarrhea and other clinical signs is unclear. Interference with intestinal sodium and chloride absorption may be involved. The cause of laminitis, which frequently develops concurrently, is not known.

Colitis X

This term does not describe a specific disease entity. Rather, it is a general syndrome that encompasses severe, typically fatal, colitis of unknown etiology. It has been suggested that clostridia, particularly certain types of *C. perfringens*, may be involved; however, colitis X can probably be caused by a variety of infectious agents.

Idiopathic colitis

Idiopathic colitis is a syndrome likely involving a variety of different bacterial organisms and mechanisms of disease. Presumably, disruption of the normal microflora allows for the proliferation of pathogenic organisms. Antimicrobial therapy, concurrent disease, transportation, diet changes, and high-grain diet are potential risk factors.

Antimicrobial-associated diarrhea

Antimicrobial-associated diarrhea is not a specific disease. Rather, it refers to cases of acute diarrhea that are temporarily associated with antimicrobial administration. Administration of any antimicrobial via any route can predispose horses to diarrhea; however, certain antimicrobials, including erythromycin and tetracycline, are considered higher risk. A variety of infectious agents such as *C. difficile*, *C. perfringens*, and *Salmonella* spp. can be involved. It is presumed that antimicrobials disrupt the normal protective bacterial microflora in the intestinal tract, permitting overgrowth of pathogenic bacteria. Drugs that have a significant impact on anaerobes and those that undergo hepatic metabolism are probably more likely to disturb the intestinal microflora.

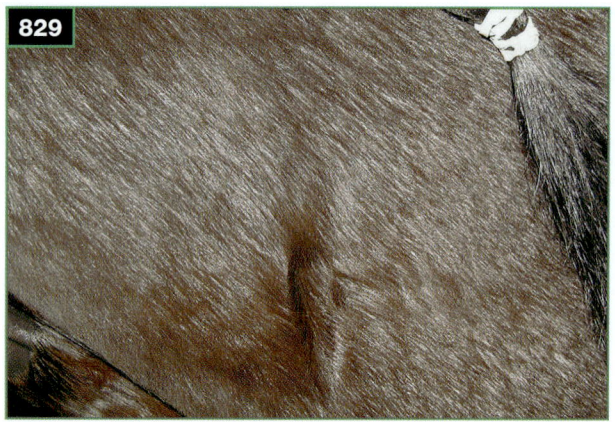

829 Prolonged skin tent in the neck of a horse estimated to be 10–12% dehydrated.

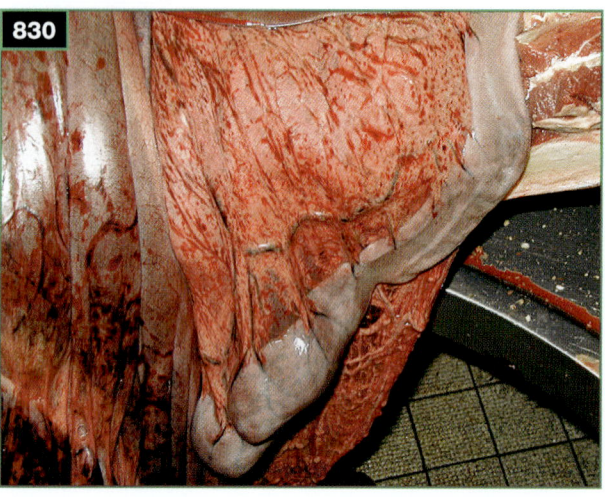

830 Small intestine and mesentery of a horse with disseminated intravascular coagulation secondary to colitis.

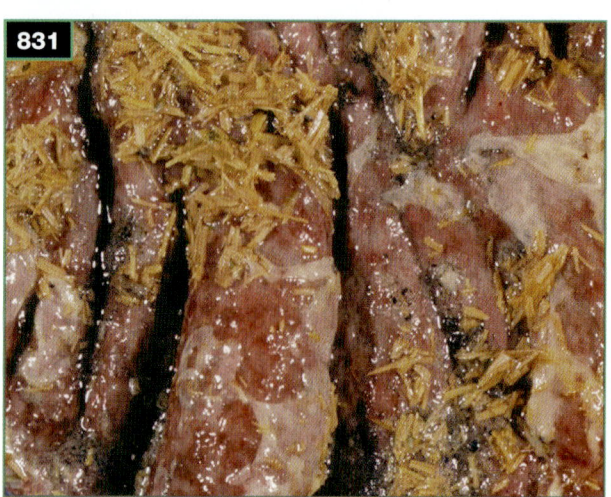

831 Intestinal mucosa of a horse with salmonellosis. Note the mucosal casts detaching from the mucosal surface.

Clinical presentation
General
The clinical presentation can be highly variable and depends on a number of factors. The spectrum of disease can range from soft feces with no other clinical abnormalities, to peracute, fatal, necrohemorrhagic enterocolitis. Diarrhea is usually present; however, clinical signs may develop before the onset of diarrhea. Varying degrees of dehydration (**829**), toxemia, depression, abdominal pain, cardiovascular compromise, and abdominal distension may be present. DIC can occur (**830**). Non-strangulating infarction of the colon from DIC should be considered in horses with colitis that deteriorate suddenly.

Salmonellosis
The 'classical' presentation of salmonellosis includes fever, depression, diarrhea, and severe toxemia; however, this combination occurs in 50% or less of affected horses. Fever of unknown origin may be the only presenting sign. Diarrhea may be mild, of short duration, or not evident in some cases. Septicemia and extraintestinal infection are of most concern in foals. Sloughing of the intestinal mucosa (**831**) may be evident as the passing of casts in the feces.

Clostridial diarrhea
The clinical presentation of CDI and *C. perfringens*-associated diarrhea is highly variable and nonspecific. Clinical presentation can range from mild disease with only soft feces, to peracute necrohemorrhagic colitis with rapid progression to death.

Potomac horse fever
PHF can have a somewhat different clinical progression. Fever can be very high (up to 41.7°C [107°F]). Usually, an initial episode of mild depression, anorexia, and fever is produced. Moderate to severe diarrhea may ensue; however, diarrhea only occurs in approximately 60% of cases. Severe toxemia and depression may accompany colic. Laminitis may develop in 25–40% of cases and may be more severe than would have been expected based on the severity of the intestinal and systemic disease. Abortion may occur several months after resolution of disease because of fetal infection.

Colitis X
The clinical presentation with colitis X is more dramatic. Typical clinical signs include severe diarrhea, severe dehydration, marked toxemia, tachycardia, abdominal distension, abdominal pain, and depression. In some cases horses will be toxemic, depressed, and dehydrated, with severe abdominal distension but no evidence of diarrhea. These cases are difficult to distinguish from acute intestinal accidents such as large-colon volvulus. DIC may be present. Diarrhea, when present, can be watery or bloody.

Some affected horses will be found dead. The progression from normalcy to death can be very rapid, occurring within 6 hours in severe cases.

Differential diagnosis

Noninfectious causes of colitis such as right dorsal colitis and sand enteropathy should be considered. Intestinal accident is a differential diagnosis in severe cases. Cantharidin toxicosis and cyathostominosis should be considered depending on the geographic location, time of year, and clinical presentation. In foals, rotavirus and *Lawsonia intracellularis* infection should also be considered. Other toxic causes of colitis such as arsenic toxicosis are uncommon, but should be considered in some situations.

Diagnosis

General

Clinical signs and hematology are nonspecific and not diagnostic. Leukopenia, neutropenia, left-shift, and toxic changes in neutrophils are common. Leukocytosis and monocytosis may occur more commonly with PHF. Urinalysis should be performed, particularly if elevations in urea and creatinine levels are present. Total plasma protein levels should be evaluated. Monitoring of plasma electrolyte concentrations is useful to guide treatment. Tests for specific pathogens are described below. Coinfection can occur, so a broad range of testing is recommended.

Palpation per rectum and passage of a nasogastric tube should be performed in all animals with abdominal pain. Abdominocentesis may be useful to differentiate colitis from intestinal accident or peritonitis, or when there is a sudden deterioration in condition.

Salmonellosis

Fecal culture is the most common diagnostic tool. Because of intermittent shedding, a single negative culture cannot rule out salmonellosis and five negative samples are required. Rectal mucosal biopsy specimens can also be submitted for culture. This is perhaps more useful in cases with chronic colic or fever of unknown origin versus fulminant colitis. The utility of PCR testing of feces in unclear.

Clostridium difficile *infection*

Detection of *C. difficile* toxins in fecal samples is diagnostic for CDI. Fecal samples should be tested for the presence of both *C. difficile* toxins A and B. Fresh, refrigerated samples are preferred; however, *C. difficile* toxins are stable *in vitro*. 'Common antigen' testing is available, usually in combination with toxin A testing. The common antigen test also reacts with nontoxigenic strains and some nonpathogenic bacteria, therefore positive common antigen results in the absence of detectable toxins in feces should be interpreted with caution. Culture is usually reserved for epidemiological purposes.

Clostridium perfringens-*associated diarrhea*

Diagnosis of *C. perfringens*-associated diarrhea can be difficult because *C. perfringens* can be isolated from the feces of a large percentage of normal horses. No correlation between numbers of *C. perfringens* or bacterial spores in feces and diarrhea has been reported. Typing of bacterial isolates to determine what toxin genes they possess can be useful, but the relevance of identification of toxigenic strains in the absence of demonstrable toxin is unclear. Type C strains are uncommonly identified in normal animals and detection of these strains is highly suggestive of disease. Similarly, identification of genes coding for the production of beta-2 toxin and *C. perfringens* enterotoxin (CPE) is suggestive. The significance of identification of type A, the most common strain, in the absence of beta-2 toxin or CPE genes is debatable. Diagnosis is best if based on identification of toxins in fecal samples. Detection of CPE in feces is highly suggestive of disease. If rapid tests to detect other *C. perfringens* toxins become available, the ability to diagnose this condition will improve.

Potomac horse fever

A presumptive diagnosis is often made based on appropriate clinical signs during the appropriate time of year in an endemic area; however, this is not definitive, as other sporadic causes of diarrhea cannot be differentiated clinically. Response to empirical treatment with oxytetracycline is suggestive, but not diagnostic. Serologic testing is available. A four-fold change in antibody titer between acute and convalescent samples is supportive, but often does not occur. PCR testing is becoming more commonly available and appears to be more useful. Early in the disease, blood samples may be PCR positive and fecal samples PCR negative. This may be reversed later in the disease, so both blood and fecal samples should be submitted.

Colitis X

Colitis X is a clinical diagnosis that is used by some in cases of severe idiopathic colitis.

Antimicrobial-associated diarrhea

Diagnosis of antimicrobial-associated diarrhea is based on a temporal association of antimicrobial administration and onset of clinical signs. Specific pathogen testing should be performed.

Idiopathic colitis

Idiopathic colitis is a diagnosis of exclusion that is made when other known causes of enterocolitis have been ruled out.

Lower gastrointestinal tract

Management

Aggressive supportive therapy, particularly fluid therapy with large volumes of balanced electrolyte solution, is the most important component of treatment. Intravenous fluid therapy is required in all but the mildest of cases. Intravenous hypertonic saline (4–6 ml/kg of 5–7% NaCl) may be useful in severely dehydrated horses, but must be followed by isotonic fluids. Supplemental potassium or calcium may be required, and supplementation should be based on monitoring of blood electrolyte levels. Ionized calcium should be measured, if possible, because total calcium levels will decrease if the horse is hypoalbuminemic, while the metabolically active total calcium may be normal. Sodium bicarbonate may be required in severely acidotic animals; however, aggressive fluid therapy will correct the acid–base status in most cases. Total protein levels should be monitored because severe hypoproteinemia can develop.

Endotoxemia is very common, regardless of the etiology. Flunixin meglumine (0.25–0.3 mg/kg i/v q8h) is often used to attenuate the response to endotoxin. Analgesic doses of flunixin (1.1 mg/kg i/v) may be required, but they should be used judiciously, particularly in dehydrated horses. Polymyxin B (6,000 IU/kg i/v q12h) may be used to bind endotoxin.

Metronidazole (15 mg/kg p/o q8h) appears to be effective in the treatment of clostridial diarrhea and many cases of idiopathic colitis. Metronidazole-resistant strains of *C. difficile* are rare, but have been reported. The use of broad-spectrum antimicrobial therapy is controversial. Parenteral antimicrobial therapy is mainly indicated to protect against bacterial translocation and is not necessary in most cases. Antimicrobial therapy (e.g. sodium penicillin/aminoglycoside) is often indicated in neonates and immunocompromised individuals. Parenteral antimicrobial administration in salmonellosis is directed at prevention and treatment of extraintestinal infection. Concerns about the use of antimicrobials include prolonging shedding of *Salmonella* (if present), development of antimicrobial resistance, and further disruption of the intestinal microflora.

Oxytetracycline (6.6 mg/kg slowly i/v q12h for 3–5 days) is indicated in cases of diagnosed or highly suspicious PHF. Typically, a response is noted within 12 hours. Abatement of fever is usually the first sign of improvement, followed by improvement in attitude and appetite. If response is not noted within 24–48 hours, the diagnosis should be reconsidered. Oxytetracycline should be used judiciously because of the potential for antimicrobial-associated colitis.

Di-tri-octahedral smectite (1.5 kg/adult horse p/o, followed by 450 g p/o q6–8h) may be useful as an adsorbent. Probiotics are widely used; however, there is no evidence of efficacy at this time.

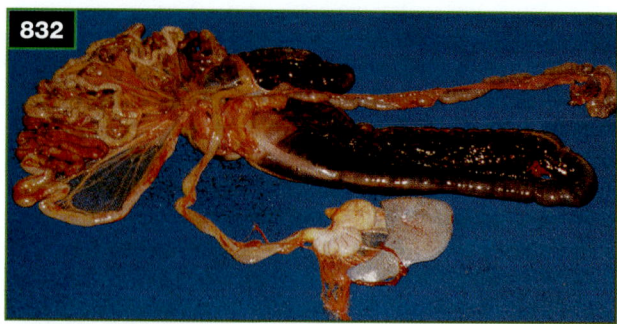

832 Infarction of the large colon in a 6-month-old foal with colitis secondary to DIC.

Whenever diarrhea occurs during antimicrobial therapy, antimicrobial administration should be discontinued if possible. If this is not possible, changing to a different drug (or combination of drugs) may be useful.

Horses that are not displaying signs of abdominal pain should be fed grass hay *ad libidum*. Small volumes of concentrates may be gradually introduced to horses that require additional caloric intake. Most horses with moderate to severe colitis will lose significant body condition, regardless of dietary intake. Parenteral nutrition may be required in cases where feeding is withheld for more than a few days.

Affected horses require intense monitoring to detect changes in clinical condition and development of complications. Laminitis, the most severe complication, is addressed elsewhere (see p. 69).

All horses with colitis should be assumed to be infectious until proven otherwise. Salmonellosis is transmissible to horses and is zoonotic. *C. difficile* can be transmitted between horses and may also be a zoonotic disease. The risk of transmission of *C. perfringens* is probably lower, but precautions should still be taken. PHF is not transmissible by horses. Idiopathic cases should be treated as infectious.

In all cases where a transmissible disease is considered possible, precautions should be taken to decrease the risk of transmission to other horses and to humans. Ideally, affected horses should be completely isolated from other animals. If this is not feasible, they should be separated as much as possible from other horses, particularly neonates. Barrier precautions, including overboots, gloves, and either disposable gowns or dedicated coveralls, should be used. Medical instruments (e.g. thermometers, nasogastric tubes) and other items (buckets, shovels, wheelbarrows) should be used only for affected horses or completely disinfected after each use. The area outside the stall should be cordoned off and disinfected frequently. Horses with colitis should not be allowed on common pasture.

Prognosis

The prognosis is variable and should be considered guarded in horses with severe, acute colitis. Death can occur as a result of severe toxemia, necrotizing enterocolitis, intestinal rupture, intestinal infarction from DIC, laminitis, or, in some cases, because of the high cost of treatment. Infarction of intestinal blood vessels, likely as a result of severe toxemia and DIC, can account for sudden deterioration (832).

Laminitis and catheter-site complications may occur in up to 25% of severe cases. If a horse recovers, long-term GI complications are uncommon; however, it may take weeks to months to return to normal body condition.

With salmonellosis, horses that recover may shed *Salmonella* for weeks to months following resolution of clinical signs. Five negative fecal cultures should be obtained before the horse is considered to no longer be infectious.

Vaccines for the prevention of *C. perfringens*-associated disease are available for ruminants. While there are anecdotal reports of administering these products to horses, particularly to mares for the prevention of neonatal diarrhea, this is not recommended because of limited evidence of efficacy and an apparent high incidence of adverse vaccine reactions.

Judicious use of antimicrobials, particularly those that tend to be associated with a higher incidence of diarrhea, is important. Antimicrobials that have not been shown to be safe in horses should be avoided.

In general, the prognosis for PHF is good if diagnosed early and appropriate therapy is started. The prognosis is worse if laminitis develops.

Sand enteropathy

Definition/overview

Sand enteropathy is an uncommon but regionally important cause of diarrhea.

Etiology/pathophysiology

Accumulation of sand in the large colon is usually associated with sand impaction; however, sand enteropathy can also result. Sand may be ingested while grazing on sandy soil or from ingestion of sand in sandy paddocks, arenas, or stalls. Horses that are underfed or kept in overstocked, closely grazed pastures may be at greater risk. Sand enteropathy is more common in areas with loose sandy soil.

It is believed that sand accumulation can result in chronic irritation of the colonic mucosa. This may result in reduction of the absorptive surface area and interference with normal intestinal motility, resulting in diarrhea. Diverticulum formation can also occur.

Clinical presentation

Diarrhea is the main presenting sign. Diarrhea may be acute or chronic. Diarrhea is usually mild and not associated with severe dehydration, toxemia, or cardiovascular compromise. Pyrexia, anorexia, weight loss, and intermittent colic may be present. 'Sand sounds' may be heard over the ventral abdomen, but they are more common with sand impaction. Colonic rupture secondary to severe inflammation and irritation is rare, but will result in the development of septic peritonitis.

Differential diagnosis

Infectious causes of colitis, including *Salmonella, C. difficile, C. perfringens*, and *N. risticii* (PHF), should be considered.

Diagnosis

Identification of large quantities of sand in feces is suggestive. Fecal sand content can be evaluated by letting a suspension of feces and water settle out in a rectal sleeve. Sedimentation of >6 mm of sand from a volume of feces of a few fecal balls is considered excessive (833). Palpation per rectum is unremarkable unless there is a concurrent sand impaction. Sand accumulation may be evident radiographically, particularly in the cranioventral abdomen. Hematology should be unremarkable, apart from changes consistent with the degree of dehydration. Total protein levels do not tend to decrease as is usually observed with enterocolitis. Peritoneal fluid is usually unremarkable unless marked colonic inflammation is present, which may result in a mild increase in total protein.

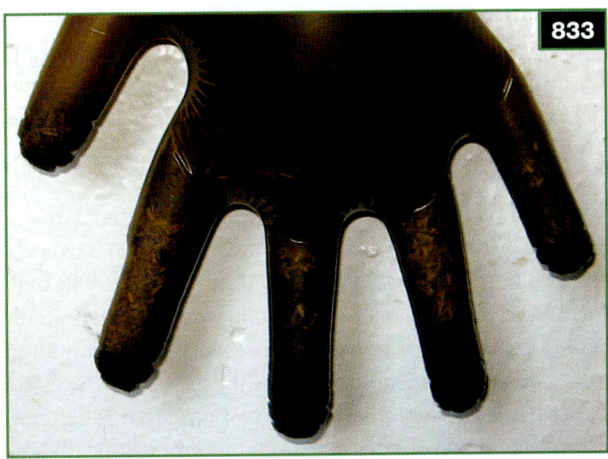

833 Fecal sand evaluation. Note the coarse sand present in the fingers indicating excessive fecal sand content. (Photo courtesy M Anderson)

Management

Oral fluid therapy may be useful in mild cases; however, considering that intestinal absorption may be impaired, intravenous fluid therapy is more effective and should be used if dehydration is clinically apparent. Analgesics should be administered as needed. The efficacy of bulk laxatives is somewhat controversial, but psyllium (0.25–0.5 kg/500 kg in 4–8 liters of water via a nasogastric tube q6–24h) is frequently used. Following resolution of clinical signs, it is prudent to continue to administer psyllium (0.25–0.5 kg/500kg) mixed with feed for 14 days and repeat the sand sedimentation test. Periodic evaluation (every 1–6 months) via a sand sedimentation test or abdominal radiography should be considered, particularly if management changes are not feasible.

Intermittent administration of psyllium may help reduce sand accumulation. Administration of 0.25 kg of psyllium/500 kg once daily for 7 days, performed monthly, has been recommended. A discussion of management practices is important.

Prognosis

Overall, the prognosis is good; however, development of peritonitis will worsen the prognosis. In a small proportion of cases, severe colon irritation may result in chronic diarrhea and ill-thrift. Management changes may be required to prevent further cases.

Right dorsal colitis

Definition/overview

Right dorsal colitis is an uncommon syndrome characterized by ulcerative inflammation of the right dorsal colon.

Etiology/pathophysiology

Chronic or excessive administration of NSAIDs is the most common risk factor; however, a history of NSAID use is not always present. Concurrent dehydration or hypotension increases the risk. Phenylbutazone use is most commonly reported, but it is unclear whether this drug is of higher risk or whether it is used more often. Performance horses are most commonly affected because of the heavy use of NSAIDs in this group.

NSAID administration results in decreased prostaglandin levels and prostaglandins are involved in local protection in the colon. With NSAID use, particularly at high levels and for prolonged periods of time, or with concurrent dehydration or hypotension, mucosal inflammation and ulceration may develop if local protective effects are overwhelmed. The inflammatory response that is generated further damages the intestinal mucosa. Clinical signs can result from intestinal inflammation, damage to the mucosal barrier with subsequent absorption of bacterial toxins, and exudation of plasma proteins.

Clinical presentation

Two general syndromes are observed. In the acute form, colic is the predominant clinical sign and is often accompanied by fever, depression, lethargy, and signs of endotoxemia. Diarrhea may also be present. In the chronic form, weakness, weight loss, depression, lethargy, intermittent colic, and peripheral edema may be observed. Diarrhea is less common.

Differential diagnosis

For the acute form, salmonellosis, clostridial enteritis, PHF, peritonitis, intestinal accident, and sand enteropathy are the main differential diagnoses. For the chronic form, inflammatory bowel disease, intestinal neoplasia, cyathostominosis, protein losing nephropathy, and *Lawsonia intracellularis* infection (weanlings) should be considered.

Diagnosis

Right dorsal colitis can only be definitively diagnosed via surgical biopsies or necropsy. Clinically, right dorsal colitis is a presumptive diagnosis. A complete blood cell count and serum biochemical profile should be submitted, with hypoproteinemia being the main abnormality. A thickened right dorsal colon may be observed ultrasonographically; however, this may be difficult to identify. Urinalysis should be performed to rule out renal protein loss. Abdominocentesis should be performed to identify other causes of disease. Gastroscopy may be useful because concurrent, NSAID-associated gastric ulceration might be present. A presumptive diagnosis is usually made in horses with appropriate clinical signs, severe hypoproteinemia, exclusion of other causes, and a history of NSAID administration.

Management

NSAID administration should be ceased if possible. If analgesia is required, alternative options such as transdermal fentanyl, epidural opioids, or parenteral opioids should be considered.

In horses with acute disease, intravenous fluid therapy with a balanced electrolyte solution is often required. Aggressive fluid therapy should be avoided if possible, particularly in hypoproteinemic animals. With chronic disease, fluid therapy is usually not indicated.

In horses with acute or chronic disease, transfusion of plasma or synthetic colloids is required in severely hypoproteinemic animals. Sucralfate (20–40 mg/kg p/o q6h) may be useful, although it is unclear whether significant drug levels are achieved in the right dorsal colon. Administration of the synthetic prostaglandin misoprostol (2 µg/kg p/o q6h) has been used; however, its effect is not known and adverse effects can be encountered.

Long-stem roughage (hay) should be withheld and a complete pelleted diet should be fed until resolution of all clinical and hematologic abnormalities. Pasture should be avoided. Affected horses should be fed small meals frequently. If body weight cannot be maintained, dietary fat should be increased via addition of a high-fat concentrate diet or supplementation with corn oil (250 ml q12h). It has been suggested that addition of psyllium (50–100g/500kg/day, divided into 1–4 doses) could be useful because it is hydrolyzed to short-chain fatty acids, which are an important energy source for colonic enterocytes.

Prognosis
Overall, the prognosis is guarded, although in some cases cessation of NSAID therapy and basic supportive care is all that is required. The prognosis for return to normality is better in horses with acute disease and when NSAID cessation is possible. The prognosis is poor in horses with severe, chronic hypoproteinemia. Serial monitoring of blood albumin levels, with gradual but steady elevation in albumin, is a good prognostic indicator. Full recovery may take months. Laminitis is a possible complication, particularly in acute cases.

Cyathostominosis
Definition/overview
Small strongyles (cyathostomes) are important GI parasites worldwide. Small-strongyle infection can cause a range of signs including inapparent infection, ill-thrift, and severe protein-losing enteropathy and diarrhea (larval cyathostominosis). In some areas (e.g. the UK), larval cyathostominosis is considered to be the most common cause of diarrhea in adult horses.

Etiology/pathophysiology
The small-strongyle group consists of approximately 50 different species. There are some differences in prevalence, pathogenicity, and life cycle between some of these species; however, speciation is rarely performed. Multiple species are often present.

Younger horses are more likely to be infected with large numbers of small strongyles, and may be more likely to develop clinical disease with lower numbers compared with adults. High stock density, inappropriate deworming programs, poor manure management, and overgrazing of pastures are risk factors for small-strongyle infection.

Larval cyathostominosis is typically a seasonal problem and is more common during the late winter and spring in most temperate areas, but in some areas cases are more common in late fall and winter. Horses 1–3 years of age are

most commonly affected. Recent anthelmintic treatment is also a risk factor. Anthelmintic treatment may trigger disease by removing the negative feedback of adult worms in the intestinal lumen, thereby resulting in excysting of larvae.

Small-strongyle eggs are shed in feces and develop into infective L3 on pasture. After ingestion, the L3 enter the mucosa of the large colon and cecum, where they encyst. Encysted larvae may remain hypobiotic for up to 2 years. At any point, L3 can develop into L4, excyst, and migrate back to the intestinal lumen, where they mature into adults. The prepatent period varies with different strongyle species, and ranges from 5 to 18 weeks.

Encysted larvae may incite a granulomatous reaction; however, the main problem occurs during emergence of hypobiotic larvae. A marked inflammatory response can ensue, characterized by edema, ulceration, and protein exudation. Nutrient and fluid absorption and intestinal motility can be affected. This syndrome is termed 'larval cyathostominosis'.

Encysted larvae are more common in the cecum and ventral colon and represent the majority of small-strongyle burden, although this may vary with geographic region and time of year. The ventral colon is the main site for adult worms, followed by the dorsal colon and cecum.

Adult worms in the intestinal lumen may cause disease, but this is of lesser importance. Pinpoint mucosal ulceration may be produced and vague signs such as ill-thrift may be present. An increased risk of colic may also be present. An association with the development of cecocecal and cecocolic intussusceptions has been reported.

Clinical presentation
Infection with adult small strongyles may produce mild and vague signs, such as weight loss or ill-thrift, and may predispose to the development of colic. This may be seasonal, recurrent, or sporadic. Chronic weight loss and chronic diarrhea have also been reported.

The main concern is larval cyathostominosis. Affected horses may present with severe diarrhea, weight loss, depression, and peripheral edema. Diarrhea is not present in all cases, and weight loss, depression, and severe hypoproteinemia may be the only clinical abnormalities.

Differential diagnosis
Protein-losing enteropathy, acute infectious colitis of a variety of etiologies, and right dorsal colitis should be considered. Various differential diagnoses exist for the mild, general disease that may be caused by adult small strongyles.

TABLE 28 Anthelmintic treatment options for cyathostominosis

DRUG	DOSE	FREQUENCY	COMMENTS
Ivermectin	0.2 mg/kg p/o	Once	Effective against adults
Moxidectin	0.4 mg/kg p/o	Once	Effective against adults and encysted larvae
Fenbendazole	50 mg/kg p/o 10 mg/kg p/o	Once q24h for 5 days	Effective against adults; resistance is a concern
Oxfendazole	10 mg/kg p/o	Once	Effective against adults; resistance is a concern
Pyrantel tartrate	2.2 mg/kg p/o	Daily	Effective against ingested larvae; resistance is a concern

Diagnosis

Diagnosis of larval cyathostominosis is difficult. Fecal egg counts are often low when clinical disease is present, largely because disease is most common in the winter months. Furthermore, disease may be triggered by recent anthelmintic therapy, therefore eggs and adult worms would be less commonly present. Hematology is nonspecific and peripheral eosinophilia is uncommon, even in severe cases. Hypoalbuminemia is common and may be severe. The degree of hypoalbuminemia is often more severe than would be expected from the severity and duration of the diarrhea. Elevations in alpha-2 and beta-1 globulins have been reported. Late L4 larvae are occasionally evident on fecal smears or on rectal gloves following palpation. Thickening of the large colon wall may be evident ultrasonographically; however, all these findings are nonspecific for larval cyathostominosis. Diagnosis involves identification of large numbers of encysted and/or emerging larvae in the large colon. Encysted cyathostomes can sometimes be detected on rectal mucosal biopsy. Exploratory laparatomy can be diagnostic, but affected animals are often poor surgical candidates, particularly if severely hypoproteinemic. Antigen-specific serologic tests for identification of encysted larvae have been evaluated, but at the time of writing none are commercially available.

Definitive diagnosis is often achieved at necropsy, where edema and thickening of the intestinal wall are evident. Encysted cyathostomes may be evident grossly in the intestinal mucosa (**834,835**).

Management

There are two aspects of management: treatment of horses with overt enteric disease (diarrhea and/or hypoproteinemia), and reduction of parasite burdens.

Treatment of horses with diarrhea and/or hypoproteinemia is largely supportive in nature. Correction of fluid and electrolyte imbalances is important, and intravenous fluid therapy is often required. Plasma or synthetic colloids may be required in severely hypoproteinemic animals.

Different treatment regimens have been proposed to reduce the parasite burden. One includes administration of fenbendazole (10 mg/kg) on days 1–5, 16–20, and 31–35, with ivermectin on days 6, 21, and 36. Concurrent administration of anti-inflammatories may also be useful because of the inflammatory response associated with the emergence or death or larvae. Corticosteroids (e.g. prednisolone, 1 mg/kg p/o q24 h for 20 days then 1 mg/kg q48h for 20 days) may be useful. Some authors have recommended a shorter duration of prednisolone (3–7 days) or the use of NSAIDs (e.g. flunixin meglumine, 1.1 mg/kg i/v or p/o q12–24h). Others recommend a single course of fenbendazole (10 mg/kg p/o q24h for 5 days). Moxidectin (0.4 mg/kg p/o once) has good efficacy against encysted larvae; however, it may not be desirable to have a rapid, effective kill of encysted larvae in horses with a large burden (*Table 28*).

Because of the difficulty in diagnosing and managing cyathostominosis, routine control is critical. Few drugs are effective against encysted larvae. As for any intestinal parasite, optimal deworming programs vary between farms based on a variety of factors. The period of highest risk for infection should be considered when designing a deworming program. Horses are more likely to be exposed in spring and fall in temperate climates, and winter in subtropical climates. Annual or biannual deworming may suffice on farms with a reasonable stocking density and

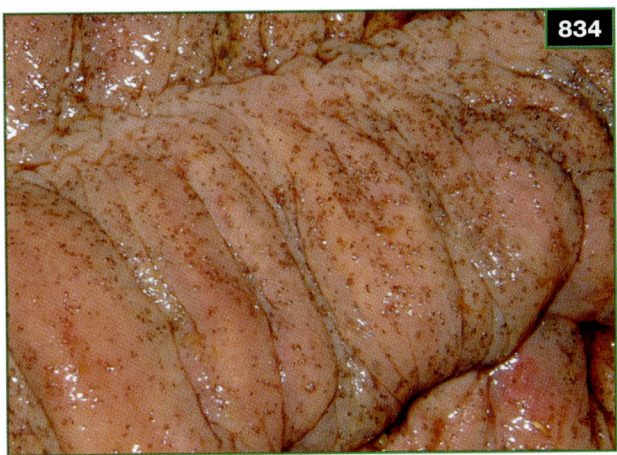

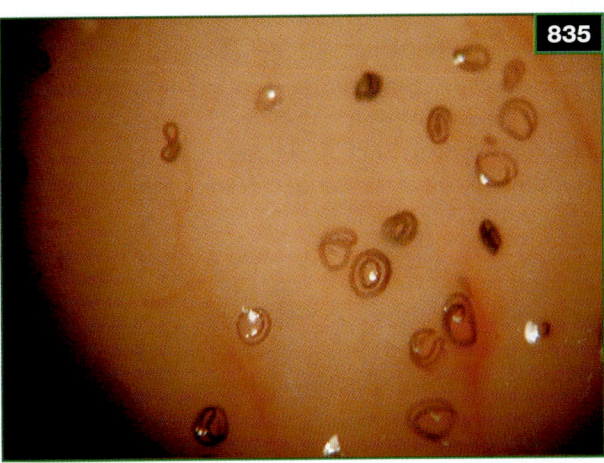

834 Mucosal surface of the large colon from a foal with severe cyathostominosis. Note the numerous small larvae in the mucosal wall.

835 Magnified view of cyathostome larvae in the intestinal wall.

good manure management. Other farms may require more frequent deworming. A targeted deworming program consisting of administration of ivermectin to adult horses with fecal egg counts of >200 epg and horses less than 2 years of age with >100 epg has been shown to be effective. With this method, fecal egg counts should be performed on all horses every few months. If sampling of all horses is not practical, a representative sample of 10% of horses (at least 10 horses in total) is a viable option. Ideally, fecal egg counts should also be performed approximately 14 days after treatment to assess response. Multiple-anthelmintic-resistant small strongyles are a serious concern.

Management factors such as stocking density, manure management, and pasture rotation need to be assessed. Ideally, manure should be removed from pastures twice weekly to prevent accumulation of infective larvae. Harrowing of pastures may also be effective in hot and dry weather as the infective larvae are susceptible to dessication. Ruminants are resistant to small strongyles, so pasture rotation with these species is useful if practical.

Prognosis
It has been reported that approximately 40% of horses with larval cyathostominosis will survive if given appropriate treatment. Some horses will die within 2–4 weeks of initial clinical signs; however, this is complicated by the difficulty in diagnosing cases. A prolonged recovery period may be required in some cases depending on the degree of mucosal damage. The prognosis is poorer if clinical signs have been present for more than 3 weeks.

Chronic diarrhea
Definition/overview
Chronic diarrhea is the continuous or intermittent passage of soft or watery feces for a prolonged period of time. Horses of all ages can be affected. It is a relatively common and often frustrating problem.

Etiology/pathophysiology
There are a variety of possible causes and most cases are idiopathic. Inflammatory, infectious, neoplastic, and nutritional causes are all possible.

The pathophysiology is variable, depending on the specific etiology. The net result is intermittent or continuous passage of soft feces because of a disruption of the normal fluid homeostasis mechanisms in the large colon. Small-intestinal disease may be present concurrently, but small-intestinal disease alone should not produce diarrhea in an adult horse.

Clinical presentation
Intermittent or continuous passage of soft feces is often the only clinical complaint. Other clinical abnormalities, including weight loss, ill-thrift, anorexia, peripheral edema, depression, and fever, may be present.

Differential diagnosis
A variety of infectious, inflammatory, neoplastic, and nutritional causes exist. Specific diseases are covered under their appropriate sections. Occasionally, non-intestinal diseases such as liver disease, Cushing's disease, and hyperlipidemia may cause chronic diarrhea.

573

Diagnosis

A thorough history should be obtained in order to characterize the changes in fecal consistency, in particular to try to make an association between diarrhea and certain management areas such as feeding, exercise, travel, or drug therapy. A variety of diagnostic tests can be performed to identify the etiology (*Table 29*).

Management

In the absence of a specific diagnosis, a variety of treatments can be tried. Diet change may be useful. Specific dietary recommendations cannot be made because of the variability in response. In general, a diet consisting of mainly, or exclusively, hay or pasture grass can be beneficial; however, some horses will respond to provision of a hay-free diet. Fenbendazole (10 mg/kg p/o q24h for 5 days) is often prescribed. Metronidazole (15 mg/kg p/o q8h for 5 days) is also often used. Probiotics are widely used, but no beneficial effect has yet been demonstrated. Yogurt is unlikely to be effective because it contains low viable bacteria numbers and does not contain organisms with any known benefit in horses. Treatment for sand enteropathy may be attempted in certain areas. Corticosteroids such as dexamethasone (40 mg/450 kg i/m q4d for 28 days, then tapering) or prednisolone (1 mg/kg p/o q12–24h, for 2 weeks, then tapering) are often used after other treatments have failed. Administration of psyllium (0.25–0.5 kg/500 kg via nasogastric tube q6–24h, accompanied by 4–8 liters of water) may be useful in some cases.

Prognosis

In general, the prognosis is poor if diarrhea is accompanied by other clinical abnormalities such as weight loss or hypoproteinemia. If diarrhea is the only complaint, then the prognosis for survival and normal function is often good, despite the fact that diarrhea may persist.

TABLE 29 Diagnostic options for chronic diarrhea

- Hematology
  - Complete blood cell count
  - Serum biochemical profile
  - Plasma fibrinogen
- Fecal analysis
  - *Salmonella* culture
  - *Clostridium difficile* toxin A/B ELISA
  - *Clostridium perfringens* enterotoxin ELISA
  - Fecal float and smear
  - Fecal sand analysis
- Abdominocentesis
- Abdominal ultrasonographic examination
- Rectal mucosal biopsy
  - Culture
  - Histology
- Exploratory laparotomy/laparoscopy with biopsies
- Carbohydrate absorption tests

Colonic tympany (gas colic)

Definition/overview

Intestinal tympany, also known as gas colic, is a common cause of colic.

Etiology/pathophysiology

A variety of risk factors have been suggested including diet change, feeding of highly fermentable substrates (grain, lush grass, wilted grass), rapid eating, electrolyte abnormalities, and dental abnormalities.

Excessive production of intestinal gas and/or alterations in colonic motility may result in colonic tympany if the rate of gas production exceeds the rate of elimination. As the intestine distends with gas, signs of pain may develop. Colonic tympany that develops secondary to obstructive lesions is covered under the specific obstruction. Cecal tympany is often present concurrently.

Clinical presentation

Signs of abdominal pain (rolling, pawing, flank-watching, stretching, recumbency, anorexia) will vary with the degree of abdominal distension. Pain can range from mild and intermittent to continuous and severe. Heart rate is usually elevated consistent with the degree of pain. Gross abdominal distension may be present. Distension is usually bilateral (as opposed to cecal tympany) and marked distension may result in tachypnea via pressure on the diaphragm. Mucous membranes are usually normal unless severe distension is present. Borborygmi may be normal, increased, or decreased. High-pitched tympanic sounds may be heard during simultaneous auscultation and percussion of the abdomen.

Differential diagnosis

A variety of signs of colic must be considered, particularly spasmodic colic, large-colon impaction, and large-colon displacement.

Diagnosis

The most important factor in the diagnosis of colonic tympany is ruling out the presence of surgical disorders such as large-colon volvulus or displacement. Distension of the large colon may be palpable per rectum. A thorough examination is required to try to identify a lesion that may be the cause of the distension. A nasogastric tube must be passed. Gaseous distension of the stomach may be present concurrently. Ultrasonographic examination of the abdomen is unremarkable. Peritoneal fluid analysis and hematology should be unremarkable.

Management

Analgesic administration is usually required. Aggressive analgesic administration should be avoided so that progression of signs, particularly any associated with a surgical lesion, is not missed. Drugs affecting intestinal motility should be used judiciously and only when required. Mineral oil (4 liters via nasogastric tube) may coat fermentable substrates, but its efficacy is unclear. Feed should be withheld. Frequent walking may be useful to simulate intestinal motility. Short periods of more intense exercise such as trotting on a lunge line may also be useful, particularly in more severe cases.

In horses with severe abdominal distension also involving the cecum, cecal trocarization may be required (see Cecal tympany, p. 562). With severe, uncontrollable pain, severe abdominal distension, or progression of clinical signs, surgical intervention may be required to decompress the intestine and rule out the presence of a concurrent surgical lesion.

Prognosis

Most cases respond well to conservative therapy. If the clinical condition deteriorates or there is a poor response to treatment, the horse should be re-evaluated to ensure that another problem is not present. It is possible that large-colon displacement or volvulus could occur secondary to gaseous distension of the large colon. Management should be reviewed to identify and address any risk factors that might be present.

Colonic volvulus

Definition/overview

Large-colon volvulus is a relatively common cause of severe, life-threatening colic. Both nonstrangulated and strangulated volvulus may occur, with the latter being more frequent. Strangulated large-colon volvulus rapidly induces hypovolemic and endotoxemic shock and affected horses require emergency surgical treatment. The prognosis for survival for horses with strangulated large-colon volvulus is guarded to poor.

Etiology/pathophysiology

The precise cause of large-colon volvulus in horses is not currently known, but broodmares just before or after parturition appear to be at increased risk for this condition. Changes in digestion and/or visceral positioning during pregnancy may predispose mares to large-colon volvulus. The condition is not restricted to broodmares and any changes in large-colon motility may predispose horses to the development of large-colon volvulus.

The equine large colon has only two fixed attachment points: the cecocolic ligament and the transverse colon. In most cases of large-colon volvulus, the right ventral colon displaces dorsomedially when viewed from behind (clockwise rotation). The pathophysiology of large colon volvulus depends on the degree of rotation of the colon. If the rotation is <270 degrees, the blood supply to the large colon is usually not compromised and only the colonic lumen is obstructed. Such large-colon rotations result in obstruction of normal passage of gas and ingesta. If the rotation is >270 degrees, the lumen of the large colon is obstructed and the blood supply (venous or arterial and venous) is compromised, resulting in a strangulating lesion. In most cases, venous occlusion and hemorrhagic strangulating obstruction occur. This results in sequestration of blood in the strangulated portions of the colon and ischemic lesions of the mucosa. The latter dies off within a few hours of ischemia and intraluminal leakage of plasmatic fluids and absorption of endotoxin occur. Affected horses rapidly develop both hypovolemic and endotoxemic shock.

Clinical presentation

Clinical signs of colonic volvulus vary with the degree of colonic rotation. Horses with nonstrangulated large-colon volvulus (rotation <270 degrees) display clinical signs similar to those associated with large-colon impaction or nonstrangulating displacements. Horses with strangulated large-colon volvulus experience peracute colic and severe, intractable abdominal pain as the most common clinical findings. Moderate to severe abdominal distension causing respiratory compromise is also frequently observed. Signs of toxemia and cardiovascular compromise may be present and can be severe.

575

Differential diagnosis

Differential diagnoses for nonstrangulated large-colon volvulus include large-colon impaction and large-colon displacement such as right and left dorsal displacement. Strangulated large-colon volvulus is probably the condition that induces the most acute and violent signs of colic in horses. The only other conditions that can induce such signs are incarcerated internal hernia (diaphragmatic hernia, epiploic foramen entrapment, incarceration in the gastrosplenic ligament, and strangulated inguinal hernia).

Diagnosis

A history of imminent or recent parturition or previous management changes is typical of horses with large-colon volvulus. Severe colic associated with abdominal distension that is nonresponsive to analgesics is characteristic of strangulated large-colon volvulus. On rectal palpation, large-colon distension with tight teniae can be identified. In horses with strangulated volvulus, edema of the large-colon wall, reflecting compromised venous blood return, is occasionally palpable.

Management

Rarely, nonstrangulated volvulus responds to conservative medical treatment; however, most horses require surgical treatment. Strangulated volvulus is a surgical emergency. Correction of equine large-colon volvulus is performed through a midline celiotomy. The large colon is identified and exteriorized. A pelvic flexure enterotomy is performed to evacuate the accumulated gas and digesta. The volvulus is then corrected. Large-colon resection is indicated if the strangulated tissues appear devitalized.

Large-colon volvulus recurrence is only about 5% in nonbreeding mares and males, but broodmares are at a higher risk. After one episode, a broodmare has a 15% chance of developing a second large-colon volvulus. After two episodes, the risk is increased to 80%. Colopexy or large-colon resection is indicated to prevent recurrence in broodmares after two episodes of large-colon volvulus.

Prognosis

The prognosis for nonstrangulated large-colon volvulus is guarded to good, whereas strangulated volvulus is associated with fatality rates of approximately 70%. The time from development of volvulus to surgical intervention is critical.

Strongyloides westeri infection

Definition/overview

Strongyloides westeri, also known as 'threadworm', is a common parasite in foals, but is usually of minimal clinical significance.

Etiology/pathophysiology

Strongyloides are unique in that they are capable of both a parasitic and a free-living reproductive cycle. Only female worms are involved in the parasitic cycle, living in the small intestine and producing eggs via parthenogenesis. After hatching, larvae usually mature into free-living adult worms. Under certain conditions the L3 can be infective and infect horses via skin penetration or ingestion, followed by development of adult worms in the small intestine. Foals may also be infected from larvae present in the tissues of mares. These larvae mobilize from arrested states in tissues of the abdominal wall and are subsequently excreted in milk. This route of infection is believed to account for the uncommon cases of clinical *S. westeri* infection in young foals. Infections tend to peak within 4–6 weeks of age and are eliminated naturally by 20–25 weeks.

Clinical presentation

Infection is usually inapparent. Disease is characterized by acute diarrhea in foals in the first few weeks of life.

Differential diagnosis

Other causes of neonatal diarrhea including foal heat diarrhea, clostridial diarrhea, salmonellosis, and rotavirus should be considered.

Diagnosis

Eggs may be evident on fecal flotation. Fresh feces should be used to avoid confusion with larvated strongyle-type eggs. Identification of eggs in feces is not diagnostic by itself because high fecal egg counts can be present in healthy foals.

Management

Specific treatment is rarely indicated because *S. westeri* is rarely a cause of disease. Transmission of *S. westeri* from mares to foals can be markedly reduced by treatment of mares with ivermectin (0.2 mg/kg p/o) within 24 hours of parturition. Treatment of foals with ivermectin at 1–2 weeks of age can hasten the elimination of *S. westeri*.

Prognosis

Excellent.

Large-strongyle infestation

Definition/overview

Large strongyles are of significant importance in areas where routine deworming is not performed. Prior to the widespread availability of ivermectin, large strongyles were a common cause of severe colic.

Etiology/pathophysiology

Strongylus vulgaris, *S. edentatus*, and *S. equinus* may be involved; however, *S. vulgaris* is of the greatest clinical importance.

Adult strongyles live in the large intestine and cecum. They are reddish, thick, and up to 4 cm in length. Eggs are passed in the feces and infective L3 develop in the environment. Following ingestion, *S. vulgaris* L3 penetrate the intestinal mucosa and molt to L4 in the submucosa. They then invade small arteries and arterioles and migrate to the cranial mesenteric artery and its main branches. After several months, they molt and L5 migrate to the intestinal wall. Nodules form around them and subsequently rupture into the intestinal lumen, releasing young adults. Inflammation of the cranial mesenteric arteries can develop in response to the larvae. Thrombosis can cause ischemia in areas of the intestinal tract. Thromboemboli may also develop and cause ischemic necrosis of other areas of the intestinal tract. Intestinal aneurysms are less common.

After ingestion, *S. edentatus* penetrates the intestinal mucosa and reaches the liver via the portal circulation. Further migration in the liver occurs, then larvae travel under the peritoneum and eventually reach the intestinal lumen.

The migratory route of *S. equinus* is less well understood. L4 larvae form in the intestinal wall, enter the peritoneal cavity, migrate into the liver, then molt in the pancreas and return to the large intestine.

Strongyle migration has also been suggested to be the cause of hemomelasma ilei, a typically benign condition (836).

Clinical presentation

Few clinical signs are produced by the presence of adult worms in the GI tract. Mild diarrhea, ill-thrift, and anemia are possible with chronic, severe burdens. Migration of *S. edentatus* and *S. equinus* larvae can produce hemorrhagic tracts in the liver and nodule formation in the gut wall or peritoneum, but clinical signs are rare. Pancreatitis has been reported, but is rare or rarely identified.

Intestinal infarction is more serious. Clinical presentation varies, depending on the degree of intestinal ischemia, duration of disease, and location of the lesion. Pain may be mild to severe. Heart rate will be elevated and can exceed 100 bpm. Respiratory rate may also be elevated. Horses may sweat profusely and appear anxious. Mucous membranes may be congested and hyperemic, with a prolonged CRT if significant intestinal ischemia or septic peritonitis is present. Borborygmi are decreased to absent.

Differential diagnosis

Strangulating intestinal infarction, severe enterocolitis, and peritonitis are the main differential diagnoses. Other clinical syndromes are uncommon and vague.

Diagnosis

Eggs are usually readily identifiable on a fecal flotation test. Large-strongyle eggs cannot be differentiated from small-strongyle eggs, therefore they are generally classified as 'strongyle-type' eggs. Absence of identifiable eggs does not rule out infection.

It is virtually impossible definitively to identify a nonstrangulating infarction without surgery or necropsy. Diagnostic findings may be suggestive of infarcted colon; however, differentiation between a strangulating and nonstrangulating etiology is not possible. Definitive diagnosis is made at surgery.

Management

Large strongyles are generally susceptible to ivermectin (0.2 mg/kg p/o), moxidectin (0.4 mg/kg p/o), or fenbendazole (10 mg/kg p/o q24h for 5 days, or 60 mg/kg single dose). Resistance to pyrantel has been reported. Pasture management, including provision of adequate stocking density, routine (twice weekly) removal of feces, and pasture rotation, is important.

If intestinal infarction is present, prompt surgical intervention is required. The affected area of intestine must be resected. Often, resection of the entire affected intestine is not possible and euthanasia is required.

Prognosis

The prognosis is excellent unless intestinal infarction is present, in which case the prognosis is guarded with surgical intervention and hopeless if surgery is not an option.

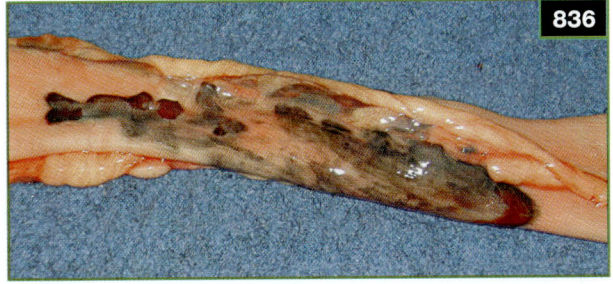

836 Characteristic appearance of hemomelasma ilei, a benign condition.

Lower gastrointestinal tract

Displacement of the large colon

Definition/overview

Movement of the large colon is only restricted by its attachment to the cecum and transverse colon, and it is therefore relatively mobile. A variety of displacements of the large colon can occur and result in abdominal distension and pain.

Etiology/pathophysiology

The etiology is unknown and likely variable. Reported risk factors for displacements include advancing age (>7 years), large size, foaling, and diet changes. Presumably, anything that results in excessive production or accumulation of gas within the large colon could predispose to development of a displacement. Two common displacements are nephrosplenic entrapment (left dorsal displacement) and right dorsal displacement.

It is presumed that gaseous distension is the inciting cause for most displacements. Often, a mild to moderate large-colon impaction is present and is presumably associated with the development of gaseous distension. Right dorsal displacements can occur in two directions: clockwise and counterclockwise. Clockwise displacements are more common and occur when the pelvic flexure is displaced between the cecum and body wall in a cranial-to-caudal direction. Counterclockwise displacements occur when the pelvic flexure travels in a caudal-to-cranial direction. Once the colon is displaced, the normal flow of ingesta and/or gas may be restricted, resulting in abdominal distension and pain. The vascular supply to the colon is minimally affected.

Clinical presentation

Clinically, signs of mild to severe abdominal pain may be evident, depending on the degree of abdominal distension. Presentation may be acute or chronic. Moderate to severe abdominal tympany may be present. Pain can be continuous or intermittent. Heart rate will be elevated according to the degree of pain. Signs of toxemia or cardiovascular compromise should not be evident. Occasionally, horses with a nephrosplenic entrapment may appear to be in pain, yet the heart rate may not be correspondingly elevated, presumably because of vagal effects.

Differential diagnosis

Any condition causing colic, particularly with gaseous distension of the large colon, should be considered.

Diagnosis

Displacements may be difficult to diagnose at times and may be difficult to differentiate from large-colon impaction or volvulus. Displacement should be suspected when there is progressive gaseous distension with a large-colon impaction.

Palpation per rectum is useful for a presumptive diagnosis of right dorsal displacement. Typically, distended colon is palpable on the right side of the abdomen and the cecum is not palpable. The colon may be palpable between the cecum and body wall. A large-colon impaction may be palpable concurrently.

Diagnosis of a nephrosplenic entrapment can be difficult at times. The nephrosplenic space can be difficult to palpate in large horses. Sometimes, a nephrosplenic entrapment can be suspected based on medial displacement of the spleen. It is not unusual to detect loops of small colon in the nephrosplenic space. These are typically incidental and must be differentiated from tightly entrapped large colon.

Transabdominal ultrasonographic examination can be useful to rule out a nephrospenic entrapment. If the left kidney and spleen can be visualized in direct apposition, then an entrapment is very unlikely. Conversely, identification of a gas-filled viscus obliterating visualization of the dorsal border of the spleen suggests the presence of a nephrosplenic entrapment. An inability to visualize the left kidney is not, in itself, diagnostic. If the displaced colon is not gas filled, a displacement may not be identified ultrasonographically.

Nasogastric reflux is rarely present with displacement of the large colon. Abdominocentesis can be a useful technique when deciding whether surgical intervention is required. Peritoneal fluid analysis is usually normal in an uncomplicated displacement.

Management

Often, medical therapy will be successful. Feed should be withheld. Fluid therapy is useful for softening an impaction, if present, and to stimulate intestinal motility. Intravenous fluid therapy is preferred, but oral therapy (up to 8–10 liters q30min) can be useful in milder cases. It is not unusual for horses to experience more pain after fluid therapy has been initiated as a result of increased colonic distension. Analgesics should be provided as required, but excessive analgesia should be avoided.

If the clinical condition deteriorates, the horse should be re-examined frequently to ensure that a more severe intestinal accident such as a large-colon volvulus has not developed. In some cases, horses will have severe, progressive abdominal distension and intractable pain. Surgical intervention is indicated in these cases.

It is unlikely that a displacement will correct spontaneously if marked tympany is present. If surgery is not an option in such cases, trocarization of the abdomen may temporarily relieve intestinal tympany.

Feed should be withheld until the displacement resolves. Occasionally, horses will improve clinically, gaseous distension will abate, an impaction (if present) will resolve, yet the colon will remain displaced after a few days of medical therapy. Very conservative feeding might be beneficial to stimulate intestinal motility and resolve the displacement. Sometimes, however, surgical correction will be required.

Left dorsal displacement of the colon lateral to the spleen but without entrapment in the nephrosplenic space will often correct with conservative therapy. If nephrosplenic entrapment is present, specific measures can be taken. Administration of phenylephrine (3–5 µg/kg/minute for 15 minutes), followed by 15–20 minutes of lunging or jogging is sometimes effective at correcting the displacement. Phenylephrine causes splenic contraction, making it easier for the entrapped colon to return to its normal position. The effects of phenylephrine are short term and administration can be repeated. Rolling under general anesthesia is another treatment option. The affected horse should be anesthetized, placed in right lateral recumbency, rolled into dorsal recumbency, and the hindquarters elevated. The horse should then be rocked from side-to-side for 5 minutes, dropped into left lateral recumbency and then sternal recumbency, at which point palpation should be repeated. Rolling can be repeated numerous times. Phenylephrine can be administered following induction of anesthesia as described above. Rolling can be successful in >50% of cases; however, the success rate is likely to be lower in horses with marked gaseous distension. Surgery may be required in severely painful cases, those that do not respond to medical treatment, or cases in which rolling has been attempted but has been unsuccessful. Midline celiotomy is most commonly performed; however, a standing left flank approach has been used successfully. While less expensive and associated with a shorter recovery period, the standing approach is limited by the fact that the surgeon is not able fully to explore the abdomen or correct any other abnormality that may be present, such as a large-colon impaction.

Prognosis
Overall, the prognosis is very good, with the vast majority of cases responding to medical treatment. While uncommon, some horses will develop repeated displacements. Techniques such as colopexy or large-colon resection should be considered in horses that develop recurrent displacements requiring surgical correction. Dietary and management changes should be attempted prior to colopexy or large-colon resection.

Large-colon impaction
Definition/overview
Impaction of the large colon with ingesta is a common cause of colic.

Etiology/pathophysiology
Large-colon impactions occur from accumulation of dehydrated and densely packed ingesta, often at a site where the large colon narrows, such as the pelvic flexure or right dorsal colon (837). The most common site is the pelvic flexure.

Factors affecting hydration of the colonic contents and intestinal motility may predispose to the development of impactions. These include dental abnormalities, ingestion of highly fibrous grass or hay, poor diet, decreased water intake (restricted access, excessively cold water, change in water source), management changes, transportation, sudden exercise restriction, pain, and gastric ulcers. Many cases occur in the absence of these factors. As firm ingesta accumulates in the affected area, colonic distension from ingesta and altered movement of intestinal gas cause variable signs of pain.

Clinical presentation
Nonspecific signs of abdominal pain, including anorexia, flank-watching, pawing, rolling, tail-swishing, straining to defecate, and sweating, are commonly observed. Intermittent pain over a few days may be reported. Pain can range from mild and intermittent to severe and continuous. Heart rate will be correspondingly elevated. Borborygmi are often decreased. Signs of systemic compromise or toxemia should not be evident. Intestinal tympany may be present. Sometimes, a decrease in fecal production or passage of firm, dry feces is reported. Feces may be covered in mucus, indicating delayed intestinal transit. Dehydration may be present, depending on the duration of signs.

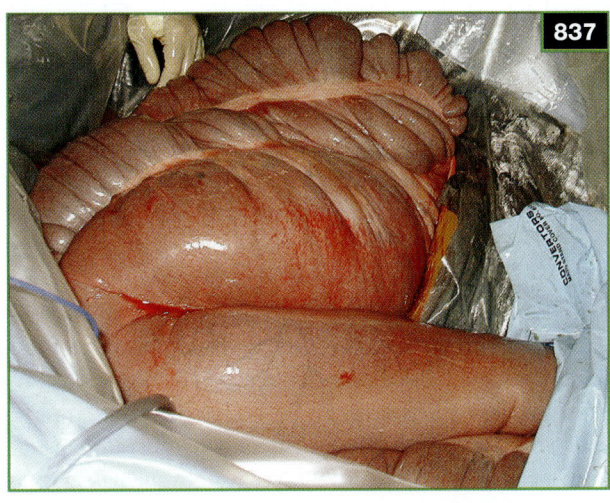

837 Severe impaction of the right dorsal colon that required surgical intervention.

Differential diagnosis

Other causes of mild to moderate colic without intestinal compromise should be considered. These include spasmodic colic, intestinal tympany, sand impaction, enteroliths, and large-colon displacement. Extraintestinal diseases such as laminitis, pleuritis, peritonitis, exertional rhabdomyolysis, urinary obstruction, and reproductive tract lesions should also be considered.

Diagnosis

Most impactions of the large colon are palpable per rectum by identification of a section of ingesta-filled and distended large colon. Pelvic flexure impactions are the most obvious and they sometimes extend into the pelvic canal. The size and texture of the impaction should be noted. Occasionally, an impaction may lie beyond reach of the examiner. Gastric reflux is unusual with large-colon impactions, but it can occur, presumably as a result of small-intestinal compression by the distended large colon or pain-induced ileus. Fluoroscopy or transabdominal ultrasonography can be useful in horses that are too small for per-rectum palpation.

Peritoneal fluid is normal in the vast majority of impactions. If abdominocentesis is performed, care should be taken to avoid penetrating a markedly distended, friable large colon. Abdominocentesis should be performed in horses that deteriorate acutely in order to determine whether colonic rupture may have occurred.

Management

Feed should be withheld, and can be restricted from otherwise healthy adult horses for a week without adverse consequences in most cases. Analgesics will usually be required. The goal of analgesic therapy should be to control pain, but not mask progression of disease.

Treatment via nasogastric tube may be useful in horses without gastric reflux. Mineral oil (4 liters) has traditionally been used; however, its efficacy has not been proven. Mineral oil can pass around dense impactions without any beneficial effect and is probably more useful in mild impactions. DSS can also be administered orally, but a beneficial effect has not been demonstrated. Repeated administration of DSS should be avoided because it can be irritating and toxicity can develop. Osmotic cathartics can be more useful. Sodium sulfate (0.15–0.5 g/kg p/o) appears to be more effective than magnesium sulfate (1 g/kg) and does not carry the risk of magnesium toxicity with repeated administration. It may be wise not to use high doses of cathartics when very large, firm, and potentially obstructive impactions are present because of the potential for the development of marked colonic distension. In these cases it might be preferable to attempt to soften the impaction with fluid therapy prior to administration of cathartics. Administration of water via a nasogastric

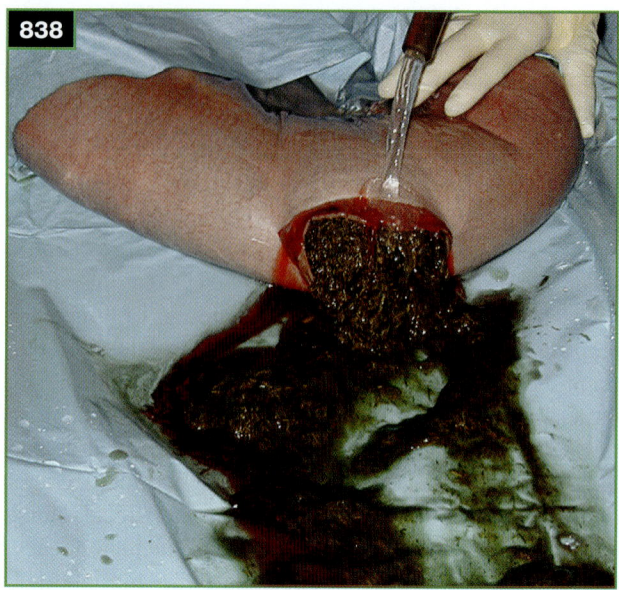

838 Pelvic flexure enterotomy.

tube is cost-effective and can be used successfully. With proper observation, and having first checked that it is positioned correctly, a nasogastric tube can be left in place and water (8 liters up to q30min) can be administered. Water administration should be stopped until the horse is re-evaluated if signs of colic progress or if gastric reflux develops. Intravenous fluid therapy may be required for more severe cases, or those that are refractory to oral therapy, and is very effective at resolving large-colon impactions.

Administration of large volumes of intravenous fluids can result in increased influx of fluid into the colon to help soften the impaction, as well as counteract any adverse effects of dehydration or electrolyte imbalance on intestinal motility.

Most impactions will resolve with medical treatment, but very large impactions that do not respond to medical treatment, or cases with severe intractable pain, may require surgical intervention (**838**). Rupture of the colon during exteriorization is a risk of surgery because the intestinal wall can be thin and friable.

Following resolution of the impaction, it is important that feeding be reintroduced gradually. Small volumes of hay, hay cube slurries, grass, or bran mashes should be used initially. Small volumes should be offered every few hours, with volume increasing over time so that a normal hay or grass ration is offered by 24–48 hours. Grain should not be fed during the first few days and should be reintroduced gradually. Risk factors for impaction, including management and dental disease, should be evaluated to help prevent recurrence.

Prognosis

In general the prognosis is very good, but worse if surgery is required. It is suspected that severe and/or long-standing impactions may damage stretch receptors in the intestinal wall, predisposing to recurrence. Rupture of the large colon during exteriorization is a concern if surgical correction is needed. Large-colon rupture is invariably fatal.

Sand impaction

Definition/overview

Accumulation of large volumes of sand in the large colon is a common cause of colic in some geographic areas.

Etiology/pathophysiology

Sand may be ingested while grazing on sandy soil, or from ingestion of sand in sandy paddocks, arenas, or stalls. Horses that are underfed or kept in overstocked, closely grazed pastures may be at greater risk. Some horses, particularly foals, may intentionally ingest sand (pica).

Following ingestion, sand can settle in the large colon. Over time, and with continued ingestion, sand can accumulate to such a degree than partial or complete obstruction occurs and signs of colic develop. The right dorsal colon is the most common site of sand accumulation, but impactions can develop in all sections of the large colon, and multiple sites may be involved.

Clinical presentation

Signs of mild to severe colic may be observed. This can be accompanied by varying degrees of anorexia, depression, and abdominal distension. Fecal production may be decreased and soft feces may be present. Signs of pain can be intermittent or continuous. Concurrent large-colon displacement or volvulus may be present and affect the clinical presentation.

Differential diagnosis

Other causes of mild to moderate colic should be considered, including large-colon impaction or displacement, intestinal tympany, gastric ulceration, and enterolithiasis.

Diagnosis

A history of potential exposure to sand is usually present; however, sand impaction can be difficult to differentiate from other causes of colic. During abdominal auscultation, characteristic 'sand sounds' can be heard, particularly over the ventral abdomen. Sand sounds are similar to friction rubs or movement of sand in a paper bag. Identification of these sounds is a relatively sensitive and specific indicator of sand accumulation. Hematologic changes are uncommon, nonspecific, and not diagnostic for sand impaction. It is often difficult to detect sand impactions per rectum because they tend to be located cranially. Gaseous distension of the large colon and cecum is often palpable with sand impactions, but this may also indicate a large-colon displacement or volvulus.

Abdominocentesis should only be performed if it is an important part of the diagnostic plan and should be done with care because of concerns about lacerating the distended colon. If enterocentesis occurs and sand is present, then a sand impaction is almost invariably present.

Sand accumulation may be evident radiographically, particularly in the cranioventral abdomen. Radiography is more sensitive in foals, ponies, and small horses. Sand may also be evident ultrasonographically within the large colon in the cranioventral abdomen.

Sand accumulation in the colon can be inferred from detection of sand in feces via a sand sedimentation test. A few fecal balls collected per rectum should be placed in a rectal sleeve, mixed with water to form a slurry, then suspended to allow the sand to settle. It has been stated that sedimentation of >6 mm of sand indicates excessive sand in the feces (833). Similarly, it has been stated that settling of >5 g (1 teaspoon) of sand after suspending six fecal balls indicates fecal passage of excessive sand.

Management

Mild impactions may respond to intragastric administration of water (6–10 liters) or mineral oil (4 liters), withholding feed and analgesic therapy. The efficacy of bulk laxatives is somewhat controversial, but psyllium (0.25–0.5 kg/500 kg in 4–8 liters of water p/o q6–24h) is frequently used. Analgesics will typically be required. Intravenous fluid therapy at 2–3 times maintenance rates (120–180 ml/kg/day) may be required in more severe impactions. Following resolution of clinical signs, it may be prudent to continue to administer psyllium (0.25–0.5 kg/500 kg) mixed with feed for 14 days and repeat the sand sedimentation test. Periodic evaluation (every 1–6 months) should be considered, particularly if management changes are not feasible. Radiography of the cranioventral abdomen can also be used to monitor resolution of sand accumulation.

Intermittent administration of psyllium may help reduce sand accumulation. Administration of 0.25 kg of psyllium/500 kg once daily for 7 days, performed monthly, has been recommended. Medical treatment is usually effective, but surgical intervention may be required in horses with intractable pain, poor response to medical therapy, or deteriorating cardiovascular status. Feed should be gradually reintroduced after the impaction has resolved. A discussion of management practices is important to avoid further sand impactions.

Prognosis

The prognosis is good; however, compared with ingesta impactions, sand impactions tend to be more difficult to treat, are more likely to require surgery, and have a higher mortality rate.

Intramural lesions of the large colon

Definition/overview

Intramural lesions (lesions within the wall) of the large colon include lymphosarcoma, adenocarcinoma, segmental eosiniphilic colitis, and intestinal wall abscess (839). They are uncommon and usually lead to mild to moderate intermittent colic. Treatment is surgical and the prognosis varies with the etiology of the lesions.

Etiology/pathophysiology

Multicentric and intestinal lymphosarcoma and adenocarcinoma have been reported as the cause of intramural lesions of the large colon in a limited number of horses. Segmental eosinophilic colitis is an uncommon disease that results in a local thickening and obstructive lesion of the colon in horses. The precise etiology is not known, but parasite involvement is suspected. In rare cases abdominal abscessation limited to the wall of the large colon can be the cause.

Local thickening and obstructive lesion of the colonic wall result regardless of whether the etiology of the lesions is neoplastic, bacterial, or inflammatory, with potential partial or complete obstruction of the colonic lumen.

Clinical presentation

The clinical signs are nonspecific. The most common clinical signs are mild to moderate recurrent colic episodes associated with abdominal distension and pelvic flexure impaction. Lethargy, weight loss, pyrexia, and diarrhea may be observed in horses with intramural lesions of the large colon.

Differential diagnosis

Causes of simple colon obstruction (food and foreign body impaction) and primary large-colon tympany are the major differential diagnoses for intramural lesions of the large colon.

Diagnosis

An abdominal mass attached to the large colon and/or large-colon distension may be palpable per rectum in horses with intramural lesions of the large colon. Ultrasonographic examination of the large colon may show an increased wall thickness or confirm the presence of an abdominal mass. Peritoneal fluid total nucleated cell count and protein concentration are usually increased, but exfoliated tumor cells are only rarely observed. A definitive diagnosis is usually made on exploratory laparotomy, during which biopsies are taken.

Management

Horses with intramural colonic lesions are usually initially treated in a supportive manner using a restricted diet, analgesics, intravenous and/or oral fluids, and laxatives. Clinical signs are often temporarily responsive to this medical treatment, but they recur as food is reintroduced or the action of the analgesics abates.

Affected horses are eventually managed using an exploratory laparotomy. Identification of the lesion and differentiation between intestinal neoplasia and an abscess may be possible grossly or after histopathology of biopsy material. If discrete areas of neoplasia or eosinophilic colitis are identified, the affected areas can be resected. Intestinal abscesses are treated using drainage with or without marsupialization, intestinal bypass or resection and anastomosis, and long-term postoperative antimicrobial administration.

Prognosis

The prognosis for intestinal neoplasia is guarded to poor as the tumor may extend to other organs. Based on one retrospective study of 22 cases, horses with segmental eosinophilic colitis treated surgically had a good prognosis for survival. Horses with abdominal abscesses that require treatment in addition to long-term antimicrobial administration also have a poor to guarded prognosis.

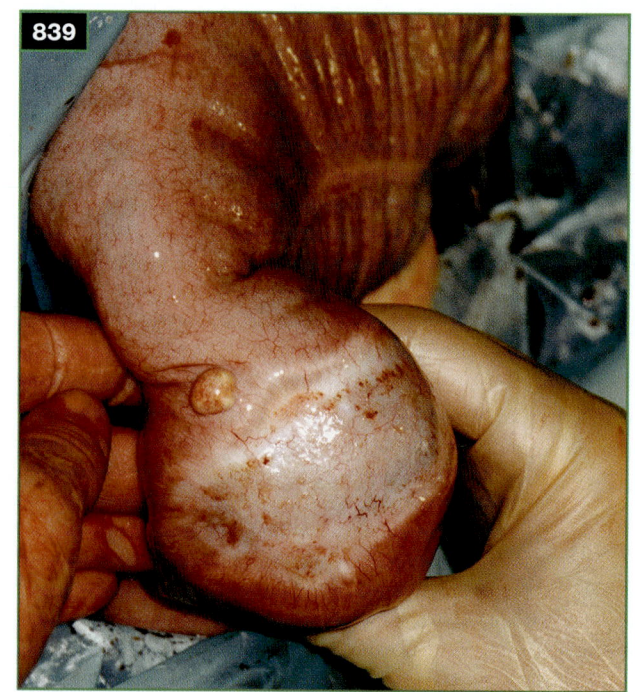

839 A large intramural abscess found in the large colon of a horse presented for exploratory laparotomy for investigation of chronic abdominal pain. (Photo courtesy GA Munroe)

Gastrointestinal system

Disorders of the small colon and rectum

Small-colon impaction

Definition/overview

Impaction is the most common disorder of the small colon. This portion of the intestine seems to be predisposed to impaction as the lumen of the large colon narrows acutely through the transverse colon into the small colon. Ponies, American miniature horses, and Arabian horses appear to develop small-colon impactions more frequently than other breeds.

Etiology/pathophysiology

The etiology of small colon-impaction includes ingestion of poor-quality roughage, poor dentition, parasitism, dehydration, and motility disorders. Older horses seem to be more frequently affected than younger horses, probably due to deteriorated dentition and decreased small colon motility. Small-colon impactions occur more frequently during the fall and winter, as access to water may be decreased and consumption of coarse roughage material is increased.

Impaction causes an intraluminal obstruction of the small colon and, as a result, ingesta, fluid, and gas accumulate in segments of the GI tract proximal to the impaction. Horses with small-colon impaction deteriorate slowly because of the aboral location of the small colon and the large space for the ingesta, fluid, and gas to accumulate orad to the impaction. As the impaction persists, the intestinal segments proximal to the obstruction, mainly large colon and cecum, become more and more distended and the affected horse experiences colic.

Clinical presentation

Horses with impaction of the small colon present initially with only mild signs of colic and reduced fecal output. As the condition progresses, they develop abdominal distension and exhibit moderate to severe signs of abdominal pain. Nasogastric reflux is an inconsistent finding.

Differential diagnosis

Differential diagnoses for this condition include any intraluminal obstruction of the large intestine in horses. This includes large-colon and cecal impactions and foreign-body, enterolith, and fecalith obstructions.

Diagnosis

Diagnosis of impaction of the small colon is based on the observation of clinical signs and rectal palpation. By the time horses with impaction of the small colon are presented to a veterinarian, they usually have decreased fecal production and a distended abdomen and exhibit moderate to severe signs of colic. On rectal examination, one or several firm, tubular, and digesta-filled loops of small colon can be palpated. The thickness of the wall and palpation of a single, free tenial band help identify the small colon.

Management

Medical conservative management is often successful in the treatment of horses with mild to moderate impactions. Aggressive enteral and/or parenteral fluid therapy is used to overhydrate the horse, stimulate intestinal secretion production, and break the impaction down. Analgesics are used to control abdominal pain and exercise is used to stimulate intestinal motility. Administration of an enema in standing horses is not recommended unless the impaction is located in the distal portion of the small colon near the rectum and the horse tolerates them well. This procedure can be associated with traumatic rupture of the small colon.

Surgical treatment is recommended in horses with severe impactions or when the impaction fails to respond to medical treatment. A celiotomy is performed, the impacted portion of the small colon is identified, and a combination of manual massage and intraluminal irrigation is used to break the impaction down and evacuate the ingesta through the anus. Intraluminal irrigation is performed by inserting a long rubber hose through the anus and infusing warm water into the small-colon lumen.

Anecdotally, horses with small-colon impaction seem to have a high incidence of developing salmonellosis in some areas. The reason for this is unclear, but this possibility should be considered during the management of affected horses, particularly if diarrhea develops.

Prognosis

Horses that respond to medical conservative treatment have a good prognosis for survival, whereas horses undergoing surgery commonly develop postoperative complications such as fever, diarrhea, salmonellosis, and laminitis. The prognosis for these horses is guarded.

Small-colon strangulation

Definition/overview

Small-colon strangulation consists of obstruction to the vasculature of the small colon and ischemic damage to the intestinal tissue. This may occur due to a strangulating lipoma, volvulus, or entrapment of the small colon through a congenital or acquired defect. Strangulating lipomas (see pp. 550) and small-colon volvulus are covered elsewhere.

Etiology/pathophysiology

The etiology considered here is small-colon strangulation secondary to herniation or incarceration in a congenital or acquired mesenteric or ligamentous rent. The small colon has a short mesentery compared with the distal small intestine, which accounts for the lower incidence of strangulation. However, the small colon can become entrapped in the gastrosplenic ligament, broad ligament, cecocolic fold, and mesocolon and through a vaginal tear. Inguinal and umbilical herniation of the small colon have also been reported.

Anatomic differences in the size and shape of intra-abdominal ligaments have been identified, and there may be a predisposition for horses to acquire defects. Congenital defects including vitelloumbilical anomalies contribute to abnormal spaces through which the small colon can become incarcerated.

Once entrapped, the vascular supply to the small colon becomes obstructed and the tissues become edematous and turgid. Further swelling of the entrapped intestine obstructs arterial supply to the intestine, resulting in ischemic damage to the intestine.

Orad distension of the small colon, transverse colon, and ascending colon is a consequence of intraluminal obstruction.

Clinical presentation

Horses with strangulating obstruction can present with signs ranging from mild to moderate abdominal discomfort to acute severe abdominal pain. Nasogastric reflux is an inconsistent finding.

Differential diagnosis

Differential diagnoses for this condition include any strangulating obstruction of the intestine in horses. This includes strangulating lipomas, inguinal and other hernias, volvulus, epiploic foramen entrapment, and entrapment of other segments of bowel in mesenteric or ligamentous rents. Small-intestinal strangulations tend to occur more acutely and with a more rapid deterioration in clinical signs and hematologic parameters.

Diagnosis

The variable location of the strangulating obstruction can lead to inconclusive rectal findings, but a common finding is impaction within the cranial small colon and, in chronic cases, colonic distension. Transrectal ultrasound is useful for diagnosing small colon impactions.

Peritoneal fluid is often serosanguineous with an elevated protein concentration and nucleated cell count. An elevated blood lactate level may be useful for demonstrating tissue ischemia.

Ultrasonographic findings include a distended, amotile small colon with a thickened wall (>3–4 mm). Normal wall thickness of the colon and small intestine may help localize the lesion to the small colon.

Management

As with all intestinal strangulations, surgical management consisting of relieving the strangulation and assessing the viability of the lesion is critical. Intestine considered to be nonviable should be resected.

Several techniques for anastomosis of the small colon are acceptable, but a common technique is a sutured, two-layered, end-to-end anastomosis. The first layer consists of a non-mucosa-penetrating, simple interrupted apposing pattern. The second layer consists of an inverting pattern (e.g. continuous Cushing suture pattern interrupted at 180 degrees).

Pelvic flexure enterotomy may be considered to decrease the load of ingesta passing by the surgical site in the immediate postoperative period.

Prognosis

It is well recognized that strangulating intestinal obstructions have a poorer prognosis than nonstrangulating lesions. Furthermore, resection and anastomosis of the small colon is considered to have a higher complication rate than more proximal sites due to increased bacterial loads of the ingesta, greater mechanical abrasion due to the passage of feces of lower water content, a higher collagenase activity, and supposedly poorer vascularity to the healing tissues. However, recent reports suggest that the prognosis may be better than previously thought.

The most proximal and distal aspects of the small colon may not be able to be completely exteriorized at the time of surgery, which may hinder surgical repair or increase the risk of fecal contamination. Taken together, a prognosis of approximately 50% for these cases is reasonable.

Small-colon obstruction

Definition/overview

Small-colon obstruction can be intraluminal or extraluminal in origin. Causes for intraluminal obstructions include impaction, foreign bodies, enteroliths, fecaliths, and bezoars (840) (see Small-colon impaction, p. 583). Causes for extraluminal obstruction include intramural hematoma and, rarely, neoplasms such as leiomyomas.

Etiology/pathophysiology

Foreign bodies involved in small-colon obstructions are usually nylon, plastic, or rubber material from halters, hay nets, bale twines, synthetic fencing material, and plastic trashcan liners. After ingestion, foreign bodies reach the large colon, in particular the right dorsal colon, where they can remain for an extended period of time. They become covered with mineral precipitate, which increases their bulk. Eventually, they pass into the transverse/small colon and cause obstructions. Foreign-body obstructions occur mostly in horses less than 3 years of age, probably because they are not as discriminative as older horses in their eating habits.

Intramural hematomas are caused by hemorrhage between the small-colon mucosal and muscularis layers. The etiology of the hemorrhage remains to this date unknown, but the condition is observed mainly in older horses.

Foreign bodies covered with mineral concretions usually have an irregular shape, often containing sharp projections. Once passed from the right dorsal colon into the transverse/small colon, they can become wedged and completely obstruct the intestinal lumen. Their sharp projections may cause pressure necrosis of the intestinal wall. Horses with an intramural hematoma are prone to develop small-colon obstruction as hemorrhage occludes the intestinal lumen and dissects along the intestine and produces intestinal necrosis.

Clinical presentation

Signs of moderate to severe colic, mild to moderate abdominal distension, and reduced or lack of fecal production are usually present.

Differential diagnosis

Differential diagnoses include any obstructive conditions of the large intestine such as fecal impaction of the cecum and the large and small colon. Although it is sometime difficult to differentiate one condition from the other, small-colon obstruction from a foreign body tends to occur more acutely, with a more rapid deterioration in clinical signs, than small-colon fecal impaction. Differential diagnosis also includes obstruction of the large colon due to foreign bodies, enteroliths, and fecaliths.

Diagnosis

Diagnosis of small-colon obstruction on the basis of clinical signs and rectal palpation is frequently difficult. On rectal palpation, one or several firm, tubular, and digesta-filled loops of small colon can be identified. Rarely, a foreign body is palpable. Definitive diagnosis and differentiation with fecal impaction are made during exploratory celiotomy.

Management

Surgical treatment is recommended in horses with complete obstruction of the small colon. With foreign-body obstruction, small-colon impaction orad to the foreign body is identified during an exploratory celiotomy. A pelvic flexure enterotomy is performed to evacuate the content of the large and small colons. Based on the location and diameter of the foreign body, it can be either massaged back into the large colon and removed through the pelvic enterotomy, or removed through a small-colon enterotomy performed through the antimesenteric tenia. Horses with a small-colon intramural hematoma also require surgical treatment. The affected portion of the small colon is identified and resection and anastomosis are performed during an exploratory celiotomy.

Prognosis

The prognosis for horses with small-colon obstruction due to a foreign body or an intramural hematoma is guarded, as postoperative complications such as diarrhea, laminitis, and leakage at the anastomosis site may occur.

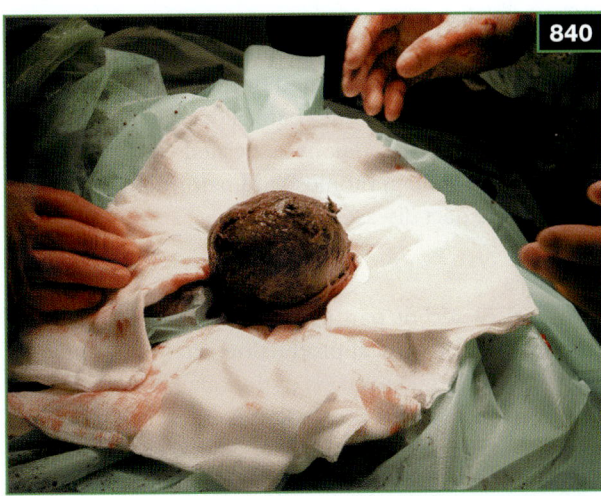

840 A large trichobezoar is being removed from the small colon at exploratory laparotomy via a flank incision. Note the careful draping around the colon to minimize contamination of the abdomen. (Photo courtesy GA Munroe)

585

Small-colon segmental ischemic necrosis

Definition/overview
Segmental ischemic necrosis of the small colon is a rare condition usually observed in broodmares.

Etiology/pathophysiology
Disruption of the caudal mesenteric artery, which is the main source of blood supply to the small colon, occurs rarely in horses. Mesocolon rupture is the main cause of disruption of the mesocolonic vasculature and of small-colon segmental ischemic necrosis in horses.

Disruption of the mesocolonic vasculature resulting from mesocolon rupture can either occur during parturition or result from type 3 or 4 rectal prolapse. During the first stage of labor, the small colon may get trapped between the uterus and the body wall as the foal vigorously positions itself and rotates from a ventral to a dorsal position. The mesocolon may stretch and rupture during this maneuver. During type 3 or 4 rectal prolapses, the mesocolon vasculature becomes disrupted if >30 cm of the distal small colon and rectum prolapse. Rupture of the mesocolon and mesocolonic vasculature results in infarction, causing segmental ischemic necrosis and functional obstruction of the small colon. Progressive signs of colic and septic peritonitis occur as a consequence.

Clinical presentation
In the broodmare affected with segmental ischemic necrosis of the small colon, mild signs of colic occur within 24 hours of parturition. Affected horses fail to pass feces. If the condition is not treated, cardiovascular status slowly deteriorates and signs of septic peritonitis and shock develop.

Differential diagnosis
Early signs of segmental ischemic necrosis of the small colon need to be differentiated from the mild abdominal pain associated with uterine contractions. Differential diagnoses also include conditions associated with small-colon obstruction, septic peritonitis, and parturition-associated reproductive tract disease.

Diagnosis
A history of recent parturition or rectal prolapse with reduced or lack of fecal production can be indicative of segmental ischemic necrosis of the small colon in horses displaying mild signs of colic. Rectal examination may not be initially diagnostic, but as the condition progresses, one or several firm, tubular, and digesta-filled loops of small colon can be palpated. Abdominocentesis initially reveals abdominal hemorrhage, with an increased WBC count and protein level as the condition progresses. Exploratory celiotomy will often be the only way definitively to diagnose the condition (**841**).

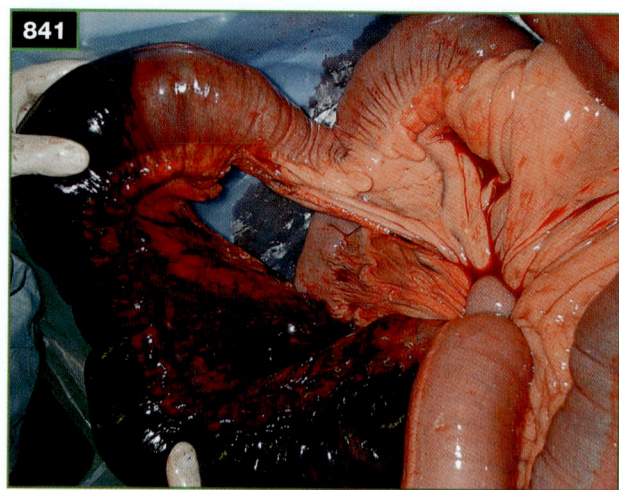

841 Typical postmortem appearance of an infarct lesion of the peritoneal rectum and distal small colon. The lesion in this broodmare resulted from a rupture of the mesocolon, which had occurred during parturition.

Management
Exploratory celiotomy and resection of the ischemic segment of the small colon and anastomosis should be performed. However, because of the location of the lesion, this procedure is rarely feasible and end colostomy is the only procedure that may be attempted to save the life of the affected horse.

Prognosis
The prognosis is directly correlated with the location of the lesion: if it is orad enough that resection and anastomosis can be performed, the prognosis is fair; if the lesion is too aborad for an anastomosis to be performed, the prognosis is grave.

Rectal tears

Definition/overview
A rectal tear occurs when at least one of the rectal wall layers is disrupted. Most rectal tears occur during transrectal palpation; they are generally located 20–30 cm from the anus, in the dorsal portion of the rectum, and have a longitudinal direction. Young horses, males, and Arabian horses are more frequently affected than other horses.

Etiology/pathophysiology
Rectal tears are most commonly iatrogenic in origin. The etiology includes transrectal palpation, enema administration, and reproductive complications such as dystocia and breeding injury. Spontaneous tears are rare, but they have been described and, presumably, result from thromboembolism of the caudal mesenteric artery.

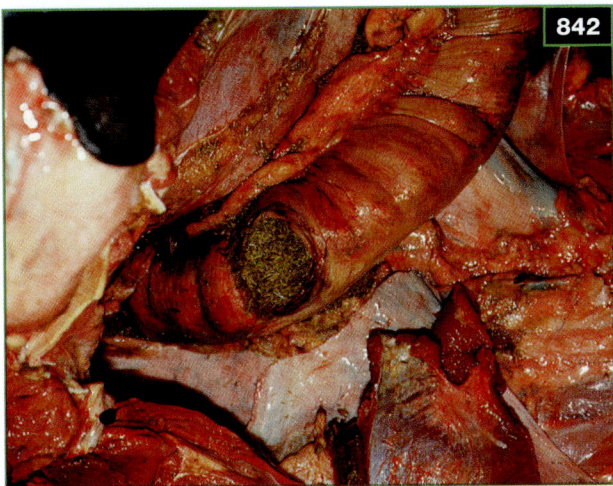

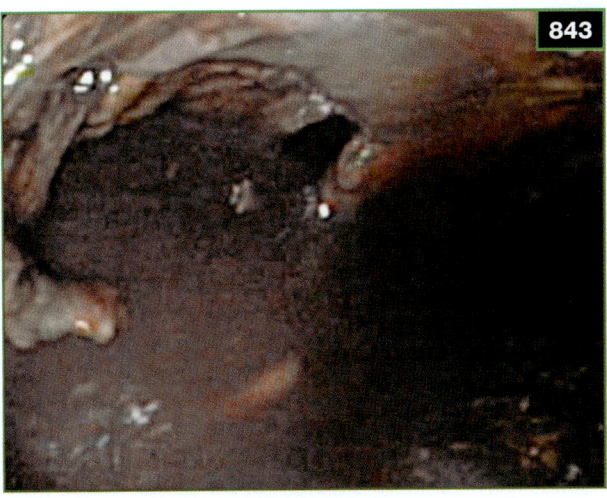

842 Typical postmortem appearance of an iatrogenic grade 4 rectal tear. Note the obvious fecal contamination of the peritoneal cavity.

843 Endoscopic image of a mare with a grade 4 rectal tear that occurred following palpation for routine reproductive evaluation.

Pathophysiology varies with the location and the degree of severity of the tears. The rectum is approximately 30 cm long in a 450 kg horse, with its oral half being in the peritoneal cavity and the aboral portion retroperitoneal. Most tears are located 20–30 cm from the anus and therefore are within the peritoneal cavity. A classification reflecting degree of severity has been established:

+ *Grade 1 tears:* only the rectal mucosa and submucosa are torn.
+ *Grade 2 tears:* the rectal muscularis layer is torn, causing the mucosa and submucosa to form a diverticulum as they protrude through the defect.
+ *Grade 3 tears:* In grade 3a tears, all the layers are affected except the serosa and in grade 3b tears all the layers are affected except the mesorectum.
+ *Grade 4 tears:* these are complete tears involving all the rectal wall layers.

Grade 1 tears are usually not associated with complications. In grade 2 and 3 tears, fecal material becomes impacted in the defect, leading to the development of a perirectal or retroperitoneal abscess, dissecting cellulitis, or rectal-wall necrosis that can eventually result in abdominal fecal contamination. Grade 4 tears usually result in massive fecal contamination of the abdominal cavity, which leads to septic peritonitis, septic shock, and ultimately death (**842**).

Clinical presentation

The presence of whole fresh blood on the rectal examination sleeve or sudden relaxation of the rectum during examination is suggestive of a serious rectal injury. Clinical signs may not be present in the short term even after serious tears. Tenesmus, abdominal pain, tachycardia, pyrexia, and ileus may develop within hours after the injury. Horses with grade 4 rectal tears develop septic shock and peritonitis very shortly after the injury.

Diagnosis

The aim of evaluating horses with rectal tears is to determine immediately the location, size, and depth of the tear. This is performed after the horse is well sedated and epidural anesthesia has been administered. The rectum should be carefully evacuated. Digital palpation with bare hands is the most valuable procedure for assessing the location, size, and depth of the tear. Endoscopic evaluation of the rectum is useful for the assessment of the tear (**843**). Care should be used to prevent excessive insufflation of the rectum during the procedure in order to reduce the risk of causing further tearing of the defect. Abdominocentesis should be performed if a grade 4 tear is suspected.

Management

The management varies with the grade of tear. Horses with grade 1 tears are treated conservatively with the administration of systemic broad-spectrum antimicrobials, NSAIDs, and laxatives. The same management is used in horses with grade 2 tears except that the administration of antibiotics is not necessary. Grade 3 and 4 tears should be referred to a hospital facility for further evaluation and treatment. In order to prevent fecal contamination of the abdomen, a well-lubricated stockinet packed with cotton should be inserted into the rectum to a level approximately 10 cm cranial to the tear. The anus is then closed using towel clamps or a purse-string suture and intravenous systemic broad-spectrum antibiotics and NSAIDs are administered. Soaking of cotton in povidone–iodine prior to insertion has been recommended.

Recent, clean grade 3 tears should be closed primarily using either a rectal or an abdominal approach through an antimesenteric small colon enterotomy. In both cases, a pelvic enterotomy should be performed to evacuate the contents of the large colon. Long-duration grade 3 tears are treated medically using frequent and careful evacuation of the rectum or, optimally, large-colon evacuation through a pelvic enterotomy.

Grade 4 tears should be closed primarily and either fecal diversion through a colostomy or the application of a temporary, indwelling rectal liner should be performed.

Prognosis

The prognosis for survival of horses with a grade 1 rectal tear is good. Grade 3 tears warrant a poor prognosis and grade 4 tears a grave prognosis.

Rectal prolapse

Definition/overview

Rectal prolapse occurs when rectal tissue evaginates and protrudes through the anus. It is rare in horses, but can be associated with any condition causing tenesmus.

Etiology/pathophysiology

Any condition causing tenesmus may lead to rectal prolapse in horses. It has been associated with diarrhea, constipation, intestinal parasitism, proctatitis, colic and rectal foreign body, and tumor. Type 4 prolapse usually occurs in mares during foaling or dystocia.

The anal sphincter applies pressure on the protruded rectal tissue and impinges on the venous return. The protruded tissue eventually becomes edematous and necrotic and is prone to irritation and trauma.

Clinical presentation

Four degrees of rectal prolapse have been described in the equine. In type 1, only the rectal mucosa (or part of it) protrudes through the anus (**844**). Type 2 prolapse occurs when there is an eversion of the entire ampula recti (**845**). Type 3 prolapse is also a complete eversion of the ampula recti, but it is complicated by an intussusception of the peritoneal portion of the rectum. Type 4 prolapse is an intussusception of the peritoneal rectum and a variable length of the small colon, both protruding through the anus (**846**).

844 Type 1 rectal prolapse.

845 Type 2 rectal prolapse.

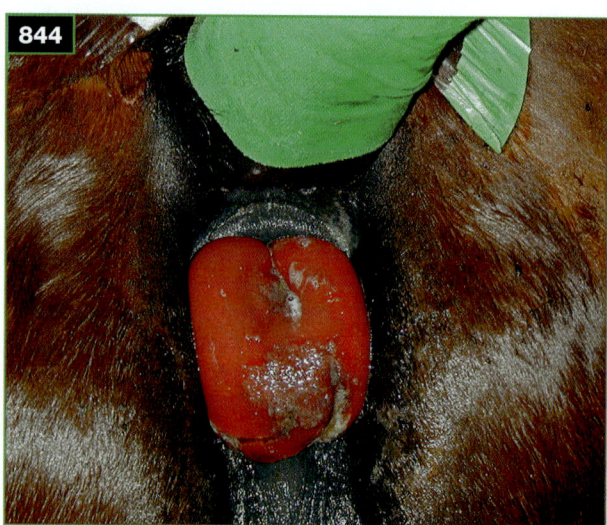

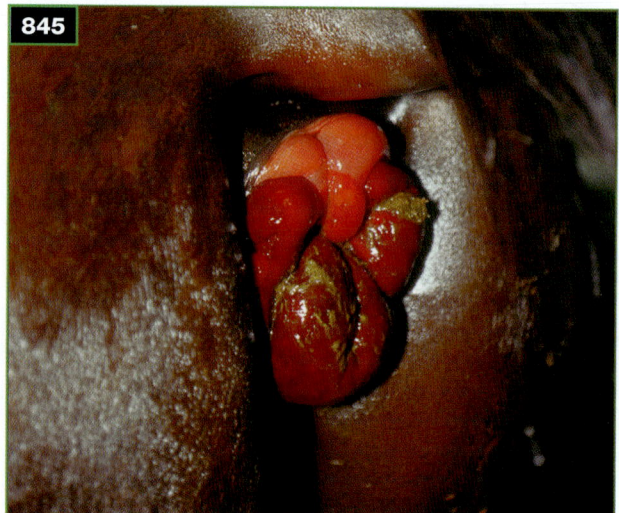

846 Type 4 rectal prolapse.

847 Purse-string suture correction of a type 1 rectal prolapse.

848 Submucosal resection technique for treatment of long-standing or recurrent type 1 or 2 prolapse.

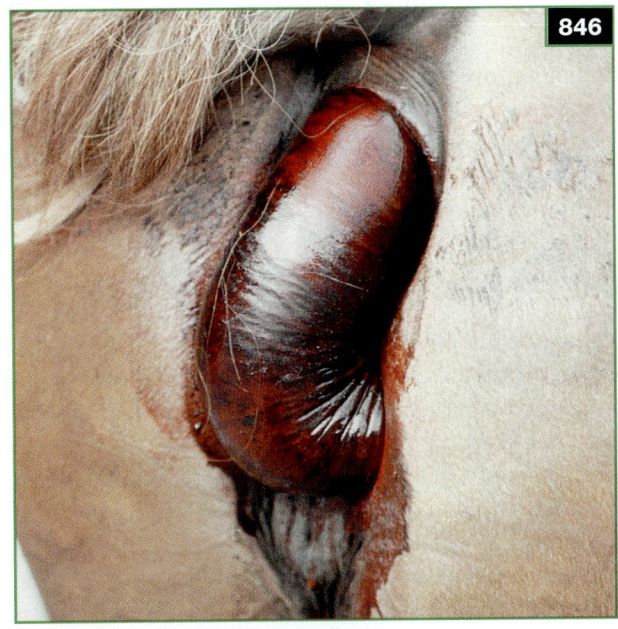

Diagnosis

The initial diagnosis of rectal prolapse is made by the observation of an abnormal mass of tissue protruding beyond the anus. The tissue is usually inflamed and cyanotic. The degree of trauma and necrosis is variable. Rectal palpation should be performed and will help with the differentiation between types 2 and 3 rectal prolapse cases. Horses with a type 3 or 4 rectal prolapse may develop septic peritonitis, therefore abdominocentesis should be performed in these cases.

Management

Acute and circumscribed types 1 and 2 rectal prolapses should be treated conservatively. The treatment involves topical application of lidocaine jelly onto the protruded tissue, repeated administration of epidural anesthesia to reduce straining, and placement of a purse-string suture for 48–72 hours. This suture is made of a double strand of 6 mm (1/4 inch) umbilical tape applied 1–2 cm lateral to the anus with four wide bites (**847**). The suture should be opened every 2–4 hours in order manually to remove the feces from the rectum. The horse should receive mineral oil and be fasted for 24 hours. A laxative diet should be fed for 10 days following purse-string removal. Most importantly, the primary cause for straining should be treated. Long-standing or recurring types 1 and 2 rectal prolapses are treated surgically using a submucosal resection technique (**848**).

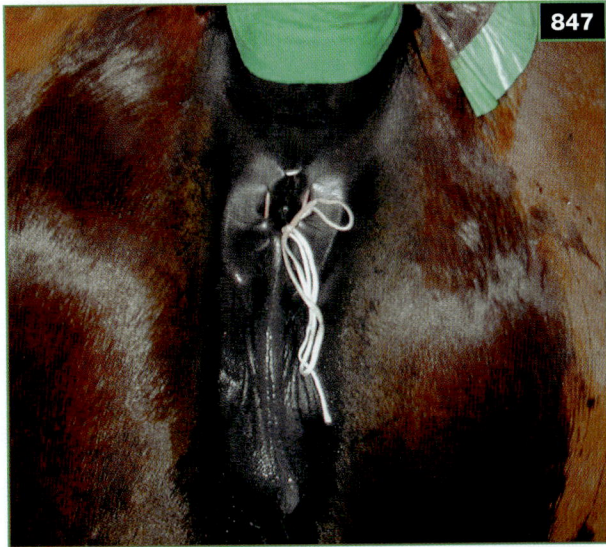

Types 3 and 4 rectal prolapses should be manually reduced immediately after they occur. However, they are usually associated with severe vascular injury to the rectum and/or distal small colon and an exploratory laparotomy is recommended. If rupture of the mesocolon and vascular supply has occurred, the affected segment has to be resected. Most often, anastomosis between two consecutive viable segments is not possible and the only surgical option is to perform a permanent end colostomy.

Prognosis

The prognosis for types 1 and 2 prolapses is good. It is poor to grave for types 3 and 4 prolapses as they are usually associated with severe injuries to the vascular supply and mesentery disruption.

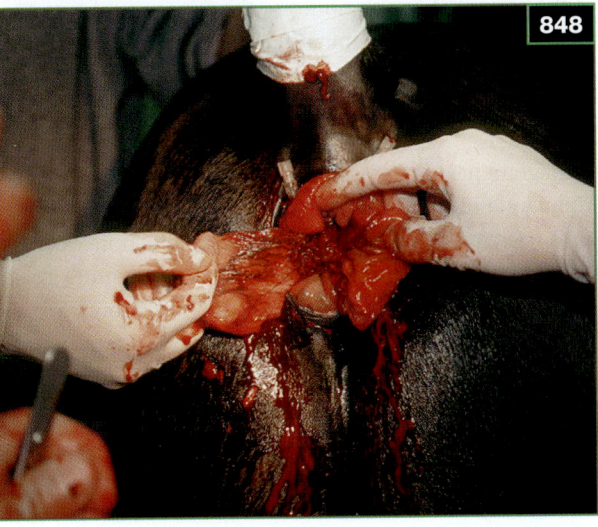

589

Anorectal lymphadenopathy/perirectal abscess

Definition/overview

Anorectal lymphadenopathy/perirectal abscess is an uncommon condition that affects mostly young horses and results in extraluminal obstruction of the rectum. Treatment involves the administration of systemic antimicrobials and anti-inflammatories, prevention of rectal impaction, and drainage of the abscess when present.

Etiology/pathophysiology

In most cases the cause is unknown, but anorectal lymphadenopathy/perirectal abscess may develop following rectal or vaginal puncture or trauma or be secondary to gravitation of a gluteal abscess following an intramuscular injection. *Streptococcus zooepidemicus* and *Escherichia coli* are most commonly implicated.

Anorectal lymph nodes are located dorsally in the retroperitoneal tissue surrounding the rectum. Sepsis causes these nodes to enlarge, which may result in an extraluminal obstruction of the rectum. Rarely, the infection progresses in the abdominal cavity and induces a septic peritonitis.

Clinical presentation

Affected horses display signs of mild abdominal pain, depression, anorexia, reduced fecal output, tenesmus, and fever.

Differential diagnosis

Perirectal abscesses need to be differentiated from the few neoplasms that develop in perirectal tissue. Extensive perineal melanoma and melanosarcoma may produce clinical signs similar to those of a perirectal abscess.

Diagnosis

Diagnosis is based on palpation of a firm perianal mass per rectum. Transrectal ultrasonography reveals enlargement of the anorectal lymph nodes or the presence of a mature abscess. Cytologic examination and bacteriologic culture of aspirates collected percutaneously or through the rectal wall confirm sepsis of the anorectal lymph nodes.

Management

Management of horses with anorectal lymphadenopathy aims to treat the anorectal lymph node infection, decreasing perirectal swelling and pain, and preventing rectal obstruction. NSAIDs, a prolonged course of antimicrobials, and oral laxatives should therefore be administered.

Perirectal abscesses should be drained based on their location either rectally or perianally. This procedure is performed under epidural anesthesia with the horse standing. Postoperatively, drained abscesses are flushed twice daily with antiseptic solution.

Prognosis

The prognosis is good to excellent unless there is extension of the septic process into the abdominal cavity.

Disorders of the peritoneum

Hemoperitoneum

Definition/overview

Blood loss into the abdominal cavity is an uncommon but potentially life-threatening problem. It is most common in multiparous mares over 11 years of age.

Etiology/pathophysiology

Hemoperitoneum occurs most commonly in broodmares as a result of ruptured uterine vessels during or after parturition (see p. 287). Rupture of ovarian granulosa cell tumors (849) or ovarian follicular hematomas, uterine leiomyomas, or leiomyosarcomas may also be associated with hemoperitoneum in mares. Pheochromocytoma is another possible cause. Less frequently, intra-abdominal hemorrhage originates from the GI tract. Splenic rupture secondary to blunt trauma or neoplasia, entrapment of the small intestine within the epiploic foramen and subsequent rupture of the caudal vena cava, and rupture of mesenteric arteries secondary to *Strongylus vulgaris* larval migration can all induce intra-abdominal hemorrhage in horses. Hemorrhage secondary to coagulopathy is uncommon but can occur.

Clinical presentation

Clinical manifestations are frequently nonspecific. Initial clinical sign include depression, lethargy, partial or complete anorexia, and colic. As the anemia and hypovolemia intensify, signs of hypovolemic shock (tachycardia, tachypnea, weak peripheral pulses, pale mucous membranes) are observed. Ileus and abdominal distension may occur if a large volume of blood accumulates.

Differential diagnosis

All conditions resulting in colic in horses should be included in the differential diagnosis. In broodmares, uterine torsion, uterine rupture, and dystocia should also be considered.

Diagnosis

Abdominal fluid accumulation, abdominal masses, or reproductive tract abnormalities may be palpable per rectum. Abdominal ultrasonography reveals the presence of hyperechoic fluid within the abdomen (786). The origin of the hemorrhage is rarely identified. Abdominocentesis is used to diagnose hemoperitoneum definitively; however, care must be taken to ensure that iatrogenic hemorrhage during abdominocentesis or centesis of the spleen is not

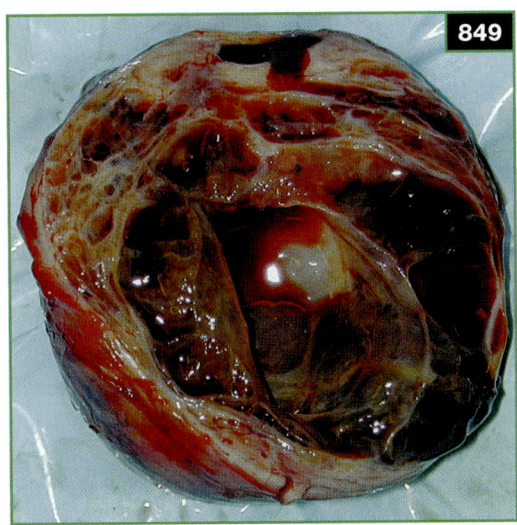

849 Ruptured capsule of ovarian granulosa cell tumors can be the source of abdominal hemorrhage.

interpreted as hemoperitoneum. In the early stages of hemoperitoneum, the erythrocyte count is generally less than or equal to the peripheral blood erythrocyte count. In chronic intra-abdominal hemorrhage the erythrocyte count is usually equal to or greater than the peripheral blood erythrocyte count due to protein and fluid resorption. On cytologic examination, platelets are not typically present unless the hemorrhage is peracute. Evidence of erythrophagocytosis suggests that the hemorrhage is subacute or chronic. In chronic hemorrhage, hypersegmented pyknotic neutrophils and hemosiderophages are observed. Hematologic abnormalities associated with acute blood loss will be seen after the initial 24 hours and include anemia and decreased total plasma protein.

Hypoproteinemia is usually observed prior to the decline in hematocrit. If there is no obvious explanation for the hemorrhage, a coagulation profile should be assessed to rule out coagulopathy. Thrombocytopenia is common and usually secondary to blood loss; however, immune-mediated thrombocytopenia (IMTP) can occur.

Management
The initial treatment of abdominal blood loss should be directed toward the treatment of hypovolemic shock. Intravenous fluid therapy with isotonic crystalloid solutions to increase vascular volume is indicated. The required fluid rate varies depending on the cardiovascular status and the volume of blood loss. In general, about three times the volume of blood loss should be replaced with crystalloids. If hypovolemic shock is present, shock-rate fluid administration (20–40 ml/kg/hour) is indicated initially. Replacement of intravascular volume may also be accomplished with hypertonic saline (4–6 ml/kg of 5.0–7.5% NaCl), followed by administration of isotonic fluids. However, when blood loss is not controlled, hypertonic saline administration is contraindicated. When the hematocrit is 0.15 l/l (15%) or lower or when the hemoglobin concentration is <50 g/l (5 g/dl), whole blood transfusion is usually required; however, with chronic blood loss horses may better tolerate a low hematocrit. Clinical signs should be taken into consideration when deciding whether transfusion is required. The volume of blood transfusion will depend on the rate and quantity of blood loss.

Abdominal surgery may be required to control hemorrhage from tumors, rupture of a viscus, or leaking GI vessels.

The opioid antagonist naloxone (one treatment of 8 mg i/v) or 10% buffered neutral formalin (10–30 ml added to 500 ml of 0.09% NaCl) has been anecdotally reported as being used to control hemorrhages in horses; however, objective evaluation of efficacy is unavailable and some clinicians oppose the rather drastic measure of formalin administration.

Prognosis
The prognosis is variable but often poor, and depends on the cause of hemorrhage.

Penetrating abdominal wounds
Definition/overview
A wound that breaches the abdominal skin, musculature, and peritoneum, potentially causing damage to the underlying abdominal organs, may be classified as a penetrating abdominal wound. The behavior of horses makes penetrating wounds more common compared to other species.

Etiology/pathophysiology
Impalement of the horse's abdomen on a sharp object such as a fence post or part of a tree branch is a common cause of penetrating wounds. Occasionally, a horse may sustain a penetrating wound (see **1280**) to the abdomen when landing on an object over which it is jumping, such as in equestrian sports. There have also been reports of shotgun wounds to the abdomen.

The pathophysiology associated with penetrating abdominal wounds will vary depending on the extent of damage to the underlying abdominal organs and whether the inciting object has left debris or is still contained within the wound. Although the skin wound may be fairly insignificant, there is often a significantly larger amount of damage to the underlying organs.

591

Most of the damage created by deeply penetrating wounds affects the spleen and GI tract. Splenic damage is usually associated with marked hemorrhage and subsequent cardiovascular compromise. There is potential for intestinal perforation and leakage with subsequent peritonitis, and a large rent in the abdominal wall may lead to evisceration. The penetrating object is usually contaminated and, therefore, even if the acute trauma is overcome, there is a high probability of infection during the healing process. Any foreign material left in the wound may cause a persistent infection and draining sinus or may result in abscess formation.

Clinical presentation

There are usually obvious signs of an open abdominal wound; however, the severity of the clinical signs may not correspond with the size of the external wound. There may be abdominal contents visible or palpable through the wound. When associated with damage to major abdominal organs, there are usually accompanying signs of shock. Even with severe internal damage such as intestinal perforation, affected horses may not initially appear significantly compromised. Signs of hypovolemic shock, endotoxemia, sepsis, or peritonitis may develop hours after the incident.

Differential diagnosis

Penetrating abdominal wounds may be confused with deep wounds to the abdominal musculature that have failed to penetrate the peritoneum and have therefore not penetrated the abdomen.

Diagnosis

Diagnosis is usually made by physical examination. Any wound over the abdominal region should be explored carefully to determine whether abdominal penetration has occurred, regardless of the size. Ultrasonographic examination of the abdomen may be useful in determining the organ damage that has occurred and whether there is hemoperitoneum or peritonitis present. Abdominocentesis is important to determine whether there has been intestinal leakage or hemoperitoneum.

Management

In the acutely injured horse, attention must be paid to stabilizing any cardiovascular compensation, especially in those cases where there has been splenic trauma, as is discussed for hemoperitoneum (see p. 590).

Broad-spectrum antimicrobials (e.g. sodium/potassium penicillin 20,000 IU/kg i/v q6h/procaine penicillin 20,000 IU/kg i/m q12h and gentamicin 6.6 mg/kg i/v q24h) should be administered immediately and should be continued until after the abdominal wound has closed. Tetanus prophylaxis must also be considered.

The presence and extent of intestinal damage may only be determined by performing an exploratory laparotomy. Thorough abdominal lavage can also be performed during surgery. Peritoneal lavage can be performed in the awake horse through indwelling drains; however, these often quickly become blocked.

Prognosis

The prognosis for penetrating wounds of the abdomen will vary according to the extent of damage to the underlying organs. If hemorrhage and infection are controlled, splenic trauma may have a fair to guarded prognosis. Cases in which there has been perforation of the bowel or evisceration have a grave prognosis.

If the injury to the abdomen has not traumatized the abdominal organs, the prognosis is improved. The wound in the abdominal wall usually heals well, but there is a high risk of infection, abscess formation, and peritonitis during the healing stages.

Diaphragmatic hernia

Definition/overview

Diaphragmatic hernia results from herniation of abdominal viscera into the thoracic cavity through a diaphragmatic defect (850). It usually leads to hypoventilation and/or simple or strangulated intestinal obstruction.

Etiology/pathophysiology

Diaphragmatic hernia only occurs when a diaphragmatic defect is present. This defect can be congenital or acquired. Congenital defects result from incomplete fusion of the pleuroperitoneal folds, causing an enlarged esophageal hiatus. External trauma, strenuous exercise, GI distension, or pregnancy can increase the intrathoracic or intra-abdominal pressure enough to create an acquired diaphragmatic defect.

Herniated viscera decrease thoracic volume and induce thoracic pain, often resulting in hypoventilation. Herniation through a diaphragmatic defect may result in simple or strangulating intestinal obstruction.

Clinical presentation

Diaphragmatic hernias are most frequently observed in mature horses with a history of trauma, strenuous exercise, breeding, or parturition. Clinical manifestations are frequently nonspecific and may include colic, exercise intolerance, and dyspnea.

Differential diagnosis

All disorders resulting in acute abdominal pain in the horse should be included in the differential diagnosis. Horses with a diaphragmatic hernia may be exercise intolerant. Any disorder of the respiratory, circulatory, and musculoskeletal systems that results in exercise intolerance must be

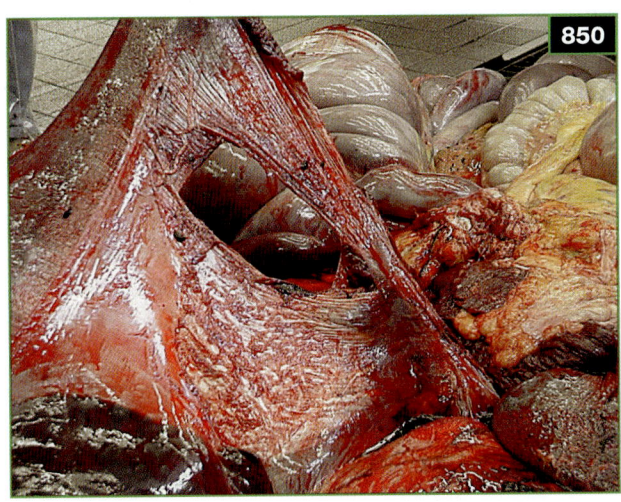

850 Postmortem view of the thoracic surface of an equine diaphragm. Note the very large defect in the ligamentous portion of this diaphragm. In this case both the small intestine and the large colon were herniated into the thoracic cavity.

851, 852 Dorsoventral (851) and lateral (852) thoracic radiographs of a horse with a diaphragmatic hernia. The large colon is within the thoracic cavity. Ingesta in the colon obscures the ventral thoracic viscera. Colonic-wall sacculations are visible dorsally because of gaseous distension.

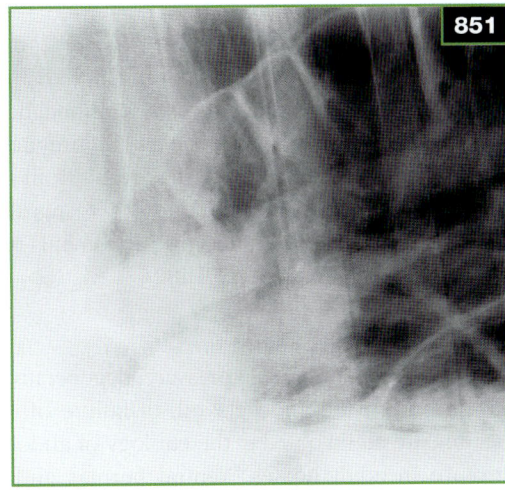

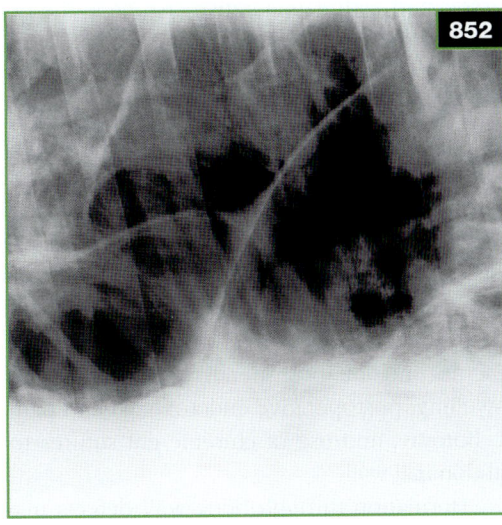

included in the differential diagnosis. Pneumonia and pleuritis should also be included in the differential diagnosis. Horses with diaphragmatic hernias are not usually pyrexic, depressed, or have an inflammatory leukogram.

Diagnosis

Even with careful examination, diagnosis of diaphragmatic hernia can be difficult and is sometimes only made at the time of surgery or necropsy. Careful thoracic auscultation and percussion should be performed in all horses with colic, particularly those with a history of trauma or parturition. Areas of thoracic dullness or reduced cardiac sounds may be identified during thoracic auscultation or percussion. Referred GI sounds are frequently heard over the caudoventral thorax in normal horses and thus cannot be used for definitive diagnosis. Perception of an empty caudal abdomen may occur during palpation per rectum. Standing lateral thoracic radiographs are used to diagnose diaphragmatic hernia. Radiographic signs include gas-filled intestinal loops in the thoracic cavity, increased ventral thoracic density, and absence of the cardiac shadow (851, 852). Loss of the diaphragmatic shadow in the area of the hernia is the most consistently observed radiographic sign. Thoracic ultrasonography may show the presence of pleural fluid and abdominal viscera in the thoracic cavity.

Hypercapnea, as a result of hypoventilation, may be present. Respiratory acidosis or uncompensated metabolic acidosis is usually observed in horses with a diaphragmatic hernia, whereas the most common acid–base derangement in horses with colic is metabolic acidosis with respiratory compensation. Abdominocentesis is usually normal; however, hemorrhagic fluid may be obtained with an acute acquired diaphragm defect and serosanguineous, turbid fluid may be present if intestinal strangulation has occurred.

593

Management

Horses with intractable abdominal pain or respiratory distress require an emergency exploratory celiotomy with assisted positive-pressure ventilation. Surgical treatment consists of reduction of the herniated viscera, resection of devitalized intestine and intestinal anastomosis, and repair of the diaphragmatic defect. In horses with acute diaphragmatic defects secondary to trauma, surgery may be delayed if the animal's condition is stable. Delay allows for the development of fibrosis of the edges of the defect and easier surgical closure.

Prognosis

Horses with diaphragmatic hernia have a poor to guarded prognosis for survival.

Abdominal hernia and prepubic tendon rupture

Definition/overview

Abdominal viscera may herniate through an anatomic opening or a defect in the abdominal wall. Abdominal herniation includes ventral hernias, incisional hernias, and acquired inguinal/scrotal hernias. In pregnant mares, defects in the abdominal wall may result from stretching/tearing of the abdominal wall muscles (rectus abdominus, oblique abdominal, and transverse abdominus muscles) or the prepubic tendon (see 477–482).

Etiology/pathophysiology

Increased intra-abdominal pressure, degenerative changes in the body wall, and delayed, or failure of, linea alba healing are all involved in the etiology of abdominal-wall rupture in adult horses. Ventral hernias and prepubic tendon ruptures usually occur in pregnant mares and are associated with degenerative change in the body wall in old broodmares, twin gestation, hydroallantois, and/or trauma.

Incisional herniation is a complication of ventral celiotomy that is reported to occur in 0.7–15% of horses that undergo this procedure. In the author's experience, incisional hernia is a rare (<5%) complication of ventral celiotomy. No breed or sex predilection exists. Dehiscence (acute incisional disruption) usually develops within 8 days after surgery. Incisional herniation can develop up to 3 months after ventral celiotomy. Incisional hernia risk factors include postoperative incisional infection and swelling, postoperative endotoxemia and pain, repeated celiotomy, and use of chromic gut sutures to close the abdominal wall.

Herniation through body-wall defects may result in simple or strangulated intestinal obstruction.

Clinical presentation

Horses with ventral herniation or prepubic tendon rupture display severe ventral abdominal swelling/edema and are reluctant to walk. They often lie down and are commonly distressed with increased heart and respiratory rates. Signs of abdominal pain may be present if the herniated contents are compromised.

Ventral swelling developing over the abdominal incision site is observed in horses with incisional herniation. In these horses, a brown serosanguineous discharge from the incision and a progressive increase in drainage of peritoneal fluid are commonly observed prior to dehiscence.

Differential diagnosis

Ventral herniation should be differentiated from prepubic tendon rupture because generally the latter is not correctable surgically. In mares with ventral herniation, the orientation of the pelvis and the mammary gland is normal. In horses with prepubic tendon rupture, the pelvis rotates cranioventrally as the prepubic tendon tension is lost from the cranial aspect of the pelvis. Lordosis may also be noticed because the pelvis and vertebral column cannot maintain normal alignment. Cranioventral displacement of the udder resulting from the tipping of the pelvis can lead to rupture of the blood supply. Blood may be observed in the milk of mares with prebubic tendon rupture.

Postoperative wound infection, severe peri-incisional edema, seroma, and sinus formation are easily differentiated from incisional hernias, with the abdominal wall being intact on palpation.

Diagnosis

External palpation and palpation per rectum are helpful to diagnose these conditions. In ventral and incisional herniation, external palpation of the abdominal wall may define the hernia ring and hernia contents. When there is extensive abdominal edema this procedure is difficult. Commonly, mares with a ventral hernia resent deep palpation of the affected area. In ventral hernia, rectal palpation may help to differentiate the condition from prepubic tendon rupture. However, per rectum palpation of the abdominal wall defect can be difficult depending on the defect's location and on the size of the fetus. Palpation of distended loops of intestine associated with abdominal pain warrants immediate exploratory laparotomy.

Transcutaneous ultrasonographic examination with a 3.5 or 5-MHz transducer is helpful to rule in herniation and to evaluate the extent of the abdominal-wall defect (see 479–482).

Management

Ventral hernia

Surgical herniorrhaphy is advocated. If the mare is close to term (at least 330 days pregnant), parturition should be induced prior to surgery. Delivery should be assisted because abdominal contractions are often insufficient. When acute herniation occurs without clinical evidence of intestinal obstruction, the surgical treatment should be delayed to allow formation of fibrosis within the hernia ring. In this case, management consists of the application of an abdominal support bandage (see **483**), the use of anti-inflammatory drugs to decrease swelling, and feeding a low-residue pelleted ration to decrease intestinal bulk volume. Once clinical signs of intestinal obstruction are present, surgical treatment should be performed without delay. Suture or mesh herniorrhaphy is performed depending on the diameter of the hernia ring.

Pre-pubic tendon rupture

This condition usually cannot be surgically corrected. Conservative treatment may be attempted. Parturition should be induced if the mare is close to term. The mare should be rested in a box stall for several months and abdominal support should be applied. If severe edema is present initially, anti-inflammatory medications should be administered. Low-bulk pelleted food should be offered to the mare to decrease the volume of digesta.

Incisional hernia

In general, surgical herniorrhaphy is postponed for 4–6 months to allow for resolution of any infection and the development of hernia ring fibrosis. Initially, an abdominal support bandage is applied and antimicrobials are administered based on wound culture and sensitivity. Ventral drainage is established and the infected wound is lavaged with a diluted antiseptic solution. Suture or mesh herniorrhaphy is performed when incisional infection has resolved.

Prognosis

The prognosis for successful correction of a ventral hernia is guarded. Incisional herniations warrant a favorable prognosis. Three to 5 months of rest are required after surgical correction of both ventral and incisional hernias. The prognosis for prepubic tendon rupture is poor.

Septic peritonitis

Definition/overview

Peritonitis is inflammation of the mesothelial lining of the peritoneal cavity. While any inflammatory stimulus can cause peritonitis, septic peritonitis is the most common in horses.

Etiology/pathophysiology

Leakage or translocation of intestinal bacteria is the most common cause. Gastric rupture, intestinal rupture, rectal tear, bacterial translocation in cases of severe enterocolitis, abdominal perforation by foreign bodies, and breeding injury in mares are most commonly implicated. A hematogenous source is uncommon in adult horses, but may occur in septic neonates. Rupture of an abdominal abscess may also cause peritonitis. A small percentage of horses develop peritonitis after colic surgery.

Clinical presentation

Clinical signs are variable and depend on the duration of disease and degree of intestinal contamination. Signs in horses with acute colonic rupture and gross contamination of the abdomen usually progress rapidly. With slowly leaking intestinal viscera or a lower level of contamination from bacterial translocation or hematogenous spread, the clinical progression may be more gradual. If intestinal rupture has occurred and septic peritonitis is developing, affected animals may actually appear to improve initially as signs of colic abate. Fever and depression may be present initially, but the condition typically progresses rapidly as septic shock develops. Body temperature may be elevated, normal, or decreased. Heart rate is almost invariably elevated and can be very high (>100 bpm). Respiratory rate is usually elevated. Mucous membranes progress from normal to hyperemic to cyanotic. GI sounds decrease and dehydration develops as fluid is sequestered in the abdomen. A variable degree of colic may be evident. Sweating and anxiety are common.

Differential diagnosis

Colitis, pleuritis, strangulating intestinal lesions, and other causes of sepsis or endotoxemia may appear similar.

Diagnosis

Physical examination is suggestive but not definitive. Neutropenia with toxic changes in neutrophils is almost always present, but is nonspecific. Total protein levels tend to decrease rapidly and hematologic changes consistent with dehydration and metabolic acidosis may be present. Occasionally, the intestinal viscera will feel 'gritty' per rectum. Sometimes, the abdomen will feel abnormally empty following intestinal rupture. A large volume of

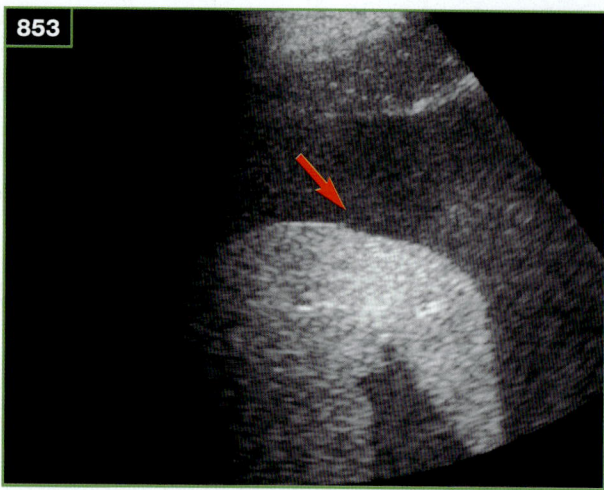

853 Excessive hyperechoic free abdominal fluid (arrowed) is evident in this horse with septic peritonitis.

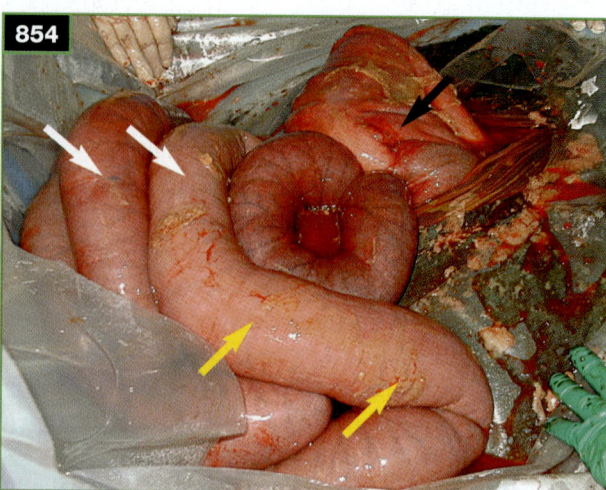

854 Distended small intestine (white arrows) and cecum (black arrow) with patches of fibrin (yellow arrows) in a horse with septic peritonitis.

hyperechoic abdominal fluid is usually evident ultrasono-graphically (**853**). Abdominocentesis is invaluable. With peritonitis, abdominal fluid may range from serosan-guineous and turbid to brownish with the presence of ingesta. Typically, marked increases in cell count (15–800 x 10^9/l) with degenerative changes in neutrophils and an increased total protein level are present. Intracellular bacteria are often evident cytologically. Bacterial culture of abdominal fluid is particularly useful if a ruptured abdominal abscess is suspected. Occasionally, normal abdominal fluid is obtained because of pocketing of fluid, particularly early in the disease, so abdominocentesis should be repeated in a horse with suspected septic peri-tonitis, but a normal initial tap, if clinical signs progress.

Management

Aggressive and early therapy is required. The inciting cause must be identified and addressed whenever possi-ble. Exploratory laparotomy is often indicated (**854**). Surgery allows for identification of the inciting cause as well as thorough abdominal lavage and placement of abdominal drains.

Intravenous fluid therapy is required. High fluid rates are often necessary early in the disease because of dehy-dration and cardiovascular compromise. Plasma trans-fusion may be required. Broad-spectrum antimicrobial therapy, including adequate anaerobic coverage (e.g. sodium/potassium penicillin 20,000 IU/kg i/v q6h and gentamicin 6.6 mg/kg i/v q24h), should be instituted immediately. Metronidazole (20–25 mg/kg p/o q6–8h) is

sometimes added for its additional anaerobic spectrum. Treatment can be changed if necessary based on culture and sensitivity results. Flunixin meglumine is typically used for its anti-inflammatory/analgesic (1.1 mg/kg i/v q12h) or anti-endotoxin (0.25–0.5 mg/kg q8h) effects.

Lavage of the abdomen is essential. Lavage can consist of a single ventral drain or a combination of dorsal ingress and ventral egress drains. Drains can be placed in standing sedated horses, ideally with ultrasonographic guidance. Horses should be stabilized before drainage and intra-venous fluid therapy should be administered to compen-sate for any fluid shifts that may occur. For lavage in adult horses, 10–20 liters of balanced electrolyte solution should be infused, then the drain(s) should be clamped and the horse walked for 10–20 minutes to distribute the fluid, after which the drain is opened. Further walking can facilitate drainage. Intraperitoneal administration of antimicrobials is not usually indicated. Infusion of other substances such as heparin has been used to decrease adhesion formation, but its efficacy has not been proven.

Prognosis

The prognosis depends on the cause of the peritonitis and the severity of the disease. If the underlying cause cannot be identified and promptly corrected, the prognosis is grave. Peritonitis caused by intestinal rupture is almost invariably fatal. With rapid and aggressive therapy, overall survival rates of 40–70% have been reported. Complica-tions are common and include intestinal adhesions and laminitis. Treatment can be prolonged and expensive.

5

Liver

Thomas Koch, Anthony Knight, and Scott Weese

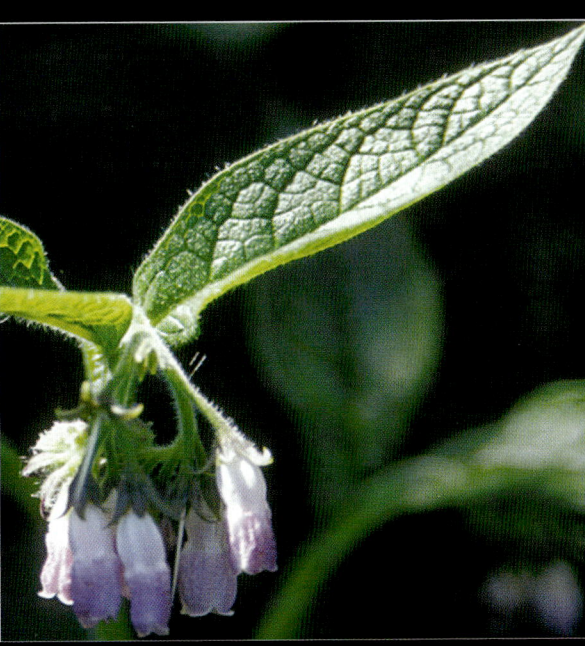

Liver

Most equine practitioners will at some point in their career encounter an equid with liver problems. Signs of liver problems can vary from ill-thrift to severe CNS disease. Significant, but poorly understood, metabolic differences seem to exist between horses and ponies, miniature horses and donkeys, resulting in differences in susceptibility and incidence of certain diseases. The prognosis varies greatly depending on the nature of the liver disease and underlying diseases, but is often guarded.

General considerations

Clinical signs of liver disease

There are no pathognomonic signs associated with liver disease or liver failure. Liver disease can be inapparent or manifested by an impressive array of clinical signs, including depression, anorexia, abdominal pain, encephalopathy, weight loss, jaundice/icterus (**855**), abnormal intestinal motility, abnormal fecal consistency, dehydration, photosensitization, bilateral laryngeal paralysis with dyspnea or severe inspiratory stridor, coagulopathy, dermatitis and pruritus, peripheral edema, oral ulceration, tenesmus, penile prolapse, hemoglobinuria due to a severe hemolytic crisis, pain on deep palpation under the right abdominal rib curvature, fever, and discolored feces in foals. Common neurologic signs are nonspecific and include ataxia, dysmetria, stupor, coma, compulsive circling, head pressing, and prolonged mastication of food without swallowing. Deep palpation of the abdomen in very small horses and foals might reveal abnormal liver size or an infected and pus-filled umbilical vein. Palpation with the hands flat (as opposed to using the fingertips) against the abdominal wall allows optimal exploration due to improved patient compliance. Palpation of foals placed in different positions might also be beneficial. Clinical signs can be acute or chronic and primary or secondary in nature and reflect damage to the biliary system, hepatocytes, or fibrosis of the liver.

Icterus/jaundice (hyperbilirubinemia)

Icterus generally reflects increased levels (2–3 times normal) of unconjugated (indirect reacting) bilirubin. Icterus does not always indicate liver disease and can be present in normal horses under certain circumstances. This is termed physiologic icterus and can occur for one of three reasons: a high basal concentration of unconjugated bilirubin despite normal liver function; increased serum carotene levels as may be present in some grazing horses; and decreased hepatic removal of unconjugated bilirubin and icterus associated with anorexia.

Clinicopathologic abnormalities and function testing

Complete blood count

A CBC is indicated in cases of possible liver disease, although significant changes often are absent. Anemia and a mature leucocytosis might indicate chronic inflammatory disease. Leukopenia, especially if accompanied by increased band-formed neutrophils and toxic changes, might indicate acute severe infection or inflammation. Cytologic evaluation of a blood smear is important to identify abnormal blood cells. Erythrocyte abnormalities that might be noted in a cytologic examination include toxic insults such as Heinz body formation and erythroid parasites such as *Babesia* spp. Neutrophils should be evaluated for toxic changes and possible infectious agents such as *Anaplasma phagocytophila*. Circulating macrophages should be evaluated for possible intracellular morulas indicative of *Neorickettsia risticii*.

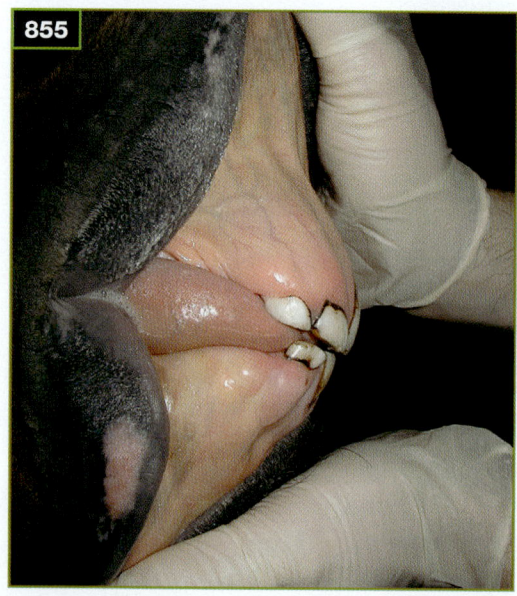

855 Icteric oral mucous membranes.

Enzymes

The most reliable diagnostic enzymatic parameter of cholestasis is elevated serum gamma-glutamyltransferase (GGT). While primarily an indicator of cholestatic disease, increases in GGT can also occur with severe and chronic hepatocellular disease. Sorbitol dehydrogenase (SDH) is very specific and has been widely used to assess hepatocellular disease. The use of this enzyme has, in the past, been largely restricted to larger referral centers due to its very labile nature and the need for special transportation precautions to obtain accurate results. Modern courier services and in-transport refrigeration might make this enzyme assay more available to practitioners. The serum glutamate dehydrogenase (GLDH) level is commonly used instead of SDH as an indicator of acute hepatocyte damage due to its specificity and *in-vitro* stability. AST elevation, although also indicative of muscle disease, is commonly seen when clinical signs of liver disease are initially noted. AST might return to within normal limits in chronic liver disease. This return of AST to within normal limits could be due to overall loss of hepatic mass with chronic liver disease. GLDH levels quickly return to normal or even below normal after an acute injury, therefore serial monitoring can be useful for evaluation of response to treatment and for prognosis. LDH elevation reflects hepatocyte damage, but is only useful if isoenzyme determination is performed because of its widespread tissue distribution. This is rarely indicated because of the availability of better options. Alkaline phosphatase (AP) is often reported as elevated in chronic liver disease, but the enzyme is not specific for liver disease and is less sensitive than GGT for cholestatic disease.

Function tests

The classic liver function test in horses is the bromsulphalein (BSP) dye clearance test where 2 mg/kg of exogenous BSP is injected intravenously and venous blood samples are obtained prior to and 5, 7, 9, and 11 minutes after injection. Dye-based function testing is rarely performed because there are few advantages over bilirubin, bile acid, and ammonia analyses.

Bilirubin

Bilirubin is a breakdown product of normal heme metabolism and increased serum concentrations are noted as icterus/jaundice on physical examination. Pathologic hyperbilirubinemia due to liver failure, cholestasis, or hemolysis must be differentiated from the physiologic hyperbilirubinemia often encountered in fasting or anorexic horses. Distinction between unconjugated (albumin-bound) and conjugated (water-soluble) bilirubin is important. Elevated levels of unconjugated bilirubin reflect physiologic hyperbilirubinemia, decreased hepatocellular function, or hepatocellular overload (i.e. hemolysis).

Elevated levels of conjugated bilirubin reflect cholestasis and reflux into the systemic circulation. Bilirubin evaluation is regarded by some as a function test since abnormal hepatocyte function, in some instances, is the cause of hyperbilirubinemia.

Bile acids

Evaluation of serum bile acids concentration is the easiest and most practical means of evaluating liver function. Elevation in serum bile acids concentration has a high sensitivity and specificity for hepatocellular damage, cholestasis, or portosystemic shunting. Since the horse has no gallbladder, a single sample unrelated to feeding can be used. Increased levels of serum bile acids reflect liver dysfunction. Reference ranges for bile acids are laboratory specific.

Nonliver-specific clinicopathologic abnormalities

Ammonia and urea

Ammonia is normally converted to urea by the liver and then excreted by the kidneys. In the face of hepatocellular compromise, inadequate conversion results in hyperammonemia. Hyperammonemia is often present in severe cases of hepatic encephalopathy, but a significant association between the two remains to be found. Decreased serum urea concentration is rarely noted. To measure ammonia, heparinized venous blood should be transported on ice to the laboratory immediately. Delays or improper storage may result in artificially low ammonia levels. Dry chemistry techniques are available. For result validation, pairing the sample with one from a normal horse is recommended.

Proteins and amino acids

Significant hypoproteinemia or hypoalbuminemia is uncommon in horses with liver disease and is typically present only in end-stage disease. A decreased albumin/globulin ratio might be noted and likely reflects increased alpha- and beta-globulin production. Liver disease causes decreased levels of short branched-chain amino acids (valine, leucine, and isoleucine) and increased levels of aromatic amino acids (phenylalanine, free tryptophan, and tyrosine). These are rarely evaluated.

Clotting factors

Clotting factors are produced in the liver and decreased levels may be present with severe liver disease. Elevations in activated partial thromboplastin time (PTT) and prothrombin time (PT) indicate coagulopathy. Laboratory reference ranges can vary greatly, so laboratory-specific ranges should be used when interpreting results. Abnormal clotting times carry a poor prognosis for survival since they are not affected until very late in disease.

Glucose

Hypoglycemia, due to decreased gluconeogenesis, may be present in horses with hypertriglyceridemia and fatty liver. Hyperglycemia may occur with other liver diseases from insulin resistance or increased cortisol from stress of disease or hospitalization.

Electrolyte and acid–base status

There are no specific electrolyte or acid–base abnormalities associated with liver disease. However, electrolyte and acid–base abnormalities are common in severely affected horses due to dehydration. Metabolic acidosis is therefore most commonly seen. Hypoproteinemia can result in alkalosis in some cases.

Urobilinogen

Urobilinogen is a water-soluble intestinal breakdown product of conjugated bilirubin that enters the porto-hepatic system and subsequently the systemic circulation, from where it is excreted in the urine. Absence of urinary urobilinogen indicates complete biliary blockage, whereas increased urinary urobilinogen indicates increased heme metabolism (hemolysis).

Diagnostic tests

Ultrasonography

The liver is normally visible by ultrasonography on the right side from the 6th to the 15th intercostal spaces (ICSs) ventral to the lung and cranioventrally on the left side between the 6th and 9th ICSs (856, 857). The left liver lobe is located medial to the spleen. In general the transducer with the highest frequency able to penetrate to the desired depth of investigation should be used. The smallest depth of field should be used and the liver should be evaluated in both dorsal and transverse planes. Normal liver parenchyma appears homogeneous and of medium echogenicity (858–861). The portal and hepatic veins are normally visible in a branching pattern. Of the two, the portal veins have the thicker and more echogenic walls. Bile ducts are not normally visible. The ventral margins of the liver should appear sharp bilaterally. The size and the visible area of the liver vary with age and conformation of the horse, but often 4–8 cm of parenchyma is visible in the young horse. The liver gradually decreases in size with age and in some older horses the right lobe cannot be visualized.

Ultrasonography can be of great value for differentiation of acute hepatocellular necrosis, chronic fibrosis, hepatic congestion, and cavities caused by hydatid cysts, polycystic liver disease, abscesses, or neoplasia. Acute hepatocellular necrosis can appear ultrasonographically as a 'collapsed liver', where the parenchyma has decreased echogenicity and the portal veins appear hyperechogenic. A cirrhotic liver also appears reduced in size, but the parenchyma is hyperechoic due to fibrosis and the portal veins are not as prominent or hyperechogenic. Iron toxicity can be associated with bile duct proliferation and cholestatic hepatopathy. Suppurative hepatitis, an uncommon condition, produces an inconsistent ultrasonographic

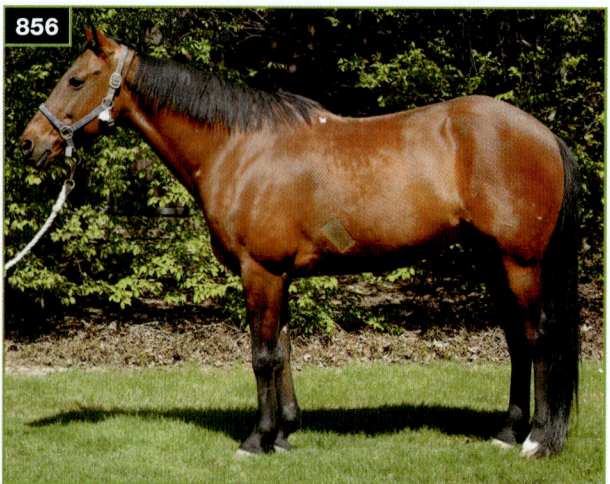

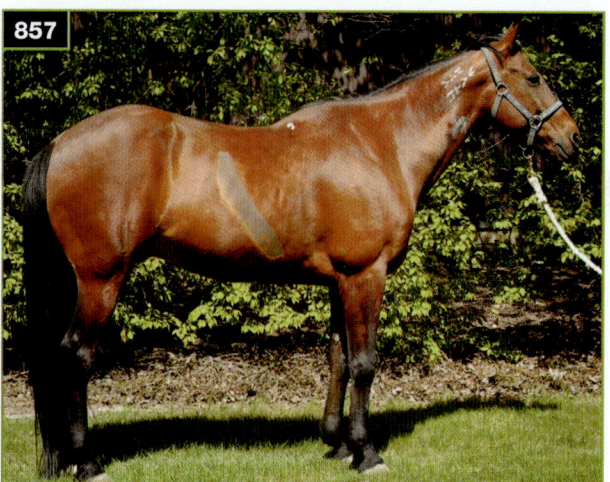

856, 857 Ultrasonography can be of great value for differentiation of acute hepatocellular necrosis, chronic fibrosis, hepatic congestion, cystic liver disease, abscesses, and neoplasia. The left liver lobe is located medial to the spleen between the 6th and 9th ICSs, as demonstrated by the clipped area (856). On the right side the liver is generally visible between the 6th and 15th ICSs ventral to the lung, as demonstrated by the clipped area (857).

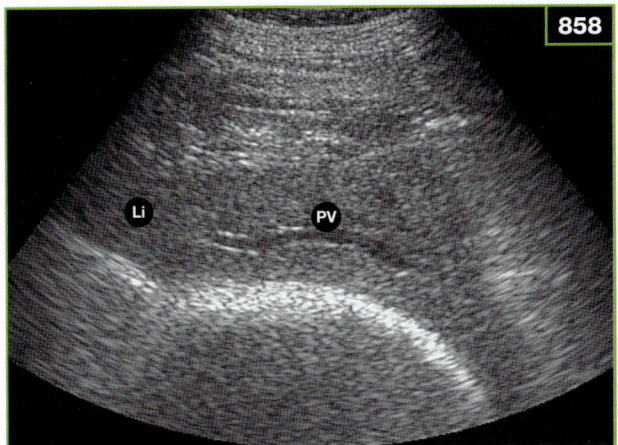

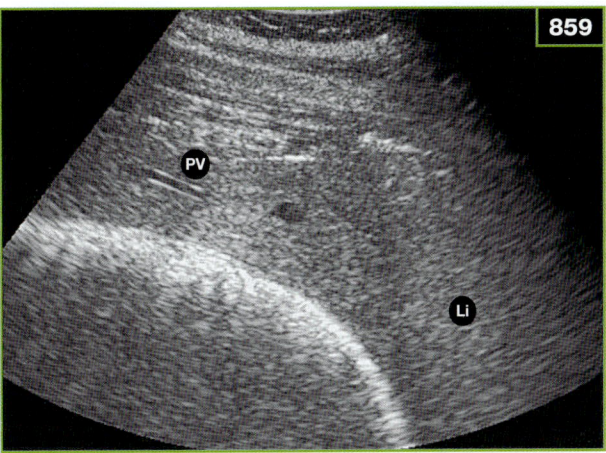

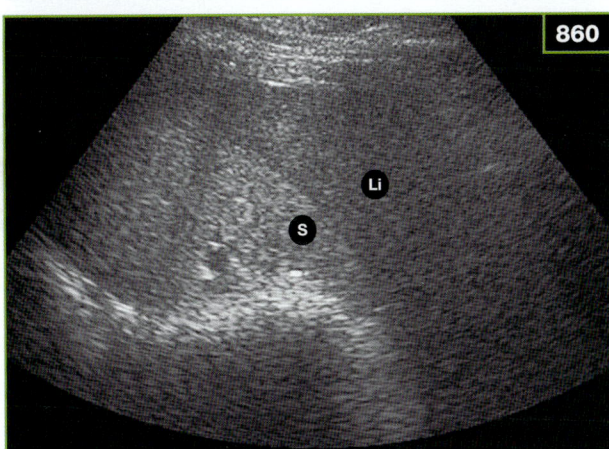

858, 859 Ultrasonographic appearance of the liver (Li) and nearby organs at the 15th (858) and 14th (859) ICSs on the right side. Note the portal vein (PV) with characteristic thick hyperechogenic walls.

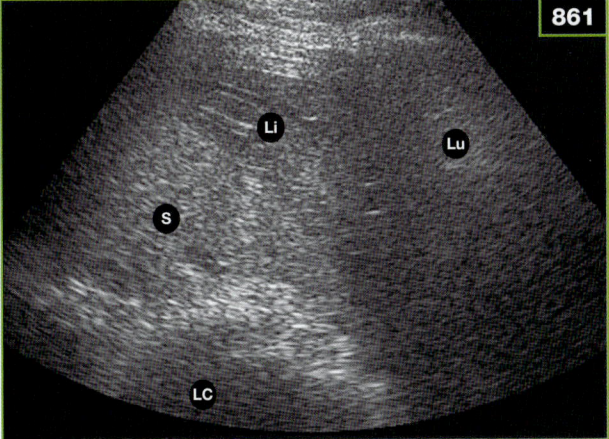

860, 861 Ultrasonographic appearance of the liver and nearby organs at the 9th ICS on the left side. Note that the splenic parenchyma is hyperechogenic compared with the hepatic parenchyma. Li, liver; Lu, lung; LC, large colon; S, spleen.

appearance ranging from a very enlarged liver with bulging capsular areas and rounded margins, to multifocal areas of hyper- or hypoechogenicity. Diffuse inflammatory diseases often appear as an overall increase in echogenicity. Dilated bile ducts are often found in cases of cholangitis, cholelithiasis, and liver fluke infestation. Dilated hepatic veins characterize hepatomegaly due to venous congestion caused by cardiac failure. Cavities with hypoechoic material might be hydatid cysts, abscesses, or neoplasia. Abscesses and neoplasia have an inconsistent appearance and often biopsies are needed to differentiate between them. However, aspiration of a liver abscess carries a high risk of septic peritonitis and is generally not recommended.

Most equine liver conditions are diffuse in nature, but focal liver disease might not be identified due to the limited visible area of the liver. Ultrasonography is very helpful in identifying suitable biopsy sites and guiding biopsy collection.

Radiography/scintigraphy

Radiographic evaluation of the liver is not possible in the adult horse and is rarely indicated in foals because other imaging modalities are superior.

Scintigraphic evaluation of the liver has been reported in limited instances. Scintigraphy offers visualization of the whole liver field, but multiple views are needed due to the thickness of the organ, and lesions less than 2.5 cm in diameter might not be visible. Comparing results with an age- and size-matched individual might be beneficial since distribution of the radio-isotope seems to differ greatly between different protocols.

Intraoperative mesenteric portography

Definitive diagnosis of portosystemic shunts can be obtained by operative mesenteric portography, in which radiographic contrast medium is injected into a mesenteric vein while radiographs of the abdomen are obtained.

Liver biopsy

Liver biopsy is a relatively easy and very useful diagnostic and prognostic tool, providing samples for culture as well as cytologic and histologic evaluation. Ultrasonography of the liver prior to biopsy is a great help in identifying an affected area suitable for biopsy and decreasing the chance of inadvertent biopsy of other structures. Aspiration of a liver abscess carries a high risk of septic peritonitis and is generally not recommended. Liver biopsies can be obtained blindly by placing the biopsy needle in the right 14th ICS on a line between the tuber coxae and the right shoulder point. However, blind biopsy carries a greater risk of complications because of the somewhat variable position of the lung and colon. Pointing the tip towards the left elbow (olecranon) increases the chance of sampling parenchyma and reduces the risk of inadvertent puncture of vessels or other organs. The biopsy needle (Vim Silverman or 'Tru-Cut') often needs to be inserted 4–8 cm before a good sample is obtained. Clotting profile evaluation is often recommended prior to liver biopsy; however, it is not always performed because of the rarity of clotting abnormalities and the importance of biopsy results. Physical and/or chemical sedation is recommended and clipping, surgical scrub, and local anesthesia are mandatory. Local anesthetic should be infused deeply. A stab incision of the skin at the insertion point greatly reduces skin drag on the biopsy needle. Multiple biopsies should be obtained.

Prognosis

The prognosis is highly variable and there are few objective guidelines. Severe hepatic encephalopathy, bilateral laryngeal dysfunction, gastric impaction, and hemolysis secondary to liver disease generally indicate a poor to grave prognosis. Other unfavorable indicators are histologic evidence of fibrosis, hypoalbuminemia (<25 g/l), hyperglobulinemia, prolonged PT (>30% of normal), and elevated GGT and AP levels in the face of normal to decreased dehydrogenase (SDH and GLDH) levels. A retrospective study of 84 horses with primary liver disease reported the following survival rates: 70% (7/10) with non-specific liver failure, 58% (11/19) with cholangiohepatitis, 24% (7/29) with pyrrolizidine alkaloid (PA) toxicity, and 8% (2/26) with serum hepatitis.

Diseases of the liver

Liver failure

Definition/overview

Liver failure is uncommon and occurs when the reserve and regenerative capacities of the liver are exceeded. The results are somewhat variable and depend on the etiology, time of onset, and signalment of the patient. In fulminant cases of liver failure, severe metabolic and/or neurologic disturbances are commonly encountered.

Etiology/pathophysiology

There are a variety of potential causes of liver failure including toxic, infectious, inflammatory, and neoplastic causes. Specific etiologies are discussed below. Often, the cause is not identified.

The reserve capacity of the liver is an amazing 70–80% and signs of liver failure are not seen until liver disease exceeds this limit. Equally astounding is the capacity of the liver to regenerate after a severe insult if a few crucial conditions are fulfilled. The three main conditions for regeneration include the presence of functional mitotic hepatocytes, an intact scaffold for the new hepatocytes, and blood supply from the portal vein. Obviously, regeneration will not occur if hepatocytes are rendered incapable of mitosis by exposure to anti-mitotic agents. Fibrosis, noted as bridging of hepatic lobules on histologic sections, prevents proper regeneration since the scaffold is interrupted and the scar tissue limits blood supply to the area.

Horses in liver failure are often presented with varying degrees of hepatic encephalopathy and many of the treatment strategies for liver failure attempt to address this condition. Understanding of the possible causes of hepatic encephalopathy is therefore important.

Clinical presentation

Clinical signs associated with liver failure are generally severe. Patients with hepatic encephalopathy may present with ataxia, dysmetria, stupor, coma, compulsive circling, head pressing against fixed objects, and prolonged mastication of food without swallowing. Bilateral laryngeal paralysis leading to dyspnea and inspiratory stridor, as well as colic due to gastric impaction caused by vagal dysfunction, may also occur. Other signs of liver failure are depression, anorexia, abdominal pain, weight loss, jaundice/icterus, abnormal intestinal motility, abnormal fecal consistency, dehydration, photosensitization of unpigmented areas, coagulopathy, dermatitis, pruritus, peripheral edema, oral ulceration, tenesmus, penile prolapse, hemoglobinuria, pain on deep palpation under the right abdominal rib curvature, fever, and discolored feces in foals.

Differential diagnosis

Common differential diagnoses for liver failure in adult horses include Theiler's disease, cholangiohepatitis/choledocholithiasis, chronic active inflammatory hepatitis, PA toxicosis, hyperlipemia (ponies and miniature horses), and toxic hepatopathies. Uncommon causes of overt liver failure include hepatic abscessation and hepatic/biliary neoplasia. Rabies should be included in the differential list of any horse with sudden CNS signs.

Foals are more likely to suffer from Tyzzer's disease, toxic hepatopathies, bacterial hepatitis secondary to septicemia, and EHV-1 hepatopathy.

Diagnosis

Liver diseases without accompanying signs of hepatic encephalopathy are often chronic, with varying degrees of hepatobiliary-specific clinicopathologic abnormalities. Horses may be presented with weight loss, anorexia, and intermittent colic signs. A CBC might reflect chronic inflammation (mature neutrophilia), anemia of chronic disease, or signs of acute inflammation such as increased band-formed neutrophils and possibly neutrophils with toxic changes in cases of acute active exacerbation of chronic disease. Increased plasma fibrinogen might also be present due to chronic ongoing inflammation.

Clinical presentation is suggestive but not diagnostic for liver failure. The presence of hepatic encephalopathy is generally the difference between horses with liver failure and horses with liver disease. A diagnosis of liver failure is made on ruling out other causes of CNS signs and demonstrating clinicopathologic and other positive diagnostic findings compatible with liver disease.

Elevations of liver enzymes, in particular GLDH and GGT, and elevated conjugated bilirubin are typically present. Enzymes such as GLDH, which are indicative of hepatocellular damage, may be normal if an acute insult was present but has passed and liver failure remains. Serum bile acids are elevated. Blood ammonia may be elevated. PT and PTT are usually normal. Elevations indicate particularly severe disease and a very poor prognosis. Blood glucose level may be decreased and should be monitored regularly. Evaluation of acid–base status is useful to guide initial therapy. Urinalysis is variable and the urine often appears dark because of high bilirubin levels.

Liver ultrasound with biopsy is important and is often the most rewarding diagnostic and prognostic tool in horses with liver disease.

Ultrasound may reveal the nature of disease (e.g. necrosis, fibrosis, venous congestion) and should be used to guide biopsies when possible. Biopsy samples should be submitted for bacterial culture, cytologic analysis, and histopathology. Biopsy can often identify the type of disease (infectious, toxic, inflammatory, neoplastic) but, partcularly if late, may not identify a specific cause.

Management

Supportive treatment is the most important aspect in most cases. If recent ingestion of a toxin is suspected, oral administration of mineral oil or activated charcoal may be useful, although the toxic insult typically occurs well before the development of clinical signs. Often, multiple problems are encountered and each must be individually addressed. If a toxic cause is suspected, changes in housing, feed, or drug administration may be useful. Drugs should be chosen with care since normal hepatic metabolism may be disturbed.

Fluid therapy is critical in most cases, at least early in treatment. Intravenous administration of isotonic crystalloids will suffice in most cases. Theoretically, fluids should not contain lactate because it requires hepatic metabolism. Lactate-containing fluids are often used because of availability, cost, and convenience. If acidosis does not respond to initial volume expansion, sodium bicarbonate supplementation (50 g/500 kg horse i/v or p/o q12h) may be necessary. Potassium chloride supplementation (up to 0.5 mEq/kg/hour i/v; 20–50 g/500 kg horse p/o q12h) is useful in anorexic horses.

Severe anemia, thrombocytopenia, and clotting abnormalities can be addressed by whole blood or plasma transfusion. Plasma is preferred if severe anemia is not present. Synthetic colloids and whole blood are best avoided since they may exacerbate hyperammonemia or potentiate coagulopathy.

Antimicrobial treatment of suspected infectious disease should be based on culture and sensitivity testing of biopsy samples. Long-term treatment (up to 3 months) is often required. While awaiting culture results, a combination of gentamicin (6.6 mg/kg i/v q24h) and either intramuscular penicillin (procaine penicillin, 20,000 IU/kg q12h), intravenous penicillin (sodium or potassium penicillin, 20,000 IU/kg q6h), or ampicillin sodium trihydrate (10–15 mg/kg i/v or i/m q6–8h) is often used. Ceftiofur (2–4 mg/kg i/v or i/m q12h) is also reasonable. Trimethoprim/sulfonamide (24–30 mg/kg i/v or p/o q12h) is often used; however, resistance amongst Enterobacteriaceae is a concern.

Nutritional support is critical. A low-protein, high-energy diet with many branched-chain amino acids (valine, leucine, isoleucine) is ideal. Oat hay or grass hay in combination with cracked corn and molasses is a reasonable first choice. However, if these first choices are rejected, then any food is better than nothing and a variety of hay and concentrates should be offered to anorexic horses, with the main goal being intake of any food. Turning the animal out to graze overnight is ideal in mild or recovering cases; however, exposure to sunlight should be restricted because of the potential for secondary photosensitization. In severely hypoglycemic patients, dextrose may be administered intravenously. Monitoring of blood and urine glucose levels (every 4–12 hours) is

603

then indicated. Feeding by nasogastric tube or parenteral nutrition may be required in some cases; however, nasogastric intubation should be avoided if coagulopathy might be present.

NSAIDs such as flunixin meglumine (1.1 mg/kg i/v or p/o q12–24h) can be used against possible inflammation. The use of corticosteroids is more controversial due to the risk of immunosuppression. Corticosteroids may be useful if significant inflammation is evident histologically and infection is not suspected. Corticosteroids are contraindicated in patients with hepatic lipidosis.

Various protocols are described aimed at reducing bacterial production of ammonia or lowering the pH in the hindgut in an attempt to reduce hyperammonemia. These include neomycin (adults: 1g q6h or 2g q12h; foals: 0.5g q6h or 1.5g q12h), metronidazole (15–25 mg/kg q6h), lactulose (0.2 ml/kg q12h), mineral oil (10 ml/kg q24h per nasogastric tube), and vinegar (0.55 ml/kg q24h). No efficacy studies are available for any of these treatments. As with any antimicrobial use, the risk of antimicrobial-induced colitis should be considered. If medication by nasogastric intubation is elected, the risk of severe nose bleeding in a horse with a possible coagulopathy should be considered.

In cases of coagulation deficiencies, treatment with vitamin K1 (phytonadione) has been advocated; however, end-stage liver disease is to be expected if coagulation abnormalities are present, warranting a poor to grave prognosis. No dosage of vitamin K1 is available for the specific treatment of liver disease, but dosages for vitamin K1 use in horses are available for treatment of warfarin toxicosis: 500 mg s/c q4–6h or 0.5–2.5 mg/kg i/m or i/v if necessary (avoid if possible), which should be diluted in saline or D_5W/saline and given very slowly (not to exceed 5 mg/minute). Substances that might interfere with vitamin K1 efficacy include oral mineral oil, phenylbutazone, chloramphenicol, sulfonamides, cimetidine, metronidazole, and erythromycin.

If neurologic abnormalities are present, the horse should be protected from self-inflicted trauma by placement in a well-bedded stall, ideally with padded walls and/or with a padded helmet. Slinging the horse might also be warranted to prevent bedsores and neuromuscular damage if prolonged recumbency is present or anticipated. Xylazine is the sedative of choice to calm a frantic horse with hepatic encephalopathy. Diazepam is contraindicated. Management of hepatic encephalopathy is described in Chapter 10 (p. 799).

Prognosis

The prognosis for horses with liver failure depends on the specific cause and any primary systemic disease leading to liver failure.

TOXIC CAUSES OF LIVER DISEASE
Plant-associated toxicities

Ingestion of a variety of plants can be associated with liver disease (*Table 30*). Knowledge of the range of toxic plants that may grow in the area, and in areas from which hay is procured, is critical. The amount of plant required to cause clinical signs and the time from exposure to onset of clinical signs are variable. Often, plant toxicities are encountered in situations where overgrazing of pasture has led to horses ingesting plants that they would otherwise avoid or when hay is contaminated with toxic plants that maintain toxicity despite drying. Adverse environmental conditions may also predispose to ingestion of toxic plants, as some are more tolerant of conditions such as drought. Plant toxicity is indistinguishable clinically and hematologically from other types of liver disease.

Pyrrolizidine alkaloid toxicity
Definition/overview

PA toxicity is a regionally important cause of hepatocellular necrosis. Multiple horses may be affected by the time the first case is identified because it is food-associated and occurs with chronic exposure. Most cases of PA toxicity occur when pastures are overgrazed and in early spring when there is a limited supply of green forage.

Etiology/pathophysiology

Examples of PA-containing plants (**862**) are tarweed and fiddleneck (*Amsinckia* spp.), rattlebox (*Crotalaria* spp.), hound's tongue (*Cynoglossum officinale*), blue weed/viper's bugloss (*Echium vulgare*), salvation Jane (Paterson's curse and Riverina bluebell in southern Australia) (*Echium plantagineum*), heliotrope (*Heliotropium* spp.), groundsels (e.g. threadleaf groundsel [*Senecio douglasii* var. *longilobus*] and broom groundsel [*Senecio riddellii*]), ragwort (*Senecio jacobaea*), butterweed (*Senecio glabellus*), and comfrey (*Symphytum officinale*). The toxicity of individual PAs varies greatly and depends on the plant and which part of the plant is ingested. PA concentrations do not change significantly during drying or storage.

PAs cause mitotic arrest of the hepatocytes, leading to delayed progressive liver damage. Mitotic arrest is caused by pyrroles (metabolites of pyrrolizidine alkaloids) binding to hepatic proteins and nucleic acids. Signs are noted when the functioning hepatocytes end their life span and replacement cells are not available, which may occur as early as 3 weeks after exposure.

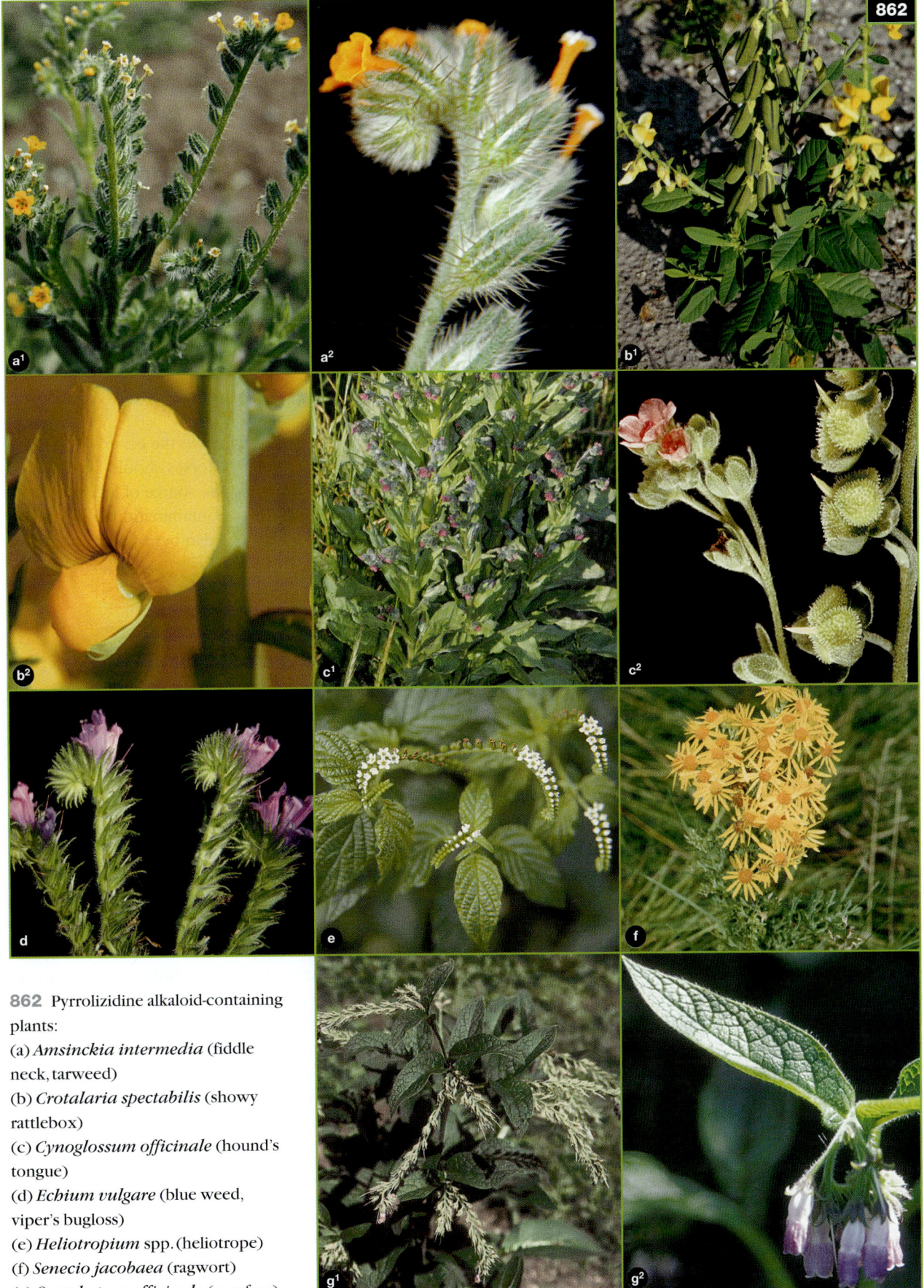

862 Pyrrolizidine alkaloid-containing plants:

(a) *Amsinckia intermedia* (fiddle neck, tarweed)

(b) *Crotalaria spectabilis* (showy rattlebox)

(c) *Cynoglossum officinale* (hound's tongue)

(d) *Echium vulgare* (blue weed, viper's bugloss)

(e) *Heliotropium* spp. (heliotrope)

(f) *Senecio jacobaea* (ragwort)

(g) *Symphytum officinale* (comfrey).

TABLE 30 Common causes of plant-associated hepatotoxicity in horses

SCIENTIFIC NAME	COMMON NAME
Pyrrolizidine alkaloid-containing plants (862)	
Amsinckia spp.	Fiddle neck, tarweed
Crotalaria spp.	Rattlebox
Crotalaria grahamiana	Chocho (Rapa Nui, Easter Islands)
Cynoglossum officinale	Hound's tongue
Echium vulgare	Blue weed, viper's bugloss
Echium plantagineum	Salvation Jane, Paterson's curse, Riverina bluebell (Australia)
Heliotropium spp.	Heliotrope
Senecio spp.	Groundsels, senecio, ragwort, butterweed
Symphytum officinale	Comfrey
Saponin-containing plants (863)	
Panicum coloratum	Kleingrass
Panicum virgatum	Switchgrass
Lantana camara	Lantana
Agave lechuguilla	Agave
Nolina texana	Bear grass
Tribulus terrestris	Puncture vine
Other hepatotoxic plants and mycotoxins (864)	
Trifolium hybridum	Alsike clover
Xanthium spp.	Cocklebur

Clinical presentation

The clinical signs vary from ill-thrift to hepatic encephalopathy and death depending on the dosage. Chronic cases may have poor haircoat, decreased appetite, weight loss, diarrhea, depression, and icterus. Photosensitization with dermatitis of white areas exposed to sunlight is common. In cases where large amounts of plants containing PAs are ingested in a short period of time, sudden onset of severe neurologic disturbances due to hepatic encephalopathy might be the initial clinical sign.

Diagnosis

Commonly GGT, AP, conjugated bilirubin, and serum bile acid levels are elevated; however, indicators of hepatocellular damage (i.e. GLDH) may be normal. In more severe cases, hypoalbuminemia and a decreased albumin/globulin ratio may be present. The ultrasonographic appearance will vary depending on the stage of disease. Hepatocellular necrosis with parenchymal collapse, seen as decreased parymchymal echogenicity and increased echogenicity of the portal veins, may be noted and in cases with fibrosis, overall increased echogenicity may be present. The intoxicated hepatocytes are seen histologically as megalocytes due to their inability to divide. Bridging fibrosis is the other characteristic histologic finding in the areas where functional hepatocytes disappear. Biliary hyperplasia is common.

Management

Treatment is supportive and follows the general guidelines for treatment of liver failure. Horses should be removed from offending pastures and the source of hay should be changed until the source of contamination is identified. Administration of intestinal adsorbents or cathartics is generally futile due to the delayed onset of signs.

Prognosis

The prognosis is based mainly on the severity of clinical signs, but evidence of bridging fibrosis indicates a poor prognosis for survival.

Saponin-containing plants (863)

Kleingrass (*Panicum coloratum*) and switchgrass (*Panicum virgatum*) are saponin-containing plants that can cause bile duct proliferation and cholestasis, leading to subsequent liver damage. The toxic potential fluctuates greatly and there are no specific recommendations except for not keeping horses on a monoculture of kleingrass. Drying does not reduce toxicity and intoxications are often due to feeding kleingrass hay.

Lantana (*Lantana camara*) causes hepatocytic necrosis, bile duct proliferation, and cholestasis due to its saponins and other unknown substances.

Agave (*Agave lechuguilla*), bear grass (*Nolina texana*), and puncture vine (*Tribulus terrestris*) are saponin-containing plants that have been associated with liver disease of sheep in particular, but are likely to be toxic to horses as well.

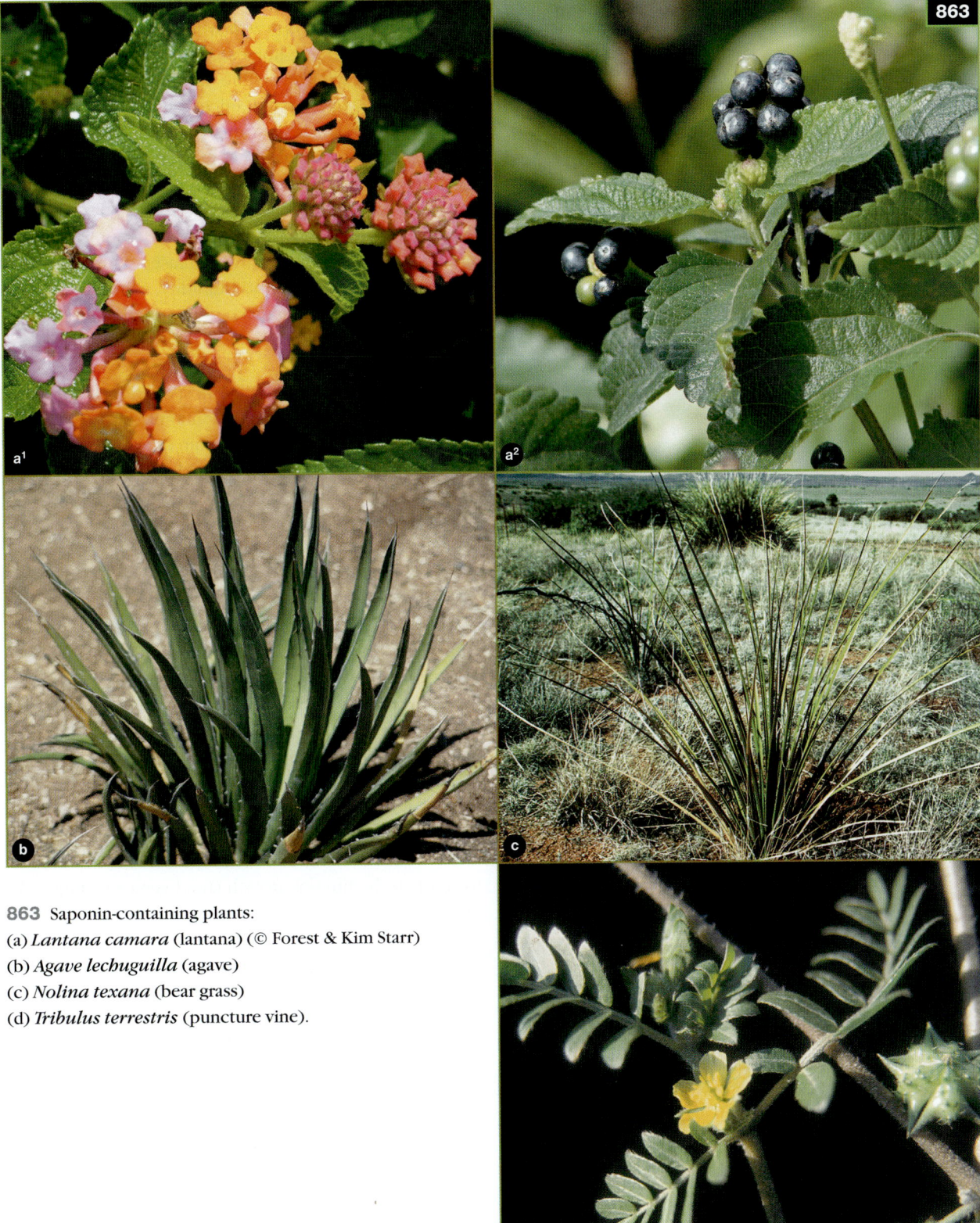

863 Saponin-containing plants:

(a) *Lantana camara* (lantana) (© Forest & Kim Starr)

(b) *Agave lechuguilla* (agave)

(c) *Nolina texana* (bear grass)

(d) *Tribulus terrestris* (puncture vine).

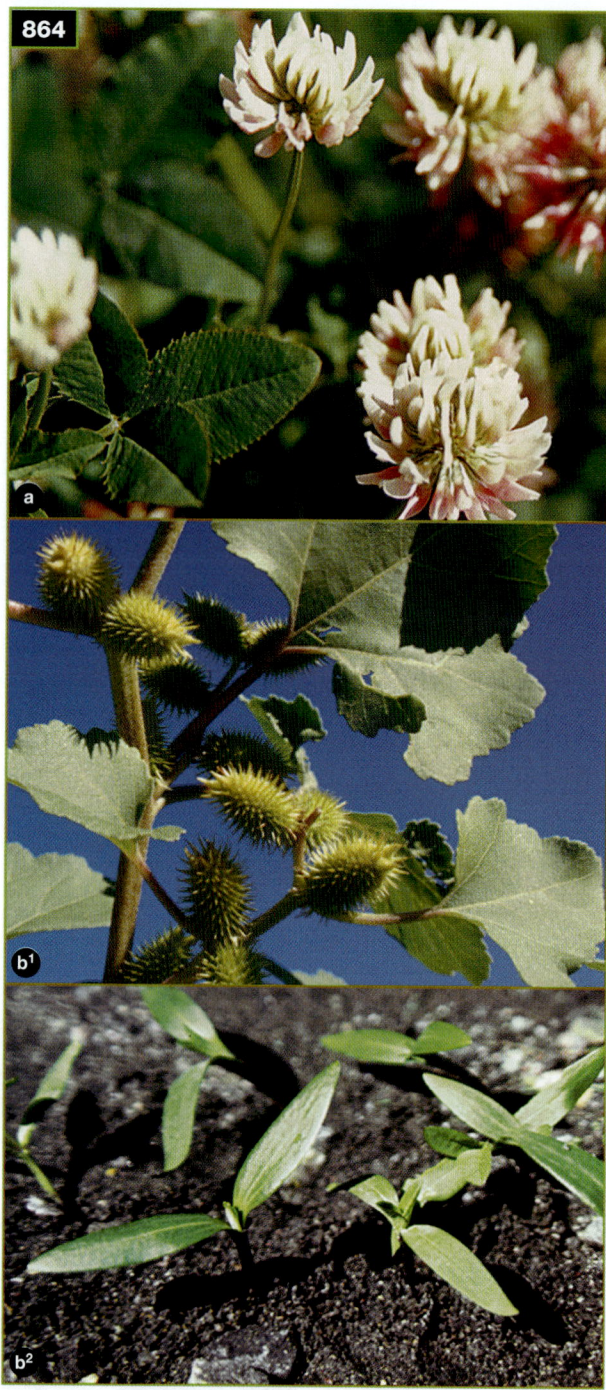

864 Other hepatotoxic plants:
(a) *Trifolium hybridum* (alsike clover)
(b) *Xanthium strumarium* (cocklebur) in mature (b¹) and cotyledonary (b²) stages.

Other hepatotoxic plants (864)

Alsike clover (*Trifolium hybridum*) is the cause of two syndromes in grazing horses. Alsike clover poisoning is characterized by irreversible liver disease, frequently accompanied by hepatic encephalopathy. The other syndrome, trifoliosis or dew poisoning, manifests as photosensitivity without apparent liver disease. The etiology of these syndromes is undetermined, but a toxic cause is suspected due to the close association of the described syndromes and grazing of alsike clover. A fungal etiology has been proposed due to the increased number of cases at times of high rainfall and humidity. Chronic exposure is often needed unless alsike clover is the main forage, in which case signs can occur within a few weeks of exposure.

Cocklebur (*Xanthium* spp., most often *X. strumarium*) intoxication is due to feed contamination where the cockleburs are ground with the grain or where a horse may graze on the newly emerging cocklebur seedlings in the cotyledonary (two-leafed) stage. The clinical signs are those of hepatic encephalopathy due to hepatic necrosis induced by the carboxyatractyloside in the cotyledons of the cockleburs.

MYCOTOXICOSIS

Intoxication by mycotoxins occurs infrequently in horses and the risk varies greatly between geographic regions and year, due to weather and agricultural practices. All mycotoxins obey the dose-and-effect principle, and antidotes are not available. Treatment is generally supportive.

Mycotoxins are products of fungal activity, but notably there is no relationship between degree of fungal growth (contamination) and presence of toxins. Two classification systems exist for fungi and their mycotoxins: one based on location at the time of growth (field versus storage); the other based on their preferred growth medium (grain or forage).

Fusarium spp. (fumonsin mycotoxins) are typical field fungi, whereas *Aspergillus* spp. (aflatoxin mycotoxins) are typical storage fungi, although they can also be field fungi. Both are common grain-related species.

Fumonsins
Definition/overview

While fumonsin toxicosis is most commonly associated with equine leukoencephalomalacia (ELEM), hepatic abnormalities can also occur. Hepatic disease often precedes neurologic signs with low-level, chronic exposure, while severe hepatotoxicity in the absenceof neurologic disease can occur with acute ingestion of high doses.

Etiology/pathophysiology

Fumonsins are produced by several *Fusarium* spp., and three toxins are recognized: fumonsin B1, B2, and B3

(FB1, FB2, and FB3). As opposed to aflatoxins, fumonsins are generally produced during the growth of corn. Drought followed by cool and moist weather is the main risk factor, although damage by insects and handling are additional predisposing factors.

The exact mechanism of fumonsin toxicity is unknown, but inhibition of proper sphinganine conversion to sphingosine is reported. This altered sphingolipid metabolism seems to affect both hepatocytes and cells of the central white matter. The horse appears to be the most susceptible domestic animal species and ingestion of 8–10 ppm of fumonsin for more than 30 days has been associated with ELEM.

Clinical presentation

Low-dose exposure of fumonsins is likely to present as ELEM, with signs of a rapid progressing neurotoxicosis. Moderate- to high-dose exposure is more likely to produce signs of liver failure ranging from depression, anorexia, and icterus to hepatic encephalopathy.

Diagnosis

Diagnosis of fumonsin toxicosis is largely based on a history of exposure and on excluding other causes. An elevated sphinganine/sphingosine ratio is the most indicative serum parameter of fumonsin toxicosis because other serum biochemical abnormalities are nonspecific. Direct tissue and urine analysis at the time of clinical signs is generally unrewarding because fumonsin seems to be quickly excreted in urine and bile after exposure. Grossly, the liver is swollen with rounded edges and a brownish discoloration. Histologically, hepatocyte vacuolation, fatty changes and loss of parenchymal architecture with portal fibrosis, bile stasis, and bile duct proliferation are characteristic.

Management

Treatment is supportive as for liver failure of other etiologies described above. Administration of intestinal adsorbents or cathartics is generally futile due to the delayed onset of signs. It is possible to clean contaminated feedstuffs prior to feeding. If feeding contaminated feedstuffs, it has been recommended that the potentially contaminated feedstuff does not exceed 20% of the total diet and that no more than 5 ppm of fumonsin is present in the contaminated feedstuff.

Prognosis

If ELEM is present, the prognosis is grave. The prognosis for liver failure is best judged by severity of disease and evaluation of liver biopsies for signs of bridging fibrosis and other lesions as described earlier.

Aflatoxins
Definition/overview
Aflatoxicosis is a cause of liver failure that can occur worldwide, but is found mainly in warm and humid regions. It is primarily associated with corn, but can involve other grains.

Etiology/pathophysiology
Aflatoxins are produced by *Aspergillus* spp. Seed-coat damage from environmental stressors such as drought, insects, or handling during harvesting are predisposing factors. Humid climates or warm storage conditions favor fungal growth. Aflatoxins can be an annual problem in areas with high humidity and temperatures constantly above 21°C (69.8°F).

Aflatoxin metabolites such as epoxide interfere with nucleic acids and proteins in multiple organs, causing organ dysfunction due to mitotic arrest of cells. The main target organs are liver, kidney, and intestinal tract. Hepatic injuries include fatty liver, hepatocytic necrosis, and fibrosis. Carcinogenic properties of aflatoxins have been proposed in cases of hepatic neoplasia. Nephritis, hemorrhagic enteritis, and cerebral edema have also been reported in field cases of aflatoxicosis; however, other non-identified toxins might have confounded these cases.

The exact toxic dosage of aflatoxins is unknown, but concentrations between 5,500 and 6,500 ppb were found in grain fed to clinical cases. Experimental studies have shown that ingestion of 0.075 mg/kg and 2 mg/kg can cause chronic and acute signs of toxicity, respectively.

Clinical presentation
Dosage and effect seem to be correlated and clinical signs vary from weight loss and ill-thrift to severe hepatic encephalopathy and death. Signs related to compromised liver function predominate, but intestinal hemorrhage, nephritis, or CNS disease can also develop. Sudden severe cases likely represent the 'tip of the iceberg' and chronic exposure to low dosages, manifesting as chronic liver disease, is more common.

Diagnosis
A detailed history is critical. Exposure to moldy grain, grain with a known history of seed-coat damage, or a history of herd mates with signs of liver disease should place aflatoxicosis on the differential diagnosis list, particularly in regions where aflatoxicosis is periodically or commonly encountered.

Hematologic changes are nonspecific and consistent with liver failure of any etiology. Ultrasonographic examination of the liver might reveal findings consistent with acute hepatocellular necrosis in acute cases or changes consistent with fibrosis in chronic cases. Histologic changes include hepatocellular necrosis, periportal

609

fibrosis, centrilobular fatty change, and bile duct proliferation. Hepatic megalocytosis, as often seen with PA toxicosis, might also be present.

Testing for aflatoxins is available at many laboratories. In an outbreak situation with potential legal consequences, feed samples should be obtained, sealed, and labeled carefully. Multiple samples or pooled samples are recommended since only a small section of the grain might be affected. Serum, urine, and stomach contents should be obtained and saved from as many exposed horses as possible. Analysis of liver aflatoxin content might be useful in acute cases with known recent exposure to aflatoxins.

Management
There is no specific treatment or antidote for aflatoxicosis. Access to potentially contaminated grain should be restricted to prevent further damage and exposure of other horses. Treatment should be supportive and based on physical examination and ancillary tests. Hydrated sodium calcium aluminosilicate, a clay-based product, has been experimentally administered to pigs, poultry, lambs, and cows as an enterosorbent agent preventing GI uptake of the aflatoxins. No studies or dosages are available for horses. All other horses in the at-risk group should be evaluated for signs of subclinical liver disease.

Prognosis
There are no specific prognostic parameters for aflatoxicosis and a prognosis has to be based on severity of clinical signs and histologic changes.

Blue-green algae poisoning
Blue-green algae or cyanobacteria can exert neurotoxic or hepatotoxic effects in horses. In cases of liver failure, secondary photosensitization is often present. Growth of cyanobacteria generally occurs in late summer when the temperature and the mineral and organic matter content of stagnant water in dams and ponds are high.

Iron toxicity
Definition/overview
Iron toxicity causing liver failure and subsequent hepatic encephalopathy can occur in both adult horses and neonatal foals. It is an uncommon condition, typically associated with inappropriate iron supplementation.

Etiology/pathophysiology
Iron toxicosis can be primary, due to a defective iron metabolism, or secondary due to excess supplementation. Most iron toxicities are secondary. Iron toxicity in foals has been associated with ferrous fumarate supplementation in the first 3 days of life. This product is no longer available commercially and is mainly of historical interest.

Foals who have not nursed prior to iron supplementation appear at increased risk of liver failure. Currently, there are no evidence-based data to support the routine administration of iron to newborn foals. If iron supplementation to a neonate appears indicated, then the foal should be allowed to nurse or be administered colostrum prior to iron supplementation in order to reduce the risk of iron toxicity.

Adult horses have been intoxicated by ferrous fumarate or ferrous sulfate, but are less susceptible than foals. Adult horses have been intoxicated by oral vitamin products containing ferrous sulfate given daily at concentrations of 0.6 mg/kg body weight.

Clinical presentation
Clinical signs in foals are usually noted 2–5 days after birth, are typical of hepatic encephalopathy, and include severely depressed demeanor to somnolence, seizure activity, head pressing, aimless wandering, anorexia, and abnormal behavior. Icterus is a common finding, but should be interpreted cautiously in neonates since they often exhibit physiologic hyperbilirubinemia. Adult horses develop similar signs and might also have petechial hemorrhages. Hemorrhages may be noted in the GI system and the bladder, likely reflecting underlying coagulopathy.

Diagnosis
Diagnosis is based on clinical signs and a history of iron exposure. Serum biochemistry changes include the usual abnormalities associated with liver failure such as increased concentrations of GGT, AP, GLDH, AST, bile acids, and bilirubin, and coagulopathy. Serum iron levels or liver iron levels can be evaluated, but increased free iron serum levels are not consistently found. Liver iron levels might be within the normal range or above. An increased liver iron level due to overzealous supplementation should be differentiated from that of hemolysis or hepatic blood congestion. At necropsy, the liver may be friable, smaller or larger than usual, and discolored (tan or mottled red-brown). Histologic abnormalities include parenchyma necrosis, bile duct proliferation, and fibrosis.

Management
Treatment is generally restricted to supportive treatment. Specific treatment with chelating agents such as deferoxamine does not appear to be as successful as in human and small-animal medicine. Phlebotomy has been recommended, but there is no information regarding efficacy.

Prognosis
Foals affected with iron hepatopathy generally die within 3–5 days of birth. In other patients the general prognostic indicators that have been described earlier apply.

Miscellaneous diseases of the liver

Theiler's disease

Definition/overview

Theiler's disease has multiple synonyms including acute hepatitis, idiopathic acute hepatic disease, serum hepatitis, postvaccinal hepatitis, and acute liver atrophy. The condition is characterized by acute hepatocellular necrosis. The exact etiology and pathophysiologic mechanism remain poorly understood, although it is highly associated with administration of equine-based biological products such as tetanus antitoxin.

Etiology/pathophysiology

Any equine-based biological product seems capable of causing acute hepatitis due to a potential immune complex-mediated (type III) hypersensitivity. Administration of tetanus antitoxin is most commonly associated with increased risk of Theiler's disease, but transfusion of plasma (including commercial products) or whole blood has also been implicated. Cases have also been reported where no recent serum-based products were administered, raising the question of a possible viral etiology.

Regardless of the cause and exact mechanism of action, the result is severe hepatocellular necrosis. Inflammatory cells may be present in the periportal areas, whereas the necrotic cells are replaced with an eosinophilic granular mass.

Clinical presentation

Clinical cases can range from mild to peracute, with most cases being very severe liver failure cases. Fever is uncommon. Respiratory distress and hemoglobinuria due to intravascular hemolysis have been reported. Subclinical serum enzyme abnormalities are possible after tetanus antitoxin treatment of lactating mares.

Differential diagnosis

Differential diagnoses are as for liver failure.

Diagnosis

Diagnosis is based on clinical signs, serum biochemistry abnormalities (marked elevation in hepatocellular enzymes), and liver biopsy. History of exposure to a biological product should be queried. Ultrasound examination of the liver may support a diagnosis of acute hepatocellular necrosis.

Management

Management of the affected horse follows the general principles of treatment of liver failure. Often, herdmates have been exposed as well and physical examination and liver enzyme screening is then warranted to detect early or subclinical cases.

Prognosis

The prognosis is based on severity of clinical signs, response to treatment, and liver biopsy results, but in general the prognosis is poor.

Chronic active hepatitis

Definition/overview

Chronic active hepatitis is an idiopathic syndrome characterized by sustained hepatic inflammation.

Etiology/pathophysiology

The histologic diagnosis is often cholangiohepatitis, but the exact etiology is unknown and might involve bacterial infections, immune-mediated processes, parasitic infestations, or toxic insults.

Clinical presentation

Clinical signs are often nonspecific and include weight loss, fever, icterus, decreased appetite, altered demeanor, and possibly signs of colic. A moist exfoliating dermatitis may be noted at the coronary bands and some horses develop areas of necrotic, leathery skin.

Differential diagnosis

Differential diagnoses for liver failure have been outlined previously. In cases of low-grade recurrent colic, a variety of differential diagnoses relating to the GI, urogenital, and respiratory systems must be considered.

Diagnosis

Serum biochemical abnormalities reflect active hepatitis. AP, GGT, bilirubin, dehydrogenase, and bile acid concentrations are all commonly elevated and the BSP dye test is prolonged. Liver biopsies should be obtained for bacterial culture, Gram staining, cytology, and histology. Histologic evidence of inflammatory and/or fibrotic changes in the bile ducts and/or periportal areas can often be grouped into a mononuclear (lymphocytes and plasma cells) or a neutrophilic response, presumably reflecting the underlying etiology (i.e. immune-mediated versus bacterial infection). Grossly, the liver may be smaller than normal and firm, and cut surfaces may have obvious irregular markings.

Management

Supportive treatment as described for liver failure is important. Proper nutrition is particularly important. Corticosteroid therapy is often used and a variety of treatment regimens have been described. Before instituting corticosteroid treatment, the likelihood of a bacterial infection should be evaluated by liver biopsy culture. Antimicrobial treatment is often used concurrently, but the actual need for antimicrobials is unclear. Ideally, treatment should be based on culture and sensitivity testing since

611

various enteric bacteria may be encountered. Dexamethasone can be given (0.05–0.075 mg/kg i/m or i/v q24h for 4–7 days, then tapered off over the next 2–3 weeks depending on the response to treatment). Prednisolone (1 mg/kg p/o q24h) may be administered for an additional 2–6 weeks based on response to treatment and severity of the inflammation. Alternatively, prednisolone can be used as the initial therapy.

Prognosis

The prognosis is poor if there is histologic evidence of periportal bridging (fibrosis). The prognosis is most favorable in a horse with mild inflammation characterized by lymphocyte and plasma cell infiltration. Response to initial treatment provides a good general assessment of long-term prognosis. One study reported a survival rate of 58%.

Cholelithiasis and choledocholithiasis
Definition/overview

Cholelithiasis is the broad term used for stones in the bile ducts (**865**), whereas choledocholithiasis describes stones in the common bile duct, these being more common in horses. Biliary stones are uncommon, but are potential causes of recurrent colic and fever of unknown origin.

Etiology/pathophysiology

The etiology is undetermined, but has been associated with parasites, ascending infection or inflammation of the bile ducts, biliary stasis, changed composition of the bile, and foreign bodies. Several enteric bacteria have been cultured from gallstones, but the cause-and-effect relationship is undetermined. Most stones have a mixed composition of normally occurring bile products such as bilirubin, cholesterol esters, bile pigment, esters of cholic and carboxylic acid, calcium phosphate, and sodium taurodeoxycholate. Clinical signs may be caused by complete biliary obstruction leading to increased hepatic pressure and dysfunction. Increased serum concentration of conjugated bilirubin causing icterus is common in cases of complete biliary obstruction. The stone(s) itself is/are likely also to cause direct pain, resulting in colic signs in some cases.

Clinical presentation

Cinical signs of cholelithiasis include pyrexia, colic (often recurring and low-grade) and icterus. Liver failure is rare.

Diagnosis

Hepatic serum enzyme activity may be elevated and a neutrophilic leukocytosis is common. Typically, GGT and AP are more significantly increased than AST and GLDH, reflecting predominantly biliary versus hepatocellular damage. Bile acids are often markedly elevated in cases of obstructive biliary conditions.

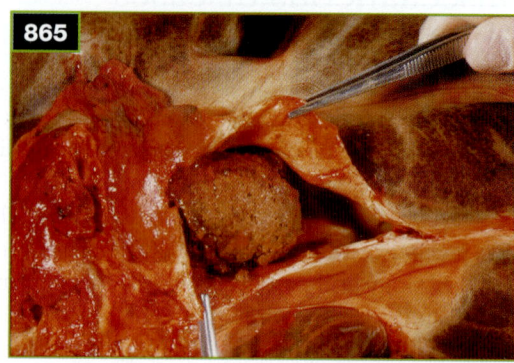

865 Cholelith *in situ*. (Photo courtesy Department of Pathobiology, Ontario Veterinary College)

Transcutanous hepatic ultrasonographic examination is the diagnostic tool of choice. In experienced hands it can identify stones in 75% of cases. If the stones are not directly visualized, supporting findings include hepatomegaly, bile duct distension, and the 'parallel channel or shotgun signs', where distended bile ducts are seen next to the portal vein.

Liver biopsy might determine the underlying cause of stone formation and guide the prognosis.

Management

Treatment of cholelithiasis is often unrewarding and restricted to nutritional management of offering a low-fat diet. Surgical removal of gallstones has proved unrewarding in most cases and, if attempted, should be preceded by broad-spectrum antimicrobial therapy.

Cholangitis and cholangiohepatitis
Definition/overview

Bile duct obstruction is most commonly due to inflammation of the bile ducts (cholangitis) and can be associated with cholangiohepatitis, where inflammation is present both in the bile ducts and the hepatic parenchyma. Cholangitis is thought to be the most common cause of biliary obstruction in horses.

Etiology/pathophysiology

Bacterial infections or foreign bodies, such as grain, sticks, stones, and sand, can cause cholangitis. Cholangiohepatitis can be a primary entity or secondary to cholelithiasis, intestinal inflammation or obstruction, parasitism, neoplasia, or toxins, and is often present in cases of chronic active hepatitis.

Foreign bodies are thought to enter the biliary tract by retrograde motion from the small intestine. Ascending infection of the biliary tract is one recognized mechanism of cholangitis and cholangiohepatitis. Suppurative cholangiohepatitis might also be caused by portal contents of bacteria, bacterial products, and/or inflammatory mediators secondary to impairment of the intestinal mucosal barrier. Duodenitis/proximal jejunitis in horses can predispose to hepatic injury through ascending infection.

Clinical presentation

Clinical signs are nonspecific and include colic, fever, anorexia, weight loss, abnormal behavior, and other signs associated with liver disease.

Diagnosis

Increases in GGT, AP, total and conjugated bilirubin, and bile acid concentrations are expected. GLDH, AST, and other indicators of hepatocellular damage are more likely to be elevated with cholangiohepatitis than with cholangitis. A neutrophilic leukocytosis is commonly present, particularly with cholangiohepatitis.

Ultrasonographic evaluation may reveal thickened or dilated biliary ducts. Biliary ducts are normally not visible on ultrasound and repeated evaluations are useful in evaluating response to treatment and formulating a prognosis.

Liver biopsies for histologic examination and bacterial culture are imperative in making the diagnosis, providing a prognosis, and formulating a rational therapeutic plan.

Management

Treatment of cholangitis or cholangiohepatitis should include prolonged antimicrobial therapy until GGT levels are within normal reference ranges. GGT levels might temporarily increase at the beginning of treatment. Antimicrobial choice should ideally be based on culture and sensitivity testing, but successful treatment has been reported using ceftiofur (2 mg/kg i/v or i/m q12h), trimethoprim/sulfadiazine (30 mg/kg p/o q12h), procaine penicillin (20,000 IU/kg i/m q12h), or enrofloxacin (7.5 mg/kg p/o or i/v q24h). Initial treatment might also include supportive intravenous crystalloids and anti-inflammatory drugs such as flunixin meglumine (1.1 mg/kg i/v q12h).

Prognosis

Recent reports indicate that prolonged antimicrobial therapy, until the GGT level is within reference ranges, carries a favorable prognosis for survival in cases of cholangiohepatitis and cholelithiasis. Severe bridging fibrosis at the time of initial assessment is an unfavorable prognostic sign.

866 Umbilical vein abscessation with extension into the liver. Note the purulent material in the enlarged umbilical vein.

Liver abscesses

Liver abscesses are uncommon, but can occur in both foals and adult horses. The route of entry is either the portal vein, the hepatic artery, or the umbilical vein in foals (**866**). Common isolated pathogens are *Rhodococcus equi* (foals, weanlings, and yearlings), α-hemolytic *Streptococcus* spp., *E. coli, Klebsiella* spp., *Bacteriodes* spp., *Clostridium* spp., *Acinetobacter* spp., and *Streptococcus zooepidemicus.*

Clinical signs are often indistinct from other abdominal abscesses and include weight loss, intermittent fever, and colic. Ultrasonographic examination may be adequate for diagnosis, particularly in foals, but exploratory laparotomy is sometimes required for definitive diagnosis.

The location of the abscess means that drainage is generally not an option, thereby complicating treatment. In foals, resection or marsupialization of the infected umbilical vein, in combination with long-term antimicrobial treatment, may be a viable option, although the prognosis is guarded.

Antimicrobial treatment should ideally be based on culture and sensitivity testing. Potential initial antimicrobial protocols include ceftiofur (2 mg/kg i/v q12h) or trimethoprim/sulfadiazine (30 mg/kg p/o q12h). These antimicrobials might be combined with metronidazole (15–25 mg/kg p/o q6–8h) and/or rifampin (5–10 mg/kg p/o q12h). Erythromycin phosphate (37.5 mg/kg p/o q12h) or estolate (25 mg/kg p/o q6h) and rifampin are indicated if *R. equi* is suspected. Other macrolide antimicrobials such as azithromycin (10 mg/kg p/o q24h) and clarithromycin (7.5 mg/kg p/o q12h), in combination with rifampin, might also be reasonable choices in selected cases.

The prognosis is poor, but long-term antimicrobial treatment has been successful in some cases.

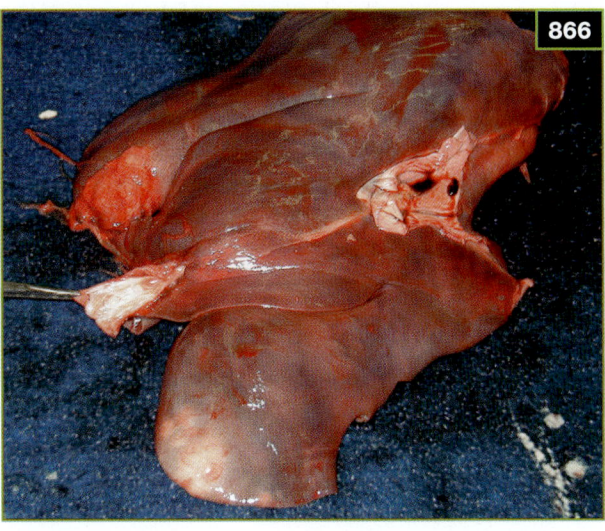

866

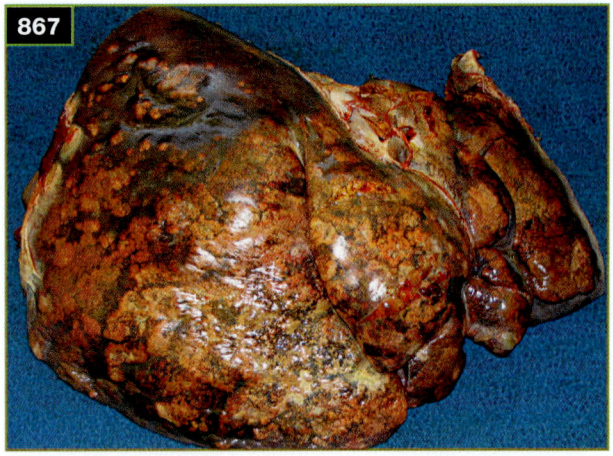

867 Hepatocellular carcinoma in a 6-year-old Thoroughbred mare.

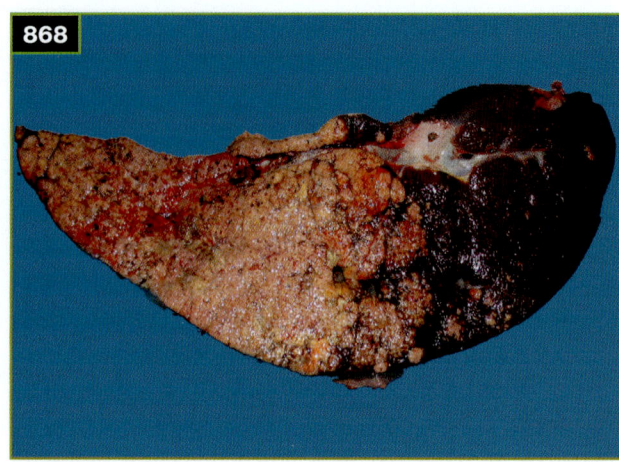

868 Cut section of the tumor shown in 867.

Neoplasia

Definition/overview

Primary hepatic or biliary neoplasia is rare in horses, constituting less than 1% of equine neoplasia (867, 868). Secondary neoplasia due to metastasis is much more common.

Etiology/pathophysiology

Primary hepatobiliary tumors are most commonly identified in geriatric horses, with cholangiocarcinoma being the most common. Other primary tumors include hepatocellular carcinoma, hepatoblastoma, mixed hamartoma, hepatosplenic lymphoma, and hepatic biliary adenofibroma. Hepatocellular carcinomas have been reported in a small number of horses and appear to occur mainly in horses under 3 years of age. Similarly, hepatoblastomas have also been reported in several young horses. Metastatic tumors can also develop because of the liver's role as a major filter organ. Common metastatic tumors include multicentric lymphoma and melanoma.

Clinical presentation

Clinical presentation is variable, but weight loss, anorexia, weakness, and lethargy are common complaints.

Diagnosis

Hematology may reveal valuable information in some cases. Erythrocytosis as a paraneoplastic syndrome has been reported in a case of hepatoblastoma. Other hematologic findings may be anemia of chronic disease, thrombocytopenia, and leukopenia. Serum biochemical abnormalities depend on the tumor location and involvement of hepatobiliary tissue.

Cytologic or histologic examination of liver biopsies is used for definitive diagnosis. Ultrasonographic guidance is useful for identifying affected areas for biopsy, as the tumor can be diffuse, regional, or multifocal.

Management

Due to the generally advanced state of disease at the time of diagnosis, treatment is palliative and supportive in nature. There appear to be no reports of successful surgical and/or chemotherapeutic treatment.

Prognosis

The prognosis is grave for any hepatobiliary tumor because disease is typically advanced by the time of diagnosis and there are few viable therapeutic options.

Parasites

Primary liver disease caused by parasites is uncommon, but various parasites may be a predisposing or contributing factor in some cases of liver disease. Incidental identification of gross or histologic hepatic changes from migrating larvae is common (869), but typically of minimal to no significance. Migrating *Parascaris equorum* larvae may cause focal or diffuse fibrosis in the liver. Hepatic AA amyloidosis was reported in a horse with severe mixed strongylid infestation.

Equine hydatidosis caused by *Echinococcus granulosus* subsp. *equinus* has historically been a disease of horses in the UK and Ireland. Clinical signs are uncommon and it is mainly an incidental postmortem diagnosis. Foxhounds are considered the main host and horses are the intermediate host. Feeding raw horse offal to foxhounds was considered the main cause of sustaining the disease.

In the US, hepatic hydatid cysts have been incidental post-mortem findings in several horses, but all these horses had been imported from the UK or Ireland.

Multilocular echinococcosis due to natural infection with *Echinococcus multilocularis* has been reported in a Japanese horse. It was an incidental finding during necropsy.

Sarcocystis-associated hepatitis has been reported in one horse. The exact *Sarcocystis* species could not be determined, but is was different from *S. neurona*.

Liver flukes

Horses are generally very resistant to *Fasciola hepatica*. In one study, adult flukes could only be found in the liver of one of 10 horses experimentally infected with high doses of metacercariae per os. Infestation of British horses with *F. hepatica* was reported in the 1970s. The horses shared pastures with diary cattle that were endemically infected. Poor performance, weight loss, lethargy, and variable appetite were the main findings in affected horses. Diagnosis was made by fecal examination for fluke ova. In Egypt, *F. hepatica* infestation of horses has also been reported.

Recently, natural infection with *Fascioloides magna* was reported as an incidental finding during necropsy of a 25-year-old Quarterhorse in Minnesota, USA.

Tyzzer's disease

Definition/overview

Tyzzer's disease is a sporadic cause of peracute or acute hepatic failure and sudden death in foals. Affected foals are typically 6–45 days of age with no history of dystocia, failure of passive transfer, or previous medical conditions.

Etiology/pathophysiology

Clostridium piliformis is a spore-forming anaerobic bacterium found in soil and manure. The bacterium can be endemic in certain areas or on certain farms. Spores are passed to the liver through the portal circulation after ingestion. Germination of the spores in the liver leads to acute necrotizing hepatitis by the vegetative bacteria. Myocarditis, colitis, and pulmonary hemorrhage are common complications of bacteremia/septicemia.

Clinical presentation

Affected foals are often found dead or in a grave condition. There are no consistent prodromal signs. Lethargy, recumbency with or without seizures, fever, icterus, diarrhea, and anorexia may be observed alone or in any combination.

Differential diagnosis

Toxic hepatopathies, bacterial hepatitis secondary to septicemia, or EHV-1 hepatopathy should be considered.

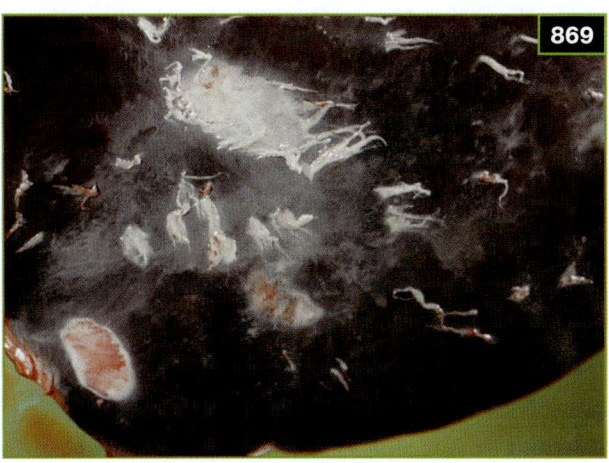

869 Scarring of the diaphragmatic surface of the liver due to parasite migration by *Strongylus edentatus*. (Photo courtesy Department of Pathobiology, Ontario Veterinary College)

Diagnosis

Antemortem diagnosis is rare because of the peracute fatal nature of the disease. A PCR technique has been described that allows antemortem as well as postmortem diagnosis of Tyzzer's disease on liver biopsy specimens. Serum biochemical abnormalities are characteristic of severe hepatocellular disease. Until the PCR technique gains widespread acceptance, postmortem examination will be needed to make a definitive diagnosis. Multifocal areas of necrosis are seen histologically. Routine stains such as hematoxylin and eosin or hemacolor often fail to illustrate the organism, but Warthin–Starry-stained sections of liver may reveal long, slender bacteria consistent with *C. piliformis*.

Management

Successful treatment of a single confirmed case of Tyzzer's disease has recently been reported. This one reported case was a 16-day-old foal Paint Horse filly who, prior to referral, was treated with lactated Ringer's solution, dextrose solution in sterile water, DMSO, diazepam, xylazine, ampicillin, gentamicin, dexamethasone, and dipyrone. The foal was comatose on arrival at the tertiary facility and received very intensive treatment, including total parenteral nutrition, before it was discharged after 4 days of hospitalization. Upon discharge from the hospital, trimethoprim/sulfamethoxazole (30 mg/kg p/o q12h) was prescribed for 7 days. The relative usefulness of these treatments is unclear. There are no known means of prevention.

Prognosis

This condition is almost invariably fatal.

Fatty liver syndrome (hepatic lipidosis and hyperlipemia, hyperlipidemia, and severe hypertriglyceridemia)

Definition/overview

Fatty liver syndrome is a condition of animals under catabolic stress caused by either reduced energy intake and/or increased energy demands such as during gestation. The negative energy balance triggers an overwhelming release of lipids from peripheral stores, which ultimately overloads the liver, causing impaired liver function and accumulation of lipids in the liver and in the circulation. Obese animals, donkeys, ponies, and miniature horses are predisposed. The condition is reversible, but early diagnosis and intervention are crucial for a favorable outcome.

Etiology/pathophysiology

Several conditions related to metabolic energy response and adjustment at times of decreased energy intake, increased energy demands, and/or disease have been described. Significant differences in glucose and fat metabolism seem to be present in ponies, donkeys, and miniature horses compared with horses. Currently, the definition of hyperlipidemia is elevation in serum triglycerides without visibly evident lipemia. Lipemia is the lactescent (milky) appearance of serum that occurs when serum triglyceride levels exceed 5.65 mmol/l (*ca.*500 mg/dl). Severe hypertriglyceridemia is a new term defined as serum triglyceride elevation above 5.65 mmol/l (*ca.* 500 mg/dl) without lactescent serum. Fatty liver and hepatic lipidosis are synonyms describing increased hepatocyte triglyceride storage, often resulting in hepatocyte dysfunction and elevation of hepatic serum enzymes. Elevated serum concentrations of very low-density lipoproteins (VLDLs) are characteristic of these disorders.

Intentional feed restriction or disease-induced anorexia are obvious risk factors. Severe disease such as endotoxemia and shock and pregnancy are likely causes of increased energy demand. These syndromes are often noted in the late winter and early spring, when the nutritional plane may be inferior and pregnant mares in the last trimester have high energy demands. Pregnant pony mares are at higher risk than horse mares, which may be due to a decreased dam to fetal ratio (a pony fetus is larger than a horse fetus in relation to the size of its dam, potentially exerting increased metabolic stress on the dam). Animals above 4 years of age appear to be predisposed.

While most cases of hypertriglyceridemia are secondary, primary cases do occur. The mechanism in primary cases is unknown.

The main regulatory enzymes and hormones of glucose and lipid metabolism are hormone-sensitive lipase, lipoprotein lipase, glucocorticoids, insulin, and heparin. Hormone-sensitive lipase promotes the release of free fatty acids (FFAs) from peripheral adipocytes under the influence of glucocorticoids and is inhibited by insulin. Uptake of triglycerides from the circulation by peripheral tissues is catalyzed by lipoprotein lipase under the influence of insulin and to a lesser extent by heparin. Lipids from the peripheral adipocytes are mainly transported as albumin-bound nonesterified fatty acids and a smaller fraction as FFAs. Lipids intended for storage in the peripheral adipocytes are released from the liver in the form of VLDLs.

Hepatic production of VLDLs beyond the uptake capacity of peripheral adipocytes leads to increased serum levels of triglycerides. Mobilization of lipids from adipose tissues beyond the processing capacity of the hepatocytes leads to accumulation of triglycerides within hepatocytes, resulting in hepatic lipidosis (fatty liver syndrome).

The proposed mechanism of this condition is 'insulin resistance', where hormone-sensitive lipase and lipoprotein lipase in adipocytes are partly resistant to insulin, causing increased lipid mobilization and decreased uptake of VLDLs, respectively.

Clinical presentation

The most frequently reported clinical signs are anorexia and a depressed demeanor. In cases of a secondary nature, clinical signs of the primary disease may dominate. GI disturbances, particularly enterocolitis in miniature horses, are commonly the primary disease problem leading to secondary hypertriglyceridemia. Neurologic disturbances due to hepatic encephalopathy are often present.

Diagnosis

Diagnosis is generally based on the history, clinical signs, lactescent serum, elevated serum triglycerides, and, potentially, liver enzyme elevations. Hepatomegaly and increased fat content may be evident ultrasonographically. Histologic evaluation of liver biopsies is confirmatory and may be of prognostic value.

Management

Treatment is directed at resolving the primary entity, caloric supplementation, and, potentially, hormonal manipulation. Caloric supplementation may involve provision of a higher-energy ration, supplementation with high-energy compounds, force-feeding via a nasogastric tube, or partial parenteral nutrition with intravenous glucose and amino acids.

Insulin is often administered in severe cases because of its inhibitory effect on hormone-sensitive lipase and stimulatory effect on lipoprotein lipase; however, this has been questioned based on the concept of insulin resistance. Protamine zinc insulin (0.1–0.3 IU/kg s/c or i/m q12h or q24h) has traditionally been provided, but access to this formulation is now limited in many areas. Alternatively, regular insulin or ultralente insulin may be used, but dosages have not been firmly established. Dosages used in the treatment of hyperlipemic miniature horses have been reported for regular insulin (16 IU i/m q12h for 3 days) and ultralente insulin (24 IU i/m once or 2 IU s/c q24h).

The efficacy of heparin treatment is unknown, but heparin administration (40–250 IU/kg s/c or i/v q12h) has been reported for its potential lipoprotein lipase stimulatory properties. However, careful case selection is advised to minimize complications of heparin administration such as increased bleeding times, especially if using high dosages of heparin. Nasogastric intubation and other procedures that might result in hemorrhage should be avoided in animals treated with heparin.

Intravenous fluid therapy is indicated in most cases. Supplementation of fluids with glucose is a useful form of caloric support. Plasma and urine glucose levels should be monitored, with the administration rate and glucose concentration changed as needed. Partial parenteral nutrition is useful in moderate to severe cases.

Prognosis

The prognosis in cases of hyperlipidemia is good, with most cases responding well to oral carbohydrate-based caloric supplementation. Classical cases of hyperlipemia in ponies, donkeys, and miniature horses generally carry a guarded to unfavorable prognosis if the serum triglyceride concentration exceeds 13.55 mmol/l (*ca*. 1,200 mg/dl) and intensive care is required. The prognosis for horses with severe hypertriglyceridemia without hepatic lipidosis mainly depends on the primary disease condition. Serum triglyceride levels in these cases generally seem to respond very well to intravenous caloric support (dextrose plus or minus amino acids).

Miscellaneous causes of liver disease in foals

- ✦ Liver disease in the equine neonate is mainly of infectious origin, but congenital, toxic, inflammatory, and immune-mediated disorders are possible. Bile acid measurements are often unreliable in the first week of life and hypoglycemia is often present in neonates with liver disease.

- ✦ Last-trimester abortions and stillborn or nonviable foals are commonly the result of infection with EHV-1 during gestation. Live foals are often very weak, icteric, and neutropenic. Hypoxic–ischemic encephalopathy and septicemia are commonly the main differential diagnoses. Affected foals may respond to initial supportive treatment, but deterioration and death due to multi-organ failure within the first week of life are common. The prognosis is poor to grave. Antiviral treatment with acyclovir (10 mg/kg p/o q8h) has been attempted, but is probably futile in severe cases.

- ✦ *Leptospira pomona* most often causes abortion, but it may also be a rare cause of liver disease.

- ✦ *Actinobacillus equuli* is a common cause of bacteremia in foals, leading to multifocal liver disease and embolic nephritis.

- ✦ Gastroduodenal ulceration and scarring have been reported as a cause of secondary cholangiohepatitis and pancreatitis.

- ✦ Neonatal isoerythrolysis (NI) has been associated with liver disease. It is likely that the liver suffers from hypoxia due to anemia and is overloaded with iron from the severe hemolysis.

- ✦ Kernicterus, also known as bilirubin encephalopathy, is a well-recognized condition in human babies and has been recently recognized in foals. The cause of the hyperbilirubinemia is generally hemolysis due to NI, which leads to high concentrations of circulating unconjugated bilirubin that is thought to exert a neurotoxic effect on the central gray matter. However, this is a rare complication of NI. Predisposing factors in cases of kernicterus may be acidosis, septicemia, hypoalbuminemia, hypoxia, and impaired blood–brain barrier. Kernicterus should be suspected in NI foals that are severely icteric and showing signs of CNS disease. The prognosis is unfavorable and long-term dementia is likely. Treatment of human babies with kernicterus consists of exchange blood transfusions, albumin therapy, and phototherapy with emission in the blue spectrum (converts unconjugated bilirubin to a water-soluble metabolite that is readily excreted).

- An idiopathic hyperammonemia syndrome has been reported in Morgan foals. Depression and weight loss shortly after weaning due to hepatic disease with hyperammonemia has been recognized in these foals. The cause is unknown, but it may be inherited and the disease is invariably fatal.
- Portosystemic shunts have been described in several foals, but the prevalence appears to be much lower than in cats and dogs. Diagnosis is based on age, clinical signs (waxing and waning hepatic encephalopathy), history, ultrasound examination, and intraoperative mesenteric portography.

- Congenital hepatic fibrosis and cystic bile duct formation is a recessively inherited autosomal genetic defect of Swiss Freiberger horses. Signs of liver failure are noted in foals between 1 and 12 months of age (average 3.7 months). Clinical signs of liver failure occur suddenly in most cases, but in some cases weight loss precedes the signs of liver failure. The condition is invariably fatal.
- PA toxicity was diagnosed in a 2-month old foal and the case is thought to represent a rare case of congenital PA toxicity induced by the mare's ingestion of *Senecio* spp. during gestation.

Endocrine system

Babetta Breuhaus

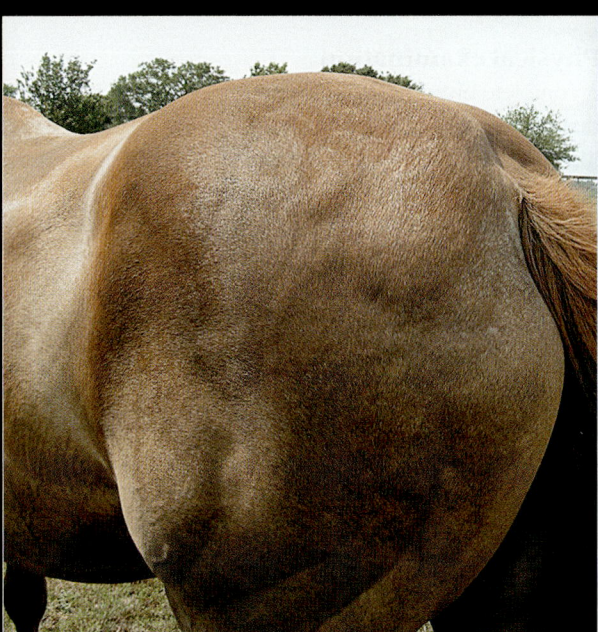

Endocrine system

The endocrine system is comprised of glands that secrete hormones into the bloodstream. These hormones act as chemical signals at distant tissues, usually to regulate their function. Proper function of endocrine systems involves a number of steps that can be regulated or controlled. Each hormone must be synthesized by the gland, stored, and secreted in response to an appropriate stimulus. Transportation in the bloodstream usually involves protein-binding, with only free fractions of hormones being metabolically active. In order to regulate target tissues, hormones must be able to diffuse into the tissues and bind to receptors. Excess hormone must be metabolized to an inactive form and either be taken back up by the gland for reprocessing and storage or be eliminated, usually through the kidneys or liver. Most endocrine systems are controlled by negative feedback, whereby products produced by the target organs inhibit further release of stimulatory or releasing hormones. Endocrine diseases usually involve problems with overproduction or underproduction of hormones, or altered tissue responses to them.

Diagnostic work-up

Physical examination

A complete physical examination is an essential part of the diagnostic work-up for all diseases. For problems that are likely to have an endocrine cause, particular attention should be paid to body weight (e.g. underweight or overweight, distribution of fat stores), haircoat (length, condition, areas of alopecia), and mental alertness and activity level (e.g. depression, lethargy, apprehension, exercise intolerance).

Hematology

A CBC and serum biochemical profile should be submitted to rule out infectious or organ system diseases that could be responsible for clinical signs. Specific or subtle changes in a CBC or chemistry panel may be typical for some endocrine diseases, as detailed in subsequent sections on those specific diseases.

Urinalysis

Endocrine-specific urinalysis is not routinely performed in horses believed to be suffering from endocrine disease. Measurement of urine concentrations of neurotransmitters or hormones may be useful in certain cases (e.g. measurement of urinary catecholamines may be useful in the diagnosis of pheochromocytoma), but these tests are not commonly performed or readily available.

Hormone analysis

Measurement of serum concentrations of hormones and response of these hormones to normal stimulants plays an important role in the diagnosis of endocrine diseases. Values of various hormones in normal healthy horses have been published, but it is important to realize that 'normal' values will vary slightly among different laboratories using different assay techniques. Therefore, it is important for clinicians to make certain that the laboratories that they are sending samples to for analysis have validated their assay techniques for horses and include a reference range of values with the results that they report.

Diseases of the thyroid and parathyroid gland

Hypothyroidism
Overview/Definition
Thyroid function plays an important role in organ growth and maturation, as well as in metabolism. Both hypothyroidism and hyperthyroidism have been described in the horse, but true thyroid gland dysfunction is probably much less common in horses than in some other species, including humans, dogs, and cats. A large number of adult horses that are administered thyroid hormones probably have normal thyroid gland function.

Etiology/pathophysiology
Two syndromes of hypothyroidism have been described in foals, but true hypothyroidism in adult horses has not been well documented. A syndrome of hypothyroidism and goiter has been observed in foals exposed to an excess or deficiency of iodine *in utero*. Another syndrome of hypothyroidism associated with thyroid gland hyperplasia and various skeletal abnormalities has been described mainly in foals born in Western Canada and the US. The etiology of this second syndrome is not known at this time, but factors such as nitrate, low iodine, low selenium, or goitrogenic plant ingestion by the mare have been suggested.

In adult horses a few cases of hypothyroidism resulting from thyroid neoplasia have been described, but most thyroid gland tumors are benign, nonfunctional adenomas. C-cell tumors and carcinomas have also been reported. Serum thyroid hormone concentrations in most horses with thyroid gland tumors are within reference ranges. The irreversible thyroid pathology that occurs with autoimmune thyroid disease in humans and dogs has not been described in the horse.

The thyroid traps and concentrates iodide, which is oxidized and bound to tyrosine, either as monoiodotyrosine or as di-iodotyrosine. Two molecules of di-iodotyrosine are combined to form thyroxine (T_4), whereas tri-iodothyronine (T_3) is formed from one molecule of monoiodotyrosine and one molecule of di-iodotyrosine. Thyroid hormones, primarily T_4, are stored within the gland bound to thyroglobulin. Control of hormone secretion occurs at three sites. Thyrotropin- releasing hormone (TRH) from the hypothalamus stimulates release of thyrotropin or thyroid-stimulating hormone (TSH) from the anterior pituitary. At the thyroid gland, TSH increases the size and activity of the epithelial cells, stimulates proteolysis of thyroglobulin, increases iodide trapping, and increases coupling of monoiodotyrosine and di-iodotyrosine. T_4 and T_3 are released into the circulation, where they bind to plasma-binding proteins. Only free (unbound) thyroid hormones are metabolically active. While the thyroid gland secretes primarily T_4, T_4 is deiodinated to T_3 (or reverse T_3) in blood and tissues. T_3 is much more active than T_4, while reverse T_3 has very little activity.

Alterations in circulating concentrations of thyroid hormones can be mediated centrally by alterations in TRH (tertiary hypothyroidism) or TSH (secondary hypothyroidism), by alterations in thyroid gland function itself (primary hypothyroidism), or by alterations in peripheral thyroid hormone metabolism or binding. Primary hypothyroidism can be caused by interference with iodine uptake by the thyroid gland or by interference with thyroid-hormone synthesis or release. Iodine deficiency or ingestion of goitrogens (e.g. sulfurated organic compounds, thiocyanates, and isothiocyanates) causes goiter in humans. Iodine deficiency also causes goiter in horses. Selenium deficiency and mustard have been suggested as potential dietary goitrogens in the horse. Excessive iodine ingestion by the mare (e.g. kelp supplements) can cause goiter and hypothyroidism in neonatal foals.

Certain drugs and various physiologic or pathologic states can alter thyroid-hormone synthesis, metabolism, or binding, resulting in altered serum concentrations of thyroid hormone. In the horse, these include phenylbutazone administration, fasting, and strenuous exercise. Diets high in energy, protein, zinc, and copper have also affected circulating concentrations of thyroid hormones. Nonthyroidal illness syndrome has not been characterized in the horse, but unpublished data of the author suggest that it is similar to the syndrome in other species.

Clinical presentation
Foals
Clinical signs in neonatal foals born to mares ingesting excessive iodine during gestation (e.g. kelp) include goiter, incoordination, hypothermia, and poor suckle and righting reflexes. Clinical signs of a syndrome of hypothyroidism described in foals in Western Canada and the US primarily involve congenital musculoskeletal abnormalities, including mandibular prognathia (**870, 871**), flexural deformities of the forelimbs, ruptured digital extensor tendons, and incomplete ossification of the carpal and

870, 871 Photograph (870) and lateral skull radiograph (871) of a foal with congenital hypothyroidism. Note the mandibular prognathia.

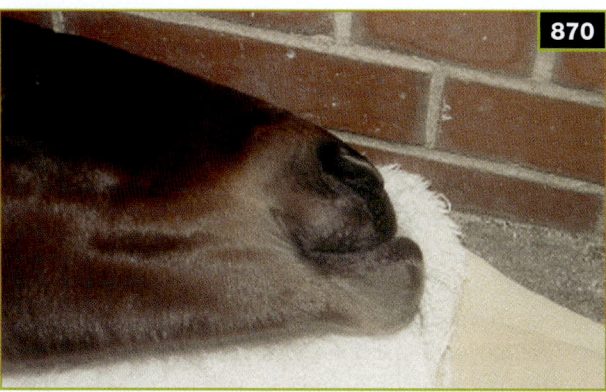
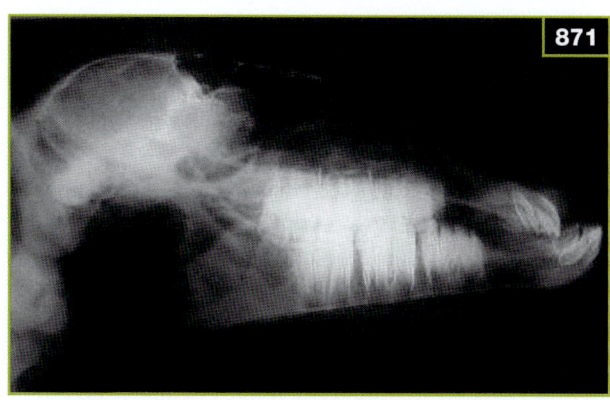

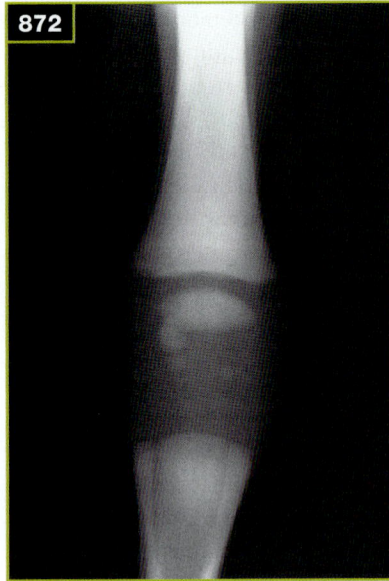

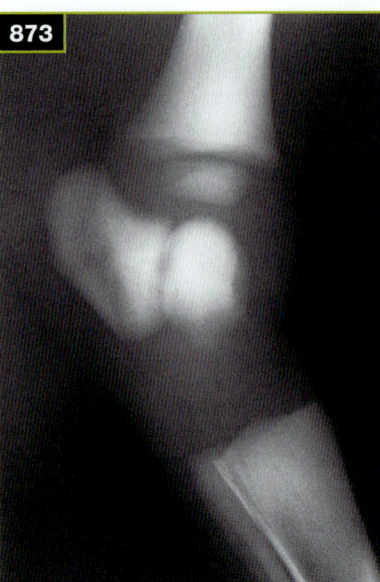

872, 873 Hypothyroidism.
(872) Dorsopalmar radiograph of incomplete ossification of cuboidal bones of the carpus in a foal with congenital hypothyroidism.
(873) Lateral radiograph of incomplete ossification of cuboidal bones of the tarsus in a foal with congenital hypothyroidism.

tarsal bones (872, 873). At birth, serum concentrations of thyroid hormones may be normal in these foals. It is thought that the musculoskeletal problems are caused by hypothyroidism during key developmental stages *in utero*.

Adults

Clinical signs of hypothyroidism in adult horses are not well defined. Overweight horses that are 'easy keepers', with cresty necks, abnormal fat pads, and a predisposition to recurrent laminitis have traditionally been described as hypothyroid. However, thyroid function tests in these horses are usually normal. Instead of hypothyroidism, some of these horses have pituitary pars intermedia dysfunction (equine Cushing's disease) or equine metabolic syndrome. Clinical signs in horses properly documented to be hypothyroid in published case reports include lethargy or work intolerance and alterations in haircoat. Horses with experimentally-induced hypothyroidism (either through surgical removal of the thyroid glands or by administration of anti-thyroid drugs) demonstrate vague clinical signs. Surgical removal of the thyroid glands of adult horses results in decreased basal heart rate, cardiac output, respiratory rate, and rectal temperature, and increased serum concentrations of triglycerides, cholesterol, and VLDLs. However, these changes are mild and do not result in resting values clearly outside reference ranges.

Hypothyroidism has been suggested as a contributing cause to several other problems in horses (in addition to laminitis) including chronic myositis, reduced fertility in broodmares, and anhidrosis, but documentation for these claims is currently lacking or incomplete. A recent study of thyroid function in anhidrotic horses demonstrated that

anhidrotic horses had normal serum thyroid hormone concentrations and responses to TRH. However, serum TSH response to TRH was mildly enhanced, suggesting that there may be some degree of subclinical hypothyroidism, or at least an altered sensitivity of the thyroid gland to TSH.

Differential diagnosis

Differential diagnoses for hypothyroidism in adult horses include pituitary pars intermedia dysfunction, equine metabolic syndrome, nonthyroidal illness syndrome, or, perhaps, overfeeding. Additional differential diagnoses for exercise intolerance could include abnormalities of the cardiovascular, respiratory, or musculoskeletal systems.

Diagnosis

Because certain drugs and pathophysiologic states can lower serum concentrations of thyroid hormones in otherwise euthyroid horses, it is important that thyroid-function tests are not performed while horses are ill, are receiving certain drugs (e.g. phenylbutazone), or are on thyroid-hormone supplementation. The author recommends that thyroid-hormone testing be performed in horses that have not received any medications for at least 2 and preferably 4 weeks prior to testing. If a horse has been receiving thyroid-hormone supplementation without prior documentation of hypothyroidism, the author recommends weaning the horse off supplementation and then testing thyroid function once the horse has not received any supplementation for at least 4 weeks.

Tests that are currently available for the assessment of thyroid function in the horse include measurement of total and free fractions of T_4 and T_3 and response of these hormones to administration of either TRH or TSH. TRH or TSH stimulation tests are considered to be superior to measurement of baseline thyroid hormone concentrations for the evaluation of thyroid function. However, these tests are not routinely performed because of the impracticality of having to take multiple blood samples over time and because TRH and TSH have not been readily available commercially or have been prohibitively expensive. Guidelines for performing a TRH stimulation test in adult horses are shown in *Table 31*.

If single point-in-time measurement of thyroid hormones is the only option available for the evaluation of thyroid status, measurement of free fractions of thyroid hormones (alone or in conjunction with measurement of total amounts) provides more useful information than does measurement of total amounts of thyroid hormones alone. Serum concentrations of free T_4 measured by equilibrium dialysis are more likely to reflect true thyroid status in ill horses, compared with other methods. Measurement of serum TSH concentrations in single samples will also aid in the diagnosis of thyroid status, once a TSH assay for the horse becomes available. Ranges for baseline serum concentrations of thyroid hormones from normal, healthy horses are shown in *Table 32* and can be used as a guideline. However, 'normal' values for serum concentrations of thyroid hormones vary from laboratory to laboratory due to differences in assay procedures, units of measurement, and populations of horses used to establish the laboratory's normal values. Therefore, when choosing a diagnostic laboratory, it is important to verify that the laboratory has validated its assays and established reference ranges in a population of normal horses.

TABLE 31 Protocol for thyrotropin-releasing hormone stimulation testing

1 Take a control serum sample.

2 Administer 1mg TRH/400–600 kg horse i/v. Administer 0.5 mg to ponies and foals. TRH (obtained from a chemical supply house) is put into solution in sterile water, and frozen in 0.5 and 1 mg aliquots for individual use.

3 Take additional serum samples 1, 2, and 4 hours following administration.

4 Submit samples for measurement of free T_3, total T_3, free T_4, and total T_4 analysis. If a TSH assay becomes available, samples can also be submitted for TSH measurement.

5 TSH should peak after 1 hour and should increase to 2.5–3 times the baseline level after TRH administration.

6 Free and total T_3 should double approximately 2 hours following TRH administration.

7 Free and total T_4 should increase by at least 1.7 times the baseline levels at 4–6 hours following TRH administration.

8 The time frame for increases in thyroid hormones in response to TRH is similar in foals to that in adults, but the amount of increase is less. In foals less than 3 days of age, total and free T_4 should increase approximately 10% 4 hours after administration of 0.5 mg TRH. Free T_4 after equilibrium dialysis should increase by approximately 30%. Total and free T_3 should increase by 40% and 60%, respectively, 2 hours after TRH administration.

TABLE 32 Examples of reference ranges for thyroid hormone and TSH concentrations in adult and neonatal horses

	TT_4 nmol/l	fT_4 pmol/l	fT_4 D pmol/l	TT_3 nmol/l	fT_3 pmol/l	TSH ng/ml
Normal adults	n = 71	n = 71	n = 71	n = 71	n = 71	n = 71
Mean	20	11	23	1.0	2.1	0.36
95% CI	18–22	10–12	21–25	0.9–1.1	1.8–2.4	0.31–0.41
Range	6–46	6–21	7–47	0.3–2.9	0.1–5.9	0.02–0.97
Normal foals, 24–36 hours old	n = 18	n = 18	n = 18	n = 18	n = 18	n = 18
Mean	249	62	92	8.4	11.3	0.28
Range	191–318	44–82	49–144	6.0–11.8	5.6–24.2	0.10–0.68
95% CI	231–268	56–68	76–107	7.5–9.3	9.0–13.5	0.21–0.36

TT_3/TT_4 = total T_3/T_4; fT_3/fT_4 = free T_3/T_4; fT_4D = free T_4 by equilibrium dialysis

Serum concentrations of thyroid hormones are much higher in neonates than they are in adults. It is thought that these high concentrations are important for perinatal organ system growth and maturation. Serum concentrations decrease gradually after birth, with free concentrations entering the adult reference range within the first few weeks of life, and total concentrations reaching adult reference ranges when foals are around 1 month old.

Management
Foals
Ensuring proper iodine concentrations in diets fed to pregnant mares can prevent neonatal goiter. Thyroid hormone supplementation may be helpful in the treatment of hypothyroid foals in terms of body-temperature regulation, suck reflex, and mental alertness. Since T_4 must be converted to T_3 for biological activity, there is a greater lag period between administration and metabolic effect for T_4 compared with T_3. Therefore, a combination of T_3 and T_4 supplementation would theoretically be more beneficial to a neonate, but appropriate dosing is unclear. Current dosing recommendations are listed in *Table 33*. Since the cause of the Western syndrome of thyroid dysfunction in foals is unknown at this time, preventive measures are also unknown.

Exercise should be restricted in foals born with incompletely ossified cuboidal bones and/or ruptured extensor tendons. Lightweight splints may be necessary to prevent foals from knuckling or to prevent collapse of the cuboidal bones on the medial sides of the joints. If used, splints must be applied carefully and monitored closely. Foals wearing splints may require help getting up to nurse and are at risk for developing decubital ulcers.

Adults
Options for thyroid-hormone supplementation in adult hypothyroid horses primarily include thyroxine and iodinated casein (*Table 33*). While 10 mg thyroxine per adult horse per day is the usual recommended dose, doses of 20–40 mg thyroxine per horse per day have been given short term to euthyroid horses without causing detectable adverse clinical effects. However, higher doses may produce agitation and hyperexcitability. Monitoring serum thyroid-hormone concentrations and maintaining them in the normal adult range can assure proper dosing.

TABLE 33 Recommended doses of T_4 and T_3 for neonatal and adult horses

Foals

- L-thyroxine: 20–50 µg/kg p/o q24h. Monitor blood T_4 to avoid overdosing.
- Tri-iodothyronine: 1 µg/kg p/o q24h.

Adults

- L-thyroxine: 20 µg/kg p/o q24h (approximately 10 mg/adult horse q24h).
- Iodinated casein: contains approximately 1% T_4 (50 mg T_4/5 g iodinated casein). Dose rate: 5–15 g/horse p/o q24h.
- Tri-iodothyronine: 1 mg/horse p/o q24h.

Prognosis
The prognosis for hypothyroid neonates is guarded. For foals born with goiter, the prognosis improves if the foal can survive the first week of life. The prognosis for foals with musculoskeletal abnormalities depends on the severity of the abnormalities. Certain problems, such as mandibular prognathia, are unlikely to correct. Incompletely ossified cuboidal bones will ossify in time, but long-term prognosis depends on whether or not the bones collapse before ossification occurs. The prognosis for adult horses with hypothyroidism is good if they are properly diagnosed and treated.

Hyperthyroidism
Hyperthyroidism is extremely rare in horses. There have only been a few cases of hyperthyroidism in adult horses properly documented in the literature, and these have been in association with thyroid hormone-producing tumors. Reported clinical signs in these horses include weight loss, tachycardia, tachypnea, hyperactive behavior, ravenous appetite, and cachexia. Circulating thyroid-hormone concentrations are also sometimes temporarily increased in horses exposed to excess iodine, such as in a topical blister.

Horses with hyperthyroidism secondary to thyroid gland neoplasia have been successfully treated with thyroidectomy or hemithyroidectomy, followed by replacement hormone therapy.

Nutritional secondary hyperparathyroidism ('big head disease', 'bran disease')

Definition/overview

Nutritional secondary hyperparathyroidism is characterized by bone demineralization caused by an imbalance of calcium and phosphorus in the diet. Young, growing horses and lactating mares are more susceptible. Primary hyperparathyroidism has also been reported in scattered case reports of parathyroid gland adenoma. Clinical signs and results of diagnostic tests in cases of primary hyperparathyroidism are similar to those of secondary hyperparathyroidism.

Etiology/pathophysiology

As the name implies, nutritional secondary hyperparathyroidism is caused by an improper diet (deficient in calcium or excessive in phosphorus). Ingestion of oxalate-containing plants that bind calcium in the GI tract can also cause this disease by decreasing calcium absorption. Specific diets that can cause nutritional secondary hyperparathyroidism are listed in *Table 34*.

Low dietary calcium or high phosphorus leads to increased parathyroid hormone release from the parathyroid gland and increased active vitamin D. The combination of increased parathyroid hormone and vitamin D promotes calcium and phosphorus resorption from the GI tract and bone, keeping serum calcium in the normal range. Serum phosphorus is unchanged (i.e. not increased), because parathyroid hormone also promotes renal tubular excretion of phosphate (although vitamin D inhibits it). Chronic stimulation of the parathyroid gland results in parathyroid gland hypertrophy and hyperplasia. The net result is maintenance of a normal serum calcium level at the expense of bone resorption.

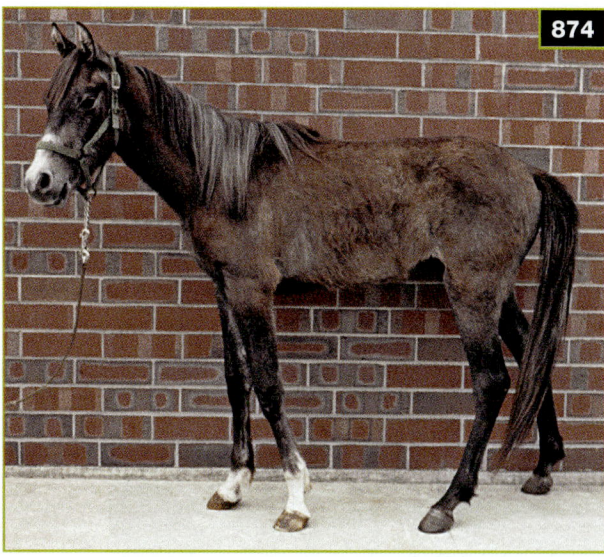

874 Young horse with nutritional secondary hyperparathyroidism. Note the thin, unthrifty appearance and the enlarged head.

Clinical presentation

Affected horses usually look unthrifty (**874**). Clinical signs mainly involve the appendicular skeleton, the teeth, and the skull. Bone demineralization results in a stiff gait, lameness, painful joints, loose teeth, and painful mastication. Pathologic fractures can occur. Demineralization and fibrous proliferation (hyperostotic fibrous osteodystrophy) in the skull result in firm enlargements of the facial bones dorsocaudal to the facial crest, thickening of the mandibles, and thickening of the nasal bones, eventually resulting in nasal obstruction.

Differential diagnosis

Differential diagnoses for hypercalcemia include renal failure, primary hyperparathyroidism, nutritional secondary hyperparathyroidism, vitamin D toxicosis, and malignancy (pseudohyperparathyroidism). Intestinal parasitism should be considered in a thin, young horse that is primarily unthrifty. Physitis should also be considered in a young horse with stiffness or pain in multiple limbs. However, if coarse facial features are present, nutritional secondary hyperparathyroidism should be strongly suspected.

TABLE 34 Diets associated with increased risk of nutritional secondary hyperparathyroidism

- Grain with high phosphorus content and poor to average hay (i.e. oats [Ca 0.07%, P 0.37%] and grass hay [Ca 0.3%, P 0.3%]).
- Increased grain to roughage ratio.
- Supplemenation with rice or wheat bran (i.e. rice bran [Ca 0.04%, P 1.8%] and wheat bran [Ca 0.12%, P 1.43%]).
- Pasture or hay with oxalate:calcium ratios >0.5% (i.e. *Setaria*, Argentine or dallas grass, and buffel grass).

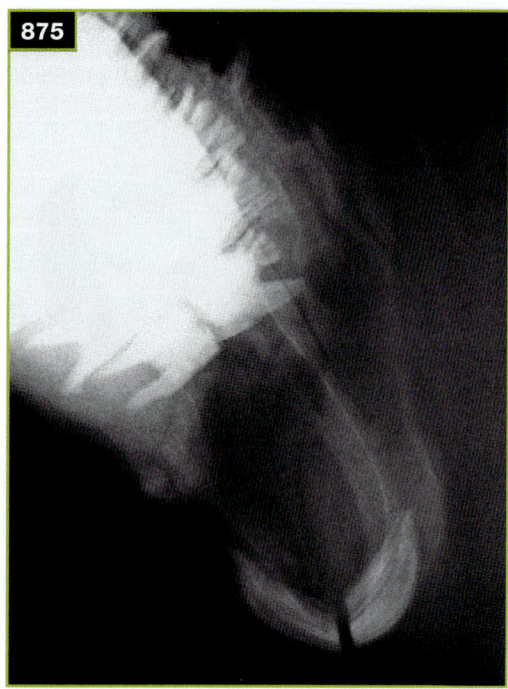

875 Lateral radiograph of the skull of the horse in 874. Demineralization of the skull is apparent by the marked difference in opacity between the bones of the skull compared with the opacity of the cheek teeth.

Diagnosis

A complete dietary history should be reviewed for evidence of a possible calcium/phosphorus imbalance. Bone demineralization can be appreciated on radiographs once the bones are at least 30% demineralized; this occurs first in the skull (**875**). Initially, there is decreased density of the laminae durae dentes, followed by decreased density of the facial bones. In less advanced cases and in the absence of concurrent renal disease, diagnosis can be made by measuring increased parathyroid hormone or increased fractional excretion of phosphorus in the urine. Normal fractional excretion of phosphorus is 0.0–0.5%. Fractional excretion of phosphorus of >0.5% is suggestive of nutritional secondary hyperparathyroidism, and fractional excretion of phosphorus of >4% is diagnostic. It is important to remember that fractional excretion of phosphorus can return to normal as quickly as 24 hours after switching to a balanced diet. Therefore, this test must be performed before the diet is changed. Serum calcium and phosphorus will be normal due to homeostatic mechanisms.

Management

Treatment includes calcium supplementation, restriction of exercise, and judicious use of NSAIDs (only as needed for moderate to severe pain or difficulty chewing). Overuse of NSAIDs could increase the risk of pathologic fractures in severely demineralized horses.

Oral calcium supplementation can be achieved with a commercial mineral mix or by addition of limestone (calcium carbonate) to the diet. Limestone is 40% calcium and contains no phosphorus. The level of calcium supplementation depends on how advanced the condition is at the time of diagnosis. If it is severe, aggressive calcium supplementation at 5 times the recommended calcium intake for the age of the horse (*Table 35*) should be started. In moderate cases, supplementation of calcium at

---

TABLE 35 Recommended daily intake of calcium for normal horses and foals

	% IN DIET		DAILY REQUIREMENT (g)	
	Ca	P	Ca	P
Foals <6 months	0.80	0.55	33	20
Weanlings	0.60	0.45	34	25
Yearlings	0.50	0.35	31	22
Two-year-olds	0.40	0.30	25	17
Mare, late pregnancy	0.45	0.30	34	23
Mare, lactation	0.45	0.30	50	34
Adults, maintenance	0.30	0.20	2.3	14

From Schryver HF, Hintz HF (1987) Minerals. In *Current Therapy in Equine Medicine 2*. (ed NE Robinson) WB Saunders, Philadelphia, p. 396.

Endocrine system

2–3 times the daily requirement is recommended. The calcium:phosphorus ratio of the total diet should be approximately 3–4:1. If the disease is mild, it may be possible to simply correct the diet to a balanced one. The calcium:phosphorus ratio of the total diet for a normal young, growing horse should be approximately 1.5–2:1.

Prognosis

The prognosis for recovery depends on how advanced the condition is at the time of diagnosis. Mild cases will probably recover completely. Moderately affected horses may become sound, but facial enlargement remains. Severely affected horses may remain lame, suffer upper respiratory obstruction necessitating tracheotomy, be unable to masticate, or suffer pathologic fractures that necessitate euthanasia.

Hypocalcemia (see also p. 801)

Definition/overview

Hypocalcemia is not a specific disease, but rather an electrolyte abnormality that can be caused by or associated with a variety of conditions, including those listed in *Table 36*.

Etiology/pathophysiology

Ionized serum calcium concentration is regulated in a narrow range by parathyroid hormone; however, certain events can influence ionized serum calcium so rapidly that this hormonal control system cannot react quickly enough. Such events can include: a sudden decrease in calcium intake; increased calcium demand (e.g. lactation); fecal, urinary, and/or sweat loss; or decreased calcium solubility. Cantharadin toxicity (caused by ingestion of blister beetles) can also cause hypocalcemia. Sepsis and hypomagnesemia are believed to cause secondary or pseudo-hypoparathyroidism. The mechanism by which endotoxemia causes hypocalcemia in the horse is unknown. It is likely that inflammatory cytokines associated with endotoxemia suppress parathyroid hormone secretion, interfere with calcium mobilization, or result in tissue or GI sequestration of calcium. In humans, sepsis is associated with increased serum concentrations of calcitonin precursors (e.g. procalcitonin) and it is thought that increased procalcitonin precipitates the hypocalcemia.

Clinical presentation

Clinical signs vary, depending on the severity of the problem. It is important to remember that clinical signs are dependent on the level of ionized calcium, not necessarily total calcium. Since calcium is protein bound in plasma, low plasma protein concentrations will result in lower measured values for total calcium, but ionized calcium may be within normal limits and true hypocalcemia is not present. With a normal serum albumin concentration,

---

TABLE 36 Conditions associated with hypocalcemia

Pregnancy/lactation
- Mid gestation
- Within 2 weeks of the end of gestation
- 10–86 days after parturition
- 1–2 days after weaning

Sweating (loss of fluid and electrolytes)
- Endurance events
- Prolonged transport, especially in heat and humidity
- Hot, humid environments

Alkalemia
- Found in association with K and Cl loss in sweat, hypokalemia associated with anorexia, hypochloremia with severe gastric reflux, or respiratory alkalosis caused by hyperventilation

Endotoxemia
- GI upsets
- Metritis
- Pleuropneumonia
- Retained placenta
- Increased procalcitonin, perhaps an inflammatory cytokine

Primary hypoparathyroidism

Secondary hypoparathyroidism

Hypomagnesemia

Acute renal failure

Acute rhabdomyolysis

Urea poisoning

Hepatitis

Blister beetle poisoning (cantharadin toxicosis)

Pancreatitis

Rapid intravenous tetracycline administration

Corticosteroids

Idiopathic (Miniature horses seem to be susceptible to this condition)

---

total serum calcium in the range of 2.0–2.5 mmol/l (8–10 mg/dl) causes mild signs, including colic, synchronous diaphragmatic flutter, or signs of hyperexcitability. Tachypnea and tachycardia, with or without arrhythmias, may be present. Total serum calcium of 1.25–2.0 mmol/l (5–8 mg/dl) may result in tetany, incoordination, stiffness of gait or goose-stepping, abnormal facial expressions ('sardonic grin'), elevation of the tail head, muscle fasciculations, laryngospasm, bruxism, and profuse sweating. Serum calcium <1.25 mmol/l (5 mg/dl) causes recumbency and stupor.

Differential diagnosis

Differentials depend on the severity of clinical signs, but can include GI upset (colic), tetanus, HPP, myositis, equine motor neuron disease, or other neurologic disease (e.g. West Nile virus (WVN) encephalitis, rabies, EPM).

Diagnosis

Definitive diagnosis is made by measurement of serum calcium concentration. Measurement of ionized calcium affords a more precise estimation of calcium status. Interpretation of total serum calcium concentration must be adjusted for serum albumin concentration (see below):

Correct total serum calcium (mg/dl) = measured serum calcium (mg/dl) – serum albumin (g/dl) + 3.5

In the absence of immediate laboratory results, diagnosis should be suspected based on clinical signs and a history of predisposing conditions.

Management

Calcium is well absorbed by the GI tract of horses. Normal adult horses should consume approximately 40 mg/kg calcium per day; pregnant or lactating mares, or horses participating in endurance exercise, may need more than this. Mild cases of hypocalcemia can be treated by oral supplementation with calcium in the form of limestone or simply by feeding alfalfa hay. Limestone (calcium carbonate) is 40% calcium and contains no phosphorus. For treatment of mild episodes of hypocalcemia, such as might occur in a horse just completing an endurance event, 20–60 g limestone can be administered orally over several hours. The limestone can be sprinkled on a small amount of grain or administered as a paste directly into the horse's mouth. It has been suggested that administration of 30 g of an electrolyte mixture comprised of 2 parts NaCl, 1 part KCl, and 1 part limestone, every 2 hours, to horses participating in heavy endurance exercise will prevent electrolyte imbalances caused by sweating.

Several products are available for intravenous administration of calcium, including calcium gluconate (available alone or in combination with dextrose and other electrolytes), calcium borogluconate, and calcium chloride.

There is no published 'safe' rate for calcium administration, as there is for potassium administration. While it is possible to administer 23% calcium gluconate slowly and directly from the bottle, it is safer and less irritating to the vein to dilute it in fluids. In severe cases of hypocalcemia, it should be safe to give approximately 500 ml of 23% calcium gluconate (diluted in fluids) over a 1-hour period. The heart rate should be monitored and the calcium infusion slowed or stopped if bradycardia or an arrhythmia develops. In general, when an exact serum calcium concentration is unknown, it is safe initially to add 100–150 ml of 23% calcium gluconate per liter of fluids and give the resulting solution as fast as 2–3 liters/hour to the average 500 kg (1,100 lb) horse. This would be the equivalent of adding 500–750 ml calcium gluconate to a 5-liter bag of fluids and giving that over a period of at least 2 hours. For prolonged calcium supplementation (e.g. 24 hours) in the absence of the facility to monitor serum calcium concentrations, it is usually safe to add 100–150 ml calcium gluconate per 5-liter bag of fluids, administered at 1–2 times the maintenance fluid rate.

Proper dietary management may help prevent hypocalcemia caused by exertion, sweat loss, or lactation. While it is important to feed high-risk horses such as pregnant mares or endurance horses a diet that meets calcium requirements, it is probably not necessary (and may be contraindicated) to feed these horses diets high in calcium before parturition or during training. It is thought that routinely feeding excessive calcium promotes pathways for calcium loss through the GI tract and kidneys. The body is then not prepared hormonally to deal with an acute demand for, or loss of, calcium. Feeding an adequate, but not excessive, amount of calcium in the diet keeps the parathyroid hormone axis more sensitive to decreases in serum calcium, allowing more rapid mobilization of calcium from bone in times of acute need. Calcium supplementation should be provided during times of acute loss (e.g. during exertion that causes profuse sweating or during early lactation).

Prognosis

If properly recognized and treated, the prognosis for recovery from hypocalcemia is excellent. However, if hypocalcemia is unrecognized in severely affected (e.g. recumbent) horses, the prognosis is poor and death may occur before the results of plasma calcium measurements are known.

Pituitary pars intermedia dysfunction (equine Cushing's disease; pituitary adenoma/hypertrophy/hyperplasia)

Definition/overview

This common condition, originally described as a benign tumor of the pituitary gland, is probably more accurately described as hypertrophy or hyperplasia of the gland. It tends to occur in older horses and is mainly an esthetic and management problem. Its chief clinical significance is that it frequently leads to certain complications such as laminitis and predisposition to infection. The latter is reflected in an increased incidence of sole abscesses, skin lesions that do not heal, dental disease, GI parasitism, and/or nonresponsive respiratory infections.

Etiology/pathophysiology

Pituitary hyperplasia is caused by a decrease in inhibitory control of the pars intermedia of the pituitary gland by dopaminergic neurons originating in the hypothalamus. The reason for the decrease in hypothalamic inhibition is currently unknown, but recent reports suggest that inflammation and oxidative stress over time lead to neurodegeneration. Certain breeds may be genetically predisposed.

The pars intermedia of the pituitary gland consists mainly of melanocytes that produce pro-opiomelanocortin (POMC), a precursor peptide that is split into adrenocorticotropic hormone (ACTH), α-melanophore-stimulating hormone (α-MSH), and β-endorphin. The traditional view of pituitary pars intermedia dysfunction is that clinical signs are caused by overproduction of ACTH, leading to excessive circulating corticosteroids. However, baseline plasma concentrations of cortisol are usually within the normal range in horses with pituitary pars intermedia dysfunction. Clinical signs may be caused by an apparent loss of the normal diurnal rhythm for cortisol. However, it is also likely that at least some of the clinical signs of pituitary pars intermedia dysfunction are caused by other metabolites and peptides that are being produced in excess (e.g. α-MSH).

Clinical presentation

The classic clinical presentation is an older horse with a long, shaggy haircoat or one that does not shed normally in spring (876). Often, the hairs at the base of the tail are bushy. There is a tendency for fat to accumulate in the crest of the neck, over the rump, in the sheath of geldings, and behind the eyes. Despite this fat accumulation, owners may complain of weight loss, which takes on an accentuated appearance due to muscle wasting, especially over the topline. Affected horses may be hyperhidrotic, secreting sweat that tends to be greasy. The long haircoat traps sweat, exacerbating skin problems, particularly *Dermatophilus congolensis* infection. Paradoxically, some horses can develop anhidrosis. A fairly uncommon manifestation is lactation in nonpregnant mares. The basis for this is unknown, but it is probably related to altered prolactin secretion. While it is possible for affected mares to carry foals to term, mares are more commonly subfertile.

876 Typical appearance of a horse with pituitary pars intermedia dysfunction (equine Cushing's disease). Note the long curly haircoat and poor muscling.

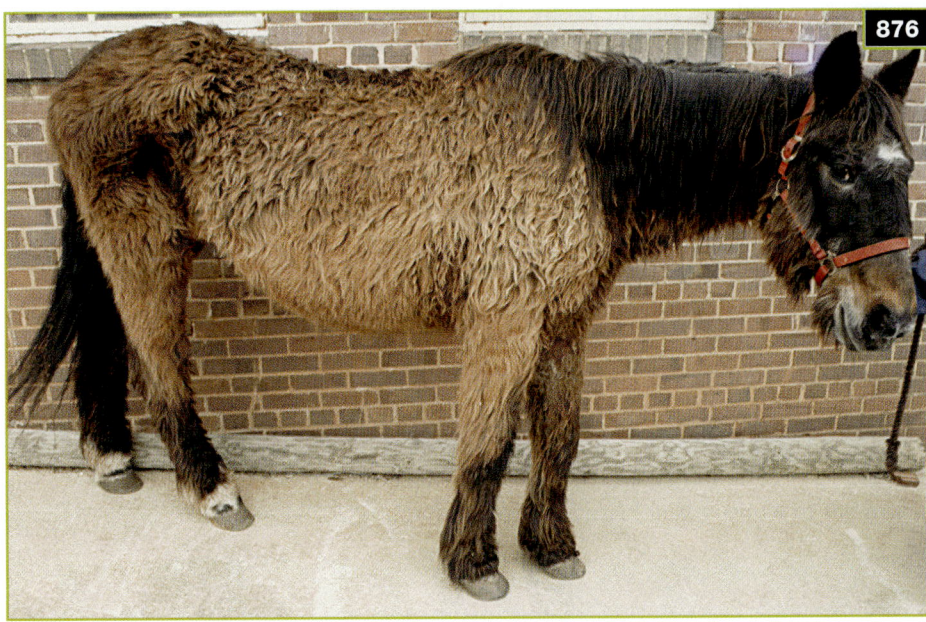

In more advanced cases, polyuria and polydipsia may be present. Possible causes for the polyuria and polydipsia include cortisol-induced thirst, osmotic diuresis secondary to hyperglycemia and glucosuria, and diabetes insipidus secondary to pars intermedia enlargement and encroachment on the neurohypophysis.

One of the most severe problems experienced by affected horses is recurrent laminitis. This is further complicated by a predisposition to develop sole abscesses. Horses may also have trouble fighting other infections such as pneumonia, tooth root abscesses, and sinusitis. Wounds tend to be slow to heal. In very advanced cases, circling, blindness, and seizure activity have been described. These clinical signs are likely caused by expansion of the pituitary gland and exertion of pressure on the optic chiasm and hypothalamus.

Differential diagnosis

The clinical appearance of horses with advanced pituitary pars intermedia dysfunction is fairly unique. However, the main differential diagnosis for horses that still have a normal haircoat would be equine metabolic disease. Haircoat abnormalities can be associated with thyroid disease, but horses with pituitary pars intermedia dysfunction have normal thyroid function.

Diagnosis

In addition to clinical signs, there are certain changes that are often present in a CBC and serum chemistry panel that support a presumptive diagnosis of pituitary pars intermedia dysfunction. These include mature neutrophilia, lymphopenia, and mild hyperglycemia. Glucosuria occurs occasionally, but is the exception rather than the rule.

The pituitary gland can be visualized by CT or MRI, but these imaging techniques are not used routinely because they require anesthesia and are costly. They also are not suited for early detection of a hyperplastic pars intermedia, before the pituitary starts to physically enlarge.

There are several endocrinologic tests that have been described for the diagnosis of pituitary pars intermedia dysfunction, but many of them have very low sensitivity and/or specificity. Measurement of serum cortisol concentration is not useful since it is usually within the reference range. It is thought that horses with pituitary pars intermedia dysfunction lose the normal diurnal variation of serum cortisol, and it has been proposed by some that pituitary pars intermedia dysfunction can be diagnosed by finding a <30% decrease in serum cortisol measured in the late afternoon relative to measurement in the early morning. However, loss of a diurnal pattern of cortisol secretion is not specific to pituitary pars intermedia dysfunction.

Other tests that have been proposed include measurement of increased fasting serum insulin concentration, increased resting plasma ACTH concentration, an accentuated ACTH stimulation test (measurement of an exaggerated plasma cortisol response to ACTH administration), a negative dexamethasone suppression test (failure of plasma cortisol to decrease in response to dexamethasone administration), TRH stimulation test (measurement of increased plasma cortisol in response to TRH administration), combinations of dexamethasone suppression with ACTH or TRH stimulation, and measurement of increased urinary corticoid:creatinine ratio. In the author's opinion, only two of these tests are useful for the diagnosis of pituitary pars intermedia dysfunction: measurement of increased resting plasma ACTH concentration and failure of plasma cortisol concentration to suppress in response to administration of dexamethasone. Measurement of elevated serum insulin concentration relative to serum glucose concentration is supportive of insulin resistance, which can be caused by pituitary pars intermedia dysfunction, but insulin resistance is not specific for this disease. Measurement of serum α-MSH concentration would likely be as useful as measurement of serum ACTH concentration, if an assay for α-MSH becomes available commercially. An advantage of α-MSH measurement over ACTH measurement is that α-MSH is more stable than ACTH, making sample handling easier, especially for ambulatory clinicians. Two recently described additional tests may prove to be useful in the diagnosis of pituitary pars intermedia dysfunction, but larger studies are needed to determine their true sensitivity and specificity. These two tests are measurement of plasma ACTH concentration in response to TRH administration (1 mg i/v) or in response to domperidone administration (3.3 mg/kg p/o). It has been reported that ACTH response to these two stimulants is exaggerated in horses with early pituitary pars intermedia dysfunction, before the resting plasma concentration of ACTH is increased.

For a number of years the most sensitive and specific antemortem test for pituitary pars intermedia dysfunction has been considered to be the dexamethasone suppression test (*Table 37*). Performance of this test may be further enhanced by addition of an injection of 1 mg TRH 3 hours after dexamethasone administration. There is some fear that administration of dexamethasone to a horse with pituitary pars intermedia dysfunction and laminitis might exacerbate the laminitis. While the risk of this appears to be low, many of the other tests listed above were developed to try to avoid administration of dexamethasone.

TABLE 37 Protocol for dexamethasone suppression testing

1 Collect baseline plasma sample for cortisol level between 4:00 and 6:00 pm.

2 Administer dexamethasone (0.04 mg/kg i/m).

3 Collect a plasma sample for cortisol level 17–19 hours later. Plasma cortisol concentration will be suppressed to <27.8 nmol/l (<1 µg/dl) in normal horses. Higher levels indicate pituitary pars intermedia dysfunction.

4 Collection of plasma samples at 15, 19, and 23 hours may be more useful, particularly in young or mildly affected horses. Some horses that are just starting to manifest clinical signs of pituitary pars intermedia dysfunction may be suppressed at 8:00 am or noon, but are no longer suppressed by noon or 4:00 pm.

If one is trying to avoid administration of dexamethasone, the next best documented test is measurement of the resting plasma concentration of ACTH. The advantages of measuring resting plasma ACTH (or α-MSH) concentration are that these tests require collection of only one blood sample and they do not require administration of dexamethasone. The primary disadvantage is that it appears that plasma ACTH (and likely α-MSH) concentrations remain normal for some unknown period of time early in the disease. Thus, false negatives are a problem. Using a cut-off value of 11–12 pmol/l (50–55 pg/ml) for ACTH (i.e. horses are not diagnosed as having pituitary pars intermedia dysfunction unless their plasma ACTH concentrations are greater than 11–12 pmol/l), the likelihood of a false positive is very low, except possibly when testing is done in the fall (see below). Additional disadvantages of ACTH measurement are that ACTH is labile and adheres to glass. Blood should be collected into EDTA (preferably in the morning), placed on ice, and processed as soon as possible (ideally within 1 hour, but certainly within 3 hours) after collection. Plasma should be stored and shipped frozen in plastic containers to prevent adherence of the ACTH to glass.

There is now evidence that the results of dexamethasone suppression tests or plasma ACTH concentrations, when performed on multiple occasions, may vary within an individual horse to the point of giving conflicting results as to whether or not a horse truly has pituitary pars intermedia dysfunction. Necropsy confirmation of diagnosis has not been performed in many of these horses, so the cause of the variation is unknown at this time. It may be

that horses that are just beginning to develop pituitary pars intermedia dysfunction have varying test results until the disease is more advanced. Seasonal variation has also been reported, with concentrations of plasma ACTH and α-MSH being higher in the fall than in the spring. It has been suggested that there is likely to be a physiologic increase in normal pars intermedia function in the fall that might be confused with disease, especially in the early stages. Therefore, testing for pituitary pars intermedia dysfunction should be avoided in the fall, if possible. If testing must be performed in the fall, it is recommended that horses testing positive be retested in the spring. Seasonally specific breakpoints for serum concentrations of α-MSH have been described, but have not been determined for ACTH.

Management

Horses without serious complications can be managed without medication. Excess hair should be removed as needed by body clipping. In addition to body temperature control, this helps to prevent sweat build up and facilitates keeping the coat clean and free of infection. In colder weather the horse can be blanketed. Regular dental and hoof care must be provided, an adequate deworming and vaccination schedule must be followed, and attention must be paid to providing an adequate diet. Horses with dental problems that cannot be resolved (e.g. multiple missing teeth, wave mouth, excessively worn teeth) may require a complete pelleted feed that has been softened so that it does not require much chewing. Care should also be taken to control the weight of horses that tend to be obese.

Horses with complications such as laminitis, respiratory or skin infections, sinusitis, or dermatitis should be treated medically, in addition to the management practices described above. It must be emphasized to owners that medications are not curative. At best, they can only be expected to improve clinical signs and, in order to remain effective, must be given for the rest of the horse's life. This is not economically feasible for all owners. The two most commonly prescribed medications are pergolide and cyproheptadine.

Pergolide is a type 2 dopamine agonist that is thought to act by inhibiting POMC production by the pituitary pars intermedia. Doses from 0.002 to 0.011 mg/kg p/o q24h (1–5.5 mg/day to a 500 kg horse) have been reported to improve clinical signs, lower plasma ACTH concentration, and improve the results of dexamethasone suppression testing. Improvements can take several months to become apparent. It is usually recommended to start a horse at a lower dose (e.g. 0.001 mg/kg), gradually increasing the dose if needed. Adverse side-effects of pergolide administration at doses of up to 0.006 mg/kg/day appear to be uncommon.

Cyproheptadine is a serotonin antagonist that is thought to act by inhibiting secretion of ACTH. There are reports that cyproheptadine (0.3–0.5 mg/kg p/o q24h) improved clinical signs in horses with pituitary pars intermedia dysfunction, particularly in those with laminitis. However, it is not clear how much concurrent management practices contributed to the reported improvements. Cyproheptadine does not appear to be as effective at lowering plasma ACTH concentration or normalizing the results of dexamethasone suppression testing as does pergolide. Some clinicians think that giving cyproheptadine in addition to pergolide is useful in horses that have not responded to pergolide alone at the maximum recommended dose.

Trilostane, a competitive inhibitor of 3β-hydroxysteroid dehydrogenase, has been studied in a limited number of horses. Given orally at 0.4–1 mg/kg once daily, trilostane decreased clinical signs of polyuria/polydipsia and improved laminitis in some horses. No adverse effects were detected over a 1–2-year treatment period. Trilostane did not alter serum insulin concentrations in treated horses.

Various dietary supplements have been proposed for the treatment of pituitary pars intermedia dysfunction, including magnesium, chromium, and vanadium. These minerals are thought to work by decreasing insulin resistance. There have been few controlled studies on the effectiveness of these supplements, although one study did find that chromium supplementation was not beneficial. Chasteberry has also been recommended as a herbal dopamine agonist.

Prognosis

The prognosis depends on the severity of clinical signs and occurrence of complications. Horses with minimal adverse complications have a good prognosis, provided basic husbandry practices as described above are followed. Skin or respiratory infections should be treated promptly. Even if owners do not want to bear the expense of pergolide therapy for the rest of the horse's life, it may be useful to initiate pergolide therapy in conjunction with antimicrobial therapy to help resolve problems such as pneumonia, chronic sinusitis or guttural pouch infections, and sole abscesses. The prognosis for horses with multiple tooth root abscesses, moderate to severe laminitis, or laminitis with recurring foot abscessation is guarded to poor.

Metabolic conditions

Equine metabolic syndrome (peripheral Cushing's syndrome)
Definition/overview
Equine metabolic syndrome is the name currently proposed for a cluster of problems in horses that are overweight, insulin resistant, and susceptible to laminitis. Other names proposed for this syndrome include peripheral Cushing's syndrome, insulin resistance syndrome, syndrome X, omental Cushing's syndrome, and central obesity. Horses with clinical signs included in this syndrome are commonly misdiagnosed as hypothyroid. There is a similar cluster of endocrine-related signs (obesity, insulin resistance, hypertension, subfertility in women, accumulation of abdominal fat) in humans. Whether this proposed syndrome in horses is pathophysiologically similar to the syndrome described in humans remains to be seen. It also remains to be seen whether this syndrome in horses truly represents a separate disease entity, or whether it merely represents a pre-cushingoid state.

Etiology/pathophysiology
A specific etiology for this syndrome is currently unknown. There is likely to be a genetic predisposition, since the syndrome is seen more commonly in certain breeds including Morgans, Paso Finos, and Mustangs, and perhaps American Saddlebreds and Arabians. It has been proposed that breeds that evolved in geographic areas where there were periods of decreased food supply developed an increased ability to store fat and an increased susceptibility to becoming insulin resistant. At this time it is unclear whether any horse, no matter what breed, could potentially become insulin resistant and develop this syndrome if it is allowed to become obese.

Although horses with equine metabolic syndrome are thought to be genetically predisposed to obesity and insulin resistance, similar to type 2 diabetes in humans, it is extremely rare for these horses to progress to overt diabetes mellitus. It has been proposed that omental adipocytes develop increased activity of 11β-hydroxysteroid dehydrogenase, an enzyme that converts inactive cortisone to active cortisol. Increased active cortisol leads to more omental obesity and dyslipidemia. In the horse it has also been proposed that insulin resistance and a local increase in active cortisol in the foot predisposes to laminitis.

Clinical presentation
Horses are described as 'easy keepers', with thick, cresty necks and fat accumulation over their rumps and, if they are geldings, in their sheaths (877,878). They tend to suffer from chronic, low-grade, recurrent laminitis.

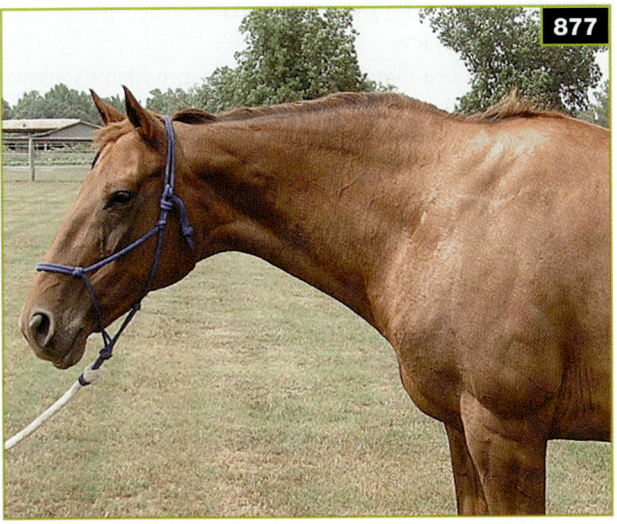

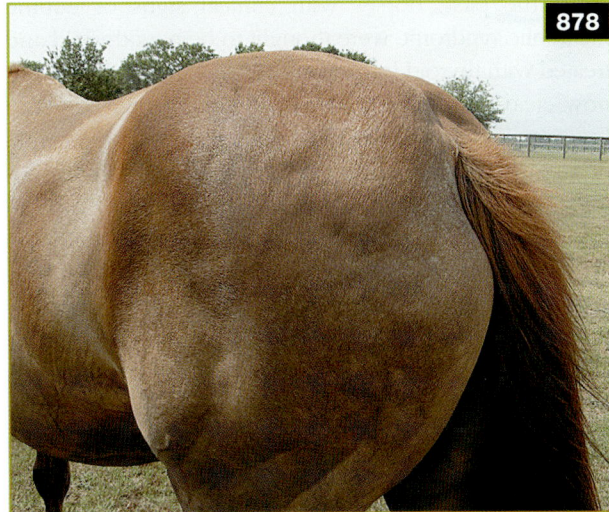

877, 878 A horse with equine metabolic syndrome having typical cresty neck (877) and excessive deposition of fat in the tailhead area (878).

Differential diagnosis

The primary differential diagnosis is pituitary pars intermedia dysfunction. The clinical signs are associated by some authors with hypothyroidism, but horses with equine metabolic syndrome have normal resting serum thyroid hormone concentrations and normal thyroid stimulation tests.

Diagnosis

There are no specific tests to diagnose equine metabolic syndrome definitively. A presumptive diagnosis is based on the presence of clinical signs (i.e. obesity, regional adiposity, tendency for laminitis) and demonstration of insulin resistance or glucose intolerance via increased serum insulin concentration with normal serum glucose concentration, slow return of serum glucose concentration to normal after administration of a glucose load, or an exaggerated insulin response to a glucose load. Several procedures for performing an intravenous glucose tolerance test have been described. When performing these tests, it is important to recognize that stress and certain disease states can alter insulin sensitivity. The syndrome is differentiated from pituitary pars intermedia dysfunction by the dexamethasone suppression test, as horses with equine metabolic syndrome have a normal response to dexamethasone administration.

Management

There are no current treatment recommendations except for weight reduction, which can be difficult to achieve. Affected horses tend to maintain body weight on very little feed. In fact, some horses remain obese when eating nothing more than pasture grass. Weight loss in these horses must be achieved by limiting access to pasture or by use of grazing muzzles. It has been suggested that horses with metabolic syndrome eat diets low in soluble carbohydrates (low glycemic index) and low in fat. Although it makes sense to avoid feeding grain to these horses (many need nothing more than a good quality hay to maintain body weight), specific dietary studies have not been performed to substantiate these recommendations. Studies in ponies that tended to be insulin resistant showed that feeding a higher percentage fat diet actually resulted in lower concentrations of serum triglycerides. However, the higher fat diets did not reduce insulin resistance. Some authors have proposed increasing magnesium or chromium in the diet, but currently there is no documented evidence to show that such supplementation is helpful, and specific dosing recommendations are lacking. Exercise has been shown to be useful for decreasing insulin resistance and for promoting weight loss, but increasing the amount of exercise may be difficult or impossible in horses with active laminitis.

In the past, horses with clinical signs of equine metabolic syndrome were thought to be hypothyroid and treated with thyroid hormone supplementation. While it is now clear that these horses have normal thyroid gland function, it is possible that thyroid hormone supplementation helps ameliorate clinical signs through a pharmacologic, rather than a physiologic, mechanism. Thyroid hormones increase metabolic rate and potentiate the action of beta-2 adrenergic agonists at their receptor sites. Therefore, induction of mild hyperthyroidism could potentiate weight loss by increasing the metabolic rate and by altering fat metabolism. In addition, beta-2 adrenergic agonists generally relax vascular smooth muscle, which could lead to increased blood flow to laminitic feet. However, potential adverse effects of prolonged hyperthyroidism have not been studied in the horse. In humans, thyrotoxicosis or oversupplementation with thyroid hormones can cause decreased bone density, increase the risk of atrial fibrillation, and perhaps increase the risk of myocardial infarction or congestive heart failure. In one recent study, normal mares were given thyroid hormones for a year. No adverse clinical signs or changes in serum chemistry panel were reported. Cardiac chamber sizes, wall thicknesses, and contractility, determined by ultrasonography, remained within reference ranges. However, prolonged ECG rhythm recordings and bone density were not measured. The mares did lose weight, as long as feed intake was controlled. Insulin sensitivity increased with weight loss, although it was not possible to determine whether this was a direct effect of thyroid hormone administration or simply due to the weight loss itself.

Although some clinical signs of this disease are similar to those of pituitary pars intermedia dysfunction, pergolide and cyproheptadine are not useful.

Prognosis
The prognosis is good for these horses if body weight and laminitis can be controlled.

Hyperlipemia/hyperlipidemia
Definition/overview
Hyperlipemia is a metabolic condition in which excessive fatty acids in the blood cause the serum to look milky. Hyperlipemia is the term used when serum triglycerides exceed 6.65 mmol/l (500 mg/dl). Hyperlipidemia refers to a milder increase in serum triglycerides that is not evident visually. Hyperlipemia occurs most commonly in ponies, donkeys, and miniature horses and is rare in other breeds.

Etiology/pathophysiology
Hyperlipemia occurs when more fatty acids are mobilized from adipose tissue than the liver can effectively utilize for energy production. The condition can be primary in certain equids (e.g. ponies, donkeys, and miniature horses), but is more commonly secondary to a disorder that incites a negative energy balance. The problem is more common in overweight individuals or in mares that are in late pregnancy or lactating. Azotemia contributes to the disease by inhibiting uptake of triglycerides by peripheral tissues, possibly by inhibiting lipoprotein lipase. Horses that are insulin resistant may be at greater risk of developing hyperlipemia during periods of anorexia or feed restriction. Other risk factors include stress, malnutrition, and intestinal parasitism.

Negative energy balance results in activation of hormone-sensitive lipase and mobilization of glycerol, FFAs, and nonesterified fatty acids from adipose tissue. These nutrients travel in the blood to the liver, where they can be converted to glucose by gluconeogenesis or oxidized to acetyl-CoA. Fatty acids can also be converted to ketones in many species, but ketogenesis does not appear to occur to a significant degree in horses. Acetyl-CoA enters the tricarboxylic acid cycle through oxaloacetate. Oxaloacetate is also needed for gluconeogenesis. If there is insufficient oxaloacetate available, FFAs are re-esterified to triglycerides and phospholipids. These accumulate in the liver (fatty liver) or are released back into the plasma as VLDLs. Fatty infiltration of the liver, when present, results in increased serum concentrations of liver enzymes.

Clinical presentation
Clinical signs include anorexia, depression, and weakness, progressing to muscle fasciculations, ataxia, head pressing, circling, recumbency, and convulsions or coma. Ventral edema may be present. Diarrhea may accompany the syndrome, either as an inciting cause of the negative energy balance or secondary to anorexia. Parasitism may contribute to poor appetite and compete for nutrients.

6

Differential diagnosis

The primary clinical signs of anorexia, depression, and weakness are nonspecific and can be caused by many diseases. Often, hyperlipemia occurs secondary to another disease process and the initial clinical signs of hyperlipidemia are either missed or ascribed to the original problem. Primary differentials for anorexia should include fever or GI problems including, but not limited to, colic, gastric ulcers, and gastric SCC. Differential diagnoses for the diarrhea include the various causes of colitis.

Diagnosis

Diagnosis is made by measurement of elevated triglycerides (>6.65 mmol/l [500 mg/dl]) in plasma or observance of lipemic plasma. Liver enzymes and function tests should be measured in cases of hyperlipemia. Additional testing to identify possible inciting causes should be undertaken.

Management

The two primary goals of treatment are (1) to identify and treat the inciting cause of the negative energy balance or the underlying disease, and (2) to improve the energy balance. Depending on the severity of the hyperlipemia, improving the energy balance may be as simple as offering palatable feeds to encourage eating. Administration of NSAIDs may improve appetite in horses with high fevers or in pain. Provision of a higher energy diet or force-feeding via nasogastric tube may also be effective in mild cases. Preparations that can be administered by nasogastric tube include solutions of glucose (or dextrose) and electrolytes, gruels made from pelleted feeds, or commercially available enteral solutions. Improperly balanced home-made solutions containing glucose and electrolytes may exacerbate metabolic acidosis or result in hyperglycemia. Commercially available enteral solutions are convenient, but may be cost prohibitive except in smaller equids. Gruels made from complete pelleted feeds have the advantage that they are nutritionally complete and relatively inexpensive, but they require co-administration of a large volume of water to keep the gruel from clogging the tube. This large volume makes it necessary to administer multiple meals (usually a minimum of six) throughout the day in order to satisfy dietary requirements without overloading the stomach. It is usually necessary to start with a smaller amount of feed (e.g. 50%) on the first day and gradually increase the amount given per feeding over a few days until either 100% of the required diet is reached or the horse begins eating voluntarily.

Moderate cases of hyperlipemia may require intravenous infusion of glucose (5 or 10%) and/or force-feeding by nasogastric tube. Concurrent administration of a balanced electrolyte solution is required to provide maintenance fluid requirements and account for any ongoing losses (i.e. diarrhea). Fluid therapy is particularly important in azotemic animals. Frequent monitoring of blood glucose levels should be performed to help maintain a steady level. At concentrations of 5–10%, intravenous glucose administration alone is not enough to meet maintenance energy requirements, but it will help stop additional fat mobilization from adipose tissue. Insulin administration may also help inhibit further fat mobilization, but hyperlipemic horses often have some degree of insulin resistance. Heparin (40–250 USP units/kg s/c q12h) stimulates lipoprotein lipase and may enhance removal of lipids from blood; however, the use of heparin is somewhat controversial because it may enhance lipid uptake into the liver and increase fat deposition in that organ. Lactulose (0.2 ml/kg p/o q12h) administration to decrease ammonia production and absorption may be useful in horses with hepatic encephalopathy. Unless absolutely required for the treatment of underlying disease, glucocorticoid administration should be avoided since steroids stimulate hormone-sensitive lipase.

Severe cases of hyperlipemia, especially in debilitated animals, may require partial or total parenteral nutrition (without the lipid component) initially. Partial or total parenteral nutrition is also useful for hyperlipidemic or hyperlipemic horses or ponies with GI disorders, such as proximal enteritis or postoperative ileus, that cannot receive enteral nutrition. Serial measurements of serum triglyceride concentrations or visual monitoring of plasma turbidity can be useful in evaluating response to treatment.

Prognosis

The prognosis is fair to poor when the syndrome has progressed to hyperlipemia. The prognosis is worse in individuals with severe underlying disease that is difficult to treat. The prognosis is better in individuals whose triglycerides return to the normal range within 3–10 days of treatment. Best results are achieved when the syndrome is recognized in at-risk individuals in the hyperlipidemia stage. Starting intravenous glucose infusions (5%) before the horse's triglycerides exceed 6.65 mmol/l (500 mg/dl) can help stop fat mobilization and prevent exacerbation of the syndrome.

Miscellaneous diseases of the endocrine system

Diabetes mellitus

In recent years there has been increasing interest and attention paid to insulin resistance and the proposed occurrence of type 2 diabetes in horses. Horses with pituitary pars intermedia dysfunction and equine metabolic syndrome may be insulin resistant and, perhaps, all obese horses have some degree of insulin resistance. However, very few horses go on to develop frank diabetes mellitus. Although case reports of diabetes mellitus exist in the older literature, descriptions of these horses are most consistent with a diagnosis of pituitary pars intermedia dysfunction. Primary clinical features include polyuria and polydipsia secondary to hyperglycemia and glucosuria. Horses that exhibit polyuria and polydipsia should be tested for pituitary pars intermedia dysfunction and have their renal function examined.

Adrenal tumors

Definition/overview

The adrenal gland is made up of the adrenal cortex (with three zones) and the adrenal medulla. The outermost zone of the adrenal cortex is the zona glomerulosa, which secretes mineralocorticoids; the middle zone is the zona fasciculata, which secretes glucocorticoids; and the innermost zone is the zona reticularis, which secretes adrenal androgens. The adrenal medulla secretes catecholamines, primarily epinephrine. Tumors of the adrenal gland are uncommon, usually nonfunctional, and generally found as incidental findings at necropsy. Tumors of the adrenal cortex include adenoma and carcinoma. Pheochromocytoma is a tumor of the adrenal medulla. The pathophysiology of functional tumors relates to oversecretion of hormones made by that particular section of the adrenal gland.

Clinical presentation

Tumors of the adrenal cortex of the horse have been associated with lethargy, abdominal pain, weight loss, hindlimb edema, and seizures. Low serum sodium concentration has also been reported. Clinical signs of pheochromocytoma, when they exist, include excessive sweating, muscle fasciculations, rapid heart rate, tachypnea, polyuria, and polydipsia. Horses may appear to be apprehensive and have dilated pupils. Recurrent bouts of colic may be encountered. Typically, the heart rate is higher than would be expected for the apparent degree of abdominal pain.

Differential diagnosis

Differential diagnoses for horses exhibiting clinical signs of pheochromocytoma could include severe endotoxemia, electrolyte abnormalities, myositis, tetanus, and equine motor neuron disease.

Diagnosis

Pheochromocytoma should be suspected based on clinical signs. Demonstration of hyperglycemia and increased blood or urinary epinephrine helps to confirm the diagnosis. Adrenal tumors may be palpable per rectum if they are large enough and on the left side. Ultrasonography may reveal a mass in the area of the right or left kidney and may provide guidance for biopsy. However, most tumors of the adrenals are diagnosed at necropsy.

Management

Surgical removal of an adrenal tumor might be possible if the tumor is unilateral and diagnosed early, while it is small. However, this would only be the case if the tumor was an incidental finding. Many are subclinical and those that do cause clinical signs are probably too extensive by the time they are diagnosed to realistically be considered candidates for surgical removal.

Prognosis

The prognosis for horses exhibiting clinical signs of pheochromocytoma is poor.

Urinary system

Modest Vengust

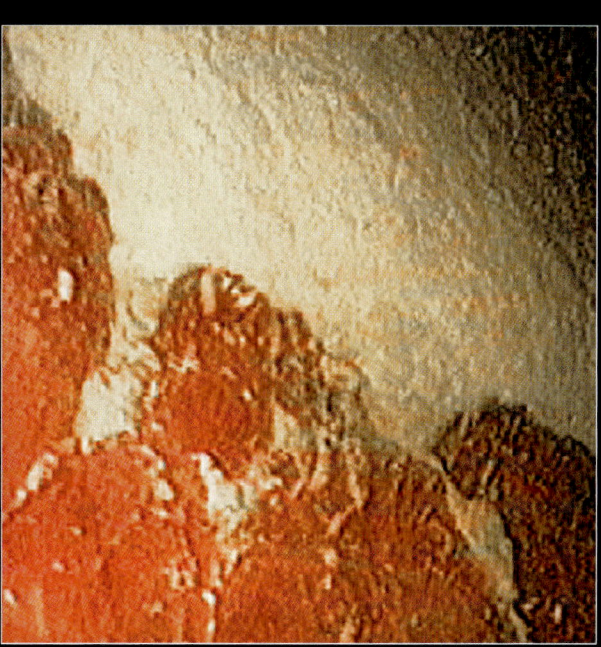

Urinary system

General physical examination

A thorough history should be taken before a physical examination is performed. The clinician should enquire about the duration and type of clinical signs, medication(s) given, response to treatment, diet, and number of animals on the premises that are affected. A full physical examination should be performed because of the potentially non-specific clinical signs of urinary tract disease. In the male patient the urethral orifice and urethra on the ventral aspect of the penis should be palpated. The vaginal opening and perineum can be readily examined in the female. In foals the umbilicus and surrounding structures of the abdomen should also be assessed. Hydration status should be assessed (879). Ideally, urination should be observed (*Table 38*).

Palpation per rectum should be performed in all animals of adequate size. The proximal urethra, bladder, ureters, and the left kidney should be evaluated. The proximal urethra is located before the brim of the pelvis. The examiner should thereafter systematically explore the bladder, ureters, and the caudal pole of the left kidney.

Physiologically, water consumption and urination vary with age and may be influenced by the climate, diet, and level of exercise. Water consumption and urine output should be assessed over a 24-hour period. A horse with normal renal function should produce 5–20 liters of urine daily (15.30 ml/kg/day [6.8–13 l/450kg horse/day]) while consuming 20–35 liters of water (15–60 ml/kg/day [6.8–27 l/450kg horse/day]). Increased water loss, either pathologic (i.e. diarrhea, hemorrhage, polyuria) or physiologic (i.e. sweating), should result in increased water intake.

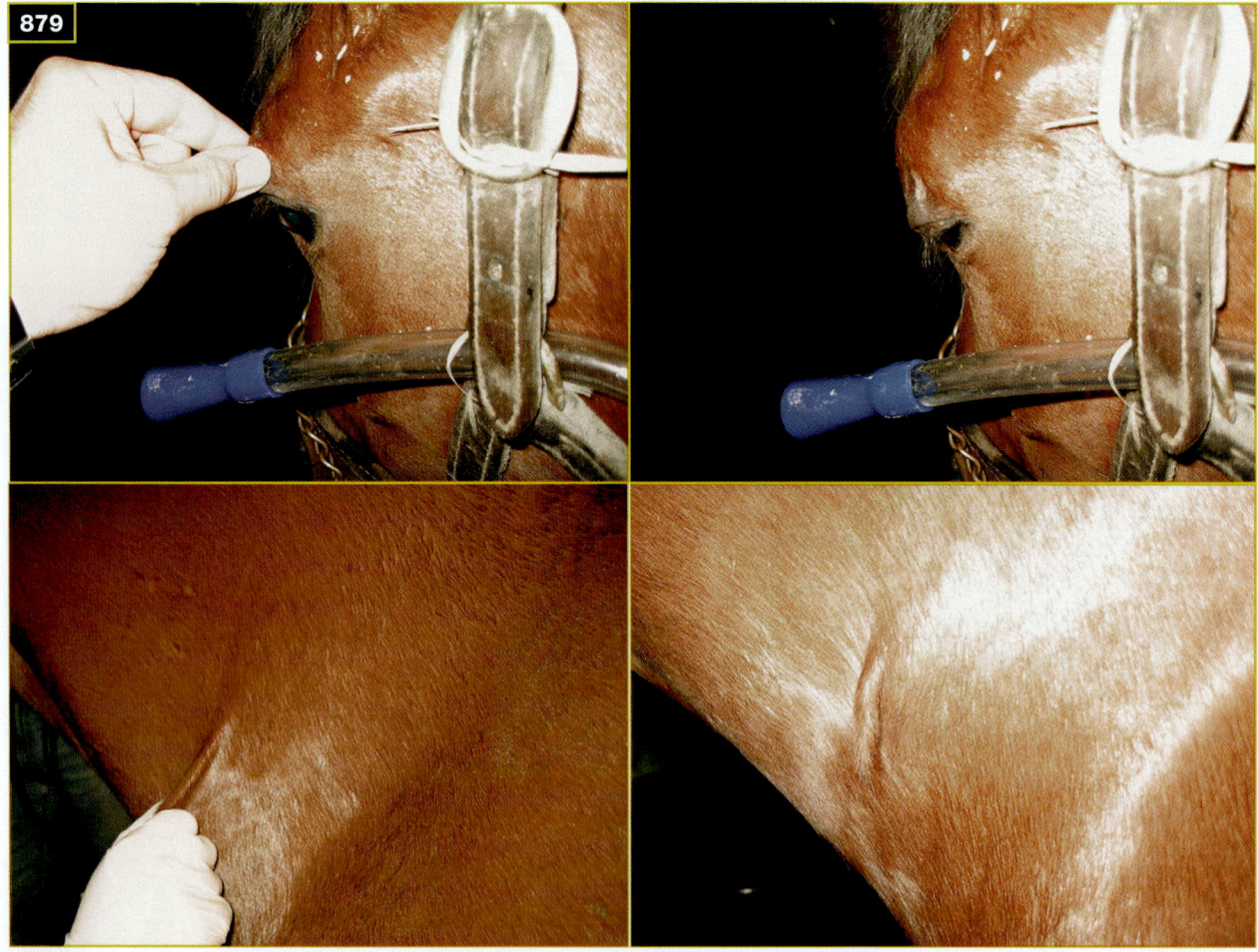

879 Altered skin turgor in a severely dehydrated horse. Skin turgor is better assessed on the eyelid (top) compared with the neck (bottom).

TABLE 38 **Terminology used in urinary tract disease**	
Stranguria	Slow and painful urination
Pollakiuria	Abnormally frequent passage of urine
Dysuria	Painful or difficult urination
Oliguria	Reduced daily urine output
Polyuria	Increased daily urine output
Anuria	Complete cessation of urine output
Azotemia	Presence of nitrogenous waste products in the blood
Isosthenuria	Urine SG between 1.008 and 1.012, indicating lack of concentration or dilution

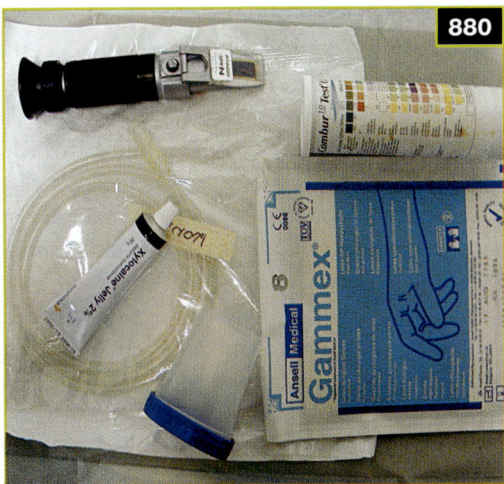

Diagnostic tests

Urinalysis

Urinalysis is required for assessment of urinary tract function. Urinalysis results may be influenced by the method used for urine collection. Voided, midstream urine samples can be readily obtained; however, contamination from the distal urethra and the genital tract makes interpretation of the results more difficult. Urethral and genital tract diseases can often be distinguished by analysis of the early stream of voided urine.

Urethral catheterization is easy to perform in most horses, with only basic equipment required (**880**). Catheterized samples should be obtained when voided urine cannot be collected or when samples for bacterial culture are required (**881, 882**). Alpha-2 adrenergic agonists (i.e. xylazine, detomidine) cause diuresis and glucosuria. Exogenous corticosteroid administration acts similarly. Trauma to the urinary tract is inevitable with catheterization, and mild increases in protein levels and the number of RBC and transitional epithelial cells are common.

880 Sterile gloves, sterile urinary catheter, sterile ointment or jelly, sterile cup, refractometer, and urine test strips are basic equipment required for aseptic urine collection.

881 Catheterization of the urinary bladder in a male.

882 Catheterization of the urinary bladder in a female.

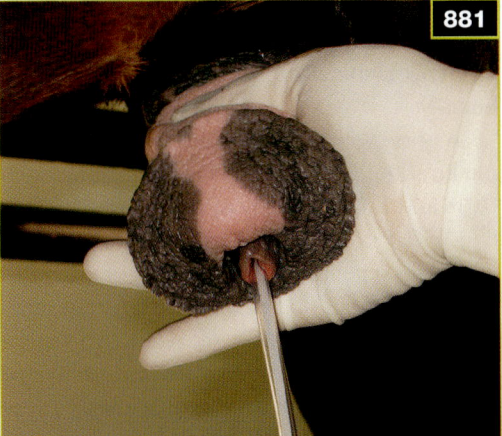

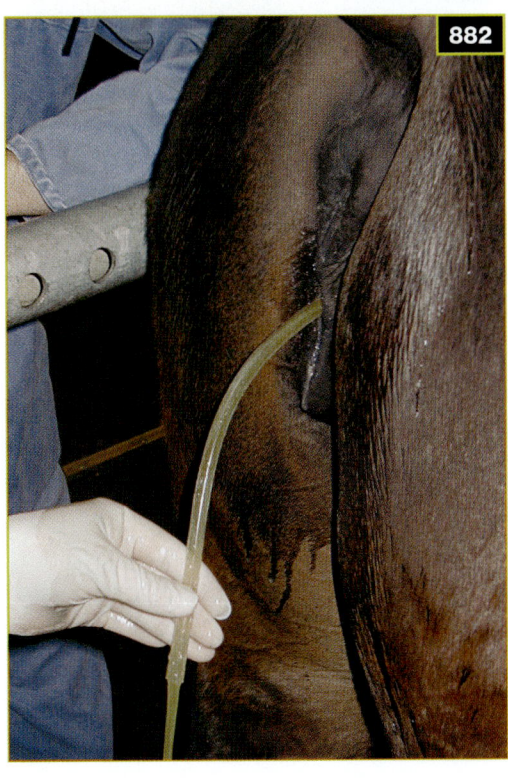

Physical and chemical properties of urine

Equine urine should be pale yellow to deep tan (**883**). Large numbers of calcium carbonate crystals and mucus may be present in normal urine, resulting in a highly turbid sample. Discoloration of the urine can be caused by pigmenturia or hematuria, neither of which should be present in normal urine samples. Pigmenturia is caused by the presence of hemoglobin or myoglobin in the urine. If discoloration of urine is present at the start or at the end of urination, the lesion may be located in the urethra or accessory sex glands. Similarly, hematuria may be more prominent at the end of urination. Hemoglobinuria, myoglobinuria, or the presence of intact erythrocytes in the urine yields a positive result on a reagent strip. Differentiation of pigmenturia is performed by evaluation of the sediment for erythrocytes and by performing the ammonium sulfate precipitation test to detect myoglobin. Protein electrophoresis may also be used to differentiate hemoglobin from myoglobin. Serum should be analyzed for concurrent hemolysis.

A horse with a normal renal function and normal water intake should concentrate the urine to an SG of between 1.018 and 1.025. When water is deprived, this may increase to 1.050 if normal renal concentrating abilities are preserved. Isosthenuria, or production of urine that is neither concentrated nor diluted (SG 1.008–1.012), may occur with disease or may be physiologic relative to water intake.

Horses usually have alkaline urine with a pH between 7.5 and 9.0. Urine may become acidic as a result of high-intensity exercise. An ammonia odor to the urine sample suggests bacterial breakdown of urea. Diluted urine usually has a neutral to slightly acidic pH.

Proteinuria may occur with pyuria, bacteriuria, and glomerular disease. Physiologically, it can be detected after exercise. Glomerular function may be temporarily altered by stress, fever, seizures, extreme environmental temperature, and venous congestion in the kidneys, resulting in reversible proteinuria. Commercial reagent strips often yield false-positive results for protein when alkaline urine is tested or when urine SG exceeds 1.035. Therefore, semi-quantitative sulfosalicylic acid precipitation or a colorimetric assay should be used to quantify the urine protein. Urine protein:creatinine ratio (UP/UC) is helpful in distinguishing primary glomerular disease (UP/UC >3; usually >5) from primary tubular disease (UP/UC <3).

Normal horse urine should not contain glucose. Dextrose-containing fluids or parenteral nutrition compounds may cause glucosuria as a result of hyperglycemia. Similarly, alpha-2 adrenergic agonists and treatment with corticosteroids may cause glucosuria. Glucosuria without hyperglycemia is usually associated with renal tubular dysfunction.

Hyperglycemia of different causes (e.g. stress, exercise, sepsis, pituitary pars intermedia dysfunction, or diabetes mellitus) produces glucosuria when blood glucose levels exceed 11 mmol/l (200 mg/dl).

Urine sediment should be evaluated for cells, bacteria, casts, and crystals (**884–886**). Evaluation should be carried out no later than 1 hour after urine collection (*Table 39*).

Urinary tract inflammation, infection, neoplasia, endotoxemia, or trauma may result in increased numbers of erythrocytes in the urine. Pyuria (>5–8 WBCs/hpf) is usually associated with urinary tract inflammation and/or infection. Bacteria can be present in the urine sediment in

883 Normal equine urine can be quite variable, ranging from clear to turbid.

TABLE 39 Characteristics of normal equine urine

pH	7.5–9.0 (concentrated feeds tend to acidify urine)
Specific gravity	1.018–1.025
Glucose	Negative
Protein	Negative*
White blood cells	<5/hpf
Red blood cells	<5/hpf
Epithelial cells	None present if voided sample
Casts	Usually negative – hyaline casts sometimes present
Crystals	Common
Hemoglobin	Negative
Myoglobin	Negative
Bacteria	Usually negative if catheterized urine

* False-positive protein result may occur on urine dipsticks with alkaline urine

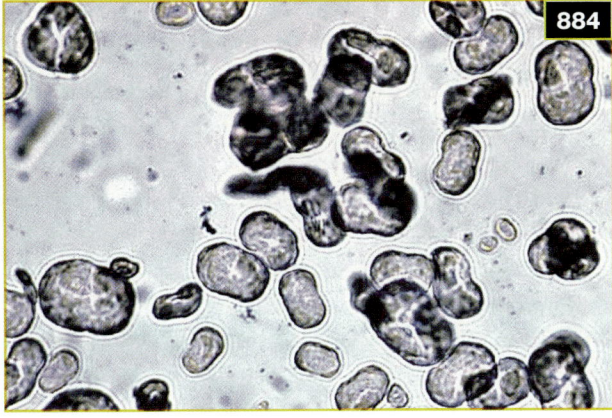

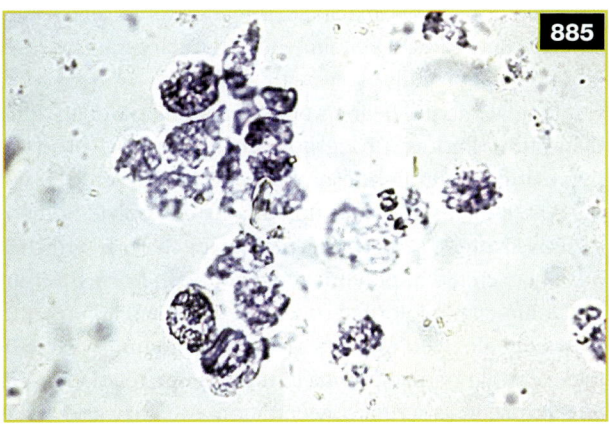

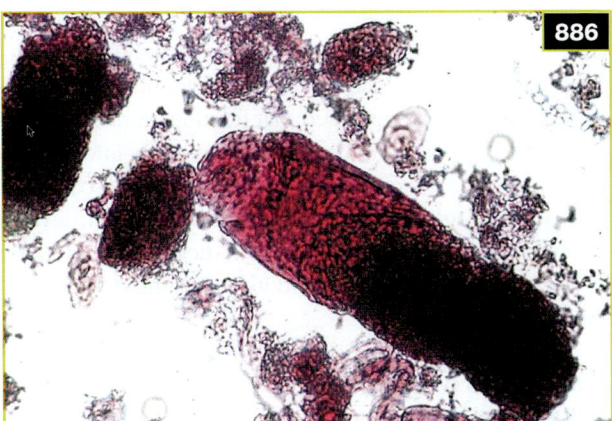

884–886 Urine sediment evalution findings. (884) Calcium carbonate crystals: a common component of equine urine. (885) Leukocytes present in the urine. (886) Granular casts. (Photos courtesy R Jacobs)

urogenital tract infection. Normally, the sediment contains no or few bacteria; however, the absence of visible bacteria does not rule out infection. Quantitative and qualitative bacterial culture should be performed on urine that was collected by catheterization or, in foals, by cystocentesis.

Casts are mucoproteineous substances that are formed within distal renal tubules. Cast formation increases when urinary tract inflammation or/and infection is/are present. Casts are rare in normal equine urine as they usually dissolve in alkaline urine; therefore, the absence of casts does not rule out renal disease. Casts are also present only transiently and may not be detected in all cases of acute renal disease.

To assess the urine sediment accurately, a small quantity of 10% acetic acid solution is added to the sample to dissolve crystals. Crystals are usually abundant in equine urine and may interfere with urine sediment evaluation. Calcium carbonate crystals are the most common crystals of equine urine, followed by triple phosphate and, rarely, calcium oxalate.

GGT is found in high concentrations in epithelial cells lining the proximal renal tubules. Physiologically, its activity in urine arises from cell turnover. Any damage to the renal tubular epithelium will increase its activity in urine. This can be expressed as a ratio of the urine GGT activity to urine creatinine concentration (urine GGT activity:urine creatinine × 0.01), with a value of above 25 being considered abnormal. The urine GGT:urine creatinine ratio, however, has been found to have a poor specificity.

Hematology and serum chemical analysis
Azotemia, an increase in serum urea, may occur with prerenal, renal, or postrenal disease. Prerenal azotemia is the most common form and is typically associated with dehydration. Renal azotemia is associated with intrinsic renal failure and does not develop until there is a functional loss of approximately 70% of nephrons. Postrenal azotemia is associated with urinary tract obstruction or rupture. Identification of the cause of azotemia is critical to the management of urinary tract disease. To define the origin of azotemia, clinical signs and laboratory analysis findings need to be assessed simultaneously. Urine SG is essential for interpretation of azotemia. The urine creatinine:serum creatinine ratio may also provide useful information in this context. A ratio of >50:1 is associated with prerenal azotemia. A ratio of <37:1 is usually associated with primary renal disease. The serum urea:creatinine ratio has been used to distinguish between acute (ARF) and chronic (CRF) renal failure; however, results are highly variable and have not proved useful in a clinical context.

Alterations in plasma and serum electrolyte levels may be encountered with certain types of urinary tract disease. Sodium is typically lost with polyuric renal failure, resulting in varying degrees of hyponatremia. Urinary tract disruption and/or uroperitoneum, however, produce hyponatremia through resorption of urine, which is lower in sodium than serum. Disrupted body electrolyte homeostasis also affects serum concentration of chloride, which is heavily excreted in polyuric renal failure in horses. Serum potassium can be normal or elevated in renal failure, and markedly elevated in cases of uroperitoneum. With ARF the excretion of phosphorus in urine is disrupted, causing an increase in its serum concentration. ARF may also result in hypocalcemia. However, hypercalcemia and hypophosphatemia are often found in CRF. Serum albumin and globulin concentrations variably decrease in chronic renal diseases. Albumin tends to be lost to a greater extent than globulin because of its low molecular weight. In cases of neoplasia, glomerulonephritis, pyelonephritis, or amyloidosis, serum globulin concentration may increase as a result of chronic antigen stimulation. Serum enzyme activity should be examined to assess the metabolism of other organs and to differentiate pigmenturia.

Mild to moderate anemia may be associated with CRF consequent to decreased erythropoietin production and a shortened erythrocyte lifespan.

Fractional excretion of electrolytes

Repeated collection of urine samples obtained by catheterization on consecutive days at the same time of day and the same stage of daily routine is the most practical way to employ fractional urinary excretion of electrolytes calculations. Volumetric urine collection during a 24-hour period is more laborious to perform, requires confinement of animals, a period during which the animal adapts to the urine collection device, and a reliable and animal-friendly urine collection device. In most instances, however, a single determination is performed.

Fractional excretion should be calculated using the following equation:

$$FE = (([Cr]_{plasma} / [Cr]_{urine}) \times ([X]_{plasma} / [X]_{urine})) \times 100$$

where $[Cr]_{plasma}$ and $[Cr]_{urine}$ are the creatinine (Cr) concentrations in the plasma and urine, respectively, and $[X]_{plasma}$ and $[X]_{urine}$ are the concentrations of a specific electrolyte or mineral in plasma and urine, respectively (*Table 40*).

TABLE 40 Reference ranges for fractional excretion of electrolytes

ELECTROLYTE	RANGE
Sodium	<1.00
Chloride	<1.50
Potassium	15–65
Phosphorus	<0.50
Calcium	<7

Urine and plasma should be collected at the same time. The suggested reference values can be influenced by diet. Concern has been expressed that fractional urinary excretion of electrolytes does not provide reliable information regarding urinary excretion of electrolytes due to considerable physiologic variation within and between days in urinary electrolyte excretion even if diet and exertion are held constant. This has limited its use in the detection of renal disease.

Water-deprivation test

The water-deprivation test is a simple test that determines whether an apparent inability to concentrate urine is caused by psychogenic polydipsia or diabetes insipidus. The bladder should be emptied by catheterization and a baseline urinalysis performed. Baseline serum urea and creatinine levels and body weight should be recorded before removal of food and water. Water-deprivation testing should never be performed in a dehydrated or azotemic horse. Urine SG is measured 12 and 24 hours after the initiation of the test. Horses should be closely monitored during water deprivation. If dehydration becomes apparent, a loss of 5% of body weight occurs, or the urine SG reaches 1.025, the test should be stopped. If the SG reaches 1.025, then the ability to concentrate urine has been proven. Horses with central or nephrogenic diabetes insipidus cannot concentrate urine. In some cases, horses with psychogenic polydipsia may also not be able to concentrate urine because of washout of the medullar interstitial osmotic gradient. In such horses a partial deprivation of water intake at 40 ml/kg/day should restore the osmotic gradient in a few days.

Urinary system

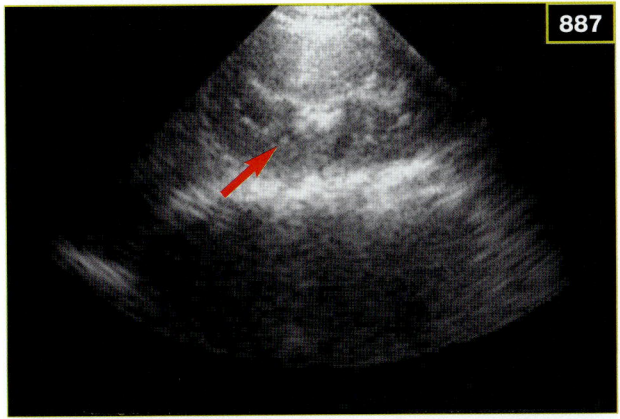

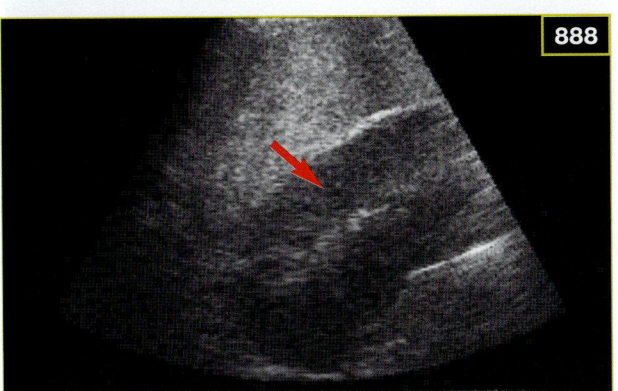

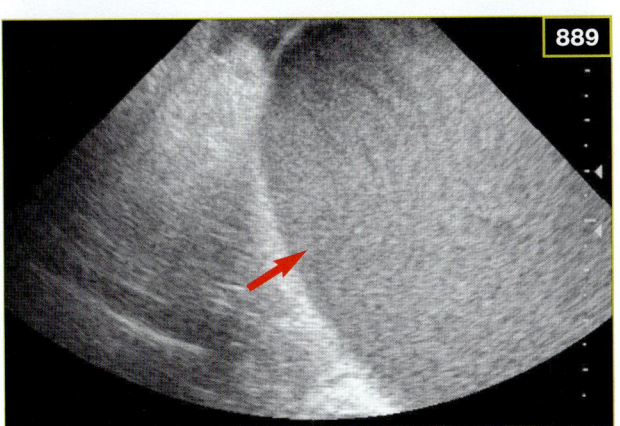

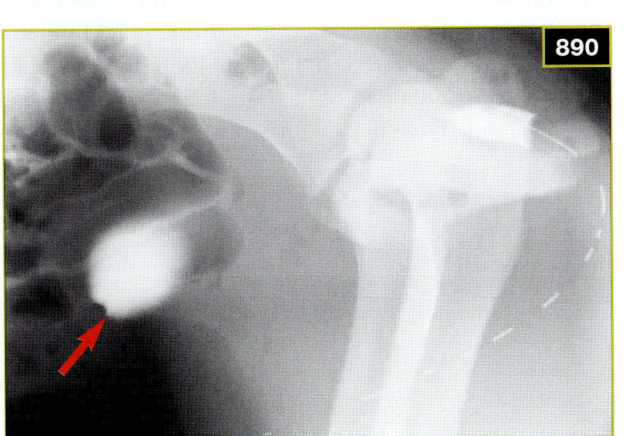

Vasopressin (antidiuretic hormone) challenge test

Diabetes insipidus is an endocrine cause of polyuria/polydipsia (PU/PD) syndrome. The lack of vasopressin secretion or the lack of response of renal collecting ducts to vasopressin distinguishes central from nephrogenic diabetes insipidus. They can be differentiated by exogenous administration of vasopressin. Intravenous administration of 20 μg desmopressin acetate should produce an increase in urine SG in normal horses and horses with central diabetes insipidus, but not horses with nephrogenic diabetes insipidus. Desmopressin acetate nasal spray had been successfully used intravenously in horses.

Ultrasonography and radiography

Kidneys can be relatively easily examined ultrasonographically. The right kidney can only be imaged transabdominally through the dorsolateral extents of the last three ICSs (887). The left kidney is imaged transabdominally in the left paralumbar fossa or transrectally (888). A good image is achieved with a 2.5- or 3-MHz probe. A 5-MHz probe is sometimes adequate to examine the right kidney. In ARF, kidneys are normal to increased in size and the corticomedullary junction may be indistinct. In CRF the kidneys are usually decreased in size with increased echogenicity. Cystic or mineralized areas can be associated with chronic renal diseases or, more often, with congenital abnormalities. Calculi within the renal pelvis are occasionally seen.

Ultrasonography of the bladder is best performed transrectally; however, the transabdominal approach may be useful in small horses and foals. Note that equine urine is not homogeneous and will have a variable echogenicity (889). The bladder wall should be assessed for masses, both ultrasonographically and by rectal palpation. Cystic calculi can also be confirmed ultrasonographically.

Urinary tract radiography is diagnostically adequate in foals and miniature horses. Excretory urography or retrograde contrast studies (890) may be performed.

887 Transabdominal ultrasonogram of the normal right kidney (arrow): long-axis cross-sectional view.

888 Transabdominal ultrasonogram of the normal left kidney (arrow): long-axis cross-sectional view. The homogeneous organ above the kidney is the spleen.

889 Transabdominal ultrasonogram of the urinary bladder (arrow). A high concentration of calcium carbonate crystals and mucus makes equine urine quite echogenic.

890 Contrast cystogram. The urinary catheter (dotted line) extends throughout the urethra into the bladder (arrow).

Urinary system

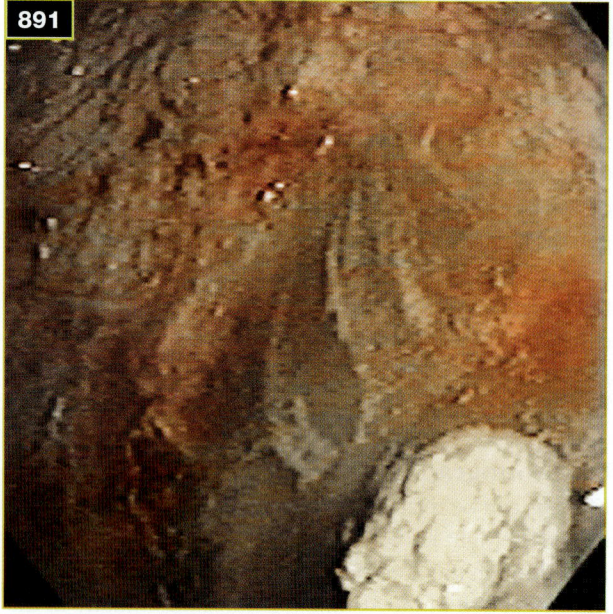

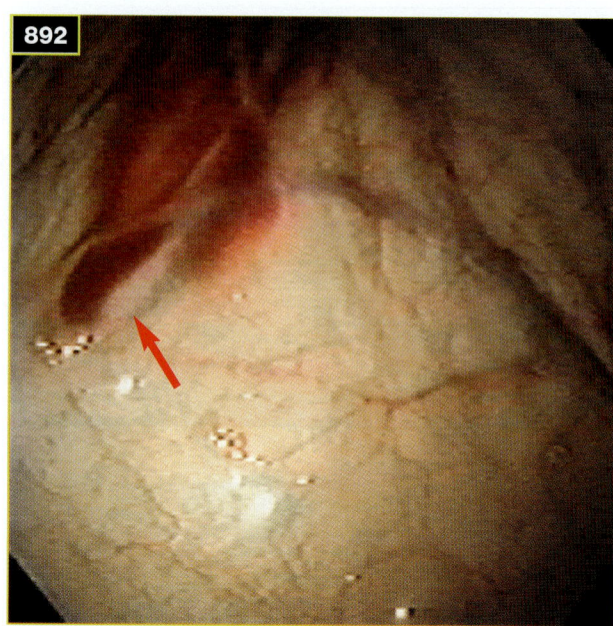

891 Cystolith. Note also bladder mucosa ulceration.

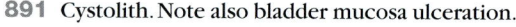

892 Ureteral opening. Note the bloody discharge (arrow).

Nuclear scintigraphic imaging in horses is available on a limited basis. It can be employed for the measurement of glomerular filtration rate (GFR) with application of radio-pharmaceuticals.

Measuring GFR as an indicator of functional renal mass assesses the excretion of endogenous or exogenous substances (creatinine, inulin, sodium sulfanilate) that are neither secreted nor resorbed after filtration into the tubular lumen. These tests are time- and labor-consuming and require specialized laboratory assays or equipment, and are not commonly used clinically. Cystometrography and urethral pressure profile analysis can be used to evaluate detrusor and urethral muscle function, but are of limited availability.

Endoscopy

Endoscopy of the urinary tract is a useful diagnostic tool. A flexible endoscope with an outside diameter of 12 mm or less should be used. An endoscope of less than 1 meter in length may not be adequate to reach the bladder in males. The procedure is identical to that of bladder catheterization. The urethra, especially its ampullar portion, colliculus seminalis, bladder, and ureteral openings should be examined. Inflammation, masses, and calculi can be visualized (**891**), as can abnormal discharges from ureters (**892**). A small amount of urine should enter the bladder from ureteral openings at least every 60 seconds. Urine can be collected from each ureter. Overinflation of the bladder causes patient discomfort and excessive straining.

Renal biopsy

Renal biopsy only occasionally offers information that is more specific than that gathered by conservative diagnostic approaches. Its use in horses with CRF, in the face of limitations and risks associated with this diagnostic technique, should be carefully considered. Interpretation of the pathologic lesions would rarely go beyond end stage renal disease with pathologic lesions of nephron or renal interstitium present.

If performed with ultrasonographic guidance, the risk for subcapsular hemorrhage and hematuria, or even bowel penetration, is small. The biopsy can also be taken without any direct ultrasonographic guidance; however, ultrasonographic evaluation is needed before the procedure to evaluate the site and depth of the kidney. Logically, the risks of the procedure become greater when renal biopsy is performed without direct ultrasonographic guidance. The horse should be sedated and properly restrained. Samples should be placed in formalin for histopathologic examination or in Michel's medium for immunofluorescence testing. Bacterial culture can be performed on samples.

Renal diseases

Acute renal failure

Definition/overview

ARF is defined as a sustained decrease in GFR leading to azotemia and fluid and acid–base disturbances. It is caused by decreased renal perfusion (prerenal or hemodynamic failure), primary renal dysfunction (intrinsic renal failure), or obstruction of urine flow (postrenal failure). Prerenal failure and renal failure are the most common.

Etiology/pathophysiology

Any cause of renal hypoperfusion such as dehydration from GI disease, heavy exercise, or blood loss may lead to prerenal ARF. Prolonged renal hypoperfusion can lead to intrinsic renal failure. Nephrotoxins such us aminoglycoside antimicrobials, oxytetracycline, NSAIDs, endogenous pigments (myoglobin or hemoglobin), heavy metals, vitamins D or K_3, and plant toxins (onions, red maple leaves, and, rarely, acorn poisoning) are often associated with intrinsic renal failure, especially in horses with concurrent renal hypoperfusion. Glomerulonephritis, interstitial nephritis, and renal microvascular thrombosis are more complex entities of intrinsic renal failure. Postrenal failure may occur from functional or mechanical urinary tract obstruction or urinary tract rupture. Other, less frequent, postrenal causes of ARF can be intraluminal (e.g. bilateral renal calculi, papillary necrosis, coagulated blood, bladder carcinoma, and fungus) or extraluminal (e.g. retroperitoneal fibrosis, colorectal tumor, and other malignant conditions).

Structural and biochemical changes that result in vasoconstriction, desquamation of tubular cells, intraluminal tubular obstruction, and transtubular backflow of the glomerular filtrate are pathophysiologic mechanisms that characterize ARF. Several clinical conditions can lead to kidney ischemia as a result of either extrarenal or intrarenal factors that compromise renal blood flow. In addition, toxins that cause tubular necrosis share many pathophysiologic features with ischemic ARF. Aminoglycoside antimicrobials and NSAIDs are the most common toxins encountered. These drugs can cause ARF by directly damaging tubular cells with consequent tubular cell necrosis.

Glomerulonephritis can also present as subacute or acute renal failure and it is characterized by intraglomerular inflammation and cellular proliferation.

Clinical presentation

The most common clinical complaints are anorexia, abdominal discomfort, dehydration, dullness, pigmenturia, and PU/PD. Concurrent disease may result in additional clinical abnormalities. Alterations in vital parameters depend on the underlying disease that caused the ARF. These may be normal, increased, or, rarely, decreased. In addition to depression and anorexia, uremia can cause encephalopathy, although this is uncommon. Urine production in horses with ARF is variable. Horses may be anuric (no urine production), oliguric (decreased urine production), normouric, or polyuric (increased urine production). Edema may be present with anuric or oliguric renal failure. Mucous membranes are usually injected or hyperemic. Laminitis may be present as a result of ARF or the underlying disease process.

Differential diagnosis

Shock; urinary tract calculi; sabulous urolithiasis; cystitis; bladder paralysis; peritonitis; visceral pain; cantharidin toxicosis.

Diagnosis

Diagnosis is based on history, clinical signs, serum biochemical analysis, and urinalysis. Palpation per rectum should be performed, where possible, to assess renal size, the presence of perirenal edema and renal pain, or the presence of obstruction in the ureters, bladder, or urethra. Typically, kidneys will be increased in size in ARF (893) and decreased in CRF.

Increases in blood urea and creatinine are invariably present. ARF can also be associated with hypocalcemia. With ARF the excretion of phosphorus with urine is disrupted, causing an increase in its serum concentration. Other changes more likely reflect underlying disease. Diagnostic samples should be collected prior to fluid therapy if possible.

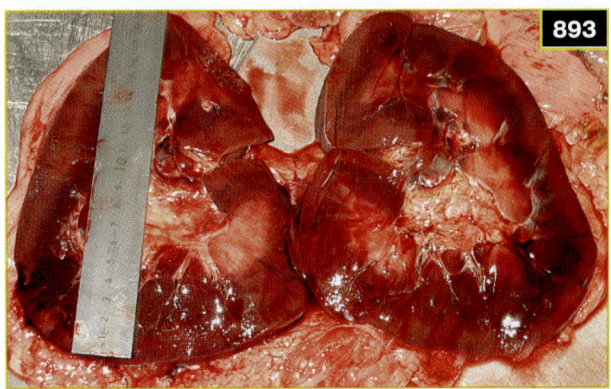

893 Enlarged kidney in a stallion (Arab) with ARF. The sagittal length of this kidney is 19 cm (7.5 inches). The normal length of the kidney is comparable to the length of 2½–3 vertebrae, which in this case should be approximately 12 cm (4.7 inches).

Urinalysis

Urinalysis is essential for differentiation of prerenal from renal failure and for characterization of the renal failure. With prerenal failure, urine should be concentrated (SG >1.018), while isosthenuria (SG 1.008–1.012) will be present with renal failure. Mild to moderate proteinuria may be present with renal failure, depending on the etiology and severity. If glomerular or tubular damage is present, changes to urine sediment such as the presence of casts and increased numbers of erythrocytes and leukocytes occur. The presence of glucosuria without hyperglycemia is strong evidence of renal tubular damage. A urinary GGT:urinary creatinine ratio of >25 is suggestive of renal tubular disease, but is not highly specific.

Fractional clearance of sodium and the urine creatinine:serum creatinine ratio can sometimes be helpful.

Renal enlargement, perirenal edema, and loss of detail at the corticomedullary junction may be evident ultrasonographically. Nephroliths may be evident. Dilation of the renal pelvis may be evident with urinary outflow obstruction (894). Renal biopsy has limited diagnostic value.

Urinary tract endoscopy may be useful if obstructive urinary tract disease is suspected.

894 Transabdominal ultrasonogram of the right kidney in a horse with suspected CRF. Note the dilation of the renal pelvis (arrow). Hydronephrosis is present on the dorsomedial part of the kidney.

Management

The primary disease should be managed accordingly. In the early evaluation of ARF it is important to rule out urinary tract obstruction, especially in patients who present with oliguria or anuria. This is done by bladder catheterization. Nephrotoxic drugs should be discontinued or, if treatment is necessary, the dosing regimen formulated at the minimal possible effective dose.

Fluid therapy is essential for the treatment of ARF, regardless of the cause. Fluid therapy will restore fluid and acid–base deficits and prevent the development of intrinsic renal lesions, if not already present. It is important to consider whether prerenal, renal, or postrenal failure and polyuria, normouria, oliguria, or anuria are present. Fluid therapy in oliguric or anuric patients should be conservative initially and set at 50% of the calculated requirements (estimated level of dehydration × body weight = amount of fluid required in liters). Pulmonary sounds and body weight should be monitored to prevent the development of overhydration and pulmonary edema. Conjunctival edema is often observed in overhydrated horses. Uremia should decrease rapidly following rehydration in cases of prerenal failure.

If hypernatremia is not present, intravenous administration of physiologic saline (0.9% NaCl solution) should be started. In acutely hypernatremic patients a 0.45% NaCl/2.5% dextrose solution should be used. A slower pace of correction is prudent in patients with hypernatremia of longer or unknown duration. In such patients, reducing the serum sodium concentration at a maximal rate of 0.5 mmol/l per hour or 10 mmol/l per day helps prevent cerebral edema. If hyperkalemia is present (serum K^+ >5.5 mmol/l), sodium bicarbonate should be given (1–2 mEq/kg i/v over 10–15 minutes). Alternatively, calcium borogluconate (0.5 ml/kg of 10% solution slowly i/v or added to 5 liters of fluids and infused over 1 hour) may be administered to counteract the cardiotoxic effects of hyperkalemia. Sodium bicarbonate is also indicated when myoglobulinuria is associated with ARF, as alkalization of the urine increases urinary myoglobin solubility and reduces intrinsic damage to the kidney.

Once the azotemia begins to resolve, fluid therapy should be continued at a rate that maintains normal hydration of the horse (maintenance rate of 55–65 ml/kg/day). It should not be discontinued until the patient's mentation is normal, creatinine values are not more than 10–15% over the high normal reference value, and other serum biochemical values are normal. Fluid therapy should be discontinued gradually and serum creatinine monitored regularly following cessation of fluid therapy.

In the later stages, during the polyuric recovery phase of ARF, intravenous or oral electrolyte/salt supplementation is required. Most horses with ARF do not require specialized dietary support. Feeding a grass forage can provide a diet low in protein, phosphorus, and calcium. Any grain may be fed at not more than 0.6–0.7 kg/100 kg of body weight per day.

If oliguria or anuria persists after rehydration, more aggressive therapy is indicated. Furosemide (1–4 mg/kg i/v q6h), mannitol (0.25–1.0 g/kg i/v as 20% solution q4–6h), and dopamine (120 mg in 1 liter of 0.9% NaCl or 5% dextrose given at the rate of 12.5 ml per minute to achieve 3 µg/kg/min) can be given in concert with fluid therapy. Treatment with mannitol and dopamine should be reserved for situations where close monitoring is available, because of the higher likelihood of adverse effects compared with furosemide administration. Mannitol is recommended, along with vigorous volume replacement and sodium bicarbonate, for the prevention and treatment of early myoglobinuric ARF. NSAIDs diminish the response to loop and thiazide diuretics, because they increase electrolyte and water resorption at the thick ascending limb of the loop of Henle.

Peritoneal dialysis may sometimes be helpful in relieving severe azotemia. The procedure is labor-intensive and usually has only a short-term benefit.

Surgical intervention may be indicated with urinary tract obstruction or rupture. Stabilization of the horse with fluid therapy and gradual drainage of peritoneal fluid are indicated if uroperitoneum is present.

Prognosis

The prognosis is affected by the duration of renal failure before the initiation of therapy. The prognosis for prerenal failure is good if the primary disease process can be controlled and appropriate fluid therapy can be provided. There is always a degree of tubular and/or interstitial damage present in ARF. Rapid resolution of azotemia (decrease in urea of 25–50% within 24 hours) is usually associated with a favorable prognosis. The prognosis becomes less favorable if azotemia does not resolve over a prolonged period of time. Horses that are oliguric for 48 hours or more before the initiation of therapy, horses that develop complications such us generalized edema, laminitis, or encephalopathy, or those that remain oliguric despite fluid therapy have a poor prognosis for recovery. Horses that have recovered from ARF are more prone to develop renal failure in the future. The prognosis for postrenal failure depends on the ability to correct the underlying problem and whether intrinsic renal failure has developed.

Specific etiologies associated with acute renal failure

Aminoglycoside toxicity

Aminoglycoside toxicity is a common cause of intrinsic ARF in horses. Neomycin is the most nephrotoxic of the aminoglycosides. Streptomycin is the least toxic aminoglycoside. Gentamicin, kanamycin, and amikacin are placed between neomycin and streptomycin. Gentamicin is most commonly associated with renal failure because of its widespread use.

Aminoglycosides may accumulate within tubular epithelial cells, disrupt metabolism, and cause tubular necrosis. Damage to the tubular epithelial cells usually develops after 3–5 days of aminoglycoside administration and most commonly occurs in dehydrated and/or hypotensive animals. Concurrent treatment with NSAIDs may aggravate the disease. Diagnosis is based on a history of aminoglycoside administration, clinical signs, and a laboratory diagnosis of intrinsic ARF as discussed above.

Nephrotoxic drugs should be promptly discontinued in horses that show any sign of ARF. Horses with aminoglycoside-associated ARF are usually polyuric. Progression to oliguric or anuric renal failure is rare and recovery occurs on discontinuing the drug and provision of supportive care in most cases.

A variety of measures can be used in an attempt to prevent aminoglycoside-associated ARF. The most important is to ensure that patients are adequately hydrated and have no underlying renal disease. Monitoring of peak and trough drug levels is very useful, where possible. The reader should refer to the renal pharmacology section at the end of this chapter (p. 668) for detailed information regarding aminoglycoside administration.

Increases in urinary GGT may be present with early tubular necrosis; however, this is not a very specific finding. Monitoring of urine for casts can be useful; however, casts are transient and urinalysis must be performed repeatedly throughout the day. Monitoring of SG and blood urea and creatinine levels can be performed, but no changes will be detected until at least 70% of renal function has been lost. Therefore, efforts are best addressed at preventing aminoglycoside-associated renal failure.

Nonsteroidal anti-inflammatory drugs

NSAID use may lead to ARF, particularly if used at excessive doses or in dehydrated or hypotensive horses. The pathologic lesion medullary crest necrosis is caused by disruption of renal synthesis of prostaglandins, which have an important function in regulating renal perfusion. Characteristic signs of renal failure are displayed. Hematuria may also be present.

If NSAID-associated ARF is suspected, NSAID administration should be ceased, if possible. If analgesia is required, alternative drugs, including alpha-2 agonists and/or opioids, given parenterally, transdermally, or via the epidural route, should be considered. If NSAIDs must be used, the lowest possible doses should be administered and normal hydration and blood pressure must be maintained. Of the NSAIDs commonly used in horses, phenylbutazone is suggested to be most nephrotoxic, followed by flunixin meglumine and ketoprofen. Treatment of NSAID-associated ARF is as described above. GI and renal toxicity of NSAIDs can occur concurrently.

Pigment nephropathy

Hemoglobin and myoglobin are potentially nephrotoxic. Horses with severe hemolysis or rhabdomyolysis are at risk of developing pigment nephropathy, particularly if dehydrated or hypotensive. Nephropathy is thought to be associated with direct tubular toxicity, tubular obstruction, and hemodynamic abnormalities. Coagulopathies that may be associated with severe hemolysis also affect renal vasculature integrity.

Identification and control of the inciting cause are essential, as is aggressive fluid therapy. Treatment of pigment nephropathy is as described for ARF. Sodium bicarbonate is indicated also when myoglobulinuria is associated with the ARF, as alkalization of the urine increases urinary myoglobin solubility and reduces intrinsic damage to the kidney.

Miscellaneous drug and other toxicities

Horses may encounter a variety of nephrotoxins, including Vitamin K_3, Vitamin D, tetracycline, polymixin B, amphotericin B, and heavy metals. Additionally, ingestion of acorns, ochratoxins, and cantharidin may induce renal failure. *Cestrum diurnum* (flowering jasmine) contains vitamin D metabolites, which may cause severe renal disease in horses through the ability to disrupt calcium metabolism. Treatment involves removal of the initiating factor and should follow general principles for the treatment of ARF. If nephrotoxins have recently been ingested, the stomach should be lavaged and charcoal administered orally (1–3 g/kg via nasogastric tube).

Chronic renal failure

Definition/overview

CRF results from irreversible loss of functional nephrons. Serious clinical signs only occur when the number of functioning nephrons decreases below 20–30%. All causes of ARF can lead to CRF; in addition, several other metabolic, immunologic, infectious, obstructive, and congenital disorders can cause CRF.

Etiology/pathophysiology

Acquired disorders are the most common cause of CRF in horses. Extensive damage to the functional nephrons usually follows ARF. Potential causes include prolonged renal hypoperfusion and exposure to nephrotoxins such as aminoglycosides, oxytetracycline, NSAIDs, endogenous pigments (myoglobin or hemoglobin), heavy metals, vitamin D or K_3, and plant toxins. Glomerulonephritis, interstitial nephritis, renal microvascular thrombosis, renal amyloidosis, renal pelvic calculi, and renal neoplasia may also cause CRF.

CRF develops when tubular and glomerular damage exceeds renal reserve capacity. As renal function decreases, surviving nephrons undergo functional changes that permit the horse to regulate water and solute homeostasis. However, if disease progresses, this compensatory mechanism may be overwhelmed.

Clinical presentation

Anorexia and weight loss are the most common presenting complaints (895). Poor athletic performance may also be detected early in the disease. With progression of uremia, depression and lethargy develop. Rough haircoat, ventral edema, and PU/PD are commonly associated with CRF, although PU/PD may not be identified in horses that are kept on pasture with free access to water. Urea may be converted to ammonia on mucosal surfaces of the GI tract, resulting in ulceration. Uremic halitosis and excessive dental tartar formation may be present (896). Encephalopathy is a possible but uncommon sequela of uremia.

Differential diagnosis

Pleuropneumonia; peritonitis; malabsorbtion/maldigestion syndrome; neurologic disorders; neoplasia; ruptured bladder; renal tubular acidosis.

Diagnosis

Diagnosis of CRF is based on clinical signs and the persistence of isosthenuria and azotemia. Palpation per rectum should be performed to investigate for masses and to evaluate the size of the left kidney and ureters. The kidney is usually normal or small in size in cases of CRF; however, with neoplasia, infection, or urinary tract obstruction, the kidney and/or ureters may be enlarged.

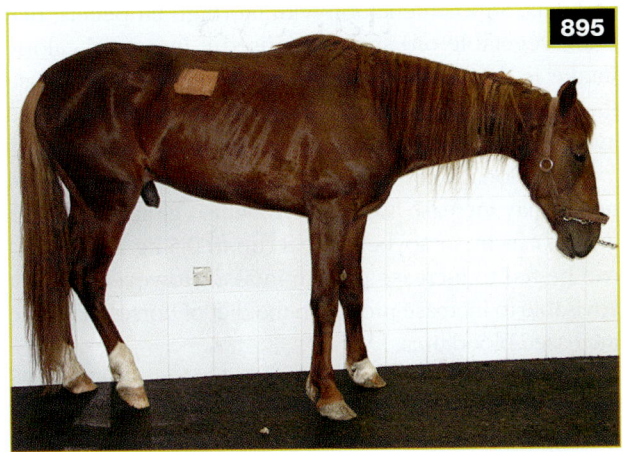

895 Anorexia and weight loss in a horse with CRF.

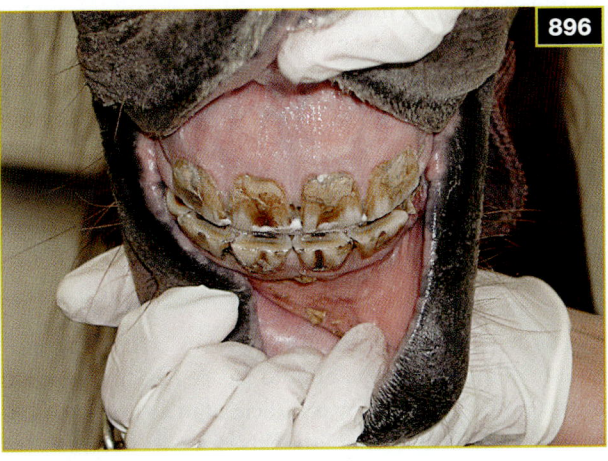

896 Excessive dental tartar in a horse with CRF.

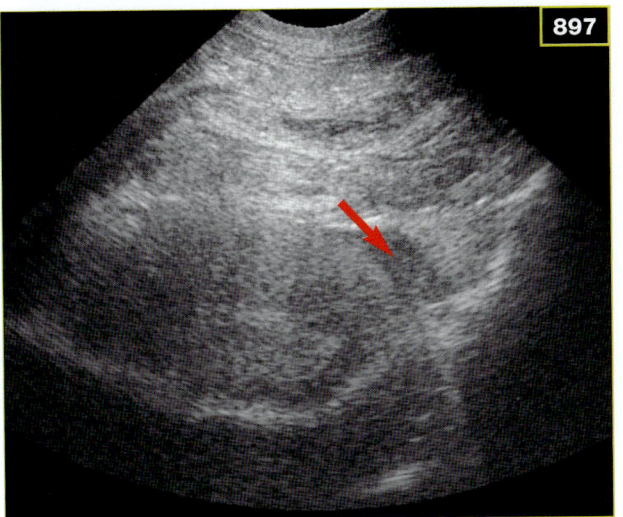

897 CRF. Note complete loss of the corticomedullary junction in the right kidney. The arrow indicates an area of mineralization.

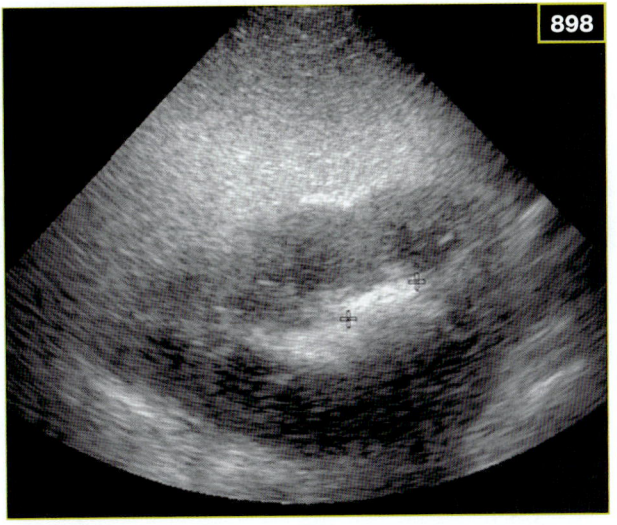

898 Transabdominal ultrasonogram of the left kidney in a horse with suspected CRF. Hypoechogenic areas between the crosses indicate mineralized debris or the presence of a renal calculus.

Increases in blood urea and creatinine are present. Normocytic, normochromic anemia, as a result of decreased erythropoietin production, may be identified. Hypoalbuminemia, which may or may not be associated with hypoproteinemia depending on the serum concentration of globulins, may also be present. Hyponatremia, hypochloremia, hypercalcemia, hypophosphatemia, and low plasma bicarbonate concentration are associated with CRF, but are variable. Excessive urinary losses of electrolytes leads to variable acid–base disturbances, which can be expressed as metabolic acidosis or, less frequently, metabolic alkalosis. Fractional clearance of electrolytes may be normal.

Isosthenuria (SG 1.008–1.012) in the presence of azotemia or dehydration confirms the presence of renal failure. If proteinuria is substantial, the SG of the urine may rise to, or exceed, 1.020 despite an inability to concentrate urine. Urine sediment is usually free of cells and casts unless CRF is associated with pyelonephritis, in which case RBCs, leukocytes, casts, and bacteria may be present. Bacterial culture of urine should be performed in all suspected cases of CRF. A catheterized sample is preferable.

Ultrasonographically, the kidneys tend to be smaller and hyperechogenic compared with normal. There may be a loss of distinction of the corticomedullary junction (**897**). Cysts or nephroliths may be visualized (**898**).

Kidney biopsy may be helpful in the diagnosis of pyelonephritis or a congenital abnormality; however, most often findings are consistent with end-stage renal disease and findings rarely influence treatment or prognosis. Immunofluorescence testing of the biopsy sample may better define the etiology of the disease. Ultrasonographic guidance is preferred because of the risk of severe hemorrhage.

Management

Any underlying disease should be addressed and administration of nephrotoxins should be ceased if possible. Intravenous fluid therapy is indicated in acute exacerbation of CRF, in azotemic animals, for the treatment of underlying or concomitant disease, or in dehydrated animals. Physiologic saline (0.9% NaCl solution) is the fluid of choice; however, a balanced electrolyte solution may be used if moderate to severe hyperkalemia is not present. Intravenous fluid therapy should replace fluid deficits and account for maintenance requirements (65 ml/kg/day) and ongoing losses. If oliguria or anuria is present, close observation is required during fluid therapy to ensure that overhydration and resultant edema do not ensue. Oliguria or anuria is uncommon; therefore, furosemide, mannitol, and/or dopamine are rarely indicated. They are more often indicated in acute exacerbation of CRF and are discussed under ARF.

Peritoneal dialysis may sometimes be helpful in relieving severe azotemia. The procedure is labor-intensive and usually has only a short-term benefit. Recovery of infused fluid is often difficult.

Supportive management is essential. A palatable diet low in protein, calcium, and phosphorus should be provided. This could consist of high-quality grass forage, corn, and oats. Supplementation with fat (high-fat pellets, rice bran, vegetable oil) should be used if increased caloric intake is desired. Legumes should be avoided because they are high in protein and calcium. Bran should also be avoided, as it is high in protein and phosphorus.

Occasionally, with severe proteinuria, dietary protein needs may increase. Corn gluten, wheat gluten, distiller's grains, casein, or soybean meal (up to 0.5 kg/horse/day) can be fed to increase protein intake. However, it is not advisable to increase protein in the diet of horses that have increased blood urea.

Vitamin supplementation should be provided to compensate for excessive polyuria-induced losses of B vitamins.

Free access to water is critical. Supplementation with oral electrolytes (NaCl 25–50 g/day p/o, sodium bicarbonate 50–100 g/day p/o) is also important. Potassium chloride (up to 50 g/day) can be administered if hypokalemia develops.

Pyelonephritis warrants specific antimicrobial therapy and is discussed elsewhere (p. 652).

Prognosis

The long-term prognosis is grave; however, proper supportive care can have significant effects on length and quality of life. The rate of deterioration is hard to predict; however, good management and regular monitoring of the disease progression may give the horse a fair short-term prognosis for life. Athletic performance and breeding capabilities are limited.

The prognosis is poor for horses with anuria or oligura, severe weight loss, severe elevations in blood urea and creatinine, or where azotemia responds poorly to fluid therapy.

Specific etiologies associated with chronic renal failure

Congenital diseases of the kidney

Renal agenesia, hypoplasia, and dysplasia are rare in horses. Unilateral renal agenesis has been identified incidentally in mature horses. Renal function of the remaining kidney is normal, but because there is less renal reserve, such horses are more prone to development of renal failure. Bilateral renal agenesis, which is not compatible with life, has been reported in a foal.

Renal hypoplasia is a condition where renal mass is at least 50% smaller than normal. Renal failure will develop if renal mass is <30% or if concurrent renal disease affects renal function.

Renal dysplasia is an abnormal differentiation of renal tissue that develops secondarily to *in-utero* exposure to teratogens. Bilateral and unilateral disease have been reported. There are no specific treatment options for any of these conditions and the long-term prognosis is poor.

Renal pelvis calculi

Nephroliths (899) that develop within or adjacent to the renal pelvis can partially or completely obstruct the upper urinary tract. As the passage of urine is obstructed, hydronephrosis develops. It is believed that a nidus of damaged renal tissue, such as may occur with CRF, is most often the initiating factor in nephrolith development. If upper urinary tract obstruction is bilateral, CRF will develop.

Diagnosis is based on history and clinical signs. In unilateral disease, azotemia may not be present; however, urinalysis may reveal pigmenturia and/or microscopic hematuria. Transabdominal and transrectal ultrasonographic examination can identify nephroliths of adequate siz. Diminished unilateral or bilateral entry of urine into the bladder from ureteral openings may be evident endoscopically. Successful dietary and/or medical procedures to dissolve nephroliths have not been reported in horses. Unilateral nephrectomy is the treatment of choice if the remaining kidney is normal.

Interstitial nephritis

Interstitial nephritis or tubulointerstitial disease is a common sequela of ARF. Depending of the degree of damage and the number of affected nephrons, CRF may develop following an episode of ARF. The degree of renal interstitial change influences the severity of clinical signs and the prognosis for short- and long-term recovery.

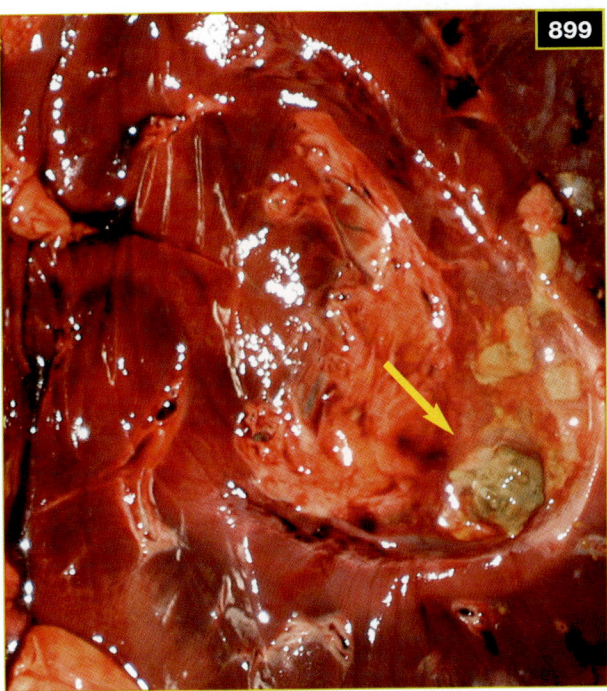

899 Nephrolith 1 cm in diameter (arrow) in the right kidney.

Immune-mediated glomerulonephritis

Glomerulonephritis can be defined as a disease characterized by intraglomerular inflammation and cellular proliferation associated with hematuria.

When antigen–antibody complexes are deposited in the glomeruli of kidneys, they cause a local inflammatory response and vasculitis. Most often it is seen following streptococcal infections. Antigens against EIA have also been associated with glomerulonephritis. However, circulating immune complexes of other chronic diseases such us leptospirosis and herpes-virus infections probably also lead to glomerular deposits. Persistent deposition of complexes leads to irreversible damage and CRF. Definitive diagnosis is via histopathologic and immunofluorescence-examination of renal biopsy or necropsy samples.

Treatment should aim at removal of the initiating cause of the glomerulonephritis and general principles of CRF treatment as described previously. Immunosuppressive therapy with corticosteroids has been successfully used in other species; however, their effect in equine glomerulonephritis has not been proven.

Pyelonephritis

Definition/overview

Pyelonephritis is a suppurative bacterial infection of the kidney (900). It is an uncommon cause of renal failure in the mature horse and most often develops as a consequence of urolithiasis, trauma, neurogenic incontinence, or bladder paralysis, which predisposes to ascending infection.

Etiology/pathophysiology

Ascending infection from the lower urinary tract is the usual source of bacterial colonization. Hematogenous spread of infection to the kidneys can also occur, although rarely. *Corynebacterium* spp., *E. coli*, *Proteus mirabilis*, *Klebsiella* spp., *Enterobacter* spp., *Actinobacillus* spp., *Salmonella* spp., *Pseudomonas* spp., and *Streptococcus* spp. are commonly implicated in ascending infections. Hematogenous infection with *Leptospira* spp., *Salmonella* spp., *Actinobacillus equuli*, and *S. equi*, among others, can occur. With long-standing pyelonephritis, progressive damage of other structures throughout the kidney occurs.

Clinical presentation

Unlike lower urinary tract infection, horses with pyelonephritis usually have signs of systemic disease. Weight loss, fever, PU/PD, generalized weakness, and depression or lethargy are frequent presenting complaints. Concurrent renal or postrenal failure may be present depending on the severity of renal damage and whether nephroliths or ureteroliths have formed and caused obstructions.

Diagnosis

Urinalysis is essential. Microscopic or macroscopic hematuria is usually present, along with pyuria. Bacteria may be evident microscopically; however, an absence of visible bacteria does not rule out infection. Urine culture must be performed, ideally from a catheterized urine sample. A neutrophilic leukocytosis is often present, as is an increase in plasma fibrinogen. Urine is usually concentrated (SG >1.020) unless renal failure is present, at which point isosthenuria will be identified. Azotemia should not be present unless renal failure has developed. Ultrasonographic examination of the bladder and kidneys should be performed, with particular attention paid to identification of nephroliths and changes in renal architecture, which may be present with pyelonephritis (901). Palpation per rectum should be performed. Possible inciting causes should be evaluated.

Management

Appropriate antimicrobial treatment is essential to treat pyelonephritis and should be based on bacterial culture and sensitivity. Beta-lactam antibiotics (procaine penicillin 20,000 IU/kg i/m q12h or ceftiofur sodium 2.2 mg/kg i/m or i/v q12h) should be used initially while awaiting bacterial culture and sensitivity results. A minimum of 14 days of therapy is required. Repeated urinalyses should be performed to assess response to treatment. Urine culture should be repeated 1 week after antimicrobial therapy is discontinued.

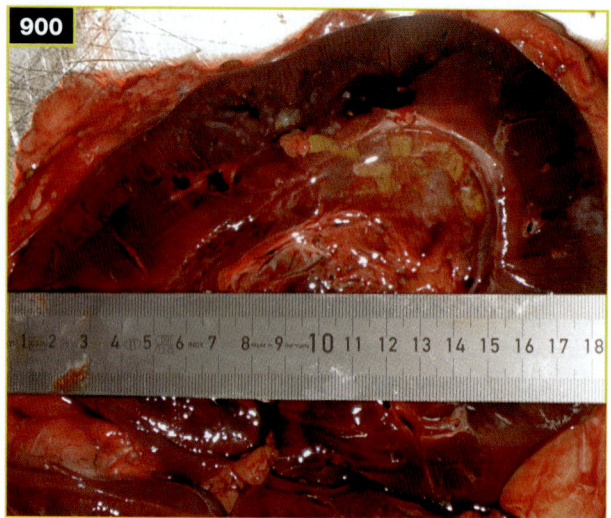

900 Pyelonephritis and renal hyperemia in the right kidney. Note the purulent debris in the renal medulla.

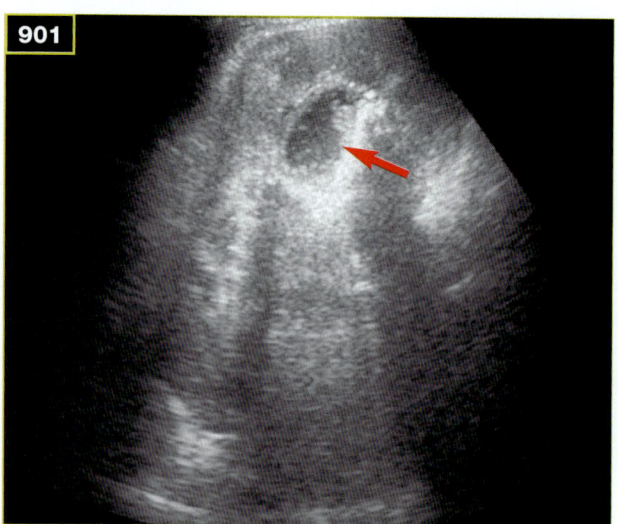

901 Transabdominal ultrasonogram of the right kidney in a horse with pyelonephritis. Note the hyperechogenic debris located in the distended renal pelvis (arrow).

Urinary system

The addition of table salt (2 tablespoons q12–24h) to the diet will encourage drinking and increase urine production. Free access to water should be provided. Nephrectomy may be considered if the disease is unilateral, severe, and poorly responsive to medical therapy. Complications such as nephrolithiasis and urinary tract obstruction must be addressed if they develop.

Prognosis
The long-term prognosis for survival is poor because pyelonephritis is often not diagnosed until disease is advanced and complications have developed.

Renal tumors
Disseminated tumors of any type, most often lymphoma and hemangiosarcoma, may localize to the kidney. Primary renal neoplasia is rare in horses. Renal cell carcinoma (adenocarcinoma) is the most frequently diagnosed renal neoplasia, followed by nephroblastoma. Renal cell carcinoma is usually diagnosed in older horses. In contrast, nephroblastoma mostly affects young animals. The treatment of choice for unilateral renal neoplasia is nephrectomy. By the time renal neoplasia is diagnosed the prognosis for recovery is already grave.

Hydronephrosis
Obstruction of urine flow from the proximal urinary tract results in progressive interstitial fibrosis and atrophy of the kidney. If unilateral, it may remain clinically inapparent for a long period of time. Dilation of the renal pelvis may be evident ultrasonographically. Ureteral distension (902) may be palpable per rectum or evident ultrasonographically depending on the location of the obstruction. Nephrolithiasis is the most common cause of hydronephrosis, followed by renal and bladder neoplasia, cystitis, acquired strictures of the urethra, or any inflammatory condition that surrounds the urinary tract. Treatment should be directed at correction of the initiating cause. Prolonged or repeated periods of obstruction cause irreversible renal damage and CRF.

Amyloidosis
Amyloidosis has been reported in horses used for antiserum production or, rarely, following chronic infection. Proteinaceous complexes are deposited in glomeruli just below the endothelium; these disturb normal renal function and cause a variable degree of renal failure. No effective treatments have been reported and the prognosis is grave by the time CRF is recognized.

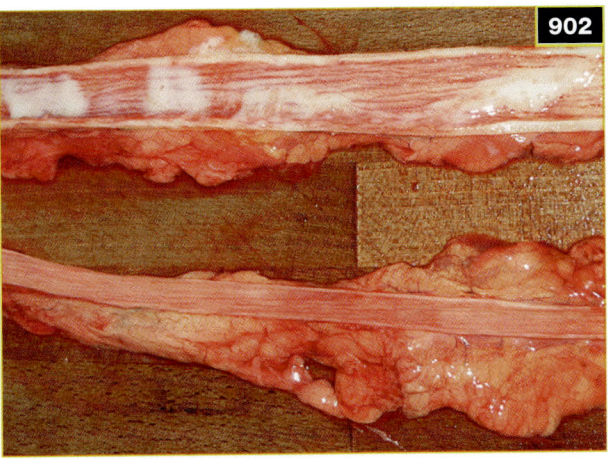

902 Distended right ureter (upper) in a horse with pyelonephritis and nephroliths. Note the purulent debris in the ureteral lumen. The left ureter (lower) is normal.

Renal tubular acidosis
Definition/overview
Renal tubular acidosis (RTA) is an uncommon condition in which the renal tubules are unable to acidify urine, resulting in a continued state of metabolic acidosis. Despite profound metabolic acidosis, urine pH remains neutral or alkaline. Normal horses have alkaline urine, which should acidify and excrete hydrogen ions in cases of acidosis.

Etiology/pathophysiology
Currently, there is no evidence that RTA is an hereditary disease; therefore, it is probably a secondary condition to renal disease. However, many cases appear to be idiopathic.

Two types of RTA have been reported in horses: type I (distal tubular acidosis), and type II (proximal tubular acidosis). Type I RTA develops when the patient is unable to acidify urine because of inadequate hydrogen ion secretion in distal renal tubules. Type II RTA is associated with an inability of the proximal renal tubules to resorb bicarbonate, which is subsequently lost in urine. Hyperchloremia and hypokalemia occur concurrently, indicating that RTA is caused by disturbances in the electrolyte homeostasis in renal tubules.

Clinical presentation
Anorexia, weight loss, depression, and weakness are the main presenting complaints. Ataxia, poor performance, ill-thrift, tachypnea, and tachycardia have also been reported.

Differential diagnosis

Renal failure; uroperitoneum; exertion; renal calculi; neurologic disorders; malabsorbtion/maldigestion syndrome.

Diagnosis

Electrolyte and acid–base disturbances are the main hematologic abnormalities. Severe hyperchloremic metabolic acidosis with a low strong ion difference is characteristic. Hyponatremia and/or hypokalemia may also be present. Fractional excretion of sodium is usually high in type I RTA, while the fractional excretion of potassium is low in type II RTA. Blood urea nitrogen and creatinine should be normal unless dehydration is present. Otherwise, elevations in blood urea and creatinine indicate concurrent renal disease. Urine pH is neutral to alkaline in type I RTA and alkaline to acidic in type II RTA.

Ammonium chloride loading has been used to detect type I RTA. Ammonium chloride delivery (0.1 g/kg in 6 liters of water given orally to a horse that has been kept off feed and water for at least 7 hours) should acidify the urine in normal horses, whereas in type I RTA the urine remains alkaline. Diagnosis of type II RTA is based on clinical and laboratory findings and following exclusion of type I RTA. The distinction between the two types of RTA is not critical, because the treatment and prognosis are similar.

Management

Treatment of RTA consists of intravenous administration of sodium bicarbonate to correct the metabolic acidosis. Initial treatment should be administered gradually to replace the estimated bicarbonate deficit ($0.3 \times$ body weight [kg] $\times$ base deficit = bicarbonate deficit in mmol/l). The initial goal is to return plasma bicarbonate concentration to values above 20 mEq/l and blood pH above 7.3, which usually does not require the administration of the whole calculated bicarbonate deficit. Thereafter, losses are controlled by oral administration of sodium bicarbonate (50–150g q12–24h). Oral potassium supplementation is often necessary during the initial stages of the treatment. Diarrhea may be observed during high-dose sodium bicarbonate administration, but usually resolves if the dose is decreased. Serum electrolyte levels and blood gases should be monitored regularly.

Prognosis

The prognosis is based on the severity of the underlying renal disorder, if present, and the duration of response to initial therapy. The short-term prognosis is usually good with proper treatment. Several horses have been reported to recover completely with bicarbonate supplementation. Relapse is not uncommon, particularly if renal disease is present.

Diabetes insipidus

Definition/overview

Diabetes insipidus is an uncommon cause of PU/PD in horses.

Etiology/pathophysiology

Antidiuretic hormone (ADH) (vasopressin) is a powerful effector of the feedback system for regulating plasma osmolarity and sodium concentration. It operates by altering renal excretion of water independently of the rate of solute excretion.

Diabetes insipidus occurs when inadequate ADH is produced (neurogenic or central diabetes insipidus) or when the distal tubules, collecting tubules, and collecting ducts are unable to respond to ADH (nephrogenic diabetes insipidus).

Central diabetes insipidus can develop secondary to head trauma, encephalomyelitis, or pituitary pars intermedia dysfunction (equine Cushing's disease). Nephrogenic diabetes insipidus can develop secondary to many types of renal disease, especially those that damage the renal medulla. A hereditary basis to the disease is possible.

Clinical presentation

PU/PD should be the sole presenting complaint, unless water intake has been restricted and dehydration has developed.

Differential diagnosis

CRF; psychogenic polydipsia; diabetes mellitus; Cushing's disease.

Diagnosis

Physical examination is unremarkable. Urinalysis should be normal apart from a lack of concentration of urine. Blood urea and creatinine levels are normal unless dehydration is present. Water-deprivation testing should be performed as described earlier. Water-deprivation testing should never be performed in a dehydrated or azotemic horse. Horses with central or nephrogenic diabetes insipidus cannot concentrate urine during water deprivation; however, psychogenic polydipsia with medullary interstitial osmotic gradient cannot be ruled out initially in horses not responding to water deprivation. In such horses, partial deprivation of water intake at 40 ml/kg/day should be performed prior to repetition of the water-deprivation test. If urine concentration still does not occur, then a diagnosis of diabetes insipidus can be made. An ADH (vasopressin) challenge test can be used to differentiate nephrogenic from central diabetes insipidus, as described earlier (p. 643).

Management

Secondary diabetes insipidus should be managed via treatment of the primary disease. Successful treatment of primary or idiopathic diabetes insipidus has not been reported; however, treatment is unnecessary provided the horse has free access to water at all times.

Prognosis

The prognosis for diabetes insipidus not associated with underlying renal or neurologic disease is excellent if access to water is available at all times. Affected horses are unable to concentrate urine and are prone to dehydration if water is restricted. The prognosis for secondary diabetes insipidus depends mainly on the prognosis of the primary disease.

Diseases of the ureters

Ectopic ureters

The presence of an ectopic ureter is rare in horses. It has been most commonly reported in fillies. It is usually noted in foals with a complaint of persistent urine dribbling and perineal dermatitis (urine scalding). There should be no other clinical or hematologic abnormalities. Endoscopic examination of the vagina and distal urinary tract may reveal the orifice of the ectopic ureter; however, visualization is often difficult. Speculum examination of the vagina can also be diagnostic. An excretory urogram may aid in diagnosis. This is most useful in young animals, as visualization decreases with the size of the animal. Depending on the location of the ectopic ureter, the severity of clinical signs, and the intended use of the animal, surgical correction may be required. Surgical relocation of the ectopic ureter into the bladder may be possible; otherwise, nephrectomy can be performed in patients with unilateral disease.

Ureterolithiasis
Definition/overview

Ureterolithiasis, the presence of calculi in one or both ureters, is a rare problem in horses.

Etiology/pathophysiology

Ureteroliths may arise as a sequela to a degenerative or inflammatory process in the kidney. Inflammatory debris serves as a nidus for calculus formation (see **902**). It is possible that nephroliths move into the ureters and cause obstruction.

Clinical presentation

With unilateral disease, a low-grade intermittent colic may be the only clinical sign present. Clinical signs in advanced cases are consistent with CRF, which may develop secondarily to ureteral obstruction.

Diagnosis

Hematology will be unremarkable unless renal failure has developed. Hematologic changes associated with renal failure have been discussed previously (p. 645). Urinalysis should be performed. Intermittent or persistent pigmenturia and increased numbers of erythrocytes are usually present. The SG can be variable depending on whether intrinsic renal failure has developed and whether disease is unilateral or bilateral. If bilateral obstructive disease is present, urine may not be obtained.

The ureterolith or enlarged ureters may be palpable per rectum. Distended ureters may be evident ultrasonographically. Urine culture should be performed, preferably from a catheterized sample. It is important to look for concurrent uroliths in the bladder and kidneys, because multifocal urolithiasis is not uncommon.

Differential diagnosis

Calculi in other parts of the urinary tract; bladder paralysis; urinary tract trauma; renal failure; sabulous urolithiasis; neoplasia.

Management

Ureterolithiasis can be treated surgically. The calculus is removed through a ureteral incision. In mares, another technique has been reported. In this technique, a Dormia basket is placed manually into the ureter to ensnare and remove the calculus. This technique may be employed in cases where calculi are ≤ 2 cm. Lithotripsy, where calculi are fragmented through the delivery of an electrical impulse/shock wave, could also be attempted, but is of limited availability. Unilateral nephrectomy may be the only possible management of ureterolithiasis in some cases. Prior to nephrectomy, it is essential that concurrent disease in the contralateral ureter and kidney are ruled out. Antimicrobial therapy and intravenous fluid therapy should support the above procedures as has been previously discussed.

Treatment of CRF is discussed elsewhere (p. 650).

Prognosis

Bilateral ureterolithiasis that advances to CRF carries a grave prognosis. Unilateral disease has a better prognosis, especially if calculi can be successfully removed. It is believed that initiating renal disease predisposes horses to develop ureteroliths. Avoiding administration of nephrotoxic agents, provision of a good diet, and ensuring adequate water consumption increase the chance for good recovery.

Diseases of the urinary bladder

Bacterial cystitis
Definition/overview
Bacterial cystitis is an inflammation of the bladder caused by bacterial infection and characterized by dysuria, stranguria, pollakiuria, and the presence of blood, inflammatory cells, and bacteria in the urine. It is rarely a primary disease.

Etiology/pathophysiology
Cystitis is most often a secondary disease that can develop from urine stasis (bladder paralysis), urinary tract catheterization, urinary tract trauma, cystic calculi, or neoplasia. *E. coli*, *Proteus* spp., *Pseudomonas* spp., *Klebsiella* spp., *Enterobacter* spp., *Streptococcus* spp., and *Staphylococcus* spp. are the most commonly identified pathogens. Dystocia predisposes mares to the development of cystitis.

When the flushing action of the voided urine cannot clear pathogenic bacteria from the bladder mucosa, infection and inflammation can develop.

Clinical presentation
Dysuria, stranguria, and pollakiuria are the most common presenting complaints. Signs of generalized disease such as fever, depression, or weight loss should not be present with uncomplicated cystitis, as opposed to pyelonephritis. Urine scalding may be observed on the perineum or hindlimbs.

Differential diagnosis
Urolithiasis; bladder paralysis; neoplasia; renal failure; colic, pyelonephritis.

Diagnosis
Physical examination findings typically suggest urinary tract disease, but are not specific for cystitis. Hematology is usually unremarkable. Diagnosis is based on urinalysis. Pyuria (more than 5 WBCs/hpf) is usually associated with cystitis. Bacteria may be evident on cytologic analysis of urine sediment, but absence of visible bacteria does not rule out an infectious cause. Microscopic or macroscopic hematuria may be present. Urine is usually concentrated (SG >1.020). Bacterial culture should be performed. A catheterized sample is preferred in order to avoid contaminants. Quantitative culture should be requested, where available, with identification of >10,000 colony forming units (CFU)/ml in a catheterized sample indicating infection. Palpation per rectum should be performed to evaluate the bladder wall and determine whether uroliths may be present. Endoscopy of the bladder via cystoscopy or ultrasonography may be helpful for investigation of primary disease.

Management
The inciting cause should be identified and treated, if possible. The use of an appropriate antimicrobial agent is essential for successful management of cystitis. The selection of the antimicrobial agent should be supported by the sensitivity of isolated bacteria, as well as the drug kinetics in the urinary tract. Procaine penicillin (20,000 IU/kg i/m q12h) or trimethoprim/sulfadiazine (24–30 mg/kg p/o q12h) is a good initial choice. If severe renal failure accompanies cystitis, trimethoprim/sulfadiazine should not be used. Other antimicrobials should be reserved for resistant infections. Cystitis requires a prolonged period of antimicrobial treatment (a minimum of 7 days). Repeated urinalysis should be performed to assess response to treatment. Urine culture should be repeated 1 week after antimicrobial therapy is discontinued. Relapses are common.

Adding 50 g of table salt daily to the diet will encourage horses to drink more; diuresis and flushing of the bladder are of benefit in cases of bacterial cystitis. Free access to water should be ensured.

Prognosis
The prognosis is good for primary cystitis. Chronic cystitis, recurrent cystitis, ascending infection into the proximal urinary tract, and neoplasia have a less favorable long-term prognosis.

Bladder tumors
Definition/overview
Bladder tumors are rarely diagnosed in horses and are associated with a very poor prognosis.

Etiology/pathophysiology
Bladder tumors are usually identified in older horses; however, fibromatous polyps are more common in younger horses. SCC is the most common bladder neoplasia diagnosed in horses, followed by transitional cell carcinoma. Non-epithelial primary bladder tumors include muscle tumors, vascular tumors, fibroblastic tumors, and lymphomas. Metastases from other common neoplasias can occasionally involve the bladder.

Clinical presentation
Clinical signs of disease are not usually evident until disease is well advanced. Weight loss and weakness are the most common presenting complaints. Appetite is usually good until advanced stages of the disease, at which point depression and lethargy may also be noted. Pollakiuria, stranguria, and hematuria may be observed. Earlier in disease, clinical signs are similar to those of cystic calculi.

Differential diagnosis

Urolithiasis; cystitis; renal failure; bladder paralysis; urinary tract trauma; colic; neoplasia of other organ systems.

Diagnosis

Physical examination is usually nonspecific. Urinalysis may be unremarkable; however, macroscopic or microscopic hematuria and neoplastic cells are often observed. SG is usually normal (>1.020).

The bladder should be palpated per rectum. If the bladder is distended with urine, it should be emptied prior to evaluation. A thickened, irregular bladder wall or obvious mass may be palpable. Transrectal ultrasonography can be used to further evaluate the bladder. Cystoscopy can be used to evaluate the bladder mucosa and to obtain a biopsy. Anemia from chronic hematuria or anemia of chronic disease may be identified on a CBC. Hypoproteinemia may be present from chronic blood loss or chronic inflammatory disease.

Management

Surgical excision and chemotherapy have had variable success in the treatment of bladder tumors. Bladder carcinomas are locally very invasive and have also been reported to metastasize to other organs. Therefore, the prognosis for recovery is grave even in the short term.

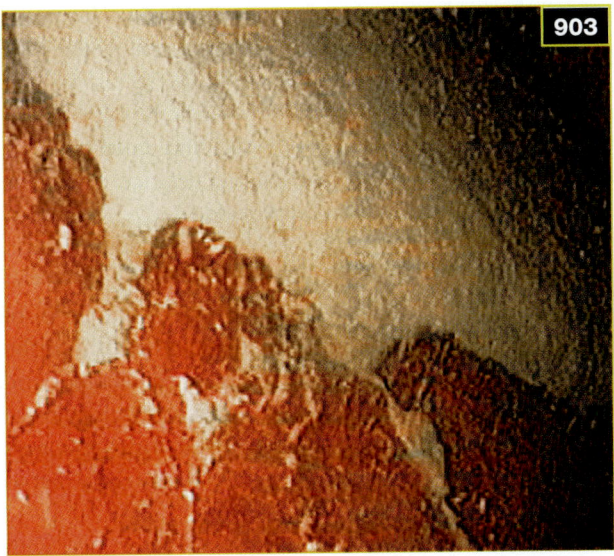

903 Sabulous urolithiasis (yellow debris) associated with cystitis.

Cystic calculi

Definition/overview

Cystic calculi (cystoliths) are the most common uroliths in horses and are usually identified in adult horses.

Etiology/pathophysiology

It is believed that a nidus in the form of organic debris is needed as a base for calculus formation. Risk factors for the development of cystic calculi are not well understood. Tissue damage, cystitis, remaining suture material, supersaturation of urine with certain minerals, and urine stasis may predispose to calculus development. A genetic predisposition is possible.

Cystic calculi are mainly composed of calcium carbonate crystals. If calcium carbonate crystals are mixed with calcium phosphate crystals, the structure of the calculus becomes stronger than that of calcium carbonate crystals alone. Most calculi are sphere-shaped stones. An accumulation of crystalloid sludge (sabulous urolithiasis) can also occur (903). The latter is usually associated with bladder paralysis and urine stasis.

Clinical presentation

Stranguria, pollakiruia, and hematuria are the most common presenting complaints. Hematuria may be more pronounced following exercise. Signs of systemic disease such as fever, depression, or anorexia should not be present. Other signs include tenesmus, colic, or incontinence and urine scalding. Urinary incontinence is common in sabulous urolithiasis.

Differential diagnosis

Cystitis; estrus; pyelonephritis; calculi in other parts of the urinary tract; renal failure; bladder rupture; neoplasia.

Diagnosis

Urinalysis, hematology, and serum biochemistry should be performed to document accompanying problems of the proximal urinary tract. The urine should be concentrated. Proteinuria, microscopic hematuria, and pyuria are common. A catheterized urine sample should be submitted for bacteriological culture, with identification of >10,000 CFU/ml indicating concurrent urinary tract infection. No hematologic abnormalities should be present with uncomplicated cases.

Calculi and/or a thickened bladder wall may be palpable per rectum. If the bladder is urine filled, it should be decompressed to allow for thorough palpation. Depending on the degree of concurrent bladder-wall inflammation, pain may be noted during palpation of the bladder. Sabulous urolithiasis consists of an accumulation

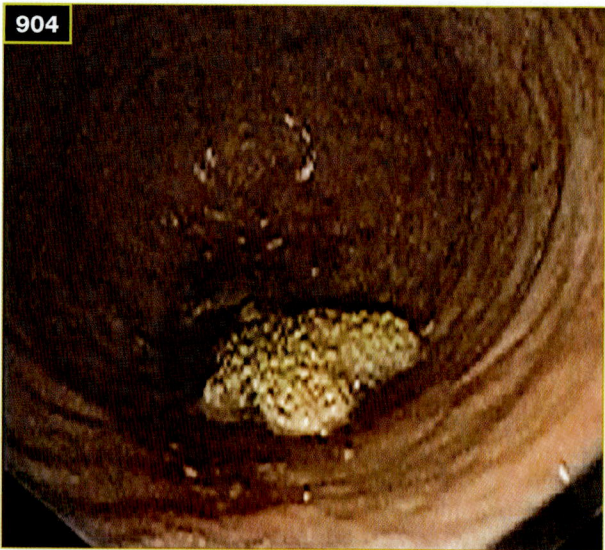

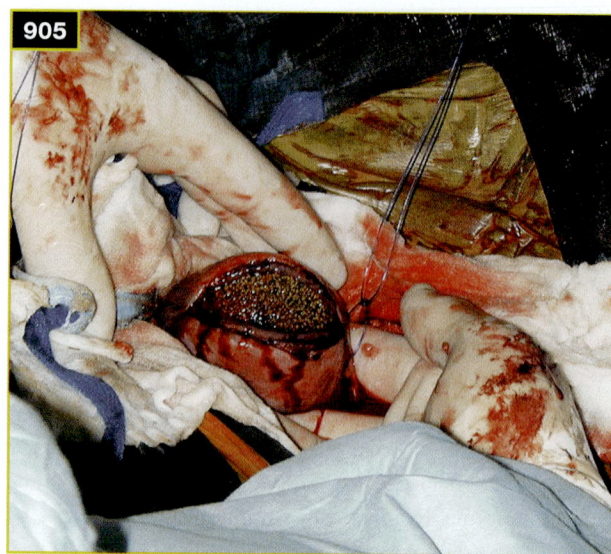

904 Solitary cystolith in the bladder of a horse with dysuria. Note the roughened surface of the cystolith and the bloody urine.

905 Laparocystotomy: surgical removal of a cystolith. (Photo courtesy A Cruz)

of sand-like debris in the bladder that may feel 'doughy' on palpation. Ultrasonographic examination of the urinary tract should be performed to exclude the presence of calculi in other locations. Cystoscopy can be used to further evaluate cystoliths (**904**) or sabulous urolithiasis.

Management

Several techniques have been described for removal of cystic calculi. Laparocystotomy or laparoscopic cystotomy are commonly performed. Subischial urethrotomy can be performed in a standing horse; however, the potential for stricture or diverticulum formation at the incision site is a disadvantage of this procedure. In mares, manual distension of the urethra may permit removal of small stones. Urethrosphincterotomy can be performed to aid the passage of fingers or a small hand into the bladder. Some stones may be crushed with forceps to facilitate removal. Sedation and epidural anesthesia are required for the procedure. Fragmentation and removal of cystic calculi by electrohydraulic lithotripsy, ballistic shock lithotripsy, and laser lithotripsy have also been reported. Pararectal cystotomy (Gökel's operation) can aid successful removal of calculi; however, postoperative complications are significant. Laparocystotomy is also indicated for surgical management of cystic calculi (**905**).

Antimicrobial therapy, as described for cystitis, should be initiated if evidence of bacterial infection is present on urinalysis and urine culture, and always when the procedure of calculi removal is performed.

Urinary acidification is used in other species to reduce urolith formation; however, it has proven to be minimally useful in horses. Oral administration of ammonium chloride (25–50 g/horse/day) or vitamin C (2 g/kg/day) has had inconsistent effects. Higher doses of ammonium chloride (520 mg/kg/day) or ammonium sulfate (175 mg/kg/day) may have more consistent effects, but are unpalatable and difficult to administer.

Bladders that contain sabulous uroliths should be irrigated with large volumes of fluid. Bladder irrigation combined with perineal urethrotomy is probably the most effective way to remove sabulous uroliths.

Oral administration of 50–75 g of table salt once or twice a day may increase water intake and diuresis, which acts therapeutically and prevents recurrence of calculi. Free access to water should be provided.

Prognosis

Approximately 41% of horses have recurrence of cystolithiasis after treatment. This depends greatly on the thoroughness of calculus removal from the bladder and whether an underlying lesion is present. High-calcium feeds (i.e. alfalfa hay) should be removed from the horse's diet and up to 70 g of table salt added to the daily diet to promote drinking and diuresis.

Sabulous cystic deposits are mostly associated with bladder paralysis and the response to treatment is poor. Unless the problem resulting in bladder paralysis can be resolved, the condition carries a poor prognosis.

Bladder paralysis/neurogenic incontinence

Definition/overview

Incontinence develops as intravesicular pressure exceeds resting urethral pressure, which results in variable degrees of urine dribbling. Incontinence and dysfunction of bladder control in horses is most often associated with neurologic disorders in the CNS or peripheral nervous system, and rarely with myogenic dysfunction in the bladder wall. Determining the origin of bladder dysfunction is important in order to plan the therapy and to establish the prognosis.

Etiology/pathophysiology

Urinary outflow is controlled by a complex activity of somatic and autonomic nerves that (1) generate sustained tone to prevent urinary leakage during bladder filling; (2) generate transient reflex increases in pressure to prevent opening of the lumen when abdominal pressure rises; and (3) undergo relaxation preceding micturition and can generate urethral opening and shortening during micturition. Normal sacral parasympathetic (pelvic nerve), somatic (pudendal nerve), lumbar sympathetic (hypogastric nerve) nerves and normal myogenic function are needed for normal micturition.

Damage to the sacral spinal cord, pelvis, and/or pudendal nerves leads to lower motor neuron (LMN) deficits. Diseases that cause LMN bladder dysfunction include EHV-1 myelitis, cauda equine syndrome, sorghum toxicosis, EPM, arboviral encephalitis, lumbosacral trauma, and neoplasia. LMN bladder dysfunction can also be caused iatrogenically with epidural administration of different pharmaceuticals. Mares are at increased risk for the development of LMN neurogenic incontinence because of the potential for trauma during breeding and parturition.

Upper motor neuron (UMN) bladder dysfunction is associated with damage to the suprasacral spinal cord or/and brainstem. Micturition is disabled via exaggerated urethral sphincter tone, despite the presence of a full bladder. Chronic UMN lesions may, through the sacral spinal reflexes, allow partial voiding of urine. This kind of incontinence is rare in horses and is caused by diseases similar to that in LMN bladder dysfunction.

Myogenic problems are rare, but have been reported in geldings. They lack a specific identifiable cause and are likely caused by a multifactorial rather than a single underlying pathologic process. It is becoming increasingly evident, however, that there is a fundamental abnormality at the level of the bladder wall.

Clinical presentation

Clinical signs include dribbling of urine and urine scalding of the perineum (mares) and medial aspect of the hindlimbs (males and females). Affected horses may frequently posture to urinate and void little or no urine.

Clinical signs of underlying neurologic diseases and their specific neurologic deficits may be evident. UMN disorders are frequently associated with recumbency and myopathy, which are often incompatible with life. Bladder distension with UMN disease may produce signs of abdominal pain or frequent posturing to urinate. Bladder rupture may occur with UMN disease.

Loss of anal and tail tone, fecal retention, hindlimb weakness and ataxia, hindlimb muscle atrophy, penile prolapse, and perineal sensory deficits are most commonly associated with UMN disease.

Hematuria may be observed if secondary infection or urolithiasis has developed. Less commonly, signs of systemic infection may be present if upper urinary tract infection has developed.

Bladder dysfunction is often associated with the accumulation of large amounts of sabulous or mucoid urinary sediment, especially so in myogenic bladder dysfunction and, less often, in LMN disease.

Severe and chronic dysfunction of the bladder wall can lead to permanent dysfunction. Ammonia accumulation in the bladder lumen causes constant irritation that damages the bladder wall and musculature further.

Differential diagnosis

Urolithiasis; cystitis; neoplasia; renal failure; cantharidin toxicosis; ectopic ureter; various neurologic diseases.

Diagnosis

A detailed neurologic evaluation is essential to localize the lesion and identify the primary cause. An LMN bladder is flaccid and easily expressible, while exaggerated sphincter tone in a UMN bladder results in firm distension. Sabulous urolithiasis may also be palpable per rectum. Transrectal ultrasonography and cystoscopy are helpful for eliminating other causes of incontinence and urine dribbling. Specific diagnostic testing for individual neurologic diseases is covered elsewhere (see Chapter 10).

Hematology is typically unremarkable unless bladder rupture occurs or secondary upper urinary tract infection is present. Urinalysis is normal unless secondary infection or urolithiasis has developed. Urine culture should be performed in all cases.

Management

Management of the underlying disease should be instituted promptly. The bladder should be regularly evacuated, which will help prevent exacerbation of bladder atony and development of sabulous urolithiasis. Nursing care, including daily cleaning of the perineum and hindlimbs, is required to reduce skin irritation. Prophylactic antimicrobial treatment is indicated in recumbent animals, if urinary tract infection is suspected or if frequent urinary catheterization is required. Procaine penicillin (20,000 IU/kg i/m q12h) or trimethoprim/sulfadiazine (24–30 mg/kg p/o q12h) is a good initial choice. Intravenous fluid therapy, if required because of concurrent disease or dysphagia, should be used conservatively, particularly if UMN bladder dysfunction is present.

It is important to consider whether UMN or LMN lesions are present. Phenoxybenzamine (0.7 mg/kg p/o q6h) can be used in cases of UMN disease to decrease urethral sphincter tone; however, the effectiveness of this treatment is unclear. Bethanecol chloride (0.025–0.075 mg/kg s/c or 0.2–0.4 mg/kg p/o q8h) can be administered to improve detrusor muscle tone and strength of bladder contraction. Response to bethanecol is usually poor with long-standing disease, and it should be discontinued if there is no response within 3–5 days. Bethanecol has no effect when the bladder is completely atonic or areflexic. Acepromazine (0.02–0.05 mg/kg i/m q8h) and diazepam (0.02–0.1 mg/kg; slow i/v administration) may decrease urethral tone and help to void urine.

Prognosis

The prognosis is guarded and depends on the ability to treat the primary disease and prevent complications such as urinary tract infection or sabulous urolithiasis.

Nonneurogenic and nonmyogenic incontinence

Cystitis and chronic urethritis can cause apparent incontinence through irritation of stretch receptors in the bladder wall. In cases of urine retention, bacteria can break down urea to ammonia, which acts as an irritant on the bladder mucosa and musculature, causing incontinence. Ectopic ureters, urethral or vaginal injury, and vaginal polyps have been associated with incontinence. Hypoestrogenism in mares has also been reported as a possible cause of incontinence.

The pathophysiology, clinical signs, and management of nonneurogenic and nonmyogenic incontinence are outlined under their respective primary causes elsewhere in this chapter.

In cases of urinary incontinence where primary disease can be managed successfully, the prognosis is reasonably good. Urine scalding can be avoided by routine cleaning. In cases of suspected estrogen-associated incontinence in mares, estradiol cypionate (4 mg/kg i/m q48h) can be administered.

Diseases of the urethra

Urethral trauma and urethral defects

Definition/overview

Urethral trauma and defects have become increasingly recognized in male horses. Mild cases express themselves only with hematuria. Breeding disability and urinary tract obstruction are possible in complicated cases.

Etiology/pathophysiology

Trauma to the penis (906), breeding injuries, dystocia, masturbation control devices (stallion rings), postsurgical scar tissue, prolonged and traumatic urinary catheterization, endoscopy of the distal urinary tract, and urethral calculi can lead to urethral trauma.

Tears of the proximal urethra at the level of the ischial arch have recently been given a more significant role. It is possible that the condition is the result of corpus spongiosum penis damage due to dramatic pressure changes during ejaculation. Hemorrhage from varicosities has also been recently more often reported.

Clinical presentation

Urethral trauma typically results in hematuria at the end of urination and hemospermia in stallions. Pollakiuria may be present in some cases. Penile, vaginal, or perineal trauma may be apparent.

Differential diagnosis

Urolithiasis; urethritis; cystitis; bladder paralysis; neoplasia; sabulous urolithiasis.

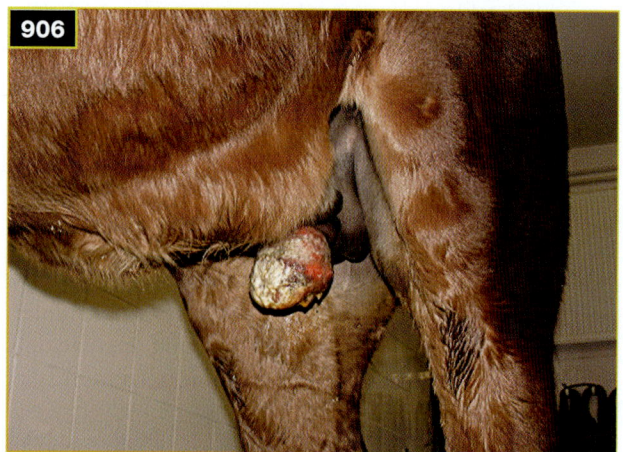

906 Penile trauma. This stallion injured himself jumping over a fence with an erect penis. Note the edema around the genitals, which may also be caused by urethral rupture and urine leakage.

907 Severe urethritis and mucosal erosions present throughout the urethra.

908 Severe urethritis.

909 Contrast urethrogram in a foal. Note the contrast material starting from the tip of the catheter and following the lumen of the urethra and bladder.

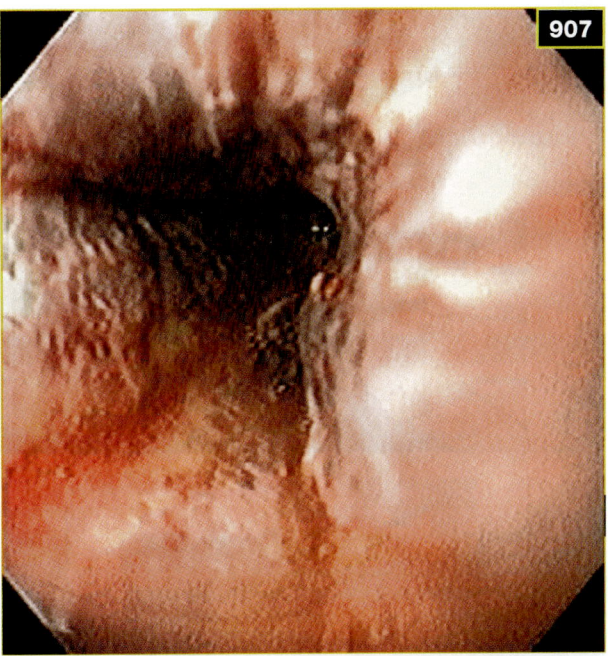

Diagnosis

No obvious clinical signs are usually present except for hematuria. Close examination should be performed to look for signs of trauma. The penis should be extruded, examined visually, and carefully palpated. The bladder should be palpated per rectum. Cystoscopy and urethroscopy should be carried out to confirm the urethral lesion (907, 908). Care should be taken during urethroscopy to prevent exacerbation of a urethral lesion. If there is a question about the patency of the penile urethra, a retrograde urethrogram can be performed (909). Ultrasonography can be useful in the examination of surrounding tissue for any evidence of foreign bodies, scars, and hematomas.

Urinalysis and urine culture should be performed. These are usually unremarkable, with hematuria being the only abnormality. Anemia may be present if urethral bleeding is prolonged or severe.

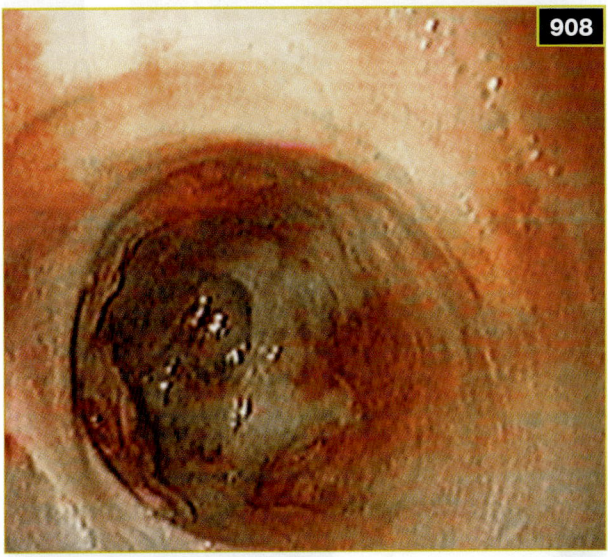

Management

Most minor lesions to the urethra will resolve spontaneously. If lesions communicate with the adjacent corpus spongiosum penis, spontaneous resolution is less likely and ischial urethrotomy, which will circumvent intraurethral bleeding to allow adequate healing, may be required. Management of calculi lodged within the urethra is discussed elsewhere (p. 663).

In cases of trauma, topical wound therapy is necessary. Systemic antimicrobials (procaine penicillin 20,000 IU/kg i/m q12h or trimethoprim/sulfadiazine 24–30 mg/kg p/o q12h) should be administered in cases where infection is suspected or therapeutic procedures are invasive. Anti-inflammatory treatment may also be necessary (flunixin meglumine 0.5–1.1 mg/kg p/o, i/m, or i/v q12–24h; ketoprofen 2.2 mg/kg i/v or i/m q24h).

Prognosis

The prognosis depends on the severity of the urethral defect. Severe trauma may obstruct urine flow primarily or secondarily with scar tissue formation and urethral stricture. In such cases, urethrotomy is necessary to bypass the stricture.

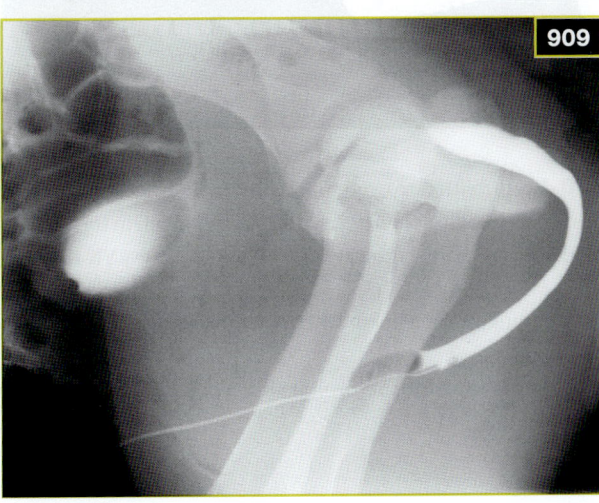

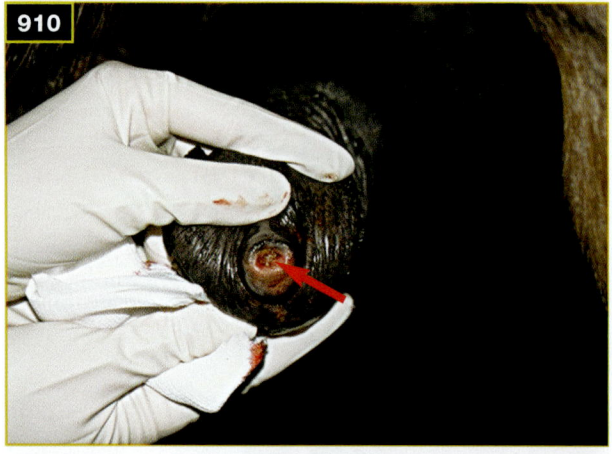

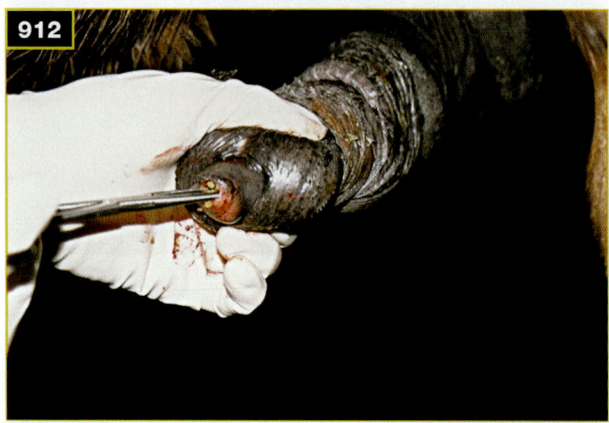

910 Urethrolith (arrowed) in the urethral orifice. Urethrolithiasis is usually associated with urinary calculi in the bladder or proximal urinary tract. (Photo courtesy VK Kos)

911 Stranguria in a horse with urethrolithiasis.

912 Removal of the urethrolith with a hemostat. (Photo courtesy VK Kos)

Urethrolithiasis

Definition/overview

Urethral calculi develop mostly in male horses. Urethrolithiasis in females is an uncommon condition. Calculi are flushed from the bladder and lodge in the urethra (910). It is highly unusual for calculi to develop in an intact urethra. The outcome of the disease depends on the degree of trauma to the urethra and surrounding tissues.

Etiology/pathophysiology

Most calculi initially lodge where the urethra narrows over the ischial arch. Some of them may move more distally and completely obstruct the urethra, causing signs of renal colic. If not treated, bladder rupture, uroperitoneum, and postrenal ARF may ensue.

Clinical presentation

Frequent posturing to urinate, pollakiuria, stranguria (911), and nonspecific signs of abdominal pain are common signs of urethrolithiasis. Blood may be seen at the end of the urethral orifice. The severity of clinical signs depends on whether complete urethral obstruction is present. With complete obstruction, signs of severe abdominal pain will develop as bladder distension progresses. If the bladder ruptures, signs of uroperitoneum develop.

Differential diagnosis

Urethral trauma; neoplasia; urethritis; cystitis; sabulous urolithiasis; bladder paralysis; colic.

Diagnosis

The penis should be extended and carefully palpated. Urethroliths may be palpable, depending on the location. The bladder should be palpated per rectum to assess bladder size. The bladder may be turgid and distended. If signs consistent with abdominal pain are present, thorough palpation of the intestinal viscera should be performed. An inability to pass a urinary catheter is suggestive of urethral obstruction; however, urethral spasm can also inhibit advancement of a catheter. Urethroscopy usually provides a definitive diagnosis.

Urinalysis, if urine can be obtained, is consistent with signs of postrenal ARF. Bacterial culture of the urine should also be performed.

Blood can occasionally be seen on the end of the urethra; however, urethral defects mostly result in hematuria at the end of urination. Initially, hematology should be unremarkable. If bladder rupture ensues, the horse becomes depressed and anorexic because of acid–base alterations and azotemia. The rest of the urinary tract should be examined for the presence of other uroliths.

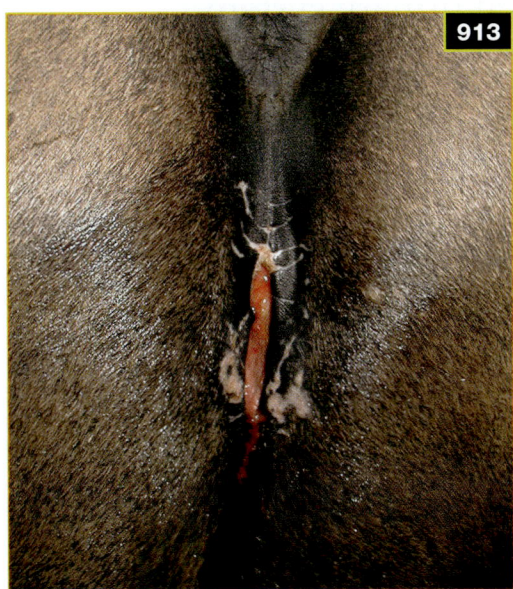

913 Perineal urethrostomy site in a stallion with urethral obstruction and subsequent bladder rupture.

Management

Calculi that are present in the distal urethra may be removed with hemostats (912). Calculi lodged further up the urethra can be removed via a urethrostomy (913). Those lodged at the ischial arch can be removed through a perineal urethrostomy (ischial urethrostomy, subischial urethrostomy). Calculi can be crushed and then removed from the urethra. However, trauma can be sustained by the urethra and bladder during stone crushing and removal. Calculi lodged in less accessible parts of the urethra may require a urethrotomy performed under general anesthesia.

Antimicrobials (procaine penicillin 20,000 IU/kg i/m q12h or trimethoprim/sulfadiazine 24–30 mg/kg p/o q12h) are necessary in most cases of urolithiasis, especially in cases where the therapeutic procedures are invasive. If concurrent infection is present, antibiotic treatment should be based on urine culture and sensitivity results.

Prognosis

The prognosis depends on the severity of the urethral lesion and secondary complications. Excessive tissue trauma increases the risk of urethral stricture.

Urethritis

Definition/overview

Urethritis is an inflammatory condition of the urethra that can be infectious or traumatic in origin. It usually develops secondary to cystitis, urethral trauma (also post catheterization), calculi, or accessory-gland infection. Idiopathic urethritis is a possible but uncommon disease in horses.

Etiology/pathophysiology

The urethra may provide a favorable environment for colonization by pathogens if its powerful defense mechanisms are defeated. Gram-negative organisms predominantly cause urethritis. *Candida* infection may occur in foals that undergo intensive antimicrobial therapy. *Habronema megastoma* may also invade the urethral process, causing granulomas (914).

Clinical presentation

Hematuria, hemospermia, and stranguria are common presenting complaints. Resentment of manual manipulation of the penis and sheath may be observed.

Differential diagnosis

Urethrolithiasis; urethral trauma; bladder paralysis; cantharidin toxicosis; neoplasia; vaginitis.

Diagnosis

Diagnosis is based on the demonstration of the lesions by palpation and endoscopic examination. Ultrasonography may be helpful in excluding involvement of the accessory sex glands. Fractionation and examination of the ejaculate may provide similar information. Bacterial culture of a urethral swab, urine, and semen should be performed. Hematology and urinalysis are not specific in primary urethritis.

Management

Treatment involves sheath cleaning and topical treatment with anti-inflammatory and antibacterial agents. Any primary disease causing the urethritis should be managed accordingly. Systemic antimicrobials are occasionally indicated. In severe cases of urethritis, oil-based antibiotic

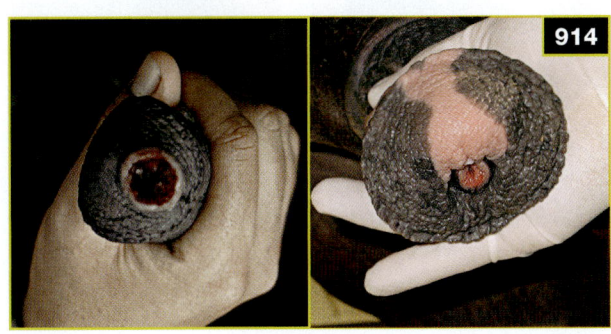

914 *Habronema* granuloma (left) and normal urethral process (right). Redness of the urethral process was caused by catheterization (right).

preparations can be infused via a urinary catheter into the pelvic urethra. Oil-based antibiotic preparations can also be used topically on the urethral process.

Habronema granulomas should be managed with ivermectin, topical insecticides, and, in advanced cases, surgical excision.

Prognosis

Urethral inflammation may result in fibrous strictures, which carries a less favorable prognosis. In cases of permanent damage to the urethra, recurrences and chronic urethritis are possible.

Urethroplasty (urethral extension)

Urethroplasty (**915**) is a surgical extension of the urethra. It is performed in mares that pool urine in the cranial vaginal vault (vesiculovaginal reflux). Vaginitis, cervicitis, endometritis, and infertility are common sequelae to urine pooling.

Urethroplasty surgically creates a mucosal shelf from the urethra to the mucocutaneous junction of the vulva, which prevents the flow of urine back into the cranial vaginal vault. The most common complication of the procedure is fistula formation along the suture line; however, for most patients the outcome is favorable.

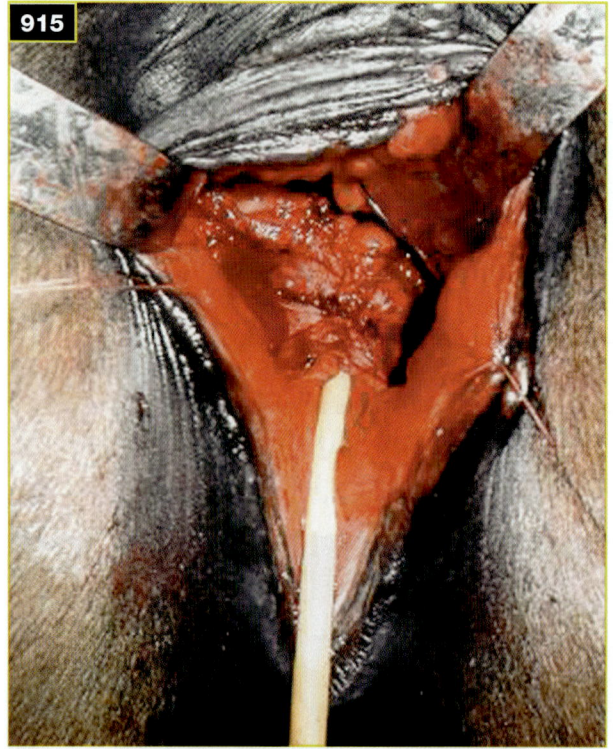

915 Urethroplasty in a mare to prevent urine pooling.

General urinary system disorders

Uroperitoneum

Definition/overview

Uroperitoneum (the presence of free urine in the abdominal cavity) is a syndrome most commonly recognized in foals between 24 and 48 hours old. Male foals and septic foals are more likely to be affected. Urinary calculi can be associated with rupture of any part of the urinary tract and with urine leakage into the abdominal cavity in older horses. Rupture of the bladder is most common.

The continuity of the urinary tract must be restored or metabolic abnormalities caused by uroperitoneum are fatal for the animal.

Etiology/pathophysiology

It is possible that the anatomy of the urethra in colts predisposes them to bladder rupture during parturition, when high pressures are applied focally or circumferentially around the bladder. The long and narrow urethra in colts resists the pressure that is put on the bladder during parturition and predisposes the weak bladder wall of the neonate to rupture. Urachal infection may also predispose to uroperitoneum.

In adult horses, uroperitoneum develops secondary to urethral obstruction, trauma, urinary catheterization, and, in mares, during dystocia.

Rupture of the bladder (**916**), urachus, ureter, or renal pelvis may result in leakage of urine into the peritoneal cavity. As urine accumulates in the abdomen, azotemia, hyperkalemia, hyponatremia, hypochloremia, and metabolic acidosis develop. These abnormalities arise from the equilibration of urine electrolytes and water across the peritoneal membrane, allowing for loss of sodium and chloride, which move into the abdominal fluid/urine; and retention of potassium, which diffuses from the abdominal fluid/urine. Urea readily diffuses across the peritoneal surface. Creatinine is a larger molecule and diffuses much more slowly across the peritoneal surface. The presence of urine in the peritoneal cavity also causes chemical peritonitis.

Clinical presentation

Abdominal discomfort, abdominal distension (**917**), and straining to urinate are often observed (**918**). Little to no urine is passed. Voiding of a small amount of urine does not exclude urinary tract rupture and uroperitoneum. A fluid wave may be felt on succussion of the abdomen. Acid–base disturbance produces depression, anorexia, tachycardia, and tachypnea. Respiratory distress can develop with severe abdominal distension, particularly in foals. If the disease is not treated, shock and collapse will develop. Severe tachycardia may be present with severe hyperkalemia.

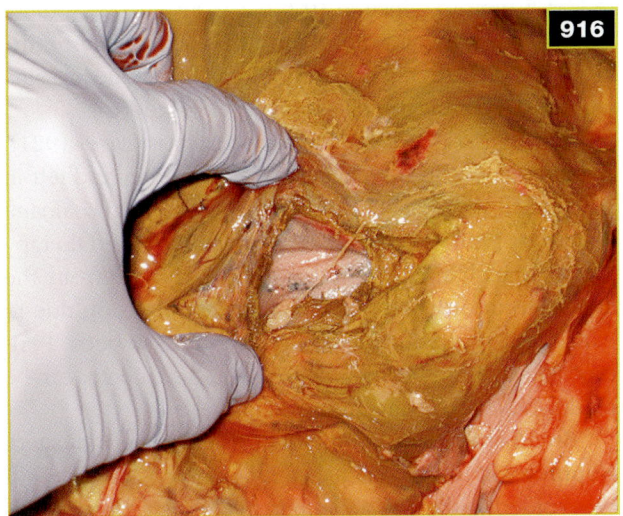

916 Bladder rupture in a foal. Note other erosions on the bladder mucosa caused by cystitis.

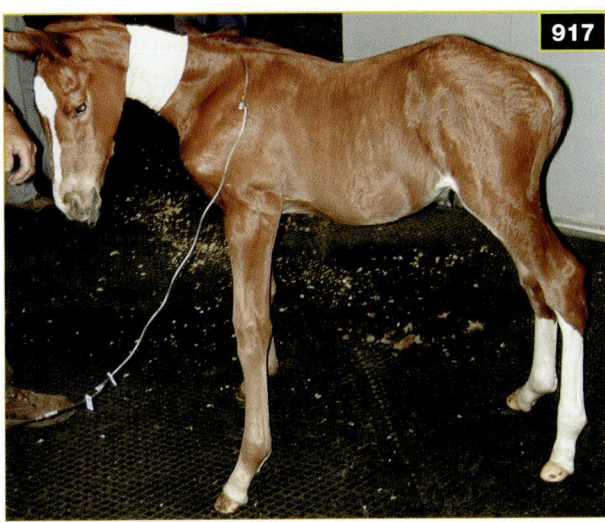

917 Abdominal distension in a foal with uroperitoneum. The foal's acid–base status is severely affected, causing depression.

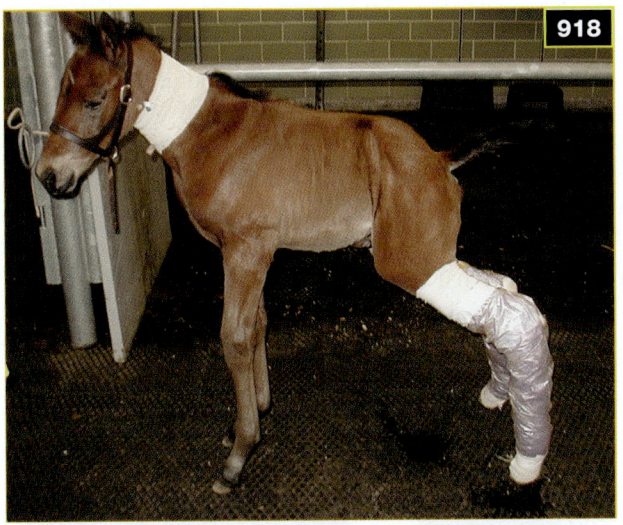

918 A foal with uroperitoneum strains to urinate. Other diseases, prematurity, sex, hospitalization, and frequent handling predispose foals to bladder rupture.

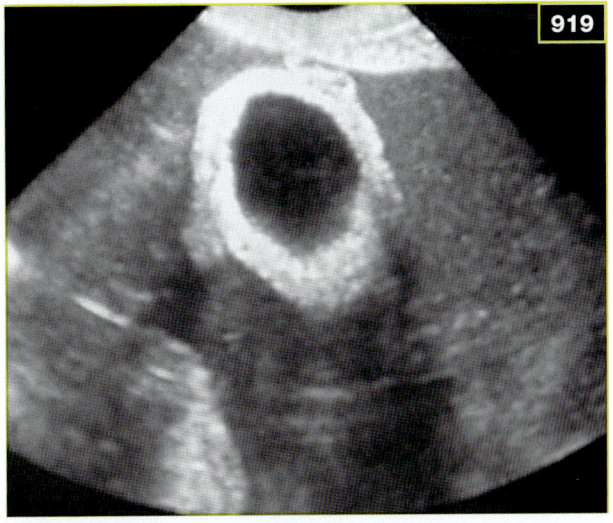

919 Transabdominal ultrasonogram of a foal with uroperitoneum. The echogenic circular structure is the bladder surrounded by a large amount of free fluid in the peritoneal cavity.

Foals may also show signs of concurrent infection and sepsis, which most often include fever, weakness, injected mucous membranes, diarrhea, and septic arthritis. Severe electrolyte disturbances can cause neurologic abnormalities.

Differential diagnosis
Colic; pleuropneumonia; sepsis; endotoxemia; renal failure; neoplasia; intestinal rupture; renal tubular acidosis.

Diagnosis
A bladder wall defect may be visualized ultrasonographically; however, often the only abnormal finding is the presence of excessive free abdominal fluid (919). Abdominocentesis should be performed. With uroperitoneum, peritoneal fluid usually contains a low cell count and may smell like urine. A peritoneal creatinine concentration of at least twice that of a concurrently obtained serum sample is diagnostic for uroperitoneum.

Peritoneal urea determination is less useful because it readily diffuses and equilibrates with serum urea. Infusion of new methylene blue into the bladder, followed by abdominocentesis 5–10 minutes later, may be used as a confirmatory test. If the peritoneal fluid is blue-tinged, bladder or urachal rupture is confirmed. The procedure is less reliable if the rupture is present in other parts of the urinary tract. Abdominal radiography only indicates free fluid in the abdomen (920). A contrast cystogram can be performed in foals to confirm the site of urinary tract rupture. Diagnostic procedures to detect concomitant diseases, such as sepsis and bacterial peritonitis, should be implemented. A blood culture should be performed.

Urinalysis, if urine can be obtained, is nonspecific. Gross or microscopic hematuria is often present.

CBC results are usually normal if concurrent disease is not present. Serum biochemical abnormalities usually include azotemia, hyperkalemia, hyponatremia, hypochloremia, and metabolic acidosis. These abnormalities may be severe. Serum chemical analysis can be influenced by intravenous fluid administration.

Cytologic and bacteriologic evaluation of peritoneal fluid is crucial to identify and define peritonitis. In foals, passive transfer of maternal antibodies should be evaluated and the umbilicus should be examined ultrasonographically.

Management

Initial treatment should be directed at stabilizing the patient. Hydration should be maintained and acid–base and electrolyte abnormalities should be corrected with intravenous fluid therapy (0.9% or 0.45% saline should be used). In hyperkalemic animals, dextrose-containing fluids are indicated (4–8 mg/kg/day). With severe hyperkalemia (K^+ >5.5 mmol/l), insulin (0.1–0.2 U/kg s/c) or sodium bicarbonate (1–2 mEq/kg) may be used concurrently, although fluid therapy and abdominal drainage are successful in reducing the potassium level in most cases.

Abdominal drainage is required in most cases (921). A catheter should be placed in the abdomen and left in place until the defect is corrected. Abdominal drainage should be performed gradually. Intravenous fluid therapy should match the amount of fluid removed from the abdomen in order to prevent acute hypotension due to expansion of previously collapsed capillary beds. Peritoneal lavage can be helpful; however, the catheter can be readily blocked by omentum and fibrin.

Broad-spectrum antimicrobial therapy is indicated. Nephrotoxic drugs such as aminoglycosides should be avoided initially in azotemic, hypotensive, and dehydrated animals. Ceftiofur sodium (2.2 mg/kg i/m or i/v q12h) is a reasonable first choice. A combination of penicillin (sodium penicillin 20,000 IU/kg i/v q6h or procaine penicillin 20,000 IU/kg i/m q12h) and an aminoglycoside (gentamicin 6.6 mg/kg i/v q24h or amikacin 15 (adults)–21 (foals) mg/kg i/v q24h) can be used when there is no concern about renal function. Alternatively, an aminoglycoside could be combined with ceftiofur postoperatively if there is a concern about Gram-negative sepsis.

Surgical repair of the bladder defect should be performed after the animal's metabolic status has been corrected (922). The abdomen should be lavaged, especially if cytology of peritoneal fluid suggests infection. In foals, internal umbilical remnants are often a source of infection and should be removed during surgery. Laparoscopic repair of a bladder defect can also be performed successfully (923).

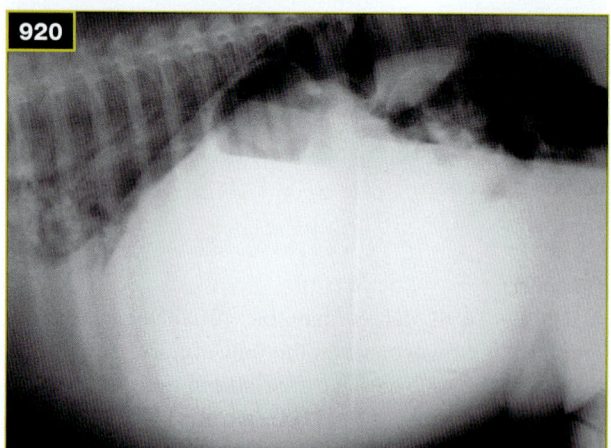

920 Abdominal radiography of a foal with uroperitoneum. The fluid line indicates the presence of free fluid in the abdomen.

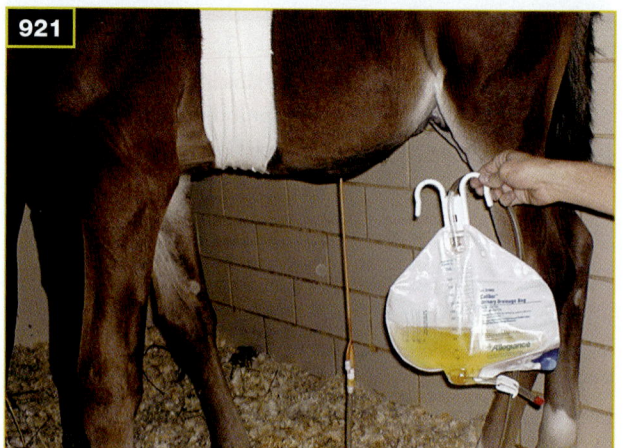

921 Drainage of urine from the abdomen in a foal with uroperitoneum.

Urinary system

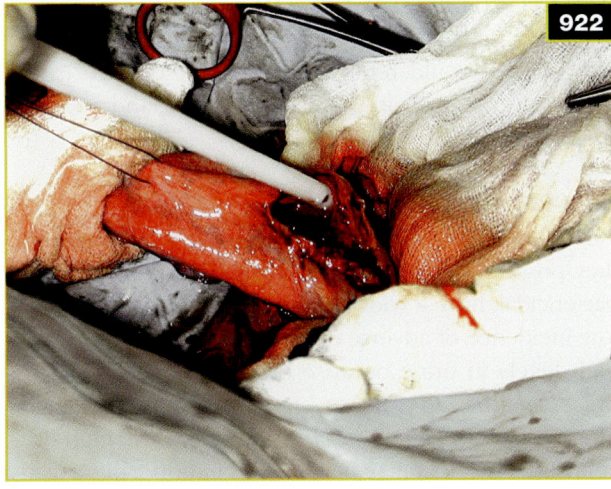

922 Surgical repair of the bladder wall tear via laparotomy.

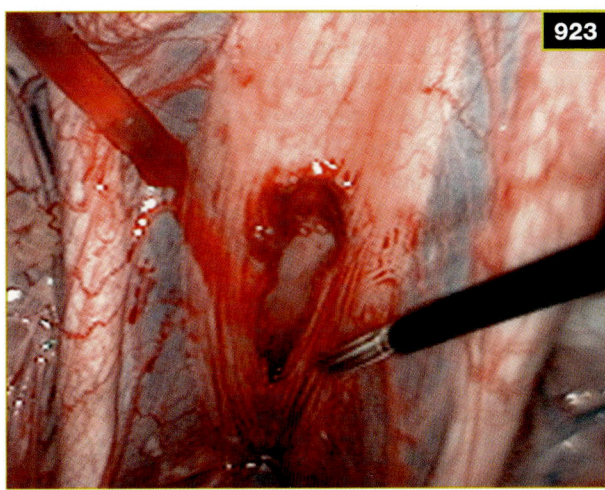

923 Laparoscopic repair of a bladder wall tear in a foal.

Uroperitoneum should be managed similarly in adult animals. Significant urine leakage from the ureters or kidneys is difficult to manage in horses. If the defect persists, nephrectomy should be considered.

Prognosis
The prognosis for recovery in foals is usually good. Concomitant infection or sepsis significantly decreases the chance of a favorable outcome.

In adults, or in cases of urine leakage from the kidney or ureters, the prognosis is less favorable.

Cantharidin toxicosis (blister beetle toxicosis)
Definition/overview
Cantharidin is a highly irritable substance that causes acantholysis and vesicle formation when in contact with skin or mucous membranes. The compound is contained in beetles belonging to the family *Meloidae*. Different species of blister beetles are found from southern Canada to Mexico, and from the Atlantic coast to Utah, Texas, and New Mexico. Even though there are approximately 2,500 known species of blister beetle worldwide, cantharidin toxicosis is a common event only in the US.

Etiology/pathophysiology
Cantharidin toxicosis occurs when horses ingest food contaminated with blister beetles (*Epicauta* spp.). The most common source is alfalfa hay. Outbreaks can occur elsewhere mostly because of shipment of contaminated alfalfa hay from the midwestern United States.

Cantharidin is reported to stimulate DNA synthesis, which increases the mitotic rate of epithelial cells. Acantholysis and vesicle formation occur as a result of disruption of cell membranes. These lead to urinary tract irritation and renal insufficiency. Hemodynamic changes due to generalized disease may contribute to the renal damage.

Clinical presentation
Typical clinical signs are those referable to shock, GI and urinary tract irritation, renal insufficiency, myocardial failure, and hypocalcemia. Extensive inflammation in the urinary tract, hemorrhage, and pseudomembrane formation are associated with stranguria, pollakiuria, and hematuria. In some cases, sudden death with few prodromal signs may occur.

Differential diagnosis
Cystitis; pyelonephritis; urolithiasis; renal failure; neoplasia; bladder paralysis; NSAID toxicity; mercury toxicosis.

Diagnosis
Concurrent signs of urinary tract and GI disease, particularly severe mucosal irritation, are suggestive of cantharidin toxicosis. Hay should be examined for the presence of blister beetles; however, failure to identify beetles does not eliminate the possibility of cantharidin toxicosis.

Urinalysis
The urine SG is low (isosthenuria) even in the face of dehydration. Macroscopic hematuria is usually present. Epithelial cells are occasionally seen in the urine, but casts are rarely present.

667

Hematology and serum chemical analysis

Clinical laboratory abnormalities that are commonly encountered include hypocalcemia, hypomagnesemia, hypoproteinemia, and mild azotemia. Chemical analysis for cantharidin is accomplished by evaluation of urine or stomach contents. Samples should be submitted as soon as cantharidin toxicosis is suspected because cantharidin is eliminated within 3–4 days.

Management

Treatment is supportive. The source of toxin must be removed. Potentially exposed animals should be treated orally with mineral oil (4–6 liters via nasogastric tube) or activated charcoal (1–3 g/kg via nasogastric tube). Mineral oil acts as a mild laxative and absorbs lipid-soluble cantharidin, which aids in the elimination of cantharidin from the intestine. Mineral oil and activated charcoal should not be administered concurrently.

Intravenous balanced electrolyte solution administration (120–180 ml/kg/day) should be commenced. Administration of diuretics (furosemide 1 mg/kg i/v or i/m q6h) has been recommended to increase cantharidin excretion after the patient is rehydrated. Supplementation of intravenous fluids with calcium borogluconate may be required and is ideally based on repeated evaluation of serum ionized calcium level. Magnesium supplementation is less commonly required, but can be achieved by administration of magnesium sulfate (0.2–1.0 g/kg dissolved in 4 liters of warm water q12h).

Analgesics are usually required and should be administrated sparingly. NSAIDs should be avoided if possible or given at reduced doses (flunixin meglumine $\leq$ 0.5 mg/kg i/v q12h; ketoprofen $\leq$ 1.1 mg/kg i/v or i/m q24h) and only after intravenous fluid therapy is initiated. Alpha-2 agonists and opioids are good alternatives for short-term analgesia.

Prophylactic treatment with appropriate antibiotics to prevent the development of secondary cystitis has been recommended, but may not be necessary in most cases. If antimicrobials are used, nephrotoxic drugs should be avoided.

Prognosis

The prognosis is variable and depends on the amount of cantharidin that was ingested and the time from the onset of signs to the start of appropriate treatment. Laminitis has occasionally been associated with cantharidin toxicosis.

Renal pharmacology

The reader should refer to the specific disease in the text for drug use, drug selection, dose, and route of administration.

Beta-lactam antibiotics

Penicillins are often used in the urinary tract because they possess a number of beneficial properties. They are bactericidal, have a wide margin of safety, and a relatively low incidence of adverse effects, and many achieve very high levels in urine because of renal excretion. Micro-organisms that are reported to be resistant *in vitro* are often, in fact, sensitive *in vivo* because of the high drug concentrations that may be achieved in urine, particularly alkaline urine. Acidification of the urine may affect the pharmacokinetic variables of penicillin. Intravenous administration of ampicillin, however, can be combined with urinary acidifiers.

Cephalosporins have the same mechanism of action as penicillins and also achieve very high concentrations in urine. In general, cephalosporins have a broader spectrum with enhanced Gram-negative activity compared to penicillins. Both penicillins and cephalosporins are effective against most anaerobes.

Sulfonamides

Sulfonamides are typically used in combination with trimethoprim, which provides broad-spectrum bactericidal activity. They are eliminated by a combination of renal excretion and metabolism in the liver. The trimethoprim/ sulfadiazine combination is more suitable for treatment of urinary tract infection than trimethoprim/sulfamethoxazole; sulfamethoxazole is largely metabolized before urinary excretion. Alkaline urine improves the solubility of sulfonamides after they undergo acetylization. They should not be given in combination with urine acidifiers. Crystalluria, hematuria, and obstruction of renal tubules, although rare, have been reported after administration of sulfonamides. Acidic urine and dehydration may predispose to the development of the above problems.

Aminoglycosides

Aminoglycoside antimicrobials have an excellent Gram-negative spectrum, but less Gram-positive activity and no activity against anaerobes. Aminoglycosides are excreted by glomerular filtration and they achieve high concentrations in urine, which may result in activity against certain organisms that are resistant *in vitro*, including Gram-positive organisms, but not anaerobes. The main concern about the use of aminoglycosides in urinary tract disease is the potential for nephrotoxicity. The accumulation of aminoglycosides in proximal tubular cells interferes with normal cell lysosomal activity and causes cell death. Aminoglycosides should not be used routinely in urinary tract infection because of their nephrotoxic activity.

Traditionally, the recommended dosing regimen of aminoglycosides was set up as a multiple-day dosing based on the peak and trough serum concentrations achieved in response to administration. Recently, once-daily administration (single daily dosing, pulse dosing) has gained acceptance for the treatment of horses. Once-daily aminoglycoside administration, compared with the traditional multiple-day dosing, exhibits:

+ Longer postantibiotic effect (continued suppression of bacterial growth despite decline of the antimicrobial concentration).
+ Enhanced bactericidal action, which in aminoglycosides is concentration dependent.
+ Reduced bacterial adaptive postexposure resistance (multiple-day dosing tends to reduce aminoglycoside uptake into the bacterial cell).
+ Reduced aminoglycoside nephrotoxicity.

Other antimicrobials

Tetracyclines have been associated with renal toxicity, do not achieve levels similar to penicillins, cephalosporins, or trimethoprim/sulfonamides in the urine, and are not used routinely in urinary tract infection.

Fluoroquinolones (enrofloxacin: 2.5–5 mg/kg i/v or i/m q24h, or 7.5–10 mg/kg p/o q24h; orbifloxacin: 2.5–5 mg/kg p/o q24h) are bactericidal and effective against many Gram-negative and Gram-positive organisms. However, based on the importance of fluoroquinolones in human medicine, they should be considered second-line drugs and used only when there is resistance to first-line drugs. Fluoroquinolones should not be used in growing animals because of effects on cartilage development.

Nonsteroidal anti-inflammatory drugs

NSAIDs, especially when given to hypotensive or dehydrated patients, may induce medullary ischemia and renal papillary necrosis. Therefore, NSAIDs should be used judiciously in urinary tract disease. Their use should be reserved for animals that are not hypovolemic, hypotensive, or dehydrated.

Mannitol

Mannitol is an osmotic diuretic that is used in some cases of acute, oliguric renal failure. Mannitol is filtered into the tubular space, where it increases tubular fluid osmolality. This impairs fluid resorption, with resultant increased excretion primarily of water, although modest amounts of sodium and potassium are also excreted. Mannitol should only be given intravenously via a blood filter administration set.

The major potential adverse effects of mannitol administration are consequences of increased plasma osmolality. When GFR is reduced, as in renal failure or congestive heart failure, mannitol cannot move into cells and is retained within the extracellular fluid. Water moves out of cells into the extracellular fluid, causing hyponatremia and tissue congestion. Volume overload may result in systemic and pulmonary edema.

Mannitol has been used for prophylaxis against renal dysfunction: however, the benefit of its administration is questionable. Mannitol is contraindicated in patients with anuria secondary to renal disease, severe dehydration, pulmonary congestion, and congestive heart failure.

Furosemide

Furosemide is a loop diuretic that blocks the nephron site responsible for urinary concentration and increases urinary water, sodium, potassium, calcium, and magnesium excretion. Loop diuretics may cause electrolyte disturbances such as hypokalemia, hypocalcemia, hypomagnesemia, metabolic alkalosis, and volume contraction. Furosemide can be useful in patients with renal insufficiency. However, factors that limit proximal tubule secretory activity (e.g. decreased renal blood flow or renal failure) reduce the effectiveness of furosemide and other diuretics.

NSAIDs diminish the response to loop and thiazide diuretics because they increase electrolyte and water resorption at the thick ascending limb of the loop of Henle.

Concomitant use of furosemide and aminoglycosides may produce severe ototoxicity, especially in young animals.

Dopamine

The use of dopamine may improve renal blood flow in horses with ARF. Dopamine dilates renal arterioles and increases renal blood flow and the GFR. Cardiac dysrhythmias are the most common adverse effects recognized in horses.

Sodium bicarbonate

Sodium bicarbonate has been successfully used in myoglobin-induced toxic nephropathy. Alkalization of urine diminishes renal retention of myoglobin. This is probably achieved with better solubility of myoglobin in the alkaline medium. Therefore, horses affected by rhabdomyolysis benefit from bicarbonate administration.

Other drugs

Ammonium chloride (60–520 mg/kg p/o q24h), ammonium sulfate (175 mg/kg p/o q24h), and ascorbic acid (1–2 g/kg p/o q24h) are used for urine acidification. Horses do not find ammonium salts palatable and will rarely voluntarily ingest the volume required to acidify urine.

Phenoxybenzamine (0.7 mg/kg p/o q6h), an alpha-adrenergic blocker, can be used to diminish urethral resistance in UMN bladder dysfunction.

Bethanecol chloride (0.025–0.075 mg/kg s/c q8h) exerts stimulatory effects on the smooth muscle of the bladder. It is a drug of choice in cases of detrusor atony. Side-effects include abdominal discomfort, excessive salivation, and lacrimation.

Cardiovascular system

Kim McGurrin

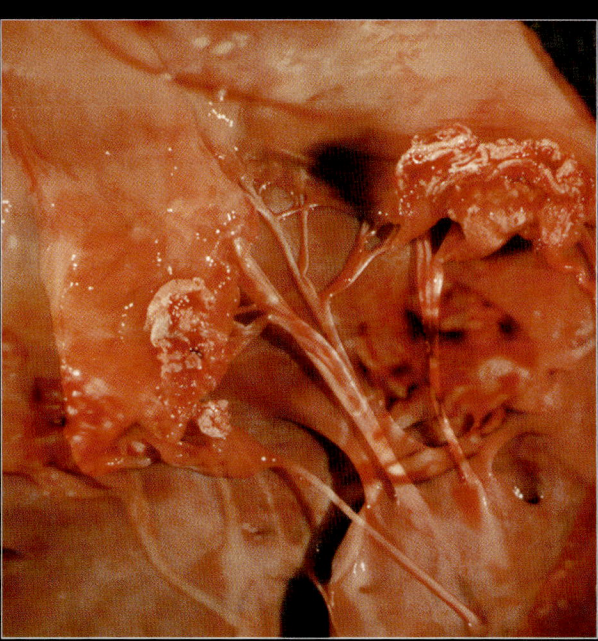

Cardiovascular system

In most instances the horse is first and foremost a performance animal and the potential impact of cardiovascular disease on performance and resale value is important. Cardiovascular abnormalities of variable clinical significance are frequently encountered in the horse. Heart murmurs and arrhythmias are common. Congenital anomalies are infrequent in the horse compared with small animal species.

Cardiology examination

Evaluation of the cardiovascular system involves, at minimum, acquiring a detailed history and performing a complete physical examination. Additional diagnostic modalities such as electrocardiography, echocardiography, and radiotelemetry may be necessary. More invasive diagnostic techniques such as cardiac catheterization are infrequently performed in the horse and are usually limited to referral facilities.

History

A detailed history is particularly important. Overt heart failure is relatively uncommon and horses are often presented with relatively mild disease when compared with small animal species. Frequently, an abnormality is detected during either routine or prepurchase examinations. The veterinarian is often faced with the task of determining the significance of such findings. In a high-level performance animal, even a slight deterioration in performance may precipitate a request for cardiovascular examination.

The signalment of the animal may aid in assessing cardiac disease. With the exception of congenital heart disease in the Arabian horse, breed association with specific cardiac disease is uncommon. Aortic root rupture most commonly occurs in aged breeding stallions.

The past, present, and future use of the horse is critical in determining the significance of a finding and in planning future action. An abnormality that is unlikely to produce overt clinical signs in a pleasure animal may result in drastic performance limitations in a racehorse. For example, atrial fibrillation (AF) may be unrecognized for an extended period of time in a pleasure horse, but results in immediate inadequate performance in a racehorse.

Performance data may be used to assess the impact of an abnormality. This is of benefit in determining whether suboptimal performance has been present and, if so, whether the animal has ever performed to expectations. Performance records can also be used to assess whether deterioration in performance has been sudden in onset or progressive. In racehorses they are used to assess what stage of the race was affected. Knowledge of the past use of a horse is an asset in assessing clinical findings. For example, large cardiac size on echocardiography would be considered as a normal finding in a horse that has undergone intensive training, but it may be suggestive of disease in an animal with no performance history. The proposed future use of the horse is essential in determining the potential impact of an abnormal finding.

It is important to determine the extent and nature of the clinical signs observed. An exact description of the owner's complaint is beneficial. The past medical history of the animal may help determine the role of current clinical findings. Documentation of a murmur over time and concurrent performance history may help elucidate the significance of the murmur. Respiratory and musculoskeletal diseases are other potential causes of suboptimal performance. While respiratory signs may indicate underlying heart failure, primary respiratory disease is considerably more common.

The age of the animal is of value in considering the relative importance and potential effect of an abnormal finding. Congenital heart disease is most frequently detected in the neonatal animal. Functional murmurs are common in fit, young performance animals. Valvular disease has an increased prevalence in older animals. The detection of a murmur consistent with aortic valvular regurgitation may be of greater significance in a young animal than it would be in an aged horse, where such murmurs are relatively common.

General examination

The general appearance of an animal may indicate the extent and duration of disease. Poor body condition may indicate advanced or chronic disease. Mucous membrane evaluation can be used to assess peripheral circulation and hydration status. Mucous membranes in the normal animal should be pale pink, with a CRT of less than 2 seconds. Alterations in mucous membrane color or CRT are not specific to cardiac disease.

The jugular veins in a horse can be used to assess cardiovascular status. First, the patency of the jugular veins should be assessed. Partial or complete obstruction from thrombosis secondary to repetitive or traumatic intravenous injection is common in the horse, and both jugular veins must be assessed. Symmetry between the jugular veins should be assessed. The jugular veins should also be assessed for extent of fill. A distended jugular vein indicates obstruction to venous return, either because of external compression of the jugular vein or because of right-sided heart failure. Slight pulsations at the thoracic inlet are normal findings. The extent of the pulsation should be assessed. In a standing horse with normal head positioning the pulsations generally extend less than one-third of the way up the jugular vein. The rate and rhythm of the jugular pulsations can be assessed and an arrhythmia can often be detected simply from such observations. A variable extent and rate of jugular fill are findings suggestive of arrhythmia. The jugular vein should be obstructed at the base of the neck and the rate of fill all the way to the jawline assessed. Slow jugular fill may indicate poor venous return because of either poor hydration or cardiac failure. The vein should be then obstructed at the top and allowed to empty. Emptying should occur within a single cardiac cycle. Poor emptying or persistence of pulsations within the jugular vein, once emptied, is abnormal. A true jugular pulse, where reflux of blood into the jugular vein from the right heart occurs, is uncommon except in advanced right-sided heart disease/failure.

Peripheral pulses should be assessed. The most common sites are at the facial or transverse facial arteries (924). The rate and the rhythm of pulsation should be assessed as well as the pulse strength. The pulse rate should be compared with the auscultated heart rate to evaluate for pulse deficits. Saphenous arterial pulses should be compared when aortoiliac thrombosis is a concern. Palpation per rectum is also indicated to assess the aortic quadrification in these cases.

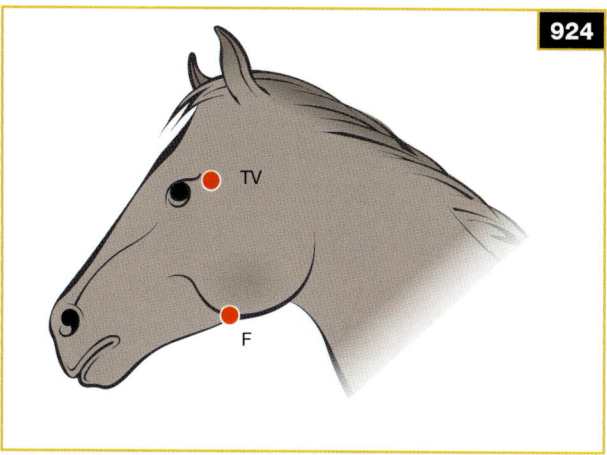

924 Areas on the head for palpation of the peripheral pulse. The transverse facial artery (TV) is palpable caudoventral to the eye (this vessel is also useful for arterial blood sampling in adults). The facial artery (F) is palpable over the mandible rostral to the masseter muscle.

The presence and extent of edema should be assessed. Limb edema is relatively common in the horse and is not usually associated with cardiac disease. While ventral edema occurs in heart failure, differential diagnoses such as hypoproteinemia and pleural effusion should be considered.

Careful auscultation of the lung fields should be performed as part of the cardiovascular examination because respiratory signs occur in left-sided heart failure and respiratory disease is a differential diagnosis for sub-optimal performance.

Thoracic percussion should be performed both to assess the location and distribution of the apex beat and to detect the presence of a cardiac thrill. The cardiac impulse is normally palpable on the left side of the thorax at the 5th or 6th ICS, above the elbow. On the right side the cardiac impulse is slightly further forward and lower, and is normally weaker than on the left. An intrathoracic mass or cardiac enlargement should be suspected if the apex beat is abnormally located. A cardiac thrill is a palpable vibration through the thoracic wall as a result of an intense murmur.

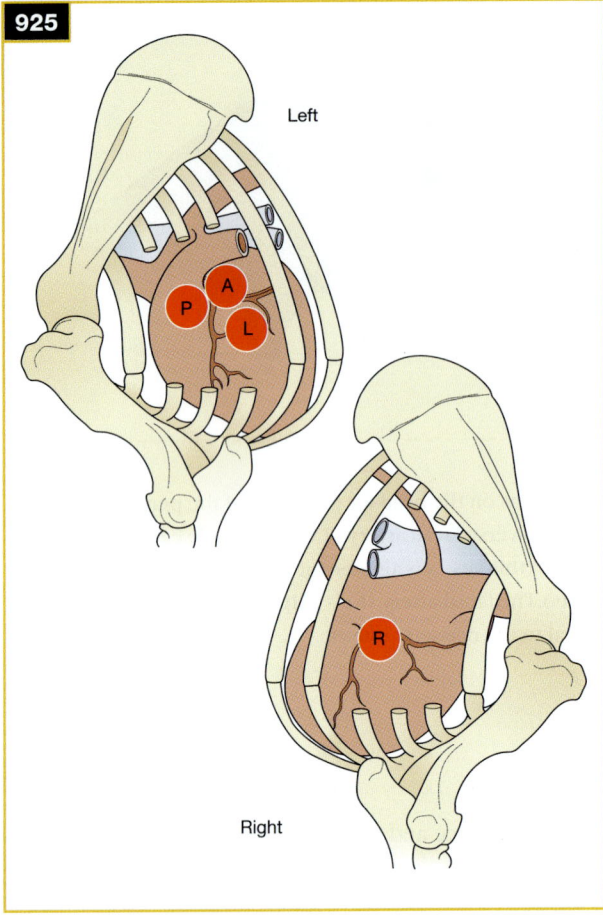

925

Left

Right

925 Location of heart valves and area of auscultation for each valve. The pulmonic valve (P) is auscultated well forward under the triceps muscle on the left side of the thorax in the area of the 3rd ICS. The aortic valve (A) is auscultated well under the triceps muscle on the left side of the thorax in the area of the 4th ICS just dorsal and caudal to the pulmonic valve. The left AV valve (L) is auscultated slightly under and just caudal to the triceps muscle on the left side of the thorax. The right AV valve (R) is auscultated under the triceps muscle on the right side of the thorax.

Cardiac auscultation

Cardiac auscultation should be the last part of the cardiac examination. The heart rate and rhythm should be evaluated and compared with those determined during pulse palpation. Simultaneous palpation and auscultation aids in determining the presence of pulse deficits and in determining the stage of cycle for cardiac murmurs. The entire cardiac area should be auscultated on both sides of the thorax, with an emphasis on detecting the location of both transient cardiac sounds and the location and distribution of cardiac murmurs, should they be present. Heart rate and rhythm and the intensity of the transient heart sounds should be assessed. Heart sounds may be muffled in obese animals or in those with pleural effusion or diaphragmatic hernia. The heart sounds, while muffled, often radiate widely if pleural effusion is present. Heart sounds are often intensified in tachycardia, such as that associated with excitement and anemia, and also in thin animals.

Heart sounds

Two to four transient heart sounds are present in the normal horse. The first and second heart sounds (S1 and S2) are present in all animals. S1 is associated with the closure of the atrioventricular (AV) valves and the beginning of systole. S2 is associated with closure of the semilunar valve and the end of systole. While the presence of the other transients, S3 and S4, is generally considered pathologic in small animals, these sounds are commonly detected in the normal horse. In many horses the fourth heart sound, corresponding to atrial contraction, is detected just before the first heart sound. The third heart sound is also often present, corresponding to rapid ventricular filling, and follows S2. Valve locations and corresponding heart sounds are outlined in **925** and *Table 41*.

Heart murmurs

Heart murmurs are generated when flow disturbances in the heart or major blood vessels cause vibrations in surrounding tissues. Once detected, a murmur should be characterized in terms of timing within the cardiac cycle, intensity (grade), character, and point of maximal intensity. Terms used to describe heart murmurs are outlined in *Table 42*. Common murmurs and their characteristics are outlined in *Table 43*.

TABLE 41	**Location of heart valves**	
VALVE	**LOCATION**	**HEART SOUNDS**
Pulmonic	Left 3rd ICS	S2 loudest
Aortic	Left 4th ICS	S2 loudest
Left atrioventricular (mitral)	Left 5th ICS	S1 loudest
Right atrioventricular (tricuspid)	Right 3rd–4th ICS	S1 loudest

TABLE 42 Murmur characterization

TERM	DEFINITION	DESCRIPTIONS
Timing	When it occurs in the cardiac cycle	• Systolic: between S1 and S2 ° Holosystolic: throughout systole, S1 and S2 audible ° Pansystolic: throughout systole. S1 and S2 obscured ° Early systolic ° Mid systolic • Diastolic: occurs after S2 ° Holodiastolic ° Early diastolic • Continuous: present throughout all phases
Intensity	Ease of detection; graded from 1 to 6	• Grade 1: not easily detected • Grade 2: soft, but easily detected • Grade 3: easily detected • Grade 4: intense sound, louder than transients • Grade 5: loud murmur with palpable thrill • Grade 6: palpable thrill, murmur heard when stethoscope held away from body wall
Character	Shape of sound	• Crescendo–decrescendo: sound appears to intensify and then decrease in intensity • Band/plateau: smooth/uniform intensity • Decrescendo: sound appears to decrease in intensity • Musical: variable high-pitch components • Coarse: not smooth sounding, but intensity stable • Complex: sounds vary or multiple sounds present

Diagnostic tools

Once the physical examination and specific cardiac examination are complete, ancillary diagnostic tools may be required to further characterize and evaluate the significance of findings.

Radiography

Thoracic radiography is of limited value for cardiac evaluation in the adult horse. Firstly, the equipment necessary to generate sufficient-quality images of an equine thorax is typically limited to referral centers. Secondly, only lateral radiography is possible in adult animals. Thirdly, many performance-limiting cardiac diseases are not radiographically apparent. There are limited data providing normal ranges for cardiac size on equine thoracic radiographs. Usually, only the caudal border of the heart is readily visible. Radiography may be of benefit in evaluating pulmonary or pleural abnormalities that may accompany, confound, or be differential diagnoses for cardiac disease.

Electrocardiography

Multiple-lead systems have been developed for use in human and small-animal electrocardiography. This allows the evaluation of cardiac rhythm, cardiac dimensions, and the cardiac conduction system. In hoofed animals the elaborate branching of the Purkinje system allows the ventricles to depolarize almost instantaneously. Such anatomy precludes the use of electrocardiography in the horse as a measure of diagnosing cardiac enlargement or conduction abnormalities, such as bundle branch block. A single lead can therefore be used in the horse. The electrocardiogram (ECG) is used to assess cardiac rate and rhythm and to evaluate the generated complexes.

TABLE 43 Murmur types and causes

PHASE OF CYCLE	TIMING	CHARACTER	INTENSITY (GRADE)	POINT OF MAXIMAL INTENSITY	RADIATION	LESION
Systolic	Early to midsystolic	Crescendo–decrescendo or band/plateau	1–3	Heart base	No	Functional
	Holo-pansystolic	Band/plateau; complex if valve prolapse	2–6	LAVV	Yes; dorsally valve variable extent	LAVVR
	Holosystolic	Band/plateau; complex if valve prolapse	2–6	RAVV	Yes; dorsally valve variable extent	RAVVR
	Pansystolic	Band/plateau; may be coarse	3–6	Variable; right sternal border; left sternal border; less common	Yes; often widely and may radiate to the left	VSD
Diastolic	Early to midsystolic	Whoop or decrescendo	1–3	Heart base	No	Functional
	Holodiastolic	Decrescendo or musical	1–6	Left heart base	Yes	AR
	Holodiastolic	Variable	1–4	Right heart base	Variable	Aortic root rupture
Continuous	Throughout; diastolic quieter	Variable	1–4	Left heart base	Variable	PDA
	Throughout	Variable, often complex	1–4	Heart base Often on right	Variable	Aortic root rupture
	Throughout	Variable	1–6	Right heart base	Variable	Arteriovenous fistula

LAVV = left atrioventricular valve; RAVV = right atrioventricular valve; LAVVR = left atrioventricular valve regurgitation; RAVVR = right atrioventricular valve regurgitation; VSD = ventricular septal defect; AR = aortic regurgitation; PDA = patent ductus arteriosus.

A standardized system should be used for electrocardiography in order to allow comparison. In general, a base–apex electrocardiogram is used, with some variation in the exact electrode positioning. Large complexes are usually generated and are therefore easily evaluated. With the Y-lead (base–apex) lead system the negative electrode (right arm) is placed at the manubrium and the positive electrode (left arm) is placed at the xyphoid. The ground electrode (right limb) is placed on either side at the shoulder (926). Alternatively, the positive electrode can be positioned at the right side of the withers and the negative electrode at the ventral midline.

Electrocardiography should be performed in the resting animal to demonstrate resting rhythm. Electrocardiography is indicated in any animal in which an arrhythmia is detected during physical examination. In the horse the ECG should be recorded at 25 mm/s and at a sensitivity of 1 mV/cm for several minutes to allow for evaluation of baseline cardiac rhythm. The short duration of ECG recording means that only those arrhythmias that are present either continuously or at the time the recording is generated can be evaluated. If cardiac arrhythmia or sporadic abnormal complexes are considered as potential causes of poor performance, weakness, or collapse, either 24-hour ambulatory recording (Holter monitor) or exercise ECG (telemetry) may be indicated. This is of particular importance when considering the possible effect on future performance and when assessing the safety of rider or driver.

Cardiovascular system

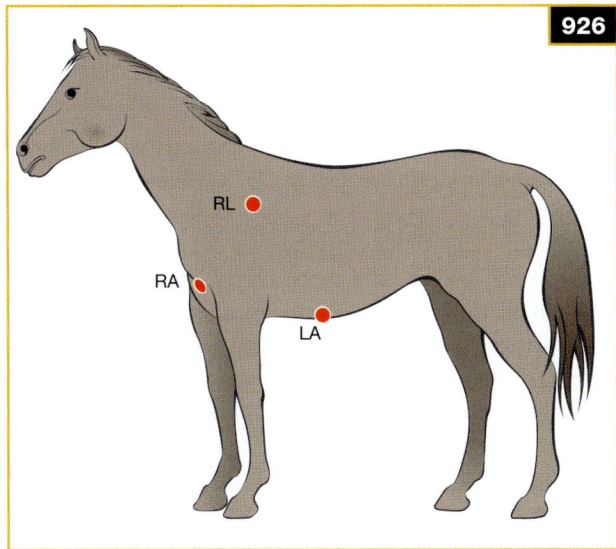

926 Locations for electrode placement for Y-lead ECG recording in the horse. The right limb (RL) is used as the ground lead and is here placed over the left shoulder. The right arm (RA) is attached over the manubrium and the left arm (LA) is attached over the xyphoid.

The waveforms generated on an ECG represent different phases of the cardiac cycle (927). The P wave represents atrial depolarization. In the horse the P wave is often bifid (having two peaks). These two positive peaks are often considered to represent the two atria, although the correspondence is not as well correlated as it is in small animals. The P wave may, alternatively, have a positive and a negative peak, or may spontaneously change in character during the ECG recording. Change in appearance of the P wave in the horse is a variation of normal. This is termed a wandering atrial pacemaker and is thought to represent variation in the pattern of depolarization within the atria.

Changes in QRS morphology are used to evaluate the ventricular conduction system and ventricular dimensions in humans and small animals, but not in horses. The QRS complex is variable in appearance between horses and is generally negative. The QRS morphology should be consistent in the same animal on successive recordings.

T wave morphology is labile. It may be positive, negative, or biphasic in nature and may vary within the same recording.

ECG interpretation

The heart rate is readily evaluated by assessing the number of complexes within a given time. The heart rhythm should then be assessed. The cardiac rhythm can be evaluated by assessing intervals between successive complexes (e.g. P to P and R to R intervals). The cardiac rhythm should essentially be regular; however, perfect regularity is as abnormal as an arrhythmia and indicates loss of autonomic control of the heart. The complexes should then be evaluated. The presence of P waves and their association with QRS complexes should be evaluated, as should the conformation of recorded complexes.

A wide range of arrhythmias has been documented in the horse. These arrhythmias are for the most part benign in nature, with some notable exceptions. Differentiation of arrhythmias based on auscultation alone can lead to confusion. In particular, second-degree heart block and AF may be similar upon auscultation in the resting horse. The clinical consequences are, however, drastically different. Electrocardiography is indicated to determine the clinical significance of any arrhythmia detected.

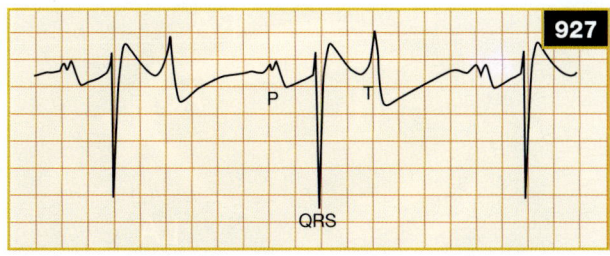

927 Base-apex (Y-lead) ECG recording from a horse in normal sinus rhythm. Bifid P wave is normal in the horse. A typical QRS complex with only an R (positive deflection) and an S (negative deflection) is present. The T wave is highly volatile in the horse and can be a positive or negative (or both) wave form. The slight negative deflection following the P wave is due to atrial repolarization (atrial T wave).

Echocardiography

Ultrasonography has provided a noninvasive procedure for the evaluation of cardiac structure, dimensions, and function. In horses, echocardiography provides the only means of assessing chamber enlargement. Echocardiography allows the clinician to identify structural anomalies and to assess the cardiovascular effects of these findings. Low-frequency probes (2–4 MHz) are required. While a decrease in image resolution is associated with such low-frequency probes, these frequencies are necessary to attain sufficient depth of penetration (24–30 cm). In all instances, simultaneous ECG recording (displayed on the ultrasound screen) during echocardiography is indicated to allow assessment of the timing of cardiac events.

Echocardiographic examination is indicated in any situation where cardiac disease is suspected. Echocardiography provides additional information whenever a cardiac murmur not considered to be a functional murmur is detected. It is also indicated to assess underlying cardiac function when a potentially pathologic arrhythmia is detected and when myocardial disease or pericardial disease is suspected. Echocardiography is of value when congenital heart disease is suspected, because of either a cardiac murmur or cyanosis.

Echocardiography may also be indicated when pyrexia of unknown origin is present (e.g. endocarditis), when exposure to a known cardiotoxin such as monensin has been detected (in the assessment of ventricular function),

and in any case of unexplained poor performance. Once an abnormality has been demonstrated, repeated echocardiography can be used to assess the progression of the lesion and its cardiovascular effects over time.

Echocardiography should be performed in a systematic way using routine images (928–931). Most evaluation is performed on the right side, provided the machine used has sufficient capabilities to achieve a depth of penetration of 27–30 cm. Additional imaging on the left side is indicated when the depth of penetration is not sufficient to image the left heart from the right side and when any murmurs attributable to left-heart disease are detected.

With M-mode imaging (932), chamber size and functional indices can be assessed. The timing of valve or wall motion relative to the ECG recording can be assessed. M-mode is most frequently used to assess left ventricular functional indices. Reference ranges have been published for Standardbred and Thoroughbred racehorses. Heart size is poorly correlated with body weight in the horse and a comparison with reference ranges should be done with due consideration to the breed of the horse and to the individual animal's performance history. Larger cardiac dimensions would be likely in an animal with a prolonged history of a high level of exercise.

Doppler imaging can be used to assess blood flow. Accurate assessment of flow velocities with pulsed-wave or continuous-wave (933) Doppler echocardiography necessitates that the ultrasound beam be as close to

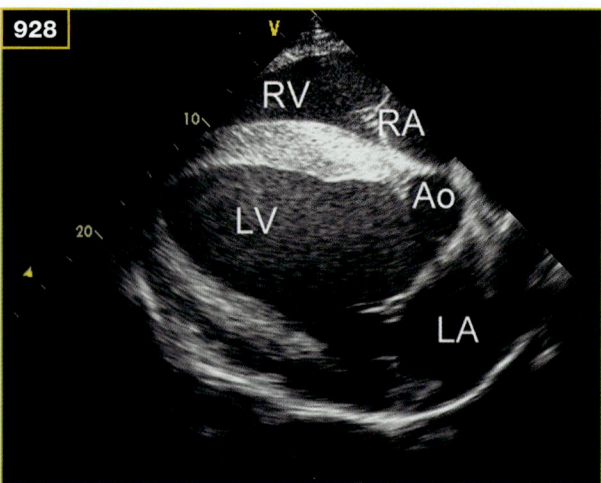

928 Right-sided, long-axis, four-chamber view. Image taken from the right 4th ICS. The probe is angled slightly caudally until all four cardiac chambers are visible. RV = right ventricle; RA = right atrium; LV = left ventricle; LA = left atrium; Ao = aorta.

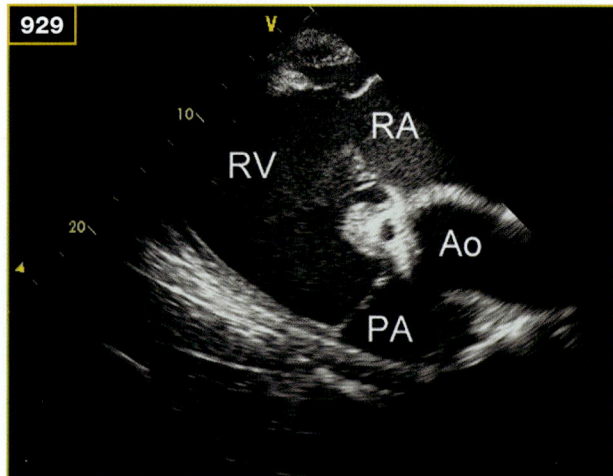

929 Right-sided, long-axis, outflow tract view highlighting the pulmonic valve. Image taken from the right 4th ICS. The probe is angled cranially until the pulmonary artery is visualized. RV = right ventricle; RA = right atrium; Ao = aorta; PA = pulmonary artery.

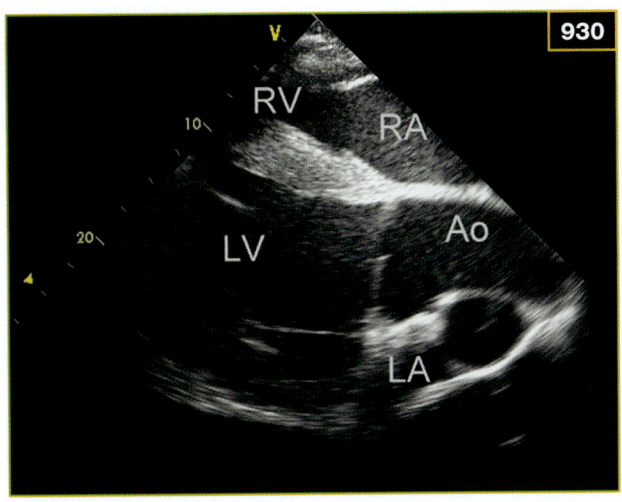

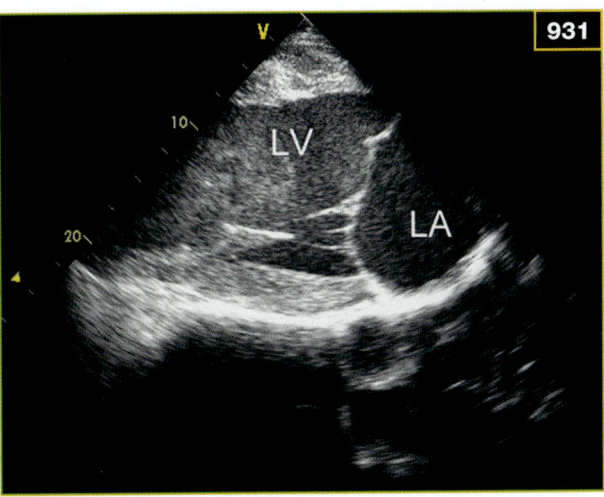

930 Right-sided, long-axis view, highlighting the aorta. Image taken from the right 4th ICS aiming across the thorax. Slight rotation of the probe is necessary to have a true long-axis view of the aorta. RV = right ventricle; RA = right atrium; LV = left ventricle; Ao = aorta; LA = left atrium.

931 Left-sided, long-axis view. Image taken from the left 5th ICS aiming across the thorax. LV = left ventricle; LA = left atrium.

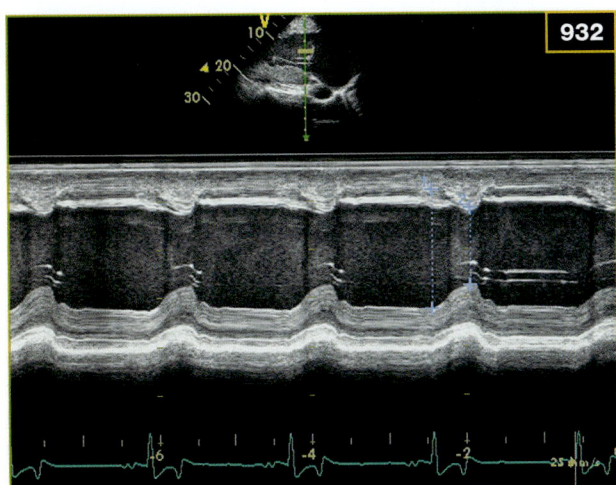

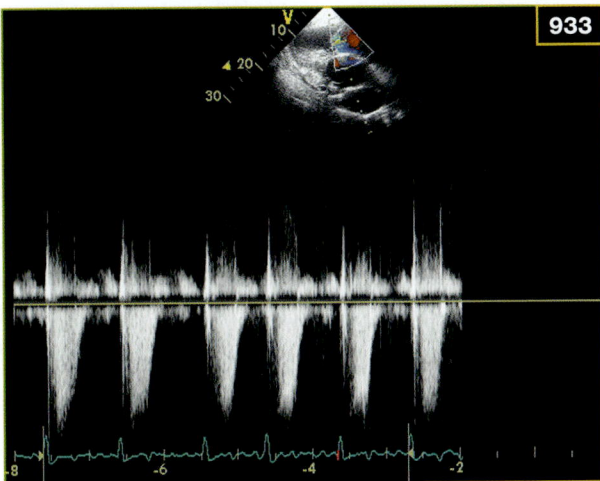

932 M-mode image of a left ventricle. Image taken from the left 5th ICS in a normal horse. The small image shows the long-axis view from which the M-mode image was collected. In this case, M-mode of the left ventricle was collected for the evaluation of left ventricular function. Left ventricular internal dimensions in diastole (LVIDd) and systole (LVIDs) were collected and then ejection fraction (EF) and fractional shortening (FS) were calculated.

933 Continuous-wave Doppler image of right AV valvular regurgitation (RAVVR). Image taken from the right 4th ICS of a 4-year-old Standardbred gelding with moderate RAVVR. Color-flow Doppler is used to locate the most intense regurgitant jet and then continuous-wave Doppler to assess the flow velocity. This can then be used to calculate pressure differential across the valve.

parallel to the measured flow as possible. This is difficult or impossible to obtain in most instances where valvular regurgitation has been detected. A fairly accurate assessment of flow velocity is possible with ventricular septal defects (VSDs) because parallel positioning of the ultrasound beam is possible. Without accurate assessment of flow velocity, pressure gradients cannot be determined. Pulsed-wave or color-flow Doppler echocardiography is used to assess the extent and direction of intracardiac and extracardiac shunts as well as valvular regurgitation. Valvular stenosis is extremely uncommon in the horse.

Contrast echocardiography, injecting a dye or agitated saline solution, allows for the evaluation of the direction of flow across shunts and across valves. This is less commonly performed now, as color-flow imaging is available on many ultrasound machines.

In a fractious animal, sedation may be required to allow for safe examination. It is important to recognize, however, that functional assessment will not be possible. Alpha-2 agonists have been shown to dramatically reduce systolic function.

Laboratory evaluation of cardiac disease

Routine serum biochemistry and hematology may be beneficial. A murmur detected in a dehydrated or anemic animal may relate to the underlying cause of the hematologic abnormality rather than to cardiac disease. Electrolyte disturbances may be the cause of arrhythmias. Hematologic and biochemical evidence of inflammation, such as increased WBC count, fibrinogen, or globulins, may raise suspicion of bacterial endocarditis as a cause for a sudden-onset cardiac murmur. Laboratory assays may be of value for assessing the systemic effects of heart failure (e.g. azotemia due to poor renal perfusion). Arterial blood gas analysis may aid reaching a diagnosis (e.g. low values [<40 mmHg] in congenital shunting).

Most antiarrhythmic medications have narrow therapeutic ranges, therefore serial analysis of serum levels of these medications is needed to optimize therapy. For example, blood levels of quinidine should be assessed repeatedly during administration; this is to minimize the risks associated with quinidine toxicity in addition to determining whether therapeutic levels have been attained.

Elevations in serum CK and LDH levels are often associated with muscular damage. In humans, CK and LDH isoenzymes specific to myocardial tissue have been used to assess myocardial injury. In horses, myocardial disease is significantly less common than in humans, and skeletal muscular damage is common. The myocardial isoenzymes are also present in skeletal muscle; therefore, any skeletal muscle damage may confound detection of myocardial injury because of the skeletal origin of isoenzyme elevations. In the absence of skeletal muscle injury, CK and LDH isoenzyme elevation may be suggestive of myocardial injury.

More recently, troponin protein assays have been developed to assess myocardial disease in humans. Cardiac troponin T (cTnT) and I (cTnI) subunits are distinct from those of skeletal origin. Specific assays have been developed and have been evaluated in the horse. Cardiac troponin I has been considered more sensitive and specific to myocardial tissue than earlier assays for troponin T because of the relatively higher concentration in cardiac muscle when compared with skeletal muscle. New (3rd-generation) cTnT are considered to be of similar diagnostic sensitivity as cTnI assays. Troponin assays should be performed when myocardial disease or myocardial damage is suspected. High conservation across species means that tests designed for human use should be capable of detecting troponin proteins in equine samples. There are many different cTnI tests, each targeting a separate portion of the cTnI protein. As much as a 100-fold variation in the reported value is possible. It is essential, therefore, that the tests are compared only with themselves and normal values established for each test.

Cardiac catheterization

Cardiac catheterization may provide additional information regarding the direction of flow across a shunt and the cardiovascular effects of an abnormal finding. This technique has declined in popularity with the increased availability of ultrasonography and is limited to referral centers, where personnel familiar with the procedure and specialized equipment are available. Interventional procedures (such as coil placement in persistent ductus arteriosus or transvenous pacemaker placement) involving cardiac catheterization are uncommon in the horse. Angiography is infrequently used in horses. More often, it is used to evaluate limb perfusion, particularly distal limb perfusion, rather than as part of a cardiac examination. Echocardiography has replaced angiography in many cases.

Arrhythmias

A wide range of arrhythmias has been documented in the horse. These arrhythmias are for the most part benign in nature, although there are some notable exceptions. Differentiation of arrhythmias based on auscultation alone can lead to confusion. In particular, second-degree heart block and AF may be similar on auscultation in the resting horse, but the clinical consequences are drastically different. Electrocardiography is indicated to determine the clinical significance of any arrhythmia detected on clinical examination.

The clinical consequences of relevant arrhythmias are, for the most part, a result of their hemodynamic effects. Suboptimal ventricular performance and cardiac output are often encountered. Syncope is uncommon, but may occur during episodes of profound bradycardia or tachycardia. Syncope is of particular concern in horses, as opposed to other species, because of the potential for injury to riders or people handling affected horses.

A number of commonly encountered benign arrhythmias, as well as some clinically significant arrhythmias, are discussed in this section. AF, because of its clinical implications and common occurrence in horses, is described in greater detail.

Atrial fibrillation

Definition/overview
AF is the most common clinically relevant dysrhythmia in the horse, with an estimated incidence ranging from 0.3–2.5% of the equine population.

Etiology/pathophysiology
The initiating event is not known in the horse. Factors such as electrolyte abnormalities and premature atrial contractions may be contributory. Horses may be predisposed to AF because of high vagal tone and large atrial dimension. Vagal tone leads to variability in action potential duration in the atrial tissue. The large atrial dimension in horses allows conduction through multiple pathways within the atria. This may lead to an increased number of re-entrant wavelets (electrical signals conducting around a self-perpetuating circuit), increasing the propensity for AF maintenance.

AF occurs as a result of a loss of coordinated electrical and mechanical function within the atria. Multiple paths of depolarization occur simultaneously. It is considered to be a re-entrant arrhythmia if the arrhythmia is self-sustaining.

Clinical presentation
AF is not usually associated with any underlying cardiovascular or systemic disease in the horse (lone AF). However, it is also commonly encountered in horses with extensive heart disease and in association with heart failure. The heart rate at rest is usually normal, except in animals with advanced heart failure. The clinical consequences of AF are also not commonly encountered at rest. The heart rhythm, however, is absolutely irregular and the peripheral pulse is variable both in rhythm and in quality. Unlike second-degree heart block, there is no predictability to the cardiac rhythm and the rhythm remains irregular during excitement or exercise. AF has significant clinical consequences at elevated heart rates and it profoundly limits performance. The classical presentation for a horse in AF is one of poor performance. A tendency to tire during exercise is common. Sudden fading during a race is a common finding associated with the onset of AF in racehorses. Syncopal episodes are uncommon. Exercise-induced pulmonary hemorrhage has been associated with AF by some authors; however, the relationship has not been closely examined. Elevated heart rates at rest, peripheral edema, and venous distension are not encountered in lone AF. These findings in horses with AF are related to the underlying cardiac disease rather than to the AF, and the arrhythmia should be considered a consequence of the underlying heart failure.

In most instances, AF is persistent once initiated. However, in some horses, short episodes of AF may occur with spontaneous onset and resolution. This is known as paroxysmal AF, and episodes are often associated with exercise. In humans, paroxysms gradually increase in duration and persistent AF often develops. Such an association has not been documented in horses. The differences in mechanism and maintenance between paroxysmal and persistent AF have not been identified in horses.

Differential diagnosis
Second-degree AV block, atrial flutter, atrial tachycardia with variable AV response, sinus arrhythmia, third-degree AV block, and AV dissociation should be considered.

Diagnosis
Physical examination should identify an arrhythmia that has no pattern of irregularity. The arrhythmia is therefore described as being irregularly irregular. Increasing the heart rate through exercise or excitement does not result in a return to regularity. Signs of heart failure are not present unless AF is secondary.

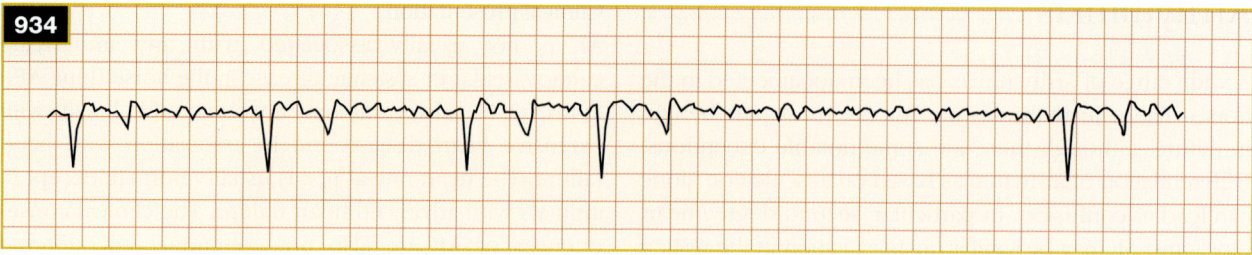

934 Atrial fibrillation. Base–apex lead recorded from an 8-year-old Standardbred gelding with sudden onset of poor performance during a race. Absence of P waves, presence of fibrillatory (f) waves, normal ventricular complexes, and irregular ventricular rhythm are seen. The ventricular rate of 40/minute is within normal limits.

AF is an electrocardiographic diagnosis (934). The criteria are absence of P waves, irregular ventricular rhythm, and irregular undulating baseline waveforms (f waves) (irregular atrial electrical activity). In contrast, in atrial flutter the baseline undulations have a repeatable appearance. Holter monitor testing or radiotelemetry are indicated if paroxysmal AF is suspected (due to resting sinus rhythm).

Except in cases with advance heart failure where increased cardiac dimensions or increased pulmonary patterns may be encountered, no radiographic abnormalities are present.

Echocardiography is indicated in all cases where AF has been diagnosed. While echocardiographic changes are uncommon, if present they have a significant impact on therapeutic management and prognosis. In particular, AV valve function, left atrial dimension, and left ventricular performance indices should be evaluated.

Management

In cases of lone AF, restoration of sinus rhythm should result in complete resolution of clinical signs. If underlying cardiac disease is present, the prognosis for restoration and maintenance of sinus rhythm is poor and treatment may be contraindicated.

Traditional management has involved the administration of quinidine salts, either orally or intravenously. Oral therapy involves the administration of multiple doses of quinidine sulfate via nasogastric tube. A common protocol is the administration of 10 g quinidine sulfate orally every 2 hours until restoration of sinus rhythm. Alternatively, a total dose of 60 g can be administered. If AF persists, the dosing interval may be increased to every 6 hours for an additional 24–48 hours. Close monitoring (i.e. hourly) of physical and ECG parameters is necessary. Administration should be under veterinary guidance and not left to the owner. Quinidine absorption rate and half-life are variable. Adverse effects are common and may range from tolerable (depression, mild tachycardia, mild hypotension) to severe and potentially life-threatening (tachyarrhythmias, neurologic abnormalities, severe hypotension, collapse). Therapy should be discontinued if the heart rate exceeds 80 bpm or if the QRS duration exceeds 1.25 times the duration of the resting QRS. Intravenous therapy with quinidine gluconate (0.5–2.2 mg/kg i/v q5–10 minutes to a maximum of 12 mg/kg) and other formulations has also been described. This is most effective in recent-onset AF. Intravenous administration may be followed by oral administration if AF persists, as long as toxicity is not observed.

Magnesium sulfate is the agent of choice for quinidine-associated Torsades de pointes (*Table 44*). In cases of quinidine toxicity, sodium bicarbonate administration is beneficial in decreasing free quinidine levels by increasing protein binding.

Quinidine is a negative inotrope (decreases force of contraction) and a positive chronotrope (increases heart rate), therefore it should be administered with caution in animals that are tachycardic at rest or have poor cardiac function. The administration of digoxin prior to and during therapy may counter some of these effects. Quinidine administration is contraindicated in congestive heart failure.

The prognosis for restoration and maintenance of sinus rhythm is considerably reduced in older horses, larger horses, when underlying cardiac disease is present, and when the duration of AF exceeds 4 months.

Recently, electrical cardioversion of AF has been described in the horse. External cardioversion with biphasic defibrillator waveform was successful in one horse with AF duration of 3 weeks and concurrent antiarrhythmic medication administration. A technique for transvenous electrical cardioversion, where catheter-mounted electrodes are placed within the right atrium and left pulmonary artery through a jugular-vein approach, has recently been developed and this technique appears to be more effective than drug therapy. Additionally, the technique has proven successful in horses with a duration of AF up to 7 years. The requirement for specialized equipment will limit this procedure to referral centers.

TABLE 44 Common drugs used in the management of cardiovascular disease

DIGOXIN

- **Main application.** Slow heart rate during heart failure. Increases cardiac output. Also used in the management of supraventricular tachyarrhythmia. Does not treat arrhythmia directly, but slows rate through decreased AV nodal conduction.

- **Toxic effects.** Depression, anorexia, and colic are common. Bradycardia, total AV block, ventricular tachyarrhythmias are all possible. Interaction with quinidine may increase potential for toxic effects. Predisposed by hypokalemia, hypoprotein-emia, dehydration, and renal disease.

- **Dose.** 0.011 mg/kg p/o or 0.0022 mg/kg i/v q12–24h. An initial i/v dose is often recommended. I/v administration is indicated if used to treat quinidine-associated tachycardia. Dose should be reduced by up to 50% if used concurrently with quinidine. Low therapeutic index, therefore monitoring of blood levels is indicated. Therapeutic range 1–2 ng/ml.

QUINIDINE

- **Main application.** Most commonly used in the management of AF. Also used in treatment of other supraventricular and ventricular arrhythmias. Quinidine sulfate (oral) is administered via nasogastric tube and is used mainly in the management of AF. Quinidine gluconate is administered intravenously and used in the management of acute AF (<4 weeks) or ventricular arrhythmias.

- **Toxic effects.** Variable. Mild signs such as depression, nasal edema, and increased frequency of defecation are common and are often tolerated. More severe signs such as marked hypotension, ataxia, colic, diarrhea, laminitis, sustained tachycardia, syncope, and sudden death have been reported. Idiosyncratic responses may occur with first dose. Torsades de pointes may be more likely in hypokalemic patients.

- **Dose.** Quinidine gluconate: 0.5–2.2 mg/kg i/v bolus q5–10 minutes to effect, maximum dose 12 mg/kg. Often conversion of ventricular tachycardia occurs with one dose at 0.5 mg/kg. Quinidine sulfate: 22 mg/kg via nasogastric tube q2h until conversion, toxic effects, therapeutic levels, or six doses. Continue administration every 6 hours until conversion or adverse effects. Monitor ECG closely during treatment. Heart rate >80 bpm, widening of QRS complexes to 125% of the pretreatment width, and abnormal complexes are all indicators to cease medication. Therapeutic range 3–5 μg/ml.

LIDOCAINE (WITHOUT EPINEPHRINE)

- **Main application.** Emergency treatment for ventricular arrhythmias. Does not have effects on supraventricular arrhythmias. Intravenous boluses are used in acute cases, while slow i/v administration is used in subacute cases. Short duration of action

- **Toxic effects.** Horses are very susceptible to lidocaine-induced CNS signs. Excitability, muscle fasciculations, and convulsions may occur after i/v bolus. Ventricular tachycardia and sudden death have been reported.

- **Dose.** 0.25 mg/kg bolus. 0.5–1.0 mg/kg slowly to effect. Can repeat in 5–10 minutes. 20–50 mg/kg/minute CRI. Therapeutic concentrations 1.5–5.0 μg/ml.

MAGNESIUM SULFATE

- **Main application.** Treatment of quinidine-induced Torsades de pointes. Has been used in the management of ventricular arrhythmias that were not responsive to other antiarrhythmic medications.

- **Toxic effects.** Colic and syncope have been reported.

- **Dose.** 1.0–2.5 g/450kg/minute over 20–30 minutes. Do not exceed 25 g total dose.

FUROSEMIDE

- **Main application.** Used in the management of heart failure to decrease volume overload and therefore decrease vascular volume and cardiac workload. Will only have effect if cardiac output is sufficient for adequate renal perfusion.

- **Toxic effects.** Prolonged or aggressive use will cause dehydration, azotemia, electrolyte abnormalities, and metabolic alkalosis.

- **Dose.** 0.5–1.0 mg/kg i/v, i/m, or p/o q12h.

PROCAINAMIDE

- **Main application.** Has been used in the management of AF, but is considerably less effective than quinidine. Also has been used in the management of ventricular tachycardia.

- **Toxic effects.** Similar to quinidine. Death due to ventricular arrhythmia has occurred during treatment for AF.

- **Dose.** 1 mg/kg/minute i/v, not exceeding a 20 mg/kg total dose; 25–35 mg/kg p/o q8h.

PROPRANOLOL

- **Main application.** Has been used in the management of ventricular tachycardia. Decreases ventricular rate.

- **Toxic effects.** Bradycardia, AV block, and arrhythmias may occur. It is a negative inotrope and may cause hypotension. Use with caution in animals with airway disease, as it may exacerbate bronchospasm.

- **Dose.** 0.03 mg/kg i/v; 0.38–0.78 mg/kg p/o q8h.

ATROPINE AND GLYCOPYRROLATE

- **Main application.** Used for the treatment of bradycardia, most commonly during anesthesia. Have been used as a diagnostic tool in heart block and sinus arrhythmia (removal of parasympathetic tone should remove these arrhythmias).

- **Toxic effects.** Mydriasis and decreased intestinal secretions and motility are possible even at therapeutic levels. Ileus and colic may develop. Tachycardia without increased contractility and arrhythmias may also occur.

- **Dose (therapeutic).** 0.005–0.01 mg/kg for bradycardia (both agents).

(Continues)

TABLE 44 Common drugs used in the management of cardiovascular disease *(continued)*

Enalapril

- **Main application.** Inhibits ACE, decreasing afterload. May be beneficial in management of horses with aortic regurgitation or aortic root rupture/aneurism. Considered potentially to slow progression of disease in aortic regurgitation. Must be withdrawn prior to competition.

- **Toxic effects.** Hypotension, diarrhea, and anorexia may develop.

- **Dose.** 0.25–0.5 mg/kg p/o q24h.

Other agents

A number of other medications have reportedly been used in the management of equine cardiac arrhythmias, but much of the information available on these is anecdotal.

Hydralazine (0.5 mg/kg i/v q12h) has been used as a vasodilator to reduce afterload.

The use of **flecainide** in the management of experimental equine AF has been reported. Anecdotal reports and one published report on the use of this medication in clinical cases have not been favorable.

Prognosis

The prognosis for horses with lone AF that respond to conversion therapy is excellent and these horses should return to their normal level of performance. Recurrence of AF is not uncommon, and horses previously diagnosed with AF that experience a sudden decline in performance should be evaluated for recurrence. The prognosis for horses with AF secondary to underlying heart disease is guarded.

First-degree heart block

Overview/etiology/pathophysiology
Normal finding in horses. The condition is associated with high vagal tone, and it may be more prevalent in fit horses.

Diagnosis/clinical presentation
Normal sinus rhythm. P waves and QRS complexes have normal conformation (935). Prolongation of PR interval beyond 0.425 to 0.47 ms.

Management
No treatment is required.

Second-degree heart block

Overview/etiology/pathophysiology
Most often a normal finding in horses. The condition is associated with high vagal tone. This results in decreased conduction through the AV node. It may be more prevalent in fit horses. Advanced block (multiple cycles at a time) may be due to myocardial inflammation.

Diagnosis/clinical presentation
Normal or slightly slow ventricular rate. P waves occur without associated QRS complexes. PP interval is consistent. QRS complexes are normal in appearance (935). Mobitz type I is more common and is characterized by gradual lengthening of PR intervals until a P wave is not followed by a QRS. Mobitz type II is characterized by a constant PR interval with intermittent block and is not as common in the horse. Advanced block may be associated with pronounced bradycardia and collapse.

On auscultation the heart rhythm is irregular. However, the blocked interval is a multiple (i.e. usually twice) of the basal interbeat interval. The predictable length of the blocked interval means that this arrhythmia is usually identified as being regularly irregular.

The arrhythmia should abate with increased heart rate or with decreased vagal tone, and it should therefore resolve with light exercise or excitation.

Management
No treatment is required. Mobitz type II may be associated with atrial myocardial disease. With advanced block, corticosteroids (dexamethasone) may be of benefit, but caution is indicated if ongoing viral infection is suspected.

Third-degree heart block

Etiology
The etiology is variable. This condition has been associated with myocarditis, pericarditis, and aortic aneurysms.

Diagnosis/clinical presentation
No relationship exists between P and QRS complexes. P waves may be lost in the QRS tracing. Bradycardia with ventricular rate of 10–20 bpm. QRS complex conformation may be normal or wide and bizarre.

Management
Treatment is not usually attempted. Pacemaker implantation is possible. Pharmacologic therapy is of limited value. Atropine administration is usually unsuccessful. The use of sympathomimetics (e.g. isoproterenol) has been reported; however, caution should be used due to the risk of ventricular tachyarrhythmias. Corticosteroids may be of benefit to treat inflammation, but caution is indicated if active viral infection is suspected.

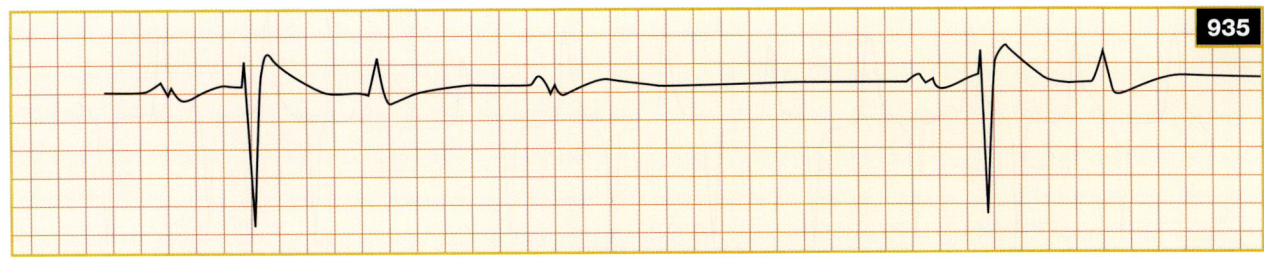

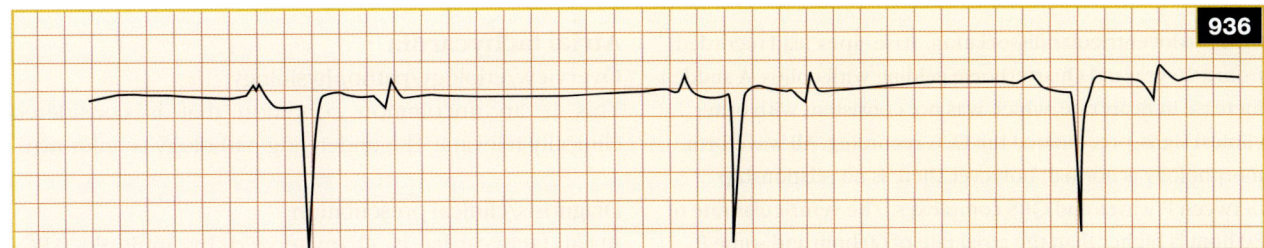

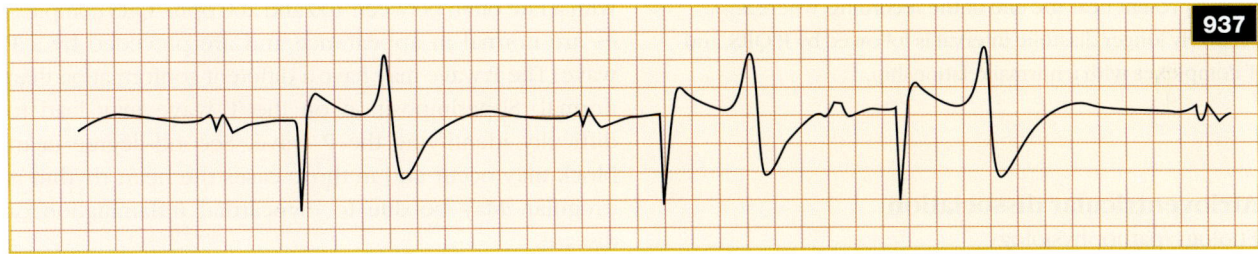

935 Base–apex lead recorded from a clinically normal Standardbred gelding at rest, with both first-degree and second-degree heart block. The PR interval is >0.42 seconds (1st-degree block). The next P wave is not followed by a QRS complex (second-degree block). All complexes are normal in conformation. P waves followed by QRS and T are present either side of a blocked beat, where only the P wave is present. PR interval is variable, therefore this is a Mobitz type I second-degree block.

936 Wandering atrial pacemaker. Base–apex lead recorded from a clinically normal Standardbred gelding at rest. Two different P wave morphologies are present. One P wave has a single peak and two are bifid P waves.

937 Atrial premature contraction. Base–apex lead recorded from a clinically normal 10-year-old Standardbred gelding at rest. Two normal cycles are followed by an APC. The APC is characterized by early occurrence of altered waveform P wave, followed by a normal ventricular complex.

Wandering atrial pacemaker

Overview
Normal finding in horses.

Diagnosis/clinical presentation
There is variable morphology to the P wave, normal QRS complexes, and a normal association between P wave and ventricular complexes (936).

Management
No treatment is required.

Atrial premature contraction

Overview/etiology/pathophysiology
Atrial premature contraction (APC) is usually a single event. Persistent or high frequency may be caused by atrial myocardial disease or inflammation.

Diagnosis/clinical presentation
There is a shortened PP interval and changes in conformation of the P wave. The QRS complex conformation is generally normal (937).

Management
Usually no treatment is required. Dexamethasone may be of benefit to control inflammation. Digoxin may be necessary to control rate if severe tachycardia is present.

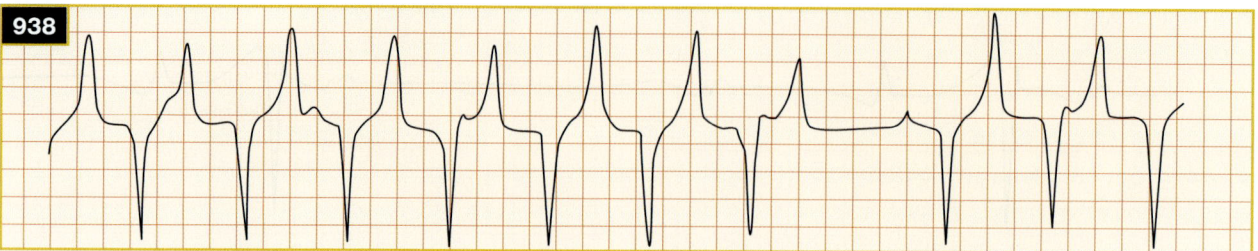

938

938 Atrioventricular dissociation. Base–apex lead recorded from a 16-year-old Quarterhorse gelding with colitis. A sudden increase in heart rate, which was not consistent with other clinical signs, precipitated the ECG recording. All waveform morphology is normal; however, there is no relationship between P waves and QRS complexes. The ventricular rate of 80 bpm is higher than the atrial rate of 60 bpm and some P waves are obscured by the ventricular waveforms. A capture beat is present near the end of the recording, where a relatively longer diastolic interval is followed by P, QRS, and T complexes with a normal relationship.

Atrioventricular dissociation

Etiology/pathophysiology
The etiology is variable. Myocardial irritation or inflammation is most common. This may be associated with systemic toxemia. An ectopic focus in ventricular tissue has a higher intrinsic rate than the SA node, consequently the atria and ventricles function as independent entities. Technically, this occurs in all cases of ventricular tachycardia, but AV dissociation is considered a separate entity when the ventricular rate is <100 bpm.

Diagnosis/clinical presentation
There is no relationship between P waves and ventricular complexes (938). The ventricular rate is higher than the atrial rate (in contrast to third-degree heart block). Ventricular and atrial complexes are often normal in conformation.

Management
The underlying disease or electrolyte imbalance should be treated.

Atrial tachycardia

Overview/etiology/pathophysiology
This is an uncommon condition that is considered clinically relevant. The underlying pathology is unknown.

Diagnosis/clinical presentation
Atrial tachycardia is characterized by multiple APCs (four or more in a row) and supraventricular tachycardia with a rate often between 100 and 200 bpm. QRS complexes are normal in appearance and are preceded by a P wave. The P wave may have a different conformation than normal. Superimposition on the T wave may lead to difficulty identifying the P wave. Second-degree heart block may occur and in those cases the heart rhythm is irregular. May be due to myocardial inflammation or disease.

Management
Identification and removal or treatment of the underlying cause, such as electrolyte imbalance or inflammation, are the most important aspects. Antiarrhythmic medication may be indicated. Quinidine has been used; however, it should be used cautiously, especially if second-degree block is present. Quinidine increases conduction through the AV node and conduction of previously blocked P waves will increase ventricular rate. Digoxin can be used to slow the ventricular rate and limit AV nodal conduction (*Table 44*).

Sinus arrhythmia

Overview/etiology/pathophysiology

Sinus arrhythmia is characterized by minor fluctuations in cardiac rhythm associated with respiration-induced changes in vagal tone (respiratory sinus arrhythmia). The term is also used to describe fluctuations in cardiac rhythm associated with exercise (exercise-associated arrhythmia). This arrhythmia is commonly found in fit horses during cardiac deceleration following submaximal exercise, and is likely to be associated with a variation in autonomic feedback. Respiratory sinus arrhythmia is not commonly found in the resting horse.

Diagnosis/clinical presentation

Respiratory sinus arrhythmia is characterized by variations in RR interval associated with respiration (939). With exercise-associated arrhythmia, the heart rate slows suddenly then rises gradually such that the cardiac deceleration has a step-like appearance.

Management

No treatment is required.

Sinus arrest/block

Overview/etiology/pathophysiology

Sinus block is considered a normal variation in resting horses. It is often associated with variations in vagal tone. Persistence at elevated heart rates may indicate a pathologic basis. Prolonged (4 seconds or greater) blocked intervals or those associated with syncope are also clinically relevant.

Diagnosis/clinical presentation

Sinus block is characterized by a normal cardiac rhythm, with periods when neither P waves nor QRS complexes occur. During these 'blocked beats' the RR interval is usually twice the normal RR interval (940). In contrast, with sinus arrest the periods of electrical silence are variable.

Management

No treatment is required for the benign form. Pacemaker implantation would be the only option for advanced block.

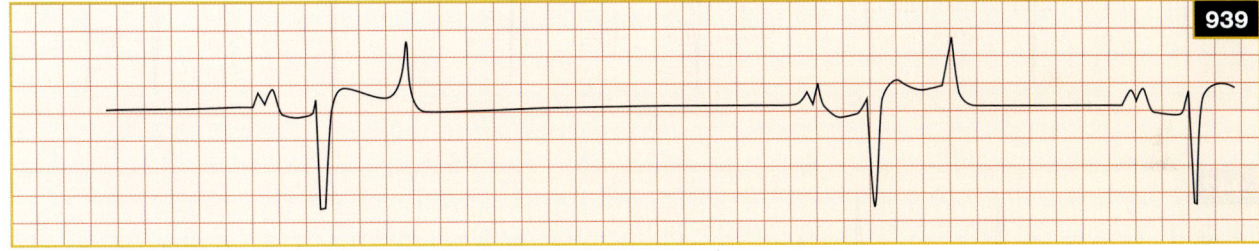

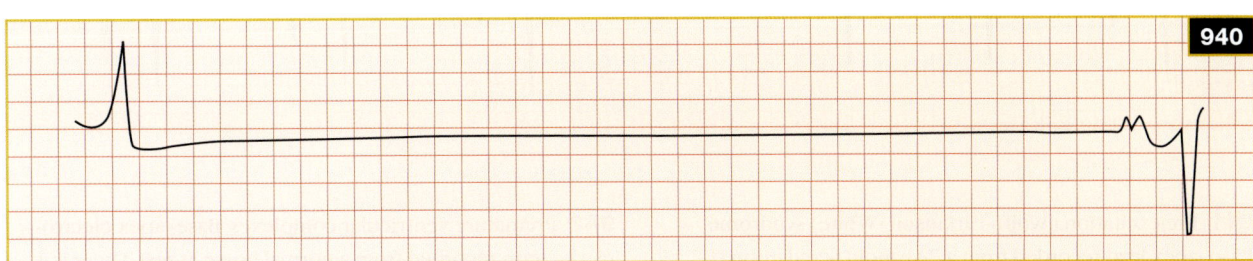

939 Sinus arrhythmia. Base–apex lead recorded from a clinically normal Standardbred gelding presented for evaluation of arrhythmia detected at routine physical examination. Normal P, QRS, and T complexes with normal temporal relationship (sinus rhythm) occurring at irregular intervals. An association with respiration was not detected and the arrhythmia abated with exercise.

940 Sinus arrest/block. Base–apex lead recorded from the same horse as in 937. A 6-second interval between complexes is present in this recording, and pauses of up to 8 seconds were detected. No clinical abnormalities were detected, the cardiac rhythm was normal at exercise, and the horse was performing to expectations. The cause of the arrhythmia in this horse was unknown.

Pre-excitation syndrome (Wolff–Parkinson–White syndrome)

Overview/etiology/pathophysiology

Pre-excitation syndrome is caused by an accessory conduction pathway between the atria and the ventricles or bundle of Hiss and surrounding tissue, and is rare in the horse. It is associated with poor performance and may result in periodic collapse. It may also predispose to paroxysmal atrial fibrillation.

Diagnosis/clinical presentation

An abnormally short PR interval combined with a prolonged QRS is present. It may appear for a couple of cycles and then disappear. QRS conformation may be variable. A delta wave (slurring of the R wave upstroke) is found at the beginning of QRS (941).

Management

There are no treatment options.

Premature ventricular complexes

Overview/etiology/pathophysiology

Premature ventricular complexes are common and are variable in their clinical significance. Single ectopic complexes are likely to be clinically insignificant. Long trains or frequent occurrence of complexes may be associated with myocardial inflammation or disease.

Diagnosis/clinical presentation

Ventricular contraction occurs prematurely in relation to the sinus complexes. QRS conformation is often bizarre (942). Heart rate is normal. Premature contractions may be single or in trains. The ectopic beat is often followed by a pause before the next sinus beat.

Management

No treatment is required for single beats or for short trains of 2–3 complexes. Some horses may respond to rest and corticosteroid administration.

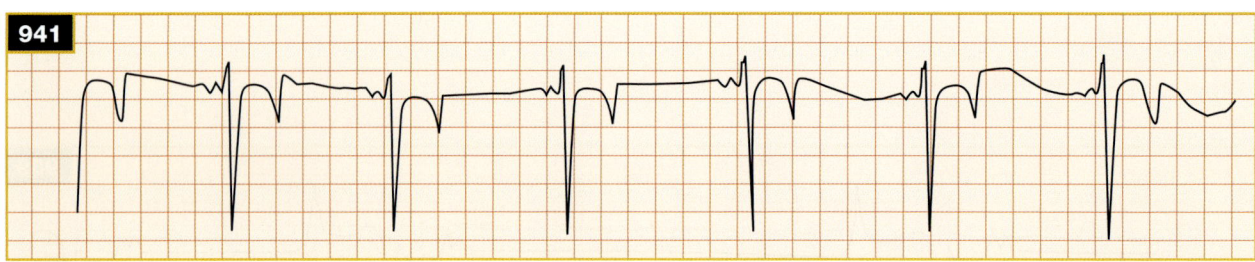

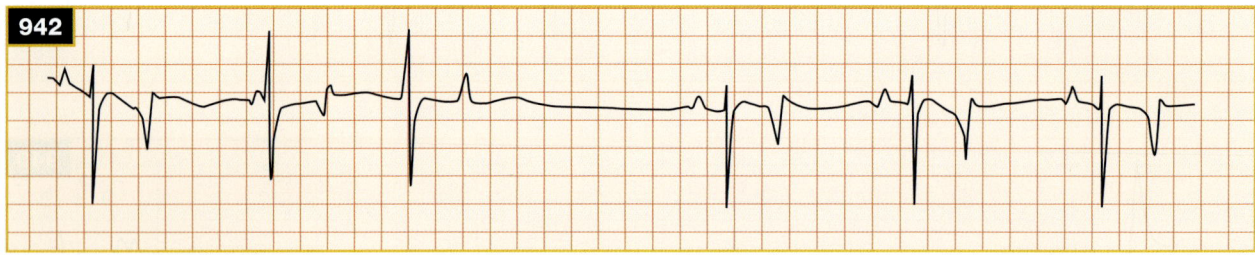

941 Pre-excitation (Wolff–Parkinson–White) syndrome. Base–apex lead recorded from a 7-year-old Standardbred gelding with a variable performance record. An extremely short PR interval and a positive delta wave are present at the beginning of the QRS complex, giving it a widened appearance. Variable conduction with some normal sinus complexes was present at elevated heart rates during treadmill exercise. The horse continued to race following this diagnosis, with variable results.

942 Premature ventricular complexes. Base–apex electrocardiogram recorded from a normal horse at rest. There is a normal PQRST (note negative deflection of QRS complex), followed by a P wave with an abnormal QRS almost obliterating the P wave. This premature ventricular complex is followed by another with the same conformation (note the absence of a P wave with this complex). A compensatory pause is then present, followed by normal complexes.

Ventricular tachycardia
Overview/etiology/pathophysiology
Ventricular tachycardia is a clinically significant condition that usually involves underlying myocardial or systemic disease.

Diagnosis/clinical presentation
Heart sounds are pounding. Pulsations in the jugular vein occur when the right atrium contracts during ventricular systole. Syncope may occur. Persistence may lead to heart failure due to myocardial fatigue. Trains of abnormal ventricular beats are present and the QRS conformation is bizarre. QRS complexes occur without a preceding P wave and the P wave may be obscured. The T wave is often long. Capture beats, when a P wave is followed by a QRS, may occur. Heart rate is high, often over 100 bpm (943). Ectopic complexes may be monoform or multiform. Multiform ventricular tachycardia is at increased risk of degenerating into ventricular fibrillation.

Management
Correction of any underlying conditions, such as electrolyte imbalances, is critical. If pulmonary edema is present, treatment should include the administration of nasal oxygen and furosemide. Administration of intravenous lidocaine may be corrective. Excitement and seizure activity have been associated with lidocaine administration. Other medications, such as quinidine, procainamide, magnesium sulfate, and propafenone have been used (*Table 44*).

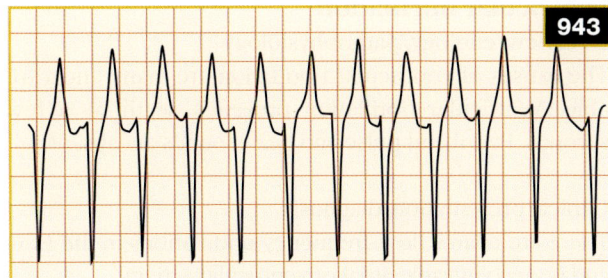

943 Ventricular tachycardia. Base–apex electrocardiogram recorded from a horse undergoing treatment for AF with the oral medication quinidine. Quinidine intoxication resulted in monomorphic ventricular tachycardia. The ventricular rate is 140 bpm. All the QRS complexes have a similar appearance.

Torsades de pointes ('twisting of the points')
Overview/etiology/pathophysiology
Torsades de pointes is uncommonly encountered during quinidine treatment for AF and is more likely in potassium-deficient animals. Sudden death during quinidine therapy may be due to development of torsades de pointes, with rapid deterioration into ventricular fibrillation.

Diagnosis/clinical presentation
Wide polymorphic ventricular tachycardia, with twisting of complexes around the baseline is present (944). This may progress to ventricular fibrillation.

Management
Quinidine administration should be ceased immediately. Lidocaine administration may be of benefit. Magnesium sulfate administration has also been used (*Table 44*). Intravenous sodium bicarbonate administration increases protein binding of quinidine and decreases the amount of the active form.

944 Torsades de pointes. Base–apex lead recorded from a 2-year-old Standardbred colt undergoing quinidine therapy for AF. Polymorphic ventricular tachycardia with twisting around the baseline is present in this recording. A ventricular rate of 240 bpm is present in the latter third of the recording.

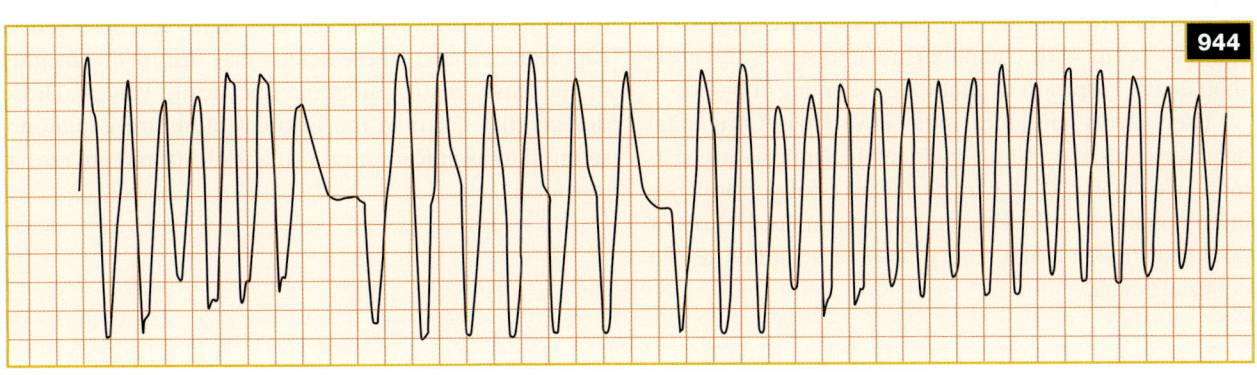

Ventricular fibrillation

Overview/etiology/pathophysiology

The causes of ventricular fibrillation are many and variable. Ventricular fibrillation precedes death by a few seconds. Peripheral pulse and heart sounds are absent.

Clinical presentation/diagnosis

There are coarse, low-frequency undulations in the ECG and no recognizable atrial or ventricular activity.

Management

Therapeutic options are limited. There is often inadequate time to respond unless the horse is under general anesthesia, when immediate recognition may occur. Electrical defibrillation may be attempted, but success is uncommon. Biphasic defibrillators are indicated if treatment is to be attempted.

Congenital cardiac disease ⸺

Congenital cardiac disease is uncommon in the horse. It may occur as single or complex anomalies. The most common congenital cardiac anomaly is VSD. Other defects, such as patent ductus arteriosus (PDA), persistent truncus arteriosus, and tetralogy of Fallot, have also been reported. Isolated anomalies involving the AV or pulmonic valves are infrequent in the horse. Complex congenital disease or severe single defects are more likely to present at an early age. In contrast, a small VSD may be an incidental finding in a mature horse.

The causes for congenital heart disease are not known in the horse and there is no proven heritability, although congenital heart disease has been more commonly reported in Arabians. Contributory factors may include maternal infection, hypoxia due to placental insufficiency, fetal infection, or toxin exposure.

Suspicion of congenital cardiac disease should be raised if a continuous holosystolic or holodiastolic murmur is detected in a foal. Innocent murmurs are common in the neonatal period, therefore detection of a quiet, soft murmur in a foal might not indicate congenital disease. Early investigation is indicated when a palpable thrill is detected or when the murmur radiates widely. Cyanosis at rest may occur with complex cardiac disease. Cyanosis should raise suspicion of right-to-left shunting of blood.

The severity of clinical signs is variable. Congenital heart disease may be an incidental diagnosis at postmortem examination. It may present as poor performance in an animal of sufficient age to perform, as ill-thrift or poor growth in a foal, or as cyanosis or heart failure in a neonatal animal.

A full physical examination should be performed, with particular attention paid to mucous membranes, jugular veins, arterial pulses, and cardiac and thoracic auscultation.

Electrocardiography does not often provide additional information aside from cardiac rate and rhythm and waveform morphology. It does not provide details of chamber dimensions or enlargement in the horse. Thoracic radiography may indicate evidence of pulmonary changes associated with cardiac disease or may provide evidence of cardiac enlargement.

2-D echocardiography, as well as Doppler and contrast echocardiography, are the most valuable tools for determining the site and extent of a lesion. Arterial blood-gas analysis may aid in determining if right-to-left shunting occurs.

Ventricular septal defect

Definition/overview

VSD is the most commonly reported congenital cardiac anomaly in the horse. It occurs both as a lone anomaly and as part of a complex of anomalies. The following discussion addresses VSD as it occurs alone. Complex congenital defects will be addressed separately. Breed predispositions for VSD have not been well documented in the horse, although the Arabian breed appears overrepresented, and in one study, an increased incidence was reported in Welsh mountain ponies when compared with Thoroughbreds. No gender predilection has been identified.

Etiology/pathophysiology

VSD is a result of failure of complete formation of the interventricular septum during embryogenesis. The interventricular septum forms by several processes, a failure of any of which results in a VSD. Several possible locations of a VSD are therefore possible (945). Membranous septal defects lie just below the septal cusp of the tricuspid valve at the top of the septum. Those defects occurring just below this area result from failure of formation of the smooth septum. Large defects involving both the smooth and membranous septa have been reported. Infundibular defects involve the ridge of muscle that divides the inflow from the outflow tracts of the right ventricle (crista supraventricularis). These defects may disrupt the integrity of the base of the pulmonic and aortic valves. Those defects that occur in the lower septum are commonly referred to as apical or trabecular defects and are rare in the horse.

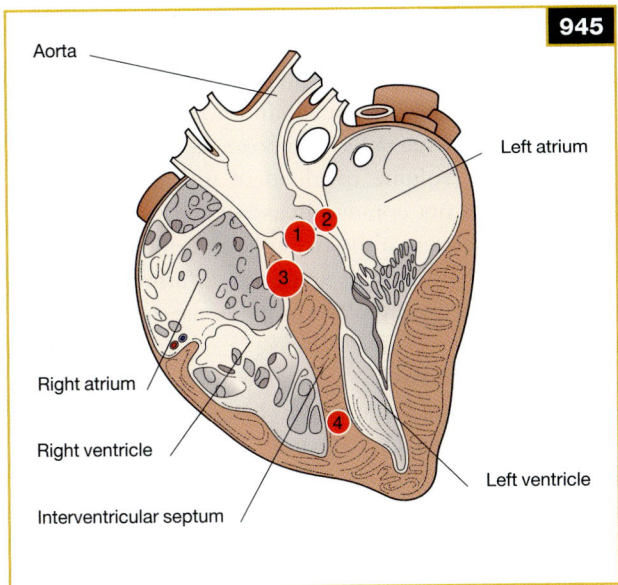

945

Aorta

Left atrium

1 2

3

Right atrium

Right ventricle

4

Left ventricle

Interventricular septum

945 Representation of the equine heart opened to visualize the interventricular septum. Membranous defects (1) lie just below the septal cusp of the right AV valve. Infundibular defects (2) occur just below the outflow tracts. Smooth septum defects (3) occur in the muscular portion of the septum just below the membranous septum. Apical defects (4) are rare in the horse.

Most VSDs are located in the membranous or smooth septum at the base of the ventricles. Because of the significantly higher pressure in the systemic circulation, the direction of blood flow across the VSD is usually from left to right during systole. In most cases, the exception being apical defects, the shunted blood flows directly from the left ventricle to the right heart outflow tract during systole, without increasing the right ventricular volume. This results in overcirculation of the pulmonary vasculature. Consequently, the left atrium and left ventricle become volume overloaded. Over time, progressive pulmonary vasculature hypertension results in pressure overload of the right ventricle and progressive hypertrophy occurs. Progressive instability of the aortic valve may be associated with infundibular defects, resulting in aortic regurgitation. Thickening of the septal cusp of the tricuspid valve has been associated with repetitive trauma by shunted flow across membranous defects.

Right-to-left shunting may occur following pulmonary overload and hypertension, resulting in increased right-sided pressure and a loss of the left-to-right pressure gradient. This is referred to as Eisenmenger's complex. Eisenmenger's complex has not been reported in horses with smaller defects (<4 cm) or in animals less than 2 years of age. Cyanosis is common with right-to-left shunting.

Clinical presentation

A coarse or harsh holosystolic to pansystolic plateau-shaped murmur, audible on both sides of the thorax, is typical of a VSD. A palpable thrill may also be present. The characteristic of the murmur aids in determining the position of the defect within the septum. With membranous defects, the point of maximal intensity (PMI) is far forward on the right side of the thorax. The murmur is often also audible well forward on the left side. With infundibular defects, the PMI is loudest on the left side at the area of the outflow tracts. The grade of the murmur does not necessarily correlate well with either the extent of the defect or its hemodynamic significance. Frequently, small defects generate louder murmurs. For example, a large defect with pressure equalization across the VSD would generate a very soft murmur, but would be hemodynamically significant.

The clinical signs associated with VSD may vary from cyanosis at birth and performance reduction, to no hemodynamic effect at all. The severity of clinical signs is associated with the location and size of the VSD. Large defects are more commonly associated with severe clinical signs, which result from volume overload and congestive heart failure. Pulmonary edema may result in dyspnea. Small defects may have no hemodynamic effects.

Cardiac arrhythmia, most commonly AF, may be present when atrial enlargement has occurred.

Diagnosis

Radiographic changes in cardiac silhouette are uncommon with VSDs in the horse. Radiographs are useful, however, in determining the hemodynamic effects (based on pulmonary edema). No characteristic ECG changes have been associated with VSDs in the horse.

Definitive diagnosis can be reached in many cases with echocardiography. Small defects may be difficult to see unless careful examination of the septum in both short- and long-axis views is performed. Infundibular defects are particularly difficult to evaluate. They may be slit-like, so are only present on one view. Color-flow Doppler can assist in identifying a defect and in demonstrating the direction of flow. Contrast echocardiography with agitated saline may be of benefit, especially when Doppler echocardiography is not available.

Management/prognosis

The prognosis with VSD is variable. With small defects the only abnormality detected may be the heart murmur and the animal may be able to lead a normal productive career. A poor prognosis is associated with large defects and those in which the aortic valve is disrupted. With time, volume overload may lead to congestive heart failure. No treatment exists for VSD in the horse. Supportive treatment is indicated if signs of congestive heart failure are present. Repeated echocardiographic examination allows assessment of progression.

Horses have been reported to be able to race with defects of <25 mm in diameter and peak shunt velocities of >4 m/s. Congestive heart failure often occurs before 5 years of age in those animals with peak shunt velocity of <3 m/s (lower velocity is suggestive of a lower pressure differential across the defect, and therefore indicates increased right heart pressures).

Horses with a VSD are considered to be at higher risk for bacterial endocarditis because of disturbed blood flow and increased probability of endocardial damage.

Atrial septal defect

Definition/overview

An atrial septal defect (ASD) is a communication between the left and right atria. This may be due to abnormal septation, true ASD, or due to failure of closure of the foramen ovale at birth (persistent foramen ovale). ASDs are rare.

Etiology/pathophysiology

No familial or breed predispositions have been identified. Most commonly, ASD occurs in combination with other defects in complex congenital anomalies. The cause is unknown.

In ASDs, blood flow shunts from left to right due to the pressure gradient between the atria. The pressure gradient is much smaller than that for the ventricles. Left-to-right flow results in increased volume in the right heart; however, unless the defect is large, the hemodynamic consequences are minimal. With large defects, volume overload of the right heart may occur. Over time, right-to-left shunting may develop, resulting in hypoxemia.

The foramen ovale is essential for fetal blood circulation. With the increased left-heart pressures present after birth, the foramen ovale normally closes. Functional closure occurs, followed by adhesion of the valve to the crista dividens, such that the structure cannot be re-opened. This anatomic closure takes several days to occur, and therefore persistent foramen ovale would be expected in any foal that dies soon after birth from any cause.

Clinical presentation

The severity of clinical signs varies with the size of the defect and the presence of additional congenital defects. In most cases the defect is small and no clinical signs are observed. With large defects, hypoxemia and heart failure may develop. Volume overload of the left heart then occurs. ASD is not commonly associated with a cardiac murmur; however, a holosystolic murmur has been described in the pulmonic valve area. Murmurs may also result from tricuspid dysplasia or pulmonic stenosis.

Differential diagnosis

With ASD as a sole abnormality, clinical signs are rare and no murmur is usually detected. Differential diagnoses include pulmonic stenosis and aortic stenosis (both rare). Differential diagnoses for complex congenital anomalies (tricuspid or pulmonic atresia) are variable and depend on the cardiac structures involved.

Diagnosis

There are no radiographic or electrocardiographic changes that are characteristic of ASD. AF has been associated with ASD when congestive heart failure has developed. Increased pulmonary vascularity and cardiac enlargement are not specific.

ASD is diagnosed echocardiographically. Careful examination of the interatrial septum is necessary. Contrast or color-flow Doppler echocardiography is of value in determining the presence of shunting. It is important to evaluate closely and to differentiate true ASD from echocardiographic drop-out. If an ASD is detected, careful examination for additional cardiac malformations is indicated. Pulmonary artery dilatation is evidence of right-heart overload.

While uncommonly performed, cardiac catheterization may demonstrate increased right heart/pulmonary pressure and increased oxygen saturation in pulmonary and right-heart blood.

Management

There is no treatment for ASD and in most cases no therapy is required. There are no therapeutic options for complex congenital deformities, and euthanasia is often indicated.

Prognosis

In cases of lone ASD of relatively small size, a reasonable level of performance may be expected. The degree of blood shunted across the defect decreases during exercise due to the increased right-heart pressure and resultant decrease in pressure gradient from left to right. The prognosis for complex congenital heart disease is grave and neonatal death is common.

Patent ductus arteriosus

Definition/overview

True PDA is a rare defect in the foal and is most often associated with complex congenital heart disease. It is important to know that the ductus arteriosus does not close immediately at birth, and a diagnosis of PDA should not be made in the early neonatal period (<4 days).

Etiology/pathophysiology

In the fetus the ductus arteriosus allows blood to pass from the pulmonary artery to the aorta, allowing oxygenated blood to access the systemic circulation. At birth the pressure gradient reverses and the ductus arteriosus normally closes. With complex congenital cardiac deformities, abnormal pressure gradients often result in PDA.

As part of the fetal circulation, the ductus arteriosus usually narrows near birth and then constricts rapidly as systemic vascular pressures increase and pulmonary vascular pressures decrease. If the ductus remains large, left-to-right flow may occur due to the development of a pressure differential. This results in volume overload that may progress to pulmonary hypertension, right ventricular hypertrophy, and heart failure. If the pulmonary pressure increases sufficiently, right-to-left shunting may occur.

Clinical presentation

Clinical signs are variable and range from none to severe. The size of the PDA, as well as the presence of other congenital deformities, contribute to the severity of clinical signs. Cyanosis may occur if the shunt reverses. Caudal cyanosis may be noted if the PDA enters the aorta distal to the brachiocephalic trunk.

Differential diagnosis

The typical 'machinery murmur' in the immediate postnatal period may be detected in the normal foal and it usually disappears over the first 96 hours. Continuous murmurs are otherwise rare in the foal. Complex cardiac abnormalities should be considered. Both systolic and diastolic murmurs may occur in animals with VSDs that disrupt the aorta. Systolic murmurs (usually physiologic flow murmurs) are common in the foal and may be normal during the first 2–3 months of life.

Diagnosis

A continuous machinery murmur loudest over the left side is usually present. The diastolic component may be quiet to inaudible. Enlargement of the cardiac silhouette may be evident radiographically. Pulmonary overcirculation and edema may also be present. There are no radiographic changes to aid in the differentiation of PDA from more complex congenital deformities. Similarly, no identifying changes are present on ECG.

Echocardiography is required for diagnosis. Direct visualization of the PDA may be possible far forward in the left cardiac window. Left atrial enlargement and left ventricular volume overload are common. Doppler echocardiography may show disturbed flow within the PDA and in the pulmonary artery.

Management/prognosis

The condition has not been thoroughly evaluated in the horse. The prognosis is grave if other defects are present. Surgical correction is possible. Pharmacologic closure with prostaglandin inhibitors (indomethacin, ibuprofen) has been described in other species.

Valvular deformities

Definition/overview

Congenital valvular deformities are uncommon in the horse. Rare cases of pulmonic-valve stenosis, tricuspid atresia, congenital mitral chordal rupture, papillary muscle deformity, and parachute valve have been described.

Etiology/pathophysiology

All valvular deformities are developmental. Tricuspid atresia and pulmonary valve stenosis are components of complex congenital deformities. Mitral-valve dysplasia and parachute valve have been described as sole anomalies. For foals to survive beyond the fetal stages with tricuspid atresia, concurrent VSDs and ASDs must also be present. Obstruction to blood flow occurs in the right heart and the ASD allows right-to-left blood flow. The blood flows from the right atrium into the left atrium, then into the left ventricle and into the right ventricle (across the VSD). This results in volume overload of the left heart.

Clinical presentation

With tricuspid atresia the foal may die suddenly in the neonatal period or may survive for only a few months. Cyanosis is common. Tachycardia and collapse are also common. A grade 4–6/6 pansystolic murmur is present with the PMI on the left side of the thorax. Heart failure may result from volume overload of the left heart. Foals with pulmonic valve stenosis or tricuspid atresia are often severely stunted. Foals with left AV valve deformities are variably stunted depending on the severity of the stenosis or regurgitation. With severe regurgitation, chamber failure may ensue. A loud systolic murmur is common.

Differential diagnosis

Acquired valvular disease, bacterial endocarditis, and complex congenital cardiac disease must also be considered.

Diagnosis

There are often no characteristic radiographic changes; however, chamber enlargement may be identified. Similarly, there are often no characteristic ECG changes. Echocardiography may demonstrate stenosis or atresia. A single papillary muscle is present with a parachute left AV valve. Doppler and color-flow Doppler are useful in order to demonstrate blood flow, direction, and the extent of the regurgitation.

Management/prognosis

There are no therapeutic options for these diseases and euthanasia is often indicated because of the severity of clinical signs.

Tetralogy of Fallot

Definition/overview

By definition, four congenital cardiac anomalies are present in tetralogy of Fallot: overriding aorta (aorta sitting over both ventricular outflow tracts), pulmonic stenosis, VSD, and right ventricular hypertrophy. If there is also an ASD, the term pentalogy is used.

Etiology/pathophysiology

The conal septum, involved in the development of the right heart outflow tract and in the septation of the ventricles, develops abnormally. This results in narrowing of the right ventricular outflow tract and an inability to complete the ventricular septum. The aorta overrides both outflow tracts as a result of the pulmonic stenosis. Pulmonic stenosis results in right ventricular pressure overload and therefore right ventricular hypertrophy.

Systemic hypoxia occurs because of mixing of oxygenated and unoxygenated blood in the aorta. Pulmonic stenosis results in decreased pulmonary perfusion. Equalization of pressure may occur across the VSD. Cyanosis is more profound if the obstruction to the right heart outflow tract is great.

Clinical presentation

Resting cyanosis is uncommon, but cyanosis following exercise is common. A loud pansystolic murmur, often with a thrill, is present over the left 3rd to 4th ICS. The murmur may be complex due to the presence of multiple anomalies. Severe exercise intolerance is common. Cyanosis is not responsive to oxygen therapy, in contrast to that associated with respiratory disease.

Differential diagnosis

Other causes of cyanosis include respiratory disease and heart failure with pulmonary edema. Other congenital cardiac anomalies, such as right ventricular hypoplasia or persistent truncus arteriosus, may be associated with similar clinical signs.

Diagnosis

Clinical pathology may be of some value. Polycythemia may occur with prolonged hypoxia. Cardiac catheterization could be used to demonstrate equalization of pressure across the VSD. Decreased pulmonary vascularity may be observed radiographically. There are no characteristic ECG findings. Echocardiography is required for a definitive diagnosis and all four components of the condition are often readily visualized. The VSD is often large, making it easy to identify, and the aorta is observed sitting above the VSD. The right ventricular wall is sufficiently thickened to be evident on echocardiography. Doppler or contrast echocardiography may be of benefit for characterizing blood flow and direction.

Management/prognosis

There are no treatment options. The prognosis for survival is poor and euthanasia is often indicated.

Acquired cardiac disease ————

Acquired cardiovascular disease is significantly more common in the horse than congenital heart disease. The majority of conditions involve the heart valves and degenerative valve disease is common. Myocardial disease, pericardial disease, and peripheral vascular disease are less common. Acquired arrhythmias are addressed in a separate section (see p. 681).

There is no particular breed predisposition. Certain conditions are more common in certain age groups. Knowledge of the age, breed, performance history, and desired future use are important in determining the significance of a finding and issuing a prognosis.

VALVULAR DISEASE

In the horse, most cases of valvular heart disease are acquired. Acquired valvular disease may be a result of degenerative changes, damage or rupture of chordae tendinae, or bacterial endocarditis. Degenerative valve disease is most common. Aortic and left AV valve changes have been reported commonly. Valvular insufficiency is a common cause of heart murmur in the horse and may or may not be associated with degenerative changes in the valve. The extent of regurgitation determines the hemodynamic significance. Valvular insufficiency of moderate to severe extent will influence performance and could be of concern if the horse has to undergo general anesthesia.

Left atrioventricular valve disease

Definition/overview

Murmurs associated with left AV valve disease are relatively common in the horse, occurring in an estimated 3.5% of the equine population, and are the most common cause for referral for cardiac evaluation. Insufficiency of this valve is more commonly associated with performance limitations than that of the right AV valve, and it is the most likely valvular insufficiency to lead to congestive heart failure.

Etiology/pathophysiology

There is no breed predilection for left AV valve disease. Structural changes in the left AV valve may contribute to regurgitation. Valvular thickening, fenestration, and cystic changes have been reported. Pathologic changes similar to those of endocardiosis in other species have also been reported.

With valvular insufficiency, blood leaks from the left ventricle to the left atrium during systole. This increases the volume load on the left atrium. With time, atrial dilatation may occur, which predisposes to the development of AF. Left-sided heart failure may occur. This progresses to pulmonary hypertension and right-sided pressure overload. Right-sided heart failure may then occur.

Clinical presentation

Typically, no clinical signs are apparent and the murmur is detected during routine examination. With severe regurgitation, respiratory signs such as labored breathing, increased respiratory effort and rate, prolonged recovery following exercise, and a tendency to cough may be detected. Overt pulmonary edema may develop in cases with chordae tendinae rupture. Frequently, the left-sided heart failure signs are overlooked as primary respiratory disease, and the horse is not presented to the veterinarian until signs of right-sided heart failure develop.

Differential diagnosis

Outflow tract murmurs (innocent flow murmurs), VSD, or endocarditis involving the left AV valve should be considered. Respiratory diseases such as heaves may also have similar clinical signs if left-sided heart failure is present.

Diagnosis

The most common clinical finding is a band-shaped, soft, blowing, holosystolic murmur over the left heart base just above the area of the left AV valve. A mid-systolic crescendo murmur may be detected in cases with valve prolapse. In those cases a beat-to-beat variability in the murmur characteristics may be present. The correlation between intensity of murmur and severity of regurgitation is poor. Usually, no other clinical signs are apparent.

There are no characteristic radiographic changes. Atrial enlargement is difficult to discern in equine thoracic radiographs. There are no characteristic ECG changes. AF in the face of moderate to severe left AV valve insufficiency should raise concern of atrial enlargement.

Echocardiography is required for diagnosis (946). Thickened AV valve margins may be detected on 2-D echocardiography. Prolapse of a valve leaflet may also be visible in some cases. Careful examination of the papillary muscles and chordal attachments is indicated, especially in those cases with sudden onset of left-heart signs. M-mode evaluation can be used to assess left ventricular dimensions and functional indices. Atrial dimensions should be assessed. Color-flow and pulsed-wave Doppler examinations are beneficial in determining the extent of regurgitation. If the jet is extensive or if there are signs of atrial enlargement, the diameter of the pulmonary artery should be compared with that of the aorta. Dilatation of the pulmonary artery such that it is larger than the aorta is an indication of pulmonary hypertension.

Management/prognosis

There is no treatment for correcting left AV valvular regurgitation. In horses with small focal jets of regurgitation, the prognosis for life and for performance is excellent without any treatment. In those horses with valve thickening or more extensive regurgitation, the prognosis is less favorable. The regurgitant fraction tends to increase with time. This may result in a gradual decrease in performance capacity. Chordal rupture is rare and usually results in sudden onset of heart failure, pulmonary edema, and respiratory distress. The case mortality rate with chordal rupture is high. Cardioversion of AF may be attempted; however, the prognosis for restoration and maintenance of sinus rhythm is guarded in cases with evidence of atrial dilatation. The onset of signs of congestive heart failure is a poor prognostic indicator. Clinical signs of heart failure should be treated as outlined on p. 706.

Right atrioventricular valve disease
Definition/overview

Murmurs associated with right AV valvular regurgitation are common in the horse; however, pathology of the right AV valve is seldom detected and right AV valvular regurgitation is not commonly associated with any clinical signs or performance effects. An incidence of 9% has been reported, with a higher incidence in Thoroughbred and Standardbred racehorses. This increased incidence is considered to be associated with hypertrophic changes following intensive training rather than with hereditary factors.

Etiology/pathophysiology

Deformities of the right AV valve are uncommon at postmortem examination, but regurgitation through the right AV valve is common. The three-valve leaflet conformation may predispose the valve to incomplete closure. Regurgitation of blood into the right atrium during systole may result in volume overload.

Right AV valvular regurgitation may be primary or may occur secondarily to left-sided heart failure. Signs of right-sided heart failure are most commonly associated with left-sided heart disease and left-sided heart failure. Pulmonary hypertension causes pressure overload of the right heart and results in right-sided failure. Chordal rupture is less common than in the left heart.

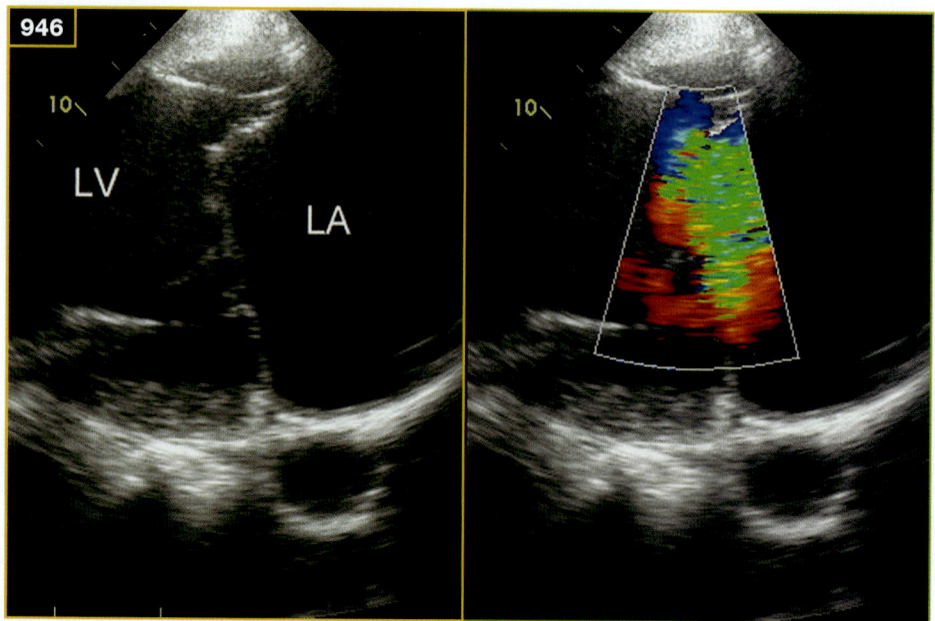

946 Left AV (mitral) valvular regurgitation (LAVVR). Left-heart long-axis view taken from the left 5th ICS. Two-year-old Standardbred colt with poor performance and a grade 5/6 left-sided holosystolic murmur. Color-flow Doppler echocardiography reveals high-velocity regurgitant flow at the left AV valve in green in the right-hand image. LV = left ventricle; LA = left atrium.

947 Right AV (tricuspid) valvular regurgitation (RAVVR). Right-heart long-axis view taken from the right 4th ICS, highlighting the AV valve. This horse had a history of poor performance, AF, and a grade 2/6 right-sided holosystolic murmur. Color-flow Doppler echo-cardiography reveals high-velocity regurgitant flow in green. RV = right ventricle; RA = right atrium; Ao = aorta; PA = pulmonary artery.

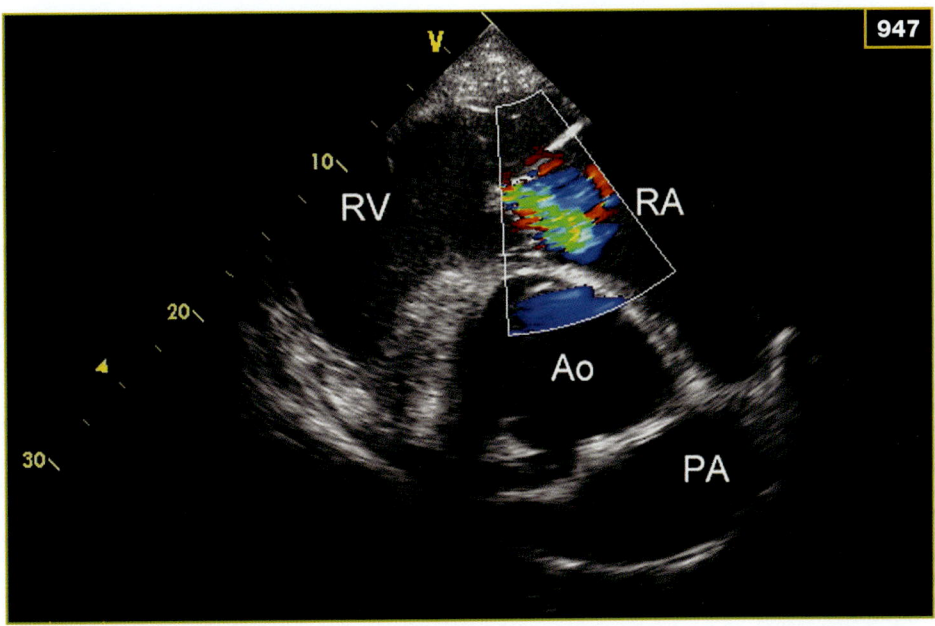

Clinical presentation

There are usually no clinical signs associated with right AV valvular regurgitation. The murmur is classically holosystolic to pansystolic, band-shaped, soft, and blowing. The PMI is on the right side of the chest, usually in the 4th ICS. Crescendo, mid-systolic murmurs associated with valve prolapse are uncommon. More intense murmurs are likely to be associated with larger defects. A murmur of intensity 3/6 or higher is generally clinically significant. AF is less commonly associated with right AV valve insufficiency than with left AV valve insufficiency, but it may develop in the face of atrial dilatation. Right-sided congestive heart failure may develop in severe cases.

Differential diagnosis

Endocarditis and functional murmurs may produce similar signs.

Diagnosis

The murmur is typically identified during routine auscultation. Location and characteristics of the murmur can be suggestive of right AV insufficiency, but echocardiography is required for confirmation (947). 2-D echocardiography is of value in determining the extent of the regurgitation, assessing any valvular changes, and assessing cardiac chamber dilatation. Color flow Doppler analysis is valuable for assessing the regurgitant jet. Right-sided chamber dimensions are difficult to evaluate. Evidence of right AV valvular regurgitation is more common than are associated murmurs.

There are no characteristic radiographic or ECG changes associated with right AV valve disease in the horse. AF in association with evidence of moderate to severe right AV valvular insufficiency may indicate right atrial dilatation.

Management

No treatment is indicated unless clinical signs of congestive heart failure develop.

Prognosis

The prognosis is excellent and clinical signs, including performance effects, are uncommon. Mild to moderate regurgitation has been documented in animals that were performing well.

Aortic valve disease
Definition/overview
Valvular pathology in the horse is most commonly found at the aortic valve. Degenerative changes consisting of nodules, fenestrations, and valve-cusp thickening are common. Fenestrations may be seen in normal animals. Aortic insufficiency is most commonly diagnosed in older animals.

Etiology/pathophysiology
With aortic insufficiency, the aortic valve fails to close completely and blood flows backwards into the left ventricle during diastole. If extensive, left ventricular volume overload may result.

Clinical presentation
Clinical signs associated with aortic valve insufficiency are commonly limited to the presence of a diastolic heart murmur.

Differential diagnosis
Diastolic flow murmur is the most common differential diagnosis. A similar murmur can occur with pulmonic valvular regurgitation, but is very rare.

Diagnosis
The presence of a holodiastolic murmur should be considered an indication of aortic regurgitation until proven otherwise. This murmur is usually crescendo–decrescendo in character, although musical or 'honking' murmurs have also been described. With severe regurgitation the peripheral pulse becomes bounding in character because of the rapid diastolic drop-off in pressure. The intensity of the murmur does not correlate well with the severity of regurgitation. AF may develop as a result of volume overload of the left heart and subsequent chamber enlargement.

There are no characteristic radiographic or ECG findings associated with aortic insufficiency in the horse. Echocardiography is used to confirm the diagnosis. Valvular regurgitation on echocardiography is more common than the associated murmur (948).

Management/prognosis
There is no treatment for aortic valvular insufficiency. In most cases the prognosis is good, both for performance and for survival. Aortic insufficiency does tend to progress, therefore repeated evaluations are indicated. The use of angiotensin converting enzyme (ACE) inhibitors, such as enalapril, has been proposed. This is an attempt to slow progression and allow the animal to continue performance (*Table 44*). The effects of this treatment are not well documented. Signs of heart failure indicate a poor prognosis and treatment only temporarily alleviates clinical signs.

Bacterial endocarditis
Definition/overview
Bacterial endocarditis is an uncommon acute or chronic disease associated with bacterial colonization and development of vegetative lesions either on the valves or on the nonvalvular endocardium. In the horse the aortic valve is most commonly affected, followed by the left AV valve and then the right AV valve. Involvement of the pulmonic valve is uncommon.

Etiology/pathophysiology
It is speculated that bacterial infection follows trauma to the valve, such as in cases of valvular insufficiency or VSD, where turbulent blood flow develops. Injury to the endocardium has been documented in stressed pigs, and may also occur in other animal species when stressed. Endocarditis has been initiated experimentally by the

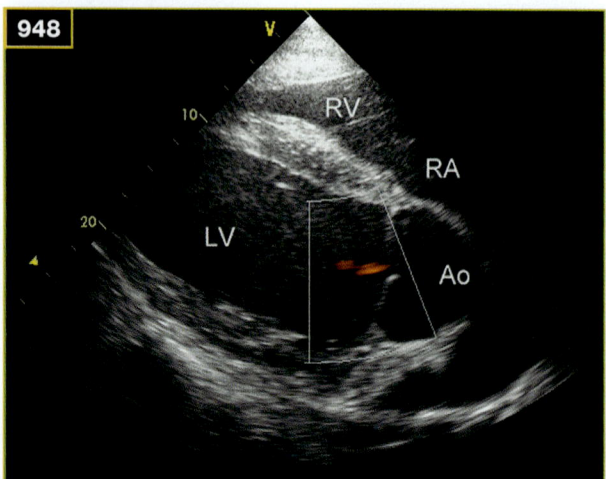

948 Aortic regurgitation. Right-heart long-axis view highlighting the aortic valve taken from the right 4th ICS. Color-flow Doppler echocardiography reveals aortic regurgitation as a red flame-like flow present during diastole. No murmurs were associated with this finding. RV = right ventricle; RA = right atrium; LV = left ventricle; Ao = aorta.

inoculation of bacteria in animals with no evidence of prior endocardial damage. Damage to the valve may be such that even if the infection is eliminated, the valve is no longer capable of normal function due to deformation. The source of infection is often unknown. Jugular-vein thrombosis has been reported as a predisposing factor. There appears to be no age or breed predilection. An increased incidence in males has been reported.

Prior injury, or that initiated by bacteria, results in platelet aggregation and fibrin deposition on the endocardial surface. This results in the formation of vegetative lesions consisting of platelets, bacteria, and fibrin at the site of infection (949). Damage to valvular endocardium results in insufficiency and, when extensive, can precipitate cardiac failure. Vegetative lesions are often friable and thromboemboli might develop. Thromboemboli from the aortic or left AV valve may cause obstruction of vital vessels such as those supplying the kidney, the brain, or even the heart itself. Immune-complex deposition may also be associated with systemic disease such as polyarthritis.

Clinical presentation

A common presentation in the horse is fever, which is often intermittent. Tachypnea, tachycardia, weight loss, anorexia, and depression are also common. A variable lameness may also be present. Cardiac murmurs are not always present with endocarditis, but suspicion should be raised when a new-onset murmur is associated with pyrexia and ill-thrift. Lesions on the left side of the heart are more likely to result in murmurs due to higher pressure differences across the valves than on the right side. Mural lesions are unlikely to be associated with a murmur. Cardiac arrhythmia secondary to bacterial emboli to the myocardium has been reported. With extensive damage to valves, valvular insufficiency may lead to heart failure. Clinical signs may also be associated with the sequelae of endocarditis, such as renal infarction.

Differential diagnosis

Parasitic endocarditis (uncommon, aortic valve), congenital heart disease, acquired valve insufficiency, abscessation, neoplasia, septicemia, and polyarthritis should be considered.

Diagnosis

Clinical signs are often unremarkable; however, sudden onset of a murmur associated with pyrexia should raise concern. A CBC and blood culture are valuable tools in the diagnosis of endocarditis. Leukocytosis with neutrophilia is common. Nonregenerative anemia consistent with anemia of chronic disease may also be present. Hyperfibrinogenemia is also common. Blood culture may be unrewarding,

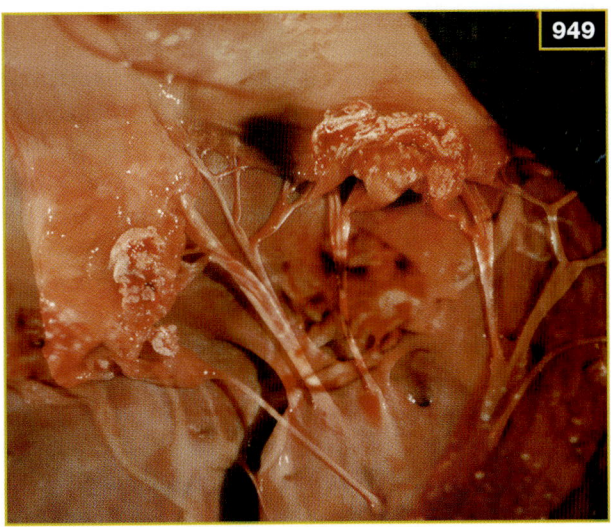

949 Gross postmortem specimen from a horse with valvular endocarditis. Photograph of left AV valve. Proliferative vegetative lesions are present on both valve cusps. Echocardiography in such a case would reveal irregular thickening of the valve margins. Color-flow Doppler examination would reveal severe valvular regurgitation.

often because of previous antimicrobial administration and low levels of circulating microbes, but should be performed. Serial blood cultures may be of benefit (e.g. every 2 hours for three cultures). Collection of blood culture during periods of pyrexia or immediately prior to a febrile period may be more useful. The organisms most commonly identified in endocarditis in the horse are *Streptococcus zooepidemicus, Actinobacillus equuli*, and staphylococci. *E. coli* has also been identified.

Echocardiography is the most useful tool in the diagnosis of endocarditis. Valvular deformity and vegetative lesions are relatively easy to visualize. Nonvalvular endocarditis is more difficult to identify. Usually there are no radiographic abnormalities. Arrhythmias are possible with endocarditis. Premature ventricular contractions or ventricular tachycardia are possible if bacterial emboli to the myocardium have occurred. The heart rate may be increased.

8

Management

Initial broad-spectrum bactericidal antimicrobial therapy is recommended. Combinations of penicillin (20,000 IU/kg i/v q6h [sodium/potassium penicillin] or q12h [procaine penicillin]) and gentamicin (6.6 mg/kg i/v q24h) provide good initial broad-spectrum coverage. Antimicrobial therapy should be re-evaluated once culture and sensitivity reports are available. Failure to improve clinically within 5 days should result in re-evaluation of antimicrobial therapy. NSAID therapy may also be of benefit, particularly in depressed or pyrexic animals. Repeated clinical examination, ultrasonography, and hematology are recommended. Resolution of clinical signs, decreased size or smoother appearance of lesions on echocardiography, a normal leukogram, and resolution of hyperfibrinogenemia are indications of response to therapy. Antimicrobials should be continued for at least 4 weeks or for 2 weeks beyond the time that fibrinogen levels return to normal. Potential sequelae are relapse on withdrawal of antimicrobials and scarring and deformity of valves, resulting in stenosis or insufficiency.

Prognosis

The prognosis in horses with endocarditis is poor both for survival and for return to performance. The onset of heart failure is a poor prognostic indicator and euthanasia should be considered in such animals.

MYOCARDIAL DISEASES

Cardiomyopathies, where cardiac dysfunction is associated with myocardial disease, are not extensively documented in horses. Heritable cardiomyopathies, such as those documented in cattle, have not been reported. However, changes in the myocardium (e.g. focal fibrosis) have been well documented at necropsy in horses. Myocardial disease or damage may occur as a result of a toxic insult, an infectious process, neoplasia, trauma, degeneration, or inflammation. Cardiomyopathy as a result of vitamin E/selenium deficiency has not been well documented in the horse. The occurrence of systolic failure (poor contractility) or diastolic failure (increased stiffness) has not been explored in the horse. True structural anomalies, such as VSD, are addressed elsewhere (see p. 690).

Clinical signs associated with myocardial disease (not including congenital anomalies) consist of tachycardia, arrhythmias, and heart failure. In all instances, cardiac function is affected. Focal lesions are more likely to be associated with arrhythmias, while extensive lesions more commonly lead to heart failure.

Primary myocarditis

Definition/overview

Myocarditis is defined as inflammation of the cardiac muscle. This inflammation is characterized by myocardial cell damage/death and infiltration by inflammatory cells. A definitive diagnosis can only be reached through histologic examination. Therefore, in clinical cases, only a suspicion of myocarditis can be reached.

Etiology/pathophysiology

Primary myocarditis occurs as a consequence of viral or bacterial respiratory disease. Inflammation and infiltration of myocardial cells disrupt cell function, myocardial contraction, and the conduction of electrical signals.

Clinical presentation

Reduced myocardial contractility and arrhythmias are the main abnormalities. Exercise intolerance, respiratory signs, congestive heart failure, and collapse are possible. Recent respiratory disease, fever, or anorexia may precede signs.

Differential diagnosis

Ionophore toxicity, cantharidin toxicity, vitamin D toxicity, and chronic respiratory disease have a similar appearance.

Diagnosis

A history of recent viral/bacterial disease and potential exposure to toxic agents should be investigated. Cardiac isoenzyme or cardiac troponin analysis may suggest active myocardial inflammation. No radiographic abnormalities are present. Electrocardiography results are variable, ranging from no abnormalities to premature ventricular contractions and ventricular tachycardia. Echocardiography may be unremarkable, although a reduction in ventricular function may be present.

Management

Underlying disease should be diagnosed and treated if possible. Supportive therapy is indicated. This may include anti-inflammatory therapy with flunixin meglumine (0.5–1.0 mg/kg i/v or p/o q12h) or dexamethasone (0.05–0.2 mg/kg i/v or i/m q24h). Corticosteroids should be administered with caution if active viral infection is suspected. Broad-spectrum antimicrobials may be of benefit if bacterial infection is suspected. Strict stall rest is indicated to limit cardiac workload. This period of rest should continue until clinical signs have resolved. Horses should be re-examined prior to return to any form of exercise because of the risk of syncope associated with arrhythmias. Exercise intolerance may persist due to myocardial damage.

Toxic myocarditis

Defintion/overview

The most commonly reported cause for toxin-induced myocardial disease in horses is exposure to ionophores. Ionophores are antibiotics that facilitate the movement of cations across biological membranes. These agents are used as growth promoters in cattle feeds and as coccidiostats in poultry feeds. Horses are exquisitely sensitive to ionophores and exposure to minute amounts can cause clinical signs. The LD_{50} for salinomycin, monensin, and lasalocid are 0.6 mg/kg, 2–3 mg/kg, and 21.5 mg/kg, respectively, in horses. Cantharidin (blister beetle) toxicosis and exposure to plants containing cardiac glycosides (e.g. oleander, milkweed, foxglove) may also cause similar signs.

Etiology/pathophysiology

Toxic insults to the myocardium may result in acute cellular necrosis, leading to fibrosis. The mechanism of action of the toxins is variable. Ionophores damage cells by altering cation distribution across the cell membrane. Facilitation of movement of cations such as calcium into the cardiac cell may result in calcium overload and cellular damage or death. Acutely, this may result in cell dysfunction. Over time, myodegeneration, loss of myocytes, and replacement with fibrosis may occur. Decreased cardiac function may result. Additionally, arrhythmias are potentiated due to regional variation in signal conduction and blockage, resulting in aberrant conduction.

Clinical presentation

Clinical signs are variable and dependent in part on the extent and duration of exposure to toxins. Signs range from mild depression to sudden death. Ataxia, weakness, intermittent profuse sweating, difficulty rising, and eventual recumbency are common in acute toxicity. Congestive heart failure, tachycardia, and arrhythmias have been documented. Severe dyspnea relating to either cardiogenic pulmonary edema or diaphragm failure may occur. Death in acute cases occurs within 24–48 hours of exposure. Hepatic, renal, and skeletal muscle abnormalities may also be present. The onset of clinical signs may occur immediately postexposure, but can be delayed for weeks. Delayed signs may occur in horses that recover from the acute phase or have experienced subacute or chronic low-level exposure. Subacute signs include depression, cardiac arrhythmia, tachycardia, and heart failure. Poor performance may be a result of acute intoxication and may be the sole clinical sign.

Differential diagnosis

Viral myocarditis, cantharidin toxicosis, idiopathic cardiomyopathy, and vitamin D toxicosis may produce similar signs.

Diagnosis

Toxin-associated disease should be suspected when multiple animals are affected. Recent feeding of a new source or new shipment of feed should be queried and, if present, provides further suspicion. The feed should be inspected and samples saved. Failure of several animals to consume feeds should also prompt investigation of the feed. Definitive diagnosis is based on detection within the feed of ionophores or cardiac glycosides or the detection of blister beetles within the hay. Gastric-content analysis is important in animals that die suddenly.

Elevations in CK and AST may be present on a serum biochemical profile. CTnI should be tested. Hypocalcemia and hypokalemia may also be present. Elevations in urea, creatinine, and bilirubin have been reported.

Multiple arrhythmias may be noted on ECG. Electrocardiographic abnormalities are not consistent, but signs of left ventricular volume overload may be evident. Left ventricular functional indices are not consistently abnormal.

Management

No specific treatments are available. If contaminated feed is suspected, an alternative source should be provided. Nasogastric administration of activated charcoal (0.75–2 g/kg) or mineral oil (4 liters/450 kg horse) may delay and decrease further absorption if recent ingestion has occurred. Intravenous fluid therapy is indicated in acute cases. Strict stall rest is of the highest importance. Vitamin E may provide some protection in acute cases via free-radical scavenging. Corticosteroids (dexamethasone 0.05–0.2 mg/kg i/v, i/m, or p/o q24h) may decrease the incidence and severity of arrhythmias. Antiarrhythmic therapy is indicated only if the arrhythmia is life-threatening because it will have effects on cardiac function. Digoxin is contraindicated if ionophore toxicosis is suspected because of exacerbation of the effects of monensin.

Prognosis

The immediate prognosis is dependent on the dose ingested and the severity of clinical signs. Some horses, especially those with high exposure, develop severe clinical signs and have a grave prognosis for survival. Multiple organ involvement also warrants a poor prognosis. Myodegeneration and replacement with fibrous tissue may lead to long-term abnormal cardiac impulse conduction and the potential for arrhythmias. Due to the potentially late onset of clinical signs, the prognosis for exposed horses is guarded regardless of the initial clinical signs, especially for return to performance.

PERICARDIAL DISEASE

Congenital pericardial disease is very rare and acquired pericardial disease is uncommon in the horse. Pericardial disease is usually caused by inflammation of the pericardial sac and pericarditis, and is classified as effusive, fibrinous, or constrictive. Benign pericardial effusion may be present during disturbances of fluid homeostasis, such as congestive heart failure or hypoproteinemia.

Pericarditis

Definition/overview
Pericarditis is inflammation of the pericardial sac.

Etiology/pathophysiology
The etiology is usually unknown and the condition is classified as idiopathic. Bacterial pericarditis may occur. Neoplastic pericarditis is rare in the horse. Fibrinous pericarditis was reported in mares during 2001 in association with the mare reproductive loss syndrome (MRLS). The pathophysiologic mechanism for pericarditis with this condition has not been elucidated.

As the volume of fluid within the pericardial sac increases, so does the pressure within the pericardial sac. When this pressure equals or exceeds that for the right heart, signs of right-sided heart failure ensue. Initially, compression of the right atrium results in decreased venous return. Venous congestion follows. As the pressure within the pericardial sac increases, more pressure is required to fill the right heart. Signs are more severe with sudden-onset pericardial effusion because the pericardial sac does not have time to stretch.

Clinical presentation
Tachycardia, a weak, rapid pulse, muffled heart sounds, venous hypertension, jugular-vein distension, and ventral edema are common. Peripheral perfusion is decreased and, therefore, the extremities are cool and CRT is prolonged. Early in the disease the heart sounds may be easily auscultated along with friction rubs. Once effusion has developed, heart sounds are muffled. Splashing sounds are unlikely to be heard unless gas-producing bacteria are present. Pyrexia is not consistent. Depression and colic signs have been reported, but are inconsistent.

Differential diagnosis
Pleuropneumonia, neoplasia, congestive heart failure, and benign effusion secondary to hypoproteinemia should be considered.

Diagnosis
An inflammatory leukogram and increased plasma fibrinogen are common. An increased cardiac silhouette and rounding of the cardiac silhouette are often evident on lateral thoracic radiographs. A gas cap may be present in the occasional case. ECG is useful and decreased QRS amplitude is a hallmark of pericardial effusion. Electrical alternans (variable size of complexes with altering large and small complexes) may also be present. Echocardiography is an invaluable tool both for initial evaluation and for monitoring progression and response to therapy. It is also valuable in guiding pericardiocentesis. Fluid within the pericardial space may be anechoic or of variable echogenicity. Air may be present in anaerobic infections. The right heart may have a flattened compressed appearance. Functional indices may be reduced.

Pericardiocentesis may be used as a diagnostic aid (*Table 45*). Samples should be submitted for cytologic examination and bacterial culture.

Management
Pericarditis with cardiac tamponade should be considered a severe life-threatening condition that requires immediate aggressive management. Mild effusion is not an emergency. Stall rest is indicated in all cases.

Antimicrobial therapy is usually indicated. Bacterial culture and sensitivity testing should be performed. However, in advance of these results, broad-spectrum bactericidal antimicrobials (e.g. penicillin in combination with an aminoglycoside) are often necessary. Echocardiography may be beneficial for guiding drug selection. The presence of air indicates a possible anaerobic infection. The presence of increased echogenicity or fibrin tags is suggestive of active inflammation and infection. Hypoechoic fluid may be due to idiopathic or benign effusion and antimicrobials may not be indicated. Idiopathic cases may benefit from the administration of corticosteroids (dexamethasone, 0.05–0.2 mg/kg i/v or i/m q24h). NSAID therapy (flunixin meglumine, 1.1 mg/kg i/v q12h) is indicated for both its anti-inflammatory and analgesic effects. Pericardiocentesis is the treatment of choice for pericardial effusion-induced congestive heart failure. Diuretics have been used in some cases, but their efficacy has not been well documented.

Prognosis
The prognosis is generally poor, but aggressive therapy has met with some success.

Constrictive pericarditis may be a sequela to effusive pericarditis. With constrictive pericarditis, diastolic filling is limited. Diagnosis is more complicated because of the absence of abnormal sounds or effusion. The clinical signs are similar. Echocardiography is of value to evaluate the thickness of the pericardium as well as cardiac function. Diastolic filling may appear normal until the elastic capacity of the pericardium is reached. A sudden ending to diastolic filling is observed. The prognosis is grave.

TABLE 45 Techniques for performing pericardiocentesis

Indications	• Cardiac tamponade • Guide therapy (culture, cytology
Contraindications	• Small amount of fluid (risk of cardiac/coronary laceration) • If echogenic pleural fluid present (risk of contamination of pericardial space)
Adverse effects	• Vessel laceration (thoracic or coronary) may lead to death • Ventricular ectopy if epicardium contacted • Extension of infection from pleural space
Cautions	• Pericardiocentesis without ultrasound guidance should be performed with great caution • Left side preferred due to lower risk of coronary artery laceration • Indwelling drains risk ascending infection and pneumopericardium
Equipment	• Ultrasound machine (optimal) • 10–12 gauge intravenous catheter • Alternatively, small-bore chest tube (if large volume)
Location	• Fifth ICS on the left side (right side only if large volume of fluid present, due to increased risk of coronary artery laceration. • Variable level, between costochondral junction and shoulde. • Avoid lateral thoracic vein
Technique	• Surgical preparation • Local anesthetic • Scalpel incision – size dependent on catheter choice • Gentle force needed to penetrate thoracic cavit. • One hand used to advance catheter • Stabilize catheter with second hand near skin to control depth of advancement • Advance catheter cautiously until slight pop detected or fluid aspirated • Sudden loss of resistance as catheter enters thoracic cavity/pericardium necessitates controlled advancement to avoid laceration • Allow fluid to drain • Aspirate with caution – risk of myocardial contact • Avoid pneumopericardium by use of one-way valve • Indwelling drain possible

Pericardial neoplasia

Definition/overview

Pericardial neoplasia is extremely rare in the horse and, if present, is often secondary to extension of another intrathoracic neoplasm. Primary mesothelioma has been reported, as has hemangiosarcoma.

Etiology/pathophysiology

Restriction of cardiac filling may develop as a result of extensive fluid accumulation in the pericardial sac.

Clinical presentation

The clinical presentation is similar to that for pericarditis, consisting primarily of tachycardia, a weak, rapid pulse, muffled heart sounds, venous hypertension, jugular-vein distension, and ventral edema. Decreased peripheral perfusion results in cool extremities and prolonged CRT. Intermittent pyrexia may be present.

Differential diagnosis

Bacterial, viral or idiopathic pericarditis, pleural effusion, and other intrathoracic neoplasia may be similar.

Diagnosis

The diagnostic process is similar to that described for pericarditis. Echocardiography and cytologic examination of pericardial fluid are the most important components. Identification of neoplastic cells in pericardial effusion is diagnostic. Hematologic changes are variable and nonspecific. Decreased QRS amplitude may be present on ECG if significant pericardial effusion is present.

Management

There are few therapeutic options. Supportive therapy, particularly pericardiocentesis, may provide short-term improvement.

Prognosis

The prognosis is poor and euthanasia is often indicated.

Heart failure

Definition/overview

While many cardiac diseases progress over time to heart failure, horses have a large cardiac reserve and overt heart failure is uncommon. Heart failure is the inability of the heart to pump adequately, resulting in circulatory failure. The presence of circulatory failure alone does not necessarily indicate heart failure, because other factors can produce evidence of circulatory failure. For example, poor venous return secondary to a thoracic mass may produce similar clinical signs.

Etiology/pathophysiology

A number of primary cardiac pathologic processes may result in the development of heart failure. Bacterial endocarditis, chordae tendinae rupture, cardiomyopathy, myocarditis, developmental defects, and pericarditis are amongst potential initiating events. Right-sided heart failure may occur secondary to chronic respiratory disease, such as severe small-airway disease. Pulmonary hypertension develops over time in response to alveolar hypoxia. This eventually results in pressure overload of the right heart, which leads to failure. This condition is known as cor pulmonale.

Heart failure should be considered as a dynamic condition that is not necessarily present in the animal at all times. An animal with cardiac disease may have sufficient cardiac reserve such that no clinical signs of heart failure are evident at rest. The same animal may, at elevated heart rates, exceed its cardiac reserve and show signs of heart failure.

Concentric hypertrophy (muscular hypertrophy without dilatation) is the typical response to pressure overload, while eccentric hypertrophy (muscular hypertrophy combined with chamber dilatation) is the typical response to volume overload and is more commonly observed in the horse.

Heart failure may be either acute or chronic. In acute heart failure, the initiating event is sudden in occurrence. Examples are acute severe blood loss leading to hypoxia, chordae tendinae rupture, and cardiac tamponade. Signs of acute left-sided heart failure are primarily respiratory, due to acute pulmonary edema. Acute right-sided heart failure is vague and peripheral edema tends to develop over 3–4 days.

In chronic heart failure the underlying lesion will have been present for weeks or even longer. Gradual decompensation occurs. Clinical signs are therefore slower in onset. When compensatory mechanisms are overloaded, however, decompensation develops rapidly.

Clinical presentation

With acute left-sided heart failure the clinical signs are of respiratory distress and severe pulmonary edema, often with large volumes of frothy fluid emanating from both nostrils. Chronic left-sided heart failure is often not obvious, as the lungs have substantial lymphatic reserve and the edema is absorbed. Mild respiratory signs might initially be attributed to respiratory diseases such as heaves. Weight loss is common. Tachycardia is almost always present. The peripheral pulse may become weak. Unsteadiness and syncopal episodes may develop. Pulmonary venous pressures become increased and, with time, the right side of the heart may become overloaded and clinical signs of heart failure become evident.

Right-sided heart failure causes elevation of systemic venous pressure. Decreased cardiac output results in decreased renal blood flow and salt and water retention. This increases body water content and, when combined with increased systemic venous pressures, peripheral edema (**950**) and venous engorgement result. Ascites, a common occurrence during heart failure in small animals, is an uncommon finding in horses.

Decreased peripheral perfusion may result from left- or right-sided failure, therefore weight loss, lethargy, renal or hepatic signs, and diarrhea may result. Dilatation of the atria often occurs in heart failure and AF is common.

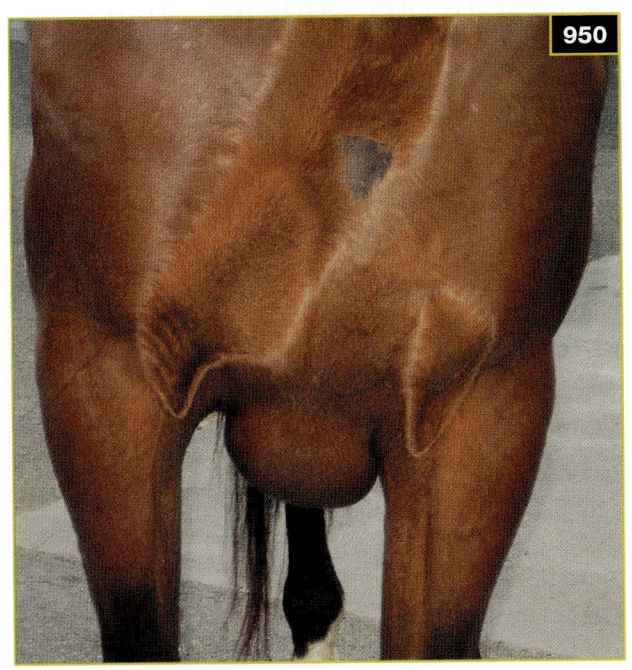

950 Ventral edema. Severe ventral edema in a 7-year-old Standardbred mare in heart failure. The mare was tachycardic, had venous distension, AF, cardiac dilatation, reduced functional indices, and severe left AV valve regurgitation. The ventral edema resolved following 1 week of therapy with furosemide and digoxin.

Differential diagnosis

Acute left-sided heart failure: acute pneumonia, anaphylaxis, pulmonary abscess rupture. Chronic failure: other causes of emaciation (neoplasia, malabsorption), other causes of peripheral edema. Acute right-sided heart failure: overly aggressive fluid therapy, particularly in neonates and in animals with compromised renal function.

Diagnosis

Clinical signs are suggestive of heart failure, but are not diagnostic. Enlargement of the heart may not be easily identified on thoracic radiographs. An increased pulmonary interstitial pattern may be present, but is nonspecific.

ECG should be performed. Tachycardia is present, although the extent is variable. AF is a common finding in horses with heart failure. Ventricular and supraventricular ectopic activity may also occur.

Enlargement of multiple chambers may be evident (951) on echocardiography. The left ventricle often has a globoid rather than a tapered appearance. Multiple valvular insufficiencies may be present. If pulmonary hypertension is a component, the pulmonary artery will be enlarged, approaching or exceeding the measurements for the aorta. With chordae tendinae rupture, part of the AV valve may appear to flail.

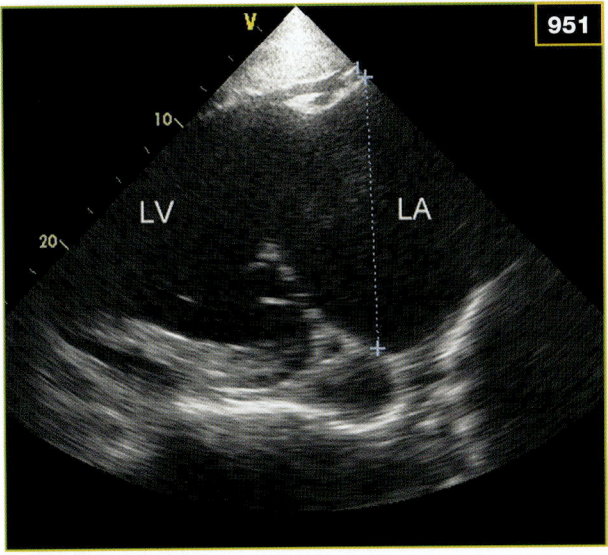

951 Left atrial dilatation. Left-sided long-axis view taken from the left 5th ICS. Two-year-old Standardbred colt with a history of poor performance and a grade 5/6 left-sided holosystolic murmur. Left atrial measurements indicated left atrial dilatation with a diameter of 16.05 cm. The horse was in sinus rhythm, with no signs of heart failure. LV = left ventricle; LA = left atrium.

Management

Since heart failure is dynamic, the goal of therapy is to restore cardiac function sufficiently, such that failure is abated. Decreasing cardiovascular demands by placing the horse in a stall is advised. Initially, administration of furosemide (0.5–2 mg/kg i/v, i/m, or p/o q8–12h) is indicated to decrease pulmonary fluids. Bronchodilators (e.g. salbutamol) may improve respiratory function. Salt supplementation should cease, but salt restriction is not indicated. Adequate hydration is indicated to avoid exacerbation of reduced renal perfusion. Fluid therapy, however, should be judicious, because of the risk of volume overload. Digoxin is of benefit due to its positive inotropic and negative chronotropic effects, thereby improving cardiac output (*Table 44*). Digoxin has a narrow therapeutic index (1–2 ng/ml), however, and digoxin levels should be monitored. Once stabilized, diuretics should only be administered as needed, as excessive or prolonged diuretic therapy may result in dehydration and reduced cardiac output. Furosemide may result in potassium depletion, which may potentiate digoxin toxicity. Venous vasodilatation is a common therapy in humans and small animals. ACE inhibitors have proven beneficial in those species and may be useful in the horse; however, financial concerns often preclude their use. Hydralazine is an arterial dilator and has proven to be of some value in other species in cases of left AV valve disease. Nitroglycerin or nitroprusside, which are venodilators, have been of value in the management of pulmonary edema in other species, but they have not been fully evaluated in horses. All vasodilators have the potential for hypotension, and the risk of collapse should be considered.

Prognosis

Once signs of heart failure have developed, it is unlikely that cardiac function can be restored sufficiently that the animal is able to perform adequately. Appropriate management may, in some cases, result in an animal that is capable of pasture turnout and of reproductive service for a limited period. Euthanasia is often appropriate, due to the poor prognosis.

Miscellaneous cardiovascular diseases

Aortic root disease
Definition/overview
Rupture of the aortic ring, or root, is an uncommon condition that is most commonly reported in aged stallions.

Etiology/pathophysiology
The etiology is uncertain; however, necrosis of the aortic wall connective tissue has been implicated. The rupture usually dissects through the right coronary sinus into the interventricular septum. Sinus of Valsalva aneurysm may have a similar etiology. In these cases there may be an abnormal appearance at the junction between the aortic root and the junction of the right ventricle and right atrium, which may appear similar to a VSD on echocardiography.

Clinical presentation
The horse may die acutely or present in acute heart failure. Tachycardia, distress, and discomfort are common. A continuous murmur over the right ventricle is characteristic. The presence of the diastolic component of the murmur on the right side is almost diagnostic.

Differential diagnosis
VSD and aortic regurgitation are the main differential diagnoses for the echocardiographic findings. In cases of sudden collapse or death, pulmonary artery rupture, various arrhythmias, and noncardiac disease should be considered.

Diagnosis
Clinical examination, including careful auscultation, is very important. Clinical pathology such as cTnI levels and cardiac isoenzymes may be of benefit in identifying active myocardial inflammation. No radiographic abnormalities typify this condition, but if acute left-heart failure is a component, increased pulmonary opacity may be observed.

Sinus tachycardia is commonly observed on ECG. Other arrhythmias may also occur. These may be junctional or ventricular in origin. In chronic cases, atrial dilatation may predispose to the development of AF.

Echocardiography is important for a definitive diagnosis (**952**). An area of hypoechogenicity may be present at the aortic root or into the intraventricular septum. Color-flow Doppler is particularly useful. In some cases, abnormal flow from the aortic root may be observed. With dissection into both ventricles, an acquired VSD may be observed. Flow would not be observed across an aneurysm unless it was ruptured. Valvular regurgitation may also be present. The rupture is often near the right coronary cusp of the aortic valve and extension into the right ventricle is common.

952 Aortic root rupture in a 7-year-old Thoroughbred stallion with a history of sudden onset of colic signs and a new right-sided continuous murmur. Right-sided long-axis view, taken from the right 4th ICS, showing the right heart and aorta in magnification. Color-flow Doppler reveals diastolic flow in red from the aorta into the right ventricle due to rupture of the aortic root, dissection into the interventricular septum, and creation of an AV fistula. RV = right ventricle; RA = right atrium; Ao = aorta; LV = left ventricle.

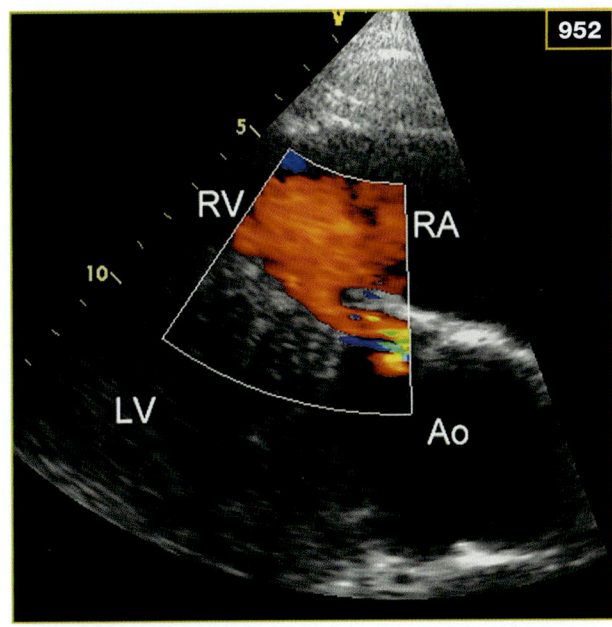

Management/prognosis

The prognosis is poor. For those animals that do not die suddenly, temporary recovery may occur; however, signs may recur or the horse may die suddenly at a later date. The owners should be informed of the danger posed by the condition. Horses with sinus of Valsalva aneurysms should be considered unsafe and at risk of rupture.

Aortoiliac thrombosis

Definition/overview

Thrombosis of the terminal aorta, the aortic quadrification, or any portion thereof may cause ischemic myopathy of the supplied muscles of the hindlimbs.

Etiology/pathophysiology

This event is of uncertain etiology. In some cases an association with *Strongylus vulgaris* larval migration has been made.

Clinical presentation

Clinical signs are variable. One or both limbs may be involved. A vague hindlimb lameness that is potentiated by exercise is common. Limb examination may reveal a slightly decreased temperature in the affected limb, a slight decrease in peripheral pulse, or reduced filling in the saphenous vein. These signs may be more pronounced following exercise. Sweating and tachypnea or colic-like signs may be present.

Differential diagnosis

Any cause of hindlimb lameness, colic, or exertional myopathy can produce similar signs.

Diagnosis

Palpation per rectum is indicated. The aorta and aortic quadrification should be carefully palpated. Pulsations in the vessels should be evaluated. Thrombi are more commonly identified in the terminal aorta. The pulse quality may be reduced. Ultrasonography of the aortic quadrification is useful in identifying thrombi (953). Variable echogenicity within the vessel is suggestive of a thrombus. Color Doppler evaluation of blood flow provides a more objective evaluation.

Management/prognosis

Stall rest and anti-inflammatory therapy is indicated. Larvicidal anthelmintics are indicated if larval migration is suspected. The prognosis is guarded to poor.

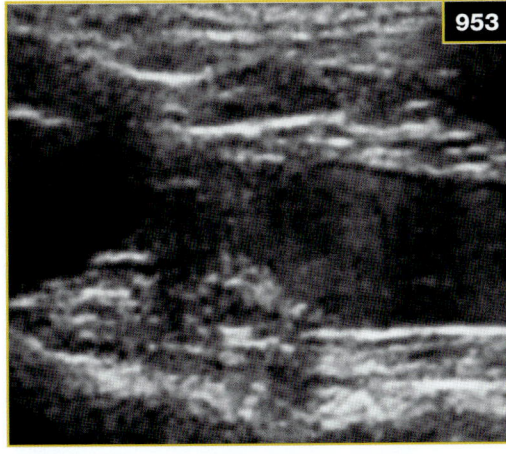

953 Transrectal ultrasound picture of a horse with aortoiliac thrombosis showing a large thrombus attached to the ventral wall of the terminal aorta, which is causing interruption of the blood flow downstream of the mass (hyperechoic area on right side of vessel). (Photo courtesy GA Munroe)

Thrombophlebitis

Definition/overview

Thrombus formation following venous catheterization or injection is a relatively common complication. The jugular vein is most commonly affected, primarily due to its predominant use for venous access. Often, the thrombus is relatively small and only affects functioning of the catheter. In some cases the vein becomes completely occluded and abscessation may develop.

Etiology/pathophysiology

While thrombophlebitis may be preceded by poor aseptic technique or irritant medication administration, it often occurs in systemically ill animals despite careful catheter management. In these cases (e.g. horses with severe colitis) a hypercoagulable state may predispose to the condition. In some cases, pulmonary thromboembolism or endocarditis may be a sequela to jugular thrombophlebitis. Thrombophlebitis may also occur following a single intravenous injection, particularly of an irritating substance.

Clinical presentation

In early cases, increased resistance to infusion through the catheter may be the only sign. This progresses to increased vessel distension distal to the thrombus. The thrombus may be palpable as a cylindrical firm structure within the vascular lumen. Distension of the facial veins may be evident. Facial swelling is not often observed unless both jugular veins are involved, in which case the swelling may be severe. Respiratory distress can develop with severe pharyngeal edema from bilateral thrombosis. Pain and heat on palpation are suggestive of thrombophlebitis. Discharge may become present at the skin surface.

Diagnosis

Clinical examination is often sufficient (954). Ultrasonography is beneficial for assessing the extent of the thrombus and for determining if any pockets of fluid or gas are present. Partial thrombosis may also be detected in a vein that empties slowly. Plasma fibrinogen assay and hematology should be performed if thrombophlebitis is suspected. If abnormalities are detected while a catheter is in place, the catheter should be removed and the tip submitted for bacterial culture.

Management

Removal of the indwelling catheter, if present, is indicated. If the thrombus is very small, catheterization of the same vein lower down on the neck may be performed. If venous access is still required, catheterization of a remote vessel, such as the lateral thoracic, cephalic, or saphenous vein is indicated. Catheterization of the other jugular vein is contraindicated due to the risk of thrombosis and the sequela of severe head swelling. The jugular veins should also be avoided when venous sampling is required. Antimicrobial therapy is indicated if infection is suspected. Mild cases may resolve spontaneously, but more severe cases may result in permanent occlusion of the vein or abscessation. Collateral circulation in time results in resolution of the edema. In rare cases, surgical resection of the affected vein or marsupialization of an abscessed vein may be necessary.

Prognosis

The prognosis is very good. Most cases resolve with conservative therapy. Development of a collateral circulation means that complete occlusion of a jugular vein does not necessarily result in long-term side-effects. Bilateral involvement is more likely to affect performance. Venous abscessation may be difficult to treat, requiring prolonged and sometimes aggressive care. Dissemination or extension of infection is uncommon, but can occur.

954 This horse had undergone recent colic surgery and long-term placement of a jugular-vein catheter. It developed jugular-vein thrombophlebitis, which clinically palpated as a hot, thready, and fibrous vein proximal and distal to the skin puncture site, which was moist and swollen. (Photo courtesy GA Munroe)

Hemolymphatic system

Darren Wood and Sonya Keller

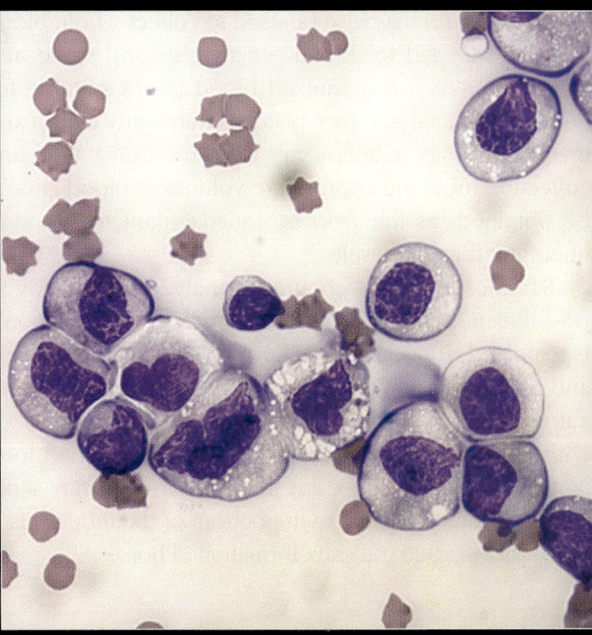

Hemolymphatic system

Diseases or abnormalities of the hemolymphatic system are often encountered in equine medicine. Evaluation of the blood-forming organs and lymphatic tissues can provide information as diverse as bone-marrow integrity, cellular response to infection, hemostasis competency, and immune-system status. A thorough evaluation of the system using blood and tissue samples may result in a definitive diagnosis or give useful therapeutic and prognostic guidance for systemic diseases secondarily affecting these tissues.

Diagnostic tests

Blood collection

The large size of blood vessels in the horse makes collection of blood samples relatively easy, even in foals. The jugular vein is most commonly used. Other veins that may be accessed include the saphenous, lateral thoracic, and cephalic veins. Blood should be taken only when the animal is calm, as excitement may induce physiologic alterations in cell counts.

Anticoagulated whole blood is required for evaluation of the hematologic system. Blood for this purpose is most commonly collected in evacuated tubes containing EDTA, which binds calcium, making it unavailable for the blood clotting process. Citrate, which is also a calcium-chelating agent, is the preferred anticoagulant for coagulation assays. Heparin may also be used to collect whole blood and can be used for blood-gas analysis and some biochemical assays. Heparinized blood is not suitable for hematologic analysis since platelets frequently clump and the morphology of leukocytes is altered (955). With any collection tube, the appropriate volume of blood should be obtained, as the ratio of anticoagulant to blood is important for valid results.

Samples for a CBC should be analyzed as quickly as possible and refrigerated at 4°C if a delay beyond 2 hours is expected. Blood smears should be made immediately and submitted with the remaining blood on cold packs for automated analysis. Refrigerated blood should be analyzed within 24 hours. After collection, tubes of equine blood that are allowed to sit for any length of time quickly separate and RBCs sediment to the bottom of the tube. This is due to the marked rouleaux formation in horses.

Samples for hemostasis evaluation must be collected very carefully to prevent any platelet activation or tissue thromboplastin-induced activation of the clotting mechanism. The initial 1–2 ml of blood collected should be discarded to avoid this problem. Unless the sample can reach the laboratory within 1 hour and be tested within 4 hours, plasma should be harvested, shipped on ice, and frozen at –20° C until analysis can be performed.

Blood-cell enumeration

Manual enumeration of platelets, RBCs, and leukocytes in the horse has largely been replaced with automated analysis. Both small in-practice and larger high-throughput instruments are available for quantifying equine blood cells. Technology utilized to enumerate cells may be based on impedance (Coulter counters), optical or laser cytometry (CELL-DYN, Advia), or on centrifugation of buffy coat cells (QBC Vetautoread). Other measured values include hemoglobin concentration, mean corpuscular volume (MCV), and mean platelet volume (MPV). From these measured parameters, hematocrit, mean corpuscular hemoglobin (MCH), mean corpuscular hemoglobin concentration (MCHC), and red cell distribution width (RDW) are calculated.

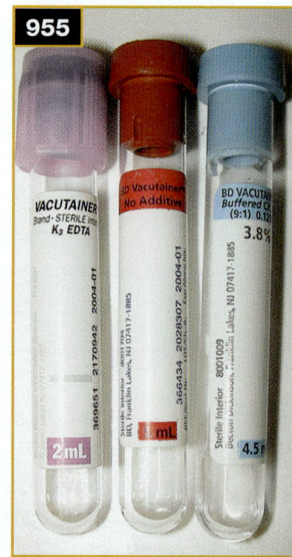

955 Three blood tubes. From left to right: purple top tube (EDTA), red top tube (no anticoagulant), blue top tube (citrate).

Blood-smear evaluation

Microscopic evaluation of a well-made blood smear is a
necessary part of a complete hematologic analysis, even
with the advent of automated differentials. Blood smears
should be prepared so that there is a feathered edge and
monolayer, an ideal area to evaluate blood cell morphology. A complete scan at low magnification is first performed
to evaluate the overall distribution of cells on the smear
and examine for the presence of platelet clumps or unusually large cells. On completion of a low-magnification
scan, higher magnification should be used to further evaluate individual cell lines. A systematic approach should be
adopted that is used each time a blood smear is evaluated
(956). It is important to make sure that all cell lines are
represented, as an absence of platelets could easily be
missed if not specifically evaluated.

Equine platelets are round to oval structures and are
the smallest blood cells present. They are anucleate and
stain very palely with commonly used Romanowsky-type
stains (Wright's, Diff-Quik). Occasional very fine stippling
of red- to purple-colored granules may be observed.
Sometimes, elongated forms can be found. Platelets may
aggregate together and be found along the feathered edge
or in the body of the smear itself.

Equine RBCs are round, stain orange to red with
Romanowsky-type stains, and exhibit minimal central
pallor. These cells are quite uniform in size in health.
Polychromatophilic RBCs or reticulocytes are not readily
observed in the horse in health or during a response to
anemia. As mentioned above, equine RBCs frequently
exhibit rouleaux formation, which is observed microscopically as rows or 'stacks of coins' of RBCs (957).
This arrangement of cells must be distinguished from
pathologic agglutination.

Equine leukocytes are examined at ×400 to ×1000
magnification for optimal evaluation. A differential examination of a minimum of 100 cells is performed to determine the percentages and then absolute numbers of
individual cell types present (958).

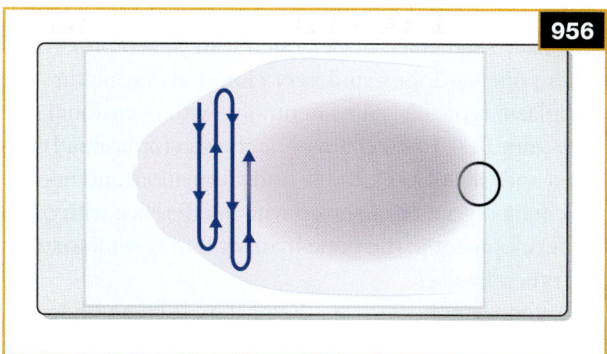

956 Wright's-stained blood smear. The arrows indicate a
systematic approach for performing a leukocyte differential
in the monolayer of the slide.

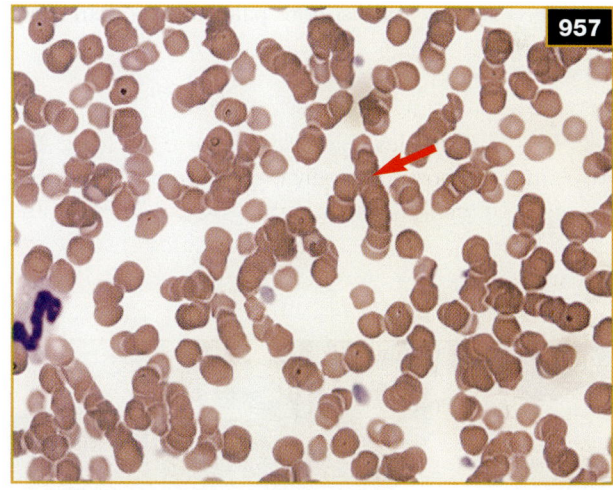

957 Normal equine blood smear. The arrow indicates RBC
rouleaux formation. (Wright's stain)

958 Blood smear demonstrating morphology of normal
WBCs and platelets: (a) neutrophil with an eosinophil below;
(b) basophil; (c) neutrophil; (d) monocyte with two lymphocyte below. The arrows indicate clusters of platelets.
(Wright's stain)

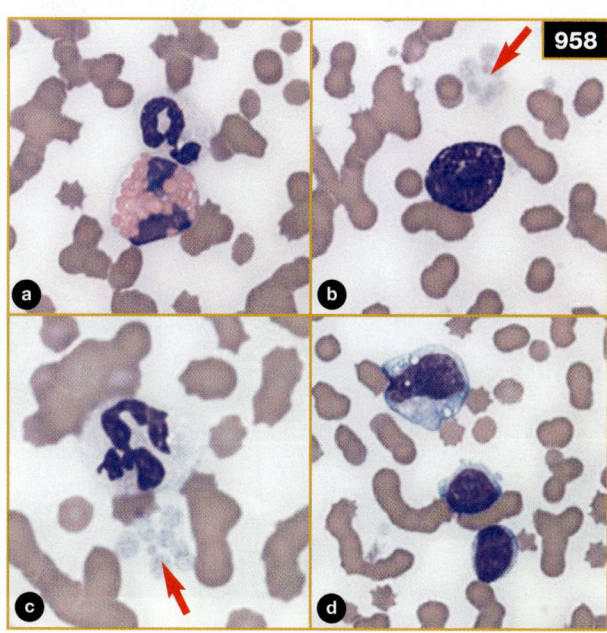

Equine neutrophils, the most abundant blood leukocyte, have segmented nuclei, often with jagged projections off the nuclear lobes, and very clumped chromatin. The cytoplasm typically stains neutrally, with occasional fine pink granules. Toxic changes such as cytoplasmic basophilia and vacuolation, Dohle body formation, and nuclear degeneration can be observed with interference with cellular development in the bone marrow during endotoxemia and other diseases.

Equine lymphocytes are the next most common leukocyte. They are small round cells with round nuclei. Only scant, slightly basophilic cytoplasm is commonly observed. Nuclear chromatin is clumped and nucleoli are typically not present.

Monocytes are infrequently observed on equine blood smears, but they are the largest leukocyte. They have abundant gray-blue cytoplasm that frequently contains small discrete vacuoles. Nuclei can be any shape except round and are not segmented. Nuclear chromatin is often described as 'lacy' and is more pale staining than other cell types.

Equine eosinophils are uncommonly observed, but are the most distinctive leukocyte. Nuclei are segmented and similar to neutrophils, but nuclear detail is often obscured by the numerous large round pink-orange granules that fill the cytoplasm.

Equine basophils are rare leukocytes, but again they have a segmented nucleus with clumped nuclear chromatin and few to many small purple cytoplasmic granules. The cytoplasm, when visible, tends to be slightly basophilic.

Collection and evaluation of bone marrow

Bone marrow is most commonly collected from the wing of the ilium or sternebrae in the horse (959). Bone marrow can be aspirated for cytologic evaluation, or a core of bone marrow tissue can be removed and fixed in formalin for histopathologic evaluation. Ideally, both specimens are collected and evaluated, as results are usually complementary. Bone marrow samples are usually interpreted by pathologists and are evaluated for cellularity, synchronous maturation, and adequate proportions of developing erythrocytic, granulocytic, and megakaryocytic cells.

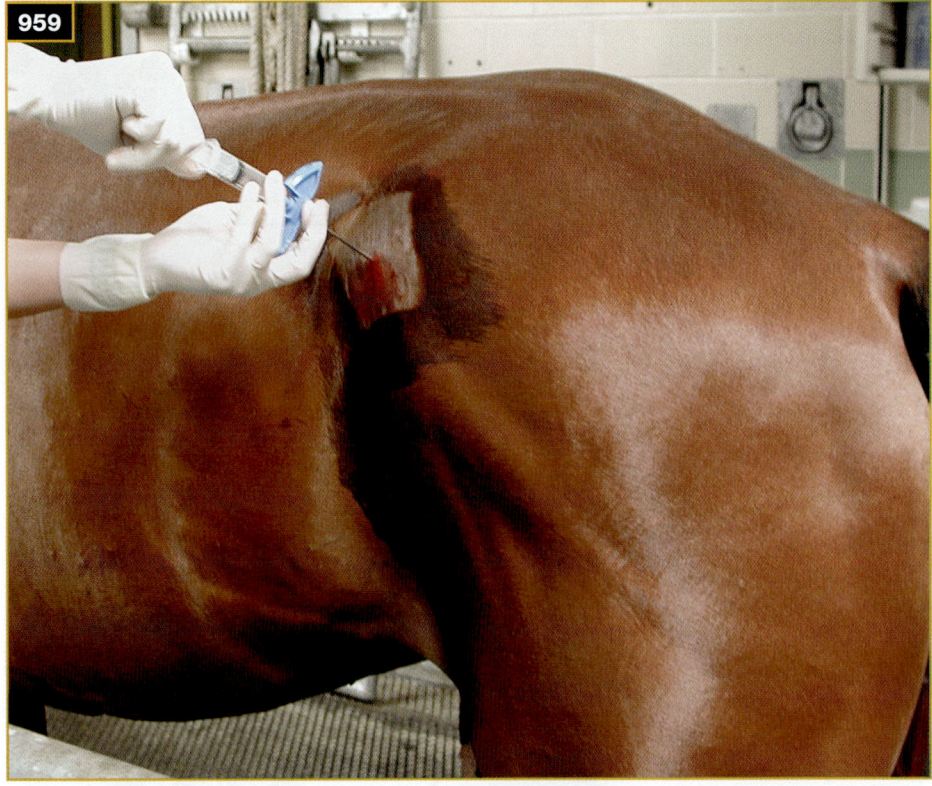

959 Collection of bone marrow from the wing of the ilium using an 11 gauge, 4 inch Jamshidi needle and a heparinized 12 ml syringe.

Hemolymphatic system

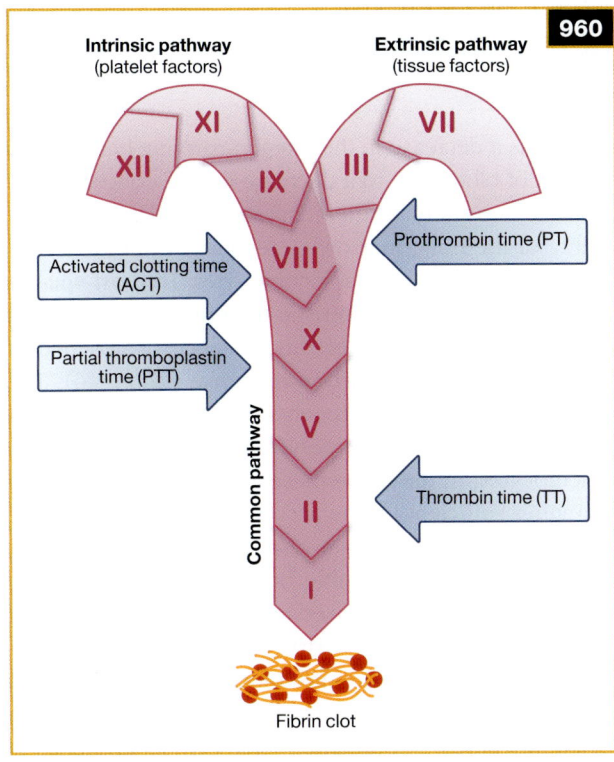

960 Diagram of the coagulation pathways, clotting factors, and routine tests used to assess the system.

Immunohematology

A crossmatch is a laboratory procedure that determines the compatibility of donor and recipient cells. Crossmatching is most often performed for horses requiring a transfusion of RBCs because of severe anemia. A major crossmatch determines whether the recipient has naturally occurring serum antibodies to antigens on the donor's RBCs. Antibody binding is indicated by agglutination (**961**), hemolysis, or a Coombs test. A minor crossmatch assesses whether the recipient's erythrocytes form complexes with the donor's serum, and is not often performed.

Blood typing is an assessment of the antigens present or absent on the surface of an individual's RBCs or lymphocytes. There are several RBC groups (or systems) in the horse that define alloantigens for this species, including A, C, D, K, P, Q, and U. Blood typing is used for predicting the occurrence of NI, analyzing pedigree, and identifying animals.

The Coombs test is performed to confirm the presence of antibody on the surface of RBCs (**962**). The Coombs reagent is composed of antibodies to species-specific immunoglobulins and complement C3. A positive test can be observed in animals with IMHA, NI, and EIA virus infection. The test is performed on EDTA anticoagulated blood.

Evaluation of coagulation

Citrated plasma is used to undertake routine functional assessments of coagulation (**960**). PT (prothrombin time) and activated PTT (partial thromboplastin time) are the most common tests performed. A normal PT indicates the presence of adequate functional proteins of the tissue factor (extrinsic) and common pathways of the coagulation cascade to form an *in-vitro* clot. A normal activated PTT indicates the presence of adequate functional proteins of the contact activation (intrinsic) and common pathways to form an *in-vitro* clot. Other assays include fibrinogen quantitation, thrombin clotting time, and indicators of fibrinolysis, such as fibrin degradation products (FDPs) and d-dimers.

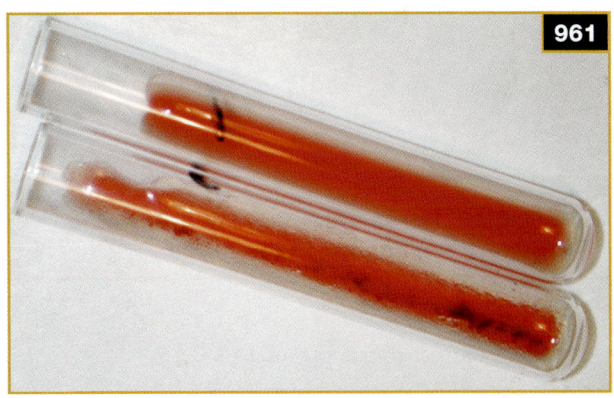

961 Major crossmatch. The upper test tube is the negative control (no agglutination) and the lower test tube is a strongly positive result (agglutination present), indicating an incompatible crossmatch.

962 Positive Coombs test with 1:64 titer (negative <1:16). Test performed in a 96-well plate with progressive dilutions of the sample. Well number 1 (far left well) is the negative control, well numbers 2 to 7 are positive (lattice formation, best observed in wells 5–7), and well numbers 8 to 12 are negative (RBCs fall to the bottom of the well to form a pellet).

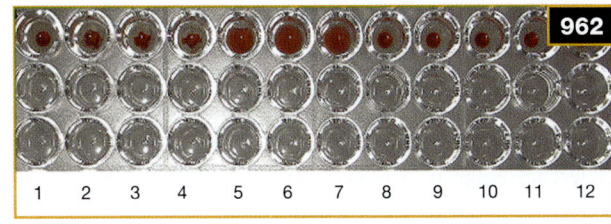

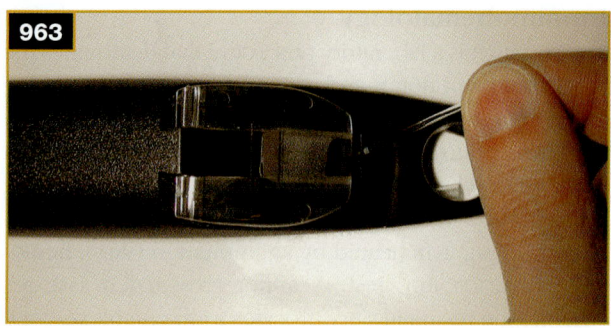

963 Technique used to transfer plasma from a micro-hematocrit tube to a refractometer to measure plasma protein concentration.

Protein determination

Total protein concentration or a more detailed assessment of individual proteins can be determined by various methods. Total plasma protein determination by refractometry is the simplest method available and provides a reasonable estimate of all the proteins in a clear specimen (963). Excess turbidity or lipemia may interfere with the refractive index, producing a falsely elevated result. Serum protein is typically measured using the biuret colorimetric assay on automated chemistry analyzers. Individual proteins can be separated by serum protein electrophoresis for a more detailed analysis of increased protein concentration.

Disorders of the hemolymphatic system

ANEMIA

Anemia is a decrease in the oxygen-carrying hemoglobin content of blood due to a decrease in RBC concentration. Anemia is usually further characterized based on the ability of the bone marrow to respond to the deficit by expanding production of erythrocytes. In most species there are several characteristic features in the CBC that facilitate determination of the presence or absence of a regenerative bone marrow response (*Table 46*). The hallmark of erythrocyte regeneration is the presence of increased numbers of polychromatophilic RBCs or reticulocytes. In the horse these cells are not released in quantities sufficient for the accurate determination of the presence of a regenerative response by most methods. Other indicators of possible bone-marrow erythrocytic hyperplasia include increased anisocytosis, macrocytosis, and a larger RDW (964). However, these features can be observed in other circumstances and cannot be used to confirm the presence of a regenerative response in isolation. Therefore, evaluating serial hemograms tends to be the best method for establishing the presence of a bone-marrow response in the horse. Examination of bone-marrow aspirates or core biopsies is another technique that can be used to facilitate this determination (965).

TABLE 46 **Parameters used to determine regenerative anemia in the horse**

- Serial hemograms
- Increased mean corpuscular volume (MCV)
- Increased RBC distribution width (RDW)
- Decreased mean corpuscular hemoglobin concentration (MCHC)
- Bone marrow evaluation

964 Blood smear from a horse with regenerative anemia showing marked anisocytosis. Hematocrit, 0.09 l/l [9%] (reference range: 0.28–0.44 l/l [28–44%]); RDW, 38.5 (reference range: 18–21). (Wright's stain)

965 Bonemarrow aspirate from the horse in 964. The sample confirms that the anemia is regenerative, as indicated by the presence of marked erythrocytic hyperplasia. Red arrows indicate developing nucleated RBCs and black arrows indicate polychromatophilic cells. (Wright's stain)

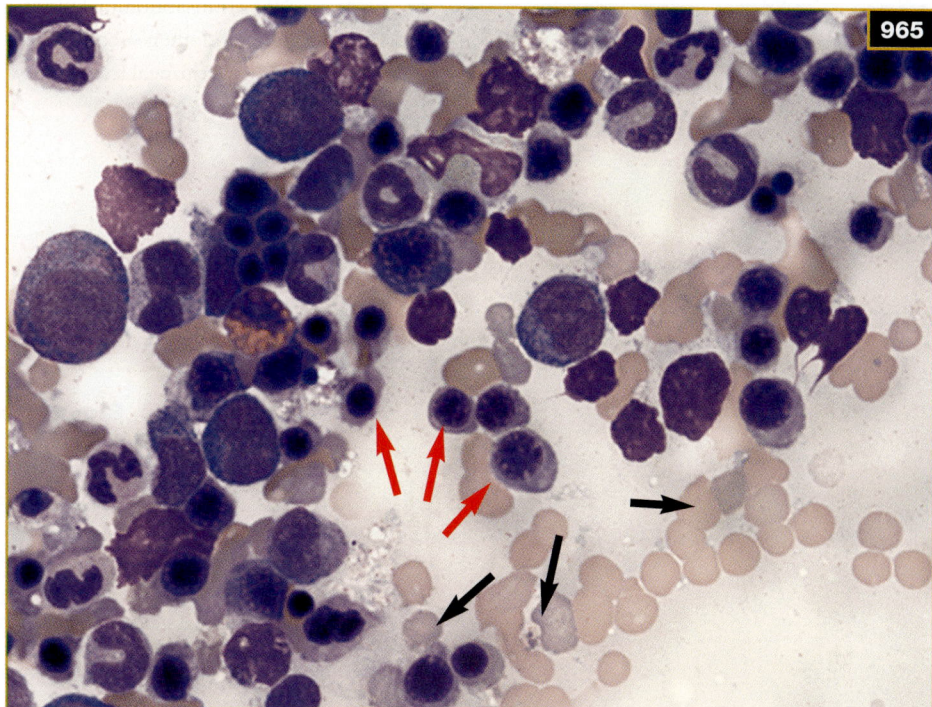

Traumatic hemorrhage

Definition/overview

Trauma to an area of the body that contains high concentrations of small blood vessels or a single large blood vessel often results in overt blood loss. The amount of blood lost determines morbidity and whether or not the animal will survive. Lacerations of major arteries can result in severe hypovolemic shock and death within minutes.

Etiology/pathophysiology

Trauma to vascularized tissue or laceration of major blood vessels results in sometimes life-threatening hemorrhage. Rapid loss of large quantities of blood may result in hypovolemic shock and death. Otherwise, animals will develop anemia once extravascular fluids move into the vascular space to replace lost volume. Over the next several days to weeks, erythrocytic hyperplasia in the bone marrow will replace the RBC deficit, as long as hemorrhage does not persist.

Clinical presentation

Trauma is usually readily recognized and frequently includes overt cutaneous lesions. The source of hemorrhage is often obvious. Other signs of trauma may include bruising and lameness. Internal hemorrhage into cavities, such as the thorax, abdomen, or uterus, may be less obvious (966). Clinical signs of blood loss depend on the volume of blood lost and whether concurrent abnormalities are present. Pale mucous membranes, tachycardia, tachypnea, weakness, and lethargy are common.

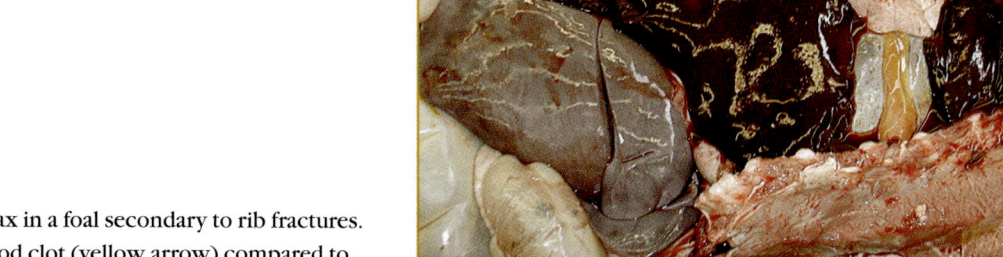

966 Severe hemothorax in a foal secondary to rib fractures. Note the size of the blood clot (yellow arrow) compared to the lung (red arrow).

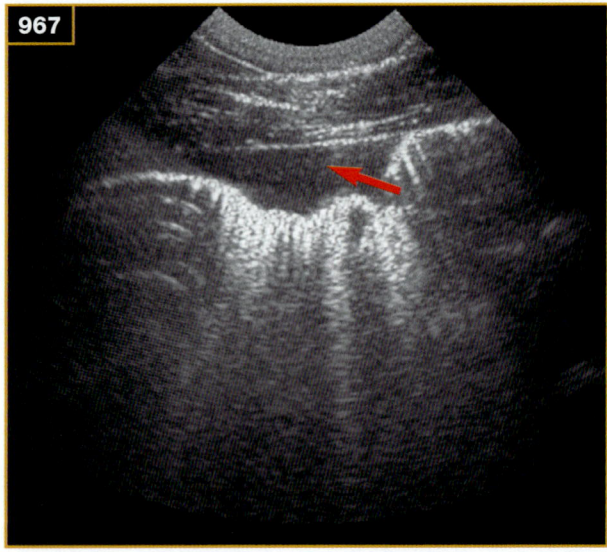

967

967 Transabdominal ultrasound image of a foal with hemoabdomen secondary to trauma. Note the echogenicity of the peritoneal fluid (arrow), which is suggestive of hemoabdomen.

TABLE 47 Blood transfusion protocol

- Select an appropriate donor. A clinically normal adult horse should be chosen. The horse should be negative for EIAV, have never received a blood or plasma transfusion, never foaled, and have a normal PCV.

- Crossmatching is ideal, particularly if the animal has had a prior transfusion. A major crossmatch identifies incompatibility of donor RBCs with recipient serum. A minor crossmatch evaluates the inverse.

- Blood should be collected into sterile containers with anticoagulant (acid-citrate-dextrose [ACD] or citrate-phosphate-dextrose [CPD]). The anticoagulant/blood ratio should be 1:9.

- Blood should be collected using sterile technique. A healthy horse can donate up to 20% of its blood volume (approximately 8 liters for a 500 kg horse) every 30 days. Blood should be used immediately if possible, but whole blood can be stored refrigerated for up to 3 weeks.

- An intravenous catheter should be placed in the recipient. Blood must be given via a transfusion filter set to remove any clots.

- Baseline heart rate, respiratory rate, and temperature should be obtained. Blood should be administered at a rate of 0.1 ml/kg over the first 15 minutes, then increased to 20 ml/kg/hour if no adverse reactions are observed. Adverse reactions include tachypnea, tachycardia, restlessness, urticaria, muscle fasciculation, and collapse.

- If adverse reactions are encountered, the transfusion should be ceased and flunixin meglumine (1.1 mg/kg i/v) given. If anaphylaxis is encountered, epinephrine (0.01–0.02 mg/kg of 1:1,000 i/v) should be administered, along with aggressive intravenous fluid therapy. Corticosteroids (prednisolone sodium succinate, 4.5 mg/kg i/v) are often administered concurrently. If the reaction was mild, transfusion can be recommenced 15–30 minutes after flunixin administration. If adverse reactions redevelop or the reaction was severe, the blood should be discarded and another source obtained.

- Transfused RBCs have a short life-span (4–6 days), so the beneficial effects of blood transfusion will be transient. Icterus and an increase in free bilirubin will be expected within a few days of transfusion.

Differential diagnosis

Hemorrhage from trauma must be distinguished from other reasons for bleeding including coagulopathy, DIC, neoplasia, and immune-mediated thrombocytopenia (IMTP).

Diagnosis

History and clinical signs are often sufficient to confirm trauma as the cause of the hemorrhage. An estimation of blood loss should be performed whenever possible, but care should be taken in interpreting client estimates of blood loss, as they are often excessive. A CBC taken immediately may not reflect blood loss, but in the ensuing hours the hematocrit declines as extravascular fluid enters the vascular space to replace lost volume. Over the next several days, if hemorrhage has ceased, the hematocrit and MCV should increase and the MCHC should decrease as younger RBCs are released into circulation. Horses do not release sufficient numbers of polychromatophils to determine easily the presence of regeneration, therefore serial hemograms should be used to follow the progress. Total protein concentration should decrease approximately in proportion with RBC concentration if external blood loss has occurred. If not, internal hemorrhage should be suspected. Additional diagnostic tools might include ultrasonography, radiography, abdominocentesis, thoracocentesis, or palpation per rectum (967). Excessive blood loss with minor trauma should prompt evaluation of hemostasis.

Management

Cessation of hemorrhage is the primary goal. If active bleeding is still present, direct pressure should be applied. Surgical intervention may be required for internal hemorrhage, severe trauma, or uncontrollable arterial bleeding. Replacement of lost blood volume is achieved by administration of fluid therapy and blood products if required. Replacement with a balanced electrolyte solution is most often indicated. Blood transfusion should be considered with severe hemorrhage and clinical signs of anemia (tachycardia, tachypnea, pale mucous membranes, weakness) (*Table 47*). Severely anemic animals may benefit from intranasal oxygen therapy. Affected animals should be rested if anemia is present.

Prognosis

The prognosis is favorable if blood loss is not life-threatening or can be stopped prior to the development of hypovolemic shock.

Chronic hemorrhage

Definition/overview

Chronic hemorrhage is bleeding that occurs slowly over an extended period of time, often several weeks to months. The presence of bleeding may not be apparent until the horse begins to exhibit clinical signs related to worsening anemia. Identification of the source of bleeding may be difficult antemortem.

Etiology/pathophysiology

Causes of chronic hemorrhage include gastric SCC, ulceration from NSAID therapy, blood-sucking parasites, and coagulopathies. Chronic blood loss from severe gastric ulceration is uncommon in horses.

At first, the bone marrow responds appropriately to the RBC deficit with erythrocytic hyperplasia. As hemorrhage continues, iron stores necessary for efficient hemoglobin production become limited and the animal enters a state of iron-limiting erythropoiesis with insufficient replacement of lost cells. Eventually, iron stores become depleted and a nonregenerative iron deficiency anemia develops.

Clinical presentation

Horses may be weak and lethargic, with mucosal pallor if the anemia is severe. Tarry feces or hematochezia may be evident. Dermatologic lesions may exist if external parasites are the source of blood loss. If a coagulopathy is present, petechial, mucosal, or body-cavity hemorrhage may be identified.

Differential diagnosis

Other causes of nonregenerative anemia, such as anemia of inflammatory disease and primary bone-marrow disorders, need to be considered.

Diagnosis

Signs or history of overt hemorrhage for an extended period of time are supportive. Characteristic findings on a CBC include a nonregenerative or poorly regenerative microcytic, hypochromic anemia. RBCs on the smear have an increased amount of central pallor due to insufficient hemoglobin production. Fragmented red cells may be observed and thrombocytosis may be present. Documentation of decreased iron stores by measuring serum iron and ferritin or examining bone marrow for iron storage, is supportive. Gastroscopy should be performed to detect gastric tumors. Care should be taken not to overestimate the role of gastric ulcers, if present, because gastric ulcers are an uncommon cause of anemia in horses. Feces should be evaluated for the presence of occult blood and parasites. Examination for cutaneous ectoparasites should also be performed.

Management

Resolution of the underlying cause of bleeding is integral to resolution of the anemia. Concurrent oral or parenteral iron supplementation may help replace iron needed for erythropoiesis in the interim. Blood transfusion should be considered if clinical signs of anemia (tachycardia, tachypnea, pale mucous membranes, weakness) are present.

Prognosis

The prognosis is poor if the cause of bleeding is a tumor, but is more favorable if parasites can be treated successfully or NSAIDs can be discontinued.

Inherited bleeding disorders

Definition/overview

Inherited deficiencies of hemostasis are rare in horses. Prekallikrein deficiency in miniature and Belgian horses, factor VIII deficiency (hemophilia A), factor IX deficiency (hemophilia B), factor XI deficiency, and von Willebrand's disease have been described in horses.

Etiology/pathophysiology

These diseases occur as a result of inheritance of a specific genetic defect that produces partial or absolute deficiency of the protein. Prekallikrein deficiency is inherited in an autosomal recessive manner and hemophilia A is sex-linked (males only) and recessive.

Individual clotting factor deficiencies, if sufficient to cause clinical signs, result in bleeding into muscle, joints, or body cavities. However, affected animals frequently do not hemorrhage spontaneously and the abnormality may only be noted after trauma, surgery, or venipuncture.

Clinical presentation

Horses with prekallikrein deficiency may be presented with prolonged bleeding after castration, but frequently they are able to clot normally. Hemophilia A patients do not usually exhibit spontaneous bleeding unless factor VIII activity is <5%.

Differential diagnosis

Other diseases that may need to be considered include DIC, anticoagulant poisoning, moldy sweet clover intoxication, and liver disease.

Diagnosis

Since many of these factors are part of the contact activation (or intrinsic) pathway, the activated PTT may be prolonged. A definitive diagnosis of which protein is affected is then made by demonstrating deficiency or absence of specific factor activity.

Management

The only potential treatment for these deficiencies, if anemia from the blood loss is severe, is replacement with blood products. This is not usually practical.

Prognosis

Successful treatment is not possible, but clinical signs are usually absent or minor. In some cases of hemophilia A, where there is complete absence of factor activity, the animal may repeatedly bleed spontaneously, warranting a poorer prognosis.

Anticoagulant toxicity

Definition/overview

Horses being treated with warfarin are at risk of hemorrhage, especially if the diet contains less vitamin K or there is concurrent administration of highly protein-bound drugs. Ingestion of moldy sweet clover (*Melitotus* spp.) or anticoagulant rodenticide may also rarely result in a similar condition that occurs by the same mechanism (968).

Etiology/pathophysiology

Coumarin, other coumarin-derivative products found in moldy sweet clover, and anticoagulant rodenticides interfere with activation of the vitamin K-dependent coagulation proteins. Sweet clover may be found in hay and pasture over a wide geographic range. Grazing of sweet clover has not been associated with coagulopathy.

Moldy sweet clover and anticoagulant rodenticides cause hemorrhage because they antagonize the effects of vitamin K. Vitamin K is required for activation of procoagulant factors II, VII, IX, and X and anticoagulant factors proteins C and S. Without proper activation, inactive factors accumulate that cannot participate in forming a fibrin clot. Subsequently, affected animals cannot form clots well and therefore bleed. Rarely, if the diet is deficient in vitamin K, the effect may be exacerbated. Additionally, the presence of protein-bound drugs (e.g. phenylbutazone) or hypoalbuminemia can increase the proportion of free (active) toxin.

Clinical presentation

Clinical signs are typically observed within 3–8 weeks of ingestion of moldy sweet clover and 3–5 days of ingestion of anticoagulant rodenticides. Affected animals are usually presented with multiple-site bleeding, often from the nose (969), GI tract, and urinary tract. Bleeding into body cavities and joint spaces may occur. Subcutaneous hematomas may occur with relatively mild trauma. Clinical signs of hypovolemia and shock may ensue if hemorrhage is severe.

Differential diagnosis

Other causes of multiple-site hemorrhage including DIC and, rarely, severe trauma or inherited hemostatic defect.

Diagnosis

The combination of clinical signs and history of exposure to the toxin is often highly suggestive. The diet should be evaluated for the presence of moldy sweet clover, and owners should be queried about the use of rodenticides in the vicinity. Lack of a history of rodenticide use does not exclude rodenticide toxicosis as a cause, because malicious poisoning may have occurred. PT and activated PTT are frequently prolonged. Factor VII has the shortest

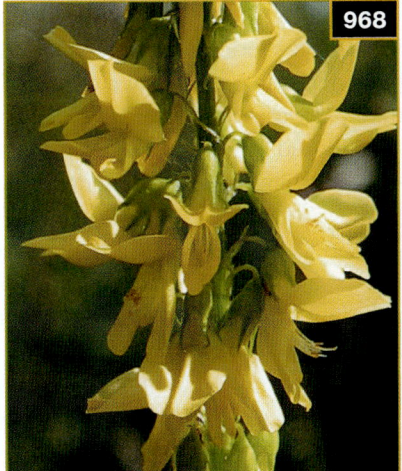

968 Flowers of sweet clover. (Photo © Kristian Peters)

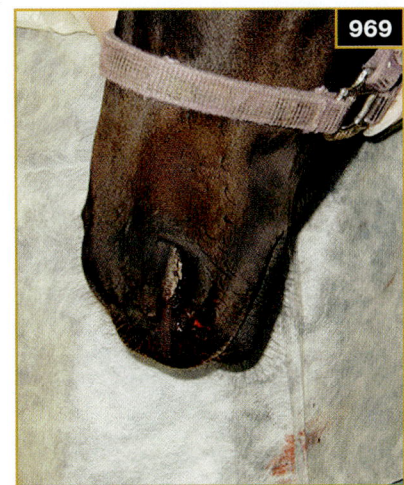

969 Horse with mild nasal hemorrhage. (Photo courtesy JS Weese)

half-life, so the PT may initially be the only abnormal test. Response to vitamin K therapy may also support the diagnosis. If hemorrhage is severe enough, anemia and hypoproteinemia may also be present. Hypoxic damage to the liver may result in elevations in hepatocellular enzyme activity.

Management
Therapeutic measures include removing the animal from the source of toxin, volume replacement, and vitamin K administration. Restoration of circulating volume may be accomplished with intravenous fluids or blood products if the anemia and hypoproteinemia are severe. Administration of fresh plasma also provides active clotting factors and may be useful if ongoing hemorrhage is present or suspected. Vitamin K1 (1.0–1.5 mg/kg s/c or i/m q4–12h for 3 days until PT has returned to reference range) should be administered. The PT and activated PTT can be used to monitor for successful therapy. Improvement in PT is often observed within 24 hours of treatment. As there is a risk of significant hemorrhage, nothing should be administered via a nasogastric tube. Severely anemic animals may benefit from intranasal oxygen therapy. Alfalfa is rich in vitamin K1 and may be fed if there are no concurrent reasons to avoid this type of feed. Vitamin K3 should not be administered because of its lower efficacy and risk for nephrotoxicity. If moldy sweet clover toxicosis is suspected, all hay should be examined prior to feeding or be discarded.

Prognosis
Horses often recover fully if the problem is recognized early, proper therapy is instituted, and hemorrhage is not life-threatening.

Immune-mediated hemolytic anemia
Definition/overview
IMHA is caused by destruction of erythrocytes by the immune system. This can be a truly autoimmune phenomenon (primary IMHA) when the process is directed against a self-antigen, or it can be induced secondarily to infectious, inflammatory, neoplastic, or drug-related stimuli (secondary IMHA).

Etiology/pathophysiology
Destruction of RBCs occurs because antigen–antibody complexes on the surface of the cells are recognized as foreign by the immune system and are removed from circulation. This can be due to loss of tolerance of a self-antigen or to unmasking of an existing antigen and presence of a new antigenic molecule. Complement-mediated cell lysis can also occur in some instances. IMHA has been reported as a sequela to lymphoma in horses. Infectious causes include EIA and acute viral and bacterial infections. Drugs, particularly penicillins, cephalosporins, and sulfonamides, have also been associated with IMHA.

Hemolysis can occur extravascularly (i.e. in macrophages in the spleen, liver, and/or bone marrow) or intravascularly. Extravascular hemolysis results in increased unconjugated bilirubin and, eventually, conjugated bilirubin, resulting in clinical icterus. Intravascular hemolysis as a primary mechanism causes hemoglobinemia and hemoglobinuria. There may be cases where both types of hemolysis exist concurrently.

Hemolymphatic system

Clinical presentation

Horses present as weak and with pale and/or icteric mucous membranes. Tachycardia and tachypnea may be present, depending on the severity and rapidity of onset of anemia. Urine may be discolored brown to dark red from hemoglobinuria. There may be a history of recent illness, drug treatment, or lymphadenopathy.

Differential diagnosis

Other causes of hemolytic anemia, including Heinz-body-induced hemolysis and parasitic hemolysis, should be considered.

Diagnosis

Diagnosis is based on suggestive clinical signs and laboratory evidence of hemolysis, including potentially severe anemia that increasingly becomes macrocytic, hypochromic with anisocytosis, and an increasing RBC distribution width. Agglutination may be present grossly and/or microscopically (970, 971). RBC ghosts may be observed on the blood smear if intravascular hemolysis is present. Spherocytes are often present, but are difficult to detect in horses. Hemoglobinemia and hemoglobinuria may also be present. The direct antiglobulin (Coombs) test is often positive. The most consistent finding on a serum biochemical profile is an increase in unconjugated bilirubin; conjugated bilirubin is often concurrently elevated to a lesser degree. Elevations in urea and creatinine will be present if pigment-associated renal failure has developed. Hypoxic damage to the liver may result in elevations in hepatocellular enzyme activity. Macroscopic or microscopic hemoglobinuria is usually present. Diagnostic testing to identify an underlying cause is important. Primary IMHA is typically identified by exclusion of known causes of secondary IMHA.

Management

Treatment of the underlying disease (if identified) and discontinuation of ongoing drug therapy are critical. If drug treatment is required, the specific drug should be changed if possible. If the anemia is severe, supportive therapy in the form of blood transfusion may be required (see *Table 47*). Immunosuppressive drugs are used to minimize further antibody formation. Corticosteriods (dexamethasone 0.05–0.2 mg/kg i/v or i/m q12–24h, tapering based on response to treatment) are most commonly used. Azathioprine (3 mg/kg p/o q24h) may be useful in refractory cases. The initial goal is to stabilize the PCV within 24–48 hours. Intravenous fluid therapy with a balanced electrolyte solution may be useful in reducing the risk of hemoglobin-associated renal damage. Severely anemic animals may benefit from intranasal oxygen therapy. Exercise should be restricted until hemolysis has ceased and the PCV has returned to normal.

Prognosis

The prognosis is good if the underlying problem can be identified and addressed. The best prognosis is with drug-associated IMHA, provided that treatment can be discontinued. If the underlying disease cannot be identified or effectively treated, the prognosis is poor to grave. The prognosis is particularly poor if lymphoma is present. The severity of hemolysis and presence of other organ damage determines the outcome.

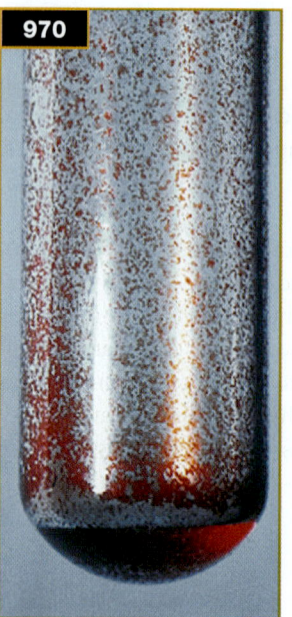

970 Grossly visible agglutination of RBCs. (Photo courtesy RM Jacobs)

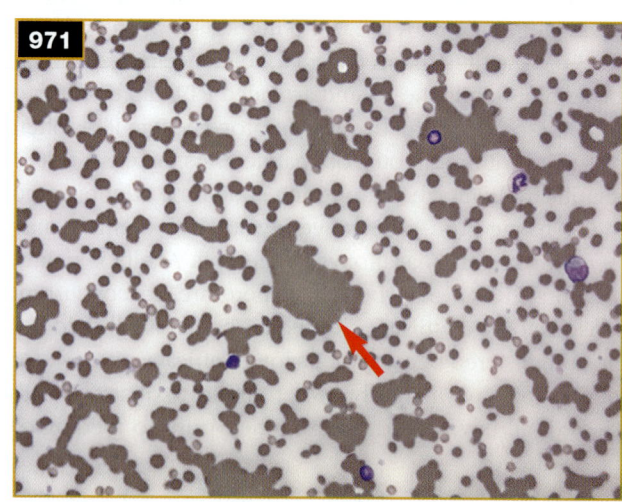

971 Blood smear with an arrow indicating RBCs in a large grape-like cluster indicative of microagglutination. (Wright's stain)

Red maple leaf toxicosis

Definition/overview

The dried leaves of the red maple tree (*Acer rubrum*) (972), if consumed in sufficient quantity, can cause Heinz body hemolytic anemia. As such, horses often are presented in the fall season when leaves drop onto pastures where animals are grazing. The quantity of leaves necessary to incite hemolysis is variable and depends on the individual horse and the amount of the toxic compound in the leaves in a given season.

Etiology/pathophysiology

Dried red maple leaves contain an undetermined toxic compound that causes oxidative damage to RBCs. Leaves eaten directly from a tree or freshly fallen leaves do not produce a similar outcome.

The toxin causes rapid depletion of glutathione, producing oxidative damage to RBCs and subsequent Heinz body formation. Hemolysis is primarily intravascular. Methemoglobinemia may also develop when oxidation of hemoglobin iron to a non-oxygen-carrying state occurs.

Clinical presentation

Clinical presentation can be highly variable, ranging from acute death to gradual development of disease. Weakness, lethargy, anorexia, pale mucous membranes, and icterus or cyanosis are common. Cyanosis may not develop if anemia is severe. Urine is frequently red-tinged due to hemoglobinuria.

Differential diagnosis

Other causes of Heinz body hemolytic anemia include onion ingestion, phenothiazine toxicosis, and lymphoma.

Diagnosis

A history of exposure to dried red maple leaves and clinical signs of acute onset of anemia are suggestive. The pasture should be examined for the presence of red maple trees. Evidence of hemolytic anemia on the CBC and finding Heinz bodies on the blood smear are other supportive findings, as are hemoglobinemia and hemoglobinuria. Plasma methemoglobin concentration may be increased, resulting in a chocolate brown discoloration of the blood. Elevations in bilirubin, predominantly the unconjugated form, are present on a serum biochemical profile. Elevations in urea and creatinine will be present if pigment-associated renal failure has developed. Hypoxic damage to the liver may result in elevations in hepatocellular enzyme activity. Microscopic or macroscopic hemoglobinura may be present (973).

Management

There is no specific treatment for this disease. Further exposure to wilted red maple leaves should be prevented. Intravenous fluid therapy may be useful in dehydrated animals and for diuresis to prevent hemoglobin-associated renal damage. Blood transfusion may be required, depending on clinical signs and PCV. Exercise should be restricted. Severely anemic animals may benefit from

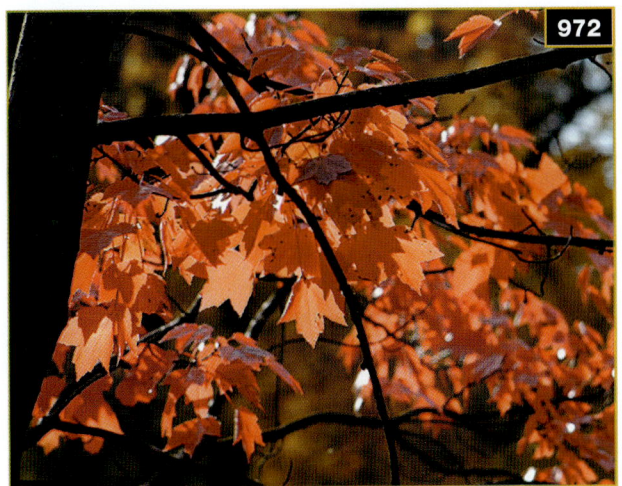

972 Red maple (*Acer rubrum*). (Photo © Jeff Dean)

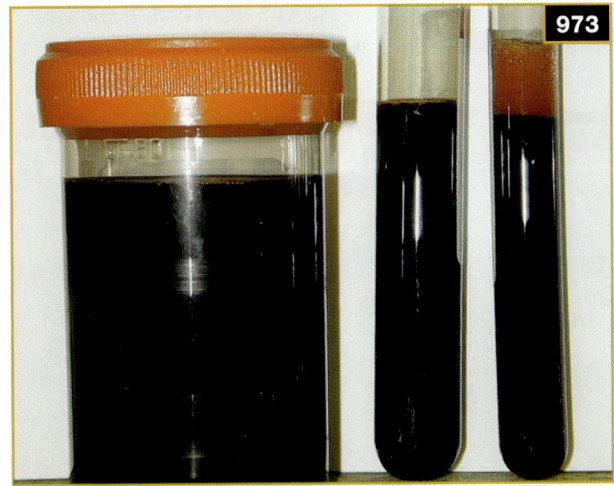

973 Left: dark brown-black urine due to methemoglobinuria. Right: two blood tubes with similar discoloration due to methemoglobinemia from a horse with red maple toxicosis. (Photo courtesy L Arroyo)

intranasal oxygen therapy. Addition of ascorbic acid (30–50 mg/kg i/v q12h) may be useful as an antioxidant. Oral ascorbic acid is less useful because of the time required to achieve therapeutic tissue levels. Methemoglobinemia resulting from wilted red maple toxicosis should not be treated with methylene blue because of the limited efficacy and potential for further Heinz body formation. Affected horses should be closely monitored for complications such as laminitis.

Red maple trees should not be accessible to horses and existing trees should be removed or adequate fencing provided so that horses do not have access to leaves. Horses should also not have access to leaves and branches from pruned red maples.

Prognosis

Intravascular hemolysis for any reason warrants a guarded to poor prognosis. If the disease is detected early and the dose of toxin was minimal, then the animal may recover. Tissue hypoxia and the effects of hemoglobin on renal function are possible complications, as is DIC.

974 Blood smear from a horse with Heinz body hemolytic anemia. The arrows indicate Heinz bodies. (Wright's stain)

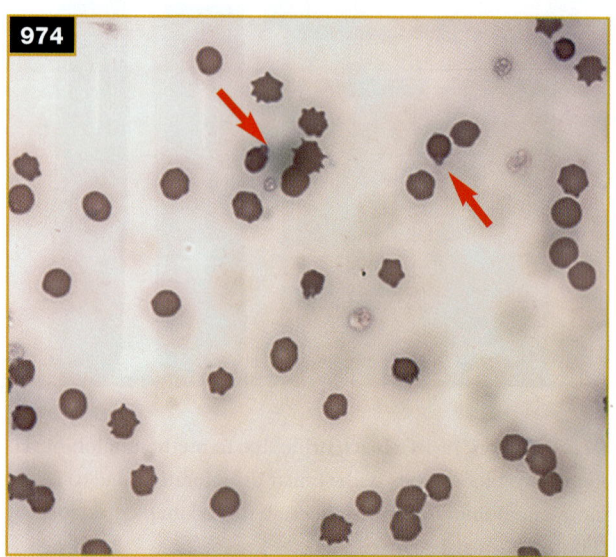

Other causes of Heinz body hemolytic anemia

Definition/overview

Although red maple leaf toxicosis is the most common cause of Heinz body hemolytic anemia in horses, other oxidant compounds also have the capacity to denature hemoglobin. These include onions and garlic and the drug phenothiazine.

Etiology/pathophysiology

Onions contain compounds that if consumed in sufficient quantity can result in Heinz body formation and subsequent hemolysis. Suspect compounds include allyl-propyl disulfide, di-n-propyl disulfide and phenol. Garlic belongs to the same genus as onions and probably has similar toxic components. High doses of phenothiazine result in oxidative damage due to production of phenothiazine disulfide in the intestinal tract.

The toxic compounds cause oxidative damage to equine RBCs. Oxidation denatures hemoglobin, with subsequent Heinz body formation. Cells with Heinz bodies are removed by macrophages in the spleen or lysed intravascularly.

Clinical presentation

Horses may be presented with pale mucous membranes and may be depressed and weak if anemia is severe. Urine may be red-tinged due to hemoglobinuria if there is sufficient intravascular hemolysis.

Differential diagnosis

Red maple toxicosis.

Diagnosis

A history of onion or garlic ingestion or administration of phenothiazine, together with laboratory evidence supportive of hemolytic anemia, including finding Heinz bodies on the blood smear, confirms the diagnosis (974). Heinz bodies can be difficult to see on Wright's-stained smears, but will be more evident when stained with new methylene blue. Other findings are similar to those described for red maple toxicosis.

Management

Administration of toxic substances should be ceased. Supportive therapy is important. (See Management of red maple leaf toxicosis.) If anemia is severe, transfusion with blood products may be required.

Prognosis

The prognosis depends on the severity of the anemia and the presence of secondary organ damage from hypoxia. In general, the prognosis is good if high levels of toxins have not been ingested and appropriate supportive care is provided.

975 Pathogenesis of equine infectious anemia. Insect vectors transmit EIAV from an infected horse to susceptible horses. Iatrogenic infection through reuse of needles or other cross-contamination of blood can also occur. Acute, subacute, and chronic (carrier) forms may ensue.

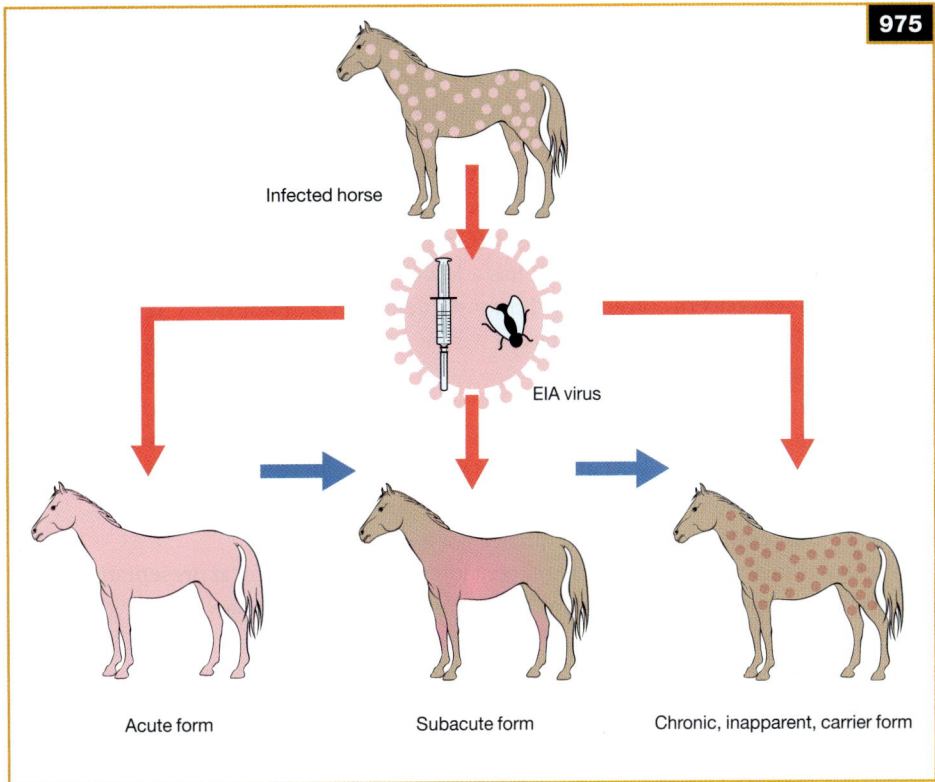

975

Infected horse

EIA virus

Acute form

Subacute form

Chronic, inapparent, carrier form

Equine infectious anemia

Definition/overview
EIA, also known as swamp fever, is a viral infection causing disease in all equids including horses, mules, donkeys, and ponies. It occurs worldwide.

Etiology/pathophysiology
EIA is caused by equine infectious anemia virus (EIAV), a nononcogenic retrovirus. The virus can exhibit latency, and recrudescence can occur intermittently.

EIAV is transmitted to a susceptible host by an insect vector (tabanid flies, deer flies, stable flies, and mosquitoes) or fomite (blood-contaminated needles, syringes, surgical instruments, blood products) and enters cells of the mononuclear–phagocytic system and endothelial cells. The disease is characterized by three distinct stages: acute, chronic, and inapparent (975). Hematologic abnormalities exist because of immune-mediated erythrocyte destruction and suppressed production of cells in the bone marrow.

Clinical presentation
The acute form is characterized by fever, depression, ventral edema, and mucosal petechiation (a result of thrombocytopenia). Life-threatening epistaxis can occur, but is uncommon. This form usually occurs within 1–4 weeks after infection and is associated with a high-level viremia. It usually persists for approximately 1 week and may not be identified in mild cases. The subacute and chronic forms are characterized by anorexia, ventral edema, weight loss, hemolytic anemia, and intermittent pyrexia. These signs are associated with recurrent episodes of viral replication. Horses will be normal between episodes and, over time (usually within 1 year) the severity of infection will wane and the inapparent carrier stage will develop. These animals are clinically normal, but are reservoirs of infection.

Differential diagnosis
Other causes of anemia and thrombocytopenia, including EVA, immune-mediated disease, ehrlichiosis, and purpura hemorrhagica need to be considered. Chronic forms may need to be differentiated from lymphocytic neoplasia and persistent inflammatory diseases.

Diagnosis

When clinical infection is present, animals usually have fever, hemolytic anemia, and thrombocytopenia. Anemia is most severe during the subacute to chronic stages. Leukopenia, lymphocytosis, and monocytosis may be observed. The Coombs test may be positive. Definitive diagnosis is achieved by detecting EIAV-specific antibody p26 in an agar-gel immunodiffusion assay (Coggins test). An ELISA is also available; however, it has a lower specificity, which is of concern considering the consequences of a positive result. Typically, the Coggins test will be positive within 45 days of acute infection.

Management

There is no specific treatment available for EIA. Supportive therapy may facilitate clinical recovery. EIA is a reportable disease in most countries. The consequences of a positive EIAV test may include euthanasia, permanent identification as EIAV infected, or life-long quarantine a minimum distance (i.e. 200 meters) away from other equids. Demonstration of EIAV-negative status is required for interregional transportation and for entering sales or competitive events in most countries. Iatrogenic transmission of EIAV can be prevented by not reusing needles and syringes and by proper cleaning and disinfection of surgical equipment. Fly control is an important management tool in endemic areas.

Prognosis

The prognosis is poor since no specific antiviral treatment is available and because of regulatory demands. Death from natural disease is uncommon and the inapparent carrier stage is usually the final outcome.

Babesiosis (piroplasmosis)

Definition/overview

Babesiosis is caused by infection with intraerythrocytic protozoal organisms of the *Babesia* and *Theileria* genera. It tends to occur in tropical and subtropical regions of the world where the *Dermacentor*, *Hyalomma*, and *Rhipicephalus* ticks that transmit the parasites are found.

Etiology/pathophysiology

Babesiosis is caused by the hemoparasites *Theileria equi* (formerly *Babesia equi*) and *Babesia caballi*. *T. equi* tends to be more pathogenic.

Babesia and *Theileria* spp. enter mature erythrocytes and cause disease by producing intravascular hemolysis. *B. caballi* infects only erythrocytes, while *T. equi* also infects lymphocytes.

Clinical presentation

The severity of clinical signs depends on the immune status of the animal. One to 4 weeks after infection in a naïve animal, fever, depression, lethargy, anemia, icterus, and petechial hemorrhages are observed. Hemoglobinuria may be present with *T. equi* infection. Death may occur, usually within 48 hours of infection. The most serious cases occur when a naïve horse has been introduced into an endemic area. A chronic carrier state may develop after acute infection. If the horse has been previously exposed, clinical disease is uncommon. Mild infections may cause exercise intolerance. Persistent infection may occur and be clinically inapparent.

Differential diagnosis

Other causes of hemolytic anemia including IMHA, EIA, and Heinz body hemolytic anemia need to be considered.

Diagnosis

Observation of characteristic protozoa in RBCs in a horse with fever, hemolytic anemia, and hemoglobinuria confirms the diagnosis. Serologic and molecular tests are available for both organisms. Serologic diagnosis depends on identification of a four-fold rise in antibody titer. A complement fixation test is the standard in many countries.

Management

B. caballi infections may be successfully treated with imidocarb (2.2 mg/kg i/m q24h for 2 doses). *T. equi* is more difficult to treat and a different treatment regimen is often used (imidocarb 4 mg/kg i/m q72h for 4–6 doses); however, infection is rarely eliminated. Injections should be divided into at least four different sites of administration. Treatment with imidocarb may prevent the development of natural immunity (particularly with *B. caballi*) and animals may be prone to reinfection in endemic areas.

Animals treated with imidocarb should be closely monitored for signs of anticholinesterase effects, including colic, hypersalivation, and diarrhea. Donkeys are particularly sensitive to imidocarb and it should either not be used or be used at the lower dose. Supportive therapy may include administration of fluids and blood products. Exercise should be restricted. This disease is reportable in many countries. Animals that survive may be persistently infected and be a reservoir of infection.

Prognosis

The prognosis for *B. caballi* infection is favorable if the diagnosis is made early and correct therapy instituted. It is difficult to successfully eliminate some *T. equi* infections even if recognized quickly. Regulatory concerns may limit the movement of infected animals. In some countries, positive horses must be euthanized or exported to a region where the disease is endemic.

Anemia of inflammatory disease

Definition/overview

Also referred to as anemia of chronic disease, this is a mild-to-moderate decrease in RBCs that occurs in response to an inflammatory condition. Anemia of inflammatory disease (AID) is perhaps a more appropriate term than anemia of chronic disease, as it is inflammatory cytokines that cause the anemia to develop, and this can be observed within 3–10 days. However, AID frequently develops insidiously.

Etiology/pathophysiology

An underlying inflammatory process such as an abscess, a systemic infection, an immune-mediated disease, or inflammation associated with neoplasia results in the release of cytokines that suppress RBC production.

Anemia develops as a result of cytokine-induced enhanced sequestration of iron in macrophages of the bone marrow and liver, decreased erythrocyte survival time, and bone marrow hyporesponsiveness to erythropoietin. The primary mechanism is decreased availability of iron for erythrocyte production. This may be an innate response by the body to make iron less available for bacterial metabolism and proliferation (**976**).

Clinical presentation

AID is often identified during investigation of the underlying disease. Clinical signs are usually attributable to the underlying inflammatory process and not to anemia.

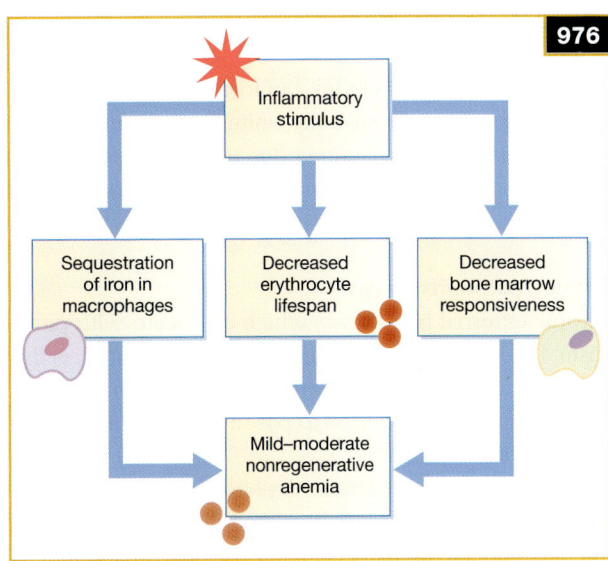

976 Pathogenesis of anemia of inflammatory disease.

Differential diagnosis

Iron-deficiency anemia.

Diagnosis

Diagnosis of AID is made by documenting a mild-to-moderate, normocytic, normochromic, nonregenerative anemia in the presence of an underlying inflammatory or neoplastic disease. Microcytosis can rarely be present. In addition, decreased serum iron and normal to slightly low TIBC, but normal to increased ferritin and bone marrow iron stores, help differentiate AID from iron deficiency. Changes in the leukogram and acute phase proteins may also be observed. Other clinical and hematologic changes reflect the underlying disease.

Management

Treatment and resolution of the underlying inflammatory lesion will result in a return to a normal hematocrit. Specific treatment for anemia is not usually required due to its mild-to-moderate nature. Iron supplementation is not effective.

Prognosis

The prognosis depends on the nature of the underlying disease. If this can be successfully treated, the anemia should resolve.

Iron-deficiency anemia

Definition/overview

Iron is important for hemoglobin formation within RBCs. Without proper iron availability, animals, especially young animals, may develop anemia due to inadequate stores. Iron-deficiency is uncommon in adult horses and is most often associated with chronic external blood loss.

Etiology/pathophysiology

Chronic external blood loss, which can occur with parasitism, bleeding GI ulcers, masses, or coagulopathy, is the most common cause. Poor iron intake in neonates on a milk diet and without access to pasture dirt may also result in iron-deficiency anemia.

When iron stores become depleted, developing RBCs in the bone marrow do not become fully hemoglobinized and may undergo an extra cellular division in an attempt to remain in bone marrow longer in order to complete hemoglobin formation. Initially, the bone marrow is able to respond to the RBC deficit, but as iron becomes a limiting factor, erythropoiesis becomes less efficient and eventually lost red cells are not replaced, resulting in worsening nonregenerative anemia.

Clinical presentation

Anemia may be inapparent until severe. Lethargy, exercise intolerance, and pale mucous membranes are common initial signs. Clinically evident hemorrhage or parasitism may or may not be apparent.

Differential diagnosis

The main differential is AID, which in rare circumstances can produce microcytic RBCs.

Diagnosis

The presence of a microcytic, hypochromic anemia is almost pathognomonic for iron deficiency. Serum iron is decreased and TIBC, which is essentially a measure of transferrin, is normal to increased. Bone-marrow iron stores are usually sparse or absent and the M:E ratio may be decreased due to accumulation of the later stages of developing RBCs that cannot complete maturation because of insufficient iron (977, 978). Total protein levels may be decreased with chronic external blood loss. Additional diagnostic testing should be directed at identifying the reason for the iron deficiency.

Management

The inciting cause should be identified and treated, if possible. Supplemental iron is required in the interim. Oral iron supplementation is preferred (ferrous sulfate 1.0–4.0 g/450 kg p/o q24h). If intravenous iron supplementation is required, iron cacodylate (1 g/adult horse) should be given slowly. Iron dextran should not be administered because of the high incidence of adverse reactions, including anaphylaxis and death. Iron should not be administered to foals in the first 2 days of life. PCV should be monitored 1–3 times weekly during initial treatment. Serum iron and TIBC should be evaluated every 2 weeks. Iron supplementation can be ceased when serum iron, TIBC, and PCV are within reference ranges. Weeks of supplementation may be required in severely iron-depleted animals.

Prognosis

The prognosis is good if the reason for the iron depletion can be discovered and eliminated.

977 Bone marrow core biopsy from a horse with iron-deficiency anemia. The lack of blue staining indicates negative staining for iron. (Perl's iron stain)

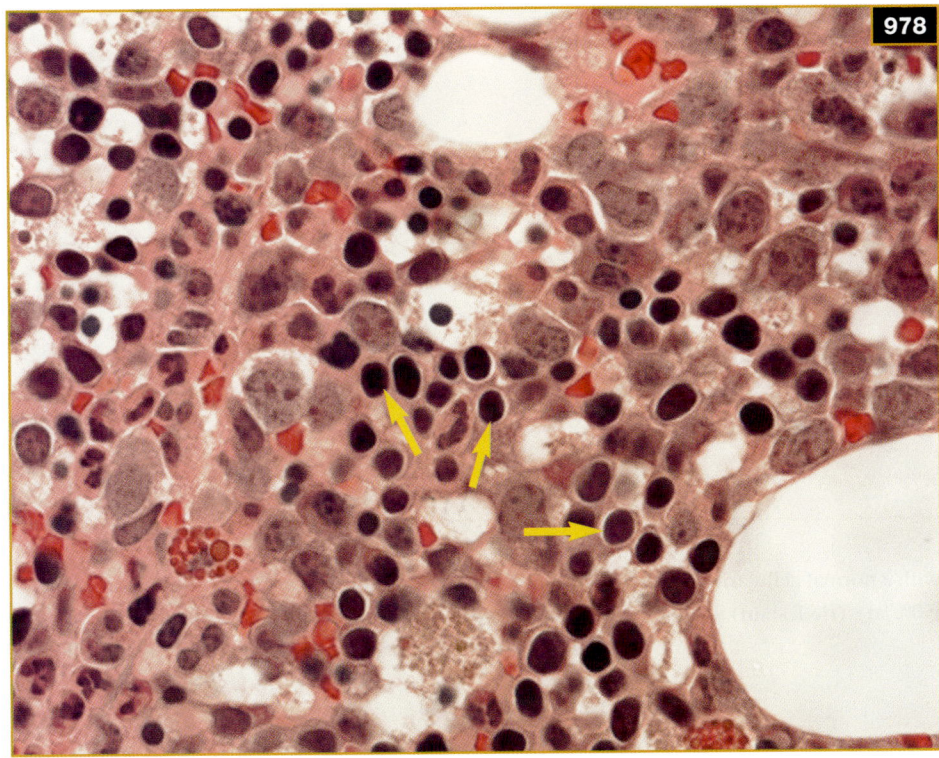

978 Bone-marrow core biopsy from a horse with iron-deficiency anemia. There are increased numbers of late-developing erythrocytic cells (arrows) and no stainable iron. Polychromatophils are not present due to the lack of iron required for complete maturation. (H&E stain)

Aplastic anemia and pure red cell aplasia

Definition/overview

Aplastic anemia (AA) is a bone-marrow stem-cell disorder characterized by decreased production of all blood cell types and replacement of normal hematopoietic tissue with adipose tissue. Pure red cell aplasia (PRCA) is characterized by a severe nonregenerative anemia due to a depletion of developing erythrocytic precursors in the bone marrow. Leukocytes and platelets tend to be unaffected in PRCA. These diseases occur rarely in the horse.

Etiology/pathophysiology

The inciting cause is often unknown, but immune-mediated phenomena and idiosyncratic drug reaction should be considered. Most cases are idiopathic. Administration of recombinant human erythropoietin has also been reported to result in PRCA in horses.

In AA it is suspected that immune-mediated mechanisms are induced subsequent to exposure to an infectious agent or drug. It is thought that antibodies develop to unknown antigens on the surface of developing stem cells in the bone marrow, and these cells are removed, resulting in lack of production of mature cell types. In PRCA, similar mechanisms are suspected, but the lesion is limited to developing erythrocytes. With recombinant human erythropoietin administration, an immune response develops to the foreign protein, which cross-reacts and removes both administered and endogenous erythropoietin.

Clinical presentation

In AA the animal is initially presented with petechial hemorrhages and epistaxis, or intermittent fever and weight loss reflecting loss of platelets and neutrophils, respectively. In PRCA the anemia is usually moderate to severe and animals develop pallor, weakness, decreased exercise tolerance, and lethargy.

Differential diagnosis

Other causes of pancytopenia or nonregenerative anemia, including iron deficiency and AID, should be considered, although the latter tends to be less severe.

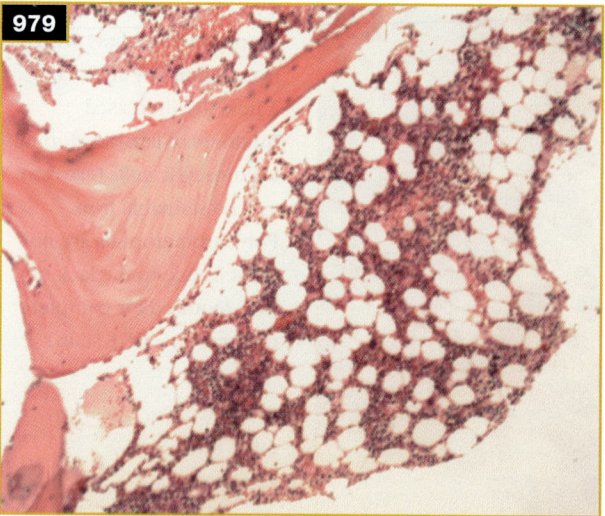

979 Bone marrow core biopsy with a normal cellularity (approximately 50% cellular and 50% fat). (H&E stain)

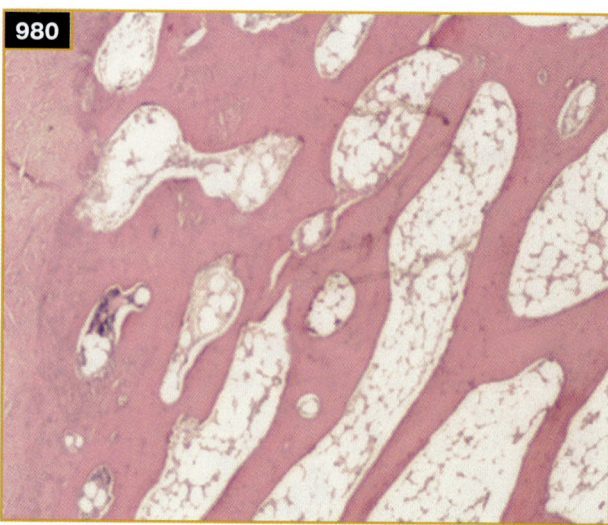

980 Bone marrow core biopsy from a horse with aplastic anemia. There is complete absence of all hematopoietic cells, with only fat remaining. (H&E stain)

Diagnosis

Diagnosis is made by documenting hematologic abnormalities (pancytopenia with AA and nonregenerative anemia with PRCA) on repeated CBCs, and examination of bone marrow demonstrating marked hypoplasia to aplasia and replacement with adipose tissue (AA) or severely decreased or absent developing erythrocytic precursors (PRCA) (979, 980).

Management

If an underlying disease process can be documented, appropriate therapy should be administered. Otherwise, supportive care, administration of broad-spectrum antibiotics, and blood product transfusions are appropriate. Bone-marrow transplantation could provide a cure, but has not been evaluated and is not available for horses.

Prognosis

The prognosis for AA or PRCA is generally guarded to poor, but there may be a response to immunosuppressive therapy. Recovery may take several weeks to months.

Immune-mediated thrombocytopenia

Definition/overview

IMTP is inappropriate destruction of mature platelets because of the presence or exposure of a perceived foreign antigen on the surface of the cell, with subsequent removal of these cells by the mononuclear phagocytic system.

Etiology/pathophysiology

IMTP may be truly autoimmune (meaning the perceived foreign antigen is a self-antigen), secondary due to the ability of some drugs to act as haptens, or because an infectious agent exposes or has a cross-reactive antigen. IMTP secondary to lymphoma has been reported. Neonatal alloimmune thrombocytopenia may also occur in foals from multiparous mares.

Thrombocytopenia develops because of the formation of antigen–antibody complexes on the platelet surface, with subsequent removal by the mononuclear phagocytic system in the spleen and liver. Hemostatic abnormalities may develop depending on the severity of thrombocytopenia. In general, spontaneous hemorrhage will not occur until $<30 \times 10^9$/l platelets are present. Most clinically affected animals have platelet counts $<10 \times 10^9$/l.

Clinical presentation

Horses present with bleeding from multiple mucosal surfaces and often have petechial or ecchymotic hemorrhages. Epistaxis, melena, and hyphema may be present, and excessive bleeding following trauma, surgery, or venipuncture may be noted. Other clinical signs are not usually present and horses are alert and afebrile unless severe hemorrhage has occurred or IMTP is secondary to an underlying disease.

Differential diagnosis

Other causes of petechial hemorrhage from thrombocytopenia, including DIC and infectious diseases, need to be ruled out.

Diagnosis

Diagnosis is made by observing appropriate clinical signs in conjunction with typical CBC findings, including severe thrombocytopenia. Platelets may be noted by the time clinical signs are identified, indicating bone marrow release of younger platelets (981). Since platelets are usually destroyed outside the bone marrow, megakaryocytes should be hyperplastic. Tests documenting the presence of antibody on platelets and megakaryocytes exist, but are not widely available.

Management

If an underlying cause is found and is treatable, this is the primary mode of therapy. Any ongoing drug therapy should be ceased, if possible. If ongoing treatment is required, then drug classes (i.e. antimicrobial classes) should ideally be switched. Immunosuppressive drugs to reduce antigen–antibody complexes are usually required, often for a minimum of 3 weeks. The most common initial treatment is administration of dexamethasone (0.05–0.2 mg/kg i/v or i/m q12–24h, tapered gradually based on response to treatment). Azathioprine (3 mg/kg p/o q24h) has been used in refractory cases or where complications of dexamethasone therapy (e.g. laminitis) have developed. Recurrent bouts of thrombocytopenia after cessation of therapy have been reported.

Prognosis

The prognosis depends on existing predisposing causes. If IMTP is secondary to lymphoma, the prognosis is poor. Idiopathic cases and those secondary to drug administration often respond to therapy. Laminitis is a risk when using high doses of corticosteroids.

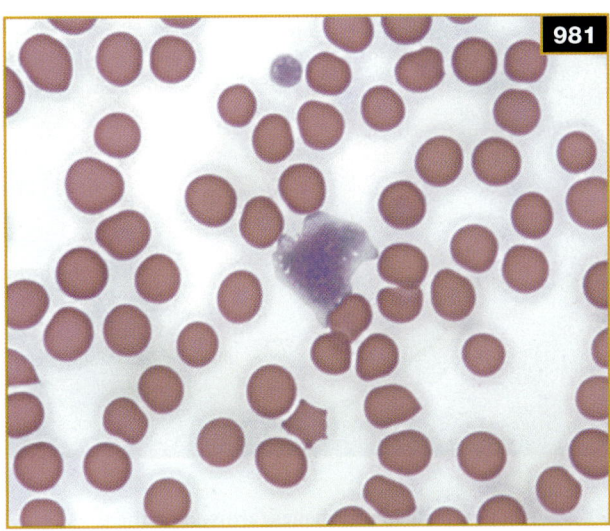

981 Blood smear from a horse recovering from thrombocytopenia. Note the large platelet (shift platelet) in the center of the field with a normal platelet above. (Wright's stain)

Disseminated intravascular coagulopathy

Definition/overview

DIC is a potential complication of many serious illnesses, particularly intestinal accident, metastatic neoplasia, and Gram-negative sepsis. With an appropriate inciting stimulus, simultaneous activation of the clotting process and consumption of clotting factors may lead to concurrent formation of thrombi and a tendency to bleed, respectively.

Etiology/pathophysiology

DIC may accompany many serious diseases including GI accidents, endotoxemia, neoplasia, severe burns, liver disease, IMHA, and snake envenomation.

Widespread or localized endothelial injury (e.g. vasculitis) results in the initiation of both platelet plug formation and thrombin generation. Platelets are consumed in the formation of numerous platelet plugs. Widespread thrombin generation ensues, with deposition of fibrin strands in vascular spaces. Pro- and anticoagulant factors rapidly become limited and fibrinolysis can predominate.

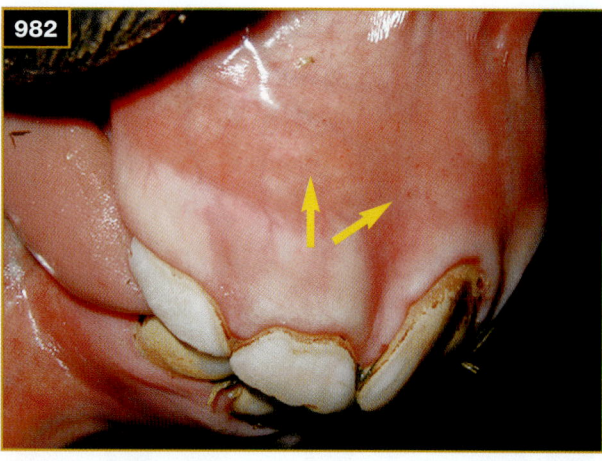

982 Small petechial hemorrhages (arrows) on the oral mucous membranes of a horse with thrombocytopenia. (Photo courtesy JS Weese)

Clinical presentation

Horses are presented with clinical signs of the primary underlying disease process and multiple-site hemorrhage. Bleeding from the nose and other mucosal surfaces is possible, and petechial and ecchymotic hemorrhages may be observed (**982**). If thrombi develop, clinical signs related to dysfunction of the affected organ will occur (e.g. dyspnea with pulmonary thrombi).

Differential diagnosis

Other hemostasis disorders presenting with mucosal surface bleeding, such as IMTP, warfarin toxicosis, and inherited or acquired platelet function defects, need to be considered.

Diagnosis

A diagnosis of DIC is usually accomplished when several supportive laboratory features are present in an animal that has a serious illness associated with its development (*Table 48*). Laboratory findings may include thrombocytopenia, fragmented RBCs (schistocytes) on the blood smear, decreased fibrinogen concentration, prolongation of PT and activated PTT, decreased antithrombin activity, and increased FDPs or d-dimers.

Management

Treatment of the underlying disease is imperative. Specific treatments for DIC include heparin administration to minimize further clot formation and plasma transfusion to replace consumed clotting factors. Administration of heparin alone may not be useful because heparin requires adequate antithrombin III levels to be effective.

Prognosis

DIC is a serious complication that can be difficult to treat and warrants a guarded to grave prognosis. Additionally, the underlying disease process tends to be serious and often difficult to treat.

Equine granulocytic ehrlichiosis

Definition/overview

Equine granulocytic ehrlichiosis (EGE) is a seasonal rickettsial disease characterized by hematologic, GI, and/or neurologic signs. It has been reported in the US, Canada, northern Europe, and Brazil.

Etiology/pathophysiology

EGE is caused by infection with a rickettsial organism called *Anaplasma phagocytophila*. The organism causing disease in horses was formerly called *Ehrlichia equi.* This is the same organism responsible for human granulocytic ehrlichiosis and ehrlichiosis of small ruminants in Europe. While being classified as the same species, it is apparent that the strain causing disease in ruminants does not affect horses.

A. phagocytophila is transmitted to the horse via tick (*Ixodes* spp.) bites. The organism has a tropism for granulocytes, predominantly neutrophils. Through a combination of increased demand, possible immune-mediated destruction, and altered bone marrow microenvironment, decreases in WBCs, platelets, and occasionally RBCs occur. The disease may also produce vasculitis.

TABLE 48 Laboratory abnormalities that support the diagnosis of disseminated intravascular coagulopathy

- Thrombocytopenia
- Prolonged prothrombin time (PT)
- Prolonged activated partial thromboplastin time (aPTT)
- Fragmented RBCs (shistocytes)
- Increased fibrin degradation products (FDPs) or d-dimers
- Decreased antithrombin
- Decreased specific factor activity
- Hypofibrinogenemia
- Prolonged thrombin clotting time (TCT)

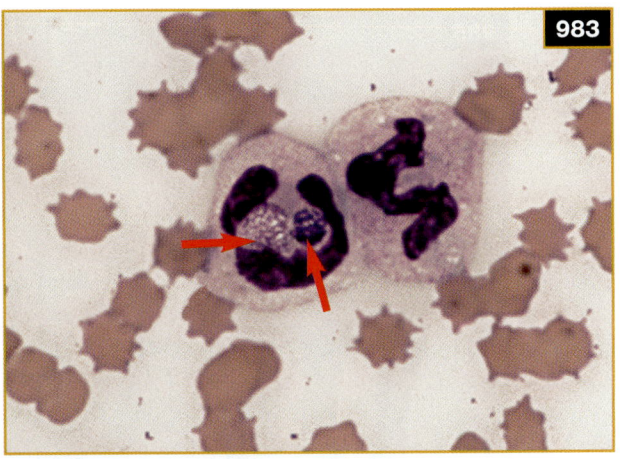

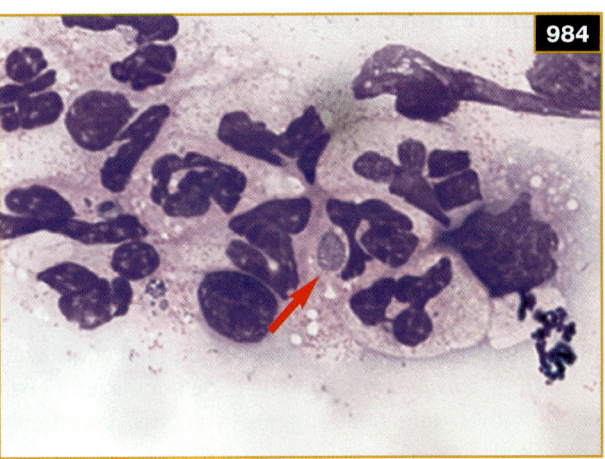

983 Blood smear from a horse with equine granulocytic ehrlichiosis. The arrows indicate the infectious agent, *Anaplasma phagocytophila*, present in a neutrophil. (Wright's stain)

984 Peritoneal fluid from a horse with equine granulocytic erhlichiosis. The arrow indicates a morula of *Anaplasma phagocytophila* in a neutrophil. (Wright's stain)

Clinical presentation

Clinical signs develop within 14 days of exposure and may be vague and nonspecific. Horses over 4 years of age tend to develop progressive fever, depression, anorexia, icterus, limb edema, and ataxia. Horses under 4 years of age tend to develop milder signs, and fever may be the only abnormality present in horses under 1 year of age. Fever is often the first sign and early infection may be assumed to be viral in origin. Signs typically peak by days 3–5, and may persist for 14–16 days. Trauma occurring because of ataxia is not infrequent.

Differential diagnosis

A variety of other causes of vasculitis, icterus, and ataxia should be considered. Other infectious organisms causing similar hematologic abnormalities, such as *Babesia equi* and EIAV, need to be considered.

Diagnosis

Physical examination findings are nonspecific. EGE should be considered in geographic areas where it has been recognized and during the appropriate season for tick-borne disease. Leukopenia and thrombocytopenia are often present on a CBC. Hyperbilirubinemia is common. Anemia is usually not present. Diagnosis can be made by observing characteristic rickettsial morulae within granulo-cytes on a blood smear or peritoneal fluid smear (**983**, **984**). Morulae are always visible in the middle of the febrile period, where they may be found in 20–75% of neutrophils. Serologic confirmation can be made by observing a four-fold rise in antibody titer, but sero-conversion may take several weeks. Molecular assays are available and are quite specific.

Management

Oxytetracycline (7 mg/kg i/v q24h for 5–7 days) is most commonly used. Doxycycline (7 mg/kg i/v q24h for 3–7 days) may also be used. Response to treatment is usually prompt and improvement may be noted in 12–24 hours. Relapse is uncommon, but has been reported within 30 days of treatment.

Supportive care is important. Ataxic horses should be restricted to a stall where the risk of injury is lessened. NSAIDs (flunixin meglumine 1.1 mg/kg i/v q12h) can be useful in pyrexic horses. Intravenous administration of a balanced electrolyte solution may be useful in dehydrated and anorexic horses. Horses with limb edema should be walked frequently if ataxia is not present. Cold hosing of affected limbs and application of limb bandages can be helpful.

Tick repellents should be used when horses are to enter *Ixodes*-infested areas. Horses should be inspected for ticks after return from infested areas.

Prognosis

Most animals recover completely, with clinical signs often improving within a few days of instituting appropriate therapy. Without treatment the infection is self-limiting and should resolve within 2–3 weeks. The main problem is development of complications such as injury from severe ataxia.

Purpura hemorrhagica

Definition/overview

Equine purpura hemorrhagica (EPH) is a potentially serious sequela to recent respiratory infection and is observed most frequently following *Streptococcus equi* infection (strangles). The reason EPH develops following such infections is uncertain, but an allergic reaction is suspected.

Etiology/pathophysiology

EPH usually develops 2–4 weeks after infection with *S. equi*, *S. zooepidemicus*, EHV-1, or equine influenza virus. Other infectious agents are less commonly implicated.

Hypersensitivity to infectious antigens is suspected as the cause of this phenomenon. As a result, vasculitis occurs and this leads to most of the clinical and laboratory abnormalities.

Clinical presentation

Clinical signs can be variable and include head, ventral body, and limb edema, petechiation, ecchymosis, fever, and anorexia (985). Heart rate is often elevated consistent with the severity of disease. Rapid weight loss may occur, presumably because of an advanced catabolic state in severe cases. Respiratory stridor and dysphagia may occur with pharyngeal edema and inflammation. Edema may be severe, with oozing of serum and sloughing of skin. Inflammation of the GI mucosa, while less common, can cause abdominal pain and ileus. Renal failure may develop.

Differential diagnosis

The main differentials include other causes of petechial hemorrhage and vasculitis including EVA, EIA, and EGE.

Diagnosis

EPH can be suspected based on a clinical history of recent *S. equi* infection or vaccination, or infection with other respiratory pathogens and appropriate clinical signs. Histologic evidence and identification of globulin deposition along vessel walls via immunofluorescence testing in a skin or mucous membrane biopsy is confirmatory. CBC abnormalities may include neutrophilia, mild anemia, and hyperfibrinogenemia. Thrombocytopenia is not often present. Testing should also be directed at identifying the inciting cause.

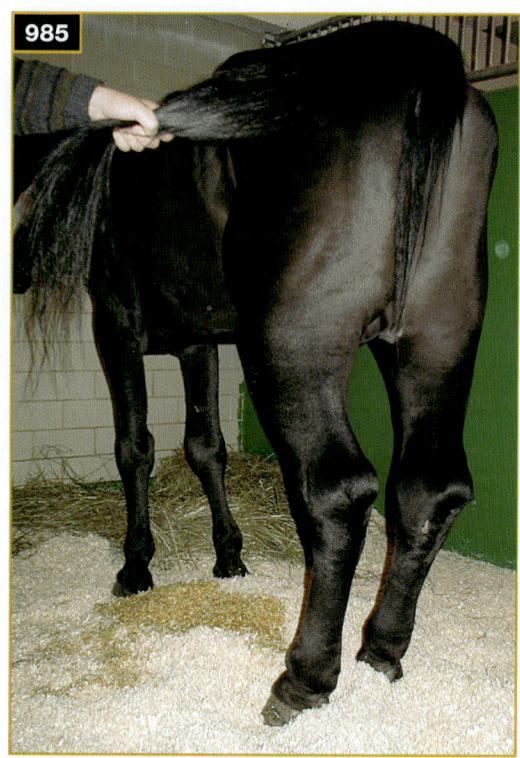

985 Severe limb edema in a horse with purpura hemorrhagica.

Management

Early and aggressive therapy is required to treat EPH. Corticosteroids (dexamethasone 0.05–0.2 mg/kg i/m or i/v q24h or prednisolone 0.5–1.0 mg/kg p/o q12–24h) are almost always used. Dexamethasone may be more effective than prednisolone early in the disease. Corticosteroids should be tapered gradually and treatment for 14–21 days is often provided. Antimicrobials (sodium penicillin, 20,000 IU/kg i/v q6h; procaine penicillin, 20,000 IU/kg i/m q12h; ceftiofur sodium, 2.2 mg/kg i/v/or i/m q12h; or trimethoprim/sulfa, 24–30 mg/kg p/o or i/v q12h) are indicated to help prevent bacteremia and sepsis and to eliminate any remaining inciting bacterial antigenic stimulus. With severe vasculitis and tissue sloughing, adequate gram-negative coverage should be provided by using ceftiofur or combining penicillin with an aminoglycoside (gentamicin, 6.6 mg/kg i/v q24h) provided hydration, perfusion, and renal function are adequate. Intravenous fluid therapy may be required in severe cases. Provision of soft feed may be required in dysphagic animals. Rarely, tracheostomy will be required. Frequent walking, cold water hosing, and application of support wraps are useful for controlling limb edema. Fluids, analgesics, and NSAIDs are required to correct dehydration, reduce pain, and decrease inflammation, respectively.

Prognosis
Successful treatment of EPH depends on aggressive early therapy and absence of secondary organ damage and sepsis. A mortality rate of 30% has been reported. With significant skin sloughing, the prognosis is poor. The recovery period can be quite long, depending on the occurrence of complications, and the prognosis becomes poor if the initial response to therapy is inadequate.

Lead toxicity
Definition/overview
Lead poisoning can occur when animals graze pastures contaminated by nearby lead smelters or other sources of lead including old batteries, discarded motor oil, machinery grease, and roofing materials. Although hematologic abnormalities occur, neurologic signs tend to predominate.

Etiology/pathophysiology
Absorbed lead inhibits certain enzymatic reactions and interferes with zinc-containing metalloproteins. Enzymes involved in heme synthesis are especially sensitive to the effects of lead. Interference with ALA dehydratase, ferrochelatase, and 5′-nucleotidase results in an accumulation of porphyrins, decreased erythrocyte lifespan, and basophilic stippling of RBCs.

Clinical presentation
Neurologic signs, including ataxia, dysphagia, laryngeal and facial paralysis, proprioceptive deficits, and masticatory problems, predominate. Dysphagia and pharyngeal paralysis may result in aspiration pneumonia. Hyperesthesia, muscle fasciculations, blindness, and head pressing may occur, but are more common in other species. Weight loss can be a prominent feature and the animal may terminally have seizures.

Differential diagnosis
Other neurologic diseases, such as botulism, tetanus, and other neurotoxins, need to be ruled out.

Diagnosis
Definitive diagnosis is made by identifying abnormally high levels of lead in blood or tissues (liver, kidney, bone). In chronically poisoned animals, however, blood lead concentrations may be within the reference interval because of deposition in bone. In these instances, measurement of free erythrocyte porphyrins or aminolevulinic acid concentrations may be useful. Determination of lead concentration in soil, pastures, or other contaminated materials to which animals had access could also facilitate diagnosis. Although anemia is usually not present, abnormal features on the blood smear may include poikilocytosis, anisocytosis, basophilic stippling, and metarubricytosis (986).

Management
The source of contamination should be removed to eliminate further poisoning. Specific treatment requires chelation with calcium disodium EDTA (75 mg/kg slow i/v in D_5W or saline divided into 2–3 daily doses for 4–5 days, stop treatment for 2 days, then repeat for 4–5 days). Thiamine (0.5–5.0 mg/kg i/m q24h) may also have a beneficial effect. Supportive care, including anticonvulsants, intravenous fluids, and nutritional support, may be required. Broad-spectrum antimicrobial therapy is indicated if aspiration pneumonia is present or suspected.

Prognosis
Affected horses may recover with appropriate therapy.

986 Lead toxicity. Basophilic stippling in RBCs (arrows). (Wright's stain)

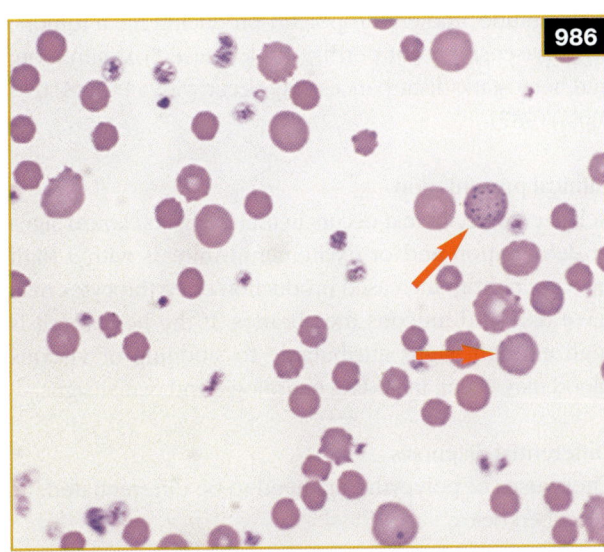

Hemolymphatic system

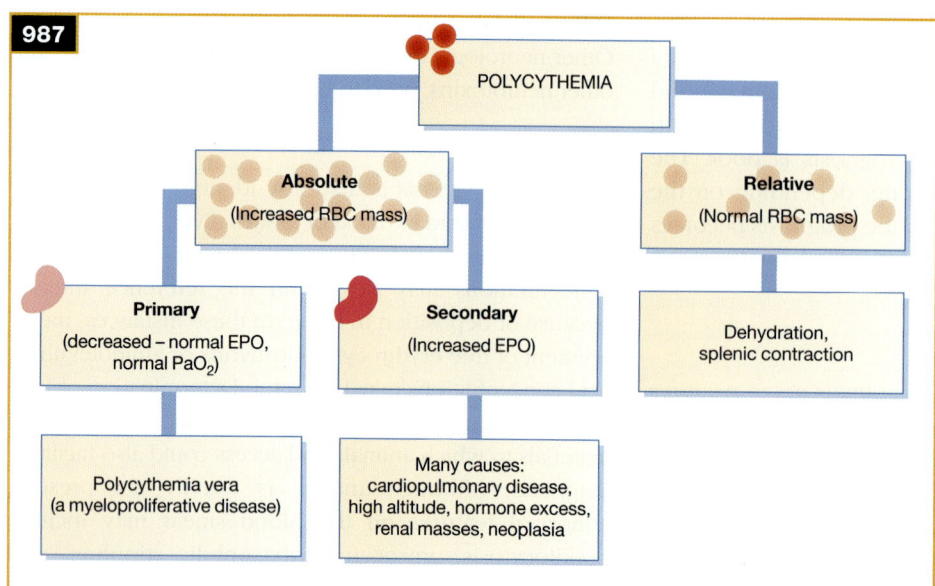

987 Causes of poly-cythemia in the horse. Polycythemia is classified as either relative (commonly a result of dehydration) or absolute (either primary, a myeloproliferative disease, or secondary, because of increased erythropoietin concentrations).

Polycythemia
Definition/overview
Polycythemia (erythrocytosis) refers to an increase in RBC count, hemoglobin concentration, or hematocrit. All three of these parameters are usually increased concurrently.

Etiology/pathophysiology
Dehydration results in lowered plasma volume, producing a relative increase in RBC and protein concentrations. Relative polycythemia can also develop in horses when epinephrine-induced splenic contraction occurs, such as with excitement, resulting in a transient increase in RBC concentration only. Absolute polycythemia may be observed with a neoplastic proliferation of mature RBCs that is erythropoietin independent (polycythemia vera), or be secondary to conditions causing hypoxemia sufficient to elevate erythropoietin production. Conditions in the latter category include cardiopulmonary disease, living at high altitude, and erythropoietin-producing renal tumors. Hyperviscosity, poor perfusion, decreased oxygenation, and hemostatic disturbances may occur with a PCV >0.6 l/l (60%) (987).

Clinical presentation
Relative polycythemia occurs in animals with clinical signs of dehydration and/or excitement. Animals with a high hematocrit from increased production of erythrocytes may have dark red mucous membranes. If the hematocrit is high enough, signs attributable to sludging of viscous blood may occur, including neurologic and ocular signs.

Differential diagnosis
The causes of polycythemia need to be differentiated, as described below.

Diagnosis
Diagnosis is made using clinical and historical information in combination with laboratory evidence of increased RBC concentration, hemoglobin, and/or hematocrit. Hydration status should be assessed clinically. Serial measurements of RBC parameters, especially following rehydration therapy, can be used to identify relative polycythemia. Causes of absolute polycythemia can be further defined by measurement of erythropoietin concentration and arterial partial pressure of oxygen (PaO$_2$). Animals with poly-cythemia vera have normal to low erythropoietin and normal PaO$_2$. Animals with a secondary absolute poly-cythemia have increased erythropoietin and may have low PaO$_2$.

Management
Treatment of dehydration with appropriate fluid replace-ment therapy will resolve dehydration-associated relative polycythemia. Causes of absolute polycythemia are usually more difficult to treat and may involve periodic blood removal (phlebotomy). Removal of 10 ml/kg of blood every 2–3 days should be performed until the PCV is <0.5 l/l (50%). If phlebotomy is performed, concurrent adminis-tration of a balanced electrolyte solution is preferred. Further blood removal should be determined based on regular monitoring of PCV. Initially, PCV should be monitored every few days. The goal should be to maintain a PCV of <0.5 l/l (50%). Secondary polycythemia caused by hypoxia should not be treated by aggressive phlebotomy because the increased PCV is a compensatory mechanism. If the PCV is not markedly elevated (<0.6 l/l [<60%]), removal of smaller volumes of blood is indicated. The primary cause of hypoxia must be addressed. In humans and small animals, hydroxyurea has been used to induce

reversible bone-marrow suppression; however, its use has not been reported in horses.

Prognosis
The prognosis for relative polycythemia is good if appropriate fluid therapy is administered and the cause of dehydration can be addressed. Cases of secondary polycythemia carry a more guarded prognosis, especially those due to neoplasia.

Myeloproliferative disorders

Definition/overview
Myeloproliferative disorders (MPDs) are neoplasms of developing nonlymphocytic hematopoietic cells including tumors of RBCs, granulocytic cells, monocytic cells, and platelets. These diseases are often referred to as leukemias and are rare in horses.

Etiology/pathophysiology
Neoplastic transformation of any cell line may occur, but the underlying cause is usually unknown in horses.

Unregulated proliferation of a cell line at a certain stage of development results in the increased autonomous production of these cells in bone marrow, which can then infiltrate other tissues and be found in circulating blood. The tumor replaces normal hematopoietic cells, resulting in cytopenias in other cell lines due to lack of production. Neoplastic cells are often observed in circulation, as they are released from bone marrow. Other tissues affected may include the spleen, liver, and lymph nodes.

Clinical presentation
Horses are typically presented with vague signs of disease that may include poor performance, lethargy, inappetence, weight loss, and weakness. More specific signs indicating hematologic involvement may include pale mucous membranes and petechial or ecchymotic hemorrhages. Intermittent fever may be present when opportunistic infections occur due to neutropenia.

Differential diagnosis
If the presence of circulating atypical cells is confirmed, the primary differential diagnoses are myeloproliferative and lymphoproliferative disorders.

Diagnosis
Diagnosis of leukemia is based on the observation of atypical cells on blood smears or in bone marrow (**988**). Further characterization of the cell type of origin can be difficult based on morphology alone. Cytochemistry can be attempted, but results can be difficult to interpret. The increased availability of cell lineage-specific markers for individual species will result in a better ability to characterize these rare tumors in horses using immunohistochemical and flow-cytometric techniques.

Management and prognosis
The prognosis for leukemia is poor to grave in horses. The uncommon occurrence of these diseases has resulted in little study and therapeutic investigation. Chemotherapeutic options for large animals tend to be very expensive and are unproven.

988 Blood smear from a horse with myelomonocytic leukemia. A monotypic population of large round cells with round-to-indented nuclei and multiple prominent nucleoli is pictured. (Wright's stain) (Photo courtesy RM Jacobs)

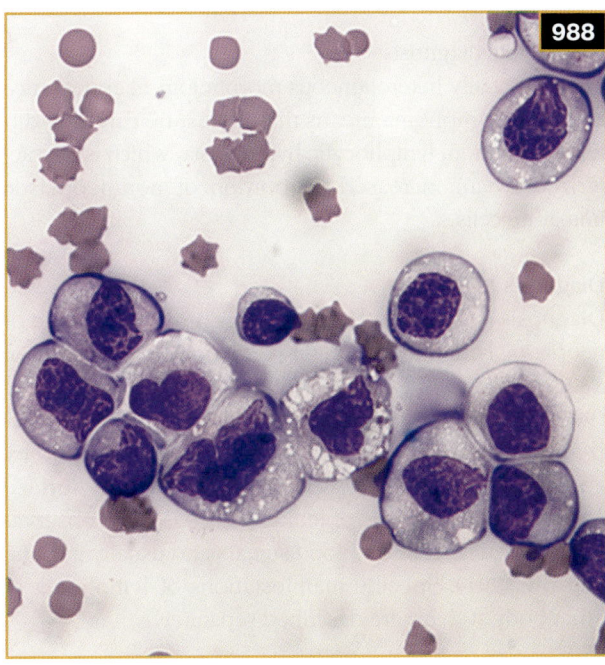

Lymphoma and lymphocytic leukemia
Definition/overview
Lymphoma is characterized by infiltration of solid tissues with neoplastic lymphocytes. Lymphoma has different clinical manifestations in the horse. Only rarely does lymphoma become leukemic, with neoplastic cells found in circulating blood. This tends to be observed in horses with generalized or multicentric lymphoma. Other forms include cutaneous, mediastinal, and intestinal disease. Unlike many other types of neoplasia, lymphoma is not uncommon in young horses and may even occur in foals.

Etiology/pathophysiology
Unregulated proliferation of a cell line at a certain stage of development results in an increased proportion of these cells in hemolymphatic tissues. The infiltrative nature of the tumor may result in replacement of normal hematopoietic cells, which will create cytopenias of other cell lines. Neoplastic cells are rarely observed in circulation. Tissues most commonly affected include the lymph nodes, spleen, and liver.

Clinical presentation
Horses are often presented because of weight loss, lethargy, and enlarged lymph nodes (989). Other features may include dyspnea, colic, and neurologic and ocular signs, depending on the localization of the tumor. Splenic enlargement or internal masses may be palpable per rectum. Horses with the cutaneous form have few to many firm nodules scattered over the body, sometimes with peripheral lymph-node involvement. The intestinal form has been associated with the development of IMHA and so horses may be presented for weakness, icterus, and pale mucous membranes.

Differential diagnosis
The potentially heterogeneous morphological appearance of equine lymphoma means that it must be carefully differentiated from lymphocytic hyperplasia, which is characterized by an increased proportion of non-neoplastic immature cells.

Diagnosis
Diagnosis is confirmed by observing a predominance of neoplastic lymphocytes altering the normal architecture of a solid tissue on fine-needle aspiration or excisional biopsy (990). The subtype of lymphoma may be further characterized on the basis of the morphology of the cells and by application of cell type-specific (i.e. T or B) surface markers. The diagnosis of leukemia is based on observation of atypical cells on blood smears and usually in bone marrow (991). Specific manifestations of lymphoma in other body systems are described separately.

Management
Cutaneous lymphoma may respond to corticosteroid therapy, but may recur after cessation of treatment. The prolonged and relatively benign nature of this form of the disease means that treatment may not be required at all. Other forms of lymphoma do not respond well to treatment; however, the recent adaptation of chemotherapeutic protocols from other species has had promising results on a limited basis. Specific treatments for lymphoma of different body systems are covered elsewhere.

Prognosis
The prognosis for lymphoma and lymphocytic leukemia is poor to grave in horses. The uncommon occurrence of these diseases has resulted in little study and therapeutic investigation. Chemotherapeutic options for large animals tend to be very expensive and unrewarding. The prognosis for horses with cutaneous lymphoma is much better, with some horses living for long periods without treatment. Some degree of palliation may be achieved with corticosteroid treatment in some other forms of lymphoma, but remission will not be achieved.

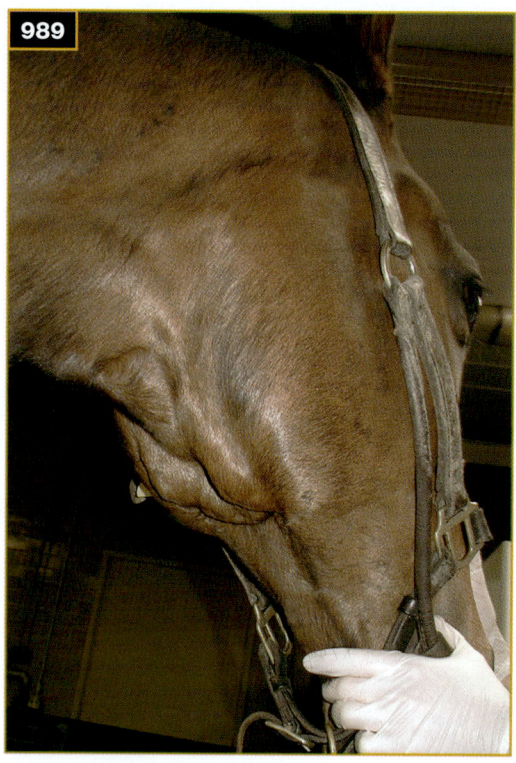

989 Enlarged submandibular lymph nodes in a horse with lymphoma.

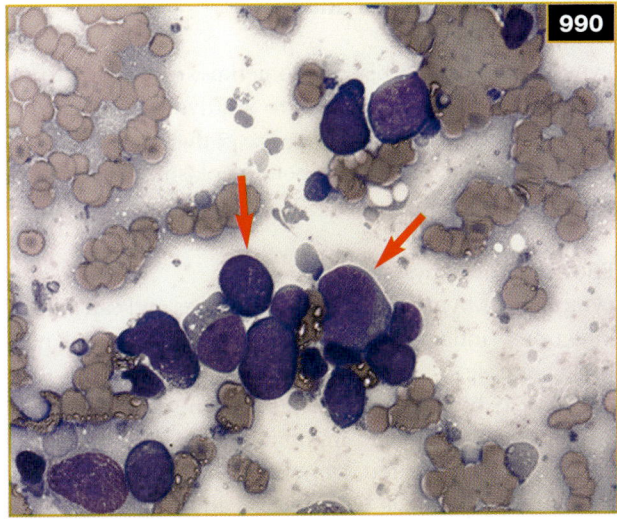

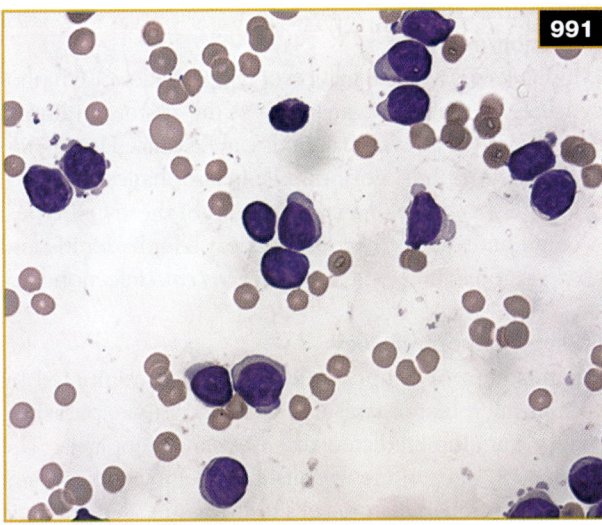

990 Lymph-node fine-needle aspirate from a horse with lymphoma. There is a heterogeneous population of small, medium, and large lymphocytes; however, the arrows indicate medium to large lymphocytes with atypical morphology (multiple prominent nucleoli). (Wright's stain)

991 Bone-marrow aspirate from a horse with lymphocytic leukemia. There is a monotypic population of neoplastic lymphocytes present. Normal hematopoietic tissue is absent due to complete effacement by neoplastic cells. (Wright's stain)

Lymph node diseases

Neoplasia

The most common neoplasm of lymphatic tissue is lymphoma (see above). Secondary or metastatic neoplasia may also occur in lymph nodes (**992**). Carcinomas, sarcomas, and other round-cell tumors, such as plasma cell myeloma, have all been reported to spread from primary sites to lymphatic tissue. Clinical signs often relate to organ dysfunction caused by the primary tumor. Neoplasia that has metastasized carries a very poor prognosis.

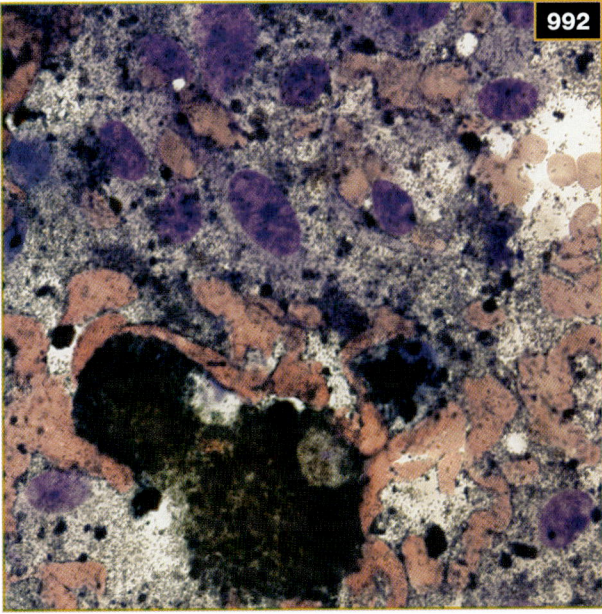

992 Fine-needle aspirate of a prescapular lymph node from a horse with metastatic malignant melanoma. The neoplastic cells have replaced the normal lymphocytic tissue. (Wright's stain) (Photo courtesy RM Jacobs)

Lymphadenitis

Definition/overview

Lymphadenitis is inflammation of lymph nodes or lymphocytic tissue in other organs such as the spleen, intestinal tract, and thymus. Lymphadenitis can be caused by infiltration of neutrophils, eosinophils, macrophages, lymphocytes, plasma cells, or a combination of these cell types. A common cause of retropharyngeal lymphadenitis and abscessation in horses is *Streptococcus equi* infection.

Etiology/pathophysiology

Inflammation of lymphocytic tissue can be initiated by various microbial organisms (bacteria, viruses, parasites, fungi), immune-mediated diseases, and neoplasia. The production of cytokines results in a chemotactic gradient that attracts inflammatory cells to the tissue. The etiologic agent, cytokine milieu, and chronicity of the process influence the populations of inflammatory cells that are present in the tissue.

Clinical presentation

Palpable lymph nodes are enlarged and may be warm and painful. Fever may be present. Other clinical signs may be present if the etiology of the inflammatory response induces pathology in other organs.

Differential diagnosis

Lymph-node enlargement due to inflammation must be differentiated from lymphocytic neoplasia and hyperplasia. The specific type of inflammation can usually be characterized based on cytologic or histologic observation of the populations of inflammatory cells present.

Diagnosis

Diagnosis is made by observing inflammation in aspiration or excisional biopsies of affected tissues.

Management

Lymphadenitis is frequently part of a systemic disease process. Treatment of the primary disease process (often with specific antimicrobials), in conjunction with anti-inflammatory drugs, should resolve the inflammation.

Prognosis

The prognosis depends on the ability to eliminate the inciting inflammatory stimulus.

Lymphocytic hyperplasia

Definition/overview

Lymphocytic hyperplasia, sometimes referred to as 'reactive' lymph node, refers to any lymphocytic tissue characterized by an increase in size of the node due to the presence of increased numbers of plasma cells and/or immature lymphocytes.

Etiology/pathophysiology

Lymphocytic hyperplasia has many causes and can include infectious, inflammatory, immune-mediated, and neoplastic disease.

Diverse disease processes result in the development of a lymphocyte-mediated immune response that is T cell and/or B cell mediated. Depending on the nature of the stimulus, lymphocytic hyperplasia can result in increases in immature lymphocytes and/or plasma cells.

Clinical presentation

Horses usually present with palpably enlarged lymph nodes, although any lymphocytic tissue can be affected. There are usually signs of systemic disease as well and these may include fever, lethargy, and anorexia.

Differential diagnosis

Other conditions to consider include lymphoma and lymphadenitis.

Diagnosis

Diagnosis is made by confirming the presence of increased numbers of immature lymphocytes and/or plasma cells on cytologic or histologic samples. There is usually a remaining heterogeneous mixture of lymphocytes, but it may be difficult to distinguish hyperplasia from lymphoma. Follicular architecture should be maintained in lymphocytic hyperplasia.

Management

Treatment of the underlying disease process is necessary for resolution of enlarged lymph nodes.

Prognosis

The prognosis depends on the ability to successfully treat the underlying disease process.

Hyperproteinemia

Hemoconcentration

Definition/overview
Hemoconcentration occurs because of loss of plasma volume due to dehydration, resulting in an apparent, or relative, increase in measured protein indices. Many equine diseases, especially those that cause diarrhea, may lead to excess loss of body fluids resulting in hemoconcentration.

Etiology/pathophysiology
Diseases in the horse that result in excess loss of body fluids can lead to dehydration and relative hyperproteinemia. Excess fluids can be lost with intestinal disease, renal disease, salivation, and sweating. Water restriction is a less common cause of hemoconcentration.

Hyperproteinemia is due to a decrease in plasma volume and not an increase in the production of proteins. Replacement of lost fluid volume restores the protein concentration to homeostatic levels.

Clinical presentation
Depending on the degree of clinical dehydration, hemoconcentrated horses may have prolonged tenting of skin, sunken eyeballs, and tacky mucous membranes. If serial weight measurements are being taken, weight loss is another clinical sign.

Differential diagnosis
Relative hyperproteinemia must be differentiated from pathologic causes for increased protein, which are usually due to an increase in globulins (see below).

Diagnosis
Relative hyperproteinemia is confirmed if the horse has clinical signs supportive of dehydration and biochemical or refractometric measurement of total protein concentration is increased.

Management
Hyperproteinemia from lost plasma volume is corrected by restoration of body volume via fluid therapy. Oral fluid therapy may be used in mild hemoconcentration, but intravenous administration of a balanced electrolyte solution is required in moderate to severe cases. The reason for the hemoconcentration needs to be addressed and ongoing fluid losses, if present, must be accounted for in the treatment plan. The underlying disease must be addressed appropriately.

Prognosis
The prognosis depends on the ability successfully to treat the underlying disease process that is causing excessive loss of fluids.

Hyperglobulinemia

Definition/overview
Hyperglobulinemia exists when there is a relative or absolute increase in the globulin fraction of total protein measurement. Globulins are not routinely measured directly, but are calculated as the remaining fraction after subtracting albumin from total protein concentration. Globulins are a diverse group of proteins that include acute-phase proteins, transport proteins, and immunoglobulins. The globulins are divided into alpha, beta, and gamma fractions based on electrophoretic separation.

Etiology/pathophysiology
Relative hyperglobulinemia can occur due to a decrease in plasma volume (usually because of dehydration), or there can be an absolute increase when production of one (a monoclonal gammopathy) or more (a polyclonal gammopathy) globulin proteins is increased. The occurrence of an absolute increase in globulins depends on the inciting stimulus. Chronic inflammatory disease results in increased production of many globulin proteins, creating a polyclonal gammopathy. Lymphocytic tumors, especially plasma cell tumors, have the capacity to produce excessive amounts of a single immunoglobulin clone, resulting in a monoclonal gammopathy (993).

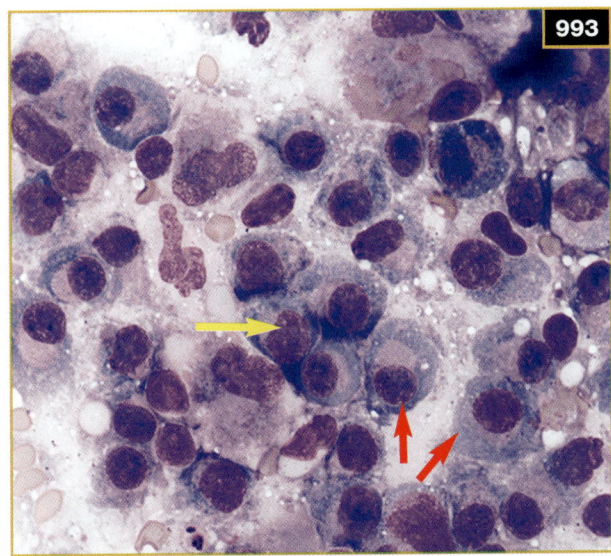

993 Fine-needle aspirate from a cutaneous mass in a horse with multiple myeloma and a monoclonal gammopathy. The red arrows indicate the monotypic population of plasma cells. The asterisk indicates the clear Golgi zone present in several of these cells. The yellow arrow indicates a single prominent nucleolus present in an atypical plasma cell. (Wright's stain)

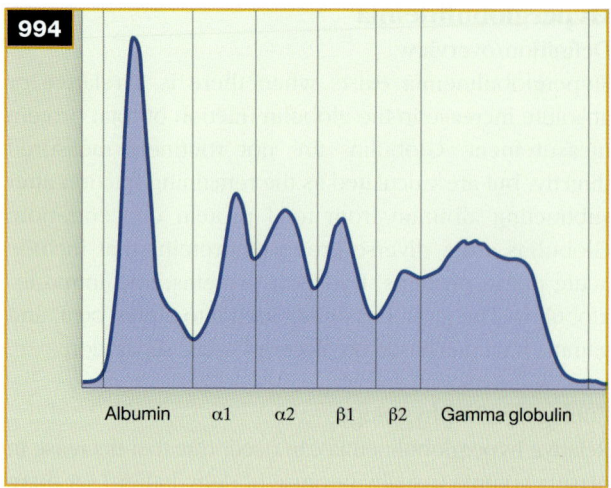

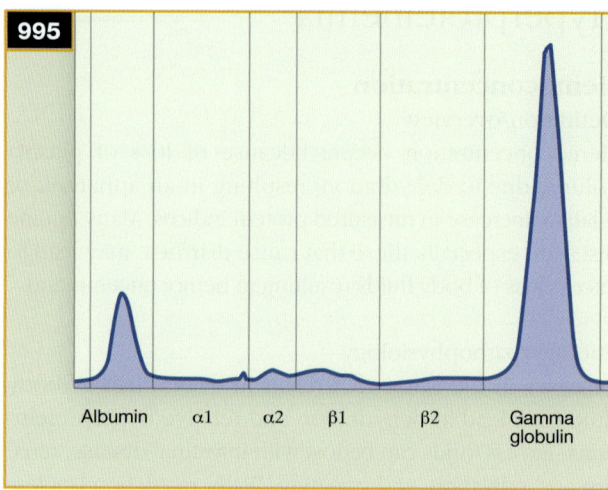

994 Serum protein electrophoresis. Polyclonal gammopathy (increase in alpha, beta, and gamma globulins). This is observed with chronic inflammation or infection.

995 Serum protein electrophoresis. Monoclonal gammopathy from a horse with B cell lymphoma. The sharp, narrow-based peak represents the clonal production of a single gamma globulin from the tumor cells.

Clinical presentation

The clinical signs vary with the cause of the hyperglobulinemia. Hyperglobulinemia itself, if severe enough, can cause sludging of blood flow to vital organs including the brain, heart, lungs, kidneys, and liver. Clinical signs related to dysfunction of these organs can be observed.

Differential diagnosis

All causes of hyperglobulinemia need to be considered and additional historical, clinical, and laboratory findings used to determine which is the cause in an individual animal.

Diagnosis

Diagnosis is made by demonstrating an increase in globulins using biochemical measurements of total protein and albumin concentration, followed by protein electrophoresis to determine if globulins are polyclonal or monoclonal in nature (994, 995). Relative hyperglobulinemia is usually accompanied by hyperalbuminemia and clinical signs of dehydration.

Management

The underlying disorder responsible for increased globulin production must be identified and treated to resolve the hyperglobulinemia.

Prognosis

The prognosis for relative hyperglobulinemia is good if lost fluids can be replaced. Other causes are more difficult to treat, especially neoplasia.

Splenic diseases

The spleen is an important organ that filters the blood, acts as a secondary lymph organ, serves as a reservoir of RBCs, WBCs, and platelets, and is a location for extramedullary hematopoiesis. In normal animals the size of the spleen is highly variable. On average, the spleen weighs approximately 1 kg and has a somewhat smooth surface. Ultrasonographically, the spleen has a relatively homogeneous character (996). Disorders of the spleen are uncommon.

Splenic rupture

Definition/overview
Rupture of the spleen is an uncommon condition in the horse that can be life-threatening because of the potential for severe intra-abdominal hemorrhage.

Etiology/pathophysiology
Splenic rupture most often occurs secondary to trauma, such as from a kick over the left abdominal wall. Rupture of a splenic hematoma, tumor, or abscess may also occur. Idiopathic splenic rupture has been reported.

Trauma to the abdominal wall overlying the spleen may cause laceration of the spleen and associated large blood vessels (997). Bleeding may be contained within the splenic capsule if minor, but significant trauma may cause splenic rupture and hemorrhage into the abdominal cavity. Severe blood loss can occur rapidly, resulting in hemorrhagic shock and potentially death. Clinical signs may be apparent with acute loss of 30% of blood volume. Acute loss of 40% of blood volume may cause ataxia or unconsciousness, while loss of 50% of blood volume usually results in death.

Clinical presentation
Clinical signs will depend on the amount of hemorrhage that has occurred. Mild bleeding may be inapparent or interpreted as mild colic. In more severe cases, tachycardia, tachypnea, weakness, pale mucous membranes, cold extremities, and abdominal distension may be observed as a consequence of hemorrhagic shock. A systolic hemodynamic heart murmur may be present. While signs similar to those of colic may be observed, the degree of pain does not correspond with the severity of other clinical signs, especially the elevation in heart rate.

Differential diagnosis
Colic of GI origin, peritonitis, septicemia, endotoxemia, and a variety of intoxications should be considered.

Diagnosis
Physical examination findings may be nonspecific unless gross abdominal distension is apparent. Evidence of hypovolemic/hemorrhagic shock of unknown origin, particularly with a history of recent trauma, suggests splenic rupture. Ultrasonographic examination of the abdomen should be performed. The volume and character of the abdominal fluid should be examined. Free blood is typically homogeneously hyperechoic, with a swirling character. The spleen should be examined carefully for changes in architecture as well as the presence of masses; however, the site of trauma is not usually identified.

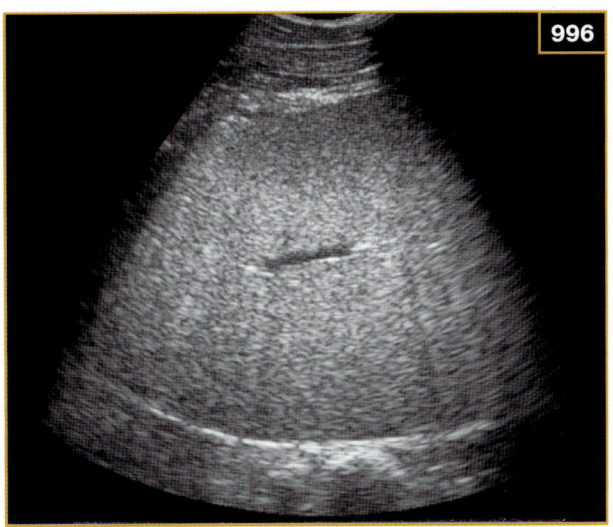

996 Ultrasonographic appearance of a normal spleen.

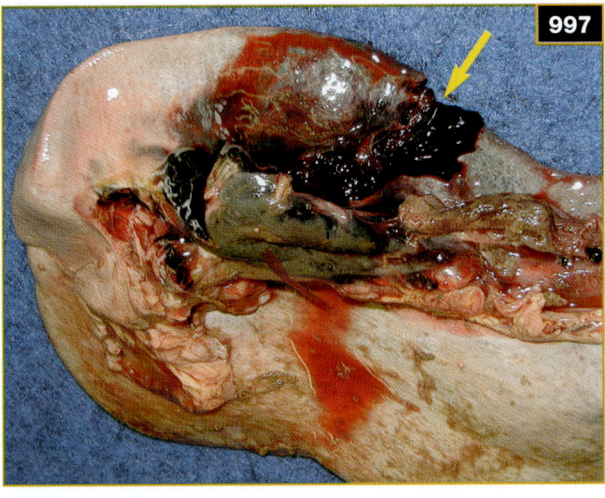

997 Splenic laceration in a foal, caused by a kick.

Other abdominal organs should be examined as possible sources of blood loss. Abdominocentesis is used to confirm the presence of blood in the abdomen. Ultrasonographic guidance is useful to avoid splenic puncture and misinterpretation of results. If only a small volume of blood is obtained on abdominocentesis and ultrasonography has not been performed, the possibility of laceration of a body wall blood vessel or splenic puncture should be considered, as opposed to hemoabdomen. Cytologic analysis is not usually able to differentiate blood contamination from hemoabdomen after acute hemorrhage. Centrifugation of the sample may be useful because plasma will often be hemolyzed with hemoabdomen but not with blood contamination. Hematology is not useful in acute hemorrhage because blood, protein, and fluid are lost concurrently. Over time, anemia and hypoproteinemia will be present, particularly if fluid therapy is provided.

Management

The treatment plan depends on the cause and severity of the bleeding and the severity of the clinical signs. Fluid therapy should be provided, particularly if hemorrhagic shock is present. Intravenous administration of a balanced electrolyte solution should be started initially at a volume of three times the estimated blood loss. Hypertonic (5–7%) saline may be useful initially, particularly when large volumes of fluids are not readily available. Hypertonic saline must be followed by administration of isotonic fluids. Synthetic colloids may inhibit platelet aggregation and alter coagulation, and should be avoided. A blood transfusion should be considered with signs of shock (i.e. heart rate >80 bpm, weakness, severe hypotension) or if the PCV is <0.2 l/l (20%) with acute bleeding. Alternatively, bovine-source polymerized hemoglobin products (i.e. Oxyglobin™, 7.5–10 ml/kg i/v at up to 10 ml/kg/hour) may be used; however, this is expensive in an adult horse. Surgical intervention may need to be considered with severe, uncontrolled bleeding, but in such cases, horses are usually an anesthetic risk. Emergency stabilization must be performed prior to surgery. A variety of methods of decreasing intra-abdominal hemorrhage have been attempted, including administration of venodilatory drugs, antifibrinolytic agents (aminocaproic acid), opioid antagonists (naloxone), and buffered formalin. There is little to no objective evidence supporting these treatments and each has potential adverse effects.

Prognosis

If bleeding can be controlled, the prognosis is good with trauma-associated splenic rupture. The prognosis is poor if rupture is from splenic neoplasia.

Splenomegaly

Definition/overview

Splenomegaly is the presence of an abnormally large spleen. It is a difficult condition to diagnose because of the inherent variability in spleen size in healthy animals. The clinical significance of apparent splenomegaly is often unclear.

Etiology/pathophysiology

Splenomegaly may be caused by obstruction of venous return (e.g. nephrosplenic entrapment of the large colon, right heart failure), acute splenitis, hemolytic anemia, purpura hemorrhagica, infiltrative disease (i.e. neoplasia), or infarction.

Cellular infiltration, congestion, and inflammation may result in an increase in splenic size.

Clinical presentation

The clinical signs are highly variable, depending on the cause. They may range from inapparent to signs of colic, anorexia, icterus, depression, weight loss, pyrexia, ventral edema, and tachycardia. In general, obstruction of venous return by left colon displacement will be manifested as acute colic. Acute splenitis will cause fever, mild colic, and potentially tachycardia. Signs of hemolytic anemia have been discussed earlier in this chapter. Splenic neoplasia is discussed below.

Differential diagnosis

A wide range of differential diagnoses must be considered, depending on the cause of the splenomegaly.

Diagnosis

Depending on the clinical presentation, an evaluation of localized and systemic infection, neoplasia, hemolytic anemia, and colic should be performed. Hematology results are highly variable, depending on the cause. Ultrasonography is used to assess splenic size and architecture. Palpation per rectum should be performed to assess spleen size, location, and texture. The presence of an irregular surface or masses should be evaluated.

Management

Treatment is variable, depending on the inciting cause, which should be addressed, if possible. Successful treatment of primary splenomegaly with splenectomy has been reported.

Prognosis

The prognosis is good with nephrosplenic entrapment of the large colon, but guarded with other causes. The prognosis with neoplasia is poor because advanced disease is usually present by the time it is diagnosed.

Splenic neoplasia

Definition/overview

Splenic neoplasia may be primary or secondary. It is uncommon in the horse.

Etiology/pathophysiology

Splenic lymphoma is most common, although melanoma and hemangiosarcoma have also been reported. Lymphoma can occur in horses of any age, but is more common in horses 2–8 years of age. Splenic tumors may be primary or secondary (metastatic).

Clinical presentation

Weight loss, intermittent colic, depression, and anorexia may be the initial signs. If splenic neoplasia is secondary, clinical signs relating to the location of the primary tumor may be present.

Differential diagnosis

The vague clinical signs mean that a number of other diseases must be considered. If a splenic abnormality can be visualized or palpated, splenic abscess or splenic hematoma should be considered.

Diagnosis

Hypoproteinemia is common but nonspecific. Serum IgM may be low, but this is an inconsistent finding. Anemia of inflammatory disease or IMHA may be present. An irregular or enlarged spleen may be palpable per rectum. The spleen can be visualized ultrasonographically over the caudal left abdomen. Depending on the type of neoplasia, increased echogenicity, abnormal shape, or the presence of focal masses may be evident (**998**). Abdominocentesis should be performed, but it is uncommon to identify neoplastic cells cytologically due to poor exfoliation. A fine-needle aspirate may be diagnostic. Ultrasonographic guidance is preferred because of the high vascularity of the spleen and the potential for focal or multifocal lesions. Splenic biopsy can be performed, but presents a higher risk for hemorrhage. Laparoscopy can also be used to visualize the spleen and obtain diagnostic samples.

If splenic neoplasia is considered, a thorough diagnostic work-up should be considered to identify the primary location (if present) and determine whether additional metastatic lesions are present.

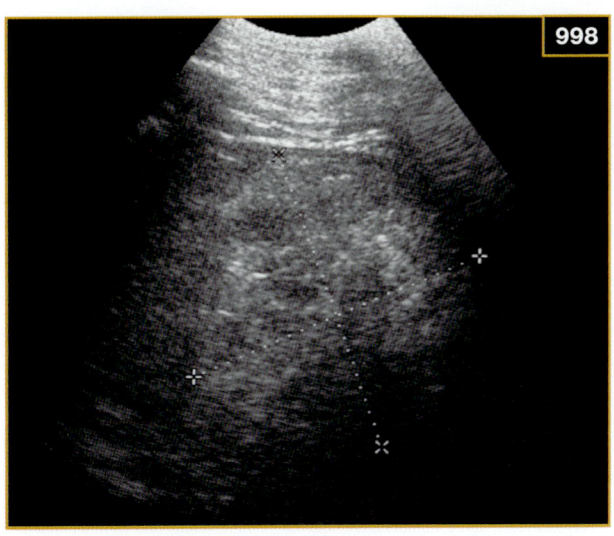

998 Transabdominal ultrasound image of a splenic lymphoma. Note the large splenic mass delineated by the caliper marks.

Management

By the time splenic neoplasia is diagnosed, advanced disease is usually present. Tumors are usually present in other locations, therefore splenectomy is rarely a viable option. If a solitary tumor with no evidence of metastasis, primary disease, or significant abdominal adhesions is identified, splenectomy could be considered. Chemotherapeutic agents have not been adequately evaluated and are cost prohibitive in most situations. Dexamethasone (40 mg i/m q4days for 4 weeks, tapered over time) has been used with anecdotal success for short-term palliation in splenic lymphoma.

Prognosis

The prognosis for splenic neoplasia is grave. A diagnosis is often not made until late in the disease and treatment is usually unrewarding.

10

Nervous system

Siobhan McAuliffe and Nathan Slovis

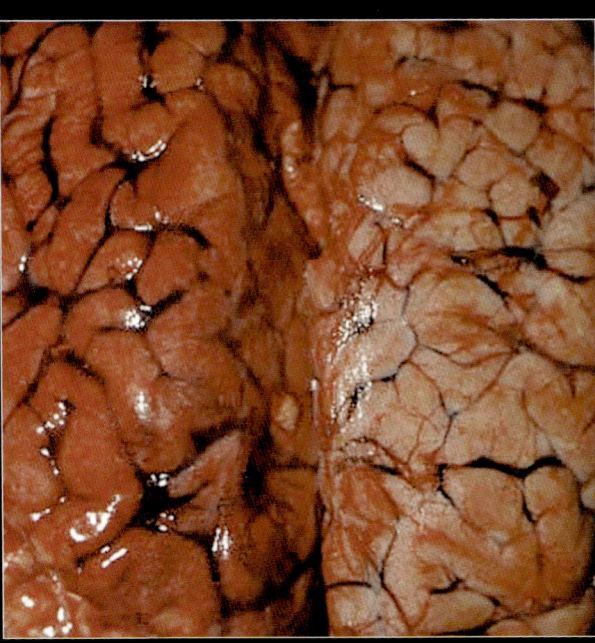

Nervous system

Neurologic examination

The aim of the neurologic examination is to determine if a neurologic disorder exists and, if so, where the lesion or lesions is/are located. Lesion location determines the differential diagnoses and allows formulation of a diagnostic plan. Several important components of the neurologic examination, such as behavior, mental status, head posture, vision, pupillary light reflexes (PLRs), and inspection for muscular symmetry, can be noted in the general physical examination that should precede the detailed neurologic examination. A thorough physical examination is important, as disease of other systems or organs may account for the neurologic signs that are seen (e.g. hepatoencephalopathy) or may take precedence for diagnosis or treatment (e.g. shock). The neurologic examination should be performed as a systematic search for defects and asymmetries. The exact order of the examination is not important, but a common principle is to start at the head and progress caudally to the tail. Procedures that may cause pain, such as spinal palpation, should be left until last. The sequence of the neurologic examination is as follows: head (behavior, mental status, head posture and coordination, cranial nerves); gait and posture; neck and forelimbs; back and hindlimbs; tail and perineum.

Behavior

The owner should be questioned about the patient's behavior and response patterns. In addition, the owner should be questioned to determine if there has been progression of the syndrome over time. Most congenital disorders are evident early in life and are progressive, whereas those related to physical injury have a sudden onset and may stabilize or improve. The patient's age, breed, or sex may influence its behavior. A horse that is recumbent as a result of cervical spinal cord or musculoskeletal disease will not have altered behavior unless it becomes frantic in its struggling, dehydrated, exhausted, or frightened.

Close observation may be required to detect seizures. A seizure is a manifestation of cerebral cortex dysfunction characterized by altered behavior, states of consciousness, and/or involuntary motor activities. A seizure may be generalized, focal, or focal with secondary generalization. Generalized seizures are commonly characterized by complete loss of consciousness and variable degrees of involuntary motor activity including flailing of limbs, passage of urine and feces, nystagmus, and vocalization. Focal seizures can take two forms. The first is characterized by localized involuntary movements and may not be accompanied by an obvious alteration of consciousness. The second may result in momentary lapses of consciousness without collapse or significant motor activity. A focal seizure with secondary generalization has a focal onset, but subsequent seizure activity spreads throughout the cerebral cortex, resulting in generalized signs. These animals may show initial head turning or focal tremors, followed by a loss of consciousness and generalized involuntary motor activity.

Bizarre and inappropriate behaviors, such as head pressing, licking objects, or compulsive wandering, may be associated with cerebral disease and are easy to recognize. Animals with cerebral lesions that circle have a tendency to circle towards the side of the lesion.

Mental status

Mental status is assessed based on the patient's level of consciousness or awareness. The animal's responsiveness to the internal and external environment is affected by the cerebral cortex and the ascending reticular activating system (ARAS). These can be affected by stimuli from the sensory nervous system and thus responses to sensory stimuli should be considered (e.g. visual, tactile, auditory, painful). Loss of awareness can be described as depression, lethargy, somnolence, obtundation, and stupor. The most profound loss of awareness is described as coma. This is a state of complete unresponsiveness to noxious stimuli. The deepest comas are usually related to brainstem, particularly midbrain, lesions.

Head posture and coordination

Normal animals maintain their heads in a certain posture and are capable of quick and smooth head movement. The most obvious abnormality of head posture is head tilt or turn. Unilateral, mild central and peripheral vestibular lesions frequently result in a head tilt that is characterized by a laterally deviated poll, with the caudal neck and muzzle remaining on the midline. The head tilt in this case is described by the direction of the poll deviation (999). A horse with a cerebral lesion that continually turns in circles often has the head and neck deviated to one side, but the head itself is not tilted. A severe unilateral vestibular lesion can result in a marked head tilt in addition to a head and neck turn, both usually away from the side of the lesion. Bilateral peripheral vestibular disease can result in wide swinging movements of the head and neck.

The cerebellum acts to modulate movements of the head, neck, and limbs. Fine control of head positioning and movement is often lost, with cerebellar disease resulting in awkward jerky movements and head tremor that is

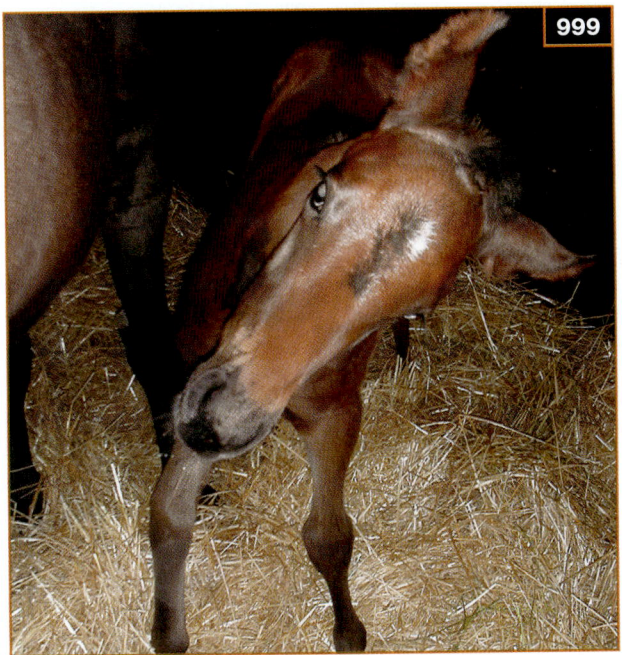

999 Three-week-old foal with a left-sided head tilt secondary to trauma. The foal was diagnosed with vestibular disease secondary to hemorrhage within the petrous temporal bone.

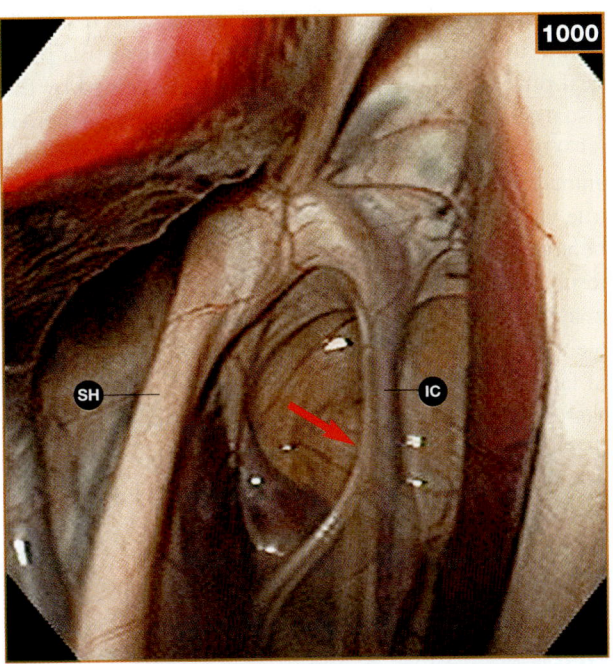

1000 Normal guttural pouch; medial compartment. The glossopharyngeal (CN IX), vagus (CN X), and hypoglossal (CN XII) nerves (arrow) lie caudomedial to the internal carotid artery (IC). The stylohyoid bone (SH) separates the medial compartment from the smaller lateral compartment.

seen at rest. Increasing voluntary effort exaggerates the abnormality and the resulting fine, jerky movements of the head are called an intention tremor. Such animals frequently have difficulty with head positioning when performing acts such as prehension, and often 'overshoot'.

Cranial nerves

Cranial nerve (CN) examination assists in localizing a lesion near or within the brainstem. The examination should start with the most rostral nerve and proceed caudally. Generally, the more distal a CN lesion, the fewer clinical signs are seen, and when more than one CN is involved, a more central lesion is likely. The anatomic relationship of CN nuclei and their peripheral pathways should be considered when interpreting findings. The cell bodies of CNs III (oculomotor), IV (trochlear), V (trigeminal), and VI (abducens) are closely related in the brain and, at their points of exit, form the cranial vault. CNs VII (facial) and VIII (vestibulocochlear) are closely related at their point of exit from the cranium and are frequently damaged by disorders of the petrous temporal bone, with which they are closely related. CNs IX (glossopharyngeal),

X (vagus), XI (accessory), and XII (hypoglossal) are found in close association adjacent to the dorsal wall of the medial compartment of the guttural pouch (**1000**).

Olfactory (CN I)

Clinical deficit of smell (anosmia) is difficult to assess and is more frequently caused by disease within the nasal passages rather than by a cranial nerve lesion. A crude estimation is the patient's ability to smell and track feed. Irritating substances such as ammonia should not be used to determine sense of smell, as these stimulate nociceptors in the nasal mucosa, which are the dendrites of the maxillary nerve (CN V).

Optic (CN II)

Vision is the function of CN II. A good initial assessment is the animal's response to its environment (e.g. walking into objects). Depressed patients or those with vestibular disease (loss of balance) may be incorrectly reported as blind by their owners because they may stumble over objects. The visual pathway can be indirectly tested by the menace response. The hand is moved rapidly toward the

747

eye in a threatening gesture (1001, 1002). This results in eyelid closure and the head may be jerked away. For practical purposes the vision in one eye is perceived by the visual cortex of the contralateral cerebral cortex, as there is 80–90% crossing of optic fibers at the optic chiasma. Some animals may not respond to a menace response test and a true visual deficiency may be detected by observing their behavior in a maze test. Menace deficit can also be the result of facial nerve paralysis. In these cases the animal is unable to blink, but usually will show avoidance movements of the head. Such animals will also have other signs of facial nerve involvement (e.g. facial drooping on the same side). Animals with cerebellar disease may also display a menace deficit, yet possess normal vision. The precise mechanism by which the cerebellum affects this pathway is not known, but is thought to involve UMN

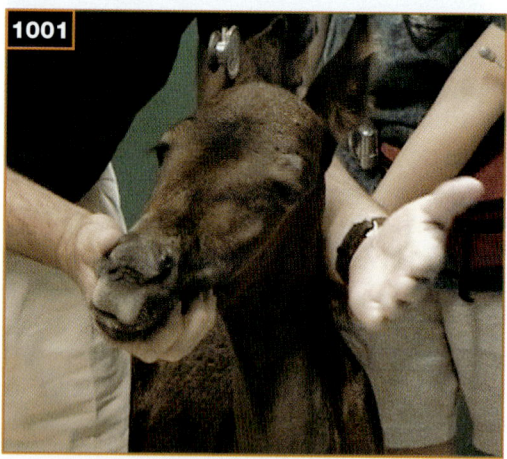

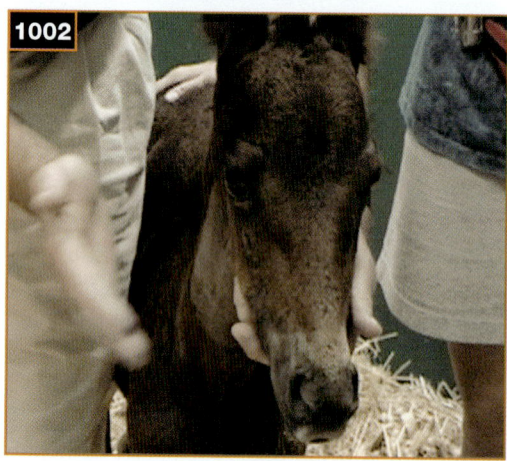

1001, 1002 (1001) Two-week-old foal with dementia and normal menace response in the left eye. (1002) Same foal with no menace response to the right eye. The foal was also noted continually to circle to the left. The foal was diagnosed with a left-sided cortical lesion. (Photos courtesy FT Bain)

control of the facial nerve. These animals retain visual acuity and will be able to perform a maze test. The motor component is mediated through the facial nerve and its nucleus is in the medulla. The afferent side of the response is extensive and involves a cerebral pathway, which implies a learned response. It is usually present by 5–7 days of age in foals. Therefore, testing the menace response in a neonatal foal will be unrewarding.

Unilateral blindness (hemianopia) can be difficult to assess, and it may take repeated efforts, such as blindfolding each eye in turn, to detect it.

An ophthalmologic examination should be included in the neurologic examination. Lesions of the eye and optic nerve result in ipsilateral blindness. Lesions of the optic tracts and lateral geniculate nucleus cause contralateral blindness. Space-occupying lesions of the brain frequently produce blindness by either direct involvement of the visual pathways or pressure of the mass and cerebral edema forcing the occipital lobes caudally. The resultant blindness is contralateral to the lesion, but often bilateral because of associated diffuse brain swelling.

Oculomotor (CN III)

The diameter of the pupillary aperture is controlled by two muscle groups, the constrictor muscles of the pupil, which are innervated by the parasympathetic fibers in the oculomotor nerve, and dilator muscles of the pupil, which are innervated by the sympathetic fibers from the cranial cervical ganglion. These autonomic innervations originate in the brainstem and change pupil diameter in response to light (oculomotor) and fear or excitement (sympathetic). The response of the pupils to light directed into the eye should be noted. The normal response to light directed into one eye is constriction of both pupils. This is as a result of a direct response in the ipsilateral or illuminated eye and an indirect response in the contralateral or non-illuminated eye. Response to this test should take into account the ambient light and emotional status of the animal. It may be necessary to decrease the ambient light to allow for pupillary dilation before this test is performed.

The PLR occurs within the brainstem and thus is not affected by lesions in the visual cortex. Thus, a widely dilated (mydriatic) pupil that is unresponsive to direct light in an eye with normal vision suggests an oculomotor lesion. If the contralateral eye has normal oculomotor function, it will respond to both ipsilateral (direct) and contralateral (indirect) illumination. A retrobulbar lesion involving the optic and oculomotor nerves will appear as a mydriatic pupil unresponsive to light shone in either eye, in addition to a menace deficit.

The oculomotor nerves can be damaged by edema and space-occupying lesions in the forebrain, resulting in pressure ventrally on the brainstem. Asymmetric swelling of cerebral tissue may exert greater pressure on one nerve, causing unequal pupil size (anisocoria). Severe brainstem lesions can produce pupillary abnormalities in association with changes in mental status such as coma. Progressive, bilateral pupillary dilation in a recumbent patient warrants a grave prognosis.

Oculomotor (CN III), trochlear (CN IV), abducens (CN VI)

In addition to innervation of pupillary constrictor muscles, the oculomotor nerve, in combination with the trochlear and abducens nerves, also innervates extraocular muscles, thus controlling the position of the globe. Dysfunction of these nerves results in deviation of the globe that is constant in all head positions:

- ✦ Oculomotor dysfunction results in a ventrolateral strabismus.
- ✦ Trochlear nerve dysfunction results in a dorsomedial strabismus. It should be noted that trochlear nerve lesions can result in ipsilateral or contralateral strabismus, depending on the location of the lesion in the brainstem, as the trochlear nerve crosses the midline twice in the area of the midbrain before exiting the cranial vault.
- ✦ Abducens nerve dysfunction results in medial strabismus and an inability to retract the globe, which is best assessed by applying a tactile stimulus to the cornea.

When determining the function of these nerves, consideration should also be given to normal responses of the eyes to head posture and movement. When the head is elevated, the eyes tend to remain horizontal and thus move ventrally in the orbits. When the head is moved from side to side, the eyes do not stay fixed but move rhythmically, with a slow phase movement in the direction opposite to the direction of the head, followed by a fast phase movement in the direction of the head. When the head ceases to move, the eyes return to the center of the orbits. These eye movements are regarded as normal vestibular nystagmus and result from the connection between the vestibular nuclei and those of the three CNs controlling eye movement (III, IV, and VI). It can therefore be deduced that normal vestibular nystagmus requires an intact vestibular system, intact CNs III, IV, and VI, and an intact connection between them. Lesions of the vestibular system can result in abnormal eye position (strabismus) or movement (nystagmus). Vestibular lesions can also result in a strabismus that changes when the head and neck are moved rather than the constant deviation that is seen with direct lesions to CNs III, IV, and VI. In addition, vestibular dysfunction also results in spontaneous nystagmus.

Congenitally blind horses may have abnormal globe position and movement, and periorbital lesions often cause mechanical globe deviations.

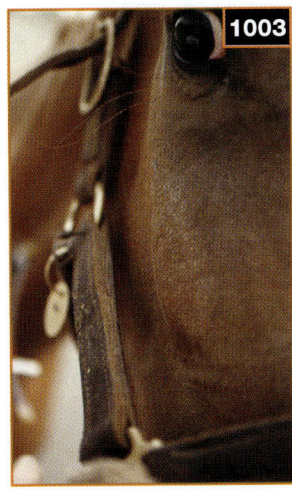

1003 Unilateral masseter muscle atrophy in a horse with equine protozoal myelitis.

Trigeminal (CN V)

The trigeminal nerve provides sensation to the face through all three branches (mandibular, maxillary, and ophthalmic) and motor stimulus to the muscles of mastication via the mandibular branch. Sensory functions are assessed by lightly stimulating the skin of the face using a closed hemostat or fingers. Some areas, such as the periorbital region, nasal planum, and lips, are more sensitive than others. Lightly brushing the ears, eyelids, external nares, and lips results in movement that is mediated through the sensory branches of the trigeminal nerve and motor branches of the facial nerve. These reflexes thus require an intact brainstem and trigeminal and facial nuclei, but do not require the animal to be consciously aware of the stimulus. Unilateral loss of facial sensation most commonly results from damage to the peripheral portion of the trigeminal nerve, the trigeminal ganglion in the petrosal bone of the skull, or the contralateral cerebral cortex. Lesions affecting the spinal tract of the trigeminal nerve in the medulla and midbrain tend to be fatal, as they usually affect the adjacent cardiovascular and respiratory centers in the brainstem. Patients with bilateral facial hypoesthesia most likely have bilateral cerebral cortex disease.

Loss of motor function of the mandibular nerve bilaterally results in a dropped jaw and inability to chew. The tongue may appear to protrude as it moves rostrally in the mouth, but it can be retracted normally when stimulated. Animals with dropped jaws also exhibit sialosis as a result of a lack of jaw movement. Unilateral lesions of the trigeminal nerve produce asymmetric jaw closure, with a slight gap between the occlusal surfaces of the teeth on the affected side; however, it is the accompanying muscle atrophy that is usually most apparent (**1003**).

Facial (CN VII)

The facial nerve provides motor innervation to the muscles of facial expression. The facial nerve is the motor pathway for many of the reflexes that have already been tested in the neurologic examination. General inspection for facial symmetry is useful, but some animals may have a subtle deviation of the nostrils or muzzle to one side. Comparison of tone in the ears, lips, eyelids, muzzle, and nostrils on each side may aid in detecting subtle weakness. Facial paralysis is generally seen as a drooping of the ear and lips, with retraction of the nose toward the unaffected side (1004). There may also be tongue protrusion from the unaffected side. In chronic paralysis the face may be deviated towards the affected side because of atrophy and contracture of the denervated musculature. Ptosis of the upper eyelid occurs as a result of paralysis of one of the muscles that raise the upper lid. Lesions of the middle and inner ear causing vestibular signs often have accompanying facial paralysis. This is because the facial nerve lies in the petrous temporal bone and is separated from the tympanic cavity of the middle ear by only a thin membrane.

Some cerebral and focal thalamic lesions may result in hypertonia and hyperreflexia of facial muscles, resulting in 'grimacing'. This can occur spontaneously or may be reflex initiated. It occurs because of involvement of the higher motor centers of UMNs controlling facial movement that normally have an inhibitory effect on the facial muscles. Grimacing can also be caused by irritative lesions such as peracute encephalitides.

Vestibulocochlear (CN VIII)

The auditory or cochlear division of this nerve is responsible for the sense of hearing. Bilateral middle ear disease can cause deafness, but unilateral hearing loss is difficult to detect.

The vestibular system comprises the sensory structures in the inner ear (semicircular canals, utricles, and saccules), the vestibular portion of CN VIII, and the central components of the vestibular system in the medulla oblongata and cerebellum. The vestibular system controls orientation of the head, body, limbs, and eyes in space with respect to gravity and motion. Dysfunction of the vestibular system results in signs such as a staggering gait, circling, falling, head tilt (1005), and spontaneous nystagmus. Signs of vestibular disease can be classified as peripheral, central, or paradoxical. Peripheral lesions affect the inner ear or CN VIII; central lesions affect vestibular structures in the medulla oblongata; paradoxical lesions affect the vestibular structures in the cerebellum. The direction of nystagmus may help in determining the site of the lesion and is always described by referring to the fast phase. In peripheral vestibular disorders the nystagmus (fast phase) is always directed away from the side of the lesion, and thus the side of the head tilt, and is usually horizontal. Central vestibular disorders result in spontaneous and positional nystagmus, which can be horizontal, vertical, or rotary and may change direction with changes in head posture. Central lesions can affect adjacent structures such as the reticular formation and pathways for voluntary limb movement, resulting in concomitant depression and ataxia. Blindfolding affected animal results in a worsening of clinical signs due to the removal of compensatory mechanisms from the optic centers (1006). Recumbent animals with vestibular lesions tend to lie with the side of the lesion down and may resist attempts to turn them. When turned, many of these animals spontaneously rotate back to the lesion-down position. Such animals may experience great difficulty in rising. Signs of peripheral vestibular disease often improve markedly within several days as the patient accommodates.

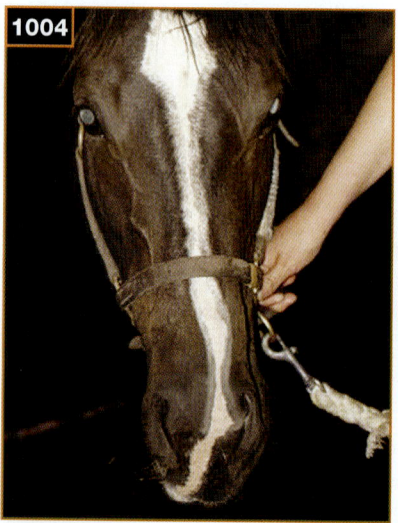

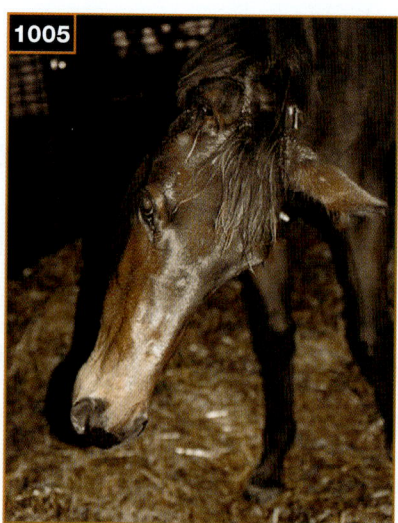

1004 Left-sided facial nerve injury. Note how the muzzle is deviated to the unaffected side (right).

1005 Horse with head tilt to the left secondary to trauma on the left aspect of the calvarium.

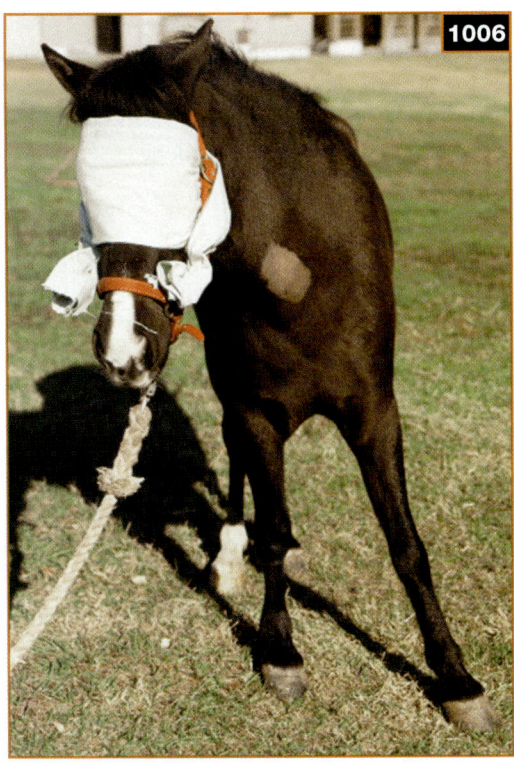

1006 Blindfolding of a horse with exaggeration of vestibular disease. Note the leaning to the right.

Glossopharyngeal (CN IX), vagus (CN X), accessory (CN XI)

The major function of these three nerves is the innervation of the pharynx and larynx with sensory and motor fibers. The most important clinical sign associated with lesions of these CNs is paralysis of the pharynx and larynx, with the severity of signs depending on whether lesions are unilateral or bilateral. The function of these nerves can be tested by listening for normal laryngeal sounds (laryngeal hemiplegia results in 'roaring'), observing normal swallowing, and inspection of the pharynx and larynx with an endoscope if necessary. The 'slap test' is a test of function of vagal innervation of the larynx. It is performed by slapping the skin in the area of the withers (caudal to the dorsal scapula) while the larynx is observed with an endoscope or the dorsolateral larynx is palpated. The normal response is for the contralateral arytenoid cartilage to adduct briefly, resulting in a palpable twitch at the laryngeal musculature. The afferent pathway is via segmental thoracic nerves, cranially via the contralateral cervical spinal cord white matter, and finally to the contralateral vagal nucleus in the medulla oblongata. The efferent pathway is via the vagus nerve to the cranial thorax, then back up the neck via the recurrent laryngeal nerve to the larynx. This reflex can be interrupted at any of these sites.

Many severe, diffuse brain diseases may cause dysphagia with an absence of lesions in the medulla oblongata. This is a result of disruption of higher motor control of swallowing. Dysphagia can also be seen with diffuse LMN and neuromuscular paralysis (e.g. botulism).

The accessory nerve provides the motor supply to at least part of the trapezius, the cranial part of the sternocephalicus, and the brachiocephalicus muscles. Signs of dysfunction are rare.

Hypoglossal (CN XII)

The hypoglossal nerve provides motor innervation to the muscles of the tongue and the geniohyoideus muscle. The function of this nerve is tested by examining the tongue for symmetry and normal movement. A normal horse will resist its tongue being withdrawn from the mouth. A unilateral lesion usually results in unilateral atrophy and weak retraction, although the tongue does not usually protrude from the mouth. If retracted, however, it may stay out. Bilateral involvement interferes with prehension and swallowing, with protrusion of the tongue and an inability to draw it back into the mouth. Severe cerebral lesions may result in tongue protrusion and slow retraction as a result of interference with voluntary control pathways. An example of this is the impaired tongue, jaw, and lip movement seen with the UMN (basal nuclei) lesion in nigropallidal encephalomalacia (yellow star thistle poisoning, see p. 790).

Gait and posture

Evaluation of the gait acts as a general assessment of brainstem, cerebellum, spinal cord, peripheral nerve, and muscle function. Firstly, it determines which limbs have an abnormal gait, and secondly, whether there is any apparent musculoskeletal abnormality. Differentiation of neurologic versus musculoskeletal lesions may be difficult. Gait abnormalities can present as weakness (interruption of motor pathways) or ataxia (interruption of proprioceptive sensory pathways). Ataxia can be further characterized as hypometria or hypermetria. Gait evaluation should be carried out while the animal is walking, trotting, turning tightly, and backing. Evaluation of more involved tasks, such as walking up and down a slope, walking with the neck extended, walking blindfolded, and running free in a field, is also useful. More subtle signs that would not normally be apparent may appear as consistent mistakes when performing these more involved tasks or when the horse becomes fatigued.

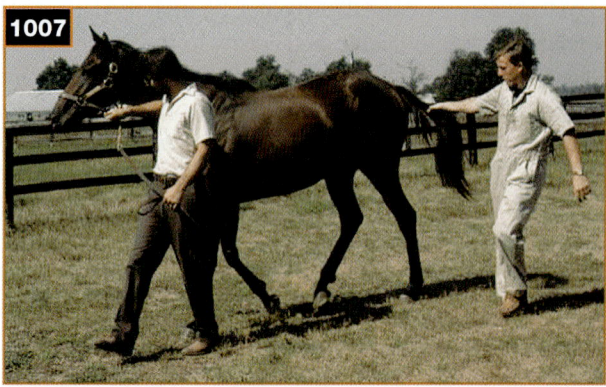

1007 Tail pull to assess weakness in the pelvic limbs. (Photo courtesy TD Byars)

Weakness

UMN lesions can cause flexor weakness in the limbs on the same side and caudal to the lesion. This weakness is evident as limb dragging, worn hooves, and a low arc to the swing phase of the stride. Weight bearing on a weak limb may result in trembling or collapse of that limb. When performing more involved tasks, the animal may stumble on a weak limb and knuckle over at the fetlock. Weakness in the hindlimbs can be assessed by pulling the tail laterally while the animal is walking to determine the degree of resistance (**1007**). Animals with UMN weakness can be pulled over while walking, but they resist strongly (extensor thrust reflex) when pulled while standing square.

Severe weakness in all four limbs without ataxia and spasticity suggests neuromuscular disease. Profound weakness in one limb is suggestive of a peripheral nerve or LMN (muscle) lesion in that limb. Peracute peripheral vestibular syndrome may result in apparent weakness in the limbs on the same side as the lesion because of the tendency to fall in that direction.

Ataxia

Ataxia is incordination and is seen as a swaying of the pelvis, trunk, and even the whole body, or as a weaving of the affected limb during the swing phase. It is an unconscious general proprioceptive deficit that results in poor coordination during movement. Ataxia results in crossing of the limbs, stepping on the opposite foot, and abducted or adducted foot placement, especially while the animal is turning tightly. Circumduction of the outside limbs when turning and circling is also regarded as a proprioceptive deficit. Tightly turning a weak and ataxic animal results in the affected limb being left in place, with the animal pivoting around it. When required to stop suddenly, ataxic animals often adopt an abnormal stance (**1008**).

Hypermetria

Hypermetria is defined as exaggerated movement and range of motion. Overreaching of the limbs and excessive joint movement are seen. It is prominent in cerebellar disease and some peripheral nerve disorders.

Hypometria

Hypometria means decreased movement and range of motion. It is evident as a stiff or spastic gait in which there is little joint flexion. The lack of flexion is usually most notable in the carpal and tarsal joints. This can be seen best by backing the animal or walking up a slope with the head elevated.

Grading gait abnormalities

Grading the degree of weakness, ataxia, hypometria, or hypermetria for each limb is important, especially in terms of determining improvement at subsequent examinations. An arbitrary scale of 0 to 5 has been described, but like many grading systems it is subject to variability depending on the examiner (*Table 49*).

A grading system can also help localize a lesion. For example, compressive lesions in the cranial cervical spinal cord (C1–C6) generally result in neurologic signs that are one grade more severe in the hindlimbs than in the fore-limbs, although they can be of the same grade.

Severe hindlimb signs (grade 3+ or 4+) without any detectable abnormality in the forelimbs is consistent with a thoracolumbar spinal cord lesion. Such signs in the hindlimbs when accompanied by mild forelimb signs (grade1+) could represent a severe thoracolumbar lesion plus a mild cervical lesion, a focal cervical lesion or even

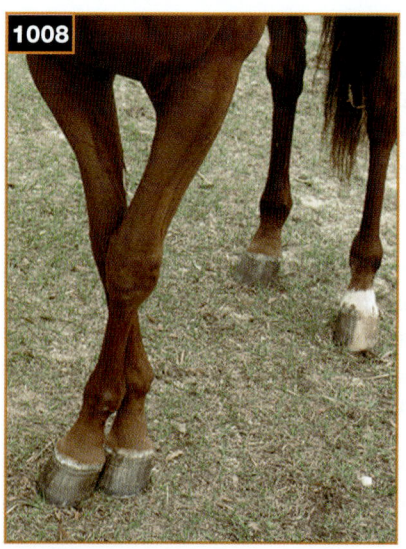

1008 Ataxia secondary to proprioceptive deficits in both of the forelimbs. This animal was diagnosed with cervical vertebral instability.

TABLE 49 System for grading of neurologic gait deficits

GRADE	DESCRIPTION
0	No gait deficit.
1	Deficit barely detectable at walk or trot, but present with special tests.
2	Deficit detected during walk and trot; exaggerated by special tests.
3	Deficit prominent at walk or trot; may fall during special tests.
4	Stumbling, tripping, or falling spontaneously at normal gait.
5	Down, cannot rise.

Evaluating recumbent patients

Recumbent animals that can attain a dog sitting posture or use their forelimbs well in attempts to rise are most likely to have a lesion caudal to T2. If the forelimbs cannot be used, the lesion is likely to be located in the cervical spinal cord. If the head but not the neck can be lifted off the ground, the lesion is in the cranial cervical area. If the head and neck can be lifted off the ground, but forelimb function is decreased such that the animal cannot maintain sternal recumbency or attain a dog sitting posture, there is likely to be a severe caudal cervical lesion.

Muscle tone can be assessed by manipulating each limb. Lower motor lesions result in a flaccid limb with decreased to absent motor activity. Caution should be used in interpreting tone in heavy animals or in limbs that have been lain upon. Increased muscle tone with decreased or absent voluntary effort may occur with a severe UMN lesion to the forelimbs (cranial to C6). This is the result of the loss of the calming influences of the descending UMN pathways. This spastic paralysis can also be seen with lesions from C6–T2 if little or no gray matter is affected.

Spinal reflexes should be tested in the forelimbs, but it is important to note that a spinal reflex can be intact without the animal perceiving the stimulus and demonstrating a related behavioral response, as perception involves intact ascending sensory pathways to the forebrain. Pinching the skin of the distal forelimb results in flexion of the fetlock, knee, elbow, and shoulder. If the reflex is absent and cannot be accounted for by decubital changes, the lesion most likely involves the C6–T2 gray matter, peripheral nerves, or flexor muscles of the forelimb. Lesions cranial to C7 may result in an exaggerated response.

The biceps reflex is performed by placing two or three fingers firmly on the biceps and brachialis muscles on the cranial aspect of the elbow joint, feeling for contraction of these muscles, and observing for flexion of the elbow while balloting the muscles with a plexor. This reflex, which has its afferent and efferent pathways in the musculocutaneous nerve and involves spinal cord segments C7 and C8, is difficult to evoke, except in small foals.

The triceps reflex is tested by holding the relaxed limb slightly flexed and balloting first the distal portion of the long head of the triceps and then the insertion of the tendon. Contraction of the triceps muscle, which causes extension of the elbow, should be observed and palpated. This reflex has afferent and efferent pathways in the radial nerve and involves spinal cord segments C7–T1. The triceps reflex is normally difficult to demonstrate in adult horses and is often most useful when easily elicited, indicating a UMN lesion.

diffuse spinal cord disease. Severe signs in the forelimbs (grade 4+) and mild hindlimb signs (grade 1+) is consistent with diffuse spinal cord disease or a lesion of the brachial intumescence (C6–T2), with involvement of the gray matter supplying the forelimbs. Severe signs in one or both forelimbs with normal hindlimbs indicate LMN involvement of the forelimbs.

Lesions of the white matter of the caudal brainstem can also result in gait abnormalities in all four limbs. However, there will usually be concurrent head signs such as cranial nerve abnormalities, which can be used to define the site of the lesion.

Evaluating the neck and forelimbs

Observation and palpation of the neck and forelimbs should be performed. Abnormalities that may be noted are skeletal defects, asymmetry, and muscle atrophy. Involvement of peripheral sympathetic neurons causes local sweating, which can be an extremely helpful localizing sign. The neck may be manipulated to determine normal range of movement, with consideration being given to other causes of neck pain or stiffness such as cervical vertebral arthrosis. Local cervical (contraction of cutaneous and brachiocephalicus muscles) and cervicofacial (ear flicking, eyelid blinking, and contracture of labial muscles) responses are assessed by tapping the skin of the lateral neck with a probe.

Other tests that may help in detecting an asymmetric forelimb abnormality are hopping (rarely done in anything other than foals), sway reaction to detect weakness or lack of resistance to lateral shoulder pressure, or a lack of resistance to withers pinching.

Voluntary effort and muscle tone are assessed by observing the animal's attempts to rise or its response to stimuli while in lateral recumbency. Asymmetry in voluntary effort may also help to localize a lesion. The hindlimb spinal reflexes should be assessed in recumbent animals and in animals that can be safely restrained in lateral recumbency (usually only foals).

The patellar reflex is assessed by supporting the limb in a partly flexed position, tapping the middle patellar ligament, and observing for reflex contraction of the quadriceps muscle and extension of the stifle. This reflex involves sensory and motor fibers in the femoral nerve and spinal cord segments at L4 and L5.

The flexor reflex is assessed by pinching the skin of the distal limb and observing for flexion. This may be difficult to assess in larger horses, especially those that have been recumbent for some time. This reflex involves sensory and motor fibers in the sciatic nerve and spinal cord segments L5–S2.

At this point in the examination the presence and location of lesions in the brain, spinal cord cranial to T3, and peripheral nerves or muscles of the forelimbs should have been identified.

Evaluating the trunk and hindlimbs

The trunk and hindlimbs should be observed and palpated for malformation and asymmetry. Asymmetric myelopathies can cause scoliosis of the thoracolumbar vertebral column, with the concave side opposite the lesion. Other useful localizing signs are sweating and sensation over the trunk and hindlimbs (1009, 1010). Sweating indicates involvement of descending sympathetic tracts in the spinal cord, whereas hypalgesia and analgesia have been detected caudal to severe thoracolumbar spinal cord lesions. Contraction of the cutaneous trunci muscle can be elicited in response to gentle pricking of the skin over the lateral trunk. Absence of this response indicates a lesion in the thoracolumbar spinal nerves, C8–T1 spinal cord segments, or lateral thoracic nerves.

Alternately pushing laterally against the pelvis and pulling laterally on the tail while the horse is standing and while walking determines the sway reaction in the hindlimbs. An animal with weak hindlimbs is easily pushed and pulled laterally. Extensor weakness (associated with LMN disease) results in little resistance to pushing or pulling the hindquarters while the horse is standing still. Flexor weakness (associated with UMN disease) results in a horse that resists lateral pressure at rest, but is easily moved off stride while moving. This is also a very useful test for detecting asymmetry in weakness or ataxia of the hindlimbs.

Buckling of the hindlimbs or overextension of the back ventrally on applying pressure to the thoracolumbar or sacral paravertebral muscles indicates weakness.

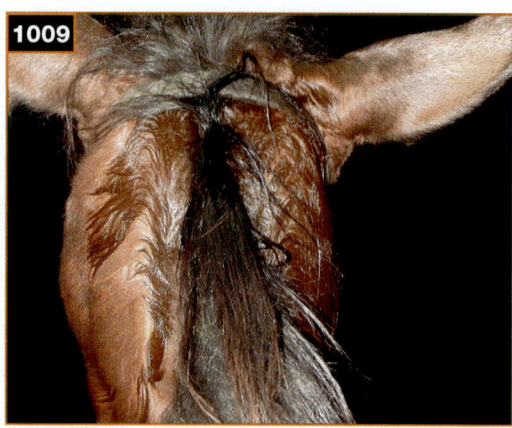

1009 A foal with a fracture of the atlas. Note the localized sweating at the region of the injury.

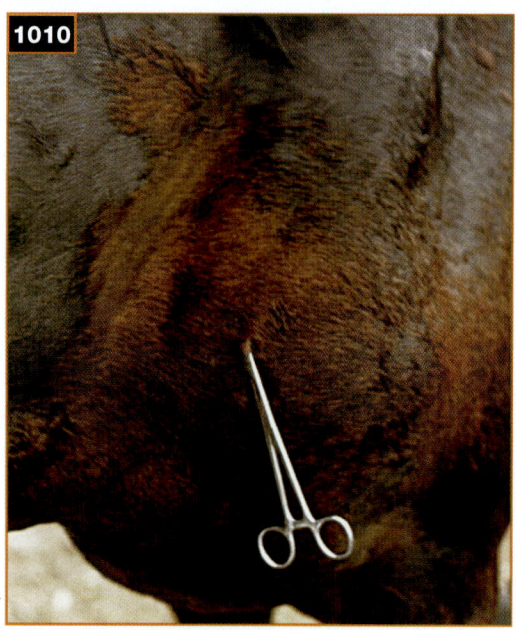

1010 Fracture of C7 and T1, with hypalgesia.

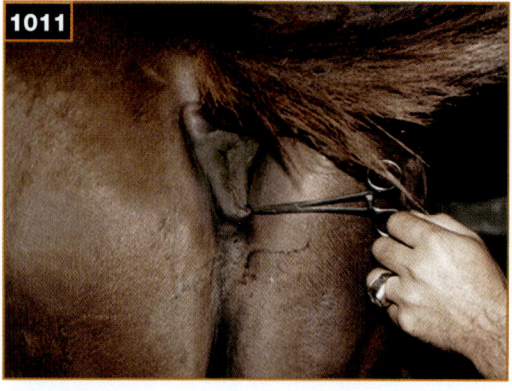

1011 No anal tone is noted in a horse suffering from EHV-1 myelitis.

Nervous system

Evaluating the tail and anus

The final component of the neurologic examination involves assessment of structures innervated by nerves from the sacral and coccygeal spinal cord segments. Tail tone should be assessed before testing the perineal reflex. A flaccid tail with no voluntary movement indicates a lesion of the sacrococcygeal segments or nerves.

The perineal reflex is elicited by lightly pricking or pinching the skin of the perineum and observing reflex contraction of the anal sphincter and flexion (clamping down) of the tail. Sensory fibers are within the perineal branches of the pudendal nerve (S1–S3). Motor fibers for contraction of the anal sphincter are within the caudal rectal branch of the pudendal nerve, while tail flexion is mediated through the sacral and coccygeal segments and nerves (S1–Co).

The spinal cord ends at the level of the first or second sacral vertebra. Focal lesions of the last lumbar, sacral, and coccygeal vertebrae may involve the cauda equina and LMNs from many sacrococcygeal spinal cord segments. Depending on the level at which the lesion is located, varying degrees of hypalgesia, hyporeflexia, hypotonia, and muscle atrophy will result (**1011**). It is also important to assess urinary bladder volume and tone in addition to rectal tone, as these may be affected by lesions involving the cauda equina.

Evidence of lesions in this area is an important finding, because abnormalities such as hypotonia, hyporeflexia, and hypalgesia of the tail and anal areas may be secondary to contusion or injury sustained in attempts to rise by a paraplegic animal.

After completing the neurologic examination, the clinician should be able to localize the lesion accurately and attempt to explain the clinical signs seen. After localizing the lesion, possible causes can be considered.

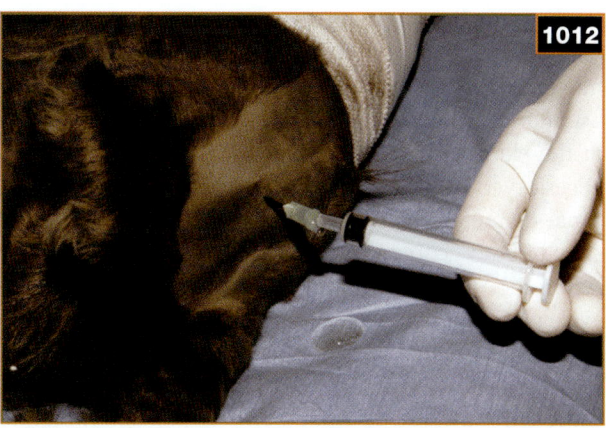

1012 Location for atlanto-occipital CSF collection.

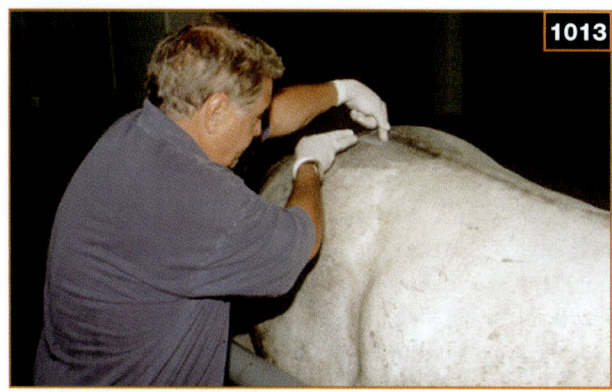

1013 Lumbosacral CSF collection. The clinician's left hand is placed at the site for needle puncture and the fingers of the right hand are at the right tuber sacrale.

Diagnostic tests

Cerebrospinal fluid collection and analysis

Cerebrospinal fluid (CSF) samples can be obtained from the lumbosacral or atlanto-occipital areas. Lumbosacral CSF collection can be performed in a standing or recumbent horse, while atlanto-occipital samples are obtained from recumbent horses. Sedation can facilitate collection at the lumbosacral site and anesthesia is generally required at the atlanto-occipital site.

Atlanto-occipital spinal tap

A CSF sample can be obtained from the atlanto-occipital area by needle insertion on the dorsal midline at the middle of an imaginary line drawn between the cranial borders of the wings of the atlas (**1012**). A 20 gauge 90 × 0.9 mm spinal needle is used in adults, while a 19 gauge 40 × 1.1 mm disposable needle with a plastic hub is preferred in foals. On entering the subarachnoid space, CSF is immediately seen in the clear hub of the needle.

Lumbosacral spinal tap

The site for needle insertion to obtain a lumbosacral CSF sample is the palpable depression on the dorsal midline just caudal to the spine of L6, cranial to the spinous process of S1, and between the paired tuber sacrale (**1013**). An 18 gauge 15–18 cm (6–7 inch) spinal needle is used in adults and an 18 or 20 gauge 9 cm (3.5 inch) spinal needle is used in foals. On entering the subarachnoid space there is a palpable change in resistance and usually some (occasionally violent) response by the horse. Gentle aspiration helps prevent soft tissues from obstructing the bevel at the tip of the needle.

Nervous system

Radiography

Plain radiography is necessary for the documentation of fractures, luxations, and malformations. It can also be useful for the demonstration of infections and neoplasms of the skull and vertebral column. Radiography is also necessary to allow objective measurements of the vertebral canal diameter in order to determine the likelihood of spinal cord compression in horses with wobbler syndrome. The use of positive contrast myelography in evaluating spinal cord disease has become more common. This procedure may be associated with potentially severe complications and should only be used when there is sufficient expertise to both perform and interpret the myelogram. Additionally, a myelogram should only be performed when the results could significantly alter the management of the case, and it should always be performed prior to spinal cord surgery in order to confirm the site, extent, and nature of the lesion.

Electrodiagnostic testing

Electromyography

Needle EMG is a useful diagnostic test to help localize a nervous system lesion (see **42**, p.29). It does not provide a definitive diagnosis of the disease process that is present, but it can provide useful information for selecting further diagnostic tests, such as the most suitable site for nerve or muscle biopsy. It can usually be carried out on a conscious animal with the use of physical or chemical restraint. Commonly used sedatives, such as xylazine and acepromazine do not interfere with EMG results. The procedure involves placing needle electrodes in muscles to detect muscle fibers displaying abnormal insertional activity on insertion of the needle into the muscle to be studied, and spontaneous activity during a nonstimulating period. Approximately 1 week after injury, denervated muscle fibers develop spontaneous electrical discharges that are collectively termed denervation potentials and include excessive insertional activity, positive sharp waves, fibrillation potentials, and bizarre high-frequency discharges.

Electroencephalography

Electroencephalography is a method of recording the electrical activity of the brain. An understanding of normal patterns allows identification of abnormal patterns, some of which are compatible with lesions such as hydrocephalus, encephalitis, and space-occupying lesions.

Congenital disorders

Hydrocephalus

Definition/overview

Hydrocephalus is an increase in CSF volume within the ventricular system (internal hydrocephalus) or subarachnoid space (external hydrocephalus). It is rare in horses. Hydrocephalus is most often seen in neonatal foals as a congenital malformation.

Etiology/pathophysiology

An inherited defect has been proposed in some cases, but the mode of inheritance has not been established. Hydrocephalus can also be acquired following conditions such as meningitis or following hemorrhage.

Hydrocephalus can be classified as normotensive or hypertensive. Normotensive hydrocephalus usually is incidental to hypoplasia or loss of brain parenchyma after destructive prenatal or postnatal infection or injury. The CSF volume expands passively to fill the space that is normally occupied by the brain tissue.

Hypertensive hydrocephalus is a result of obstruction of the CSF conduit between the sites of production, in the third and lateral ventricles, and the sites of absorption by the arachnoid villi in the subarachnoid space. Blockage may be due to hypoplasia or aplasia of a part of this system or it may be acquired. The increased CSF pressure results in dilation of the third and lateral ventricles, with resulting tissue damage.

Clinical presentation

Hydrocephalic animals are often born dead or weak and die shortly after birth. Animals that survive may have a varied presentation. Abnormalities relate to compression of the cerebral cortex. In neonates, poor suckle reflex, blindness, lack of affinity for the mare, depression, ill-thrift, and growth retardation may be present (**1014**). The head may be grossly enlarged and dome shaped, but this is not consistent or always apparent (**1015**). A mildly dome-shaped skull can more commonly be the result of intra-uterine growth retardation or immaturity.

Differential diagnosis

Hypoxic–ischemic encephalopathy; electrolyte imbalances; meningitis; hypoglycemia; premature weak foal; septicemia.

Diagnosis

Presumptive diagnosis of congenital hydrocephalus is commonly based on clinical signs of impaired mental function and a domed skull. CT and MRI could also be used for diagnosis in neonates. Without advanced imaging, necropsy is required for a definitive diagnosis (**1016**).

1014 Hydrocephalus in a 6-week-old foal. The foal was not able to lift his head and pull his tongue into the mouth. The foal suffered from severe perinatal asphyxia and developed necrosis of the cerebrum. CSF took the place of the lost parenchyma. This was a case of compensatory hydrocephalus. (Photo courtesy FT Bain)

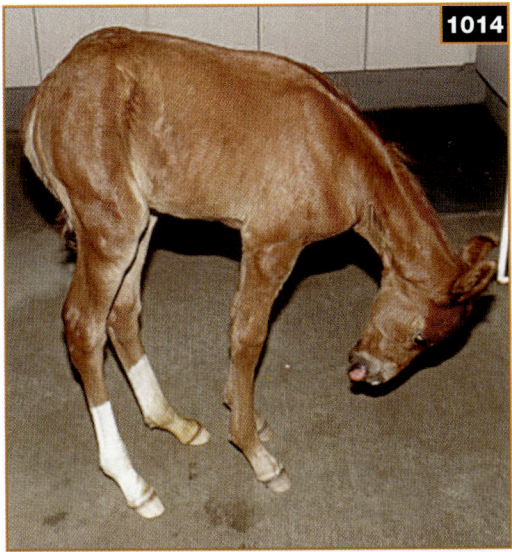

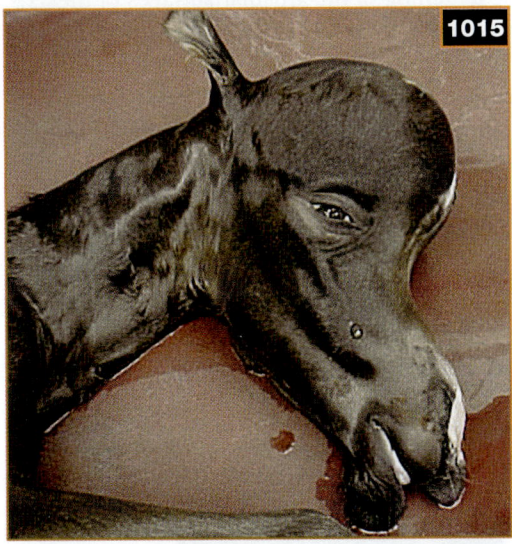

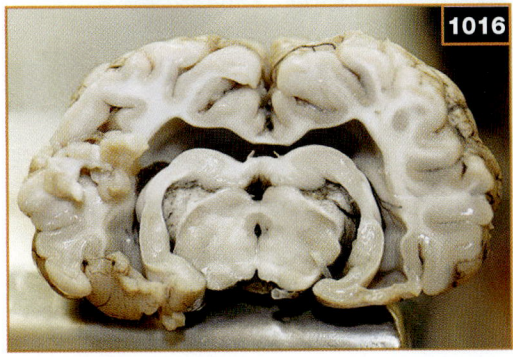

Management
Specific medical or surgical treatment for hydrocephalus is not recommended, and euthanasia must be considered depending on the severity of the signs.

Prognosis
The prognosis is grave. Surviving animals will have residual neurologic deficits.

Cerebellar hypoplasia
Cerebellar hypoplasia is commonly associated with *in-utero* viral infections in ruminants. Other causes include genetic, toxic, and degenerative diseases. Toxins or viruses have not been linked with abnormalities of cerebellar development in foals, and congenital malformation or hypoplasia of the cerebellum appears to be rare. Cerebellar syndromes and degenerative lesions are seen in Thoroughbred and Paso Fino foals. Signs, including dysmetria and ataxia, are evident as soon as the foal attempts to stand and walk.

Cerebellar abiotrophy
Definition/overview
Cerebellar abiotrophy is a familial disease that occurs in purebred Arabian or Arabian crossbred horses as well as in the Oldenburg, Gotland, and Eriskay ponies.

Etiology/pathophysiology
The cause of cerebellar abiotrophy is unknown, but there is a familial occurrence. It is assumed that an inherited defect of Purkinje cells in the cerebellum is involved.

Clinical presentation
Animals may be normal at birth, but abnormal clinical signs usually develop in the first 6 months of life. Signs range from mild ataxia to complete diffuse cerebellar dysfunction. Head tremor is a commonly recognized sign and may occur in a vertical or horizontal direction. Signs usually appear suddenly and may remain static

1015 Congenital hydrocephalus in an aborted foal. Note the domed appearance of the skull.

1016 Gross examination of the distension of the lateral ventricles from the hydrocephalic foal pictured in 1014. (Photo courtesy M Saulez)

or gradually progress and then plateau. Affected foals develop a hypertonic and hypermetric (goose-stepping) gait, especially of the forelimbs (1017). These deficits can be exaggerated by turning the animal sharply, stepping up and down a curb, or walking on an incline. Most animals have a decreased menace response despite normal visual and facial nerve function. Foals with normal menace responses have been reported.

Differential diagnosis

Meningitis; equine protozoal myeloencephalitis (EPM); hypoxic–ischemic encephalopathy; cerebellar abscess; parasitic migrans in the cerebellum; West Nile virus (WNV) encephalitis.

Diagnosis

A tentative diagnosis can be made on history and clinical signs. Ancillary examinations have not detected any specific abnormalities. The CSF values in affected foals are usually normal, although increased CK has been reported in a number of cases.

Management/prognosis

There is no effective treatment and these animals are unsafe for riding. On recognition, the owner should be counseled with regard to the suspected inherited nature of the disorder and discouraged from future breeding of the parents or affected animal.

Occipitoatlantoaxial malformation

Definition/overview

Occipitoatlantoaxial malformation (OAAM) is an uncommon problem in horses and appears to be not one single defect, but rather a spectrum of cervical spinal abnormalities.

Etiology/pathophysiology

The five different types that have been described in horses are:

- Symmetric atlanto-occipital fusion, atlantalization of the axis, and hypoplasia of the atlantal wings. This has been described as a heritable condition in Arabians and has also been described in an Arabian-cross colt.
- Spinal lesions similar to those found in Arabians have been reported as a nonfamilial disease of Quarterhorses.
- Asymmetric malformations of the occipitoatlantoaxial area in Morgan horses and Standardbred foals.
- Atlantal duplication of Arabian crossbred horses.
- Asymmetric occipitalization of the atlas and symmetric atlantalization of the axis.

Macroscopic changes that are common to all five forms include loss or flattening of the occipital condyles, asymmetric flattening of the articular surfaces of the axis, and shortened dens.

Clinical presentation

There is a wide range of clinical signs from normal neurologic function, with or without torticollis, to brainstem compression, sudden death, and stillbirth (1018). Signs such as tetraparesis or tetraplegia are usually seen soon after birth. Ataxia may be progressive. In rare cases, signs

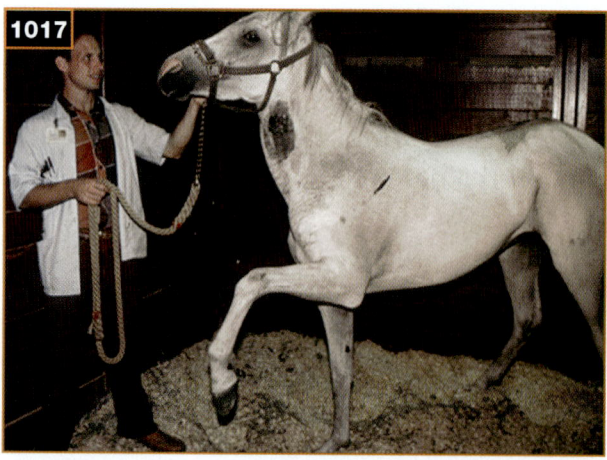

1017 Cerebellar abiotrophy in an Arabian. Note the hypermetria of the forelimb. (Photo courtesy FT Bain)

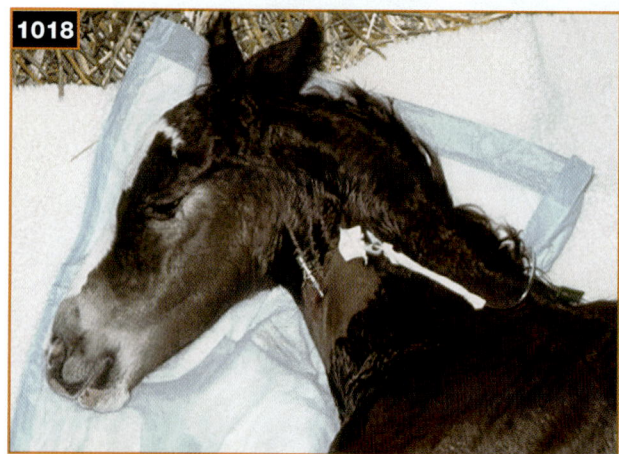

1018 Atlanto-occipital malformation in an Arabian foal. Note the exaggerated dorsal flexion of the proximal cervical vertebrae. (Photo courtesy FT Bain)

Nervous system

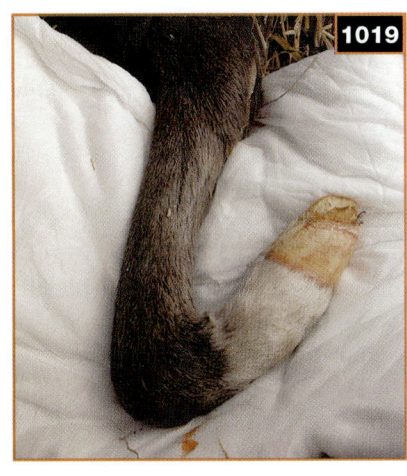

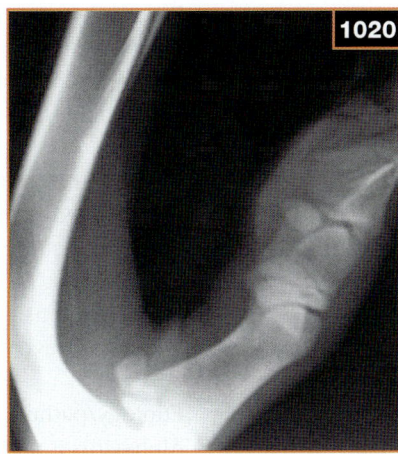

1019 Arthrogryposis of the hind fetlock of a foal. The foal was a dystocia delivery.

1020 Radiographic view of the arthrogryposis in 1019. Note the deformation of the 3rd metatarsal bone (bowing).

have not been seen until the animals are a few years old. Movement of the head may result in a clicking noise or crepitation, and some animals show a reluctance to move the head and neck. Abnormal head and neck carriage may be evident.

Differential diagnosis
Atlanto-occipital luxation; cervical trauma.

Diagnosis
In horses with neurologic deficits, the neurologic examination will localize the lesion to the cervical spine. Some abnormalities of the atlas and axis may be palpable. Characteristic clinical signs and observation or palpation of the malformation is highly suggestive of OAAM, but radiography is required for confirmation. The bony lesions are apparent on radiographs.

Management
Laminectomy has been used to alleviate spinal cord compression and clinical signs. It has been suggested that surgical fusion of the atlantoaxial joints, with or without laminectomy, could be used as a treatment. Arabian horses should not be treated because of the heritable nature of the disorder in that breed.

Arthrogryposis
Definition/overview
Arthrogryposis is an uncommon congenital developmental defect that is characterized by fixation of multiple joints and severe muscle contracture. It may be accompanied by other flexural limb deformities (see p. 44).

Etiology/pathophysiology
The primary defect is believed to be in the skeletal or nervous system in the majority of cases and is often accompanied by other anatomic and neurologic defects. The primary defect may also occur in the muscles.

Distinguishing between a neurogenic defect and a muscular one can be difficult because muscular atrophy, with an increase in fibrous and adipose tissue, can be seen in both. This has led to the term neuromuscular arthrogryposis. Lesions in both muscles and nerves have been demonstrated in individual cases. In humans the majority of cases are neurogenic in origin, with undefined disturbances of the anterior horn cells thought to be responsible.

The cause of the primary abnormality in the horse is unknown. Genetic and environmental factors, such as uterine malpositioning and maternal ingestion of locoweed (*Astragalus* spp.) or hybrid Sudan pasture, have been suggested. Detailed examination of neuromuscular tissue has rarely been carried out and the majority of cases are simply suggested to be skeletal in origin.

Clinical presentation
The condition can involve one to four limbs and the axial skeleton. Dystocia is a frequent complaint and the more severely affected animals are commonly born dead. Milder cases can occur with, for example, an inability to straighten one fetlock (**1019, 1020**). The affected muscles in these cases appear to have lost sarcomeres from the end of the myofibers. The use of constant tension seems to result in the restoration of these sarcomeres.

Management
Milder cases may be treated symptomatically with the use of splints, casts, and physiotherapy.

Prognosis
A reasonable prognosis for normal function is reserved for foals that are mildly affected, delivered normally, and respond to treatment. Death, from dystocia or complications associated with inability to ambulate, is more common. Surviving animals should not be bred because a genetic component cannot be ruled out.

Spinal cord vascular abnormalities

Hemangioma, hematoma, hamartoma, and aneurysm are rare vascular abnormalities that have caused signs of focal spinal cord compression in horses. Lesions increase in size by growth or vascular degeneration and hemorrhage, and result in compression of neural tissue as they enlarge within the CNS.

Infectious diseases

Borna disease (Near Eastern encephalitis)

Definition/overview

Borna disease is a rare cause of encephalitis in horses, humans, sheep, goats, cattle, and rabbits. Outbreaks have been reported in many countries across Europe and the Middle East.

Etiology/pathophysiology

Borna disease is an encephalitic disease of mammals caused by a member of the Flaviviridae family of viruses. The viruses of Borna disease and Near Eastern encephalitis are indistinguishable.

Borna virus is transmitted between birds by the tick *Hyalomma anatolicum*. It is thought that outbreaks of the disease in the Middle East may represent transmission from a dense population of infected wild birds. The Borna disease virus is shed through nasal secretions and urine from infected animals. It is resistant to drying and adverse environmental conditions.

Clinical presentation

Clinical signs are similar to those seen with other viral encephalitides (i.e. depression, ataxia, head pressing, head tilt, compulsive movements, and muscular tremors). Severe encephalitis causing death is common.

Differential diagnosis

A variety of other viral causes of encephalitis should be considered, depending on the geographic area.

Diagnosis

Clinical findings are not diagnostic for Borna disease. Antemortem diagnosis is based on the identification of antibodies in the serum and CSF. Gross pathology is usually unremarkable. Histologically, the characteristic lesion is the Joest–Degen inclusion body in the neuronal nucleus.

Management

Specific treatment is not available. Supportive care should be provided.

Prognosis

The mortality rate is very high and most affected horses are euthanized because of the severity of the disease and the potential for latent and persistent infection.

Alphavirus encephalitis of horses

Definition/overview

Western equine encephalitis (WEE), Eastern equine encephalitis (EEE), and Venezuelan equine encephalitis (VEE) are seasonal, geographically important causes of potentially severe encephalitis in horses.

Etiology/pathophysiology

Alphavirus is the most prominent genus of the Togaviridae family, which causes WEE, EEE, and VEE. Traditionally, alphavirus encephalitis of horses has been clinically more important than other arbovirus encephalitides of horses. In recent years, however, WNV encephalomyelitis has become clinically more significant in North America.

Eastern equine encephalitis. There is one EEE virus with two antigenic variants based on hemagglutination inhibition tests: North American and South American. EEE is recognized primarily in the US east of the Mississippi river and has been sporadically reported in southeastern Canada. It has also been recognized in the Caribbean and Central and South America. Enzootic cycles in North America involve a mosquito vector *Culiseta melanura* and passerine birds as amplifying hosts. *Culiseta* spp. are essentially ornithophilic and thus epizootics involve mosquito species that feed on birds as well as other animals (e.g. *Aedes* and *Coquilleltidia* spp.). There is a seasonal variation in disease, with peak incidence in late summer or early fall. Infected horses and humans are regarded as dead-end hosts, as the level of viremia that develops is insufficient to infect epizootic hosts.

Western equine encephalitis. The WEE complex contains seven virus species: WEE, Highland 1, Sindbis, Aura, Fort Morgan, Buggy creek, and Y62-33. WEE occurs throughout most of the Americas, with extensive epizootics in Argentina. The disease has also been reported in Canada. The principal enzootic vector is *Culex tarsalis* and the epizootic mosquito vector is an *Aedes* species. At intervals of 5–10 years the level of viral transmission within the maintenance cycle is more intense, with epidemics occurring in horses and humans. Equine cases usually precede human cases by several weeks and thus act as a sentinel for human infection. Similar to EEE, humans and horses are regarded as dead-end hosts for WEE infection.

Venezuelan equine encephalitis. The VEE complex is one virus with six antigenic subtypes (I–VI). Serotypes IAB and IC are responsible for epizootics. The geographic range is primarily South America with extension into Central America. However, epizootics have extended as far north as Texas. Enzootic cycles are maintained via *Culex* spp. and small vertebrate hosts. *Aedes* and *Psorophora* mosquito species transmit epizootic viruses IAB and IC in association with many different vertebrates, leading to high mortality in both humans and horses. Unlike EEE and WEE, horses with VEE develop a sufficient viremia to act as an amplifier of the disease.

Clinical presentation

Infection with alphavirus is associated with an initial incubation period of approximately 1 week during which a biphasic viremia takes place. This is associated with biphasic fever in EEE and WEE, although the first fever spike may not be noticed. Horses with VEE usually have a consistently elevated temperature during the disease. Other nonspecific signs such as lethargy and stiffness are seen during the viremic phase. As the disease progresses, neurologic abnormalities become more evident, with the severity of signs dependent on the virus involved and the extent of CNS lesions. EEE and WEE usually have a similar clinical appearance, with ataxia, somnolence, conscious proprioceptive deficits, stiff neck, and compulsive walking or chewing. WEE does not usually progress beyond nonspecific initial signs or, less seldom, mild CNS signs such as those above. EEE typically progresses to severe CNS deficits that occur secondary to diffuse cerebrocortical disease. Signs associated with more severe disease in EEE include apparent blindness and circling, excitement and aggressive behavior, laryngeal, pharyngeal, and tongue paralysis, dysphagia (**1021**), and signs of brainstem dysfunction such as head tilt, nystagmus, strabismus, and pupil dilation (**1022**). VEE may also cause inapparent infections, signs similar to those of other encephalitis viruses, or produce signs such as epistaxis, pulmonary hemorrhage, oral ulcers, and diarrhea that may be unrelated to CNS damage. Seizures can occur with any of the alphavirus infections and sudden death may also occur despite seemingly insignificant clinical signs.

Differential diagnosis

Other viral causes of encephalitis should be considered depending on the geographic incidence of individual diseases and time of year.

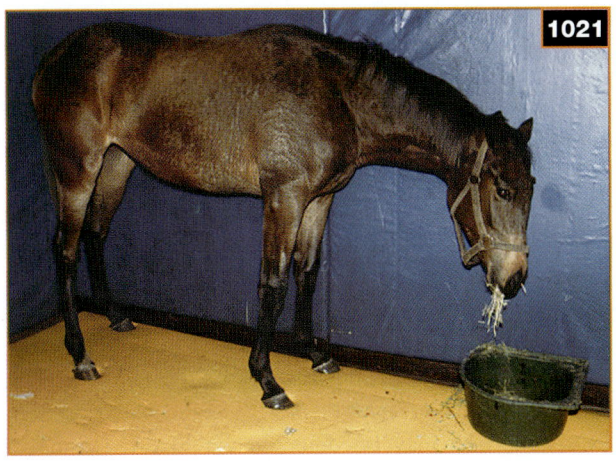

1021 Dysphagia and dementia associated with EEE. (Photo courtesy FT Bain)

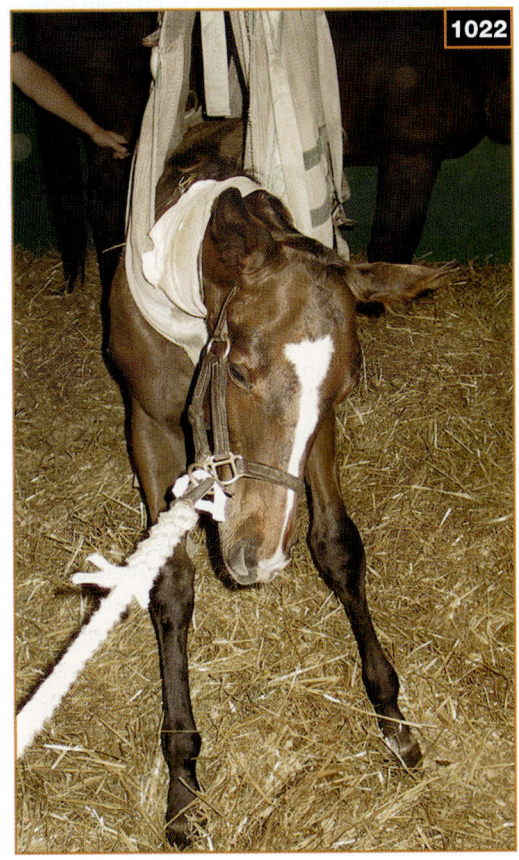

1022 Severe ataxia and recumbency in a sling of a horse infected with EEE. The horse eventually died.

Diagnosis

Establishing a definitive diagnosis is important to allow implementation of control measures, but it can be challenging. Clinical signs are nonspecific or similar to those of other encephalitides. Serologic testing is helpful, with a four-fold rise in antibody titers being diagnostic. However, a four- fold rise may not be detected as antibody levels rise rapidly after infection and a delay in taking the acute sample frequently results in sampling during the peak antibody titer. Another problem frequently encountered with serologic testing is that horses with EEE often do not live long enough for comparison of paired samples. High immunoglobulin M (IgM) titers suggest recent exposure to EEE virus and may be detected via ELISA. Definitive antemortem diagnosis can also be made based on viral isolation or identification of viral nucleic acid by reverse transcription- (RT-) PCR. RT-PCR is a sensitive and specific test for detection of viral nucleic acid in CNS tissue or CSF. EEE, WEE, or VEE viruses can be isolated from brain tissue of infected horses via Vero-cell culture or mouse inoculation. Immunohistochemistry testing can also be performed on brain tissue. Virus isolation from serum is usually unsuccessful.

Other findings that are not specific for alphaviruses are peripheral leukocytosis and increased cellularity and elevated protein concentration of CSF.

Management

There is no specific treatment available and current therapy is based on supportive care. Anti-inflammatory drugs (flunixin meglumine [1 mg/kg i/v or p/o q12–24h] or DMSO [1 g/kg administered as a 10% solution i/v or via nasogastric tube q12–24h]) are commonly used to reduce CNS inflammation. In addition, good nursing care, monitoring of hydration status, and protection from self-induced trauma are important. In many regions these diseases must be reported to governmental authorities.

Prevention is based on vaccination and limiting exposure to vectors. Monovalent, bivalent, and trivalent killed vaccines are available. Recommendations vary depending on the region, with vaccination 2–4 times annually recommended in temperate areas where vectors may survive all year round. In areas bordering Central America or for horses traveling to endemic areas, twice-yearly vaccination against VEE is recommended. Foals from vaccinated dams are generally protected for 6–7 months. Vaccination of foals against EEE should be started at 4 months of age in endemic areas and repeated at 6 and 12 months of age.

Limiting exposure to vectors involves efforts to eliminate mosquitoes or their habitats, use of repellants, and stabling at dawn and dusk when mosquitoes are most active.

Prognosis

Prognosis varies greatly between the different diseases. In general the prognosis for EEE is grave, with mortality rates of 75–100% being reported. Mortality rates for VEE and WEE of 40–80% and 25–50%, respectively, have been reported. Residual neurologic deficits may be present in survivors.

West Nile virus encephalomyelitis
Definition/overview
WNV is a geographically important cause of encephalitis in horses. It is endemic in certain regions of the Middle East and has made periodic incursions into wider geographic areas, including Africa, Asia, and Europe. Recently, WNV has emerged as an important cause of encephalitis in horses and other species in North America.

Etiology/pathophysiology
WNV is a flavivirus of the Japanese encephalitis virus antigenic complex that also includes St. Louis encephalitis virus, Murray Valley encephalitis virus, and Kunjin virus. WNV encephalomyelitis is a mosquito-borne disease that affects a broad range of animals including birds, cats, dogs, horses, and humans.

The virus cycles between bird reservoir hosts and mosquitoes. Competent bird reservoir hosts sustain an infectious viremia for 1–4 days following exposure and then develop lifelong immunity. Susceptible birds may become ill or die from myeloencephalitis. Horses become infected via the bites of infected mosquitoes, particularly those of the *Culex* genus. Humans, horses, and most other mammals are considered dead-end hosts, as they do not develop a sufficient viremia to complete the cycle. Many species can develop an immune response without demonstrating signs of disease. Cases are most commonly seen in late summer to early fall, but may be observed year round in areas with prolonged vector seasons. No significant age or breed disposition has been identified. More males than females were affected in one report.

Clinical presentation
Only a small percentage of infected horses develop clinical signs. In those with signs, the onset is generally acute following an incubation period of 6–10 days. A range of clinical syndromes exists, from mild peripheral neuritis to encephalitis. Signs include pyrexia in approximately one third to one half of cases, ataxia that is most prominent in the hindlimbs, muscle fasciculations, and hypersensitivity to touch. Muscle fasciculations may be more common with WNV encephalomyelitis than with other causes of encephalitis. A narcolepsy-like syndrome has also been reported. Lethargy is associated with subclinical cases and a case of neurogenic diabetes insipidus was thought to be related to WNV encephalomyelitis.

Differential diagnosis

Other viral causes of encephalitis should be considered, depending on the geographic region and time of year.

Diagnosis

WNV encephalomyelitis should be suspected in any horse showing signs of neurologic disease in an area where WNV activity has been documented. Confirmation of a positive case of WNV encephalitis has been based on IgM-capture ELISA on serum or CSF, plaque reduction neutralization test (PRNT) on serum, viral isolation, or PCR performed on brain tissue. IgM-capture ELISA serum titers greater than or equal to 1:400 suggest recent exposure to the virus. High IgM titers decline within less than 2 months after exposure. In contrast, single determination of IgG level via ELISA is not useful diagnostically because the longer persistence of IgG may represent previous exposure or vaccination. PRNT with titers greater than or equal to 1:10 indicate an IgG response, but may not be present in the acute phase of the disease and may persist for 15 months. Cytologic examination of the CSF is variable. A wide variety of nonspecific changes in cell count and protein concentration may be present.

Vaccination does not interfere with the ability to diagnose acute cases because no IgM is detectable in vaccinated horses.

Management

As with the Alphavirus encephalitides, there is no specific treatment and therapy is based on supportive care. The focus of therapy is to decrease brain inflammation, treat fevers, and provide supportive care. Anti-inflammatory treatment (flunixin meglumine [0.5–1 mg/kg i/v q12h] or DMSO [1 g/kg as a 10% solution i/v q12–24h for 3 days]) is thought to be very important. Anti-edema therapy with mannitol (0.5–1.0 g/kg as a 20% solution i/v via a blood filter q12–24h for 2–3 days) is generally reserved for rapidly progressing neurologic signs. Commercial hyperimmune serum or plasma products are available. Neutralizing antibody is the predominant antibody response and appears important in the blocking of intracellular infection *in vitro*. At the time of writing, the clinical efficacy of these products had not yet been proven. The hypothesis is that the administration of neutralizing antibody against WNV early in the course of the disease will reduce the severity and shorten the duration of clinical signs in the horse. Interferon alpha (3 million units diluted in 250 ml saline s/c or i/v q12h [recumbent horses] or q24h [standing horses] for 5–7 days) has been used with anecdotal success.

Prevention is also based on limiting exposure to mosquito vectors and vaccination. Killed vaccine, recombinant DNA, and chimera vaccines are available and have proved to be both safe and efficacious. Vaccine recommendation for the killed and recombinant DNA products is a 1 ml dose by intramuscular injection and a second 1 ml dose 3–6 weeks after the first dose, with annual or bi-annual revaccination. The chimera product is unique in that it only needs a single intramuscular dose for a full 12 months of protection. The chimera vaccine is currently labeled for use in animals 5 months of age and older. Vaccination guidelines for foals have not been fully investigated, but can only be speculated at this time. Common recommendations involve administration of three doses to foals 4–6 weeks apart, starting at 4–5 months of age. No West Nile virus vaccines have been approved for use in pregnant animals.

Prognosis

Approximately 30% of horses with neurologic disease die or are euthanized 3–4 days after the onset of clinical signs. The prognosis is reasonable in animals that remain standing. The prognosis is poor in horses that are unable to stand because of hindlimb paralysis or that have signs of cerebral lesions (e.g. seizures or coma). The 70% that recover usually have a complete resolution of clinical signs in weeks to months; however, persistent neurologic deficits have been reported.

Other arboviral diseases

Equine encephalosis is an acute arthropod-borne viral disease caused by the equine encephalosis virus, which is classified in the genus Orbivirus of the family Reoviridae. It is endemic in most parts of South Africa, with *Culicoides* spp. the presumed vector of the disease. Most infections are subclinical, with clinical cases developing ataxia, stiffness, and facial swelling that is similar to AHS. Infected horses are viremic for 4–7 days and can be infective for vectors during this time. There is no evidence that horses become carriers of the disease.

EIA is another arboviral infection of horses that may result in neuropathologic changes. EIA virus is a member of the Retroviridae family. The most common neurologic abnormality is symmetric ataxia of the trunk and limbs. Other reported abnormalities include circling, gait alterations, and behavioral changes. Hydrocephalus has also been found at necropsy. These signs may rarely occur alone, but usually are present with clinical signs related to hemolymphatic dysfunction. (See also p. 723.)

Other than those discussed above, there is a variety of neurotropic arboviruses that have been reported to infect horses, leading to seroconversion and occasional disease. These include louping ill, Japanese B, St. Louis, Murray valley, Semliki forest, Russian spring-summer, Powassan, and Ross River encephalitis viruses, which are all members of the family Flaviviridae. Members of the family Bunyaviridae such as Main Drain viruses and California group viruses may also cause neurologic disease in horses.

Rabies

Definition/overview

Rabies is a fatal neurologic disease of mammals. Disease in horses is rare, but is of concern because of the severity of disease and risk to humans. Rabies has been identified in horses in many parts of the world.

Etiology/pathophysiology

Rabies virus is highly neurotropic Lyssavirus (Rhabdoviridae) with strain differences in pathogenicity and host range.

Rabies has two classic cycles: canine (urban) rabies and wildlife (sylvatic) rabies. The majority of wildlife vectors are small to medium sized omnivores such as skunks and raccoons. Dogs may be higher risk in certain countries with higher levels of endemic rabies in the feral canine population. Domestic animals are generally regarded as dead-end hosts and are usually infected following contact with the wildlife vectors. Rabies is most commonly transmitted by salivary contamination of a bite wound, although infection by inhalation, oral, or transplacental routes has been demonstrated in some species. The incubation period varies from 2 weeks to several months depending on the site of inoculation and the dose and pathogenicity of the strain. Following inoculation, the rabies virus replicates locally and after several days attaches to peripheral nerve receptors. The virus is then passed to the CNS via retrograde axoplasmic transport. Rabies virus has a predilection for replication in the cell bodies (gray matter) of the CNS, with subsequent dysfunction of these neurons leading to behavioral changes and abnormalities of the cranial and peripheral nerves. The cause of death may be respiratory paralysis as a result of infection of the medulla. Shedding of the virus in nasal and salivary secretions has been shown to predate the onset of clinical signs by up to 29 days.

Clinical presentation

The presentation can be highly variable and rabies should be considered in any horse with neurologic abnormalities in endemic areas, particularly in acute and progressive cases. The presenting signs and clinical course are extremely variable. Reported signs have included any of the following: anorexia, depression, blindness, mania, hyperesthesia, muscle twitching, lameness, paresis, ataxia, colic, urinary incontinence, and sudden death. The most commonly reported signs in horses are hyperesthesia and recumbency. Sometimes, neurologic abnormalities are not evident early in disease, and early rabies may mimic other conditions such as an acute abdominal viral infection. The disease is normally rapidly progressive once signs are seen and results in death in 3–10 days. Evidence of a recent animal bite is rarely present.

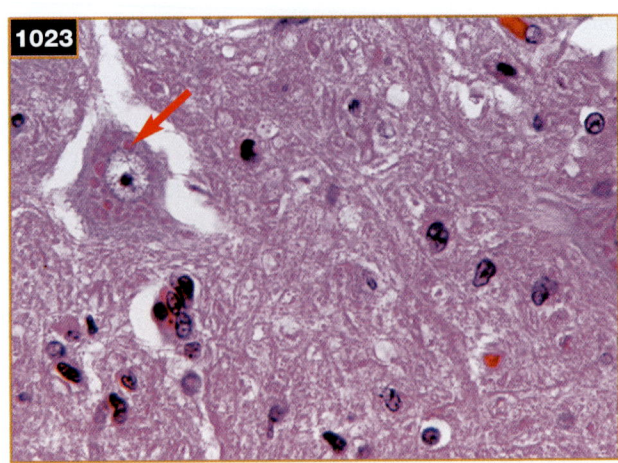

1023 Histopathological changes associated with rabies virus infection. Note the Negri bodies (arrow), cellular inclusions that are present in neuronal cell cytoplasm. (Photo courtesy D Perl [CDC])

Differential diagnosis

Rabies has many differential diagnoses, including other conditions with signs of gray-matter disease such as polyneuritis equi, herpesvirus myeloencephalitis, EPM, and sorghum-Sudan grass poisoning. Cerebral diseases, such as hepatoencephalopathy, leukoencephalomalacia, alphavirus encephalitides, space-occupying masses, and meningitis, should be considered in some cases.

Diagnosis

Antemortem diagnosis of rabies is difficult. Differentiation of rabies from other encephalitides on the basis of clinical signs is impossible. CSF findings are usually nonspecific and can include moderate increases in protein, mononuclear cells, and occasionally neutrophils. An antigen-capture enzyme immunodiagnostic technique is available for antemortem diagnosis using salivary gland specimens, but has not gained widespread clinical use. The gold standard for diagnosis is an indirect fluorescent antibody test on brain tissue that accurately diagnoses 98% of clinical cases. Microscopic examination of hematoxylin and eosin-stained brain sections may reveal nonsuppurative encephalitis and Negri bodies, which are diagnostic (1023). Intracerebral inoculation of mice is also considered an accurate method of diagnosis.

Management

Other than recovery in a presumptive case of experimentally produced rabies in a donkey, the disease is invariably fatal. In the rare situation where an antemortem diagnosis is reached, the animal should be euthanized to avoid further human contact. Transmission from horses to humans has never been reported, but should nonetheless be regarded as a possibility and all necessary precautions should be taken when dealing with animals demonstrating neurologic signs in an endemic area. Affected horses should be handled as little as possible and only by experienced (and ideally vaccinated) personnel. Barrier precautions, including gowns, gloves, and overboots, should be worn. Eye protection should be considered depending on the clinical presentation and procedure to be performed. Rabies suspects should be quarantined and prominently identified. Government authorities should be contacted, where applicable. Public health authorities should be contacted to coordinate management of exposed humans.

Inactivated annual vaccines are used for protection of horses in endemic areas. Foals in endemic areas should be vaccinated at 4–6 months of age with two doses administered 3–4 weeks apart, followed by a booster at 1 year of age. If a previously immunized animal is bitten by a suspected rabid animal, it can be given three booster immunizations over 1 week and quarantined for at least 90 days. Exposed, unvaccinated animals of low economic value should be euthanized immediately. If the animal is valuable, confinement and close observation for at least 6 months is necessary. Primary immunization can be administered 1 month before release from quarantine.

Prognosis
Rabies is always fatal in horses. Death usually occurs 3–10 days following development of neurologic abnormalities.

Equine herpesvirus myeloencephalopathy
Definition/overview
Equine herpesvirus myeloencephalopathy (EHM) is a relatively common cause of CNS disease in the horse. It has a worldwide distribution. Neurologic disease is an uncommon sequela to EHV infection, but it can occur and outbreaks have been widely reported. Adult horses are more commonly affected.

Etiology/pathophysiology
EHV-1 is the only herpesvirus that has been consistently associated with neurologic disease and a neuropathogenic form has recently been identified. EHM has been described in many countries and has occurred with or without other recognized EHV-1 syndromes. Disease has also been reported in nondomestic Equidae including zebras, but has not been reported in infected donkeys or mules.

Viremia results from inhalation of virus and infection of respiratory epithelium or recrudescence of latent viral infection. Subsequent infection of CNS vascular endothelium results in vasculitis, thrombosis, and ischemic myeloencephalopathy. An immune-mediated Arthus-type reaction is suspected.

Clinical presentation
Multiple horses in a herd may be affected, although sporadic individual cases are not uncommon. The history often, but not always, includes contact with horses demonstrating signs of herpesvirus disease (fever, depression, cough, nasal discharge). Outbreaks may occur following introduction of new horses onto the farm. The onset of neurologic signs is usually preceded by fever, lethargy, and inappetence of 1–3 days' duration. The signs that are most frequently seen are symmetric hindlimb ataxia and paresis, bladder atony, fecal retention, and recumbency. Many other signs have been reported and there is a wide range in the severity of signs seen. If recumbency occurs, it is usually within the first 24 hours and is associated with a much poorer prognosis. Those horses that remain standing usually show stabilization of signs in 24–48 hours and then slowly improve over the following weeks to months.

Differential diagnosis
Equine degenerative myelitis; EPM; WNV encephalomyelitis; trauma; aberrant parasite migration (*Halicephalobus deletrix*); equine motor neuron disease; cervical vertebral stenotic myelopathy; hyperammonemia; metabolic derangement; spinal cord impingement secondary to neoplasia.

Diagnosis
A presumptive diagnosis of EHM is often made in horses with characteristic neurologic signs and a related history of other signs of active EHV-1 infection. The CSF frequently has an increased total protein with little or no change in nucleated cell count. Xanthochromia (associated with red-cell breakdown) is frequently noted. Attempts to isolate the virus from the CSF have been largely unsuccessful. CSF changes bear no correlation with the severity of clinical signs and cannot be used as a prognostic indicator.

Confirmation of the diagnosis can be difficult and requires either isolation of the virus from nasopharyngeal swabs and buffy coats, or demonstration of a four-fold rise in virus neutralizing or complement fixing antibody titers between acute and convalescent samples taken 7–10 days apart. Isolation of the virus from CNS tissue and differentiation between antibodies to EHV-1 and EHV-4 is difficult, making a definitive diagnosis difficult to achieve. Complement fixation antibody titers are preferable, as many horses have high levels of virus neutralizing antibody, which is long lived. Many cases have high levels of complement fixation antibodies (>1:160) at the onset of clinical signs. Identification of seroconversion of other horses on the farm with respiratory or neurologic disease is suggestive. Recently, a PCR assay has been developed to differentiate the neuropathogenic form of EHV-1 from non-neuropathogenic strains.

Management

The main feature of treatment is supportive care including evacuation of the bladder and rectum as needed. Maintenance of adequate nutrition and hydration is important. Other controversial therapies include administration of corticosteroids and antiviral agents. The use of corticosteroids (dexamethasone, 0.05–0.1 mg/kg i/v q24h) has been based on the theory that there may be an immune component to the neurologic manifestations. This is still a controversial issue and evaluating the efficacy of corticosteroids is difficult given the natural course of the disease. Administration of antiviral agents such as acyclovir (20 mg/kg p/o q8h or 10 mg/kg p/o 5 times daily for 7–10 days) is a rational, affordable, and potentially useful therapy, although objective data are lacking. Other treatments that are widely used include flunixin meglumine (1.1 mg/kg i/v q12h) for treatment of vasculitis and DMSO (1 g/kg i/v as a 10% solution q12h) for platelet inhibition and scavenging of free radicals.

At present there are no proven methods for preventing EHM. Vaccines that are currently used to prevent EHV-1 respiratory disease and abortion do not offer protection against myeloencephalopathy. Routine vaccination may reduce the likelihood of exposure to the virus by reducing the incidence of other EHV-1 diseases. Vaccination during an outbreak is controversial, as previous exposure to EHV-1 or EHV-4 may be a risk factor for development of neurologic signs. Most authors do not recommend vaccination during an outbreak, but this continues to be an area of active research.

Management practices are important in helping to prevent the introduction and subsequent dissemination of EHV-1 infection (e.g. isolating new animals for 3 weeks and maintaining distinct herd groups according to age, gender, and occupation). Pregnant mares should not have access to the general population and stress should be minimized. The ability of EHV-1 to remain latent for prolonged periods of time and then re-emerge complicates infection-control measures.

Prognosis

The prognosis is reasonable provided horses remain standing. Often, there will be good improvement within the first 48 hours of treatment. More gradual improvement is then typically seen. Full recovery is possible, but weeks to months may be required. The prognosis is poor if there is clinical deterioration or no improvement over the first week of treatment.

Listeriosis

Listeriosis is rare in horses, although seroprevalence was reported as 68% of animals in one study. It can be manifested as septicemia, abortion, or meningoencephalomyelitis. The neurologic form resembles the disease in ruminants, with signs of cauda equina involvement. CSF analysis in these cases has not been reported, but elevated protein levels and pleocytosis is likely. *Listeria monocytogenes* has been isolated from blood cultures. Infection has been associated with immunosuppression and ingestion of improperly prepared corn silage. Most antimicrobials that are routinely used in horses, with the exception of ceftiofur, should be effective against *L. monocytogenes*.

Meningoencephalomyelitis

Definition/overview

Bacterial meningitis is a highly fatal disease that is rare in adult horses, but more common in neonatal foals.

Etiology/pathophysiology

Escherichia coli, Actinobacillus equuli, and *Klebsiella* spp., common causes of septicemia in neonatal foals, are most commonly implicated. Staphylococci and hemolytic streptococci may also be involved. *Salmonella* spp. meningitis may occur in foals and adults, although meningitis is a rare sequela to colitis in adult horses.

Meningitis in the horse is usually bacterial in origin and commonly occurs in one of three ways: (1) hematogenous spread from other sites; (2) direct extension of a suppurative process in or around the head; and (3) secondary to penetrating wounds. Neonatal septicemia is the most common cause of bacterial meningitis. Septic meningitis is the most common form and results in profound neurologic signs due to involvement of the superficial parenchyma and nerve roots of the brain and spinal cord. As the condition progresses, secondary CNS edema and obstructive hydrocephalus may lead to a worsening of clinical signs.

Clinical presentation

The initial clinical signs, such as aimless wandering, depression, loss of affinity for the dam, and abnormal vocalization, are not specific for meningitis, although they do indicate neurologic disease (**1024, 1025**). These signs are typical of those seen in hypoxic–ischemic encephalopathy in young foals and can cause misdiagnosis in the early stages. Sometimes, fever of unknown origin is the first abnormality that is detected. As meningitis progresses, other signs such as hyperesthesia, muscular rigidity, blindness, CN deficits, ataxia, and paresis of all limbs are seen. Without treatment, recumbency, coma, seizures, and death can occur.

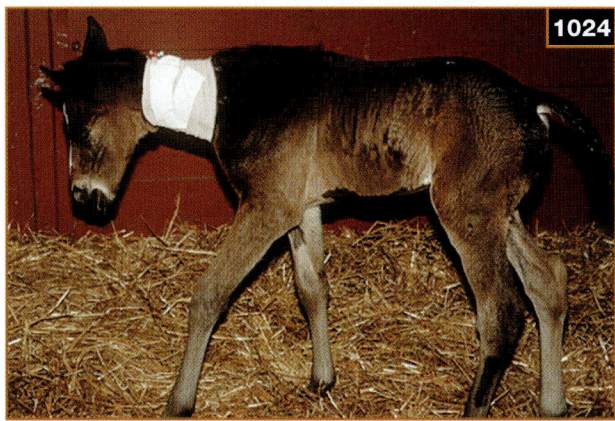

1024 A foal with meningitis wandering aimlessly.

1025 Seizuring and head pressing in a horse with meningitis.

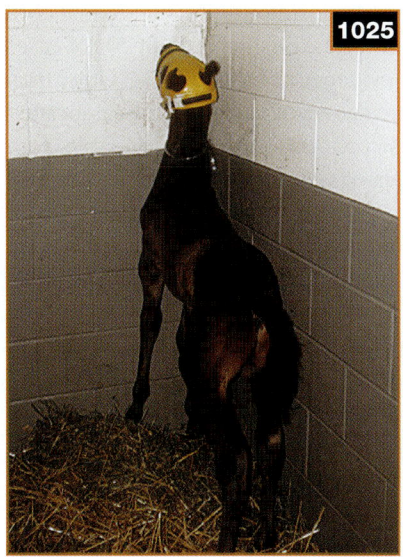

Differential diagnosis
EPM; hypoxic–ischemic encephalopathy; viral encephalitis (EEE, WEE, WNV); leukoencephalomalacia; cholesterol granuloma of the choroid plexus; trauma; aberrant parasite migration (*Halicephalobus deletrix*); hyperammonemia; metabolic derangement.

Diagnosis
Meningitis in foals should be regarded as a clinical emergency and early confirmation of the diagnosis is essential. This can be done by demonstrating bacteria or increased numbers of inflammatory cells with high protein and low glucose concentration in the CSF. Culture and cytology of CSF in addition to blood culture and culture of any other available septic sites should be performed in an attempt to isolate the causative organism. PCR may also be useful for identification of certain pathogens in the CSF.

Management
Without bacterial isolation and sensitivity patterns, or identification of an organism on cytology, treatment with broad-spectrum or combination antimicrobials is required. Commonly used treatments include aminoglycoside and penicillin combinations, potentiated sulfonamides, third-generation cephalosporins, and chloramphenicol. Meningeal inflammation considerably improves penetration of drugs into the CSF. Duration of antimicrobial therapy should be a minimum of 14 days, with therapy continuing for 7 days after the resolution of clinical signs. Other therapy includes the use of DMSO (1g/kg i/v given as a 10% solution) for its reduction of cerebral edema and free radical scavenging effects. If a septic focus is present, it should be addressed if possible. Aggressive supportive care, including nutritional support, may be required.

Prognosis
The prognosis for bacterial meningitis is poor. Even with aggressive supportive care, >50% of foals with bacterial meningitis die despite appropriate treatment. Early identification of disease and early treatment with appropriate antimicrobials are critical.

Borreliosis (Lyme disease)
Definition/overview
Lyme disease, an immune-mediated disorder caused by *Borrelia burgdorferi*, may occasionally cause brainstem encephalitis in horses in certain geographic areas. The true incidence of disease in the equine population is poorly understood.

Etiology/pathophysiology
B. burgdorferi is a spirochete that is maintained in a 2-year enzootic cycle involving *Ixodes* spp. ticks and mammals. Transmission to horses is known to occur during feeding activity of adult female ticks in the summer, fall, or late winter. Serologic studies have demonstrated a high incidence of seropositivity in horses in certain regions.

Clinical presentation
Clinical signs of Lyme disease in horses are variable, the most common including low-grade fever, stiffness and lameness in more than one limb, swollen joints, hyperesthesia, lethargy, and behavioral changes. Neurologic dysfunction and panuveitis have also been reported.

Differential diagnosis
Meningitis; exertional rhabdomyolysis; septic arthritis; laminitis; WNV encephalitis; fractured pelvis; trauma.

Diagnosis

Diagnosis is based on geographic area, clinical signs, ruling out other causes for the clinical signs, and finding a high (>300 KELA units) ELISA titer or a positive Western blot test for *B. burgdorferi*. The time from infection to seroconversion is 3–10 weeks, the great limitation of serologic tests being that they are unable to distinguish between active infection and subclinical exposure. Therefore, positive test results should be interpreted with caution. A PCR test is available for detecting the spirochete. It can be performed on tissue (including skin and muscle), ticks, synovial fluid, or whole blood.

Management

Treatment consists of oxytetracycline (6.6 mg/kg i/v q12h for 7 days) or oral doxycycline (10 mg/kg p/o q12h for 7 days). Treatment is often continued for a month, but this is empirical. Recurrence of clinical signs is often reported after treatment is discontinued. Other supportive treatments, including chondroprotective agents and NSAIDs, should also be considered.

Prevention in endemic areas involves the prevention of tick exposure and prolonged tick attachment, together with early antimicrobial treatment following *Ixodes* exposure. Insecticidal sprays are not approved for use in horses and there is no commercially available vaccine at this time, although ponies have been protected against experimental infection by the use of a vaccine.

Prognosis

The prognosis is good if appropriate treatment is provided.

Equine protozoal myeloencephalitis

Definition/overview

EPM is a common cause of neurologic disease in certain areas. A diverse range of clinical signs can be encountered.

Etiology/pathophysiology

Sarcocystis neurona appears to be the causative agent in most cases, although some cases have been linked to *Neospora hughesi*. The Virginia opossum (*Didelphis virginiana*) is the only definitive host for *S. neurona* in the US, while a related opossum (*Didelphis albiventris*) carries *S. neurona* in South America. Armadillos, raccoons, and the striped skunk have been identified as natural intermediate hosts. No definitive host has yet been identified for *N. hughesi*. The disease occurs in areas in which the causative organism and its host are found (i.e. North and South America). Cases have occurred all over the world in horses that have been imported from the US, often many months to years after arrival. The seroprevalance of the disease has been reported at 26–60%, but the incidence of new disease has been reported to be up to 0.51%, indicating that development of disease is uncommon following exposure to the causative agent. A number of risk factors have been associated with the development of clinical disease. One study noted a higher incidence in the spring, summer, and fall, and increased incidences in animals less than 5 years of age, animals living in wooded terrain, and if EPM had been diagnosed on the property previously.

Horses are infected by ingestion of sporocysts in food or water that has been contaminated by feces from the definitive host. Sporocysts may excyst in the small intestine, resulting in the release of sporozoites into the bloodstream. Uncommonly, the organism may penetrate the blood–brain barrier and multiply within neurons and leukocytes. This results in neuronal inflammation and death. A wide range of clinical signs may be evident depending on the location of infected neurons.

Clinical presentation

EPM is noted for its diversity of clinical signs, as a result of lesions of varying size and severity in any part of the CNS. The onset of signs may be insidious or acute. Spinal cord involvement occurs in most cases, while only 5% of cases are reported to show evidence of brain disease. Other than neurologic signs, there are no other syndromes associated with EPM. The disease course is also highly variable, with progression over hours or years possible, or a waxing and waning of signs over extended periods.

Signs of spinal cord disease that are seen include gait abnormalities (toe-dragging, cross cantering, interference between limbs, asymmetry of stride length), weakness and ataxia in the limbs or trunk, but usually most prominent in the hindlimbs, and abnormal proprioception. Signs are usually asymmetric and a small proportion (5–10%) of cases will demonstrate severe neurogenic atrophy of muscles of the trunk or limbs. The spectrum of clinical signs reported has also included cauda equina syndrome (paralysis of the bladder, rectum, anus, and penis; sensory loss of the tail and perineum), Sweeney, stringhalt, and a radial nerve-type syndrome.

Signs of brain disease are usually one of three forms:
+ Acute-onset asymmetric brainstem disease commonly involving dysfunction of CN VII (facial) and CN VIII (vestibulocochlear). Animals demonstrate signs of vestibular disease, with head tilt/turn, circling in one direction, and abnormal eye positions and nystagmus. Other CNs can be affected with associated clinical signs.
+ Atrophy of the lingual or masticatory muscles (**1003**). This is usually of an insidious onset and may appear as a singular syndrome. These cases do not normally progress beyond complete and permanent atrophy of the muscle affected.
+ A cerebral syndrome, with horses showing signs of dysfunction of the visual or sensory centers, such as blindness or facial hypalgesia.

Other less frequent signs that have been recorded are head pressing, demented behavior, and seizures.

Differential diagnosis
As EPM may mimic almost any other neurologic disease, the list of diagnostic rule-outs is extensive.

Diagnosis
A definitive antemortem diagnosis cannot be achieved by clinicopathologic means and most often a clinical diagnosis of EPM is reached based on an accumulation of data. Important considerations in reaching a diagnosis are relevant history and compatible clinical signs, clinical progression, laboratory and other diagnostic aids, exclusion of other possible causes, and response to treatment. Laboratory and other diagnostic aids have been divided into three categories: (1) positive immunoblot for *S. neurona* antibodies, which supports the diagnosis; (2) negative immunoblot, which tends to exclude the diagnosis; and (3) tests that support alternative diagnoses and thus indirectly exclude a diagnosis of EPM. Serum and CSF immunoblots for *S. neurona* antibodies have a high sensitivity (horses that have the disease test positive about 87% of the time) but a poor specificity (about 44% of horses that do not have the disease also test positive) and therefore should not be used alone for diagnosis. The main problem with CSF antibody detection is that inadvertent contamination of the sample with serum antibodies is common and can produce false-positive results. Detection of *S. neurona* antigen by PCR is highly suggestive; however, positive results are uncommon in affected animals because of the intracellular nature of the organism.

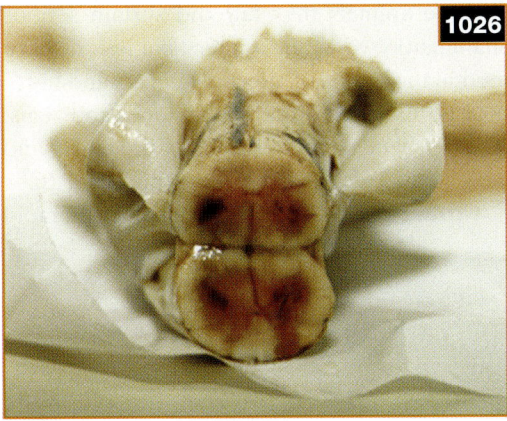

1026 Gross lesions of EPM in the spinal cord of a horse. Grossly hemorrhagic regions are visible. (Photo courtesy FT Bain)

A positive serum immunoblot test is also only indicative of exposure and not necessarily reflective of active disease. However, because of the high sensitivity, a negative result is often considered more significant, making it highly unlikely that the horse has the disease. Because of the poor specificity of the serum and CSF immunoblot tests, many clinicians use other criteria, such as a response to treatment, to allow them to make a retrospective diagnosis. Postmortem analysis may be required for a convincing diagnosis (**1026**).

Management
Antiprotozoal drugs are the most important feature of therapy. Other treatments that may be considered in individual cases are anti-inflammatories, antioxidants, biological response modifiers, and physical therapy. Traditional treatment has centered around the use of combinations of pyrimethamine (1 mg/kg p/o q24h for 3–6 months) and sulfonamides (20–30 mg/kg p/o q12h for 3–6 months). These sequentially inhibit folic acid synthesis in the protozoa. Originally, pyrimethamine was administered with trimethoprim/sulfonamide tablets, but many compounding pharmacies now produce sulfadiazine/pyrimethamine solutions/suspensions. It is recommended that the horse is not fed for 1 hour before and after administration.

Diclazuril, toltrazuril, and ponazuril are triazine-based agents that are effective against coccidia in birds and mammals and are also reported to be effective against *S. neurona*. Toltrazuril and diclazuril are licensed for use in poultry in some countries, but efficacy against EPM is unclear. Ponazuril is a metabolite of toltrazuril and is currently approved in the US for the treatment of EPM at a dose rate of 5 mg/kg p/o q24h for 28 days.

Recently, nitazoxanide has been approved for the treatment of EPM in the US. The recommended dosing regimen is 25 mg/kg p/o q24h for days 1–5 then 50 mg/kg p/o q24h for days 6–28.

The comparative effectiveness of ponazuril and nitazoxanide is not objectively known; the opinion of many clinicians is that they have similar efficacy.

Antioxidant therapy with vitamin E (10,000 IU p/o q24h for 30 days) can be used as adjunctive treatment. Anti-inflammatory therapy (e.g. flunixin meglumine, 1 mg/kg i/v or p/o q12–24h) may be warranted.

An EPM vaccine is available, but currently there are no scientific data supporting the efficacy of the vaccine.

Prognosis
The prognosis can be good if ataxia of grade 2 or less is present. If the animal becomes recumbent, the prognosis is considered poor. Some animals recover from the initial event, but have sustained permanent nerve injury resulting in residual nerve deficits.

Trypanosomiasis

Trypanosomes are blood-borne protozoa that cause disease in many mammals, including horses. There are numerous species with different modes of transmission and strains with differing virulence. Tsetse fly-transmitted trypanosomes cause disease in Africa. *Trypanosoma evansi* is transmitted by hematophagous flies and vampire bats, resulting in Surra, an important disease of economic importance in Asia and South America. Dourine is caused by *T. equiperdum* in Asia, South Africa, India, and Russia. This is the only trypanosome that is vertically transmitted. This disease has been eradicated from North America. Clinical signs of trypanosomiasis are variable, but include pyrexia, anemia, weight loss, lymphadenopathy, and often death. Signs of meningoencephalomyelitis that can be seen include muscle atrophy, facial nerve paralysis, and limb ataxia and weakness that is worse in the hindlimbs. Treatment involves the use of various trypanosomides, but resistance may be encountered. Treatment of animals with dourine is not recommended, as they may become carriers.

Verminous meningoencephalomyelitis

Definition/overview
Verminous meningoencephalomyelitis is a rare and sporadic disorder caused by the aberrant migration of parasites through the CNS.

Etiology/pathophysiology
Several parasites have been reported including *Strongylus*, *Hypoderma*, *Habronema*, *Draschia*, *Halicephalobus*, and *Setaria* species. Transmission of *Halicephalobus gingivalis* from mare to dam has been reported. *S. vulgaris* thromboarteritis may rarely lead to embolic showering of the cerebrum.

Clinical presentation
The spectrum of clinical signs is variable and depends on the area of the CNS that is involved. Diffuse, focal, or multifocal disease may be evident. Cerebral, cerebellar, brainstem, or spinal cord signs may be observed.

Diagnosis
Diagnosis is usually based on clinical signs and necropsy findings. CSF changes are not specific or consistent, with some hemorrhage and an increased numbers of inflammatory cells, such as eosinophils and neutrophils, to be expected. CSF eosinophilia suggests the possibility of parasitic disease, but is neither highly sensitive nor highly specific. Uncommonly, larvae may be evident in the CSF. Peripheral eosinophilia is uncommon.

Management
Therapy should include the use of anthelmintics (fenbendazole, 50 mg/kg p/o q24h for 3 days) and anti-inflammatories (flunixin meglumine, DMSO, vitamin E, and/or dexamethasone). Avermectins may not be effective because of the drugs' gamma aminobutyric acid (GABA)-inhibiting method of destroying parasites. It is also theoretically toxic to mammals due to the GABA inhibition if it crosses the blood–brain barrier.

Recently, prominent cervical scoliosis with minimal ataxia in adult horses has been described in the northeastern US. This syndrome appears to be due to *Parelaphastrongylus tenuis* (meningeal worm of white-tailed deer) entering the cervical spinal cord via the dorsal nerve roots and causing a selective myelitis in the dorsal gray columns. There are no localizing signs of motor or sensory loss and no denervation muscle atrophy associated with this syndrome. The scoliosis may be the result of disafferentiation of cervical musculature. The signs are permanent.

Prognosis
Overall, the prognosis is guarded. In animals that do not become recumbent and only display mild abnormalities, the prognosis is fair to good.

Equine ehrlichiosis

Horses infected with the tick-borne pathogen *Anaplasma phagocytophila* (formerly *Ehrlichia equi*) often have transient truncal and limb ataxia. These animals may also display weakness. The weakness and ataxia seen can be severe and these animals may fall and sustain serious injuries. Inflammatory vascular or interstitial lesions have been reported in the brains of affected animals and histologically there is inflammation of small arteries and veins, primarily in the subcutis, fascia, nerves of the limbs, and reproductive organs. Treatment with oxytetracycline (6.6–7.5 mg/kg i/v q12–24h for 3–7 days) often results in rapid improvement.

Tetanus

Definition/overview

Tetanus is a highly fatal infectious disease caused by *Clostridium tetani*. The disease is characterized by muscular rigidity and hyperesthesia in horses of all ages. While the causative agent is relatively ubiquitous, disease is uncommon in developed countries because of widespread vaccination, but common in areas where vaccination is less widely used.

Etiology/pathophysiology

C. tetani is a spore-forming anaerobic bacterium that is widespread in the environment. Spores of *C. tetani* may be found in soil and feces worldwide.

Inoculation of *C. tetani* from spores in soil or feces into wounds can lead to growth of the organism if the proper local conditions are present. Specifically, an anaerobic environment, produced by local tissue necrosis or contamination with facultative anaerobic bacteria, allows *C. tetani* spores to germinate, proliferate, and produce toxins. Three main toxins are produced:

✦ Tetanolysin causes tissue necrosis, allowing for continued proliferation of *C. tetani*.

✦ Tetanospasmin spreads hematogenously to the CNS by passage along peripheral nerves. It localizes in the ventral horn of gray matter of the spinal cord and brainstem, binding irreversibly to gangliosides within synaptic membranes. The main action of the toxin is to block the release of inhibitory neurotransmitter. Thus, reflexes normally inhibited by descending inhibitory motor tracts or by inhibitory interneurons are greatly facilitated, resulting in tetanic contractions of muscle following normal sensory stimuli.

✦ A nonspasmogenic toxin is also produced, and may produce excessive sympathetic stimulation.

Horses are particularly sensitive to the effects of tetanus toxins.

Clinical presentation

There is a wide variability between the time of wound contamination and onset of signs of tetanus, as the spores are viable for many months and may germinate long after a wound has apparently healed if the conditions are appropriate (i.e. re-injury). The incubation period is generally 1–3 weeks, but can be several months, and there may be no history or evidence of a wound.

The severity of signs and rate of progression of the disease depend on the dose of toxin and the size and age of the animal. The signs that are seen are reflective of spasticity of striated and smooth muscle and initially include a stiff gait and hyperesthesia. Spasm of the muscles of mastication results in difficulty opening the mouth ('lockjaw'). Facial muscle spasm results in an 'anxious' expression with retracted lips, flared nostrils, and erect ears. Extraocular muscle contraction causes retraction of the eyeball, with resulting prolapse of the nictitating membranes (**1027**). A tap on the forehead or other stimulus frequently results in marked spasm of cervical, facial, masticatory, and extraocular muscles. The striated muscles are progressively affected, causing rigid extension of the neck, limbs, and tail (saw-horse stance) (**1028**).

If an affected mature horse falls, it is usually unable to rise because of rigid extension of the extremities and further muscle spasms as a result of attempts to rise. Foals that fall may be helped to stand. Death from respiratory arrest or aspiration pneumonia usually occurs within 5–7 days of the onset of clinical signs. Other complications of recumbency and intense muscle spasm such as fractures can also be lethal.

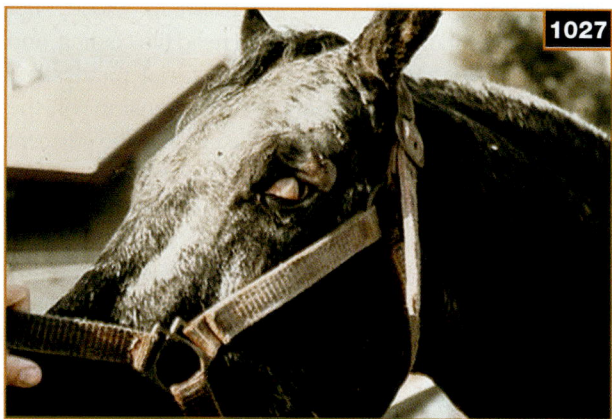

1027 Prolapse of the nictitating membrane in a horse with tetanus.

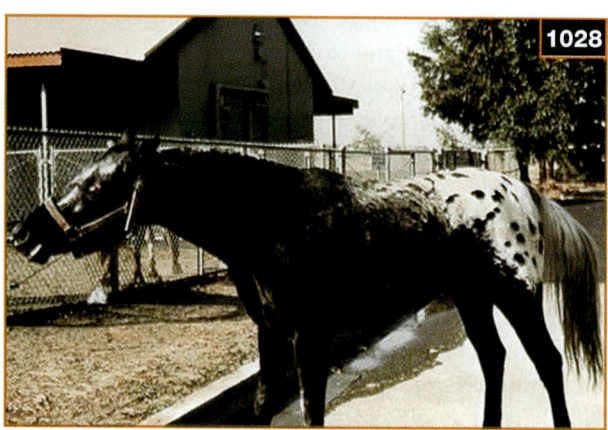

1028 Saw-horse muscle rigidity noted in a horse with tetanus.

Management

Treatment is based on the knowledge that the toxin–gangliosides bond is irreversible and that gradual replacement of altered gangliosides by normal metabolic processes will lead to recovery and is thus primarily symptomatic and supportive. The primary objectives of therapy are destruction of *C. tetani* organisms, neutralization of unbound toxin, control of muscle spasm, and general supportive care. Neutralization involves the administration of large amounts of tetanus antitoxin (TAT). The recommended doses and frequency of administration of TAT vary widely. The dose given should be based on the history of the case and influenced by factors such as a delay in treatment of several hours after injury, lack of aggressive debridement, or no history of vaccination. Recommended doses range from 5,000–20,000 IU i/v and/or 5000–20000 IU intrathecally. Intrathecal administration of tetanus antitoxin has been used with variable success. In addition to TAT administration, tetanus toxoid should also be administered because protective humoral immunity is not induced by natural disease. Penicillin (sodium penicillin [20,000–40,000 IU/kg i/v q6h] or procaine penicillin [20,000–40,000 IU/kg i/m q12h]) should be administered. Wound care, including debridement, is important. Sedation (acepromazine, 0.05–0.1 mg/kg i/m or i/v q4–6h) may be useful to reduce anxiety and provide muscle relaxation. Muscle-relaxing drugs such as guaifenesin should not be used.

Supportive care is important. Horses should be placed in a dark, quiet environment with minimal stimulation. Ear plugs may be useful. Intravenous fluid therapy will be required in dysphagic horses. Nutritional care, including feeding via a nasogastric tube or parenteral nutrition, may be necessary. Frequent passage of a nasogastric tube should be avoided to reduce stimuli.

Horses that are presented in lateral recumbency have little chance of recovery and euthanasia should be considered.

Active immunization is reliably achieved with readily available toxoid vaccines. Current recommendations are administration of tetanus toxoid at 3, 4, and 6 months of age, followed by annual vaccination, although there is evidence that protective titers persist for years after the first booster. Unvaccinated horses are commonly given TAT after injury, but there is an association between the administration of TAT and the development of an acute fatal hepatic necrosis (Theiler's disease), and the owner should be informed of this risk if it is necessary to administer TAT (e.g. previously unvaccinated animal). It is reasonable to administer tetanus toxoid rather than antitoxin to an animal that has sustained an injury but has been vaccinated with tetanus toxoid in the previous year. Circulating tetanus antitoxin may interfere with the immune response to later tetanus toxoid administration, and for this reason any foals that have received colostrum from mares that have been vaccinated within 30 days of foaling or, alternatively, received TAT at birth should not be vaccinated until 3–6 months of age. Routine administration of TAT to foals from vaccinated mares in not warranted.

Prognosis

The prognosis depends on the severity of clinical signs, but is poor overall. Mortality rates of 50–75% in treated animals have been reported. Prolonged treatment is often required, and financial concerns may preclude treatment in some cases.

Otitis media-interna/temporohyoid osteoarthropathy

Definition/overview

Otitis media-interna is uncommon in horses compared with other species.

Etiology/pathophysiology

Streptococcus spp., *Staphylococcus* spp., *Actinobacillus* spp., and *Aspergillus* spp., have been implicated, but the causative agent is often not identified.

It is assumed that infection of the middle ear arises as a result of hematogenous spread or direct extension of infectious processes in the pharynx, guttural pouch, or external ear. In some cases, osteoarthropahy of the petrous temporal bone and stylohyoid bone may result in fusion of the temporohyoid articulation. The vestibular and facial nerves may be affected as bony proliferation progresses. In some situations, fracture of the stylohyoid bone may occur as a result of immobility of the temporohyoid joint. Stylohyoid fracture typically produces a sudden onset or worsening of clinical signs, particularly those involving the facial and vestibular nerves. The hypoglossal and vagal nerves may also be affected.

Clinical presentation

Clinical signs that are seen are normally those of a peripheral vestibular syndrome, with head tilt, circling, and ataxia (**1029**). Concurrent ipsilateral facial paralysis is common and usually results from extension of the suppurative process from the middle ear into the adjacent facial canal or internal acoustic meatus containing CN VII. Signs of facial nerve damage such as exposure keratitis may precede the vestibular signs. Discharge from the external ear following rupture of the tympanic membrane is occasionally seen. Head shaking has been reported as another rare clinical sign in cases of primary otitis media.

Differential diagnosis

EPM; WNV encephalitis; trauma; ear ticks; polyneuritis equi.

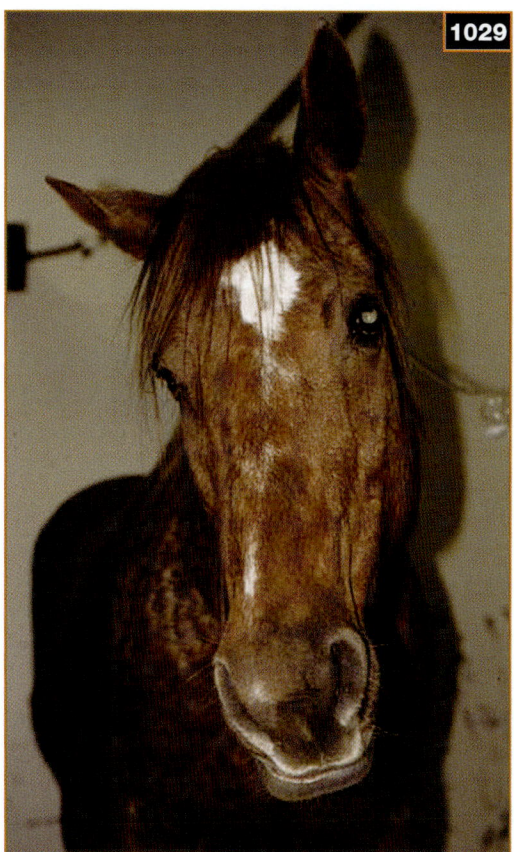

1029 Right-side head tilt and facial and vestibulo-cochlear nerve deficits with right-sided otitis interna/media and temporohyoid osteoarthropathy. Note the muzzle deviation to the left.

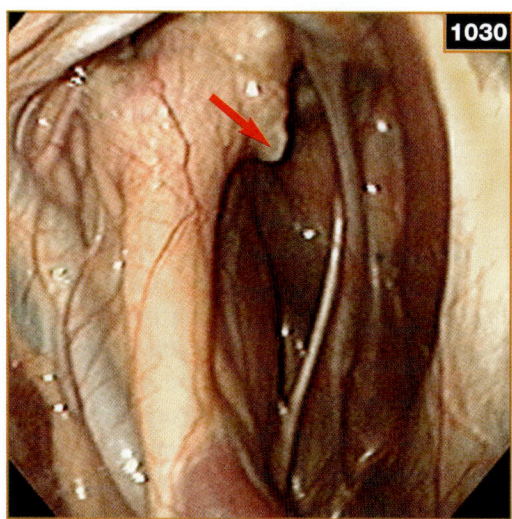

1030 Right-sided temporohyoid osteoarthropathy. Note the osseous proliferation of the temporohyoid joint (arrow).

Diagnosis

The neurologic examination should identify vestibular and facial-nerve involvement. Diagnosis is based on clinical signs, endoscopy, and radiography with or without isolation and culture of an infectious organism. Endoscopy may demonstrate pharyngitis, guttural pouch disease, or proliferative lesions involving the petrous temporal bone and proximal portion of the stylohyoid bone (1030). Sclerosis of the affected tympanic bulla may be evident radiographically even in acute cases, with thickening and sclerosis of the stylohyoid and petrous temporal bones. Exudates from the ear, guttural pouch, or pharynx should be cultured. CSF is usually normal. Flushing sterile fluid through the middle ear via tympanocentesis can confirm the presence of sepsis. Many cases that are diagnosed as otitis media or otitis interna are in fact secondary manifestations of temporohyoid joint disease without middle ear infection.

Management

While not all cases are bacterial in origin, antibiotic treatment is justified in all suspected cases of middle ear infection. Prolonged antimicrobial therapy (trimethoprim/sulfamethoxazole, 30 mg/kg p/o q24h for 30 days) is usually required in addition to anti-inflammatory treatment (flunixin meglumine, 1.1 mg/kg i/v or p/o q12–24h; phenylbutazone, 2.2–4.4 mg/kg p/o q12h for 3–7 days). Short-term corticosteroids (dexamethasone 0.05 mg/kg i/v q24h for 24–48h) may be useful. If fusion of the temporohyoid articulation is evident, removal of a section of the affected stylohyoid bone may minimize mechanical stresses resulting from ankylosis of the temporohyoid joint. Sequelae to facial nerve paralysis (e.g. corneal ulceration) should be treated promptly.

Prognosis

The prognosis is fair to good. Facial nerve paresis and compensated vestibular function may remain following functional recovery.

Central nervous system trauma/accidents

Lightning strike

Signs from mild ataxia to sudden death may be seen. Evidence such as singed lines in the coat or evidence of lightning strike on nearby trees may be present. Multiple animals may be affected, particularly if they have taken shelter under the same tree during a storm. Commonly, no evidence is found and there is simply a history of a thunderstorm in the area. Also, animals may on occasion become frightened in a storm and collide with fixed objects, resulting in spinal injuries and death.

Cerebral trauma

Definition/overview

Signs related to cerebral trauma most frequently occur following trauma to the frontal or parietal regions of the head. Horses are susceptible to such injuries because of their size, behavior, and relatively thin calvarium.

Etiology/pathophysiology

Abnormal neurologic signs may be the result of mechanical injury to the brain, cerebral edema, parenchymal hemorrhage, and ischemia produced by brain swelling and intravascular clotting. Mechanical injury and cerebral edema are the most important factors in animals with cerebral trauma with fractures. Compound fractures of the frontal and parietal bones are likely to cause cerebral laceration and hemorrhage. Intracranial bleeding is more common in neonates.

Clinical presentation

In severe cases an initial period of unconsciousness of variable length may be encountered. Fluctuating neurologic signs, which are dependent on the degree of intracranial hypertension associated with cerebral edema and hemorrhage, are displayed. Wandering towards the side of the lesion and depression are common clinical signs. Ataxia is not usually seen unless there is progressive involvement of other parts of the brain. PLRs are usually brisk, but there may be some asymmetry of the pupils and miosis. Characteristically there is central blindness and depressed menace responses.

Swelling of the cerebral hemispheres may cause herniation caudally against the midbrain (subtentorial herniation) and lead to signs such as dilated unresponsive pupils (1031) and tetraparesis.

Diagnosis

A history of head trauma or clinical evidence of trauma (abrasions, lacerations) is often present. If head trauma is known or highly suspected, the diagnostic plan should be

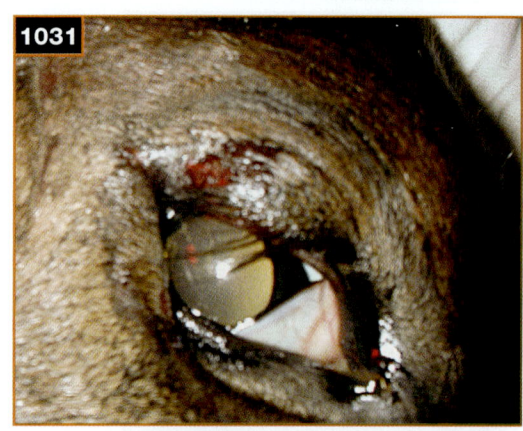

1031 Foal that was found down in the pasture. The foal had nonresponsive pupillary light reflexes and was obtunded. It made a full recovery from the cerebral trauma after 5 days of treatment.

to localize the lesion and establish a baseline neurologic examination to monitor progression of the disease. If a history of trauma is less clear, testing to rule out other conditions may be warranted.

Management

In most cases (i.e. those that do not require immediate surgical intervention because of depressed skull fractures), early management is supportive and medical. Any other life-threatening conditions should be attended to first, as the trauma associated with the cerebral injury may have caused other more immediate problems such as cardiac arrhythmias. Seizures or excessive, difficult to manage thrashing may require sedation or short-term anesthesia. Diazepam (5 mg [foal] and 50–100 mg [adult] i/v or i/m) can be repeated as necessary to control seizures. Phenobarbital (12 mg/kg i/v loading dose followed by 6 mg/kg i/v q12h) or pentobarbital (150–1,000 mg i/v for foals; for adults slow increments of 500–1,000 mg i/v to effect) may also be used to control seizures. Care should be used with these drugs, as they are highly protein bound and can be displaced by other drugs, leading to a larger amount of free or active drug. Repeated seizures may require long-term therapy and more than one anti-seizure drug may be required if there is a poor initial response. Treatment should always begin at the lowest dose possible, which can then be increased daily if required until the seizures have been controlled. Alpha-2 agonists (e.g. xylazine, detomidine) should be avoided for the treatment of seizures in the acute stages as they can cause transient hypertension, exacerbating CNS hemorrhage, and can suppress ventilation.

After the establishment of proper respiratory function and control of seizures, the general medical principles for the treatment of CNS trauma are administration of osmotic diuretics, nutritional and fluid support, and protection from the self-inflicted trauma effects of prolonged recumbency. Many consequences of cranial trauma, such as hemorrhage, laceration necrosis, secondary ischemia, and midbrain injury, are inaccessible to therapy. However, the presence of some of these lesions is difficult to diagnose and failure to improve or a deterioration in neurologic condition may be the only clue to their existence.

The use of corticosteroids in horses with CNS signs is controversial. Some clinicians administer dexamethasone (0.1–0.25 mg/kg i/v q4–6h) for 1–4 days. (**Note:** The administration of dexamethasone for the treatment of supratentorial intracerebral hemorrhage in humans has failed to show a beneficial effect.) Studies in humans with methylprednisolone (30 mg/kg bolus followed by CRI 4 mg/kg/hour) have shown beneficial effects, which is thought to be derived from the stoichiometric antioxidant activity of the steroid. However, it requires frequent administration and the benefits should be weighed against the possible complications of steroid administration in the horse. Intravenous administration of 20% mannitol (0.25–1.0 g/kg via a blood filter) has been used for the treatment of increased intracranial pressure. Mannitol is thought to decrease CSF pressure due to vasoconstrictive effects, in addition to acting as an osmotic diuretic. Response to mannitol is usually noted within 1 hour and if a response is noted, mannitol administration should be repeated every 4–6 hours for the first day. DMSO (1 g/kg slowly i/v as a 10% solution) has several potentially beneficial pharmacologic effects including diuresis, free-radical scavenging, inhibition of platelet aggregation, vasodilation, and increased penetration of steroids and antimicrobials into the brain. There are many anecdotal reports of successful treatment with DMSO, but clinical trials in other species have not shown a clear benefit in treating CNS trauma. Adverse effects include intravascular hemolysis, which has been associated with too rapid administration or administration of a more concentrated solution. DMSO administration can be repeated every 12 hours for 3–4 days if clinical improvement is seen.

Hypoxemia and hypercapnia should be avoided, as hypoxia exacerbates brain swelling and hypercapnia increases intracranial blood volume and pressure. Recumbent horses should be rolled every 4–6 hours to minimize pulmonary arteriovenous shunting and ventilation perfusion mismatching. Ideally, the head should also be maintained at heart-base level or higher to avoid hypostatic intracranial congestion. Maintenance of hydration is important, but overhydration should be avoided, as it can exacerbate brain edema.

Close monitoring and good nursing care are essential. If an improvement is noted in 6–8 hours, treatment should be repeated. If no improvement is seen, more aggressive treatment may be warranted, including exploratory craniotomy. If no improvement is seen or deterioration is noted in a comatose patient 36 hours after surgery or anesthesia, euthanasia may be indicated.

Prognosis

The prognosis is highly variable. Recumbency is a poor prognostic indicator. Ideally, stabilization of neurologic abnormalities should occur within 24–48 hours, with gradual improvement over the next week and slower improvement from then on. Once a plateau in improvement is encountered, there will usually be minimal further recovery. The development of a midbrain syndrome warrants a poor prognosis, whereas an uncomplicated cerebral syndrome usually has a good prognosis, as response to treatment for brain swelling can be good.

Intracarotid injection

Inadvertent intracarotid injection in horses is common because of the close apposition of the jugular vein and carotid artery in the caudal third of the neck. It commonly results in an acute seizure, followed by recumbency and degrees of coma. Contralateral facial twitching and a wide-eyed apprehensive appearance may precede the seizure. Animals may rear or strike violently. The onset of signs is rapid with viscous or irritant drugs. With water-soluble drugs, such as xylazine or acetylpromazine, recovery usually occurs, with the horse standing in 5–60 minutes and completely normal in 1–7 days. With insoluble and oil-based drugs, recovery is usually unsatisfactory, with epilepsy, stupor, or coma as common sequelae that necessitate euthanasia.

Treatment is not usually necessary with the tranquilizers and water-soluble drugs because effects are self-limiting and of reasonably short duration. Violent horses should be sedated with diazepam (50–100 mg to an adult horse i/v), placed in a padded stall, and treated with dexamethasone (0.02–0.05 mg/kg i/v). Administration of mannitol or other osmotic diuretics should be avoided in the first 24 hours because of potential damage to the blood–brain barrier or active bleeding in the CNS. The use of proper injection techniques should greatly reduce the risk of intracarotid injection.

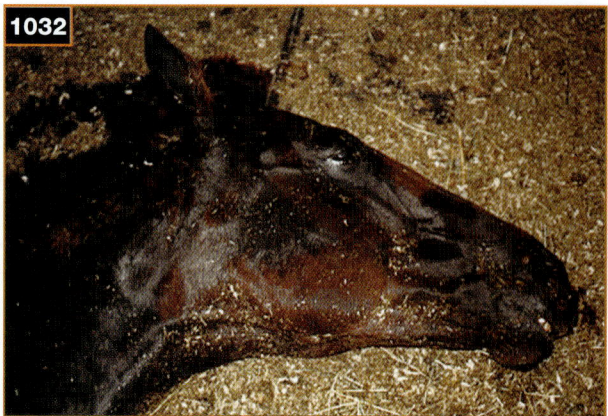

1032 Horse with a basisphenoid fracture.

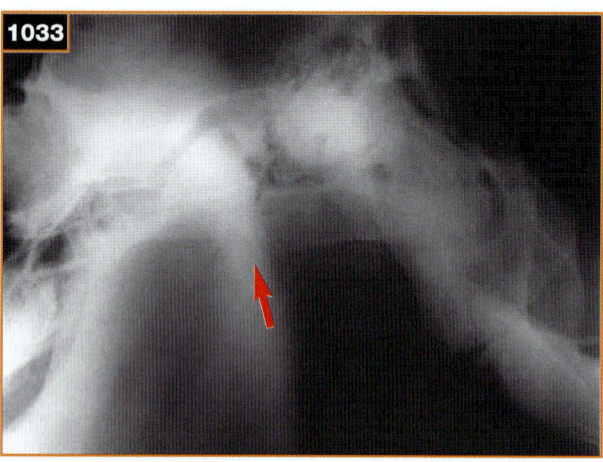

1033 Radiographic film depicting a basioccipital fracture (arrow). Note the displacement ventrally of the basisphenoid bone. This horse reared up and flipped over when a bridle was being placed.

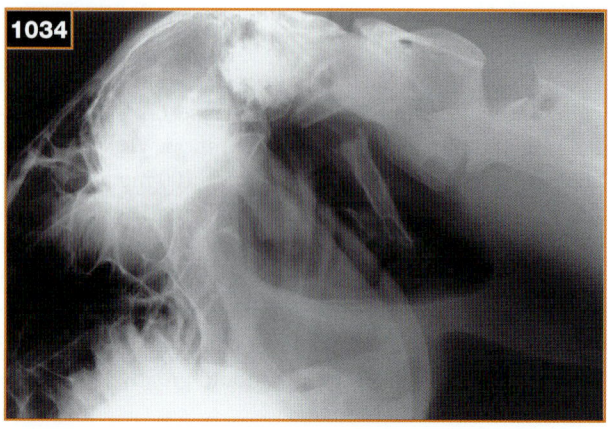

1034 Radiograph of a displaced fracture of the basisphenoid bone. The horse had reared up and flipped over in the show ring, resulting in temporary unconsciousness followed by seizures, ataxia, and bilateral epistaxis.

Brainstem trauma

Trauma to the poll by rearing and hitting an overhead obstruction or falling over backwards and striking the head on the ground is the most common cause of brainstem injury, which may occur with or without skull fractures. Commonly recognized syndromes in horses following poll trauma are midbrain syndrome, optic nerve injury, and, most commonly, medullary inner ear syndrome.

Midbrain syndrome can arise as a result of basisphenoid/basioccipital bone fracture and associated hemorrhage causing severe brainstem injury (**1032–1034**). Cerebral edema may also compress this area. Profound neurologic signs and a poor prognosis accompany injury to the midbrain and sudden death can occur. Sub-basilar hemorrhage may also result in life-threatening inspiratory dyspnea or cardiac arrhythmias.

Optic nerve trauma results from stretching of the optic nerves due to the sudden backward movement of the brain against the fixed canalicular portion of the optic nerves when the head strikes the ground. Tearing of optic fibers results in immediate and irreversible blindness and can affect one or both eyes. Suppressed menace responses and degrees of pupillary dilation are noted immediately. Signs of optic nerve atrophy (loss of vascularity and color change in the optic disk) are apparent after approximately 2 weeks. Treatment as described for cerebral trauma should be attempted (see p. 774). The prognosis is usually guarded.

Vestibular and cerebellar injury

Trauma to the back of the head may cause hemorrhage around the medulla or into the middle or inner ear. This may be complicated by fractures of the occipital and petrosal bones, separation of these bones, or separation of the basioccipital and basisphenoid bones ventral to the pons and medulla (**1035**). Pre-existing osteoarthrosis and ankylosis of the temporohyoid joint(s), which may or may not be associated with otitis interna, predispose to fractures of the hyoid bone and through the osseous bulla and adjacent petrous temporal bone. The neurologic signs that result are often quite variable and asymmetric, depending on which CNs are affected and the extent of medullary parenchymal damage. Hemorrhage into the middle and inner ear cavities causes vestibular and facial nerve signs such as head tilt, circling, ipsilateral facial paralysis, and spontaneous horizontal or rotary nystagmus, with the fast phase away from the side of the lesion. Vestibular nystagmus may be abnormal or absent. Additional signs associated with hemorrhage in or around the medulla and into the CSF (e.g. depression and ataxia) are

1035 Comminuted, displaced fracture of the occipital protruberance (arrow) as a result of falling over backwards.

1036 Skull fracture causing trauma to the left facial nerve. Note the muzzle deviation to the right.

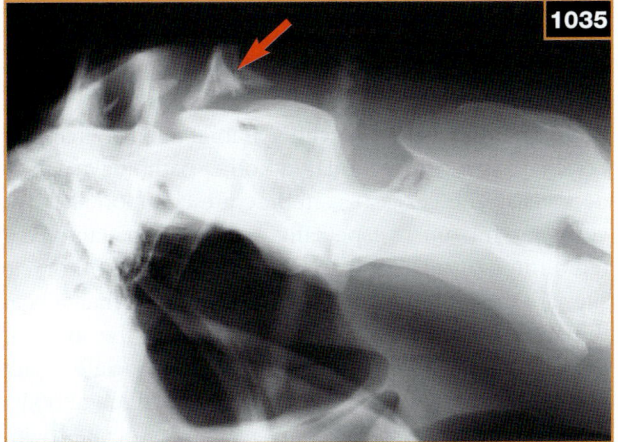

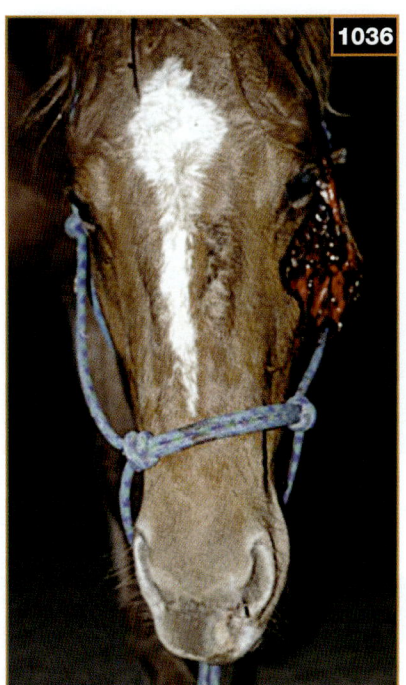

often seen. Horses suffering a blow to the poll occasionally develop a head nod or coarse head tremor that is especially obvious during eating or drinking. This is probably due to direct cerebellar injury. Treatment is similar to that described for cerebral trauma (see p. 774). The prognosis is fair.

Facial nerve trauma

The facial nerve (CN VII) innervates the muscles of facial expression. Facial paralysis is common in horses and, depending on the site of damage, some or all of the facial muscles may be affected. Unilateral facial paralysis is more common and is evident as deviation of the muzzle towards the normal side, ipsilateral ear, eyelid, and lip drooping, in addition to reduced flaring of the ipsilateral nostril during inspiration. Inability to close the eyelid causes exposure keratitis. There may also be damage to the secretomotor fibers of the facial nerve, leading to reduced tear production. These fibers may be damaged at or proximal to the geniculate ganglion. Bilateral facial nerve paralysis can result in signs of dysphagia, with dropping of feed and accumulation of feed between teeth and cheeks. It is important to determine the site of the lesion, as it determines the prognosis. Full facial paralysis occurs if the facial nerve is injured proximal to the vertical ramus of the mandible. These injuries are seen with fractures of the

vertical ramus of the mandible, the stylohyoid bone, or the petrous temporal bone. Other causes of unilateral facial paralysis without direct injury to the facial nerve are medullary lesions involving the facial nucleus, polyneuritis equi, idiopathic facial paralysis, hemorrhage into the middle or inner ear, guttural pouch mycosis, and parotid lymph-node abscessation.

Distal facial nerve damage is most commonly caused by direct injury from a blow and can be caused by prolonged lateral recumbency (**1036**). A frequent site of damage is where the nerve or its branches cross(es) the mandible or zygomatic arch.

Treatment consists of either NSAIDS (phenylbutazone [2–4 mg/kg i/v or p/o q12h] or flunixin meglumine [1.1 mg/kg i/v or p/o q12h for 3–5 days]) or corticosteroids (dexamethasone, 0.05–0.1 mg/kg i/v, i/m or p/o q24h for 48–72 hours). The use of a topical anti-inflammatory cream, such as 1% diclofenac sodium, may also be indicated to control inflammation associated with the facial nerve. The prognosis for the return of facial nerve function depends on the site and severity of the lesion. Without severe skin laceration, the prognosis for peripheral facial paralysis is good, although recovery may take several weeks to months. If there is section of the nerve and the ends can be identified, immediate surgical repair is indicated.

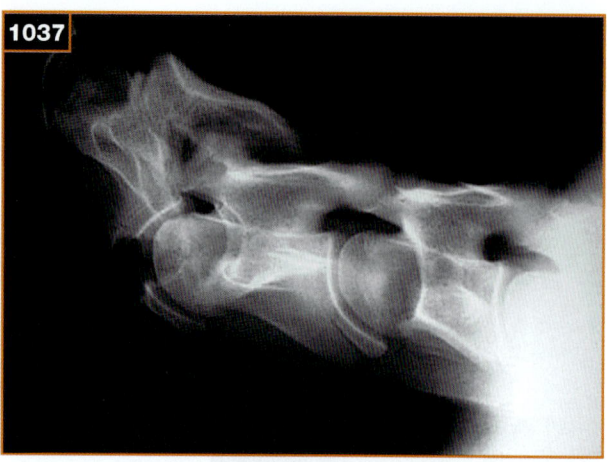

1037 Displaced cervical (C5) fracture.

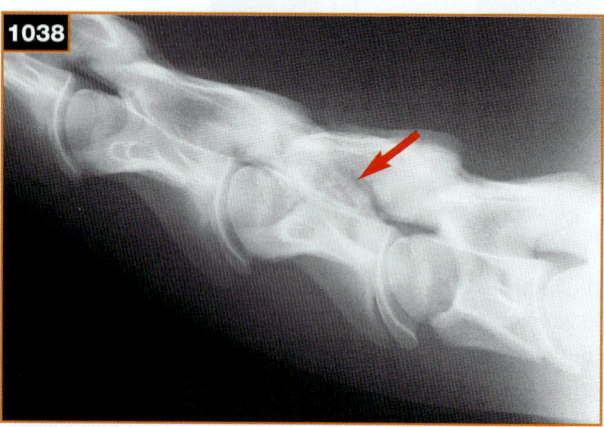

1038 Fracture of the cervical body of C5 that occurred as a result of a fall.

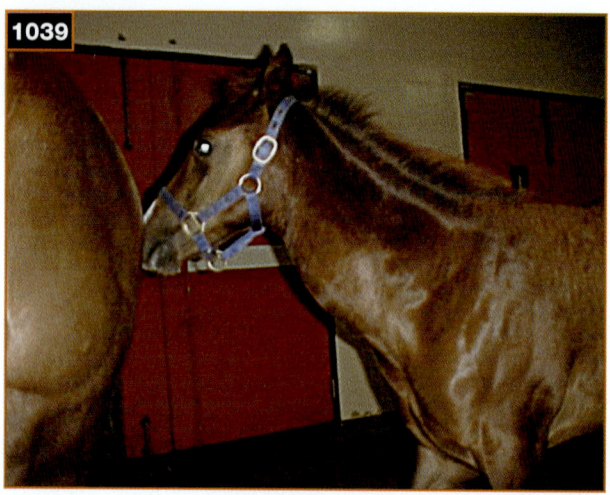

1039 Foal with symmetrical grade 3 ataxia in all four limbs. Note the swelling in the mid-caudal neck. The foal had a fracture of C5, as displayed in figure 1037.

Spinal cord trauma

Definition/overview
Suspected spinal cord trauma is one of the most common neurologic disorders presented to equine practitioners. Musculoskeletal and/or neurologic abnormalities may be encountered.

Etiology/pathophysiology
Many cases of vertebral trauma with or without neurologic signs have been reported. Spinal cord trauma typically occurs following a traumatic incident (e.g. a fall) and may or may not be associated with vertebral trauma. Fractures occasionally occur secondary to other pathology such as neoplasia. The cervical vertebrae are common sites for vertebral fractures, especially the occipitoatlantoaxial region in foals. The lower cervical and cranial thoracic sites are the most common areas for vertebral fractures in the adult horse (1037, 1038). Fractures of the thoracic dorsal spinous process are not usually associated with neurologic signs, whereas fractures of the vertebral body, arch, or articular processes are usually associated with neurologic signs.

Clinical presentation
Neurologic abnormalities are not always present in cases of vertebral trauma. There is much variability in the syndromes that result from trauma, depending on the area affected and the severity of the lesion.

Cervical spine. A recumbent horse with a lesion at C1–C3 has difficulty raising its head off the ground, whereas a recumbent horse with a lesion at C4–T2 should be able to lift its head and cranial neck. C1–T2 lesions may not result in tetraplegia, but they may present as tetraparesis and ataxia. Spinal cord lesions above C6 will result in normal to increased muscular tone and spinal reflexes (panniculus, triceps, and biceps) in all limbs. If the lesion is located at the C6–C8, the forelimb reflexes are diminished or absent and those of the hindlimbs are normal or increased (1039).

Thoracic spine. Lesions of T3–T6 may cause paraplegia or paraparesis and ataxia. A paraplegic horse that 'dog sits' usually has a lesion caudal to T2. Most animals with thoracic spinal cord injury have normal to exaggerated spinal reflexes and hypertonia of the hindlimbs. Some degree of asymmetry may be present with spinal cord trauma, but signs are almost always bilateral. The level of hypalgesia on the neck or back indicates the cranial extent

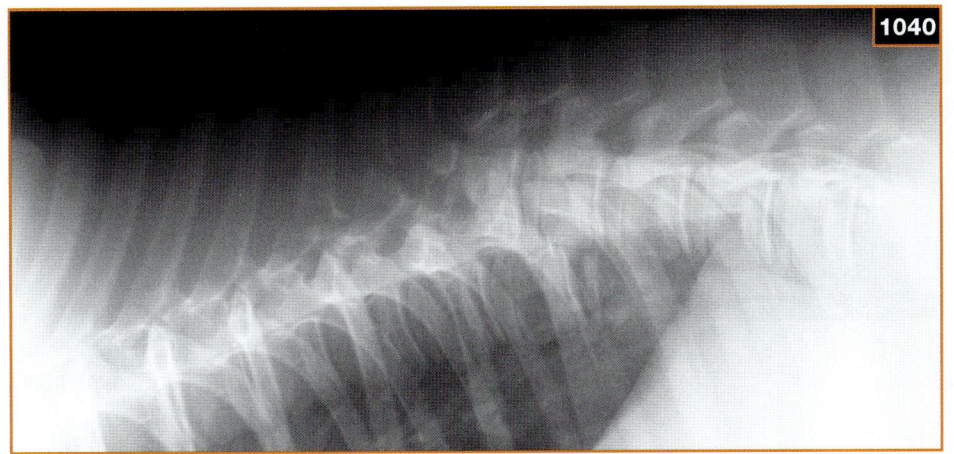

1040 A markedly displaced fracture of the thoracic spine secondary to a high-speed collision.

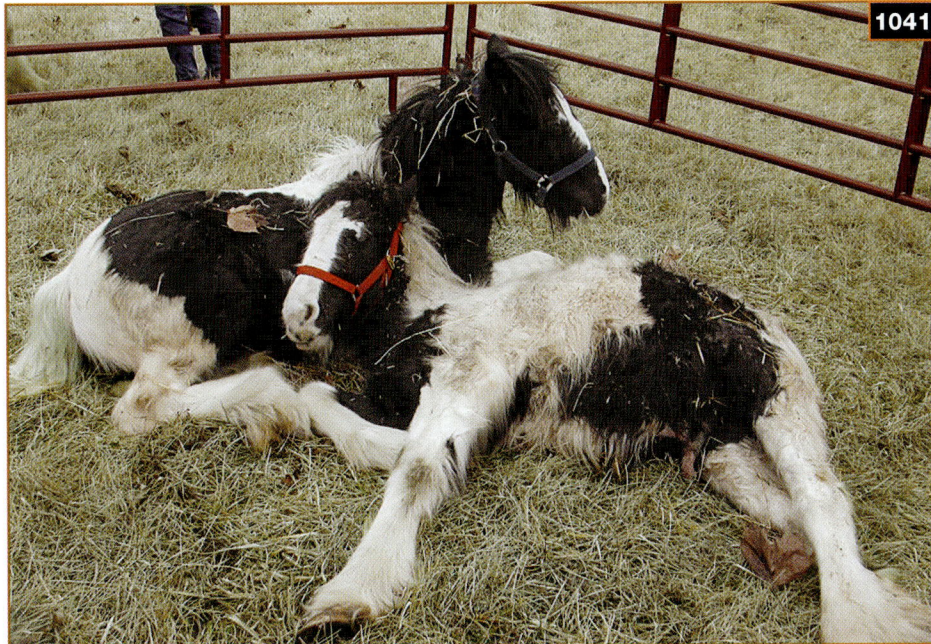

1041 Two foals that were in a trailer accident and unable to stand. Note the paraphimosis of the foal in the foreground. This foal had a fracture of the 3rd lumbar vertebra (see 1042). The foal in the background is sitting sternal and was able to 'dog sit'. This foal had a fracture of the 8th thoracic vertebra.

of the lesion. In the early post-trauma phase, a region of hyperesthesia may be detected just cranial to the lesion. Strip patches of sweating may occur when thoracolumbar spinal nerve roots are damaged. Whole-body sweating, seen frequently in horses with a broken neck or back, may be due to involvement of pain pathways and sympathetic spinal cord pathways (1040).

Lumbar spine. Lesions at L1–L3 result in normal or hypertonic and hyperreflexic hindlimbs and lesions at L4–S2 may result in hypotonia and hyporeflexia of the hindlimbs. The bladder is distended, but sphincter tone is normal. Tail and anal tone are normal (1041, 1042).

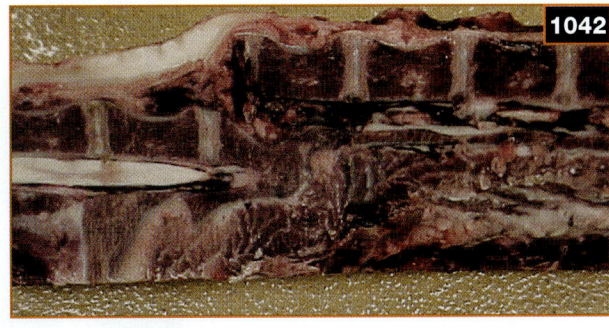

1042 Transection of the spinal cord at the 3rd lumbar vertebra.

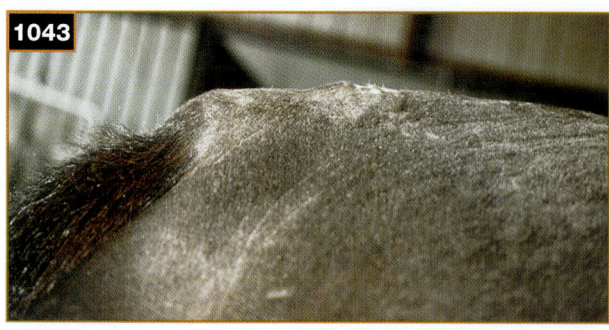

1043 Stallion with sacral trauma. Note the bony protuberances on the sacrum.

Sacrococcygeal spine

Lesions of S1–S2 result in decreased conscious proprioceptive responses of the hindlimbs and diminished flexor reflexes of those limbs. Anal tone is diminished to absent and the bladder is distended and hypotonic. Atony of the urethral sphincter results in incontinence and urine scalding. The tail is flaccid and paralyzed (1043). Paraphimosis may also result (1044).

Diagnosis

The neurologic examination should be used to localize the lesion. Plain radiography is the most helpful aid in confirming vertebral trauma, but does not directly evaluate the presence or extent of spinal cord damage. Abnormalities seen that indicate injury are displacements of vertebral components, shortened or abnormally shaped vertebrae, slipped physeal plates, and fractures.

Fracture-induced changes in the CSF may be useful for ancillary diagnosis. These changes can be classified as acute (<24 hours) or chronic (>24 hours). The acute changes include diffuse blood contamination, a high RBC count, a normal to high WBC count, and a high protein concentration. Chronic CSF changes include a normal to slightly increased WBC count, normal to increased RBC count, increased protein concentration, and xanthochromia.

Management

It is arguable whether drug administration hastens recovery, but recommendations are similar to those for cerebral trauma (see p. 774), with many authors recommending the administration of DMSO and dexamethasone, although the efficacy of these is unclear. Pain should be managed with NSAIDs. Caution should be used when administering analgesics or tranquilizers to ataxic patients, as the animal may fall and worsen the lesion. Good nursing care is essential, especially for recumbent patients, and should include bladder and rectal evacuation as necessary.

If the spinal fracture appears stable and the animal can stand with assistance, it may be placed in a water tank and supported for long periods. Other methods of support include slings (1045), but these should not be used for animals that cannot support themselves, as severe respiratory compromise or compressive myopathy may result. Slinging of animals with mild neurologic signs may help minimize secondary complications, improve extensor tone, and hasten recovery.

Prognosis

The prognosis for horses with spinal cord trauma associated with luxations or fractures of the vertebral body, arch, or articular processes must remain guarded to poor for return to use. Healing of these fractures frequently results in vertebral malalignment. Delayed callus formation and degenerative changes in adjacent articulations can result in delayed permanent spinal cord compression even after apparent resolution of clinical signs. The prognosis is best

1044 Paraphimosis in a stallion secondary to sacral trauma. The paraphimosis never resolved.

1045 Use of a sling in the management of a yearling with a fracture at C7.

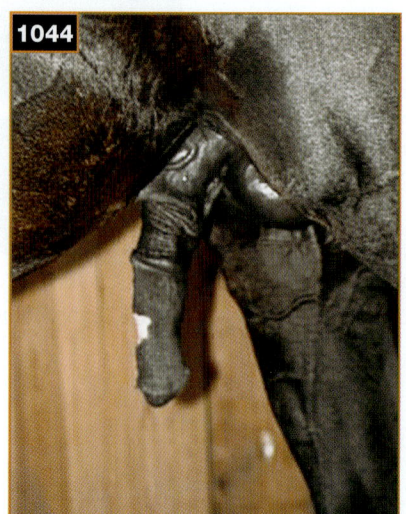
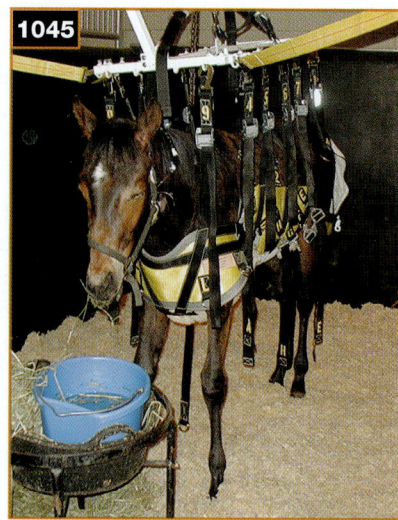

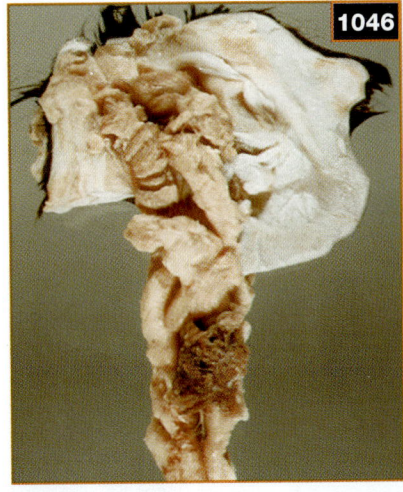

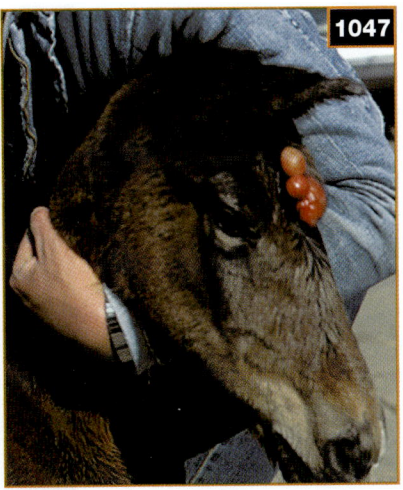

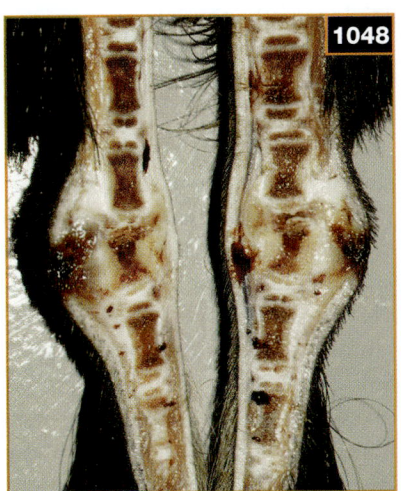

1046 Anencephaly. (Photo courtesy FT Bain)

1047 Encephalocele. (Photo courtesy FT Bain)

1048 A tail abscess that resulted in severe osteomyelitis of the caudal vertebrae.

judged on the basis of repeated neurologic examinations. The longer a patient remains recumbent and neurologically impaired, the poorer the prognosis.

Myelodysplasias
Myelodysplasias are developmental anomalies of the spinal cord that may result in clinical neurologic disease. Gross malformations of the axial skeleton tend to accompany severe anomalies of the spinal cord. An example that is occasionally seen in horses is spina bifida. This results from failure of fusion of the halves of the dorsal arch, which includes the spinous processes. This may or may not be accompanied by protrusion through the vertebral defect of cystic dilations of the spinal cord (myelocele), meninges (meningocele), or both (meningomyelocele). Other forms of myelodysplasia may occur with or without vertebral anomalies. These may include varying degrees of syringomyelia (tubular cavitations), hydromyelia (dilation of the central canal), or diplomyelia (spinal cord duplication). Similarly, vertebral malformations and vertebral column defects may occur without myelodysplasia and are not normally associated with neurologic deficits.

Myelodysplasia may be clinically evident at birth or manifested soon after as stable neurologic abnormalities such as paraparesis. A 'bunny-hopping' gait and bilaterally active reflexes in the limbs at the level of the defect are prominent features. Progressive neurologic defects resulting from spinal cord compression are associated with severe vertebral anomalies.

Anencephaly
Anencephaly is a rare, invariably fatal condition characterized by an absence of brain tissue that results from failure of the cranial neural folds to fuse (**1046**).

Encephalocele
Herniation of any part of the brain may occur if mesenchyme forming any of the skeletal components of the calvaria fails to develop properly (**1047**).

Fibrocartilagenous emboli
Focal spinal cord infarction resulting from fibrocartilaginous emboli is very rare, but has been reported. The emboli are believed to originate from the nucleus pulposus of the intervertebral disks, but the exact cause and mechanism by which they occur are unknown. There is no effective treatment and affected animals have not recovered, although improvement over time has been noted. The prognosis for this condition in dogs is good, with partial to complete recovery seen over weeks to months, therefore if this condition is suspected hasty euthanasia should be discouraged.

Tail injuries
Lifting heavy horses by the tail may result in damage to coccygeal nerves. Sacrococcygeal dislocation results in severe stretching and tearing of the cauda equina and will often result in permanent neurologic dysfunction. If there is no luxation of the tail, the lesion is more likely to be a neuropraxia and this should resolve with time.

Peripheral nerve disorders
Definition/overview
Trauma is the primary cause of peripheral nerve disorders, but injections, tumors, abscesses (**1048**), or parasitic invasion of the nerves can also be seen.

Etiology/pathophysiology

Suprascapular. Trauma to this nerve commonly occurs when horses collide with each other or, more commonly, with inanimate objects. Tension on the nerve can also be caused by the animal stumbling with the limb stretched backwards. Damage to the nerve results in paralysis of the infraspinatus and supraspinatus muscles. Early denervation is characterized by an outward bowing of the scapulohumeral joint when the animal is weight bearing. This is followed by neurogenic atrophy over a number of months, resulting in prominence of the scapular spine. Some horses circumduct the limb during protraction to avoid dragging the toe. These horses are unsound for athletic purposes. This condition is commonly known as 'Sweeney' (**1049**).

Radial nerve. The radial nerve provides motor innervation to the extensor muscles of the forelimbs. It is most vulnerable to trauma over the lateral aspect of the elbow joint. Injury most commonly arises from direct trauma to the nerve during prolonged anesthesia or recumbency without sufficient padding. Radial paralysis can also accompany humoral fractures or fractures of the first rib, and function of this nerve should be evaluated before fracture repair because of the poor prognosis that accompanies radial nerve damage. The limb position varies depending on the location of the lesion in the radial nerve. A lesion at or near the elbow joint results in a high radial nerve paralysis, with a dropped elbow, failure of limb protraction, and flexion of all distal limb joints. The animal is unable to bear weight on the limb and the foot is knuckled over at rest. Distal radial nerve lesions will result in flexion of the carpus, fetlock, and pastern joints. The animal can support weight on the affected limb if the metacarpus and distal limb are held in extension. The triceps reflex in affected patients will be decreased to absent. Sensory deficits are variable between patients (**1050**).

Brachial plexus. Lesions of the brachial plexus can be caused by shoulder trauma, deep penetrating axillary wounds, and traction on fetal forelimbs during dystocia relief. Nerves of the brachial plexus supply motor innervation to the biceps, coracobrachialis (musculocutaneous), pectoral, subscapularis, and triceps muscles, therefore severe lesions result in complete flaccidity of the forelimb, with the animal unable to bear weight. Triceps and biceps reflexes are absent. Pectoral nerve dysfunction results in elbow abduction and a dropped shoulder results from subscapular nerve paralysis. Inability to flex the elbow, with hyperextension at rest, results from musculocutaneous nerve paralysis. Signs of radial nerve paralysis will also be present, as will complete desensitization of the entire forelimb.

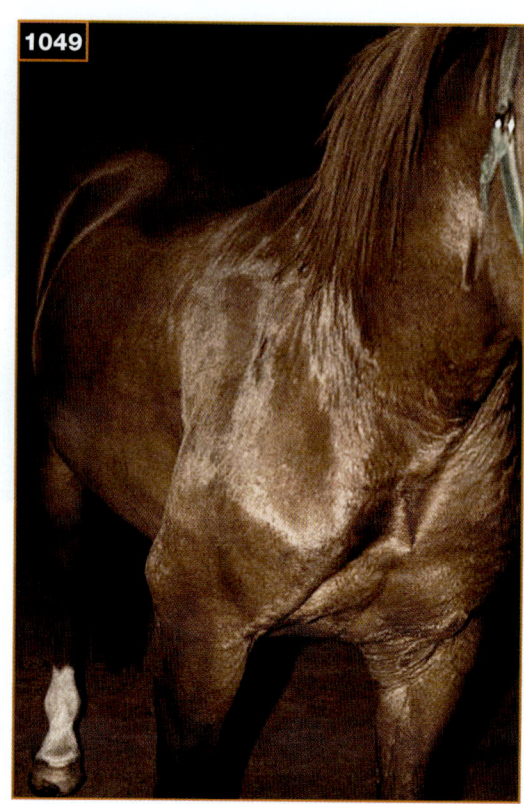

1049 Suprascapular nerve injury secondary to a collision with another horse.

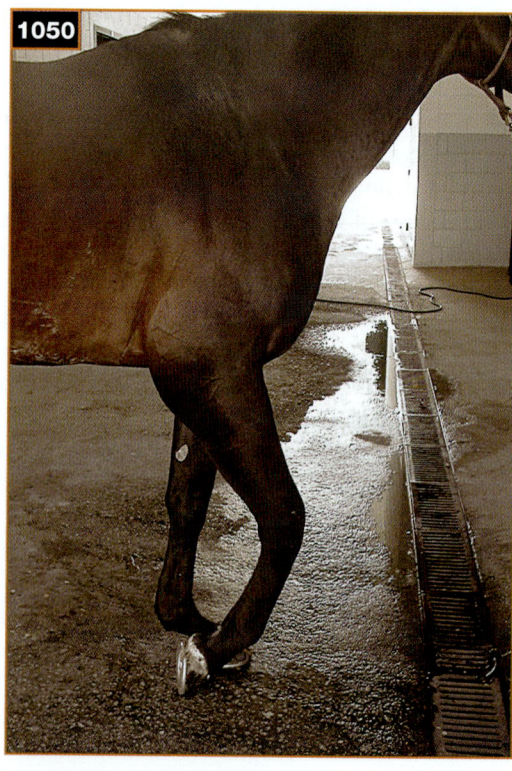

1050 Radial nerve paralysis.

Musculocutaneous, median, ulnar. These nerves innervate the flexor muscles of the elbow, carpus, and digit. Dysfunction most commonly occurs as a result of brachial plexus injuries, but it can also be seen with spinal cord lesions involving the gray matter of the brachial intumescence. Gait alterations can occur with injury to the individual nerves, but these may disappear or be very subtle after approximately 3 months. Ulnar neurectomy results in the most pronounced abnormalities, with decreased flexion of the carpus and fetlock, and residual effects such as stumbling are common. The improvement that can be seen over time, particularly with musculocutaneous and median nerve injuries, may be due in part to crossing of fibers from one nerve to the other.

Femoral. Femoral nerve paralysis can be caused by abscesses, tumors, and aneurysms in the region of the external iliac arteries, in addition to penetrating wounds of the caudal flank. Fractures of the pelvis and femur may be associated with femoral nerve damage and in such cases the integrity of the nerve should be determined before fracture repair. Damage to this nerve may also be associated with prolonged anesthesia or recumbency, although myopathy may complicate the clinical picture. Spinal cord lesions of the ventral gray matter or nerve roots at L4 and L5 can also result in femoral nerve paralysis and these have been seen in horses with EPM.

The femoral nerve innervates the quadriceps femoris, which is the major extensor muscle of the stifle, in addition to providing sensory innervation via the saphenous nerve to the medial aspect of the limb. Paralysis of this nerve results in an inability to extend the stifle. Reciprocal flexion of the tarsus and digits when the stifle flexes means that femoral nerve damage results in extensor paralysis, with the affected limb resting in a flexed position and the ipsilateral hip in a lower position than the contralateral hip. There is no weight bearing on the affected limb during locomotion. Bilateral involvement results in a horse that has great difficulty rising from a recumbent position and has a crouching posture when standing because of flexion of the joints of both hindlimbs. The patellar reflex will be depressed or absent, but a normal flexor reflex will be present if the sciatic nerve is intact. The prognosis is guarded in cases of femoral nerve paralysis unless the nerve can be repaired.

Tibial. Tibial nerve paralysis is uncommon because the nerve is well protected by the muscles and bones of the limb. This branch of the sciatic nerve provides motor innervation to the gastrocnemius and digital flexor muscles. Paralysis causes the limb to be held with the tarsus flexed and the fetlock resting in a flexed or partly knuckled position. This results in the hip being held lower on the affected side. Flexion of the hock and extension of the digits is unopposed and results in overflexion of the limb when walking, with the foot raised higher than normal. Controlled extension of the hock is absent at the completion of the advancing phase of the stride and results in the foot being dropped straight to the ground. This gives the gait a similar appearance to 'stringhalt'. There is anesthesia of the caudomedian aspect of the leg.

Peroneal. This branch of the sciatic nerve is most vulnerable to injury where it crosses the lateral condyle of the femur. Injury from kicks and lateral recumbency is most common, but the nerve is not usually severed and these horses eventually improve.

The peroneal nerve supplies the flexor muscles of the tarsus and extensor muscles of the digits. Paralysis results in extension of the tarsus and flexion of the fetlock and interphalangeal joints. At rest this results in a horse that holds the limb extended caudally, with the dorsum of the hoof resting on the ground. During locomotion the hoof is dragged along the ground. If the limb is advanced manually and the toe extended, the horse can bear weight on the limb. It is important to support and protect the limb while the animal is given time to improve. Hypalgesia is reported to occur on the craniolateral aspect of the hock and metatarsal regions.

Sciatic. The sciatic nerve has a close relationship with the pelvis and may be damaged by pelvic fractures, especially ischial fractures. In foals, deep injection reactions caudal to the proximal femur and osteomyelitis of the sacrum and pelvis have resulted in sciatic paralysis. Treatment of primary problems may resolve the sciatic paralysis, but if the nerve is severed the prognosis is poor even with surgical anastomosis, as there is a great distance over which fiber regeneration must occur. Sciatic palsy can also occur with spinal cord lesions affecting the L5–S3 ventral gray matter or nerve roots. Other signs such as urinary bladder paralysis, gluteal atrophy, and extensor weakness may also be present.

The sciatic nerve supplies the main extensor muscles of the hip and flexor muscles of the stifle and divides into peroneal and tibial branches. Total sciatic paralysis results in an abnormal gait and posture. At rest, extension of the stifle and hock results in the limb hanging behind the horse with the fetlock and interphalangeal joints partly flexed and the dorsum of the hoof on the ground. If the foot is manually advanced and placed on the ground ventral to the pelvis, the horse can support weight with some flexion of the hock and take a stride. Muscles of the caudal thigh and the entire limb distal to the stifle atrophy. Degrees of hypalgesia over most of the limb, except for the medial thigh, have been reported.

Post-foaling paralysis. The obturator nerve innervates the adductors of the thigh and paralysis is an infrequent sequela to foaling. Signs may be seen without a history of dystocia. This nerve courses along the medial aspect of the shaft of the ilium and is vulnerable to compression by the foal impinging on this region during parturition. Depending on the severity of damage, signs may range from mild stiffness to paraplegia. Unilateral damage may be apparent as abduction and circumduction of the affected limb at a walk. Bilaterally affected animals have great difficulty rising and may require the support of a body sling.

Hemorrhage in and around the femoral nerves has also been associated with foaling and results in extensor weakness.

The prognosis for survival in post-foaling paralysis is fair, with a recovery rate of approximately 50%. Complications of prolonged recumbency (ischemic neuropathy, decubital ulcers), frequently necessitate euthanasia.

Management

Medical management of peripheral nerve injuries involves reduction of inflammation, relief of musculoskeletal pain, prevention of secondary medical disorders, and provision of adequate nutrition. Systemic administration of dexamethasone (0.05–0.20 mg/kg i/v q12h), flunixin meglumine (1.1 mg/kg i/v q24h), or phenylbutazone (2.2 mg/kg p/o q12h) for 3 days may help suppress local inflammation that can further damage nerve fibers. Confinement in deeply bedded stalls is appropriate and application of cold water or ice packs in the first 24 hours may be beneficial. Recumbent animals should be turned 6–8 times daily to prevent decubital ulcers and pressure myopathy. Support of some patients in slings may be useful and helps maintain strength in the opposite limbs.

Toxin-associated disorders

Mercury

Mercury toxicity is a rare cause of neurologic disease in horses. Organic fungicides used to treat seed grain and inorganic mercury found in blistering agents are both hazardous and accessible to horses. The toxicokinetics of elemental, organic, and inorganic mercury are distinctly different, with a varied effect on the target organ of toxicosis. Chronic exposure to elemental mercury vapor causes CNS dysfunction, but this type of toxicosis is unlikely. The organic mercurial compounds, such as methyl mercury, are neurotoxic to central and peripheral nerves. Inorganic mercury salts are corrosive to the GI tract and the absorbed fraction is nephrotoxic. This is the most common type of toxicosis reported and has been associated with ingestion of blistering compounds.

Urea and nonprotein nitrogen sources

Urea has been used as a nonprotein nitrogen source for adult horses, but it has no advantage over more common sources. Horses are not as efficient in the utilization of urea as cattle, with toxicity being much less likely, as urea is absorbed by the GI tract and excreted in urine before reaching the hindgut, where it is hydrolyzed by the microbial population to ammonia. Horses are more susceptible to toxicosis by the ingestion of ammonium salts, which can occur following accidental exposure. The lethal dose of urea when ingested orally is 4 g/kg and the lethal dose of ammonium salts is about 1.5 g/kg when ingested orally. Clinical signs are confined to the nervous system, with muscle tremor, incoordination, and weakness. Death is the result of ammonia intoxication. The exact mechanism of ammonia toxicosis is not known, but is thought to involve

1051 Mycotoxicosis. This horse was one of six affected horses on a farm. When asked to walk the animals had a marked hypermetric gait of the hindlimbs only. The animals would always stand with all four limbs underneath themselves. A new batch of hay had recently been purchased and mold was noted in two of the bales that were fed to these horses. The horses improved with supportive care within 72 hours. No residual neurologic effects were noted and mycotoxin ingestion was presumed.

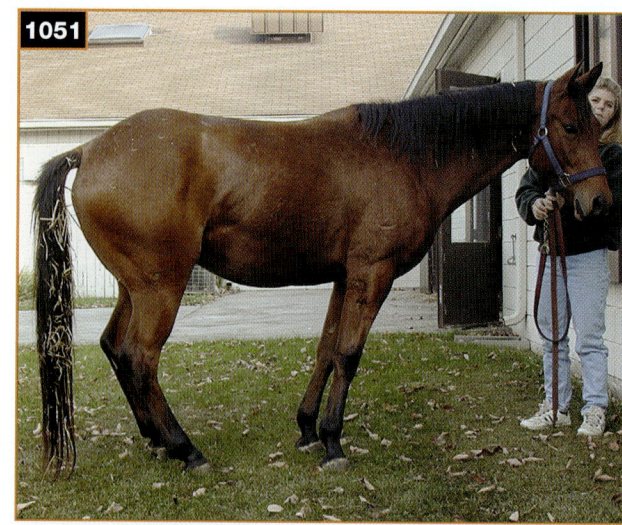

inhibition of the citric acid cycle. Animals that die of ammonia toxicosis exhibit no characteristic lesions. Clinical signs and history may be useful in establishing a diagnosis. Blood ammonia may be evaluated, but many factors influence the levels found and results should be interpreted with caution. Treatment with lactulose (200 ml p/o or per rectum q4–6h) may be attempted.

Monensin

Monensin is an ionophore antibiotic that is used as a feed additive for its growth-promoting and coccidiostatic effects in cattle and poultry, respectively. The primary action of monensin is selective transport of sodium and potassium ions between the intracellular and extracellular spaces. It is thought that toxicity results from abnormal levels of potassium or calcium within the cell leading to cell death. The heart is the primary organ of toxicity. Horses are the most sensitive domestic animal to monensin toxicosis, with an LD_{50} of 2–3 mg/kg. Inadvertent consumption has resulted in several syndromes of toxicity, which are dose related. Peracute toxicity may result in progressive severe hemoconcentration, hypovolemic shock, and death within a few hours of ingestion. These cases are commonly found dead. The acute form results in ataxia, progressive muscle weakness, tachycardia, hypotension, dyspnea, polyuria, anorexia, abdominal pain, and intermittent profuse sweating. These may show signs for 1–4 days before death. Horses surviving sublethal doses show signs of unthriftiness, decreased athletic performance, and cardiac failure. Cardiac arrhythmias and pleural and pericardial effusion may also be seen. Clinicopathologic findings are not pathognomonic and toxicity should be suspected on the basis of clinical signs and exposure to contaminated feed. As the LD_{50} is so low for horses, feed contamination may not be immediately apparent.

There is no specific antidote for monensin. Early and aggressive treatment with fluids to combat hemoconcentration and hypovolemic shock is warranted in patients with known ingestion. Correction of acid–base and electrolyte abnormalities is essential. The use of mineral oil and activated charcoal to evacuate the bowel and decrease absorption, respectively, is also warranted.

There are two important treatment contraindications in horses that have ingested monensin. The first is that digitalis glycosides should never be used acutely in affected horses, as they have been shown to be synergistic with monensin and immediately fatal to cardiac cells. The second is that calcium should not be administered to acutely affected horses, as it can be irritating to an injured myocardium and the hypocalcemia that is seen is transitory, with serum calcium levels usually returning to normal in 24 hours. Affected horses are very susceptible to cardiac damage, which is often permanent.

Organophosphates

Organophosphate poisoning in horses is usually due to overzealous application of insecticides, acaricides, or anthelmintics, or accidental contamination of feed or water. The clinical signs that are seen are the result of inhibition of acetylcholinesterase activity, leading to uncontrolled muscarinic, nicotinic, and CNS effects of acetylcholine. Hyperexcitability, frequent urination, sweating, muscle tremors, and colic are followed by weakness, recumbency, and death due to respiratory insufficiency.

Treatment consists of atropine (0.1 mg/kg, half slowly i/v and half i/m) and pralidoxime chloride (2-PAM) (20 mg/kg i/m). Skin washing and saline purgation can be used to remove residual organophosphates. Horses are said to be highly resistant to delayed neurotoxicity caused by organophosphates, but transient laryngeal paralysis has been reported.

Chlorinated hydrocarbons

Chlorinated hydrocarbons were once widely used in industry, horticulture, and agriculture. They are now highly restricted because of environmental persistence of the parent compound and contaminating dioxins. There are few credible reports of exposure of horses to toxic levels of the parent compounds, but neurotoxicity related to exposure of dioxins has been reported. Dioxin is present in waste oil sludge, which has previously been used to keep down dust in riding arenas. Of 85 horses exposed to dioxins in this way, 48 died over weeks to years. In addition to clinical signs of emaciation, colic, and laminitis, cerebral edema was noted at necropsy. Chronic accumulation of chlorinated hydrocarbons may cause a wide array of central and peripheral neuropathies, in addition to degeneration of other tissues.

Mycotoxicosis

Mycotoxins are secondary metabolites of molds produced during mold growth in grains or forages. They are not produced consistently and may result from stresses or limitations to mold growth, such as unusual temperature, humidity, or drought. There is little correlation between spore counts or fungal growth amount and mycotoxin contamination. Similarly, the absence of mold growth does not mean that a food or forage is free from mycotoxins (**1051**). Mycotoxins can persist in mold-free feed as the common mycotoxins are resistant to the temperatures and drying that destroy fungi. There are many mycotoxins that are of concern, including aflatoxin, fumonisin, and ergot alkaloids. The syndromes of ryegrass staggers, paspalum staggers, and leukoencephalomalacia are examples of mycotoxicosis in horses and are discussed below.

Tremorgenic mycotoxicosis

Definition/overview

The ingestion of several tremorgenic mycotoxins can result in syndromes that are characterized by staggering. Ryegrass staggers is the best described and has been reported in the US, Australia, New Zealand, and Europe.

Etiology/pathophysiology

Perennial ryegrass (*Lolium perenne*) is the major forage supporting the endophytic growth of *Neotyphodium lolii*, which produces tremorgenic mycotoxins known as lolitrems A, B, C, and D. Lolitrem B is considered the major toxin and is characterized by an indole moiety. The toxin is highest in the seed and the syndrome is most commonly seen in the late summer or fall, as the concentration of lolitrems varies seasonally.

Paspalum staggers results from ingestion of Dallis grass (*Paspalum dilatatum*) that has been invaded by *Claviceps paspali,* which subsequently produces an ergot sclerotium. The sclerotium contains alkaloids produced by *C. paspali* and includes indole compounds, which are derivatives of lysergic acid and known as paspalitrems. Inhibition of GABA, which is one of several inhibitory neurotransmitters, is the probable mechanism of toxicosis. Dallis grass is grown in the south central and southeastern regions of the US and the sclerotia may be consumed on pasture or in hay.

Staggers has occurred in Florida in horses fed coastal Bermuda grass hay and may be comparable to Bermuda grass tremor of ruminants. A fungal tremorgen is thought to be responsible.

Tremorgenic mycotoxins are associated with reduced effects of inhibitory amino acids, which result in increased presynaptic neurotransmitter release and prolonged depolarization. Synaptic transmission at the motor end plate is facilitated, providing a probable mechanism for the uncontrolled tremors and incoordination observed clinically.

Clinical presentation

Initially, there is a diffuse, intermittent, mild muscle tremor that progresses to varying degrees of ataxia, with a head nod and a wide-based rocking stance. An uncoordinated and swaying gait is common and affected animals may stumble and fall. If undisturbed, recumbent horses usually recover and regain their feet within a short time. Excitement and blindfolding markedly exacerbate signs. The condition itself is not usually fatal, but accidents associated with falling have resulted in death.

Differential diagnosis

Fluphenazine reaction; reserpine reaction; EPM; WNV encephalitis; lead toxicosis; equine LMN disease; trauma; hyperammonemia; metabolic derangement (hypocalcemia); spinal cord impingement secondary to neoplasia.

Diagnosis

Ruling out other potential neurologic disorders and/or the detection of these toxins in the pasture environment are used for diagnosis.

Management

There is no antidote for either perennial ryegrass staggers or paspalum staggers, but removal from the suspect forage results in recovery in 3–7 days or 1–3 weeks, respectively. The animals should be placed in a quiet secure place during recovery and provided with nursing care.

Prognosis

The prognosis is good provided the source of the toxin is removed and supportive care is provided. With chronic ryegrass staggers, residual defects from degenerative CNS lesions may be present.

Leukoencephalomalacia

Definition/overview

Leukoencephalomalacia is a highly fatal neurologic disease caused by ingestion of mycotoxins.

Etiology/pathophysiology

Intoxication of horses is caused by ingestion of corn contaminated with *Fusarium moniliforme* and, occasionally, *Fusarium tricinctum*. Cool humid conditions favor the growth of the fungus and therefore this intoxication is most common in the late fall and early spring, with a worldwide occurrence. The fungi produce the toxins (B1, B2, and B3) that are thought to be responsible for the condition.

The pathophysiology is not fully understood, but it is thought that fumonisin (B1) plays a major role. This toxin interferes with sphingolipid metabolism, disrupting endothelial cell walls and basement membranes. Liquefactive necrosis and malacia of the white matter of one or both cerebral hemispheres results. Lesions can be seen in other organs, primarily the liver. Fumonisins have also been implicated in the etiology of porcine pulmonary edema, human esophageal cancer, hepatotoxicity in animals, and disease in poultry.

Clinical presentation

Clinical signs are seen on average 3 weeks after initial ingestion of contaminated corn. Initial signs are referable to cerebral disease and include depression, circling, aimless wandering, blindness, and finally recumbency, paddling, coma, and death. Morbidity in outbreaks has been reported as 14–100%. The clinical course is usually short (1–3 days), but may be prolonged in animals that recover and survivors usually have permanent neurologic dysfunction. Horses with uncomplicated leukoencephalomalacia are not usually febrile, which helps distinguish them from those affected by arboviral encephalomyelitides.

Differential diagnosis

EPM, verminous migrans, hepatic encephalopathy, rabies, metabolic derangements, trauma, lightning strike, and cerebral abscess should be considered, depending on the presentation.

Diagnosis

Clinical presentation and history of possible exposure to contaminated feed should raise suspicion of leuko-encephalomalacia, particularly if multiple animals are affected. Definitive diagnosis is difficult antemortem. Hematology is usually unremarkable, although signs of hepatic dysfunction may be present. Results of CSF analysis are frequently normal; elevations in protein and cell count are sometimes present. The liquefactive necrosis seen grossly at necropsy is usually diagnostic.

Management

There is no specific treatment. Supportive care, removal from contaminated feed, and elimination of toxin by use of activated charcoal (2.2 kg/500 kg body weight in 4 liters of water q12h for 24–36 hours) are recommended.

Prognosis

The prognosis is poor. Mortality rates of 40–84% have been reported.

Metaldehyde toxicosis

Definition/overview

Metaldehyde toxicosis is uncommon in horses and may result from inadvertent ingestion or malicious poisoning.

Etiology/pathophysiology

Metaldehyde is a polycyclic polymer of acetaldehyde and is an ingredient in slug and snail baits. These baits usually contain oats, bran, rice, soybeans, sorghum, or apples in addition to metaldehyde, and are readily consumed by horses. The CNS is primarily affected, but the exact mechanism of action is unknown. Studies in mice have indicated that excitatory neurotransmitter levels are increased and inhibitory neurotransmitter levels are decreased. The exact toxic dose in horses is not known. The reported oral lethal dose in horses ranges from 60–100 mg/kg, which is less than the lethal dose reported for other species including ruminants, dogs, laboratory animals, and poultry.

Clinical presentation

Clinical signs are reported to begin within 15 minutes of ingestion in the horse and include ataxia, hyperesthesia, muscular twitching, and agitation. Convulsive spasms are commonly seen. Limb movements resembling stringhalt, tachycardia, tachypnea, weak pulse, and profuse sweating are other signs that have been seen. Death can occur within a few hours of the onset of clinical signs and is often accompanied by violent convulsions.

Diagnosis

Diagnosis is based on clinical signs and known exposure to metaldehyde. Clinical pathologic tests, including CSF analysis, are nondiagnostic and postmortem lesions are nonspecific. Metalehyde testing can be done on stomach contents or serum.

Management

The primary aim of treatment is to control convulsions, as there is no antidote available. Mineral oil or activated charcoal may be beneficial soon after ingestion to minimize absorption. Supportive care in addition to treatment for any dehydration or acidosis is also warranted.

Prognosis

Horses that do recover do not seem to suffer from any sequelae.

Lead toxicosis

Definition/overview

Lead toxicosis is a rare cause of neurologic disease in horses and is associated with inadvertent ingestion of lead.

Etiology/pathophysiology

Lead is regarded as a global contaminant. The most likely sources of lead for horses are contamination from nearby mines and smelting operations, discarded lead-acid batteries, and ashes remaining after combustion of older buildings. Lead-based paints on buildings were a major source of contamination, but these are only likely to be found on buildings built before 1960 in most countries.

Most ingested lead is finely divided and highly available. It is solubilized in the acidic environment of the stomach and readily absorbed from the proximal small intestine. Atomic similarities mean that bivalent lead acts like calcium once absorbed. In mammals, most lead from chronic exposure is dynamically bound in the bone matrix. The toxic dose depends on the age of the animal, with younger animals absorbing 10–20% of absorbed lead versus 1–2% in adults, based on the increased calcium requirement of younger animals. Ingestion of forage containing more than 80 ppm lead may cause chronic lead poisoning. Chronic lead exposure results in slowly developing toxic manifestations, which are primarily neurologic (peripheral neuropathy) or hematopoietic (anemia). Exposure to high levels of lead may result in overt CNS toxicity, as lead enters the brain at a dose-dependent rate following absorption. Lead deposition in the CNS results in acute cerebellar hemorrhage and edema from capillary dysfunction.

Clinical presentation

In horses, lead poisoning is manifested as a combination of central and peripheral nerve dysfunction, GI upset, and interference with hematopoiesis. Clinical signs commonly seen are laryngeal hemiplegia, dysphagia (with associated secondary aspiration pneumonia), ataxia, muscle fasciculations, hyperesthesia, weight loss, and depression. The mild to moderate anemia seen with chronic poisoning is primarily due to disruption of hemoglobin synthesis. An increase in nucleated RBCs out of proportion to the anemia suggests lead poisoning, especially when accompanied by basophilic stippling.

Differential diagnosis

Equine motor neuron disease; anticholinesterase insecticide toxicity (organophosphates and carbamates).

Diagnosis

Definitive diagnosis of lead poisoning is based on detection of blood lead concentration greater than 0.35 ppm in an animal with appropriate clinical signs. Greater than 10 ppm lead in liver and kidney samples is also compatible with lead poisoning. Supportive analyses include urinary lead concentrations before and 6–12 hours after chelation therapy is initiated.

Management

Treatment is aimed at enhancing urinary excretion with chelation therapy. Calcium disodium EDTA will accelerate excretion from blood and soft tissues, but does little to lead that is stored in bone. A 6.6% solution of calcium disodium EDTA is prepared in 5% dextrose or normal saline and administered at 75 mg/kg/ day i/v divided into three doses. A therapeutic protocol of 4 days treatment, 2 days off, and 4 days treatment should be followed. The days between treatment allow for equilibrium of the lead out of the bone and other body stores so that it is available for chelation. Concurrent intravenous fluid therapy is preferred because it facilitates excretion of the water-soluble chelate and also aids dehydrated animals. The effectiveness of the chelation therapy can be evaluated by changes in the lead concentrations of urine and blood. Blood levels should be stable below 0.2 ppm following treatment, whereas urinary concentrations are expected to increase 2–30 times above baseline during treatment. The blood concentration should be checked within 2 weeks of final chelation and if it has rebounded to exceed 0.35 ppm, a second course of chelation therapy is recommended. Thiamine therapy (1 mg/kg i/v) is also used in ruminants with lead poisoning and has proved an effective adjunctive treatment with EDTA. The nature of the protective effect of thiamine is unclear. Supportive care should also be instituted while patients are undergoing chelation therapy. Identification of lead toxicosis in a horse should prompt an environmental investigation to identify the source of contamination.

Prognosis

The prognosis is good if chelation therapy is started and the animal's lead levels decrease.

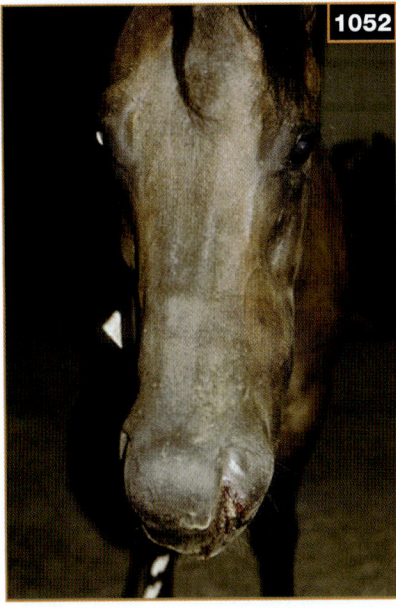

1052 Rattlesnake bite on the nares of a mare in Arizona, USA.

Snakebite

Bites from a wide variety of venomous snakes have been reported in horses. Most reports involve snakes from the families Crotalidae (pit vipers) and Elapidae (cobras). The majority of venomous snakebites are inflicted by rattlesnakes, copperheads, and water mocassins. These usually cause local effects, with swelling and edema at the bite site. Usually the head and muzzle are affected, but bites can occur in other areas such as the limbs. The venom of members of the family Elapidae is mainly neurotoxic, with minimal local effects. This family includes cobras, mambas, and coral snakes. These snakes, however, frequently require prolonged contact (30 seconds or longer) to work the venom into the skin of its prey, so envenomation is extremely uncommon. When it occurs there is an initial period of excitement and hyperesthesia, followed by generalized weakness. Snakebites are not usually fatal to adult horses, but can be fatal in young foals. Treatment includes supportive care, tetanus prophylaxis, broad-spectrum antimicrobials, and local treatment of wounds (1052).

Tick paralysis

Definition/overview
Tick paralysis is a rare condition in horses. It causes progressive, ascending LMN paralysis.

Etiology/pathophysiology
The ticks *Ixodes holocyclus* and *Dermacentor andersoni* have a toxin present in their saliva that can cause neuromuscular junction dysfunction. *Ixodes* paralysis has been reported in horses in Australia. *Dermacentor* is a cause of tick paralysis in a variety of animal species in North America; however, its role in equine disease is less clear. Inhibition of acetylcholine release at the neuromuscular junction results in signs of generalized flaccid paralysis.

Clinical presentation
Tick paralysis is characterized by ascending paresis followed by paralysis. The progression of disease can be rapid and horses may die within 24 hours in some cases.

Differential diagnosis
The main differential diagnosis is botulism. Differentiation based on clinical signs is impossible.

Diagnosis
Diagnosis is based on characteristic clinical signs and identification of ticks on the body. There is no other means of diagnosis.

Management
If tick paralysis is suspected based on clinical signs and geographic region, a thorough search should be performed for the presence of ticks on the body. All ticks must be removed. It is very easy to overlook a small number of ticks, so careful examination is required. Heavily haired areas should be very closely examined. Clipping may be required. Supportive care beyond tick removal is similar to that described for botulism (see p. 792). Prevention of disease involves avoiding tick infested areas and inspection and prompt removal of ticks from horses that have had access to potentially infested areas.

Prognosis
The prognosis is good with *Dermacentor* infestations, provided ticks are identified and removed, but poor with *Ixodes* infestation.

Locoweed intoxication

Definition/overview
Locoweed intoxication is a geographically important cause of neurologic disease associated with chronic ingestion of locoweeds, plants of the *Astragalus* and *Oxytropis* genera.

Etiology/pathophysiology
Astragalus and *Oxytropis* spp. are found in the rangelands of western North America and Australia. These are perennial plants that contain a variety of toxic compounds.

Swainsonine and swainsonine N-oxide inhibit the lysosomal enzyme mannosidase, resulting in lysosomal accumulation of mannose-rich oligosaccharides. The cellular vacuolation that results from the inhibition of mannosidase leads to cellular dysfunction, comparable to hereditary mannosidosis of humans and cattle. Locoweed is initially ingested when other foodstuffs are scarce, but horses apparently acquire a taste for the plant once ingestion has started. Horses are more susceptible to the effects of locoweeds compared with other species.

Clinical presentation
Clinical signs appear 2 weeks to 2 months after ingestion commences. Continuous ingestion is required to cause disease. The signs can appear abruptly and are indicative of a diffuse CNS disorder. Periods of depression alternating with frenzy and overreaction to stimulation are common features. Other signs that can be seen are gait abnormalities (including a stringhalt-like gait), head nodding, visual impairment, and dysphagia. Weight loss occurs quickly and can lead to emaciation and death. Other organs are frequently affected and reproductive problems such as abortion and limb deformities in foals are common.

Differential diagnosis
EPM; WNV encephalitis; trauma; aberrant parasite migration (*Halicephalobus deletrix*); metabolic derangement; hepatic encephalopathy; rabies; drug reaction (reserpine, fluphenazine).

Diagnosis
Clinical presentation and a history of possible chronic ingestion of locoweeds are suggestive. Identification of cytoplasmic vacuolation in lymphocytes is supportive of locoweed intoxication.

Management
There is no effective treatment for chronic locoweed intoxication. Sedation is usually ineffective in hyperexcitable horses.

Prognosis
Mildly affected horses recover in 1–2 weeks if the source of locoweed is removed. However, there is no recovery from chronic locoweed poisoning and these animals continue to show signs of neurologic disease when excited.

Nigropallidal encephalomalacia

Definition/overview
Nigropallidal encephalomalacia is a plant toxicosis that has only been reported in horses, although donkeys and mules may also be susceptible.

Etiology/pathophysiology
Yellow star thistle (**1053**) (*Centaurea solstitialis*) and Russian knapweed (*C. repens*) are capable of causing this disease. Malta star thistle (*C. melitensis*) may also be capable of causing this disease, but has not yet been confirmed. Yellow star thistle is an aggressive weed found mainly in the US in California, Oregon, and Idaho. Russian knapweed has a broader distribution throughout the intermountain states. These plants are not considered palatable, but some animals appear to develop a taste for the plant and will consume it preferentially. Most poisonings occur in the spring when the plant is young and green, but it remains toxic when dry and thus poisoning can occur as a result of ingestion of contaminated hay. Up to twice the horse's bodyweight has to be consumed before signs of toxicity develop and as a result, the animal has usually been ingesting the plant for weeks to months prior to the appearance of signs.

The toxic agent of these plants is known as repin, a sesquiterpene lactone with high affinity for neural tissue. Studies in rats suggest that repin exerts its neurotoxic effect by inhibiting dopamine release. Other neurotoxic compounds, including glutamic and aspartic acids, have also been isolated from *Centaurea* plants.

Clinical presentation
Young horses (<3 years old) appear to be more frequently affected, but it is not apparent if this relates to age susceptibility or more frequent ingestion of the plants. The onset of signs is acute and a sudden lack of coordination of facial and oral movements is most apparent. Effective eating or drinking is not possible, although many affected horses display ineffective chewing movements (**1054**). Other signs are head edema, yawning, ataxia, muscle tremors, hypertonicity of the lips and tongue giving a fixed facial expression, and involuntary lip twitching. Death, if it occurs naturally, is usually a result of starvation, dehydration, or aspiration pneumonia.

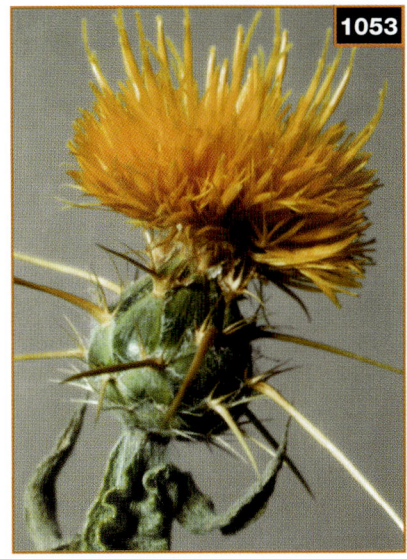

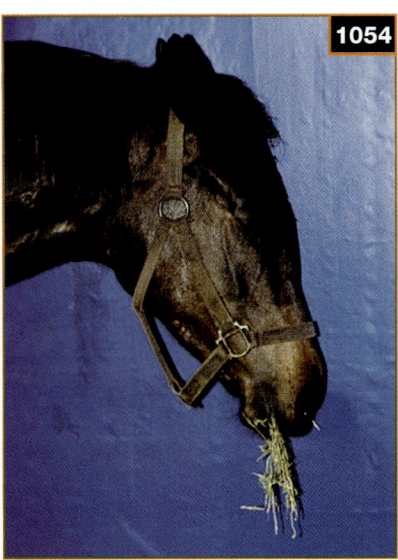

1053 Yellow star thistle (*Centaurea solstitialis*). (Photo courtesy WA State Noxious Weed Control Board)

1054 Horse with dysphagia secondary to yellow star thistle ingestion.

Differential diagnosis
EPM; dental abnormalities; fractured jaw; glossitis; pharyngeal abscess/neosplasia; esophageal obstruction; guttural pouch pathology; lead toxicosis; botulism; arboviral encephalitis.

Diagnosis
Diagnosis is usually based on clinical signs and history of chronic exposure to the toxic plant. The pasture should be evaluated, as should multiple bales of hay. MRI has been successfully used for antemortem diagnosis, but is not readily available. Focal necrosis and malacia of the globus pallidus and/or the substantia nigra are characteristic lesions of this disease and are usually seen bilaterally.

Management
There is no specific treatment for the disease other than supportive care. Horses should be removed from the pasture if this is the suspected source. Otherwise, the hay source should be changed.

Prognosis
Complete recovery is not seen.

Other plant poisonings
Bracken fern and horsetail poisoning
Ingestion of either *Pteridium* (bracken fern) or *Equisetum* (horsetail) species causes neurologic disease in horses. These plants are not usually eaten by horses, but can be in times of shortage of more palatable forage or if the plants have been incorporated into hay. These plants contain a thiaminase that, after repeated exposure, causes thiamine deficiency. Clinical signs occur weeks after ingestion begins and may continue after removal of the source. Anorexia, bradycardia, and ataxia are frequently seen,

while signs of forebrain disease, such as blindness and head pressing, are more infrequent. Ataxia may be severe and involve all four limbs. Thiamine administration (0.5–1 g p/o q12h) results in a rapid resolution of clinical signs.

Grove poisoning
Grove poisoning occurs in areas of southern Florida with intensive horticultural activity and has been associated with plants of the *Indigofera* genus. The clinical syndrome seen indicates diffuse cerebral, vestibulocerebellar, and spinal cord disease; however, there has been no consistent neuropathologic lesion. The signs may fluctuate in severity, but are progressive over time and poisoning usually results in death.

Solanaceous plants
Members of the family Solanaceae contain either the tropane (atropine-like) or solanum groups of alkaloids and cause signs of neurotoxicity when ingested by horses. *Datura spp.* (thornapple, jimsonweed), *Atropa belladonna* (deadly nightshade), and *Dubosia spp.* (corkwoods) contain the tropone alkaloids. These plants are widely distributed, but are unpalatable to horses. Poisoning may occur when these plants are included in hay or grain. Associated signs are anorexia, depression, excessive urination and thirst, diarrhea, mydriasis, muscle spasms, and convulsions. Physostigmine or neostigmine (a short acting cholinesterase) (1–5 mg s/c q1–4h) is the treatment of choice and should be used to effect. *Solanum nigram* (black nightshade) is the most toxic of the solanum alkaloid-containing plants. Colic, ataxia, weakness, tremors, and convulsions are associated with black nightshade poisoning. *Solanum tuberosum* (common potato) may also be toxic when green.

791

Toxic alcohols

Umbelliferous plants (hemlock-type) contain higher alcohols, including enanthotoxin and cicutoxin, and are amongst the most poisonous plants known. The toxins are concentrated in the root and stem and these plants are found throughout the US and in many other countries, especially in Europe, growing in wet or swampy areas. Signs of poisoning include salivation, mydriasis, colic, delirium, and convulsions.

Botulism

Definition/overview

Botulism is a neuromuscular disease characterized by flaccid paralysis caused by neurotoxins produced by strains of *Clostridium botulinum*. Horses are one of the most susceptible species, with both individual and group outbreaks reported.

Etiology/pathophysiology

C. botulinum is a Gram-positive, spore-forming anaerobic bacterium. Spores are found in the soil throughout most of the world, with the distribution of strains dependent on temperature and soil pH. Eight serotypes of botulinum neurotoxin exist (A, B, C_1, C_2, D, E, F, and G), all of which have similar toxicity. There is geographic variation in the predominant serotypes. In North America, botulism in horses is most often caused by type B toxin and less often by types A and C_1.

There are two main forms of botulism. Toxicoinfectious botulism, also known as 'shaker-foal syndrome', occurs almost exclusively in foals as a result of overgrowth of *C. botulinum* in the intestinal tract, followed by production of neurotoxins. The disease most often affects fast-growing foals from 1–2 months of age, although cases outside this age range have been seen. The mature, protective GI microflora of adult horses typically prevents overgrowth of *C. botulinum* following ingestion. In adult horses, botulism occurs following ingestion of preformed toxins in feed. Spoiled hay or silage is most commonly implicated in botulism caused by types A and B. Silage with a pH greater than 4.5 is favorable for sporulation and toxin production. This is known as 'forage poisoning'. It has also been suggested that birds may be able to carry preformed toxin from carrion to the feed of horses. Type C botulism is associated with ingestion of feed or water contaminated by the carcass of a rodent or other small animal. Less commonly, botulism can occur when neurotoxins are produced in wounds infected with *C. botulinum*. Proliferation of *C. botulinum* type B organisms in gastric ulcers, foci of hepatic necrosis, abscesses in the navel or lungs, and wounds in skin and muscle have been associated with toxicoinfectious botulism.

Botulinum neurotoxins bind to presynaptic membranes at neuromuscular junctions, irreversibly blocking the release of the neurotransmitter acetylcholine and resulting in flaccid paralysis. Botulinum neurotoxin has also been linked to equine grass sickness.

Clinical presentation

The clinical picture of symmetrical flaccid paralysis is consistent, with the onset and rate of progression dependent on the amount of toxin that is absorbed. The initial clinical signs include dysphagia with apparent excess salivation, weak eyelid, tail and tongue tone, and exercise intolerance (1055). Affected animals also spend increased amounts of time resting due to generalized muscle weakness, which is also associated with tremors, carpal buckling, and ataxia. Pharyngeal and lingual paralysis causes marked dysphagia and predisposes to aspiration pneumonia (1056). Affected animals tend to quid their food. Paralysis of the diaphragm and intercostal muscles results in an increased respiratory rate and decreased chest wall expansion. Severely affected animals die from respiratory paralysis and cardiac failure.

Differential diagnosis

Differential diagnoses for botulism include viral causes of encephalitis, protozoal causes of encephalomyelitis, and toxic causes of sudden death or neurologic dysfunction.

Diagnosis

Botulism should be suspected in animals with flaccid paralysis displaying the above clinical signs. Botulinum toxin does not affect the CNS, but does affect the CNs, therefore symmetrical CN deficits in an animal with normal mentation can help differentiate botulism from other disorders. Botulism is often a clinical diagnosis. Definitive diagnosis can be achieved by the mouse inoculation test using serum or GI contents. However, horses are extremely sensitive to the toxin and this test is often negative. If the toxin is demonstrated with mouse inoculation, the serotype can be determined through inoculation of mice passively protected with different serotypes of antitoxin. Detection of antibody titers in a recovering unvaccinated horse is also evidence for the diagnosis of botulism. Demonstration of spores in the intestine is not diagnostic, as they can be ingested and observed as contaminants.

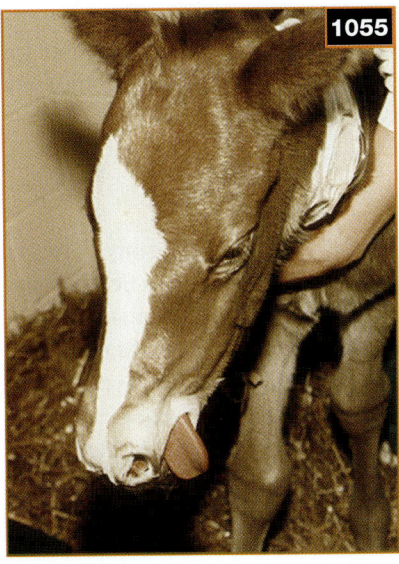

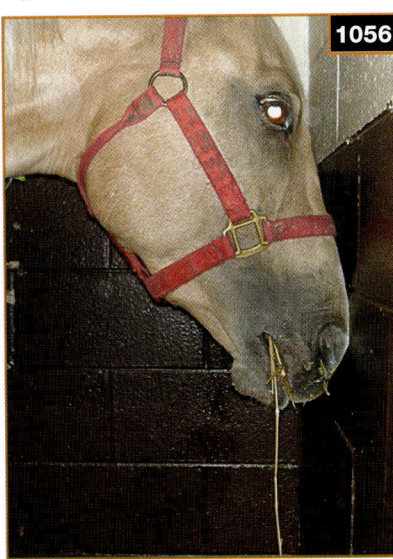

1055 Weak tongue tone and dysphagia in a foal with type B botulism.

1056 A mare that was dysphagic and had weak palpebral tone. The mare had botulism secondary to forage poisoning. Eight other horses on the farm were affected.

Management

Immediate treatment with a polyvalent antitoxin prevents binding of the toxin to presynaptic membranes, but antitoxin cannot reactivate neuromuscular junctions that have already been affected. Therefore, antitoxin administration may have little effect in animals that are severely affected. Generally, only one dose (200 ml of antiserum to foals [30,000 IU] or 500 ml [75,000 IU] to adults) of antitoxin is needed and provides passive protection for up to 2 months.

Antimicrobials should be administered if toxicoinfectious botulism is suspected or if there are secondary lesions such as aspiration pneumonia or decubital ulcers. Antimicrobials that can cause neuromuscular blockade and possibly exacerbate clinical signs (e.g. aminoglycosides) should be avoided and neurostimulants such as neostigmine should not be used. Good nursing care, including the provision of a deep bed and a quiet environment, is essential. Frequent turning of recumbent animals, nasogastric feeding and fluid support for animals with pharyngeal and lingual paralysis, frequent catheterization of the urinary bladder, application of ophthalmic ointments, and ventilatory support may all be required.

If botulism is suspected to have been caused by ingestion of preformed toxin in feed, an alternative feed source should be provided while the origin is investigated.

Prevention

Type B toxoid is available and should be used in areas in which type B botulism is endemic. Vaccination is particularly important in areas where neonatal botulism occurs. Widespread vaccination of mares in certain high-risk areas has dramatically decreased the incidence of neonatal botulism. An initial series of three vaccinations 1 month apart followed by annual boosters has been recommended. Pregnant mares should receive a booster 4 weeks prior to foaling to ensure adequate antibody levels in colostrum. Type B vaccine only provides protection against type B toxin. There is no cross protection against type C toxin, and type C toxoid is not licensed for use in North America.

Silage and other fermented feeds should not be fed to horses because of the risk of botulism.

Prognosis

A survival rate of 88% has been reported in foals with toxicoinfectious botulism that were provided with intensive nursing care (including mechanical ventilation and botulism antitoxin). However, this type of treatment is not available in all areas and is quite expensive. Without aggressive supportive care the mortality rate is high, with death usually occurring 1–3 days after the onset of clinical signs.

The prognosis is variable in adult horses that have ingested preformed toxin, depending on the amount of toxin absorbed and the severity of clinical signs. Mildly affected animals may recover with minimal treatment, while severely affected animals that become recumbent have a poor prognosis. The mortality rate has been reported to be as high as 90% in recumbent adult horses, with death occurring within hours of the appearance of signs. In animals that survive, complete recovery is most common. Development of full muscular strength takes weeks to months. Persistent tongue weakness not affecting the ability to eat has been reported.

Miscellaneous neurologic conditions

Cerebral abscess

Definition/overview
Cerebral abscesses are rare and sporadic in horses.

Etiology/pathophysiology
Cerebral abscesses may develop secondary to bacterial infection elsewhere in the body or via extension of local disease processes such as sinusitis, rhinitis, dental disease, and periocular lesions (1057, 1058). *Streptococcus equi* has been most commonly implicated; however, a variety of species, including *S. zooepidemicus*, *Actinobacillus equuli*, *Klebsiella* spp., and *Pasteurella* spp., may be involved. Bacterial meningitis may be present concurrently.

Clinical presentation
Signs become apparent with sufficient compression of cerebral tissue, the onset being insidious or acute depending on the rate of growth of the abscess. The clinical course is often characterized by marked fluctuations in the severity of signs. Fever is not always present. Behavioral changes such as depression, wandering, or unprovoked excitement are most obvious. Contralateral impaired vision, deficient menace response, and decreased facial sensation are consistent early findings. Affected horses frequently circle or stand with the head and neck turned towards the side of the lesion. Progression leads to recumbency, unconsciousness, seizures, and signs of brainstem compression such as asymmetric pupils, ataxia, and weakness.

1057 Right cerebral abscess in a horse. The horse was displaying belligerent behavior and had difficulty rising. The peripheral WBC count was normal, with normal fibrinogen.

Differential diagnosis
EPM; trauma; arboviral encephalitis; leukoencephalomalacia; hepatoencephalopathy; cholesterol granuloma of the choroid plexus of the lateral ventricle; uremic encephalopathy; rabies.

Diagnosis
Antemortem diagnosis can be difficult. A history of recent bacterial infection, particularly *S. equi* infection, should prompt further investigation of cerebral abscessation, although other causes of asymmetric cerebral disease should be ruled out. Hyperfibrinogenemia, hyperglobulinemia, and leucocytosis may be present, but are not consistent. Changes in the CSF depend on the degree of meningeal or ependymal involvement. Most cases exhibit xanthochromia and a moderate elevation of CSF protein levels reflective of cerebral damage and compression. CT can be very useful for diagnosis, but is currently of limited availability. The horse should be evaluated for the presence of a septic focus elsewhere in the body. Appropriate diagnostic specimens, including blood, should be submitted for bacterial culture in an attempt to identify the causative organism.

Management
If the signs are acute, severe, and rapidly progressive, it is likely that brain edema is also present. Corticosteroids (dexamethasone, 0.1–0.5 mg/kg i/v q24h) are controversial, but used by some clinicians. Osmotic agents (mannitol, 0.5–1.0 mg/kg as a 20% solution i/v over 15 minutes q12–24h) and diuretics (furosemide, 0.75–1.0 mg/kg i/v q12–24h; DMSO, 1 g/kg as a 10–20% solution q12–24h) are often used to try to counteract life-threatening increases in intracranial pressure (ICP). In addition to the treatment of increased ICP, prolonged antimicrobial administration is required. Based on pathogen(s) isolated from cerebral

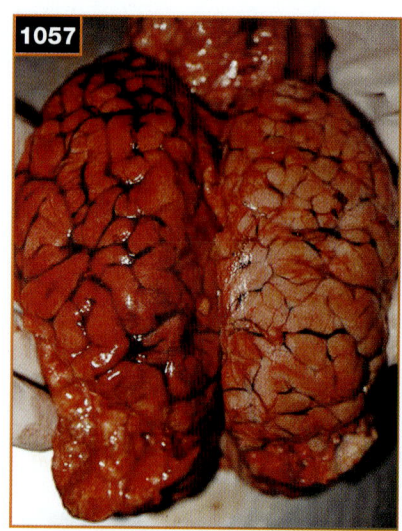

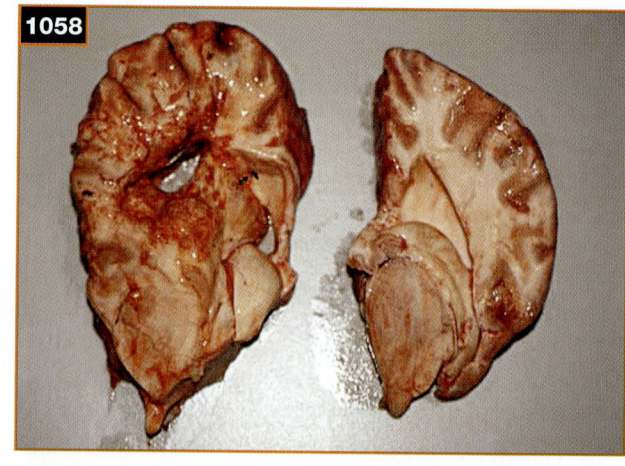

1058 Cerebral abscess caused by *Streptococcus equi.*

abscesses in horses, the use of potassium or sodium penicillin (20,000 IU/kg i/v q6h) and gentamicin (6.6 mg/kg i/v q24h) would seem to be a good initial choice. Surgical evacuation of the lesion is another approach that has been used successfully in a limited number of cases.

Prognosis
The prognosis is poor. Medical therapy alone is unlikely to successfully treat a cerebral abscess. Horses that recover may have residual deficits such as impaired vision.

Vertebral osteomyelitis

Definition/overview
Vertebral osteomyelitis (spondylitis) is an infectious or inflammatory degenerative disease of one or more vertebrae. When an adjacent intervertebral disc is involved, the condition is termed discospondylitis. These are rare but serious conditions of the horse.

Etiology/pathophysiology
Vertebral osteomyelitis has been related to hematogenous spread of infectious agents in the newborn and extension from local wounds. Progression of the vertebral infection leads to paravertebral abscess, meningitis, vertebral collapse, and spinal cord compression. Many pathogens have been isolated including *Streptococcus equi* and *Rhodococcus equi* in foals (**1059**).

Clinical presentation
The initial signs of localized spinal pain usually go unnoticed. Fever, stiffness, and sensory deficits with variable paresis are the signs that are noted. There may be rapid progress to recumbency.

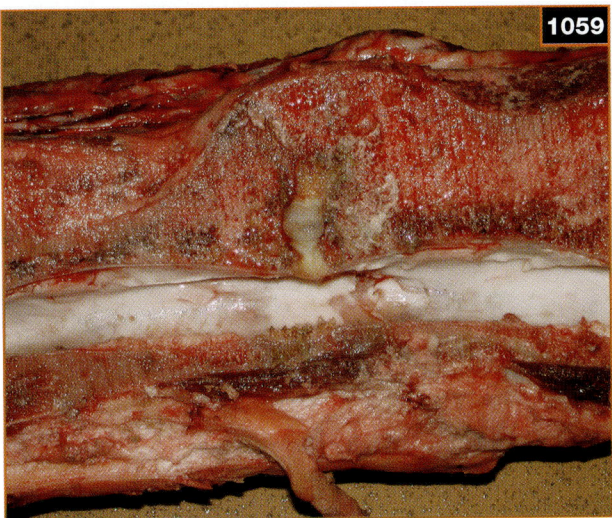

Differential diagnosis
Spinal trauma or neoplasia, meningitis, and arboviral encephalitis should be considered.

Diagnosis
Diagnosis is based on clinical signs, history, and positive findings on radiography, scintigraphy, CT, or ultrasonography. Hematology findings are usually consistent with inflammation and CSF analysis may be normal or consistent with spinal cord compression. Blood culture may be useful for identifying the offending pathogen. Repeated blood cultures may be required. Ideally, blood cultures are taken during periods of pyrexia. Culture of possible septic foci should also be attempted, ideally prior to initiation of antimicrobial therapy. Possible useful tests should be borne in mind in animals with other clinical signs; for example, tracheal wash cultures and cytology in foals suspected of *Rhodococcus equi* infections. Nuclear scintigraphy or myelography may be useful in some cases to identify a lesion or evaluate the degree of spinal cord compression.

Management
Long-term (3–6 months) antibiotic therapy is required and relapses are common. In the absence of culture and sensitivity data, broad-spectrum antimicrobial therapy is required.

Prognosis
The prognosis is poor if neurologic abnormalities are present. The success of treatment depends on the severity of signs at presentation and the presence and severity of concurrent disease.

Polyneuritis equi (neuritis of the cauda equina)

Definition/overview
Polyneuritis equi refers to a condition of neuritis of the cauda equina in addition to CN deficits. The facial, trigeminal, and vestibulocochlear nerves are most commonly affected.

Etiology/pathophysiology
Polyneuritis equi is considered to be a disease of the adult horse and is thought to involve an autoimmune response against the myelin of the cranial and sacrococcygeal extradural nerve roots. Prior bacterial and viral infections have been implicated in this response.

1059 Vertebral osteomyelitis causing spinal cord compression. *Streptococcus equi* was isolated from the bone.

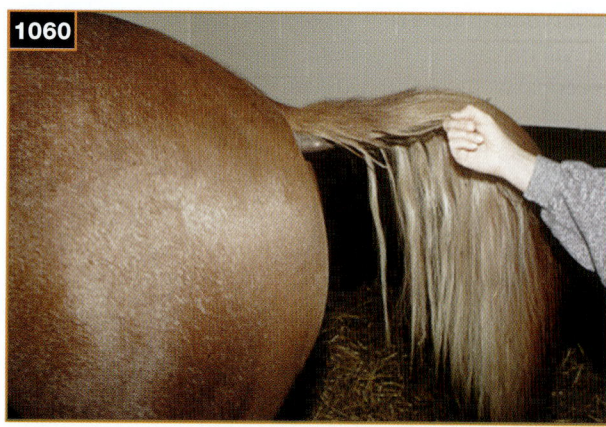

1060 Poor tail tone secondary to polyneuritis equi.

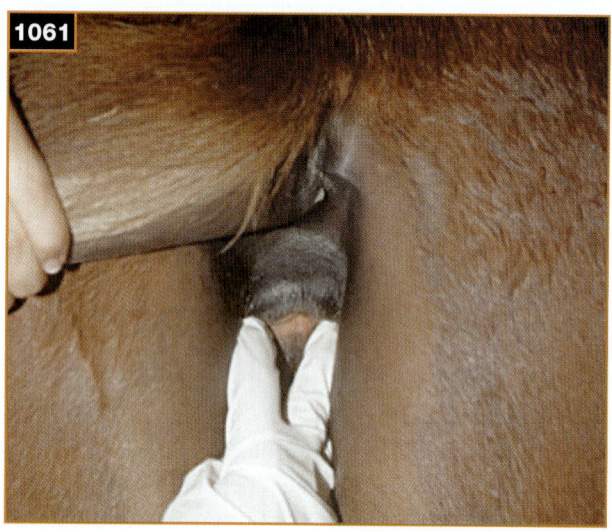

1061 Poor anal tone secondary to polyneuritis equi.

Clinical presentation
The neurologic deficits primarily reflect LMN deficits at the level of the cauda equina and most notably include obstipation and urinary incontinence. The tail hangs limply without tone (1060), and the anal sphincter (1061), rectum, bladder, urethral sphincter, and vulva or penis are paralyzed. There is usually an insidious onset, with progression over several weeks. The condition is usually progressive, but signs may remain static after attaining a certain level of severity. CN signs are not always present, but when they are, they help distinguish this disease from other conditions that result in damage to the structures of the cauda equina such as sacral trauma.

Differential diagnosis
EHV encephalomyelitis, arboviral encephalitis, rabies, EPM, trauma, and equine motor neuron disease should be considered.

Diagnosis
Polyneuritis equi is often diagnosed after excluding other possible causes. Hematology and CSF cytology are usually unremarkable. Mild increases in protein and leukocytes may be present in the CSF. Antimyelin antibodies can be detected in CSF; however, the usefulness of this test is debatable. Definitive diagnosis can only be obtained at necropsy.

Management
There is no specific treatment. Supportive therapy may include manual evacuation of the rectum, provision of a soft diet, and urinary bladder decompression. Corticosteroids (dexamethasone [0.05–0.2 mg/kg q24h] or prednisolone [1 mg/kg p/o q12h]) are commonly used. Affected horses should be monitored closely for complications such as intestinal tract impactions, esophageal obstruction, and urinary tract infections. Antimicrobial therapy may be required to treat secondary urinary tract infections.

Prognosis
The prognosis is poor because this is a progressive disease that rarely responds to treatment.

Cholesterol granuloma (cholesteatoma)
Cholesterol granulomas, also known as cholesteatomas, are found incidentally in the choroid plexuses of up to 20% of older horses. They occur more commonly in the fourth ventricle, but usually reach a larger size in the lateral ventricles and are thus more likely to cause clinical signs. They appear as brownish nodular thickenings and microscopically consist of abundant cholesterol crystals interspersed with hemosiderin, empty clefts, and an inflammatory reaction consisting of giant cells and macrophages (1062). Compression of brain tissue or an obstructive hydrocephalus may result in a minority of cases. Clinical signs are insidious in onset and include altered behavior, depression, somnolence, seizures, ataxia, weakness, and unconsciousness. There is no effective treatment.

Gomen disease
Gomen disease is a progressive degenerative cerebellar disease recognized in the northwest part of New Caledonia in the South Pacific that causes mild to severe ataxia. It occurs in indigenous and introduced horses that are allowed to roam free, with confined horses generally unaffected. Signs may take 1–2 years to develop following introduction to an endemic area. Prominent signs include ataxia and a wide-based stance referable to cerebellar involvement and weakness likely due to brainstem or spinal cord involvement. The condition is progressive, with most horses dying or being euthanized within 3–4 years.

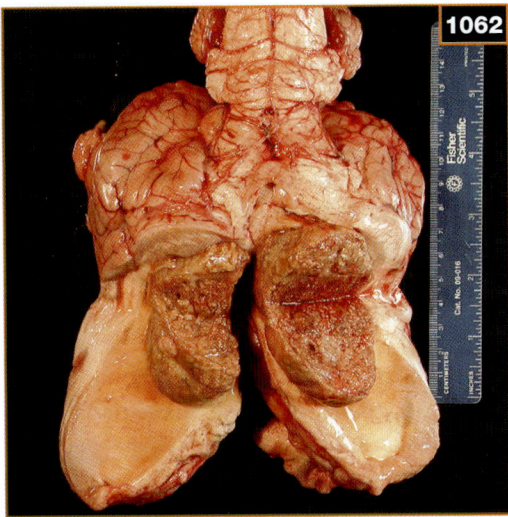

1062 Cholesterol granulomas in the lateral ventricles of a 20-year-old mare. The mare had a history of seizures. (Photo courtesy M Saulez)

Gross examination of the brain reveals cerebellar atrophy, with severe depletion of Purkinje neurons visible histologically. There is moderate to severe lipofuscin pigmentation of neuron cell bodies throughout the brain and spinal cord. This is considered greater than normally expected in horses of a similar age. The pathogenesis is unknown, but is thought to involve a metabolic disorder, perhaps resulting from toxicity.

Postanesthetic myelopathy

Postanesthetic myelopathy has been reported in young, heavy horses, although there have been reports of cases in Thoroughbreds. Halothane anesthesia was used in all cases. Signs ranged from difficulty standing to tetraplegia with flaccid paralysis and anesthesia of the hindlimbs. Affected horses became recumbent or remained in lateral recumbency until euthanasia 1–8 days later. Necropsy revealed hemorrhage and congestion of the meninges and spinal cord, and degrees of malacia of gray matter over at least several spinal cord segments at sites anywhere from the caudal cervical to caudal sacral spinal cord. These changes are consistent with hypoxic and ischemic neuronal damage. The syndrome is thought to involve a number of factors including systemic arterial hypotension, local venous congestion caused by halothane anesthesia, and compression of the caudal vena cava by abdominal viscera. The prognosis is hopeless in the cases that have been described, but milder cases may not be recognized.

Stringhalt
Definition/overview

Stringhalt is a disorder that is characterized by an abnormal gait with involuntary and exaggerated flexion of the hock and stifle of one or both hindlimbs, usually at a walk. Adult horses of any breed may be affected. Stringhalt is usually an individual disorder with one limb affected. It can occur as outbreaks, known as 'Australian stringhalt', although these have been recorded in New Zealand and North and South America in addition to Australia. In these cases, both hindlimbs are commonly affected, although one limb may be more severely affected. Forelimb cases have also been recorded.

Etiology/pathophysiology

The etiology of sporadic stringhalt is unclear. It has been suggested that damage to the reflex arc or its connections, perhaps from trauma, may lead to the abnormal and characteristic hock flexion that is seen. Thus, a sensory or motor neuropathy, spinal cord disease, or myopathy may be responsible. In some cases, injury to the metatarsus and tarsus has preceded the development of clinical signs by several months. Injury may interrupt control of the muscle spindle trigger mechanism. The epidemic form is thought to involve fungal or plant toxicity. It has been associated with the ingestion of certain plants, particularly *Hypochoeris radicata*, and with certain environmental conditions such as drought and overgrazing of poor-quality pasture.

Clinical presentation

The condition is easily recognized by the characteristic gait. The disorder varies in severity from a grade 1 affected horse with only mild exaggeration of flexion during backing and turning, that may be inapparent during exercise, to a grade 5 in which the affected limb may strike the abdomen during movement.

In outbreaks the onset is sudden, with several horses that are grazing the pasture affected, and the severity of signs increasing in the first days to weeks. In contrast to the sporadic cases, these horses usually recover without treatment, although the recovery time may be prolonged. Clinical and neurologic examinations are usually unremarkable in both the sporadic and epidemic form; however, it should be noted, especially in sporadic cases, that stringhalt may also have a central cause and ruling out other CNS conditions, such as EPM, is important.

Management

In the epidemic form most horses recover in weeks to months. A toxic etiology is suspected and horses should be removed from the pasture they were grazing at the time of onset of clinical signs. The administration of phenytoin (15 mg/kg p/o q24h; q12h in severe cases) for 2 weeks may result in a more rapid resolution of clinical signs. Treatment may have to be extended if clinical signs become worse.

In the sporadic form, exercise, intra-articular administration of steroids in trauma cases, and surgical therapy by tenotomy or tenectomy of the lateral digital extensor tendon have been attempted with variable success.

Prognosis

Full recovery is rare in cases of sporadic stringhalt. Immediate improvement may be noted in some horses following surgical intervention, although response is variable. The prognosis is good with the epidemic form. Most horses recover fully, although weeks to months may be required.

Shivers

Definition/overview

Shivering is a condition of unknown etiology with a suspected genetic origin that has been long recognized in draft breeds.

Etiology/pathophysiology

Both etiology and pathophysiology are unclear. It has been speculated that 'shivers' could be associated with PSSM (see p. 229).

Clinical presentation

Shivering is characterized by spasmodic muscle tremors affecting the hindlimbs and tail and is most commonly observed if the horse is asked to back, turn, or lift a hindlimb. Typically, one limb is held in a flexed and abducted position, with muscle trembling for a few moments, and it is then slowly lowered to a normal position. Elevation and tremor of the tail are also commonly observed.

Differential diagnosis

Hindlimb laminitis, trauma, EHV-1 neuralgia, and idiopathic neuralgia should be considered.

Diagnosis

Diagnosis is based on clinical signs, but these may be subtle. Forced flexion of the hock may produce signs in an otherwise normal appearing animal. Muscle biopsy is indicated if PSSM is suspected.

Management

There is no effective treatment. Treatment of PSSM can be attempted.

Prognosis

The long-term prognosis is guarded. This condition is slowly progressive, although in some cases the signs may plateau. Horses may stabilize or improve with rest; however, signs may return when exercise is resumed.

Hepatic encephalopathy

Definition/overview

Hepatic encephalopathy is a clinical syndrome that is characterized by an abnormal mental status that occurs secondary to hepatic insufficiency, acute hepatic necrosis, idiopathic hyperammonemia, portosystemic shunts, and hyperammonemia due to renal or GI disease.

Etiology/pathophysiology

Liver failure of any origin may result in development of hepatic encephalopathy. Portosystemic shunts are another potential cause, but are uncommon in horses. Persistent hyperammonemia of Morgan foals could also be included in this category, as the defect is believed to be at the level of the hepatic mitochondria.

The precise pathophysiology of hepatic encephalopathy remains undefined, but it is thought to be multifactorial, with three major mechanisms proposed: (1) accumulation of synergistic neurotoxins such as ammonia, mercaptans, or short chain fatty acids; (2) accumulation of false neurotransmitters due to decreased metabolism of aromatic amino acids such as tyrosine, phenylalanine, and free tryptophan; and (3) increased activity of the inhibitory neurotransmitter GABA.

Clinical presentation

Clinical signs are often subtle and reflect cerebral dysfunction. The most prominent early sign is a change in behavior such as depression. Other animals become maniacal or exhibit erratic behavior. Additional signs that can be seen are compulsive walking/circling, yawning, head pressing, inspiratory stridor secondary to laryngeal paralysis, and coma.

Differential diagnosis

A variety of neurologic diseases should be considered including aboviral encephalitis, rabies, EHV encephalitis, EPM, and head trauma.

Diagnosis

Diagnosis is suspected from clinical signs and is confirmed by laboratory changes indicative of liver failure, including elevated levels of blood ammonia. Evaluation of liver failure is covered elsewhere (see p. 602).

Management

Treatment is as for liver failure. Specific treatment of hepatic encephalopathy is supportive in nature. Animals may be dangerous to themselves and humans and should be handled carefully. Ideally, they should be in an environment where there is a lesser chance of injuring themselves (e.g. a large, padded stall without permanent fixtures). Sedation may be required, although diazepam should be avoided because it may potentiate the neurologic signs. Lactulose (0.2–0.3 ml/kg p/o q6–8h) may be used to decrease GI ammonia production and absorption. Treatment of hepatic failure is covered elsewhere (see p. 603).

Prognosis

The prognosis is poor and depends on the ability to address the inciting cause. In general, advanced liver failure is present by the time signs of hepatic encephalopathy are observed. The prognosis is best when hyperlipidemia/hyperlipemia is the inciting cause and can be corrected.

Hypoglycemia

Definition/overview

Hypoglycemia can cause a variety of neurologic abnormalities. It is most commonly encountered in neonatal foals.

Etiology/pathophysiology

A variety of possible causes are recognized. Hypoglycemia may result from increased uptake (sepsis or exhaustion), inadequate intake (starvation), reduced production and mobilization (glycogen depletion or inadequate gluconeogenesis), or disordered regulation of blood glucose. In neonates, anorexia and sepsis are the most common causes. It has also been seen in insulin overdose, whether nonintentional, associated with treatment of hyperlipemia, or intentional, associated with insurance fraud. End-stage liver disease and withdrawal of corticosteroid administration have also been reported to cause hypoglycemia. Clinical signs are not usually evident until blood glucose is less than 2.2–2.8 mmol/l (40–50 mg/dl).

The principal lesion of hypoglycemia is ischemic neuronal cell change similar to that of cerebral hypoxia, with neurons of the cerebral cortex most severely affected.

Clinical presentation

Hypoglycemia results in weakness, depression, and ataxia that may progress to loss of consciousness. Hypoglycemia is not normally associated with seizure activity except in neonates.

Management

Signs are readily reversible with oral or intravenous administration of glucose. Bolus administration of hypertonic glucose solutions should be avoided, as rapid changes in serum osmolality may exacerbate CNS derangements. The cause of the hypoglycemia should be assessed and continued intravenous glucose therapy should be guided by serial measurements of serum glucose. Blood glucose measurement should be performed frequently to assess response to treatment and ensure that hyperglycemia does not result.

Prognosis

The prognosis depends on the severity of, and ability to address, the underlying problem. If untreated, hypoglycemia may result in irreversible brain damage.

Nervous tissue hypoxia/ischemia

Nervous tissue has a high and continuous demand for oxygen and is thus vulnerable to impaired oxygen delivery resulting from hypoxia or ischemia. The major effect is altered carbohydrate and energy metabolism, with a switch from aerobic to anaerobic glycolysis. This leads to depletion of brain glucose, decreased energy production, and localized lactic acidosis. The resulting neuronal swelling may exacerbate ischemia, with progression leading to further edema, neuronal necrosis, and cavitation. The clinical manifestations depend on the extent of the area affected. Localized interruption of blood supply can occur with fibrocartilaginous emboli, intracarotid injections, verminous thromboembolism, and aortic thrombosis. When there is acute deprivation of oxygen to the entire CNS, the first signs that are seen are referable to impaired cerebral function, with depression leading to coma and seizures (**1063**). Most cases result from respiratory insufficiency that may arise from a variety of

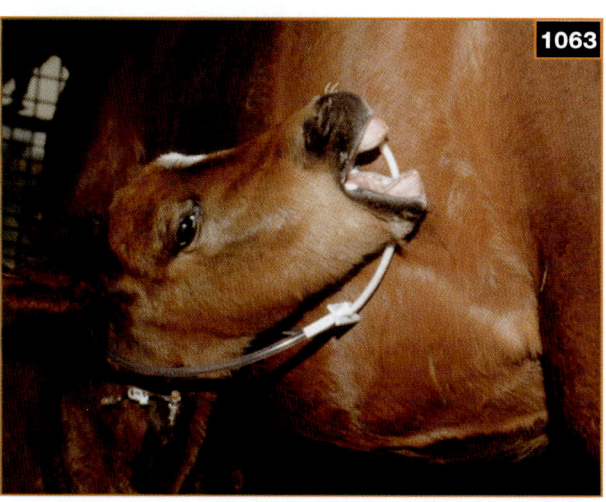

1063 Foal with chewing seizures secondary to hypoxic–ischemic encephalopathy.

TABLE 50 Options for the treatment of hypoxic–ischemic encephalopathy

Allopurinol: 40 mg/kg p/o within 2–3 hours of birth.

Ascorbic acid: 100 mg/kg/day i/v. The optimal dosage of ascorbic acid for neuroprotection is not known. In high risk human premature infants a dose of 100 mg/kg/day has been found to be safe.

Vitamin E: 4,000 IU p/o q24h (neonate) or 10,000 IU p/o q24h (dam). Vitamin E is an antioxidant that is synergistic with ascorbic acid. For an effective dose to reach the brain or circulation, vitamin E needs to be given for some days before the ischemic insult. There may be a role in early fetal distress, with vitamin E supplementation given to the mare.

Magnesium sulfate: 50 mg/kg i/v infusion for first hour then 25 mg/kg/hour CRI. There is a lack of consensus in human medicine regarding the use of magnesium in the treatment of infants with hypoxic–ischemic encephalopathy. The current dose regimen has been noted to be safe in foals when infused over 3 days.

Thiamine: 1 g i/v in 1 liter of fluids q12h. Thiamine is thought to be neuroprotective due to its action of increasing activity of the adenosine triphosphate-dependent sodium pump, thereby regulating ion uptake and decreasing cellular water.

DMSO: 0.25–1.0 g/kg i/v q6–12h as 10% solution. Used as a treatment for cerebral edema and suspected increase in ICP (osmotic diuretic). DMSO is also a hydroxyl radical scavenger and may theoretically prevent some cellular damage attributed to oxygen radical generation.

Mannitol: 0.25–1.0 g as a 20% solution q6–12h as an i/v bolus over 15–20 minutes. Osmotic agent, which has been specifically used for the treatment of cerebral edema. It also has some neuroprotective properties.

Diazepam and phenobarbital: diazepam (0.11–0.44 mg/kg i/v) or phenobarbital (12 mg/kg i/v loading dose then 2–7 mg/kg i/v q12h). Give slowly, monitor serum concentrations (maintain serum levels 15–40 mcg/ml). Use for seizure activity.

Hyperbaric oxygen therapy: 1.5–2.0 ATM for 45 minutes to 1 hour q8–12h.

causes, a few examples being neonatal respiratory distress syndrome, pulmonary edema, intracardiac or extracardiac shunts, pneumonia, airway obstruction, pneumothorax, botulism, and severe hypotension. Hypoxic or ischemic brain damage is thought to be one of the principal factors in the development of neonatal maladjustment syndrome (see p. 977).

Effective management depends on treatment of the underlying disorder, with most cases benefiting from insufflation of nasal oxygen. Dexamethasone and DMSO (previously discussed under cerebral trauma, p. 774) should be considered for treatment of the edema and inflammation associated with CNS hypoxia and ischemia (*Table 50*).

Hyponatremia

Hyponatremia is most commonly associated with conditions such as diarrhea, excessive sweat loss, and adrenal insufficiency, which cause sodium depletion. Other conditions that may lead to hyponatremia are rapid accumulations of sodium-containing fluids in body cavities or the gut lumen, leading to plasma volume reduction and decreased serum sodium concentration as compensating renal responses cause water retention. An example of this is rupture of the bladder in neonatal foals. Rhabdomyolysis in neonatal foals may also cause hyponatremia. Iatrogenic hyponatremia may occur if excessive amounts of free water are delivered to patients with renal compromise. The neurologic signs that are seen are a result of the rapidly developing hypotonic hyponatremia and include depression, convulsions, and coma. Progressively severe disturbances can be seen as the serum sodium concentration falls below 115 mmol/l (115 mEq/l). The severity of signs depends not only on the degree of hyponatremia, but also on how quickly it develops.

Hypernatremia (salt poisoning)

Clinically significant hypernatremia is uncommon in horses. Hypernatremia may occur in the initial stages of diarrhea, vomiting, or renal disease if water loss exceeds electrolyte loss. Food and water deprivation is associated with decreased urine and fecal output, but continued cutaneous and respiratory insensible water losses may result in hypernatremia. The hypernatremia that is observed in salt poisoning of ruminants and swine is associated with water restriction in animals that have been maintained on a high salt diet. Inappropriate oral electrolyte supplementation, particularly in foals, may also cause hypernatremia. Salt poisoning is associated with severe GI and neurologic signs including head and neck extension, blindness, aggressiveness, hyperexcitability, ataxia, proprioceptive deficits, and head pressing. The pathophysiology involves deposition of sodium ions in the CNS, which when followed by access to ion-free water results in cerebral edema, with death occurring by respiratory failure. Treatment involves gradual reduction of serum sodium over a few days, along with supportive care and treatment of the cerebral edema.

Hypocalcemia (see also p. 627)

Definition/overview
Hypocalcemia is a relatively uncommon cause of weakness in the horse.

Etiology/pathophysiology
Hypocalcemia in horses may occur in a number of situations. Lactation tetany in mares, transit tetany associated with transportation over long distances, idiopathic hypocalcemia, exhausted horse syndrome associated with endurance competitions, sepsis/endotoxemia, malabsorption syndromes, renal disease, severe rhabdomyolysis, and other causes including cantharidin toxicosis have been reported.

Clinical presentation
The clinical signs that are seen are related to an increase in membrane excitability of excitable tissues such as the heart and skeletal muscle. The signs are variable and related to the degree of calcium depletion. Signs include a stiff gait, muscle fasciculations, tachycardia, sweating, cardiac dysrhythmias, convulsions, coma, and death. Synchronous diaphragmatic flutter is a sign that is also frequently seen and is thought to occur as a result of altered membrane potential of the phrenic nerve, which passes directly over the atrium, resulting in nerve discharges in response to atrial depolarization. Total calcium values of 1.25–2.0 mmol/l (5–8 mg/dl) may produce tetanic spasms, while values of below 1.25 mmol/l (5 mg/dl) result in recumbency.

Diagnosis
Diagnosis is based on the recognition of characteristic clinical signs in affected horses combined with laboratory demonstration of hypocalcemia. Other abnormalities that can be seen in association with hypocalcemia are metabolic alkalosis, hypo/hypermagnesemia, and hypo/hyperphosphatemia. Total serum calcium is approximately 50% ionized, 40% is protein bound, especially to albumin, and 10% is complexed with anions such as citrate and phosphate. Only ionized calcium is biologically active and therefore the measurement of ionized calcium is preferred. Acid–base status should also be determined because alkalosis decreases ionized calcium levels, while acidosis increases the ionized calcium level. The protein-bound fraction will decrease with hypoalbuminemia. This hypocalcemia secondary to hypoalbuminemia is usually clinically irrelevant because the ionized calcium remains normal.

Management
This condition can be life-threatening and warrants immediate treatment in most cases. Treatment involves the administration of intravenous calcium solutions such as 20% calcium borogluconate (0.25–1.0 ml/kg of 23% calcium gluconate slowly i/v diluted 1:4 with saline or dextrose). Administration should be closely monitored via the cardiovascular response. The infusion should be suspended or the rate decreased if signs of cardiotoxicity (bradycardia or arrhythmias) develop. Resolution of clinical signs can occur within minutes to hours of calcium infusion. High calcium forages, such as alfalfa, should be fed to horses with recurrent hypocalcemia.

Prognosis
The prognosis depends on the ability to correct the underlying condition. Idiopathic hypocalcemia in foals carries a poor prognosis.

Neoplasia of nervous tissue
Neoplasms of the CNS of the horse, with the exception of the pituitary adenoma, are extremely rare. For the purposes of this discussion, only nonpituitary CNS neoplasms will be discussed.

The prevalence of neurologic disease related to neoplasms has been estimated at 2%, with tumors of lymphoid origin being the most common. Primary neoplasms of the nervous system are very rare and in a survey of North American university veterinary hospitals, all nervous tissue tumors found in horses involved peripheral nerves. Neurofibromas and neurofibrosarcomas were the most common, with the former frequently being found cutaneously in the pectoral region, neck, face, and abdomen. Secondary neoplasms may reach the nervous system by vascular spread, growing through osseous foramina or penetration of the cranial vault or vertebrae.

Lymphoma is the most common secondary tumor affecting the nervous system of horses and has been found in the epidural space as a cause of compressive myelopathy, in the brain and olfactory tracts, and infiltrated into various peripheral nerves.

Melanomas in white or gray horses occasionally invade the CNS and have been found in the epidural space following contiguous spread from melanomatous sublumbar lymph nodes. Cutaneous melanomas have also metastasized to spinal meninges, spinal cord, and brain.

Other reported secondary nervous system tumors in horses are hemangiosarcoma, adenocarcinoma, osteosarcoma, and plasma cell myeloma.

The clinical signs seen are usually related to the area of the brain or spinal cord involved and are most often due to compression from the expanding tumor mass.

Juvenile idiopathic epilepsy

Definition/overview

Juvenile idiopathic epilepsy, also known as benign epilepsy of foals, is a cause of seizures in foals of a few days to several months of age. Most affected foals are Arabians or Arabian crosses.

Etiology/pathophysiology

The etiology is unknown. The disorder may reflect a low seizure threshold that increases sensitivity to many temporary stimuli.

Clinical presentation

Seizure activity can be quite variable in foals. Often, focal seizures characterized by abnormal mouth movements are observed. Facial tremors and head twitching may occur with mild localized seizures. Generalized seizures with muscle spasms over the entire body, recumbency, and rhythmic thrashing may also occur. With generalized seizures, blindness may persist for hours to days.

Differential diagnosis

Meningitis, hypoglycemia, and arboviral encephalitis are the most common differential diagnoses.

Management

Although this disorder disappears with age, anticonvulsant therapy should be initiated at the first signs and maintained for several weeks to months. The use of phenobarbital (12 mg/kg p/o or i/v loading dose and then 6 mg/kg p/o or i/v q12h) has been clinically rewarding. Phenobarbital induces microsomal enzymes, which may alter the metabolism of the drug with repeated administration. Serum phenobarbital concentrations should be monitored and maintained between 10 and 30 µg/ml. Failure to treat these animals may result in neuronal death and further, possibly permanent, seizure foci. Foals with uncontrolled disease should be housed in an area where they are less likely to be injured should a seizure occur. Underlying problems such as fever that may initiate further seizures should be corrected.

Prognosis

Juvenile idiopathic epilepsy usually resolves with age.

Acquired epilepsy

Definition/overview

Acquired epilepsy is characterized by adult onset of seizure activity.

Etiology/pathophysiology

There is no evidence of familial adult-onset epilepsy in horses. It is therefore assumed to be acquired and caused by an intracranial epileptogenic focus or foci acquired during postnatal life. Foci may become active following recovery from a cerebral insult, although the interval from brain disease to the onset of seizure activity may be several years and is referred to as epileptogenic ripening. Foci are the nucleating sites for the spreading of paroxysmal neuronal changes that are evident clinically as seizures.

Clinical presentation

Transient changes in the horse's behavior usually precede attacks. Seizures may be partial, such as facial twitching on one side, or generalized, with recumbency and convulsive movements of the limbs.

Management

A generalized seizure is potentially dangerous, although usually short in duration. Thus, it is safer to prevent the next seizure rather than try to treat the current one, unless the horse is in status epilepticus. If seizures are mild, infrequent, or declining in frequency, no treatment may be required. The history may indicate if a particular activity induces seizures and if so this activity should be avoided. When management changes do not result in a decreasing frequency or severity of seizures, or if these are increasing, antiepileptic treatment should be instituted and maintained. Acute treatment should consist of diazepam (0.1–0.2 mg/kg i/v in foals and 0.02–0.08 mg/kg i/v in adults), which may be repeated after 30 minutes. Phenobarbital can be considered for long-term treatment (see Juvenile idiopathic epilepsy, above). For cases that are refractory to phenobarbital, potassium bromide (30–40 mg/kg p/o q24h) may be added. A general recommendation is that the doses of these drugs can be reduced gradually after 2 months without attacks, and the horse should not be ridden until it has been seizure-free without medication for a minimum of 6 months. When making this recommendation it is important to consider the possible consequences of an unexpected seizure, especially with a child's pony.

Prognosis

The prognosis is highly variable because of the idiopathic nature of the disease. A fair prognosis should be given; however, some horses will not respond well to treatment. Horses with uncontrolled intermittent seizure activity should be considered unsafe to ride, even if the seizures are very infrequent.

Narcolepsy–cataplexy

Definition/overview

Narcolepsy is a sudden onset of excessive daytime sleepiness. It is usually accompanied by cataplexy, a sudden and profound loss of muscle tone. Both have been recognized in several breeds and are classified as two different syndromes. The first is a fairly common transient condition affecting primarily foals of light breeds and is frequently induced by restraint. The second is a rare but persistent form that appears to be familial in miniature horses and has also been seen in ponies and Suffolk horses.

Etiology/pathophysiology

The etiology is unclear. A familial predisposition is suspected in certain breeds. Often a specific stimulus is associated with initiation of an episode. In rare cases, signs have been reported in association with EPM. The pathogenesis of the condition is not fully understood, but is suspected to involve abnormalities of the neuropeptides (hypocretins and orexins) that are linked to the regulation of sleep.

Clinical presentation

The intermittent episodes are characterized by lowering of the head and buckling of the fetlocks, with occasional collapse and rapid eye movement (REM) sleep. Between episodes, animals are clinically normal.

Differential diagnosis

Differential diagnoses include other causes of collapse, such as syncope or seizures, and any disorder that may prevent a horse from lying down, leading to excessive sleepiness (e.g. a musculoskeletal problem).

Diagnosis

Diagnosis is based on history, clinical signs, and exclusion of other problems. Affected horses are normal between episodes and routine clinicopathologic evaluation is normal. Intravenous administration of physostigmine salicylate (0.1 mg/kg i/v) may elicit signs of narcolepsy within minutes in some individuals, but this response is not consistently found in all animals with narcolepsy.

Management

If an inciting cause can be identified, it should be avoided. The signs of adult-onset narcolepsy usually persist for life. Treatment with the tricyclic antidepressant imipramine (0.5–2.0 mg/kg i/m, i/v, or p/o q6–12h) may improve clinical signs in some animals. Oral absorption is poor and the oral route of administration may not provide an acceptable response.

1064 Symmetrical ataxia of the hindlimbs in a horse with EDM.

Prognosis

Narcolepsy–cataplexy is not a life-threatening condition; however, affected horses are not safe to ride, even when being treated. Some foals may outgrow the condition and would be safe for use provided a long period (at least 6 months) has passed since the last episode.

Equine degenerative myeloencephalopathy

Definition/overview

Equine degenerative myeloencephalopathy (EDM) is a diffuse degenerative disease of the spinal cord and brainstem. Its incidence has been reported to be as high as 23–45% of horses that present with spinal cord disease in some areas. The disease usually occurs in foals of either sex, but may affect horses up to 3 years of age.

Etiology/pathophysiology

The disease has been shown to have a familial hereditary basis in some breeds including Morgans, Appaloosa, Standardbreds, and Paso Finos. An hereditary basis is suspected in a number of other breeds.

Vitamin E deficiency early in life has been implicated as a causative factor, although the exact pathogenesis is not known. By the time clinical signs become apparent, the vitamin E levels may be normal. Free radical damage to nerve tissue is the most likely cause of neurologic damage.

Clinical presentation

The disease may occur in an individual or may affect groups of young horses (usually related). The onset of signs may be abrupt or insidious. Symmetrical ataxia, paresis, and dysmetria are seen, with hindlimb signs worse than forelimb signs (1064). Clinical signs may stabilize for several months or may progress to cause recumbency.

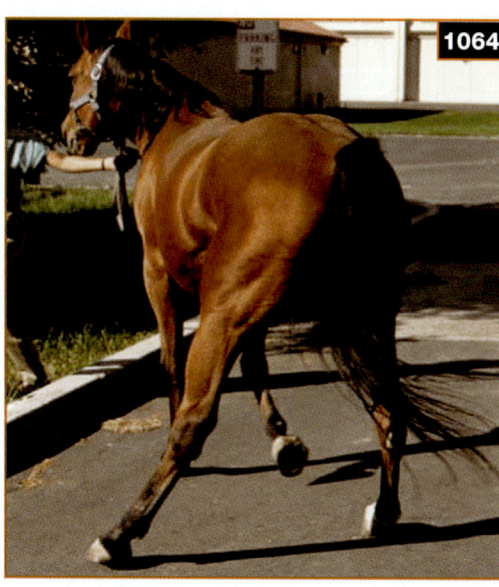

1064

Other signs that are reported include marked hyporeflexia over the neck and trunk, including an absent slap test, cutaneous trunci reflex, and cervicofacial reflex, indicating thoracic spinal cord disease. It is difficult to differentiate this disease from other differential diagnoses, especially wobbler syndrome.

Differential diagnosis
Cervical vertebral instability/stenosis, EPM, WNV encephalitis, trauma, equine LMN disease, hyperammonemia, hypocalcemia, and spinal cord impingement secondary to neoplasia may produce similar signs.

Diagnosis
Diagnosis is often made based on clinical presentation and exclusion of other possible causes. Low serum vitamin E levels may be present, but this is an inconsistent finding with a low sensitivity and specificity, and results are difficult to interpret. If vitamin E levels are tested, it is useful to compare results with those of herdmates of similar ages and on the same diet. An increase in CSF CK may be present, but this is not diagnostic. A definitive diagnosis can only be made by histopathologic evaluation of the spinal cord, which demonstrates diffuse axonal degeneration, myelin digestion, and astrocytosis.

Management
Treatment should include oral supplementation of vitamin E (5,000–7,000 IU/day p/o) in addition to ample green forage.

Prognosis
Remission or recovery has not been reported and treatment is aimed at stabilizing clinical signs. Some mild improvement may occur over time; however, it is unclear whether this represents healing or compensation. Affected animals and their parents should not be bred because of the suspected heritable nature of the disease.

Equine motor neuron disease
Definition/overview
Equine motor neuron disease (EMND) is a neurodegenerative disorder of the somatic LMNs of horses that clinically and pathologically bears resemblance to the human disorder amyotrophic lateral sclerosis (Lou Gehrig's disease). Mature horses are affected, with a mean age of 9 years.

Etiology/pathophysiology
The etiology is unclear. Absence of access to pasture is regarded as a significant risk factor, with most cases appearing to be related to chronic vitamin E deficiency. Most cases have been reported from the northeastern US, although cases have been reported from a variety of other countries.

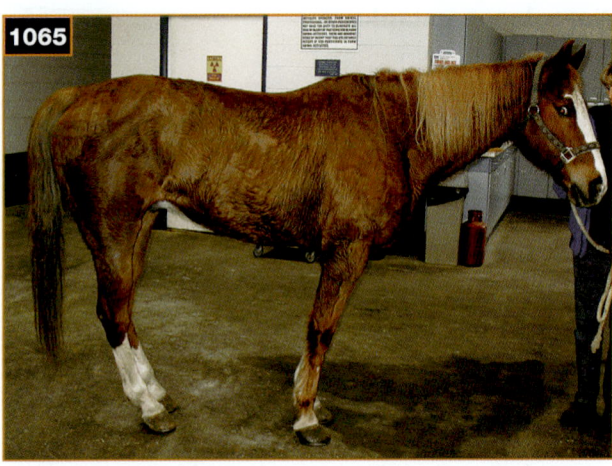

1065 EMND in a Tennessee Walking Horse. Note the 'camped under' posture and full-body sweating. This horse was very weak in all four limbs and muscle fasciculations were noted before the animal would lie down.

Clinical signs are the result of oxidative damage to the somatic ventral motor neuron cells. Parent motor neurons that supply type 1 motor fibers (high oxidative muscle groups) are preferentially affected. Neurogenic atrophy of the affected muscles occurs and because of the large contribution of type 1 muscle fibers to the postural muscles, the horse appears to have difficulty in fixing its 'stay-apparatus'. This neurogenic atrophy and fibrosis of the sacrocaudalis dorsalis medialis muscle results in elevation of the tail head. Signs are only seen when 30% of motor neuron cells die or become dysfunctional.

Clinical presentation
The clinical signs vary depending on the duration of the disease and are best described by dividing EMND into a subacute and a chronic form. Horses with the subacute form develop an acute onset of trembling, muscle fasciculations, shifting of weight in the hindlimbs, and abnormal sweating, and they appear to lie down frequently (**1065**). There may be a gradual loss of muscle mass noted for 1 month prior to the development of clinical signs. Appetite and gait are not usually affected, but the head carriage may be abnormally low. Horses with the chronic form are usually, but not always, those that have stabilized from the subacute form. Poor performance, fatigue, and abnormal

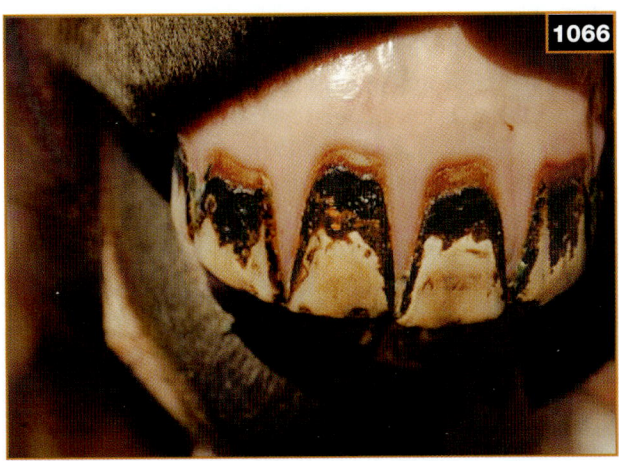

1066 Black tartar on the incisors of a horse with EMND.

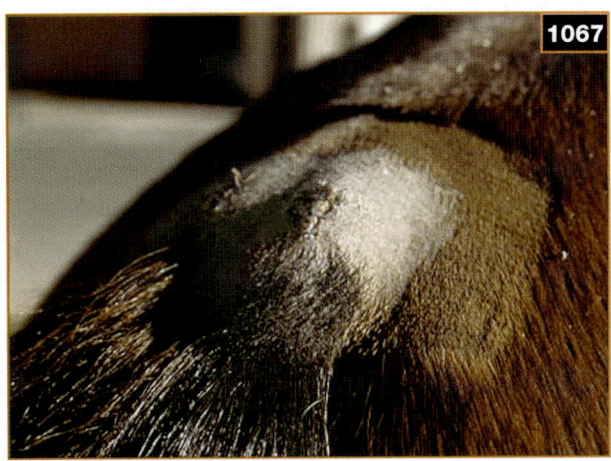

1067 Biopsy site of the sacrocaudalis dorsalis medialis muscle.

gaits are the most frequently recognized signs in the chronic form. Muscle fasciculations and excessive time lying down are not prominent features of the chronic form. Muscle atrophy is common in the chronic form and the tail head is frequently raised in both forms of the disease. In 30% of cases, abnormal brown pigment deposits may be seen in the fundus on ophthalmoscopic examination. Black dental tartar has been noted on the incisors of several horses, and analysis of the tartar has revealed high concentrations of copper, iron, and phosphorus (**1066**).

Differential diagnosis
Lead toxicosis, mycotoxin ingestion, trauma, metabolic derangements, laminitis, and colic may produce similar clinical signs.

Diagnosis
The disorder may be suspected on the basis of clinical signs and laboratory findings. In the subacute form, muscle enzymes may be moderately elevated. Plasma vitamin E levels are low (<1.0 µg/ml) in subacute cases, with corresponding low levels in the CNS, peripheral nerves, muscle, liver, and adipose tissue. Serum ferritin and hepatic iron are elevated in the majority of cases and copper levels in the spinal cord, but not the liver, are also elevated.

Confirmation of EMND is achieved by examination of a muscle biopsy of the sacrocaudalis dorsalis medialis muscle (**1067**) or by a biopsy of a ventral branch of the spinal accessory nerve. Both of these tests have a sensitivity and specificity of 90% when interpreted by an experienced pathologist.

Management
Currently, there is no treatment that influences the course of the disease. Based on the suspected chronic vitamin E deficiency, supplementation with this vitamin may be beneficial. Current recommendations are 5,000–7,000 IU/horse/day p/o combined with an increase in green forage. If one horse in a stable develops EMND, vitamin E supplementation should be provided to all other horses in the stable that have had a similar diet.

Prognosis
Approximately 40% of horses will show an improvement with vitamin E supplementation and may look normal within 3 months. However, return to work frequently results in rapid clinical deterioration. Of the remainder, 40% stabilize, but are permanently disfigured, and 20% will have continual progression resulting in eventual euthanasia. Affected horses should not be ridden.

Cervical vertebral instability and stenosis (wobbler syndrome)

Definition/overview

Cervical vertebral instability and stenosis (wobbler syndrome) is a neurologic syndrome characterized by progressive ataxia that occurs as a result of spinal cord compression. There are two manifestations of the disease: dynamic stenosis and static stenosis of the cervical vertebral canal.

Dynamic stenosis or cervical instability occurs when the neck is flexed or extended, and results in a transient decrease in the diameter of the cervical vertebral canal. Dynamic lesions are usually found at ICSs C3–C4 and C4–C5 of young horses 6–18 months of age (1068).

Cervical static stenosis is a vertebral canal narrowing that is present regardless of the position of the neck. This type of lesion occurs more frequently at ICSc C5–C6 and C6–C7. Affected horses may be of any age. In some cases the onset of disease may be late in life as a result of slowly progressive degenerative joint disease of the articular facets.

With either form of the syndrome, more than one vertebral space may be involved and osteochondrosis or degenerative joint disease of the dorsal articular facets of the affected vertebrae may be radiographically evident.

Etiology/pathophysiology

The etiology of wobbler syndrome is not clear. It is likely that interactions between diet, the rate of bone growth and development, abnormal biomechanical forces, and trauma produce deformities of the cervical vertebrae, the result of which is compression of the cervical spinal cord. Osteochondrosis and osteoarthritis have also been implicated in this disorder. There is circumstantial evidence that the disease could be inherited.

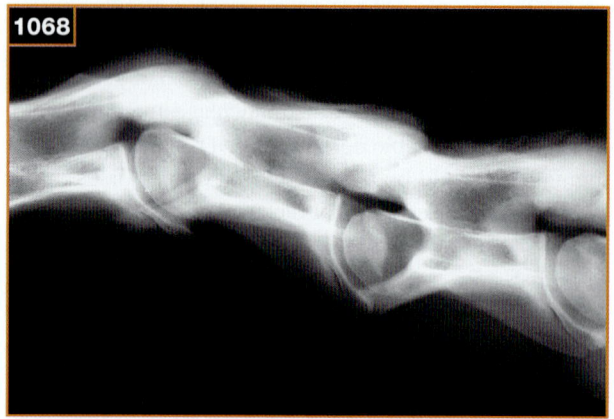

1068 Cervical vertebral instability of C3–C4. Note the abnormal angulation.

Clinical presentation

Ataxia, typically involving all four limbs, is the most obvious clinical sign in most cases. Physical examination may reveal abrasions around the heels and medial aspect of the forelimbs due to interference, and short, squared hooves due to excessive toe dragging. Neurologic examination reveals UMN signs and general proprioceptive deficits compatible with deficits expected from symmetrical compression and damage of the cervical spinal cord white matter. In a standing horse, proprioceptive deficits, such as abnormal wide-based stance, abnormal limb placement, and delayed positioning reflexes, will be noted, as will signs of hypermetria, such as exaggerated limb movements and spasticity. Neck stiffness and pain, as evidenced by a reluctance to move the neck or eat off the ground, may be present. Neurologic deficits are usually slowly progressive; however, in some cases a sudden onset or severe deterioration may be observed.

While most commonly identified in horses between 1 and 3 years of age, a wide range of ages can be affected. wobbler syndrome in older horses (>13 years of age) is usually the result of degenerative joint disease in the articular facets. This is most commonly seen in Warmbloods and Warmblood crosses.

Differential diagnosis

The most important differential diagnoses for spinal cord ataxia in a young horse other than cervical vertebral instability/stenosis are equine protozoal myeloencephalitis, trauma, EDM, EHV myeloencephalopathy, rabies, and viral encephalitis (Eastern, Western, Venezuelan).

Diagnosis

The neurologic examination should localize the lesion to the cervical spinal cord. Standing radiographs of the cervical spine are diagnostic in many cases (1069). A semiquantitative scoring system is used by some clinicians to assess spinal radiographs. This system evaluates angulation of the cervical articulations, minimum sagittal diameter, encroachment of the caudal vertebral physis into the vertebral canal ('ski-jump' lesion), abnormal ossification of the physis, caudal extension of the dorsal arch, and the presence of degenerative joint disease. Alternatively, sagittal ratios of the vertebral canal diameter (minimal sagittal diameter) to the sagittal width of the vertebral body (maximum sagittal diameter) can be used with plain survey radiographs to assess the likelihood that a horse has a cervical vertebral stenosis. Sagittal ratios less than or equal to 0.50 at C4–C6 or less than 0.52 at C7 are highly suggestive of a stenotic lesion. The sensitivity and specificity of this ratio method are >89% at each vertebral site. Often, radiographic changes are present, but the clinical relevance is unclear. Additionally, dynamic lesions may be the cause of disease, but will not be apparent on standing radiographs.

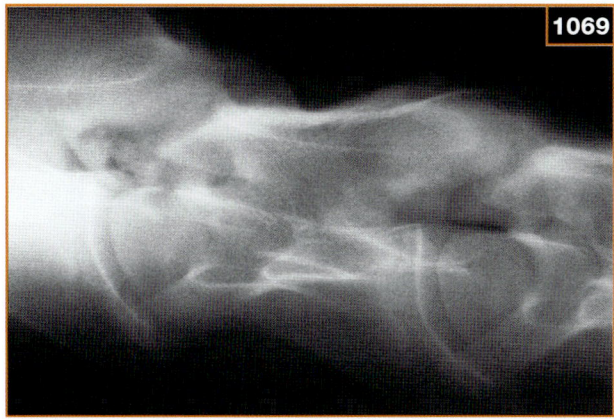

1069 Osteochondrosis at C2/C3, with fracture of the articular facets.

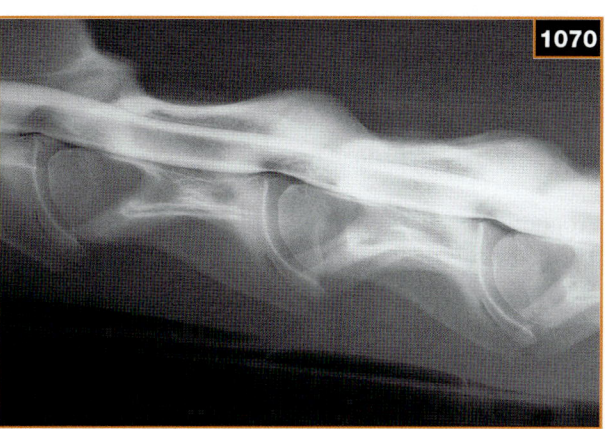

1070 Myelogram performed in a horse with dynamic cervical vertebral instability. Note the thickness of the ventral and dorsal dye column at C3 and C4. No compression is noted in this neutral view.

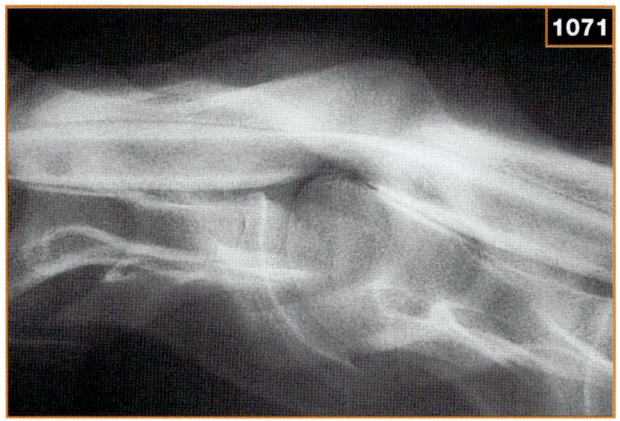

1071 A flexed view revealed dorsal contrast narrowed more than 50% compared with the same site in the neutral view in 1070. This myelogram confirms a compressive lesion at C3 and C4.

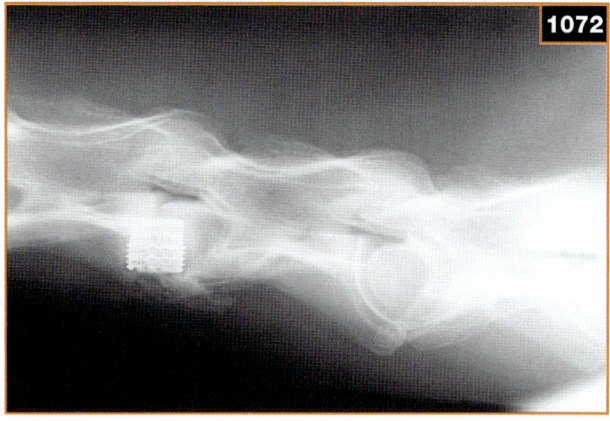

1072 Fusion of the vertebral bodies of C3/C4 in a horse with wobbler syndrome.

Myelography is sometimes required to confirm a diagnosis, particularly with dynamic lesions (1070, 1071).

Management

Medical therapy is aimed at reducing cell swelling and edema formation around the spinal cord. Treatment with anti-inflammatory drugs (e.g. flunixin meglumine, 1.1 mg/kg i/v q12h; and DMSO, 0.5–1.0 g/kg i/v as a 10% solution) is most common. Osmotic diuretics (mannitol, 0.5–1.0 g/kg i/v q12h) can also be used to help reduce edema. Injecting cervical articular joints with cortico-steroids and/or hyaluronic acid can be beneficial in horses that demonstrate mild to moderate neurologic deficits (grade 2–3/5) and moderate to significant degenerative changes.

In horses less than 1 year old, changes in management such as restricted exercise and diet are recommended. This is achieved by feeding grass hay and a vitamin/mineral supplement and keeping the foal confined to a stall for a period of several months, with periodic re-evaluation. Carbohydrate excess in the diet is thought to contribute to developmental orthopedic disease through endocrine imbalance involving the elevation of serum insulin concentrations and decreased serum thyroxine concentra-tions, resulting in a lack of cartilage maturation.

The use of surgical treatment is controversial. The ventral interbody fusion (Bagby Basket) has resulted in osseous remodeling of the articular processes and regres-sion of associated soft tissue swelling at the treated site (1072). Following surgery, an improvement of one to grades out of five is expected, but not guaranteed. There is a low probability that a horse will improve by more than three grades post surgery and therefore this surgery should not be performed on horses with severe ataxia or with compression of more than two sites.

Prognosis

The prognosis depends on the severity of the neurologic deficits, degenerative joint changes, and the age of the animal. Generally, horses with cervical instability or stenosis will be able to live; however, their performance may be impaired and horses may pose a risk to themselves and handlers depending on the severity of ataxia. Without treatment, the prognosis for all types of instability is poor to guarded.

11

Eyes

Heather Gray

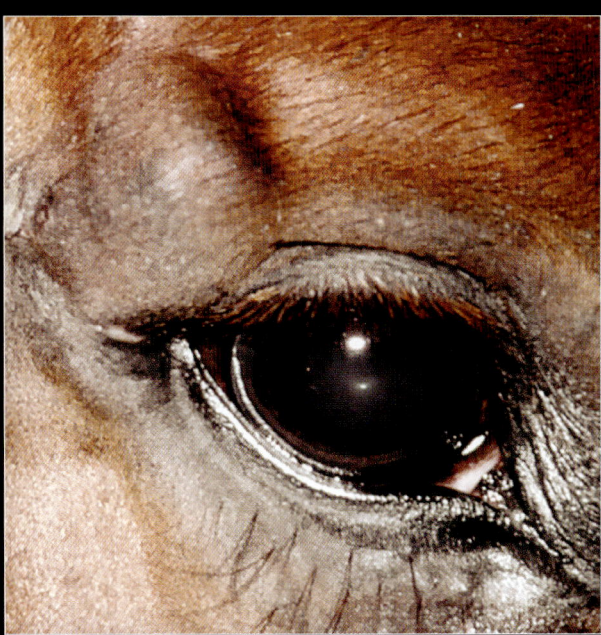

The horse has the largest eye of any land mammal. The lateral globe placement and horizontal ovoid pupil allow a total visual field of 350 degrees. Narrow blind spots exist immediately in front of the nose and directly behind the hindquarters. A horse needs to lower its head to see objects that are far away and lift its head to see close-up objects. Both eyes are used to look at a distant object until it comes within 1.0–1.3 meters (3–4 feet), which forces the horse to turn its head and look with only one eye. The mean refractive error is –1.0 diopters (D).

Anatomy of the equine eye

Horses have a number of unique anatomic differences compared with the dog and cat. These include a complete bony orbit, which gives added protection to the eye, and well-developed extraocular muscles, which make manipulation of the eyelids and globe challenging. The globe is slightly deviated medially and ventrally (mild medioventral strabismus) in the neonatal foal; however, it attains the normal adult position by 1 month of age. The iridocorneal angle (ICA) in the horse is easily visible temporally and nasally without the use of a goniolens. The equine pupil is bordered by a granula iridica (corpora nigra), an exaggerated prominence of the posterior pigmented epithelium layers of the iris (1073). The granula iridica is more prominent on the dorsal pupillary margin than ventrally.

This structure is believed to play a role in the filtration of light through the pupil. The normal equine lens has prominent Y sutures and needs to accommodate less than 2D to maintain a focused image on the retina. Persistent hyaloid artery remnants are common in the equine neonate and may contain blood in the first few hours after birth; however, they usually disappear by 3–4 months of age.

The horse has a paurangiotic fundus that contains 40–60 small retinal vessels that radiate from the edge of the optic nerve head (ONH) and extend only 1.0–2.5 disk diameters from the optic disk. The variations in the normal equine fundus are numerous and are primarily related to coat and eye color. The optic disk appears as a horizontal oval to round, salmon pink structure that is located slightly temporally in the nontapetal region (1074). It is approximately 5–7 mm horizontally and 3.5–5 mm vertically and is used to estimate the size of fundic lesions in terms of optic disk diameters. A physiologic cup is generally not apparent and the ONH is only rarely myelinated. When present, myelin may appear as white to gray streaks radiating from the ONH and following the course of the retinal vessels nasal and temporal to the disk. The normal tapetum may be yellow, green, or blue, with small reddish-brown dots that represent end-on views of choroidal capillaries, or 'Stars of Winslow' (1075). The nontapetal fundus is typically heavily pigmented, appearing dark brown or chocolate. The fundus may appear reddish in horses devoid of retinal pigment epithelium (RPE) pigment, tapetal cells, and choroidal pigmentation (1076). This lack of pigment is often seen in horses with blue irises. There are two types of cones present in the equine retina, suggesting that they have the capacity to see color. Although controversial, behavior tests have indicated that horses can distinguish red or blue from gray with little difficulty, but research on the ability to distinguish green from yellow has had mixed results.

An ophthalmic examination should be completed in all horses undergoing prepurchase examination, as well as those exhibiting signs of ocular and/or systemic disease. Visual impairment may be dangerous to the animals themselves and to humans who come into contact with them. Horses with sudden-onset blindness are more likely to be dangerous (*Table 51*). Ocular disease may also affect the use of the animal, with even mild vision deficits impacting negatively on the high-performance athlete. However, a recent retrospective study reported that 31/33 horses that underwent unilateral enucleation returned to their previous performance level immediately postoperatively (including flat racing, eventing, steeplechase, jumping, dressage, driving, and pleasure horses).

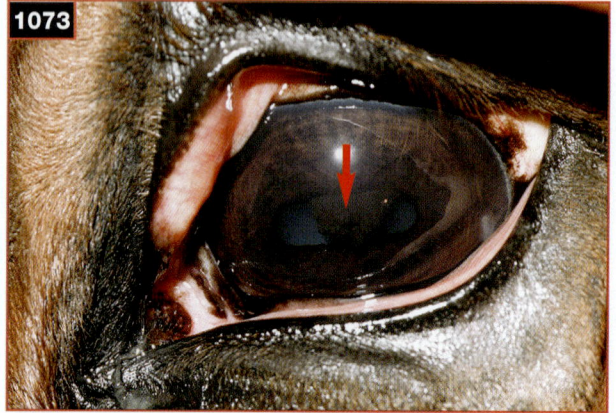

1073 The granula iridica (arrow) is most prominent dorsally.

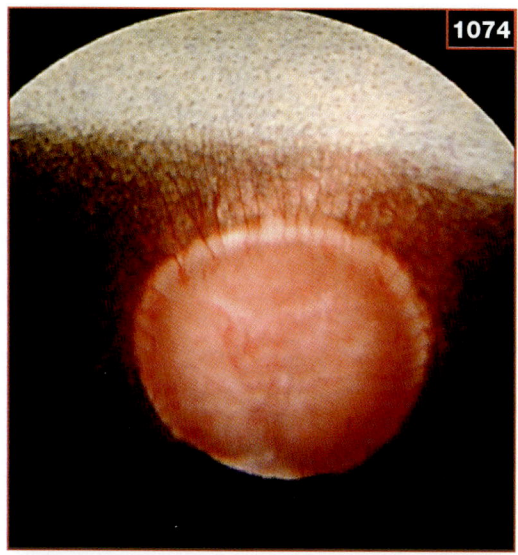

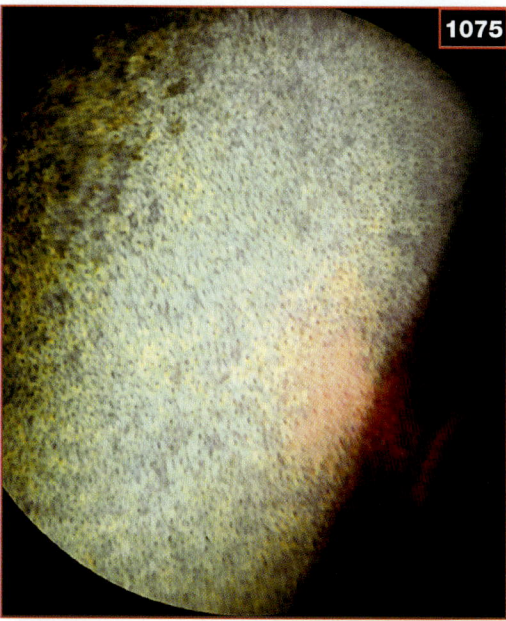

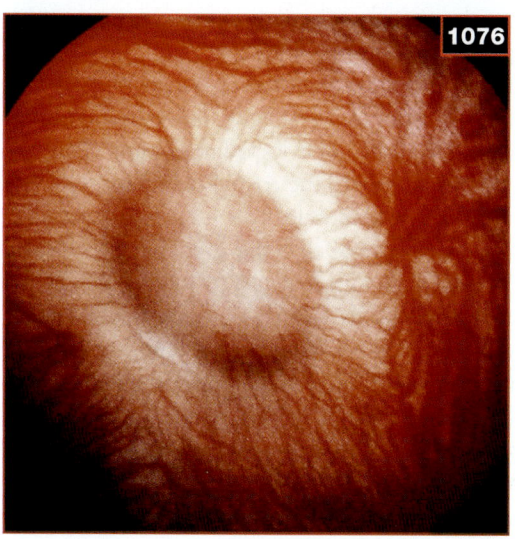

1074 Normal equine fundus. The area illustrated is approximately what one would expect examining the fundus with direct ophthalmoscopy.

1075 Equine fundus, tapetal region. The dark foci, called 'Stars of Winslow', are end-on choroidal vessels penetrating the tapetum.

1076 Normal, subalbinotic fundus. This fundus is characterized by lack of both choroidal pigment and tapetum lucidum. The anatomy of the extensive choroidal vasculature is readily viewed.

TABLE 51 **Differential diagnoses for sudden blindness**

ABNORMAL PUPILLARY REFLEXES (peripheral blindness)

- Optic neuritis
- Retinal detachments
- Equine recurrent uveitis
- Glaucoma
- Exudative optic neuritis
- Head trauma – optic nerve avulsion
- Ocular trauma/intraocular hemorrhage
- Retrobulbar granuloma/neoplasia (i.e. cryptococcosis)
- Viral encephalomyelitis (i.e. Eastern, Western or Venezuelan equine encephalitis, Borna disease)

NORMAL PUPILARY REFLEXES (CNS/cortical blindness)

- Cataracts
- Congenital (hydrocephalus, storage disease)
- Metabolic diseases (hypoglycemia, hepatic encephalopathy)
- Toxins (lead poisoning; fiddleneck, horsetail ingestion)
- Nutritional (thiamine deficiency)
- Head traumatic/vascular (embolus)
- Hypoxic – postictal, respiratory or cardiac arrest
- Infections (toxoplasmosis)
- CNS neoplasia or other space-occupying lesions
- Idiopathic

Examination of the eye

Ocular examination

A quiet area that can be darkened appropriately is critical for the ophthalmic examination. Chemical restraint, pharmacologic mydriasis and auriculopalpebral nerve blocks may be required. A diffuse and focal light source, such as a transilluminator and direct ophthalmoscope, respectively, are essential equipment.

When performing an ophthalmic examination, a thorough and systematic technique must be used in order to ensure that all areas of the adnexa, eye, and orbit are examined (*Table 52*). It is important to obtain a full history and perform a general inspection and neuro-ophthalmic examination before sedation, nerve blocks, or other diagnostic ophthalmic tests are performed. A detailed history should include the duration of the problem as well as any treatment that the animal has received and its response. Additionally, questions that are designed to determine if the problem is a primary ocular disease or secondary to a systemic disorder should be integrated into the history. This is followed by examination of the adnexal structures, the anterior segment of the eye (conjunctiva, cornea, anterior sclera, anterior chamber, iris, lens, and ciliary body) and, finally, evaluation of the posterior segment (vitreous and retina) of the eye. Selection of other diagnostic tests, such as a Schirmer tear test (STT), fluorescein staining, and tonometry, depends on information obtained from the history, general inspection, and ophthalmic examination.

Neuro-ophthalmic examination

A neuro-ophthalmic examination should be completed in the horse prior to sedation and/or nerve blocks. The palpebral reflexes should be elicited by touching the eyelids and observing a blink response (1077, 1078). This reflex involves branches of the trigeminal nerve (CN V) for the sensory afferent pathway and branches of the facial nerve (CN VII) as well as the orbicularis oculi muscle for the motor efferent pathway. The menace response is then elicited by making a quick threatening motion towards the eye and observing a blink or flinch (1079). Proper technique is important as false-positive results can occur in blind eyes if the vibrissae are touched or if an air current is produced. The retina and the optic nerve (CN II) provide the sensory afferent pathway, and branches of the facial nerve and the orbicularis oculi muscle are involved in the motor efferent pathway for this reflex. The PLRs evaluate retinal function, CN II, and the midbrain for the sensory afferent pathway and the oculomotor nerve (CN III) and iris sphincter muscle for the motor efferent pathway. A beam of focal light is shone into the eye and the normal pupillary response involves constriction of the pupil. This test is called the direct pupillary light response

---

TABLE 52 Main causes of enophthalmos and exophthalmos

ENOPHTHALMOS

- Globe rupture/perforation
- Dehydration
- Horner's syndrome
- Orbital fat loss – starvation
- Phthisis bulbi

EXOPHTHALMOS

- Orbital abscess – bacterial
- Orbital granuloma – fungal (i.e. cryptococcosis)
- Orbital tumor
- Glaucoma – buphthalmos?
- Orbital trauma
- Retrobulbar extra-adrenal paraganglioma

(1080, 1081). Constriction of the contralateral pupil should occur simultaneously and is termed the indirect or consensual pupillary light response. Evaluation of the consensual pupillary light response in the horse requires the use of an assistant, with one person observing the contralateral pupil while the other shines a bright light in the ipsilateral pupil (1082). This test can be extremely helpful in the crude evaluation of the retinal and optic nerve integrity in an eye with opacities that prevent direct viewing of the posterior segment (corneal edema, cataract, intraocular hemorrhage).

The 'dazzle' reflex, a subcortical response, may also be performed using a bright, focal light source that is shone into the eye, causing the horse to squint or blink. This test evaluates the retina, CN II, the rostral colliculus, CN VII, and the orbicularis oculi muscle.

It is important to note that the menace response is absent in normal newborn foals up to 14 days of age. In addition, normal foals are born with circular pupils and sluggish PLRs. By 3–5 days post birth the pupils become more ovoid and the PLRs more rapid. Atropine administration, synechiation, iridal colobomas, and iris atrophy may also affect the PLRs.

Following the neuro-ophthalmic examination, sedation and/or nerve blocks may be performed.

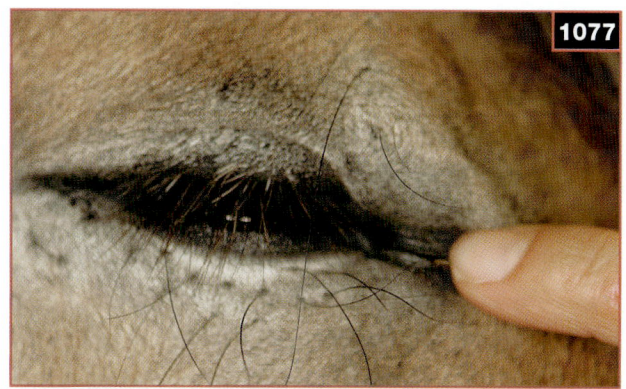

1077, 1078 Palpebral response. Gently tapping the medial (1077) or lateral (1078) canthus will stimulate the sensory branches of CN V and generate the afferent stimulus. The efferent motor branch of the reflex is mediated by CN VII.

1079 Menace response. A threatening gesture is made near the eye; the expected response is eyelid closure, often accompanied by movement of the head away from the stimulus. Care must be taken to avoid producing air currents or inadvertently touching the vibrissae while performing this test.

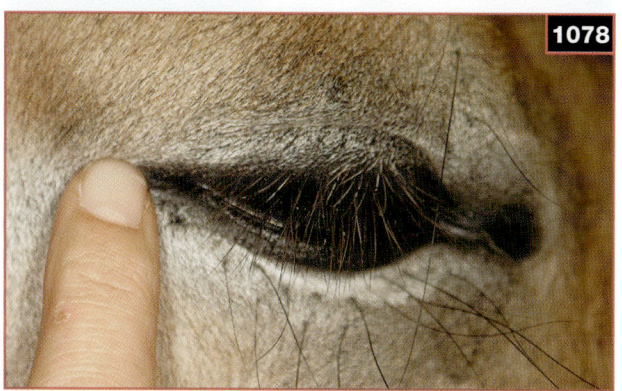

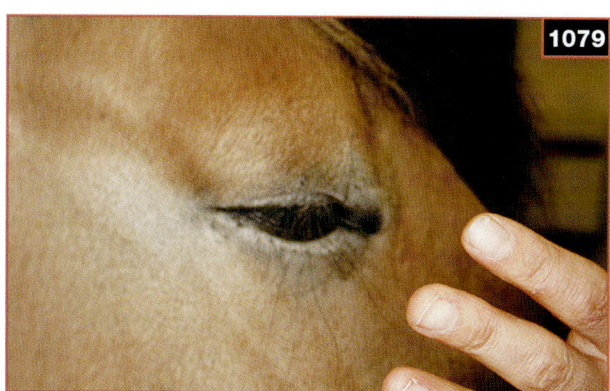

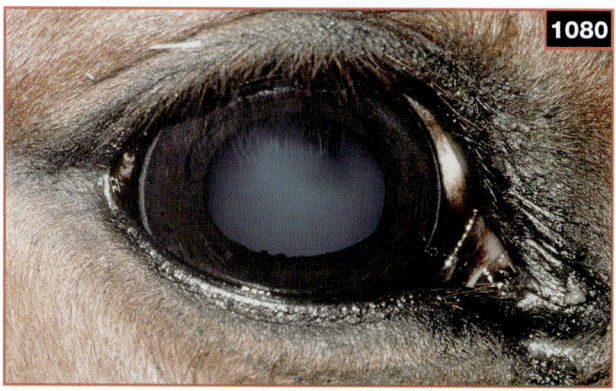

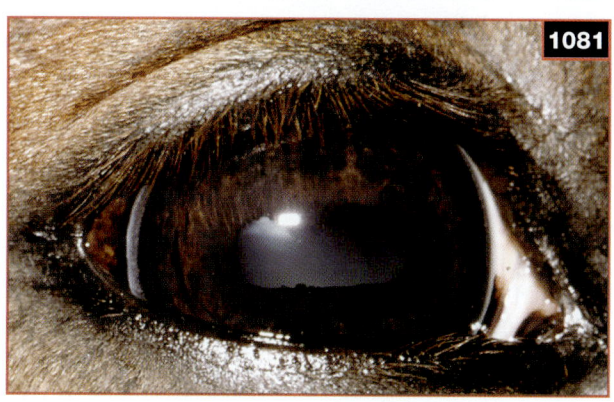

1080, 1081 Pupillary light response. (1080) Normal pupil in ambient light. (1081) Pupil under effect of direct bright light stimulus. The retina, CN II, and the midbrain mediate the afferent arm of this reflex, whereas the efferent motor pathway is through CN III and the iris sphincter muscle.

1082 Evaluation of the indirect pupillary light response. An assistant is required to shine a bright focal light into one eye while the examiner evaluates the response of the contralateral pupil by diffusely illuminating that eye.

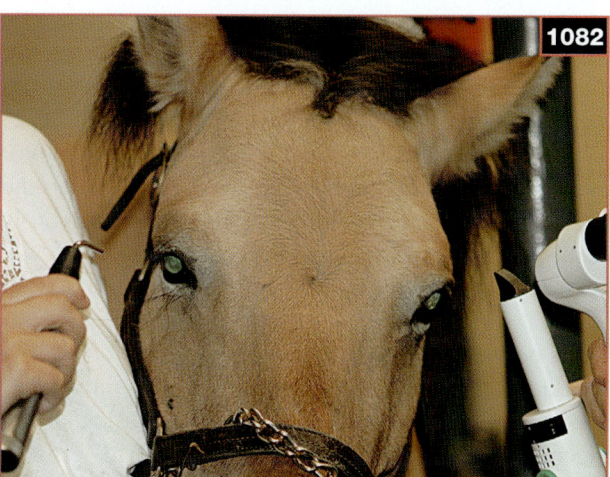

Diagnostic procedures

Techniques to aid in ophthalmic procedures
Chemical restraint

Sedation may be required to facilitate evaluation because of the temperament of the patient or as a result of ocular pain. Alpha-2 adrenoreceptor agonists, including xylazine (0.3–1.1 mg/kg i/m or i/v), romifidine (12.5–50 μg/kg i/m or i/v) and detomidine (10–40 μg/kg i/m or i/v) are used most commonly when performing ophthalmic examination in the horse. Additional medications, such as butorphanol (0.02–0.05 mg/kg i/m or i/v) or acepromazine (0.02–0.05 mg/kg i/m or i/v), may be necessary to obtain the appropriate level of analgesia and sedation. Physical restraint techniques, including a nose, ear or skin twitch, and stocks, may also be required.

Topical anesthetic

Topical anesthetic (e.g. 1% proparacaine) is applied to desensitize the ocular surface before conjunctival or corneal scrapings or biopsies are collected, irrigation of the nasolacrimal system, manipulation of the third eyelid, tonometry, or to facilitate the examination of a painful eye. Topical anesthetic impedes corneal healing and should never be used to treat ophthalmic disorders. Topical anesthetic can be drawn into a tuberculin syringe (0.1–0.2 ml) and applied directly onto the corneal and conjunctival surface (1083). Alternatively, the solution can be sprayed onto the corneal surface from a tuberculin syringe with the hub of a needle attached. Always break off the needle when choosing this method, and avoid getting too close to the eye, as the hub tip is still sharp enough to damage the cornea.

Auriculopalpebral nerve block

The equine eyelids are very strong and paralysis of the orbicularis oculi muscle is usually required in order to allow eyelid manipulation for ocular examination and sample collection, especially when the eyes are painful. It is also used when placing a subpalpebral lavage system (SPL) or when the nasolacrimal system is cannulated or catheterized. The auriculopalpebral branch of the facial nerve supplies the ipsilateral orbicularis oculi muscle. It may be blocked by injecting local anesthetic over the nerve as it exits the skull at the base of the ear just caudal to the posterior ramus of the mandible and the zygomatic arch. A depression can be appreciated in this area, but the nerve cannot be palpated. A 21–23 gauge 5/8–1 inch needle is inserted into the depression in a dorsal direction, and 5–6 ml of 2% lidocaine hydrochloride injected (1084). The facial nerve may also be blocked where it can be palpated as it traverses the dorsal zygomatic arch, using a 3 ml syringe with a 25 gauge 5/8 inch needle and 1–3 ml of 2% lidocaine injected subcutaneously. The area of injection

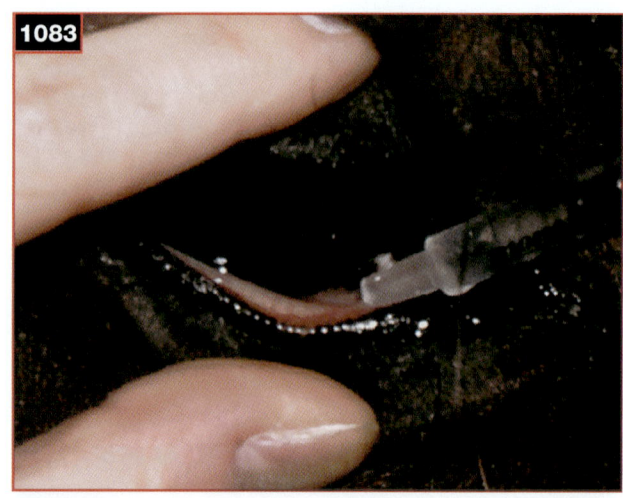

1083 Topical liquid medication administration.

may be massaged to facilitate diffusion of the drug. Sedation may be required in order to complete this nerve block. When successfully performed, a narrowed palpebral fissure, mild ptosis, and eyelid paralysis will be produced within 5 minutes. The eyelids may remain paralyzed for up to 1–2 hours. It is important to remember that this block does not provide any sensory nerve analgesia to the eyelid.

Supraorbital nerve block

The frontal or supraorbital nerve is a branch of the ophthalmic division of the trigeminal nerve (CN V). It is blocked as it exits the supraorbital foramen, which can be palpated superior to the orbit in the supraorbital process of the frontal bone, and provides sensory denervation to the majority (middle two thirds) of the upper eyelid. A 22–25 gauge 5/8–1 inch needle is introduced 0.5–2.0 cm into or over the supraorbital foramen and 2–3 ml of 2% lidocaine is infiltrated. Another 2–3 ml is deposited subcutaneously as the needle is withdrawn (1084). This nerve block will also achieve some motor paralysis of the upper lid.

Other nerve blocks

Blocking of the lacrimal, zygomatic, and infratrochlear nerves, all branches of the ophthalmic division of the trigeminal nerve, is occasionally used to provide sensory denervation to the lower eyelid.

Retrobulbar nerve block

Retrobulbar injection of local anesthetic is frequently used as an adjunct to general anesthesia, allowing a lower depth of anesthesia to be used, and for postoperative analgesic purposes. It helps control nystagmus and enophthalmos during light anesthesia and reduces the need for neuromuscular blockage. It also reduces the risk of brady-arrhythmia and hypotension associated with the oculocardiac reflex. Retrobulbar nerve blocks may be performed using a number of techniques including direct injection into the orbital cone using a 6.25 cm (2.5 inch), 22 gauge needle inserted perpendicular to the skin in the orbital fossa just posterior to the dorsal orbital rim. Alternatively, a 10 cm (4 inch), 18 gauge needle may be inserted 1 cm caudal to the lateral canthus and advanced in a ventromedial direction parallel to the medial canthus. In all cases the syringe is first aspirated to ensure that the needle is not in a blood vessel prior to injecting 10–12 ml of 2% lidocaine hydrochloride (or other local anesthetic). Cycloplegia occurs and ocular reflexes are lost within 5 minutes. A four-point block may also be used, which involves the use of a 7.5 cm (3 inch), 20 gauge needle that is inserted into each quadrant followed by injection of 5–10 ml of 2% lidocaine hydrochloride per site. Retrobulbar injection can pose a risk of orbital hemorrhage, optic nerve damage or neuritis, and globe penetration.

Basic ophthalmic tests

Schirmer tear test

The STT measures both basal and reflex tear production and must be conducted before instilling fluorescein stain, topical anesthetic, or ocular medication. To perform an STT the commercially available strip is placed in the middle to lateral third of the inferior conjunctival fornix for 1 minute. The strip is then removed and the amount of tear-wetting is measured in mm/minute. Dye-impregnated strips, with their own scales, are also available and can facilitate this measurement (1085). Results may vary; however, the horse generally produces large volumes of tears and the strip is often saturated within 30 seconds. An STT value of <10 mm/minute is considered abnormal.

Fluorescein staining

Sodium fluorescein stain is used to evaluate the eye for corneal epithelial defects or ulcerations. Fluorescein will not stain the normal corneal epithelium or Descemet's membrane, but will stain the hydrophilic corneal stroma following a disruption in the epithelium. This test is performed by first wetting the fluorescein strip with sterile saline or eyewash solution and then touching it to the dorsal bulbar conjunctiva and allowing the horse to blink. Touching the strip directly to the cornea can lead to false-positive results. Alternatively, fluorescein solution in

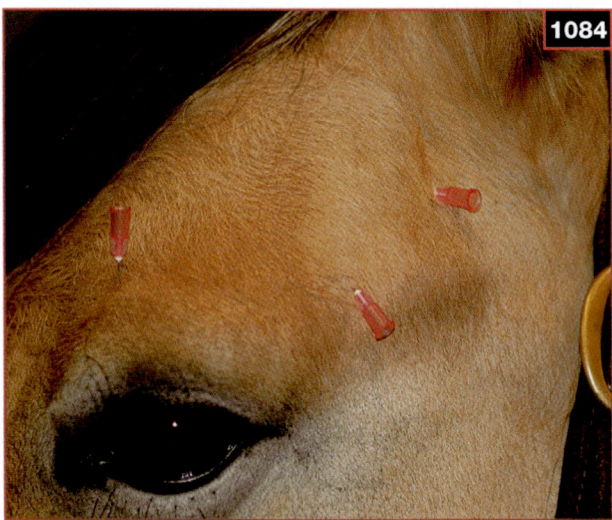

1084 Location of common peripheral nerve blocks. Sites shown from left to right: supraorbital nerve block; palpebral nerve block; auriculopalpebral nerve block.

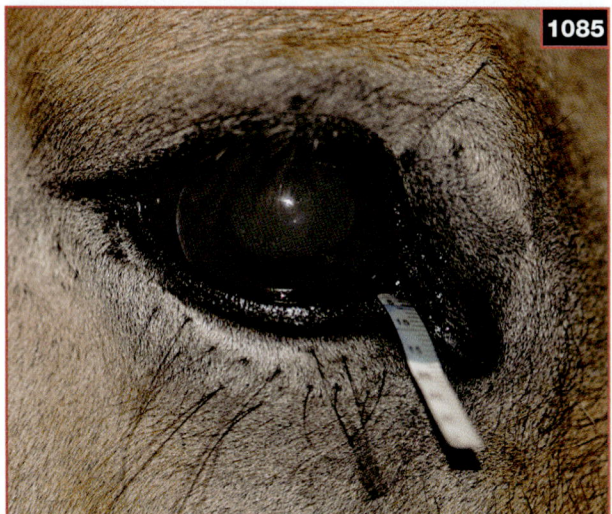

1085 Schirmer tear test. The test strip is placed in the inferior conjunctival cul-de-sac. The test strip shown contains a convenient millimeter ruler and is impregnated with a blue dye, which travels along the strip with the tears for accurate measurement.

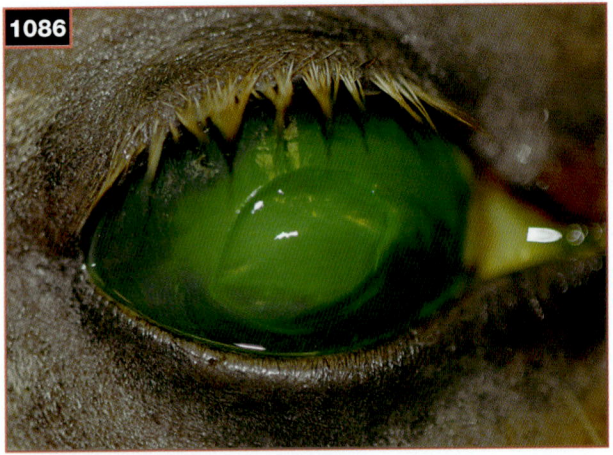

1086 Corneal ulcer stained with sodium fluorescein stain. The stain can be excited by a cobalt blue light, better delineating the extent of corneal damage. This horse has a central stromal defect as well as a more superficial ulcer involving the dorsal aspect of the cornea.

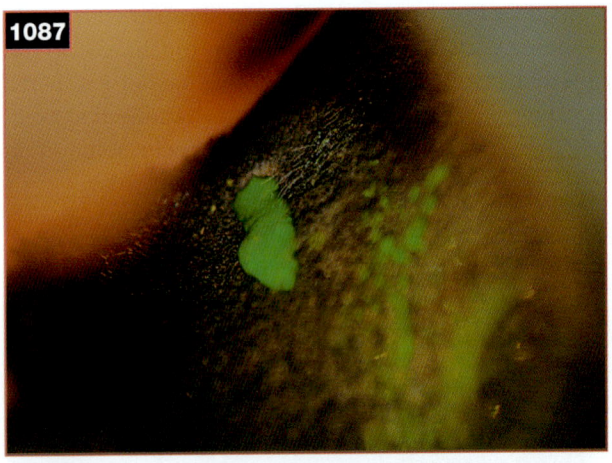

1087 Close-up photograph of the nasal lacrimal punctum at the floor of the opening of the nares. The opening is highlighted by fluorescein.

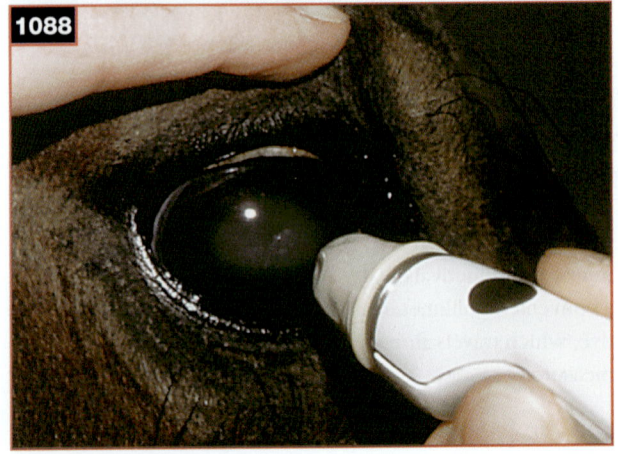

single-dose disposable ampoules or made by irrigating a fluorescein strip with saline eyewash can be applied to the superior palpebral conjunctiva. It is important not to dilute the fluorescein stain too much as that may result in a false-negative result. Occasionally, it is necessary to irrigate the eye with sterile saline to rinse out any remaining fluorescein. A cobalt blue light source is used to illuminate the eye. Any areas of ulceration will appear as an apple-green fluorescent lesion (**1086**). An indication of nasolacrimal patency may be obtained if fluorescein appears in the nostril after traversing the nasolacrimal system following topical instillation (**1087**). Fluorescein can also be used to determine tear film break-up time (average 21.8 seconds +/− 10 seconds), which may be helpful in diagnosing qualitative tear film disorders in horses.

Tonometry

Topical anesthetic is first applied to the cornea. The intraocular pressures are then measured indirectly using an applanation tonometer such as the Tonopen™ or Tonovet™. Applanation tonometers are relatively expensive; however, they are portable, easy to use, accurate, and allow the patient's head to be held in any position. The tip of the applanation tonometer is gently and repeatedly touched perpendicular to the corneal surface until an IOP reading is obtained. A disposable rubber membrane covers the tip of the tonometer and should be replaced between animals to prevent the spread of infectious disease (**1088**). The normal IOP range in the horse is 15–32 mmHg.

Lighted ocular examination

The horse is initially evaluated in a lighted environment. A general distance examination looking for evidence of facial asymmetry, globe positioning, size and movement, abnormal ocular signs, and vision loss is performed. A photopic (in ambient light) obstacle course, or maze test, may be considered to further evaluate vision in those animals suspected of having deficits. The neuro-ophthalmic examination and basic diagnostic tests are then completed, followed by palpation of the orbital rim and globe retropulsion. Examination of the adnexa and anterior segment, using diffuse or 'wide-beam' illumination (transilluminator, penlight, direct ophthalmoscope, or slit lamp biomicroscope) is then performed. A head loupe, surgical glasses, direct ophthalmoscope, or a slit lamp will provide magnification to aid in the identification of lesions.

1088 Applanation tonometry. Care must be taken to avoid digitally compressing the globe during tonometry, which can inadvertently increase eye pressure. When holding the eyelids open for this test, the fingers should rest on the surrounding orbital bones rather than on the globe.

1089 Direct ophthalmoscopy. With the dial set at zero, bring the fundic reflex into view at arm's length, then move in to approximately 2–3 cm from the eye, at which point the diopter setting can be adjusted for clearer focus.

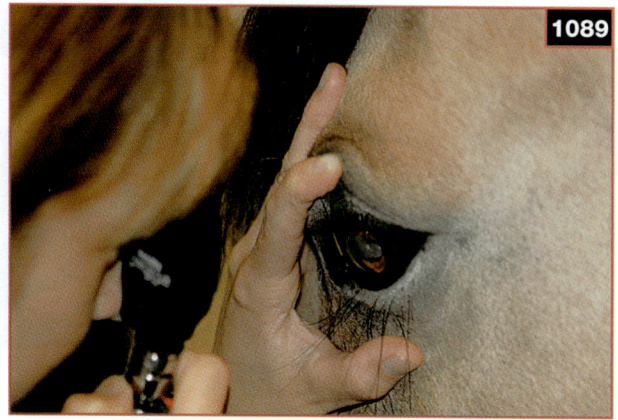

Dark ocular examination

The lights are dimmed and examination of the adnexa and anterior segment is accomplished with diffuse illumination. Diffuse light will detect gross lesions involving the eyelid, conjunctiva, cornea, anterior chamber, iris, lens, and anterior vitreous. A focal light source, narrowed slit beam, and magnification are then used to further identify and evaluate lesions. Slit apertures may be found on many direct ophthalmoscopes and, occasionally, penlights. A slit lamp biomicroscope provides stereopsis and excellent magnification and may also be used; however, they are expensive and require training to use properly. A slit beam will produce three images inside the eye as it strikes the anterior corneal surface, the anterior lens capsule, and the posterior lens capsule. These Purkinje–Sanson images are used to determine the depth of ocular lesions.

Following adnexal and anterior segment examination, the posterior segment is examined. Pupil dilation with 1% tropicamide can facilitate examination of the posterior segment. Tropicamide is the mydriatic of choice, as it provides dilation within 20–25 minutes and persists for up to 8 hours following application in the horse. Topical mydriasis should not be administered until the neuro-ophthalmic examination, the STT, and diagnostic sample collection for culture and sensitivity are completed. A direct or indirect ophthalmoscope may be used to evaluate the posterior segment in the horse.

Direct ophthalmoscopy (distant and close)

To use a direct ophthalmoscope, the examiner should hold the instrument to their eye at arm's length from the patient (approximately 50–75 cm), and first view the tapetal reflex. A dial allows the observer to set the diopteric power, with green or black numbers representing convex or converging lenses and red numbers representing concave or diverging lenses. A distant examination is performed using a diopter setting of 0 as a quick screening test of the eye to look for any opacity that may be present between the observer and the ocular fundus. The examiner should then move to within 2–3 cm of the eye to view the fundus (**1089**). The hand holding the instrument should rest on the horse's head, so that any sudden movement does not injure the eyes of the horse or the examiner, or damage the instrument.

It is recommended that the examiner use his or her left eye when examining the animal's left eye, and vice versa, for ease of examination. The rheostat should be positioned so that the light intensity is at a comfortable level for examination and one that illuminates subtle lesions. The direct ophthalmoscope provides a real, erect image magnified up to eight times. The fundus should be in focus using a diopter setting of 0 to −3 on a direct ophthalmoscope. The ONH should be examined closely, followed by the rest of the fundus, which is examined in quadrants. Progressively higher positive diopter strengths are then used as the examiner proceeds to examine the more anterior structures of the eye. A direct ophthalmoscope is generally set at +12 D to +8 D for examination of the lens, +15 D to +12 D to evaluate the iris, and +20 D to +15 D to examine the external eye and adnexa. Compared with indirect ophthalmoscopy, direct ophthalmoscopy has the advantage of greater magnification, the availability of a slit aperture, and the ability to alter the dioptric strength without the need for additional equipment. The disadvantages include the availability of only one hand to manipulate the eyelids, the small field of view, the lack of stereopsis, the difficulty in visualizing the peripheral fundus, and the short working distance from the patient's face, which increases the likelihood of injury to the examiner, the animal, and the ophthalmoscope.

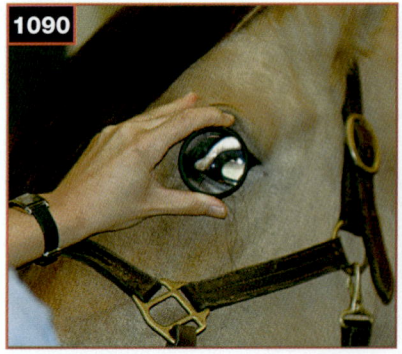

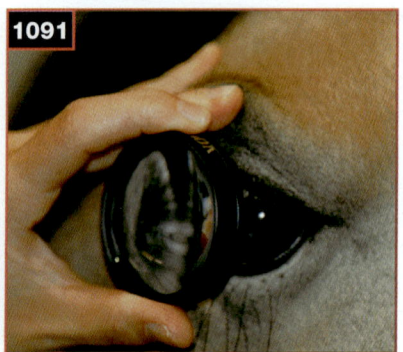

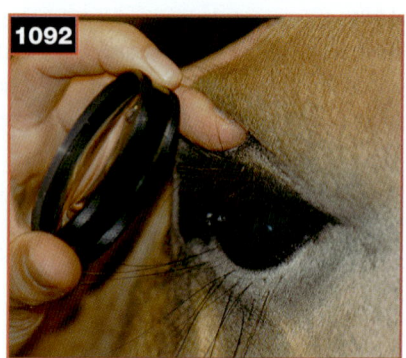

1090–1092 Indirect ophthalmoscopy. (1090) With the examiner positioned approximately an arm's length from the eye, the fundic reflex is established with a light source held near the examiner's eye. (1091) The lens is positioned in front of the eye in such a fashion that the upper eyelid can be retracted with the examiner's middle finger. (1092) The lens can be lifted up out of the direct path of the light to re-establish the fundic reflex without taking the finger off the eyelid.

Indirect ophthalmoscopy

Indirect ophthalmoscopy can be performed using a 20 D convex lens and a transilluminator or penlight to produce a virtual image of the fundus. The light source (transilluminator or penlight) is held near the examiner's eye an arm's length away from the horse's eye (approximately 50–75 cm) and shone through the pupil to obtain a tapetal reflex (1090). Once a fundic reflection is visible, the lens is inserted into the beam approximately 3–5 cm away from the surface of the horse's cornea (1091, 1092). The fingers of the hand holding the lens should rest lightly on the animal's head to prevent injury to the eye in case of any sudden movement. The fundic image will appear inverted and reversed. A 14 D lens can be used to get a more magnified view of the ONH or any retinal lesions. The magnification provided is significantly less than that obtained by direct ophthalmoscopy (approximately 0.8–2 times) and the technique is more difficult to master; however, the indirect method allows a greater field of view, the examiner may be farther away from the patient, and the equipment is relatively inexpensive. An indirect ophthalmoscope headset (binocular indirect ophthalmoscopy) may be used to provide stereopsis and allow both hands to be used to manipulate the adnexa; however, this technique can be even more difficult to master and the instrument is expensive.

Special diagnostic tests
Culture and sensitivity testing

Culture is used routinely to diagnose infectious disease and the antimicrobial sensitivity results are essential when determining the appropriate antimicrobial therapy. Samples for bacterial or fungal cultures must be collected prior to fluorescein staining and topical anesthetic administration, as these solutions may inhibit the growth of microorganisms or cause contamination of the sample. Corneal cultures are indicated in suspected cases of bacterial or fungal keratitis. Samples should be taken from the center and edge of the corneal lesions (1093). Conjunctival cultures are rarely indicated because large numbers of potential pathogens are present in the conjunctiva as normal flora. The normal flora of the equine conjunctival sac varies depending on season and geographic location, but can include the bacteria *Staphylococcus epidermidis*, *Corynebacterium* spp., and *Bacillus cereus*, as well as the fungi *Aspergillus, Penicillium, Alternaria*, and *Cladosporium* spp.

1093 Cellular collection for culture and sensitivity. A sterile culturette can be used to swab the cornea for microbes. Care should be taken to avoid inadvertent contamination by the eyelids and samples should be collected prior to use of topical anesthetics in order to maximize yield.

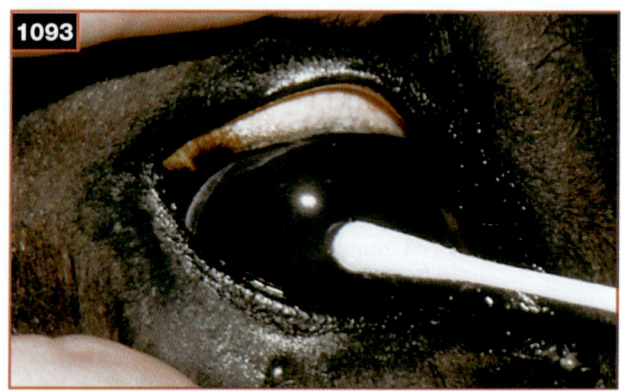

Corneal/conjunctival cytology

Samples for cytology may be collected following the application of a topical anesthetic. A Dacron swab, cytobrush, stainless steel spatula (e.g. Kimura spatula), or the blunt end of a scalpel blade may be used to collect scrapings for cytologic evaluation. Fungal organisms have an affinity for Descemet's membrane and the deeper layers of the corneal stroma; therefore, when collecting material for evaluation of corneal ulcers or abscesses, deep scrapings from the center of the lesion as well as from the periphery are required. These samples are placed on microscope slides and Gram or Wright–Giemsa stains are routinely used to evaluate the types of cells and organisms present. More specialized stains such as periodic acid–Schiff (PAS) stain and Gomori's methenamine silver stain may be used when fungal infection is suspected.

Nasolacrimal system cannulation and lavage

If an obstruction or abnormality in the nasolacrimal system (NLS) is suspected, a nasolacrimal flush may be performed. The NLS is normally easily catheterized and flushed in a retrograde manner with 20–60 ml of physiologic saline, using a soft #5 or #6 French feeding tube, tom cat catheter or polyethylene tubing (1094, 1095). Alternatively, the upper or lower punctum may be cannulated with a small urinary catheter, or an intravenous catheter with the stylet removed, and flushed with 20–30 ml of physiologic saline in an anterograde fashion (1096). The addition of a small amount of fluorescein dye will facilitate identification of the fluid as it exits the nasal or lacrimal puncta. Any debris flushed from the NLS should be collected for cytology as well as for culture and sensitivity testing.

Anterior and posterior chamber paracentesis

Anterior chamber paracentesis (aqueocentesis) and posterior chamber paracentesis (vitreocentesis) are very rarely indicated, but may be performed in the sedated animal with appropriate physical restraint, an auriculopalpebral nerve block, and topical anesthesia. These procedures should only be performed by a specialist. Following application of dilute povidone–iodine solution and sterile saline, an eyelid speculum is placed and the bulbar conjunctiva grasped near the site of entry using tissue forceps (e.g. Bishop Harmon). To perform an aqueocentesis a 25–30 gauge needle attached to a 3 ml syringe is first

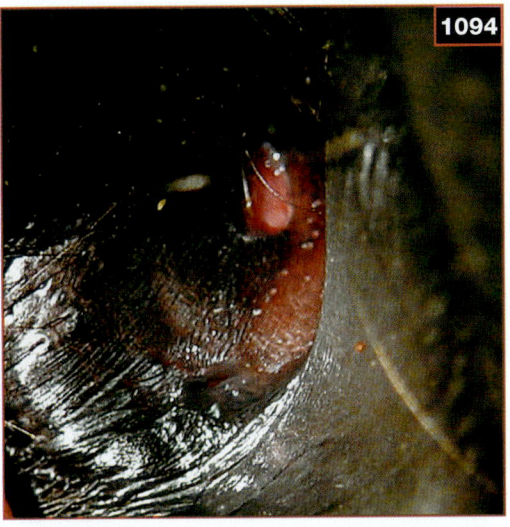

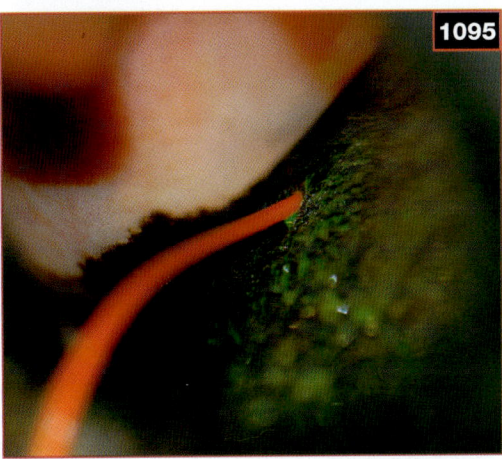

1094, 1095 Retrograde flushing of the nasolacrimal system. (1094) The distal opening is on the floor of the nasal vestibule. After administration of an anesthetic gel over the distal duct, the opening can be cannulated with a variety of catheters, such as the #5 Fr feeding tube shown (1095).

1096 Anterograde flushing of the nasolacrimal system. The proximal openings to the nasolacrimal duct (puncta) are located just inside the eyelid margin of the superior and inferior eyelids. Following application of topical anesthetic to the area, the puncta can be cannulated with an open-ended tomcat catheter or an intravenous catheter (without interior needle) as shown here.

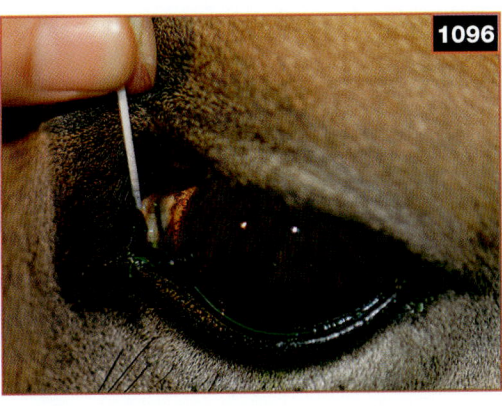

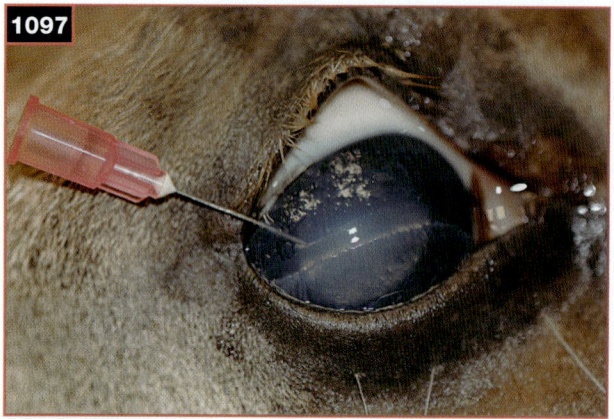

1097 Aqueous paracentesis. The anterior chamber is entered at the limbus using a small bore (25–30 gauge) needle. The bevel should be up and the needle should be positioned parallel to the surface of the iris.

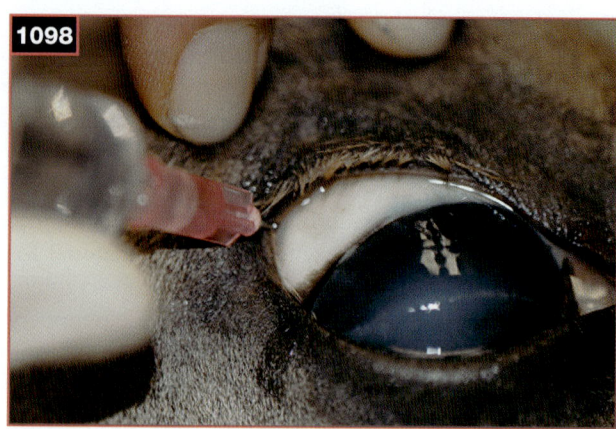

1098 Vitreous paracentesis. Vitreous is removed from the eye using a 22–23 gauge needle. If approaching the dorsal sclera (usually well exposed in a sedated or anesthetized horse), the sclera can be entered approximately 10 mm posterior to the limbus. The needle should be angled posteriorly toward the optic nerve to avoid hitting the lens.

tunneled under 2–3 mm of bulbar conjunctiva in order to help decrease globe leakage. The needle is then introduced into the anterior chamber at the limbus parallel to the iris face (**1097**). A small amount (i.e. 0.25 ml) of aqueous humor is slowly aspirated. A vitreocentesis requires the use of a 22–23 gauge needle attached to a 3 ml syringe. This needle should be introduced 8–10 mm posterior to the limbus and aimed at the center of the vitreous body (**1098**). If the vitreous is degenerated (liquefied), 0.25 ml may be slowly aspirated. If the vitreous is intact, three or four quick aspirations (as with lymph node aspirates) are required to obtain a sample. As the needle is withdrawn, a cotton swab may be placed firmly over the exit site or the bulbar conjunctiva may be grasped with forceps to decrease leakage. The aqueous or vitreous may be removed for cytologic evaluation or determination of certain infectious disease titers. Complications of anterior or posterior paracentesis include hyphema, anterior uveitis, uveal edema and hemorrhage, lens capsule rupture with phacoclastic uveitis, corneal endothelial damage resulting in edema, glaucoma, and retinal detachment.

Electroretinography

Electroretinography (ERG) is a test of retinal, not visual, function. It is the study of electrical potentials produced by the retina when it is stimulated by light of varying intensity, wavelength, and flash duration. Electrodes implanted onto a contact lens amplify and record these electrical potentials on paper. ERG is used to diagnose retinal dysfunction (e.g. Appaloosas suspected of congenital stationary night blindness [CSNB]) and to ensure retinal function prior to cataract extraction.

Radiography

Survey radiographs may be useful when there is an abnormality involving bone or there is the possibility of a radio-opaque foreign body. A Flieringa ring may be placed at the limbus to establish a landmark for orientation. Radiography can also be used with contrast for a variety of procedures, including dacryocystorhinography, to establish the extent of a congenital or an acquired NLS abnormality. To perform a dacryocystorhinogram, the upper lacrimal punctum is cannulated or catheterized, as previously described, and approximately 5 ml of iodine-based contrast medium is injected to outline the nasolacrimal system.

Ocular ultrasonography

Ultrasonography is a valuable, noninvasive diagnostic technique for evaluating the eye. Sedation and local anesthesia may be required. Use of a 7.5–10-MHz probe is ideal. The probe should be applied directly to the cornea, with or without a stand-off or a transpalpebral technique may be used. Horizontal and vertical sections of both eyes should be evaluated and compared. Ultrasonography may be useful when attempting to define characteristics of retrobulbar disease, intraocular cysts, lens subluxation or luxation, intraocular hemorrhage, retinal detachment, and intraocular masses or foreign bodies.

Computed tomography/magnetic resonance imaging

CT is used primarily for evaluating retrobulbar disease. MRI provides excellent visualization of the eye and orbit. Unfortunately, CT and MRI are only available for horses at a few large referral centers.

Methods of medicating the equine eye

Treatment of ocular disease in the horse may require topical application, subconjunctival injection, and/or systemic administration of medications.

Topical administration

Topical application provides high concentrations of the medication to the anterior segment of the eye, while decreasing the likelihood of their associated systemic side-effects. Topical ophthalmic medications are used for treating diseases of the conjunctiva, cornea, anterior part of the sclera, anterior chamber, iris, or ciliary body, but will not establish therapeutic drug levels in the posterior segment tissues or eyelids. Topical medications are available in ointment, suspension, and solution form. Topical ophthalmic ointments may be applied to the conjunctival sac of the eye. Ointments have a longer contact time in the eye than solutions or suspensions and have a lower rate of systemic absorption, but they may have a greater ability to impair corneal healing. Ointments should not be used in the presence of, or when there is a high risk of, globe rupture, globe perforation, or intraocular surgery, as they are irritating and damaging to the internal structures of the eye. Application of topical ophthalmic solutions or suspensions may be facilitated by using a tuberculin syringe and a 25 gauge needle with the tip broken off at the hub to gently spray the medication into the eye. This technique will help avoid contamination of the medication bottle and decrease the likelihood of globe perforation or damage. Ophthalmic solutions and suspensions have the shortest contact time, as topically applied medications mix readily with tears and wash away rapidly. Frequent therapy is normally required to maintain high therapeutic drug levels. Unfortunately, even with adequate physical restraint the application of topical ophthalmic medication can be difficult, if not impossible, in the horse because of the strength of their orbicularis oculi muscle. Often horses become resistant to, and even violent during, administration of ocular medications, posing a danger to themselves and others. For these reasons, an SPL system is recommended in horses with ocular disease requiring frequent or long-term administration of topical medications or in those animals that are becoming resistant to therapy.

Subpalpebral lavage system

Placement of an SPL system is an excellent means of facilitating administration of ocular medications. SPL systems ensure that medications get into the eye in a safe and efficacious manner, with decreased risk of damage to the cornea and decreased risk of injury to the medicator. Adequate chemical and physical restraint, an auriculopalpebral nerve block, regional anesthesia, and topical anesthetic instilled into the conjunctival fornix are necessary for safe placement of SPL systems. Alternatively, an SPL system may be placed postoperatively under general anesthesia. SPL systems should be placed aseptically with sterile gloves, after the site of placement is clipped and prepped with dilute povidone–iodine solution and sterile saline or eyewash in a routine manner. Various modifications exist for the placement of these systems, including the use of various types of tubing (e.g. silastic, polyethylene, or a #5 French feeding tube) and systems (e.g. through-and-through or single-entry, and those that are open-ended, fenestrated, or have an attached footplate). SPL kits are available commercially for ease of use. Traditionally, SPL systems have been placed in the dorsal or superior conjunctival fornix in the upper eyelid (1099–1101). Dorsally placed SPL systems require the use of a supraorbital nerve

1099–1101 Dorsal subpalpebral lavage system placement. (1099) The needle is tunneled under the eyelid through the palpebral conjunctival fornix. The lavage tubing is fed through the needle and both needle and tubing are pulled through the hole in the eyelid. (1100) The footplate is shown as it is pulled up under the dorsal eyelid. (1101) The lavage entry hole should be at the highest point possible through the conjunctival fornix in order to avoid inadvertent corneal contact with the lavage footplate.

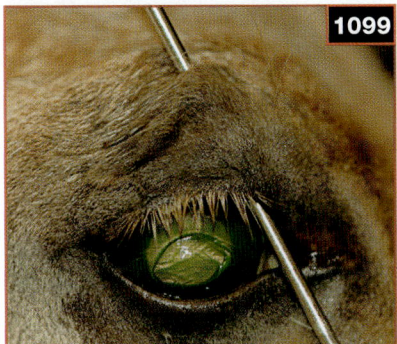
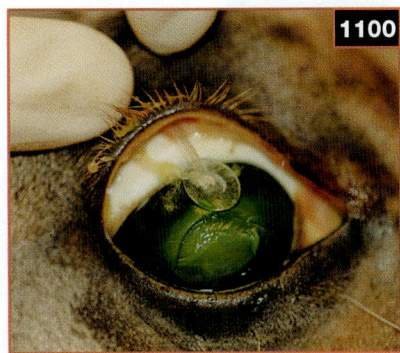
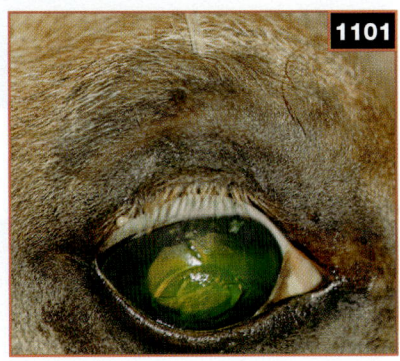

821

block for sensory denervation of the upper eyelid. More recently, inferomedial placement of a single-entry subpalpebral lavage (SSPL) tube has been reported, and is preferred over dorsal placement as it is associated with a lower incidence of complications. The chief advantage involves the location of the footplate between the less mobile inferior eyelid and the anterior aspect of the nictitating membrane, which helps protect the cornea from the SSPL tube and makes the tube less apt to migrate out. Proper positioning is relatively easy and gravity helps maintain the appropriate position. SSPL tube systems are

positioned by first introducing a 12 or 14 gauge needle with the hub removed into the inferomedial conjunctival fornix and pushing through the eyelid in a ventronasal direction (1102). Hemostats placed over the exit site will provide counter pressure and help the needle exit the skin. Commercially available silastic tubing, with an attached footplate, may then be threaded through the needle going from the conjunctival surface to the skin surface. Once the tubing exits the sharp end of the needle, both the needle and the tubing are pulled through the eyelid. The footplate is positioned deep in the medial aspect of the inferior

1102–1106 Ventromedial subpalpebral lavage system placement. (1102) The needle is tunneled through the medial aspect of the ventral eyelid. Care is taken to avoid the inferior nasolacrimal punctum. (1103) The lavage footplate is pulled into position. (1104) The juxtaposition of the nictitating membrane in this region reduces the risk of corneal contact with the footplate. (1105) The lavage system in place with tubing secured to facial skin at several points in order to minimize movement. (1106) The distal aspect of the lavage system showing the injection port of the tubing secured to a tongue depressor for added support.

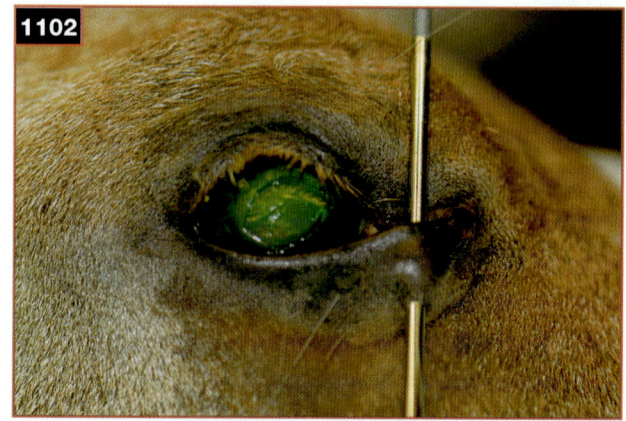

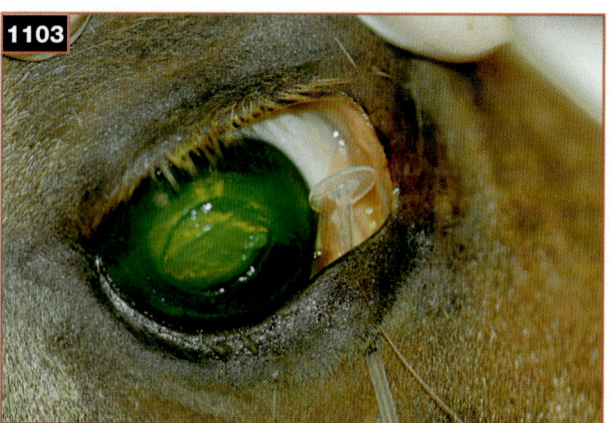

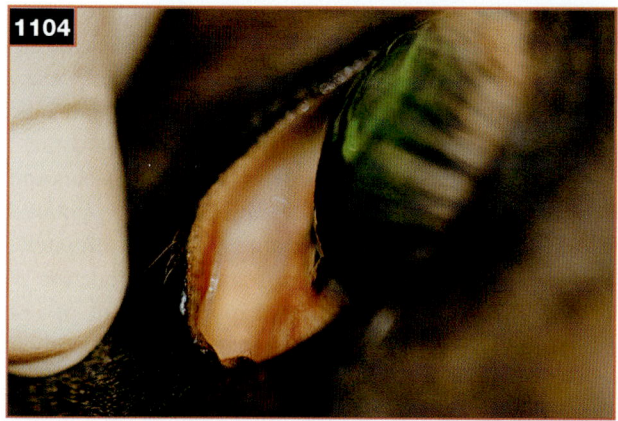

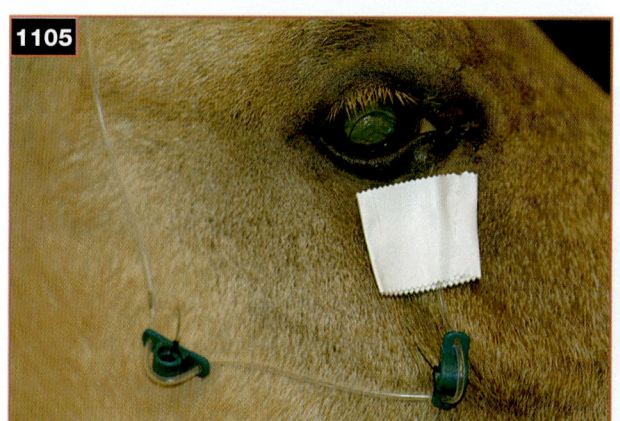

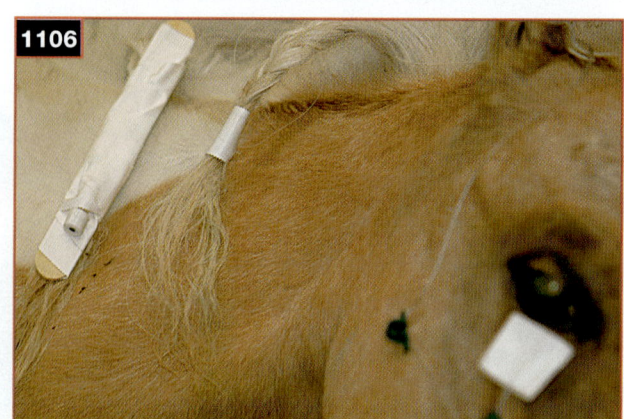

conjunctival fornix so that it lies flat between the lower eyelid and the anterior surface of the nictitating membrane (1103, 1104). A piece of tape is then attached to the tubing flush with the exit point from the skin to prevent the tube from sliding back (1105). The tubing is brought over the poll and braided into the mane and is secured to the horse using tape and skin sutures. An injection port, for manual injection, can then be attached to the free end of the tubing, secured to a tongue depressor and wrapped in gauze and tape to make it less likely for the end to bend or kink (1106). Manual delivery involves injecting approximately 0.15–0.2 ml of medication into the tubing system at the injection port and flushing the drug into the eye using 3 ml of air. The air must be injected slowly to avoid irritation to the corneal or conjunctival surface, thereby decreasing the likelihood of patient discomfort. Although manual injection is most often used to deliver the treatment solution through the SPL system, continuous drip or pump systems have also been employed. Complications associated with SPL systems include infection of the eyelid, loss of the footplate in the eyelid (although no long-term problems have been reported), conjunctival granuloma, endophthalmitis, iatrogenic trauma to the globe during insertion, plugging or breakage of the tubing, tube displacement or premature removal by the horse, suture loss, and injection port damage or loss. Poorly placed tubing or tube slippage can quickly produce corneal irritation or ulceration or allow topical medications to leak into the subcutaneous tissue, leading rapidly to eyelid swelling (chemosis) and severe inflammation. SPL systems should be checked daily for complications associated with their use and to ensure patency. SPL systems are generally easily placed and well-tolerated for extended periods of time. Topical ophthalmic suspensions and ointments should not be used in an SPL, as they will clog the tubing.

Nasolacrimal lavage system

A nasolacrimal lavage system has also been described for delivering drugs to the eye. This system may also be placed under sedation and local anesthesia using a technique similar to NLS cannulation and lavage, as previously described. A #8 French, 42-inch feeding tube or polyethylene tubing is introduced into the nasal punctum and passed to the level of the nasolacrimal sac. Tape is placed around the tubing at the point of entry into the nasal punctum and secured to the nose before the tubing is run up the head and along the neck and attached in a similar manner to the SPL system. Larger volumes of drug are required in this type of delivery system, making systemic absorption more likely. The tubing may also slip or kink and, as the tubing does not completely occlude the nasolacrimal duct, the medication may drain down around the tubing.

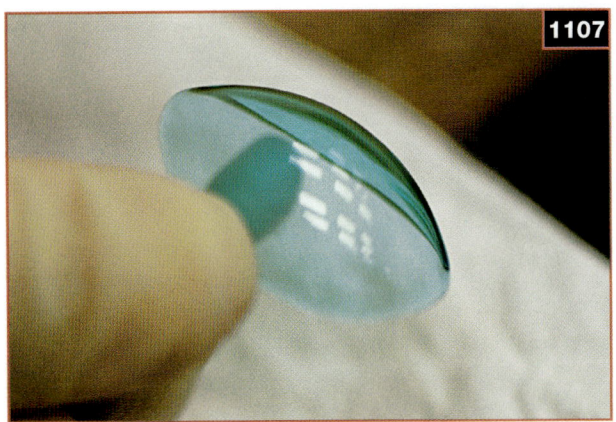

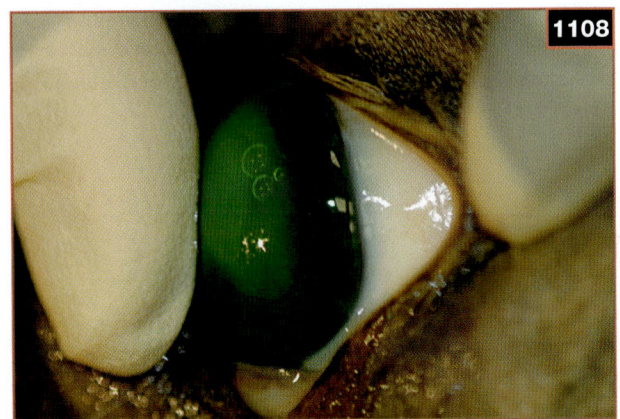

1107, 1108 Contact lens. (1107) A tinted contact lens may be easier to work with and identify on the eye. (1108) The ideally sized contact lens will not extend onto the sclera.

Topical drug reservoirs

Drug-impregnated collagen shields and contact lenses can also be used as drug delivery devices, providing prolonged therapeutic drug levels, but avoiding frequent administration (1107, 1108). Collagen shields and contact lenses should be pre-soaked in the chosen drug for 10 minutes and 30 minutes, respectively, to ensure saturation of the medication. Initial corneal drug levels may be high, but they deplete rapidly, thereby limiting their apparent benefit over topical therapy. Their use as drug reservoirs tends to be limited to emergency treatment to help establish high drug levels rapidly.

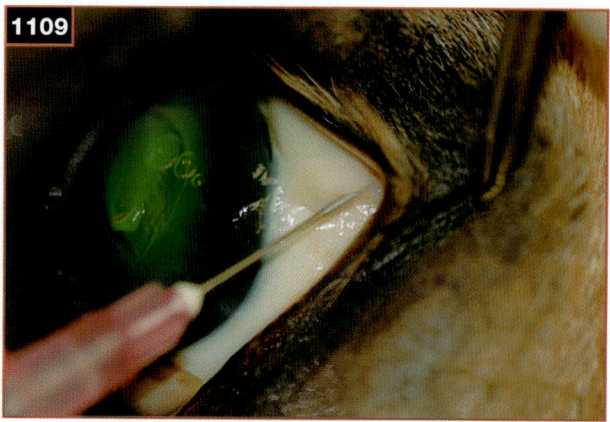

1109

1109 Subconjunctival administration of a drug. Using a fine-gauge needle (25–30 gauge), the conjunctiva is tented with the needle tip and the subconjunctival space is then expanded with drug.

Subconjunctival administration

Subconjunctival injection can be facilitated by the use of topical anesthesia and an auriculopalpebral nerve block. A maximum volume of 1 ml may be injected under the bulbar conjunctiva using a 25–27 gauge needle. The bevel of the needle should remain up and the hand holding the syringe should rest on the horse's head when injecting in order to decrease the risk of inadvertent globe perforation or trauma (1109). The dorsolateral quadrant is the easiest place to inject; however, it is important to inject as close to the lesion site as possible, as drug levels are highest in the region immediately adjacent to the injection site. Subconjunctival injection may establish much higher medication levels in tissues for a longer period of time than that attained with occasional topical application. It is beneficial in emergency situations requiring the need to establish high tissue levels of antimicrobials or when using repository corticosteroids, as therapeutic levels may be maintained for several days. Low intravitreal drug levels may be achieved. They are often used to augment topical therapy.

Intraocular administration

Intracameral (into the anterior chamber) or intravitreal (into the vitreous) administration is also used occasionally. Intracameral injections are performed at the limbus using a 25–30 gauge 5/8-inch needle that is first tunneled under the conjunctiva for a few millimeters before entering the eye, parallel to the iris face, in order to decrease the chance of aqueous humor leakage. Intravitreal injections are performed by stabilizing the globe with forceps and introducing a 25 gauge needle into the eye 8–10 mm from the limbus and angling it towards the center of the vitreous. Intraocular injection may be useful in cases of endophthalmitis, but can be damaging, irritating, or toxic to the intraocular tissues. Not all ophthalmic medications are safe to inject into the eye. This is a specialist procedure and this route is rarely indicated. It may be associated with a number of severe complications and side-effects.

Parenteral therapy

The ability of most drugs to cross the blood–ocular barrier (BOB) may limit the usefulness of this route for intraocular disease. Chloramphenicol and sulfonamides penetrate the BOB adequately. Inflammatory conditions may facilitate penetration of antimicrobials not normally able to penetrate the BOB. Intravenous administration is preferred to intramuscular or subcutaneous routes because the higher plasma levels attained by this route will lead to higher intraocular concentrations. There is no advantage to continuous infusion over pulsed therapy. The major drawback involves the relatively higher risk of associated systemic side-effects.

Neonatal and congenital ocular disorders

Ocular diseases of the foal may be congenital or acquired. Congenital ocular defects have a reported incidence of 0.5–3% in the horse. Foals may be born with single or multiple ocular defects including NLS atresia, entropion, eyelid, iris or fundic colobomas, anterior segment dysgenesis, cataracts, microphthalmia, retinal dysplasia, retinal detachment, and CSNB. Cataracts are the most frequently reported congenital lesion in foals. Congenital defects must be differentiated from acquired lesions or disorders such as ocular trauma, globe perforation, and phthisis bulbi.

Normal foals have decreased corneal sensitivity and lower tear production than adult horses. Additionally, their menace reflex may not appear until 7–14 days postpartum. These factors make foals prone to acquired ocular disease, especially those that are systemically ill and/or recumbent. All compromised neonatal foals should be examined daily for signs of ocular disease or ulceration. Ophthalmic lubricant ointments should be administered regularly to help protect the cornea from damage.

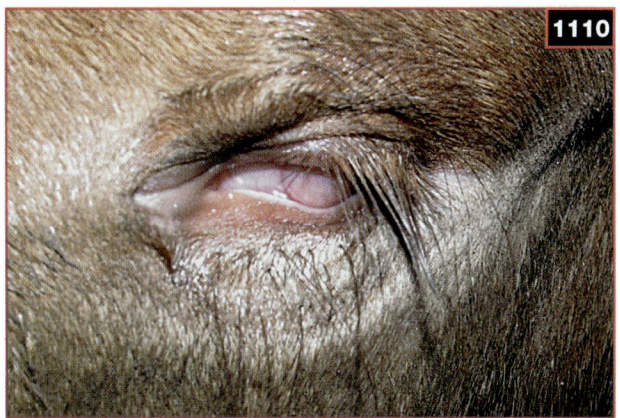

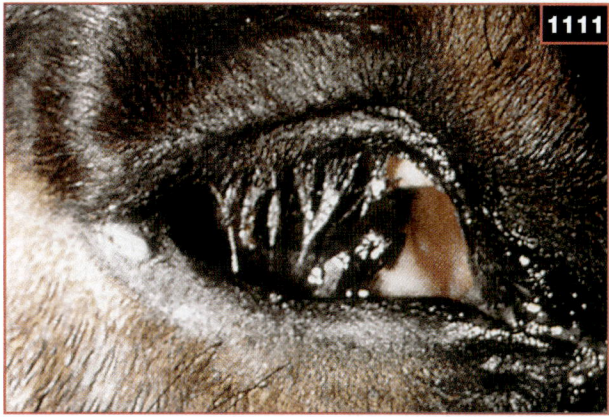

1110 This neonatal Thoroughbred foal was born with bilateral microphthalmos and was blind. The left eye shows a smaller than normal orbit, prolapsed nictitans, and small, pink, residual globe. (Photo courtesy GA Munroe)

1111 Phthisis bulbi (shrunken globe), typically associated with severe chronic intraocular inflammation, must be distinguished from microphthalmos in the horse.

Anophthalmos and microphthalmos

Definition/overview
Anophthalmos is a very rare condition that involves the complete absence of ocular tissues, resulting in blindness. Microphthalmos is a congenitally small globe that can be subdivided into simple or pure microphthalmos (or nanophthalmos) and complicated microphthalmos. Pure microphthalmos involves a small but otherwise normal and visual globe. Complicated microphthalmos is more common and involves a congenitally small globe in combination with multiple anterior and/or posterior segment defects that may have an effect on vision. One or both eyes may be affected.

Etiology/pathophysiology
Anophthalmos and microphthalmos are congenital anomalies with unknown etiologies. Most cases are considered to be spontaneous and idiopathic; however, a variety of underlying causes have been suggested including intra-uterine maternal infections and exposure to toxins during gestation. Thoroughbreds have been reported to be at higher risk, although an inherited component has yet to be confirmed.

These anomalies occur when the neuroectoderm of the primary optic vesicle fails to develop properly from the anterior neural plate of the neural tube during embryonic development. Disfigurement of the orbit may occur secondary to an absent or smaller than normal-sized globe.

Clinical presentation
Affected foals are born with an apparent absence of ocular tissue or a small eye, which is usually obvious on examination. A small palpebral fissure, an elevated/prominent nictitating membrane, conjunctivitis, and facial asymmetry may also be noted (1110). Entropion may occur secondary to failure of the smaller than normal globe to support the eyelids, and may result in mild keratitis to severe corneal ulceration. Vision may be present, but usually the eye is blind. Multiple ocular anomalies may also be present, including colobomas, cataracts, retinal dysplasia, and/or retinal detachment.

Differential diagnosis
Globe perforation, globe rupture, and phthisis bulbi (a normal-sized globe that atrophies secondary to severe ocular disease) (1111) are acquired conditions that may be confused with anophthalmos or microphthalmos.

Diagnosis
A thorough history and ocular examination should allow the practitioner to differentiate between congenital anophthalmos or microphthalmos and acquired diseases. Differentiating anophthalmos from microphthalmos may require histopathologic examination; however, this is rarely indicated, as the distinction is not often clinically relevant.

Management
There is no treatment. In cases where secondary entropion is present and the eye is uncomfortable, surgical correction may be required. In unilateral cases of chronic ocular irritation or discomfort, where the eye is blind, enucleation may be the treatment of choice. In cases of bilateral involvement causing severe visual deficits or blindness, euthanasia may be indicated.

Prognosis
Anophthalmos and microphthalmos are congenital non-progressive lesions with a variable effect on vision.

Strabismus

Definition/overview

Strabismus is a deviation of the globe from its normal position that may be congenital or acquired and unilateral or bilateral. It may be present continually or intermittently. Normal neonatal foals have a slight medioventral strabismus that will change to the normal adult position by 1 month of age. Bilateral convergent strabismus ('cross-eyed') is termed esotropia, while divergent strabismus is exotropia. Vertical upward deviation is termed hypertropia and downward deviation is hypotropia.

Etiology/pathophysiology

Congenital lesions may be inherited, as with the dorso-medial strabismus and hypertropia seen in horses with CSNB. Saddlebreds have an increased incidence of eso-tropia. Strabismus may occur as a result of congenital anomalies or trauma to, or atrophy of, the extraocular muscles. Periorbital abscesses or tumors can also cause deviation of the globe. Central or peripheral neurologic disease may lead to strabismus.

Clinical presentation

Deviation of one or both globes from the normal position is noted on examination as excessive scleral exposure. Dorsomedial displacement of the globe may be associated with dim-light vision deficits in animals with CSNB. Spontaneously resolving medioventral strabismus is seen in otherwise normal neonatal foals. Ambylopia (vision loss in the deviated eye leading to a lack of true stereopsis) may be present in congenital or early-onset cases.

Differential diagnosis

Primary congenital strabismus and the cause of acquired strabismus must be differentiated for purposes of management and prognosis.

Diagnosis

Clinical appearance will readily lead to a diagnosis of strabismus. History and/or additional diagnostic tests such as ultrasonography may be required to help differentiate the cause of the strabismus.

Management

Surgical therapy to repair strabismus can be attempted; however, it is technically challenging and often unsuccessful. In cases of acquired strabismus, the underlying cause should be treated. Horses with strabismus associated with CSNB should not be bred.

Prognosis

The prognosis is excellent for normal neonates with medioventral strabismus, which will spontaneously resolve. The prognosis is guarded for other causes.

Entropion

Definition/overview

Entropion, or inversion of the eyelid, may occur as a primary ocular disorder or, more commonly, secondary to another ocular disease. It may occur in one (typically the lower) or both eyelids and may be unilateral or bilateral. Entropion may be categorized as congenital or acquired. It may occur as a primary anatomic condition or be secondary to the enophthalmos resulting from microphthalmos, and is a relatively common condition in premature, dysmature, or systemically ill foals. Although a high incidence has been reported in certain Thoroughbred and Quarter horse families, inheritance has not been proven. Acquired entropion also occurs occasionally in adults secondary to trauma and severe scarring of the eyelids (cicatricial), prolonged blepharospasm (spastic), enophthalmos, or phthisis bulbi.

Etiology/pathophysiology

Common causes of entropion are listed in *Table 53*. Primary entropion (hereditary) may occur due to weakness of the tarsal plate, abnormal positioning of the globe, or micropalpebral fissure (abnormally small eyelids). Trauma to the eyelid may lead to fibrosis of the orbicularis oculi muscle, resulting in cicatricial entropion. Spastic entropion is caused by chronically painful conditions of the conjunctiva and cornea, which frequently lead to, or exacerbate, entropion due to blepharospasm. Regardless of the type of entropion, the rolling in of the eyelids may cause cilia and facial hairs to contact the conjunctiva

TABLE 53 **Common causes of entropion**

PRIMARY

- Spontaneous/idiopathic
- Inherited – Thoroughbred, Quarter horse

SECONDARY

- Failure of passive transfer
- Prematurity/dysmaturity
- Dehydration
- Malnutrition/weight loss
- Microphthalmos
- Enophthalmos
- Phthisis bulbi
- Eyelid or surgical trauma (cicatricial entropion)
- Blepharospasm from ocular pain (spastic entropion)

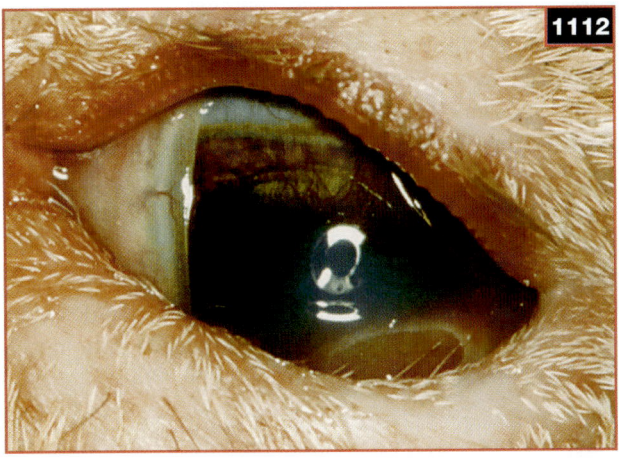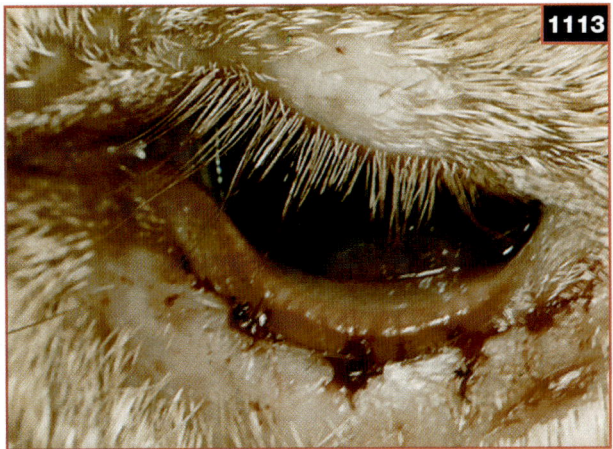

1112, 1113 Entropion in a foal as a result of microphthalmos. Note the corneal ulcer present in the ventral aspect of the cornea (1112). Inferior entropion has been resolved following a Hotz–Celsus surgical eversion technique (1113) .

and/or cornea (trichiasis), leading to corneal irritation and increased lacrimation, blepharospasm, conjunctivitis, keratitis, and/or cornea ulceration. Most cases in foals are the result of systemic illness and orbital fat loss (cachexia) or dehydration due to systemic illness or maladjustment. Blepharospasm can exacerbate the entropion.

Clinical presentation
The lower and/or upper eyelid is inverted (**1112**). Excessive lacrimation, blepharospasm, photophobia, conjunctivitis, keratitis, and corneal ulceration may be observed if trichiasis is present. Additional congenital eyelid abnormalities may be present in cases of primary entropion (i.e. ankyloblepharon, coloboma, dermoid, and cilia abnormalities). Other ocular abnormalities may be present in cases of cicatricial or spastic entropion.

Differential diagnosis
Other causes of ocular pain or irritation such as conjunctivitis, keratitis, keratoconjunctivitis sicca (KCS), foreign bodies, and corneal ulceration.

Diagnosis
Diagnosis is based on clinical examination, which confirms inversion of the eyelid margin. It is important to determine if the entropion is primary or secondary. Spastic entropion will resolve when topical anesthesia is applied. Positive fluorescein staining will be present when spastic entropion occurs secondary to corneal ulceration. Cicatricial entropion is normally diagnosed based on a history of trauma or eyelid surgery.

Management
Treatment of entropion will vary with cause, severity, and chronicity. Primary entropion may be self-correcting in foals. In young animals exhibiting clinical signs, treatment to temporarily evert the eyelid margin and eliminate the corneal irritation should be undertaken. Temporary tacking may be accomplished by using either nonabsorbable suture material (e.g. 4–0 silk) in a vertical mattress pattern or surgical staples to create a normal conformation. These are maintained until orbital growth establishes normal eyelid conformation or the cause of the entropion has resolved. Subcutaneous injection of procaine penicillin G (up to 3 ml) into the area adjacent to the affected eyelid margin can also be used until the lid returns to a normal position; however, repeated injections are often required, which can lead to inflammation and scarring. Adjunctive medical management typically includes topical eye lubrication. For those cases in which ulceration is present, topical antimicrobials and atropine should be administered as described under the discussion for corneal ulceration. Secondary uveitis or any other underlying cause should also be treated if present. If the entropion persists, surgical repair via a modified Hotz–Celsus procedure may be required (**1113**).

Prognosis
The prognosis is good.

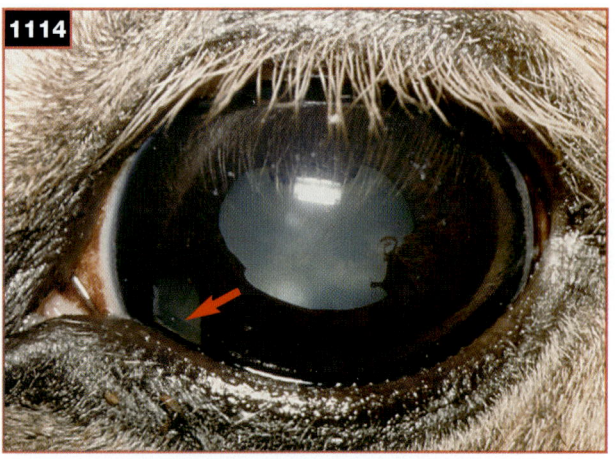

1114 A coloboma (arrow) is present in the ventromedial iris of this foal. Additional anomalies in this eye include cataract, iris hypolasia, and a dysplastic corpora nigra. (Photo courtesy D Ramsey)

Coloboma

Definition/overview
Colobomas involve the congenital absence of tissue that is normally present. They may be defined by location, with those found in the 6 o'clock position, along the line of closure of the optic fissure, categorized as typical, and those found in other areas as atypical. The eyelids, iris, ciliary body, lens, choroid, retina, and/or optic disk may be affected. Colobomas are rare in the horse, but when they do occur they are often seen in combination with other ocular disorders or individually as incidental findings in blue-eyed or incompletely albinotic horses.

Etiology/pathophysiology
The cause is unknown and the occurrence sporadic. Colobomas occur very early in embryogenesis and are related to defective closure of the embryonic fissure (typical coloboma) or lack of development of tissue due to a variety of early embryonic stresses or toxins (atypical coloboma).

Clinical presentation
Colobomas can vary in appearance from small notches in, to an almost complete absence of, tissue in the eyelid, iris, ciliary body, lens, choroid, retina, and/or ONH. Trichiasis, leading to keratitis and blepharospasm, may be present secondary to an eyelid coloboma. Dyscoria (abnormal pupil shape) may be noted in cases of iris colobomas (1114). Partial or complete retinal detachment, as well as decreased or absent vision, may be found with retinal or optic nerve colobomas. Scleral ectasia is occasionally observed, as are other congenital ocular abnormalities such as microphthalmos. Cataract and retinal dysplasia may also be present.

Differential diagnosis
Eyelid lacerations may resemble eyelid colobomas, and synechiae may appear similar to iris colobomas. Lens luxation may mimic lens colobomas. Other causes of retinal detachment (*Table 54*) must be ruled out. Glaucoma with optic nerve cupping should be easily differentiated from optic nerve colobomas.

Diagnosis
Diagnosis is based on clinical identification of a defect in the eyelid, iris, lens, choroid, retina, and/or optic nerve that has been present since birth.

Management
In cases where clinical signs are associated with an eyelid coloboma, blepharoplasty using advancing skin and/or conjunctival flaps can be used to close the defect. Cryoepilation of eyelashes or facial hair contributing to corneal irritation and ocular lubrication may also provide relief. There is no therapy for intraocular colobomas; however, in cases of partial serous retinal detachment related to fundic colobomas, laser therapy may prevent complete detachment.

TABLE 54 Etiologies of retinal detachment

- Congenital/inherited
  - Associated with retinal dysplasia and/or cataracts
- Systemic infectious diseases (mycoses, lymphosarcoma, toxoplasmosis)
- Neoplasia
- Vitreoretinal traction bands/adhesions (traction detachment)
- Trauma
- Vitreal degeneration
- Cataracts (i.e. uveitic, traumatic or idiopathic)
- Sudden decreases in intraocular pressure
- Serous or fluid detachments (vasculitis, uremia, vascular hypertension)
- Glaucoma
- Extraocular pressure
- Retinal tears/holes (rhegmatogenous detachment)
- Equine recurrent uveitis
- Head trauma or perforating globe wounds
- Idiopathic
- Postoperative complication of phacoemulsification

Prognosis

Colobomas are typically nonprogressive, although there is an associated risk of retinal detachment with optic nerve or retinal colobomas. A coloboma that directly or indirectly causes visual loss will render the horse unsound unless surgical correction is possible.

Dermoids

Definition/overview

Dermoids are relatively uncommon focal congenital masses consisting of displaced normal skin tissue that can involve the eyelid, nictitating membrane, conjunctiva, and/or cornea. These teratomas most often affect the temporal limbus and involve the neighboring bulbar conjunctiva and cornea. Coarse hairs commonly grow from these masses and can cause irritation to the conjunctiva or cornea depending on location and the tissues involved.

Etiology/pathophysiology

The etiology of dermoids is unknown. There is an association of limbal dermoids with iris hypoplasia and cataracts in Quarter horses. They have also been reported in a French Saddle filly in conjunction with corneal staphylomas.

Dermoids may occur as a result of abnormal differentiation of isolated groups of cells early in development or abnormal invagination of ectodermal tissue later in gestation. They may interfere with blinking, which may lead to exposure keratopathy. The hair that grows from the surface of these masses often causes mechanical irritation of the cornea, leading to keratitis. The degree of visual impairment depends on the extent of corneal involvement and the occurrence or absence of disease secondary to corneal problems.

Clinical presentation

A dermoid may appear as a pigmented mass with or without hair growth involving the eyelid, nictitating membrane, conjunctiva, and/or cornea (1115). The hair that grows from the surface of these masses often causes mechanical irritation of the cornea, which leads to epiphora and keratitis. Vision can be variable. Quarter horses may have iridal hypoplasia and cataracts, as well as limbal dermoids.

Differential diagnosis

Aberrant pigmentation and ocular melanomas, as well as other eyelid, conjunctival, and corneal neoplasms, may have a similar appearance to dermoids.

Diagnosis

Clinical appearance is usually adequate. Histopathologic evaluation is confirmatory.

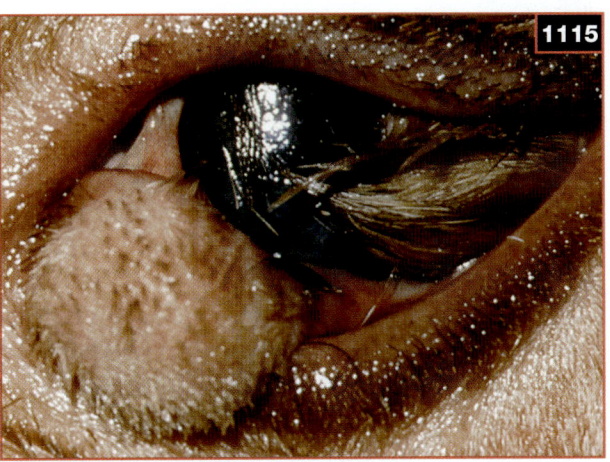

1115 Dermoid in a foal involving the temporal cornea and conjunctiva, and separately on the palpebral surface of the nictitating membrane.

Management

Dermoids may be left untreated if they are not causing clinical signs. If abnormal ocular signs are present, the treatment of choice is surgical resection of the aberrant tissue. Depending on the location, eyelid resection, conjunctivotomy, and/or a superficial to deep keratectomy may be necessary. Resection may be followed by reconstructive blepharoplasty and/or medical therapy as for corneal ulcer management (see p. 850). Dermoids involving the deeper layers of the corneal stroma, although rare, may require corneal mechanical support with a contact lens, collagen shield, or surgical grafting procedure.

Prognosis

The prognosis for vision is good.

Nasolacrimal system atresia

Definition/overview

NLS atresia is a congenital absence of part of the NSL pathway. The upper or lower eyelid puncta, part of the nasolacrimal duct itself and/or the nasal punctum, may be involved. An imperforate nasal punctum is the most common abnormality. It may be unilateral or bilateral.

Etiology/pathophysiology

The cause is unknown. Clinical signs may not develop until 1–2 years of age, once dacryocystitis has developed and copious amounts of mucopurulent ocular discharge are present. Chronic epiphora can lead to dermatitis, poor cosmesis, and infectious keratoconjunctivitis.

Clinical presentation

Absence of the eyelid punctum or nasal meatus punctum may be evident on clinical examination. Epiphora is typically noted by 4–6 months of age. This is followed by severe chronic mucoid or mucopurulent (secondary to dacryocystitis) ocular discharge. Dermatitis, conjunctivitis, and keratitis may also be present.

Differential diagnosis

Acquired NLS obstruction due to trauma, chronic dacryocystitis, foreign body, parasites, respiratory infection, and neoplasia should be differentiated from NLS atresia.

Diagnosis

NLS atresia may be confirmed by noting visually absent eyelid or nasal punctal openings on ophthalmic examination. Failure of fluorescein solution to exit the nasal punctum after application to the surface of the globe may suggest a blockage in the NLS. An inability to cannulate or flush the NLS and/or distention of the floor of the conjunctiva overlying the imperforate nasal punctum in response to irrigation will confirm an NLS abnormality. Samples for culture and sensitivity are recommended due to the frequency of secondary infection (dacryocystitis). Contrast radiography (dacryocystorhinography) may be useful to determine if there is associated nasolacrimal duct agenesis. CT can also be helpful in diagnosing NLS atresia.

Management

Treatment involves surgery to relieve the obstruction by creating a new opening and medical management to treat secondary bacterial infection and prevent re-obstruction. In the case of an imperforate punctum, the patent punctum is first cannulated and, occasionally, the tip of the catheter may be palpated slightly proximal or distal to the expected location of the punctum. The NLS is flushed, which often causes the eyelid conjunctival or nasal mucous membrane overlying the site of the atretic puncta to dilate. Once the atretic site is identified, a cutdown through the palpebral conjunctiva or nasal mucosa will establish patency. Electrocautery may be necessary for hemostasis. The catheter tip is then grasped with a hemostat and the catheter pulled through the new punctal opening. A stent of polyethylene tubing or silicone is sutured in place for 3–8 weeks to prevent closure of the new opening while the new duct and punctum becomes epithelialized and the dacryocystitis resolves. After surgery, topical antimicrobials or antimicrobial/corticosteroid preparations (e.g. triple antibiotic solution or triple antibiotic/steroid combination solution) and systemic antimicrobials should be used for several weeks to allow the dacryocystitis to resolve. The antimicrobial selected should be based on culture and sensitivity results. Nasolacrimal duct agenesis may also accompany the eyelid or nasal puncta atresia. Depending on the location of the NLS obstruction, a more complicated surgical correction such as canaliculorhinostomy, dacryocystorhinostomy, conjunctivobuccostomy, or conjunctivorhinostomy may be required.

Prognosis

The prognosis will depend on the extent of the atresia. Surgery can be challenging and relapses can occur.

Heterochromia iridis

Definition/overview

Heterochromia is the term used to describe iris color variation. Congenital heterochromia iridis is seen clinically as an iris with more than one color or two different colored irides in an individual. This lack of iris stromal pigmentation is a normal variation present from birth in Appaloosa, palomino, chestnut, gray, spotted, and white horses. Lay terms for this condition include 'wall-eye' (white and blue iris color with a brown corpora nigra) and 'china eye' (white iridal color with brown corpora nigra).

Etiology/pathophysiology

Heterochromia iridis and heterochromia iridum are inherited conditions. In these cases the iris is normal except for incomplete development of the pigment granules in the cytoplasm of the stromal cells. Pigment failure may occur in one iris or a portion of one iris. Uveal stromal cysts may be associated with heterochromia irides. The tapetum of affected eyes is often poorly developed or even absent and areas of the fundus may be deficient in pigment (subalbinotic fundus).

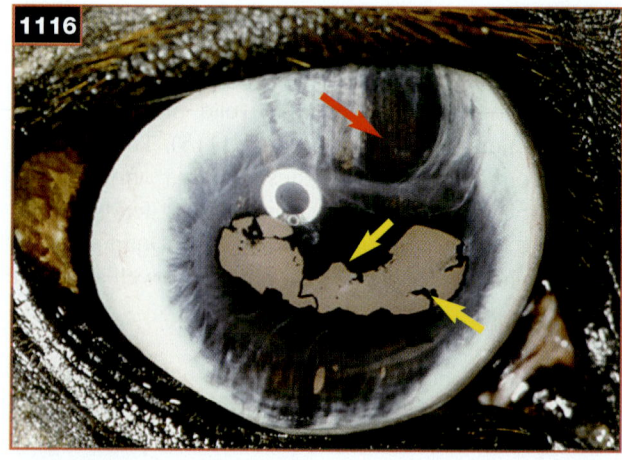

1116 Heterochromia and iris stromal hypoplasia are apparent in this horse. The 12 o'clock location is typical for iris stromal hypoplasia (red arrow). This eye also has an incidental finding of several areas of posterior synechiae (yellow arrows).

1117, 1118 (1117) Cystic dilation of the ventral corpora nigra. Large uveal cysts in this location can impair vision, particularly when the pupil is constricted. (1118) The same eye following ablation of the cyst with a diode laser.

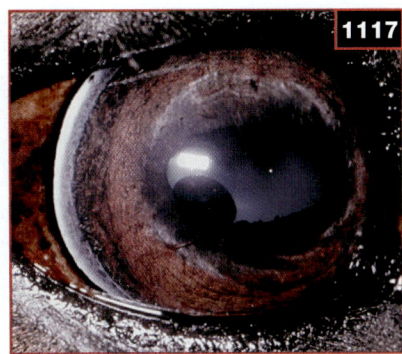 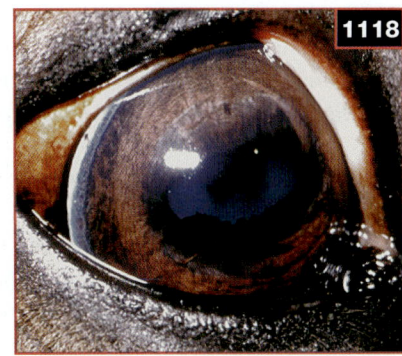

Clinical presentation

In cases of heterochromia iridis, on examination the iris is partially or completely blue or white and the corpora nigra is brown (**1116**). The affected area of the iris may bow into the anterior chamber. Uveal stromal cysts may also be present. The fundus may be subalbinotic, with nontapetal hypopigmentation and tapetal hypoplasia. In some horses with heterochromia there is accompanying iris hypoplasia. In Rocky Mountain horses and other breeds with partial albinism, heterochromia iridis can be associated with multiple ocular defects.

Differential diagnosis

Chronic uveitis causing increased pigmentation (or uveal melanoma) should be differentiated.

Diagnosis

History and clinical appearance should identify heterochromia iridis.

Management

There is no treatment for this condition.

Prognosis

Heterochromia iridis is congenital and nonprogressive.

Uveal cysts

Definition/overview

Uveal cysts are pigmented cysts arising from the posterior epithelium of the iris or granula iridica. Pigmented cysts are found free floating in the anterior chamber or attached at the pupillary margin. Uveal stromal cysts may be associated with iris hypoplasia and heterochromia iridis. They may be unilateral or bilateral.

Etiology/pathophysiology

The cause of uveal cyst formation is unknown. They involve the posterior pigmented epithelium of the iris and/or the granula iridica, which are extensions of the posterior pigmented epithelium of the iris. Cystic granula iridica are

most likely to cause clinical problems. Uveal stromal cysts may also occur in the thinned iris stroma of horses with blue irides and iris hypoplasia. They bulge out into the anterior chamber and can distort the pupil (dyscoria).

Clinical presentation

Uveal cysts appear as pigmented spherical, smooth-surfaced structures free floating in the anterior chamber or attached to the pupillary margin (**1117**). They may only be lightly pigmented and appear translucent or darkly pigmented with a solid appearance. There may be some fluctuation in size over time; however, there are usually no associated clinical signs. Rarely, they may obstruct the pupil and affect vision, causing visual impairment, decreased performance level, and head shaking. They may also rupture, leaving a circular area of benign pigment on the corneal endothelium. Uveal cysts in the stroma of horses with blue irides and iris hypoplasia tend to occur at the 12 o'clock position where the iris appears to bow into the anterior chamber and may cause dyscoria. They are more common in older horses and ponies.

Differential diagnosis

Intraocular neoplasia (e.g. uveal melanoma) and hypertrophic granula iridica should be differentiated from uveal cysts.

Diagnosis

Uveal cysts can be differentiated in some instances from other pigmented iridial masses on the basis of gross appearance alone. They may be transilluminated using a focused light source, but this is inconsistent and, in some cases, ultrasonography may be necessary.

Management

Treatment is usually unnecessary as uveal cysts rarely have clinical significance. Uveal cysts may be aspirated or treated with a Nd:YAG or diode laser if they are large enough to obstruct vision, occlude the pupil, or compromise the ICA (**1118**).

Prognosis
Uveal cysts have an excellent prognosis, although occasionally they are associated with other ophthalmic abnormalities.

Aniridia and iris hypoplasia
Definition/overview
Iris hypoplasia is usually severe and bilateral, with most cases described clinically as aniridia (the complete absence of the iris tissue). True aniridia may be seen alone in the American Quarter horse and Belgian draft horse, or it may be seen associated with limbal dermoids and/or cataracts. Aniridia has also been reported in Thoroughbreds, along with congenital cataracts. Iridal hypoplasia is common in Appaloosas and eyes with heterochromia iridis.

Etiology/pathophysiology
The cause of iris hypoplasia is usually unknown. Aniridia is inherited in the Belgian draft horse, and suspected of being inherited in the American Quarter horse, as an autosomal dominant trait.

Iris hypoplasia involves the failure of ingrowth of the third wave mesenchyme and disorderly differentiation of neuroectodermal tissue. The lens of affected eyes is often cataractous, although it may occasionally be ectopic or hypoplastic. The trabecular meshwork within the ICA may be malformed and glaucoma may be present.

Clinical presentation
Horses with iris hypoplasia or aniridia may present with blepharospasm, photophobia, or reduced vision, and the PLR may be marginal or absent. They may exhibit ocular discharge, perilimbal keratitis, and/or cataract formation. The iris hypoplasia can be so severe that the affected iris bulges anteriorly. The hypoplastic or absent iris may also allow the lens equator and ciliary processes of the ciliary body to be visible on ophthalmic examination in some cases (1119). The affected areas are often readily trans-illuminated. Vision may be degraded. Iris hypoplasia may be seen alone or associated with multiple ocular anomalies. In Belgian draft horses and Quarter horses anterior cortical cataracts and/or conjunctival dermoids may also be present.

Differential diagnosis
Any cause of an abnormally large pupil (mydriasis) or lens subluxation may be confused with aniridia or iris hypoplasia.

Diagnosis
History and clinical appearance are usually sufficient to confirm the diagnosis.

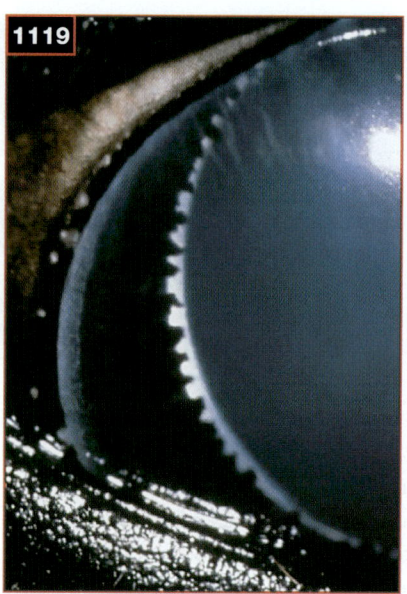

1119 Aniridia. The almost complete absence of iris exposes the normally hidden ciliary processes attached to the periphery of the lens.

Management
There is no specific treatment available, although supportive measures may be useful, such as using facemasks or dark-tinted contact lenses to decrease ambient light and increase patient comfort.

Prognosis
This congenital condition is nonprogressive. Affected horses are considered unsound.

Congenital ocular anomalies in Rocky Mountain horses
Definition/overview
This is an inherited syndrome of ocular lesions in the Rocky Mountain horse that can manifest as cysts of the iris, ciliary body, or peripheral retina with or without proliferation of the RPE, retinal dysplasia, and retinal detachment, or as multiple ocular anomalies. An increased prevalence of these anomalies is found in those horses with a chocolate coat color and a white or flaxen-colored mane and tail (partial albinism). A comparable set of congenital ophthalmic lesions has also been seen in the Kentucky Mountain Saddle horse, Mountain Pleasure horse, Morgan horse, and pony and miniature breeds in animals with similar color combinations. The disease is bilateral, but often asymmetrical.

Etiology/pathophysiology

This is a semidominant, inherited trait. Interestingly, the same founder stallion was used to produce the Kentucky Mountain Saddle horse, Mountain Pleasure horse and Rocky Mountain horse breeds.

A genetic mutation, closely linked to the dominant gene found at the Silver Dapple locus in horses with a chocolate coat and white or flaxen-colored mane and tail, is thought to be responsible for this syndrome.

Clinical presentation

Large, translucent, cystic structures arising from the posterior surface of the iris, ciliary body, or the peripheral retina are seen most frequently and are usually located in the temporal region (1120). Single to multiple well-delineated, darkly pigmented curvilinear streaks may be seen in the temporal part of the peripheral tapetal fundus (1121). These curvilinear streaks are frequently bilateral, but are not symmetrical. Unilateral or bilateral retinal dysplasia, characterized clinically as linear folds or vermiform streaks, is seen most often in the temporal peripheral retina.

Additional ocular abnormalities may also be noted, including megalocornea, macropalpebral fissures, abnormal corneal contour with excessive protrusion, an excessively deep anterior chamber, miosis, dyscoria, iris stromal hypoplasia, and the absence of a discernible collarette. A readily visible pupillary sphincter muscle, appearing as radially oriented deep stromal strands of iris tissue extending from the pupillary ruff, may also be visible (1122). The granula iridica may be hypoplastic and appear flattened and circumferentially oriented at the pupil margin. The PLRs can be decreased or absent, and there may be no, or minimal, response to mydriatics in eyes with iris abnormalities. There may be areas of poorly developed or absent pectinate ligaments in the ICA or even areas where multiple strands of pigmented tissue extend from

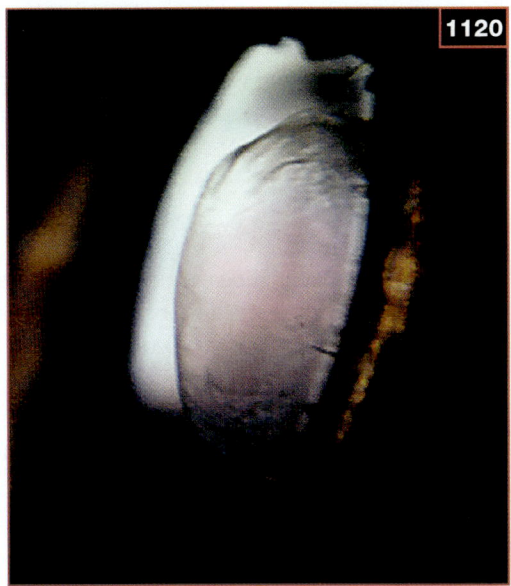

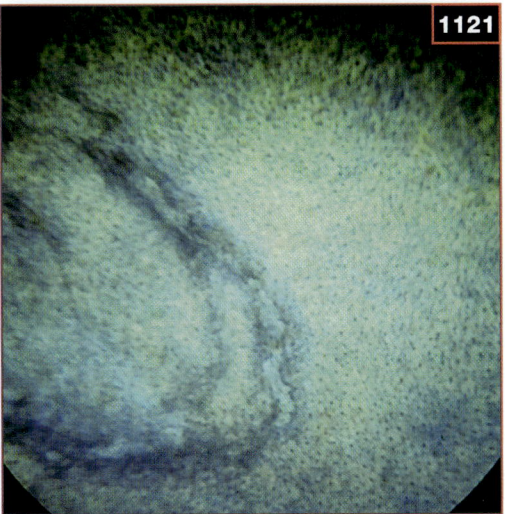

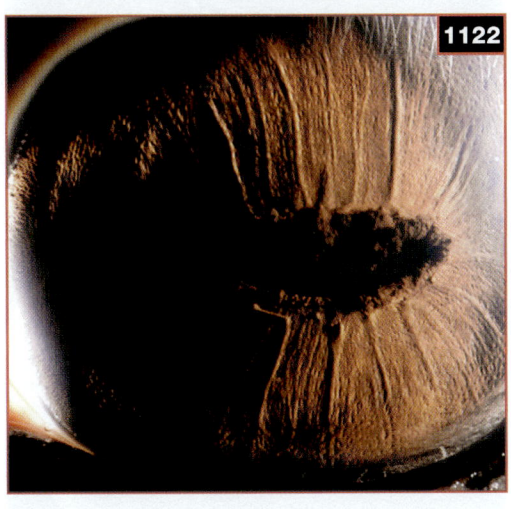

1120 Ciliary body cyst in a Rocky Mountain horse. These are typically located in the medial or lateral aspects of the ciliary body and can be very large. (Photo courtesy D Ramsey)

1121 Fundus of a young Rocky Mountain horse demonstrating curvilinear retinal lesions, possibly associated with previous detachment. (Photo courtesy D Ramsey)

1122 Rocky Mountain horse with hypolastic granula iridica, miosis, circumferential corpora nigra, visible sphincter muscle, and an absent iris collarette. (Photo courtesy D Ramsey)

the temporal peripheral iris to the peripheral cornea (goniosynechiae) (1123). Immature lenticular nuclear opacities (cataracts) and ventral subluxation of the temporal part of the lens (1124), an abnormal prominence of the anterior orbital rim, and/or microphthalmos may also be visible.

Differential diagnosis
Noninherited congenital ocular defects, causes of chronic uveitis, acquired cataracts, and other retinal diseases, as well as ocular trauma, should be considered.

Diagnosis
Diagnosis is based on signalment, history, and ophthalmic examination.

Management
There is no treatment available. As this is an inherited condition, affected animals should not be bred.

Prognosis
This is considered a nonprogressive disease.

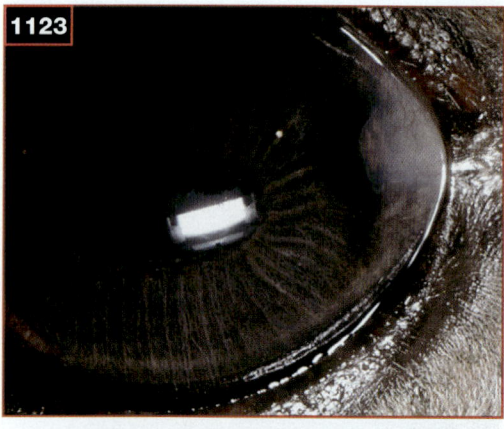

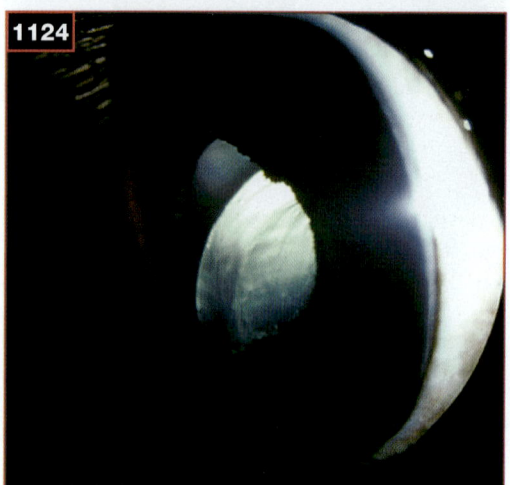

Congenital cataracts
Definition/overview
A cataract is a focal or diffuse opacification of the lens that may involve the capsule, cortex, and/or lens nucleus. Cataracts may be unilateral or bilateral, symmetrical or asymmetrical, stationary or progressive, and congenital, inherited, or acquired. They have a variable effect on vision. Congenital cataracts are present at birth, most being bilateral. They may occur alone or in association with multiple ocular anomalies. They are the most common congenital anomaly in the horse and are believed to be the most common cause of visual impairment or blindness in foals.

Etiology/pathophysiology
Cataracts may be inherited, or develop as a result of *in-utero* stresses. They may also occur secondary to other developmental abnormalities. Congenital cataracts are inherited in the Belgian draft horse and possibly in the Thoroughbred as a dominant trait. In most cases the underlying cause is unknown.

Abnormal lens vesicle invagination, separation, or defects in lens epithelium or capsule may result in congenital peripheral cataract formation. Those associated with mild microphthalmos may result from early abnormalities in the lens placode and involve the lens nucleus, cortex, or both. Persistence of a portion of the perilenticular mesoderm (tunica vasculosa lentis and/or hyaloid artery) can also lead to congenital cataract formation.

Clinical presentation
Cataracts will appear as a lens opacity (cloudy lens) and can vary in shape, size, and location within the lens (1125, 1126). The level of vision compromise is dependent on the degree of opacification. Congenital cataracts may be associated with multiple ocular anomalies. Other ocular lesions that may be associated with cataract formation include synechiae, uveitis, lens luxation, and/or retinal disease. They are seen as part of the anterior segment dysgenesis/multiple ocular anomaly syndrome in Rocky Mountain horses. Nonprogressive, nuclear, bilaterally symmetrical cataracts that do not seriously affect vision are seen in Morgan horses (1127).

1123 Goniosynechiae in the periphery of the anterior chamber of a Rocky Mountain horse. (Photo courtesy D Ramsey)

1124 Lens subluxation with ventral displacement in a Rocky Mountain horse. (Photo courtesy D Ramsey)

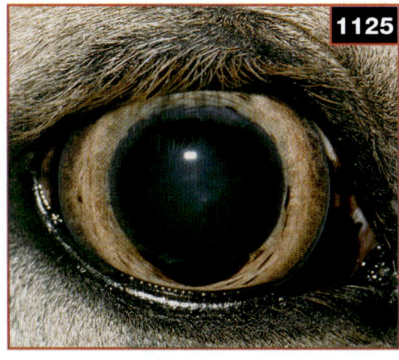 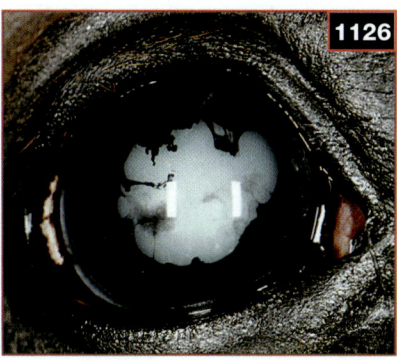 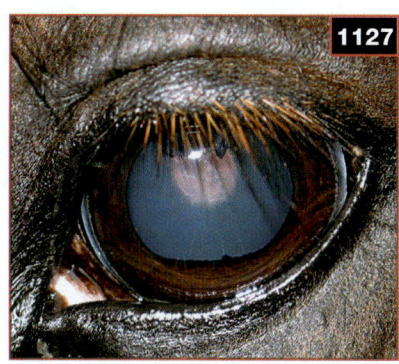

1125 The faint anterior cortical incipient cataract present in this horse was identified on prepurchase examination and was not associated with apparent visual compromise. The cause was undetermined.

1126 This mature cataract was associated with chronic bouts of recurrent uveitis. Note the posterior synechiae, a typical postinflammatory finding.

1127 Nuclear cataracts, present in the center of the lens, are hereditary in the Morgan breed. Although nuclear cataracts are usually nonprogressive, their central position can create vision distortion, particularly when bright light causes pupillary constriction.

TABLE 55 **Main causes of cataracts**

CONGENITAL

- *In utero* infections/toxins/ocular inflammation/trauma/stresses/faulty nutrition
- Persistent hyperplastic tunica vasculosa lentis, persistent hyperplastic primary vitreous, persistent pupillary membranes

INHERITED

- Belgian, Thoroughbred, Morgan, Rocky Mountain horse, Quarter horse, Arabian

ACQUIRED

- Chronic uveitis
- Glaucoma
- Traumatic – blunt or penetrating; whiplash injury
- Iatrogenic from surgical trauma/laser therapy
- Lens subluxation/luxation
- Retinal disease/degeneration/detachment
- Neoplasia
- Senility >18 years old
- Exposure to toxins
- Systemic metabolic disease
- Nutritional
- Electrical (i.e. lightning)
- Radiation

Differential diagnosis

Congenital cataracts need to be differentiated from prominent posterior Y sutures, which are present in the majority of foals. Other differentials should include inherited or acquired cataracts and any other cause of vision deficits in the horse (*Table 55*).

Diagnosis

Cataracts are diagnosed based on identification of a unilateral or bilateral lenticular opacity. The menace response may be absent if the cataract is severe. Ocular ultrasonography and ERG will help identify posterior segment abnormalities, if present, prior to cataract surgery.

Management

Foals with unilateral or bilateral immature or mature cataracts that interfere with vision should be referred to a veterinary ophthalmologist promptly for evaluation. Removal by phacoemulsification is the treatment of choice for cataracts in animals with visual impairment, good PLRs, good dazzle reflexes, and no other ocular abnormalities or diseases that may interfere with vision. Absence of retinal detachment, based on ophthalmoscopy or ultrasonography, a normal ERG (in Appaloosas), no systemic disease, and absent or controlled preoperative uveitis, are also required. The patient must be healthy and amenable to the level of postoperative medical care necessary following intraocular surgery. Potential intraoperative complications include corneal edema, collapse of the anterior chamber due to vitreous pressure, iris prolapse through the corneal incision, hyphema, and posterior lens capsular tears. Postoperative complications include, but are not limited to, self-trauma, periorbital edema, corneal edema, corneal ulceration (**1128**), fibrin formation, uveitis, synechiae, posterior lens capsule tear enlargement, posterior capsular opacifications, preiridal fibrovascular membrane (PIFM) formation, vitreous presentation, retinal degeneration, retinal detachment, endophthalmitis, and phthisis bulbi.

Prognosis

The age of the patient influences the postoperative success rate. Cataract surgery in foals less than 6 months of age typically has very good results (approximately 80% success rate); however, the success rate is lower in older animals. Following phacoemulsification, foals should be monitored daily for corneal ulcers and other postoperative complications. In foals with subclinical systemic disease, postoperative endophthalmitis may occur. Horses are far-sighted following cataract surgery. In an attempt to improve vision, intraocular lenses have been developed for use in horses and research into their placement is ongoing.

Congenital glaucoma

Definition/overview

Glaucoma is an elevation in IOP caused by obstruction to the outflow of aqueous humor that is detrimental to normal ocular function. Glaucoma will eventually result in optic nerve damage and blindness. Congenital glaucoma occurs rarely in horses and, when it is seen, it is often associated with multiple congenital anomalies. There is no particular breed predisposition.

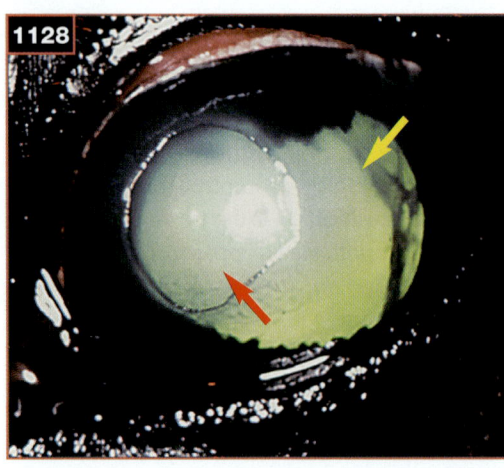

1128 Chronic corneal ulcer (red arrow) in a horse following phacoemulsification of cataracts. Note the edge of the lens capsule adjacent to the medial border of the iris (yellow arrow). (Photo courtesy American College of Veterinary Ophthalmologists)

Etiology/pathophysiology

The causes of congenital glaucoma include idiopathic/ spontaneous, inherited, or secondary to trauma that occurs prenatally or at the time of birth. The condition results from an abnormal development of the ICA (goniodysgenesis), resulting in poor drainage of fluid in the fetal eye and an increase in IOP.

Clinical presentation

A fixed dilated pupil, vision impairment/blindness, buphthalmia, corneal edema, Haab's striae (stretch marks or breaks in Descemet's membrane that appear as deep linear corneal opacities), lens subluxation/luxation, tapetal hyperreflectivity, retinal degeneration/atrophy, and/or optic nerve degeneration/cupping may be found in horses with congenital glaucoma. The condition may be seen with other developmental ocular anomalies such as iris hypoplasia, microphakia, cataract, abnormal ICA, and retinal dysplasia (anterior segment dysgenesis).

Differential diagnosis

Primary glaucoma, secondary glaucoma, and other causes of vision deficits in foals.

Diagnosis

History, clinical appearance, and tonometry results indicating an elevation in IOP can be used to diagnose glaucoma. Examination of the ICAmay show malformations, with failure of tissue to undergo rarefaction to form pectinate ligaments during the first few weeks postnatally.

Management

Medical treatment may include 0.5% timolol maleate (q12h) and topical carbonic anhydrase inhibitors (e.g. 2% dorzolamide or 1% brinzolamide) either alone or in combination (e.g. Cosopt) (q8h). Oral NSAIDs such as flunixin meglumine may be used to help control intraocular inflammation and increase patient comfort. Early surgical intervention has been suggested as the best option for foals with congenital glaucoma. Cyclocryotherapy with nitrous oxide or laser cyclophotocoagulation can be used to decrease the amount of aqueous humor produced by the ciliary body in eyes in an attempt to preserve vision. Intraocular inflammation must be controlled prior to these procedures. Gonioimplants have also been used in foals with some success. Often, affected eyes will become blind and chronically painful. Enucleation or evisceration with intrascleral prosthesis is the treatment of choice in these cases.

Prognosis

Early detection and treatment are vital; however, the prognosis remains poor for vision.

Retinal dysplasia

Definition/overview

Retinal dysplasia is a defective development of the fundus where folds occur in the neurosensory retina. It may be seen as an isolated finding or, more often, be associated with other congenital ocular abnormalities. Single or multiple linear or larger regions may be affected. Retinal dysplasia is usually bilateral. Although the Thoroughbred may have an increased incidence, retinal dysplasia is not an inherited condition in the horse.

Etiology/pathophysiology

Retinal dysplasia can be caused by problems with in-utero ocular development or inflammation or it may be seen with perinatal trauma.

Abnormal induction by an inherently defective RPE or from necrosis of the developing retina can result in the failure of proper apposition of the two layers of the optic cup. Abnormal neurosensory differentiation by dysplastic RPE and abnormal attempts at regeneration in a retina that has undergone necrosis can lead to the formation of rosette-like structures or multifocal disorganization in the neurosensory retina. Retinal nonattachment or complete retinal detachment occurs early in embryogenesis due to an abnormal involution of the optic vesicle. This severe failure of contact between the two layers of the optic cup tends to be associated with multiple and severe congenital ocular anomalies.

Clinical presentation

Retinal dysplasia may be seen as single or multiple gray, linear, vermiform-like streaks or larger lesions in the tapetal or nontapetal fundus. A detached retina may also be present, observed as a floating gray veil of opaque tissue in the vitreous behind a typically dilated pupil in severe cases. Other congenital ocular anomalies may also be present.

Differential diagnosis

Active chorioretinitis (seen in foals born to mares suffering from systemic disease during late gestation), retinal scars (that will appear as small, circular lesions with a hyper-pigmented center and a depigmented peripheral ring), and retinal hemorrhages (usually incidental and due to a difficult birth) should be easily differentiated from retinal dysplasia.

Diagnosis

Definitive diagnosis is based on clinical identification on ophthalmoscopy and/or histopathologic evaluation revealing rosettes of neural tissue.

Management

There is no treatment.

Prognosis

Vision is usually not impaired with this condition (except in severe cases, such as those with retinal detachment).

Congenital stationary night blindness

Definition/overview

CSNB is an inherited condition in the Appaloosa and possibly in the Thoroughbred, Paso Fino, Standardbred, and Quarter horse. Affected animals have limited vision in the dark (scotopic); daylight (photopic) vision is usually unaffected. No lesions are visible on ophthalmic examination.

Etiology/pathophysiology

CSNB is an inherited autosomal or sex-linked recessive trait in affected breeds. CSNB in the Appaloosa is associated with leopard complex coat-spotting patterns, which are determined by a single autosomal dominant locus, the leopard complex locus (LP). Appaloosas that are homozygous (LP/LP) are affected with CSNB, whereas heterozygous (LP/lp) and wild type horses (lp/lp) are not affected by CSNB. Appaloosa horses with a chocolate coat color are most often affected.

A defect in neural transmission between the photoreceptors and the bipolar cells within the retina has been suggested as the cause of vision problems in horses with CSNB. It has been suggested that down-regulation of the gene TRPM1 may be responsible for CSNB and leopard-spotting patterns in the Appaloosa.

Clinical presentation

Animals with CSNB usually exhibit visual impairment or blindness in reduced illumination, with normal vision in light conditions, although day vision may also be absent in the most severe cases. A normal ophthalmoscopic examination, including fundic evaluation, is present. Affected animals may appear disoriented, stare off into space, seek lighted conditions, and may have bilateral dorsomedial strabismus, nystagmus, and/or subtle microphthalmos.

Differential diagnosis

Other causes of visual deficits or blindness in the horse must be ruled out (e.g. corneal disease, cataracts, glaucoma, retinal disease, CNS disease).

Diagnosis

Diagnosis of CSNB is made on history, observing visual impairment in a poorly lit (scotopic) obstacle course, and a normal ophthalmoscopic examination. The diagnosis is confirmed with an ERG that shows a large negative a wave.

Management
There is currently no treatment available for CSNB. Affected animals are unsound and should not be used for breeding.

Prognosis
CSNB is typically a static, nonprogressive disease.

Optic nerve hypoplasia
Definition/overview
Optic nerve hypoplasia involves underdevelopment of the optic nerve and is seen clinically as a smaller than normal optic disk. Optic nerve hypoplasia is rare, but when it occurs it is most often seen in the Quarter horse or Appaloosa breeds. It may be unilateral or bilateral, with animals exhibiting near normal vision to total blindness depending on the severity. It may occasionally be diagnosed as a single entity, but is usually seen with other ocular abnormalities.

Etiology/pathophysiology
The cause is unknown. Optic nerve hypoplasia is believed to result from a congenital lack of proper development and differentiation or severe destruction of the retinal ganglion cells. This may occur as a result of viral, toxic, genetic, or idiopathic retinal disease.

Clinical presentation
Smaller optic disks, either unilateral or bilateral, are noted on fundic examination. Mydriasis may be noted, with slow or absent PLRs. Usually, the hypoplasia is mild and vision appears unaffected; however, horses with extensive lesions may be visually impaired or blind. A searching nystagmus can be seen and other ocular defects (multiple ocular anomalies), such as retinal dysplasia and microphthalmia, may be observed.

Differential diagnosis
The differential diagnosis for this condition in the older animal is optic nerve atrophy due to previous optic neuritis or optic nerve trauma.

Diagnosis
Optic nerve hypoplasia is diagnosed based on fundoscopic identification of a small optic disk, which is often pale or dark gray. If the condition is unilateral, the diagnosis is made by direct comparison with the contralateral optic nerve.

Management
There is no treatment.

Prognosis
This disease is nonprogressive.

Ocular manifestations of neonatal septicemia
Definition/overview
Foals with septicemia may exhibit associated ocular signs including anterior uveitis, chorioretinitis, and panuveitis. Neonatal septicemia is covered in depth elsewhere (see p. 970).

Etiology/pathophysiology
A number of microorganisms have been reported to cause neonatal septicemia in the horse, in particular *Escherichia coli, Streptococcus* spp., *Pasteurella* spp., *Salmonella* spp., *Actinobacillus equuli,* and *Klebsiella* spp.

Pathophysiology
Ocular lesions occur following breakdown of the BOB and entry of bacteria into the ocular tissues.

Clinical presentation
Ocular lesions may include anterior uveitis, chorioretinitis, endophthalmitis, and panophthalmitis (1129). Multifocal hemorrhages, exudates, and focal detachments may be seen in the retina.

Differential diagnosis
Other etiologies of secondary ocular abnormalities should be considered.

Diagnosis
A clinical diagnosis of the ocular lesions is made based on a thorough ophthalmic examination. The ocular lesions are nonspecific and additional testing is required for a definitive diagnosis of sepsis.

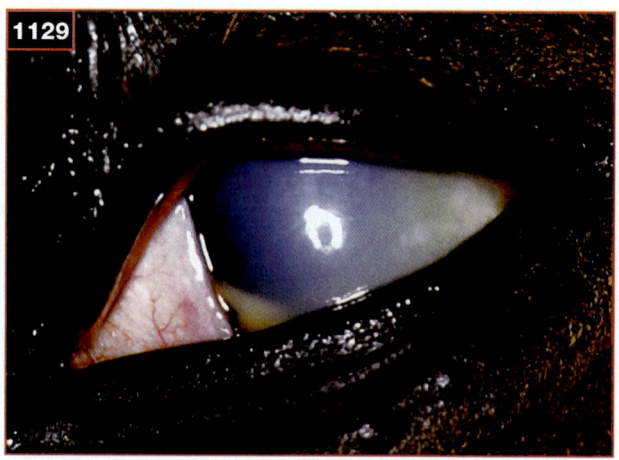

1129 Endophthalmitis in a septicemic neonatal foal. Corneal edema and hypopyon are present in this severely inflamed eye.

Management

Topical prednisolone acetate (or dexamethasone), atropine sulfate, and antimicrobials (with good corneal penetration) are administered if anterior uveitis is present. Systemic antimicrobials should be used based ideally on culture and sensitivity testing results. Systemic NSAIDs should be given to help control inflammation and counteract the changes associated with endotoxemic and septic shock. Other components of therapy are discussed elsewhere (see p. 971).

Prognosis

The prognosis for foals with neonatal septicemia is guarded. In those animals that survive, ocular lesions such as posterior synechiae and chorioretinal scars may be observed.

Tumors of the eye, orbit, and adnexa

Periocular sarcoids

Definition/overview

Sarcoids are the most common tumor in horses and the second most common tumor of the equine eye and adnexa. They may present as solitary or, more often, multiple masses and may be typed clinically as occult, verrucous (hyperkeratotic fibropapilloma), nodular types A and B, fibroblastic types A and B, mixed, or malignant. The medial canthus and/or upper eyelid are the most often affected, with a lower incidence in the lateral canthus and/or lower eyelid. Sarcoids are locally aggressive, but they are only very rarely malignant. They usually affect horses 7 years of age or less with no gender or coat color predilection. There is reported to be a higher incidence in Arabians, Appaloosas, Thoroughbreds, and Quarter horses.

Etiology/pathophysiology

The cause of equine sarcoids is uncertain; however, bovine papilloma virus and C-type retrovirus have been implicated. Sarcoids may occur at the site of previous trauma and areas that come into contact with pre-existing sarcoids. There is also a strong familial predisposition, but a genetic or inherited component has not been established. Direct contact, an arthropod vector (e.g. flies), or fomites may play a role in transmission by translocating sarcoid cells into open wounds. The fibroblastic types are especially aggressive locally and verrucous tumors can convert to fibroblastic types following intervention.

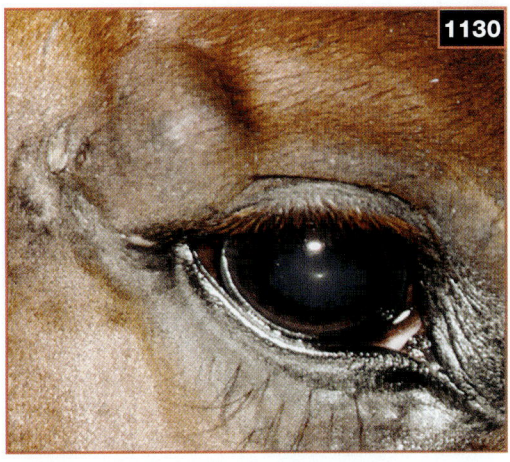

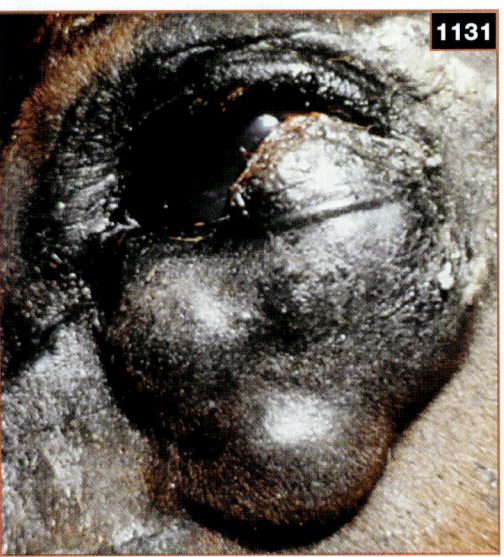

1130, 1131 Nodular sarcoids are common in the periocular region of the horse (1130) and can be extensive (1131). (Photos courtesy A Gemensky-Metzler [1130] and American College of Veterinary Ophthalmologists [1131])

Clinical presentation

Equine sarcoids have a variable appearance. Occult sarcoids can appear as small, subepidermal, miliary nodules or plaques that are hairless or have altered hair. Verrucous sarcoids can appear partially or totally hairless, rough, and wart- or cauliflower-like, with miliary nodules and/or thickened areas that may be ulcerated. Nodular sarcoids are typically solid, smooth, and spherical or ovoid, with a well-defined outline (1130, 1131). They may be entirely subcutaneous or a variable amount of the overlying skin may be involved. Fibroblastic sarcoids are fleshy masses that resemble granulation tissue ('proud flesh'). They may be pedunculated or have a broader base with ill-defined margins, and they can be ulcerated. Mixed sarcoids encompass the characteristics of a combination of two or more of the above lesion types. Malignant sarcoids are very rare. They may be characterized by nodules and cords of abnormal tissue and typically grow at a much faster rate. Periocular sarcoids may cause secondary corneal ulceration or nasolacrimal duct obstruction. The tumors themselves are not painful or pruritic.

Differential diagnosis

Differential diagnoses for periorbital sarcoids include other neoplasms such as SCC, papilloma, fibroma, fibrosarcoma, neurofibroma, neurofibrosarcoma, schwannoma, melanoma, myxosarcoma, fibromyxosarcoma, and dermoids, as well as cutaneous habronemiasis (parasitic granuloma), any non-neoplastic granulation tissue (e.g. exuberant granulation tissue/'proud flesh', bacterial granuloma, foreign body reaction), dermatophilosis (rain scald), subcutaneous or deep fungal infections, dermatophytosis (ringworm), abscesses, traumatic superficial abrasions or scratches, rub marks, scarring, sebaceous cysts, alopecia areata, and idiopathic periorbital vitiligo.

Diagnosis

The clinical appearance of the tumor may be suggestive. Although it can be challenging for pathologists, definitive diagnosis is made based on histopathology examination following tumor removal. Partial excision or biopsy is contraindicated because it may activate the lesion.

Management

Treatment will depend on the size, location, and type of the sarcoid, with consideration of the equipment available and the financial constraints of the owner. Benign neglect may be chosen, as some lesions will spontaneously regress, but this may take years. Sarcoids may be removed with a scalpel or via carbon dioxide laser excision; however, periorbital sarcoids are highly infiltrative, resulting in a high rate of recurrence when treated with excision alone. This infiltrative nature also contributes to aggressive tumor regrowth when sarcoids are partially excised or biopsied. Surgical debulking or excision should, therefore, be accompanied by adjunctive therapy such as cryotherapy, radiofrequency hyperthermia, immunomodulation, chemotherapy, or radiation.

Cryotherapy is simple, rapid, and inexpensive. It typically involves the application of 2–3 rapid freeze–thaw cycles using nitrous oxide or a liquid nitrogen cryoprobe or spray. Thermocouple needles are placed 0.5 cm from the tumor margin and below the base of the tumor to monitor the tissue temperature. The tissue temperature must reach $-20°$ to $-30°C$ and be followed by a slow thaw to be most effective. Cryotherapy has been shown to be useful for verrucous or occult sarcoids that are <2 cm^2; however, a high overall recurrence rate has also been reported. Treated tissue typically becomes edematous, necrotic, and sloughs. This is followed by second-intention healing over several weeks. Depigmentation of the treated area is also expected after cryosurgery.

Radiofrequency hyperthermia involves heating the tumor tissue to 50°C for 30 seconds at 4-day intervals for a total of four treatments. Radiofrequency hyperthermia has only a limited ability to treat deeper tissues.

Bacillus Calmette–Guérin (BCG) immunomodulation requires treatment using 25 gauge needles to inject 1 ml/cm^3 BCG into the tumor tissue. This is repeated every 2–4 weeks for up to six injections. A mild to severe inflammatory tissue reaction may occur and anaphylaxis has also been reported. Pretreatment with intravenous flunixin meglumine (1.1 mg/kg i/v) and systemic corticosteroids can minimize these effects. There have been reports of 100% success rates when surgical debulking is followed by intralesional BCG administration.

Intralesional cisplatin or 5-fluorouracil (5-FU) chemotherapy may be useful for fibroblastic or nodular lesions. Intralesional cisplatin chemotherapy is administered at a dose of 1 mg/cm^3 for up to four doses at 2-week intervals. 5-FU (50 mg/ml with 1:1 sesame oil) may be administered at a dose of 1 ml/cm^3 lesion. Topical 5-FU and mitomycin have also been used to treat sarcoids, although anaphylaxis has been reported.

Interstitial brachytherapy irradiation using iridium^{192} implants can be administered over 10–14 days for a total dose of 7,000–9,000 rads. Cesium^{137}, radon^{222}, gold^{198}, iodine^{125}, and cobalt^{60} have also been used with varying success. Beta strontium^{90} irradiation can be applied to smaller tumors twice daily over 5 days for a total dose of 10,000 rads. Generally, radiation treatment appears to have an excellent outcome, but it does not penetrate tissue deeper than 1–2 mm, is expensive, and is potentially dangerous for handlers.

Enucleation or exenteration may be required for extensive periocular tumors. Sliding H-plasty advancement flaps, partial orbital rim resection, mesh skin expansion, and second-intention healing are a few of the options available for closing large periocular wounds.

Prognosis

The prognosis for equine periorbital sarcoids is variable depending on the size, location, and type of sarcoid, as well as the treatment modality chosen. While some regress spontaneously, the prognosis is generally guarded.

Although they only rarely metastasize, it is often impossible to remove periocular sarcoids completely while allowing for wound closure. This leads to high rates of recurrence, especially with excision alone. Extensive occult and verrucous or mixed sarcoids are the most difficult to treat. Cases that are unsuccessfully treated several times have a poorer prognosis regardless of tumor type or the treatment modality used. Research has shown that there is a significantly greater probability of local recurrence when the surgical margins are positive for bovine papilloma virus DNA. The lowest recurrence rate has been reported in those cases of periocular sarcoids treated with immunotherapy or brachytherapy intralesionally.

Periocular/cutaneous squamous cell carcinomas

Definition/overview
Cutaneous SCCs are the second most common tumor in the horse and the most common tumor of the equine eye and adnexa. The prevalence increases with age, with Appaloosas, Paints, Pintos, and draft horses (e.g. Belgians, Clydesdales) at higher risk. Horses with white, gray, and palomino coat colors are predisposed. SCCs occur predominately in middle-aged to older horses. Tumors are commonly located on the eyelid, nictitating membrane, conjunctiva, cornea, and/or limbus, in one or both eyes. They are locally invasive and, rarely, will metastasize to regional lymph nodes, salivary glands, and the lungs.

Etiology/pathophysiology
The cause of ocular SCCs is unknown, but it is likely multifactorial. Prolonged exposure to ultraviolet (UV) radiation, increased altitude and latitude, and nonpigmented or lightly pigmented ocular and periocular structures appear to increase susceptibility to SCC. Other pathogenic factors include exposure to mechanical irritants and papillomavirus

Although the pathophysiology is unknown, lesions typically progress from noncancerous plaques to papillomas to carcinomas *in situ* prior to transforming into SCC. These SCC tumors can then invade locally and/or metastasize.

Clinical presentation
Clinical signs will depend on the anatomic location and stage of development. Tumors may appear as well-circumscribed, small, white, elevated, hyperplastic plaques. Ocular SCCs may also appear as raised, rough, irregular pinkish-white warty or cauliflower-like structures with a broad base of attachment. They can appear ulcerated and necrotic, with lesions that may bleed easily (1132–1134). They can also be invasive or infiltrative. Tumors involving the nictitating membrane may present as

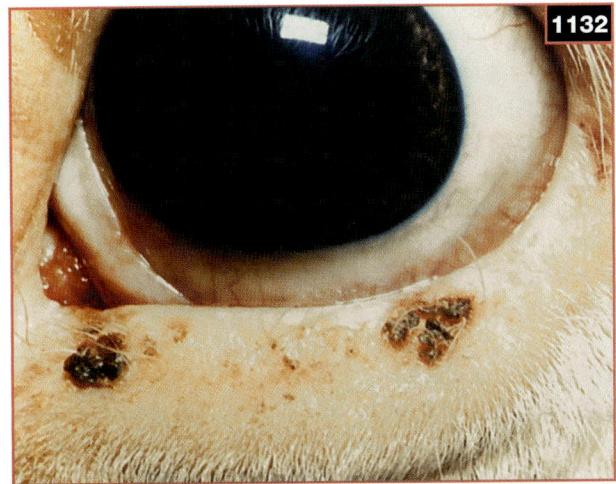

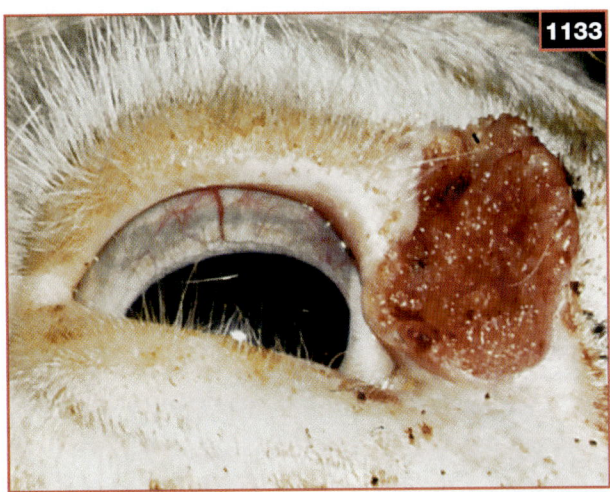

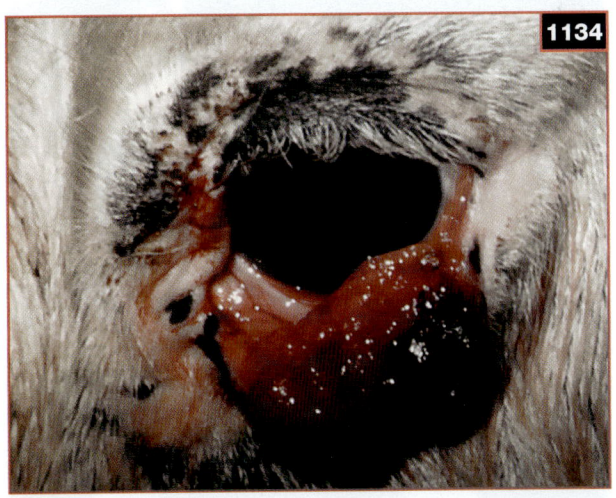

1132–1134 Squamous cell carcinoma of the eyelid. (1132) Early, superficial lesions can be categorized as plaques or squamous cell carcinoma *in situ*. (1133, 1134) Advanced eyelid lesions have deeper involvement and are consequently more challenging to treat.

inconspicuous, small lesions on the leading edge (1135). Extension of the mass to involve deeper aspects of the third eyelid is common and can only be appreciated by retropulsing the globe to expose the surface of the nictitans (1136). Limbal SCCs often appear as a raised, vascularized, gray-white corneal opacity with associated conjunctival hyperemia and thickening (1137). SCCs may also invade the orbit, leading to signs associated with retrobulbar masses (e.g. exophthalmos, lagophthalmos, exposure keratitis).

Differential diagnosis

Depending on the location, differential diagnoses should include granulation tissue, abscesses, habronemiasis, cutaneous onchocerciasis, *Thelazia* infestation, bacterial and fungal granulomas, foreign body reactions, dermoids, and other neoplasms such as sarcoids, papillomas, adenomas, adenocarcinomas, melanomas, mast cell tumors, basal cell tumors, fibromas, fibrosarcomas, lymphomas, lymphosarcomas, histiocytomas, schwannomas, angiosarcomas, neurofibromas, trichoepitheliomas, hemangiomas, hemangiosarcomas, myxosarcomas, and plasma cell tumors.

Diagnosis

SCC should be considered with any persistent proliferative or ulcerative eyelid lesion. The clinical appearance may be suggestive, but definitive diagnosis is based on cytology (fine-needle aspirate [FNA] or scrapings) or histology (incisional/wedge or excisional biopsy). This typically shows cords and/or islands of polyhedral cells with intercellular bridges, lack of basal lamina, keratinized 'pearls',

1135, 1136 Squamous cell carcinoma of the nictitans. (1135) Only the leading edge of the nictitans appears affected. (1136) With retropulsion of the globe, the nictitans is elevated, demonstrating deeper tissue involvement.

1137 The temporal corneoscleral limbus is a predisposed location for squamous cell carcinoma. A pink, fleshy mass is apparent laterally, invading the cornea.

1138 An eye with limbal squamous cell carcinoma following debulking, superficial keratectomy, and CO_2 laser ablation as adjunctive therapy to increase the likelihood of destroying any neoplastic cells not removed by debulking.

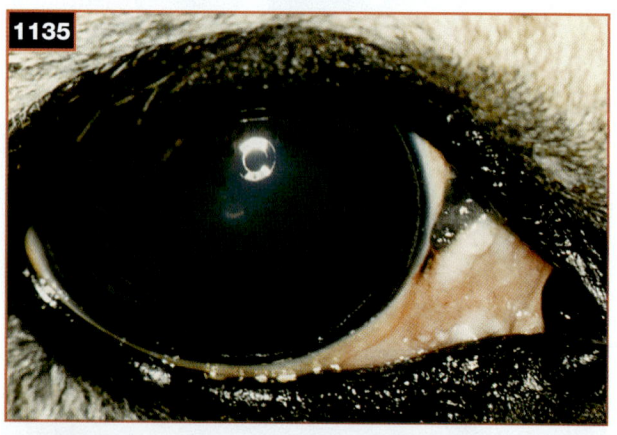

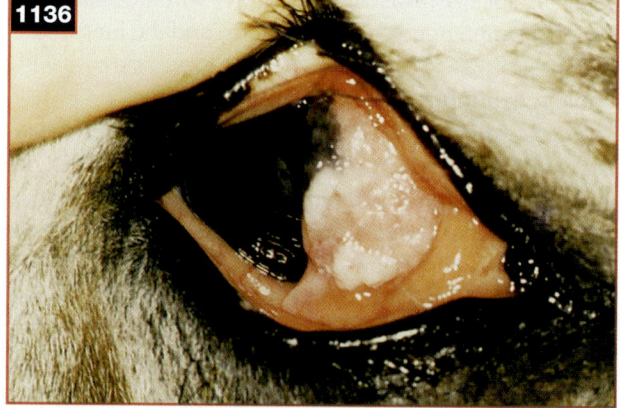

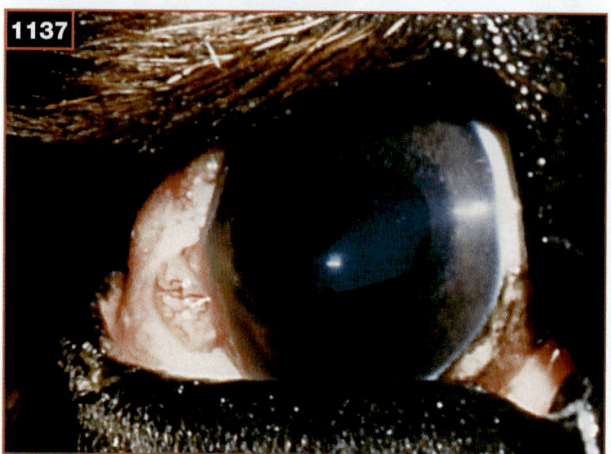

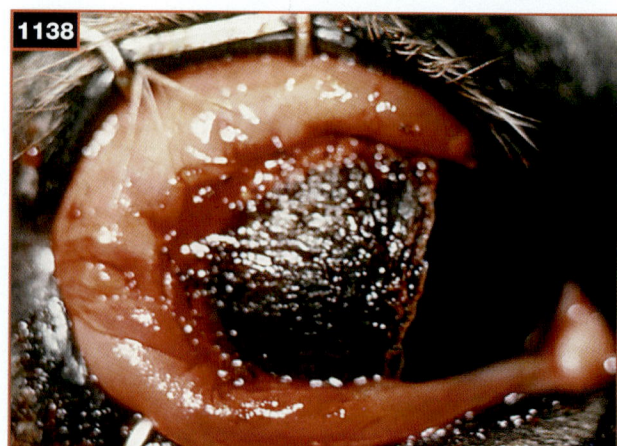

and mitotic figures. The use of urinalysis test strips to detect occult blood in the tears in order to differentiate corneal and/or conjunctival SCC from granulation tissue has also been advocated.

Management

Therapy varies with tumor size, location, extent of invasion, visual status, intended use of the animal, the equipment available, and financial constraints. Surgical debulking or excision followed by cryotherapy, radiofrequency hyperthermia, immunomodulation (i.e. Bacillus Calmette–Guérin or BCG), intralesional chemotherapy (i.e. cisplatin), and radiation therapy may be performed. For extensive cases involving the eyelids, globe, and/or orbit, exenteration (surgical removal of all orbital contents) is recommended. Beta radiation is most beneficial, following keratectomy or penetrating keratoplasty, in superficial SCC of the cornea and/or limbus. Carbon dioxide laser ablation may also be used for limbal SCCs (**1138**).

Prognosis

The prognosis is variable depending on the size and location of the tumor, as well as the treatment modality selected. In general there is a good overall prognosis for survival; however, SCCs are usually locally aggressive and may invade orbital soft tissues and/or bone. They can also metastasize to regional lymph nodes, salivary glands, and the thorax. Tumor size is inversely related to survival, with more extensive tumors carrying a poorer prognosis. Tumor location influences survival, with eyelid and orbital SCCs carrying a poorer prognosis than those located on the third eyelid or limbus. Recurrence can be high (>30%), especially when the eyelid or nictating membrane is affected, and one or more recurrences of SCC following therapy also markedly decreases the survival time; therefore, early follow-up is recommended, with repeated treatment as necessary. The incidence and recurrence of ocular SCC can be reduced by decreasing exposure to UV radiation, using sports sunscreen, and using hoods or protective fly masks. Tattooing nonpigmented eyelids and margins of the third eyelid has been shown not to be effective in preventing or decreasing the incidence of SCC, as the ink is subepithelial and does not provide any protection to the epithelial cells from UV light.

Melanoma
Definition/overview

Melanomas are primary neoplasms of the equine eye and adnexa that involve neoplastic melanocytes. They may present as single or multiple, usually darkly pigmented, dense masses. They most commonly affect the ocular adnexa, but may also affect the orbit, epibulbar tissue, conjunctiva, cornea, and uveal tissue (iris, ciliary body, or choroid). Most are slow growing and benign, but they may, after years, transform into malignant tumors. Malignant melanomas grow rapidly and will metastasize to regional lymph nodes, lungs, spleen, and liver. Hematogenous spread may also occur.

Etiology/pathophysiology

The cause is uncertain. The incidence increases with age, with melanomas being rare in horses less than 6 years old. They usually occur in gray or white horses, with Arabians, Lipizzaners, and Percherons exhibiting an increased risk. Melanomas rarely occur in horses with colored haircoats. Approximately 80% of gray horses older than 15 years of age are affected by melanomas.

The pathophysiology appears to be related to lightly pigmented or nonpigmented ocular and periocular tissues. It has been suggested that a disturbance in melanin metabolism, possibly associated with graying, may lead to tumor formation. An aberrant immune response or cytotoxic reaction with subsequent local destruction of normal melanocytes has been implicated. Intraocular melanomas may cause uveitis with secondary cataract formation and/or secondary glaucoma due to their interference with the ICA.

Clinical presentation

Melanomas may appear as firm or soft, dome-shaped, hairless, gray or black pigmented masses on the eyelid (**1139**), conjunctiva, and cornea, or, rarely, intraocularly. They may occasionally be unpigmented. Solitary or multiple masses

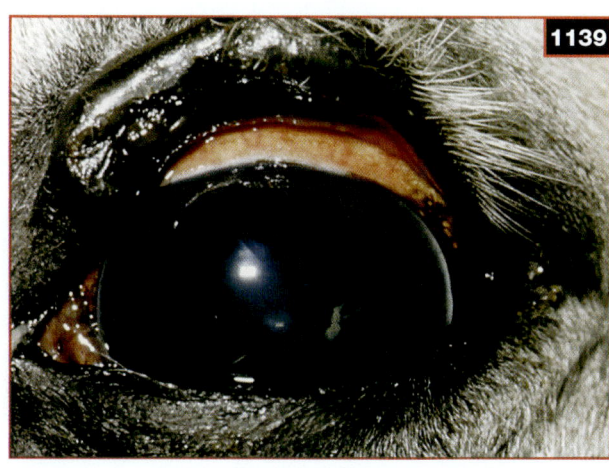

1139 Melanoma involving the upper eyelid in a gray horse. There are several coalescing nodules. (Photo courtesy R Morreale)

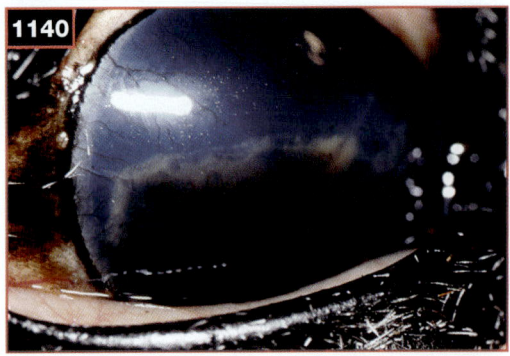

1140 Uveal melanoma with secondary glaucoma. The mass can be seen as it conforms to the back of the cornea. Glaucoma was present, associated with diffuse mass extension into the iridocorneal angle.

may be found and they may be ulcerated and infected. They are most frequently reported as locally expansive and destructive. They may be slowly or rapidly expanding. Anterior uveal melanomas may cause secondary pupil distortion or obliterate the anterior chamber (**1140**). Uveitis, cataract formation, and secondary glaucoma may develop.

Differential diagnosis
Extraocular melanomas must be differentiated from sarcoids, hemangiomas, hemangiosarcomas, dermoids, SCCs, granulomas, and abscesses. Orbital melanomas must be differentiated from other orbital neoplasms and other causes of retrobulbar disease. Differential diagnoses for intraocular melanomas include uveal cysts.

Diagnosis
Melanomas are diagnosed based on the history, ophthalmic examination, cytology (from scrapings or FNA), and histopathology. They may be categorized as benign or malignant, using the mitotic index. Intraocular melanomas may be differentiated from anterior uveal cysts by using a focused beam of light (e.g. transilluminator) and/or high-frequency ultrasonography.

Management
Surgical excision may be used alone or in combination with adjunctive therapies, including cryosurgery, radiofrequency hyperthermia, immunotherapy, radiation, and intralesional chemotherapy, depending on tumor size and location as well as the equipment available and financial constraints. Surgical excision may be curative for small extraocular melanomas. Intratumoral chemotherapy with cisplatin is best given at the time of, or immediately after, surgical resection in order to limit the amount of tumor repopulation that may occur during the treatment interval

and improve overall efficacy. Long-term cimetidine (2.5 mg/kg p/o q8h) has also been used, alone and in combination, in the treatment of cutaneous melanomas to limit or stop the progression of the tumor. It has been shown to be beneficial in some horses by decreasing the size or number of melanomas. If clinical improvement does not occur within 3 months, the cimetidine may be discontinued.

Intraocular melanomas may be monitored for progression or surgically excised via iridocyclectomy. Enucleation or exenteration is recommended in certain cases where the tumor is extensive or secondary intraocular changes cause blindness or chronic pain.

Prognosis
The prognosis will depend on the location, size, and extent of the melanoma as well as the treatment modality chosen. Generally, melanomas have a good prognosis, as they are typically slow growing and benign; however, they can be locally aggressive and metastasize. In contrast to epibulbar melanomas, conjunctival melanomas are often aggressive and should be considered potentially malignant. An increase in length of the surgical scar, generally associated with an increase in tumor size, is associated with a poorer prognosis. In general, the longer the interval between surgery and intralesional cisplatin chemotherapy treatment, the more opportunity is provided for tumor regrowth to occur. It is therefore advantageous to keep the interval between surgery and intralesional cisplatin therapy as short as possible.

Lymphosarcoma
Definition/overview
Lymphosarcoma (LSA) is the most common systemic neoplasm affecting the equine eye or adnexa. LSA is a life-threatening neoplastic disease of the lymphoreticular tissue capable of involving any system or body organ, alone or in combination. Approximately one quarter of horses with systemic LSA will develop lesions of the eye or ocular adnexa.

Etiology/pathophysiology
This is a metastatic neoplastic disease of the adnexa and eye. The cause is unknown. Systemic involvement typically may proceed or accompany ocular lymphosarcoma.

Clinical presentation
Ocular manifestations of lymphosarcoma include: serous or mucopurulent discharge; diffuse retrobulbar infiltrates leading to exophthalmos, lagophthalmos, and exposure keratitis; third eyelid masses; neoplastic infiltrate of the palpebral conjunctiva; conjunctivitis; chemosis; conjunctival hemorrhage; corneoscleral masses; corneal neovascularization; edema and/or ulceration; anterior uveitis; hyphema; hypopyon; secondary glaucoma; chorioretinitis;

and retinal detachment. Lymph node enlargement and signs of visceral involvement may also be present.

Differential diagnosis
Other causes of conjunctivitis, corneal ulceration, anterior uveitis, hyphema, retinal detachment, chorioretinitis, glaucoma, and orbital disease should be considered.

Diagnosis
The history and clinical presentation can be suggestive for LSA. Cytologic samples provided via FNAs or histopathology of biopsy samples of affected periocular tissues, regional or enlarged lymph nodes, and/or bone marrow can provide a definitive diagnosis.

Management
There is no specific treatment for LSA, therefore affected horses are only treated supportively. Palliative care may involve enucleation or exenteration.

Prognosis
The overall prognosis for survival is poor. The majority of affected horses die within 6–12 months.

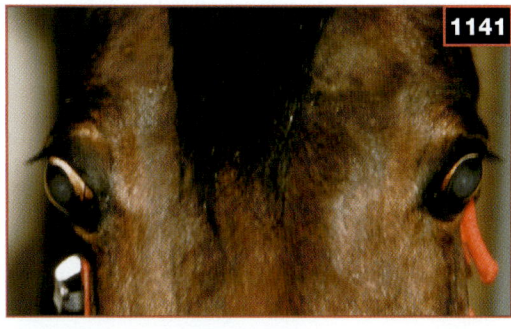

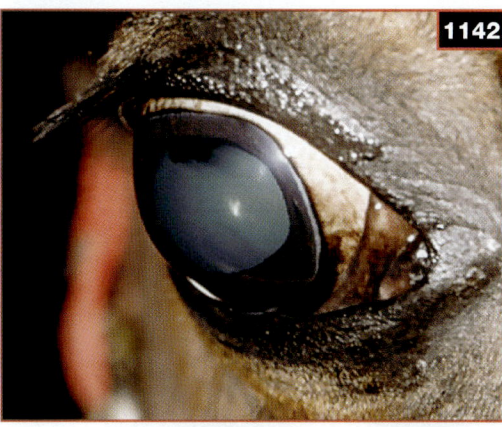

1141, 1142 Exophthalmos affecting the right eye (1141). The affected eye has globe protrusion, increased exposure of the sclera, mild lateral strabismus, and a fixed, dilated pupil (1142).

TABLE 56 **Types of orbital neoplasia**
• Sarcoid
• Squamous cell carcinoma
• Adenocarcinoma
• Multilobular osteoma
• Lymphosarcoma
• Fibroma/Fibrosarcoma
• Hemangioma/hemangiosarcoma
• Melanoma
• Lipoma
• Angiosarcoma
• Granulocytic carcinoma
• Neuroendocrine tumor
• Microglioma
• Medulloepithelioma
• Neuroepithelial carcinoma
• Osteoclastoma
• Extra-adrenal paraganglioma
• Neurofibromas (schwannoma, neurilemmoma)
• Undifferentiated carcinomas
• Mast cell tumor

Orbital neoplasia

Definition/overview
Orbital neoplasia may be primary, secondary, or metastatic. Primary orbital tumors may arise from any orbital tissue and are typically malignant. Secondary orbital neoplasia can involve local extension of masses from adjacent structures. Metastatic and multicentric neoplasia of the orbit can also occur in horses. Orbital neoplasia is usually unilateral, although bilateral tumors do occur occasionally.

Etiology/pathophysiology
The cause is largely unknown. Most orbital tumors are primary and highly malignant (*Table 56*). Primary malignant cell types predominate. Orbital neoplasia may also result from invasion by neoplasms of the nasal or paranasal sinuses, extension from adjacent structures, or metastases from distant sites.

Clinical presentation
Orbital neoplasms in the horse typically manifest as slowly progressive, often painless, unilateral exophthalmos, with varying amounts of globe displacement (strabismus), lagophthalmos, and secondary exposure keratitis (1141, 1142). Conjunctival hyperemia, blepharedema, elevated third eyelid, mydriatic pupil, and resistance to retropulsion

845

may be present. Facial and/or periorbital swelling, decreased air passage through the nostril(s), serosanguineous nasal discharge, and vision impairment may also be seen. The menace response and/or PLR may be normal, decreased, or absent. A soft tissue mass may be detected in the retrobulbar space when the orbit is palpated over the supraorbital fossa. There is often a decreased or absent ability to retropulse the globe. Occasionally, scleral indentation is visible on ophthalmoscopy.

Differential diagnosis

Orbital abscesses, orbital cellulitis, chronic sinusitis, salivary gland mucoceles, trauma, retrobulbar hemorrhage/hematoma, orbital foreign body, guttural pouch mycosis, guttural pouch empyema, retrobulbar hydatid cyst, fungal granuloma, orbital varixes, and EIA should be considered as differential diagnoses.

Diagnosis

Diagnosis is based on history, clinical presentation, cytologic examination and culture and sensitivity of discharge or FNA from the orbit, biopsy of masses, survey radiography, orbital angiography, dacryocystorhinography, and/or ultrasonography. When available, MRI and CT are invaluable when evaluating orbital disease.

Management

Early exenteration is generally the therapy of choice unless the orbital tumor is well circumscribed.

Prognosis

The prognosis is generally poor to guarded because most orbital tumors in horses are primary and highly malignant.

Infectious/inflammatory disorders of the eye

Conjunctivitis

Definition/overview

Inflammation of the conjunctiva is called conjunctivitis. It may be caused by a variety of primary etiologies or be secondary to systemic disease.

Etiology/pathophysiology

The causes of conjunctivitis are wide and varied (*Table 57*). The normal microflora of the equine conjunctiva is variable depending on the season and geographic location, and includes bacterial and fungal organisms such as *Staphylococcus aureus*, *Moraxella equi*, and *Streptococcus zooepidemicus*, and *Corynebacterium*, *Bacillus*, *Aspergillus*, *Penicillium*, *Alternaria*, and *Cladosporium* spp. Conjunctivitis can occur when there is a change in the normal conjunctival flora that allows either opportunistic commensal or pathologic organisms to cause disease; however, not all causes are infectious.

Clinical presentation

Epiphora, conjunctival hyperemia, conjunctival edema (chemosis), conjunctival thickening, and follicles on the palpebral and/or bulbar conjunctiva or third eyelid may be present (**1143**).

Differential diagnosis

Other causes of conjunctival hyperemia or 'red eye' should be considered.

Diagnosis

Conjunctival cytology and/or culture and sensitivity, as well as STT results can be used to diagnosis various causes of conjunctivitis. A full ophthalmic and clinical examination is important because conjunctivitis can occur as a component of other ocular abnormalities and/or systemic disease.

1143 This right eye had a chronic foreign body in the lower conjunctival fornix, which led to chronic conjunctivitis with lower eyelid swelling, generalized conjunctival hyperemia and edema (chemosis), and a mucopurulent ocular discharge. (Photo courtesy GA Munroe)

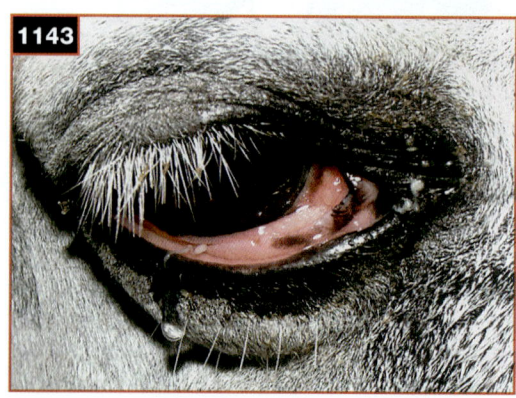

Management

Specific treatment will vary depending on the underlying cause of the conjunctivitis. Topical corticosteroids may be used if no corneal ulcer is present. Topical antimicrobials may also be used alone or in combination with corticosteroids. The NLS should be flushed to ensure normal patency, as dacryocystitis can exacerbate conjunctivitis.

Prognosis

The prognosis is poor to excellent depending on the cause.

Keratoconjunctivitis sicca

Definition/overview

KCS is uncommon in the horse. Clinical signs are similar to those found in other species with this disease.

Etiology/pathophysiology

The cause of KCS in most cases is unknown, but trauma to the head or orbital region leading to facial nerve paralysis is the most common cause of equine KCS. It may also be caused by lacrimal gland dysfunction via toxic effects on lacrimal glandular tissue because of locoweed poisoning or chemical exposure. Eosinophilic dacryoadenitis has also been reported. Topical atropine and other medications can also temporarily decrease lacrimation.

Regardless of the etiology, KCS involves a reduction in tear production, which can result in superficial corneal damage, delayed epithelial healing, and exposure of the corneal stroma. Secondary infections can occur.

Clinical presentation

Blepharospasm, mucopurulent ocular discharge, conjunctivitis, keratitis, corneal ulcers, corneal perforations, and panophthalmitis are common.

Differential diagnosis

Any cause of chronic keratitis and/or conjunctivitis should be considered.

Diagnosis

History, clinical signs, and STT should be diagnostic.

Management

The underlying cause should be treated if possible. Any sequelae (e.g. corneal ulceration) must also be treated appropriately. An antimicrobial/steroid combination topical medication may be helpful to treat the inflammation and secondary bacterial invaders in some cases (e.g. neomycin sulfate/polymyxin B sulfate/dexamethasone 0.1% [or triple antibiotic/steroid combination solution or ointment] q4–12h). It is vital that corneal ulceration is ruled out prior to using corticosteroids. A topically applied tear lubricant should be used frequently to prevent the

conjunctiva and cornea from drying out. Topical cyclosporine is a lacrimomimetic in horses. Parotid duct transpositions have been attempted in horses.

Prognosis

If KCS is acute and the only disease process present, the prognosis is favorable, as most cases are transient and of unknown etiology. Appropriate management of the condition to ensure the maintenance of corneal health is paramount, but this can lead to problems with owner and/or patient noncompliance. A poor prognosis is given to those horses with KCS secondary to facial paralysis. Panophthalmitis after perforation of the globe due to decreased tear production has a poor prognosis.

TABLE 57 Common etiologies of conjunctivitis

- Bacterial
  - *Streptococcus equi, Actinobacillus* spp., *Chlamydia, Rhodococcus* spp., *Moraxella equi, Leptospira* spp.
- Viral
  - Adenovirus, EHV-1 (rhinopneumonitis), EHV-2 (cytomegalovirus), EHV4?, EIA, EVA, equine influenza type A2, parainfluenza, African horse sickness (reovirus)
- Mycotic
  - *Histoplasma capsulatum* var. *farciminosum* (also called called *H. farciminosum*), *H. capsulatum*, sporotrichosis, blastomycosis
- Parasitic
  - *Habronema muscae, H. microstoma, Draschia megastoma, Onchocerca cervicalis*
- Allergic
- Follicular
- Systemic causes
  - Pneumonia, equine protozoal myeloencephalitis, polyneuritis equi, vestibular disease syndrome, epizootic lymphangitis
- Eosinophilic keratoconjunctivitis
- Trauma
- Foreign body
- Entropion
- Dacryocystitis
- Environmental irritants/chemical irritation
- Neonatal maladjustment syndrome, neonatal septicemia, immune-mediated hemolytic anemia
- Keratoconjunctivitis sicca
- Lymphosarcoma
- Idiopathic/immune-mediated

Corneal ulcers/ulcerative keratitis

Definition/overview

The large, prominent, laterally placed equine eye, the behavioral tendencies of the horse, and an environment rich in bacterial and fungal organisms predispose to traumatic corneal injury and secondary infection. Breaks in the corneal epithelium (corneal ulcers) are very common in the horse. Corneal ulcers are typically classified based on etiology, depth, the presence of complicating factors such as infection or collagenase activity, and the rate of progression. Melting ulcers are rapidly deepening ulcers caused by collagenase enzymes that destroy the corneal stroma. Ulcers that have progressed to the level of Descemet's membrane and are on the verge of perforating are called descemetoceles. Corneal ulcers can be sight threatening, requiring early diagnosis and appropriate, prompt medical and surgical management to avoid serious complications.

TABLE 58 Etiologies of corneal ulcers

- Trauma
- Anaerobic and aerobic bacterial infection
  - *Pseudomonas* spp., *Enterobacter* spp., *Actinobacter* spp., *Streptococcus zooepidemicus*, *S. equi*, *Staphylococcus aureus*, *Corynebacterium* spp., *Bacillus cereus*, *Klebsiella* spp., *Moraxella equi*, *Bacillus* spp., *Streptomyces* spp., *Neisseria* spp.
- Fungal infection
  - *Aspergillus* spp., *Fusarium* spp., *Penicillium* spp., *Alternaria* spp., *Cladosporium* spp., *Pseudoallescheria* spp., *Geotrichum* spp., *Candida* spp., *Mucor* spp., *Exophiala* spp., *Torulopsis glabrak*, *Hanseniaspora euvarum*, *Drechslera* spp., *Cylindrocarpon destructans*, *Curvularia* spp., *Trichosporin cutaneum*, *Phycomyces* spp., *Paecilomyces* spp.
- EHV-2 infection
- Eosinophilic keratoconjunctivitis
- Indolent-like ulcers
- Immune-mediated keratitis/limbal keratopathy
- Conformational – entropion; lagophthalmos
- Abnormal hair growth – trichiasis; distichia; ectopic cilia
- Keratoconjunctivitis sicca
- Ocular foreign body
- Corneal degeneration/calcium deposition/band keratopathy
- Corneal sequestration
- Exposure to caustic substances/chemical irritants (i.e. alcohol, soaps, insect repellent), heat or radiation
- Exposure keratopathy due to CN deficits (i.e. facial paralysis or corneal hypoesthesia), inadequate eyelid function, buphthalmos or exophthalmos

---

Etiology/pathophysiology

Most ulcers in horses are initiated by trauma; however, a variety of other causes may also be involved (*Table 58*). The most common pathogens will vary, based on geographic location and season. *S. zooepidemicus*, alpha-hemolytic streptococci, and *Staphylococcus aureus* are common Gram-positive organisms involved, while *Pseudomonas* spp. and *Actinobacillus* spp. are often reported as the most common Gram-negative organisms.

The intact corneal epithelium acts as a protective barrier to invasion by normal microbial inhabitants of the equine environment as well as by corneal and conjunctival microflora. A partial or full-thickness defect in this barrier, usually the result of trauma, allows opportunistic and pathogenic bacterial and fungal organisms to readily adhere to, invade, and replicate in the injured or diseased corneal surface, thus initiating infection. The level of pathogenicity of an organism is related to its ability to resist the natural ocular defense mechanisms, adhere to the injured cornea, and colonize the surface. Fungi have a predilection for invading the deep stroma or Descemet's membrane. Activation and/or production of excessive proteinolytic enzymes such as MMP-2, MMP-9, and neutrophil elastase by the corneal epithelial cells, leukocytes, and certain microbial organisms (especially *Pseudomonas* and beta-hemolytic streptococci) results in sudden, rapid degeneration of collagen and other components of the stroma, inducing corneal liquefaction or keratomalacia (corneal 'melting'). Keratomalacia can lead to globe rupture in less than 12 hours if it is not controlled.

The presence of anterior uveitis secondary to corneal disease is common in horses. Anterior uveitis can lead to scarring and/or blockage of the ICA and/or uveoscleral outflow pathway and cause an elevation in the IOP or glaucoma.

Predisposing factors for corneal ulceration include prolonged topical antimicrobial, corticosteroid, or corticosteroid/antimicrobial combination drugs, which may inhibit the growth of normal bacteria and predispose to mycotic infection.

Clinical presentation

Corneal ulcers can range in appearance from simple, superficial breaks or abrasions in the corneal epithelium not visible to the naked eye, to deep stromal ulcers, to full-thickness corneal perforations with iris prolapse (**1144**). Associated ocular signs vary considerably, but can include blepharospasm, photophobia, epiphora, serous to mucopurulent ocular discharge, conjunctival hyperemia, chemosis, conjunctivitis, corneal edema, variable corneal neovascularization (superficial and/or deep), white to gray to brown plaque adhered to the corneal surface (fungal infections) (**1145, 1146**), interstitial keratitis, and white-yellow or gray gelatinous corneal opacity or exudate (stromal necrosis/liquefaction or keratomalacia). Signs of corneal ulcers can be quite subtle, especially in sick or hospitalized foals, as they have significantly less sensitive corneas than normal foals or adult horses. Clinical signs of secondary anterior uveitis, ranging in severity, are also commonly seen in horses with corneal disease (i.e. miosis, aqueous flare, hypopyon). Other associated complications of corneal ulceration include scarring, pigmentation, anterior and posterior synechiae, cataract formation, endophthalmitis, phthisis bulbi, and blindness.

Differential diagnosis

A corneal facet (an ulcer that has re-epithelialized), stromal abscess, uveitis, glaucoma, and other causes of a red or cloudy eye should be included in the list of differential diagnoses for corneal ulceration.

Diagnosis

Visual examination and fluorescein staining can identify corneal ulceration (see 1086). In an effort to determine the underlying etiology, corneal swabs should be collected from the central and peripheral aspects of the ulcer for culture and sensitivity testing. This should be followed by corneal scrapings for cytology, collected using a sterilized Kimura spatula or the blunt end of a scalpel blade, unless perforation is imminent. Corneal tissue samples must be collected carefully using appropriate instrumentation in order to avoid inadvertent corneal rupture. Mixed bacterial and fungal infections can occur. Fungal isolates have a predilection for Descemet's membrane, so aggressive and repeated scrapings are often required. Specialized stains, such as modified Wright–Giemsa, Gomori methenamine silver, and PAS, may be useful in the detection of fungal organisms. Corneal samples for histopathology may also be collected, usually at the time of surgery. PCR has been shown to be invaluable in research settings in the identification of fungal and viral agents, and is being used increasingly on clinical cases of equine ulcerative keratitis.

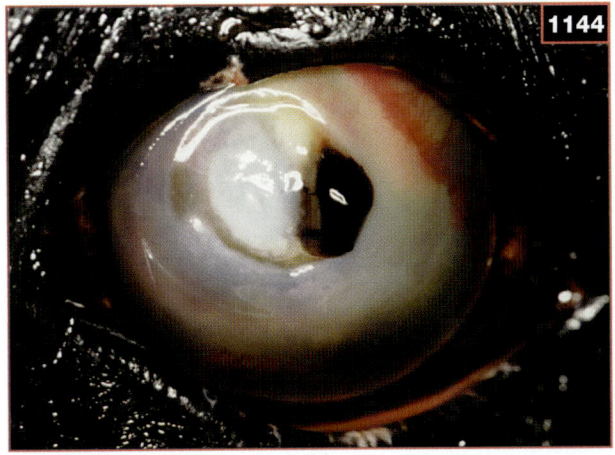

1144 Iris prolapse. This horse has a descemetocele with dark iris prolapsing through a perforation at the temporal aspect of the lesion. With focal perforations in the horse eye, it is common for the corneal defect to become 'plugged' with iris. The incarcerated iris tissue then becomes a wick from the exterior to the interior of the eye, increasing the risk of intraocular microbial contamination.

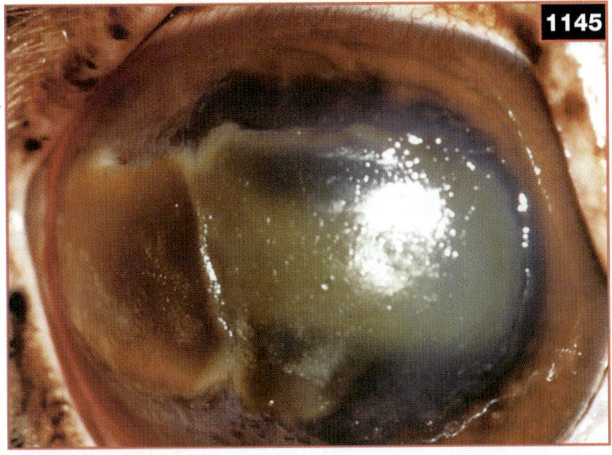

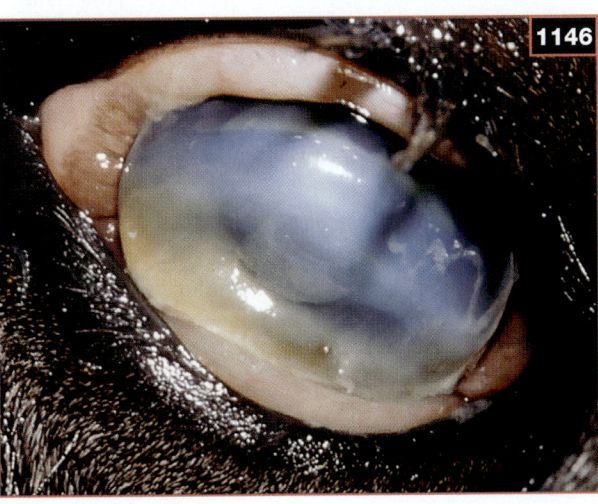

1145, 1146 Fungal keratitis. Fungal organisms can affect the superficial cornea, but they also have a predilection for colonizing the deeper cornea. (1145) Chronic superficial fungal keratitis produced this necrotic plaque of corneal tissue, referred to as a corneal sequestrum. When the plaque was removed, the fungal organisms were recovered cytologically from the underlying corneal stroma. (1146) This foal developed severe, progressive keratitis and secondary uveitis, determined to be associated with colonization by *Fusarium* spp. Note the reactive conjunctival chemosis, diffuse corneal edema, undulating corneal topography indicating stromal loss, and intraocular hypopyon.

Management

Early consultation with an ophthalmologist is highly recommended to establish appropriate diagnostic procedures, therapy, and criteria for referral. Aggressive medical therapy may reduce the likelihood of requiring surgical intervention. As administration of medications may be as often as hourly, hospitalization is often required for successful management. The use of SPL systems is invaluable in these cases in order to facilitate administration of topical medications; however, treatment can be very time consuming and expensive.

Therapy is based on the underlying etiology, depth of the ulcer, the presence of complicating factors, the rate of progression, and the response to treatment. It is therefore vital to identify and remove or treat the cause. Regardless of etiology, all ulcers should be treated initially and aggressively with topical and/or subconjunctival broad-spectrum antimicrobials to prevent or control infection, as well as topical atropine to help control ciliary body spasm and make the horse more comfortable.

Broad-spectrum antimicrobials, preferably those that are bactericidal, should be instituted based initially on cytology staining, pending culture and sensitivity results. Triple antibiotic (neomycin–polymyxin–bacitracin/gramicidin) or chloramphenicol q4–12h is a good choice for initial treatment of simple ulcers while awaiting laboratory results. When cytology reveals Gram-positive organisms, ciprofloxacin, ofloxacin, and erythromycin can also be considered. For gram-negative organisms, gentamicin, tobramycin (0.3%), and amikacin are examples of topical medications that may be selected. In deep, complicated, or melting ulcers, combination medications such as cefazolin (5.5%) and ciprofloxacin or triple antibiotic and ciprofloxacin are excellent choices for initial therapy.

Antifungals should also be instituted in endemic areas, or in those cases where mycotic infection is suspected, pending laboratory results. Fungal involvement should be suspected if there is a history of corneal injury with vegetative material, or if a corneal ulcer has received prolonged antimicrobial and/or corticosteroid therapy with minimal or no improvement. Miconazole (1%), natamycin (3.33%), itraconazole, and voriconazole are some examples of topical antifungal medications that may be selected. Frequency of application of topical antimicrobials should be aggressive and will vary from hourly to every 8 hours. Many ophthalmologists suggest that topical antifungals should not be administered more often than every 4 hours due to the severe inflammation produced by dead and dying fungal organisms. In cases where perforation or surgery is imminent, only ophthalmic solutions should be used as the vehicles in ophthalmic ointments can incite severe endophthalmitis if they enter the globe.

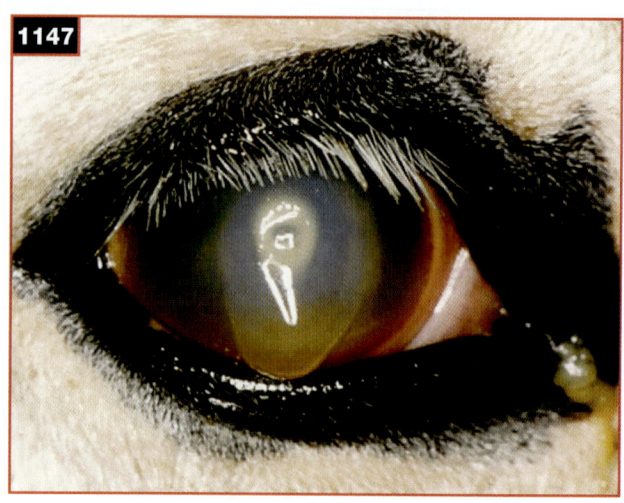

1147 Keratomalacia, or 'corneal melting' is associated with the establishment of collagenase activity and can result in rapid deterioration of the cornea. There is a tendency for such wounds to progress in a circumferential pattern from the initial stimulus, in this case presumed to be a sharp penetrating wound from something in the foal's environment.

Systemic antibiotics such as trimethoprim sulfadiazine (24–30 mg/kg p/o or i/v q12h), penicillin (sodium/potassium penicillin, 20,000 IU/kg i/v q6h; procaine penicillin, 20,000 IU/kg i/m q12h) and gentamicin (6.6 mg/kg i/v q24h), as well as systemic antifungals such as itraconazole (3 mg/kg p/o q12h), ketoconazole, and fluconazole (1 mg/kg p/o q12h), may also be indicated in certain cases (e.g. when corneal perforation or surgery is present or impending), as well as when the disease process extends to the eyelids or orbit.

As keratomalacia (**1147**) may lead to perforation in as little as 12 hours, topical antiproteinases, such as acetylcysteine, Na EDTA, Ca EDTA, heparin, and/or autogenous serum, should be used to help inhibit stromal necrosis (melting). Serum can be administered topically as often as possible, but it requires refrigeration and has a short shelf life (replace with new serum every 72 hours, with strict attention to reducing contamination). Tetracycline family drugs, especially doxycycline, have strong anti-MMP effects and may also be selected in cases of keratomalacia.

Uveitis is present in all types of corneal ulceration and must be controlled in order to prevent associated complications and preserve vision. Topically applied atropine sulfate is effective in stabilizing the blood–aqueous barrier, (BAB) reducing vascular protein leakage, minimizing pain from ciliary muscle spasm, and reducing the chance of synechiae formation by causing mydriasis. It should be used to effect (as often as every 4 hours), with the frequency of administration reduced as soon as the pupil dilates. Pupil size should be evaluated closely, as it is a good indicator of clinical improvement or control of intraocular inflammation. Topical atropine has been shown to prolong intestinal transit time and decrease or eliminate intestinal sounds. For this reason, horses receiving atropine should be monitored closely for signs of colic and for changes in GI sounds via abdominal auscultation, especially when it is being administered at higher frequencies. Limited exercise (e.g. hand walking) and grazing should be permitted several times each day. NSAIDs, such as flunixin meglumine (1.1 mg/kg i/v or p/o q12–24h) or phenylbutazone (2.2–4.4 mg/kg i/v or p/o), will help reduce ocular inflammation, relieve ocular discomfort, prevent further injury, and limit complications. In cases receiving high doses of systemic NSAIDs for extended periods of time, systemic gastroprotectants may also be administered. Topical or systemic corticosteroid therapy is contraindicated in the treatment of corneal ulcerations.

Soft contact lenses or collagen shields can be used as corneal bandages to help encourage ulcers to heal (1107). Cyanoacrylate adhesive (tissue glue) may also be used in some cases of corneal ulceration; however, it can be expensive, is infrequently indicated, and application can be difficult. It should not be used to seal leaking corneal perforations and is not recommended for use in descemetoceles, as perforation may result from the resulting heat and contraction. The use of a well fitting hood with a hard eye-cup, cross-tying, or constant supervision may be required to prevent self-trauma in a painful eye or perforation in an eye with a severely compromised cornea.

When treating horses with corneal ulceration, frequent re-evaluations are required to determine how rapidly the ulcer is changing, and treatment should be modified according to the response to therapy. In addition to the depth of the corneal ulcer, the eye should be evaluated closely at each examination for evidence of corneal melting. In general, if goals of therapy are not met on target, adjustments to medications should be made accordingly and the need for surgical intervention and referral ascertained. Sequential photographs or detailed drawings can be very helpful in documenting changes.

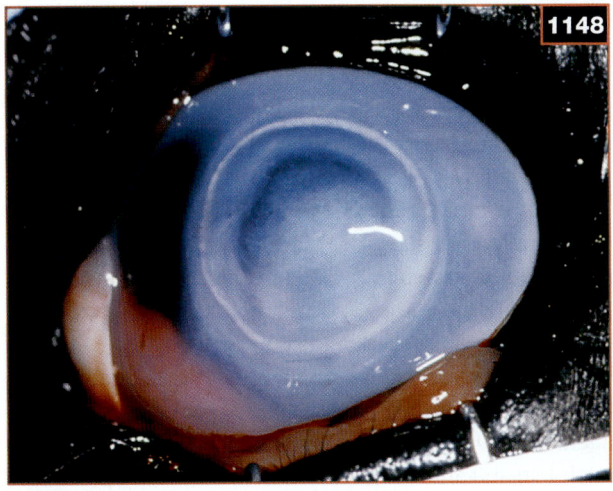

1148 A lamellar keratectomy is initiated with a partial depth incision several millimeters beyond the area of active disease. In this case the cornea is diffusely edematous, but the active collagenolysis (corneal 'melting') is confined to the area inside the initial incision. The stroma within the outlined incision is then removed in a lamellar fashion, ideally reaching just beyond and beneath the diseased portion, leaving any healthy underlying tissue. This eye has hyphema, an anterior uveal reaction to the acute nature of the corneal damage.

Unfortunately, surgery may be necessary in addition to medical management, and in these cases expedient referral to an ophthalmic specialist is vital. Surgical intervention can help by decreasing the dose, length of time, and frequency at which medications are administered more quickly than with medical management alone. In general, surgery is recommended in those cases where the ulcer is greater than 50% of the corneal depth, stromal necrosis (melting) is present, or the ulcer is progressing despite appropriate medical management. A lamellar keratectomy, in which the anterior stroma and epithelium are surgically removed, is performed to eliminate diseased tissue (necrotic stroma), shorten the course of the disease, and acquire tissues for diagnostic testing (1148). The keratectomy site may be repaired with placement of a conjunctival pedicle graft (CPG); free conjunctival island graft; tarsoconjunctival graft; porcine small-intestinal submucosa, corneoscleral, or corneoconjunctival transposition; or corneal autograft, allograft, or heterograft.

These measures are aimed at increasing the patient's comfort and preserving ocular integrity. Porcine small-intestinal submucosa is a collagen-based material that is safe, relatively inexpensive, commercially available in individual packages, easy to handle, and resistant to anticollagenase activity.

With lesions deeper than 50% of the corneal depth, CPGs and corneoscleral or corneoconjunctival transpositions are recommended. CPGs provide mechanical reinforcement of the cornea and facilitate healing by providing tectonic support, providing fibrovascular tissue to fill the stromal defect, and delivering a direct vascular supply to the lesion, including antiproteolytic and antimicrobial agents (1149, 1150). Vascular grafts offer significant antimicrobial and anticollagenase activity, which helps control bacterial infections and corneal liquefaction. They provide a cornea compatible with useful vision, allow postoperative inspection of the cornea, permit the administration and absorption of topical medications, increase patient comfort postoperatively, and reduce the chance of recurrence. The main disadvantage of conjunctival grafts is the residual corneal scarring that can impair vision, especially when located axially. This disadvantage can be minimized by trimming the graft pedicle 6–8 weeks postoperatively once the corneal condition has resolved.

Corneoscleral or corneoconjunctival transpositions may be preferred in cases of axial corneal ulceration, as they minimize scarring in the central visual axis. Due to the autologous nature of the graft, no rejection of the graft is seen and no postoperative trimming of the graft base is necessary. They are not recommended in the presence of severely weakened corneal stroma or when the size of the

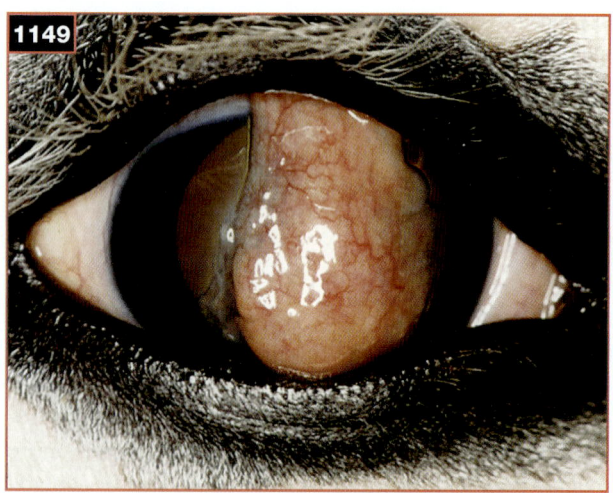

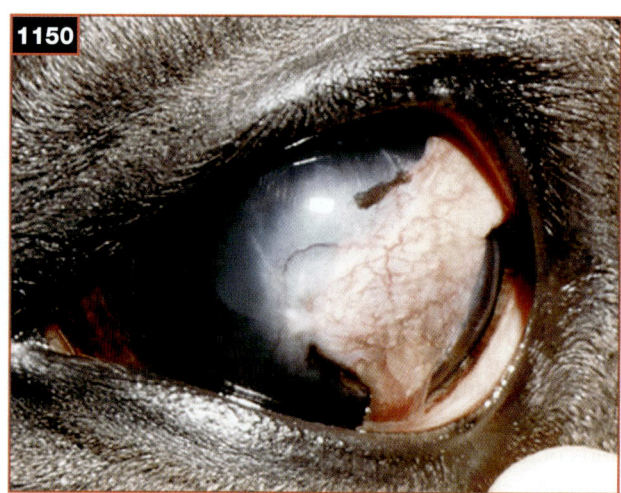

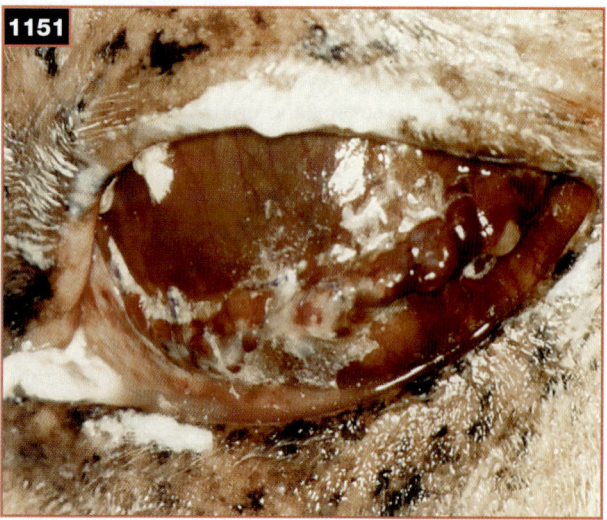

1149–1151 Conjunctival grafts. Pedicle grafts may have a single vascular base or can be based in two locations 180° apart. (1149) A pedicle graft used to treat the eye shown in 1140. The graft had been in place for approximately 1 month and was ready to have its blood supply trimmed. This allows for scar modification and contraction, hopefully increasing the functional peripheral vision in this eye. The advantage of a bi-pedicle or bridge graft (1150) is a blood supply from two sources, theoretically increasing the integrity of the graft vasculature. This is particularly useful for very large central ulcers. (1151) A 360° conjunctival graft was performed on this horse with a diffuse, rapidly progressing deep corneal ulcer. Topical medication is present on the surface of the graft. Although the resultant axial scar was large, the eye was preserved and some vision was retained.

lesion is greater than 25% of the corneal diameter because there is insufficient tissue present for an autologous sliding graft. Advanced surgical skills are required. Corneal transplantation has also been used in horses to restore vision, to control medically refractory disease, to provide mechanical or tectonic support, and to improve cosmesis. A functional and clear corneal transplant does not often occur, because of graft rejection, seen clinically as scarring and vascularization, and the absence of viable endothelial cells. In cases of perforation, the lesion may be repaired using primary closure with or without a conjunctival graft if it is <3 mm in diameter. Aggressive medical therapy and monitoring are still warranted for the first few days following surgery, particularly if keratomalacia was present.

A variation on the conjunctival pedicle graft is the 360° conjunctival graft (1151). The conjunctiva is elevated a few millimeters from the limbus in an encircling fashion, and the dorsal and ventral conjunctival tissues are advanced centrally and sutured together over the center of the cornea. It is typically used when the entire cornea is affected with severe ulcerative keratitis and the availability of microsurgical instruments and magnification is limited; however, it should not be considered as a first-choice procedure. The main advantages of this technique are the relative speed with which the graft can be harvested and closed, and the fact that actual corneal suturing is not required. The major disadvantages are inability to view the eye while the graft is in place and loss of the ability for the horse to see through or around the graft during healing. Following resolution of the disease process there is a need to trim these grafts diligently to ensure minimal permanent scarring.

Enucleation may also be considered based on financial constraints, the inability to heal or the progression of corneal ulceration, and the animal's inability to tolerate long-term frequent application of topical medication.

Prognosis

The prognosis is variable (good to guarded) depending on the underlying etiology, corneal depth, rate of ulcer progression, the presence of stromal necrosis (melting), and the therapy selected. Mycotic infections can be very difficult to heal medically and keratomalacia can be difficult to control.

Corneal stromal abscess
Definition/overview

A corneal abscess is an intrastromal accumulation of bacteria and/or inflammatory cell debris (sterile abscess) beneath an intact epithelium. Corneal abscesses usually occur in horses following trauma to the cornea. There may be a history of previous ulceration or clinical signs of ocular discomfort. Corneal abscesses can be difficult to treat and may require weeks to months of medical therapy and/or surgical intervention to assist with healing.

Etiology/pathophysiology

As with corneal ulcers, corneal abscesses may be bacterial, fungal, or sterile in origin (see *Table 58*).

Corneal stromal abscesses develop following focal trauma to the cornea that allows opportunistic pathogens and debris into the stroma beneath the corneal epithelium. Subsequent healing or re-epithelialization of this ulcer or epithelial micropuncture forms a barrier that protects the bacteria or fungi from topically administered antimicrobial medications, sealing in the microorganisms and allowing ongoing infection. Alternatively, the initial treatment may kill the microorganisms, but subsequent release of toxins by dying bacteria and fungi, as well as degenerating leukocytes, continues the stimulus for abscessation. Topical antimicrobial/corticosteroid combination therapy can predispose horses to developing corneal abscessation. Fungi appear to have a predilection for the deep corneal stroma and/or Descemet's membrane. Concurrent anterior uveitis occurs due to corneal sensory nerve irritation (oculopupillary reflex). Anterior uveitis is the main cause of posterior synechia, cataract, and fibrin formation.

The normally avascular equine cornea vascularizes at an extremely slow rate with stromal abscesses. This contributes to the long recovery periods for horses with corneal abscesses, as vascularization is necessary for abscesses to heal.

Clinical presentation

Corneal stromal abscesses may appear as single or multiple, focal, white to yellow, stromal infiltrates or opacities with associated corneal edema and variable corneal neovascularization (1152, 1153). They can occur at all depths of the cornea from superficial to deep and may even rupture into the anterior chamber. They can occur axially, paraxially, or peripherally and can be very small to quite large in diameter. Associated clinical signs can also include lacrimation, blepharospasm, photophobia, enophthalmos, third eyelid elevation, conjunctival hyperemia, corneal edema, miosis, and signs associated with anterior uveitis.

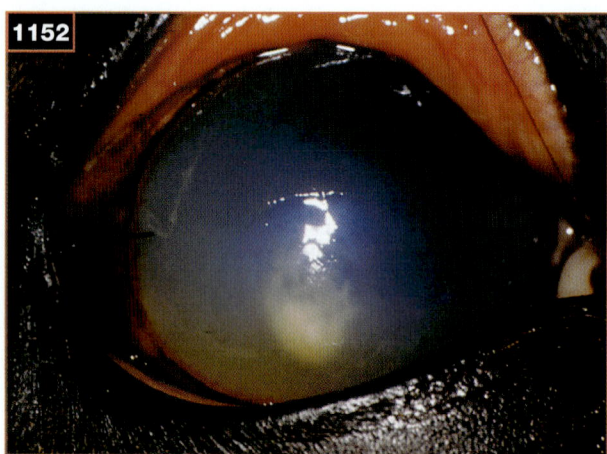

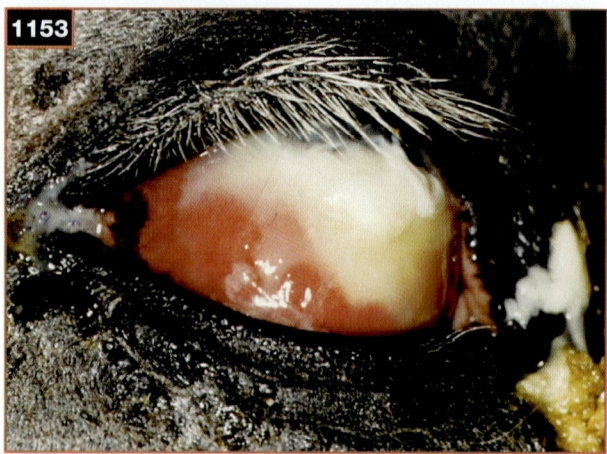

1152, 1153 Stromal abscesses (1152) appear as creamy white to yellow focal areas in the cornea and are usually accompanied by corneal edema, corneal vascularization, and varying degrees of reflex uveitis. (1153) If left untreated, or if treated inappropriately, a focal abscess can progress to involve the entire cornea, as in this eye treated for a suspected inflammatory problem with topical steroids.

Differential diagnosis

Ulcerative keratitis, corneal degeneration, calcific band keratopathy, neoplasia (e.g. SCC, hemangioma, angiosarcoma), corneal foreign body, granulation tissue, parasitic infestation (e.g. *Onchocerca*), eosinophilic keratitis/keratoconjunctivitis, nonulcerative keratouveitis, beta-radiation, leukoma, and anterior segment dysgenesis should be differentiated from corneal abscessation.

Diagnosis

A history of previous trauma and/or evidence of ulceration, the clinical appearance of a yellow-white corneal stromal infiltrate, and negative fluorescein staining over the site of the abscess are normally sufficient for a clinical diagnosis of corneal abscessation. Samples for cytology, culture and sensitivity, and histopathology should be collected following epithelial debridement. Preoperative sample collection can be difficult due to the presence of an intact epithelium and the deep location of most abscesses. Fungal isolates have a predilection for Descemet's membrane, so aggressive and repeated scrapings are often required in order to obtain diagnostic samples. Specialized stains such as modified Wright–Giemsa, Gomori methenamine silver, and PAS may be useful in the detection of fungal organisms. Corneal samples are often collected at the time of surgery to aid in the etiologic diagnosis.

Management

The medical therapy for corneal abscessation is similar to that for corneal ulceration, consisting of aggressive use of topical and systemic antimicrobials (antibiotics and antimycotics), topical atropine, and systemic NSAIDs. Careful selection of topical medication is required, as only certain drugs can penetrate an intact epithelium satisfactorily (e.g. ciprofloxacin, chloramphenicol). It may be necessary in cases of superficial abscesses periodically to debride the cornea and remove the epithelium in order to allow topical medications to penetrate the cornea more effectively. As diagnostic samples for culture and sensitivity can be difficult to obtain and the etiologic agent is often unknown, empirical therapy targeting both bacteria and fungal agents is often recommended. Placement of an SPL system can facilitate treatment. Vascularization, either in the form of corneal neovascularization or surgical placement of a conjunctival graft, is required for stromal abscesses to heal. NSAIDs significantly inhibit corneal vascularization, so when they are being used without placement of a conjunctival graft, care must be taken. Topical steroids are contraindicated in the presence of corneal ulceration or abscessation.

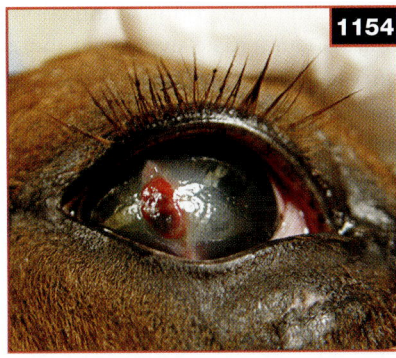
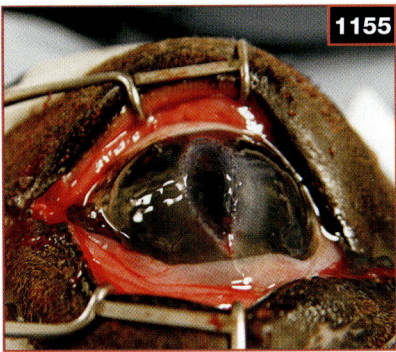
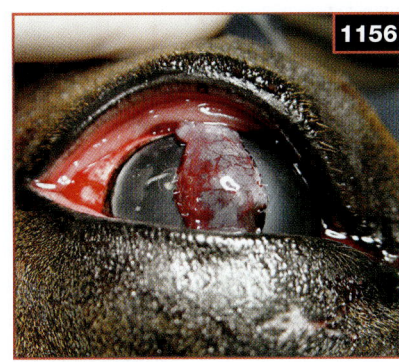

If significant improvement does not occur within the first few days of intensive medical therapy, or there is deterioration following an initial improvement, surgery should be considered. Although controversial, it is believed by some ophthalmologists that early surgery will improve the overall prognosis and may speed recovery in certain cases when compared with medical management alone. It also allows for collection of additional tissue samples that will aid in obtaining a definitive etiologic diagnosis and determining the appropriate antimicrobial therapy. A keratectomy can be performed on superficial abscesses to remove sequestered microbes and necrotic debris, shorten the course of the disease, and acquire tissues for diagnostic testing. The resulting lesion may be left to heal on its own or it may be covered by a conjunctival pedicle graft to provide an immediate vascular supply.

Deep stromal abscesses respond poorly to medical therapy and most tend to involve Descemet's membrane. In these cases a full-thickness keratoplasty (therapeutic penetrating keratoplasty [TPK]) can be used to remove the diseased tissue in conjunction with a corneal transplantation (fresh or frozen donor cornea), conjunctival graft, and/or porcine small-intestinal submucosa (1154–1156). A posterior lamellar keratoplasty (PLK) has also been reported to be successful in horses for abscesses located in the posterior third of the stroma. Reports have stated that PLK involves considerably shorter surgery and healing times than those observed with TPK (57.2 +/− 14.2 days versus 23.7 +/− 5.2 days). If an ulcer is present preoperatively, the PLK flap tends to be slow to heal and results in more significant anterior uveitis and larger scars. Therefore, it is recommended that surgery is delayed, if possible, until the ulcers are healed or until a CPG can be positioned over the flap. Complications of TPK and PLK may include stromal hemorrhage, corneal edema, corneal vascularization, granulation tissue, aqueous leakage, anterior uveitis, fibrin in the anterior chamber, anterior and/or posterior synechiae, corneal ulceration, cataract formation, globe rupture, and corneal scarring. Aqueous leakage may be seen following an inadequate number of sutures or inappropriate suture placement, or from conjunctival flap

1154–1156 Penetrating keratoplasty and conjunctival grafting. (1154) A perforating corneal wound with iris prolapse is present in this eye, indicated by the dark area within the lesion. The chronicity of the corneal disease is evidenced by the attempted vascular ingrowth of the wound. (1155) Following full-thickness resection of the diseased cornea and amputation of the entrapped iris, a corneal allograft is shown sutured in position. Fresh or frozen corneal allografts or heterografts can provide exceptional tectonic support. The addition of a conjunctival graft (1156) over the corneal graft provides the benefits of an immediate diffuse blood supply to assist in wound stabilization and immunologic support. (Photos courtesy I Jurk)

dehiscence due to self-trauma, uncontrolled infections, or excessive restraint during application of medications. Anterior synechiae may occur secondary to aqueous humor leakage and/or presurgical or postsurgical uveitis. A corneoscleral or corneoconjunctival transposition may also be used. A deep lamellar endothelial keratoplasty has recently been reported.

Prognosis
The prognosis is variable, depending on the depth, rate of progression, and therapy chosen. Corneal abscesses can reportedly heal by vascularization in anything from 1 week to as much as 2–3 months. In general, the prognosis has been reported to be good with surgical intervention. Progression, imminent or pre-existing rupture into the anterior chamber, and endophthalmitis are indications for a poor visual outcome.

There is a poorer prognosis, due to the association with increased rejection rates, when using corneal grafts in the presence of uncontrolled anterior uveitis if the corneal graft site location is close to the limbus, if there is neovascularization, and/or when the keratoplasty is >8.0 mm in diameter.

Uveitis

Definition/overview

Inflammation of the iris and/or ciliary body is termed anterior uveitis, whereas posterior uveitis involves inflammation of the choroid. Inflammation of all structures of the uvea is termed panuveitis. Reported worldwide, equine uveitis can be incited by a wide variety of causes; however, the underlying cause is often not identified. Uveitis is usually associated with systemic disease in the foal. In adults it is most often immune mediated or due to direct invasion of microorganisms into the eye. Regardless of the etiology, cases of equine uveitis share common clinical features and should be treated symptomatically. Cataracts and pupillary seclusion are the most frequent causes of blindness in horses suffering from uveitis. Appaloosas appear predisposed, whereas Standardbreds may have a reduced risk. Horses that are seropositive to *Leptospira* serovar *pomona* are 13 times more likely than seronegative horses to have signs of uveitis. Uveitis may occur unilaterally or bilaterally.

Etiology/pathophysiology

Proposed causes have included trauma, neoplasia, infectious disease, and other systemic diseases (*Table 59*). The underlying initial insult in any case of uveitis is tissue damage and breakdown of the BAB. Trauma, infection, inflammation, or neoplasia can initiate uveitis via these mechanisms. Leptospirosis is the most commonly implicated infectious cause of equine uveitis. In naturally occurring and experimental infections, clinical uveitis does not occur until months or years after primary infection with leptospirosis. Antigen mimicry between *Leptospira* spp. and equine ocular tissues has been demonstrated, supporting an immune-mediated process in the pathophysiology of equine recurrent uveitis. Aberrant ocular migration of *Onchocerca cervicalis* microfilariae is the most commonly implicated parasitic cause of recurrent uveitis. Live *Onchocerca* microfilariae can be identified as an incidental finding in normal equine eyes; therefore, it is believed that only certain individuals will develop uveal inflammation in response to dying microfilariae.

Decreased IOP typically occurs due to a decrease in production of aqueous humor as a result of ciliary body inflammation. Aqueous flare is caused by exudation of protein and inflammatory cells from the uveal tissue, which may accumulate in large amounts as hypopyon and cause synechiae. These adhesions of the iris to the lens and the presence of products of inflammation that interfere with lens metabolism lead to secondary cataract formation. Secondary lens luxation may result from the effect of inflammation on the lens zonules or because of traction by fibrous adhesions. Vitreal haze can occur secondary to inflammatory cell infiltrate and exudation of protein from the uveal tract. This exudate in the vitreous may organize to form bands of tissue that adhere to the retina and may contract to produce retinal detachment. In chronic uveitis, corneal degeneration can occur secondary to pathologic changes within the cornea such as accumulation of calcium in the corneal epithelial basement membrane, which may cause disruption of the epithelium resulting in ulceration. Anterior uveitis may also lead to PIFM formation that may limit aqueous absorption by the iris and lead to physical and functional obstruction of the ICA. Other lesions that cause glaucoma with subsequent buphthalmos by interfering with the flow of aqueous humor include, lens luxation, anterior synechiae, iris bombé, or pupillary seclusion. In end-stage uveitis, fibrosis of the uveal tract results in phthisis bulbi.

Clinical presentation

Clinical signs can vary depending on the severity of inflammation, the area(s) of the uvea involved, and the duration of the problem. They may include variable vision deficits, lacrimation, blepharospasm, photophobia, enophthalmos, conjunctival/episcleral congestion, corneal edema, corneal neovascularization/ciliary flush, keratic precipitates, aqueous flare, fibrin in the anterior chamber, hypopyon, hyphema, miosis, cellular debris and/or

---

TABLE 59　Main causes of uveitis

- Equine Recurrent uveitis
- Trauma – blunt or penetrating
- Iatrogenic from surgical trauma i.e. intraocular surgery
- Systemic infections
  - Bacteria – *Leptospira* spp., *Brucella abortus*, *B. melitensis*, *Borrelia burgdorferi*, *Salmonella* spp., *Streptococcus equi*, *Escherichia coli*, *Rhodococcus (Corynebacterium) equi*, *Actinobacillus equuli.*, *Salmonella* spp., leishmaniasis, tuberculosis
  - Parasites – *Onchocerca cervicalis, Halicephalobus deletrix,* intestinal strongyles*, Dirofilaria immitis*
  - Viruses – Equine viral arteritis, equine infectious anemia virus, equine herpes virus Types 1 and 4, equine influenza virus
  - Protozoal – *Toxoplasma gondii, Neospora* spp.
  - Fungal – *Cryptococcus*
- Keratitis-associated axonal reflex uveitis
- Immune-mediated/idiopathic
- Neoplasia
- Lens-induced uveitis

---

pigment on the anterior lens capsule, edematous and/or hyperemic iris, yellow-green discoloration/vitreal haze, peripapillary chorioretinitis, and retinal detachment. Possible sequelae include band keratopathy (white chalky speculated opacities in the cornea), dyscoria, anterior and posterior synechiae, iris bombé, iris color change, corpora nigra atrophy, cataract formation, secondary glaucoma, lens subluxation/luxation, pigment changes in the iris, vitreal liquefaction/floaters, vitreal traction bands, retinal detachment, depigmentation of the peripapillary region in a focal or alar pattern/butterfly lesions, and phthisis bulbi (1157–1160). In many cases, posterior segment lesions cannot be appreciated due to the severe anterior segment abnormalities.

Differential diagnosis
Other causes of red eye, cloudy eye, glaucoma, lens luxation, keratitis, and conjunctivitis should be ruled out.

Diagnosis
A definitive diagnosis of the cause of uveitis is often elusive. A CBC, biochemistry panel, urinalysis, fecal float, urine, fecal and vitreal cultures, serum *Brucella*, leptospirosis and toxoplasmosis titers, conjunctival biopsy for *Onchocerca*, leptospiral microscopic agglutination test, vitreal leptospiral titers, and PCR may all be used in an attempt to determine the underlying cause of the uveitis.

Management
The underlying cause should be treated if one is identified. Regardless of the etiology, uveitis requires aggressive treatment to reduce or control ocular inflammation in order to decrease pain, minimize the progression of ocular lesions, decrease the incidence of postinflammatory sequelae, and preserve vision. Topical, subconjunctival, and/or systemic anti-inflammatory therapy is vital regardless of the suspected cause in order to inhibit BAB breakdown. Prednisolone acetate (1%) is the anti-inflammatory of choice due to its ability to penetrate an

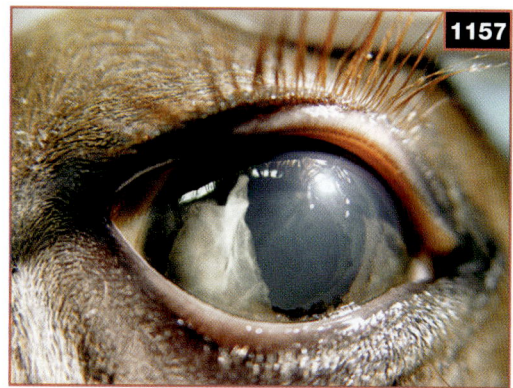

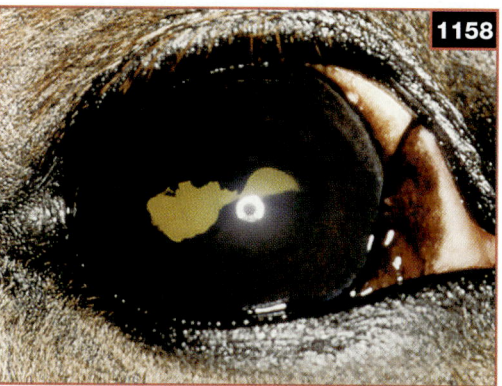

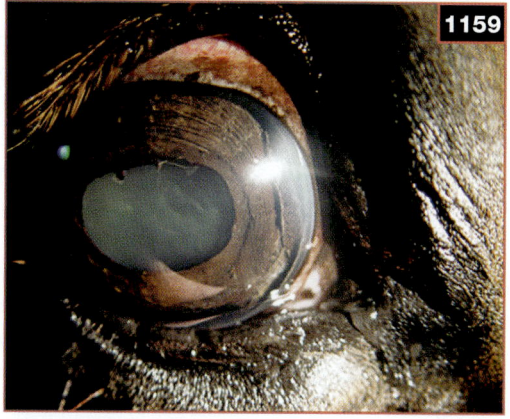

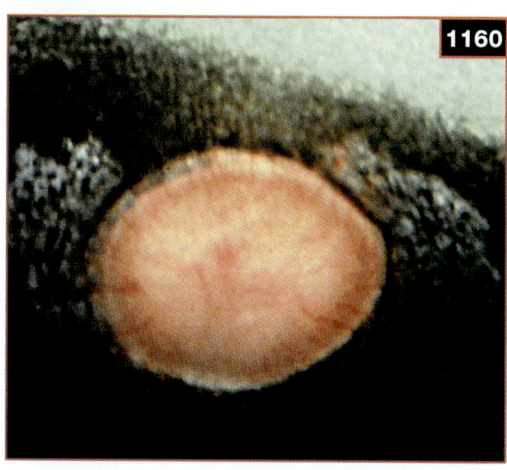

1157–1160 Uveitis can present acutely, in which case the anterior chamber may contain fibrin (as seen in this horse), inflammatory cells, or blood (1157). With recurrent bouts of inflammation, sequelae include yellow staining in the vitreous due to protein accumulation, and posterior synechiae (1158). Cataract and polishing or atrophy of the corpora nigra are common sequelae of uveitis (1159). 'Butterfly lesions' are associated with chorioretinal scarring around the peripapillary retinal vasculature (1160). (Photos 1157 and 1159 courtesy I Jurk)

intact corneal epithelium. Topical 0.1% dexamethasone is also an acceptable choice. Topical corticosteroids may be applied every 2–6 hours based on the severity of inflammation. Subconjunctival injections of corticosteroids such as methylprednisolone acetate (20–40 mg) or betamethasone (5–15 mg) may also be helpful. Steroids should not be used in the presence of corneal ulceration. Instead, topical NSAIDs such as diclofenac, flurbiprofen, or suprofen can be applied every 6–12 hours as needed. Topical NSAIDs not only act as anti-inflammatories, but their antiprostaglandin action facilitates mydriasis. The frequency of topical anti-inflammatory medication is gradually reduced once clinical improvement of the uveitis occurs. Systemic NSAIDs such as flunixin meglumine (1.1 mg/kg i/v or p/o q12–24h) or phenylbutazone (2.2–4.4 mg/kg p/o or i/v q12–24h) may be used to provide analgesia and inhibit the prostaglandin production associated with uveitis. They are typically initiated at higher dosages and then gradually reduced once the inflammation subsides. Topical atropine sulfate (1%) administration is essential for pupillary dilation, to prevent or decrease the risk of posterior synechiae formation, to provide analgesia by eliminating ciliary body spasm (cycloplegic), and to stabilize the BAB. Atropine may last several days to weeks in the normal equine eye, but only a few hours in an inflamed eye. It should be administered topically to effect. The frequency of administration may range from 2–6 times each day. GI motility should be monitored. Topical tropicamide may be used for short-term mydriasis to prevent the risk of inducing GI ileus or colic with frequent atropine administration. Topical or subconjunctival phenylephrine (2.5–10% or 5 mg per eye, respectively) may also be used to help dilate the pupil. Tissue plasminogen activator (TPA) may be used intraocularly to help clear fibrin.

In cases of band keratopathy, a superficial keratectomy may be performed and/or calcium-chelating drugs (e.g. 0.05% sodium or potassium EDTA) may be administered.

Topical or systemic antimicrobials are not usually indicated unless corneal ulceration is present or the uveitis appears to be septic, the horse is pyrexic, or a systemic disease responsive to antimicrobials (e.g. leptospirosis, Lyme disease) has been identified as the cause. In uveitis induced by *Onchocerca cervicalis*, larvicidal medication is indicated once the active inflammation has been controlled (e.g. ivermectin, 0.2 mg/kg ivermectin once, or diethylcarbamazine, 4.4–6.6 mg/kg p/o for 21 days).

In eyes that are blind and chronically painful, an enucleation or evisceration should be performed.

Immunization of horses against leptospirosis when *L. pomona* has been implicated as the cause of endemic outbreaks is controversial. Administration of a multivalent *Leptospira* vaccine to a seropositive horse with uveitis may exacerbate the inflammation due to immunologic stimulation. Therefore, immunization should be limited to seronegative horses at increased risk for uveitis associated with leptospirosis.

Prognosis

The prognosis is guarded due to the likelihood of recurrence and possible vision-threatening sequelae (e.g. cataracts, secondary glaucoma). In peracute cases, if therapy is prompt, intensive, and prolonged, the prognosis for preserving vision is fair to good. Unfortunately, uveitis is often recurring.

Equine recurrent uveitis

Definition/overview

Equine recurrent uveitis (ERU) is a painful, chronic, ocular condition characterized by clinical manifestation of recurrent and increasingly severe episodes of active inflammation of the uveal tract (iris, ciliary body, and/or choroid), separated by variable lengths of quiescence. Initial ocular injury or infection associated with ocular inflammation leads to the establishment of immunologically sensitized cells. As the uvea can function as an accessory lymph node, systemic re-exposure to similar circulating antigens (molecular mimicry) that enter the eye through a destroyed BAB, or native ocular antigens, will cause a nonspecific, immune-mediated, delayed hypersensitivity reaction and recurrent bouts of uveitis. The recurrent inflammation causes progressive ocular destruction with potential loss of vision. Also called periodic ophthalmia, recurrent iridocyclitis, and moonblindness, ERU is a frustrating disease to treat as recurrence can be frequent and long-term medication is often required. The disease is bilateral in approximately 20% of cases. It is the leading cause of vision impairment and blindness in adult horses, and a major cause of economic loss worldwide. Appaloosas appear predisposed (more than eight times more likely to have uveitis compared with other breeds), suggesting a possible genetic link. Treatment is expensive and time consuming. An enucleation or evisceration may be required to remove a chronically painful nonvisual eye.

Etiology/pathophysiology

While the pathogenesis appears immune-mediated, the specific causes of ERU are unknown. Proposed causes have included trauma and bacterial, viral, fungal, parasitic, and other systemic diseases. In most cases an etiologic agent cannot be identified. One theory suggests that periodic episodes of inflammation can be directly induced and maintained by the persistence of a specific antigen in the ocular tissues. *Leptospira interrogens* is considered the most important infectious agent associated with ERU. However, definitive evidence for this theory is lacking. A second theory implicating an immune-mediated, delayed-type hypersensitivity reaction to self or sequestered antigen (antigen mimicry) in the uveal tract in ERU is supported clinically by the recurring nature of the disease, the lack of response to antimicrobials and/or deworming programs, the common absence of an identifiable infectious agent, and the positive response to anti-inflammatory therapy.

Intraocular inflammation occurs due to BAB breakdown, which results in infiltration of inflammatory cells and protein and the clinical signs of anterior uveitis. Active episodes of inflammation may last days to weeks, gradually resolving to a relatively comfortable quiescent period. Recurrent episodes of uveitis are associated with progression of irreversible ocular damage. Cataracts and pupillary seclusion are the most frequent causes of blindness in horses suffering from uveitis. Cataracts may occur secondary to chronic uveitis, as decreased aqueous production and diffusion of inflammatory mediators across the lens capsule and subsequent alterations in the metabolism of the lens can cause cataractous changes. Occasionally, glaucoma with buphthalmos develops secondary to anterior synechiae, lens luxation, or pupillary seclusion. The vitreous may appear yellow-green in color due to the presence of fibrin and porphyrin metabolites. Vitreal fibrin may form vitreoretinal traction bands, which can lead to retinal detachment. Fibrosis can lead to phthisis bulbi in end-stage disease.

Differential diagnosis
Previous ocular trauma and inflammation, as well as the other causes of equine uveitis, should be considered. Alternative causes of a cloudy, red, or painful eye must also be ruled out.

Clinical presentation
Clinical signs can vary depending on the severity of inflammation, the area(s) of uvea involved, and the duration of the problem, but may include variable vision, lacrimation, blepharospasm, photophobia, enophthalmos, conjunctival hyperemia, conjunctivitis, corneal edema, corneal neovascularization, keratic precipitates, aqueous flare, hypopyon, hyphema, miosis, dyscoria, peripheral and/or posterior synechiae, iris bombé, corpora nigra atrophy, debris and/or pigment on the anterior lens capsule, edematous and/or hyperemic iris, cataract formation, lens subluxation/luxation, yellow vitreal haze, vitreal degeneration/liquefaction, peripapillary chorioretinitis, butterfly lesions/retinal scarring, and/or retinal detachment (1161). Associated lesions may also include corneal degeneration, corneal ulceration, secondary glaucoma, retinal degeneration/atrophy, and phthisis bulbi. In many instances, vitreal or retinal lesions cannot be appreciated due to severe inflammation of the anterior segment or its sequelae. Lesions may be unilateral or bilateral.

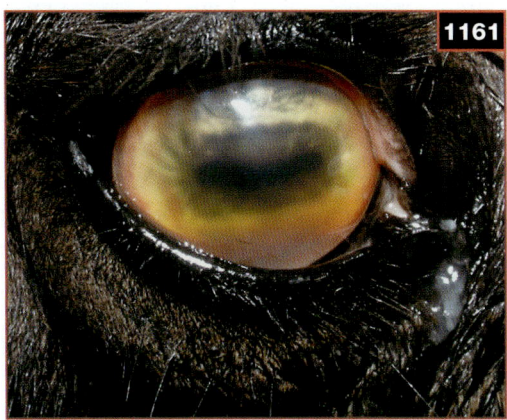

1161 The right eye of a horse with acute anterior uveitis showing increased lacrimation, miosis, aqueous flare, swelling and discoloration of the iris, circumlimbal corneal vascularization, mild corneal edema and hypopyon. (Photo courtesy GA Munroe)

Diagnosis
Ophthalmic signs suffice for a diagnosis in most cases. A presumptive diagnosis of ERU can be made based on a history of previous, recurring episodes of inflammation that responded to anti-inflammatory agents, examination findings consistent with chronic uveitis, no significant laboratory findings, and no signs of systemic disease.

Management
The major goals of treatment for each inflammatory episode are to preserve vision, decrease pain, minimize ocular tissue damage, and prevent or decrease the recurrence of attacks of uveitis. The extent of damage depends on the severity and duration of the acute uveitis attack, and the promptness and effectiveness of therapy. Specific prevention and therapy are often difficult, as the etiology is not identified in each case. Treatment is, therefore, nearly always symptomatic, involving the intense use of anti-inflammatory and mydriatic/cycloplegic drugs. Anti-inflammatory medications, to control the intraocular inflammation that can lead to blindness, have been the most important factor in the treatment of ERU to date. Usually, corticosteroids are used topically and/or subconjunctivally and NSAIDs are given systemically. Prednisolone acetate or dexamethasone is an excellent choice for topical therapy. When the horse is not cooperative or the frequent application of topical steroids is not practical, subconjunctival corticosteroids (20–40 mg methylprednisolone acetate or 5–15 mg betamethazone) may be used. Systemic corticosteroids may be beneficial in

859

severe, refractory cases of ERU, but should be used with caution due to their side-effects and potential complications (i.e. laminitis). Horses that experience frequent recurrence may benefit from long-term, low-dose corticosteroid therapy. Unfortunately, long-term use of topical steroids for prophylaxis can cause serious side-effects (e.g. predispose to corneal infection), require owner and animal compliance, and is not always effective. The use of corticosteroids is contraindicated in the presence of a corneal ulcer. NSAIDs may be used and are effective at reducing the intraocular inflammation when a corneal ulcer is present. Flunixin meglumine and phenylbutazone are frequently used systemically to control intraocular inflammation. Some horses become refractory to these medications and substituting another NSAID may be necessary. Topical atropine sulfate has been used to minimize synechiae formation by inducing mydriasis and to alleviate some of the pain of ERU by relieving spasm of the ciliary body; however, mydriasis can increase the IOP. Tropicamide may, therefore, be safer than atropine for use in uveitis as it carries the same beneficial effects as atropine, yet its duration of action is shorter. If the IOP increases following mydriasis, tropicamide administration may be stopped and its effects will wear off within a day. Medications should be slowly reduced in frequency once clinical signs abate. Therapy can last for weeks or months and should not be stopped abruptly or recurrence may occur. Often, medical treatment can be ineffective, time consuming, and expensive, with life-long therapy often required.

A polyvinyl alcohol/silicone-coated intravitreal sustained-delivery device that can deliver 4 µg/day of cyclosporine A (CsA) for up to 5 years has been developed for the treatment of ERU in horses. It has been shown to be safe for long-term use and appears to be effective in decreasing the frequency, duration, and severity of future inflammatory episodes, minimizing progression of ocular lesions, and improving the response time to therapy during future attacks. Studies report that it can provide excellent control of the disease, reducing the rate of recurrent episodes from an average of 7.5 episodes each year to 0.36, and maintaining vision in almost 90% of eyes over a 14-month period. However, in some cases, progression of cataracts occurred despite a decrease in number or complete elimination of recurrent episodes of uveitis. Additional complications such as intraocular hemorrhage, glaucoma, retinal detachment, phthisis bulbi, and blindness may also occur. A suprachoroidal implant has been developed and preliminary data indicate a significant decrease in the severity and frequency of recurrence, with a very low rate of complications, making it a superior procedure to intravitreal devices. CsA implantation may be

considered if the documented history and ocular signs are consistent with ERU (i.e. the frequent multiple episodes of uveitis, the progression of the ocular disease despite appropriate medication, the presence of adequate retinal function [as determined by a normal direct PLR, positive menace and visibly normal retina, normal photopic and sceptic maze testing, ERG], and the lack of cataract formation or other vision-threatening complications). Formation and progression of cataracts have been seen in a small number of ERU cases with intravitreal CsA, although most of these were the result of surgical trauma.

Pars plana vitrectomy has been used to treat ERU in European warmbloods, with high success rates reported and with stable vision in the majority of cases. Removal of uveitis-induced 'immunologic memory' or organisms causing persistent infection in the vitreous by vitrectomy may reduce adverse interaction between the vitreous and the uveal tract, and therefore reduce the recurrence of ERU. For unknown reasons, attempts to perform this surgery in North America have been fraught with complications, including vitreal hemorrhage, postoperative uveitis, and a high rate of vision-threatening cataract formation (46%). Both groups had a high rate of vision-threatening cataract formation and/or progression even when the inflammation appeared controlled. Retinal detachment can also occur post vitrectomy.

In cases of band keratopathy, apart from treating the underlying disease, corneal scrapings or superficial keratectomy may be performed, followed by topical EDTA.

Management practices aimed at reducing exposure to potential antigens through parasite-control programs, eliminating environmental contact with cattle and wildlife, excluding horses from ponds and swampy areas, limiting rodent access, decreasing incidence of respiratory and systemic infections, and maintaining good-quality feed should be implemented.

Prognosis

The long-term prognosis for vision in horses with recurrent uveitis is generally poor, as sequelae are inevitable and vision loss occurs in one or both eyes in 44% of cases. The prognosis is affected by breed and leptospiral seroactivity. Appaloosas with uveitis are approximately four times more likely to become blind in one or both eyes compared with other breeds, and horses with uveitis associated with leptospiral seropositivity are over four times more likely to lose vision than are horses with uveitis attributable to other causes. The long-term prognosis for horses with ERU on suprachoroidal CsA therapy has not yet been determined, as its use is still limited; however, the short-term results from published and ongoing studies are encouraging.

Neurologic disorders of the eye

Horner's syndrome

Definition/overview

Horner's syndrome is not a specific disease, but a syndrome that involves the loss or disruption of sympathetic innervation to the eye and adnexa. It is characterized in the horse by ptosis of the upper eyelid, ipsilateral facial sweating, mild miosis, enophthalmos, and regional hyperthermia. It may be unilateral or bilateral and may or may not be permanent.

Etiology/pathophysiology

There are a number of possible causes of Horner's syndrome in the horse (*Table 60*).

Sympathetic innervation to the eye and adnexa may be divided into three neuroanatomic sections: central, preganglionic, and postganglionic. The sympathetic pathway begins with the central component, which consists of fibers descending from the brainstem, down the tecto-tegmentospinal tract to synapse at spinal cord segments T1–T3. The axons leave the spinal cord and enter the sympathetic trunk in the dorsal thorax. These preganglionic sympathetic axons then travel through the cervicothoracic and middle cervical ganglia and continue up the neck, in the vagosympathetic trunk, to synapse in the cranial cervical ganglion. The postganglionic sympathetic axons then continue forward, where they pass through the middle ear, join the ophthalmic branch of the trigeminal nerve, and distribute to the sweat glands of the head, smooth muscles of the periorbita, eyelids, and the iris dilator muscle.

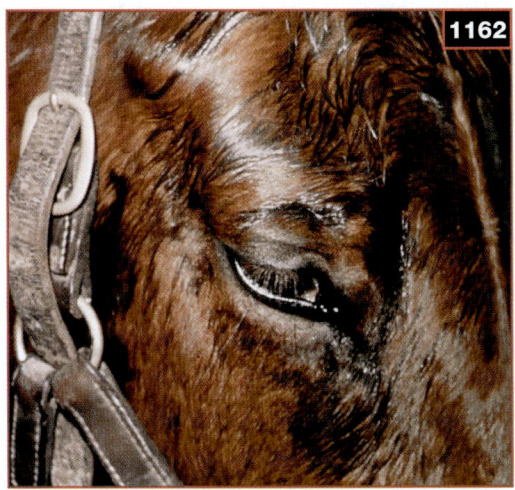

1162 Horner's syndrome in horses is characterized by ipsilateral sweating of the face and neck, as well as enophthalmos, miosis, and ptosis.

TABLE 60 **Causes of Horner's syndrome**
• Severe head, neck and chest trauma
• Cranial thoracic neoplasia/space-occupying masses
• Otitis media/interna
• Cervical neoplasia or abscesses
• Intracarotid artery or jugular vein drug injection
• Guttural pouch disease or surgery i.e. carotid artery ligation for facial surgery or guttural pouch epistaxsis
• Esophageal rupture, obstruction or surgery
• Periorbital abscesses or tumors
• Postanesthetic myopathy
• EPM
• Cauda equine neuritis/polyneuritis equi
• Systemic aspergillosis
• Central nervous system infection or neoplasia

Lesions causing cranial sympathetic denervation, and thus leading to Horner's syndrome, can occur anywhere along this pathway. Loss of sympathetic innervation to Muller's muscle of the upper eyelid and tissue of the lower eyelid results in narrowing of the palpebral fissure and ptosis (drooping of the upper eyelid). Ipsilateral facial sweating and regional hyperthermia are believed to be caused by vasodilation and increased cutaneous blood flow that occur due to loss of sympathetic innervation to the sweat glands of the head. Lack of tone in the orbital smooth muscle causes the eye to retract slightly, leading to enophthalmos. Loss of normal sympathetic tone to the iris dilator muscle results in ipsilateral miosis and anisocoria.

Clinical presentation

The clinical signs in horses are variable and often subtle, but can include increased lacrimation; hyperemia of nasal and conjunctival mucosa; ipsilateral sweating at the base of the ear, face, and neck; increased cutaneous temperature on the affected side; ptosis; miosis; anisocoria; enophthalmos; inspiratory stridor; and dermatitis due to chronic sweating (**1162**). Prolapse of the third eyelid, commonly seen in small animals with Horner's syndrome, is rare in horses with the syndrome.

Differential diagnosis

Anterior uveitis, corneal ulceration, and other causes of anisocoria should be considered as differentials for Horner's syndrome.

Diagnosis

Diagnosis is based on history as well as a complete physical, neurologic, and ophthalmologic examination. In dim lighting, dilation of the affected side will occur; however, it will not be as extensive as in the normal eye. Pharmacologic testing using topical phenylephrine, a direct-acting sympathomimetic agent, may help determine if the lesion is pre- or postganglionic. Both eyes need to be treated for comparison. Dilute topical phenylephrine will cause more rapid and extensive pupil dilation on the affected side due to denervation hypersensitivity. In horses with postganglionic lesions, mydriasis will occur within 20 minutes of administration, whereas the onset of dilation is 30–50 minutes in animals with preganglionic lesions. The guttural pouches and the pharynx of all patients should be examined endoscopically and the jugular furrows should be palpated for swellings. A history of recent intravenous or intramuscular injections in the neck should be obtained. Radiographs of the cervical vertebrae or thorax may also be indicated.

Management

Treatment will vary depending on the underlying cause. There is no specific treatment for Horner's syndrome; however, topical phenylephrine may be used therapeutically to alleviate temporarily the associated clinical signs.

Prognosis

The prognosis depends on the underlying cause; however, it is generally guarded as the neurologic signs are often irreversible even when the primary cause has been treated and eliminated.

Photic headshaking

Definition/overview

This is an uncommon condition, characterized by uncontrollable, spontaneous, and repetitive shaking movement of the head and neck in the absence of obvious stimulus. It is induced by exposure to light and eliminated by blindfolding, a darkened environment, or tinted contact lenses. Photic headshaking may be accompanied by sneezing, snorting, and nasal rubbing. The cause of this condition has been attributed to optic–trigeminal nerve summation, or to neuropathic pain summation in which optic nerve stimulation produces referred sensation to the nasal cavity. Headshaking behavior may be so frequent and violent that the horse can become dangerous to ride or handle. The condition is seasonal, with clinical signs typically beginning in the spring and ending in the late summer or fall. Most animals are clinically normal in the winter when light levels are lower. There is no breed or gender predilection. The mean age of onset is 9 years old. Stimulation or worsening of the clinical signs is typically seen with exposure to sunlight, stress, excitement, or exercise.

Etiology/pathophysiology

The underlying etiology for photic headshaking is unclear. It has been suggested that a latent viral infection (e.g. EHV-1) in the trigeminal nerve ganglia may be the inciting cause.

The infraorbital nerve and maxillary branch of the trigeminal nerve supply sensory innervation to the ipsilateral upper lip, cheek, nostril, and gums to the level of the first cheek tooth in the horse. Photic headshaking may occur when exposure to sunlight stimulates parasympathetic activity in the infraorbital nerve or sensory branch of the trigeminal nerve, causing an irritating nasal sensation to the horse that leads to sneezing, rubbing, flipping of the nose and head, and other clinical signs. Inflammation of the trigeminal nerve from latent viral infection may contribute to the irritability of the infraorbital nerve (a branch of the trigeminal nerve).

Clinical presentation

Horses with photic headshaking make sudden, spontaneous, and repetitive violent vertical, horizontal, or rotary movements of the head and neck in the absence of obvious external stimuli. Affected animals may appear to have an anxious expression and seem to seek shade to avoid light, warmth, or wind on the face. They will often snort or sneeze excessively, rub their muzzles on objects or the ground, strike at their nose with their forelimbs, and/or head press. Clinical signs may occur with light as the triggering factor and appear to worsen with exercise or excitement. Clinical signs are often seasonal, beginning in the spring and resolving in the fall or winter. Ophthalmologic examination findings are normal.

Differential diagnosis

There are numerous differential diagnoses for headshaking behavior. They include otitis media/interna, parasitic infestation (e.g. ear mites), guttural pouch disease, foreign body, URT disease, dental disease, ocular disease (e.g. melanotic iris cyst, vitreal floaters), progressive ethmoidal hematoma, allergic rhinitis or sinusitis, vasomotor rhinitis, osteoma of the paranasal sinuses, partial asphyxia, and stereotypical behavior.

Diagnosis

A thorough history and complete physical examination, including ophthalmic, otic, and oral assessments, are required in order to eliminate other causes of headshaking behavior. A blindfold, dim lighting, or use of certain shaded masks may relieve the clinical signs. Radiography of the head and cervical spine and/or nasopharyngeal endoscopy, including guttural pouch evaluation, will also help rule out other potential causes of headshaking.

Management

Currently, medical management with cyproheptadine (0.2–0.5 mg/kg p/o q12–24h), an antihistamine (H1-blocker) serotonin antagonist, in combination with carbamazepine (4 mg/kg p/o q6–8h), a sodium channel blocker and anticonvulsant, is usually recommended initially in cases of photic headshaking. Clinical improvement may be seen within 24–48 hours; however, carbamazepine is short acting and the horse must be exercised within 2 hours of treatment. Continuous therapy is required during the times of year when symptoms are seen, which can be expensive and may be impractical. Melatonin therapy (12 mg/450 kg) has also been used in horses with the syndrome. Topical anesthetic creams and/or nebulized steroids (e.g. betamethazone) may be effective by temporarily numbing the infraorbital nerve.

Management practices such as riding with a gauze veil or nylon stocking over the muzzle, the use of goggles or other eye protectors, and riding in the early morning or late evening under dim lighting conditions may help reduce the severity of the clinical signs temporarily. Reducing sunlight exposure by providing shelter/shade or a face mask while on pasture, turning the affected animal out in the evening rather than the daytime, and housing the horse in the darkest area of the stable during the daytime may also be helpful.

The response of photic headshakers to medical therapy is variable and, when effective, may be transient. Bilateral infraorbital neurectomy has been used in medically refractory cases when infraorbital nerve blocks reduce or eliminate the behavior; however, it is often ineffective and potential complications include the formation of painful neuromas. Posterior ethmoidal nerve blocks have also been reported to be successful in temporarily resolving headshaking symptoms in some horses.

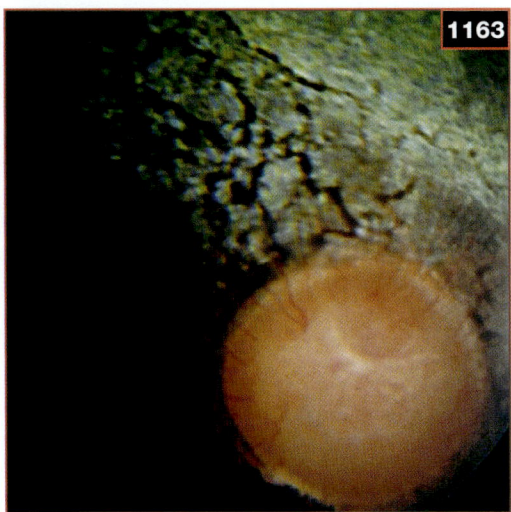

Prognosis

The prognosis is guarded as no treatment has proven consistently effective; however, medical management with cyproheptadine and carbamazepine appears to have the highest likelihood of success in relieving symptoms. Occasionally, headshaking resolves spontaneously.

Equine motor neuron disease

Definition/overview

EMND is an oxidative neurodegenerative disorder of the somatic LMNs in horses deprived of adequate dietary vitamin E for an extended period of time. While the neurologic disease is the primary complaint in most cases, ophthalmologic disease can occur concurrently. Non-ophthalmic aspects are covered elsewhere.

Etiology/pathophysiology

Vitamin E is an endogenous fat-soluble antioxidant that counteracts the harmful free radicals normally produced during metabolism in animals. A deficiency in these protective antioxidants is believed to predispose animals to neurotoxic and/or oxidative injury. The photoreceptor outer segments in the neurosensory retina have a high proportion of polyunsaturated fatty acids in their lipids, which are extremely susceptible to oxidative stress. In cases of EMND, accumulation of ceroid-lipofuscin in the retinal pigmented epithelial cells over the tapetal and nontapetal fundus is likely the result of light-generated oxidative injury to the retina. This accumulation leads to the increased retinal pigmentation visible on fundoscopy in affected animals. The remaining clinical findings of EMND are the result of dysfunction and/or death of somatic efferent motor neurons, which leads to axonal degeneration in the ventral roots and peripheral and cranial nerves.

Clinical presentation

Retinal lesions are very common (50%) and may be seen on fundoscopic examination as yellow-brown to black pigmentation found in an irregular mosaic (reticulated) pattern and/or horizontal band at the tapetal–nontapetal junction or generalized throughout the fundus (1163). The effect on vision appears variable, with most cases not reporting obvious deficits; however, a 50% decrease in b-wave amplitude has been documented in the electroretinogram of horses with EMND. The PLRs may be abnormal.

1163 A pigmented mosaic pattern is apparent in the peripapillary region of this fundus and is typical of the lesions seen in equine motor neuron disease. (Photo courtesy A Gemesky-Metzler)

Differential diagnosis

Equine protozoal meningitis (EPM), equine grass sickness/dysautonomia, lead toxicosis, botulism, laminitis, and other causes of lameness, colic, rhabdomyolysis, PSSM and other chronic myopathies, iliac thrombosis, and senile retinopathy should be considered.

Diagnosis

The diagnosis should be based on history, clinical appearance (i.e. musculoskeletal signs), fundoscopy, muscle biopsies, and laboratory results. Fundic lesions alone can be suggestive of EMND. In some cases, ERG may show decreased or extinguished b wave amplitudes despite the apparent lack of visual impairment. EMG may also be performed and will frequently reveal denervation.

Definitive diagnosis of EMND can be made post mortem with retinal histopathology revealing retinal pigmented epithelial cell congestion with ceroid-lipofuscin. Ceroid-lipofuscin deposition is also always observed in the endothelial capillaries in the spinal cord and, occasionally, in the liver and GI tract.

Management

Treatment for horses with EMND involves dietary supplementation with vitamin E and access to pasture or fresh forage.

Prognosis

The prognosis is variable. In 40% of cases, marked improvement in clinical signs is seen within 4–6 weeks after relocation to another stable and/or administration of dietary antioxidants. However, 40% of horses are euthanized or die due to continual deterioration (i.e. inability to stand or respiratory distress) within 4 weeks of the onset of clinical signs. Some horses survive and regain weight and the disease progression is arrested, although they may never fully compensate for the irreversible loss of motor neurons and often suffer permanent chronic debilitation.

Traumatic optic neuropathy

Definition/overview

Traumatic optic neuropathy occurs following severe blunt head trauma, when concussive cranial injuries cause damage to the optic nerve(s) or chiasm. The result is an acute onset of unilateral or bilateral blindness immediately following or soon after injury. Optic nerve atrophy occurs within a few weeks and will manifest itself as a pale ONH. Peripapillary chorioretinitis may also occur with chronicity.

Etiology/pathophysiology

The optic nerves are contained within the dural sheaths, which are continuous with the periosteum of the optic canal, thus fixing their position. Severe blunt head trauma caused by rearing up or falling over backwards and striking the occipital region, can allow posterior movement of the brain away from the fixed intracanalicular portion of the optic nerves. This can cause stretching, shearing, and/or avulsion of the retinal ganglion cell axons/optic nerve(s) or chiasm, resulting in optic nerve atrophy and sudden blindness. Partial or complete visual loss occurs in the affected eye(s) within 24 hours of injury.

Clinical presentation

Horses with traumatic optic neuropathy present with a history of sudden onset of blindness with or without a known history of trauma. The pupil(s) is (are) fixed and dilated with sluggish to absent PLRs in the affected eye(s). Ophthalmic lesions are not usually seen initially because of the often retrobulbar nature of the injury.

Ophthalmoscopic lesions, including peripapillary and/or ONH edema or hemorrhage, and exudate into the vitreous may be present within 24–48 hours of injury (1164). With chronicity, the lamina cribrosa becomes more prominent, the ONH will appear pale and atrophied, the peripapillary retinal vessels will appear diminished/attenuated, and focal gray patches medial, lateral, and ventral to the ONH, indicating choroidal degeneration, may also be seen.

1164 Traumatic optic neuropathy. This horse presented blind and was suspected to have fallen backward after rearing up. Note the peripapillary and ONH hemorrhages, as well as hemorrhagic streaming into the vitreous.

Differential diagnosis

Optic nerve and retinal degeneration in the horse has been reported to develop secondary to ERU, glaucoma, hypovolemia/blood loss, exposure to toxins, progressive retinal atrophy, and carotid artery ligation. Brain injuries should also be considered in the list of differential diagnoses for traumatic optic neuropathy.

Diagnosis

Diagnosis should be based on history and findings on physical and ophthalmic examination. A failure to navigate photopic and scotopic maze tests is also present.

Management

Treatment when cases are presented acutely traditionally involves high doses of anti-inflammatories such as systemic corticosteroids (e.g. dexamethasone), NSAIDs, and DMSO in order to help decrease optic nerve swelling and inflammation. There is no treatment available for chronic cases.

Prognosis

The prognosis for restoration of vision is guarded to poor, as it is often a permanent condition.

Exudative optic neuritis/neuropathy

Definition/overview

Exudative optic neuritis is seen as a sudden onset of bilateral blindness in older horses. The most prominent finding is marked exudate present over the surface of the ONH.

Etiology/pathophysiology

The cause is unknown. It may represent a more extensive form of traumatic optic neuropathy and, likewise, have a mechanical cause. The pathophysiology is unclear. The exudate contains proliferating astrocytes and lipid-laden phagocytic cells.

Clinical presentation

Acute blindness is seen in affected animals. The retinal lesions seen on fundoscopy may vary, but are typically seen as white to gray exudates that radiate from the ONH and are raised into the vitreous. The exudate may obscure the ONH completely. If the ONH is visible, edema and multiple small hemorrhages are often present. With chronicity the ONH will appear atrophied.

Differential diagnosis

Sepsis and other causes of optic neuritis (*Table 61*), traumatic optic neuropathy, benign exudative/proliferative optic neuropathy, and ONH tumors should be included in the list of differentials for exudative optic neuritis.

TABLE 61 Causes of optic neuritis

- Idiopathic/immune-mediated
- Fungal
  - Systemic aspergillosis, *Cryptococcus neoformans*
- *Toxoplasma gondii*
- *Onchocerca cervicalis*
- *Leptospira* spp.
- Neoplasia
- Toxins
  - Lead, arsenic, thallium, ethyl/methyl alcohol, chlorinated hydrocarbon?
- Septicemia
- Bacterial
  - *Streptococcus equi, Actinomyces* spp., Borna disease, toxoplasmosis, *Actinobacillus equuli, Rhodococcus equi*
- Vitamin A deficiency?
- Orbital inflammation
- Trauma
- Vascular embarrassment/ischemia
- Borna disease
- Parasite migration
- Brain abscess/meningitis i.e. *Pseudomonas mallei* (glanders), *Streptococcus equi,* Cryptococcosis
- Equine protozoal encephalomyelitis
- Hepatoencephalopathy, leukoencephalomalacia, hydrocephalus, idiopathic epilepsy
- Verminous migration
- Profound blood loss
- Rabies

Diagnosis

Diagnosis is based on history and clinical findings.

Management

Treatment is not successful.

Prognosis

The prognosis is generally poor as the ONH lesions will typically progress to atrophy.

Benign exudative/proliferative optic neuropathy

Definition/overview

Benign exudative neuropathy and proliferative optic neuropathy are terms that describe white or gray material protruding anterior to the optic disk and into the vitreous in an otherwise normal fundus. The exudate may slowly enlarge over months or years; however, there is no or minimal effect on vision (unless it becomes large enough to obscure portions of the retina) and it is generally considered to be a benign lesion. This incidental finding is seen unilaterally, primarily in older horses (>15 years old).

Etiology/pathophysiology

The cause is not known and the pathophysiology is unclear. The mass has a similar appearance to a schwannoma/astrocytoma on histopathology.

Clinical presentation

Vision is not affected. Proliferative optic neuropathy is seen as white or gray masses on or near the optic disk and protruding into the vitreous humor in middle-aged or older horses. They are typically attached at the periphery of the optic disk, are vascularized, and can be pedunculated or multilobular.

Differential diagnosis

This disease should be differentiated from exudative optic neuritis, traumatic optic neuropathy, and optic nerve neoplasia.

Diagnosis

Diagnosis is based on history and clinical appearance.

Management

No therapy is available. Vision is not affected clinically and the lesions appear to be stable, so treatment appears unnecessary.

Prognosis

Benign exudative/proliferative optic neuropathy is usually an incidental finding. In the absence of other changes, this condition is considered benign and nonprogressive and the prognosis for vision is excellent.

Parasitic diseases of the eye

Onchocerciasis

Definition/overview

Onchocerciasis is caused by the aberrant migration of the microfilariae of the parasite *Onchocerca cervicalis* into the conjunctiva, eyelids, cornea, and sclera, and/or intraocularly. It is a nonseasonal and nonpruritic disease, with the incidence increasing with age.

Etiology/pathophysiology

The parasite *O. cervicalis* is responsible for the disease. The adult form of *O. cervicalis* resides harmlessly in the ligamentum nuchae. The microfilariae migrate through the subcutaneous tissues to the dermis and become ingested by the intermediate host, a biting midge (*Culicoides* spp.). The microfilariae are then transmitted to the horse by a bite and develop into adults. Aberrant migration of the microfilariae may involve the eyelids, conjunctiva, cornea, sclera, anterior chamber, uvea, and/or fundus, producing ocular signs of the disease.

Clinical presentation

Ocular signs include lacrimation, blepharospasm, conjunctival thickening (**1165**) and depigmentation of the temporal limbus (vitiligo) (**1166**), conjunctivitis, corneal edema, vascularization and stromal cellular infiltration (keratitis), small nodules and corneal opacities, anterior uveitis, and peripapillary chorioretinitis. Other clinical signs may include lesions of diffuse, patchy alopecia, erythema, and scaling along the ventral midline, face, base of the mane, and craniomedial forearm, and a cranial pectoral 'bull's eye' lesion in the center of the forehead.

Differential diagnosis

SCC, habronemiasis, mycotic infection, and other causes of keratitis, uveitis, and chorioretinitis should be considered.

Diagnosis

A presumptive diagnosis may be made based on history, clinical signs, exclusion of other differential diagnoses, and response to therapy. Conjunctival biopsy illustrating free microfilariae (**1167**), eosinophils, and lymphocytes is diagnostic.

Management

The microfilariae may be eliminated using ivermectin (0.2 mg/kg p/o). Minor adverse reactions (fever and swelling) occur in 25% of horses treated with ivermectin. Unfortunately, there is no treatment for the adults, so recurrence is possible. Topical and/or systemic anti-inflammatories may help control the inflammation incited by the dying microfilariae. The ocular signs should also be treated

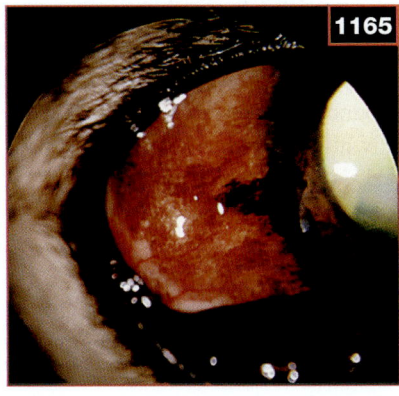

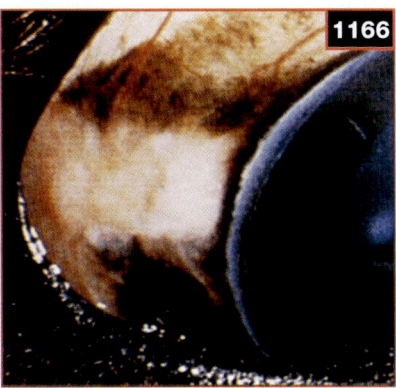

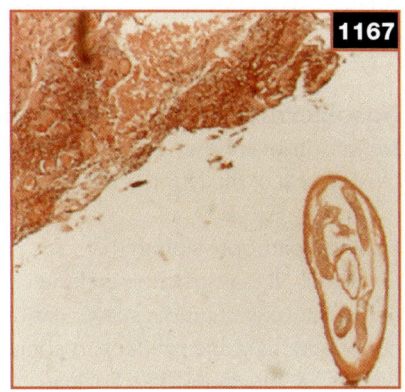

symptomatically (i.e. corneal ulcers should be treated with topical antimicrobials and atropine; uveitis with topical and/or systemic anti-inflammatories and atropine).

Prognosis
Most horses will improve within 2–3 weeks of treatment. As adult worms are not affected, the disease may recur in 2 months. Routine deworming practices are therefore recommended for all horses.

Habronemiasis
Definition/overview
Habronemiasis is caused by the aberrant migration of nematode larvae. It tends to occur in the warmer summer months and is also called 'summer sores'.

Etiology/pathophysiology
Habronemiasis is caused by the aberrant migration of nematode larvae of the species *Habronema muscae*, *H. microstoma*, and *Draschia megastoma*. The adult parasite resides in the stomach of the horse. The eggs or larvae are passed in the feces and ingested by the larvae of the intermediate host (either the house fly *Musca domestica* or the stable fly *Stomoxys calcitrans*). Horses are infected following ingestion of an infected adult fly, or infectious L3 larvae may be deposited on wounds around the eye or near the mouth. Larval migration through tissue incites a granulomatous inflammatory response, which can become walled off into discrete nodules or multilobulated masses that become caseous and necrotic. They can occasionally be mineralized and ulcerated. Lesions of the skin of the medial canthus are the result of inflammation and ulceration caused by larval migration into the NLS.

Clinical presentation
Ocular signs of habronemiasis include raised, irregular, proliferative wounds or nodular masses on the medial canthus that may be ulcerated, conjunctivitis, pruritus, and lesions associated with self-trauma.

1165–1167 Onchocerciasis. (1165) Active conjunctival hyperemia and chemosis. (1166) Vitiligo at the lateral limbus is a sequela to *Onchocerca*-related inflammation. (1167) *O. cervicalis* was recovered from a biopsy of the conjunctiva at the lateral limbus. (Photos courtesy American College of Veterinary Ophthalmologists)

Differential diagnosis
SCC, sarcoids, onchocerciasis, phycomycosis, foreign body reaction, and exuberant granulation tissue are all differential diagnoses to consider.

Diagnosis
History and clinical signs are suggestive. Definitive diagnosis is sometimes difficult as the larvae are easily missed on conjunctival scraping and/or fecal examination. Conjunctival biopsy may reveal eosinophilic infiltrates, mast cells, granulation tissue, and/or gritty caseated lesions that are almost pathognomonic for the disease ('sulfur granules'). Gastric lavage may reveal eggs or larvae.

Management
Systemic ivermectin (0.2 mg/kg p/o) or moxidectin (0.4 mg/kg p/o) is the treatment of choice. Topical (e.g. flurbiprofen) and/or systemic (e.g. flunixin meglumine or phenylbutazone) NSAIDS can help decrease the inflammatory reaction associated with treatment. Surgical debulking or removal of lesions may be performed for large granulomas prior to ivermectin therapy.

Preventive measures should include fly control, regular removal of manure, an appropriate anthelmintic treatment regime, and topical organophosphates.

Prognosis
The overall prognosis is good. Routine deworming is recommended in all horses.

Eyes

Miscellaneous conditions of the eye

Nasolacrimal system obstruction

Definition/overview
Obstruction of the NLS is common in horses.

Etiology/pathophysiology
Causes of NLS obstruction include chronic dacryocystitis, neoplasia (e.g. cutaneous SCC, nasal and paranasal sinus neoplasia), habronema blepharoconjunctivitis, and foreign bodies. A blocked NLS can lead to dacryocystitis and associated ocular signs.

Clinical presentation
NLS obstruction in horses is typically nonpainful, with epiphora or mucopurulent ocular discharge (if dacryocystitis is present). Facial dermatitis and conjunctivitis are other clinical signs that may be present.

Differential diagnosis
Congenital NLS anomalies and other causes of chronic epiphora should be considered as differentials.

Diagnosis
Diagnosis is based on failure of fluorescein dye to exit the nostril after application to the eye and an inability to flush or cannulate the nasolacrimal duct. Dacryocystorhinography will confirm the diagnosis (1168).

Management
The NLS should be flushed and the nasolacrimal duct catheterized. The need for additional surgical procedures will vary based on the cause and location of the obstruction. Topical and systemic antimicrobials and anti-inflammatories are helpful in preventing or treating infection and inflammation associated with the obstruction. The antimicrobial selected is ideally based on culture and sensitivity results.

Prognosis
The prognosis is poor to excellent depending on the underlying cause. NLS obstruction secondary to neoplasia typically has a poor prognosis. Obstruction due to foreign body material is usually given an excellent prognosis for resolution of the clinical signs following removal.

Iris prolapse

Definition/overview
Corneal perforation with iris prolapse may be a sequela to a traumatic insult to the globe or orbit, as well as to ulcerative disease of the cornea.

Etiology/pathophysiology
There is an equal prevalence of traumatic lacerations and perforations associated with ulcerative disease leading to iris prolapse. Blunt trauma most often causes globe rupture at the limbus or equator where the sclera is thinnest and, therefore, the most fragile, resulting in protrusion of uveal tissue through the corneal rupture site and hyphema. Sharp trauma can cause rupture of the cornea, limbus and/or sclera. Corneal perforation can also occur secondary to rapid enzymatic degradation of stromal collagen and ground substance caused by infectious and noninfectious ulcerative keratitis. Deep stromal abscessation in the horse can also progress to full-thickness corneal rupture in rare cases. Globe rupture may also occur during examination of deep corneal ulcers or descemetoceles if the horse is not amenable to examination. Globe rupture results in hyphema, fibrin formation, and uveal prolapse. Perforations may initially seal, but are unstable and may leak intermittently.

Clinical presentation
An iris prolapse typically appears as a focal red to brown or tan corneal mass bulging from the surface and associated with corneal edema and fibrin formation (1169). A very soft globe may be noted if the prolapse has not resealed and the globe reinflated. Obvious fluid leakage from the

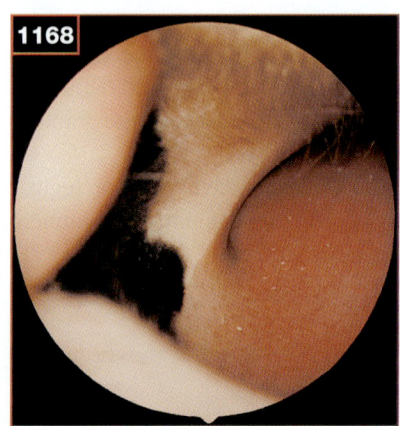

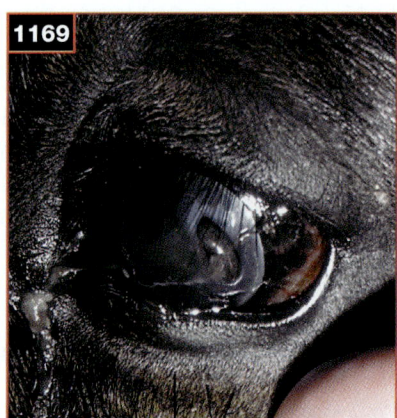

1168 View inside the nostril of a 2-year-old Clydesdale cross with chronic bilateral ocular discharge, which was due to a congenital absence of the distal nasolacrimal duct puncta.

1169 Prolapse of iris through a defect in the centrolateral cornea following corneal laceration. Note the dark brown mass (staphyloma) with surrounding corneal edema and a distorted pupil. (Photos courtesy GA Munroe)

globe may be present. Clinical signs may include lacrimation, red-tinged serous ocular discharge, mucopurulent ocular discharge, blepharospasm, photophobia, enophthalmos, blepharoedema, chemosis, keratomalacia, miosis, dyscoria, shallow or absent anterior chamber, hyphema/intraocular hemorrhage, and anterior synechiae.

Differential diagnosis

Phthisis bulbi, ulcerative keratitis, and corneal/conjunctival masses are differential diagnoses for iris prolapse.

Diagnosis

The history and clinical appearance are usually enough to make a diagnosis. Fluid leakage may be confirmed by a positive Seidel test in which 2% sodium fluorescein is applied to the eye, causing a stream of aqueous humor to fluoresce bright green when viewed under cobalt blue light. In cases of perforation following corneal ulceration, samples for cytology, culture and sensitivity, and histopathology should be collected at the time of surgery in an attempt to determine the underlying etiology. With appropriate restraint and care, transpalpebral ultrasonography may be performed to evaluate the posterior segment as well as identify possible intraocular foreign bodies. Gentle handling is required to prevent worsening of the injuries. Radiography is helpful for orbital disease (e.g. fracture) or when a radio-opaque foreign body is present or suspected.

Management

Immediate referral for surgical repair is recommended in cases of corneal perforation. The presence of an indirect PLR to the other eye implies that retinal function persists in the eye with the iris prolapse and is a positive sign that vision may be saved. An absent PLR may reflect severe intraocular disease or intense miosis of the pupil and opacity of the intraocular fluids. All criteria should be examined critically to determine if therapy should be aimed at saving vision, establishing a cosmetic globe, or removing a blind and chronically painful eye. As contamination may occur at the time of injury, aggressive topical and systemic antimicrobial therapy is warranted.

Prognosis

The prognosis in cases of iris prolapse will depend on its duration, size, and location, as well as the intraocular structures involved; however it is generally guarded for vision as approximately one third of eyes are blind at the time of discharge and over half of these eventually develop phthisis bulbi. The visual outcome is slightly better if the prolapse is the result of ulcerative keratitis rather than laceration (40% versus 33%); however, the overall rate of ocular survival is better in cases of laceration compared with ulcerative keratitis (80% versus 67%). Eyes with corneal perforations or lacerations present for more than

15 days, as well as those measuring 15 mm or more in length and extending to, along, or beyond the limbus, tend to have a poor visual outcome and usually require enucleation. Perforation as a result of blunt trauma has a worse prognosis than that due to sharp trauma as it is often accompanied by greater damage to tissues. The presence of keratomalacia or mixed infections can lead to endophthalmitis and these cases have a worse overall prognosis. Performing an iridectomy (removal of necrotic iris) does not appear to exacerbate postoperative anterior uveitis or adversely affect the visual outcome, and it may facilitate postoperative mydriasis and prevent septic endophthalmitis. The chances of retaining vision are substantially reduced in cases of iris prolapse accompanied by hyphema where 10% or more of the anterior chamber is affected.

Common sequelae following iris prolapse may include endophthalmitis, persistent intraocular inflammation, the formation of PIFMs, anterior and posterior synechiae, cataract formation, phthisis bulbi, blindness, and enucleation.

Cataracts

Definition/overview

Cataracts in horses may present as focal or diffuse, unilateral or bilateral, symmetrical or asymmetrical, and stationary or progressive lenticular opacities. They can involve the lens capsule, cortex, and/or nucleus. Cataracts may be present at birth (congenital) or acquired in early neonatal or in later adult life. Acquired cataracts may be primary/inherited or secondary to another ocular disease process. Approximately 5–7% of horses have cataracts. Cataracts are most often acquired in the horse, with chronic inflammation of the anterior uvea, especially ERU, being the most common cause. The risk of developing cataracts secondary to chronic anterior uveitis is higher in Appaloosas. Cataracts are the most frequent congenital ocular defect in foals. Very small incipient lens opacities are common and not associated with blindness. As the cataracts mature and become more opaque, the degree of blindness increases. Most veterinary ophthalmologists recommend surgical removal of cataracts in foals less than 6 months of age if the foal is healthy, no uveitis or other ocular problems are present, and the animal's personality will tolerate aggressive topical medical therapy.

Etiology/pathophysiology

The majority of adult equine cataracts are acquired, with chronic uveitis being the most common cause (see *Table 55*). The lens is nourished by the aqueous humor and any alteration in its production, composition, or flow can have adverse affects on lens metabolism and result in cataract formation. Acquired cataracts can occur secondary to chronic uveitis, as diffusion of harmful

869

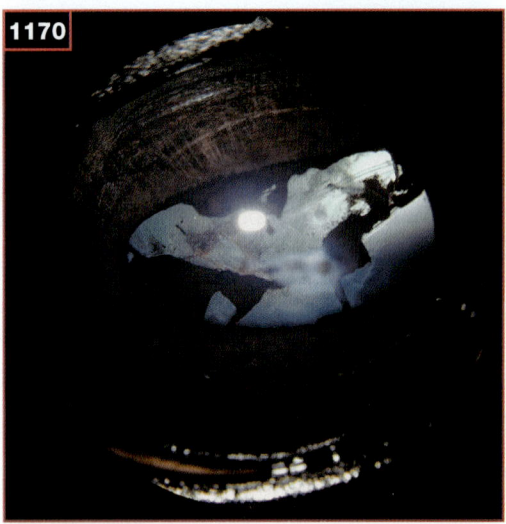

1170 Chronic uveitic eye with multiple posterior synechiae and iris rests, leading to a number of anterior capsular and cortical cataracts of varying density. (Photo courtesy GA Munroe)

inflammatory mediators across the lens capsule can occur, with subsequent alterations in the metabolism of the lens causing cataractous changes.

Clinical presentation

Cataracts will appear as an opacity in the lens (see **1125**, **1126**). Cataracts can have variable effects on the menace response and vision, depending on the extent of the cataract as well as the underlying etiology and possible sequelae. Other ocular lesions that may be associated with cataract formation include conjunctival hyperemia, corneal ulceration, uveitis (**1170**), synechiae, glaucoma, lens luxation/subluxation (see **1124**), and retinal disease or detachment. Horses with cataracts causing visual impairment are prone to traumatic injury.

Differential diagnosis

Differential diagnoses include any other cause of vision deficits in the horse.

Diagnosis

Cataracts are diagnosed based on documentation of a unilateral or bilateral opacity in the lens. Ocular ultrasonography and ERG are useful in diagnosing posterior segment abnormalities.

Management

Horses with cataracts may become visually impaired to the extent that they cannot be ridden or used for their intended purpose. They may be dangerous and prone to self-injury. Horses with unilateral or bilateral immature or mature cataracts that interfere with vision should be referred to a veterinary ophthalmologist promptly for evaluation to confirm the diagnosis and discuss treatment options. Where appropriate, surgical removal by phacoemulsification is recommended to restore functional vision in healthy animals with visual impairment, good PLRs, good dazzle reflexes, and no other ocular abnormalities or diseases that may affect vision. Recent investigation into the use of a foldable +14D intraocular lens in horses has shown that pseudophakic equine patients can be successfully returned to within 1D of emmetropia. Absence of retinal detachment based on ophthalmoscopy or ultrasonography, a normal ERG (in Appaloosas), no systemic disease, and absent or controlled preoperative uveitis are also required. The patient must be amenable to the level of postoperative medical care necessary following intraocular surgery. Cataracts secondary to uveitis are poor candidates for cataract surgery.

Potential intraoperative complications in the horse include corneal edema, collapse of the anterior chamber, iris prolapse through the corneal incision, hyphema, and posterior lens capsule tears. Postoperative complications include, but are not limited to, self-trauma, periorbital edema, corneal edema, corneal ulceration (see **1128**), fibrin formation, uveitis, synechiae, posterior lens capsule tear enlargement, posterior capsular opacifications, PIFM formation, vitreal presentation, retinal degeneration, retinal detachment, endophthalmitis, and phthisis bulbi (see **1111**). Enucleation or intrascleral silicone prosthesis, a more cosmetic alternative to enucleation, may be performed in horses with painful, nonvisual eyes in which cataract surgery is contraindicated.

Prognosis

The age of the patient influences the postoperative success rate. Cataract surgery results by experienced veterinary ophthalmologists in foals less than 6 months of age are very good (approximately 80% success rate); however, the success rate is lower in older animals (approximately 50%). Although functional vision can be restored in some cases in adult horses with cataracts secondary to ERU, generally success is less likely compared with what is typically possible in young horses and adult animals without ERU.

Glaucoma

Definition/overview

Glaucoma is an elevation in the IOP that is too high for normal retinal ganglion cell and optic nerve axon function. It is caused by a decrease or reduction in the outflow of aqueous humor, which eventually results in optic nerve damage and blindness.

Etiology/pathophysiology

Glaucoma may be categorized as congenital, primary, or secondary. Congenital glaucoma occurs rarely in horses, but it has been reported in Thoroughbred, Arabian, and Standardbred foals. When it is seen, it is often associated with multiple congenital ocular anomalies and may be unilateral or bilateral. Acquired glaucoma may be categorized as primary, due to an abnormal aqueous drainage pathway, or secondary, as a result of other ocular diseases that cause mechanical blockage of the pupil and/or ICA or functional obstruction of the ICA and/or uveoscleral pathway. Primary glaucoma is uncommon and often bilateral. Secondary glaucoma is most frequently found and is often a sequela to anterior uveitis, but it may also occur as a result of trauma or lens luxation/subluxation. Horses with previous or concurrent ERU, those older than 15 years, and Appaloosas are at increased risk of developing glaucoma. Bilateral involvement does occur in horses with secondary glaucoma in some cases of bilateral ERU.

Aqueous humor is produced constantly and must flow from the posterior chamber into the anterior chamber between the lens and iris. It drains from the eye through the ICA and uveoscleral outflow pathways. Primary glaucoma results from abnormal development of the ICA predisposing to poor fluid drainage and an increase in IOP. Horses with primary glaucoma in one eye are predisposed to developing it in the other eye. Secondary glaucoma occurs through damage to the ICA or uveoscleral outflow pathway from scarring, vascularization, or accumulation of inflammatory cells and debris. This is the result of another ocular disease such as chronic uveitis, intraocular neoplasia, lens luxation, or trauma. This obstruction leads to retention of aqueous humor and subsequent increase in the pressure within the eye, which decreases retinal ganglion cell function, causing optic nerve axon degeneration and progressive visual deterioration.

Clinical presentation

Vision impairment or blindness, buphthalmos, blepharospasm, mydriasis, epiphora, conjunctival hyperemia, episcleral congestion, corneal edema, Haab's striae (breaks in Descemet's membrane), uveitis, lens subluxation/luxation, tapetal hyperreflectivity, retinal degeneration/atrophy, and optic nerve cupping/atrophy may be found in horses with glaucoma (1171). Congenital glaucoma may be seen with other developmental ocular anomalies such as iris hypoplasia, microphakia, cataract, goniodysgenesis, and retinal dysplasia (anterior segment dysgenesis). Secondary glaucoma most often occurs as a result of chronic or recurrent uveitis. Historically, these horses have multiple episodes of intraocular inflammation with bouts of ocular cloudiness/edema and discomfort as well as clinical signs of uveitis. In horses with secondary glaucoma, associated clinical signs may include posterior synechiae (adhesions), a miotic pupil, and cataract formation. These eyes may be enlarged (buphthalmos), possibly with an ulcerative exposure keratitis, and lens subluxation/luxation can also occur late in the disease (1172). These eyes may or may not be painful.

1171, 1172 Glaucoma. Pressure on the corneal endothelium with glaucoma creates corneal striae (Haab's striae), linear track-like lesions that can also become edematous (1171). Posterior luxation with the dorsal edge of the lens visible in the ventromedial aspect of the pupil in a horse with glaucoma (1172).

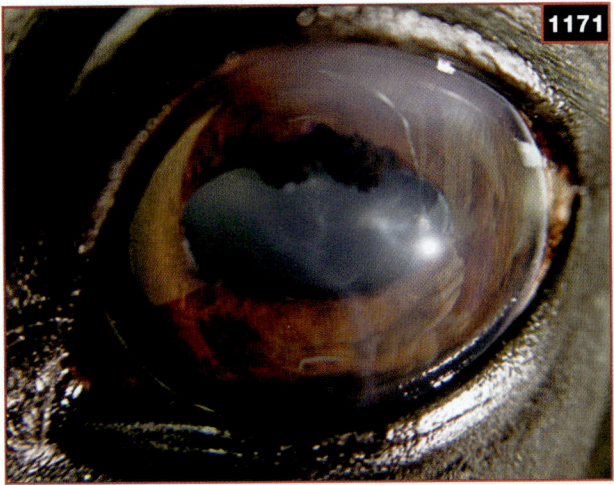

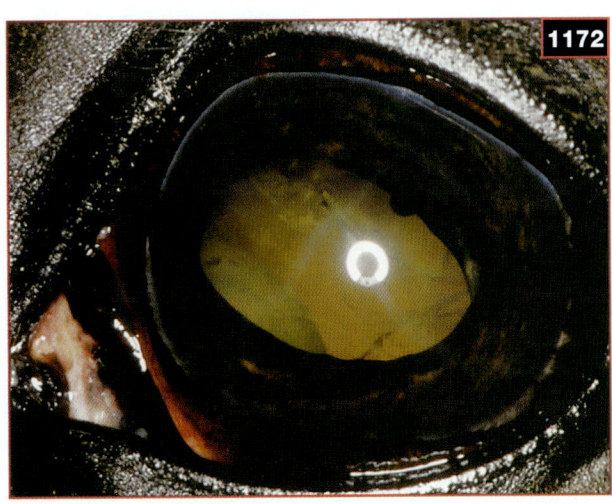

Differential diagnosis

Glaucoma should be considered in any case of unexplained corneal edema, vision impairment, or severe unrelenting ocular inflammation.

Diagnosis

Diagnosis of glaucoma can be made based on the history, clinical appearance, and applanation tonometry illustrating an elevation in IOP. Historically, these horses have multiple episodes of intraocular inflammation followed by a severe unrelenting bout of ocular cloudiness and discomfort (as a result of the development of glaucoma) that does not respond to traditional uveitis therapy. A thorough and complete ophthalmic examination is vital to help rule out other causes of corneal edema, vision impairment, and ocular pain, and to determine if the glaucoma is primary or secondary. The IOP averages 23 mmHg in the horse eye (normal range 17–28.6 mmHg). A Tonopen measurement greater than 30 mmHg is consistent with a diagnosis of glaucoma. Examination of the ICA may show abnormalities. Ocular ultrasonography may be used to help rule out other intraocular diseases (e.g. intraocular tumor).

Management

It is essential to determine the cause of the glaucoma because therapy will vary according to etiology; however, the most common cause in horses is ERU. There is inconsistent response to antiglaucoma medications. Treatment of glaucoma is centered on decreasing the production of aqueous humor or increasing outflow. Medical treatment may include topical beta adrenergic blockers (e.g. 0.5% timolol maleate q12h) and topical carbonic anhydrase inhibitors (e.g. 2% dorzolamide or 1% brinzolamide q8–12h). A timolol/dorzolamide combination medication is offered for use in the horse to help decrease the number of medications necessary. Systemic carbonic anhydrase inhibitors are also available (e.g. acetazolamide, 2–3 mg/kg p/o q6–12h; dichlorphenamide, 1 mg/kg p/o q12h; methazolamide, 0.25 mg/kg p/o q24h), but potassium supplementation is typically required. Topical and systemic anti-inflammatory medications should be used initially to help control intraocular inflammation and increase patient comfort.

Laser cyclophotoablation can be used to decrease the amount of aqueous humor produced by the ciliary body in eyes with the potential for vision that do not respond to antiglaucoma medications. Existing intraocular inflammation must be controlled prior to treatment and other intraocular diseases such as neoplasia should be ruled out. If corneal ulcers are present, they should be treated prior to laser surgery. Systemic anti-inflammatory medications are required for 7–10 days following laser therapy. Lasers appear to be very effective at controlling IOP and helping to preserve vision, with over 50% of eyes remaining sighted. However, antiglaucoma medications are usually required indefinitely after surgery. Postsurgical complications include continued or recurring elevation in IOP, hypotony, blepharoedema, chemosis, corneal edema, ocular hemorrhage, corneal ulceration, cataract formation, vitreal fibrin and hemorrhage, and decreased vision or blindness. Many eyes need to be treated again in 6–12 months. Similarly, cyclocryoablation has also been used; however, some clinicians suggest that it should be reserved for use in blind eyes only. Again, any decrease in aqueous production may only be temporary.

Surgical techniques to increase aqueous outflow (e.g. gonioimplants, sclerostomies, and iridectomies) have also been used in horses with glaucoma with varying success. Horses with glaucoma should have their IOP measured regularly in order to monitor the response to therapy. Often, affected eyes will become blind and chronically painful. Enucleation or evisceration with intrascleral prosthesis is the treatment of choice in these cases. In horses with unilateral primary glaucoma, preventive antiglaucoma medications should be used in the unaffected eye. Repeated measurements of the IOP should be taken in the predisposed eye 3–4 times per year for life or until the eye becomes glaucomatous.

Prognosis

The prognosis for vision is guarded. The most effective long-term therapy currently available appears to be cyclophotoablation in combination with topical antiglaucoma medications.

12

Skin

Reginald Pascoe

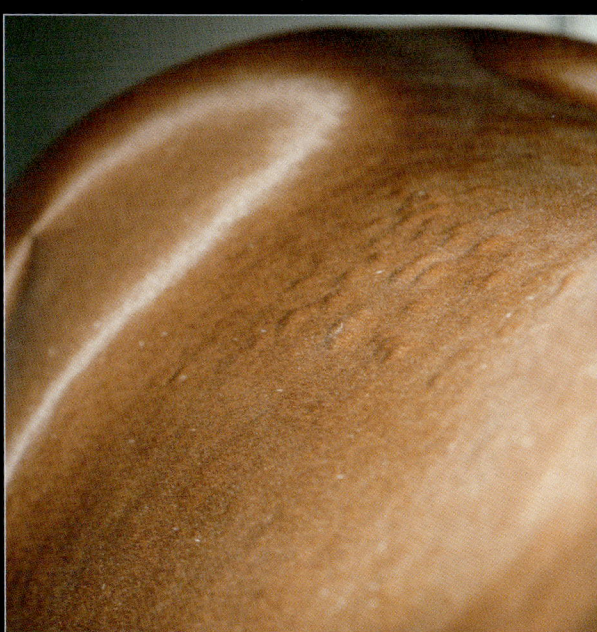

The skin is recognized as the body's largest organ and among its more important tasks are protection of the horse against the environment, thermo-regulation (sweating and heat conservation), sensory perception, secretory function, pigmentation, and as an indicator of the horse's general health. The careful assessment of clinical signs, understanding their significance in relation to a disease process, and a basic understanding of skin morphology and function allow the accumulation of sets of indicators of disease that help the clinician to reach an accurate diagnosis.

The initial approach is to determine the predominant clinical signs. The three most common components of skin disease are pruritus, hair loss, and nodular lesions. Secondary changes include dry dermatosis (scaling and crusting), moist dermatosis (weeping and seeping), and pigmentary changes. The history of the disease, any treatment already given, the owner's views, and then the appearance of the horse should be examined to see if these three important signs, plus any or all of the three secondary conditions, are part of the disease pattern. While it may be more scientifically 'correct' to make an approach based on the causal agent or agents, these may not be clear until tests are taken and the diagnostic process begun.

Examination

History

The historical record should cover the clinical history of the disease process, an extensive review of the horse's environment and feeding regimens, and should identify any outside source(s) of causal agents to eliminate these early in the course of the investigation. The use of a formulated examination sheet allows a structured and thorough approach. With long-standing cases it is helpful to list the following in chronological order: (1) notes of the disease's progress; (2) changes in feed; (3) location; (4) events; and (5) other riders or tack that have been used. A list should also be made of all or any previous medications, not only for the skin condition itself, but also for any other medical or surgical condition that the horse has had in the past. The results of any tests and follow-up treatments should also be listed.

Clinical examination

The clinical appraisal of the horse involves looking at its general health and bodily condition and visually assessing the obvious sites of the skin problem, which may be localized or generalized. A complete clinical examination should be performed, as there may be indicators suggesting that organ function tests should be carried out. Some examples are endocrine diseases such as equine Cushing's disease and anhidrosis, both of which have marked effects on the hair coat. Immune-mediated diseases are rare, but diseases such as systemic lupus erythematosus (SLE) also have multisystemic effects and their diagnosis requires the combination of skin biopsy, clinical signs and positive antinuclear antibody (ANA) and lupus erythematosus (LE) cell tests. Fungal organisms, such as *Phycomycetes,* can show both generalized and cutaneous forms. Liver toxicosis due to feed toxins or poisonous plants may show skin changes.

The skin lesions should be carefully evaluated. Various diagnostic skin tests are available for use and contact should be made with a pathology laboratory to enable discussion of the clinical features of a case and to receive advice on the most appropriate samples to collect.

Diagnostic tests

The identification of the condition into one or more of the major categories of skin disease allows a logical pathway of diagnosis to be followed. Flowcharts can be used to facilitate the process by narrowing the list of suspect diseases and directing the clinician towards individual disease descriptions.

After recording a complete history of the horse's condition and a thorough clinical examination, it is necessary to choose appropriate tests that will confirm the diagnosis or eliminate possible differential diagnoses.

Samples should be taken in the following order:
1. Skin sampling for parasites.
2. Hair and scab scraping for fungi and bacteria.
3. Swabs for bacterial and fungal culture.
4. Biopsy for histopathology:
   - ✦ Special tests:
     - ◇ Immunofluorescence testing.
     - ◇ Culture swab from biopsy site (deep mycosis lesions).
5. Needle aspirate for cytology: nodules and subcutaneous masses.
6. Serum for ANA testing.

Skin sampling

All horses with pruritic skin disease or evidence of a papular or crusting dermatitis should be carefully checked for the presence of ectoparasites. A flea comb, a hand lens, and a strong pencil-light torch are very useful for the collection of lice and mites. Superficial scrapings using a fixed-blade dull scalpel are made to collect hair skin scurf and the superficial layer of skin and do not cause bleeding. *Psoroptes* spp., *Pymotes* mites, *Dermanyssus gallinae* (poultry red mite), and lice may be found in these samples. Deep scrapings collect material from the intrafollicular space and superficial dermis, and are deep enough for bleeding to occur. *Demodex, Sarcoptes, Chorioptes* spp., *Pelodera* spp., or *Strongyloides* spp. may be found in these samples. Samples should be taken from as many fresh areas as possible, as there is difficulty in obtaining mites in all samples. There is no finite number of samples to take. In most instances positive findings are indicators of a positive diagnosis. Care should be taken when *Demodex* is found because it can be a normal finding in clinically normal horses. Unless a sufficiently large sample has been taken, negative findings may not necessarily indicate an irrefutable negative result.

Clear acetate tape preparation

This was originally a technique to detect *Oxyuris equi* eggs around the anus, vulva, and perineum. Is it now also used for other free-moving skin parasites such as chigger mites,

poultry red mites, *Psoroptes equi*, lice, and *Trombiculid* mites. The hair should be clipped with scissors to allow the acetate tape to be applied firmly to the skin and base of the hairs. After removal from the skin site the tape is placed on a microscope slide and examined by hand lens and microscope. A hand lens is used for closer examination initially of ears, base of mane and tail, muzzle, and limbs in the search for *Psoroptes equi*.

Hair sampling

Indications for the use of this technique are altered hair growth patterns, broken hairs, crusts, scales, and actual loss of hair, or where *Dermatophilus* spp. or dermatophytes are suspected. Hair and associated scabs are plucked from a number of fresh lesions and placed in sterile containers. Samples are examined by direct or impression smears and stained appropriately to allow identification of the organisms. Hair samples taken from potential dermatophyte cases are cultured on special medium (Sabouraud's dextrose agar plus a variety of additives) for up to 14 days to confirm smear findings.

Swabs for bacterial and fungal culture

The horse's skin abounds with commensal and contaminating bacteria that decrease the usefulness of skin culture. Swabs taken from the surface of lesions are likely to be unreliable. Needle aspiration of pus and debris from the deeper layer of the diseased area is more likely to give a pure culture of pathogens. An intact pustule or recently infected area should be sampled before any other sampling is carried out. The deep portion of a biopsy can be used to obtain a swab for culture, or a small portion should be aseptically removed and placed in transport medium for culture. A positive culture and the use of sensitivity disks is a well-practiced laboratory procedure, but it is important to remember that drugs applied topically may reach lower levels than those used systemically. Parenteral use of suitable antibiotics, as identified by sensitivity testing, may be inappropriate in skin infections.

Skin biopsy

The response of skin to a variety of conditions can give identical histopathology, which is often why biopsy results are disappointing to both clinician and pathologist. Skin biopsies are taken for the following reasons: to establish a specific diagnosis; to eliminate other clinical diagnoses; to follow the course of the disease; and to confirm the completeness of excision of a tumor. It is unlikely that a single biopsy will give answers to all these questions. If a primary diagnosis is required, it is usual to biopsy a representative mature lesion, except in the case of any vesicular disease, which should be biopsied as early as possible to decrease the likelihood of secondary, self-inflicted lesions.

Biopsies are useful for the diagnosis of the following diseases:

+ Biopsies of granulomas are often specially stained to show the presence of bacteria, fungi, and parasites, and in such diseases as onchocerciasis and habronemiasis.
+ Staphylococci, streptococci, *Dermatophilus* spp., and dermatophytes may be obtained from very early fresh lesions by swabbing, but culture from the inside of the sterile biopsy punch after biopsy is taken is more useful.
+ Autoimmune diseases such as pemphigus foliaceus and bullous pemphigoid require biopsies taken for both histopathology and immunofluorescence.

The biopsy is usually taken under sedation and local anesthetic infiltration. Samples are placed in 10% buffered neutral formal saline (10 × volume of fixative to specimen) and/or swabbed for bacterial or fungal culture. The skin must not be stretched during biopsy. A scalpel and a fine-toothed forceps or needle is used to remove the biopsy. Ideally, the specimen size should be reduced to <1 cm to allow for proper fixation. Multiple biopsies are desirable. Small specimens (<4 mm) may be barely adequate, especially if distorted by stretch, compression, or crushing in sampling. Large specimens need to be handled carefully to prevent curling and distortion of the specimen in the fixative. The pathologist should be consulted before taking samples to ensure the best site samples are selected and properly fixed for transport.

The following types of biopsy can be taken:

+ A shave biopsy is a thin slice of epidermis and small portion of dermis. Suturing is not required.
+ Punch biopsy. A disposable sterile 6 mm punch is the most commonly used biopsy for collection of epidermis, dermis, subcutaneous fat, and panniculus muscle. Suturing is not usually required.
+ A wedge biopsy is a full- thickness section cut through the abnormal tissue and includes a small piece of normal skin on one edge of the wedge for comparison and to orientate the lesion for the pathologist. Suturing may be necessary.
+ An excision biopsy is used where small lesions are excised whole, with an elliptical incision using a scalpel, and including all tissue down to the panniculus muscle. One or more sutures are placed to close the skin.

Smears and needle aspirates

Smears taken from erosive or ulcerating masses, nodules, and draining lesions can be of value for fresh *Dermatophilus* lesions, section of tumors, and subcutaneous nodules. They are taken directly from the lesion or from the cut surface of a lesion.

FNAs can be obtained from the contents of a nodule or mass with a 1–2 ml syringe with a 23-gauge needle. The contents are extruded onto a slide and a smear is made, stained, and examined. The horse's skin has many contaminants and, due to the density of nodules, this test is both time consuming and often unrewarding. The use of a biopsy punch is a more practical and reliable technique.

Immunofluorescence

Tests using these techniques are available in specialized pathology laboratories. Some pathologists question the value of direct immunofluorescence in horses, preferring the use of histopathology. Biopsy samples should be placed in 10% formal saline for routine histopathology and in Michel's medium for immunofluorescence testing.

Antinuclear antibody testing

The ANA titer and LE cell preparation assist in the diagnosis of SLE, which is a rare multisystem autoimmune disease. ANA titer detects the component of the cell nucleus, whereas LE preparation detects antibody to nucleoprotein. While neither test is specific for SLE, a positive result (titers exceeding 1/160) serves to indicate a possible autoimmune dysfunction.

Allergy testing

Intradermal skin testing in horses is fairly restricted. Both false-negative and false-positive tests occur. Many substances, such as grass, tree and weed pollens, molds, stable dust, dust mites, feathers, and dander, cause inhalant allergies. If skin testing is to be carried out, the horse must not have been recently treated with drugs such as corticosteroids, antihistamines, some tranquillizers, or anesthetics. Lyophilized allergen panels are available for horses, but, once reconstituted, they must be used within 3 months. Small amounts of various allergens are injected intradermally, usually on the neck. To avoid clipper rashes, clipping should be carried out a day or two previously. Controls used are histamine for positive responses and normal saline for negative responses. Reaction to allergens can then be compared with the two test reaction sites.

In-vitro allergy tests

Commercially available tests on serum use either the radioallergosorbent test (RAST) that uses radioactively labeled antiserum, or an ELISA that uses antibody coupled to enzymes. Both tests require serum samples for incubation. Very careful evaluation of results is necessary, as many tests lack specificity and results can vary widely from laboratory to laboratory. Sufficient data regarding reported testing and its results have yet to be published to allow evaluation of their efficacy in equine dermatology.

Pruritic diseases

Pruritus is itching/scratching and is the most common clinical sign of skin disease. It may be related to insect bites, be a manifestation of a systemic disease, or it may be a hypersensitivity reaction (immediate or delayed). A very detailed history of the case is required:

✦ Is it seasonal or always present?
✦ Is the condition localized or generalized?
✦ Are all animals in the group affected?
✦ What treatments have been previously given?
✦ Were they topical or systemic, successful or not, and a prescribed treatment?
✦ What is the location of the horse, including its proximity to poultry, tall grass, forest, or scrub, and is there new stable bedding?
✦ Are lesions due to self-trauma?
✦ Are there some primary changes such as urticaria?
✦ Are there pigmentary changes?
✦ Are in-contact animals affected?
✦ Are in-contact humans also itchy?
✦ Are there insects/visible eggs present?

Pruritus can be a self-regenerating disease triggered by a moment of intense itchiness, followed by rubbing, biting, and self-mutilation that initiate a vicious circle, with the possibility that the initial trigger has gone. Pruritus is common to many skin disorders, especially allergic inflammation and parasite infections. Pruritus is entirely epidermal in origin and does not occur in deep ulcerations, although they may be painful.

Physical and chemical pruritus

Definition/overview
This is a condition where physical or chemical damage to superficial layers of skin leads to dermatitis and pruritus (1173).

Etiology/pathophysiology
Chemically-induced dermatitis results from the application of chemicals at normal strength to horses with sensitive skins, or accidental application of overstrength or irritant substances to skin.

Physical damage related to burns, freezing, trauma, and pressure necrosis from harness results in mild to severe injury to the superficial to deep layers of the epidermis, with progressive loss of skin and deeper vascular structures causing necrosis and skin death.

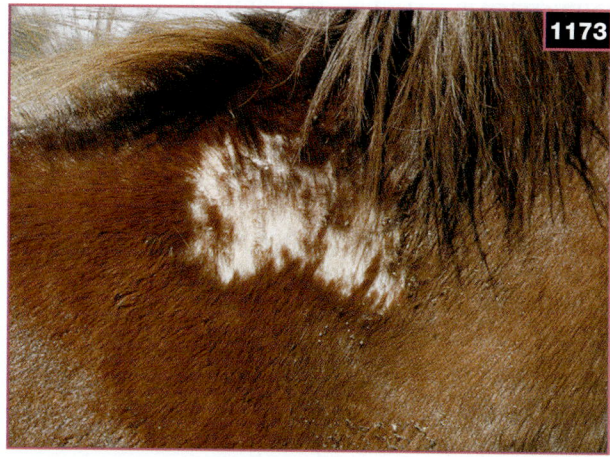

1173 Chemical-induced dermatitis following the application of overstrength insecticides. There is severe pruritus, alopecia with crusts, and folding of skin over the withers. (Reprinted from Pascoe RR and Knottenbelt DC (1999) *Manual of Equine Dermatology*, WB Saunders, with permission)

Clinical presentation
The condition presents as fine to coarse scale and patchy alopecia, with moist exudative dermatitis that may be painful to touch. Pruritus may be severe with self-mutilation. Chronic injury may result in scar tissue followed by lichenification.

Differential diagnosis
Inappropriate medication; early sweet itch; pediculosis; poultry red mite infestation; *Psoroptes* spp. infestation.

Diagnosis
Visible physical dermatitis with a history of injury, application of irritants, or accidental application of inappropriate substances may be the only indicators. Biopsy may show superficial perivascular dermatitis.

Management
Management is empirical unless an accurate diagnosis is obtained. A mild soap or shampoo wash should be used, followed by clean water. In mild cases, a mild astringent is used. In more severe cases, corticosteroid topical ointment, oral prednisolone or pain-relieving medication may be required.

Prognosis
The prognosis is fair to good unless damage to the dermis occurs, when permanent scarring may be a long-term result.

INFECTIOUS CAUSES – BACTERIAL
Definition/overview
There are no specific bacterial diseases in horses that clinically exhibit only pruritus. Swelling and pain are the more likely indicators. Pruritus may occur secondarily to a healing lesion (e.g. a healing incised abscess).

INFECTIOUS CAUSES – FUNGAL
Malassezia spp. yeast dermatitis
Definition/overview
This may be an emerging disease in horses. It is a cutaneous, pruritic, erythematous skin condition caused by *Malassezia* spp. yeasts, which in other animals appear as potential opportunistic skin pathogens.

Etiology/pathophysiology
Malassezia spp. yeast dermatitis may be related to immunologic dysfunction associated with corticosteroid use. In one study the yeast was isolated from approximately 50% of normal horses.

Clinical presentation
Affected horses present with a scaly, erythematous, and greasy pruritic dermatitis.

Differential diagnosis
Werneckiella equi; pemphigus foliaceus; *Staphylococcus* spp.; dermatophytosis; dermatophilosis.

Diagnosis
Skin scrapings are taken from the affected area and/or impression smears from skin. On cytology, yeasts are seen in clusters or adhered to keratinocytes. Culture is attempted on Sabouraud's chloramphenicol agar (peanut-shaped cell morphology).

Management
The skin is greasy and requires a keratolytic degreasing shampoo followed by the antiyeast drug miconazole applied directly to the skin for 5–10 minutes, rinsed off with 4% chlorhexidine, and repeated twice weekly until the condition resolves.

Prognosis
The number of reported cases is still too small to enable a real indication of outcomes to be given.

Pythiosis (phycomycosis)
Definition/overview
This is a chronic subcutaneous, ulcerative, and granulomatous, subtropical and tropical skin disease caused by the fungus *Pythium insidiosum*. It affects horses of all breeds and ages, and both sexes. Other names include bursati, Florida horse leech, and swamp cancer.

Etiology/pathophysiology
Pythiosis is caused by *Pythium* spp. – free-living aquatic organisms that are not true fungi. Horses become infected by standing for long periods in stagnant water containing rotting organic material at high ambient temperatures (30–40°C). Damaged skin assists the entry of the organisms into the body.

Clinical presentation
Pruritus with biting and kicking at affected areas is followed by subsequent ulceration of skin or wounds. Sticky, serosanguineous, stringy discharge either mats hairs or hangs from the body wall and/or limbs in thick mucopurulent strands (**1174, 1175**). Large 1–2 cm aggregations of organisms ('kunkers') are found buried in the fibrous tracts. Lymphadenopathy occurs in chronic cases, and involvement of joints and tendons with sinus formation is a serious complication.

Differential diagnosis
Sarcoid; *Habronema* infestation in wounds; neoplasms; mycetoma; botryomycosis; excess granulation tissue; other zygomycetes.

Diagnosis
Pythiosis occurs where horses have access to waterlogged pasture or lagoon creeks. They exhibit characteristic clinical signs. Early lesions should be biopsied, with fresh samples taken for immediate culture (on selective medium such as Campy blood agar or Sabouraud's dextrose agar) and histopathology. If the time for arrival at the laboratory is 1–3 days, samples are better transported on ice packs and then cultured on nonselective blood agar.

Management
There are no reported cases of spontaneous remission. Surgical excision under general anesthesia is the most common and successful treatment, particularly in chronic cases. Ten percent tincture of iodine is packed into the surgical area and left *in situ* for 2–3 days, and pressure bandages are applied where possible. When granulation commences the wound can be left unbandaged. Repeat surgery is common, especially when the lesions occur around tendons and joints. Sodium iodide (7 mg/kg i/v as a 3.5% solution in normal sodium chloride solution and repeated in 7 days) should be given. This is a useful

1174 *P. insidiosum* lesion on a horse's belly. Note the thick stringy exudate. The horse exhibits severe irritation, with biting and rubbing of the affected area.

1175 Pythiosis in a chronic limb lesion. Note the characteristic numerous discharging, granulomatous lesions, with a stringy serosanguineous exudate.

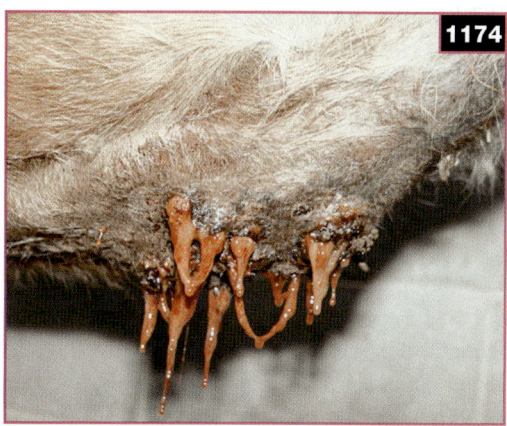

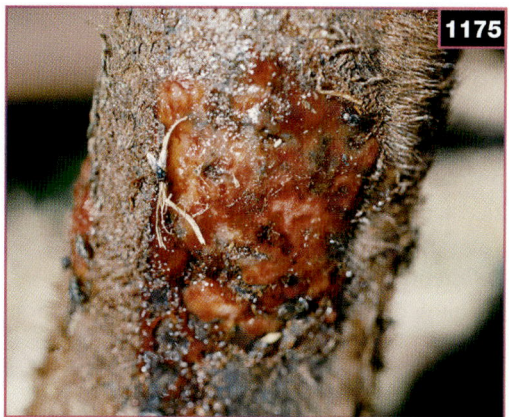

adjunct to surgery and aids in the reduction of some abdominal growths of excessive size. A phenolized vaccine has been successful in the treatment of early lesions. Successful treatment depends on the age of the horse, its general physical condition, previous treatment, age/size/site of the lesion, and whether there is bone involvement. Young fresh lesions of 2 weeks' duration respond very well to immunotherapy alone, but response is poor if lesions are older than 2 months. Infection in the bone is usually fatal.

Prognosis
The prognosis is good for body-wall lesions, but guarded for lesions involving joints and tendons.

Basidiobolus haptosporus

Definition/overview
This soil saprophyte is a member of the genus *Basidiobolus* of the Phycomycetes group of fungi. It causes lesions on the chest, abdomen, head, and neck. It is a similar disease to pythiosis, but with several important clinical differences.

Etiology/pathophysiology
Characteristically, this disease occurs in a much drier dusty environment than pythiosis. Skin injury allows entry of the saprophyte. Single lesions are common.

Clinical presentation
The clinical presentation is similar to that of pythiosis, but growths are more shallow and are confined to the neck and abdomen, with no isolations on the limbs (1176). 'Kunkers' are small to nonexistent and the pruritus is moderate to severe.

Differential diagnosis
Pythiosis; mycetoma; exuberant granulation tissue; *Habronema* infestation; neoplasms; fibroblastic sarcoids.

Diagnosis
The diagnosis is as described for pythiosis infection. 'Kunkers' are smaller and few in number. Fungal hyphae are found in foci of necrosis on biopsy samples. Biopsy punch samples should be cultured directly onto Sabouraud's dextrose agar.

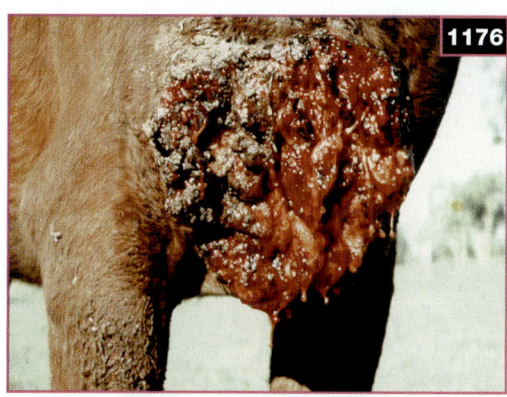

1176 *Basidiobolus haptosporus* infection. (Photo courtesy R Miller)

Management
Surgery is curative if all affected tissue is removed. Sodium iodide (7 mg/kg i/v as a 3.5% solution in normal sodium chloride solution and repeated in 7 days) should be given. No vaccine is available.

Prognosis
The prognosis is guarded to good, depending on the case.

879

Skin

INFECTIOUS CAUSES – PARASITIC (Helminths)
Larval nematode dermatitis
Definition/overview

Larval forms of *Pelodera strongyloides* and *Strongyloides westerii* have been reported to cause pruritus on the limbs of horses, resulting from being held in old, wet, holding yards.

Etiology/pathophysiology

Larval forms of *P. strongyloides* and *S. westerii* are free living and in wet weather they may invade the skin of the lower limbs of horses, particularly foals. Infestation usually occurs under poor hygienic conditions, muddy holding yards, or with contaminated bedding.

Clinical presentation

A parasitic folliculitis causes papules, pustules, ulcers, crusts, alopecia, erythema, and swelling of the limbs, ventral thorax, and abdomen, with marked to moderate pruritus, stamping feet, restlessness, and unusually frenzied activity.

Differential diagnosis

Fly bites; onchocerciasis; trombiculiasis; chorioptic mange; dermatophilosis; poultry red mite infestation.

Diagnosis

Skin scrapings may reveal motile nematode larvae on microscopic examination. On skin biopsy there is perifolliculitis, folliculitis, and furunculosis, with nematode segments present in hair follicles.

Management

Affected horses should be removed from contaminated yards, the bedding changed, the limbs cleaned, and antimicrobial creams applied topically if necessary. Severe clinical signs are reported to regress over 3–4 weeks.

Prognosis

The prognosis is very good.

Onchocercal dermatitis
Definition/overview

Onchocerca larvae can be found in the skin of normal horses; however, hypersensitivity appears to develop in some horses, affecting the skin of the ventral midline, chest, withers, face, and neck.

Etiology/pathophysiology

The adult worms live in the ligamentum nuchae, with the microfilaria circulating in the most superficial layers of the dermis. Dermatitis is related to and associated with *Onchocerca* spp. microfilaria antigen leading to the development of type 1 and type 3 hypersensitivity.

Clinical presentation

Horses exhibit pruritus and patchy alopecia, with small papules and thickened, dry, scaly skin (1177). Severe cases show marked itching and excoriation, leading to scab formation, a so-called 'bull's eye' lesion on the skin. The ventral midline shows more constant alopecia and poor regrowth of new hair (1178). Tail rubbing is rare, but there can be loss of mane hair.

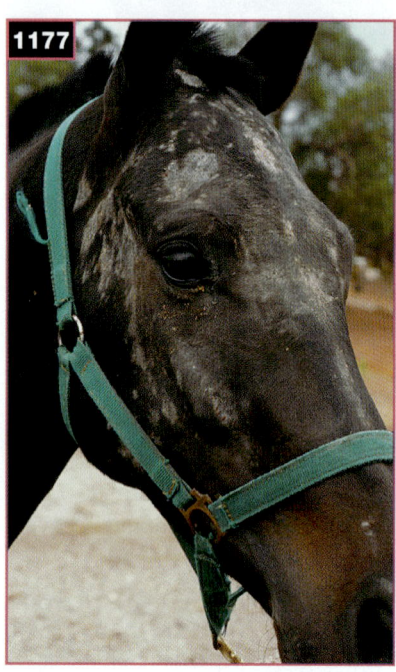

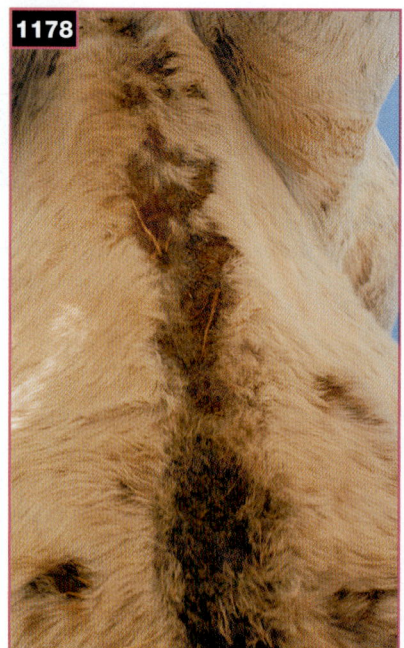

1177 *Onchocerca* infection showing typical head lesion of 4-weeks' duration with scaling, crusts, and alopecia. The horse rubbed the affected areas frequently.

1178 Ventral midline dermatitis due to *Onchocerca* infection. There is loss of hair, scaling with scattered lesions either side of the midline, and mild to severe pruritus with biting and rubbing of the thickened belly wall.

Differential diagnosis
Sweet itch; trombiculiasis; *Boophilus* infestation (cattle tick larvae); nematode dermatitis; *Simulium* spp. infestation; equine unilateral papular dermatosis; bacterial folliculitis; *Demodex* spp. infestation. Sweet itch and onchocerciasis are involved with *Culicoides* spp., therefore both conditions can exist simultaneously.

Diagnosis
The clinical picture is characteristic. Pruritus regresses in winter and returns in summer. Biopsy reveals the presence of larval worms in the skin of clinically affected horses.

Management
Treatment is with ivermectin (0.2 mg/kg) or moxidectin (0.4 mg/kg) paste given orally and repeated in 4–6 months. Most cases resolve with a single treatment. A massive kill of larvae can exacerbate the eye and skin inflammation for 3–5 days after treatment.

Prognosis
The prognosis is very good.

Oxyuriasis (pin worm)
Definition/overview
Female *Oxyuris equi* worms lay eggs on the perianal skin, causing irritation and self-induced trauma. Regular deworming with routine anthelmintics has all but eliminated this disease, which is mainly seen in stabled horses.

INSECT-INDUCED PRURITUS
Fleas
Definition/overview
Stickfast (or stick tight) fleas (*Echidnophaga gallinacea*), found in warm climates, typically cause this problem. Parasitized horses may be in contact with poultry or current/former poultry sheds.

Midges
Definition/overview
Culicoides spp. can cause irritation of the skin. Variations in the target skin area of the horse depend on the species involved. All horses are attacked by *Culicoides* spp. and show signs of irritation, which leads to restlessness and even pruritus. When climatic conditions are favorable for rapid generation of 'wave' attacks, many horses show this irritation, which rapidly abates with the passage of the 'wave' peak, leaving only those horses with hypersensitivity reactions with a serious pruritic problem.

Etiology/pathophysiology
Culicoides spp. midges occur in summer and autumn and can establish waves of large numbers under favorable weather conditions.

Clinical presentation
Irritation and restlessness are seen in the whole group of animals. Pruritus is usually more intense around the head, ears, base of the mane and tail, and over the withers, but the chest, ventral areas, and the face can also be affected when associated with outbreak numbers of *Culicoides* spp. A variable number of horses progress to typical hypersensitivity reaction (see below).

Differential diagnosis
Mosquitoes; simulid, buffalo, or horn flies.

Diagnosis
Finding large numbers of *Culicoides* spp. (use of night light trap) in the presence of appropriate clinical signs is highly suggestive.

Management
Repellents and rugs should be used. Powerful overhead fans are useful with stabled horses. With large groups of paddock horses, smudge fires may be needed.

Prognosis
The prognosis depends on the success of insect control measures.

Insect hypersensitivity
Definition/overview
By far the most common skin allergy in horses, 'sweet itch' or 'Queensland itch', is due to hypersensitivity to bites of *Culicoides* spp. midges. There is no sex, hair color, or skin color predilection. Foals appear to be unaffected up to 6–9 months of age. The condition worsens with repeated yearly attacks and with aging.

Etiology/pathophysiology
Hypersensitivity takes time to develop and it is rare to see it before 3 years of age. There may be a genetic basis that predisposes Welsh and Icelandic ponies and Shire horses. This disease represents type 1 and type 4 hypersensitivity to salivary antigens of *Culicoides* spp., *Simulium* spp., *Haematobia* spp., and *Stomoxys calcitrans*.

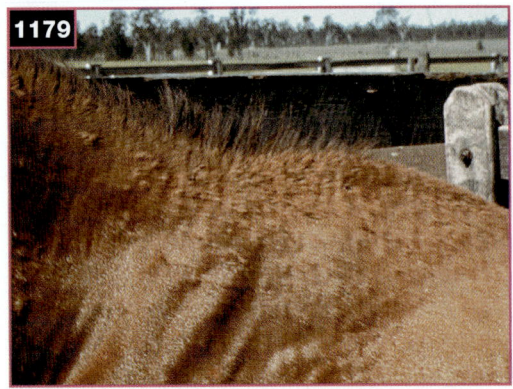

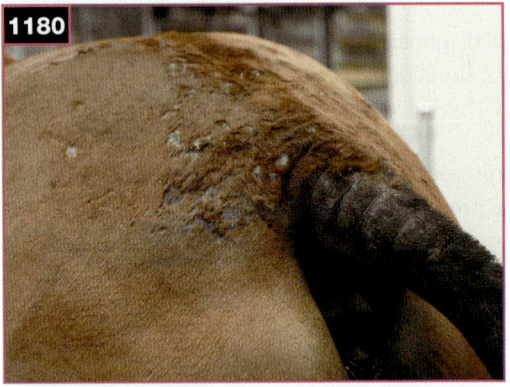

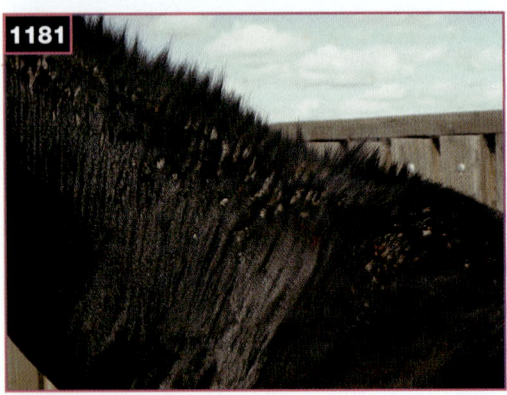

1179 Early case of *Culicoides* spp. hypersensitivity with papules, alopecia, slight scurf, and the mane extensively rubbed out due to severe pruritus. (Reprinted from Pascoe RR (1990) *Colour Atlas of Equine Dermatology*, Wolfe, with permission)

1180 *Culicoides* spp. affect rugged horses without tail protectors, resulting in rubbed-out tail hairs. These lesions had been present for over 3 weeks.

1181 Old lesions due to *Culicoides* spp. still show severe permanent damage to the skin and mane hair, and lichenification of the skin in midwinter.

Clinical presentation

Acute reactions follow a midge attack. Papules occur along the back of the horse from ears to tail, inducing rubbing of the tail, neck, head, and back (**1179, 1180**). Alternatively, depending on the geographical location and the midge species, lesions occur on the ventral midline of the affected horse. Biting and rubbing cause exfoliation, exudation of serum, patchy alopecia, crusts, and melanotrichia.

Chronic reaction shows as thickened skin rugae, which develop on the withers, neck, and tail head ('rat tails') (**1181**). A similar chronic thickening occurs on the ventral midline. Both show chronic hair loss due to mechanical irritation from rubbing. Horses may suffer loss of weight due to constant irritation. Generally, affected horses itch more in early evening (dusk) and early morning, shown by tail switching, increased rubbing, and restlessness. *Culicoides* spp. cause a primary bite irritation in all horses, but not all horses develop hypersensitivity.

Differential diagnosis

Microsporum gypseum; psoroptic mange (tail), *Oxyuris* infestation; other flies such as *Stomoxys calcitrans*, *Simulium* spp., and *Haematobia exigua*; dermatophilosis; onchocercal dermatitis; equine unilateral papular dermatosis; stick fast flea; spinose ear tick; cattle tick larvae; bee stings; horse lice; chemical irritation; anhidrosis.

Diagnosis

Clinical signs and seasonal incidence are highly suggestive. All other ectoparasitic causes should be excluded. Biopsy shows dermatitis with mild to severe eosinophilic folliculitis. Intradermal skin testing needs aqueous whole insect antigen and is reported to give reliable positive results, but is unavailable for general use. Identification of biting insects is important, as not all *Culicoides* spp. bite in the dorsal areas. Some species attack ventral areas only and cause ventral skin changes. Not all hypersensitivity is due to *Culicoides* spp. alone, as it can be associated with *Tabanid* spp. (horse flies), *Stomoxys* spp. (stable flies), *Haematobia* spp. (buffalo flies), or a mixture.

Management

Individual horses can be treated with an antihistamine such as hydroxyzine (1–2 mg/kg p/o q8–12h). For a longer lasting effect in seriously affected horses, methylprednisolone (1 mg/2.5 kg i/m at 3–4 weekly intervals) can be used. Prolonged usage is not advisable. While oral daily treatment with prednisolone granules during the high-risk season can reduce pruritus to a minimal amount, secondary effects from prolonged corticosteroid medication must be constantly reviewed.

Insect repellents (e.g. dibutyl phthalate) applied to rugs or to the backs of individual horses have been helpful. Treatment of unrugged paddock horses is extremely difficult, but an application of light oil dressing to the dorsum of the horse gives some measure of relief.

The most important control measure is the protection of the horse against further contact with *Culicoides* spp. Unless this can be accomplished, all other measures are likely to be less successful. With show horses, stabling from 16.00 hours to 08.00 hours, combined with rugging with sheets and hoods, may prevent serious skin damage. Insect proofing stables by using high velocity air fans is certainly the ultimate method of prevention, but it is difficult to achieve. Treatments include:

+ Sprays: Maldison 500g/l (malathion). Use 125 ml/ 10 liters of water initially as a spray and repeat in 7 days.
+ Wipe-ons: Coopers Fly Repellent Plus (permethrin and citronella); Deosan Dysect 5% (cypermethrin).
+ Shampoos: Radiol Insecticidal soapless shampoo (a compound mixture of pyrethrins and other synthetics). Apply as a smear to areas likely to be bitten. Must be applied daily; twice daily in wet weather.
+ Weekly body sprays of pyrethroids or organophosphates are recommended. Organophosphate residual effects do not appear to be satisfactory beyond 7 days.

All the methods/treatments available must be employed in highly susceptible horses.

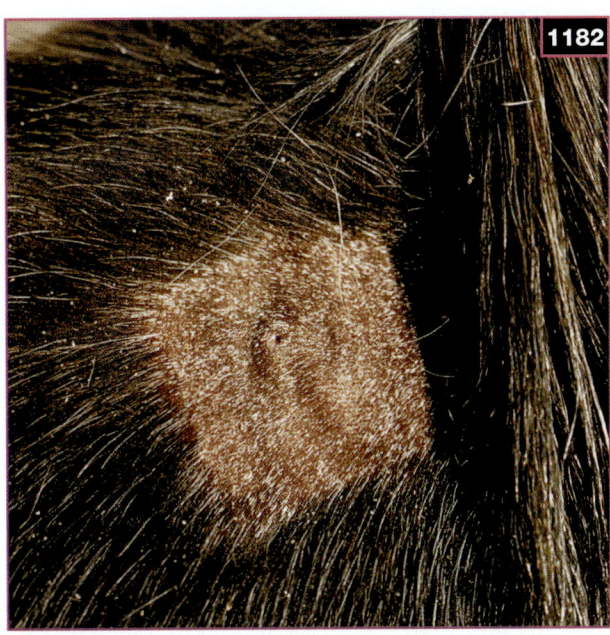

1182 Warble fly. Extrusion of L3 larvae from a nodule or cyst with a breathing 'pore'. (Photo courtesy A Waddell)

Hypodermiasis

Definition/overview
Hypodermiasis is caused by *Hypoderma* (warble) fly larvae. They belong to a genus of flies whose larvae invade tissues and then damage the tissue, as well as the skin, when they emerge (**1182**). Horses in the northern hemisphere are only occasionally affected.

Etiology/pathophysiology
Adult flies attach eggs in a row to horse hair. The larvae hatch and crawl down to the skin and then penetrate and wander in the subcutaneous tissues as L1 larvae. L2 larvae migrate to the withers, where their presence is shown by subcutaneous swellings.

Clinical presentation
Subcutaneous nodules and cysts are seen located over the withers, some with the development of a breathing 'pore' over the cyst. Pruritus may be present during development of the larvae. If larvae die or are ruptured, the horse may show an anaphylactic reaction.

Differential diagnosis
Infectious granulomas; epidermoid and dermoid cysts; neoplasms; equine eosinophilic granuloma.

Diagnosis
It is important to assess the horse's geographical location and origin of travel/movement. Physical examination of the lesion and demonstration of the presence of larvae is diagnostic.

Management
Surgical removal of the entire nodule is required. Routine deworming with ivermectin or moxidectin orally should prevent larval migration and growth, but anaphylactic reactions to dead larvae have been reported.

Prognosis
The prognosis is fair. Scarring may result if secondary infection occurs at the breathing hole site.

Insect bites or stings

Definition/overview
These are many and varied and a complete clinical history will be necessary to eliminate the possibility of many of the likely agents. With most free-living *Diptera,* the adult female only requires one blood feed to lay eggs and is therefore difficult to control.

Clinical presentation
Most bites show a central bite mark surrounded by a small circular edematous plaque. The larger the fly, the larger will be the bite puncture and area of edema. Irritability of the horse (e.g. stamping feet, restless movements, rubbing and galloping around the paddock) is due to pain and annoyance caused by the presence of biting insects.

Diagnosis
The history must be carefully analyzed. Most biting insects are more prevalent in warm months and after rain. The presence of flies, midges, bee swarm, wasps, or contact with insect nests (e.g. gardens, stables) should be noted. Stable flies are usually found only around buildings, in spider webs in the corners and roofs of stables, and in tropical and subtropical areas. The presence of cattle accompanied by *Haematobia* spp. in proximity to horses is significant.

Management
Removal of the causal agent is required.

Prognosis
A good to excellent prognosis can be given.

Horse flies (*Tabanid* spp.)

Definition/overview
These flies vary in size from 9–33 mm and feed at 3–4 day intervals, allowing continued egg laying. They are mechanical vectors of many diseases.

Etiology/pathophysiology
Horse flies are blood feeders and inflict a painful bite while drawing blood. They can transmit EIA as well as other viral, bacterial, protozoan, and filarid diseases.

Clinical presentation
The main presenting sign is a large fly associated with a very severe bite. Blood loss can amount to 0.5 ml per fly feeding, with more blood loss from oozing of the wound.

Differential diagnosis
Stomoxys calcitrans bites.

Diagnosis
Observation of actual fly bites and the presence of flies is used for diagnosis.

Management
Tabanids are difficult to control, but treatment should include frequent use of residual sprays, such as synthetic pyrethroids (e.g. permethrin or cypermethrin), applied to the limbs, abdomen, and neck. Antibiotic/corticosteroid ointment can be used for local treatment. All rank vegetation and brush should be removed from the horses' vicinity, and they should be kept housed during daytime. An insect light trap can be used inside the stable at night.

Prognosis
The prognosis is excellent with fly removal.

Stable flies

Definition/overview
Adult *Stomoxys calcitrans* flies resemble the common house fly (*Musca domestica*), the bush fly (*M. vetustissima*), and the face fly (*M. autumnalis*).

Etiology/pathophysiology
Eggs are deposited in manure and moist decaying vegetable matter. *Stomoxys calcitrans* flies are of great annoyance to horses and in some susceptible yearlings can cause edematous plaques to develop. The most common bite sites are the neck, back, chest, and limbs. The flies can cause hypersensitivity and can mechanically transmit *Microsporum gypseum* spores.

Clinical presentation
Flies cause extreme irritation, limb stamping, cow kicking, and tail twitching. Bites show as small papules with raised hair (5–10 mm) and a small central scab (**1183**). The skin around the bite can develop edema. Self-mutilation is seen in hypersensitive horses.

Differential diagnosis
Tick worry; wasp stings; mosquito bites; spider bites; poultry red mite infestation; *Culicoides* spp. bites; *Tabanid* spp. flies; trombiculid mites; bee stings; buffalo and horn flies.

Diagnosis
The presence of *Stomoxys* spp. should be observed. Bites occur in daylight, and they can also attack humans.

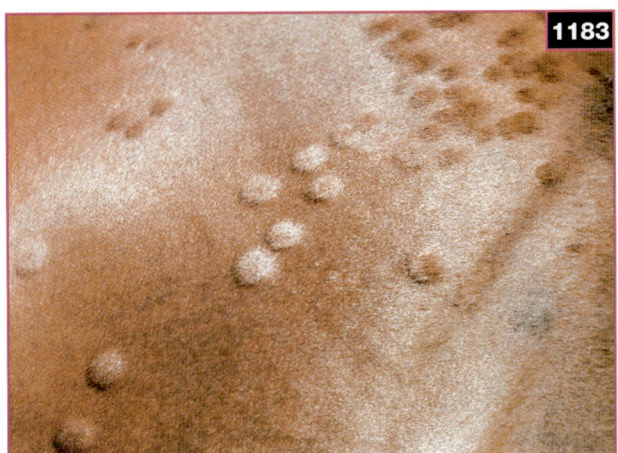

1183 *Stomoxys calcitrans* attack in a 2-year-old Thoroughbred filly causing numbers of 3–4 mm raised nodules with central bite marks.

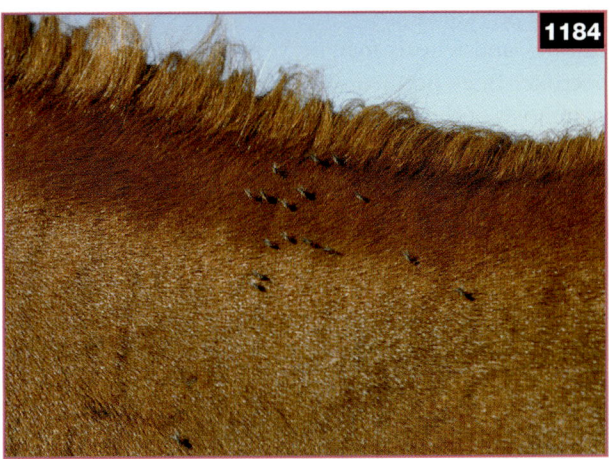

1184 Buffalo and horn flies. *Haematobia* spp. tend to feed head down in small groups on upper portions of horses and can cause severe annoyance.

Management

Individual treatment of a horse agitated by flies is by sedating with acepromazine (10 mg/125 kg i/m). Analgesic creams (e.g. calamine lotion or cream with lidocaine) should be applied to the bitten area. Manure disposal, slashing long grass, and removing rotting vegetation are important, and the stables, walls, and yard rails should be sprayed with diazinon or crotoxyphos.

Prognosis

The prognosis is good.

Buffalo and horn flies
Definition/overview

Haematobia exigua and *H. irritans* are small (4 mm in length) flies that are mainly found in subtropical to tropical areas. They are identified on the horse by their head-down body position, feeding in small or large groups, and by aggregating around the shoulders, neck, withers, flanks, and abdomen of the horse (1184).

Etiology/pathophysiology

Larvae develop in fresh manure, principally bovine. Both male and female flies are blood feeders, taking up to 20–30 meals daily.

Clinical presentation

H. exigua causes scaling, ulcers, and crusts on the neck and shoulders. *H. irritans* can cause seasonal ventral midline dermatitis, very similar to that observed in onchocerciasis.

Differential diagnosis

Culicoides spp. infestation; *Simulid* spp. infestation; mosquitoes.

Diagnosis

The presence of numerous small feeding flies in groups, with ulceration of the skin, is used for diagnosis.

Management

Paddock horses are given some relief by the provision of smudge fires, which flies will not penetrate. As the flies need cattle manure to breed successfully, removal of horses from the vicinity of cattle reduces the numbers of flies to manageable proportions. Residual insecticidal sprays should be used at regular intervals.

Prognosis

Paddock horses are difficult to protect.

Black flies
Definition/overview

Small black flies lay their eggs in running water (*Simulium* spp.) or still water (buffalo gnat). The eggs hatch in 6–12 days. They can travel long distances and be blown up to 100 km by wind currents.

Etiology/pathophysiology

Flies are active in the morning and evening in spring and summer and usually reach plague proportions following long rainy periods. They cause extreme irritation and inflict painful bites as well as transmit viral (e.g. papillomavirus [see p. 903]), bacterial, protozoan, and filarid diseases. Their saliva contains allergens and toxins that cause increased capillary permeability.

Clinical presentation

Papules and wheals may be vesicular, hemorrhagic, or necrotic. Bites occur on the head, ears (with papillary acanthosis of the pinnae and aural plaques), and ventral abdomen. Swarm attacks can induce death in individual horses from toxin release. Hypersensitivity can occur.

Differential diagnosis

Culicoides spp. infestation (may occur simultaneously); *Haematobia* spp. infestation; onchocerciasis; mosquitoes.

Diagnosis

Identification of the presence of swarms of black flies (humped thorax) and numerous skin lesions.

Management

Stabling horses during periods of high fly density can be useful. Sedatives such as xylazine (0.6–1.0 mg/kg slow i/v) and application of skin relief products, such as calamine lotion, may be helpful. Severe cases may require systemic glucocorticoids. Residual sprays of synthetic pyrethroids (e.g. deltamethrin) may be required.

Prognosis

The prognosis is good except in swarm attacks, when shock can result in death.

Mosquitoes

Definition/overview

Mosquitoes rely on the availability of water for their breeding cycle. Eggs are laid and larvae develop in permanent, preferably stagnant, water. Most attacks are at dusk and early evening, but, where insects reach plague proportions, they can also occur in daylight hours.

Etiology/pathophysiology

The breeding cycle is complete in 7 days in warm weather, therefore explosive populations occur rapidly. They are responsible for the transmission of viral diseases such as Eastern, Western, Venezuelan, and Murray River encephalitis and Ross River virus.

Clinical presentation

All affected horses show multiple fine papules (1185), restlessness at night, irritable behavior, and edema of the eyelids. Urticarial plaques appear on some horses.

Differential diagnosis

Bee stings; wasp stings; feed allergy; urticaria; buffalo and horn flies; *Stomoxys* spp. and *Simulium* spp. bites.

Diagnosis

The presence of very large numbers of mosquitoes can be diagnostic.

Management

Severely irritated horses should be sedated using acepromazine injection (0.03–0.10 mg/kg i/m). Selenium sulfide shampoo gives relief from the pruritus and edema. Swelling regresses in 2–3 days. Antihistamines give some relief in more severe cases. All horses should be rugged and hooded, smudge fires should be used around the stables, and residual insecticidal sprays applied to the horses. Dibutyl phthalate is used on rugs and on horses to reduce self-mutilation and rubbing in individual cases. If horses in paddocks show severe irritation, smudge fires are used.

Prognosis

Horses usually recover from physical damage quickly, but there may be a residual problem with vector diseases.

Bees

Definition/overview

The honey bee (*Apis mellifera*) has been reported to attack horses in the spring and summer, producing edematous wheals and plaques.

Wasps

Definition/overview

Various species inhabit and nest in shrubs, trees, and brick and stone-wall buildings, particularly under eaves. Accidental damage to a nest usually precipitates an attack.

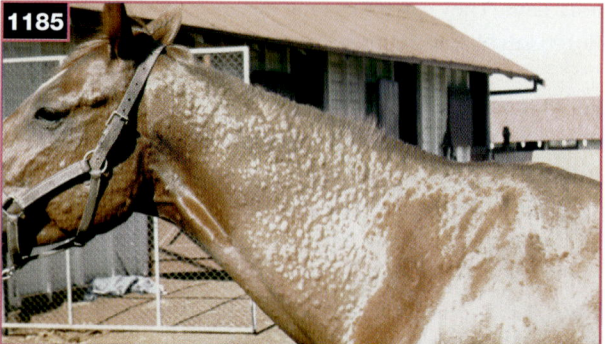

1185 Mosquito bites leading to numerous papules of varying size on the neck up to the edge of the rug margin. The presence of mosquitoes aids diagnosis.

Myiasis (hypodermiasis)

Definition/overview
Infestation of tissue by living fly larvae can be caused by *Hypoderma bovis*, *H. lineatum*, or blow fly strike (*Calliphora* spp.).

Etiology/pathophysiology
The larvae cause infestation of neglected smelly wounds, plaster casts, dirty bandages, necrotic neoplasm, and sarcoids. A more serious disease occurs when infestation is by screw-worm larvae in fresh wounds and tumors due to *Callitroga hominivorax* and *C. macellaria* in North, Central, and South America, and *Chrysomyia bezziana* in Africa and Asia.

Clinical presentation
Irritation is shown by the horse, with increased odor and discharge, chewing at wounds and bandages, and the presence of the breathing pore end of larvae within wounds (**1186**).

Differential diagnosis
Secondary fly strike by blow flies.

Diagnosis
Diagnosis is based on close examination of wounds and seeing the breathing pore end of fly larvae.

Management
Bandages, casts, and other items should be removed. Pure Dettol should be applied to remove larvae. An insecticide mixed with pine oil (1:1) can be used as a topical dressing.

Prognosis
The prognosis is good provided debridement and follow-up prevention are carried out.

Pediculosis (lice)

Definition/overview
Werneckiella (Damalinia) equi lice (1–2 mm in size) can be found on the head, neck, and dorsolateral trunk (**1187**). *Haematopinus asini* lice are larger (3 mm in size) and more numerous and are found on the body, limbs, mane, and base of the tail. Both species cause irritation, dermatitis, and unthriftiness and they are one of the most common causes of pruritus during colder months (**1188**).

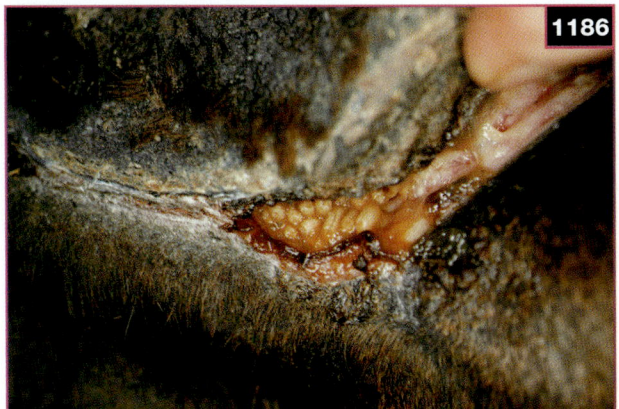

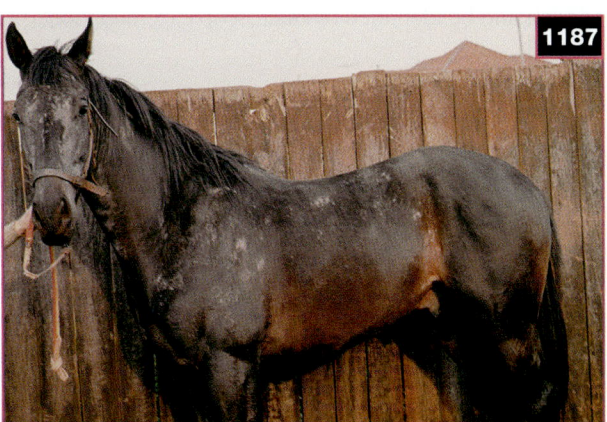

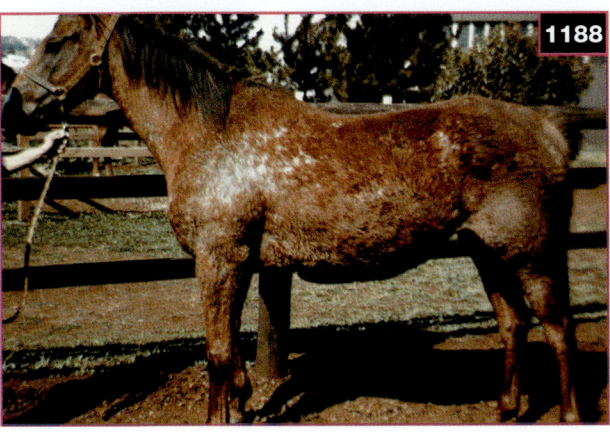

1186 Myiasis due to *Calliphora* spp. larvae in a wound.

1187 Pediculosis. *Werneckiella (Damalinia) equi* on a 4-year-old racing horse with patchy alopecia, loss of head hair from rubbing, some scurf, and severe pruritus.

1188 Pediculosis. *Haematopinus asini* all over the body, with alopecia and increased scurf in a longhaired winter coat.

Etiology/pathophysiology

Lice are highly contagious. They do not breed at temperatures above 38°C (100.4°F) and they die at 50°C (122°F). Some survive hot months by hiding on cooler parts of the horse's body, but they cannot survive off the host for more than 3 weeks.

Clinical presentation

Pruritus with patchy alopecia, irritation, rubbing, and biting is characteristically present. Physical injury to the skin with serum exudation occurs, and there is loss of condition, particularly in poorer horses. Occasionally, anemia develops.

Differential diagnosis

Psoroptic mange; *Culicoides*; trombiculosis; oxyuris infestation (tail rubbing); *Dermanyssus gallinae*; *Tyroglyphus* spp.; microsporosis; stick fast fleas; spinose ear tick; foal diarrhea scalding; overstrength insecticides.

Diagnosis

Diagnosis is based on the presence of lice or nits glued to the hair shafts. Use of a hand lens may be necessary. *W. equi* may be present in small numbers present and they can be very difficult to find; horses bite and rub affected areas. *H. asini* are seen in larger numbers and are readily found over the entire horse in severe infestations. Lice and eggs should be identified by microscopic examination.

Management

Because lice are highly contagious, contact between horses, horse gear, and rugs should be restricted. Lice are killed by heat, so steam cleaning rugs, brushes, and other fomites should be considered.

    H. asini, a sucking louse, is treated efficiently with oral ivermectin (0.2 mg/kg twice at 14-day intervals). Otherwise, sprays and powders can be used for both species (i.e. fipronil, permethrin, and cypermethrin powders and washes, or 1% selenium sulfide shampoo, all applied weekly). Body spraying requires 5–10 liters per horse. (*Note*: Follow the manufacturer's instructions, dosage and concentration implicitly for all sprays.)

Prognosis

The prognosis is good. Lice are usually self-limiting with the onset of hot weather.

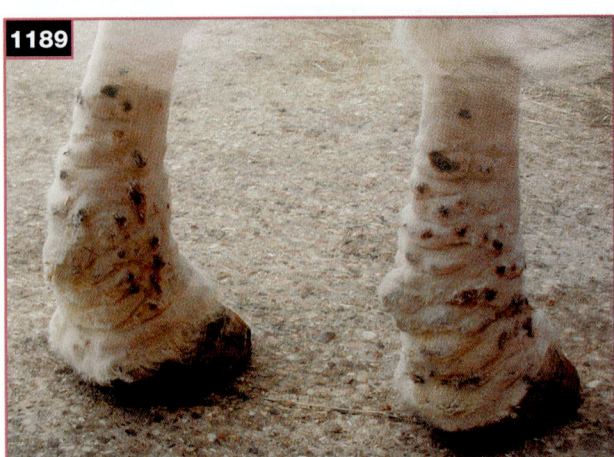

1189 Chorioptic mange in a draft horse presenting with severe irritation, stamping, rubbing, and biting at the lower limbs. The hair on the back of the limbs has been clipped to reveal raised scabs and areas of dried exudate. Lack of owner compliance to remove this hair often prevents proper treatment. (Photo courtesy GA Munroe)

Mites
Chorioptic mange
Definition/overview

Chorioptes equi is a surface feeding mite that causes pruritus and dermatitis, particularly on the lower limbs of feathered-legged draft horses.

Etiology/pathophysiology

C. equi feed on the epidermal debris. A life cycle of 3 weeks is completed on the host. Mites can live for up to 70 days off a horse. Transmission is by direct and indirect contact and is more common in cold weather. The lower limbs are mainly affected, but it can extend to the belly, axilla, and groin.

Clinical presentation

Pruritus with irritation and restlessness, stamping and biting at limbs, exudation of serum, matting of limb hair, alopecia and scabs, and rubbing on rails, fences, and posts (**1189**) will be observed.

Differential diagnosis

Dermatophilus; trombiculidiasis; *Strongyloides westerii*; sarcoptic mange; greasy heel; cattle tick and larval forms; pastern folliculitis.

Diagnosis

Deep skin scraping from the edge of a fresh lesion is required for microscopic identification of mites. There is a breed predilection, the condition mostly occurring on heavy-coated draft horses.

Management

Initially, long hair and scabs should be removed and all affected areas scrubbed with permethrin, selenium sulfide, or fipronil. These reduce the number of mites and give temporary remission of clinical signs. Other insecticides, such as oral ivermectin paste (0.3 mg/kg weekly for 4 weeks), have not been as successful. The use of 0.25% fipronil as a general body spray is best (or 125 ml of product applied to each limb, particularly from the elbow and stifle down), repeated in 3–4 weeks.

Isolation of all infected horses from foals and yearlings may help control the spread of mites.

Prognosis

The prognosis is often guarded due to poor owner compliance in maintaining clipping of limb hair.

Poultry red mite
Definition/overview

Dermanyssus gallinae is a nocturnal mite that emerges only at night to feed on the host. It has eight legs and is white, gray, or black, becoming bright red after feeding. Horses are attacked when stabled in or near poultry houses. Mites can live for up to 4–5 months in disused buildings without feeding.

Etiology/pathophysiology

This blood-sucking mite lives and lays egg in cracks in the walls and ceilings of poultry houses. Contact is made when horses are kept in proximity to poultry sheds or when sheds are converted into stables for horses.

Clinical presentation

The mite causes severe pruritus and irritation, leading to stamping and biting of limbs and body (1190). Small red mobile mites may be located.

Differential diagnosis

Horse lice; larval ticks; *Stomoxys calcitrans*; scrub itch mites; harvest mite; *Trombiculid* spp. mites; overstrength insecticides; larval nematode dermatitis.

Diagnosis

Sampling should be performed at night, in or near poultry sheds. Mites are free moving and need careful microscopic examination of shallow skin scrapings to find them.

Management

Horses should be sprayed with 0.25% Maldison and removed from proximity to poultry. The poultry shed should be power sprayed with 0.5% Maldison. Treatment is repeated in 7 days in summer and 10–14 days in winter.

Prognosis

The prognosis is good if spray is used effectively to eliminate mites.

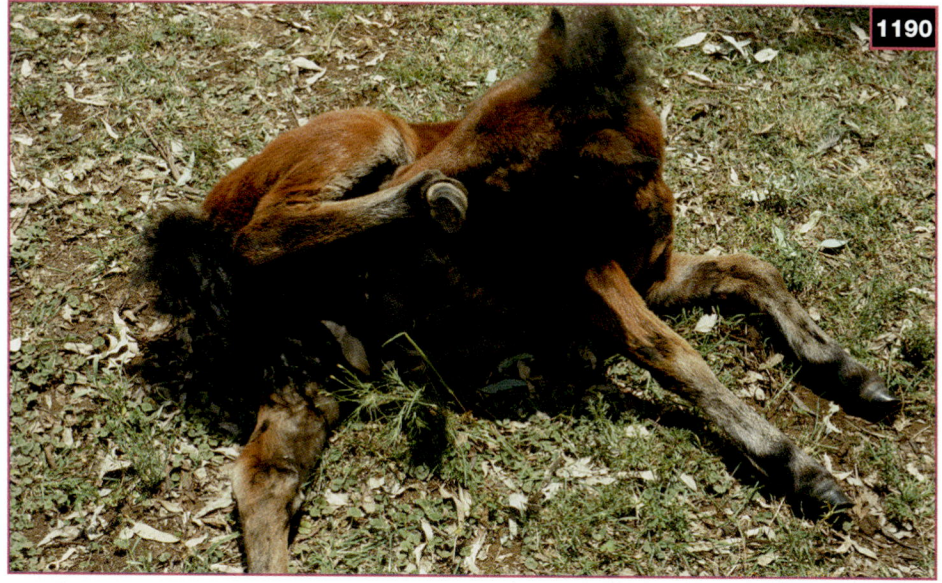

1190 *Dermanyssus gallinae*. A 5-week-old foal is lying down and biting its limbs. Severe pruritus and self-mutilation are common with poultry red mite infestation.

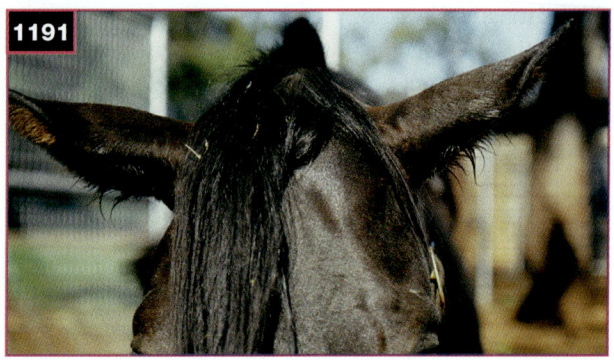

1191 Psoroptic mange in stabled horses with floppy ears due to the presence of *P. equi* mites in the ears.

Psoroptic mange

Definition/overview
Infestation with *Psoroptes* spp. mites leads to pruritus, patchy alopecia, excoriation to the head, head shaking, and tail rubbing in infested young horses. Older stabled horses can also be affected by contact with infested yearlings or contaminated stables or tack.

Etiology/pathophysiology
P. equi is a large mite that lives on tissue fluids and has a 10-day life cycle. Survival time is prolonged for up to 7–12 weeks in cool conditions. Transmission is both direct and indirect. Mites prefer areas with thick denser hair (ears, mane, tail).

Clinical presentation
Affected horses have pruritus and irritability around the head, leading to aural discharges and head rubbing. Itchiness of the tail mane and body occurs in stabled yearling horses (mites carry over from year to year in some stables). Some horses display 'droopy' ears (**1191**).

Differential diagnosis
Sweet itch; aural hematoma; conchal cyst; stick fast flea; *Tyroglyphus* spp. mites; *Oxyuris* spp. infestation; spinose ear tick; lice; cattle tick larvae; ticks; overstrength insecticides.

Diagnosis
Ear wax should be examined with a hand lens or microscope. Mites are seen as small white moving dots.

Management
Tranquillization may be necessary to clean all accumulated wax and debris from the ears. General body and tail itch in yearlings responds well to the use of Maldison washes (50–125 ml/10 liters) or oral ivermectin (0.2 mg/kg). Treat twice, at 14-day intervals.

Prognosis
A good prognosis can be given.

Sarcoptic mange

Definition/overview
Sarcoptes scabei var. *equi* has been eradicated in many locations in the world, but still occurs in some less well-developed countries where horses are used for transportation. Lesions are seen on the head, neck, and ears and may spread over the entire body. Spread is by direct and indirect contact.

Etiology/pathophysiology
Mites tunnel and feed on tissue fluid and epidermal cells. The life cycle is 2–3 weeks. Mites cannot live off horses and they are very susceptible to dehydration.

Clinical presentation
Papules and vesicles occur on the skin, with intense pruritus. Rubbing and biting of the limbs and ventral abdomen leads to excoriation, with the skin becoming very crusty and thickened. Secondary bacterial infections can occur.

Differential diagnosis
Larval cattle tick infestation; chorioptic mange; *Culicoides* hypersensitivity; onchocerciasis.

Diagnosis
Multiple deep skin scrapings should be taken for microscopic identification of *S. scabei* var. *equi*. (**Note:** Do not rule out a diagnosis on one or two negative skin scrapings.)

Management
Oral ivermectin (0.2 mg/kg twice at 14-day intervals) or 0.1% diazinon (applying sprays every 7–10 days for 3–6 treatments) can be used. All infected horses should be isolated and all potential fomites should be fumigated. Mites can live up to 3 weeks in infested stables and fomites.

Prognosis
The prognosis is good with proper treatment and isolation.

Trombiculidiasis

Definition/overview
Trombiculidiasis is caused by infestation with harvest, American chigger, or scrub itch mites. Mites infest the head and limbs of paddock horses. Stable horses may be infested over the entire body through contact with infested pasture hay used as feed or bedding.

Etiology/pathophysiology
Mites and nymphs are free-living in pastures. They will attack horses and humans if given the opportunity. Mites feed on horses in the late afternoon.

Clinical presentation
Affected horses show limb stamping and nose rubbing with small papules on the limbs, nose, and body, often with lip biting at the lower limbs. Small hairless areas develop after 2–3 days (1192).

Differential diagnosis
Poultry red mite; *Stomoxys calcitrans* bites; onchocercal dermatitis; chorioptic mange; tick larvae; horse lice; plant spikes such as thistles.

Diagnosis
This condition can be confirmed by identification of the presence of mites but, as mites fall off after feeding, this may be difficult. Multiple scrapings should be taken of the most recent lesions.

Management
Fipronil, permethrin, lime sulfur, or 0.25% Maldison as a limb and body spray can be used. 0.5% Maldison can be sprayed onto walls, floors, and sand rolls. Horses usually lose infestation quickly and so should only be treated supportively if necessary.

Prognosis
The prognosis is good.

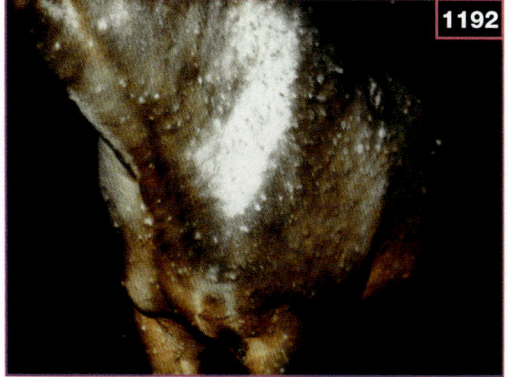

Tick infestation
Cattle ticks
Definition/overview
The cattle tick (*Boophilus microplus*), New Zealand cattle tick (*Haemaphysalis longicornis*), and similar ticks and their nymphs and larvae that infest cattle can infest horses pastured with cattle.

Etiology/pathophysiology
All forms live in pasture grass and attach to the limbs and head of horses initially, but soon spread all over the body. Hypersensitivity to *B. microplus* larvae occurs in some horses.

Clinical presentation
Severe pruritus occurs, with loss of condition. Horses become irritable and rub, bite, and stamp their limbs. Lip biting by the horse to remove adult ticks induces 'bite' injury lesions. Embedded ticks cause edema of the skin, with raised hair. Alopecia occurs from rubbing. Large numbers of ticks cause unthriftiness and scaling of the skin.

Differential diagnosis
Sweet itch; chorioptic and psoroptic mange; onchocercal dermatitis; dermatophytosis; other ticks.

Diagnosis
Skin scrapings may be used to find larval and nymph forms. A hand lens is used to identify all the parasites found on the skin. Geographical location is important, as the presence of ticks on cattle in the same locality, or pasture contamination with nymph or larval ticks from cattle usage of the paddock, could indicate a possible cause.

Management
Body sprays of 0.25% Maldison solution can be used. Stables and yards are sprayed with 0.25% Maldison in power kerosene. Amitraz causes irreversible gut stasis and death in horses and should not be used.

Prognosis
The prognosis is good if horses are regularly sprayed in high-tick areas.

1192 Trombiculid mite bites occur on horses at pasture, causing hairless areas around the head and limbs.

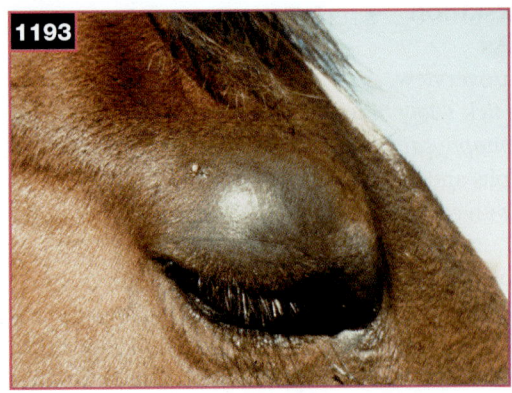

1193

Scrub ticks
Definition/overview
Ixodes holocyclus and *Dermacentor amblyomma* adults and intermediate stages can infect horses of all ages.

Etiology/pathophysiology
Eggs are laid in the ground, then hatch and larvae attach to warm animals as they graze.

Clinical presentation
Pruritus and localized scaly epidermis occurs with edema around the area where a tick or instar is embedded (**1193**). There may be signs of pus present. Staggers, along with posterior and respiratory paralysis, may occur with increasing numbers of ticks, particularly in young foals. Untreated cases can result in death of the foal.

Differential diagnosis
Cattle tick and instars; lice; mites; stickfast fleas.

Diagnosis
Diagnosis is based on being in a known 'scrub' tick area, followed by identification of the tick or instar.

Management
Body sprays should be used as described for cattle ticks. In cases of paralysis in foals, canine antiserum, plus either a glucocorticoid or flunixin meglumine to prevent serum anaphylaxis, can be attempted. Fomites and tack should be fumigated, and stables sprayed with 0.25% Maldison.

Prognosis
The prognosis is guarded if muscular paralysis and respiratory impairment are present.

Spinose ear ticks
Definition/overview
Otobius megnini is a soft-shelled tick that attaches to the external ear canal of horses.

Neoplastic disease
Primary neoplasia in the horse may cause depression and pain, but is rarely pruritic. Where pruritus occurs, examination for blow fly larvae or fungal infection, such as pythiosis, is warranted. *Habronema* spp. larvae have also been found in skin neoplasms on histopathologic examination.

Atopy
Definition/overview
Atopy is a genetically mediated pruritus and type 1 hypersensitivity.

Etiology/pathophysiology
Breed predisposition in this disease tends to indicate genetic programming. The classic description is of IgE becoming tissue-fixed, especially to skin. Mast cell-fixed IgE then reacts with its specific allergen or allergens, causing mast-cell degranulation with the release of many pharmacologically active agents. There is evidence of the role of Langerhans cells, T cells, and eosinophils in the disease process.

Clinical presentation
Recurrent, irregular, bilaterally symmetrical pruritus, with or without urticaria, which may be related or unrelated to the season of the year, is characteristic. This often occurs without any other clinical signs. Initially, there is self-mutilation, with horses biting themselves and rubbing raw areas on their body, limbs, head, and/or ears (**1194**). Secondary lesions are partly related to self-inflicted damage, leading to excoriation, alopecia, lichenification, and hyperpigmentation. Some develop a sterile eosinophilic folliculitis.

Differential diagnosis
Hypersensitivity to food, pollens, molds, dust, and many insects (ectoparasites).

Diagnosis
A careful history and a thorough clinical examination should be performed, with absolute elimination of all other causes of pruritus.

Intradermal skin testing may have limited use related to the availability of antigens (molds, pollen, and dust). Due to the lack of standardization of allergen sources, valid comparison of results is difficult to impossible. The list of possible allergens covers a very wide spectrum of molds, mites, dusts, weeds, grasses, and trees, as well as a long list of foods, mites, etc. that cause irritation in the horse.

Positive results must be analyzed very cautiously. It is important to ensure that the clinical case is completely free of glucocorticoids, antihistamines, and progestagens prior to testing. It is important to remember that the horse may have more than one condition concurrently, therefore treatment of only one of the causal agents may not resolve the pruritus or the urticaria.

Definitive diagnosis is essentially clinical. Skin biopsy shows superficial to deep perivascular dermatitis with eosinophilia (also frequently observed with insect and food hypersensitivity).

Management

A positive diagnosis of a specific allergen may require treatment for the rest of the horse's life. Multiple small causes may become additive to produce clinical atopy. All likely contributors must be evaluated, with the objective of reducing or even eliminating as many as possible. If the allergen can be determined (e.g. a food allergen) it may be possible to avoid contact and attempt to hyposensitize. Hypoallergenic shampoos and rinses, antihistamines, omega-6/omega-3 fatty acids, and, possibly, systemic glucocorticoids can be used. Prednisolone (1 mg/kg q12h) is used until control is established. Once stability is reached, the daily dose is reduced to alternate day low-dose morning therapy. This may continue for very long periods.

Allergen-specific immunotherapy (ASIT) is available at some centers; success rates approaching 70% have been obtained.

Prognosis

The prognosis is guarded. Results will be dependent on the multiplicity of causes and the possibility of reduction of these causes.

Alopecic conditions

Alopecia is deficiency of the hair caused by failure to grow, or loss after growth, and arises from a variety of primary and secondary diseases. There is a significant difference between those conditions in which grown fibers are lost, those in which stumps of fibers remain, and those in which the hair root has been shed from the follicle. The primary change is loss of hair and this may be accompanied by, or caused by, pruritus as a primary condition.

Superficial changes such as scaling and crusting can progress to erosion and ulceration of the epidermis and dermis. Scaling, either dry or greasy, is due to shedding of dead epidermal cells, while crusting is a collection of varied colored skin exudates. It may be possible during the preliminary examination to determine whether a physical, chemical, or infectious agent may be involved, allowing a subdivision into these sections, but clinical signs of scales and crusts are not diagnostic in themselves.

Erosion and ulceration are both secondary changes. Erosions are associated with loss of epidermis at varying levels down to the basement membrane, and these lesions heal without scarring. Ulceration damages tissue beyond the basement membrane and may result in scarring. Additional information will allow some further division into physical and chemical causes, infectious agents, tumors (or nodules), immune-mediated diseases, and miscellaneous diseases.

PRIMARY ALOPECIA
Physical burns
See section in Chapter 13 (p. 956).

Set-fast
Definition/overview
Areas of superficial gangrene develop from persistent chronic pressure caused by a poorly fitting saddle or other harness.

Etiology/pathophysiology
External pressure on the skin causes vascular damage and tissue anoxia and, if prolonged, dry gangrene and/or skin slough.

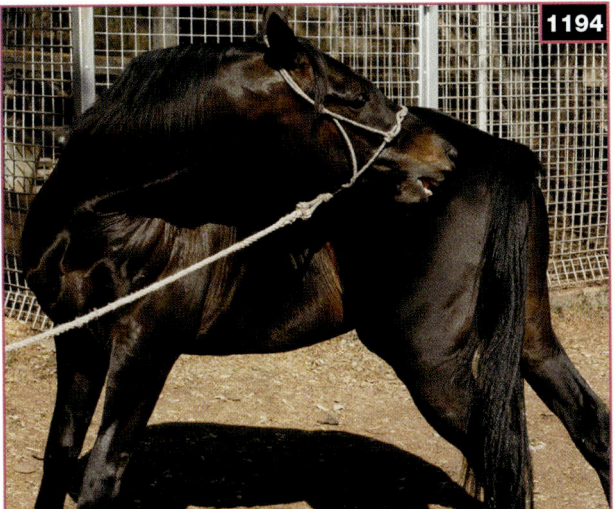

1194 Atopy. Type I hypersensitivity is genetically mediated and affected horses often bite at an apparently normal area of skin, causing severe self-mutilation.

893

Skin

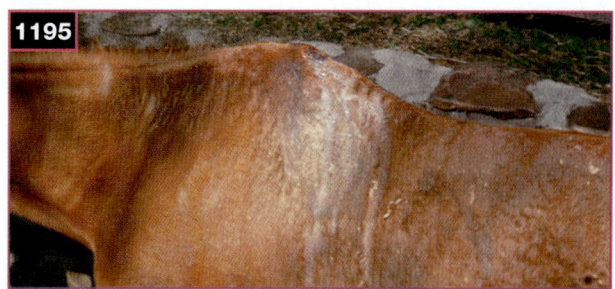

1195 'Set-fast'. The withers region of this horse became swollen, sore, and with a dried out 'cardboard'-like skin due to pressure necrosis from a poorly fitted saddle.

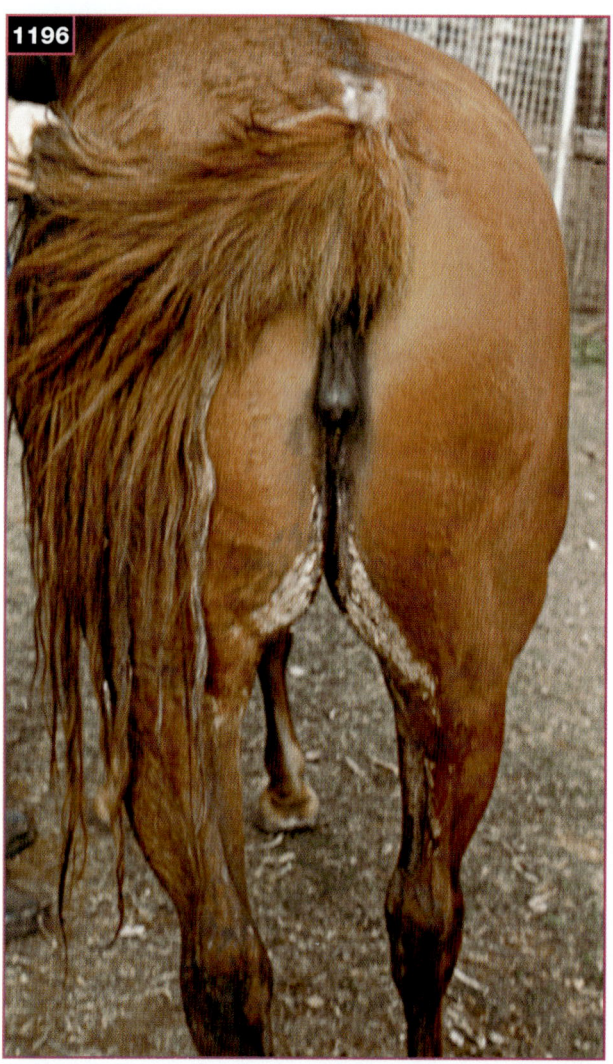

1196 Hair loss due to scalding from urinary incontinence, in this case due to *Sorghum* spp. poisoning.

Clinical presentation

Set-fast is characterized by roughly circular areas of skin that initially may be raised and painful, due to progressive damage, then lead to a cardboard-like consistency of the affected skin (1195).

Diagnosis

History and location are used for diagnosis.

Management

Saddlery should be examined and any improperly fitted areas corrected. The horse should be rested. Early cases can be treated with astringents and massage. Old cases may require surgery and skin grafting.

Prognosis

The prognosis is good with treatment for early damage. Surgical results following prolonged injury are fair.

Urine scalding

Definition/overview

Urine scalding is usually found around the skin of the caudal area of the hindlimbs of mares and the lower cranial hindlimbs of geldings with urinary incontinence.

Etiology/pathophysiology

Signs appear following foaling injury or caudal spinal trauma. Ingestion of S*orghum* spp. can cause nerve damage, leading to bladder dysfunction, with overflow showing as prolonged wetting of skin, scalding, and loss of hair.

Clinical presentation

Loss of hair may be patchy and sometimes painful (1196), obviously of urinary origin, and associated with the smell of urine on the limbs. Other neurologic signs may be present.

Diagnosis

The bladder should be examined to determine if retention and overflow is the primary cause. A previous history of feeding of improved *Sorghum* spp. pasture or hay, or a history of foaling accident or trauma to the hindquarters or sacrum, is supportive.

Management

When the cause is related to nerve damage, treatments are likely to be ineffective. Regular cleaning and greasing of the affected and other vulnerable areas of skin can limit the damage.

Prognosis

A guarded prognosis should be given, as most cases show no remission.

Wound scalding

Definition/overview

Prolonged weeping of tissue fluid or serum from wounds can cause excoriation and loss of hair. Regular cleaning and greasing of the affected and other vulnerable areas of skin can limit the damage.

Scar

Definition/overview

Severe skin injury causes loss of hair follicles and subcutaneous tissue, with fibrous tissue replacing dermis and epidermis.

Chemical agents scalding

Definition/overview

The application of overstrength pour-on agents or medications injures the superficial to deep layers of normal skin. Oversensitive skin can react in a similar manner to normal concentration levels of medication. Extreme cases occur with the application of blisters and vesicants.

INFECTIOUS CAUSES – VIRAL
Equine coital exanthema

Definition/overview

Equine coital exanthema (ECE) is a venereally transmitted viral skin disease caused by EHV-3.

Etiology/pathophysiology

EHV-3 can be transmitted during coitus or by nasal contact or contact with nasal secretions (1197).

Clinical presentation

Vesicles, which rapidly develop necrotic tops 0.15–0.5 cm in diameter, occur on the penis in males, principally in the area of the junction of parietal and visceral folds of the prepuce on the dorsal surface, with local swelling of the prepuce.

In mares they occur on the mucosal surface of the vulva and often extend to the skin of the vulva and perineum. Severe cases affect the anus and tail skin (1198). Initially, there is edematous swelling of the vulval lips. By day 4 the lesions are covered with serum and encrusted scabs and the edema regresses. Healthy granulation occurs within 10–14 days. Some lesions have depigmented areas (leukoderma) when healed. Occasionally, lesions develop around the nose and mouth.

Differential diagnosis

Equine viral papular dermatitis; equine molluscum contagiosum; leukoderma; staphlococcal dermatitis.

Diagnosis

Virus isolation is only successful when samples are taken as soon as lesions appear. Paired sera 28 days apart can be used for a serum neutralization test and complement fixation test (CFT), with titer increases indicative of recent infection.

Management

Scabs should be cleaned off with peroxide and eroded areas should be treated with iodine-based solutions. Daily treatment with antibiotic and corticosteroid ointment should be considered. Sexual rest is indicated until the lesions have healed.

Prognosis

The prognosis is good with sexual rest.

Equine viral papular dermatitis

See Nodular diseases (p. 902).

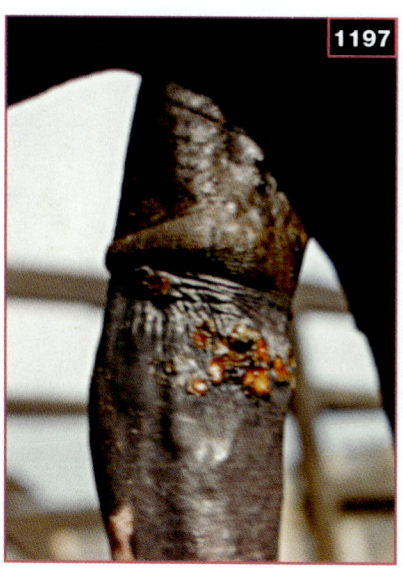

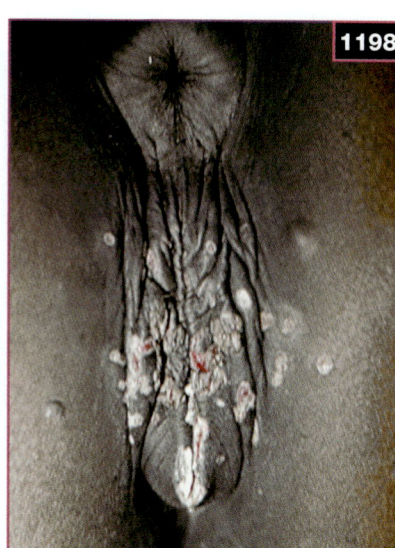

1197 Equine coital exanthema. This infection occurred in a 4-year-old maiden stallion approximately 12 days post coitus with an infected mare.

1198 Equine coital exanthema. Papules, pustules, crusts, and erosion of the skin related to the vulva, anus, and ventral surface of the tail have occurred in this mare post service.

INFECTIOUS CAUSES – BACTERIAL
Dermatophilosis
Definition/overview
Dermatophilosis is caused by *Dermatophilus congolensis* and is characterized by exudation and matted hair, with excessive scab formation.

Etiology/pathophysiology
The natural habitat of this organism is unknown and a multiplicity of factors operates, allowing the proliferation of the organism. The two most important factors are skin damage and prolonged moist conditions in the horse's haircoat.

Clinical presentation
Alopecia (1199), generalized crusting, lethargy, depression, poor appetite, weight loss, fever, and enlarged lymph nodes are observed. Crusts are often better felt than seen in the haircoat. There is little to no pruritus. Plucking of the crust leads to removal of the hair. Head and limb lesions occur more prominently on white skin areas and can have severe erythema exacerbated by a type of photodermatitis (1200).

Winter haircoat. Thick, creamy, white to yellow or green pus adheres between the skin and the overlying scab. Removal shows slightly raised moist skin with an ovoid shape. The undersurface of the plucked scab is often concave and has hair roots protruding through the scab.

Summer haircoat. Shorter hair means that the lesions tend to have smaller scabs (shot-like lumps 1–2 mm in diameter) comprising 8–10 hairs in the scab. Widespread infection (rain scald) gives a paintbrush effect (1201). With excessive moisture, eczematous lesions occur, especially on foals kept in wet unhygienic stables, and on the back of the pastern (greasy heels) in older horses (1202).

A separate clinical entity occurs on the hind cannon bone of racehorses. The lesions are typical of the summer type, with closely placed, small, matted hair patches down the front of both hind cannon bones (1203).

Differential diagnosis
Dermatophytosis; sunburn; rope burns; pemphigus foliaceus; equine viral papular dermatitis; equine sarcoidosis; pastern leukocytoclastic vasculitis; contact dermatitis; generalized granulomatous disease; pastern folliculitis; actinic dermatosis; anhidrosis; coronary band dystrophy; tick infestation; wound scalding; larval nematode dermatitis; sweet itch; chorioptic mange.

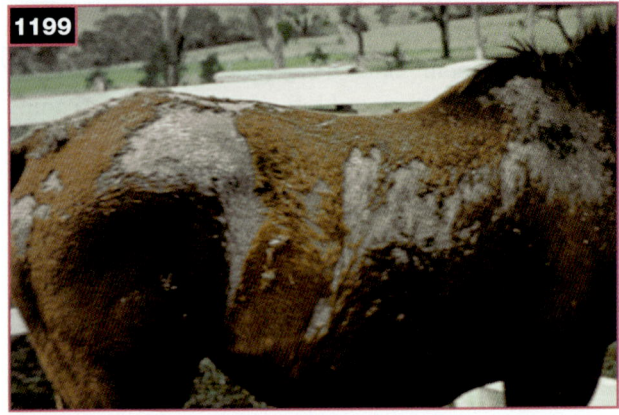

1199 Midwinter dermatophilosis after a prolonged rainy period of 10 days. The alopecia is distributed similarly to the water run-off patterns.

1200 This white-skinned nose shows a combination of signs due to sunburn and infection with *D. congolensis*.

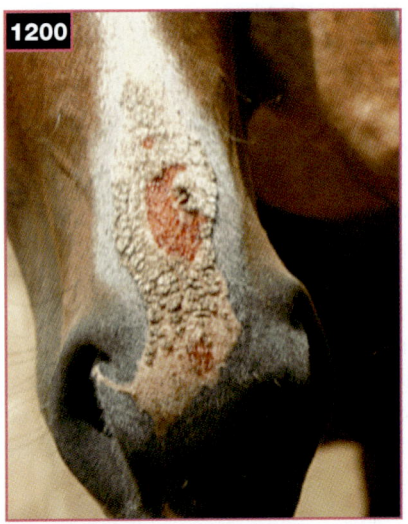

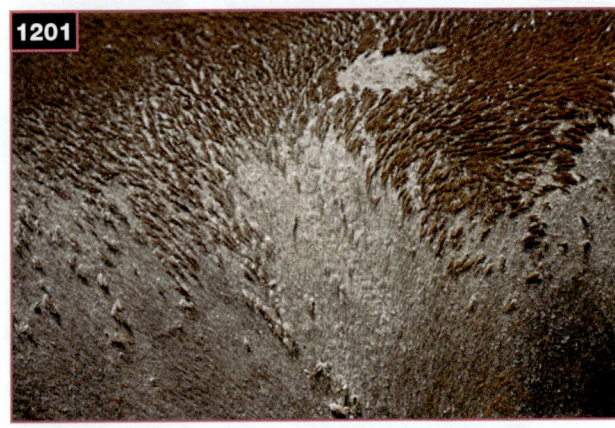

1201 'Paint-brush' effect caused by matting of small groups of hair infected with *D. congolensis*.

1202 *D. congolensis* was isolated in this horse as the cause of 'greasy heel' associated with alopecia, scabs, and cracking of the pastern skin. The condition frequently affects white limbs only.

1203 *D. congolensis* infection in this horse caused small shot-like lesions on the front of the hind cannon from working on a cinders-covered training track.

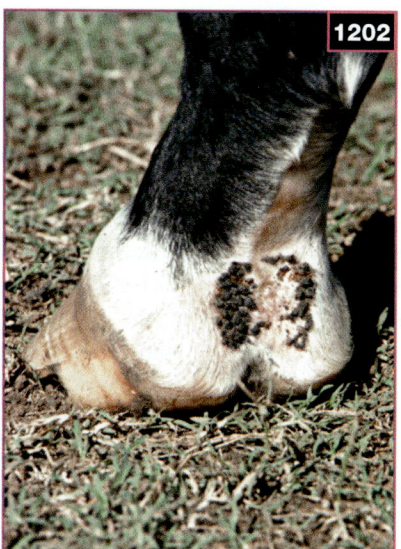

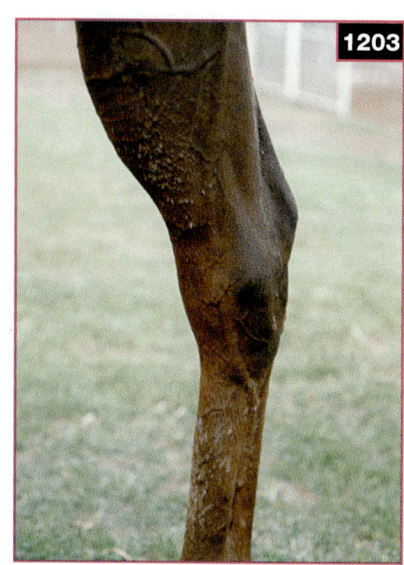

Diagnosis

The clinical appearance of matted hair encased with exudate with protrusion of hair roots is highly suggestive. Lesions may be located on the back line of the horse, the lower limbs, face, back of the pastern, and front of the hind cannon. A fresh lesion can be smeared on a microscope slide and stained.

Management

Generalized infection in large groups is not usually treated due to logistical problems. The disease under these conditions is usually self-limiting, with most horses showing regression and healing in 3–4 weeks in the winter and shorter periods in the summer, providing the wet weather has ended. In severe cases, individual treatment becomes necessary. Affected skin is gently swabbed with povidone–iodine. All infected debris is removed from the skin and the infected area is kept dry. 5% potassium permanganate in 0.5% aqueous brilliant green solution is applied daily for 3–5 days. Severe infections on white skin areas may crack or fissure. These are treated with an emollient cream of antibiotics and steroids; white lotion, zinc sulfate, and lead acetate solution are used. Sun block F20 is used where photodermatitis has occurred. In lower-limb lesions, protective bandaging must be used with caution as it may increase the severity of the disease by keeping areas moist. Contamination with wet bedding should be prevented. Skin weakness and chronic scarring occur with prolonged infections, making the skin prone to reinfection. Lameness can occur.

Systemic antibiotic treatment with procaine penicillin (20,000 IU/kg i/m q24h for 3–5 days) should be effective. Larger generalized skin infection can be treated with one of the following: aqueous 5% potassium permanganate with 0.5% brilliant green solution; 0.1% chloramine (Halamid disinfectant) solution; 1 in 1,000 benzalkonium chloride 10% solution; or 4% povidone–iodine.

Infections on white-skinned areas of the nose and limbs may be associated with a secondary photodermatitis and, despite antibiotic treatment, may continue to exhibit dermatitis due to exposure to sunlight. Stabling or protection of the affected area from sunlight is required.

Affected horses should be removed from contact with wet grass and wet stables, the bedding must be clean, nonirritating and dry, and the horse must be kept out of the rain.

Prognosis

The prognosis is generally excellent, but guarded for chronic pastern dermatitis.

Staphylococcal skin infection

Definition/overview
This is a contagious bacterial disease that causes acute folliculitis and furunculosis. *Staphylococcus aureus, S. intermedius*, and *S. hyicus* are the common isolates.

Etiology/pathophysiology
Organisms gain entry via any natural orifice, contaminated wound, or abrasion and the condition is usually associated with unhygienic conditions, dirty gear, and dusty yards.

Clinical presentation
Small (1–2 mm) extremely painful lesions rapidly enlarge, exude serum, and coalesce (**1204**). Scabs form with little pus present. Edema may develop around lesions that are principally associated with harness areas and saddle cloths and most commonly affect the skin of the back, saddle place, loins, and chest. *S. hyicus* has been isolated from 'greasy heel'-type lesions of the pastern and coronet, which may be pruritic, but tend to be severely painful.

1204 Staphylococcal folliculitis. The shoulder of a camp-draft horse with small alopecic pustules with a number of adjacent small papules due to infection following rug rub.

1205 Streptococcal infection involving the lymphatics. There is hair loss over a fulminating abscess, with rupture and discharge of yellow pus, in a typical position under the jowl.

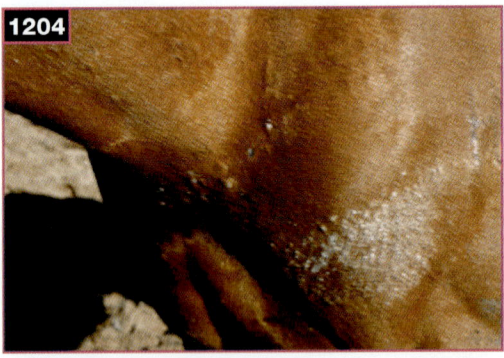

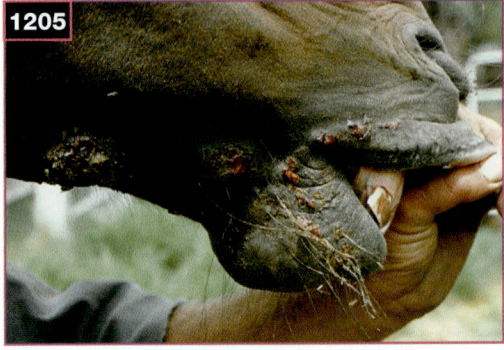

Differential diagnosis
Streptococcal folliculitis; other bacterial infections.

Diagnosis
Smear and culture from fresh lesions is used for diagnosis.

Management
Abscesses should be thoroughly cleaned with povidone–iodine twice daily. All gear should be fumigated with formalin vapor. Vaccination, which is only available in some countries, may be needed if more horses in a large stable become involved. Antibiotics have little effect.

Prognosis
The prognosis is guarded. There can be a protracted recovery.

Streptococcal skin infection

Definition/overview
This is a highly infectious skin disease, especially if due to *Streptococcus equi* (strangles), causing folliculitis, furunculosis, and ulcerative lymphangitis.

Etiology/pathophysiology
Organisms gain entry via any natural orifice, contaminated wound, or abrasion.

Clinical presentation
Small painful follicular infections occur around the mouth, vulva, and wounds, which may become generalized in cases of strangles, causing lymphadenopathy, abscess formation, and very painful, localized swellings, with exudation of serum (**1205**). Epilation of hair precedes rupture of the abscess.

Differential diagnosis
Staphylococcal folliculitis; other bacterial infections.

Diagnosis
Culture of a needle aspirate is used for diagnosis. Gram staining of an aspirate smear to detect the presence of Gram-positive cocci can be suggestive.

Management
Locally infected areas can be sanitized with iodine compounds. Abscesses should be opened whenever possible. Horses can develop vasculitis and purpura if a second infection cycle occurs. Prolonged treatment with intramuscular penicillin is controversial.

Prognosis
The prognosis is guarded when compounded by immune-mediated complications.

INFECTIOUS CAUSES – FUNGAL
Trichophytosis (ringworm)
Definition/overview
This is a common fungal infection of the hair follicles caused by *Trichophyton* spp. *T. equinum* is the most common cause of dermatophytosis in horses. It is a highly contagious disease affecting horses of all ages. It is spread by contact with a source of contaminated material or from horse to horse.

Etiology/pathophysiology
Most common are *T. equinum* var. *equinum*, *T. equinum* var. *autotrophicum*, and, less commonly, *T. verrucosum* and *T. mentagrophytes*. The organisms are found on horse hair or fomites and rarely in soil. Infection occurs more readily if the skin is abraded (e.g. rubbed by grooming brush, girth) and contaminated with the organism. The surface of the hair shaft is invaded by arthrospores, which migrate down to invade the hair follicle. Clinical disease appears 9–15 days post exposure.

Clinical presentation
Loss of hair, scaling, and scurfing of skin occur. In the early stages, hair follicles become erect in a circular area 5–20 mm in diameter (1206). Lesions can occur wherever contaminated gear contacts the horse or foal (e.g. the girth). Actively infected sites are pruritic. Initially single lesions occur, then the infected area becomes covered with multiple, often coalescing lesions (1207). The hair plucks easily 10–15 days post infection.

Differential diagnosis
Dermatophilosis; *Microsporum gypseum* infection; sweet itch; equine insect hypersensitivity; mite infestation; equine sarcoidosis; equine granulomatous enteritis; alopecia areata; anhidrosis; actinic dermatitis; wound scalding; *Malassezia* spp. infection.

Diagnosis
Hairs plucked from a fresh lesion are cleaned with chlor-lactophenol, then examined on a clear slide with warm 30% potassium hydroxide. Hyphae and large endothrix spores will be seen. The hair is cultured on Sabouraud's agar at 25°C (77°F). (*Note:* Clinically, hairs do not fluoresce under UV light.)

Management
Most horses develop resistance to dermatophytes and infection is usually self-limiting. Control is by preventing spread between horses when groups are involved. All scabs and infected hairs should be carefully removed and burnt. All lesions and surrounding hair should be scrubbed for 1–2 minutes daily for 7–10 days with one of the following treatments: 10% povidone–iodine solution;

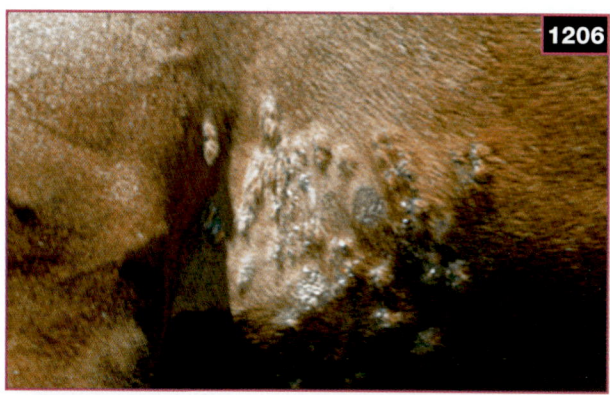

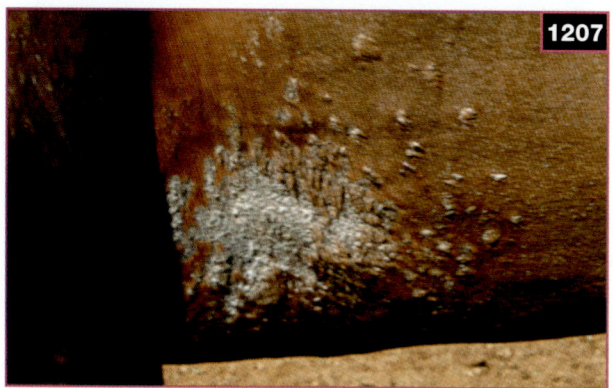

1206 Early infection with *T. equinum* var. *equinum* due to the use of a contaminated girth 14 days earlier is seen as small areas of alopecia and small papules with erect hairs.

1207 An older dermatophyte infection with a large area of alopecia. The early lesions have coalesced, with a secondary infected area of smaller peripheral lesions.

2.5% lime sulfur in water; or enilconazole 0.2% solution. Isolated lesions can be treated with 2.5–10% iodine or 0.3% Halamid. Many of the above medications cause clinical improvement, but fail to remove pathogenic fungi from the hair and skin for up to 7–28 days after treatment. In generalized lesions the affected area can be clipped and miconazole cream applied daily for 2–4 weeks; alternatively, 2–4% chlorhexidine is shampooed thoroughly into the haircoat for 15 minutes, then rinsed and repeated every 2–3 days. Miconazole 2% and enilconazole 0.2% twice weekly are recommended by the manufacturers for the removal of pathogenic fungi in horses. All tack should be fumigated to prevent spread.

Prognosis
The prognosis is good in individuals, but hygiene and quarantine must be strict to prevent spreading.

Microsporosis (ringworm)

Definition/overview
Microsporosis is a common fungal infection of the hair follicles caused by *Microsporum* spp. It is most commonly caused by *M. gypseum* and occasionally by *M. equinum*.

Etiology/pathophysiology
Microsporosis is usually spread by contact with a contaminated area (e.g. horse transport, tack, soil) and can be spread by biting insects and skin abrasion. *M. gypseum* is a soil saprophyte and invades hair similarly to *Trichophyton* spp., but it fails to destroy all the hair in the infected area so that a clean pluck rarely occurs, leaving a moth-eaten look to the haircoat.

Clinical presentation
Small hairless areas (alopecia) commonly develop on the face and limbs, but they can follow a distributed pattern of insect bites (**1208**). Not all hairs are affected or are shed. Purulent discharge associated with folliculitis may be present. Active lesions are not pruritic, but are positive to a scratch test.

Differential diagnosis
Trichophytosis; *Stomoxys* bites; sweet itch; mites; nymph ticks; lice; *Malassezia* spp. infection.

Diagnosis
Hairs plucked from a fresh lesion should be examined. Wood's light fluoresces only *M. equinum* and some *M. canis*. *M. gypseum* does not fluoresce. Culture of hair on Sabouraud's agar at 25°C (77°F) can be performed.

Management
The treatment is as for *T. equinum* infection. The response is slow and variable, but lesions heal with time. Removal of horses from contaminated yards after treatment is probably advisable. It does not appear as a yearly problem.

Griseofulvin (10 mg/kg q24h in the feed for 7 days) is a commonly used treatment for ringworm in horses, but should not be used in pregnant mares. Further research into its use is necessary to indicate its true value. Control measures should be used as described for trichophytosis.

Prognosis
The prognosis is good, but response is slower than for *Trichophyton* spp. infection.

OTHER ALOPECIC SKIN DISEASES
These diseases are loosely grouped, as one of their common clinical signs is related to loss of hair unrelated to pruritus or insect irritation.

Anhidrosis

Definition/overview
This condition is related to poor performance and an inability to sweat. It may be associated with patchy alopecia.

Etiology/pathophysiology
Anhidrosis is possibly an inappropriate response to prolonged stress, which can be evoked in about 10% of horses. It characterized by an inability to sweat in response to an adequate stimulus. The cause is unknown.

Clinical presentation
Loss of performance, exercise intolerance, alteration to respiration, an inability to sweat normally, and patchy alopecia may be observed (**1209**).

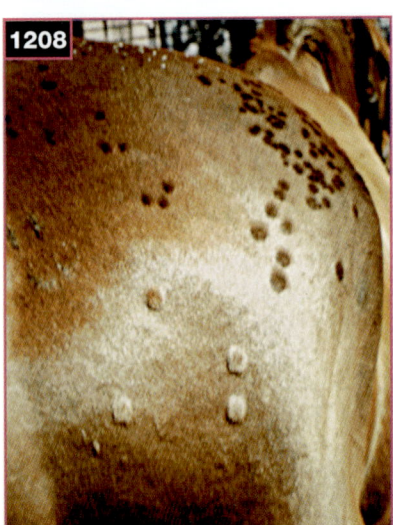

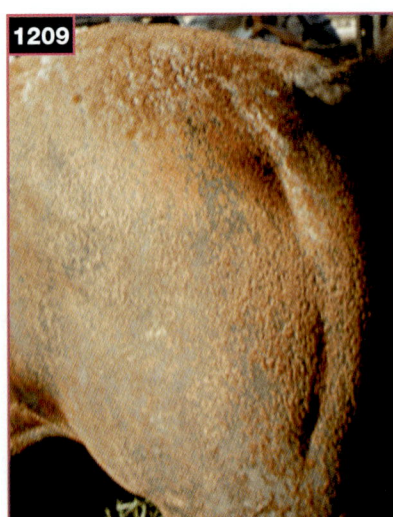

1208 *M. gypseum* spread by *Stomoxys calcitrans* flies. The distribution of infected sites corresponds to areas where *S. calcitrans* feeds on the horse.

1209 A 5-year-old race mare with loss of hair, a moth-eaten appearance of the general body coat, an inability to sweat, and with a reported loss of performance. The condition was confirmed as anhidrosis.

Differential diagnosis

Sweet itch; dermatophilosis; dermatophytosis.

Diagnosis

Affected horses have a history of loss of performance and increased respiratory effort. The adrenaline (epinephrine) skin test is used to confirm the diagniosis. The skin is injected with several dilutions of epinephrine: 0.5 ml of $1:10 \times 3$; of $1:10 \times 4$; of $1:10 \times 5$; and of $1:10 \times 6$. Anhidrotic horses have reduced sensitivity and a prolonged response time. Normal horses sweat at all dilutions.

Management

Affected horses should be moved to a colder climate for the summer months. Air conditioning should be used in stables in summer and reduction of stress can also be attempted. ACTH may give relief in very early cases.

Prognosis

The prognosis is poor unless the horse can be relocated to a cooler climate.

Anagen defluxion

Definition/overview

This is usually an acute hair loss associated with high fevers, illness, or malnutrition.

Etiology/pathophysiology

Anagen defluxion is a condition that affects the hair growth phase, resulting in abnormalities of hair follicles and hair shafts. Affected hairs break easily.

Clinical presentation

Excessive hair shedding and alopecia associated with sudden-onset systemic disease, high temperature, or malnutrition in a short time span are characteristic.

Differential diagnosis

Telogen defluvium (stressful diseases); *Leucaena* poisoning; fulminating abscesses.

Diagnosis

Changes to hairs, including irregularities of the shaft diameter (narrow and deformed), can be observed.

Management

If the inciting causes (e.g. fever) are removed, hair eventually regrows. The use of antimitotic drugs should be stopped.

Prognosis

The prognosis is cautious until regrowth commences.

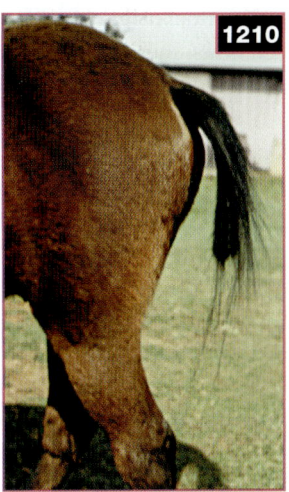

1210 Plant poisoning occurred when *Leucaena leucocephala* was fed to a group of brood mares, leading to loss of tail hairs.

Iodine poisoning

Definition/overview

Iodine poisoning may occur as a result of prolonged medication with either oral potassium iodide or intravenous sodium iodide.

Clinical presentation

Lacrimation, heavy scurf on the neck, mane, and body, and alopecia may be observed.

Differential diagnosis

Seborrhea; SLE.

Diagnosis

A history of medication, ingestion of kelp, or iodine supplementation should be evaluated.

Management

Intake of iodine should be reduced or stopped.

Poisonous plants

Definition/overview

Ingestion of some tropical and subtropical plants can cause hair loss. Among these are *Leucaena* spp. (used for forage and shade trees) and *Mimosa pudica* (a common ornamental shrub). The active principle in both plants is mimosine, a toxic nonprotein amino acid.

Etiology/pathophysiology

Mimosine has potent depilatory effects related to the quantity eaten and over what time scale.

Clinical presentation

Alopecia, particularly of the mane, tail and around the fetlock and coronary band, will be present (**1210**). Severe cases may develop laminitis, loss of appetite, and weight loss.

901

Differential diagnosis
Selenosis; mercurial poisoning; arsenical ingestion (1211); anagen defluxion malnutrition.

Diagnosis
Diagnosis is based on identification of access to *Leucaena* spp. or *Mimosa pudica* and the elimination of such diseases as equine insect hypersensitivity and *Oxyuris* infestation.

Management
Horses should be prevented from eating toxic plant material. Remedial treatment is mainly anecdotal and unreliable.

Prognosis
This condition has a slow recovery. Severe laminitis may lead to euthanasia.

Selenium toxicosis
Definition/overview
Ingestion of *Morinda reticulata* or *Neptunia amplexicaulis*, both of which accumulate selenium, may cause selenium toxicosis.

Etiology/pathophysiology
Selenium toxicosis is related to high levels of selenium in the soil or the presence of selenium-accumulating plants. Levels are highest in low-rainfall areas with alkaline soil.

Clinical presentation
Lameness including acute and chronic laminitis, loss of hooves, and loss of mane and tail hairs will be present.

Differential diagnosis
Mimosine toxicity; coronary band dystrophy; causes of laminitis; other causes of mane and tail dystrophy.

Diagnosis
Hair, hooves, liver, and kidney can be tested for selenium levels.

Management
Affected animals should be placed on a daily high-protein supplement and given 2–3 g DL methionine orally per day. Feed additives, such as sodium arsenate, arsenilic acid, and copper supplements, have been reported as treatments. Access to implicated plants should be restricted.

Prognosis
The prognosis is fair in early cases, but very poor when foot changes occur.

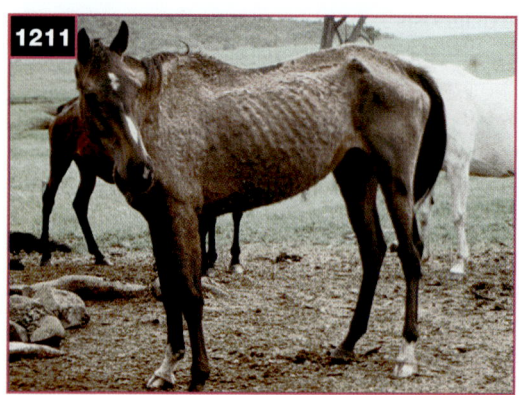

1211 Arsenical poisoning with general loss of condition, emaciation, and generalized exfoliative dermatitis.

Seborrheic diseases

Primary sebaceous gland dysfunction is rare in horses. Seborrheic disease seems more likely to be related to abnormal cornification resulting in scaling and crusting than to sebaceous gland dysfunction. Secondary seborrhea is usually related to a skin response from some other injury (e.g. 'greasy heel' in heavy horses).

Nodular diseases

Introduction
The development of a solid skin swelling of >1 cm, which exceeds the dimensions of a papule, can be included in the category of nodular skin disease. Many forms of skin disease may originate as macules or papules, but progressively increase in size, either singly or in numbers, and so become included in this category.

Nodules can be subdivided into inflammatory or neoplastic lesions. The inflammation may be due to injury or infection and the inflammatory infiltrate will vary from blood and tissue fluid through to neutrophils, lymphocytes, histiocytes, plasma cells, and eosinophils. Visible nodules develop from this substrate as the infiltrating cells begin to aggregate to wall off the injury or the infective process. As the lesion enlarges, the dermis and subcutis become completely infiltrated by the above cells and the overlying epidermis may become atrophic, leading to erosion, ulceration, and possible exudation of contents.

Most neoplasms of the skin and subcutaneous tissue originate as nodules and then usually increase by cell division. As secondary inflammatory changes occur around them, they develop into typical tumors of the skin, which may present as enlarged nodules or verrucous forms, or develop ulcerative changes and necrosis.

Swellings also include urticarial swellings, abscesses, and body swellings such as hernias and cysts. Urticaria is covered later in the chapter (see p. 928). Abscesses are localized fluid- to solid-filled lesions. They are the result of inflammatory changes, usually related to trauma and/or infection, and consist of dead cells, debris, and local tissue components that have liquefied through proteolytic and histolytic enzymes. While usually related to infection, abscesses can be sterile.

Tumors, nodules, and swellings tend to be primary disease sites and in horses are infrequent manifestations of systemic disorders. The major disease considerations in establishing a differential diagnosis are physical causes, infectious diseases, hypersensitivity reactions, sterile inflammatory diseases, and neoplasia.

Injuries to the skin and underlying tissues may result in superficial trauma to the epidermis right through to joint, bone, and muscle injury. This is manifested by an alteration to the normal contour of the skin and may lead to misdiagnosis between cellulitis, hematoma, bursitis, and hernias.

Bruising is extravasation of blood into the dermis and epidermis without severe dislocation of the external epidermal layer. Hematoma is rupture of blood vessels in subcutaneous tissues leading to extravasation of blood into the interstitial tissue. Cellulitis is extravasation of cellular fluid into tissue space, which may or may not be infected.

1212 Equine molluscum contagiosum is due to a poxvirus occurring around genital organs of mares and stallions and presents with small papules and a waxy skin surface. (Photo courtesy DW Scott) (Reprinted from Pascoe RR and Knottenbelt DC (1999) *Manual of Equine Dermatology*, WB Saunders, with permission)

1213 Three-month-old lesions of papillomatosis around the upper and lower lips of a weanling Thoroughbred filly.

INFECTIOUS CAUSES – VIRAL
Equine molluscum contagiosum (Uasin gishu disease)
Definition/overview
This is a mild contagious cutaneous infection caused by unclassified pox viruses. Lesions may occur on the penis, prepuce, scrotum, mammary glands, thighs, axillae, and muzzle (**1212**).

Equine viral arteritis (EVA)
Definition/overview
EVA is a viral disease associated with abortion, infertility, and skin disease. Some strains are relatively avirulent and infection may go unnoticed and undiagnosed (see p. 278).

Papillomatosis
Definition/overview
Papillomatosis is a viral skin disease characterized by small warts on the nose, lips, around the eyes, inside of the ear, and very occasionally on the neck and limbs.

Etiology/pathophysiology
The warts are caused by a DNA papovavirus that can produce two distinct clinical forms of papillomatosis: viral papillomatosis and aural papilloma (aural plaques).

Clinical presentation
Papillomatosis is characterized by small, cauliflower-like, warty growths that increase in number rather than size. They are predominately restricted to young horses 9–36 months of age (**1213**), but are occasionally seen affecting aged horses (>25 years). Aural plaques are also found on the internal surface of the ear.

Differential diagnosis
Sarcoid; SCC; equine molluscum contagiosum.

Diagnosis
The clinical appearance, age of the horse, and the size and number of warts are suggestive. Histopathology of biopsy specimens is confirmatory.

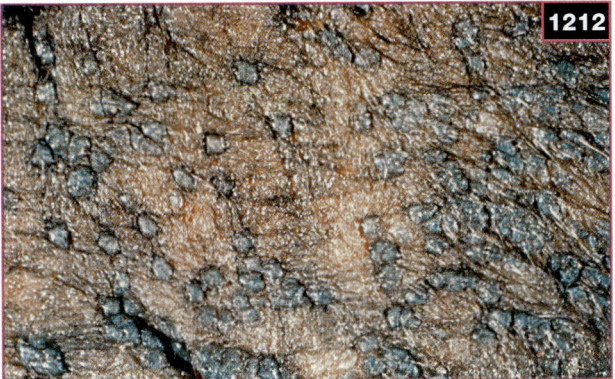
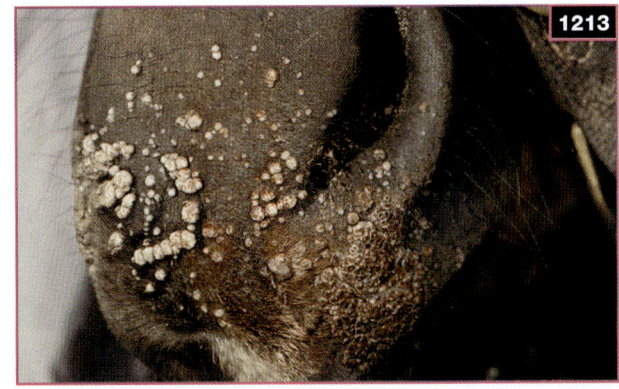

Management

In young horses most warts drop off after 3–4 months. Surgical removal of warts from around the eyes and commissure of the mouth may be needed. There may be little regression in the aged horse.

Prognosis

The prognosis is excellent.

INFECTIOUS CAUSES – BACTERIAL
Abscess
Definition/overview

An abscess is an aggregation of leukocytes and tissue debris related to skin and subcutis; it may be infected or sterile.

Etiology/pathophysiology

Infected abscesses can be caused by a variety of organisms, but those more commonly involved are *Streptococcus equi* (1214), *Corynebacterium pseudotuberculosis*, and *Clostridium* spp. They are often associated with intramuscular injections or wounds, but can be disseminated through the lymphatic system. Ectoparasites were incriminated in one outbreak of *C. pseudotuberculosis*.

Clinical presentation

Abscesses usually appear as subcutaneous swellings that may fluctuate. Acute abscesses are attached to the skin and may be hot and painful. Chronic abscesses may be walled off and may or may not be attached to the skin. Clostridial abscesses often have gas formation, acute swelling, and severe pain.

Differential diagnosis

Hematoma; cyst; acute eosinophilic granuloma; hernia.

Diagnosis

Aspiration of contents followed by culture or cytologic examination of a smear is used for diagnosis.

Management

Surgical drainage is indicated. Antibiotics may be required. Aeration of affected tissues by extensive surgical incision is important for clostridial infections.

Prognosis

The prognosis is very good if full drainage is established, but poor if pockets of infection remain.

1215 An internal injury to the buccal mucosa can lead to the formation of cheek abscesses due to *Staphylococcus* spp. This case took 3 days to point and rupture. (Reprinted from Pascoe RR and Knottenbelt DC (1999) *Manual of Equine Dermatology*, WB Saunders, with permission)

Cheek abscess
Definition/overview

This is an acute abscess formation at or around the lateral commissures of the mouth.

Etiology/pathophysiology

Cheek abscesses are caused by penetration of the buccal mucosa by grass, barley, or oat awns, or by lacerations by cheek or wolf teeth on the buccal mucosa, followed by infection.

Clinical presentation

Acute painful swelling of the 'bit' area or adjacent cheek area (1215), a small area of exudation over a pointing abscess, and hair loss (alopecia) may be observed.

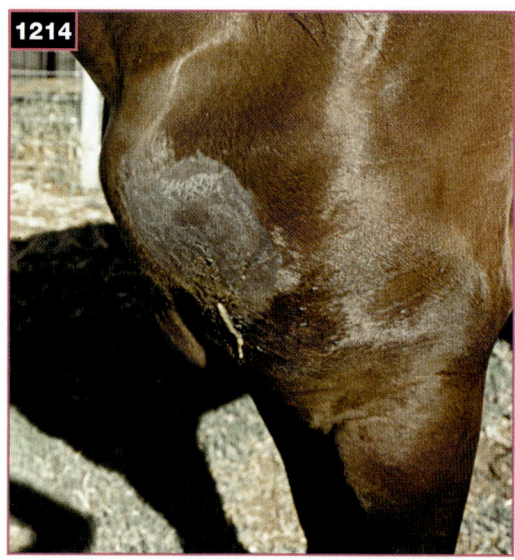

1214 *Streptococcus equi* abscess caused large alopecic area and skin slough in this unvaccinated mare during a strangles outbreak. (Reprinted from Pascoe RR and Knottenbelt DC (1999) *Manual of Equine Dermatology*, WB Saunders, with permission)

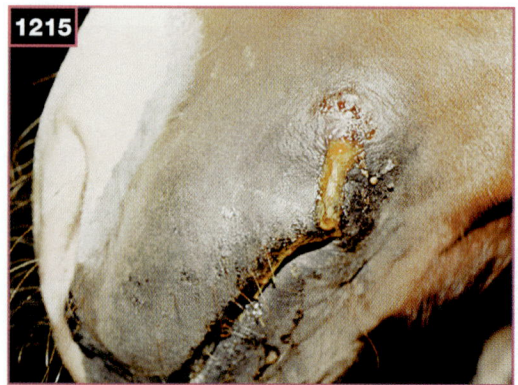

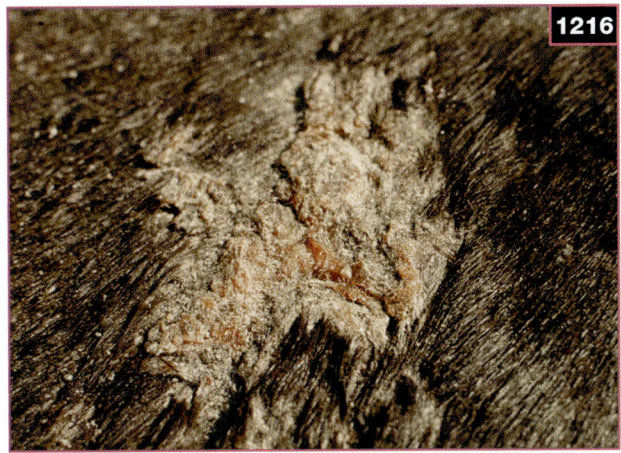

1216 Staphylococcal furunculosis. Note the heavy mat of exudate with hair slough about to occur.

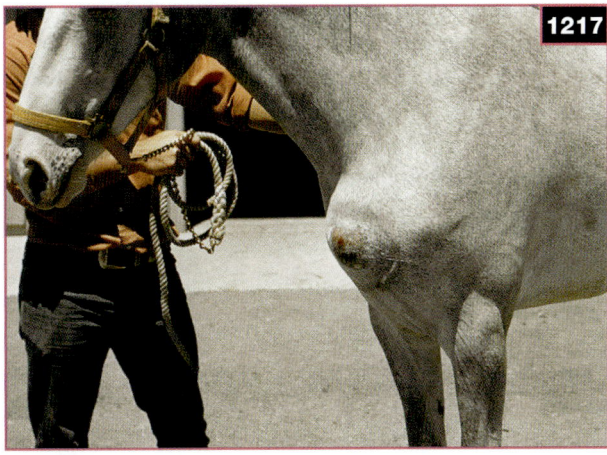

1217 *Corynebacterium pseudotuberculosis* abscess ('Wyoming strangles' or pigeon breast), which can be spread by biting flies. (Photo courtesy AA Stannard)

Differential diagnosis
Bit injury in the mouth; cuts inside the commissure; foreign bodies.

Diagnosis
The presence of cuts or wounds inside the mouth adjacent to the abscess, the presence of a 'boil' on the cheek or mouth commissure, and/or evidence of a badly fitting mouth bit should be investigated.

Management
Hot and cold fomentations may be useful. The abscess should be incised when possible. Early use of antibiotics should be avoided.

Bacterial or fungal folliculitis and furunculosis (acne)
Definition/overview
Folliculitis is an inflammation of the hair follicle with an accumulation of inflammatory cells within the follicle lumen. It can be caused by bacteria or fungi. As the infective process proceeds, degeneration of the hair follicle leads to infection of the surrounding dermis and subcutis (furunculosis) (1216). Where multiple infections sites coalesce, a carbuncle or a boil is formed. These occur in horses with saddle boils, heat rash (*Staphylococcus* spp.), cheek abscesses, and pigeon breast (Wyoming strangles [*C. pseudotuberculosis*]) (1217).

Etiology/pathophysiology
Unhygienic skin conditions, complicated by areas of friction from harnesses, rugs, or saddle cloths causing injury and infection of hair follicles, are associated with this condition. Coagulase-positive staphylococci produce endotoxins, hemolysins, leukocidins, and dermonecrotoxins, and are responsible for some cases of cellulitis and/or exfoliation.

Clinical presentation
Rapidly developing, small, painful papules followed by the presence of edema and exudation will be observed. There is an increasingly acute painful response and horses may kick or bite while being examined.

Differential diagnosis
Fungal folliculitis; dermatophytosis; dermatophilosis; onchocerciasis; other bacterial pyodermas.

Diagnosis
Deep biopsy for culture and susceptibility testing is carried out.

Management
Surgical drainage of larger lesions may be necessary. This should be followed by skin washes with povidone–iodine or chlorhexidine solution. If surgical drainage has been required, treatment with parenteral antibiotics such as penicillin (20,000 IU/kg i/m q24h for 3–5 days) or oral antibiotics such as trimethoprim/sulfadiazine (24–30 mg/kg p/o q12h for 2 weeks) may be required. All in-contact gear must be fumigated and hygiene improved.

Prognosis
The prognosis is guarded and this condition can be very slow to resolve.

Bacterial granuloma (botryomycosis)

Definition/overview
Botryomycosis is a pyogranulomatous lesion associated with skin injury.

Etiology/pathophysiology
It is caused by lacerations and puncture of the skin followed by infection, which slowly progresses to multiple miliary interlinking abscesses discharging through multiple sinuses.

Clinical presentation
Alopecia, a slowly healing wound, induration of the edges, and chronic purulent discharge from one or more sinuses, with rosette formation of granulation tissue around sinuses, may be observed (1218).

Differential diagnosis
Habronema infestation; pythiosis; foreign body sinus drainage.

Diagnosis
Diagnosis is based on the history of the type of injury and biopsy for histopathology.

Management
Surgical excision should be performed, with subsequent administration of sodium iodide solution (66 mg/kg i/v every 7 days) until signs of iodism appear.

Prognosis
The prognosis is guarded, as reinfection can occur following surgery, with a return of a similar clinical entity.

1218 Bacterial granuloma (botryomycosis lesion) showing many discharging sinuses in the granulation tissue.

Glanders (farcy)

Definition/overview
Glanders is a highly contagious disease of horses caused by *Burkholderia* (*Pseudomonas*) *mallei* infection (1219). It is usually fatal. It may be acute or chronic and has respiratory tract and skin forms. It has occurred in Eastern Europe, Asia, and North Africa. The disease can be fatal to humans and extreme care should be taken when sampling suspect cases.

Etiology/pathophysiology
B. mallei infection is transmitted from skin and nasal discharges by close contact between horses and fomites, and by ingestion of contaminated feed and water.

Clinical presentation
Glanders begins as subcutaneous nodules anywhere on the body, but particularly around the inside of the hocks. There is rapid ulceration of the skin, leading to discharge of a honey-like secretion associated with corded lymphatics, lymphangitis, and regional lymphadenopathy.

Differential diagnosis
Ulcerative lymphangitis (*Corynebacterium paratuberculosis*); epizootic lymphangitis (*Histoplasma farciminosum*); sporotrichosis (*Sporothrix schenckii*).

Diagnosis
Diagnosis may be confirmed by a mallein test, various serologic tests (CFT, immunofluorescent antibody [IFA] test, ELISA), culture, and/or histopathology.

Management
None.

Prognosis
Glanders is usually a fatal disease.

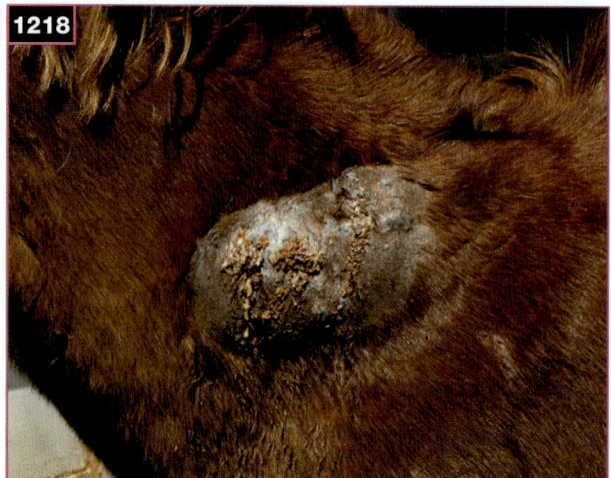

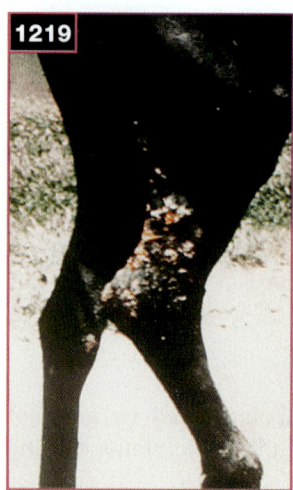

1219 Glanders (farcy). Extreme care should be exercised with all conditions resembling this case. (Photo courtesy AA Stannard) (Reprinted from Knottenbelt DC and Pascoe RR (1994) *Colour Atlas of Diseases and Disorders of the Horse*, Mosby, with permission)

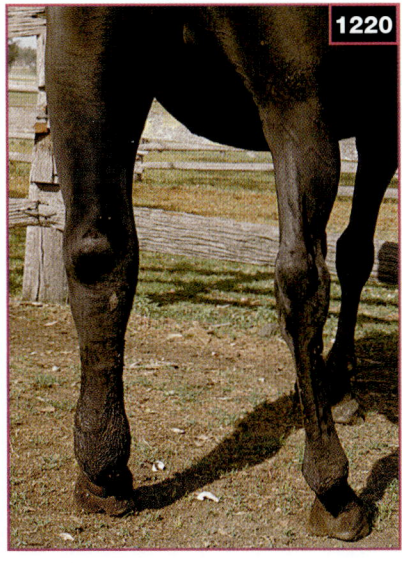

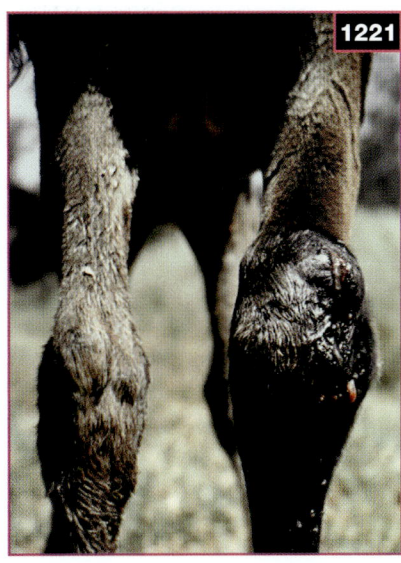

1220 Lymphangitis or 'big leg' in an 11-year-old Thoroughbred mare with an acutely hot painful swollen limb. This occurred suddenly 24 hours previously.

1221 An umbilical infection in a foal was followed by ulcerative lymphangitis, with swollen lymphatics and nodules, generalized swelling, and creamy pus discharge from sinuses above and below the hock.

Ulcerative lymphangitis

Definition/overview
Ulcerative lymphangitis is a mildly contagious disease characterized by lymphangitis of the lower limbs.

Etiology/pathophysiology
It is a bacterial infection with stasis of affected lymphatics related to poor hygiene and management, and insect transmission.

Clinical presentation
There is a sudden onset of moderate to severe edema of the lower limb. Swelling may extend to the elbow or stifle and is most common in the hindlimbs. Usually, only one limb is affected (**1220**). Serum exudate of the lower portion may occur with cording of the lymphatics of the upper limb. Ulceration and discharge of creamy, greenish pus occur very occasionally (**1221**). The limb is painful, but reaction time is slow due to bulky limb edema. Recurrence of edema is common.

Differential diagnosis
Sporotrichosis; mycetoma; systemic mycosis; enzootic lymphangitis; glanders.

Diagnosis
Clinical appearance is diagnostic, with identification of the definitive cause by culture of exudate.

Management
Depending on the culture results, treatment with appropriate antibiotics plus intravenous medication with sodium iodide (66 mg/kg every 7 days until iodism occurs) should be considered. Chronic lymphatic nodules can be removed with elastic ligatures around the base of the swelling.

Hydrotherapy and walking in hand are also useful adjunctive therapies for this condition.

Prognosis
The prognosis is guarded, as long treatment may be required.

INFECTIOUS CAUSES – FUNGAL
Cutaneous mycosis (dermatophytosis)
See under Alopecic conditions (p. 899).

Subcutaneous mycosis

Definition/overview
This disease occurs as chronic subcutaneous fungal tumors, which may cause generalized swelling, sinus and fistula formation, and tissue granules that may be colored black, white, or yellow. Most affected horses are pruritic.

Mycetoma

Definition/overview
Eumycotic mycetomas are caused by fungi and actinomycotic mycetomas are caused by bacteria such as *Actinobacillus*, *Nocardia*, and *Actinomyces* spp.

Etiology/pathophysiology
Saprophytic fungi cause the disease through wound contamination. The commonest reported fungus is *Pseudoallescheria boydii*.

Clinical presentation
Ulcerating nodules occur on the limbs, head, or ventral abdomen. There is chronic discharge from granulating sores, and pruritus is present. Some cases may present as nodules covered by ulcerated hairless skin, but with no other clinical abnormalities.

907

Differential diagnosis
Pythiosis; *Basidiobolus* infection; sporotrichosis; ulcerative lymphangitis; pastern folliculitis; phaeohypomycosis.

Diagnosis
Diagnosis is basaed on physical examination, clinical signs, biopsy, and culture with isolation of *Curvularia geniculata* or *Pseudoallescheria boydii*.

Management
Some cases respond well to surgical removal and use of systemic iodides. Some prove difficult and require repeat treatments.

Prognosis
Prolonged treatment may be unsuccessful.

Phaeohypomycosis
Definition/overview
This is a chronic subcutaneous and systemic fungal disease, often showing as small multiple subcutaneous nodules. *Drechslera spicifera* has been isolated.

Etiology/pathophysiology
Phaeohypomycosis is caused by various soil saprophytic fungi contaminating wounds.

Clinical presentation
Small, black, denuded plaques containing papules and pustules will be identified. Small, multiple, fibrotic, subcutaneous nodules can occur on the neck, body, and limbs .

Differential diagnosis
Eosinophilic granuloma; infectious granuloma; neoplasms; foreign body granuloma.

Diagnosis
Diagnosis is based on biopsy and culture on Sabouraud's agar.

Management
Systemic iodide treatment is indicated. Amphotericin B therapy is unsuccessful. Ketoconazole therapy has been suggested. Topical application of etisazole in DMSO has been reported.

Prognosis
A guarded prognosis should be given.

Pythiosis (phycomycosis)
See under Pruritus section (p. 878).

Sporotrichosis
Definition/overview
Sporotrichosis is a chronic sporadic skin and subcutaneous infection caused by *Sporotrichum (Sporothrix) schenckii*.

Etiology/pathophysiology
Organisms occur in the soil or organic debris and cause infection, usually by introduction through small skin wounds.

Clinical presentation
Hard, subcutaneous, 1–5 cm diameter nodules associated with 'corded' hardened lymphatics, ulceration, creamy pus discharge, and encrustation will be present (**1222**).

Differential diagnosis
Bacterial ulcerative lymphangitis (*C. paratuberculosis*); mycetoma; epizootic lymphangitis (*H. farciminosum*); glanders (*Burkholderia mallei*).

Diagnosis
Identification of nodules on lymphatic channels, culture on Sabouraud's agar slopes, and Gram staining of exudates are often used. Biopsy is not usually helpful.

Management
Systemic and oral iodides, topical iodine, and surgical removal should be considered.

Prognosis
The prognosis is guarded.

Systemic mycosis
Definition/overview
Occasionally, fungal disease of internal organs has skin manifestations. These causative organisms rarely cause primary skin disease.

Coccidioidomycosis
Definition/overview
Coccidioides immitis has been commonly reported as a generally chronic, debilitating, highly infectious disease in southwest USA, with spores from soil dust generally being inhaled into the respiratory tract. Very occasionally, cases manifest as a skin condition.

Histoplasmosis (epizootic lymphangitis)
Definition/overview
Histoplasmosis is a rare, chronic, contagious disease characterized by suppurative lymphangitis. It occurs on the hindlimbs, but has been reported on the neck, lips, and areas where harness abrasions occur. The condition is caused by *Histoplasma farciminosum*.

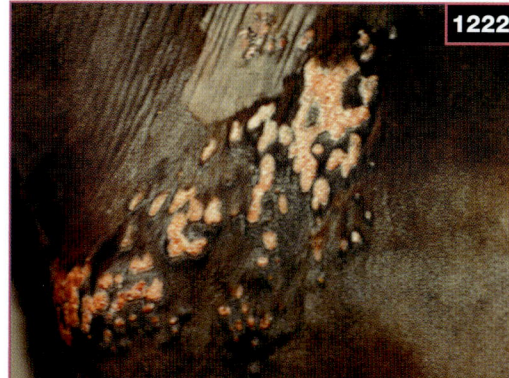

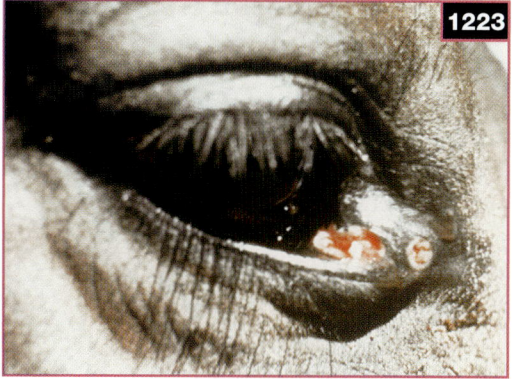

1222 Sporotrichosis. Nodules and corded lymphatics with ulceration and a creamy purulent discharge. (Photo courtesy DW Scott)

1223 Habronemiasis lesion in a tear duct.

Habronemiasis

Definition/overview

Infestation of wounds with the larval forms of the stomach nematodes *Habronema muscae*, *Draschia megastoma*, and *H. majus* commonly cause ulcerative cutaneous granulomas in horses. Larval worms are capable of penetrating intact skin. Recurrence of infection can occur on a yearly basis. It is associated with an increased fly population, poor manure collection or disposal, and moist patches of long grass. A predilection has been shown for light-colored horses.

Etiology/pathophysiology

Habronemiasis is caused by the combined presence of *Habronema* spp. stomach worms, house and/or stable flies, and poor hygiene. It is most prevalent in summer and autumn. Cutaneous habronemiasis is part hypersensitivity reaction and part seasonal, with spontaneous regression in the winter months because larvae do not overwinter in the tissues. It is a sporadic disease, with only individual horses in a herd affected on a recurring annual basis.

Clinical presentation

Affected animals have rapidly granulating sores at the medial canthus, prepuce, and urethra, or elsewhere; rapid growth of granulating wounds, with failure to heal; and cheesy sulfur-like granules in sores, especially in the medial canthus. Some sores show a stringy serosanguineous exudate. Multiple areas can be affected. Urethral process infection can lead to bleeding during covering by stallions, may reduce fertility, and produce blood-stained urine. Rubbing of eyes, very mild pruritus, and biting at lesions also occur (**1223**).

Differential diagnosis

Exuberant granulation tissue; SCC; phycomycosis; pythiosis; fibroblastic sarcoid; botryomycosis lesions.

Diagnosis

Biopsy and histopathology show the presence of yellow granules in wounds, with a nodular to diffuse dermatitis. Cheesy 'kunkers' are often present. Scrapings and smears from lesions may give false-positive results (e.g. it is not uncommon to find *Habronema* spp. larval infestations in sarcoids, in *Pythium* spp. lesions, or in SCC lesions, thus causing a multiple clinical diagnostic problem). There may be hemorrhage from the enlarged urethral process.

INFECTIOUS CAUSES – PROTOZOAL
Besnoitiosis

Definition/overview

This is a protozoal disease caused by ingestion of feed contaminated with cat feces, bites from blood-sucking insects, and parenteral injection of blood from acute cases. Cases have been reported in South Africa. Cattle are also affected in Africa, Asia, Southern Europe, and South America.

INFECTIOUS CAUSES – PARASITIC

The primary clinical sign of the majority of skin parasitic diseases is pruritus, therefore, most conditions have already been discussed under Pruritus (p. 877).

Demodicosis

Definition/overview

Demodicosis is a very uncommon clinical disease, even though mites can be demonstrated regularly (i.e. *D. caballi* from eyelids and muzzle, and *D. equi* from the body of normal horses). Clinical disease is manifested as alopecia and scaling with papules and pustules and likely only occurs in horses with lowered general immmunity. Positive skin scrapings, lack of another identifiable cause, and evidence of a compromised immune system can be used for diagnosis.

Management

Oral ivermectin paste is very efficient, but occasionally a second dose is required 3–4 weeks after the initial dose, followed by regular dosing. Surgical removal of some lesions of the medial canthus, 3rd eyelid, or urethral process is possible. Follow-up treatment of eye lesions by oral medication may also require a local application of cortisone drops plus a 50% mixture of ivermectin and artificial tears solution. Recently, it has been shown that parenteral corticosteroids (dexamethasone, 0.04 mg/kg p/o q24h; or prednisolone, 1 mg/kg p/o q24h continued and tapered off over 20–30 days) have given a better response in cases with larger mass involvement. The average recovery time was approximately 23 days.

Control of fly breeding grounds by cutting long grass, prompt and proper manure and soiled bedding disposal, and control of house and stable flies is essential.

Prognosis

The prognosis is good, but all aspects of control as well as treatment must be followed.

IMMUNE-MEDIATED NODULES OR SWELLINGS ASSOCIATED WITH CONGENITAL, DEVELOPMENTAL, AND POSSIBLY HEREDITARY DYSFUNCTIONS

Dentigerous cysts

Definition/overview

Dentigerous cysts are hard swellings that occur between the base of the ear and the eye (temporal region) and arise from tooth germ tissue (**1224**). Occasionally, they are also found on the cranial vault or maxillary sinus and contain enamel-forming tissue. They may contain one tooth or more. Drainage may occur near the ear through the skin.

1224 Dentigerous cyst.

Dermoid cysts

Definition/overview

Dermoid cysts are single or multiple, firm to fluctuant, smooth, round cysts, usually with normal overlying haired skin. They most commonly occur along the dorsal midline of the thorax and back, and while a breed predisposition has not been proven, an Australian survey indicated that they occur more frequently in Thoroughbred yearlings.

Etiology/pathophysiology

These are congenital, developmental, and possibly hereditary lesions. They are thought to be due to embryonal displacement of ectoderm into the subcutis.

Clinical presentation

Single to multiple nodules, covered with skin, 10–15 mm in diameter, and usually found on the dorsal midline from withers to rump will be observed. The nodules contain soft cheese-like gray material and coiled hairs. Young horses are usually affected between birth and 18 months.

Differential diagnosis

Epidermoid cysts; dentigerous cysts; hypodermiasis.

Diagnosis

The location and clinical picture are suggestive. Excisional biopsy shows a cyst wall lined with stratified squamous epithelium containing adnexal structures.

Management

Total surgical ablation of the cyst wall and contents is required.

Prognosis

The prognosis is very good following surgery.

Epidermoid cysts

Definition/overview

Epidermoid cysts are usually solitary cysts, 7–30 mm in diameter, occurring on the head and limbs. They are freely movable, well-circumscribed, firm to fluctuant on palpation, and contain a yellow to gray mucoid fluid.

Atheroma is a type of epidermoid cyst that occurs as a hemispherical, 10–50 mm structure located in the false nostril (**1225**).

Etiology/pathophysiology

The cause is unknown. Epidermoid cysts are classified according to differentiation of the epithelial lining.

Clinical presentation

Large nodules, usually singular and containing only a mucoid fluid and no hairs, will be present.

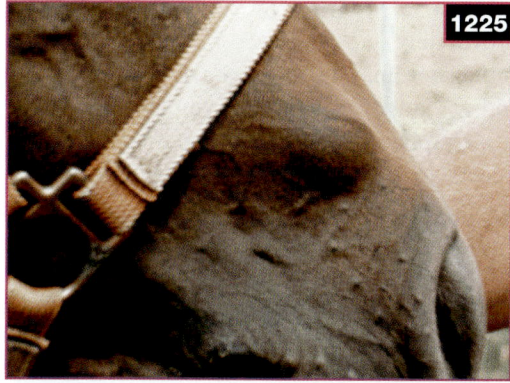

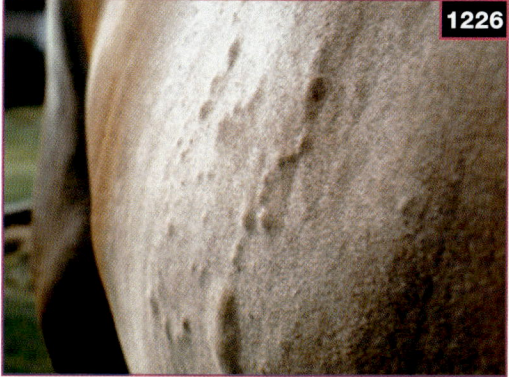

1225 Atheroma is a specific epidermoid cyst occurring in the false nostril.

1226 Equine eosinophilic granuloma. One large calcified nodule and several small hard subcutaneous nodules are present on the side of the chest.

Equine eosinophilic granuloma
(with collagen degeneration)
Definition/overview
This condition results in one to several, firm, dermal nodules occurring on the neck, withers, or back, associated with degenerative collagen. It is probably one of the most common nodular skin conditions in the horse.

Etiology/pathophysiology
The cause is unknown. It is probably multifactorial and may be related to insect hypersensitivity. Two thirds of the cases in one study occurred in spring and summer.

Clinical presentation
Fully haired, hard, subcutaneous nodules between 0.5 and 5 cm in diameter are present (1226). Single, several, or many nodules appear. They are painless and nonpruritic. Mineralization may occur in old lesions.

Differential diagnosis
Mastocytoma; epidermoid and dermoid cysts; insect bites; unilateral papular dermatosis; hypodermiasis; amyloidosis; phaeohypomycosis; panniculitis; erythema multiforme.

Diagnosis
Biopsy and histopathology, which show foci of necrobiosis of collagen fibers associated with heavy eosinophilic infiltration, are the best diagnostic techniques.

Management
Using corticosteroids is the only successful treatment apart from surgical removal. Where large numbers of nodules are present, 600–800 mg prednisolone p/o q24h for 10–14 days, followed by 500–600 mg q24h for another 10–14 days should be given; any remaining lesions are injected intra- or perilesionally with triamcinolone (3–5 mg/lesion) or methylprednisolone (5–10 mg/lesion). Many nodules are very dense and may require the use of a pressure syringe and 25 gauge needle, or perilesional injection. Surgical ablation should be considered where lesions remain after prolonged corticosteroid treatment or have become calcified.

Prognosis
New cases show a better response than chronic cases. Calcified lesions need surgical removal.

Differential diagnosis
Cysts: dentigerous, false nostril, dermoid, or conchal; hypodermiasis.

Diagnosis
Histopathology is diagnostic and identifies an epithelial lining that shows maturation and keratinization typical of the epidermis. No adnexal structures are present.

Management
Surgical removal is required.

Prognosis
The prognosis is excellent as long as all the cystic lining material is removed.

Equine calcinosis circumscripta
Definition/overview
This condition is characterized by firm nodules, commonly over the lateral stifle area and less commonly over other joints such as the carpus and tarsus.

Equine cutaneous amyloidosis
Definition/overview
This is a rare papulonodular disorder of the skin and URT mucosa. It usually occurs in older horses.

Equine unilateral papular dermatosis

Definition/overview

This condition is most frequently seen in yearlings and 2-year-old horses. Papules and nodules appear in multiple numbers, usually forming a loose group in a circular arrangement.

Etiology/pathophysiology

The etiology is unknown. It is most commonly reported in Quarter horses.

Clinical presentation

Numerous, even sized, firm, round, well-circumscribed nodules are evident. There is no alopecia or pruritus and the nodules are nonulcerative and nonpainful (**1227**). Fresh nodules may occur in almost concentric rings around the original lesions.

Differential diagnosis

Dermatophytosis (before hair is lost); *Stomoxys calcitrans* bites; sweet itch and other insect bites; onchocercal filariasis.

Diagnosis

History, clinical appearance, and the absence of any known pathogens are suggestive. A skin biopsy confirms the diagnosis.

Management

Oral prednisolone (1.1 mg/kg q24h) may help in some cases.

Prognosis

The prognosis is good. Regression occurs over a period of time.

Lymphedema

Definition/overview

The preputial area may be the primary location, with nodules and cording of lymphatics. Lymphedema can be caused by a lymphatic system disorder. Swelling of the prepuce occurs, usually unilaterally. It may be secondary to injury, infection, or neoplasia.

Etiology/pathophysiology

Lymphedema is caused by obstruction of lymphatic drainage from congenital abnormalities, trauma, inflammation, or neoplastic occlusion.

Clinical presentation

Nodules and enlarged lymphatics involving the prepuce are evident. In primary cases it is painless and rarely fluctuates, with little pitting on pressure. Secondary cases usually have other conditions involved and may be painful and pit on pressure. Lymphatic tissue may be hypoplastic, with the absence of lymphatic drainage, or be hyperplastic, with dilation of lymphatics up to 3–4 mm in diameter.

Differential diagnosis

Hemangioma; lymphangioma; other tumors; injury, post-castration swelling; schirrhous cord.

Management

Surgical treatment is required in some cases. Poor healing is common.

Prognosis

A guarded prognosis should be given.

Panniculitis

Definition/overview

Panniculitis involves multiple subcutaneous nodules and may affect the trunk, neck, and proximal limbs. Nodules may or may not be painful on palpation. It is a rare, multifactorial, inflammatory condition of the subcutaneous fat of horses. The cause of the disease is obscure. Vitamin E deficiency has been suspected in some cases.

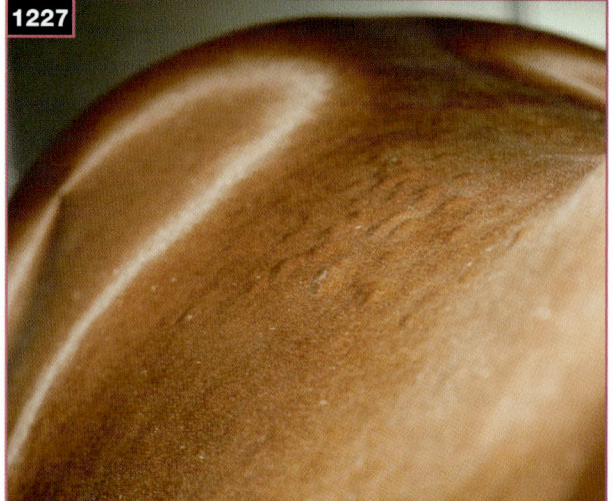

1227 Equine unilateral papular dermatosis in a 1-year-old Thoroughbred. There are groups of small nodular lesions (15–100) on the flank and saddle areas.

Neoplasia

Introduction

Certain skin tumors are very common in horses. When confronted with a lump or bump, in or under the skin, and if trauma and hematoma formation can be eliminated, the next step is confirmation of a diagnosis. Following careful history taking and a full evaluation of the tumor, needle or punch biopsy or, in the case of a small tumor, a total excisional biopsy should be undertaken. Histopathologic diagnosis will be a major determinant of how the case is managed in the future.

PARANEOPLASTIC DISEASE
Equine sarcoid
Definition/overview

A locally aggressive fibroblastic tumor, sarcoid is the most common cutaneous tumor found in horses. Recent studies indicate that there is no significant sex or age predisposition. The distribution of lesions varies with the type of sarcoid and appears to vary from one geographic location to another. For example, the paragenital region is affected the most frequently in horses in the UK, while in Australia the majority of lesions occur on the head, neck, and limbs and very rarely in the paragenital region. A recent study of sarcoid cases in the UK showed single and small numbers of sarcoids (2–8 sarcoids per horse) to be uncommon, whereas 10 to several thousand are more common (**1228**).

Six major types are described: occult, verrucous, nodular, fibroblastic, malevolent, and mixed. The distribution of these shows great variation, with a preponderance of fibroblastic tumors occurring in the paragenital area. In Australia almost all limb sarcoids are fibroblastic. Sarcoids have a high capacity to invade the dermis and subcutis. Sarcoids can occur in fresh healing wounds in previously normal horses, or recur at the same site following apparently complete surgical removal. True metastatic dissemination does not occur. Many lesions are frequently not life threatening, but they can severely limit the use of the horse and reduce its sale prospects. Euthanasia is not uncommon due to the prolonged nature of treatment, the likelihood of recrudescence of the problem, and cost.

The role of a virus, in particular bovine papillomavirus (BPV), in the cause and transmission of equine sarcoid is still uncertain. BPV has also been detected in normal skin samples from horses with sarcoids, suggesting the possibility of a latent viral phase. Viral latency may be one explanation of the high rate of recurrence following surgical removal. Population and family studies have shown an association between sarcoid susceptibility and major

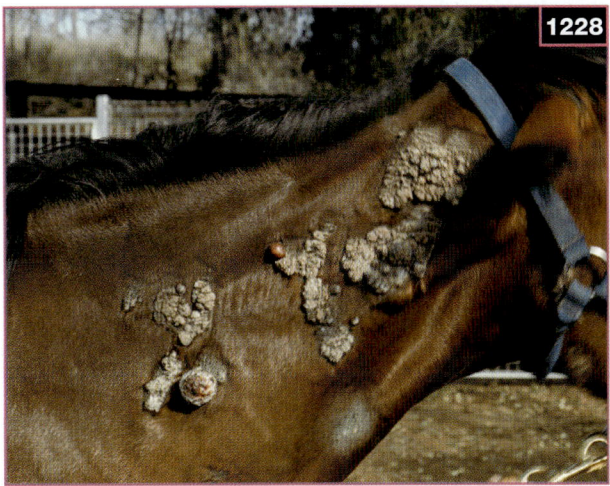

1228 Sarcoid. An 8-year-old horse with a mix of (35) sarcoids on the body and neck with verrucous, fibroblastic, mixed, and occult forms.

histocompatibility genes (class II alleles), suggesting a genetic predisposition. BPV DNA was detected in 88% and 91% of the successful swabs and scrapings from sarcoids, respectively. There are known cases of spontaneous full and permanent self-cure.

Lesions occur in locations that are prone to injury and some have a history of previous skin wounds. There is also strong presumptive evidence that sarcoids can be transmitted by biting by domestic flies that feed on sarcoid tissue and then browse on other horses with open sores, wounds, or tumors. The introduction of a horse with fibroblastic sarcoids can result in the appearance of sarcoids in other previously uninfected horses on the farm within 6–8 months. Sarcoids can multiply on individual horses, but can also remain static for long periods. There are also instances where treatment of one or several lesions has resulted in regression of other untreated lesions on the same horse.

The most important information on sarcoids is the complete unpredictability of their clinical course whether treated or not treated.

Clinically and pathologically sarcoids resemble true neoplasms, but differ markedly in that they present with at least six distinct clinical forms or entities. It is important to remember that the entities can rapidly change into another form, usually with increasing malignancy. This may be as a result of trauma, surgery, medication, or for no apparent reason, leading to a complexity of treatments and prognoses.

Occult sarcoid

Definition/overview
These are hairless areas usually containing one or more small hyperkeratotic cutaneous nodules.

Clinical presentation
Loss of hair is roughly circular and very slow spreading (until injured). One or more hard shot-like cutaneous nodules (1–5 mm) is/are present in the hair loss area (1229). These may progress to small, warty verrucous growths with the surrounding skin becoming more thickened or hyperkeratotic with time or, if injured, developing into fibroblastic lesions. Lesions are commonly found around the mouth, eyes, neck, and body.

Differential diagnosis
Dermatophytosis (ringworm); blisters; burns.

Diagnosis
The clinical picture is highly suggestive. It is important to remember that taking a biopsy sample may convert the lesion into an active fibroblastic sarcoid.

Verrucous (warty) sarcoid

Definition/overview
These tend to be slow growing and not very aggressive, hyperkeratotic, wart-like lesions, until injured in some fashion (e.g. biopsy, rubbing). They mainly occur around the face, neck, and axilla, but can occur anywhere.

Clinical presentation
Verrucous sarcoids are slow-growing, wart-like growths on and above the skin. They may be sessile or pedunculated. Trauma to the surface may convert them into a fibroblastic reaction.

Differential diagnosis
Papillomatosis; chronic blistering; hyperkeratosis (chronic sweet itch); equine sarcoidosis (chronic granulomatous disease); SCC.

Diagnosis
If a biopsy is taken, it is preferable to use total excision followed by cryotherapy.

Nodular sarcoid

Definition/overview
Nodular sarcoids occur as subcutaneous, well-defined, firm nodules. There may be single nodules, small numbers, or huge, multiple, intertwining groups of many hundreds of nodules. Where these erode overlying skin they become more aggressive, fibroblastic tumors.

Clinical presentation
Subcutaneous spherical nodules (0.5–20 cm) are evident. Two separate types are found: one type can be freely moveable in relation to both skin and subcutis; the other has more involvement with skin and the subcutis. The skin may become thin over larger nodules. The second type is more aggressive, especially following an erosion of overlying skin. They are most frequently found in the groin or eyelid area (1230).

Differential diagnosis
Fibroma; neurofibroma; equine eosinophilic granuloma; melanoma; collagen necrosis (axilla – rare); dermoid cysts.

Diagnosis
Biopsy is diagnostic. Total excision should be performed, if possible with wide margins.

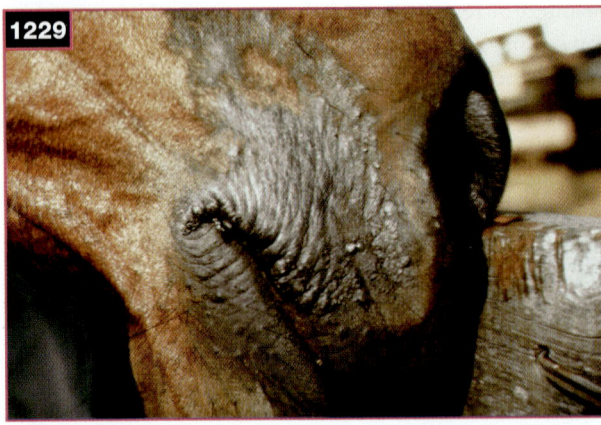

1229 Occult forms of sarcoid appear clinically as an area of alopecia containing one or more small nodules.

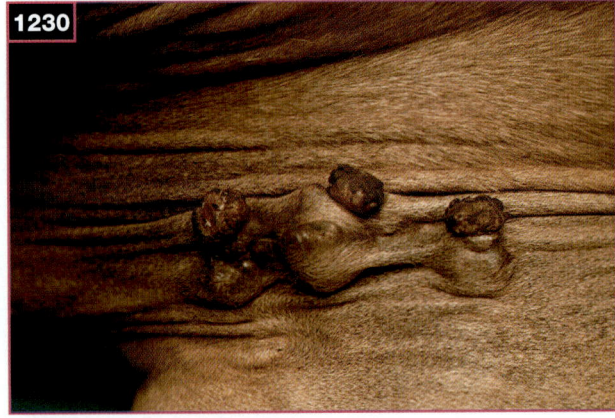

1230 Subcutaneous sarcoid nodules are often seen in and around the prepuce and scrotum. Surgical removal can be successful.

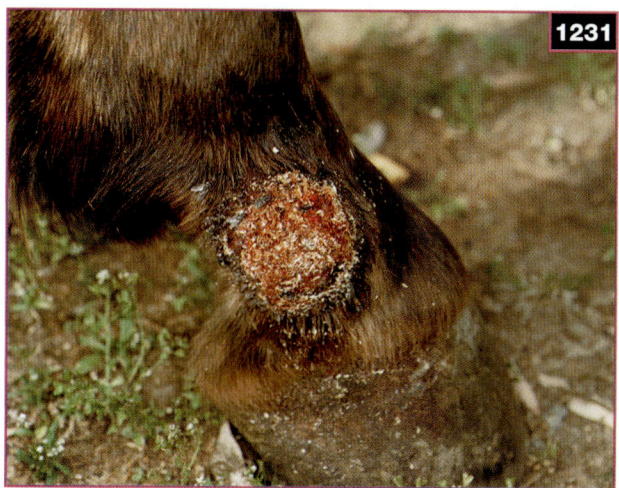

1231 Fibroblastic sarcoid limb lesions are more difficult to control and carry a less favorable prognosis.

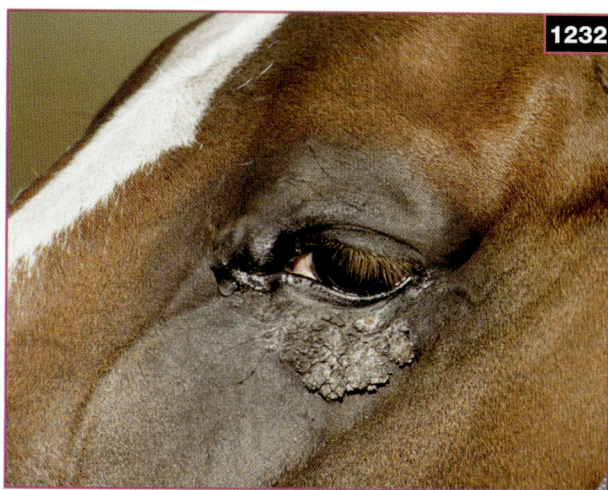

1232 Mixed, verrucous, fibroblastic, and occult forms of sarcoid occur in the periorbital region and histopathology may be necessary to distinguish them from neurofibroma.

Fibroblastic sarcoid

Definition/overview

This type has the appearance of excess granulation tissue. It is a more aggressive tumor, particularly when located on the lower limbs and coronet (**1231**). It frequently develops after skin wounds or follows injuries to other sarcoid entities.

Clinical presentation

A tumor resembling fleshy granulation tissue with erosion and exudation is evident. It may be pedunculated or sessile. The pedunculated type has two forms: one with a thin (stretched) skin only; the second with a more thickened defined neck. The sessile type may be more flattened, but still has the capacity, following injury, for rapid growth. Lateral progression is by local invasion. All types are subject to invasion by *Habronema* larvae, bacteria (*Staphylococcus* spp.), or fungi (*Pythium* spp.).

Differential diagnosis

Exuberant granulation tissue; habronemiasis; neurofibroma/neurofibrosarcoma; botryomycosis; fibrosarcoma; SCC; pythiosis; sweat gland tumor.

Diagnosis

Biopsy is used for diagnosis.

Mixed occult, verrucous, and fibroblastic sarcoid

Definition/overview

This form of sarcoid is progressively more aggressive, as changes occur from the occult and verrucous types to the fibroblastic type.

Clinical presentation

This type of sarcoid is probably a progressive state from either an occult or a verrucous type. All three entities may be evident (**1232**).

Diagnosis

The presence of more than one form of sarcoid is almost self-diagnostic.

Malevolent sarcoid

Definition/overview

This is a recent variation of sarcoid showing increased malignancy.

Clinical presentation

This sarcoid may result from other types of sarcoids subject to repetitive injury, medication, or surgery. Occasionally, with no previous history of interference, they spontaneously develop into multiple tumors locally and/or metastasize into lymphatics and lymph nodes. Cords of tumor extend into the lymphatics. This is a particularly dangerous sarcoid around the eyelids.

Differential diagnosis

SCC; subcutaneous mycosis; lymphangitis; glanders; enzootic lymphangitis; cutaneous histoplasmosis.

Diagnosis

Clinical changes to the original sarcoid are suggestive, as is invasiveness of regrowth from a previously treated sarcoid.

General management considerations

Due to the uncertain outcome, the horse owner should be made very aware of the seriousness of the problems that can arise from this disease. Treatment should involve a full discussion of treatment options, the likelihood of successful treatment, and the likelihood of prolonged or repeated treatment that, while containing the condition, may not fully resolve it.

Assesssment

An assessment should be made on the following grounds:
+ The value of the animal – actual or sentimental.
+ Previous treatment and history.
+ The cost of each avenue of treatment and the likelihood of a successful outcome to that type of treatment (i.e. repeated single local medication may eventually be much more expensive than surgical removal, radiation therapy, or cryosurgery).
+ If at all possible, the results of biopsy should be known before the final prognosis is given.
+ Likelihood of further spread of the condition if treatment is (a) not undertaken, (b) delayed, or (c) incorrect.
+ The possibility of a contagious nature of the sarcoid and the further transmission to other horses in the group.

Treatment modalities

Ligatures. Elastrator rings, lycra, or even heavy elastic bands can be used. Application is easy. This works best on single sarcoids where loose skin on the body or neck is available to allow proper placement of the ligature (i.e. skin-only pedicles).

Local medication. Moderately successful on single small sarcoids:
+ Podophyllin 50% applied daily for >30 days.
+ 10% arsenic trioxide in aqueous solution for 5 days. Causes heavy scab formation, which may be difficult to remove.
+ 5-fluorouracil cream applied under a bandage.

Vaccination or stimulation of immune system. Bovine wart vaccine has been found to be valueless. Pox vaccines injected into the actual sarcoid lesion were also unsuccessful. Autogenous vaccines have been manufactured, but results have not been good, with recovery in <25% of animals treated. Intralesional BCG therapy has been successful, particularly in eyelid lesions.

Surgery. Removal of the sarcoid, under local or general anesthetic, plus at least a 15–20 mm ring of normal tissue. Disadvantages: 50% may return; as the wound heals sarcoids may spread to other areas on the horse; removal of large areas of normal skin precludes closure and slows healing time; inability to remove this quantity of skin from limb lesions increases the risk of return.

Electrocautery. Where single small masses are involved, ordinary cautery is satisfactory, but recurrence can be expected. With large electrocautery units use a cutting current to remove the sarcoid, then treat the area, particularly the skin edges, with fulguration to desiccate the tissue.

Cryosurgery. Useful for sarcoids, but depends on a correct technique. Complications are under- or overtreatment and injury to surrounding blood vessels, nerves, bone, and tendon.

Radiation therapy. Can be either a large, distant irradiating source (teletherapy), which restricts its use to a limited number of large facilities, or treatment with implants or isotopes applied to or in the tumor (brachytherapy), which is more practical for equine treatment. SCCs, sarcoids, soft tissue sarcomas (fibrosarcoma, hemangiosarcoma, and neurofibromas), cutaneous lymphomas, and melanomas are suitable for this mode of treatment.

Advantages: less disfigurement, better therapeutic success, and as a best choice for follow-up for failed surgery, cryosurgery, or immunotherapy. Best results come from its application following debulking surgery under general anesthesia. The previous debulking leads to residual activity of dividing tumor cells, which are most susceptible to radiation, and to lowered isotope cost due to smaller treatment area.

Disadvantages: requires the presence of a specialist radiologist or radiophysicist and special secure areas for the use of hospitalized horses. Training of personnel to use care and protection around treated horses is essential. There are increased costs due to isotopes, general anesthetic, and longer hospitalization in specialized accommodation.

The isotopes strontium-90, radon-222, iodine-128, cesium-137, gold-198, and iridium-192 could be used. In practical terms, those commonly used are iridium-192 and gold-198, which are both gamma emitters. Strontium-90 is a beta particle emitter and has a limited penetration of 3 mm, so its use is restricted to treating tumors that allow very careful debulking initially or for cleaning up surface cells in conjunction with implants. When applied to the target area following surgical ablation of the tumor, strontium-90 in an applicator has been successfully used for some sarcoids and ocular SCCs.

Photodynamic therapy. The therapeutic use of the photodynamic compound hypericin has been evaluated experimentally and results suggest that it has a potential for noninvasive treatment of equine sarcoids. Intratumor injections were given every 5 days under short-acting general anesthesia. The mean dosage of hypericin was 0.7 mg/cm^3 tumor tissue. Tumors were illuminated for 30 minutes each day by a cold light source, at 1 cm distance from the surface, for a total of 25 days. An 81% reduction in tumor volume was obtained at the end of therapy, and 2 months later a 90% reduction was observed. Further experimental work is required.

Radiofrequency hyperthermia. This modality has been used in equine sarcoids and SCCs and is most successful in small tumors. Reports indicate that repeat treatments are commonly required and the method has not gained wide acceptance.

Chemotherapy. Many and varied compounds of inorganic tissue poisons have been used to treat sarcoids: podophyllin, methotrexate, 5-fluorouracil, cisplatin, mitomycin C, AW-3-LUDES cream, and, more recently, 5% imiquimod cream (Aldara 3M). All require some form of repeated administration, many on a daily basis, for as long as 30–84 days. Results from a study using AW-3-LUDES indicate that an 80% recovery rate is achievable, particularly if the drug is used as the initial treatment for the condition. Repeat treatments and previously treated unresolved lesions are likely to be less successful. Client compliance is important for higher success rates.

Electrochemotherapy. This process enhances the effectiveness of chemotherapeutic agents. All treatments are given under short-acting general anesthesia. Cisplatin in oil is injected into the lesion. After 5 minutes, two electrodes are placed over the tumor using a conductive paste, and short, intensive, electrical pulses (8 pulses 0.1 ms at 1-Hz frequency with 1.3 kV voltages) are applied to increase the permeability of the tumor cell membrane in order to achieve higher cell concentration of the injected drug. It works most satisfactorily on small tumors (<5 cm) with several successive treatments at 2-week intervals. Larger tumors (>10 cm) were found to be best treated after debulking, and were given multiple treatments simply by overlapping and shifting the electrodes. In the small number of horses treated so far, eradication has been successful with fewer than four treatments.

Prognosis
The prognosis varies from good to poor depending on the site, number, and type of lesions, plus their response to initial treatment.

NEOPLASTIC TUMORS
Basal cell carcinoma
Definition/overview
This is a rare, slow growing, well-demarcated tumor, often with an ulcerated surface, located in the neck, pectoral regions, and trunk.

Fibroma/fibrosarcoma
Definition/overview
The lesions are often single. They may be firm or soft, well-circumscribed, dermal or subcutaneous nodules, which may ulcerate or develop into a flattened verrucous-type lesion. Fibromas are benign. Fibrosarcomas may be multiple and are locally invasive.

Etiology/pathophysiology
These are uncommon tumors of the horse arising from dermal or subcutaneous fibroblasts. They usually occur in older horses.

Clinical presentation
The tumors present as dermal or subcutaneous nodules, which may ulcerate (**1233**) or develop into verrucous to cauliflower-like growths on the head, limbs, neck, and flanks. Fibroma is the most common neoplasm encountered in the horse's frog.

Differential diagnosis
Sarcoids; lymphoma; other tumors.

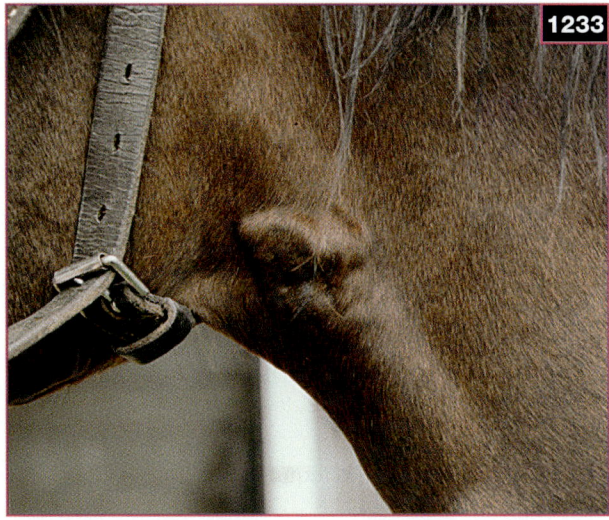

1233 Fibroma. A slow-growing, flat fibroblastic tumor on the lateral neck. Histopathology is required to confirm the diagnosis.

Diagnosis

Biopsy and histopathology are reqired for diagnosis.

Management

Total surgical excision is required. Cryotherapy is only partly successful. Radiation is more successful.

Prognosis

The prognosis is good for fibroma, but guarded for fibrosarcoma.

Hemangioma/hemangiosarcoma

Definition/overview

These are uncommon tumors of the vascular system.

Etiology/pathophysiology

They are benign or malignant neoplasms arising from the endothelial cells of blood vessels.

Clinical presentation

Numerous tortuous and enlarged blood vessels, occurring on the elbow (1234), groin, thorax, and distal limbs and which may ulcerate and bleed very easily, are observed.

Differential diagnosis

Lymphedema; other tumors.

Diagnosis

Diagnosis is based on histopathology of the lesion.

Management

Complete surgical ablation is required. This is usually best performed under general anesthetic.

Prognosis

The prognosis is fair for benign tumors, but very poor for malignant tumors.

Malignant fibrous histiocytoma

Definition/overview

This is a rare, giant-cell tumor.

Clinical presentation

Lesions are solitary, firm and poorly circumscribed. They frequently occur on the neck and proximal limbs. They are locally invasive and slow to metastasize.

Management

Radical surgical excision is required.

Prognosis

The prognosis is poor and recurrence is common due to the locally invasive nature of the tumor.

Leiomyosarcoma

Definition/overview

This is a very rare tumor arising from the smooth muscle cells of erector pili muscles or cutaneous blood vessels.

Clinical presentation

Leiomyosarcoma is an ulcerative type of tumor exhibiting moderately rapid growth (1235). The lesion is often malodorous and clinically similar to SCC.

Management

Total surgical removal is required.

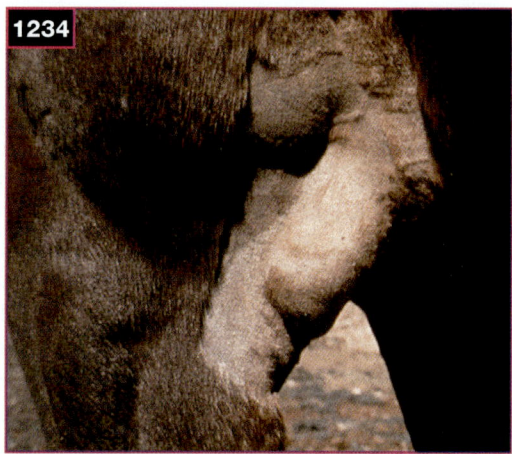

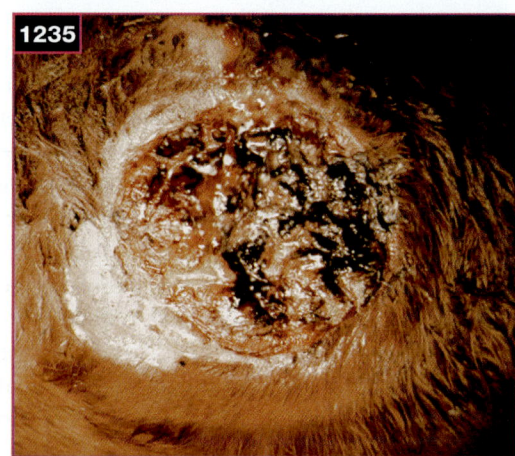

1234 Hemangioma in a 3-year-old Standardbred. A fluctuant swelling with enlarged blood vessels is seen around the elbow area.

1235 Leiomyosarcoma with moderate purulent discharge and a crust adherent to the surface of a granulating mass.

1236 Lipoma. Fatty tumors are found in many locations and can be difficult to remove because differentiation from normal fat tissue is difficult.

1237 Lymphangioma appears clinically like hemangioma, but contains lymph rather than blood. Note the enlarged vessels in the axilla region.

1238 This case of lymphoma resembles a fibroma, but has more subcutaneous spread.

1239 Lymphosarcoma in this case is manifested as multiple small nodules. (Photo courtesy DC Knottenbelt) (Reprinted from Knottenbelt DC and Pascoe RR (1994) *Colour Atlas of Diseases and Disorders of the Horse*, Mosby, with permission)

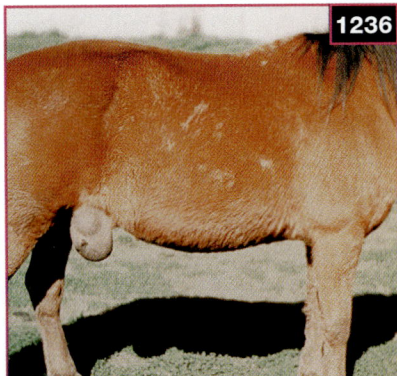

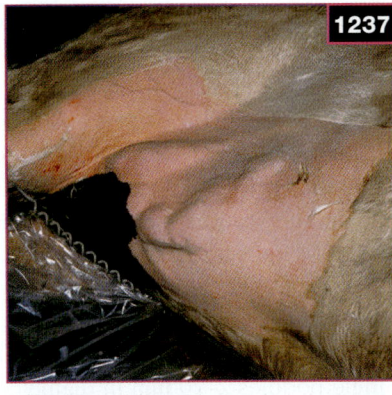

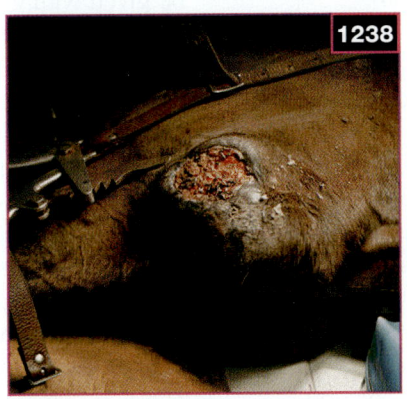

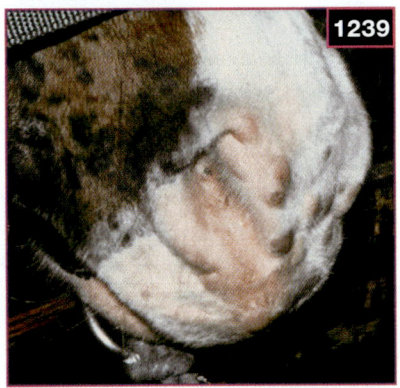

Lipoma/liposarcoma

Definition/overview
These are uncommon to rare tumors formed from subcutaneous lipoid tissue. They are usually seen in older to aged horses (1236). They also occur in the abdominal cavity, causing strangulation of the bowel and colic.

Management
Wide surgical excision is required.

Prognosis
The prognosis is very guarded for the malignant form.

Lymphangioma

Definition/overview
Lymphangioma is a rare benign tumor of lymphatic vessels (1237).

Lymphoma

Definition/overview
Lymphoma is any tumor involving the lymphoid tissue. Nonepitheliotropic or epitheliotropic lymphoma may occur. There are many variations.

Clinical presentation
Lymphoma is characterized by the presence of a depressed, ulcerated lesion with subcutaneous spread, slight discharge, and some scab formation (1238).

Management
Wide surgical removal is indicated.

Prognosis
The prognosis is guarded and size dependent.

Lymphosarcoma

Definition/overview
This tumor is infrequently seen as a skin-only neoplasm in the horse. It occurs more as a generalized thoracic or abdominal neoplasm with cutaneous lesions (1239).

Mast cell tumors/equine cutaneous mastocytoma

Definition/overview
These tumors usually present as a single cutaneous nodule characterized by a focal aggregation of mast cells and eosinophils, fibrinoid necrosis of collagen, and, occasionally, mineralization of the contents. Multiple lesions can occur and appear to be less responsive to treatment.

Clinical presentation
Male horses are more commonly affected than females. Single nodules 2–20 mm in diameter occur. The surface may be normal, hairless, or ulcerated (1240).

Differential diagnosis
Equine eosinophilic granuloma; amyloidosis.

Diagnosis
Needle biopsy, Giemsa-stained histopathology, and impression smears are used for diagnosis. Large numbers of mast cells with metachromic granules are evident.

Management
Surgical ablation is indicated. Oral cimetidine has been used as a treatment; however, results are equivocal.

Prognosis
A guarded prognosis should be given.

Melanoma/melanocytoma

Definition/overview
The nomenclature for melanotic tumors is complex. Either term describes a black-pigment tumor occurring more commonly in gray- and white-coated horses.

Etiology/pathophysiology
Melanomas are common malignant neoplasms arising from malignant proliferation of melanocytes. Melanocytomas are uncommon benign neoplasms, also arising from melanocytes.

Clinical presentation
Some families of gray horses have a higher incidence of these neoplasms. They manifest as small hard tumors in the subcutis, slowly increasing in size. They are commonly found around the anus, vulva, tail, and prepuce (1241) and less commonly in the parotid region (1242), eyelids, and lips. Melanocytomas and melanomas can occur sporadically anywhere on the body, usually as a multiple tumor, except in 'other' colored horses, where they may occur as a single tumor. They may erode through the skin and ooze black exudate. Clinically, melanocytomas are only 'depots' of melanin pigment, are noninvasive, and cause disruption by bulk. Melanomas (melanosarcomas) are rapidly invasive and often respond poorly to surgery.

Diagnosis
Melanomas are the most common tumor found in gray horses. Clinical appraisal, including location, is suggestive. Biopsy or complete removal and histopathology are diagnostic.

Management
Individual tumors on other than gray horses can be surgically removed. A slightly more cautious prognosis should be given with gray horses, even though the majority of 'black' lumps are benign. Wide surgical excision, cryotherapy, biologic response modifiers, and chemotherapy are the modalities that give the most successful response. Small or single tumors (<3 cm diameter) are usually more successfully treated by wide surgical excision or cryotherapy. Surgical excision alone in some horses can cause rapid tumor regrowth by stimulation of abnormal melanoblasts in the proximity of the surgical site. Other horses are reported to develop large sheets of melanotic tumor tissue from merging or coalescence of numerous smaller tumors (e.g. around the tail, anus, and vulva). These are more suitable for cryonecrosis with a double freeze–thaw cycle, especially those tumors that are inaccessible to total surgery (e.g. anal sphincter area). The tumor is debulked and the remaining inaccessible area treated by cryotherapy. This rarely 'cures' the problem, but it allows a further useful life span for the treated horse.

The role of histamine (H2) and the growth of tumors may be related to activation of T suppressor cells. Cimetidine is a potent H2 blocker that has been used in the treatment of melanoma, with variable results. Its successful use may be related to active growth, but where growth has been minimal or static, the response can be very poor. The normal response is a slowing of growth. If after 3 months' treatment there is either minimal or no cessation of growth, then there is no benefit from further treatment. The dosage is 2.5 mg/kg q8h; alternatively, the daily dose of 7.5 mg/kg can be given as a single dose or divided into two doses (less satisfactory). A response is indicated by a slow decline down to 50% of pretreatment size occurring during the first 6 weeks of treatment. The progression of the tumor may be halted for months to years following cessation of treatment.

The use of chemotherapy in the trreatment of melanomas has been restricted to cisplatin. Tumors >3 cm should be debulked and cisplatin injected into the base of the tumor at the rate of 1 mg/cm^3 of tissue every second week for four treatments. The drug is an irritant and the use of 22–25 gauge needles is advisable to stop back leakage following injection. The drug is injected as the

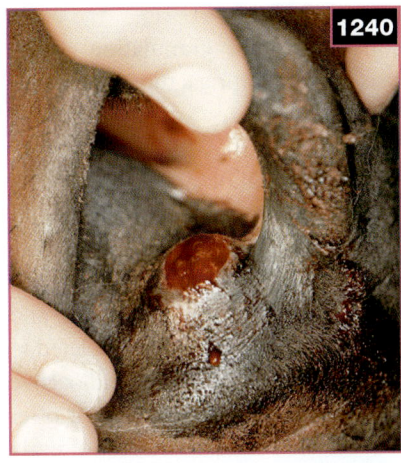

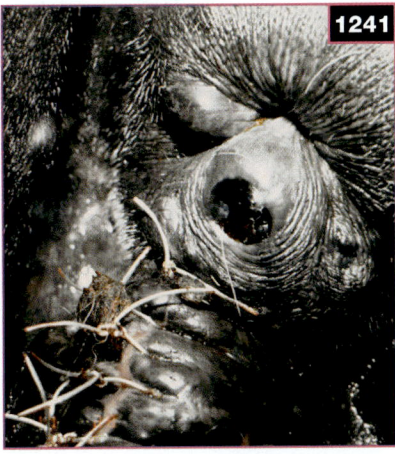

1240 Mastocytoma. There is an ulcerated lesion in the ventral nares of this horse.

1241 Melanocytoma with benign nodules around the anus and vulva exuding melanin.

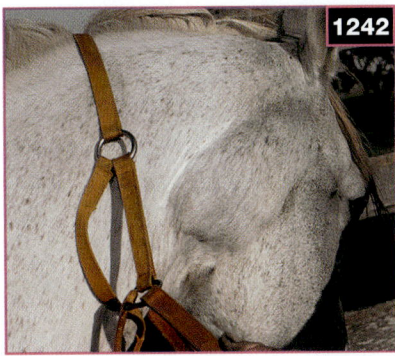

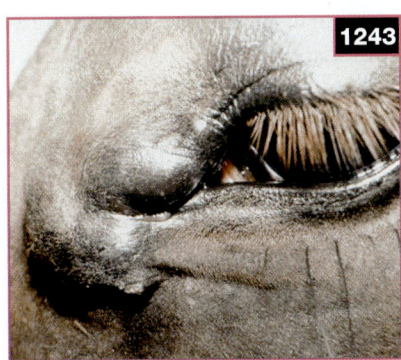

1242 Melanoma (melanosarcoma) in a 12-year-old Welsh Mountain pony with a malignant tumor in the right parotid gland area that was inoperable.

1243 Neurofibroma is most commonly found on the upper and lower eyelids as small hard subcutaneous nodules, with hairless areas around the tumor similar to sarcoid.

needle is withdrawn in order to fill the needle track. Injection sites should be spaced 5–8 mm apart, as diffusion of the drug is limited. Post-treatment therapy to minimize postinjection swelling includes the use of penicillin or potentiated sulfur drugs, plus an anti-inflammatory such as phenylbutazone. This treatment has been used on stallions and pregnant brood mares without ill effects. Recurrence in unsuccessful cases is seen 7–8 months following therapy; repeat treatment may be used following the same procedure used in the initial treatment. Cisplatin has to be freshly prepared and when reconstituted is only stable at room temperature for approximately 15 hours.

Prognosis
The prognosis is guarded.

Neurofibroma (schwannoma)
Definition/overview
Neurofibroma is a tumor of peripheral nerves. They may occur anywhere associated with nerve sheath tissue, but predominantly in the upper and lower eyelids (**1243**).

Etiology/pathophysiology
Dermal or subcutaneous Schwann cells are involved. The cause of the neoplastic change is unknown.

Clinical presentation
Small (1–10 mm), hard, subcutaneous nodules are present. Multiple nodules may be observed. Growth of the nodules causes erosion through the overlying skin, allowing development into a fibroblastic-type lesion. Hair loss is rare until ulceration occurs.

Differential diagnosis
Sarcoid.

Diagnosis
Surgical removal and histopathology are diagnostic. Depending on the pathologist, the tumor may be diagnosed as a neurofibroma or a sarcoid. A neurofibroma is clinically a distinct lesion and has a different clinical appearance to sarcoids located around the eyelids.

Management
Complete surgical removal is required. Tumors recur at a different site in the eyelid in approximately 25–50% of all operated cases. Injection of tumor with BCG (1–4 injections, 28 days apart) has shown some success.

Prognosis
The prognosis is guarded. The tumors are persistent, but multiple surgeries will prolong useful life.

Squamous cell carcinoma

Definition/overview

This is a common invasive tumor of the skin, sinuses, and GI and reproductive tracts.

Etiology/pathophysiology

SCC is a malignant tumor arising from keratinocytes. Skin exposed to actinic (solar) radiation due to increasing altitude, decreased skin pigmentation, and sparse haircoat is frequently involved. The irritant nature of equine smegma is implicated in male genital SCC (1244). Irritation due to these factors may be a trigger for accelerated growth.

Clinical presentation

SCC is characterized by a small granulating sore that may be depressed below skin level, eroding into normal tissue. There is often malodor even with early lesions. On the penis and prepuce they may vary from cauliflower-like to erosive. On the vulva and anus they are often slow growing. On the eye and eyelid they often start as white, raised plaques at the edge of the lid or corneal/scleral junction, and may progress rapidly to granulomatous and ulcerated lesions. Around the nose and mouth they appear as a depressed ulcer that progresses to a granulomatous and malodorous growth/erosion (1245, 1246).

Differential diagnosis

Sarcoids; other tumors; exuberant granulation tissue; habronemiasis; pythiosis and other fungal tumors.

Diagnosis

Total excisional biopsy for histopathologic examination is indicated.

Management

Wide surgical excision, cryotherapy, irradiation, and chemotherapy are used with degrees of success related to the invasiveness and accessibility of the tumor. Radioactive implants with gold-198, cobalt-90, or iridium-192 offer increased chances of survival. Surgical removal of early tumors is more successful, with complete remission in most cases (1247). Where wide excision can be performed, results are equally good (e.g. amputation of the tail, enucleation of the eye, complete removal of the eyelids, or amputation of the penis). Surgical removal of long-standing invasive tumors on the eyelids, prepuce, mouth, and, to a lesser extent, the vulva in mares is less successful.

Prognosis

A guarded prognosis should be given.

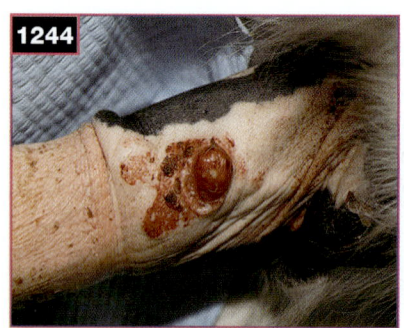

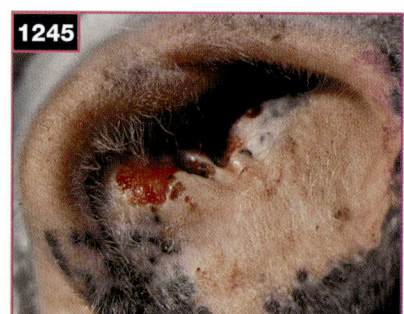

1244 Squamous cell carcinoma of the prepuce. This depigmented skin tumor was moveable with preputial skin and was completely removed surgically.

1245 Squamous cell carcinoma at the mucocutaneous junction of the nose.

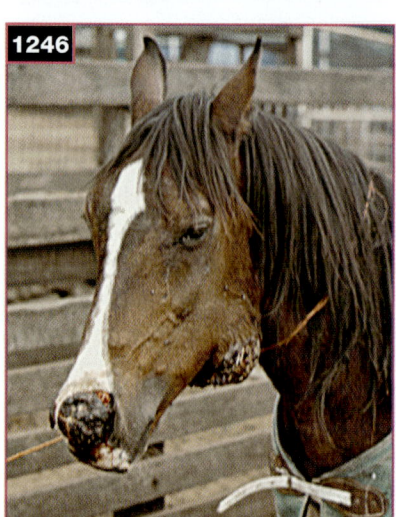

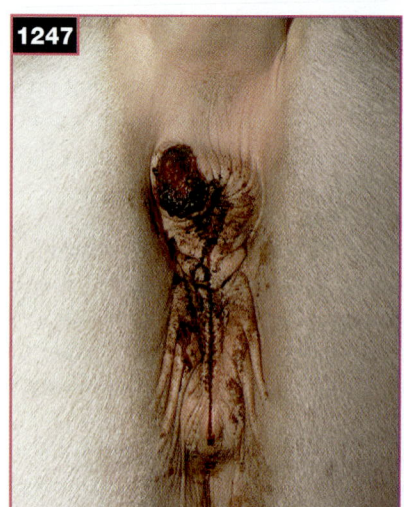

1246 Squamous cell carcinoma with metastatic spread to the jowl area from the nose of a 25-year-old Arabian stallion. The horse was euthanized.

1247 A tumor involving the anal sphincter in an 8-year-old Piebald pony that was surgically removed. There was no return in 3 years. Histopathology was required to confirm diagnosis of a slow-growing squamous cell carcinoma. (Reprinted from Pascoe RR and Knottenbelt DC (1999) *Manual of Equine Dermatology*, WB Saunders, with permission)

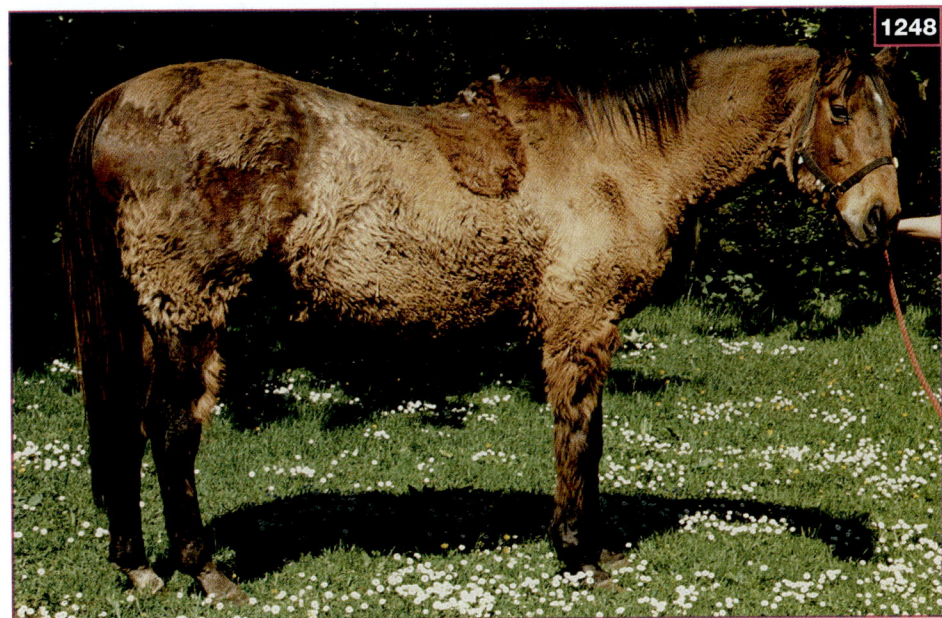

1248 Equine Cushing's disease. Note the very long haircoat. The tail and mane are unaffected. (Photo courtesy GA Munroe)

Sebaceous gland tumors

Definition/overview
These are quite rare tumors arising from sebaceous gland cells. They occur in adult to aged horses, are solitary, and vary from nodules to alopecic lobulated growths. They may occur anywhere. Treatment involves surgical excision or cryotherapy.

Sweat gland tumor

Definition/overview
Sweat gland tumor is an uncommon tumor of the apocrine sweat glands. They occur in older horses and, most commonly, around the ears and vulva. They present as single, firm to cystic, dermal nodules that are usually benign and resemble sarcoids. Complete surgical ablation is the treatment of choice. The prognosis can be good, but is related to size, rate of growth, and accessibility.

Equine Cushing's syndrome

Definition/overview
Equine pituitary adenomas of the pars intermedia clinically display signs of hirsutism due to a failure to shed body coat hair or rapid regrowth of longer than normal hair (8–10 cm long) (**1248**). The mane and tail are not affected. (See also p. 632.)

Immune-mediated skin diseases

Introduction
Inflammatory changes occur in the skin when it is injured. These changes are initially related to the inciting cause and, secondarily, may relate to autologous changes that follow the initial injury. Protection of the host is by means of a structured immune response. In a normal response this action is to restore normal body function, but under- or overactivity often leads to serious problems for the host. Under-response leads to infection and poor elimination of toxic by-products. Over-response gives an overabundant inflammatory response that may result in the production of autoimmune disease. Both these responses adversely affect the skin.

Apart from insect hypersensitivity and urticaria, immune-mediated diseases in the horse are uncommon to rare and their diagnosis may be aided by elimination of all the other more common causes of crusting and scaling. A very careful examination of the horse's history, a series of careful biopsies of recent lesions, and choice of a veterinary dermatopathologist are paramount to the success of reaching a diagnosis.

Contact hypersensitivity

Definition/overview
Contact hypersensitivity is a rare and poorly documented problem associated with skin contact with allergens, leading to a variable degree of pruritus and maculopapular or lichenified dermatitis.

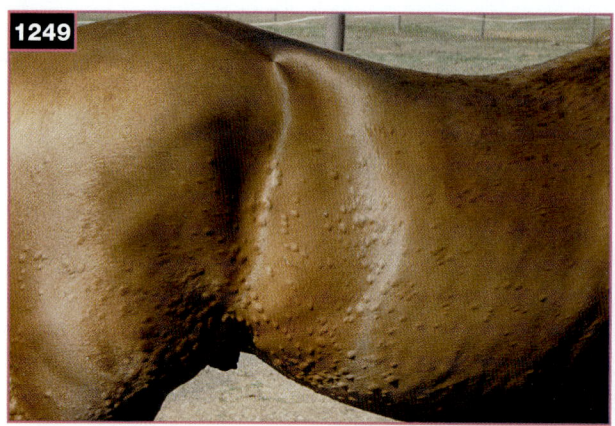

1249 Drug eruption in a 5-year-old Thoroughbred mare caused immediately by intravenous injection of pethidine and acepromazine.

Drug eruption

Definition/overview
Drugs, given by any route, including most antibiotics and many vaccines, may cause skin eruptions.

Etiology/pathophysiology
A type 4 hypersensitivity reaction develops. It can be immediate or delayed for weeks or even months after the administration of the causal drug.

Clinical presentation
A nonspecific skin eruption occurs. It may mimic urticaria, with papules, vesicles, and generalized pruritus (1249). Reactions can occur a long time after cessation of administration of the original drug.

Diagnosis
Diagnosis is very difficult unless the onset is acute. Presumptive evidence is if drugs are withdrawn and the signs disappear, then reappear with reintroduction of the suspect drug.

Management
Suspected drugs should be discontinued. If a severe reaction occurs, systemic glucocorticoids may be administered, but the response may be poor.

Prognosis
The prognosis is guarded.

1251 Equine cutaneous lupus erythematosus was diagnosed in this gray, 12-year-old, Arabian stallion with depigmentation in areas of the neck, flank, and tail. Depigmentation of skin under the tail was very clear.

Equine cutaneous lupus erythematosus

Definition/overview
Equine cutaneous lupus erythematosus (CLE) is a rare, incompletely defined, clinicopathologic entity found in the horse and differing in many instances from the classic forms seen in humans and dogs (1250).

Etiology/pathophysiology
CLE is an autoimmune disease. The pathogenesis is multifactorial.

Clinical presentation
There is a sharp demarcation between pigmented and depigmented areas. Depigmentation is seen around the eyes, lips, nostrils, vulva, anal ring, and prepuce (1251, 1252). Loss of pigment can be gradual or rapid. Erythema and scaling with alopecia occur, causing the skin of long-standing cases to look like wrinkled leather. The horse may show photosensitivity, weight loss, and fever. Occasionally, there are signs of systemic disease in the more severe CLE-type cases.

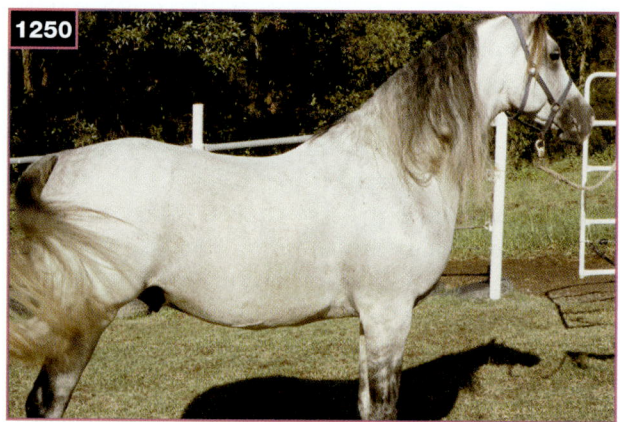

1250 Equine cutaneous lupus erythematosus.

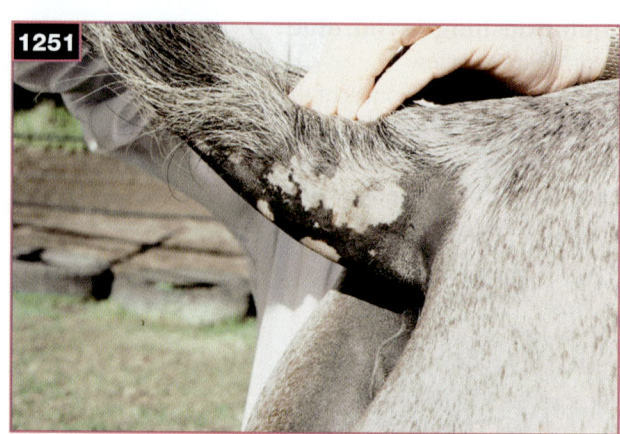

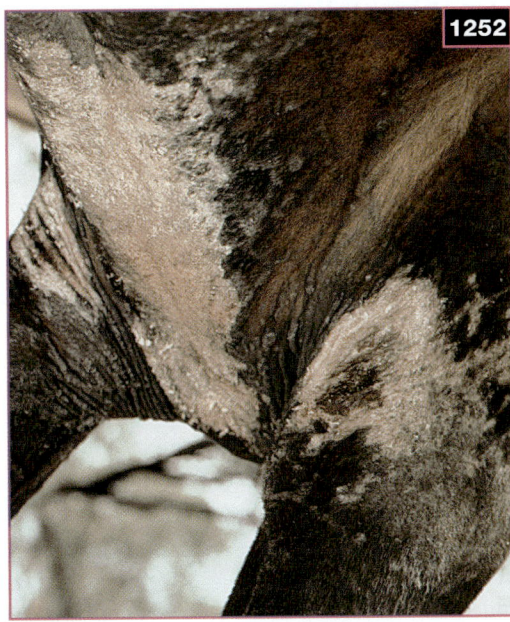

1252 Systemic lupus erythematosus in a 16-year-old stock horse that had severe exfoliation of the body, neck, and head, with marked depigmentation of the elbow area. Autopsy revealed a chronic pleuritis and abscessation on the left lateral chest wall.

Diagnosis
Skin biopsy is used for diagnosis. Specimens should be placed in formalin for conventional histopathology and Michel's medium for immunofluorescence studies. Serum for an ANA test and quantification of IgM and/or IgG may also be used.

Differential diagnosis
All other depigmentation diseases; Arabian fading syndrome; Appaloosa parentage; equine granulomatous enteritis; leukoderma.

Management
CLE is not usually successfully treated and therefore treatment is not indicated. Equine CLE may regress and recur over periods of time.

Prognosis
The prognosis is guarded to poor.

1253 Equine alopecia areata in a 13-year-old gray Arabian mare with patchy alopecia of 5 years' duration. Biopsy revealed only very small numbers of lymphocytic bulbitis in hair follicles.

Equine alopecia areata
Definition/overview
This is a cell-mediated 'autoimmune' skin disease. The condition is rare, but increased awareness of its manifestation may increase its reported incidence. Widespread alopecia areata is also named alopecia universalis.

Etiology/pathophysiology
T lymphocytes attack the hair matrix and root sheath. Early diseased hair follicles may show defective keratinization. In chronic cases, inflammation may be minimal and a section may only show small telogen follicles lacking hair. There is a possible hereditary factor, because 20% of reported cases are familial.

Clinical presentation
Diffuse thinning of the mane and tail and the presence of one or more reasonably circumscribed areas of partial to complete alopecia are observed (1253). Onset is slow to very rapid. Areas can coalesce to produce extensive alopecia without pruritus. There are no visible signs of inflammation. Spotted leukotrichia may be associated with hair loss in an affected area. Defective hoof growth may occur. Spontaneous remission has been recorded.

Differential diagnosis
Dermatophytosis; dermatophilosis; occult sarcoid.

Diagnosis
Nonspecific alopecia is present, with mane and tail dystrophy. Biopsy should be performed for histopathology.

Management
None.

Prognosis
The likelihood of complete and permanent remission is poor.

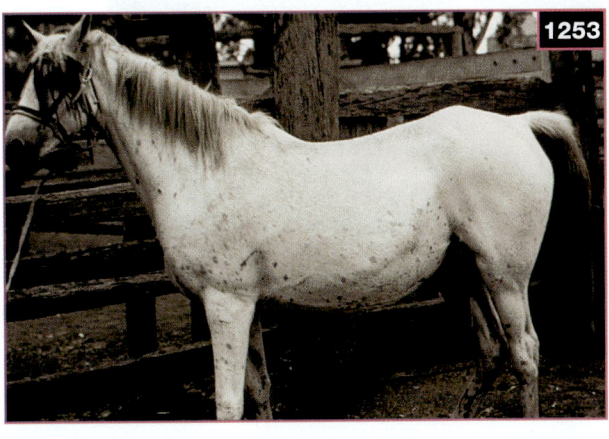

Equine linear keratosis (equine linear alopecia)

Definition/overview

This is an idiopathic, possibly inherited, dermatosis characterized by unilateral, linear, vertical bands of hyperkeratosis on the neck, thorax, and upper hindlimbs (1254).

Etiology/pathophysiology

Equine linear keratosis is an uncommon to rare, possibly inherited, dermatosis of unclear pathogenesis.

Clinical presentation

The condition occurs at between 1 and 5 years of age and is seen most commonly in Quarter horses. One or more vertically arranged bands of alopecia and hyperkeratotic papules and plaques associated with scaling/crusting are present. There is no pruritus or pain.

Differential diagnosis

Chronic hyperkeratosis from irritant drugs; dermatophilosis.

Diagnosis

Biopsy should be performed for histopathology. The primary change is a lymphocytic mural folliculitis.

Management

No treatments are satisfactory. Use of a keratolytic agent, such as 5% salicylic acid ointment, reduces the amount of hyperkeratosis. Remission ceases when treatment stops.

Prognosis

A poor prgnosis should be given.

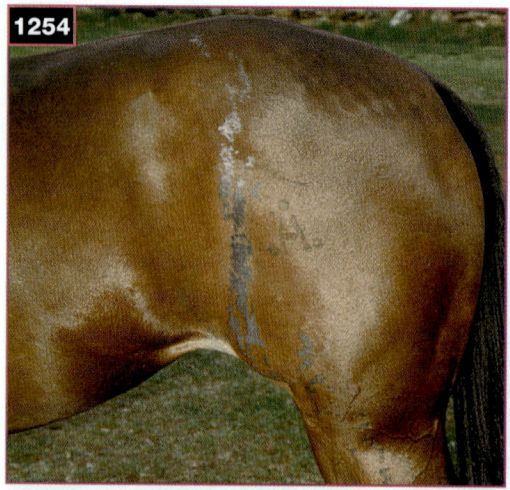

1254 Equine linear keratosis shows as vertical linear bands of hyperkeratosis.

Equine pemphigus foliaceus

Definition/overview

Pemphigus foliaceus is an autoimmune disease characterized by an exfoliative dermatitis. It is a scaling disease with the formation of heavy crusts (1255, 1256). Appaloosas may be predisposed.

Etiology/pathophysiology

A type 2 hypersensitivity is the cause.

Clinical presentation

Early cases show transient vesicles, erosion, epidermal collarettes, crusting, scaling, fever, depression, weight loss, coronary band lesions, variable pruritus, and pain. Advanced cases show severe crusting and scaling, alopecia, and poor appetite.

Differential diagnosis

Dermatophilosis; dermatophytosis; onchocerciasis; *Culicoides* dermatitis; equine granulomatous enteritis; equine viral papular dermatitis; equine sarcoidosis; epitheliogenesis imperfecta; junctional mechanobullous disease; coronary band dystrophy; seborrhea; generalized skin eruptions of unknown etiology; *Malassezia* spp. dermatitis; yeast dermatitis.

Diagnosis

History and clinical appearance are suggestive. Direct smears should be taken from intact vesicles or pustules. Multiple biopsies should be taken from multiple sites, which must always include a surface scab. The skin should not be wiped or shaved prior to biopsy. Histopathology should be performed. Direct immunofluorescence testing shows intracellular deposits of immunoglobulin in the epidermis. Perilesional skin should be sampled if vesicles or pustules are not present.

Management

High immunosuppressive doses of corticosteroids are indicated (prednisolone, 2–4 mg/kg q12h for several weeks). Attempts should then be made to change to alternate-day therapy. Treatment should be continued for the rest of the animal's life. Consideration should be given to using gold injections if there is a lack of response to corticosteroids.

Prognosis

The prognosis is very poor and recovery is rare.

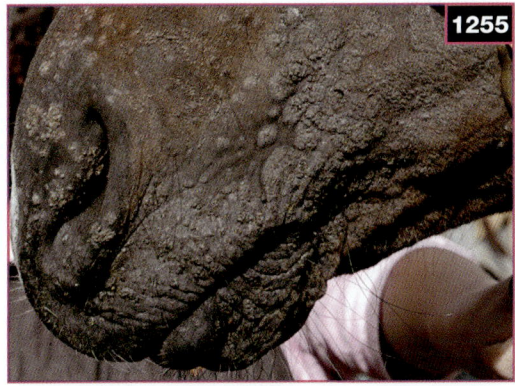

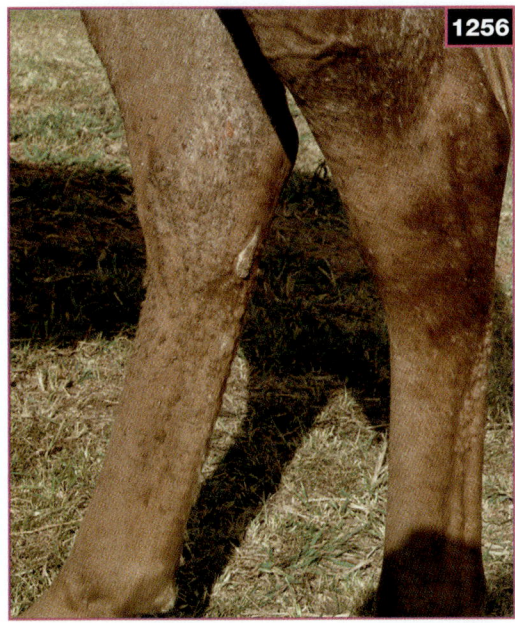

Equine pemphigus vulgaris and bullous pemphigoid
Definition/overview
These vesicobullous ulcerative diseases are extremely rare conditions in the horse. They affect the oral cavity (1257), mucocutaneous junction, or skin, or a combination of all three. They resemble type-2 hypersensitivity.

Equine sarcoidosis
Definition/overview
This is a rare systemic granulomatous disease exhibiting exfoliative dermatitis (1258), severe wasting with weight loss, poor appetite, persistent low-grade fever, and exercise intolerance. There may be sarcoidal granulomatous infection of multiple organ systems. There are no age, breed, or sex predilections.

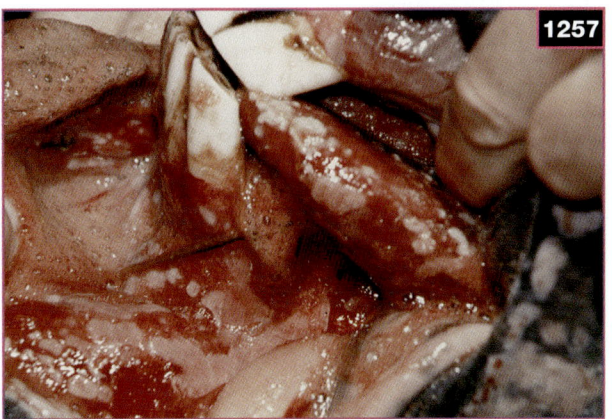

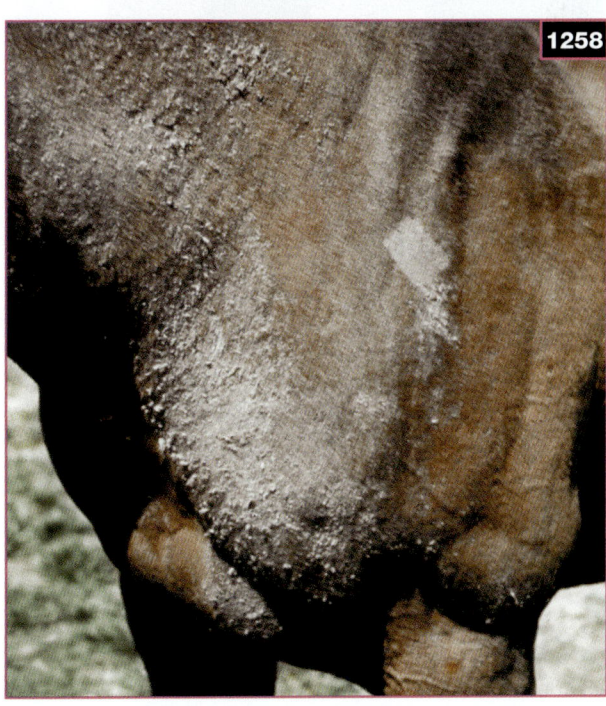

1255 Equine pemphigus foliaceus with scabs and scale on the muzzle and face.

1256 Equine pemphigus foliaceus lesion resembling dermatophilus infection on the thigh and cannon bone.

1257 Bullous pemphigoid erosion in the mouth. (Photo courtesy DW Scott)

1258 Equine sarcoidosis in a 7-year-old gelding with chronic wasting disease, marked exfoliative dermatitis, and heavy scurf on the shoulder and neck. (Photo courtesy JR Vasey)

Erythema multiforme

Definition/overview

Erythema multiforme is a rare, acute, self-limiting, urticarial, maculopapular or vesicobullous dermatosis. There are triggering influences such as drugs, infections (especially herpesvirus), and tumors (especially lymphoreticular neoplasms). Many cases are classified as idiopathic. Characteristic 'donut-like' skin urticarial lesions develop rapidly from the initial urticaria and plaques (**1259**).

Urticaria

Definition/overview

Horses show the greatest incidence of urticaria of all the species of domestic animals. Urticaria is a specific skin lesion rather than a specific disease entity. It has many different etiologies and pathogeneses. Generally, it is discussed as a single entity even though its clinical manifestations vary from a minor transitory nature to major, systemic, life-endangering problems.

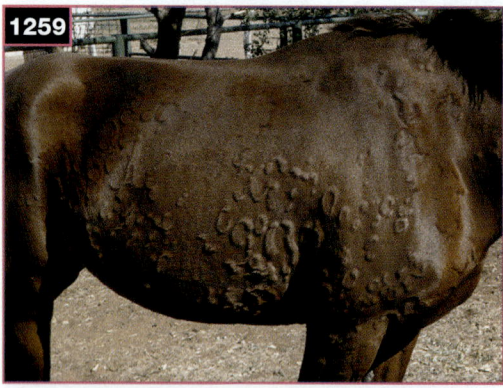

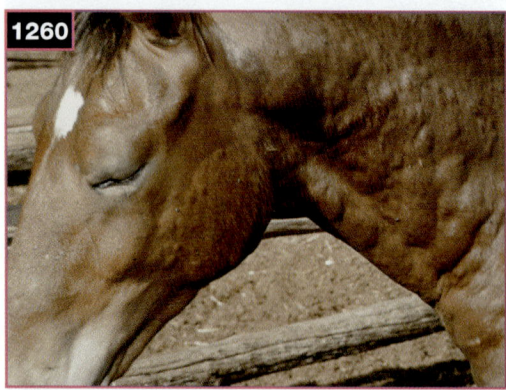

1259 Erythema multiforme. Characteristic donut-like lesions of urticarial-type swelling.

1260 Urticarial lesions of 2–5 mm diameter spread all over the body due to a change of feed. They disappeared in 48 hours.

Etiology/pathophysiology

Many causes of urticaria have been suggested:

✦ Degranulation of mast cells and basophils is presumed to be the basic pathogenesis. Liberation of chemical mediators, which cause increased vascular permeability, leads to wheal formation.

✦ *Immunologic.* Hypersensitivity where antigen/allergen probably reaches the skin via the systemic route rather than by local contact (i.e. via injection [drugs], ingestion [chemical, feeds], or inhalation [pollen, dust, chemicals, molds]).

✦ *Allergic urticaria.* Drug related, food allergy, inhaled antigens, pollens, molds, contact allergy (very rare). Must be carefully distinguished from allergic contact dermatitis.

✦ *Physical urticaria.* Nonimmunologic pathogenesis.
  ◇ Dermatographism: wheal developing from blunt scratch on skin.
  ◇ Urticaria due to cold, heat, or light.
  ◇ Exercise-induced urticaria.

Clinical presentation

The onset of the condition can be acute to peracute, with signs developing within minutes up to a few hours. An edematous lesion of the skin or mucous membrane develops, called a wheal. This is a flat-topped papule/nodule with steep walled sides, which pits on pressure. Some have slightly depressed centers. Wheals vary in size and shape and may be divided into:

✦ *Conventional.* 2–3 mm up to 3–5 mm (**1260**).

✦ *Papular.* Multiple small, uniform, 3–6 mm diameter wheals (e.g. insect bites).

✦ *Giant.* Either single or coalesced multiple wheals up to 20–30 cm diameter.

✦ *Annular.* Donut-like lesions.

The lesion may present differently depending on the location of the edema (e.g. whether it is in the upper layers of the dermis or subcutaneous tissue):

✦ *'Oozing' urticaria.* Where dermal edema is severe, oozing of serum from the skin surface may occur. Care should be taken to distinguish this from an erosive/ulcerative process or pyoderma. The lesion must still pit on pressure.

✦ *Gyrate urticaria.* This syndrome has been referred to as the dermal form of erythema multiforme, but it should be stressed that it is not related to 'true' erythema multiforme, which is primarily an epidermal disease. Drug reactions appear to be the most common cause of this form of urticaria.

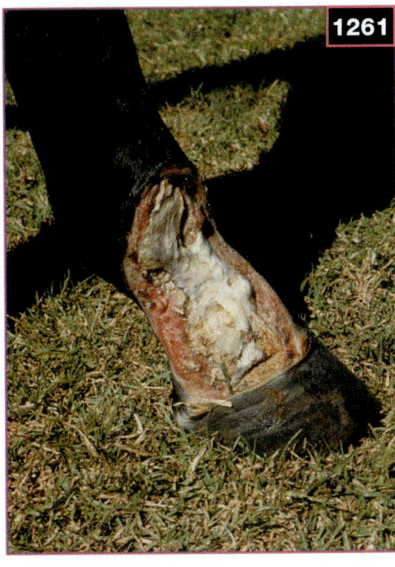

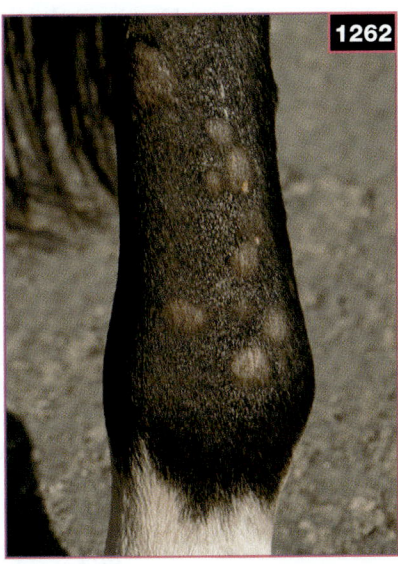

1261 Vasculitis following *S. equi* vaccination during a severe outbreak of strangles on a Standardbred farm. This yearling had lesions on all four pasterns and fetlocks.

1262 Leukocytoclastic vasculitis in a mature horse, with swelling on the black areas of the limbs. The cause was undetermined.

◆ **Angioedema** (angioneurotic edema). A subcutaneous form of urticaria that tends to be more diffuse due to lack of restraint against spread in the subcutis. It usually involves the head and extremities and is more indicative of a systemic and serious disease than urticaria. Pruritus may or may not be present.

Diagnosis

Initially, diagnosis is mostly based on clinical signs and history. Biopsy is often unrewarding or even misleading. The presence of dermatographism should be evaluated by a coarse instrument scratch, which shows a wheal in <15 minutes. For a 'cold' urticaria test, an ice cube should be applied to the skin, with development of edema within 15 minutes indicating a positive response. Inhaled antigen testing can be performed using a specific ELISA or RAST. Food allergy can only be traced by elimination diets and then challenge with suspected feed.

Differential diagnosis

Insect bites (*Stomoxys* spp. and *Culicoides* spp.); mosquito bites; bee and wasp stings; cellulitis and possibly vasculitis; purpura hemorrhagica; erythema multiforme; hematoma; lymphangitis.

Management

Initial therapy typically consists of a short course of systemic corticosteroids. Treatment can be repeated if signs recur. If urticaria is still present after 8 weeks (persistent urticaria), hyposensitization can be considered, following evaluation with a skin test for ectopic disease (IgE) or a specific ELISA or RAST for IgE. Long-term use of corticosteroids and/or antihistamines may be required in some situations. Oral administration of prednisolone at the lowest possible dose on an alternate-day basis or oral antihistamine hydroxyzine hydrochloride (1–2 mg/kg q8–12h) are options. Improvement may occur in 3–4 days, but if improvement is not seen within 2 weeks, other medication should be investigated.

Vasculitis

Definition/overview

Vasculitis is an uncommon disorder characterized by purpura, edema, necrosis, and ulceration of the lower limbs and oral mucosa.

Etiology/pathophysiology

Types 1 and 3 hypersensitivity reactions can cause vasculitis.

Clinical presentation

Vasculitis is often associated with *Streptococcus equi* and can occur 2–4 weeks after infection. The most common site is on the coronet, pastern, and fetlock (**1261**) and the lips and periorbital tissues. Edema, erythema, necrosis, and ulceration are seen. Pyrexia, depression, anorexia, and weight loss may also be present. There is no pruritus or pain, except in early scabs. Chronic or recurrent infection can develop.

Differential diagnosis

Equine granulomatous enteritis; equine leukocytoclastic vasculitis (**1262**); greasy heel.

Diagnosis

Clinical appearance is suggestive. Biopsy is used for confirmation. Diagnostic biopsies are best taken in the first 24 hours of a fresh lesion occurring.

Management

If possible, the underlying disease should be treated. Provided the diagnosis is very rapid, oral prednisolone (1–2 mg/kg) should be given twice daily until regression occurs, and then reduced to the lowest possible alternate-morning dose.

Prognosis

The prognosis is guarded.

Disorders of pigmentation

Introduction

Melanocytes in the epidermis and hair bulbs are frequently affected independently of each other. Leukoderma is where the epidermal melanocytes are affected and the skin loses pigment. Leukotrichia, or white hairs, is where pigment is lost from the hair bulb. The independent relationship between hair and skin is easily demonstrated by shaving the area and noting the discrepancy between the original white hairs and the now revealed white skin area. As more than one factor may be involved in the production of leukoderma and leukotrichia, consideration must be given to the effects of trauma, inflammation, heredity, autonomic nerve system defects, and immunologic response. Loss of pigment, loss of haircoat color, and changes in coat color are of concern and the following conditions exhibit some of these characteristics. Most can be diagnosed, but are unable to be treated.

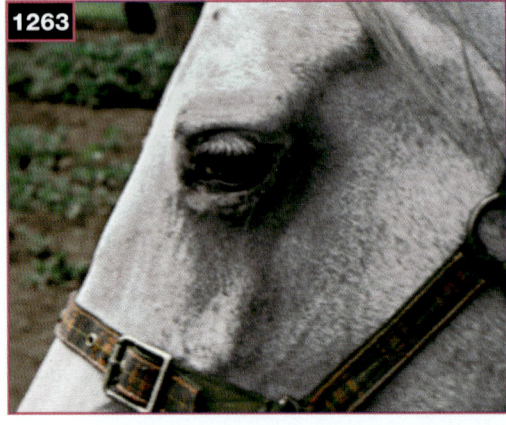

1263 Leukoderma (acquired vitiligo) that occurred in a 12-year-old mare following severe streptococcal infection of the mouth and eye region.

Hyperesthetic leukotrichia

Definition/overview

This is a rare disease characterized by the presence of single to multiple crusts along the back line of yearlings. The Quarter horse, Thoroughbred, and Standardbred breeds appear to be predisposed, suggesting a genetic cause. Examination of lesions evokes a pain response. Lesions remain for 1–3 months and then regress, followed by permanent white markings. There is no treatment.

Leukoderma (acquired vitiligo)

Definition/overview

Loss of pigment in the hair and skin can be related to various factors such as pressure sores, cryosurgery, and surgery.

Etiology/pathophysiology

Leukoderma is a complication of many different diseases that destroy melanocytes, or that inhibit or change melanogenesis.

Clinical presentation

White patches of hair and skin in irregular shapes may develop following surgery, X-ray radiation, cryosurgery, contact with irritants such as harness or rubber bits, or infection (**1263**).

Differential diagnosis

Equine coital exanthema; Arabian fading syndrome; equine SLE; leukotrichia; Appaloosa parentage.

Diagnosis

Histopathology of biopsies from affected areas reveals lack of melanocytes.

Management

None known.

Prognosis

The pigment change is permanent.

Leukotrichia (tiger stripe, variegated leukotrichia, reticulated leukotrichia)

Definition/overview

Leukotrichia is characterized by dorsal, bilateral, reticulated, white hair striping (**1264**). It may develop in yearlings, but is often seen in older horses with unknown earlier history. It has been suggested that leukotrichia could be a form of erythema multiforme.

Etiology/pathophysiology

Some breed predisposition is apparent, indicating that genetic factors may be involved. Mainly Standardbred and Quarter horses are affected.

1264 Leukotrichia in the back line of a 6-year-old Standardbred mare. The white markings appeared at 2 years of age.

1265 Vitiligo depigmentation on the chest and neck of a 5-year-old Thoroughbred gelding. The numbers had increased, but not the size, since it was a yearling.

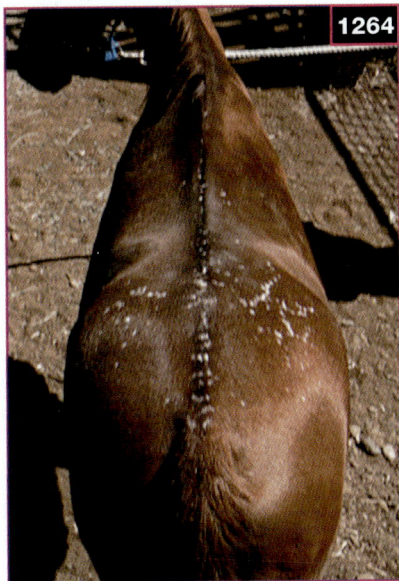 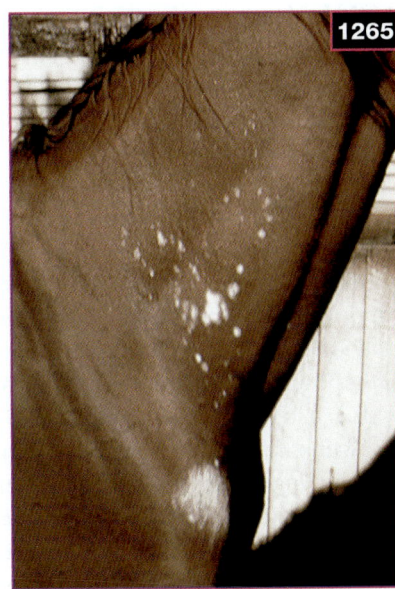

Clinical presentation
Linear dorsal crusts are arranged in a cross-hatched pattern. Temporary alopecia is present following shedding of crusts. New hair is white, but the skin remains with its original pigmentation.

Differential diagnosis
Leukoderma; vitiligo.

Diagnosis
Clinical history and examination should be performed to eliminate any other causes such as equine SLE. The possibility of a drug- or vaccine-related trigger mechanism should be evaluated.

Management
There are no known treatments.

Prognosis
The pigment change is permanent.

Vitiligo (Arabian fading syndrome)
Definition/overview
The condition appears more often in Arabians and is characterized by the presence of annular areas of macular depigmentation of the muzzle, lips, around the eyes, and occasionally around the perineum, sheath, and hooves. It can occur at any age, but is usually found in horses over 4 years of age. Occasional body patches of depigmentation have also been observed in Welsh Mountain ponies, but rarely in Thoroughbred horses. Variations show depigmentation spots appearing all over the skin.

Etiology/pathophysiology
Vitiligo is idiopathic or due to primary damage to melanocytes. It is an acquired, possibly genetically programmed, depigmentation.

Clinical presentation
Depigmented circular spots up to 1 cm diameter, which increase in number rather than size, are present (**1265**). Occasional white patches and leukoderma depigmentation may be evident. The condition may wax and wane in intensity, but is usually permanent. Alopecia occasionally occurs around the eyes.

Differential diagnosis
Copper deficiency; equine CLE; leukoderma; Appaloosa parentage.

Diagnosis
Clinical appearance and absence of injury are suggestive. Wetting the horse with water allows depigmentation to become more obvious. History may indicate Arabian or Welsh Mountain pony heritage. Leukoderma may not be synchronized with the area of associated leukotrichia. Skin biopsy can assist diagnosis.

Management
There is no reliably effective treatment. Some affected horses seem to be under stress. The use of reserpine has resulted in regression in some horses.

Prognosis
Partial spontaneous recovery has been reported, but is uncommon. The number of spots may increase over time.

Actinic dermatosis

Definition/overview
This condition is caused by UV radiation and facilitated by lack of pigment and hair. It may be acute or chronic.

Etiology/pathophysiology
Actinic dermatosis falls into two categories: (1) sunburn (excessive exposure) with expected outcome; and (2) normal exposure with unexpected outcome (photosensitization). Photosensitization is related to three factors: (1) the presence of a photodynamic agent within the skin; (2) exposure to sunlight or certain wavelengths of UV light; and (3) cutaneous absorption of this UV light.

Actinic dermatosis may be a systemic condition due to primary ingestion of a photodynamic agent from the digestive tract (e.g. 'St John's Wort' [*Hypericum perforatum*] and other plant species), with transfer into the skin via the circulation, or it may be hepatogenous due to phylloerythrin accumulating in animal tissues as a photodynamic agent.

Clinical presentation
A cutaneous lesion, usually restricted to light skin or hairless areas, is apparent. Severe cases extend into dark-skinned areas or areas well-covered in hairs. It commonly affects the lips, face, eyelids, perineum, and coronary band region. Conjunctivitis, edema, erythema, pruritus, pain, oozing, necrosis, and sloughing of skin are common.

Differential diagnosis
Dermatophilosis; dermatophytosis; greasy heel.

Diagnosis
Liver function tests should be performed. Any history of pasture grazing, treatment, and diet should be investigated. Lesions due to pasture plants, sprays, or drugs may be localized to the lip and lower limb. Plants can be tested for pyrrolizidine alkaloids. Biopsy reveals nonspecific histopathologic changes.

Management
The horse should be protected from direct sunlight by stabling, hoods, rugs, or other means. Emollient creams can be applied. Sources of photodynamic agents should be eliminated. Supportive therapy for hepatic disease should be provided if needed. Glucocorticoids and NSAIDs may be of assistance in reducing inflammation.

Prognosis
Most affected animals recover, but severe cases may have residual skin scarring.

Diseases of the pastern and coronet

Introduction
Diseases of this area may be related or linked to disease processes elsewhere in the horse, or they may be confined to the coronet and pastern alone. This part of the horse's limb is subjected to changeable environmental conditions and has diseases that are difficult to identify positively and treat. Some are found as part of a general disease pattern (e.g. dermatophilosis, occasionally dermatophytosis, and less commonly vasculitis); the remainder are open to speculation and require further investigation.

Coronary band dystrophy

Definition/overview
Mature and draft breed horses seem to be most susceptible.

Etiology/pathophysiology
Coronary band dystrophy is an idiopathic defect in the cornification of the coronary band.

Clinical presentation
All four hooves are affected, with proliferation and hyperkeratotic changes to the coronary band, ergot, and chestnut. Wall and severe coronary band changes are also seen. Cracks and fissures can bleed or ooze serum.

Differential diagnosis
Pemphigus foliaceus; dermatophilosis; chronic granulomatous disease; selenium toxicosis; pastern folliculitis.

Diagnosis
Clinical signs and the elimination of all other causes are typically used in diagnosis. Histopathology is not well documented.

Management
Palliative measures should be used. Removal of excessive horn and the application of emollient creams to the coronet may be helpful.

Prognosis
The prognosis is poor.

'Greasy heel' syndrome

Definition/overview
This is a loose conglomeration of diseases that have a clinically similar presentation of scaling, crusting, and erosion, with pyoderma of the pastern and heels. It can be associated with lameness.

Etiology/pathophysiology

Only one pastern, frequently a hindlimb, is usually involved and it may also be 'white socked'. Greasy heel syndrome is not a specific disease entity, but can be due to a variety of inflammatory skin conditions of the horse's pastern region.

Clinical presentation

Many similarities exist between different causes. The condition usually starts at the posterior aspect of the pastern, but with time and poor management it may extend up to the fetlock and around the front of the limb. Erythema, oozing, crusting, alopecia, and vasculitis lead to ulceration. With time and many and varied medications, the skin becomes thickened and develops fissures and a true dermatitis. Lesions are painful and lameness occurs. Severe chronic lesions may lead to chronic granulation tissue.

Differential diagnosis

+ *Contact dermatitis.* Primary irritant or allergic contact dermatitis: (a) irritant substances on pastern; allergic contact (clover); (b) all four extremities are usually involved (1266).
+ *Pastern folliculitis/pyoderma infections:* (a) staphylococcal infections (1267); (b) dermatophilosis (1268, 1269); (c) dermatophytosis: rare; usually due to *M. gypseum*; (d) *Fusiformis* infection (plus infection in liver) (1270). Need culture to define these infectious types.
+ *Chorioptic mange.* Mostly affects draft horses, but has been isolated in other breeds. Very pruritic. Contagious. Scraping: mites are usually easy to find.

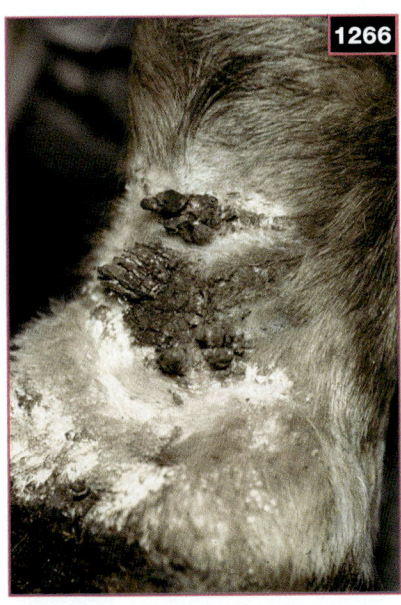

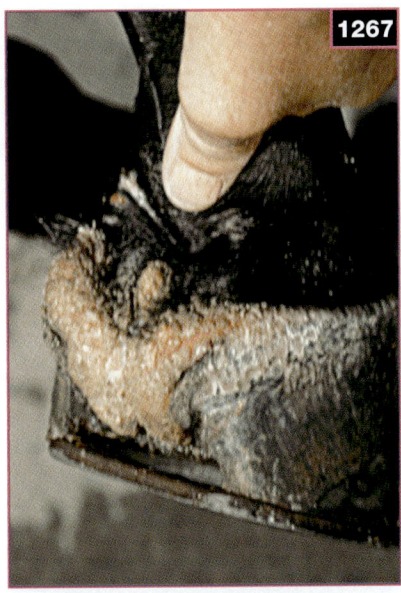

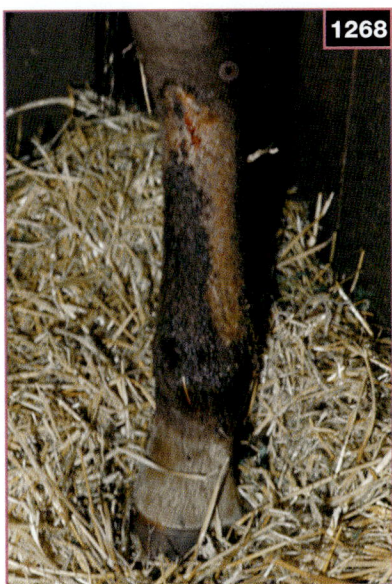

1266 Contact dermatitis with scurf, coronitis, and chronic granulation tissue at the back of the pastern.

1267 Staphylococcal infection in a 3-year-old Thoroughbred with skin erosion, alopecia, and involvement of the back of the heel.

1268 Acute *D. congolensis* scald with lameness and swelling above the fetlock.

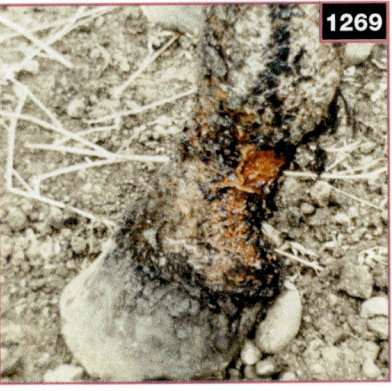
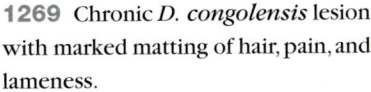

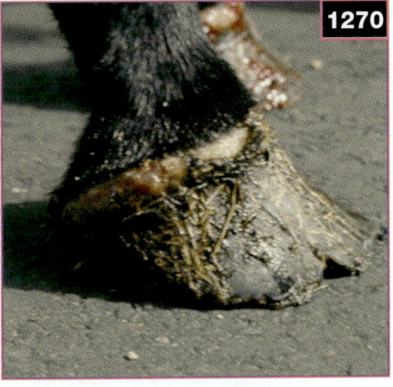

1269 Chronic *D. congolensis* lesion with marked matting of hair, pain, and lameness.

1270 *Fusiformis* infection with all four feet affected by exudative coronitis. This case also had severe liver infection.

- *Actinic dermatitis.* Systemic (phylloerythrin). Involves white pasterns and other white areas (e.g. nose and lower extremities).
- *Pastern leukocytoclastic vasculitis.*
- *Immune-complex vasculitis:* purpura hemorrhagica (**1271**) and strangles vasculitis (**1272**).
- *Mycetoma* (**1273**).
- *Idiopathic pastern dermatitis.*
- *Pastern folliculitis.*

Management
Proper management relies on a careful and correct diagnosis, which is extremely difficult with this syndrome.

Prognosis
Overall it is very difficult to give a prognosis because of the likelihood of only a partially correct diagnosis and management program.

Pastern leukocytoclastic vasculitis
Definition/overview
This is a specific clinicopathologic condition unique to horses. A sporadic disease, it may be more common than realized. It affects individual mature horses and has no sex predilection. It is almost exclusively confined to nonpigmented extremities and may only affect one limb even though other limbs are nonpigmented.

Etiology/pathophysiology
The disease usually occurs in summer in regions with plentiful sunlight. It may be caused by either immune or nonimmune mechanisms.

Clinical presentation
Medial and lateral aspects of the pastern are the most commonly affected sites. Early lesions include erythema, oozing, and crusting, and they are clearly demarcated (**1274**). Later lesions show erosions and ulceration with some edema of the affected limb, which is more extensive than expected for the lesion size. Chronic lesions develop a wart-like surface, which is resistant to removal and painful rather than pruritic. Occasionally, pigmented limbs are affected. Nonpigmented skin involvement suggests a role for UV light, but the disease is not a true photosensitization. Records of affected horses also indicate no known contact with photosensitizing compounds, and liver function has been normal.

Differential diagnosis
Photosensitization, especially due to plants (requires liver function tests and careful history taking to eliminate plants); dermatophilosis.

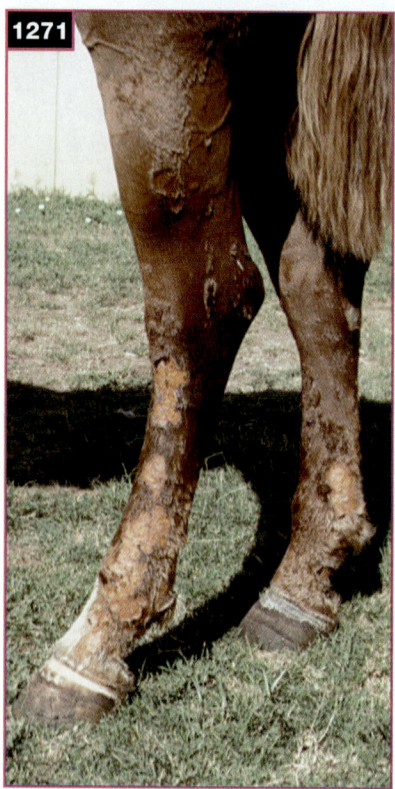
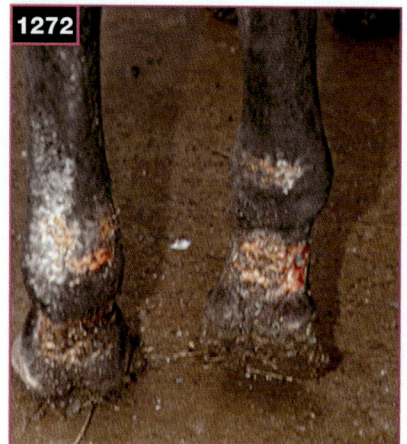
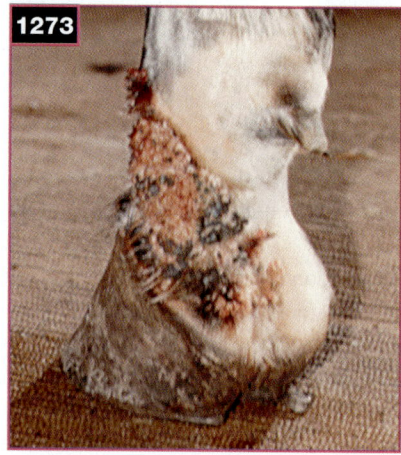

1271 Vasculitis due to purpura hemorrhagica, with hair loss, exudation on the limbs, and petechial hemorrhages in the mucosa of the eye, mouth, and vulva.

1272 Vasculitis associated with strangles infection showing swollen limbs, oozing serum, and sloughing skin.

1273 Mycetoma. A granulomatous-type lesion with subcutaneous nodules on the coronet and pastern. (Photo courtesy DW Scott)

Diagnosis

Diagnosis is based on the clinical appearance of the disease and involvement of a nonpigmented pastern. Biopsy should be performed.

Management

Affected areas should be protected from UV radiation by stabling, application of limb bandages, or use of sun block (SPF20). Large doses of corticosteroids may be required daily for up to 2 weeks, with a gradual reduction over the next 4 weeks. Emollient cream or keratolytics, such as salicylic acid, may be helpful. There may be occasional regression when treatment stops, requiring a further course of corticosteroids.

Prognosis

The prognosis is guarded. Recovery requires very good nursing and improved husbandry practices.

Idiopathic pastern dermatitis

Definition/overview

This is a chronic pastern disease of unknown origin.

Etiology/pathophysiology

Unknown.

Diagnosis

A complete history is important. Liver function tests should be carried out if lesions are limited to nonpigmented skin. Careful evaluation for dermatophytes and *Dermatophilus* should be performed. Biopsy, histopathology, and immunofluorescent studies may be useful. Bacterial and fungal culture may be of low value due to a high contamination rate of the area.

Management

Supportive therapy, including removal of crusts and thorough cleaning of the area, is an important component of treatment. Horses should be protected from unhygienic conditions, irritants, sunlight, and harsh treatment. The use of emollients containing antifungal, anti-inflammatory, and antibacterial drugs may be beneficial. Progress should be monitored very closely. High-level doses of corticosteroids may be required when immune complexes are involved. It is important to remember that previous treatment of other conditions may be the cause of the present condition.

Prognosis

This condition is characterized by a very slow recovery, with many regressions and the likelihood of permanent scarring.

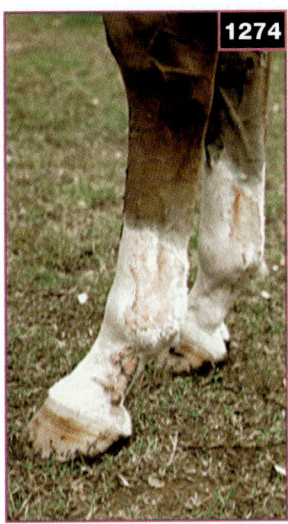

1274 Pastern leucocytoclastic vasculitis exhibits very painful small areas of alopecia, crusting, and serum exudation on the pastern.

Pastern folliculitis

Definition/overview

Pastern folliculitis is a bacterial folliculitis, with pyoderma of the pastern and coronet, caused by *Staphylococcus aureus, S. hyicus*, and possibly *S. intermedius* (see 1267).

Clinical presentation

The condition is usually limited to the posterior of the pastern and the bulbs of the heels. One or more limbs may be involved. Very early cases consist of papules that coalesce and produce large areas of ulceration and suppuration. Affected horses may exhibit lameness, but systemic effects are usually absent.

Differential diagnosis

All other forms of 'greasy heel': dermatophilus, hepatocutaneous syndrome, mycetoma, coronary band dystrophy, vasculitis, chorioptic mange, contact dermatitis.

Diagnosis

Smears or positive culture of organisms must be regarded with caution because the causative agents can also be found as skin contaminants.

Management

This condition can be painful to treat. The area should be cleaned and dressed with appropriate antimicrobial creams, ideally based on susceptibility tests. Parenteral antimicrobials may be required in severe cases.

Prognosis

The prognosis is guarded and recovery can be slow.

Skin diseases of foals

Most genetically oriented equine skin disease is manifested at birth or shortly afterwards, although some gradually develops as the foal ages (e.g. cutaneous asthenia). Foals can display signs of all types of skin disease at an early age and it is therefore important to distinguish diseases of genetic origin that are uncommon, unlikely to be treatable, and result in the majority of affected foals being euthanized. The solution for these defects lies in rearranged breeding programs or disposal of the blood lines.

Skin changes occurring from birth to 10 weeks of age are mostly from contact with irritant substances, bacteria, fungi, and some parasites. These can be managed relatively easily provided a correct diagnosis can be reached.

Aplasia cutis congenita (epitheliogenesis imperfecta)

Definition/overview
This is a rare, congenital, inherited cutaneous defect of foals seen at birth and caused by a single autosomal recessive character. There is a complete absence of epidermis and skin appendages (1275). Lesions usually occur distal to the carpus and tarsus. They bleed easily and quickly become infected, leading to septicemia and death.

Hereditary equine regional dermal asthenia (cutaneous asthenia, hyperelastosis cutis)

Definition/overview
These are a group of autosomal recessive inherited connective-tissue diseases that have also been described as Ehlers–Danlos syndrome and dermatosparaxis. The disease has occurred principally in Quarter horses.

Etiology/pathophysiology
At least nine different subtypes occur in humans and are classified on clinical, genetic, and biochemical differences. There is decreased collagen, as well as fragmentation and disorientation of collagen fibers.

Clinical presentation
Signs appear at birth or shortly afterwards. The foal has loose, wrinkled skin, which is hyperextensible, hyperfragile, tears easily, and repairs slowly. The condition may be generalized over the whole body or be sharply demarcated. Scar formation is common. Subcutaneous hematomas and abscesses occur (1276).

Diagnosis
This condition characteristically occurs in young Quarter horses. The clinical appearance of loose, hyperfragile skin is suggestive. Biopsy may indicate collagen changes, but histopathology in the horse has not been well documented.

Management
Affected horses should be removed from breeding programs. There is no treatment, apart from minimizing trauma. Breeding stock genetics should be investigated and all carriers should be culled. Inbreeding programs should be avoided.

Prognosis
The prognosis is guarded.

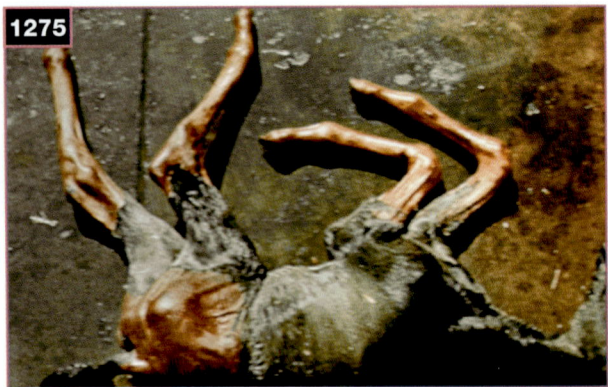

1275 Aplasia cutis congenita (epitheliogenesis imperfecta). Complete absence of epidermis and skin appendages distal to the carpus and tarsus. (Photo courtesy JP Hughes)

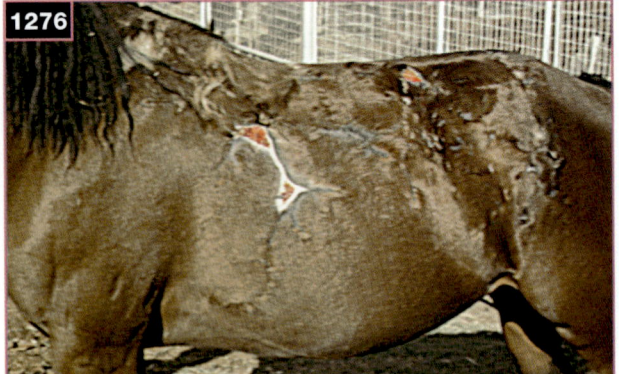

1276 Cutaneous asthenia in a 3-year-old inbred Quarter horse filly (dam × own son). There is abscessation of loosened skin and the presence of old scars from previous similar events. (Reprinted from Pascoe RR and Knottenbelt DC (1999) *Manual of Equine Dermatology*, WB Saunders, with permission)

Junctional epidermolysis bullosa

Definition/overview
This refers to a group of hereditary mechanobullous diseases characterized by the presence of blister formation following mild trauma.

Etiology/pathophysiology
Junctional epidermolysis bullosa is a hereditary disease, occurring principally in Belgian draft foals.

Clinical presentation
Both sexes can be affected. Lesions are present at birth or within 2 days. Lesions occur at skin mucocutaneous junctions and in oral mucosa (1277). Collapsed bullae may be found in the mouth. Exudation and crusting are often pronounced, with separation of hooves at the coronary band. Dystrophic teeth occur commonly. Affected foals become increasingly depressed and cachectic and are euthanized.

Management
The parents of affected foals should be tested (a DNA test is available) and, if found to be carriers, they should be stopped from further breeding.

Papillomatosis

Definition/overview
Papillomavirus has the ability to pass across the mare's placenta and is occasionally found on the skin of newborn foals.

Etiology/pathophysiology
The condition is caused by papillomavirus crossing the mare's placenta.

Clinical presentation
It can be located anywhere on the head, neck, or trunk, usually as a single cauliflower-like, flattened, wart, 5–20 mm in size, on the skin of a newborn foal (1278).

Diagnosis
Clinical appearance is suggestive. Biopsy should be performed for histopathology. Viral studies can be performed on a fresh unpreserved sample.

Management
Papillomatosis may be treated by ligature or surgical removal. Conservative treatment such as application of 50% podophyllin paste daily for 20 days can be attempted.

Prognosis
The prognosis is good and most cases respond very well to treatment.

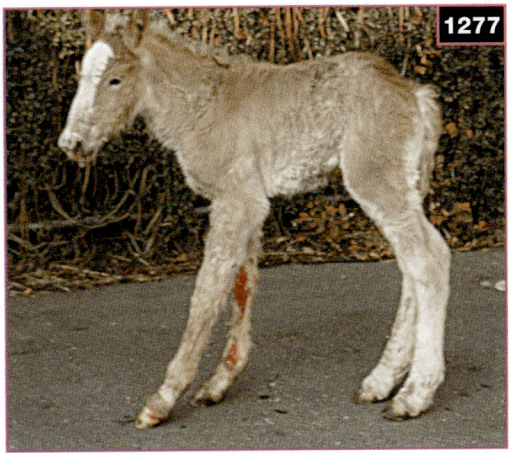

1277 Junctional epidermolysis bullosa occurs in Belgian draft foals, with lesions commonly occurring at the skin and mucocutaneous junctions. (Photo courtesy DC Knottenbelt) (Reprinted from Pascoe RR and Knottenbelt DC (1999) *Manual of Equine Dermatology*, WB Saunders, with permission)

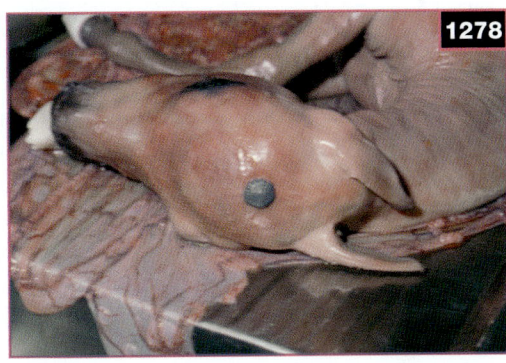

1278 Papillomatosis. A 10 mm wart on an aborted foal's head is shown.

Dermatophilosis

Definition/overview

Dermatophilosis is an uncommon disease in young foals. It tends to affect foals with long (downy) coats stabled under unhygienic conditions and subjected to higher than normal rainfall and/or warm humid weather, or foals that are immunologically compromised (1279).

Ringworm

Definition/overview

Occasionally, young foals become infected with *Trichophyton* spp. or *Microsporum gypseum*. Usually the dam is affected or the foal is immunocompromised.

Pediculosis

Definition/overview

Foals may contract lice from infested dams or other horses in a group, or from contaminated rugs and stables.

Strongyloides westerii and *Pelodera strongyloides* infestation

Definition/overview

Free-living larval strongyloid worms cause severe irritation to the limbs of foals.

Etiology/pathophysiology

Infestation usually only occurs after prolonged wet weather where foals are kept in old horse yards, on contaminated bedding, or under poor hygienic conditions.

Clinical presentation

Limb stamping, irritability, pruritus, and biting at limbs are evident. The limbs may swell if contact is prolonged.

Differential diagnosis

Stable fly bites; itch mites; poultry red mites; colic.

Diagnosis

Placing the foal's limbs in a plastic bag and washing off mud allows for examination of washings for the presence of free-living larvae.

Management

Foals should be removed from the contaminated environment and the limbs washed thoroughly.

Prognosis

The prognosis is very good.

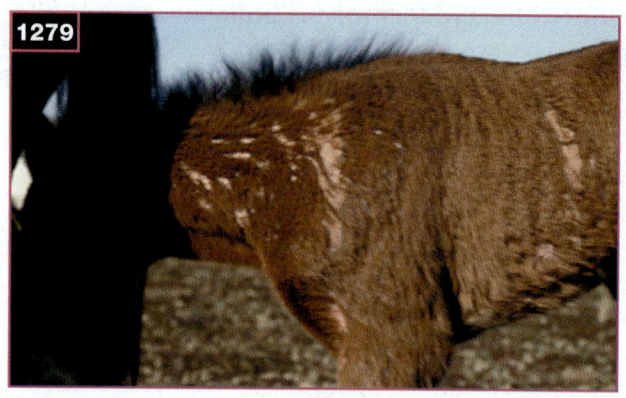

1279 *Dermatophilus* infection in a 2-week-old Arabian foal with severe combined immunodeficiency. Note the loss of hair from the head and neck, with typical rain-scald appearance.

Wound management and infections of synovial structures

Antonio Cruz and Graham Munroe

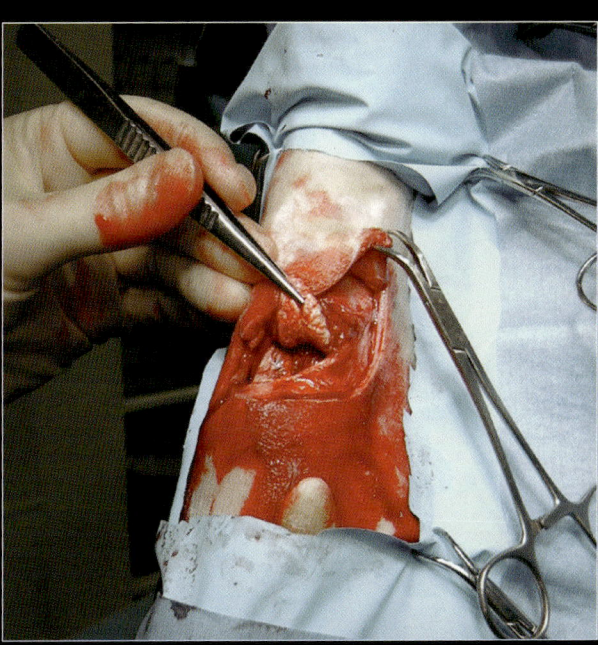

Wound management and infections of synovial structures

The behavior of horses and the presence in the environment of objects of different sizes, shapes, and materials means the practicing veterinarian has to confront a variety of traumatic injuries. A wound represents an injury to the skin (epithelium and subepithelium) where its physical integrity has been disrupted and there is exposure of the vascular elements and endothelium to the surrounding tissues. Visual disruption of skin is, however, not always present in wounds such as contusions and hematomas.

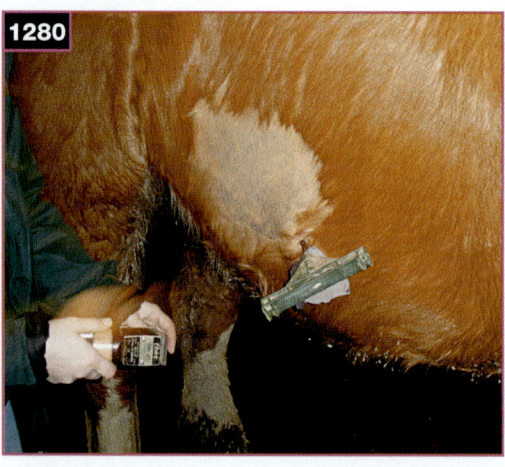

1280 A puncture wound to the right abdominal wall caused by a metal stake used to carry an electric fence wire. The object had penetrated the wall and damaged a loop of small intestine.

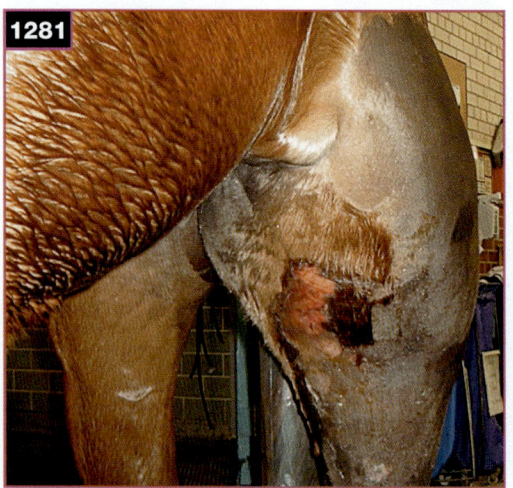

Classification of wounds

Wounds are basically classified as open (complete epithelial loss) or closed. Open wounds include lacerations, incisions, ulcers, and punctures (**1280**). Closed wounds include contusions, abrasions, and hematomas (**1281**). A wound is more importantly defined by its cause, subsequent pathophysiology, and its anatomic location. A causative classification of wounds includes mechanical, thermal, and chemical causes, or subsequent to irradiation. It is particularly important to assess the vascular supply to the damaged area, the degree of contamination, and the possibility of infection, plus the sequelae derived from the involvement of different anatomic structures.

Lacerations and puncture wounds are particularly common, especially following wire- or wood-fence injuries. Barbed wire can lead to severe loss of tissue and exposure of large amounts of connective tissue and bone (degloving injuries) (**1282**). Smooth-wire lacerations can lead to vascular strangulation of the affected extremity, with resulting catastrophic consequences.

Closed wounds such as abrasions, contusions, or hematomas are less dramatic in their appearance and most heal without further intervention. These may be the result of kicks or self-inflicted trauma during stall casting. Abrasions and erosions present with only partial epithelial loss, no dermal exposure, and an intact basement membrane. Contusions disrupt the subepithelial tissue vascular supply, predisposing them to anoxia and necrosis with secondary loss of epithelium and colonization by bacteria. Closed wounds may present with delayed and severe tissue damage (e.g. rope burns), misleading the clinician in his/her initial assessment of the injury. Adequate follow-up of these types of injury is therefore essential. Some of these injuries may result in the development of septic cellulitis, producing significant tissue damage, necrosis, and sloughing within the first 5–7 days (**1283**). The clinician must not forget that the body's natural tendency is to heal and in the absence of deleterious factors such as infection or lack of vascular supply, a wound will heal.

1281 This picture illustrates a swollen thigh as a result of a contusion and hematoma. Note the area of alopecia in the craniomedial aspect of the limb. Hair loss is one of the early signs of tissue necrosis prior to sloughing, usually seen 3–5 days after the original injury.

Stages of wound healing

Once a wound has occurred a series of events follows that constitute the healing process. The timing and cellular elements of this process characterize the different stages in each separate tissue. These stages overlap each other and occur in programmed succession to achieve a final result. The role of the veterinarian is to modulate these stages, through intervention, to facilitate and speed the healing process, to promote a quick return to proper function, and to improve the cosmetic outcome. The five stages of wound healing are described below.

Hemostasis

The extravasation of vascular elements and the exposure of the subendothelial structure lead to aggregation of platelets, which contributes to clot formation. Platelet function is also responsible for additional features of hemostasis such as the fibrin mesh network and the chemoattraction of neutrophils. The hemostatic phase may last a few minutes to a few hours.

Inflammation

The inflammatory response is characterized mostly by the presence of neutrophils, which are bactericidal and protect the body against invasion by foreign organisms or substances. The release of local chemotactic factors serves as a migration signal for the neutrophils, which begin a process of diapedesis and migration to the injury site. Other factors released at a local level (e.g. serotonin, histamine, bradykinin) are responsible for a vasodilatory response and an increase in vascular permeability, which further facilitates neutrophil migration. The acute inflammatory phase starts within minutes of a wound occurring and lasts for a few hours to days depending on the severity of the injury and degree of contamination. The activation and death of neutrophils is responsible for the release of enzymatic products and inflammatory mediators. In the absence of infection, neutrophils are not necessary for wound healing.

Debridement

The debridement phase begins within a few hours of the injury and its duration depends on the severity of the injury. It starts by the enzymatic breakdown of debris by substances released from the dead neutrophils. Monocytes are chemoattracted into the wound at the same time as neutrophils and are responsible for the elimination of debris, necrotic tissue, foreign substances, and micro-organisms. Unlike neutrophils, monocytes are necessary for wound healing to progress. They transform into macrophages once in the wound and remain there for days to weeks, regulating the progression of wound healing.

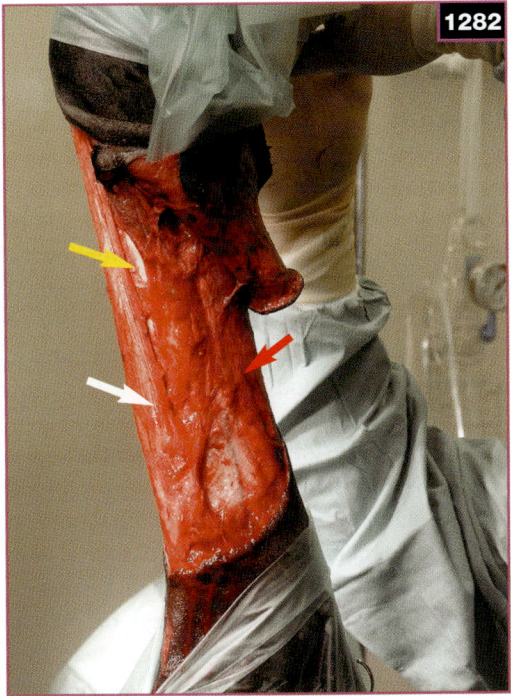

1282 Acute degloving injury of the hind cannon following the leg being trapped through the floor of a horse trailer. The long digital extensor tendon is exposed (white arrow), along with the flexor tendons (red arrow), and areas of the third metatarsus (yellow arrow). Periosteal damage in these areas can lead to bone sequestrum formation at a later date.

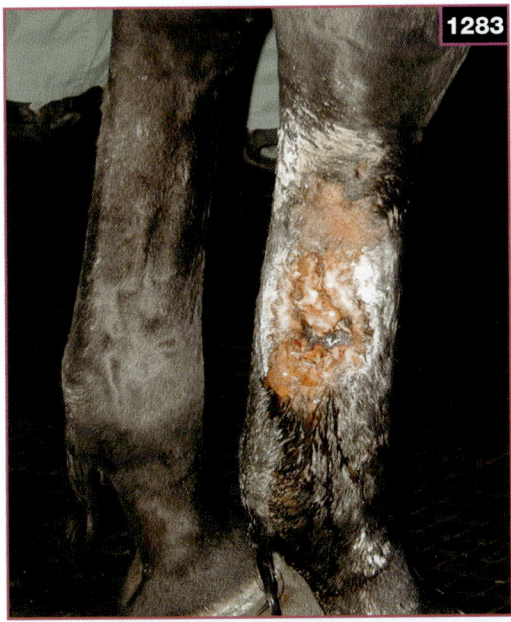

1283 Tissue sloughing on the lateral aspect of the metacarpal area as a result of a rope burn sustained 6 days previously. Similar injuries are also produced as a result of pressure sores from incorrect cast application.

Repair

The repair phase is characterized by the presence of fibroblasts, which produce collagen and connective tissue matrix (granulation tissue) and lead to wound contraction. The granulation tissue scaffold facilitates the migration of epithelial cells. During second-intention or open wound healing, epithelialization and contraction are ultimately responsible for wound repair (1284). This is only possible if the wound is clear of debris, infection, tissue necrosis, and exuberant granulation tissue. Epithelialization can begin as soon as 12 hours post wounding in primary healing or after 4 or 5 days in secondary wound healing. Wound contraction is most important in secondary wound closure and stops with contact inhibition between cells, excessive tension, exuberant granulation tissue, or if full-thickness grafts are applied before the 5th day of healing.

Maturation

The return to normal structure and function of the connective tissue is characterized by the balance between collagen synthesis and lysis, as well as the return of normal architecture with an adequate pattern of collagen fiber orientation. This leads to an increase in the wound's tensile strength to approximately 80% of the original tissue. Following the maturation phase the tissue evolves through a subclinical period of remodeling, which may last weeks to months.

Factors affecting wound healing

Nutritional status

In the horse, food deprivation and malnutrition can have a deleterious effect on wound healing. Conditions associated with a reduction in plasma protein (e.g. malnutrition) delay the repair phase of wound healing by preventing the onset of fibroplasia and diminishing the tensile strength of a wound. The poor surgical wound healing in cases of large colon torsion, where subsequent hypoproteinemia is a common occurrence, is a good example.

Hypovolemia, hypotension, and hypoxia

In cases of sudden hypovolemia due to considerable blood loss, the microcirculation is impaired due to the reduction in circulating blood volume, leading to local tissue hypoxia and reduced micronutrient delivery, which results in delayed healing. Lacerations of the palmar or plantar digital artery during heel bulb lacerations can lead to a significant amount of blood loss (1285), while local hypovolemia can occur following strangulating trauma. This may include smooth-wire injuries, overzealous use of pressure bandages, or rope wounds preventing or reducing vascular supply to the distal extremity, with the resulting hypoxic tissue damage and, possibly, necrosis leading to tissue edema and sloughing.

1284 A wound on the dorsal aspect of the upper cannon that is being treated by second-intention healing. Note the healthy granulation-tissue bed and active epithelial edges.

1285 Severe hemorrhage may occur in cases of lacerations in the palmar or plantar aspect of the pastern or heels. Laceration of the digital vessels is not uncommon in this type of injury and can cause severe blood loss.

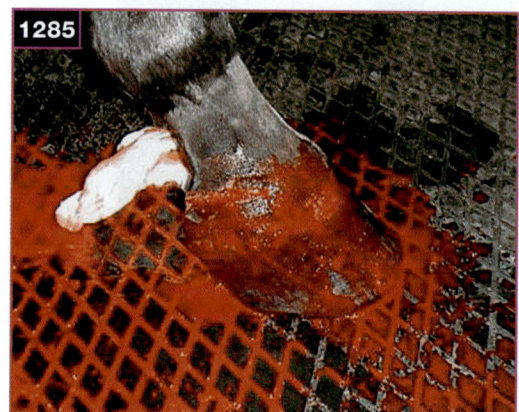

Wound management and infections of synovial structures

Hypothermia

Optimal wound healing is accomplished at environmental temperatures of around 30°C (86°F). Dropping the environmental temperature from 20°C (68°F) to 12°C (53.6°F) decreases the tensile strength of wounds by about 20% in humans. The effect of temperature changes on wound healing in horses has not been studied, but it is thought that, except in extreme temperature conditions, temperature change should have no net effect on the process of wound healing.

Infection

Severe wound contamination, lack of vascular supply, and the presence of foreign material may lead to wound infection, particularly if the wound is not promptly decontaminated and debrided. In general terms, the severity of wound contamination is directly related to its proximity to the ground. Contamination is not synonymous with infection and bacterial colonization is necessary for the latter to occur. In a properly treated wound, infection is an uncommon occurrence and the largest challenge to the veterinarian is when bone or synovial structures are involved or major tissue necrosis is present. In these circumstances, bacteria may become quickly established, with catastrophic and costly consequences. Infection interferes with and delays wound healing. It is important to consider debridement of a wound in order to eliminate necrotic tissue, foreign material, blood, and exudates and to help reduce the bacterial load to levels that can be dealt with by the host immune system. The use of systemic or topical antibiotics will depend on the clinician's assessment of the wound, but antibiotics alone will not prevent an infection in the presence of other predisposing factors.

Topical medications

Topical medications are used for several purposes, including preventing excessive granulation tissue, speeding up healing, improving the cosmetic outcome, and preventing wound infection.

There is no single product effective in all these areas and there is a lack of proper clinical trials showing unequivocal data supporting the use of a single product. Existing medications fall into the categories of antimicrobials, antiseptics, irritants, and cell-function modulators. Antimicrobials and antiseptics may be indicated in the initial stages of wound healing to reduce the bacterial load. Since granulation tissue is very resistant to infection, the use of antimicrobials is not indicated once a suitable granulation-tissue bed is present. Corticosteroids are commonly used to prevent excessive granulation-tissue production, but they have dose-dependent healing delaying effects and they have to be used cautiously.

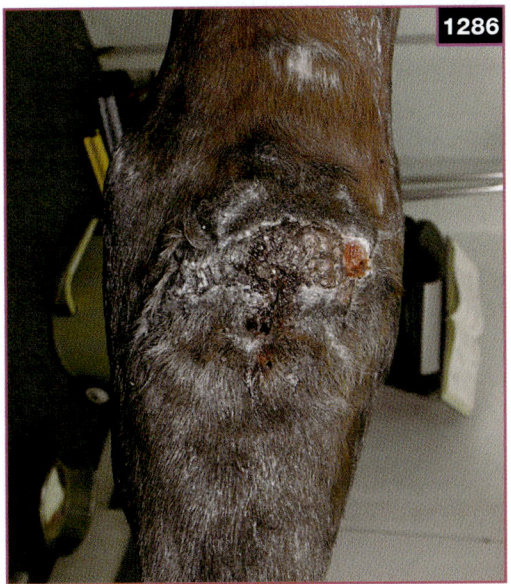

1286 Chronic wound on the dorsal aspect of the hock and upper cannon bone. This had been treated for 9 months, but because of excessive movement and difficulty in maintaining bandages in place the result was very poor, with thickening of the skin surrounding a nonhealing central area. Surgical removal of the scar and subsequent repair were required.

Movement

Excessive movement promotes exuberant granulation tissue and interrupts the process of healing (1286), particularly where there is poor local musculature, such as the distal limbs. Movement should be aggressively controlled by the use of bandages, splints, or casts. Immobilization of a high-motion area by using a fiberglass cast is a useful technique in distal limb wounds.

Necrotic tissue

Necrotic tissue delays or prevents wound healing by preventing cell proliferation and adequate vascular supply. In addition, it potentiates ongoing inflammation and wound infection. Debridement of necrotic tissue can substantially improve wound healing.

Tumors

The presence of neoplastic tissue prevents wound healing by impairing cell function and the normal contraction and epithelialization processes. A consequence of open wound healing can be metaplasia of tissues, predisposing the affected site to the development of fibroblastic sarcoid.

Types of closure

Primary closure

Primary closure refers to the apposition of the skin epithelium, with restoration of skin surface. This is the mechanism by which surgical wounds heal. Primary closure should be chosen when there is adequate vascular supply, minimal tension across the sutured wound, and none or minimal bacterial contamination (1287–1289). If these criteria are not met, dehiscence will occur (1290). Partial primary closure is also an option for wounds that may have an area of isolated tissue necrosis, excessive skin loss, or require wound drainage in cases of excessive dead space or contamination. If drainage is needed, the most dependent part of a wound should not be sutured or the use of drains should be considered (1291).

Delayed primary closure

Delayed primary closure is performed prior to the onset of fibroplasia, approximately 3–5 days after wounding. This allows the wound to drain and clear excessive debris or bacterial load before being closed, thereby decreasing the chance of dehiscence (1292, 1293). Other advantages include improved vascular supply, improved debridement, and decreased healing time when compared with second-intention wound healing. If closure is delayed, initial wound-edge retraction may increase wound tension and make wound apposition more difficult. It is imperative to practice meticulous wound care during the time that the wound is open prior to closure. Protection and debridement of the wound and removal of exudates and necrotic debris, while preventing wound desiccation and cross-contamination, are essential. This is accomplished by confining the animal, by the use of permeable bandages applied daily either as dry-to-dry or wet-to-dry modalities to debride and support the wound, wound lavage, and by the careful use of systemic antibiotics and anti-inflammatories in some cases to control infection and excessive inflammatory reaction.

Secondary or open wound closure

Due to the nature of equine wounds and the relative scarcity of skin in the distal extremities, veterinarians are frequently forced to use secondary closure to repair wounds. The physiologic processes that control this healing modality are wound contraction and epithelialization; therefore, these two functions must be preserved through proper wound care.

Secondary closure is chosen when first-intention healing is not possible because of excessive motion, tension, tissue damage, or infection (1294). This option is not without complications. The most common are the development of exuberant granulation tissue in the lower extremities and the time required for re-epithelialization (1295). Appropriate wound management during the healing stages is usually time-consuming and expensive. Much effort has been made to develop wound-dressing materials that will significantly shorten the healing period, but without significant side-effects. Secondary closure relies on the formation of an appropriate granulation-tissue bed for the wound to contract and re-epithelialize. Granulation tissue starts to form as early as 72 hours and proceeds rapidly if the wound conditions are adequate (i.e. lack of infection and immobility). The role of the clinician is to manage an open wound in such a way that facilitates the processes of wound contraction and epithelialization by maintaining an appropriate wound environment.

1287–1289 An acute laceration of the right stifle region of a Thoroughbred racehorse. (1287) The wound has been lavaged, explored, and cleaned prior to surgical debridement. (1288) The wound has been sharply debrided and lavaged prior to repair. (1289) The wound has been repaired in anatomic layers, including muscle, fascia, and subcuticular layers, before skin staples are used to close the skin.

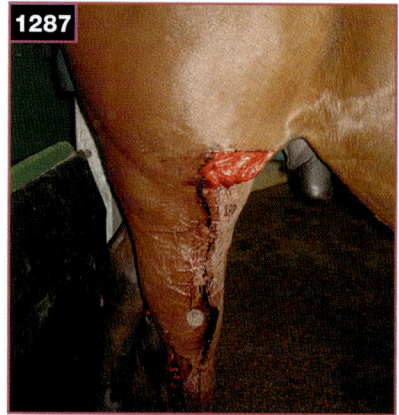

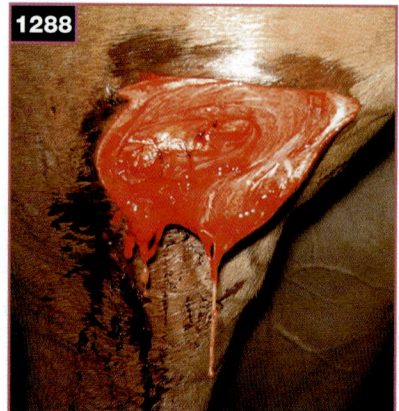

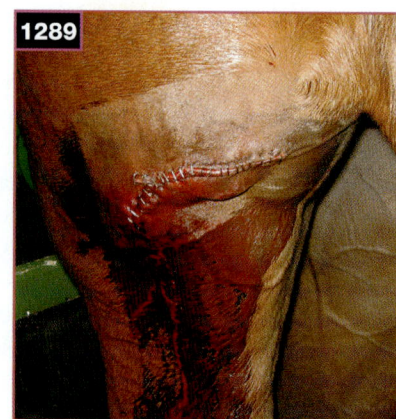

Wound management and infections of synovial structures

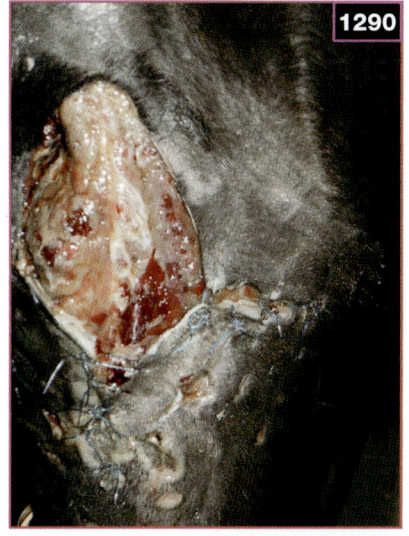

1290

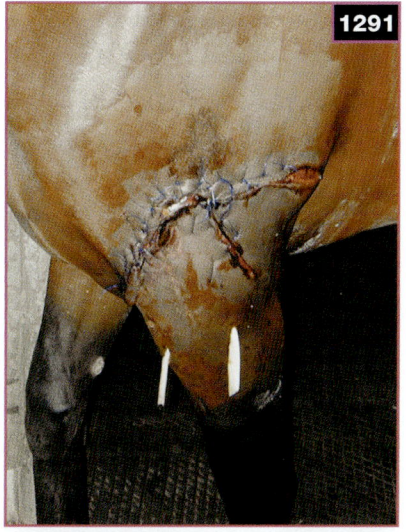

1291

1290 Wound dehiscence as a result of excessive tension, motion, and tissue necrosis. This particular wound dehisced 96 hours after primary closure.

1291 Primary wound closure after an acute laceration. Note the everting suture pattern used (horizontal mattress) and the placement of Penrose drains.

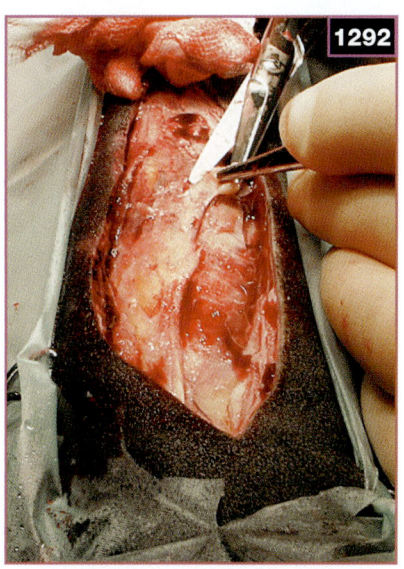

1292

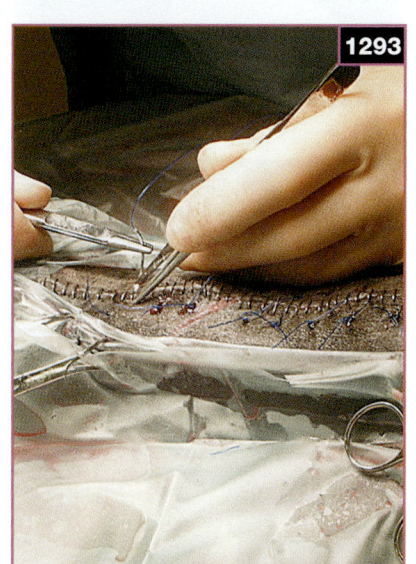

1293

1292, 1293 This horse has sustained a laceration to the dorsal mid cannon bone due to entanglement with a wire fence. It was elected to treat the wound by delayed primary closure with a regimen of daily wound lavage and cleaning, topical hydrogel application, compression bandaging, and systemic antibiotics and NSAIDs. (1292) At 5 days post injury the wound was debrided under general anesthesia prior to lavage and surgical repair. (1293) The wound edges were mobilized by undermining and closed with a combination of subcuticular sutures, skin staples, and vertical mattress bolster monofilament nylon sutures.

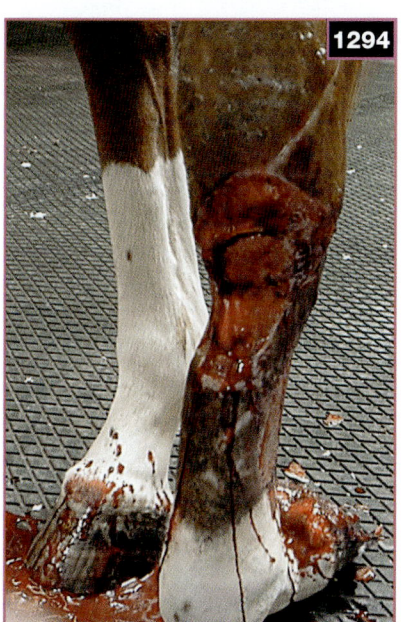

1294

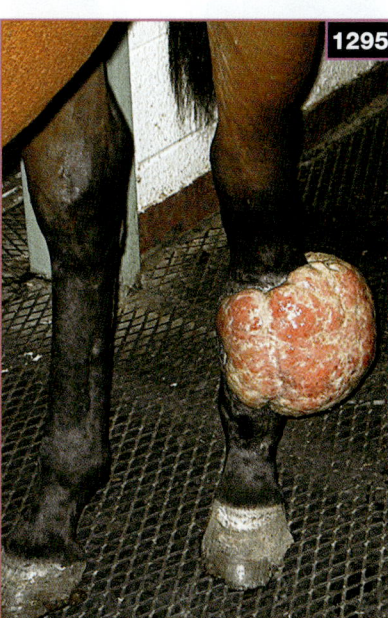

1295

1294 This picture shows an extensive wound to the dorsal aspect of the tarsal and proximal metatarsal regions, typically encountered in barbed-wire fence injuries. Due to its size and location, this wound is not amenable to primary closure and secondary closure or open wound healing was selected.

1295 Exuberant granulation tissue present after a wound in the dorso-lateral aspect of the metatarsal region of a 9-year-old Quarter horse.

Wound management and infections of synovial structures

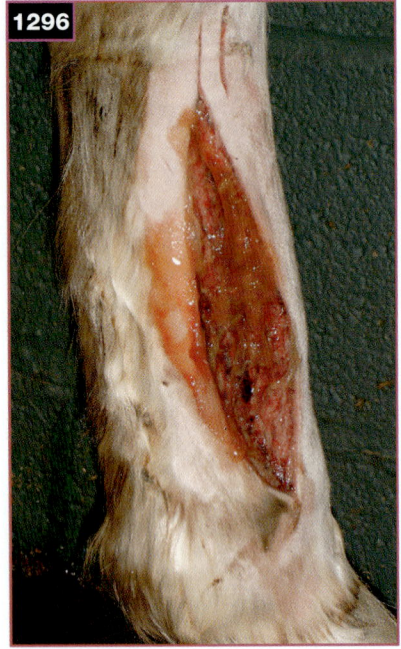

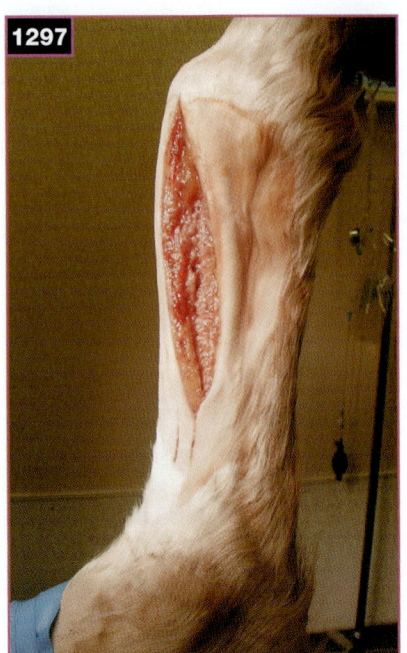

1296–1298 This horse sustained a wound of the medial cannon region 8 days previously (1296). The wound was cleaned, lavaged, and bandaged every day, and systemic antibiotics and NSAIDs were given (1297). The wound was repaired by delayed secondary closure (1298) and healed without incident.

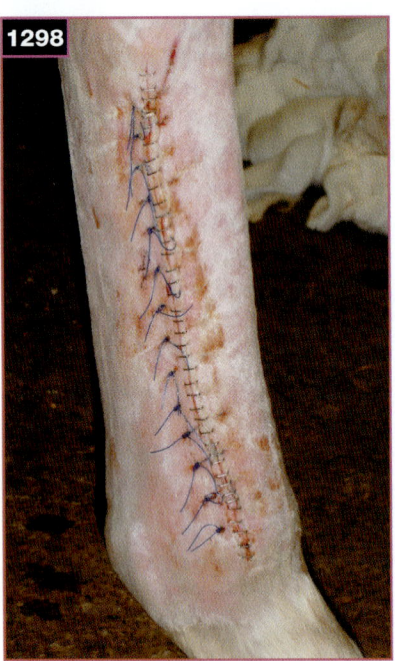

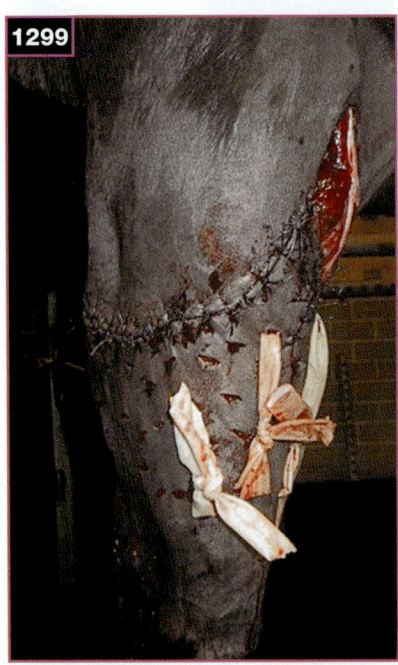

1299 The 'mesh-expansion' technique can be seen in this picture. Note the direction of the stab incisions parallel to the direction of the wound.

Delayed secondary closure

Delayed secondary closure is performed by suturing a wound after the process of fibroplasia has produced a healthy granulation-tissue bed. When applied correctly it can prevent the development of exuberant granulation tissue and considerably accelerate the horse's recovery. In preparation for delayed secondary wound healing the granulation-tissue bed must be debrided of its superficial layer and the skin edges undermined and freshened (1296–1298) to accomplish apposition with minimal tension and facilitate tissue healing. Additional tension-release techniques, such as mesh expansion (1299), can be used to decrease the likelihood of dehiscence of the suture line.

Wound closure

Preparation, lavage, and debridement

Assessment and treatment of any wound are best achieved in a quiet, clean, and well-lit environment. The whole horse should be examined thoroughly. Sedation may be necessary in some cases. Prior to the administration of any drugs the horse should be assessed particularly for signs of shock and severe blood loss (e.g. tachycardia, pale or muddy mucous membranes, prolonged CRT, skin tent). The steps towards the evaluation of a wound should include:

✦ Move the horse, if necessary, to a better environment.
✦ Make an initial assessment of the wound.
✦ Apply sterile hydrosoluble gel to the wound surface.
✦ Clip hair from the surrounding area to at least 5 cm from the wound edges.
✦ Lavage the wound with sterile saline, or hose with cold water if not available, while manually removing gross contamination (e.g. dirt, straw, hair).
✦ Protect the wound bed with additional sterile hydro-soluble gel and scrub the wound periphery with a suitable solution, such as chlorhexidine soap, avoiding contamination of the wound bed.
✦ Prepare 1 liter of 0.1% povidone–iodine solution and irrigate the wound either with a Waterpick™ or with a 60 ml syringe through a 19 gauge needle. Pressure should be used to dislodge contamination and can be helped by using sterile gauzes.
✦ Explore the wound in a sterile manner with a sterile metal probe or sterile gloved digit to assess the depth and presence of wound tracts. It is important to determine the anatomic structures involved, tissue deficits, vascular supply, level of deep contamination, dead space, and potential deep tracts that the wound may have followed.

Once wound evaluation has been completed, a therapeutic plan should be developed and a decision about primary or secondary closure reached. Surgical debridement is essential and should be performed by careful resection of necrotic tissue while preserving all vital structures. Over-debridement may potentially delay the healing process or invade and damage critical structures such as synovial cavities. Tissues with questionable viability should be preserved as much as possible. Occasionally, a skin flap may be maintained for a few days as a 'biological' dressing, only to be debrided once fibroplasia has started. It is important to understand that wound debridement is also a staged procedure that may continue for several days following initial assessment of the wound. Any interaction with the wound should be carried out with at least clean, if not sterile, gloved hands, as cross-contamination from the veterinarian's hands is possible.

Suture materials and patterns

The clinician must choose the appropriate suture material, needle, and pattern. As an overall classification, there are absorbable and nonabsorbable suture materials, which can also be mono or multifilament (*Table 62*). Ideally, the suture material used should be user-friendly, prevent a large foreign-body reaction, maintain tension and knot security until the sutured tissue has acquired enough tension of its own, and minimize the risks of harboring bacteria. This would mean that a monofilament absorbable material, such as polydioxanone, would be ideal in subcutaneous tissues, and a nonabsorbable material, such as polypropylene, in the skin. The size of the needle and suture material should be proportional to the thickness of the tissue and, except in subcutaneous tissues, where a round tip noncutting needle is preferred, a reverse cutting needle is indicated. Suture size 2/0 or 3/0 (3 or 3.5 metric) is appropriate for subcutaneous tissues and skin.

TABLE 62 **Types of suture material available to the equine clinician**

SUTURE MATERIAL	ABSORBABLE	CONFORMATION	COMMERCIAL NAME
Polydioxanone	Yes	Monofilament	PDS/Biosin
Polypropylene	No	Monofilament	Prolene
Polyglactin 910	Yes	Multifilament	Vicryl/Polysorb
Polyglycolic acid	Yes	Multifilament	Dexon
Polymerized caprolactam	No	Multifilament	Supramid
Poliglecaprone 25	Yes	Monofilament	Monocryl
Polyester	No	Multifilament	Ethibond
Polyglyconate	Yes	Monofilament	Maxon

Wound management and infections of synovial structures

If excessive tension is anticipated, a larger suture size or the use of a different suture pattern may be required. For wounds where tension is not a concern, a simple or cruciate mattress interrupted pattern is appropriate. If tension is anticipated, it is better to use a pattern that provides tension relief such as a near–far–far–near or a vertical mattress. Appositional or everting suture patterns are adequate in the skin. Where the end cosmetic result is important, a subcuticular simple continuous pattern can be chosen. The clinician must bear in mind that the holding strength of this pattern is inferior to that of a dermal pattern. Closure of dead space by suturing the subcutaneous layers will prevent the development of seromas and speed the healing process.

Wound drainage

The purpose of drainage is to remove the excess fluid generated in a wound and to minimize anatomic dead space, thereby decreasing bacterial proliferation, reducing the risk of infection, and promoting healing. In general there are two types of draining methods: passive and active.

Passive drainage mainly uses gravity to facilitate fluid elimination and this can be achieved by strategically placed incisions in a ventral location relative to the drainage area. Gentle body motion helps passive drainage and should be encouraged whenever possible without jeopardizing the wound-healing process. In addition, devices such as Penrose drains made out of latex or sterile tubing and not exiting directly through the wound, may be used to facilitate and maintain an open drainage flow (1300). The main disadvantage of passive drainage is the possibility of promoting an ascending infection. Passive drainage devices are therefore only placed for a short period of time and in situations where it is absolutely necessary. The use of passive drains in cases of synovial wounds or osteosynthesis is controversial.

Active drainage requires a suction system that provides a continuous negative pressure that will remove exudate as soon as it is produced and prevent retrograde contamination of the drained area. Active drains can be manufactured using a large syringe, some tubing, and a needle (1301). They are also commercially available. Depending on the exudate volume that is produced, careful emptying and reconnection may be necessary to maintain the closed suction system. In order to prevent disconnection or drain failure, a strategic location must be chosen for attaching the suction system to the horse. The presence of drain tubing in the wound may stimulate a foreign-body reaction and fluid production. If the fluid produced is a response to the presence of a 'foreign' object, this must be recognized by the clinician and the drain should be removed. In general, a drain should be in place for <72 hours. Proper care of drains is essential to maximize their effectiveness and reduce their complications.

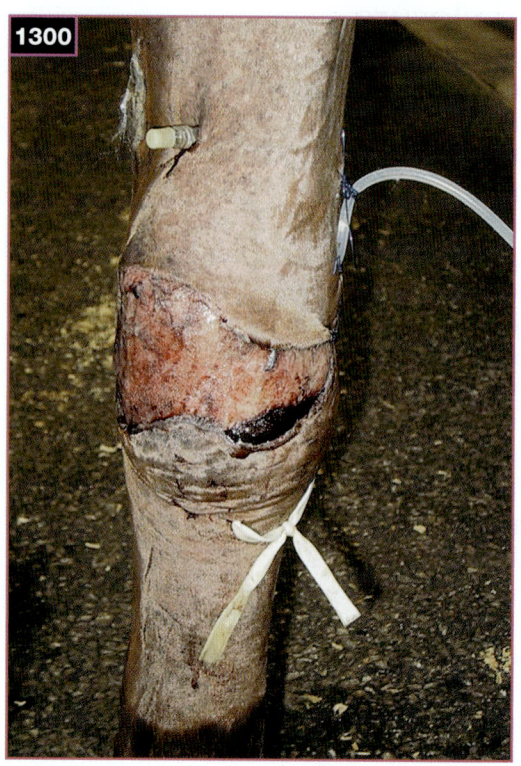

1300 A Penrose drain is shown placed away from the wound edges and into an area of dead space to facilitate wound drainage and prevent the formation of a seroma.

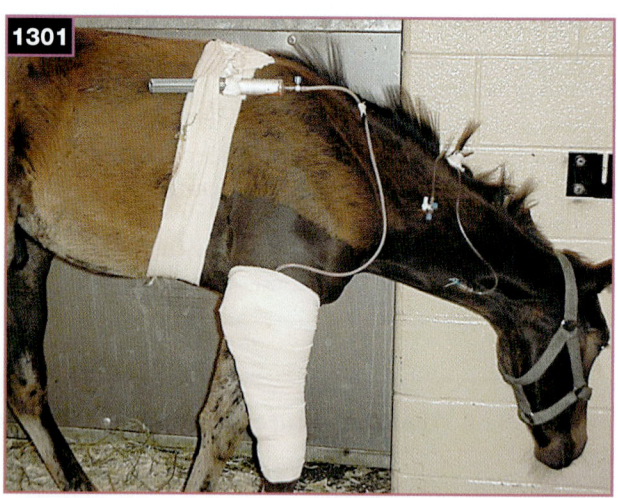

1301 An 'active' drain, following a fracture repair, is shown in this picture. Active drains maintain a constant negative suction pressure that prevents infection ascending into the affected area. Note the location of the collection chamber of the drain and its simple construction.

Wound management and infections of synovial structures

Postoperative care

Dressings and immobilization

Bandages are composed of three layers. These, according to their function, can be defined as contact, absorbent or intermediate, and protective or shell. The contact layer is the immediate layer on the wound surface and it may fulfill all or some of the functions of protection, debridement, absorption, and occlusion, and be a vehicle for topical medications. The absorption capacity of the contact and intermediate layers is determined by their hydrophilic properties. Depending on their permeability to liquid (exudates) and gas (oxygen), they can be occlusive or semi-occlusive. Occlusive dressings (*Table 63*) maintain a very high level of moisture in the wound as the exudates are not allowed to evacuate the surface. Their use may

TABLE 63 **Types of bandage and their applications according to their moisture content**

TOPICAL DRESSING	COMMENTS	INDICATIONS
Corticosteroids	Once daily; apply a clear thin layer. Prevent granulation tissue, speed healing, may decrease fibroplasia and delay wound contraction and epithelialization, perhaps dose related.	Prevents exuberant granulation tissue. Use in repair phase.
2.5% ketanserin	Once daily; apply a clear thin layer. (NB: Use gloves.) Prevents granulation tissue. No bandage needed. Experimental results equivocal; do not compare with bandaging management.	Prevents exuberant granulation tissue.
Silver sulfadiazine (1%)	Once daily; apply a clear thin layer. No effect on wound healing. Good effects as antimicrobial *in vitro*.	Infected wounds, burns.
Biological dressings	No advantages in bacterial proliferation, inflammatory reaction, wound contraction, and epithelialization. Some dressings are occlusive.	Use during repair phase.
Amniotic membrane	Decreases granulation tissue; faster healing. Time-consuming to produce; costly.	Use during repair phase.
Hydrogels	Humans: pain relief, inhibition of bacterial proliferation, debrides devitalized tissue, provides moist healing environment. Horses: no effect on contraction and epithelialization shown. Costly.	Use in the late stages of the repair phase.
Colloids	Occlusive.	Use in wounds with established granulation tissue, advanced contraction, and decreased fluid production.
Nitrofurazone	Once daily; apply a clear thin layer. Helps decrease bacterial load. Nonadherent. Conflicting results as to its effects on contraction and epithelialization.	Use when granulation tissue is present and a small amount of exudate, which would indicate a larger bacterial load.
Tri-peptide copper complex	Rats: benefits chronic ischemic wounds and accelerates contraction and epithelialization.	No horse studies are available.
Occlusive dressing	Horses: delays healing, increases inflammatory reaction, increases exudate production.	Use in the late stages of the repair phase.
Gauze	Semi-occlusive. Dry-to-dry or wet-to-dry.	Debriding wounds. Nonadhesive. Maintains wound moisture while allowing drainage.
Telfa, melolite	Semi-occlusive.	Nonadhesive. Use after granulation tissue present.
Tegaderm, Op-site	Occlusive.	Increases wound moisture.
Vigilon, NuGel, 2nd skin	Occlusive, hydrogel.	Increases wound moisture. Promotes granulation tissue.
Tegasorb, Duoderm, Intrasite	Occlusive, hydrocolloid.	Become incorporated into the wound. Promotes epithelialization and granulation.

Wound management and infections of synovial structures

promote additional exudation, exuberant granulation tissue, and an inflammatory response, which results in delayed healing. They should not be used in primary post-surgical wounds, as they may facilitate wound dehiscence by maintaining an increased level of moisture at the wound site. They are best applied once the amount of exudates is reduced and the wound is starting to granulate. Their overall use during equine wound healing is still controversial.

Semi-occlusive dressings are, in the author's opinion, more versatile and adjust better to the objectives of wound healing, particularly during open wound management. The use of a nonadherent, semi-occlusive dressing should be limited to cases of primary wound healing or secondary wound healing once there is a granulation-tissue bed. During the largely exudative stages of secondary wound healing (inflammatory and debridement) the clinician should consider the use of semi-occlusive bandages on a dry-to-dry, wet-to-dry, and wet-to-wet fashion (*Table 64*).

According to moisture gradients, bandages can be used to control their absorptive capacity and, therefore, regulate the level of moisture at the wound surface. They can be used in a dry-to-dry (dry contact layer, dry intermediate layer), wet-to-dry (wet contact, dry intermediate), or wet-to-wet (wet contact, wet intermediate) fashion. When treating open wounds, dry-to-dry bandages can be used during the first 48–72 hours when debridement is needed. As the level of exudation in the wound increases during the inflammatory and debridement phases, a wet-to-dry (or wet-to-wet if exuding excessively) bandage can be applied until a granulation-tissue bed is visible. Subsequently, a nonadherent semi-occlusive material is used.

In cases of primary wound healing where a surgical incision has been closed with minimal tension and good apposition, migration of epithelial cells across the wound margins occurs quickly and bandages have primarily a protective role. The use of nonadhesive dressings such as telfa or melolite in addition to a well placed bandage is usually sufficient .

The application of topical medications to wounds in the initial stages of wound healing is rarely necessary if the principles of adequate wound debridement, environment control, and motion control are followed. The use of topical medications to manage exuberant granulation tissue is discussed elsewhere (see p. 952).

Wound immobility is also a crucial factor and excessive motion at the wound bed not only promotes dehiscence and delays wound healing, but it also promotes exuberant granulation tissue. Inadequate wound-motion management is one of the main reasons for the exuberant granulation tissue formation seen in clinical practice. Different degrees of immobilization can be accomplished with an appropriately applied bandage with or without the use of a splint or a cast (1302). A heavily layered bandage or modified Robert Jones bandage will provide immobility directly related to the number of layers. It is important to maintain the conformation and the uniform pressure of the bandage in order to avoid complications, such as pressure sores and undue wound irritation (1303). Splints should be light, waterproof, easy to contour, strong, cheap, and without sharp edges. PVC piping is an ideal material. It is important to customize the splint so that it has the appropriate length and width and conforms well to the individual horse. Inappropriately placed or padded splints may produce large pressure sores, particularly in foals. Too little padding can lead to pressure sores, while too much padding will allow the splint to move around the horse's limb. The use of splints allows the clinician access to the wound as required, but they must be placed carefully. Application of a cast may be preferable for wounds where daily access is not required. A bivalved cast or bandage–cast combination permits the best of both worlds, allowing regular access to a wound and yet providing adequate

TABLE 64	**Types of semi-occlusive bandage**		
BANDAGE	CONTACT LAYER	INTERMEDIATE LAYER	USES
Dry-to-dry	Dry gauze, permeable	Dry, hydrophilic, permeable	Initial stages (debridement) of wound healing when mechanical debridement is needed.
Wet-to-dry	Wet gauze, permeable	Dry, hydrophilic, permeable	In wounds with moderately thick and abundant exudate.
Wet-to-wet	Wet gauze, permeable	Wet, hydrophilic, permeable	In wounds with a large amount of thick exudate.

Wound management and infections of synovial structures

1302 The use of a foot cast for the treatment of a severe heel bulb injury.

1303 This horse has a wound on the dorsal aspect of the carpus, which has been surgically repaired. The limb is bandaged post surgery in a full limb Robert Jones bandage, with splints fitted to the lateral and dorsal aspects of the limb from just distal to the elbow to just above the fetlock.

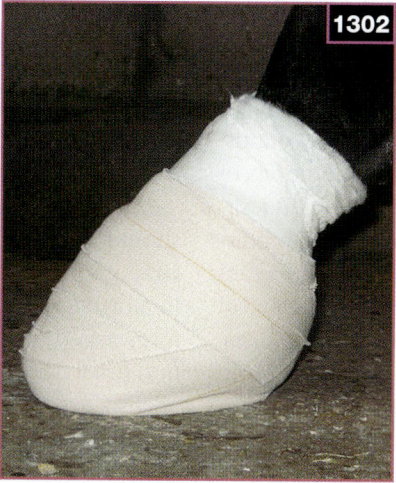

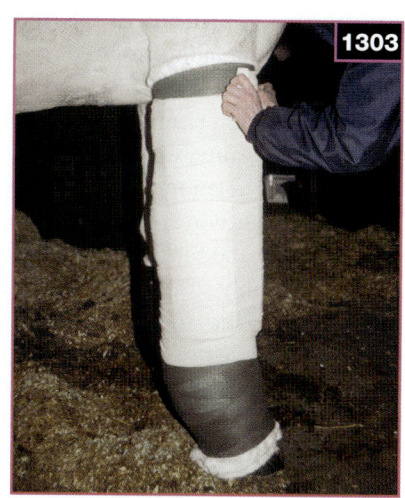

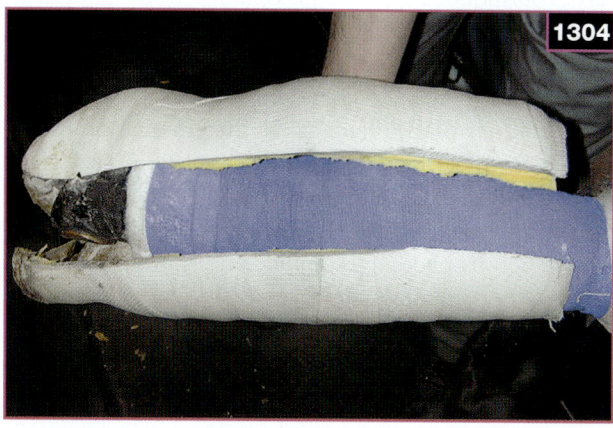

1304 A bivalved cast or cast–bandage combination is ideal to treat injuries that require immobilization and daily care. Note that the limb is not allowed to bear weight during wound therapy.

1305 A heel bulb and coronary band injury treated by surgical debridement, lavage, and stabilization in a foot cast. This is at the first change of the cast and already the wound is healthy, healing well by second intention, and showing no excessive granulation tissue.

immobilization (**1304**). This modality is extremely useful in cases of wounds affecting synovial cavities, particularly tendon lacerations involving the digital flexor tendon sheath, where the foot can be maintained in a fixed position between treatments and the wound can be accessed daily for care.

The use of casts for the treatment of open wounds, especially of the distal limb, will facilitate wound healing and prevent the formation of exuberant granulation tissue (**1305**). A cast requires daily evaluation for cracks or excessive exudates or inflammation at the top of the cast, or for lack of use by the horse or hot spots, which may indicate a pressure sore. If doubts exist pertaining to any complications, the cast should be removed and the limb evaluated. Pressure sores over areas such as the proximal sesamoids or accessory carpal bones may potentially lead to serious and expensive complications.

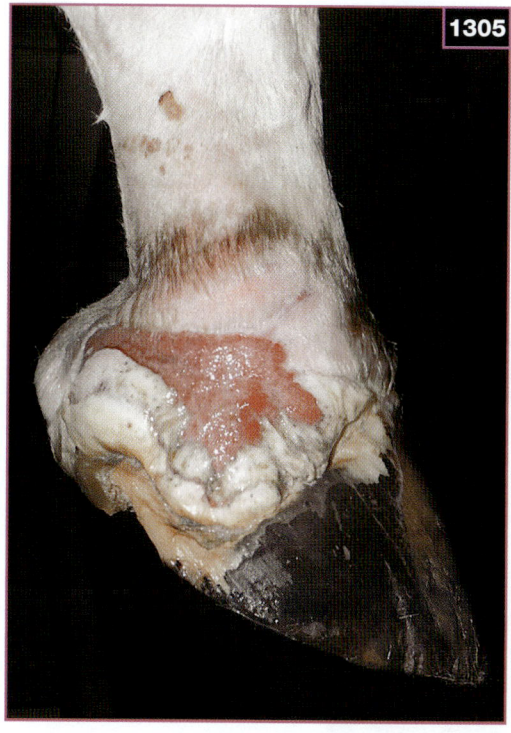

Exuberant granulation tissue management

Exuberant granulation tissue or 'proud flesh' stops the process of wound contraction and epithelialization and is the most common nonfatal complication of second-intention wound healing of equine distal extremity wounds. Exuberant granulation tissue occurs where conditions of motion and infection are present and results in an undesirable cosmetic and functional outcome. Individual predisposition is highly suspected as a risk factor for exuberant granulation tissue and it seems to be less prevalent in ponies. A complex cascade of events involving cytokines, particularly transforming growth factors β1 and β3, and their regulation may be at the origin of exuberant granulation tissue. The specific cause(s) of the development of exuberant granulation tissue remain(s) unknown.

Although a small amount of granulation tissue responds well to treatment, dealing with large amounts of exuberant granulation tissue can be a frustrating, lengthy, and costly process. Prevention of motion and infection early on in wound healing will greatly limit the incidence of proud flesh. Once exuberant granulation tissue has been identified, its management requires aggressive therapy. There are no treatments that consistently prevent or eliminate exuberant granulation tissue formation in all horses. The use of caustics and irritants, such as soda lime, turpentine, or motor oil, has not been shown to be an effective therapeutic alternative and, in fact, wound irritation may further delay wound healing.

1306 Trimming granulation tissue. The blade is maintained parallel to the wound surface and the granulation tissue is trimmed from distal to proximad. Note the amount of blood present during this procedure.

Topical corticosteroids can be beneficial, but the response is dose-dependent and in large doses they can also have undesirable side-effects. The principles of treating exuberant granulation tissue are radical surgical excision, topical use of corticosteroids, reduction of motion, elimination of wound infection, and the use of grafting techniques.

To debulk excessive granulation tissue the veterinarian should prepare the horse in a clean and well-lit area. Granulation tissue has abundant capillaries and thus hemorrhage will be profuse and the owner should be forewarned. Despite its absence of innervation, granulation tissue should be excised cautiously as the epithelial edges surrounding the patch of tissue will be sensitive to touch. Sedation is recommended in order to ensure the safety of the horse and veterinarian. Infiltration of local anesthetic into the wound periphery is not usually necessary. Tourniquet application is optional, and it should be removed as soon as the debulking is finished. Following a surgical preparation of the wound periphery and a saline wash of the granulation tissue surface, a scalpel or dermatome blade is placed flat against the granulation tissue. With a steady see-saw motion the granulation tissue is cut level with the epithelium, starting at the bottom of the wound and moving upwards (1306). A pressure bandage with generous padding is applied and left in place for 12 hours to ensure adequate hemostasis. Once hemostasis has been accomplished, bandaging, with or without topical medications, casting, or grafting, can be used to manage the wound.

Complications

The most common wound complications include the formation of exuberant granulation tissue, dehiscence, seroma formation, and infection. All of these can be related and the common result is failure to heal. It must be understood that the body always has a tendency to heal unless it is prevented from doing so by motion, infection, or self-inflicted trauma. On many occasions this will result in the formation of exuberant granulation tissue.

Wound dehiscence

Wound dehiscence may be due to wound infection, inadequate blood supply, excessive motion, or inappropriate holding power of the suture line, either tissue- or suture-related. Infection-related wound dehiscence may take several days to occur, while tension-related dehiscence may occur within the first 24 hours. The reason for the dehiscence must be identified and corrected. As long as the wound edges are healthy and strong, a dehisced wound can be resutured by treating the underlying infection for a few days and freshening the wound edges prior to closure. If the dehiscence occurs because of tension, a different closure technique may be used. Surgical techniques to reduce tension include the use of mattress suture

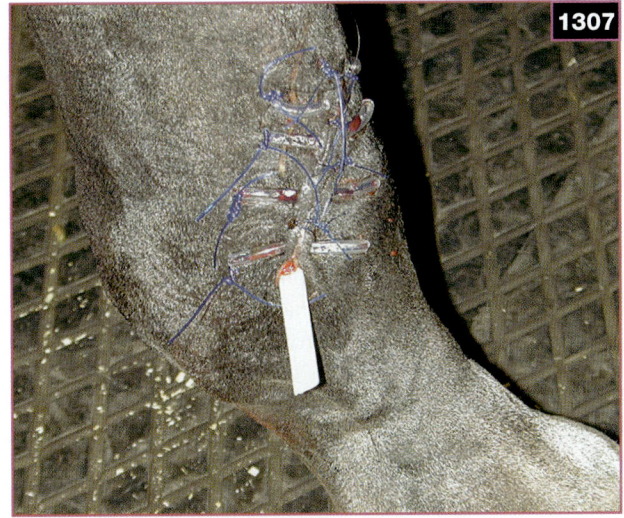

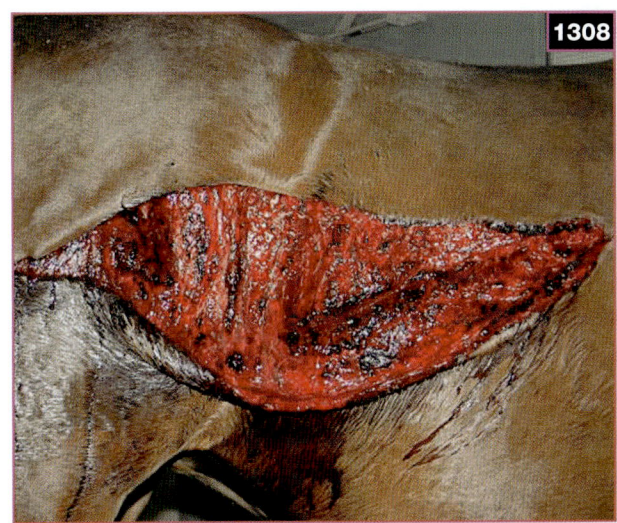

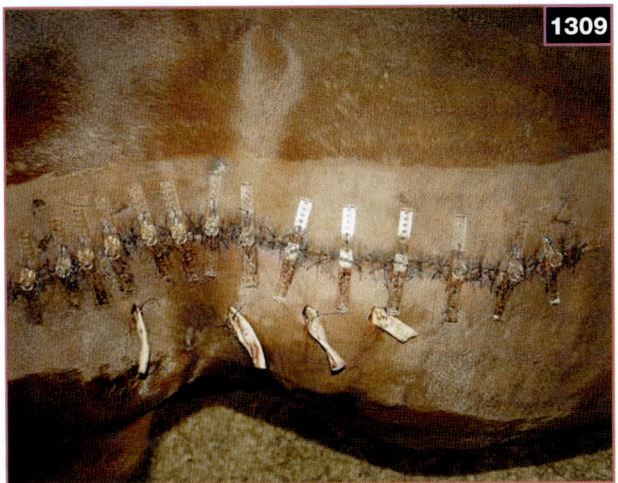

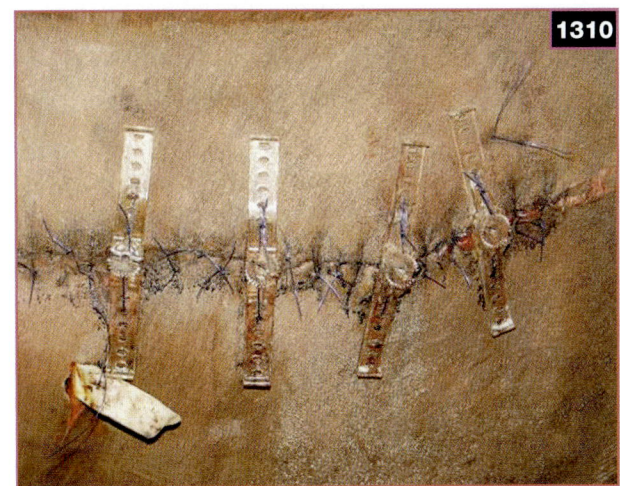

patterns, mesh-expansion techniques, stents, plastic reconstruction techniques, or tension-relief sutures. A favored technique is the use of vertical mattress sutures approximately 2.5–3.75 cm (1.0–1.5 inches) from the sutured wound. These can be placed every 5 or 7.5 cm (2 or 3 inches) in an attempt to reduce the tension on the suture line. When the suture line is under an excessive amount of tension, the suture may be threaded through a button or a small rubber sleeve to prevent the suture from cutting through the tissues (bolster sutures) (1307). Alternatively, wound edge approximators (1308–1310) have been used by the author with good results. This device allows daily approximation of the wound edges, prevents retraction of the wound, and evenly spreads the tension of each individual suture in order to minimize tissue damage. This device may require several days before apposition of wound edges is accomplished.

1307 The use of bolster sutures. Polyethylene tubing is used to distribute suture tension and minimize the chances of suture-induced tissue necrosis.

1308–1310 These three illustrations show how tissue approximators can be used in cases of large separation of skin edges. (1308) A flank wound prior to repair. (1309) The same wound repaired with the use of tissue approximators. (1310) Detail of the tissue approximators. The 'dial' piece in the center is used on a daily basis to approximate the wound edges. (Photos courtesy D Trout)

Seroma formation

Seromas usually occur due to increased subcutaneous dead space, inadequate hemostasis, the presence of foreign bodies, or severe inflammation. Small and innocuous seromas should be monitored and left alone to resolve with time. Hot compresses can also be applied to help resolution. If the seroma gets progressively larger and jeopardizes the suture line, it should be drained either by aspiration or by providing a drainage route. Prior to intervening it is recommended that an ultrasound evaluation of the seroma cavity and its contents is carried out. This will provide the clinician with information pertaining to the size of the sermoa, the volume and nature of the exudates, and potentially identify a foreign body. Careless aspiration of contents may introduce bacteria into the seroma and lead to a severe infection. In addition, it may only provide temporary relief until the seroma reforms, usually in 24–48 hours. The placement of a drain and pressure bandage is indicated in cases of large seromas.

Skin grafting

Overview

The purpose of skin grafting is (1) to accelerate and facilitate the process of wound healing; (2) to prevent the development of exuberant granulation tissue; and (3) to improve the cosmetic outcome of the healing process.

Full-thickness grafts include the entire dermis and epidermis, while partial- or split-thickness grafts include the entire epidermis and a variable portion of the dermis, depending on the thickness of the graft. Split-thickness grafts are 0.5–0.76 mm thick. Ideally they should be harvested with a dermatome (**1311**) that ensures a consistent and uniform graft thickness. Each type of graft has definite advantages and disadvantages (*Table 65*).

The healing process of a skin graft goes through a sequence of adherence and graft nutrition (48 hours), revascularization (2–4 days), firm union (7–10 days), and contraction (primary or immediate, secondary or delayed). Graft failure is usually due to infection, motion, or accumulation of fluid beneath the graft. Infection impedes vascular

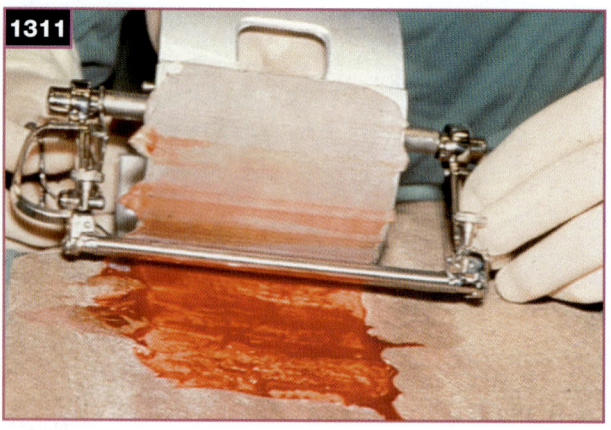

1311

1311 A drum dermatome is shown during split-thickness graft collection. (Photo courtesy S Barber)

TABLE 65 **Advantages and disadvantages of the different types of skin grafts**		
TYPE OF GRAFT	**ADVANTAGES**	**DISADVANTAGES**
Full-thickness grafts (pinch, punch, tunnel, or sheet)	• Practical in the standing horse • No specialized equipment required • Better cosmetic outcome	• Morbidity of donor site • Slower revascularization and 'graft-take' • Slower healing • Limited graft size • Greater primary contraction
Split-thickness grafts (thin, medium, or thick sheet grafts)	• Quicker revascularization and 'graft-take' • Faster healing • Abundance of donor skin	• Specialized equipment required • General anesthesia required • Poorer cosmetic outcome • More secondary contraction

954

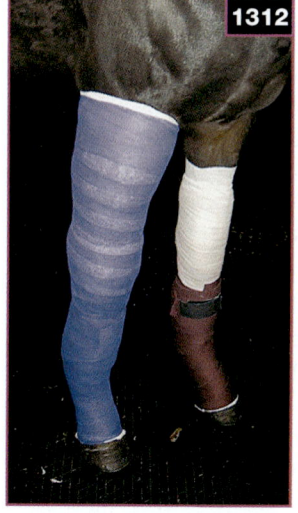
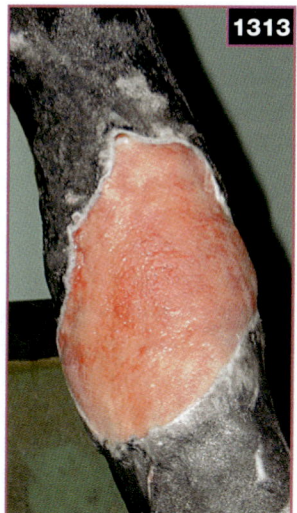
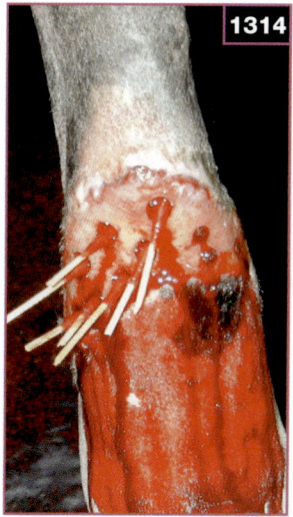
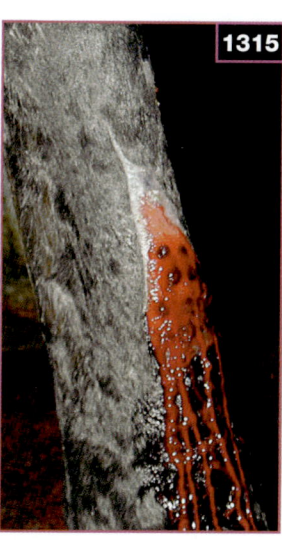

supply at the microvascular level by formation of micro-thrombi and also leads to an increased level of fibrinolytic substances, which compromise graft adherence. Fluid accumulation beneath the graft may prevent revascularization by physical separation of the donor and recipient elements, leading to graft ischemia and necrosis. Meticulous preparation of the donor graft and recipient site is essential to diminish the likelihood of graft failure. This may include wound surface antimicrobial strategies and accurate hemostasis while placing the graft. Excessive motion will compromise the graft by affecting the process of graft attachment and revascularization. The use of appropriate bandaging techniques (1312) or cast immobilization is required to prevent excessive motion, particularly in high-motion areas such as joints.

Appropriate recipient site preparation and proper grafting procedure are vital to achieve success. Grafts should be transplanted to wounds with a healthy granulation-tissue bed, which is characterized by a good vascular supply and uniform granulation tissue with absence of cracks or fissures and level with the peripheral epithelium (1313). The absence of a large bacterial load or suppurating focus is mandatory for successful grafting. Once the wound is covered by a healthy granulation-tissue bed, this should be trimmed to eliminate surface contaminants and to level it with the peripheral epithelium. Granulation tissue bleeds profusely when trimmed (see 1306) and this procedure should be avoided immediately prior to grafting. Following trimming, the wound should be bandaged in a sterile manner with a nonadherent dressing to facilitate hemostasis. The use of topical preparations (e.g. silver sulfadiazine or diluted Dakin's solution) helps to ensure a low or absent bacterial load prior to grafting. Ideally, preparation of the recipient site should be done within 24 hours of grafting.

1312 A properly applied bandage must give the impression of firmness, cleanliness, and tidiness.

1313 A granulation-tissue bed ready for grafting must be flush with the epithelial edges and appear well vascularized, with minimal exudates and no discolored tissues.

1314 Cotton buds applied to the recipient site of punch grafts to facilitate hemostasis and improve graft 'take'.

1315 Punch grafts in place. Note that the grafts are slightly below the granulation-tissue surface and are separated by about 0.5 cm.

Pinch or punch grafts

Despite their practicality, which makes them a good option under field conditions, full-thickness punch or pinch grafts require meticulous preparation and application to succeed. During and after grafting, the most important aspects to keep in mind are adequate hemostasis and elimination of motion. Hemostasis can be produced by temporarily packing cotton tips into the granulation-tissue defect created to receive the donor skin (1314). Punch grafts are maintained in place by pressure-fitting the donor graft into a smaller recipient site. Immediate graft contraction after they have been taken means that the donor graft should be at least 2 mm wider than the recipient site (1315). Pinch grafts are placed into a horizontal pocket created to ensure graft stability. Vascular invasion or 'take' of a full-thickness graft is facilitated by removing any subcutaneous fat that

955

may have been acquired with the donor graft. Pinch or punch grafts should be placed about 5 mm apart within the recipient granulation tissue. Appropriate bandaging is crucial to maximize graft survival. Excessive motion and premature bandage changes will reduce the chances of graft take. Ideally, a modified Robert Jones bandage or cast should be applied for 5 days, by which time many of the grafts would have been incorporated into the donor site. The contact layer of the bandage should be removed with extreme caution to prevent tearing grafts away from the recipient bed. It is common for only a percentage of the grafts to survive, and 70% survival would be considered a good outcome.

Tunnel grafts

Tunnel grafts can also be used in the field. They require tunneling of the granulation-tissue bed and the implantation of a full-thickness rectangular (narrow and long) graft beneath the granulation-tissue surface with the skin facing upwards (1316). The entry and exit points of the graft should be adequately identified in order to facilitate identification of the granulation tissue overlying the graft, usually 7–10 days after implantation, and allow its removal. Failure to do so may lead to inadvertent graft damage during the graft-uncovering process.

Split-thickness grafts

Split-thickness grafts include mesh grafts, which are technically more demanding and unlikely to be practical under field situations (1317). If a large area of skin needs to be grafted, it is best to refer these cases to a fully equipped hospital for application of a meshed sheet graft.

Burns

Thermal injuries in horses are most frequently due to barn or forest fires (1318). The most important aspect when evaluating burns in the horse is to provide analgesia and quickly evaluate the damage, as a poor prognosis should be an indicator for euthanasia. The prognosis is directly related to the extent and severity of the burns. The amount of body surface involved in a burn is expressed as a percentage of total body surface. Each forelimb represents 9%, each hindlimb 18%, the head and the neck 9%, and the dorsal and ventral thorax/abdomen 18% each. Severe burns involving 50% of the body surface area are associated with a high degree of mortality. The severity of burns has been classified from 1st to 4th degree (*Table 66*).

The systemic effects associated with burns depend on the severity and extent of the burn and include severe anemia, hemoglobinemia and hemoglobinuria, hypernatremia, immediate hyperkalemia, and a delayed diuretic hypokalemia. Electrolyte monitoring during the first 2 weeks post wounding is paramount to avoid serious electrolyte shifts and ensure optimal systemic management. Horses with burns are at high risk of developing a life-threatening septicemia, and systemic antibiotics are recommended. A high-calorie diet, and possibly anabolic steroids, are also required due to the catabolic state that follows burn injuries in horses. Very important, and not necessarily related to the severity of skin lesions, is pulmonary damage by smoke inhalation. This produces direct damage to the airways and lung tissue by exposure to heat, particulate matter in smoke, and the gaseous by-products of fire. Smoke inhalation injury can lead to bronchospasm

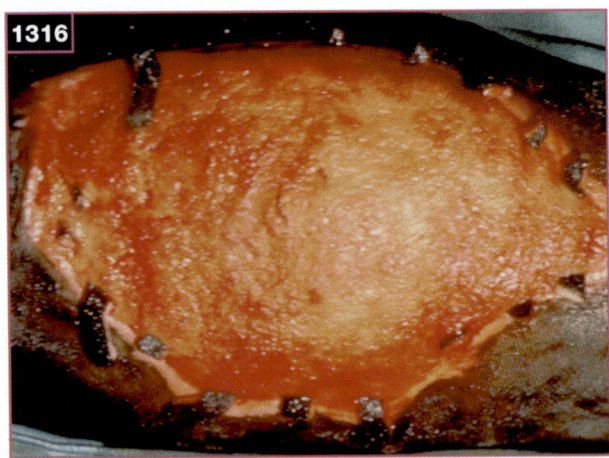

1316 Tunnel or 'strip' grafts are shown. Note that the grafts are easily identifiable. This will facilitate the location of the graft and prevent iatrogenic damage during 'de-roofing'.

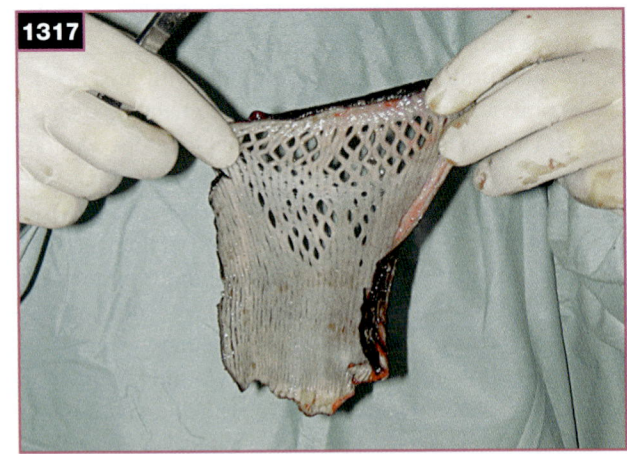

1317 A split-thickness graft following collection and meshing and ready to be applied.

Wound management and infections of synovial structures

1318 This horse was involved in a barn fire and sustained severe burns over most of the dorsum of its body. At this stage the horse has had several sessions of pinch grafting and the area affected by the burns is gradually healing by second intention.

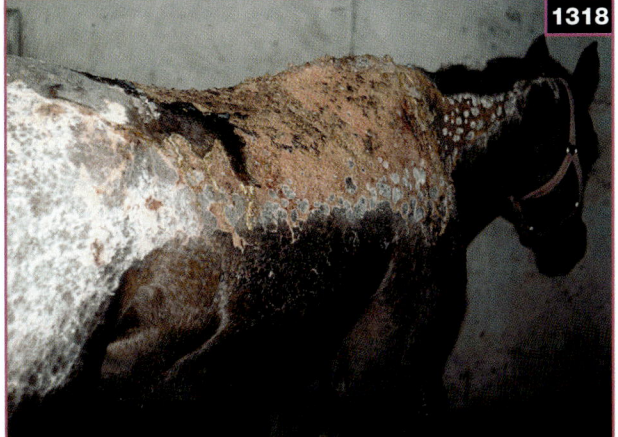

1318

TABLE 66 **Classification of burns according to the degree of tissue damage**

CLASSIFICATION	SIGNS
First degree	Erythema, edema, pain, desquamation of superficial layers
Second degree superficial	Fluid accumulation between stratum granulosum and basal cell layers (blister), moderate pain
Second degree deep	Edema fluid at epidermal–dermal junction, epidermal necrosis, increase in WBCs at basal layer, eschar production, minimal pain
Third degree	Loss of epidermal and dermal elements, fluid and cell response at the margins and deeper tissue, eschar formation, lack of pain, shock, infection
Fourth degree	Carbonization of tissue, deep tissue destruction as far down as muscle, bone, etc.

and bronchoconstriction, carbon monoxide poisoning, pulmonary edema, acute respiratory distress, and pneumonia. Treatment involves the administration of supplemental moistened oxygen (if there is difficulty in breathing) and the use of bronchodilators. The overall therapy of patients with burns should have several stages, with different goals in mind depending on their severity:

✦ 1st stage (0–4 days): systemic and respiratory stabilization of the horse, analgesia, wound protection, prevention of sepsis.
✦ 2nd stage (5–10 days): progressive wound debridement, wound protection, systemic support, prevention of sepsis.
✦ 3rd stage (10 days onwards): wound repair, protection, restoration of epithelium.

First-degree burns should be cooled with ice or cold water. In addition, prevention of infection dictates the use of a topical antibacterial preparation and the protection of the wound from further trauma. These wounds may be left uncovered. Analgesia is indicated.

Superficial second-degree burns are characterized by the formation of a blister, which should be left intact if at all possible. If the blister bursts, it is sensible to remove the tissue and clean and protect the affected area with a bandage. A scab may provide adequate initial protection

to a wound as long as it is not disturbed or does not become infected. In addition, a nonadherent dressing or a petrolatum- or antibiotic-impregnated gauze should be applied as a contact layer. This bandage needs to be changed as required depending on the extent of the wound, location, possibility of bacterial contamination, and the amount of exudate present.

Deep second-degree burns and third-degree burns require a closed technique, which includes the use of an occlusive bandage, as long as there is no infection or scab, or much exudate. The eschar technique allows the wound to be protected by the presence of the eschar and works best in small burnt areas. It is not indicated in large burns or areas where the burn may become traumatized. Since the wound is left open, the clinician must be aware that trauma and/or infection may occur. The third technique is called semi-open and involves the continuous application of moist bandages and antibacterial agents to the eschar. A moist dressing prevents heat and moisture loss, protects the eschar, and helps prevent bacterial contamination and infection. The frequent bandage changes with this technique allow frequent wound debridement and even though it is time-consuming, it controls the amount of tissue removed so healthy tissue is not accidentally or excessively removed.

Wound management and infections of synovial structures

Wounds involving synovial structures

Overview

Wounds affecting any synovial structure can be devastating and potentially life-threatening. For this reason, any wound in the vicinity of a joint or tendon sheath must be thoroughly investigated to rule out synovial involvement (1319). This may require careful sterile digital exploration or increasing the pressure of the synovial structure by instilling intrasynovial sterile lactated Ringer's solution in order to investigate communication with the wound. Relying on the pain level to diagnose synovial involvement may not be adequate, particularly in cases where the synovial structure has been opened and allowed to drain through the wound. Centesis of a potentially affected synovial structure at a remote location from the original wound is essential. The clinician must judge whether the benefits of synoviocentesis outweigh its risks. In cases where a severe cellulitis exists around the wounded area, the clinician must be careful not to seed a previously uninfected synovium by performing a synoviocentesis. In these cases, aggressive anti-inflammatory and antibiotic therapy is recommended until the inflammation calms down and a safe area to perform a synoviocentesis can be identified.

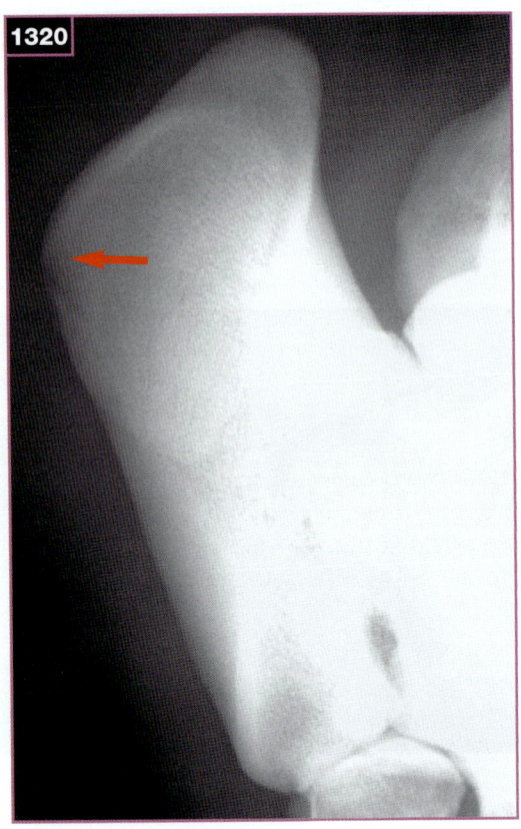

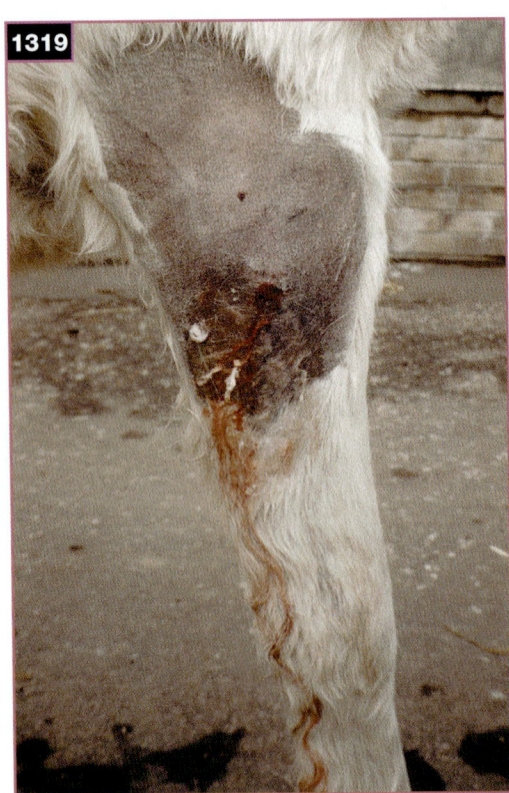

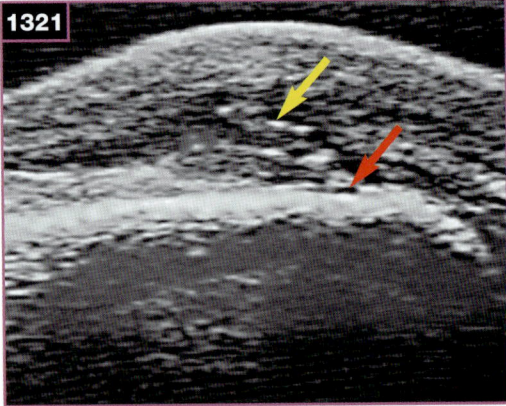

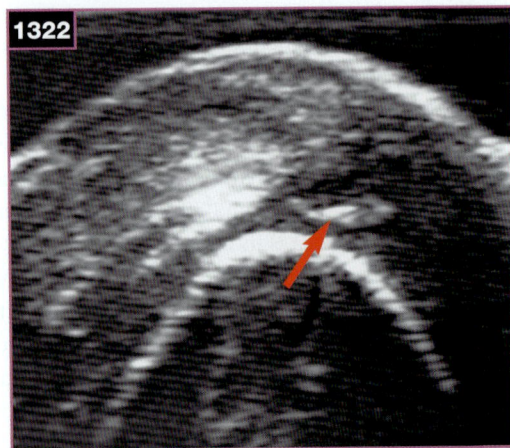

1319 This pony received a kick wound to the left lateral elbow region and penetration of the joint has occurred. Note the discharging synovial fluid.

Wound management and infections of synovial structures

1320–1322 (1320) Dorso 45° lateral/plantaromedial oblique radiograph of the calcaneus of a horse that has received a kick wound to the proximal medial aspect of the point of the hock. Note the subtle lysis of the cortical surface of the calcaneus just below the point of the hock (arrow). (1321) Longitudinal ultrasonogram of the wound area showing the superficial damage to the bone surface (red arrow), overlying soft-tissue proliferation, and mild distension of the intertendonous calcaneal bursa (yellow arrow). (1322) Transverse ultrasonogram of the wound area showing a small separate fragment of bone to the lateral (left) side of the calcaneus (arrow).

1323 A very common injury, particularly in racehorses, is a laceration in the palmar aspect of the distal metacarpal region. Most of these injuries penetrate the tendon sheath and may have a degree of tendon damage.

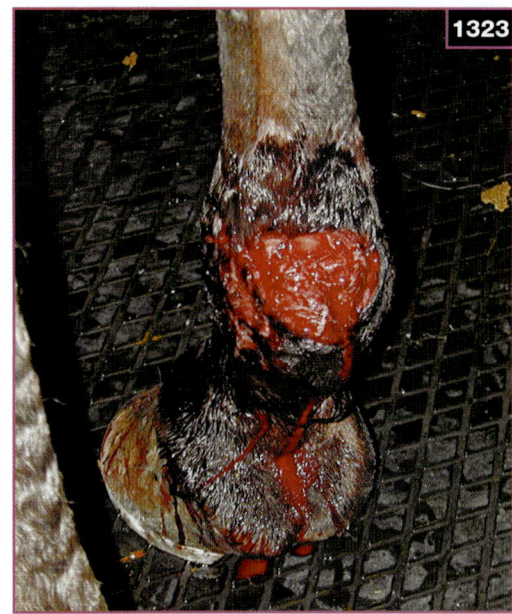

Failure to diagnose a penetrated synovial cavity promptly may delay initial therapy and jeopardize the outcome. Radiographic and ultrasonographic evaluation of the area is strongly suggested, as bone involvement or the presence of foreign bodies will dictate further courses of action and prognosis (**1320-1322**).

Two of the most commonly injured synovial structures are the fetlock joint and the digital flexor tendon sheath (**1323**), perhaps as a result of self-inflicted damage during racing or an encounter with a sharp object. Fully open synovial cavities are easier to detect and carry a better prognosis than puncture wounds. A mixed bacterial population is usually present. Broad-spectrum antimicrobial therapy should be used, with particular focus on coliforms, *Streptococcus* spp., and *Staphylococcus* spp. Meticulous initial exploration and sterile bandage changes are required when a synovial structure has been penetrated. The overall prognosis depends on prompt diagnosis and aggressive long-term (around 6 weeks) therapy with a combination of anti-inflammatory drugs, local and systemic antimicrobials, analgesia, and synovial lavage or drainage.

Management of synovial sepsis in the adult

Infection within a synovial structure produces the greatest and most dramatic joint/sheath inflammatory response and a marked synovial effusion. This effusion is easily detected except in cases where the joint is not clearly palpable, such as the hip, or where periarticular cellulitis and severe edema are present. Confirmation of an infectious synovial process is obtained through cytologic evaluation of synovial fluid. A previous intra-articular steroid injection (up to 3 weeks) is a risk factor for the development of a septic joint and may also alter the expected cytologic findings. The interpretation of synovial fluid results should include assessment of protein content, differential cell count, and cellular morphologic characteristics. The presence of 75% or more neutrophils or toxic changes to neutrophils, with a compatible medical history, should be considered evidence of synovial sepsis until proven otherwise. If any doubt exists pertaining to the diagnosis, the clinician should assume that a synovial cavity is infected and start treatment promptly. Failure to treat a synovial infection promptly may jeopardize the final outcome.

The treatment of infectious synovitis is aimed at different areas: (1) eliminating the causative organism(s); (2) diminishing the inflammatory process and providing analgesia; (3) restoring synovial homeostasis; and (4) rehabilitating the horse.

Eliminating the causative organism(s)

The organisms involved in synovial infections are generally well known. Postinjection synovial infections are most commonly caused by *Staphyloccocus aureus* and post-traumatic infections by coliforms. This may not always be the case and the sensitivity patterns vary depending on geographic location and bacterial strain. Failure to obtain a positive culture, which can happen in up to 50% of cases, should not preclude an educated guess as to what antibiotics may be most effective. Bacterial elimination from a synovial cavity is achieved by a combination of antimicrobial therapy and synovial lavage. Synovial lavage is best performed by arthroscopy, although where cost is an issue it can be carried out by a through-and-through method using needles and drip sets. In refractory cases, open joint

959

TABLE 67 **Local and regional antimicrobial therapy options for infections of synovial structures**

	INTRAOSSEUS	INTRAVENOUS	INTRASYNOVIAL
Method	Use 4.5 mm or 5.5 mm cannulated screw (custom-made or manufactured by Cook). Can be placed standing or under GA. Perfuse under sedation over 30–45 minutes.	Use a butterfly needle (18–20 gauge) or a catheter. Can be performed on saphenous, cephalic, or abaxial sesamoid vessel.	Direct daily injection or use of CRI pump.
Amikacin	Administer 1 mg/kg q24h for 3–5 days diluted in 60 ml of total saline volume. Inject slowly over a period of 2–4 minutes. Total volume in foals may be decreased to 12 ml.	Same as intraosseous.	Administer 125–250 mg by direct injection q24h for 3–5 days. If used in a CRI pump, will deliver 10 ml (2,500 mg/450 kg) of amikacin/day.
Gentamicin	Administer 1–2 mg/kg q24h for 3–5 days diluted in 60 ml of total saline volume. Inject slowly over a period of 2–4 minutes. Total volume in foals may be decreased to 12 ml.	Same as intraosseous.	Administer 100–300 mg by direct injection q24h for 3–5 days. If used in a CRI pump, will deliver 6 ml (600 mg/450 kg) of gentamicin/day.
Ceftiofur	Administer 1 mg/kg q24h for 3–5 days diluted in 60 ml of total saline volume. Inject slowly over a period of 2–4 minutes. Total volume in foals may be decreased to 12 ml.	Same as intraosseous.	Administer 150 mg by direct injection. If used in a CRI pump, make a 50% ceftiofur solution (25 mg/ml) and deliver 0.5 ml solution/hour (300 mg/day).
Vancomycin	Administer 300 mg diluted to a maximum of 5 mg/ml and give at a speed of 2 ml/minute or 10 mg/minute, q24h for 3–5 days.	Same as intraosseous.	Not recommended.
Advantages	Good concentration in synovial fluid, medullary cavity, and tendons distal to perfusion site. Concentrations persist up to 24 hours and slightly longer compared with intravenous perfusion. Very well tolerated. Minimal side-effects.	Very good concentration lasting over 24 hours.	Very good concentrations lasting over 24 hours.
Disadvantages	Need special equipment. Painful perfusion. Potential blemish over perforated bone. Avoid proximity to any tendon.	Very difficult in cases where cellulitis prevents identification of the vessel. Repeated injection necessary if catheter not placed. Catheter may kink or dislodge. Difficult to maintain in distal extremity. Sloughing of hoof possible if vascular damage occurs at the level of the distal extremity.	Daily injection needed. CRI device sometimes may not work properly.

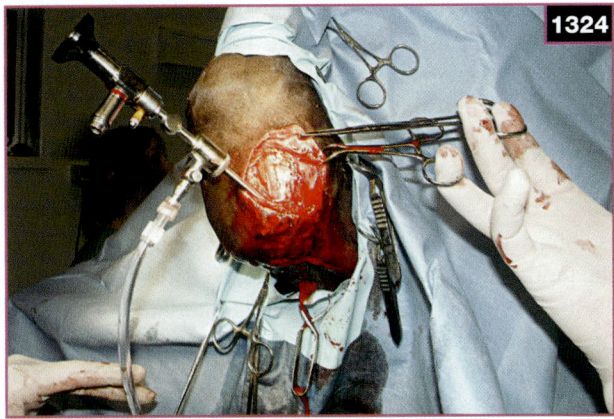

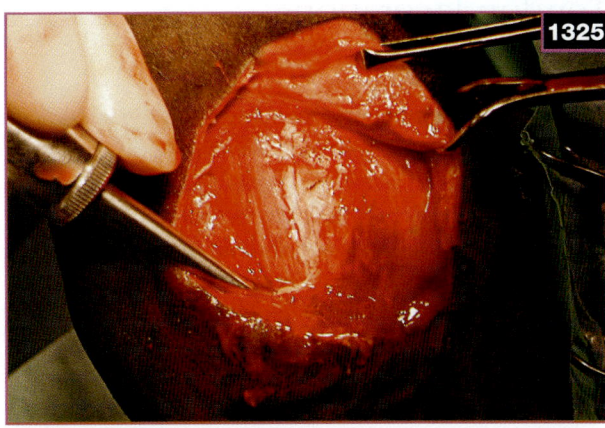

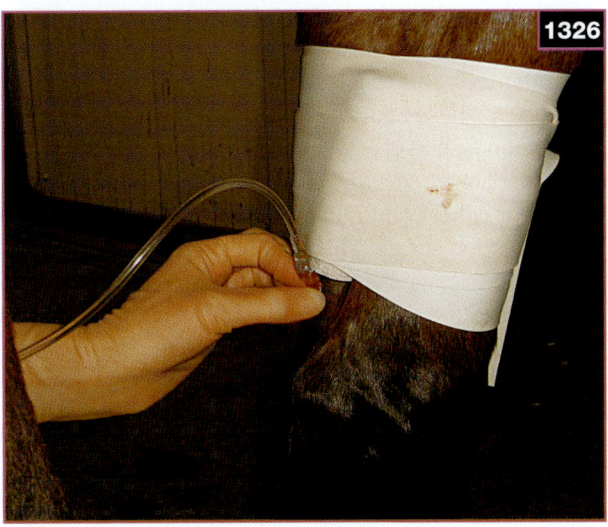

1324–1326 This horse fell on the road when at exercise, lacerated the dorsal aspect of its right carpus, and subsequently had synovial fluid draining from the wound. Under general anesthesia and after surgical debridement/exploration of the wound, a defect into the dorsolateral aspect of the antebrachiocarpal joint was detected. This allowed an arthroscope to be inserted into the joint for exploration and lavage (1324). After the joint was lavaged, the tendon sheath of the extensor carpi radialis was also lavaged, as this had been involved in the trauma and was contaminated (1325). Distal limb regional perfusion of antibiotics can be carried out in the standing sedated horse (1326). Note the tourniquet placed on the forearm proximal to the carpus and the intravenous catheter in the cephalic vein.

drainage may be necessary (1324, 1325). Currently, the most widely used antibiotic combination is either penicillin or a third-generation cephalosporin (e.g. ceftiofur, ceftazidime), together with an aminoglycoside (e.g. amikacin). Systemic and local/regional administration of antibiotics in cases of synovial sepsis has become a routine treatment. Local/regional antibiotics are very effective in eliminating bacterial infection from synovial structures, and should be included as a treatment strategy in these cases (1326, *Table 67*).

Reducing inflammation and providing analgesia
The benefits of adequate analgesia cannot be overemphasized. Comfort allows the animal to ambulate and diminishes potential complications associated with pain and lack of movement such as impaction colic, other limb overuse injuries, and adhesion formation in cases of intrathecal infections. The most common NSAIDs used are phenylbutazone, flunixin meglumine, and ketoprofen. Any of these seem to work adequately, although the authors favor the use of phenylbutazone (2.2–4.4 mg/kg q24h, depending on the response to therapy). In severely

painful cases or in those where NSAIDs may not be indicated, the use of epidural morphine (0.01–0.3 mg/kg) (hindlimbs) or fentanyl patches (2–4 10 mg patches q72h) (forelimbs) provides good analgesia and comfort superior to NSAIDs. Analgesia also permits early ambulation, which may have a very positive effect on the rehabilitation of horses affected with synovial infection. Abusing a heavy analgesic regimen could potentially mask clinical deterioration or recrudescence of the infection, and the clinician should titrate the analgesic protocol to the minimal dosage needed.

Restoring synovial homeostasis
The restoration of synovial hemostasis occurs with time once the inflammatory process has subsided. If the damage inflicted has been severe, synovial homeostasis may never be fully reached. The intrasynovial administration of hyaluronic acid provides anti-inflammatory effects and helps restore normality. Passive rest followed by hand walking, starting once the acute inflammation has subsided, is also beneficial. Systemic and/or oral glycosaminoglycans supplements may be useful.

Tendon lacerations

Flexor tendon

Flexor tendon lacerations commonly affect the superficial and/or deep digital flexor tendons and, on rare occasions, other tendonous structures as well (1327). The clinician should promptly identify the characteristic appearance of a distal limb that has lost flexor support. In cases where the suspensory ligament has also been severed or torn, the fetlock will be dramatically dropped (1328). In cases where palmar/plantar support has been lost or severely compromised, immediate support of the distal limb is mandatory, as failure to do so may predispose to hyper-extension of the limb resulting in overstretching of the palmar/plantar blood vessels and severely compromising the vascular supply. Flexor tendon lacerations in the forelimb may occur as a result of overreaching injuries in racehorses. These injuries are commonly associated with small wounds; however, wound size should not be associated with damage severity. Laceration of the flexor tendons may occur either within (intrathecal) or outside (extrathecal) the tendon sheath. This is an important distinction, as the clinical management and prognosis vary according to the location of the injury and to whether only the superficial digital flexor tendon and/or the deep digital flexor tendon and/or suspensory ligament have been involved. Intrathecal injuries have the added dimension of a contaminated synovial cavity, therefore extrathecal injuries are simpler to manage. Prompt and aggressive therapy is recommended. Management of lacerated flexor tendons requires time and money, and many horses may not return to their previous level of athletic activity. Whether tenorrhaphy is used or not, the rehabilitation period often spans an entire year. The use of tenorrhaphy is controversial. In general it is advocated in cases where the tendon edges have not been severely damaged (1329, 1330) and the injury is intrathecal. In addition, it appears that tenorrhaphy allows a quicker tensile strength gain during the first 12 weeks, thus facilitating the management of weight bearing.

Horses with lacerated tendons should be maintained in a cast for a period extending from 8–12 weeks depending on the severity of the damage and the response to treatment. If the wound needs daily care, the application of a bivalved cast or a bandage–cast combination is useful. A light bandage is placed on the limb before casting. It is important that the cast is not too snug in order to allow for daily changing of the underlying bandage. Once the cast has been set, it is split in two halves, which are secured in place with duct tape. To change the bandage, the limb should be held up and the bivalved cast opened to allow attention to the wound and application of a new bandage. The horse must not bear weight on the affected limb at this time.

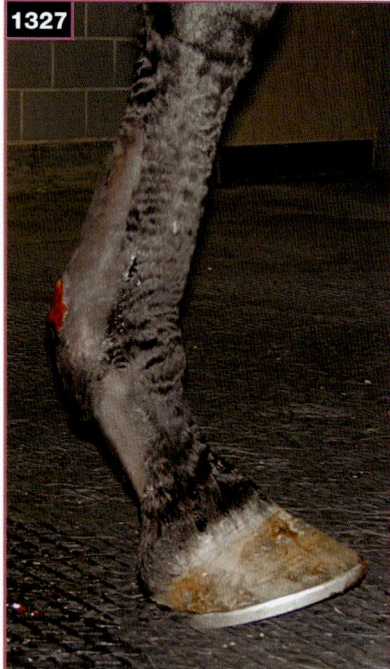

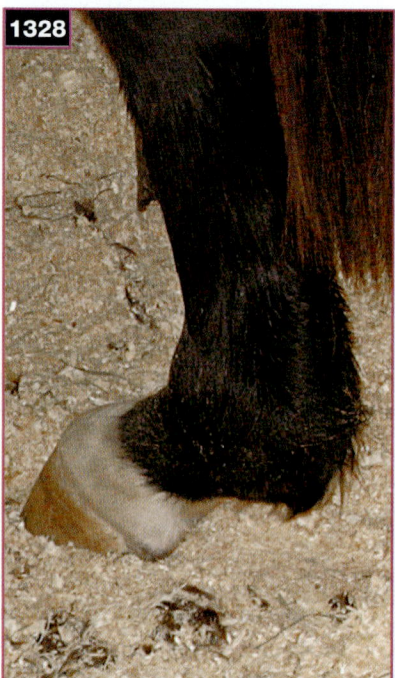

1327 The forelimb of a horse following a small laceration in the distal metacarpal area. Despite the small size of the laceration, loss of flexor tendon (deep digital flexor) support is obvious by the elevated position of the toe.

1328 This picture shows an abnormal fetlock angle as a result of 'suspensory apparatus breakdown'. Note the almost horizontal position of the first phalanx.

Wound management and infections of synovial structures

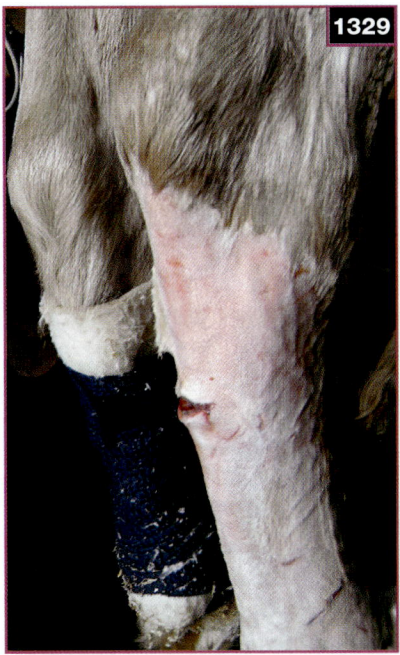

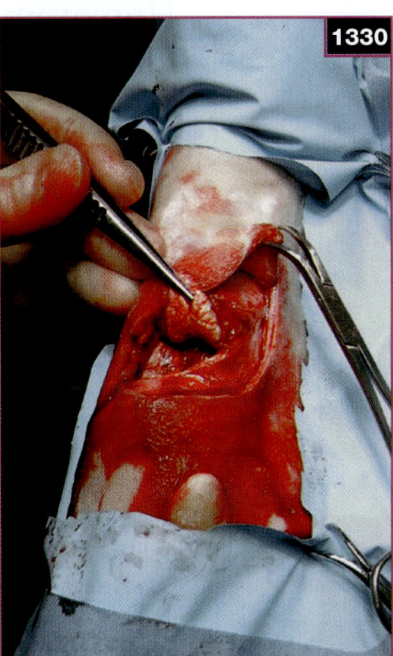

1329, 1330 There is a small laceration to the skin of the upper plantar cannon of the right hindlimb of this horse (1329). At surgical exploration of the wound there is a partial laceration of the plantar surface of the superficial digital flexor tendon, which was debrided and repaired (1330).

The weight-bearing management and rehabilitation protocol for flexor tendon lacerations includes:

✦ Weeks 1–6. Nonweight bearing. Limb in a cast or Kimzey splint. Stall rest.
✦ Weeks 6–9. As for previous six weeks or Patten shoe applied with heel elevation at approximately 30 degrees. Limb maintained in a Robert Jones bandage. Stall rest.
✦ Weeks 9–12. Patten shoe dropped at 15 degrees. Stall rest.
✦ Weeks 12–16. Patten shoe replaced by shoe with elevated heels at 12 degrees. Stall rest.
✦ Weeks 16–20. Heel elevation at 9 degrees. Hand walking for 5 minutes once daily.
✦ Weeks 20–24. Heel elevation at 9 degrees. Hand walking for 10 minutes once daily.
✦ Weeks 24–28. Heel elevation at 6 degrees. Hand walking for 5 minutes once daily.
✦ Weeks 28–32. Heel elevation at 6 degrees. Hand walking for 10 minutes once daily.
✦ Weeks 32–40. Heel elevation at 3 degrees. Hand walking for 5 minutes once daily with 5 minutes increments every week until week 40.
✦ Weeks 40–44. Heel elevation at 3 degrees. Hand walking for 20 minutes once daily. Light trot for 5 minutes once daily.
✦ Weeks 44–48. Normal shoe. Carry on exercise at 20 minutes walking exercise under saddle and 5 minutes trot on a lunge line with 5-minute weekly increments.
✦ Week 48–52. Start light flat work.

In addition, it is important that ultrasonographic evidence of healing is obtained every 8 weeks during the healing process.

Extensor tendon

Extensor tendon lacerations usually occur at the level of the cannon bone in either the fore- or hindlimbs. The common (forelimb) or long (hindlimb) extensor tendon in the distal limb lacks a synovial membrane, thus simplifying the management of lacerations. Tenorrhaphy is not necessary and maintenance of the limb in a cast, bandage, or splint is usually sufficient to encourage healing. The general principles of wound care apply to these wounds, and the edges of the tendon can be debrided to encourage fibroplasia. These lacerations are rewarding to clinicians because the associated prognosis is often excellent. Initially, the horse is unable to extend the limb and the use of a cast or splint is recommended during the healing process (6–8 weeks). It is not uncommon to find the edges of the tendon 5–7.5 cm (2–3 inches) apart, but this does not seem to affect the final outcome. Horses seem to rehabilitate from this injury very well and most of them return to their previous level of activity.

Hematomas

A hematoma is a collection of free blood in the tissues. Hematomas are usually caused by high-impact contusions. These damage blood vessels of different caliber, determining the size of the hematoma. A large hematoma constitutes an ideal area for bacteria to proliferate, resulting in abscess formation and tissue sloughing. The severity of the clinical signs and consequences associated with a hematoma depend on its size, location, and whether or not it is colonized by bacteria. Horses suffer from high-impact trauma as a result of kicks, self-inflicted during casting episodes, fence trapping, or rope burns. These injuries usually do not result in skin breakage (**1331**) and produce an ideal environment for bacterial colonization and proliferation. In addition, the accumulation of fluid beneath a rigid fascial plane may result in the development of compartment syndrome. This pressure increase is responsible for the interruption of lymphatic drainage and blood supply to the surrounding tissues, which eventually produces severe edema, inflammation, and tissue necrosis (see **1281**). Horses affected by compartment syndrome usually present with a very severe lameness and pain, with a mildly swollen and turgid affected region. This is most commonly seen in the external aspect of the thigh, affecting the quadriceps region. Due to the initial lack of skin breakage and severe and nonspecific signs, large hematomas leading to compartment syndrome are usually unnoticed. Clinicians should be aware that subsequent regional celullitis may become a serious and life-threatening injury and horses should be treated promptly. The area should be investigated by ultrasound and the clinician should exercise extreme caution if aspirating the affected region. In the initial stages of a hematoma, the area should be iced to produce vasoconstriction and stop further bleeding. After the initial 48 hours this should be followed with warm therapy to facilitate reabsorption of the hematoma. Aggressive anti-inflammatory therapy, broad-spectrum antibiotics, and diuretics should be administered to reduce the inflammation and edema present and to prevent or treat a possible infection. If compartment syndrome is diagnosed, the area should be opened and a fasciotomy performed (**1332**) to drain the tissues, release the pressure, and prevent tissue necrosis. In advanced stages of compartment syndrome, tissue necrosis and sloughing occur and the prognosis is grave even when aggressive therapy is used. Following its resolution, a large hematoma may also result in tissue fibrosis and calcification, potentially leading to gait abnormalities.

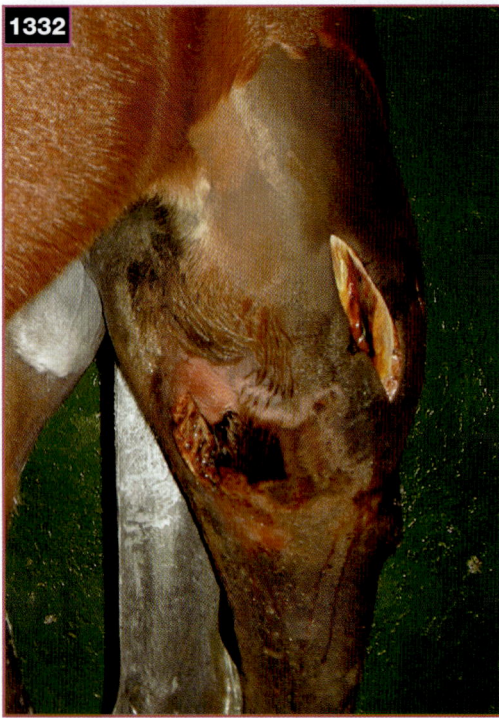

1331 A hematoma of the thigh region in a horse following a kick. Note the area of discoloration in the central aspect of the thigh. These injuries may potentially lead to compartment syndrome, with catastrophic consequences if not attended to promptly.

1332 A fasciotomy of the fascia lata has been performed in this case following a severe hematoma of the quadriceps musculature. Tissue necrosis had already occurred at the time of presentation and aggressive therapy was therefore deemed necessary.

14

The foal

Sarah Stoneham and Graham Munroe

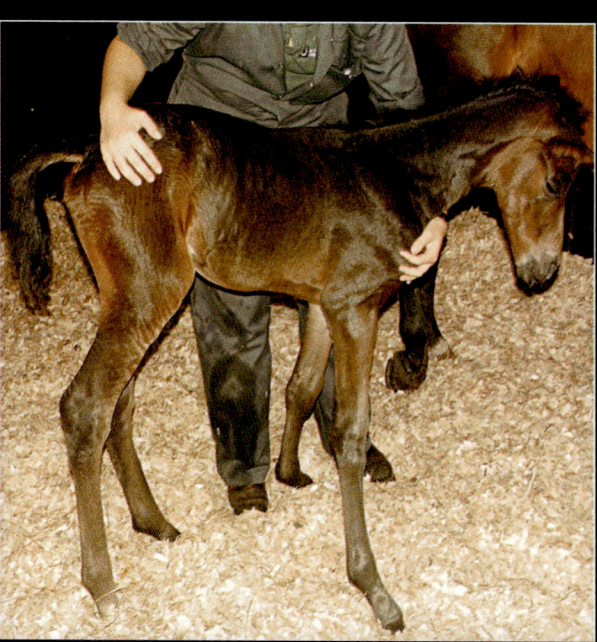

14

The foal

Examination of the neonatal foal

It is important to remember that a neonatal foal is not just a 50 kg horse. Early signs of disease tend to be nonspecific, so familiarity with the normal behavior patterns and physiologic parameters of the young foal is essential (*Table 68*). Routine examination should be systematic and thorough to ensure no subtle signs of abnormality are overlooked.

History

The history of the foal includes the history of the pregnancy and parturition. The mare's health and past breeding record should be considered. The length of gestation, history of vulval discharge, premature lactation, birth, and examination of the placenta may provide useful information when evaluating a sick foal.

Behavior

It is worth spending a few minutes evaluating the foal's behavior by watching its interaction with the mare and the environment. Normal foals have a righting and suck reflex within the first few minutes after birth, they stand within 1–2 hours and suckle from the mare within 3 hours, they feed 5–7 times an hour (less while sleeping), and frequently pass large volumes of dilute urine. They are inquisitive and active in behavior.

Physical examination

The principles of a general physical examination are the same in the foal and adult horse, but there are particular aspects that should be emphasized when examining a foal. The physical appearance should be evaluated, with close attention paid to signs of lack of maturity and intrauterine growth retardation, such as low body weight and poor body condition, floppy ears, mole-like coat, domed forehead, and generalized weakness. The foal should be examined for any congenital deformities.

The head should be examined for wry nose, parrot mouth, any facial swellings, or milk at the nostrils. Mucous membranes should be moist and pink, with rapid CRT. Jaundice may indicate NI or EHV infection. Petechiation or congestion may be observed with sepsis. Dry membranes indicate that the foal may not be feeding adequately and is dehydrated.

Entropion is a common problem and may occur as a result of dehydration or corneal ulceration (retraction of eyeball associated with pain), or be idiopathic. Scleral hemorrhage or congestion may indicate a traumatic birth, while yellowing of the sclera is associated with jaundice. Uveitis may be seen with bacteremia/sepsis. The remnant of the hyaloid artery is frequently visible and is of no significance. Fundic hemorrhages are a common finding in neonatal Thoroughbred foals and are of no clinical significance.

Respiratory rate and effort can be useful indicators of pulmonary disease. The ribs should be palpated carefully to check for fractures (**1333**). Auscultation of the lungs in the newborn foal should be performed; however, it is not a reliable indicator of pulmonary disease.

Auscultation of the heart should be performed and the rate and rhythm assessed. The heart rate is very labile in the young foal and if the rate is rapid, it is worth re-evaluating once the foal has relaxed. A grade I–IV left-sided holosystolic murmur is often audible for the first 2–3 days, associated with the PDA. A flow murmur may be audible at the base of the heart on the left side and this

TABLE 68 **Normal heart and respiratory rates and rectal temperature of the neonatal foal**

AGE	HEART RATE (beats/minute)	RESPIRATORY RATE (breaths/minute)	TEMPERATURE °C (°F)
1 minute	60–80	Gasping	37–39 (99–102)
15 minutes	120–160	40–60	37–39 (99–102)
12 hours	80–120	30–40	37–39 (99–102)
24 hours	80–100	30	37–39 (99–102)

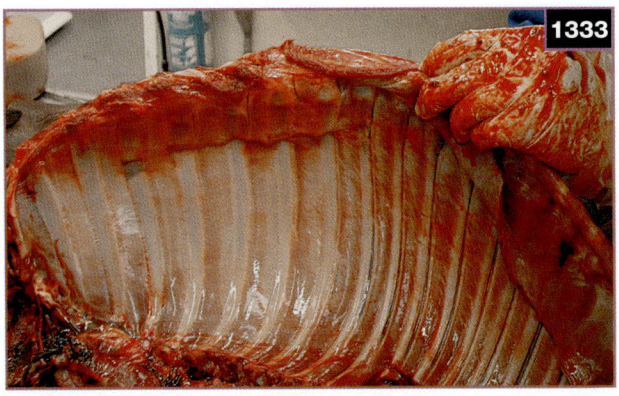

1333 Postmortem specimen illustrating fatal multiple rib fractures.

may persist for many days. It is important to check for signs of cardiovascular compromise if a murmur is detected. Any indication of cardiovascular compromise merits further investigation, including radiography and echocardiography.

The abdomen should be evaluated for distension or a 'tucked up' appearance. The umbilical remnants should be palpated for thickening or dampness. The latter may indicate a patent urachus. Any umbilical hernia should be evaluated.

There may be large quantities of meconium in normal foals and only the appearance of the paler milk feces indicates all the meconium has been passed.

Limbs should be evaluated for joint effusion and flexural and angular limb deformities.

Physiologic differences between the neonatal foal and the mature horse

There are several physiologic differences that are important when assessing and treating neonatal foals. Newborn foals have a larger total body water content (70–75% compared with 60% in the older animal) and a larger extracellular fluid volume (394 +/− 29 ml/kg) and plasma volume (94.5 +/− 8.9 ml/kg) at 2 days, falling to an extracellular fluid volume of 348 +/− 45 ml/kg and a plasma volume of 61.8 +/− 5.9 ml/kg by 4 weeks. Young foals are particularly susceptible to water loss, as they have a high surface area to volume ratio and the kidneys are less able to compensate. Hepatic function is not mature for the first

7–14 days of life, which may slow drug metabolism. There are significant differences in the pharmacokinetics of some drugs in the neonatal foal. Dose rates of some antibiotics are higher (e.g. gentamicin, 7–10 mg/kg q24h) and others have a shorter dosing interval (e.g. ceftiofur dose in young foals is 5 mg/kg q12h). Consequently, it is important to use foal-specific doses for drugs, especially antibiotics (*Table 69*). It is important to consider the age of the foal, as from approximately 1 month of age drug metabolism becomes similar to that of the adult. Foals have an immature colonic function and do not ferment food material in their hindgut. Neonatal foals are metabolically less stable, with poorly established homeostatic mechanisms, and therefore they are susceptible to disturbances in blood glucose and serum electrolyte levels. The foal is dependent on frequent ingestion of milk to maintain blood glucose, fluid, and electrolyte requirements. Thermoregulatory function is less able to compensate for changes in environmental temperature. Foals are agammaglobulinemic at birth and immunologically naïve, with reduced levels of many of the components of the nonspecific immune system. Antibody levels and effective neutrophil function are dependent on adequate passive transfer of colostral immunity.

Routine care of the neonatal foal

Instituting a preventive medicine strategy can reduce the incidence of disease in the neonatal period. Ensuring ingestion of adequate quantities of good quality colostrum is essential. Routinely checking colostral quality using refractometry can identify mares that produce poor-quality colostrum or those with premature lactation who have lost all their colostrum. These foals will require high-quality donor colostrum by bottle or stomach tube as soon after birth as possible in order to ensure adequate transfer of passive immunity. Foals that fail to suck within 3 hours should receive good-quality colostrum (a minimum of 500 ml for a 50 kg foal) by nasogastric tube. If no donor colostrum is available, a colostrum substitute may be used; however, each product should be evaluated for its immunoglobulin content and sterility. Routine blood samples taken at 12–36 hours can be used to identify early signs of disease and the efficacy of passive transfer. A profile including hematology, proteins, immunoglobulin, and inflammatory proteins will provide this information. Care of the umbilicus is important. It should be kept clean and dry. A 0.5% solution of chlorhexidine can be used for topical application.

TABLE 69	**Dosages of some drugs used in the foal**		
DRUG	**ROUTE**	**FREQUENCY** (hourly interval)	**DOSE**
Amikacin	i/v	24	21–25 mg/kg
Butorphanol	i/v	As required	0.01–0.1 mg/kg
Caffeine	p/o	24	10 mg/kg loading, then 2.5–3 mg/kg q6–12h
Ceftriaxone	i/v	12	25 mg/kg
Ceftiofur	i/m	12	5 mg/kg
Detomidine	i/v	As required	up to 10 µg/kg
Dexamethasone	i/v	24	0.1–0.2 mg/kg
Diazepam	slow i/v	Single bolus	5–15 mg/50 kg
DMSO	i/v infusion	24	1 g/kg as 10% solution
Doxycycline	p/o	12	10 mg/kg
Doxapram	i/v	Bolus	0.5 mg/kg
Erythromycin	p/o	8	25 mg/kg
Gentamicin	i/v	24	7–10 mg/kg
Imipenem	i/v	6	10 mg/kg
Metronidazole	p/o	6–8	15–25 mg/kg
Naloxone	i/v	Bolus	5 mg/foal
Oxytetracycline	i/v	12	5–10 mg/kg
Penicillin (Na or K)	i/v	6	22,000 IU/kg
Phenobarbitone	i/v	8–24	2–10 mg/kg
Phenytoin	i/v	6	5–10 mg/kg initially, 1–5 mg/kg maintenance
Rifampicin	p/o	12	5–10 mg/kg
Tetracosactide acetate (Synacthen)	i/v	6 for 3 doses	0.4 mg/foal, then 0.2 mg/foal for 2 further doses
	i/m	Single bolus	0.125 mg
Ticarcillin	i/m	8	50 mg/kg

Immunodeficiency disorders

Failure of passive transfer of immunity
Definition/overview
The most common immunodeficiency in the newborn foal is failure of passive transfer (FPT) of maternally-derived immunity. The foal is agammaglobulinemic at birth and is dependent on ingestion and absorption of adequate quantities of good-quality colostrum in the immediate postpartum period for the transfer of antibody. Failure of this process increases susceptibility to infection in the neonatal and pediatric periods. The incidence of FPT in foals is estimated to be between 2.9 and 25%.

Etiology/pathophysiology
FPT can occur because of mare and/or foal factors. Premature lactation is a common cause. If the mare drips milk in the days preceding parturition, colostrum can rapidly be lost. Poor-quality colostrum may also result in FPT. Some mares produce poor-quality colostrum and this tends to be repeated in subsequent pregnancies. The SG of the colostrum should be 1.060 or higher. On a sugar refractometer the reading should be greater than 22%.

Failure to absorb IgG from ingested colostrum is uncommon, but may occur. This may be a primary problem with intestinal absorption or, more commonly, with ingestion of colostrum after 12–24 hours of age, when immunoglobulins are no longer absorbed. Failure to ingest adequate quantities of colostrum is a major cause of FPT, and a variety of problems can prevent the foal from standing, reaching the mare, and/or successfully nursing.

The epitheliochorial structure of the equine placenta prevents the transfer of maternally-derived antibodies to the foal *in utero*. It is dependent on ingestion and the transfer of colostral immunoglobulins. Antibodies and other important factors are selectively secreted into the udder in the last few weeks of gestation. Short-lived specialized cells in the foal's small intestine pinocytose large molecules (e.g. IgG and, to a lesser extent, IgA and IgM), which pass into the lymphatics and then into the circulation. It is thought that other factors, including complement, lysozyme, lactoferrin, and B lymphocytes, may be transferred via the same mechanism and enhance the foal's naïve immune system. Failure of this process results in low levels of specific antibody and compromise of the nonspecific immune system, rendering the immunologically naïve foal susceptible to infection.

Clinical presentation
FPT may be detected on routine screening blood samples taken at 12–36 hours or when investigating newborn foals with infectious disease.

Differential diagnosis
Congenital immunodeficiences.

Diagnosis
Blood samples taken at 18–36 hours to measure serum IgG can be used to assess the efficacy of passive transfer. There are several different tests available including zinc sulfate turbidity and CITE tests, and the more accurate immuno-turbidometric and serial radial immunodiffusion (SRID) assays. In a healthy foal, serum globulin levels have been shown to be highly correlated with IgG and provide an additional check on the less accurate methods of IgG assessment. Serum IgG levels <4 g/l (0.4 g/dl) are considered to indicate FPT. Levels between 4 and 8 g/l (0.4 and 0.8 g/dl) may increase susceptibility to infection, particularly when the level of infectious challenge is high, while levels >8 g/l (>0.8 g/dl) are considered normal. The decision to treat the foal with a plasma transfusion must be based on an assessment of risk of infection and IgG level. In clinically healthy foals with normal inflammatory parameters, serum globulin levels of >12 g/l (>1.2 g/dl) are likely to correlate with IgG levels of >4 g/l (0.4 g/dl).

Management
During the first 4–6 hours after birth, administration of high-quality colostrum (IgG level >60 g/l [>6 g/dl]) via bottle or stomach tube is appropriate (1–2 liters is suggested, as necessary, but this is dependent on quality: 300–500 ml feedings q1–2h). Oral plasma is also an option, but it is relatively dilute in IgG compared with colostrum, and five times the amount is required to achieve the same effect. After closure of the specialized small intestinal transfer mechanism, which starts at 6–12 hours after birth and is complete by 24 hours, the only treatment is transfusion with plasma, preferably with high IgG (>15 g/l [1.5 g/dl]) levels. Commercially produced frozen hyperimmune plasma is available. Alternatively, fresh plasma may be harvested aseptically from a disease-screened, cross-matched donor. A 50 kg foal will typically require 1–2 liters of plasma to raise IgG levels >4 g/l (0.4 g/dl). Plasma can be administered via an aseptically placed 16 gauge jugular catheter and blood-giving set with an inline filter. The transfusion should be started very slowly and the foal monitored for signs of an adverse reaction. If it is tolerating the transfusion, the rate can be gradually increased. One liter can be administered over 20–30 minutes in a clinically healthy 50 kg foal to minimize stress. If two liters are given, the second liter should be administered at a slower rate to prevent circulatory overload. It is essential, whenever carrying out a transfusion, to monitor the foal closely for any signs of a transfusion reaction, cardiovascular overload, or anaphylaxis. When the adverse signs are mild, it may be possible to continue the transfusion at a slower rate. The IgG levels should be checked the following day to ensure that satisfactory levels have been achieved. The use of broad-spectrum antibiotic therapy may be indicated depending on the age of the foal, management, clinical signs, and other risk factors.

Simple measures, such as the use of a refractometer to measure colostral quality (1334), use of donor colostrum when the colostrum is of poor quality, and stomach-tubing foals that fail to suckle within the first 3 hours postpartum, will significantly reduce the incidence of FPT.

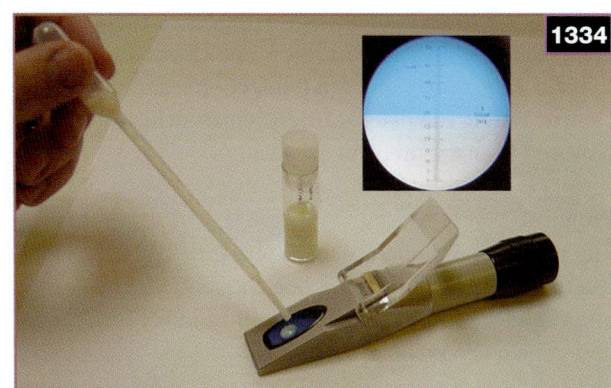

1334 A sugar refractometer being used to measure colostral quality.

Severe combined immunodeficiency

Definition/overview
Severe combined immunodeficiency (SCID) is most frequently seen in Arabians and occasionally Appaloosas. It is an inherited autosomal-recessive trait that results in failure to produce functional B and T lymphocytes.

Etiology/pathophysiology
There is an inherited 5-base-pair deletion in gene encoding of a DNA protein kinase catalytic subunit. When a foal is homozygous for this defect, it blocks the production of mature B and T lymphocytes. Heterozygous carriers of the gene are clinically normal.

Affected foals with effective transfer of colostral immunity are usually healthy for the first 1–3 months of life. When the maternally-derived antibody levels start to fall, the foal is unable to produce endogenous antibody and cell-mediated immune responses, and succumbs to recurrent infection.

Clinical presentation
Affected foals are normal at birth and suckle well, then suffer from recurrent severe infections. These often involve the respiratory system, with atypical organisms (adenovirus, *Pneumocystis jiroveci, E. coli*), within the first 2–3 months of life. The foals usually die by 6–9 months of age of bacterial pneumonia and/or enteritis.

Differential diagnosis
Other immunodeficiences such as selective IgM deficiency; bacterial pneumonia.

Diagnosis
Diagnosis is based on clinical signs, breed, and age of the foal. Once clinical signs become apparent there will be a persistent lymphopenia, absence of circulating IgM (after maternally-derived levels have waned), and lymphocytic hypoplasia of lymph nodes, spleen, and thymus seen at biopsy or postmortem examination. Diagnosis is confirmed by genetic testing at specialist laboratories.

Management
There is no specific treatment. Supportive therapy may extend life for a short period of time by treating opportunistic infections, but fatal infections are inevitable. Genetic testing can detect carrier animals, which should be removed from the breeding population.

Prognosis
The prognosis is hopeless and humane destruction is indicated once the diagnosis has been confirmed. The genetic and therefore future breeding implications for the mare and stallion should be considered.

Fell pony immune-deficiency syndrome

Definition/overview
A syndrome affecting Fell pony foals was first reported in 1998. It is thought to be an immunodeficiency with foals having low numbers of B lymphocytes, a small thymus, absence of secondary lymphoid follicles, and neuronal chromatolysis. Research into the condition – which is thought to be probably due to a single autosomal recessive gene – is ongoing.

Affected foals are healthy at birth, but usually present at 1–16 weeks of age with chronic, multiple, and severe viral/bacterial/fungal infections, often respiratory or gastrointestinal, and usually die by 2–6 months of age. Oral candidiasis is common and severe skin infections also occur.

These foals have a severe nonregenerative anemia, lymphopenia, low IgM levels and peripheral ganglionopathy. Mortality is 100%.

Immune-mediated thrombocytopenia
(See Chapter 9, Hemolymphatic System, p. 728)

Neonatal septicemia

Definition/overview
Generalized systemic septicemia is life threatening in the neonatal foal. It one of the most common causes of mortality in neonates in the US, but the incidence is variable in different geographic regions. Sepsis when untreated progresses rapidly to septic shock and multiorgan dysfunction in the neonate. Early aggressive intervention is necessary to increase the likelihood of a favorable outcome.

Etiology/pathophysiology
Bacterial infection (*E. coli, Enterobacter* spp., *Staphylococcus* spp., *Streptococcus* spp., *Actinobacillus* spp., *Klebsiella* spp., *Pasteurella* spp., *Salmonella* spp., *Clostridium* spp., and *Enterococcus* spp.) is the most common cause of septic shock. Viral (EHV-1, equine arteritis virus) and fungal infections, and/or severe hypoxic–ischemic insult can trigger the cascade of intrinsic mediators, which may predispose to bacterial infection and septic shock.

The neonatal foal is uniquely susceptible to invasion by pathogenic organisms. The immune system is naïve, dependent on passively derived antibody, and not as immune-competent as in the mature horse. Sites of entry include the 'open' gut prior to the ingestion of adequate quantities of colostrum (generally considered to be the most common site of entry), the respiratory tract, the placenta *in utero*, and the umbilicus. Following pathogen invasion, most of the changes seen in septic shock are due to a cascade of intrinsic mediators released in response to the triggering agent (e.g. bacteria and their toxins).

Firstly, the systemic inflammatory response syndrome (SIRS) is initiated. This is a cascade of proinflammatory mediators that kill invading pathogens and remove damaged tissue. SIRS is balanced by the compensatory anti-inflammatory response syndrome (CARS). When the response of these two components is balanced, only the invading organisms and damaged tissue are destroyed; however, if SIRS predominates, septic shock with multiorgan dysfunction results. If CARS predominates, the individual is overwhelmed by the invading organism. Following invasion and, usually, multisystem involvement, some bacteria may localize in organs such as the lung, abdomen, gut, joints, brain, eye, liver, and kidney.

Risk factors include:
- Maternal: placentitis; systemic illness; stress; loss of colostrum; poor nutrition; prolonged gestation.
- Parturition: dystocia; induction.
- Environment: poor stable hygiene and management; overcrowding.
- Foal: prematurity/dysmaturity; FPT or inappropriate antibodies; perinatal asphyxia syndrome.

Clinical presentation
Clinical signs are variable. They may range from subtle, nonspecific, and insidious in onset to acute and fulminant. They may include: less frequent feeding to complete anorexia; lethargy and increasing periods of recumbency; increased heart and respiratory rates; increased respiratory effort; respiratory distress; raised or subnormal temperature; congestion and petechiation of mucous membranes; altered mental status such as depression and seizures; diarrhea; colic and abdominal distension; uveitis with ocular pain; hypovolemia; bone or joint infections with joint effusion and lameness; umbilical infections and patent urachus; cardiovascular collapse; coma and death.

Differential diagnosis
Perinatal asphyxia syndrome; metabolic disturbances.

Diagnosis
Diagnosis is based on history and a thorough clinical examination combined with clinical pathology. Sepsis should always be considered until proven otherwise. If sepsis is suspected, treatment should be instituted immediately, prior to laboratory confirmation. Blood culture should be obtained aseptically, if possible prior to administration of antibiotics. A positive result is the gold standard for diagnosis; however, a negative blood culture, particularly a single sample, does not rule out sepsis. Ideally, three samples should be taken over a 24-hour period to help improve culture results. Samples can also be taken from other sources to obtain culture material, and these include joints and other synovial structures, tracheal washes, urine, feces, and CSF. The use of a sepsis scoring system may increase the accuracy of diagnosis. This involves the collection of a number of clinical and biochemical assay results and allocating them a score in a table, which then predicts the likelihood of sepsis. However, sepsis scores should only be used as an aid to diagnosis, as recent research has indicated that the accuracy of the system tends to be institution-specific. Radiography of joints and the chest, plus ultrasonography of the umbilicus and abdomen, are used as directed by the clinical findings.

Early in the course of the condition these foals are leucopenic and neutropenic, with toxic changes and band neutrophils. Serum amyloid A, an acute phase protein, typically rises dramatically over the first 12–24 hours. Fibrinogen rises more slowly and an increased concentration in a foal <36 hours old indicates in-utero pathology.

It is important to determine the efficacy of passive transfer, as there has been a failure of this process in most cases of septicemia. Hypoglycemia is common in septic foals, often from a combination of decreased nursing, inflammatory response, and bacterial consumption. As the disease process progresses, affected foals may become hyperglycemic. Renal dysfunction is a common complication and should be assessed via serum biochemical profile and urinalysis. Homeostatic mechanisms to maintain serum electrolyte levels are poorly established, so significant disturbances may develop rapidly. Blood lactate concentrations are a sensitive measure of tissue perfusion, and they increase rapidly in states of hypoperfusion. Blood gas analysis is useful, if available. Hypoxemia is common. Hypercarbia may also be present. Acidosis is common and may be respiratory, metabolic, or mixed in nature.

Management
Antibiotics. Careful selection of the most suitable antibiotics is important. Broad-spectrum bactericidal antibiotics with good penetration of affected tissues are required. Provided renal function is not significantly compromised, penicillin and an aminoglycoside (gentamicin or amikacin) is a commonly used first choice. Some third-generation cephalosporins are useful, but care must be taken to give the appropriate foal dose and, if administered intravenously, it must be given by slow infusion (10–15 minutes). If the foal fails to respond, antibiotic therapy can be changed in the light of culture and sensitivity results.

Cardiovascular support. It is important to maintain tissue perfusion and adequate oxygen delivery to the tissues. Monitoring hydration, blood pressure, mental status, and blood lactate concentrations provides useful information. Resuscitation fluid boluses (10–20 ml/kg of balanced electrolyte solution given at a higher flow rate [i.e. 1 liter/50 kg foal over 20 minutes]) will provide temporary volume expansion. Response to therapy should be monitored and further boluses may be necessary. It is important to remember that foals are more susceptible to volume overload than mature horses. Plasma and synthetic colloids may also be useful during resuscitation. Plasma is particularly useful as it contributes antibodies, metabolic nutrients, and clotting factors to the foal. Failure to respond to appropriate fluid therapy indicates the need to use ionotropes and vasopressors to support blood pressure. There are extensive, excellent reviews of the use of hemodynamic agents and cardiovascular monitoring.

Respiratory support. Prolonged periods of recumbency, poor tissue perfusion, and weakness contribute to ventilation/perfusion mismatch and atelectasis. Most sick collapsed foals benefit from humidified intranasal oxygen therapy. Maintaining the foal in sternal recumbency and coupage to encourage drainage of secretions is helpful. Some clinicians use xanthine derivatives such as caffeine (10 mg/kg p/o loading dose, 2.5–5.0 mg/kg q12–24h) to reduce hypercapnea.

Nutrition. Nutritional support is vital to recovery, but in many cases enteral feeding is poorly tolerated and parenteral nutrition should be considered at an early stage.

If enteral feeding is well tolerated, mare's milk is most appropriate. If the suck reflex is weak, an indwelling feeding tube will allow the feeding of low volumes at frequent intervals. Feeding for the first 2–3 days should be hourly, decreasing to every 2 hours by 3–4 days post partum. Volumes of milk given at each feed should be small at first (100–200 ml/feed) and gradually built up if the foal tolerates the initial feeding. A healthy foal consumes about 20–23% of its body weight per day to fulfill requirements for growth and maintenance, but the requirements of a sick foal for maintenance are about half this amount. A target of about 10% of body weight per day should be worked towards over several days. A maximum of 500 ml/per feeding is recommended. It is important that the foal is closely monitored for ileus as the volume of milk fed increases.

Other drugs. Reduced doses of flunixin meglumine (0.25 mg/kg i/v q8h) have been used in the treatment of septic shock, but the evidence for their efficacy remains controversial. The potential for causing serious side-effects, nephrotoxicity, and gastroduodenal ulceration must be considered before their use, especially in hypovolemic and collapsed foals.

The prophylactic use of antiulcer medication remains controversial and each case should be evaluated on its merits. A recent publication refutes previous suggestions that the stomach pH of sick foals may be high; however, the etiology of gastroduodenal ulceration may be different in sick neonates. Hypoperfusion of the GI mucosa may be a significant factor. Further discussion can be found in the section on gastroduodenal ulceration (p. 981).

High standards of hygiene and nursing care provide an important part of therapy and should include the careful regulation of the environmental temperature.

Prognosis
Mortality rates can be high. There is considerable variation in reported survival rates and these reflect the speed of referral to a critical-care center, the level of care available, and the financial resources available for critical care. Survival rates in the field have not been documented.

Neonatal isoerythrolysis
Definition/overview
NI is characterized by the destruction of RBCs of the foal due to the presence of alloantibodies of maternal origin that were absorbed from colostrum. NI occurs in newborn foals within the first week of life.

Etiology/pathophysiology
The disease occurs because of the presence of antibodies against RBCs that were absorbed with the mare's colostrum. There are 32 blood-group antigens in the horse. Ninety per cent of cases of NI are associated with Aa and Qa. Aa is the most antigenic, usually producing the peracute form of the disease within 12–18 hours of birth. Qa has not been associated with clinical disease, but may cause a weak false positive when tests are carried out for the condition. There is a breed difference in the occurrence of the erythrocyte antigens that affects the prevalence of the disease. It has been reported in 2% of Standardbreds and in less than 1% of Thoroughbreds. The frequency of isoimmunization is much lower than that of incompatible pregnancies, and the mechanism of this difference is unknown.

The primary isoimmunization by genetically incompatible erythrocytes occurs late in pregnancy, with antibody levels in the mare's serum peaking at 9 days post partum. First foals, therefore, do not show clinical signs. However, during subsequent pregnancies, the secondary anamnestic response produces significant antierythrocyte antibodies concentrated in the colostrum, which put the foal at risk. It is also reported that tissue vaccines or transfusions may sensitize a mare to genetically incompatible erythrocytes. Transfer of antibodies across the equine placenta is not possible. Antibodies become concentrated in the colostrum during the last weeks of pregnancy and are absorbed during the first 24 hours after birth. The antibodies pass into the foal's circulation and attach themselves to the surface of the foal's erythrocytes, causing them to agglutinate and be removed by the monocyte–phagocytic system, or hemolyse intravascularly in the presence of complement.

The disease only develops if: (1) the mare lacks certain red cell factors; (2) the mare is repeatedly exposed to that factor; (3) the mare conceives a foal that inherits that red cell factor from the sire; (4) colostrum is produced containing antierythrocyte antibody; and (5) the foal ingests and absorbs antibody, which leads to the immune-mediated destruction of its red cells.

Clinical presentation

Foals appear healthy at birth. The speed of onset and severity of clinical signs are dependent on the red-cell antigen involved (Aa and Qa being the most rapid and severe) and the efficacy of transfer of passive immunity. Clinical signs usually develop between 12 and 48 hours post partum, although occasionally up to 96 hours.

Early clinical signs may be subtle and nonspecific. Foals become lethargic and yawn, becoming depressed, spend more time recumbent, and suck less frequently. When excited or restrained, heart rate and respiratory rate increase. Examination of the mucous membranes and sclera reveals varying, but often marked, degrees of jaundice. In severe cases the urine becomes red due to the presence of hemoglobinuria. There can be a rapid progression to collapse, coma, and death in some cases. More frequently, in less severe cases, signs progress more slowly, and in unusual cases the development of signs may be delayed.

Differential diagnosis

Other causes of hemolytic anemia need to be considered, including drug administration, hemoparasites, toxin exposure, and sepsis.

Diagnosis

Diagnosis is based on clinical signs, history (multiparous mare, signs seen 12–72 hours after birth), and laboratory results. Hematologic examination reveals a marked anemia, an RBC count $<4 \times 10^{12}$/l ($<4 \times 10^{6}$/µl), hemoglobin <70 g/l (<7 g/dl) and PCV <0.20 l/l (20%). Anemia can be severe (PCV <0.1 l/l [<10%]) and thrombocytopenia is present in some cases. Plasma protein concentration remains within the reference interval. Anisocytosis and RBC ghosts may be seen on a blood smear and hemoglobinemia and hemoglobinuria may be present if sufficient intravascular hemolysis exists. Unconjugated bilirubin concentration is increased. A direct Coombs test (a nonspecific test detecting antibody or complement components on red cell surface) will be positive, although false negatives do occur. Definitive diagnosis requires demonstration of alloantibodies in the dam's blood or colostrum directed against the foal's red cells. Serum and red cells from the mare and foal are required for this test, which is offered by some commercial or specialist laboratories.

Management

Treatment is dependent on the severity of clinical signs and the degree of anemia. In mild cases the foal should have minimal handling and box rest. RBC parameters should be monitored twice daily for the first few days. Management of these foals is important and care should be taken when handling them not to excite or stress them. Exercise should be limited to short periods of nursery paddock exercise. Transfusion with donor red cells is usually considered appropriate when the PCV falls below 0.12 l/l (12%) and RBCs below 3.5×10^{12}/l (3.5×10^{6}/µl); however, should the foal become depressed, be off suck, or suffer signs of hypoxemia, transfusion should be considered earlier. Early and rapid development of clinical signs is likely to necessitate early transfusion. If the fall in RBCs is slow, the foal is better able to adapt.

The volume of RBCs required can be calculated as shown below:

$$\text{Volume} = \frac{\text{body weight (kg)} \times \text{blood volume} \times (\text{PCV desired} - \text{PCV observed})}{\text{PCV of donor}}$$

The blood volume of the foal is considered to be 7.5% of body weight. The limiting factor is usually the foal's circulating volume. It is usual to transfuse 1–2 liters of packed washed cells by slow infusion. The dam is usually the most suitable donor; however, the red cells must be washed free of plasma-containing antibody. This can be done by washing the cells three times in saline and then resuspending them in a 50% isotonic solution of saline. If it is not possible to wash the cells, or the dam is not a suitable donor, then a cross-matched gelding can be used (1335) as a source of packed cells or whole blood. Electrolyte solutions can be administered to provide diuresis and prevent hemoglobin-associated renal failure. Supportive therapy and nursing are an essential part of treatment.

The foal should be restricted to the box while showing clinical signs of disease. Once the clinical signs have regressed and the red cell picture starts to improve, then limited periods of nursery paddock exercise may be appropriate. The foal should not be stressed by temperature. In cold conditions it may be appropriate to heat the box and use rugs. In some cases where the foal is severely hypoxemic, the use of intranasal oxygen may be considered.

In the acute phase it is essential to ensure that the foal is receiving adequate quantities of milk. If it is weak, it may be necessary to supplement the foal with milk via a bottle or stomach tube to meet nutritional requirements. The use of oral hematinics may be considered.

Once a mare has been identified by blood typing or a history of previous foals with NI, preventive strategies can be used for subsequent pregnancies. It may be possible to check the dam's and sire's blood typing to assess the risk of developing NI. Alternatively, a blood sample can be taken from the mare during the last 2–3 weeks of gestation and titrated for anti-erythrocyte antibodies. It is important not to take the sample too early, because antibody levels rise late, often peaking after foaling. Once a potential case has been identified the foal must be prevented from suckling and given 500 ml of appropriate donor colostrum immediately after birth, then muzzled prior to udder-seeking behavior. It should then be bottle-fed a minimum of a further 500 ml of colostrum and then milk replacer at the appropriate rate. The foal's IgG levels should be checked at 18–24 hours post partum to ensure they are adequate. The mare's udder should be stripped frequently following parturition and the IgG concentration monitored till it falls. These strippings must be discarded. It is then considered safe to allow the foal to suckle the mare provided it has been appropriately fed, because it is thought that feeding hastens closure of the specialized absorptive mechanism in the foal's small intestine. It is usually possible to let the foal return to the mare within 24 hours of foaling.

Perinatal/young foal conditions

Prematurity/dysmaturity

Definition/overview
The normal gestation in the horse is approximately 335–345 days, with variation between breeds and individuals. Historically, gestational age has been used to define this condition: those being born at <320 days are termed premature, and those born with a normal or prolonged gestation, but having characteristics of prematurity, as dysmature. The authors consider that because of the wide normal variation in gestational length (and potential errors in breeding records), each foal should be evaluated individually, with greater reliance on clinical signs than on gestational age. Most foals born prior to 320 days require some veterinary intervention. Two hundred and eighty days is considered the cut-off for survival. The degree of maturity of the various body systems may be asynchronous.

Etiology/pathophysiology
Twin foals are almost always either premature or dysmature. Much dysmaturity in foals is caused by endocrine or placental dysfunction and/or inadequacy. These foals have immature body systems, and those born suddenly, without chronic placental pathology, frequently have not been 'switched on' in readiness for birth by the final surge

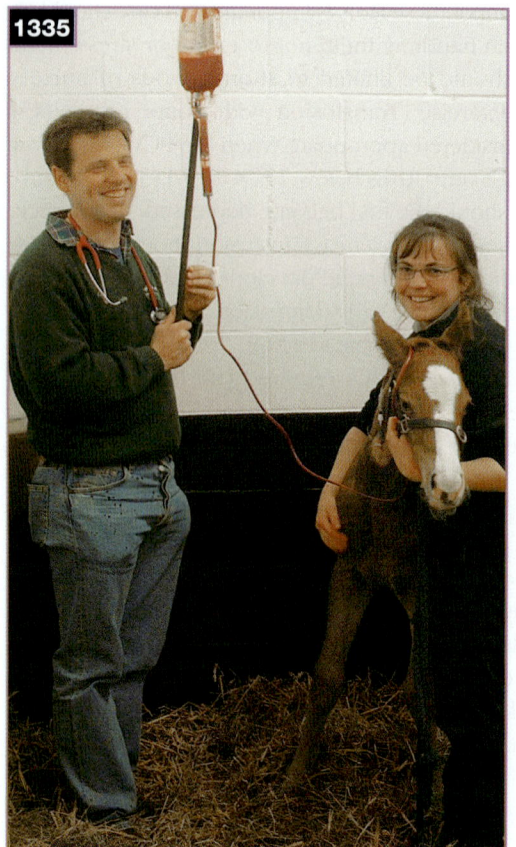

1335 A foal receiving a transfusion of packed red cells.

The foal

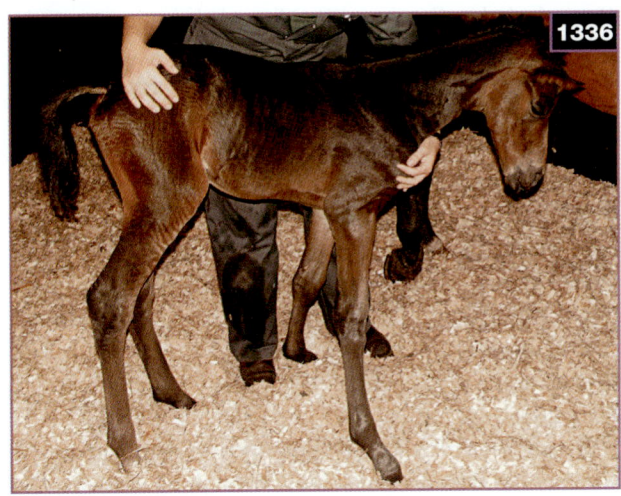

1336 A foal showing some of the classic signs of dysmaturity including a domed forehead, low body weight, silky coat, and laxity of the limbs, especially in the carpal joints. It also had a poor suck reflex and is being assisted onto the mammary gland of the mare.

of the fetal adrenocortical hormones. When there is chronic placental pathology, foals have often undergone this final vital maturation of body systems, considerably increasing their chance of survival.

Clinical presentation

Foals present with some or all of the following physical characteristics in both prematurity and dysmaturity syndromes (1336): small and underweight; slow to stand and suck; poor body condition; silky mole-like coat; domed forehead; floppy ears and discolored tongue; flexor tendon laxity and weak musculature; pale mucous membranes; weakness and occasionally incoordination; poor thermoregulation.

Further investigations may reveal: incomplete ossification of cuboidal bones and joint instability (1337); poor tolerance to enteral feeding, with colic and abdominal distension; poor respiratory function with slow rate and/or abnormal respiratory pattern; altered mentation; increased susceptibility to infection; dehydration; leukopenia and neutropenia; neutrophil:lymphocyte ratio <2:1; hypoxia and hypercapnea; acidosis.

Differential diagnosis

Sepsis; perinatal asphyxia syndrome.

Diagnosis

Diagnosis is based on the history of the pregnancy, physical appearance, degree of ossification of the cuboidal bones, and hematologic parameters. An ACTH stimulation test can be used. An initial blood sample is taken to

measure the total and differential WBC count, then 0.125 mg short-acting ACTH (Synacthen) is given intramuscularly and a blood sample taken 2 hours post injection to evaluate changes in the total and differential WBC count. Mature foals show an increase in total WBC count and an increase in the neutrophil:lymphocyte ratio (>2:1). Radiographs of the lungs are helpful in order to assess the severity and type of respiratory abnormalities (e.g. atelectasis).

Management

These foals require intensive and supportive treatment with an enormous input of nursing care. Owners of such foals need to be made aware of this at the outset.

Prenatal corticosteroids. In humans the use of prenatal betamethasone has been shown to hasten fetal maturation and improve outcome. The opportunity for their use in the mare is limited and the most appropriate dose and drug have not been established. Recently published investigations into the role of dexamethasone in the horse are, however, encouraging.

Postnatal corticosteroids. The use of corticosteroids in the newborn remains controversial. The use of 1.3 mg dexamethasone q8h or 4 mg/50 kg foal q12h i/m for the first 2 days and then gradual withdrawal has been reported to be helpful, but scientific evidence is still not available. Depot ACTH (0.26 mg total dose divided) may be used to enhance endogenous corticosteroid production, but the authors have some reservations about the effect of ACTH on the immature adrenal cortex.

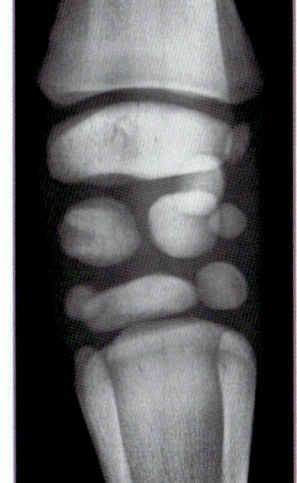

1337 Radiograph of incomplete ossification of the carpal bones of a premature foal.

Nutritional support. Premature foals may not tolerate enteral feeding due to the immaturity of the GI tract. If they are fed enterally, these foals may develop ileus and colic. In some regions, *Clostridium difficile* enterocolitis appears to be a concern in such foals; however, this is quite variable geographically. It is wise to be cautious of the enteral route until normal GI function is evident. Premature foals are often in poor body condition and prone to hypoglycemia, therefore the use of intravenous glucose, plus careful blood glucose monitoring during assessment, is appropriate. Some foals are unable to regulate blood glucose level and a continuous intravenous infusion of insulin may be required. It is challenging to maintain stable blood glucose levels between 4 and 10 mmol/l (72 and 180 mg/dl), as some degree of insulin resistance is often observed. A combination of enteral feeding and parenteral nutrition may be required in many of these cases in order to maintain calorie intake. In those cases where parenteral nutrition is necessary it is important to encourage GI maturation; therefore, 5–10 ml/hour of milk should be administered. Additionally, the use of glutamine (10 g/day in divided doses) may help enterocyte repair and function.

Metabolic support. Homeostatic mechanisms may be poorly established and electrolyte concentrations should be monitored regularly. Premature foals may be unable to maintain body temperature and this should be monitored closely. They should be warmed or the environmental temperature increased as required. Premature foals can suffer 'second day syndrome': after 24 hours of improvement they slide irreversibly into hypotension, hypoxia, septic shock, and multiorgan dysfunction syndrome.

Immunologic support. Premature foals frequently fail to absorb adequate quantities of colostral immunoglobulins and, combined with an immature immune system, they are particularly susceptible to infection. The use of broad-spectrum bactericidal antibiotics and intravenous hyperimmune plasma is helpful. The potential side-effects (e.g. nephrotoxicity) should be considered when selecting antibiotics in these foals, although the risk is low with appropriate fluid therapy.

Respiratory support. Arterial blood gases should be monitored to assess lung function. In some cases, humidified intranasal oxygen may be required. The foal should be maintained in the sternal position or regularly turned from side to side; if it can stand, it should be assisted in doing so. Failing respiratory function is a poor prognostic sign and unless it can be reversed, the foal declines to severe hypoxia and multiorgan failure. Oral caffeine (10 mg/kg followed by 2.5 mg/kg p/o q24h) may stimulate ventilation drive. Mechanical ventilation may be required.

Musculoskeletal support. The degree of ossification of the cuboidal bones is considered an indicator of maturity. Those with poorly ossified carpal and tarsal bones (grade 3 or less using the scoring system developed by Poulos and Adams) can develop severe crushing of the cuboidal bones and severe limb deformity. Restricted exercise, maintaining steady growth, and good farriery can help. In severe cases, limb splint bandages, casts, or custom made limb supports have been suggested, but evidence suggests that these individuals carry a poor prognosis for future athletic performance.

Prognosis
The prognosis for survival after 300 days is influenced by whether the pathology resulting in the premature delivery was acute or chronic. Those with chronic placental pathology have a greater chance for survival, whereas those that are born without 'switching on' have a poor prognosis. Sepsis is a particularly common and serious complication in these foals, leading often to a rapid deterioration and death 48–72 hours after birth. When undertaking treatment of immature foals it is important to consider the future use of the horse, because musculoskeletal problems may preclude an athletic future. No individual parameter is the key to the prognosis and a whole range should be considered before deciding on the best course of treatment.

Meconium aspiration syndrome
Definition/overview
This condition is usually associated with maternal or fetal stress. It is fairly uncommon. The severity of the disease can vary from mild respiratory compromise to fatal respiratory distress.

Etiology/pathophysiology
The fetus can pass meconium during periods of stress. If either the fetus gasps *in utero* or the fluids are not cleared from the airways prior to the first breath, meconium-contaminated amniotic fluid is aspirated into the lungs (1338). This produces a chemical pneumonitis.

Clinical presentation
The foal is born covered in liquid brown meconium and the amniotic fluid is stained brown. Foals often have brown-stained fluid at the nostrils immediately after birth. The foals develop respiratory distress within the first few days of life and some may also exhibit signs of perinatal asphyxia syndrome. Foals often have increased respiratory effort. The degree of hypoxemia and respiratory acidosis is dependent on the quantity of fluid aspirated and the degree of lung injury. Signs of respiratory disease are not always apparent initially, and they may develop over time as pneumonitis worsens.

Diagnosis

History and clinical signs can provide a presumptive diagnosis. Visualization of brown-stained fluid in the trachea with endoscopy, or a granular appearance of the caudoventral lungs on radiographs, provides further evidence. Confirmation is based on histologic examination of the lungs.

Management

If diagnosed early, attempts should be made to suction as much meconium-contaminated fluid from the airways as possible, but care must be taken not to induce further lung damage. Arterial blood gas analysis will determine the requirement for humidified intranasal oxygen or mechanical ventilation. The use of corticosteroids remains controversial. There is some evidence in children that a single dose of dexamethasone early in the course of the condition may be beneficial. When economics permit, the use of a surfactant is indicated, but costs can be very substantial because the dosing interval is very short. High levels of supportive care may be required and broad-spectrum bactericidal antibiotics should be given.

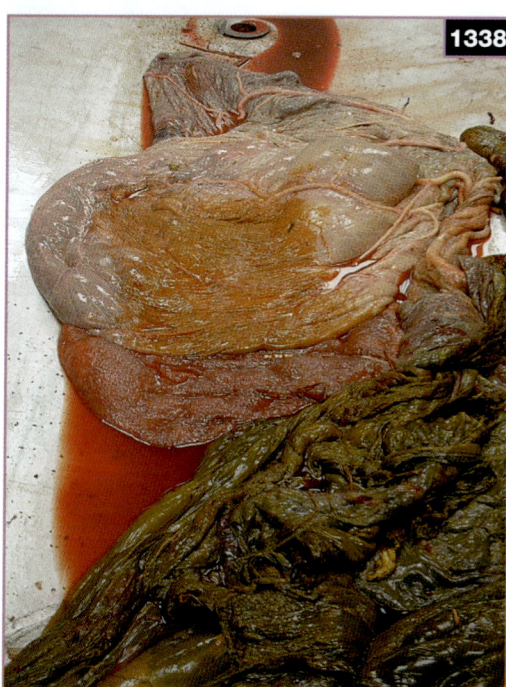

1338 A meconium-stained placenta from a mare where the foal suffered meconium inhalation.

Perinatal asphyxia syndrome (neonatal maladjustment syndrome, neonatal encephalopathy, hypoxic/ischemic encephalopathy, 'barker' foals, 'dummy' foals, convulsive foals)

Definition/overview

Perinatal asphyxia syndrome is a noninfectious syndrome of newborn foals (usually <3 days old) leading to a wide range of signs due to behavioral disturbance and neurologic and multiorgan dysfunction. It is often accompanied by some degree of respiratory compromise. The range and severity of clinical signs are highly variable.

Etiology/pathophysiology

The cause of this syndrome is still obscure, but it is most common in foals that are thought to have suffered an episode of hypoxic–ischemic injury either pre- or intranatally. It is often associated with foals that have had: resuscitation at birth; a Cesarean section; an excessively rapid, slow, or difficult delivery; an early delivery of the placenta indicating premature placental separation; abnormalities of the placenta; meconium aspiration. Maternal factors such as anemia, endotoxemia, and pulmonary disease have also been implicated and the condition is common following induced parturition. In some cases, birth trauma resulting in thoracic trauma and rib fractures is a feature. Cerebral hemorrhage and edema have been reported, but are uncommon features of the condition. These hypoxic–ischemic insults produce cellular damage to a variety of organ systems, particularly those with high blood flow. The CNS, kidney, and gut tend to be most severely affected.

The pathophysiology of this condition is not completely understood. Evidence available from other species has implicated an hypoxic–ischemic insult affecting various organ systems (e.g. cerebrum, renal, and GI systems) and many of the homeostatic mechanisms required for extrauterine survival. There is often further secondary damage due to reperfusion injury, free radical formation, cell membrane damage, and cell death.

Clinical presentation

Two main types of foal are recognized with this condition: (1) foals that appear normal and are full term and suck normally, but between 6 and 24 hours post partum rapidly develop clinical signs; and (2), foals that are abnormal at birth with changes in mentation and reflexes, and are associated with abnormal parturition or placenta.

There is a range of presenting clinical signs present in these cases, often related to the degree of initial hypoxia. They are nonspecific and may include:

✦ Neurologic signs: loss of suck reflex and poor teat searching; persistent chewing movements with collection of food material in the mouth; aimless wandering and galloping; altered mentation; reduced interaction with mare/environment; sneezing; hyper-esthesia, especially when handled or stimulated; weakness, rapid exhaustion, inability to stand or stay standing; central blindness with anisocoria; opisthotonus or hypotonia; altered gait; seizures (1339); coma (1340).

✦ Respiratory signs: periods of apnea, abnormal breathing patterns, or barking vocalization (rare); shallow tachypnea and/or dyspnea.

✦ Other signs: tachycardia, prominent jugular pulse, and hypoxia; ileus/colic; meconium impactions; diarrhea and necrotizing enterocolitis; oliguria/anuria; renal dysfunction and electrolyte disturbances.

Differential diagnosis

Numerous differential diagnoses may be present. It may be difficult to differentiate this condition from neonatal sepsis. Septic meningitis, severe metabolic disturbances leading to electrolyte imbalances and renal failure, cranial trauma, hydrocephalus, and cerebellar abiotrophy may also appear similar.

Diagnosis

Diagnosis can be difficult because early signs may be subtle or obscured by concurrent diseases. History and clinical signs are very important. Clinicopathologic abnormalities should not be present unless there is concurrent disease.

Management

Control of seizures. Diazepam can be useful in an emergency situation and for initial control of seizures, but it only has a short duration of action. Midazolam is useful by continuous infusion. Phenobarbitone (3–10 mg/kg by slow i/v infusion up to q8h) reduces CNS excitability and can be used for control of frequent, more severe seizures. An oral form is available. Phenobarbitone can produce significant respiratory depression. The half-life may be considerably prolonged, therefore titration of dose to effect is necessary. Phenytoin (5 mg/kg i/m q6h) diminishes the spread and propagation of focal neural discharges. It has a relatively short half-life. It can be given orally in a syrup form, which is useful for prolonged treatment. It is important to wean foals gradually off both phenobarbitone and phenytoin, because sudden withdrawal of these two drugs can trigger seizure activity.

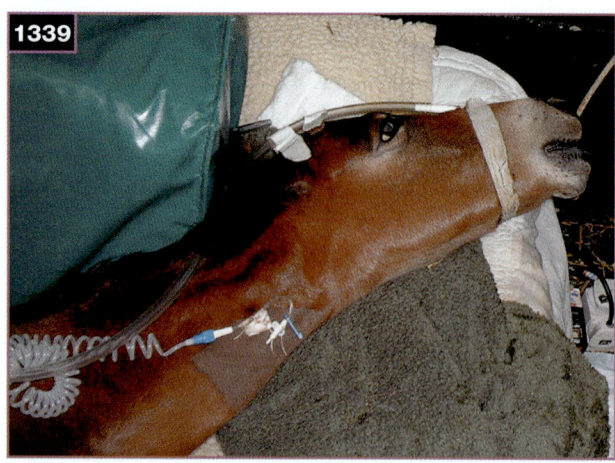

1339 A foal showing seizure activity.

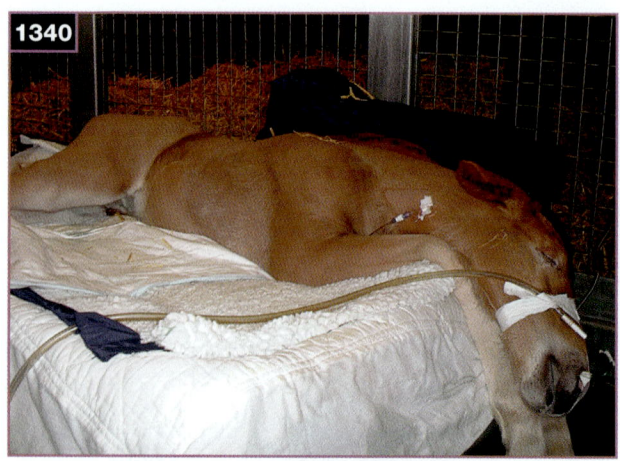

1340 A Suffolk Punch foal in a coma secondary to severe perinatal encephalopathy.

Cardiovascular support. It is important to maintain adequate tissue perfusion, which frequently involves the use of appropriate fluid therapy to restore circulating volume and ionotropes and pressors to maintain blood pressure. (See Neonatal septicemia, p. 970.)

Respiratory support. Most recumbent or heavily sedated foals with neonatal encephalopathy require respiratory support. It is important to maintain PaO_2 levels >60 mmHg or hypoxic damage will continue. This is generally possible using humidified intranasal oxygen at 2–15 liters/minute. Positioning and encouraging mobility significantly improve lung function. Oral caffeine (10 mg/kg p/o followed by 2.5 mg/kg p/o q24h) may stimulate ventilatory drive.

Nutritional support. Nutritional support is a vital part of treatment and enhances recovery. Many of these foals suffer hypoxic damage to the gut and extreme caution with enteral feeding until gut function is normal is appropriate. The use of small volumes of milk (5–10 ml/hour) and glutamine is important for normal development of the gut and recovery from hypoxic damage. Foals can be maintained on glucose solutions for 12–24 hours; however, the use of parenteral nutrition at an early stage can hasten recovery and prevent problems associated with premature enteral feeding in these compromised individuals. Discussion of enteral and parenteral nutrition is beyond the scope of this text.

Others. Vitamin E acts as a free radical scavenger. Oral administration has been shown to significantly increase vitamin E levels in sick foals, and some clinicians consider this approach safer than injecting it. Glutamine (10 g/day divided into 6 doses orally) is important for enterocyte function, therefore supplementation may have a place in the treatment of hypoxic gut damage.

Aggressive antimicrobial therapy is routine in all these cases. All cases require correction of any FPT.

Control of cerebral edema. DMSO acts as a free radical scavenger and has anti-inflammatory effects. Its use in practice is controversial. Care must be taken with administration (10% solution at a dose of 1 g/kg by slow infusion daily for up to 3 days). It can cause severe hemolysis when given at concentrations >20%, or by rapid infusion.

Mannitol (0.5–1.0 g/kg by slow infusion of a 20% solution) has been used to treat cerebral edema. It is contraindicated if hemorrhage is suspected. Dexamethasone (4 mg/50 kg foal i/v q12h) is also used, but is controversial.

Nursing. High standards of nursing care and hygiene are required. A quiet warm environment, if possible close to the mare, is essential. Manual restraint on a padded bed to prevent self-inflicted trauma is important. For the more severely affected individuals, encouragement to rise, move, regain the suck reflex, interact with the environment, and finally suck from the mare takes considerable patience, time, and skill.

Prognosis
The prognosis depends on the severity of the insult and the time taken to stabilize the foal to prevent further hypoxic damage. Foals affected by hypoxia during birth, rather than prenatal effects, often do not exhibit clinical signs until a few hours after birth, and their prognosis for recovery and future athletic use is good. For those foals suffering severe prenatal effects, with clinical signs present at birth, the prognosis tends to be poor. Early referral to a critical-care facility considerably improves the prognosis.

Atresia coli/recti/ani
Definition/overview
Atresia coli, atresia recti, and atresia ani are rare congenital abnormalities where part of the hindgut fails to develop *in utero*. Obstruction of the passage of feces leads to clinical signs of colic, usually manifest in the first 1–2 days of life. In most cases the condition is fatal.

Etiology/pathophysiology
These are developmental abnormalities of one or more segments of the GI tract. Atresia coli, and to a lesser extent atresia ani, are the most commonly seen (1341). Atresia coli is characterized by membranous occlusion of the lumen, remnants of gut connecting two blind ends (cord atresia), or the presence of blind ends with no connection. The condition may be due to vascular anomalies in the fetus. Defects are most commonly found between the left ventral and dorsal colon. Atresia ani is associated with the absence of an anus and variable parts of the rectum. Concurrent urinary tract defects may be present (rare).

Clinical presentation
Foals are normal at birth and usually stand and suck normally. They usually present within 4–24 hours with a progressive, moderate to severe colic, due to physical obstruction of the passage of gas and feces. The more caudal the defect in the gut the slower the onset of signs. In atresia ani no anus is visible or it appears grossly abnormal. In obstructions elsewhere, digital examination *per rectum* reveals no feces present or palpable. Abdominal distension, anorexia, and colic develop and progress over a period of hours.

Differential diagnosis
Meconium impaction; abdominal crisis (e.g. small intestinal volvulus); ruptured bladder; ileocolonic aganglionosis (lethal white syndrome); ileus.

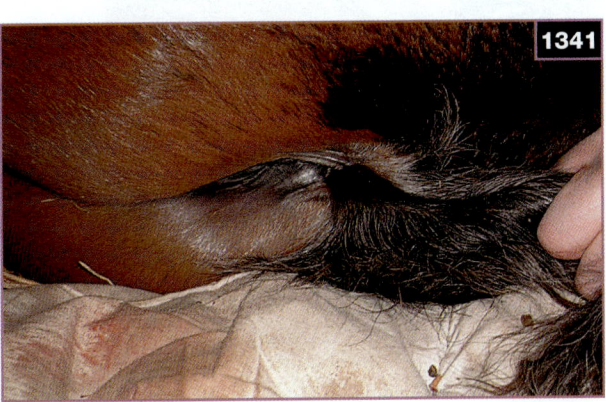

1341 A foal with atresia ani.

Diagnosis

Diagnosis is based on clinical signs, physical and digital examination, which is diagnostic for atresia ani, and diagnostic imaging. Ultrasound examination may confirm colonic obstruction or possible narrowing. Plain radiographs of the abdomen may demonstrate fecal impaction and/or gaseous distension proximal to the site of the intestinal occlusion. Contrast radiography with a barium enema can be useful for confirming the location of the atresia. Proctoscopy or colonoscopy will usually confirm the lesion. In some cases an exploratory laparotomy is required to confirm diagnosis of more proximal lesions and to determine what (if any) treatment options are available.

Management

The location of the abnormality partly determines the possibility of surgical correction. In true atresia ani, surgical reconstruction of the anus may be possible. Colostomy and anastomosis techniques have been attempted in a few published cases, but the results have been poor, particularly as many cases have extensive intestinal motility problems. Most cases are not amenable to surgery because of the degree of atresia, and the prognosis is therefore hopeless.

Meconium impaction

Definition/overview

Meconium consists of the digested amniotic fluid and cell debris accumulated during fetal life and is usually passed within 12 hours of birth. It is usually pelleted or occasionally tarry, dark brownish/green or black fecal material. It is followed by the yellowish material formed from milk products after the first sucks.

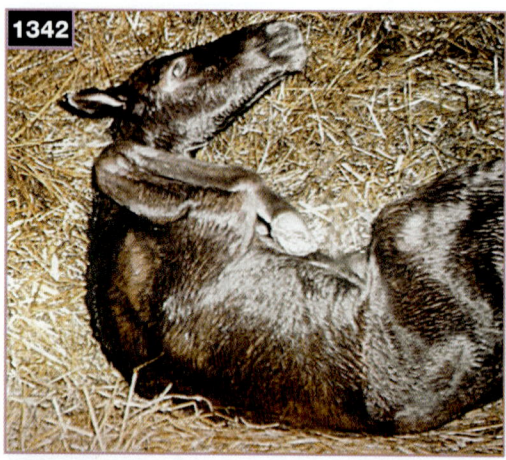

1342 A 24-hour-old foal exhibiting colic associated with meconium impaction.

Etiology/pathophysiology

Impaction may occur in the small colon, possibly more commonly in overdue foals, although the exact cause is unknown. Impaction in the rectum may be related to a narrow pelvic inlet diameter, particularly in Thoroughbred colt foals. Impactions may be seen in foals suffering from perinatal asphyxia syndrome.

Clinical presentation

Foals with meconium impaction usually present with mild to severe colic, which can be progressive, 6–36 hours post partum (**1342**). The foal may become recumbent with rolling and struggling movements. There is persistent unproductive straining to pass feces, with tail swishing or lifting, squatting, and crouching (rounded back). The foals develop progressive gas abdominal distension and are either intermittently or completely off suck. Some foals have been observed to pass small amounts of meconium, but they remain in pain.

Differential diagnosis

Congenital deformities of the GI tract where there is segmental aplasia produce similar signs. Foals with a ruptured bladder may present in a similar way, but these foals are usually older and passing milk feces. An abdominal crisis caused by an obstruction usually presents with severe unrelenting pain and sudden onset.

Diagnosis

Clinical examination and history are important. Careful digital rectal examination may palpate narrowing of the pelvis and some pellets of meconium. The full extent of the impaction is often underestimated by this technique. Ultrasonographic examination of the abdomen and barium enema radiographs may be useful to confirm the diagnosis in refractory cases.

Management

Good colostrum intake will boost nutritional and immunologic status, but it also has a laxative effect and may have benefits in preventing this condition. Primary treatment involves the use of enemas. Buffered phosphate enemas are effective in mild cases; however, repeated use may result in hyperphosphatemia and an inflamed rectal mucosa. Soap and water enemas are not recommended due to their irritancy and the large volume required. Overhydration should not be used in the foal as a treatment for impaction. The use of mineral oil by nasogastric tube should be avoided because it coats rather than rehydrates the impaction and takes some time to reach the site of impaction. In refractory cases the use of 4% buffered acetylcysteine enemas has almost eliminated the need to resort to surgery. Acetylcysteine (100–200 ml of warmed solution administered slowly via a 30 French gauge Foley catheter with the balloon inflated with 30 ml of air) is a powerful mucolytic that helps break down the meconium. It should be retained in the rectum for 30–40 minutes if possible. The enema may take several hours to work and occasionally it may be necessary to repeat the enema. The use of analgesics to control abdominal pain and ensure adequate hydration is equally important. Good nursing care is important, particularly protection against self-inflicted trauma. Surgery should be avoided if at all possible. The use of fingers or instruments to remove pellets from the rectum is contraindicated.

Prognosis
The prognosis is usually good to excellent with correct management, but it is compromised by the presence of concurrent problems such as sepsis. Colt foals with a very narrow pelvic diameter need careful monitoring for up to 14 days.

Conditions affecting older foals

Gastroduodenal ulceration syndrome
Definition/overview
This condition often develops in association with disease or stress or as a complication of diarrhea, in particular rotavirus diarrhea. Ulceration may develop in association with the use of NSAIDs in the foal. Clinical signs are frequently more obvious than in the mature horse; however, sudden death secondary to rupture of a subclinical gastric ulcer is well recognized.

Etiology/pathophysiology
Prolonged diarrhea, various types of stress or concurrent disease, and the administration of NSAIDs have all been associated with an increased incidence of ulceration.

Ulcers develop in the stomach or duodenum when there is an imbalance between the aggressive factors (e.g. gastric acid and pepsin) and the protective factors (e.g. normal GI motility, bicarbonate-rich mucus layer over the glandular mucosa, mucosal blood flow, local prostaglandins, and normal turnover of mucosal cells). The gastric environment in the young foal is highly acidic and disruption of any of the protective mechanisms is likely to result in ulceration. Many types of disease process and various stresses in the neonatal foal may disrupt this mechanism, and the antiprostaglandin effect of NSAIDs can be a significant factor. Ulceration can occur at any point within the stomach of the foal but, unlike the adult, occurs more commonly in the glandular portion. Ulceration in this position tends to lead to more severe clinical signs. In the most serious cases there is perforation of the stomach and/or a major blood vessel, which typically is fatal.

Clinical presentation
There are several syndromes associated with gastric ulceration in the foal:
+ *Type 1.* This type is characterized by the presence of small lesions visible at the margo plicatus without clinical abnormalities.
+ *Type 2.* Active. The foal is usually depressed, partly 'off suck', and may exhibit teeth grinding and increased salivation. It may exhibit signs of abdominal pain such as rolling and lying in dorsal recumbency (1343). There may be a failure to thrive or diarrhea. Ulcers are clearly visible on gastric endoscopy. Linear esophageal ulcers have been seen in severe cases and often result in spontaneous reflux.
+ *Type 3.* Perforated ulcer. May present as acute shock or sudden death or be the end result of severe active ulceration.
+ *Type 4.* Duodenal stenosis. This develops secondary to significant scarring associated with healing of duodenal ulcers. Affected foals usually present with gastric ulcers that initially respond well to treatment and then deteriorate as the stenosis develops. Clinical signs include profound salivation, spontaneous reflux, and poor growth and weight gain.

Differential diagnosis
Other causes of colic such as enteritis, septicemia, and peritonitis may produce similar signs.

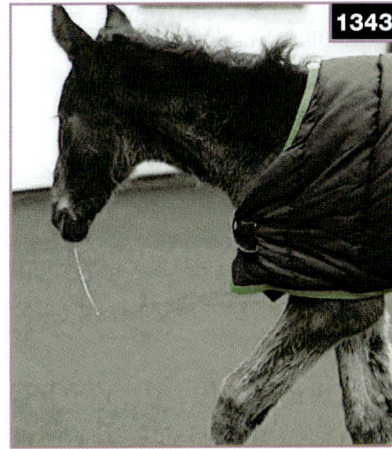

1343 A foal with gastric ulceration showing hypersalivation.

Diagnosis

History and clinical signs are often strongly suggestive of gastroduodenal ulceration. Diagnosis is confirmed with gastroscopy. Lesions are most commonly seen at the margo plicatus and glandular lesions are more frequently seen in the foal than in the mature horse. Care must be taken when interpreting mild changes in the squamous region, because increased desquamation is considered a normal finding in the young foal. Contrast radiography with barium administered by stomach tube can be performed, but may be difficult to interpret. If strictures occur in the region of the bile duct, GGT and serum alkaline phosphatase blood levels will be raised. Abdominocentesis in severe cases will reveal evidence of severe peritonitis with a perforated ulcer.

Management

Early and aggressive therapy is important, as progression of the disease can be rapid. Any underlying disease needs to be treated. Treatment should continue until all the ulceration has healed, which in some cases may be several weeks. In cases with duodenal stenosis, response to treatment is disappointing. Various drugs have been used to treat gastroduodenal ulcers:

+ **Proton pump blockers.** Research indicates that omeprazole (4 mg/kg q24h) is the drug of choice for treatment of gastric ulcers in the horse. Clinical signs often resolve within 24–48 hours; however, it is important to treat for an adequate time to allow complete resolution of the lesions. An equine paste preparation is currently available.
+ **H2 antagonists.** H2 blockers have been widely used. Research indicates that they must be given at adequate dose rates and frequency to be effective and for at least 14–21 days to allow complete healing. Oral ranitidine (6.6 mg/kg q8h) is available. Ranitidine is the only intravenous ulcer treatment (1–2 mg/kg q8h) available in many regions, and intravenous administration may be necessary when the condition of the foal precludes the use of oral drugs. Cimetidine (16–20 mg/kg p/o q6h) is also available, but is of questionable efficacy.
+ **Sucralfate.** This sulfated sugar binds to the ulcer sites, and current research in man suggests it also promotes ulcer healing and increases mucosal blood flow. In combination with a proton pump blocker it may rapidly alleviate clinical signs. It is administered orally (20 mg/kg q6h).
+ **Others.** Depending on the age of the foal and the severity of clinical signs, supportive care and the judicious use of analgesics (opioids) may be useful.

Foals with gastroduodenal stenosis will require nasogastric decompression and in severe cases may only recover with gastrojejunostomy bypass surgery.

Prevention of gastroduodenal ulceration is best achieved by allowing normal feeding habits with mare and foal, careful use of NSAIDs in the foal, and prophylactic use of antiulcer medications in foals subjected to stresses such as surgery, other drug therapy, or other illnesses. The use of prophylactic antiulcer medication in the foal remains controversial.

Prognosis

The prognosis is good with early diagnosis and effective treatment, but the prognosis is poorer if adhesions or stenotic problems occur. Perforated ulcers result in a grave prognosis.

Umbilical infections

Definition/overview

Infection of the external umbilical remnants or the internal umbilical vessels is quite common in the foal.

Etiology/pathophysiology

Infection occurs either due to contamination of the external remnants of the umbilical vessels during the peripartum period, or as a result of deposition of bacteria in thrombosed vessels from hematogenous spread. The infection can then either form a focal abscess with or without surrounding body-wall cellulitis, or extend into the clots and infect the intra-abdominal portion of the vessels and/or urachus. Many cases will involve both internal and external portions. Infection of the umbilical vein may result in abscess formation in the liver. Rarely, cases will exhibit signs of generalized septicemia or localized bacterial infection such as pneumonia and septic arthritis/osteomyelitis. The bacteria most often involved are those seen in neonatal septicemia (i.e. Enterobacteriaceae, *Streptococcus* spp., and *Staphylococcus* spp.).

Clinical presentation

Clinical presentation is variable, depending on the severity of disease and whether disseminated infection is present. Foals with involvement of the external remnants may develop significant swelling of the umbilicus, which is often hot and painful to palpate. There will be a particularly painful swelling, which will also involve the body wall if cellulitis of the latter is present. Frequently, pus can be expressed from the vessels and samples should be collected for culture and sensitivity testing. Some individuals may be pyrexic and inappetent. In some situations, signs of sepsis or its sequelae (i.e. septic arthritis) may be the initial abnormality. Umbilical infections may act as a focus of infection to seed other sites, therefore a thorough clinical examination should be carried out with particular attention paid to localized signs of infection such as septic arthritis/osteomyelitis. Infections of the internal remnants only are usually detected when a focus for infection is being sought.

Diagnosis

Diagnosis is based on clinical signs and palpation and confirmed on ultrasound examination. All foals with evidence of localized or systemic infection should have the umbilicus examined carefully, including using transabdominal ultrasonography. The internal vessels remain visible for about 4 weeks. The normal umbilical vein running cranially to the liver is <10 mm in diameter and the umbilical arteries running caudally to the bladder are normally <12 mm in diameter. Infected vessels are enlarged, contain hypoechoic, echogenic or anechoic material depending on the nature of the purulent material within the vessels, and may have thickened walls.

Blood samples for hematology (neutrophilia), differential proteins (increased plasma fibrinogen), and IgG are helpful in detecting signs of systemic involvement and determining the immune status of the foal, respectively. Some cases of localized external infection show minimal inflammatory/infectious changes in the blood picture.

Differential diagnosis

Umbilical rupture, hemorrhage or hernia; patent urachus; ventral edema or cellulitis.

Management

When infection is confined to the external remnants and there are no signs of systemic involvement, encouraging drainage of the abscess and broad-spectrum bactericidal antibiotics, preferably based on sensitivity testing, may be effective. The case should be carefully monitored and assessed ultrasonographically. Up to 14–21 days of antibiotics may be required. If there is significant involvement of the umbilical vessels (doubled or more increase in vessel size and/or multiple structures involved) or signs of systemic involvement (e.g. septic arthritis/osteomyelitis), surgical resection of the internal and external umbilical vessels should be performed without delay.

Correct care of the umbilicus at foaling is critical, as is early ingestion of high-quality colostrum. General management issues such as providing a clean foaling environment and minimizing contact of foals with sources of contamination (wash teats and udder prefoaling) should be addressed.

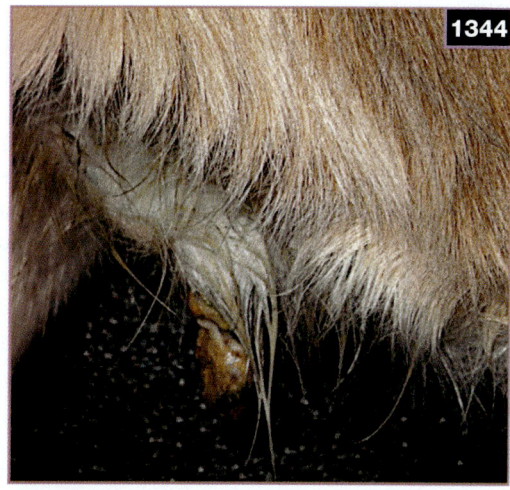

1344 A foal with an acquired patent urachus showing a moist and swollen remnant of the umbilical cord through which urine is drained intermittently.

Persistent or patent urachus
Definition/overview

Patent urachus is a condition whereby the urachus is open and urine leaks from the umbilical remnants. This may occur as a result of the urachus failing to seal at birth (persistent urachus) or when the urachus closes for a few days but then reopens.

Etiology/pathophysiology

The urachus is present in the fetus to allow urine to pass into the allantoic cavity. It normally closes at parturition and urine flow should cease within 24 hours. The exact mechanism whereby this closure mechanism goes wrong is not known, but possible causes include: umbilical disorders such as torsion, increased length, and clamping of the cord rather than natural rupture; excessive foal straining (i.e. meconium retention or ruptured bladder); localized urachal/umbilical infections; systemic infections; prolonged recumbency. Patent urachus is one of the most common complications that develop in compromised foals undergoing intensive care. It can also occur when irritant agents are applied to the umbilical remnants. These then necrose and leave the urachus and umbilical vessels exposed.

Clinical presentation

Urine is often observed leaking from the umbilical remnants continually or when the foal urinates. The umbilical area is continually wet and this may lead to urine scalding and dermatitis of the ventral abdominal skin. In some cases the umbilical remnants are necrotic (**1344**).

983

Differential diagnosis

Other umbilical disorders; ventral abdominal edema; localized cellulitis.

Diagnosis

Clinical signs are usually adequate for diagnosis. Ultrasonographic examination may reveal evidence of an umbilical infection or a dilated structure continuous with the bladder. Urinalysis and culture will identify any infection within the urinary tract. Contrast cystography has been used in more obscure cases. In compromised foals, full blood analysis and clinical work-up are required.

Management

If no other disease is present, many cases will resolve spontaneously within 24–36 hours provided the umbilicus is kept clean and dipped in 0.5% chlorhexidine solution 2–4 times a day. Prophylactic broad-spectrum antibiotics are often administered concurrently. The application of desiccating or cauterizing agents to the opening of the urachus to enhance closure remains open to debate, but may be appropriate if localized infection is not present. Various materials are used including 2% iodine solution, silver nitrate sticks, or even 4% formalin solution. These should be inserted into the urachal remnants (only 1–2 cm at most) for a few seconds 2–4 times daily for 2–4 days. Any concurrent or underlying disease needs to be treated. Surgical removal of the entire umbilicus will be necessary if it is refractory to medical treatment after 4–5 days, if it or other structures in the umbilicus are infected, if the foal has systemic signs, or if the area is abscessed or necrotic.

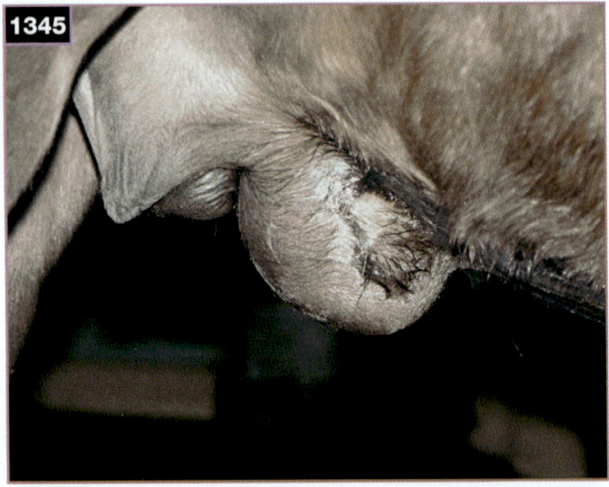

1345 A young male foal with a congenital umbilical hernia. The hernial sac could easily be replaced into the abdomen and did not contain intestine at any stage.

Umbilical hernia

Definition/overview

This is a relatively common abnormality due to failure of abdominal musculature to close around the umbilicus.

Etiology/pathophysiology

Umbilical hernia is possibly a congenital inherited disorder, especially in the Thoroughbred, where filly foals may be more commonly affected. Hernias may develop following umbilical disorders such as cord infection or inflammation. Up to 2% of the foal population can develop umbilical hernias, but intestinal incarceration is very rare. The size and contents of a hernia determine its significance as a clinical problem. Larger hernial rings are less likely to close spontaneously and have a greater chance of containing intestine or omentum.

Clinical presentation

The hernia is characterized by a visible and palpable swelling of the umbilicus, which is reducible on palpation (1345). It may be detected soon after birth but is often only identified later in life when the foal is suckling or weaned. The muscular edge of the defect is readily palpable. There are no other clinical signs unless there is abscessation or loops of bowel become incarcerated in the hernia, the latter being a rare complication. Incarcerated bowel leads to colic, local swelling, and palpable pain.

Differential diagnosis

Umbilical infection; ventral abdominal-wall injuries; ventral edema; colic.

Diagnosis

In the majority of cases palpation will determine the size of the umbilical defect and its contents, give an indication as to whether it is reducible, and rule out other umbilical disorders. Ultrasonographic examination can confirm the diagnosis in selected cases.

Management

Many hernias will reduce in size spontaneously over the first few weeks of life. Smaller hernias can be treated by careful application of elastrator bands or, in some countries, hernial clamps. Larger defects (6–8 cm) or those that persist through to 6–9 months of age should be treated surgically. Very large hernias may require repair via the insertion of a polypropylene mesh subperitoneally.

Prognosis

The prognosis is very good for small hernias that resolve spontaneously, good for hernias that require simple surgical intervention, and guarded for those that have incarcerated bowel or need mesh repairs.

1346 A foal with uroperitoneum showing persistent posturing in order to urinate.

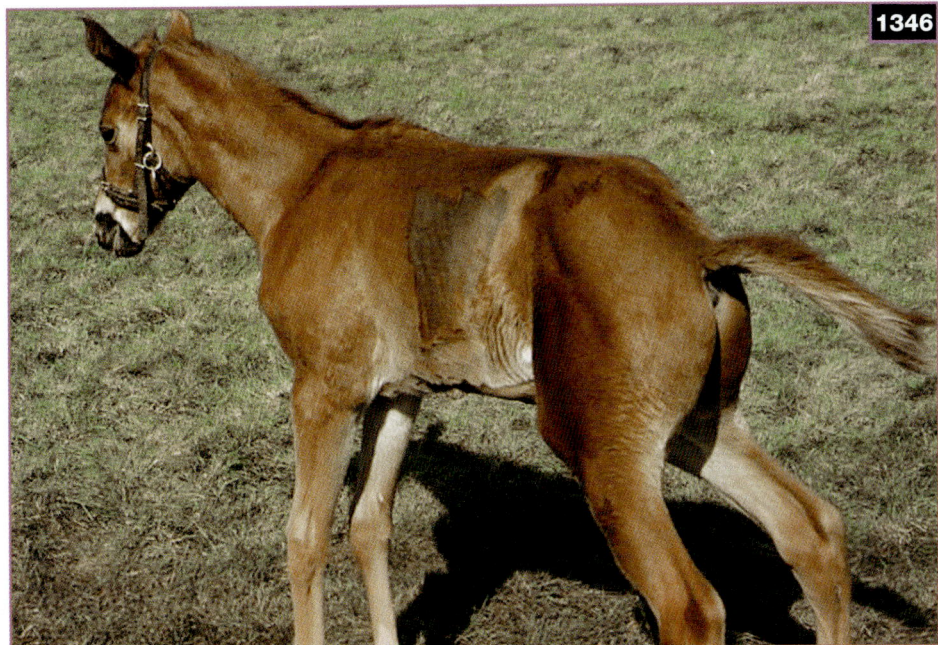

Uroperitoneum in the foal

Definition/overview

Uroperitoneum (the presence of urine in the peritoneal cavity) is a well-recognized syndrome in the young foal. Ruptured bladder is the most common cause, with clinical signs presenting in the first 2–4 days of life. Congenital defects in the bladder or other parts of the urinary tract can also occur, but are rare. Occasionally, uroperitoneum occurs slightly later secondary to a traumatic injury. Rupture of the bladder and other parts of the urinary tract, including the urachus, does occur secondary to infection in some cases ascending from the umbilicus. The presence of urine in the peritoneal cavity leads to severe metabolic and electrolyte abnormalities, which are fatal if not corrected.

Etiology/pathophysiology

Most tears in the bladder are thought to occur during the birthing process, with defects most commonly found in the dorsal wall, suggesting a predisposing weakness. The causes of ruptured bladder in the foal are currently being reconsidered. It has been suggested that the condition is more common in male foals and this was noted to be due to their longer urethra decreasing the chance of bladder emptying. Recent evidence does not support an increased incidence in males. Congenital defects in the urinary tract include failure of the dorsal bladder wall to close during gestation, ureteral ectopia with rupture, or ureteral/urethral atresia and rupture. Occasional foals are unable to detect distension of the bladder and initiate a micturition reflex. It has been suggested that this may be associated with hypoxic–ischemic insults and foals may

require catheterization for up to 7 days before function develops. Rupture of the bladder and/or urachus has been noted secondary to infection and necrosis, which may be ascending from the umbilicus. These tears are often in a more variable position at the apex of the bladder or in the urachus itself, and clinical signs occur later. Traumatic rupture of the bladder from abdominal trauma is also seen in older foals.

Clinical presentation

The foal is normal at birth and the signs are rather non-specific initially, with progression over the first 2–3 days. In foals where infection of the tract is an etiological factor, clinical signs may only become obvious as late as 5–10 days of age. Foals may be observed to pass no urine or small quantities of urine (defect is small), which can be deceptive. Straining to urinate with a hollowed back and extended hindlimbs is classically noted, sometimes associated with dribbles of small amounts of urine (**1346**). Other signs include lethargy, progressive abdominal distension, mild colic, and going off suck. Fluid waves may be felt on percussion of the abdomen. Some preputial or perineal edema may develop. This has been particularly noted in urethral and urachal ruptures. Pyrexia is not usually present in classic ruptured bladders, but it will be noted if there is infection involved. There are often increased heart and respiratory rates with, in the later stages, poor pulse quality, electrolyte-related dysrhythmias, and hypovolemia. With severe electrolyte disorders there may be CNS signs, circulatory collapse, and death.

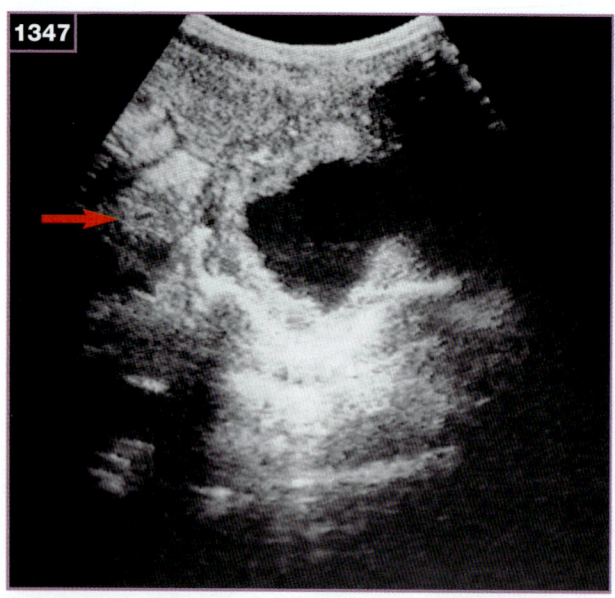

1347 Transabdominal ultrasound image of a urinary bladder (arrowed) that several days earlier had been repaired surgically for a rupture. This postoperative check clearly shows an intact and distended bladder.

Differential diagnosis

Meconium impaction; other causes of colic.

Diagnosis

History and a careful physical examination, including abdominal palpation, are important. Diagnosis is confirmed on ultrasound examination of the abdomen (**1347**). Large quantities of free fluid are seen and the bladder often appears rather shrunken. The defect in the bladder wall may be visible. Ultrasound-guided abdominocentesis can be used to collect urine from the peritoneal cavity. The umbilicus should also be examined by ultrasonography. Measurement of peritoneal and blood creatinine concentrations should be carried out: creatinine concentrations of twice that in the blood confirm that the abdominal fluid is urine. Methylene blue in sterile solution can be infused into the bladder via a urethral catheter; if there is a defect in the bladder, it is subsequently found in the peritoneal fluid. Plain and contrast urography/cystography have been used in the past, but their major use now is in the diagnosis of problems of the ureters and urethra. Typically, these foals are hyperkalemic, hyponatremic, hypochloremic, hypoglycemic, acidotic, and azotemic due to the accumulation of urine in the peritoneal cavity and the equilibration of electrolytes and fluid across the peritoneal membrane. Diagnostic tests to detect concomitant sepsis or bacterial peritonitis should be considered.

Management

Ruptured bladder is initially a medical rather than surgical emergency. It is important to stabilize foals metabolically prior to surgery, as they present a high anesthetic risk. Urine should be drained from the abdomen gradually while providing intravenous fluids to support the circulation and prevent acute hypotension due to expansion of previously collapsed capillary beds. The catheter can be left in place until the defect is corrected surgically. Hydration should be maintained, and acid–base and electrolyte abnormalities should be corrected with intravenous fluid therapy (0.9% or 0.45% saline can be used). In hyperkalemic animals, dextrose-containing fluids, such as 5% dextrose saline, are indicated (4–8 ml/kg/minute). With severe hyperkalemia (K$^+$ >5.5 mmol/l [>5.5 mEq/l]), insulin (0.1–0.5 IU/kg s/c or i/v) or sodium bicarbonate (1–2 mEq/kg) have been used concurrently by some clinicians, although fluid therapy and abdominal drainage alone may be successful in reducing potassium levels in most cases. Continuous monitoring of cardiac activity with an ECG is useful, particularly when the blood potassium concentrations are >6.0 mmol/l (>6.0 mEq/l). Broad-spectrum antibiotics are indicated, but nephrotoxic drugs such as aminoglycosides should be used with caution in these foals. Once the foal is stable, surgical repair of the bladder should be performed without delay. Umbilical remnants may be removed and peritoneal lavage is often carried out prior to surgery to repair the defect. Laparoscopic repair has been reported, but many clinicians still prefer a conventional midline laparotomy approach. Damage or problems elsewhere in the urinary tract are rare and surgical approaches are decided on a case-by-case basis.

Prognosis

In uncomplicated cases the prognosis for recovery is fair to good, although second surgeries are occasionally required. Concomitant infection worsens the prognosis.

Diarrhea
Definition/overview
Diarrhea is probably the most common problem in foals. In one survey, up to 80% of foals under 6 months of age had one or more episodes of diarrhea. Diarrhea is a clinical sign rather than an actual disease. The severity can vary from a transient self-limiting episode in an otherwise healthy foal to a life-threatening condition as a result of the disease or of secondary complications. Identification of the specific etiology in individual cases is difficult because of the extensive list of causes and limited diagnostic methods available. Treatment is often supportive in the physiologic and noninfectious forms.

Etiology/pathophysiology
In the young foal, immature colonic function is unable to compensate for small-intestinal disease and therefore many more causes of diarrhea are associated with small-intestinal disorders than are seen in the adult. The list of possible causes in the foal is extensive, but it can be split up on the basis of the pathophysiology of the individual diseases:

✦ **Physiologic.** Many foals will have a bout of mild and self-limiting diarrhea at 7–10 days old that may last for 1–7 days and is associated with the development of normal large-bowel function. 'Foal heat diarrhea' is so-called because of its association with this part of the mare's reproductive cycle. It is not related to milk changes, but is associated with the development of normal function of the large colon and establishment of the natural microflora of the colon and cecum by coprophagia and exploration of its environment by the foal. The diarrhea is profuse and watery, but the foal remains well and on suck.

✦ **Dietary.** Well-known causes include milk overload, inappropriate milk replacer feeding to orphan foals, dietary indiscretion, and lactose intolerance (see p. 548), which can be a secondary complication of infectious enteritis such as rotavirus or *Clostridium difficile* infection.

✦ **Bacterial.** *C. difficile*, *Salmonella* spp., *C. perfringens*, *E. coli*, *Campylobacter* spp., *Rhodococcus equi*, *Aeromonas hydrophilia*, and *Actinobacillus equuli* have been implicated, with varying degrees of evidence. Some bacteria, such as *E. coli*, after adhering to the gut mucosa, are able to produce enterotoxins, which are absorbed and then affect the secretory patterns in the gut, leading to watery and profuse diarrhea. Other bacteria, such as salmonella and clostridia, invade the bowel wall, causing extensive mucosal and submucosal damage and sloughing, which does not heal quickly. Because of the loss of

the mucosal barrier the foal may become more vulnerable to bacterial invasion, bacteremia, and septic shock. Inflammatory cellular infiltration and edema in the deep layers of the intestine impair absorptive and secretory functions. Protein is lost into the lumen, increasing its fluid content. Intestinal spasms may lead to colic signs or ileus. The diarrhea is profuse and fetid and may contain blood. *Lawsonia intracellularis* is a cause of protein-losing enteropathy in older foals, and is discussed in more detailed elsewhere (see p. 544).

✦ **Viral.** Rotavirus and coronavirus can cause mild mucosal cellular damage, particularly at the tips of the intestinal villi, leading to maldigestion and malabsorption. The cellular damage is transient, but osmotic drawing of fluid into the bowel leads to diarrhea in the foal because the colon and cecum in foals up to 3 months of age are unable to compensate for small-intestinal pathology. Rotavirus infections are common in suckling foals and they are highly contagious.

✦ **Protozoal.** *Cryptosporidium parvum.*

✦ **Parasitic.** *Strongyloides westeri*, *Parascaris* spp., and large and small strongyles can all cause diarrhea due to migrating larval damage, subsequent inflammation and vascular damage, motility disturbances, and significant protein leakage. Many of these diseases are more significant in the older foal and weanling.

Passive transfer of immunity is important in the protection of foals against diarrhea, particularly in infectious causes. Where the transferred local and systemic immunity is high against the local pathogens, the foal is more effectively able to withstand an infectious challenge, unless it is overwhelming.

The pathophysiologic consequences of diarrhea in the foal can be very serious, with rapid and substantial deficits and changes in fluid and electrolyte balance. These can quickly lead to circulatory shock, collapse, and death within hours.

Clinical presentation
A full clinical history of the individual and farm involved should be taken and assessed. It is important to gather data on the effectiveness of passive transfer of immunoglobulins to the foal and its health status, feeding/sucking, nutrition, and general demeanor. The epidemiology of the premises on which the foal is kept should be thoroughly explored, especially movements in or out, the preventive disease measures in place, the health status of all animals on the premises, and previous problems.

A full clinical examination should be performed including abdominal auscultation and assessment of hydration status. The diarrhea itself should be evaluated because

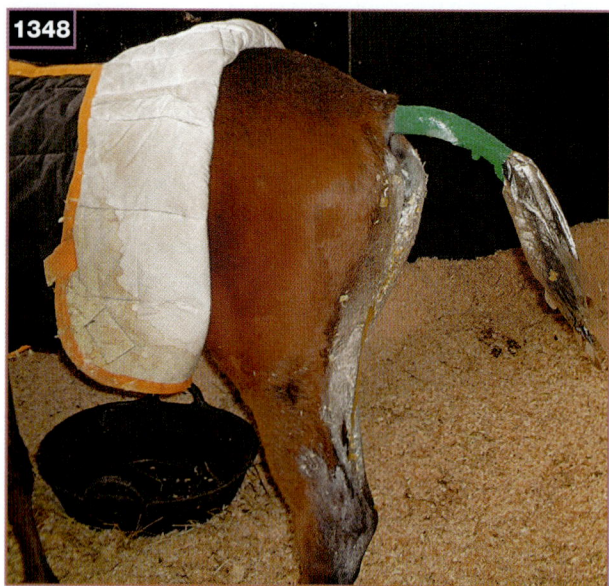

1348 A foal with severe diarrhea associated with salmonellosis.

its consistency and volume can vary considerably, and are important when calculating fluid losses (**1348**). Abdominal pain is variable and some foals with low-grade abdominal pain may be anorexic. Foals can become rapidly dehydrated and suffer significant electrolyte imbalances when the diarrhea is watery and high volume. In addition, their milk intake is reduced. Pyrexia, depression, other systemic signs of sepsis, and circulatory collapse can occur rapidly in some of the bacterial infectious types of diarrhea. Severe bacterial enteritis with septic shock can rapidly lead to acute renal failure; therefore, renal function should be monitored closely by assessment of urine output and renal enzymes. There may be a period of 12–18 hours before the foal develops diarrhea and shows colic-like signs, and this is a particular feature of rotavirus infections. Gastroduodenal ulcers are a complication of diarrhea, particularly in rotavirus infections.

Diagnosis

Despite the fact that it is only possible to make a specific diagnosis in about 50% of cases, attempts should be made to achieve this due to the infectious nature of the more common causes (e.g. rotavirus). In many cases it is appropriate to take fresh fecal samples for virology testing, bacteriology culture and sensitivity testing, clostridial toxin assays, parasitologic examination, and direct microscopy. It is important to collect adequate quantities of fecal material and place them in sterile containers.

In chronic cases, or those with severe clinical signs, blood samples are indicated. Blood cultures should be taken in all young foals with diarrhea and systemic clinical signs. Assessment of blood samples for hematology, serum electrolytes, serum proteins, inflammatory markers, and renal enzymes is useful for both diagnosis and therapy. PCV and total protein levels may help with assessment of hydration. The total and differential WBC count will vary with the type of infection, often showing dramatic decreases in *Salmonella* infections. Blood glucose concentrations are unstable in neonatal foals and can be seriously depressed in diarrhea cases. Electrolyte and acid–base status are more difficult to ascertain in the general practice situation, but are very useful in developing a rational treatment plan. All of the major electrolytes (sodium, potassium, chloride, calcium) may be reduced and there may be a metabolic acidosis. Repeated samples to indicate trends or responses are particularly useful.

Management

Treatment should be instituted as soon as possible, usually before the results of diagnostic tests are available. This is especially important in the infectious forms of the disease, which can rapidly become life threatening.

Fluid therapy. Adequate appropriate fluid therapy is the key to successful treatment. When it is necessary to give fluids, consideration should be given to the most appropriate route and composition of those fluids. This will be determined by: (1) the age of the foal; (2) the degree of mucosal damage suspected; (3) the severity of the dehydration; (4) metabolic disturbances; (5) milk intake; and (6) the complicity of the foal and the competence of its handlers.

If oral fluids are used, it is important to ensure that they have adequate quantities of sodium, chloride, glucose, potassium, and bicarbonate or its precursors. Many types of commercially produced electrolyte solutions or powders are readily available, some with the option of adding glucose. Small volumes should be given frequently (up to 500 ml q1–2h) either by stomach tube, dosing, or bucket feeding. Fresh clean water should always be available.

Intravenous fluids are extremely important in foals with diarrhea in order to restore circulatory volume rapidly and correct electrolyte imbalances. They are ideally administered by continuous infusion via an intravenous catheter. In many practice situations, intermittent boluses of fluid may be necessary. In the absence of laboratory results, isotonic balanced electrolyte solution or lactated Hartman's spiked to give 5% glucose solution is a good starting point. The first liter may be given as a resuscitation bolus in hypovolemic foals over 20 minutes, then the rate of infusion decreased to 3–5 ml/kg/hour taking into account maintenance requirements and increased losses. Additional potassium can be added to the fluids, but it is safer given as KCl (8 g/50 kg q8h). A plan for fluid therapy in the future should be made. Colloids may be used to increase oncotic pressure or correct hypovolemia. Plasma will also enhance immune function. Bicarbonate should be used with caution in fluid resuscitation/rehydration.

Anti-endotoxin hyperimmune plasma. This is commercially available and can be useful.

Antiulcer medication. This should be considered, especially in rotavirus cases.

Protectants/adsorbents. There are many protectants/adsorbents on the market, but it is important to dose with adequate quantities. The preparation used is a question of personal preference. The authors use bismuth subsalicylate (Pepto Bismol) at a dose of 1–2 ml/kg q8–12h.

Drugs that alter motility. Drugs that reduce intestinal motility are contraindicated in infectious cases of diarrhea. In chronic noninfectious cases, loperamide has proved useful (0.1 mg/kg p/o q6h, then increased incrementally to 0.2 mg/kg).

Probiotics. Many are available and they may help re-establish normal gut flora, although few scientific data are available.

Oral plasma. This has been used in foals, especially those with rotavirus diarrhea, by some clinicians for its local protective effects (50 ml q4–6h).

Analgesics and anti-inflammatory drugs. Flunixin meglumine is useful in the treatment of endotoxemia (0.25 mg/kg i/v q8–12h), but extreme care should be taken with its use because the toxic effects are increased in young foals, especially if they are collapsed and/or hypovolemic. A useful analgesic in foals is N-butylscopalammonium bromide (Buscopan™) (0.3mg/kg i/v) or butorphanol (0.01–0.04 mg/kg i/v), which is short acting and has sedative effects.

Antibiotics. In most cases of diarrhea the use of antibiotics is contraindicated; however, there are several situations when they are necessary. Young foals with sepsis and diarrhea should receive antibiotics. The combinations noted in the 'Neonatal septicemia' section (p. 970) are the best first choice. Translocation of bacteria can occur in young foals with diarrhea caused by an agent that damages the GI mucosa. Metronidazole (10–15 mg/kg p/o q6–12h) is indicated for treatment of clostridial diarrhea. Young foals with salmonellosis should be given antibiotics, because they usually have or will develop sepsis. Intracellular bacteria (e.g. *R. equi*) may respond to treatment with erythromycin (25 mg/kg p/o q8–12h) or azithromycin (10mg/kg p/o q24h) and rifampicin (5mg/kg p/o q12h). Antibiotic choice should be based on culture and sensitivity results where possible, but in many cases, due to the delay in obtaining these results, treatment is started on the basis of clinical judgement. It is important to understand the pharmacokinetics of the antibiotics that are used, because any that are excreted or secreted into the bowel after systemic administration, along with those given orally, will be more likely to cause intestinal flora upsets. The toxic side-effects of antibiotics (e.g. nephrotoxicity with aminoglycosides) are potentiated in the hypovolemic foal.

Feeding. In line with current recommendations for feeding children with diarrhea, milk is not withheld if the foal wishes to nurse. In severe cases, parenteral nutrition may be necessary, as malnutrition can significantly delay recovery. When the foal is off suck, bolus stomach tubing or, ideally, the use of an indwelling feeding tube will allow the nutritional requirements to be met via the enteral route. It is important to evaluate whether the enteral route is appropriate in foals that are off suck. In addition, as the foal's stomach is small, it must not be overloaded. A starting volume of 300–400 ml is appropriate for a Thoroughbred foal under 2 weeks of age.

Nursing. High standards of nursing and hygiene are important with sick diarrheic foals. They should be kept clean, dry, and comfortable, with regular cleaning of soiled areas and applications of barrier ointments. It is also important to advise handlers of potential zoonoses (*Salmonella, Campylobacter*) and also the highly infectious nature of some of the infectious causes of diarrhea.

Control and prevention. The use of protective clothing, gloves, and foot dips will help reduce the spread of infection. Keeping each mare and foal in a designated stable throughout has been shown to reduce the build-up of infectious disease. Stabling or using dedicated contaminated 'dirty' paddocks for scouring foals will help contain environmental build-up of infection. A rotavirus vaccine is available to vaccinate mares in the 8th, 9th, and 10th months of pregnancy. This vaccine increases antibody levels in the colostrum and IgA in the milk during lactation.

Septic arthritis/osteomyelitis

Definition/overview

Septic arthritis/osteomyelitis is a common, potentially career- or life-threatening condition seen in young foals. In one survey of Thoroughbreds, up to 1% of foals were affected. It may be part of other multifocal infections in some foals. Early diagnosis and appropriate aggressive treatment is the key to a successful outcome.

Etiology/pathophysiology

Infection via the hematogenous route is most common in foals. Infection can occur as a secondary complication in septic foals or it may develop as a result of bacteria seeding from a focal infection (e.g. the umbilical remnants) or from the digestive and respiratory systems. The increased blood flow to rapidly growing bones, the presence of trans-physeal vessels for the first few weeks, and the slow flow and low oxygen tensions in the terminal metaphyseal and synovial vessels tend to favor foci of pathogenic bacteria in the joint itself or the nearby bony epiphysis/physis. Spread can also occur into a joint from adjacent infective foci in the physis or soft tissue. Traumatic wounds involving synovial structures or iatrogenic infections after joint injections can also less commonly lead to joint sepsis. Multiple joints and/or the physes/epiphyses may be involved. The most commonly isolated bacteria are similar to those recorded in septicemic foals (i.e. *E. coli*, *Actinobacillus equuli*, *Salmonella* spp., *Klebsiella* spp., *Streptococcus* spp., and *Staphylococcus* spp.). In older foals *R. equi* may also lead to bone infection in the epiphysis and physis and/or, in some foals, to an immune-mediated nonseptic synovitis.

Foals that are described as 'high risk' with FPT of immunoglobulins, prematurity/dysmaturity, or adverse peripartum events are predisposed to septic arthritis/ osteomyelitis.

Once infection is localized and established in the joint or bone, there is a marked exudative septic inflammation leading to rapid ischemic necrosis of affected tissues. This leads to rapid bone and/or cartilage degeneration with soft tissue fibrosis and reaction and, in the bone, abscess formation.

Clinical presentation

There are five different types of disease presentation classified according to the site anatomically, the etiology of the initial infection, and the subsequent clinical signs, radiographic changes, and necropsy findings. Differentiation clinically in some cases may be difficult.

✦ *S type.* There is a septic synovitis without bone involvement. The foal is less than 14 days old, with one or more swollen and painful joints and acute-onset severe lameness. There may be systemic illness.

Minimal radiographic signs are evident initially, with typical septic synovial fluid identified on arthrocentesis.

✦ *E type.* There is infection in one or more joints and the adjacent epiphysis in slightly older foals (3–4 weeks), with acute-onset severe lameness. The stifle and tarsocrural joints are most commonly affected with joint distension, considerable periarticular swelling, and deep bone pain. Bone changes are often evident on appropriate radiographic views. These cases carry a more guarded prognosis.

✦ *P type.* Infection occurs in the physis and metaphysis, usually at a single site. The adjacent joint may become infected by local or vascular spread, or there may be sympathetic inflammation in the joint without septic changes. This is less common than the S type and can occur from 1–12 weeks of age. There may be swelling and pain on palpation over the physis with or without joint distension. Radiographic changes occur quite quickly, but repeat series may be necessary to identify some cases. In some cases there is a prior history of systemic illness such as diarrhea or pneumonia. The distal physis of the long bones appears most vulnerable to this type.

✦ *I type.* Infection enters the joint from infected periarticular soft tissues. It is a new classification and appears to affect the upper limb joints (i.e. the coxofemoral and femorotibial joints). Early detection of the soft tissue infection will help prevent this serious complication.

✦ *T type.* This is a rare form involving infection of the small cuboidal bones of the tarsus and carpus. Collapse of these bones allows the infection to spread to the joint or joints. It is a separate condition from the more common aseptic collapse of the cuboidal bones seen in premature and dysmature foals (see p. 975). There is joint swelling, moderate to severe lameness, and radiographic changes.

The clinical signs will vary depending on the type of sepsis that is involved, but signs usually include acute, moderate to severe lameness, which rapidly worsens, and some degree of joint swelling and/or soft-tissue swelling associated with a joint epiphysis or physis (**1349**). Some joints that may be involved are not always easily palpable (e.g. the shoulder or hip joint), therefore all joints should be carefully examined. Skin surfaces should be evaluated for signs of trauma or a penetrating wound. Pain and restricted movement of an affected joint, or pain on palpation of the physis, should be evaluated. A thorough clinical examination is required to identify foci of infection as well as systemic or multifocal disease.

Differential diagnosis

Other causes of lameness of both infectious and noninfectious types (i.e. fractures, foot abscess, traumatic injuries, kicks); nonseptic joint disease; hemoarthrosis. In a young foal presenting with two or more of the above clinical signs, the case should be treated as a potential infection until proven otherwise.

Diagnosis

Diagnosis is confirmed on aseptic synoviocentesis and analysis of the retrieved synovial fluid. The sample should be subjected to visual examination, total and differential WBC counts, and total protein analysis. Synovial fluid and blood culture and sensitivity testing are important, but are often disappointing in the number of positive results that are obtained. Any material obtained from bone lesions should also be cultured and examined cytologically. Radiographs of any suspicious joints or physeal regions are helpful in differentiating the types of disease, directing specific therapy, and clarifying the prognosis. In chronic cases they help detect severe damage such as osteoarthritis or osteomyelitis. Radiographs are especially helpful in cases involving bone infection (1350). False-negative radiographic findings do occur in early cases, and repeat radiographs should be considered 3–10 days later in these cases. Ultrasonographic examination of suspicious joints and swellings can yield useful information, particularly where there is considerable periarticular swelling. In both bone and joint infection, blood samples usually indicate signs of infection. The total WBC count is usually increased, with a neutrophilia, marked increase in serum amyloid A, and increased fibrinogen concentrations.

In all cases of septic arthritis/osteomyelitis it is essential to check for other disease and a focus of infection, including ultrasound evaluation of the umbilical remnants.

Management

Early instigation of treatment is essential due to the rapid and progressive degenerative changes in an infected joint and the life-threatening nature of some of these infections. There are considerable economic implications regarding treatment of these cases, and these should be discussed at the outset.

Antibiotics. Broad-spectrum, bactericidal antibiotics that reach adequate concentrations in joints and bone should be administered systemically at suitable dose rates. The choice of antibiotic(s) should be based on culture and sensitivity results if available, but there should be no delay in their use while awaiting results. It is important that antibiotics are administered for at least a week after resolution of the lameness and hematological improvement. Intra-articular antibiotics are used regularly by some clinicians to

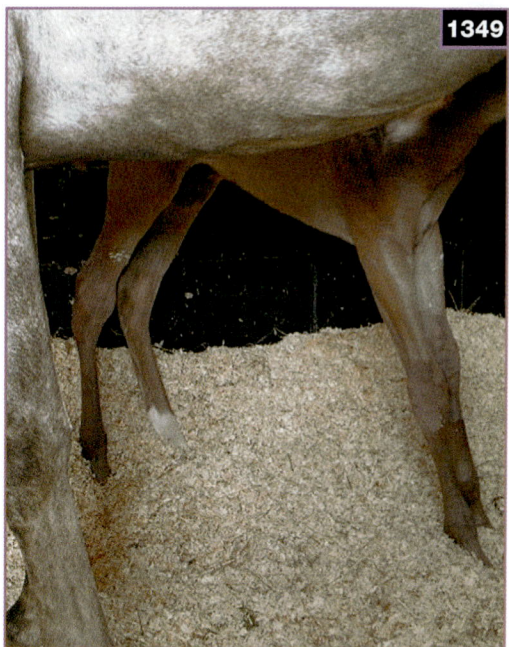

1349 A foal with distended intercarpal and tarsal joints.

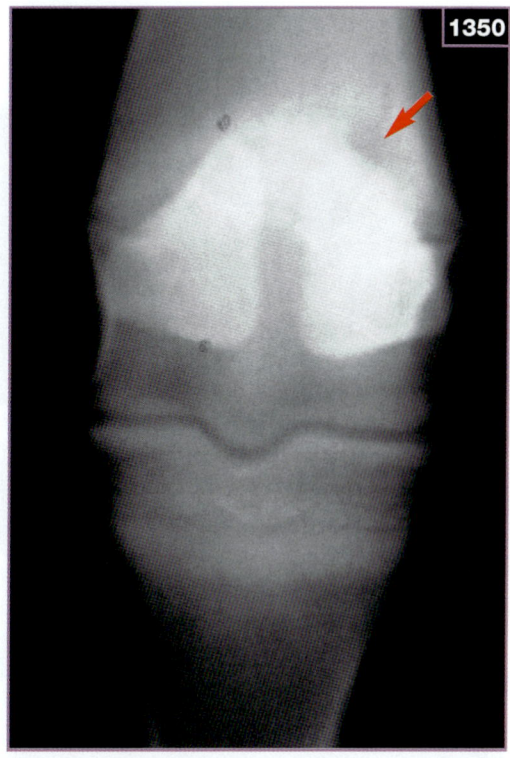

1350 Dorsopalmar radiograph of the distal 3rd metacarpal bone and metacarpophalangeal joint of a 4-week-old Thoroughbred foal with a medial metaphyseal osteomyelitic abscess of the distal 3rd metacarpus (arrow).

991

achieve very high local levels, but some antibiotics are irritant to the joint and may cause increased inflammation. Antibiotics may be injected into the joint following lavage and/or drainage (i.e. 150–300 mg gentamicin or amikacin) and subsequently repeated, or antibiotic-impregnated collagen sponges can be left in the joint to provide sustained release of the drug over a period of time. Regional perfusion with antibiotics and/or intraosseous medication is a useful technique in the treatment of septic arthritis and osteomyelitis in foals, particularly in nonresponsive cases. If aminoglycosides are used both systemically and locally, it is important to consider the total dose/day to reduce the risks of nephrotoxicity.

Lavage. Joint lavage is essential to remove inflammatory material. There are a variety of techniques to achieve this, with different advantages, disadvantages, and costs. The joint may simply be drained with a needle. Distension and irrigation of the affected joint are often achieved by a through-and-through technique with 3–5 liters of sterile polyionic fluid per joint in the sedated or anesthetized foal (1351).

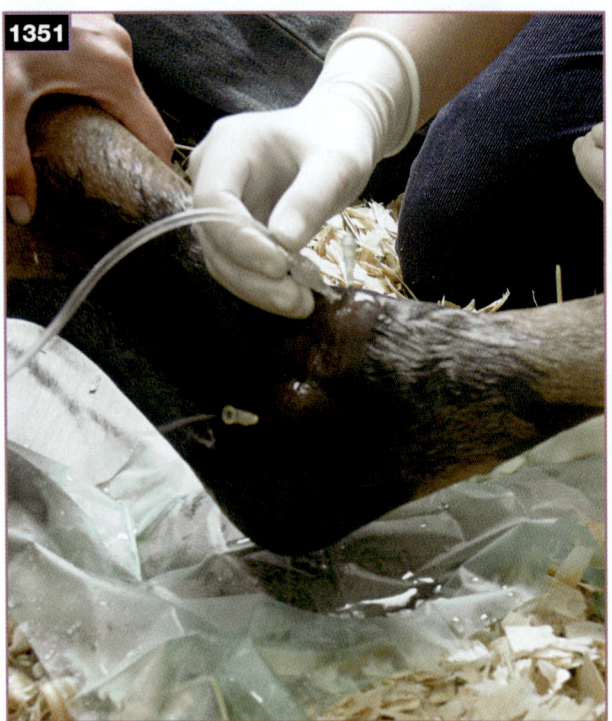

1351 The tarsocrural joint of a young Thoroughbred foal with a septic synovitis undergoing through-and-through lavage of the joint under heavy sedation and local regional analgesia.

Surgery. Lavage can most effectively be accomplished via an arthroscope. The added diagnostic advantages of this technique are the retrieval of material from within the joint and synovial biopsies for culture, plus it gives a clearer prognostication for the future of the foal. Therapeutically, the advantages are a more thorough removal of abnormal material and synovium plus the opportunity to debride cartilage and bone lesions in the joint. Postoperative drainage can be established. In chronic nonresponding or poorly responding cases arthrotomy and open drainage have been used very effectively, but the postoperative management of these cases is expensive and prolonged. Surgical curettage of bone lesions of the physis followed by open drainage and lavage has proven very successful, but it is expensive and can lead to pathologic fractures.

Other treatments. NSAIDs are useful in these cases to decrease inflammation and pain, but they can cause toxicities, especially in systemically ill foals. They can also confuse the degree of lameness as a part of assessing response to therapy. However, reduced doses of flunixin meglumine are very suitable for this purpose. The routine use of antiulcer medication is recommended in these cases, as they present with a high risk for this complication. The foal should be box rested and affected limbs bandaged. There should be aggressive treatment of any concurrent systemic problem, careful monitoring of nutritive intake, and supportive nursing. The foal should be closely monitored for response to therapy. In cases of septic arthritis, if the lameness fails to improve significantly and the synovial white cell count remains increased, repeat lavage should be carried out. In cases of osteomyelitis, serial measurement of serum amyloid A protein is useful in monitoring the response to selected antibiotics. In cases that respond to the selected treatment, serum amyloid A protein levels start to fall over 48–72 hours, often in advance of improvement in the lameness.

Prognosis

The prognosis is dependent on the number of sites of infection, the degree of damage to the joint(s), the presence of bone involvement, concurrent systemic disease, and the response to therapy. Multiple joint and/or bone involvement seriously affects the likely outcome, as does the presence of systemic illness. Chronic cases and those poorly responsive to initial aggressive treatment often require extensive and prolonged treatment, with a poor prognosis for a return to full soundness. Acute S-type cases treated quickly and aggressively carry the best prognosis. A recent study indicated that Thoroughbred foals treated for septic arthritis were less likely to start on a racecourse when compared with controls, and they were also older when they first started on a racecourse.

Behavioral problems

Katherine Houpt

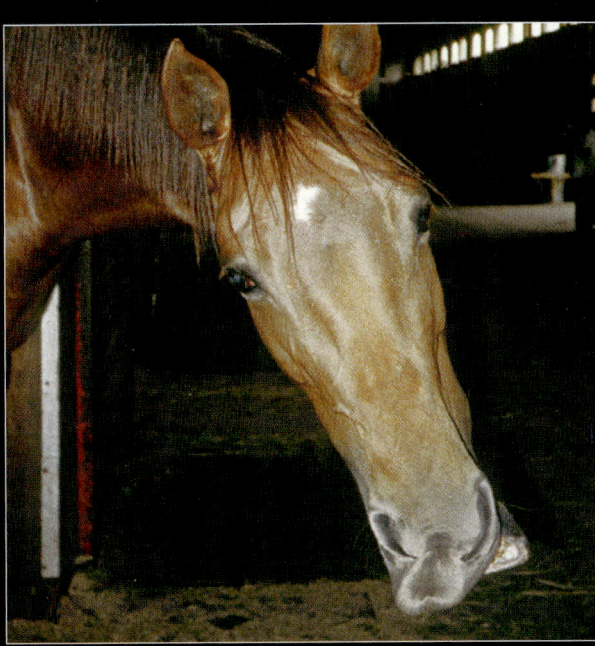

15 Behavioral problems

Behavioral problems probably contribute to the wastage (euthanasia or selling at auction) of horses as much as most medical conditions. There has not been a survey determining the prevalence of equine behavior problems, with the exception of stereotypic behaviors. Stereotypic behavior is defined as repetitive, apparently functionless behavior and includes what were once termed stable vices such as weaving, stall walking, and cribbing. Surveys in Canada, the UK, and Sweden have revealed that 0–10% of horses displayed stereotypic behavior.

The most serious type of equine behavior problem is aggression. People and other horses can be badly injured or killed. Fears or phobias that result in sudden violent movements and bolting can also result in injury to the rider. Other problems, in addition to those described here, include excessive sexual behavior in geldings, insufficient sexual behavior in stallions, escape behavior when separated from other horses, and misbehavior when loading or riding in a trailer.

Behavior assessment

An equine behavioral history form should answer six questions: (1) what is the problem behavior; (2) who performs the behavior; (3) who is the recipient; (4) what does the horse look like when performing the behavior (i.e. were his ears back, where was the tail); (5) where does the problem take place; (6) when does the behavior occur and for how long? A standardized form can be useful when performing a behavioral assessment (*Table 70*). An example is a horse presented as aggressive. The animal is a 5-year-old Thoroughbred mare. She is aggressive to people, mostly to women, and only in her stall. The behavior occurs at least weekly, but waxes and wanes. It is not related to her estrous cycle. At the time she aggresses, her tail is clamped to her rump, her ears are held sideways, and the sclera is visible. This horse is fearfully aggressive, so the treatment prescribed should reflect this.

In contrast to cats and dogs, horses are rarely owned by the same person for their entire lives. This makes determining the cause of a behavior difficult. A horse may have been sold because it had the behavior problem, but the former owners may be reluctant to admit that. Another difficulty is that owners often do not take care of the horse at their own home. If the horse is boarded, a behavior such as cribbing, that is not a problem to the owner, may become a problem because the manager believes, erroneously, that the behavior is learned. Managers may also be reluctant to offer more hay or bedding, or change turnout schedules, for an individual horse.

The history of a racehorse is even more difficult to elucidate. The horse often moves from a training facility to the track and back again. The veterinarians are different and the people who ride the horse change. The trainer may change and even the groom, who probably knows the horse best, may not be the same from season to season and facility to facility.

In addition to the signalment, an understanding of the management of the horse is important. Stall size and bedding are important for understanding stereotypies. The purpose for which the horse is kept will help to determine the prognosis. An aggressive horse should not be a child's mount, nor should a nervous horse be used for Western pleasure classes. The steps the owner has taken will determine what treatments may or may not be successful. For example, many stable managers try to 'teach horses to be patient' by forcing them to wait to be fed or to be taken outside. This only serves to teach the horses that they must paw, neigh, or pace longer before they are rewarded with food or freedom.

Videotaping is very helpful, if it can be accomplished safely, because owners may not be able to describe the horse's posture and facial expressions adequately.

Many behavioral problems first appear with an environment change. For example, a gelding may be fine in a stall with solitary turnout or with a group of geldings, but may exhibit sexual and inter-male aggression when pastured with geldings and mares. Horses usually kept outside frequently exhibit stereotypic locomotory behavior, such as weaving or stall walking, if moved to a stall.

Refusal to load, or problems while leaving trailers, require detailed information on the type and design of the trailer. The driver of the vehicle, the horse's past experience in trailers (e.g. its behavior when the trailer is parked, in motion, turning, stopped for a traffic light) should also be known.

The past behavior of a mare that rejects her foal and where the foaling took place will help to determine the prognosis for the current and future foalings.

TABLE 70 Example of a behavioral assessment form for use in horses

Owner's name: Veterinarian's name: Horse's name:

Address: Address   Breed:

                                                                         Sex, age:

Telephone: Telephone: Color:

BEHAVIOR PROBLEM

What is the main behavior problem or complaint?. . . . .

When did you <u>first</u> notice the main problem (age of horse)?. . . . .

Describe the chronology of the behavior problem
(i.e. how it developed over time).. . . . .

When did it first become a serious concern? . . . .

In what general circumstances does the horse misbehave? . . . .

How frequently does/do the problem(s) occur
(how many times daily, weekly, or monthly)?. . . . .

Describe several examples (in detail: time, place,
horse's behavior, human reaction)

1. Most recent incident . . . . .Date. . . . .

2. Second to last incident . . . . .Date. . . . .

3. Third to last incident . . . . .Date. . . . .

Other significant incidents . . . .

What have you done so far to try to correct the problem? . . . .

How do you discipline your horse for this problem?. . . . .

HORSE'S BACKGROUND

Why did you decide to get a horse? . . . .

Why this particular breed, sex, color? . . . .

Where did you get this horse (check one):   ☐ Finder   ☐ Newspaper/magazine advertisement

                                             ☐ Breeder   ☐ Friend

                                             ☐ Rescue   ☐ Other . . . .

Have you owned horses before?   ☐ Yes   ☐ No

DIET AND FEEDING

What do you feed your horse? Please be specific
(e.g. frequency, amount and brand name) . . . .

What type of hay do you feed (frequency, amount)? . . . .

Other supplements . . . .

HORSE'S ENVIRONMENT

1. Type of housing (stall, pasture, run-out shed)? . . . .

2. Exercise (hours per week ridden, hours per week in paddock)? . . . .

3. Type of bit used, martingale? . . . .

4. Other horses in environment and relations between horses (friendly, aggressive, neutral)? . . . .

5. Other animals in environment? . . . .

(Continues)

TABLE 70   **Example of a behavioral assessment form for use in horses** (continued)

EARLY HISTORY

1. Why was horse obtained? Is it still used for this purpose? ....

2. Age at weaning (if known)? ....

3. Age when obtained by present owner? ....

4. Were there previous owners? ....

5. Do related horses have similar problems? ....

EDUCATION

1. Age at halter-breaking? ....

2. Method of training to saddle or harness, age when training began? ....

3. Other types of training methods?   ❑ Driving   ❑ Jumping

    ❑ Dressage   ❑ Games

    ❑ Trail riding   ❑ Cutting

OTHER BEHAVIOR PROBLEMS

1. Shying, how often and at what? Any other problems? ....

2. Head shy? ....

3. Resentful of grooming? ....

4. Aggression toward humans or animals (dogs, cows, etc.)? ....

5. Aggression toward other horses (threatens, strikes, bites, kicks, chases)? ....

6. Misbehavior under saddle (check appropriate behavior)

    ❑ Moves while rider mounts   ❑ Backs in harness

    ❑ Bucks, rears   ❑ Wants to lead/ will only follow other horses

    ❑ Runs away   ❑ Slow to leave and quick to return to barn

    ❑ Hard to keep on right or left   ❑ Other ....

7. Barn problems (check appropriate one)

    ❑ Cribs   ❑ Chews wood

    ❑ Paws   ❑ Kicks stall

    ❑ Weaves   ❑ Stall walks

8. Sexual behavior (check one)

    ❑ Excessive   ❑ Inadequate   ❑ Abnormal

9. Maternal behavior (check one)

    ❑ Excessive   ❑ Inadequate   ❑ Abnormal

PHYSICAL HISTORY

1. Present medical problems? ....

2. Past medical problems? ....

3. Drug history? ....

4. Results of diagnostic tests? ....

Behavioral problems

The training methods and agent involved with training may explain the horse's present behavior. The tack used, the severity of bits, and the martingale will indicate how difficult the horse is to handle under saddle. The amount of exercise the horse gets, under saddle or in a paddock, can explain some behavior problems.

The horse's diet, including brand names of commercial feeds and amounts fed, should be noted. Just writing that the horse is fed hay and grain is not adequate. Many horses are overfed for the amount of work they perform and they may expend the excess energy in misbehavior rather than in deposition of adipose tissue.

The horse's schedule of turnout should be included. The substrate (grass or bare ground), social condition (alone or with another horse or horses), and frequency and length of turnout should also be evaluated.

The present owner may or may not know about the horse's early training, but that can be helpful if available. Problems under saddle, such as bolting, refusing to leave the stable, or refusal to let another horse pass, may give clues as to the horse's personality. The presence or absence of stereotypic behavior should be recorded.

Perhaps most important are the owner's goals for the horse. Although the veterinarian may feel one aspect of the horse's behavior is important, the owner may be concerned about a totally different behavior.

Environmental enrichment

Environmental enrichment has become a popular catch-phrase for those concerned with animal welfare. The phrase is used to mean anything that will improve the life of caged or confined animals from laboratory mice to zoo elephants. Although horses are considered pampered companions or recreational or performance animals, they are kept in confinement as limited in size on a body weight basis as that of laboratory mice. There are two main behaviors of horses that environment enrichment has addressed to date: locomotory and oral. Locomotory enrichment usually takes the form of 'turnout'. Turnout usually involves taking the horse on a lead line from its 3.6 × 3.6 meter (12 × 12 foot) box stall to a grassless paddock where it is released, usually alone, for a variable number of hours. Horses are usually eager to enter the paddock and they may canter and buck for a few minutes, but after 10 minutes they typically revert to the default behavior (e.g. foraging in the soil, pacing). Horses with stereotypic behavior in the stall are turned out longer than stereotype-free horses, which probably is not because turnout causes stereotypies, but because the owners are trying to enrich the environment of horses with stereotypies.

Much oral enrichment is based on the hypothesis that horses are 'bored' and want to play. For that reason, hanging toys, balls, large plastic carrots, or even empty plastic bottles, are suspended in stalls. These are usually ignored by the horse. The exceptions are young horses, usually colts, which are playful and exploratory.

Better forms of oral environmental enrichment are based on the hypothesis that horses are grazing animals that would normally spend half their time, day and night, acquiring food. The simplest form of enrichment is to provide as much roughage as the horse can ingest and a variety of roughage (i.e. hay, straw bedding, branches of nonpoisonous trees), provided there are no contraindications to exposure of a given horse to these sources (e.g. heaves). There are devices that slow ingestion, such as hay nets or weights on bales of hay in a rack, both of which force the horse to pick out the hay a bit at a time. Other devices are lollypops – sugar or molasses in gelatin-based cylinders that the horse should lick. Unfortunately, some horses bite these and, therefore, consume the lollypop quickly, sometimes resulting in obstruction. There are models that can be suspended or which force the horse to lick rather than chew. Flavored rollers have also been marketed to distract horses from wood chewing.

Natural grazing consists of grasping a stalk of grass with the prehensile lips, biting it off with the incisors, and masticating with the molars, and, after 3–6 bites, walking a step or three to the next patch. The best forms of environmental enrichment available combine this eating and walking pattern. There are cylinders or balls with holes that release pellets or grain as the device turns. The horse pushes it with its nose, harvests the feed from the floor, and takes a step or two to push the device again.

The aspect of a horse's natural situation that none of these devices address is the social one. Horses are herd animals living in the natural state with 6–10 other horses: an adult stallion, several adult mares, and immature foals. Some stables attempt to improve the social environment by turning horses out in compatible groups. The typical box stall allows no contact with other horses, but even those stalls with bars, rather than solid walls, between the horses do not permit normal interactions.

Stall companions, such as a dog, cat, chicken, goat, pony, or another horse, have all been used to enrich the environment socially. These are not always practical, so mirrors have been used. Horses, especially stallions, may attack a mirror initially, but later will usually orient themselves to it and be calmed.

The optimum environment enrichment for a horse is to live in a group of horses with forage, shelter, and water freely available. The closer we can make the domestic horse's environment to that, the more enriched it will be.

Drugs for treatment of behavioral problems

The psychoactive medications used to treat equine behavior problems fall into four categories: (1) those affecting dopamine; (2) those affecting serotonin; (3) those affecting gamma aminobutyric acid (GABA); (4) those affecting opiates. Hormones may also be used.

Dopamine

The most commonly used medications are those affecting dopamine. Dopamine receptor blockers include acepromazine and the longer-acting fluphenazine. These drugs are used to calm nervous horses and to reduce aggression. There is an ethical issue when drugs are used to enhance the performance of show horses. Apparently, acepromazine is frequently used to calm Western pleasure horses before a competition, but this should not be done because the whole point of those competitions is to demonstrate how naturally calm the horse is.

The phenothiazine tranquilizer fluphenazine is a good example of both the ethical problems involved in the use of psychopharmacologic agents in the horse and the health risk to the horse. Fluphenazine is a long-acting dopamine blocker and, as such, is valuable for reducing fractious behavior for several weeks at a time. It is difficult to detect in the blood a few days after injection so, until newer methods were used to detect fluphenazine, a horse could perform or be sold while under the influence of the drug. Although it is a more potent dopamine blocker than the more commonly used acepromazine, the risk of side-effects is greater. Dystonia and akathisia were observed in a Thoroughbred filly following 0.1 mg/kg i/m of fluphenazine. Periods of circling, pawing, and agitation alternated with periods of extreme sedation. Diphenhydramine (250 mg i/v) reverses the effects of fluphenazine. Benztropine mesylate (0.035 mg/kg p/o q12h) has also been used with anecdotal success.

Acepromazine is useful for the treatment of foal rejection. The pharmacologic explanation is that dopamine inhibits prolactin release. When dopamine is blocked by acepromazine, prolactin is released and stimulates milk production and, possibly, maternal behavior. At the least, an increase in milk production will increase udder fill and make suckling more pleasurable for the mare.

Lactation by nonpregnant mares can be induced by a 3-week course of the dopamine antagonist sulpiride. A protocol for this has been devised by Dr. Dietrich Volkmann of the Cornell University College of Veterinary Medicine (*Table 71*).

Serotonin

The drugs of most use for both aggression and stereotypic behavior are those that influence serotonin. Serotonin is released into the synaptic cleft and returned to the presynaptic neuron by a reuptake neuron and a reuptake mechanism. Blocking this mechanism can prolong serotonin activity. The nonspecific reuptake blockers, such as amitriptyline (50 mg/horse p/o q12h gradually increasing to effect or 250 mg), are used most frequently, in part because they are inexpensive.

Paroxetine (0.5 mg/kg p/o q24h) was used to suppress weaving in a single horse. She ceased weaving when her stable mates were present, but would weave as soon as she was alone.

TABLE 71 Protocol for induction of lactation in nonpregnant mares

Day 1
0.1 mg/kg estradiol benzoate i/m q24h
0.44 mg/kg regumate p/o q24h
1 mg/kg sulpiride i/m q12h

Days 2–5
0.02 mg/kg estradiol benzoate i/m q24h
0.44 mg/kg regumate p/o q24h
1 mg/kg sulpiride i/m q12h

Day 6
PGF2α (e.g. 5 mg dinoprost i/m)

Day 7
0.02 mg/kg estradiol benzoate i/m q24h
0.44 mg/kg regumate p/o q24h
1 mg/kg sulpiride i/m q12h

Day 8
Introduce foal and perform cervico-vaginal stimulation

Days 8–21
1 mg/kg sulpiride i/m q12h

Vigorous stimulation of the cervix, mimicking passage of the foal at parturition, can then be used to induce maternal behavior.

Cyproheptadine is a serotonin antagonist. It has been used to stimulate appetite and to reduce stallion-like behavior in geldings. The mode of action of the latter effect is either the anti-androgenic properties of the drug or is secondary to its serotonin antagonism, which would inhibit ACTH release. Some geldings that exhibit behavior changes in their teens may have pituitary adenomas. These produce ACTH, which in turn stimulates adrenal steroids, including adrenal androgens. The dose of cyproheptadine is 16–88 mg per horse p/o q24h. Treatment should be started using the lower dose, with a gradual increase of 8 mg/day until the behavior is improved or the highest dose level is reached.

Ejaculation has been induced in stallions using tricyclic antidepressants, either clomipramine (2.2 mg/kg i/v), or imipramine (500 mg/stallion i/v, which stimulates erection and masturbation), followed 45 minutes later by the alpha-adrenergic agonist xylazine (0.5 mg/kg i/v). Imipramine (100 mg/stallion p/o q12h) has also been used to improve sexual performance.

Hormones

The posterior pituitary hormone oxytocin has been used successfully to stimulate maternal behavior as well as milk let down in mares who are reluctant to allow their foals to nurse. It has also been used to stimulate ejaculation in impotent stallions (10–20 IU/horse i/v).

Progesterone is widely used to reduce aggressive behavior in horses. Injection of progesterone (0.4 mg/kg/day i/m) appears to be more effective than oral administration of altrenogest (0.02 ml/kg/day of a 0.22 % preparation). The mode of action is unknown, but progesterone has a depressive effect on many areas of the brain. Testosterone has been used to increase libido in stallions. Although most stallions with poor libido have testosterone levels comparable to laboratory standards for stalled stallions, stallions living in a band with mares have a much higher level and those having at least fence contact with mares have an intermediate level of testosterone. Presumably the herd stallion's level is optimal for a breeding stallion.

Gamma aminobutyric acid

Stallions that are frightened to breed due to past unpleasant experiences or lack of experience can be improved by administration of diazepam (0.05 mg/kg slowly i/v). Diazepam is a GABAergic drug that acts to inhibit neurons by its effects on chloride channels.

Opiates

Opiate blockers have been used to treat two equine behavior problems: cribbing and self-mutilation. The fact that blocking opiates with naloxone (0.02–0.04 mg/kg i/v), for example, reduces cribbing within 30 minutes may indicate that opiate release leads to cribbing and not *vice versa*.

Behavioral disorders

Coprophagia
Definition/overview
Coprophagia is the ingestion of feces, either the horse's own or those of another horse.

Etiology/pathophysiology
In adult horses the cause of coprophagia appears to be a dietary deficiency, particularly of roughage, but the behavior also occurs when horses are protein or vitamin deficient. Coprophagia is a normal behavior of foals for the first few months of life. The dam's feces are preferentially consumed. It is hypothesized that coprophagia introduces bacteria and protozoa from the GI tract of the adult horse to that of the foal. Another hypothesis is that it familiarizes the suckling foal with the foods selected by its dam.

Because it is normal behavior in foals, no pathology is involved. Presumably, parasites could be introduced, particularly if the feces were not fresh. The factors that lead to coprophagia in adult horses have not been linked to any particular lesion. It has been associated with equine motor neuron disease, probably because both are associated with management of the horse in a grassless paddock.

Clinical presentation
The horse is either observed to be ingesting feces or the owner will find that there is no longer any manure in the stall. Foals usually eat their mother's feces. Stalled horses may consume their own feces (autocoprophagia) often following an episode of diarrhea or when hay is replaced with a complete pelleted diet.

Differential diagnosis
Coprophagia must be differentiated from obstruction if the only sign is a lack of manure in a stall. Ingestion must be differentiated from sniffing of the feces, which many horses do when encountering another horse's feces. It should also be differentiated from geophagia, during which soil is consumed.

Diagnosis

Diagnosis is based on direct observation of the horse prehending, mouthing, and actually swallowing feces (1354).

Management

No treatment is necessary for foals because the behavior wanes with time, disappearing by 15 weeks of age. Provision of roughage or pasture will solve coprophagia due to a lack of fiber. Provision of browse-branches from a non-toxic tree has also been successful in eliminating coprophagia in horses that must be maintained in a grassless enclosure. Correction of underlying GI problems should reduce associated coprophagia. Correction of any other deficiency (protein or vitamin) will eliminate coprophagia.

Prognosis

The prognosis is excellent.

1354 Coprophagia. Eating feces is a normal behavior in foals. (Photo courtesy R Keiper)

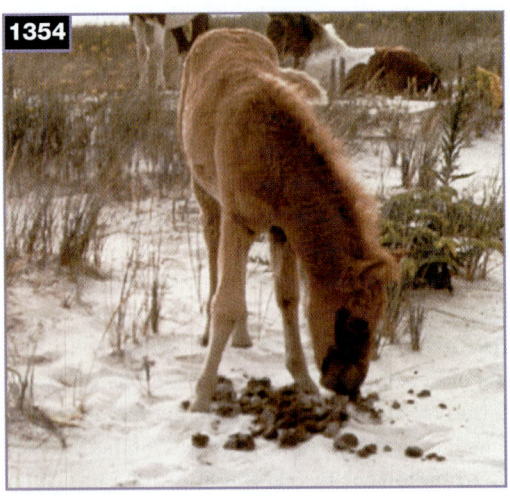

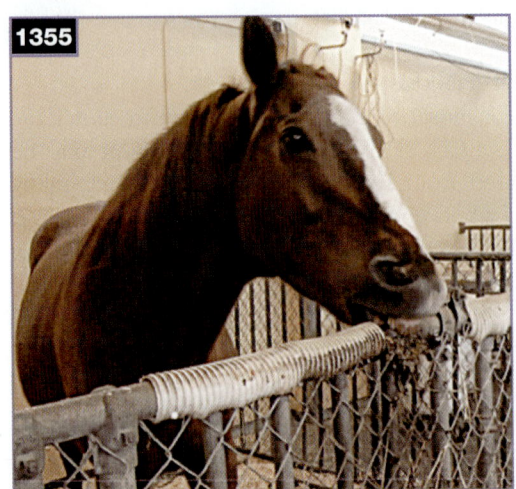

Cribbing

Definition/overview

Cribbing is the behavior in which a horse grasps a horizontal surface with its teeth, flexes its neck, and aspirates air into the esophagus, creating a low-pitched grunting sound (1355).

Etiology/pathophysiology

The cause is unknown, but it is apparently familial. It is much more common in some breeds, particularly Thoroughbreds and Warmbloods. It is also more common in horses used for dressage, eventing, and jumping than in those used for endurance riding. Cribbing is apparently stimulated by eating sweetened grain mixtures.

Although opiates may be involved, cribbing does not result in an increase in blood opiates. The pathologic consequences of cribbing are wearing of the incisor teeth, development of the musculature of the neck, and potentially colic, including epiploic foramen entrapment. Rarely, a horse will be emaciated because it cribs rather than eats.

Clinical presentation

Cribbing begins when foals are weaned into stalls and fed grain; pasture-weaned foals are less likely to crib. The owner may be concerned about the behavior because it is considered a 'vice' and is believed to be learned from other horses, although that has never been documented. Cribbing may cause damage to property if the horse pulls buckets off the wall or rails off the fence.

Differential diagnosis

Cribbing must be differentiated from wood chewing, in which wood is ingested, and from mouthing without neck flexure or aerophagia.

Diagnosis

Diagnosis is based on observation of the cribbing behavior, including the sound of air being ingested.

Management

Making the horizontal surface aversive with taste repellent is usually not successful. Electrifying surfaces is usually effective, but the horse may find another place, such as the waterer, to crib. Covering wooden surfaces with metal does not help because most horses prefer to crib on metal. Surgical treatment (accessory neurectomies and myotomies) is no longer recommended. There are a variety of collars that act by preventing the horse from flexing its neck. These do inhibit aerophagia, but they must

1355 The typical position for cribbing, with an arched neck as teeth grasp a horizontal bar.

Behavioral problems

be kept extremely tight. Cribbing muzzles prevent the horse from reaching a surface. There is a shock collar that delivers a shock when the horse flexes its neck. These are effective in some horses, but dangerous in others that are shocked repeatedly, as they throw their heads to avoid it. There is no evidence that using aversion to prevent cribbing will increase the incidence of other stereotypies, although the horse may appear depressed. Avoiding sweet feed and pasturing the horse in a compatible social group is the most effective treatment.

Prognosis
The prognosis is poor because the horse will usually crib when the collar is removed.

Noise making
(door banging, wall kicking, etc.)
Definition/overview
Noise making is any action by a horse that produces a loud noise. The noise can be produced by holding the stall door in the teeth and pulling it back and forth, by kicking the stall walls, rattling buckets, or running the teeth up the bars of the stall.

Etiology/pathophysiology
There are three possible etiologies: (1) lack of environmental stimulation, which leads the horse to produce its own aural and tactile stimulation; (2) learned behavior that has been rewarded with feed, so the horse is more likely to perform the behavior again; (3) aggression toward a neighboring horse, which is more likely if the behavior is stall kicking.

Concussive injury to the limbs can result from kicking or a minor limb problem can be aggravated. Tooth wear may result from rubbing on the bars or, possibly, from grasping the door.

Clinical presentation
Stallions are more likely to stall kick, usually as a form of aggression. Horses that apparently make a noise for stimulation are usually presented because they are annoying and/or are damaging the barn. Horses that have been 'trained' to make a noise before feeding are often fed last to 'teach them to be patient', which actually teaches them to make a noise for an even longer period of time.

Differential diagnosis
These repetitive, apparently functionless, behaviors must be differentiated from escape behavior or neurologic problems.

Diagnosis
Diagnosis is based on observation of the horse producing the noise.

Management
Reducing confinement time, providing free-choice roughage of at least two types and mirrors, can help a horse that cannot be kept outside in a group. A motivated owner could teach the horse that silence, not noise, will be rewarded by giving the horse small food treats for increasing lengths of silence, beginning with 5 seconds.

Prognosis
The prognosis is fair to poor if the behavior has been performed for many years, and excellent if the horse can be pastured, not stalled.

Pica
Definition/overview
Pica is the ingestion of nonfood objects (1356).

Etiology/pathophysiology
The cause of pica is unknown, but in some cases it may be the result of mineral or other nutrient deficiencies, in which case the eating of soil high in minerals would be nutritional wisdom. In some cases the pica is not intentional (e.g. a horse picking grain from the ground may ingest sand). Pica can result in obstruction of the GI tract.

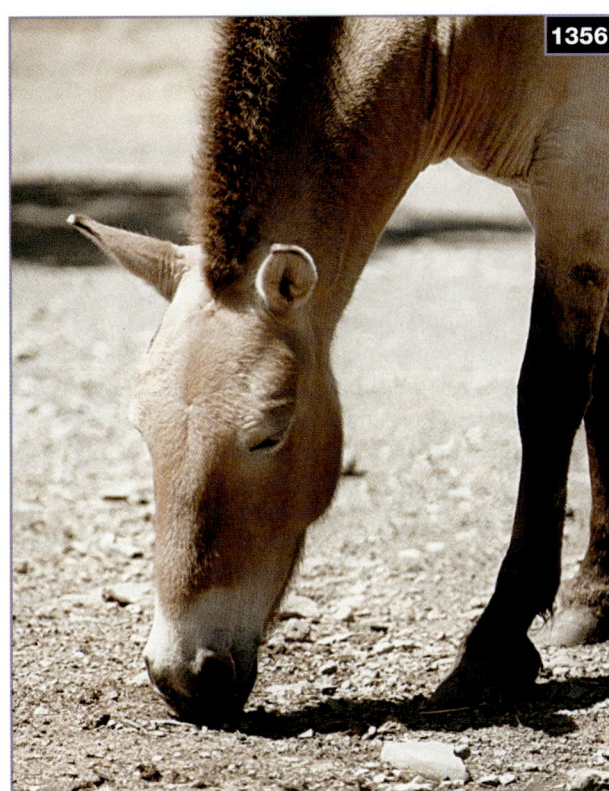

1356 Geophagia (the habit of eating clay or earth/soil) by a Przewalski's horse.

Clinical presentation

A horse with pica is usually presented because it has an indigestible object lodged in the GI tract, either the esophagus (choke) or the ileocecal valve (colic). Eating rocks seems to be more common in the late winter or early spring. Foals may ingest the objects they are exploring, especially stringy objects. This can lead to intestinal obstruction, intestinal accident, or formation of enteroliths.

Differential diagnosis

Pica must be differentiated from wood chewing and non-ingestive mouthing.

Diagnosis

Diagnosis is based on observation of the horse eating a nonfood object or discovery of the object during examination or surgery.

Management

The usual treatment is to remove the object from the horse's environment or make the surface aversive with taste repellent. If necessary, the horse can be muzzled to prevent ingestion.

Prognosis

The prognosis is fair because the horse may attempt to eat rocks or other items again. Foals usually cease the behavior as they develop.

Weaving

Definition/overview

When weaving, the horse shifts its weight from side to side for minutes to hours at a time. It is actually walking in place, but the front hooves are lifted higher than the hind ones.

Etiology/pathophysiology

Weaving occurs in confined horses that have little or no visual access to other horses. This is an escape behavior because the horse usually does it at the door.

Weaving can be so frequent that extreme hoof wear occurs. General stress on the musculoskeletal system can develop from the repetitive activity.

Clinical presentation

The horse is presented because it is spending so much time weaving that the owner is concerned about effects on performance. The behavior is worse just before feeding or if a companion horse is removed.

1357 A horse weaving in response to separation from other horses. Her head is extended out of the Dutch door. Note the lashing tail.

Differential diagnosis

Weaving should be differentiated from other types of stereotypic or pathologic walking, and from horizontal head shaking.

Diagnosis

Diagnosis is based on observation of the horse performing the behavior (1357).

Management

The best treatment is to house the horse in a compatible social group on pasture. If that is not possible, more visual contact with other horses should be provided or a mirror can be placed in the stall. Physically preventing the behavior with weaving guards is not recommended because the horse will be frustrated. The specific serotonin inhibitor paroxetine (0.5 mg/kg p/o q24h) reduced weaving in one horse.

Prognosis

The prognosis is good if management is changed; otherwise it is poor.

Head shaking

Definition/overview

Head shaking is movement of the head rapidly and frequently, either vertically or horizontally.

Etiology/pathophysiology

Most head shaking is pathologic rather than behavioral in origin, but a few horses have learned this behavior in anticipation of food or in response to rider demands.

Foreign bodies, trigeminal neuritis, guttural pouch empyema, ear mites, ethmoidal hematoma, atlanto-axial arthritis, and laryngeal hemiparalysis are some of the pathologies observed in head shakers.

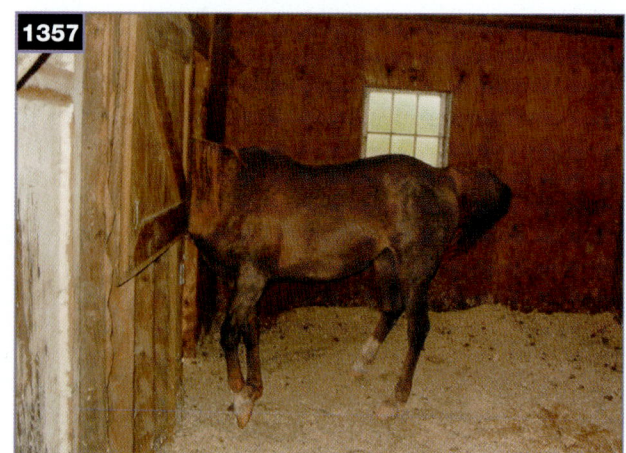

Behavioral problems

Clinical presentation

The horse is presented because the movement of its head precludes a comfortable or even a controllable ride. A few horses head shake only in their stall, but that is probably food anticipation (see Pawing, p. 1009). Shaking, a straight up-and-down or sideways movement, must be differentiated from the head twist that is usually a sign of frustration and ceases as soon as the horse can reach its goal. Head shaking can be a threat gesture, but it will be repeated only a few times in contrast to stereotypic head shaking.

Differential diagnosis

Allergies, including reaction to sunlight, intranasal foreign bodies, partial seizures, or cervical skeletal problems can all cause head shaking. Some head shaking can be a response to ill-fitting tack or a poor rider.

Diagnosis

Diagnosis is based on the repetitive movement of the head in the absence of a pathologic cause. Diagnosis of specific pathologic causes should be explored as described elsewhere.

Management

For anticipatory head shaking, the feed and the time of presentation should be manipulated to reduce frustration. The horse can be taught to lower its head on command and to maintain that position. Standing martingales can be used, although they will only restrain the horse, not change its motivation.

Prognosis

The prognosis is fair to good for behavioral head shaking; good to poor for pathologic causes.

Self-mutilation

Definition/overview

Self-mutilation is the act of a horse biting its own body, usually the flanks, but sometimes the chest or limbs. The behavior is usually accompanied by squealing and kicking. Self-mutilation is most common in stallions, but it may also occur in geldings. It is rare in mares.

Etiology/pathophysiology

If all medical causes have been eliminated, the etiology is unknown, but self-mutilation appears to be associated with frustration, particularly sexual frustration. This is probably displacement behavior. The stallion is motivated to court and breed mares or to fight other stallions. If that is not possible, he bites himself. Geldings pastured with their dams have an approach–avoidance response to their dam when she is in heat. They are motivated to breed her if they are among the 25% of geldings who retain some sexual behavior, but because of innate incest avoidance they do not. Instead, they self-mutilate (1358).

Clinical presentation

The usual presentation is a stalled stallion stabled with other stallions and with little opportunity to exercise. The pathology caused by this behavior can range from saliva-soaked hair to serious lacerations of the skin and under-lying tissue. Not only does the stallion injure himself, but his kicking can injure others.

Differential diagnosis

A painful condition of the skin or underlying organs must be eliminated as a cause. Tapeworms or other parasites should be eliminated. Colic can present as biting at the sides, but the kicking will usually be cow kicking directed at the belly. Neurologic problems must be eliminated.

1358 Self-mutilation. This colt began to bite its flanks while a suckling foal. The behavior occurred whenever the mare was removed from the stall to be ridden. It has persisted, occurring whenever the horse is aroused.

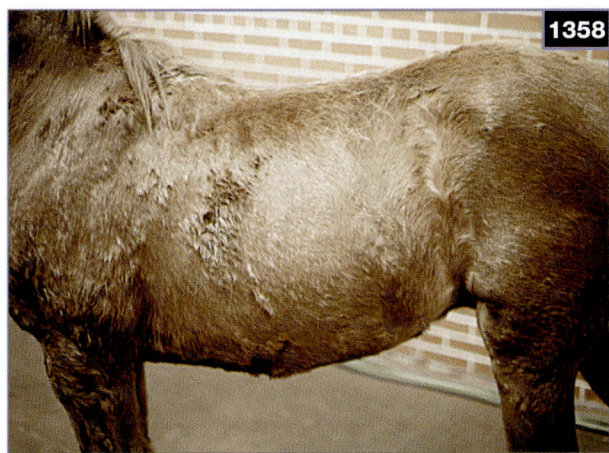

Diagnosis

If the behavior of biting at the body persists for weeks without worsening, it is unlikely to be colic. If other causes of pain or pruritus are eliminated, the diagnosis is psychogenic self-mutilation.

Management

The best treatment is to provide companionship, particularly a mare, or to isolate geldings. Exercise, a decrease in concentrates, and an increase in roughage have also been successful. A cradle on the horse's neck if he bites his flanks (or a bib if he bites his chest) can prevent tissue damage, but the horse will still swing his head to the flank in an attempt to bite and will still kick, therefore he still may injure others. Opiate blockers, such as naloxone, have been successful, as has the tricyclic antidepressant amitriptyline in a gelding.

Prognosis

The prognosis is good if social change can be effected, but fair otherwise.

Savaging

Definition/overview

Aggressive behavior, usually biting of the withers, by a stallion toward a mare is termed savaging.

Etiology/pathophysiology

The cause is usually pathologic or behavioral sexual dysfunction. It is common in stallions whose libido has become poor from overuse, or it can occur as a displacement activity in a stallion that has an approach (to breed) avoidance problem because he associates pain with erection, intromission, or ejaculation, or because he is subordinate to the mare.

Any lesion of the genital tract (e.g. embolism of the penile artery) can result in a stallion acting aggressively as a displacement activity when breeding is painful.

Clinical presentation

The horse is usually a young stallion or one in his teens who, when presented with an estrous mare, approaches the mare and rears to mount without an erection and bites at her neck, withers, or back and may kick as he dismounts.

Differential diagnosis

Savaging must be differentiated from grooming of the mare, which is part of normal courtship, or aggression not associated with sexual behavior and mounting.

Diagnosis

Observation of the behavior and a history of overuse, misuse, or injury during breeding should confirm the diagnosis.

Management

First the mare should be protected with a padded cape over her withers. The stallion can be muzzled. Treatment should take place during the natural breeding season (late spring through early summer) using first a dummy mount and then gentle mares in true estrus with which the stallion has not had bad experiences. Also, the stallion should be handled by experienced personnel in order to train him to be well mannered.

Prognosis

The prognosis is fair for older stallions and good for young ones.

Abnormal tongue movements

Definition/overview

This involves protrusion of the tongue centrally or from the side of the mouth. A variant is folding and sucking of the tongue within the oral cavity.

Etiology/pathophysiology

The etiology is unknown. In some cases the behavior has been rewarded. There is no specific pathology.

Clinical presentation

The owner complains that the horse sticks out its tongue. This, depending on the event, may be a disadvantage to the horse in the show ring. Tongue play may also precede feeding as a rewarded behavior (see Pawing, p. 1009) (1359).

Differential diagnosis

Paralysis of the tongue.

Diagnosis

If the horse voluntarily moves the tongue and has no oral pathology or nerve damage, it can be diagnosed as tongue play (1360).

Management

No treatment is necessary. A tongue tie could be used and the horse could be punished for sticking out its tongue. If the horse has been rewarded with attention or food, the reward should be withdrawn when the horse sticks out its tongue. Eventually the behavior may be extinguished.

Prognosis

The prognosis is good.

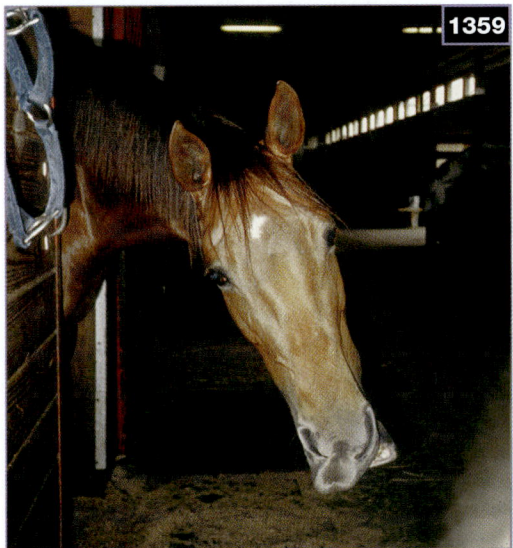

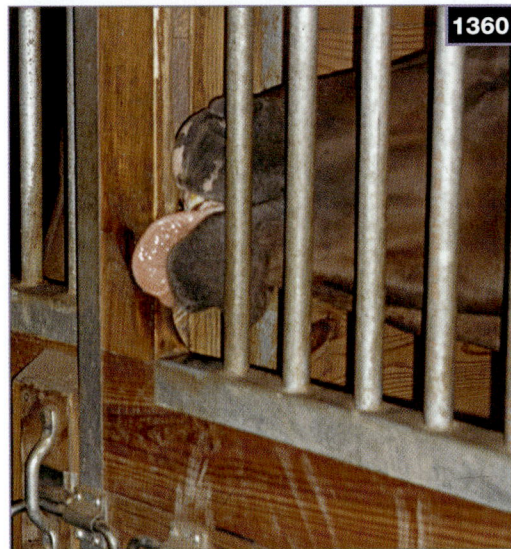

1359 Tongue movements by a horse anticipating food. (Photo courtesy SJ Diaz)

1360 Bar licking, probably as a means of oral stimulation.

Masturbation is a testosterone-dependent behavior. Testosterone exposure is necessary during fetal life to organize the brain to perform the behavior and during adulthood to activate the behavior, although, because it occurs in geldings, it is not totally dependent on circulating testosterone.

Clinical presentation
The usual clinical presentation is by an owner who is concerned that her colt will masturbate in the show ring, by an owner who believes her gelding has not been castrated because she noticed that he masturbated, or by a stallion owner who is worried that a stallion that masturbates will not have sufficient libido. A more serious presentation is the gelding that masturbates when the farrier works on his hooves, possibly because the farrier may carry mare odors on his leather apron.

Differential diagnosis
The behavior must be differentiated from paraphimosis or penile paralysis.

Diagnosis
Observation of the erect penis being flipped against the belly for 5 minutes or less with no sign of discomfort is sufficient for the diagnosis of masturbation.

Management
There is no need to treat the behavior because it is a natural one. There are many devices patented to discourage masturbation, including stallion rings that fit around the flaccid penis, but will be too tight when it is tumescent. The horse learns to avoid the pain by not masturbating. If the horse masturbates in the show ring, he could be punished. The problem with punishing erection is that the horse may be inhibited later in a breeding situation.

Prognosis
The prognosis is good if the owner can be convinced that this is a normal behavior that will not adversely affect the horse.

Masturbation
Definition/overview
Masturbation is defined as letdown and erection of the penis, which is then lifted against the ventral abdominal wall. Pelvic thrusting and ejaculation rarely take place.

Etiology/pathophysiology
Masturbation is a normal male horse behavior. Stallions normally spend half an hour a day with an erect penis, sometimes accompanied by masturbation. Geldings masturbate less frequently. Because this behavior is most apt to occur after periods of lying, which normally occur in the middle of the night, owners may not be aware of it. Stallions on pasture with mares also masturbate, usually when they are standing resting in the afternoon.

Foal rejection

Definition/overview

Foal rejection is either refusal to allow a mare's own foal to nurse, or aggression towards the foal.

Etiology/pathophysiology

The etiology is unknown, but it is familial and may be a consequence of lower than normal prepartum progesterone levels.

There is no known pathology of the mare associated with foal rejection. Trauma to the foal or FPT of maternal antibodies is a potentially life-threatening outcome.

Clinical presentation

There are four types of presentation: (1) the mare accepted the foal, licked it, and neighs when it is removed from her, but she will not accept suckling; (2) the mare appears afraid of the foal, avoids it whenever it approaches, and does not respond if the foal is removed; (3) the mare attacks the foal, usually biting it in the crest of the neck and throwing it; (4) the mare initially accepted the foal, but the foal was removed from her sight for a day or more and upon reintroduction she will not accept it. Some mares in category 1 become more overtly aggressive and develop into category 3 if not treated correctly.

Differential diagnosis

Foal rejection must be differentiated from agalactia or mastitis. If other horses are nearby, the mare may redirect aggression to the foal if she cannot reach the other horses. Any postpartum complications that have stressed the mare can interfere with bonding with the foal. If the mare refuses to let her foal nurse, bites and kicks at it, is willing to leave the foal, and does not respond when the foal is threatened by a dog or if another horse approaches, she has rejected it.

Management

The key to successful treatment is the continuous presence of the foal. The foal should be able to suckle on a normal schedule, which is at least every 15 minutes. Separating the foal and reintroducing it every few hours is rarely successful. To prevent injury to the foal, the mare should be tied and restrained behind a pole or bar so that she cannot move her hindquarters. Bales of straw or wood shavings can be used in front of and behind the mare to prevent the foal from becoming trapped. Another bale can be placed between the mare's fore- and hindlimbs to prevent her from cow kicking or squatting to prevent the foal from suckling. If necessary, the mare can be muzzled and hobbled. Acepromazine (0.01mg/kg i/m) can be used not only to sedate the mare, but also to stimulate prolactin production and thus lactation. The dose can be increased if required, but care should be taken to keep it as low as possible to avoid oversedating the foal. This drug, a dopamine inhibitor, is much better than an alpha-adrenergic drug for the treatment of foal rejection. Oral altrenogest or injectable progesterone can be used to reduce aggression further. Except for exercise to reduce edema, the mare should live in confinement for at least a week and possibly for several weeks. If there are no signs of aggression when the foal suckles or when it approaches the mare's head, the restraint can be removed, but the mare should be observed for the next hour. Initially, the restraint should be removed only during the day.

Prognosis

The prognosis for acceptance of the foal gradually decreases from category 1 to 3. Some mares have rejected 12 foals. Nevertheless, if treated correctly, the mare may accept the foal. In that case, she is highly likely to accept her next foal. The experience of mothering is an important learned component of maternal behavior.

Hay dipping

Definition/overview

Hay dipping is the behavior in which a horse carries a mouthful of hay to its water bucket, trough, or automatic waterer and places the hay in the water.

Etiology/pathophysiology

The cause is unknown, but horses with this behavior may not produce enough saliva to masticate and swallow dry hay easily. They may simply be increasing the palatability and improving the texture of the roughage.

There is no known pathology associated with this behavior, but parotid gland pathology or parotid duct obstruction might be suspected. There is no risk to the horse from the behavior, but owners dislike the soiling of the water container and the spillage of water onto the stall floor.

Clinical presentation

The horse presents with a damp stall floor and strands of hay present in the water container. The horse may be observed alternating quickly between eating hay and immediately drinking water, rather than eating for 10 or more minutes and then drinking.

Differential diagnosis

Hay dipping must be differentiated from dental problems such as quidding, dysphagia, or any pathologic condition in which hay might drop from the mouth. Finding feed in locations other than the water source would be expected in those cases.

Diagnosis
When medical causes have been ruled out, observation of the horse or a video recording of the behavior of prehending hay and then walking a few steps before expelling it into the water source should confirm the diagnosis.

Management
In mild cases, relocation of the hay farther away from the water source solves the problem. Provision of wetted hay, or maintenance of the horse on pasture, should eliminate the behavior, but clinical data are not available.

Prognosis
The prognosis is excellent if the horse can be provided with a moister ration or kept on pasture. If the horse is kept in a tie stall where the water source must be right next to the hay, the prognosis is poor.

Pawing
Definition/overview
Pawing involves scraping the hoof on the substrate, or vacuum pawing in which the hoof is kept in the air but the same movement, flexion of the forelimb, is made.

Etiology/pathophysiology
The cause of the behavior is frustration of the desire to reach a goal or perform an activity. In free-ranging horses, pawing is the action taken to uncover grass below snow or to uncover water below mud. In the domestic situation it occurs when a horse is waiting for or eating food, or if it is restrained from moving or some other activity it wishes to pursue. Pawing can occur so frequently that hoof wear occurs.

Clinical presentation
The horse is usually presented because the pawing results in holes in the ground if the stall has a dirt floor, or hoof wear and rubber mat damage if it has a concrete floor. The behavior often occurs before and during grain feeding.

Differential diagnosis
Pawing should be differentiated from striking, in which the forelimb is raised and extended (i.e. an aggressive behavior), and from an injury that causes the horse to avoid weight bearing on a forelimb.

Diagnosis
If the horse has no forelimb disorder, such as laminitis, the behavior is not directed at another horse or person (striking), and it occurs in a frustrating situation or in a situation where the horse has learned that pawing is followed by feeding, the behavior is pawing.

Management
The cause of the frustration should be identified and corrected, if possible. The horse should be taught that it will be rewarded for not pawing by requiring 2 seconds with no pawing for a handful of feed, then 10 seconds with no pawing, then 30 seconds, and so on, until the horse learns that no pawing is rewarded. Most owners do not have the time or inclination to do this counter-conditioning procedure, so to reduce pawing they should simply reduce the horse's frustration by feeding the horse first. Because horses tend to paw when eating sweet feed, the sweetness of feed can be reduced by substituting oil for carbohydrate calories and providing feed in a ball or cylinder that dispenses pellets so the horse is moving while eating.

Prognosis
The prognosis is good to fair, depending on the changes in management.

Psychogenic polydipsia
Definition/overview
Psychogenic polydipsia is the ingestion of abnormally large amounts of water, usually due to an increase in the frequency of drinking rather than an increase in intake in any one bout.

Etiology/pathophysiology
The cause is unknown, but in some cases it may be the result of confinement or lack of environmental stimulation, especially in young horses recuperating from injury. In severe cases, hemodilution can occur. Medullary washout from chronic psychogenic polydipsia can decrease the ability to concentrate urine when required, leading to a risk of rapid dehydration if the water source becomes unavailable (e.g. broken, frozen).

Clinical presentation
A horse with psychogenic polydipsia is usually presented because the horse is polyuric and its stall is wet as a result. Excessive drinking may not be detected if automatic watering systems are used.

Differential diagnosis
Psychogenic polydipsia must be differentiated from primary water loss through deficiency of vasopressin or insulin, hyperadrenocorticism, or inability of the kidneys themselves to conserve water. Other physiologic causes of thirst are a decrease in blood volume, such as occurs with lactation or administration of furosemide, and an increase in plasma osmotic pressure. Psychogenic polydipsia must also be differentiated from play behavior in which a young horse operates the automatic waterer or splashes water from his buckets for environmental stimulation.

Diagnosis

Excessive urination or drinking, or both, are observed. Psychogenic polydipsia is a diagnosis of exclusion. Pathologic causes should be investigated as described in Chapter 7 (Urinary system). A water deprivation test may be required to evaluate the ability of the kidneys to concentrate.

Management

Providing stall toys from which the horse can acquire food or transfer to a different environment may help. Water can be limited if pituitary and renal mechanisms of water conservation are intact.

Prognosis

The prognosis is unclear. Some horses spontaneously cease drinking too much.

Stall walking

Definition/overview

Stall walking is characterized by walking around or in figure of eight patterns at the front of the stall (1361). The locomotion can be rapid or slow.

Etiology/pathophysiology

The etiology is confinement or inability to reach a goal. Rapid stall walking is usually thwarted escape behavior and is accompanied by neighing and defecation. Slower stall walking appears to be a stereotypic behavior.

Clinical presentation

The horse is presented either because its arousal serves to excite the other horses in the barn or because the animal exerts itself to the point of sweating and might become chilled in colder weather. The horse that stall walks slowly is less of a disturbance, but is still using energy it might otherwise use for performance. If tied, the horse will usually weave. Often, evidence of stall walking can be seen in the stall bedding.

Differential diagnosis

Stereotypic stall walking must be differentiated from central neural damage that causes stall walking in 'dummy' foals, for example. Most stereotypically stall-walking horses will circle in either direction, as opposed to horses with central or peripheral vestibular lesions, which tend to circle in one direction only.

Diagnosis

Diagnosis is based on excluding other diseases and observation of the behavior of moving in a circular or figure of eight pattern within a stall or at a gate. A complete neurologic examination should be performed.

Management

Removal from confinement and placement in a compatible social group is the optimal treatment. Increasing visual contact with neighboring horses or installing a mirror can also reduce stall walking. Increasing solitary turnout will not help.

Prognosis

The prognosis is good if the horse can be kept in a pasture or run-out situation, but fair if the animal must be confined.

Wood chewing

Definition/overview

Wood chewing is ingestion of wood from objects such as trees, fences, or walls. It must be differentiated from cribbing, in which the horse grasps a horizontal surface with its teeth but does not ingest the substrate. Some horses do both.

Etiology/pathophysiology

Wood chewing is not a functionless behavior, so it has clear appetitive (searching for wood) and consummatory (ingestion) phases, and the horses will cease eating wood after several minutes. The cause is a lack of roughage. In addition, cold, wet weather and lack of exercise appear to be risk factors.

The consequences of wood chewing to the horse are usually minimal, although it is possible for impaction or penetration of the GI tract by a splinter to occur. Pressure-treated wood may be toxic, as are the leaves of certain plants and trees. The most important consequence to most owners is the destruction of wooden structures, to the extent that fence rails or stall walls must be replaced.

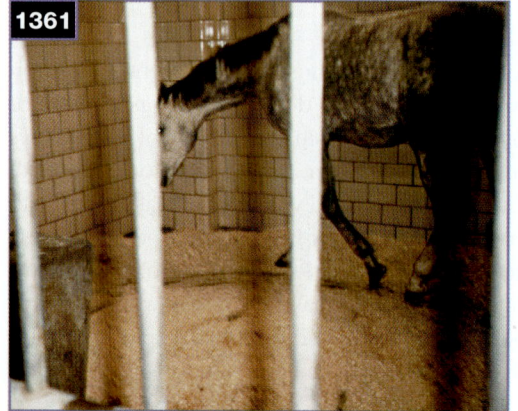

1361 Stereotypic stall walking. Note the path that has been made in the bedding.

Clinical presentation

The owner usually presents the horse in late winter when fence rails and barn walls are being destroyed.

Differential diagnosis

Cribbing, oral exploration, and aggression in which the horse bites at the barrier between it and another horse must be differentiated from wood chewing.

Diagnosis

If wood, trees, or bedding are actually being ingested, the behavior is wood chewing.

Management

Provision of free-choice roughage and a variety of roughages is the best treatment. Protecting trees and stall surfaces with metal or hardware cloth protects the wood, but does not address the horse's need. Increasing exercise may also help. A supplement to reduce wood chewing is being marketed.

Prognosis

The prognosis is good if the dietary adjustments can be made.

Further reading

1 Musculoskeletal system

1.1 Approach to the lame horse

Bramlage LR (1983) Current concepts of first aid and transportation of the equine fracture patient. *Compend Cont Educ Pract Vet* **5**:564.

Bromily MW (1991) *Physiotherapy in Veterinary Practice*. Blackwell Scientific Publications, Oxford.

Butler JA, Colles CM, Dyson SJ, Kold SE, Poulos PW (2008) *Clinical Radiology in the Horse*, 3rd edn. Wiley-Blackwell, Oxford.

Cauvin E (2010) Tenoscopy and bursoscopy. In *Diagnosis and Management of Lameness in the Horse*, 2nd edn. (eds SJ Dyson, MW Ross) WB Saunders, Philadelphia, pp. 260–265.

Clayton HM, Lanovaz JL, Schamhardt HC (2001) Net joint moments and powers in the equine hindlimb during the stance phase of the walk. *Equine Vet J* **33**:43.

Denoix J-M, Pailloux JP (2001) *Physical Therapy and Massage for the Horse*, 2nd edn. Trafalgar Square Publishing, London.

Dyson S, Pilsworth R, Twardock AR, Martinelli M (2003) *Equine Scintigraphy*. Equine Veterinary Journal Ltd, Newmarket.

Dyson S, Murray R, Schramme M, Branch M (2003) Magnetic resonance imaging of the equine foot: 15 horses. *Equine Vet J* **35(1)**:18–26.

Fackelman GE, Nunamaker DM (1994) *Equine Osteosynthesis: an Electronic Manual of the AO/ASIF Technique*. Synthes-AO/ASIF Foundation, Paoli.

Hodgeson E, Clayton HM, Lanovaz JL (2000) The forelimb in walking horses: kinematics and ground reaction forces. *Equine Vet J* **32**:287.

Kraft SL, Gavin P (2001) Physical principles and technical considerations for equine computed tomography and magnetic resonance imaging. *Vet Clin North Am Equine Pract* **17**:115.

Ledwith A, McGowan CM (2004) Muscle biopsy: a routine diagnostic procedure. *Equine Vet Educ* **16(2)**: 62–67.

McClure, SR (2010) Shockwave therapy. In *Diagnosis and Management of Lameness in the Horse*, 2nd edn. (eds MW Ross and SJ Dyson) WB Saunders, Philadelphia, pp. 914–919.

McIlwraith CW (2005) (ed) *Diagnostic and Surgical Arthroscopy in the Horse*, 3rd edn. Lea and Febiger, Philadelphia.

McIlwraith CW, Trotter GA (1996) *Joint Disease in the Horse*. WB Saunders, Philadelphia.

Mair TS, Kinns J, Jones RD, Bolas NM (2005) Magnetic resonance imaging of the distal limb of the standing horse. *Equine Vet Educ* **17(2)**:74–78.

Nixon AJ (1996) *Equine Fracture Repair*. WB Saunders, Philadelphia.

Reef VB (1998) *Equine Diagnostic Ultrasound*. WB Saunders, Philadelphia.

Reimer JM (1997) *Atlas of Equine Ultrasonography*. Mosby, Edinburgh.

Ross MW, Dyson SJ (2010) (eds) *Diagnosis and Management of Lameness in the Horse*, 2nd edn. WB Saunders, Philadelphia.

Sims MH (1983) Electrodiagnostic techniques in the evaluation of neuromuscular diseases affecting skeletal muscle. *Vet Clin North Am Small Anim Pract* **13**:145.

Stashak TS (2002) *Adams' Lameness in Horses*, 5th edn. Lea and Febiger, Philadelphia.

Tucker R L, Sande R D 2001 Computed tomography and magnetic resonance imaging in equine musculo-skeletal conditions. *Vet Clin North Am Equine Pract* **17**:145.

Tunley BV, Henson FMD (2004) Reliability and repeat-ability of thermographic examination and the normal thermographic image of the thoracolumbar region in the horse. *Equine Vet J* **36(4)**:306–312.

Turner T (1991) Thermography as an aid to the clinical lameness evaluation. *Vet Clin North Am Equine Pract* **7**:311–338.

Valberg SJ, Dyson SJ (2010) Skeletal muscle and lameness. In *Diagnosis and Management of Lameness in the Horse*, 2nd edn. (eds SJ Dyson, MW Ross) WB Saunders, Philadelphia, pp. 818-839.

Walmsley JP (1996) Management of a suspected fracture. In *A Guide to the Management of Emergencies at Equine Competitions*. Equine Veterinary Journal Ltd, Newmarket, pp. 13–20.

Wijnberg ID, Van der Kolk JH, Franssen H, Breukink HJ (2003) Needle electromyography in the horse compared with its principles in man: a review. *Equine Vet J* **35(1)**:9–17.

1.2 The foal and developing animal

Auer JA (2006) Angular limb deformities. In *Equine Surgery*, 3rd edn. (eds JA Auer, J Stick) WB Saunders, Philadelphia, pp. 1130–1150.

Bathe AP (2006) Treatment of angular limb deformities using extracorporeal shockwave therapy: a prospective clinical trial. *WEVA Congress*, Marrakesh.

Bramlage LR (1993) Osteochondrosis related bone cysts. In *Proceedings of the American Association of Equine Practitioners* **39**:83.

Bramlage LR (1993) Identification, examination, and treatment of physitis in the foal. *Proceedings of the American Association of Equine Practitioners* **39**:57.

Chan CC-H, Munroe GA (1996) Congenital defects of the equine musculoskeletal system. *Equine Vet Educ* **8(3)**:157–163.

Ellis DR (2010) Physitis. In *Diagnosis and Management of Lameness in the Horse*, 2nd edn. (eds SJ Dyson, MW Ross) WB Saunders, Philadelphia, pp. 638–639.

Kidd JA, Barr ARS (2002) Flexural deformities in foals. *Equine Vet Educ* **16(2)**:62–67.

Munroe GA, Chan CC-H (1996) Congenital flexural deformities of the foal. *Equine Vet Educ* **8(2)**:92–96.

Van Weeren PR (2006) Osteochondrosis. In *Equine Surgery*, 3rd edn. (eds JA Auer, J Stick) WB Saunders, Philadelphia, pp. 1166–1178.

Von Rechenberg B, Auer JA (2006) Subchondral cystic lesions. In *Equine Surgery,* 3rd edn. (eds JA Auer, J Stick) WB Saunders, Philadelphia, pp. 1178–1184.

Wright IM, Minshall G (2005) Diagnosis and treatment of equine osteochondrosis. *In Pract* **27**:302–309.

1.3 **The foot**

Hood DM (1999) (ed) Laminitis. *Vet Clin North Am Equine Pract* **15(2)**.

O'Grady SE (2003) (ed) Podiatry. *Vet Clin North Am Equine Pract* **19(2)**.

Pollitt CC (1995) *Color Atlas of the Horse's Foot.* Mosby Wolfe, London.

Ross MW, Dyson SJ (2003) The foot. In *Diagnosis and Management of Lameness in the Horse*, 2nd edn. (eds SJ Dyson, MW Ross) WB Saunders, Philadelphia, pp. 270–386.

Stashak TS (2002) The foot. In *Adams' Lameness in Horses*, 5th edn. (ed TS Stashak) Lea and Febiger, Philadelphia, pp. 645–733.

1.4 **The forelimb**

Auer JA, Stick JA (2006) (eds) *Equine Surgery*, 3rd edn. WB Saunders, Philadelphia.

McIlwraith CW, Robertson JT (1998) *Equine Surgery: Advanced Techniques*, 2nd edn. Williams and Wilkins, Baltimore.

Nixon AJ (1996) *Equine Fracture Repair.* WB Saunders, Philadelphia.

Ross MW, Dyson SJ (2010) (eds) *Diagnosis and Management of Lameness in the Horse*, 2nd edn. WB Saunders, Philadelphia.

White NA, Moore JN (1998) *Current Techniques in Equine Surgery and Lameness*, 2nd edn. WB Saunders, Philadelphia.

1.5 **The hindlimb**

Auer JA, Stick JA (2006) (eds) *Equine Surgery*, 3rd edn. WB Saunders, Philadelphia.

Colahan PT, Merritt AM, Moore JN, Mayhew IG (1999) (eds) *Equine Medicine and Surgery.* Mosby, St Louis.

Nixon AJ (1995) *Equine Fracture Repair.* WB Saunders, Philadelphia.

Reed SM, Bayly WM, Sellon DC (2004) *Equine Internal Medicine*, 3rd edn. WB Saunders, Philadelphia.

Robinson NE (1997) (ed) *Current Therapy in Equine Medicine*, 4th edn. WB Saunders, Philadelphia.

Ross MW, Dyson SJ (2010) (eds) *Diagnosis and Management of Lameness in the Horse*, 2nd edn. WB Saunders, Philadelphia.

Smith BP (2001) *Large Animal Internal Medicine*, 3rd edn. Mosby, St Louis.

Stashak TS (2002) *Adams' Lameness in Horses*, 5th edn. Lippincott Williams and Wilkins, Philadelphia.

White NA, Moore JN (1998) *Current Techniques in Equine Surgery and Lameness*, 2nd edn. WB Saunders, Philadelphia.

1.6 **The head**

Blythe L (1997) Otitis media and interna and temporo-hyoid osteoarthropathy. *Vet Clin North Am Equine Pract* **13**:21–42.

Henninger R, Beard W, Schneider R, Bramlage L, Burkhardt H (1999) Fractures of the rostral portion of the mandible and maxilla in horses: 89 cases (1979–1997). *J Am Vet Med Assoc* **214**:1648–1652.

Hurtig M, Barber S, Farrow C (1984) Temporomandibular joint luxation in a horse. *J Am Vet Med Assoc* **185**:78–80.

Ragle C (1993) Head trauma. *Vet Clin North Am Equine Pract* **9**:171–183.

Walker A, Sellon D, Cornelisse C, Hines M, Ragle C, Cohen N, Schott H (2002) Temporohyoid osteoarthropathy in 33 horses (1993–2000). *J Vet Int Med* **16**:697–703.

Warmerdam E, Klein W, Herpen B v (1997) Infectious temporomandibular joint disease in the horse: computed tomographic diagnosis and treatment of two cases. *Vet Rec* **141**:172–174.

1.7 **The axial skeleton**

Denoix JM (1999) Ultrasonographic evaluation of back lesions. *Vet Clin North Am Equine Pract* **15**:131–159.

Denoix JM (1996) Ligament injuries of the axial skeleton in the horse: supraspinal and sacroiliac desmopathies. In *Proceedings of the 1st Dubai International Equine Symposium*, Dubai, pp. 273–286.

Dyson S, Murray R (2003) Pain associated with the sacro-iliac joint region: a clinical study of 74 horses. *Equine Vet J* 35:240–245.

Haussler KK (1999) Osseous spinal pathology. *Vet Clin North Am Equine Pract* 15:103–112.

Haussler KK, Stover SM (1998) Stress fractures of the vertebral lamina and pelvis in Thoroughbred race-horses. *Equine Vet J* 30:374–381.

Henson FMD (2009) *Equine Back Pathology: Diagnosis and Treatment*. Wiley-Blackwell, Oxford.

Jeffcott L (1980) Disorders of the thoracolumbar spine of the horse – a survey of 443 cases. *Equine Vet J* 12:197–210.

Marks D (1997) Back pain. In: *Current Therapy in Equine Medicine*. (ed N Robinson) WB Saunders, Philadelphia, pp. 6–12.

Schweinitz DV (1999) Thermographic diagnostics in equine back pain. *Vet Clin North Am Equine Pract* 15:161–177.

Walmsley J, Pettersson H, Winberg F, McEvoy F (2002) Impingement of the dorsal spinous processes in 215 horses: case selection, surgical technique and results. *Equine Vet J* 34:23–28.

Weaver M, Jeffcott L (1999) Radiology and scintigraphy. *Vet Clin North Am Equine Pract* 15:113–129.

1.8 **Soft-tissue injuries**

Auer JA, Stick JA (2006) (eds) *Equine Surgery*, 3rd edn. WB Saunders, Philadelphia.

Dowling BA, Dart AJ, Hodgson DJ *et al.* (2000) Superficial digital flexor tendonitis in the horse. *Equine Vet J* 32:369–378.

Dranchak PK, Valberg SJ, Onan GW *et al.* (2005) Inheritance of recurrent exhertional rhabdomyolysis in thoroughbreds. *J Am Vet Med Assoc* 227:762–767.

Dyson SJ (2004) Medical management of superficial digital flexor tendonitis: a comparative study in 219 horses (1992–2000). *Equine Vet J* 36:415–419.

Koenig J, Cruz A, Genovese R *et al.* (2005) Rupture of the peroneus tertius tendon in 27 horses. *Can Vet J* 46:503–506.

McGowan CM, Fordham T, Christley RM (2002) Incidence and risk factors for exhertional rhabdomyolysis in thoroughbreed racehorses in the United Kingdom. *Vet Rec* 151:623–626.

Reef VB (1998) *Equine Diagnostic Ultrasound*. WB Saunders, Philadelphia.

Ross MW, Dyson SJ (2010) (eds) *Diagnosis and Management of Lameness in the Horse*, 2nd edn. WB Saunders, Philadelphia.

Smith MR, Wright IM (2006) Noninfected tenosynovitis of the digital flexor tendon sheath; a retrospective analysis of 76 cases. *Equine Vet J* 38:134–141.

Smith RK (2006) Stem cell technology in equine tendon and ligament injuries. *Vet Rec* 158:140.

Stashak ST (2002) *Adams' Lameness in Horses*, 5th edn. Lippincott, Williams and Wilkins, Baltimore.

Upjohn MM, Archer RM, Christley RM *et al.* (2005) Incidence and risk factors associated with exhertional rhabdomyolysis syndrome in National Hunt racehorses in Great Britain. *Vet Rec* 156:763–766.

Valberg SJ, Mickelson JR, Gallant EM *et al.* (1999) Exhertional rhabdomyolysis in Quarter horses and Thoroughbreds: one syndrome, multiple aetiologies. *Equine Vet J* Suppl 30:533–538.

Votion DM, Linden A, Saegerman C *et al.* (2007) History and clinical features of atypical myopathy in horses in Belgium 2000–2005. *J Vet Int Med* 21:1380–1391.

2 Reproductive system

2.1 **Female reproductive tract**

Carnevale EM (2007) Advances in reproduction. *Vet Clin North Am Equine Pract* 22(3):663–872.

England G (2005) *Fertility and Obstetrics in the Horse*, 3rd edn. Blackwell Scientific Publications, Oxford.

Renaudin CD, Gillis CL, Tarantal AS (1997) Transabdominal combined with transrectal ultrasonographic determination of equine fetal gender during mid gestation. *Proceedings 43rd Annual Convention of the American Association of Equine Practitioners*, pp. 252–255

Rossdale PD, Mair TS, Green RE (2002) *Equine Veterinary Education Manual 5: Reproduction – Foaling Part 1: Maternal aspects*. Equine Veterinary Journal Ltd., Newmarket.

Samper JC, McKinnon AO, Pycock J (2005) *Current Therapy in Equine Reproduction*. WB Saunders, Philadelphia.

2.2 **Male reproductive tract**

Knottenbelt DC, Le Blanc MM, Lopate C, Pascoe RR (2003) *Equine Stud Farm Medicine and Surgery*. WB Saunders, Edinburgh.

Lopate C, LeBlanc M, Knottenbelt DC (2003) The stallion. In *Equine Stud Farm Medicine and Surgery*. (eds DC Knottenbelt, RR Pascoe, M LeBlanc, C Lopate) WB Saunders, Philadelphia, pp. 43–112.

Ricketts SW (2005) *Equine Stud Medicine Course Notes 2005*. British Equine Veterinary Association, Soham.

Samper JC (2009) (ed) *Equine Breeding Management and Artificial Insemination*, 2nd edn. Saunders/Elsevier, St Louis.

1014

Samper JC, Pycock JF, McKinnon AO (2005) (eds) *Current Therapy in Equine Reproduction*. Saunders/Elsevier, St Louis.

Schumacher J (2006) Testis. In *Equine Surgery*, 3rd edn. (eds J Auer, J Stick) Saunders/Elsevier, St Louis, pp. 775–810

2.3 **Equine castration**

Searle D, Dart AJ, Dart CM, Hodgson DR (1999) Equine castration: review of anatomy, approaches, techniques and complications in normal, cryptorchid and monorchid horses. *Aust Vet J* 77:428–434.

3 Respiratory system

McGorum BC, Dixon PM, Robinson NE, *et al.* (2007) *Equine Respiratory Medicine and Surgery*. WB Saunders, Philadelphia.

Newton JR, Wood JL, Chanter N (2003) A case control study of factors and infections associated with clinically apparent respiratory disease in UK Thoroughbred racehorses. *Prev Vet Med* 60:107–32.

Robinson NE (2003) Inflammatory airway disease: defining the syndrome. Conclusions of the Havemeyer Workshop. *Equine Vet Educ* 15:61–63.

Sweeney CR, Timoney JF, Newton JR *et al.* (2005) *Streptococcus equi* infections in horses: guidelines for treatment, control and prevention of strangles. *J Vet Intern Med* 19:123–134.

Verheyen K, Newton JR, Talbot NC *et al.* (2000) Elimination of guttural pouch infection and inflammation in asymptomatic carriers of *Streptococcus equi*. *Equine Vet J* 32:527–532.

Wood JL, Newton JR, Chanter N *et al.* (2005) Association between respiratory disease and bacterial and viral infections in British racehorses. *J Clin Microbiol* 43:120–126.

4 Gastrointestinal system

4.1 **Upper gastrointestinal tract**

Dixon PM (2005) Dental anatomy. In *Equine Dentistry*, 2nd edn. (eds G Baker, J Easley) Elsevier, Philadelphia, pp. 25–47.

Dixon PM, Tremaine WH, Pickles K *et al.* (1999) Equine dental disease. Part 2. A long-term study of 400 cases: disorders of development and eruption and variations in position of the cheek teeth. *Equine Vet J* 31:519–528.

Fubini S, Starrak GS, Freeman DE (1999) The Esophagus. In *Equine Surgery*, 2nd edn. (eds JA Auer, JA Sick) WB Saunders, Philadelphia, pp. 199–212.

Greet TRC (2005) Management of oral trauma. In *Equine Dentistry*, 2nd edn. (eds G Baker, J Easley) Elsevier, Philadelphia, pp. 79–86.

4.2 **Lower gastrointestinal tract**

Cohen ND (1997) Epidemiology of colic. *Vet Clin North Am Equine Pract* 13:191–201.

Dart AJ, Hodgson DR, Snyder JR (1997) Caecal disease in equids. *Aust Vet J* 75:552–557.

Hassel DM, Langer DL, Snyder JR *et al.* (1999) Evaluation of enterolithiasis in equids: 900 cases (1973–1996). *J Am Vet Med Assoc* 214:233–237.

Love S (2003) Treatment and prevention of intestinal parasite-associated diease. *Vet Clin North Am Equine Pract* 19:791–806.

Magdesian KG (2005) Neonatal foal diarrhea. *Vet Clin North Am Equine Pract* 21:295–312.

Mair TS, Smith LJ (2005) Survival and complication rates in 300 horses undergoing surgical treatment of colic. Part 3. Long-term complications and survival. *Equine Vet J* 37:310–314.

Matthews S, Dart AJ, Reid SW *et al.* (2002) Predictive values, sensitivity and specificity of abdominal fluid variables in determining the need for surgery in horses with an acute abdominal crisis. *Aust Vet J* 80:132–136.

Murray MJ, Nout YS, Ward DL (2001) Endoscopic findings of the gastric antrum and pylorus in horses: 162 cases (1996–2000). *J Vet Int Med* 15:401–406.

5 Liver

Bain PJ (2003) Liver. In *Duncan & Prasse's Veterinary Laboratory Medicine: Clinical Pathology*, 4th edn. (eds KS Latimer, EA Mahaffey, KW Prasse) Iowa State Press, Ames, pp. 193–214.

Barr AC, Reagor JC (2001) Toxic plants. What the horse practitioner needs to know. *Vet Clin North Am Equine Pract* 17:529–46.

Guglick MA, MacAllister CG, Ely RW *et al.* (1995) Hepatic disease associated with administration of tetanus antitoxin in eight horses. *J Am Vet Med Assoc* 206:1737–40.

Knight AP, Walter RG (2001) Plants affecting the skin and liver. In *A Guide to Plant Poisoning of Animals in North America*. (eds AP Knight, RG Walter) Teton NewMedia, Jackson.

McGorum BC, Murphy D, Love S *et al.* (1999) Clinicopathological features of equine primary hepatic disease: a review of 50 cases. *Vet Rec* 145:134–9.

Mogg TD, Palmer JE (1995) Hyperlipidemia, hyperlipemia, and hepatic lipidosis in American miniature horses: 23 cases (1990–1994). *J Am Vet Med Assoc* 207:604–7.

1015

Osweiler GD (2001) Mycotoxins. *Vet Clin North Am Equine Pract* **17**:547–66, viii.

Parraga ME, Carlson GP, Thurmond M (1995) Serum protein concentrations in horses with severe liver disease: a retrospective study and review of the literature. *J Vet Intern Med* **9**:154–61.

Peek SF, Divers TJ (2000) Medical treatment of cholangiohepatitis and cholelithiasis in mature horses: 9 cases (1991–1998). *Equine Vet J* **32**:301–6.

Reef VB (1998) Adult abdominal ultrasonography. In *Equine Diagnostic Ultrasound.* (ed VB Reef) WB Saunders, Philadelphia, pp. 273–363.

6 Endocrine system

Allen AL, Townsend HG, Doige CE *et al.* (1996) A case-control study of the congenital hypothyroidism and dysmaturity syndrome of foals. *Can Vet J* **37**:349–351; 354–358.

Beech J (1998) Disorders of thyroid gland function. In *Metabolic and Endocrine Problems of Horses.* (ed TDG Watson) WB Saunders, New York, pp. 69–74.

Beech J, Boston R, Lindborg S, Russell GE. (2007) Adrenocorticotropin concentration following administration of thyrotropin-releasing hormone in healthy horses and those with pituitary pars intermedia dysfunction and pituitary gland hyperplasia. *J Am Vet Med Assoc* **231**:417–426.

Breuhaus BA (2002) Thyroid-stimulating hormone in adult euthyroid and hypothyroid horses. *J Vet Intern Med* **16**:109–115.

Donaldson MT, LaMonte BH, Morresey P *et al.* (2002) Treatment with pergolide or cyproheptadine of pituitary pars intermedia dysfunction (equine Cushing's disease). *J Vet Intern Med* **16**:742–746.

Donaldson MT, McDonnell SM, Schanbacher BJ *et al.* (2005) Variation in plasma adrenocorticotropic hormone concentration and dexamethasone suppression test results with season, age, and sex in healthy ponies and horses. *J Vet Intern Med* **19**:217–222.

Dunkel B, McKenzie HC 3rd (2003) Severe hypertriglyceridaemia in clinically ill horses: diagnosis, treatment and outcome. *Equine Vet J* **35**:590–595.

Dybdal NO, Hargreaves KM, Madigan JE *et al.* (1994) Diagnostic testing for pituitary pars intermedia dysfunction in horses. *J Am Vet Med Assoc* **204**:627–632.

Eiler H, Frank N, Andrews FM *et al.* (2005) Physiologic assessment of blood glucose homeostasis via combined intravenous glucose and insulin testing in horses. *Am J Vet Res* **66**:1598–1604.

Frank N, Elliott SB, Brandt LE *et al.* (2006) Physical characteristics, blood hormone concentrations, and plasma lipid concentrations in obese horses with insulin resistance. *J Am Vet Med Assoc* **228**:1383–1390.

Frank N, Sommardahl CS, Eiler H *et al.* (2005) Effects of oral administration of levothyroxine sodium on concentrations of plasma lipids, concentration and composition of very-low-density lipoproteins, and glucose dynamics in healthy adult mares. *Am J Vet Res* **66**:1032–1038.

Frank N, Elliott SB, Boston RC (2008) Effects of long-term oral administration of levothyroxine sodium on glucose dynamics in healthy adult horses. *Am J Vet Res* **69**:76–81.

Frank N, Buchanan BR, Elliott SB (2008) Effects of long-term oral administration of levothyroxine sodium on serum thyroid hormone concentrations, clinico-pathologic variables, and echocardiographic measurements in healthy adult horses. *Am J Vet Res* **69**:68–75.

Hughes KJ, Hodgson DR, Dart AJ (2004) Equine hyperlipaemia: a review. *Aust Vet J* **82**:136–42.

Jackson LP, Moore GE, Sojka JE (2008) Correlation of pituitary histomorphometry with adrenocorticotrophic hormone response to domperidone administration in the diagnosis of equine pituitary pars intermedia dysfunction. *Vet Pathol* **45**:26–38.

Johnson PJ (2002) The equine metabolic syndrome, peripheral Cushing's syndrome. *Vet Clin North Am Equine Pract* **18**:271–293.

Johnson PJ, Goetz TE, Foreman JH *et al.* (1995) Pheochromocytoma in two horses. *J Am Vet Med Assoc* **206**:837–841.

Mansmann RA, Carlson GP, White NA et al. (1974) Synchronous diaphragmatic flutter in horses. *J Am Vet Med Assoc* **165**:265–270.

McFarlane D, Holbrook TC (2008) Cytokine dysregulation in aged horses and horses with pituitary pars intermedia dysfunction. *J Vet Intern Med* **22**:436–442.

Ronen N, van Heerden J, van Amstel SR (1992) Clinical and biochemistry findings, and parathyroid hormone concentrations in three horses with secondary hyperparathyroidism. *J S Afr Vet Assoc* **63**:134–136.

Sommardahl CS, Frank N, Elliott SB *et al.* (2005) Effects of oral administration of levothyroxine sodium on serum concentrations of thyroid gland hormones and responses to injections of thyrotropin-releasing hormone in healthy adult mares. *Am J Vet Res* **66**:1025–1031.

Van der Kolk H (1998) Diseases of the pituitary gland, including hyperadrenocorticism. In *Metabolic and Endocrine Problems of Horses.* (ed TDG Watson) WB Saunders, New York, pp. 41–59.

Further reading

7 Urinary system _____

Aleman MR, Kuesis B, Schott HC *et al.* (2001) Renal tubular acidosis in horses (1980–1999). *J Vet Intern Med* **15**:136–143.

Bayly WM, Brobst DF, Elfers RS *et al.* (1986) Serum and urinary biochemistry and enzyme changes in ponies with acute renal failure. *Cornell Vet* **76**:306–316.

DeBowes RM (1988) Surgical management of urolithiasis. *Vet Clin North Am Equine Pract* **4**:461–471.

Edwards DJ, Brownlow MA, Hutchins DR (1990) Indices of renal function: values in eight normal foals from birth to 56 days. *Aust Vet J* **67**:251–254.

Ehnen SJ, Divers TJ, Gillette D *et al.* (1990) Obstructive nephrolithiasis and ureterolithiasis associated with chronic renal failure in horses: eight cases (1981–1987). *J Am Vet Med Assoc* **197**:249–253.

Enzerink E, van Weeren PR, van der Velden MA (2000) Closure of the abdominal wall at the umbilicus and the development of umbilical hernias in a group of foals from birth to 11 months of age. *Vet Rec* **147**:37–39.

Godber LM, Walker RD, Stein GE *et al.* (1995) Pharmacokinetics, nephrotoxicosis, and in vitro antibacterial activity associated with single versus multiple (three times) daily gentamicin treatments in horses. *Am J Vet Res* **56**:613–618.

Helman RG, Edwards WC (1997) Clinical features of blister beetle poisoning in equids: 70 cases (1983–1996). *J Am Vet Med Assoc* **211**:1018–1021.

Holt PE, Mair TS (1990) Ten cases of bladder paralysis associated with sabulous urolithiasis in horses. *Vet Rec* **127**:108–110.

Jose-Cunilleras E, Hinchcliff KW (1999) Renal pharmacology. *Vet Clin North Am Equine Pract* **15**:647–664.

Kisthardt KK, Schumacher J, Finn-Bodner ST *et al.* (1999) Severe renal hemorrhage caused by pyelonephritis in 7 horses: clinical and ultrasonographic evaluation. *Can Vet J* **40**:571–576.

Knottenbelt DC (2003) Differential diagnosis of polyuria/polydipsia. In *Current Therapy in Equine Medicine 5.* (ed NE Robinson) WB Saunders, Philadelphia, pp. 828–831.

Kohn CW, Chew DJ (1987) Laboratory diagnosis and characterization of renal disease in horses. *Vet Clin North Am Equine Pract* **3**:585–615.

Laverty S, Pascoe JR, Ling GV *et al.* (1992) Urolithiasis in 68 horses. *Vet Surg* **21**:56–62.

Rantanen NW (1986) Diseases of the kidneys. *Vet Clin North Am Equine Pract* **2**:89–103.

Robertson JT, Embertson RM (1988) Surgical management of congenital and perinatal abnormalities of the urogenital tract. *Vet Clin North Am Equine Pract* **4**:359–379.

Traub-Dargatz JL, McKinnon AO (1988) Adjunctive methods of examination of the urogenital tract. *Vet Clin North Am Equine Pract* **4**:339–358.

Ziemer EL, Parker HR, Carlson GP *et al.* (1987) Renal tubular acidosis in two horses: diagnostic studies. *J Am Vet Med Assoc* **190**:289–293.

8 Cardiovascular system _____

Fregin GF (1992) Medical evaluation of the cardiovascular system. *Vet Clin North Am Equine Pract* **8**:329–46.

Marr CM (2010) (ed) *Cardiology of the Horse*, 2nd edn. WB Saunders, New York.

McGurrin MKJ, Physick-Sheard PW, Kenney DG (2005) How to perform transvenous electrical cardioversion in horses with atrial fibrillation. *J Vet Cardiol* **7**:109–119.

Mogg TD (1999) Equine cardiac disease. Clinical pharmacology and therapeutics. *Vet Clin North Am Equine Pract* **15**:523–34.

Muir WW, McGuirk S (1987) Cardiovascular drugs. Their pharmacology and use in horses. *Vet Clin North Am Equine Pract* **3**:37–57

Patteson MW (1996) *Equine Cardiology.* Blackwell Science, Cambridge, Mass.

9 Hemolymphatic system _____

Aleman M (2008) Diseases of the hematopoietic and hemolymphatic systems. In *Large Animal Internal Medicine*, 4th edn. (ed BP Smith) Mosby, St. Louis.

Kramer JW (2000) Normal hematology of the horse. In *Schalm's Veterinary Hematology*, 5th edn. (eds BF Feldman, JG Zinkl, NC Jain) Lippincott Williams & Wilkins, Philadelphia.

Latimer KS, Rakich PM (2007) Peripheral blood smears. In *Diagnostic Cytology and Hematology of the the Horse*, 2nd edn. (eds RL Cowell, RD Tyler) Mosby, St. Louis.

McClure JT (2000) Leukoproliferative disorders in horses. *Vet Clin North Am Equine Pract* **16**:165–182.

Parry BW (2008) Clinical pathology. *Vet Clin North Am Equine Pract* **24**:225–464.

10 Nervous system

DeLahunta A (1983) Neurological examination of the horse. In *Veterinary Neuroanatomy and Clinical Neurology*, 2nd edn. WB Saunders, Philadelphia, pp. 389–401.

Fontaine-Rodgerson G (2003) Viral encephalitides. In *Current Therapy in Equine Medicine 5.* (ed NE Robinson) WB Saunders, Philadelphia, pp. 47–50.

Galey FD (2001) Botulism in the horse. *Vet Clin North Am Equine Pract* **17**:579–588.

Galey FD (2002) Disorders caused by toxicants. In *Large Animal Internal Medicine*, 3rd edn. (ed BP Smith) Mosby, St.Louis, pp. 1616–1631.

George LW (2002) Peripheral nerve disorders. In *Large Animal Internal Medicine*, 3rd edn. (ed BP Smith) Mosby, St.Louis, pp. 1013–1018

Johnson PJ, Constantinescu GM (2000) Collection of cerebrospinal fluid in horses. *Equine Vet Educ* **1**:7–12.

Johnson PJ, Constantinescu GM (2000) Analysis of cerebrospinal fluid in horses. *Equine Vet Educ* **12**:13–17.

Mayhew I (2009) Neurological examination. In *Large Animal Neurology. A Handbook for Veterinary Clinicians*, 2nd edn. Wiley-Blackwell, Oxford, pp. 11–46.

Ostlund EN, Andresen JE, Andresen M (2000) West Nile encephalitis. *Vet Clin North Am Equine Pract* **16**:427–441

Reed SM (2004) Disorders of the neurologic system. In *Equine Internal Medicine*, 2nd edn. (eds SM Reed, WM Bayly, DC Sellon) WB Saunders, Philadelphia, pp. 533–541.

Sullivan ND (1985) The nervous system. In *Pathology of Domestic Animals*, 3rd edn. (eds KVF Jubb, PC Kennedy, N Palmer) Academic Press, Orlando, pp. 201–338.

11 Eyes

Gilger BC (2005) (ed) *Equine Ophthalmology*. Elsevier Saunders, St Louis.

Gelatt KN (2007) (ed) *Veterinary Ophthalmology*, 4th edn. Volumes 1 & 2. Lippincott Williams & Wilkins, Baltimore.

Barnett KC, Crispin SM, Lavach JD, Matthews AG (2004) (eds) *Equine Ophthalmology: an Atlas and Text*, 2nd edn. Elsevier Saunders, Toronto.

Maggs DJ, Miller PE, Ofri R (2008) (eds) *Slatter's Fundamentals of Veterinary Ophthalmology*, 4th edn. Elsevier Saunders, St Louis.

12 Skin

Henson FMD, Dobson JM (2004) Use of radiation therapy in the treatment of equine neoplasia. *Equine Vet Educ* **15**:315–318

Knottenbelt DC, Kelly DF (2000) The diagnosis and treatment of periorbital sarcoid in the horse: 445 cases from 1974–1999. *Vet Ophthalmol* **3**:169–191

Pascoe RR (1990) *A Colour Atlas of Equine Dermatology*. Wolfe Publishing, London.

Pascoe RR, Knottenbelt DC (1999) *Manual of Equine Dermatology*. WB Saunders, London.

Paterson S (2003) Treatment of skin disease in the horse. *In Pract* **25**:86–91

Scott DW, Miller WH (2003) *Equine Dermatology*. Elsevier Science, Philadelphia.

13 Wound management and infections of synovial structures

Barber SM (1990) Second intention wound healing in the horse: the effect of bandages and topical corticosteroids. *Proceedings American Association of Equine Practitioners* **35**:107–116.

Bertone AL (1989) Principles of wound healing. *Vet Clin North Am Equine Pract* **5**:378–383.

Berry DB, Sullins KE (2003) Effects of topical application of antimicrobials and bandaging on healing and granulation tissue formation in wounds of the distal aspect of the limbs in horses. *Am J Vet Res* **64**:88–92.

Carrico TJ, Mehrhof AI, Cohen IK (1984) Biology of wound healing. *Surg Clin North Am* **64**:721–723.

Gomez JH, Schumacher J, Lauten SD *et al*. (2004) Effects of 3 biologic dressings on healing of cutaneous wounds on the limbs of horses. *Can J Vet Res* **68**:49–55.

Howard RD, Stashak TS, Baxter GM (1993) Evaluation of occlusive dressings for management of full-thickness excisional wounds on the distal portion of the limbs of horses. *Am J Vet Res* **54**:2150–2154.

Stashak TS, Theoret CL (2008) *Equine Wound Management*, 2nd edn. Wiley-Blackwell, Iowa.

Theoret CL (2005) The pathophysiology of wound repair. *Vet Clin North Am Equine Pract* **21**:1–13.

Wilson DA (2005) Principles of early wound management. *Vet Clin North Am Equine Pract* **21**:45–62.

Further reading

14 The foal

Cash RSG (1999) Colostral quality determined by refractometry. *Equine Vet Educ* **11**:36–38

Corley KTT (2002) Monitoring and treating haemo-dynamic disturbances in critically ill neonatal foals: Part 1: Assessment and treatment. *Equine Vet Educ* **14**:270–279.

Corley KTT (2002) Monitoring and treating haemo-dynamic disturbances in critically ill neonatal foals: Part 2: Haemodynamic monitoring. *Equine Vet Educ* **14**:328–336.

Knottenbelt DC, Holdstock N, Madigan JE (2004) *Equine Neonatology Medicine and Surgery.* WB Saunders, Philadelphia.

Palmer J (2001) Septicaemia update. www.nicuvet.com

Paradis MR (2006) (ed) *Equine Neonatal Medicine.* Elsevier Science, St Louis.

Reef VB (1998) Paediatric abdominal ultrasound. In *Equine Diagnostic Ultrasound.* (ed VB Reef) WB Saunders, Philadelphia, pp. 364–403.

Stoneham S (2001) Foal nursing. In *Equine Veterinary Nursing Manual.* (ed K Coumbe) Blackwell Science, Oxford.

15 Behavioral problems

Archer DD, Freeman DE, Doyle AJ *et al.* (2004) Association between cribbing and entrapment of the small intestine in the epiploic foramen in horses: 68 cases (1991–2002). *J Am Vet Med Assoc* **224**:562–564.

Francis-Smith K, Wood-Gush DGM (1977) Coprophagia as seen in thoroughbred foals. *Equine Vet J* **9**:155–157.

Gillham SB, Dodman NH, Shuster L *et al.* (1994) The effect of diet on cribbing behavior and plasma b-endorphin in horses. *Appl Anim Behav Sci* **41**:147–153.

Houpt KA (2004) *Domestic Animal Behavior for Veterinarians and Small Animal Science,* 4th edn. Blackwell Press, Oxford.

Krzak WE, Gonyou HW, Lawrence LM (1991) Wood chewing by stabled horses: diurnal pattern and effects of exercise. *J Anim Sci* **69**:1053–1058.

Luescher UA, McKeown DB, Dean H (1998) A cross-sectional study on compulsive behaviour (stable vices) in horses. *Equine Vet J* (Suppl) **27**:14–18.

McGreevy PD, Cripps PJ, French NP *et al.* (1995) Management factors associated with stereotypic and redirected behaviour in the Thoroughbred horse. *Equine Vet J* **27**:86–91.

McGreevy PD, French NP, Nicol CJ (1995) The prevalence of abnormal behaviours in dressage, eventing and endurance horses in relation to stabling. *Vet Rec* **137**:36–37.

McGreevy PD, Richardson JD, Nicol CJ *et al.* (1995) Radiographic and endoscopic study of horses performing an oral based stereotypy. *Equine Vet J* **27**:92–95.

Mills DM, Nankervis K (1999) *Equine Behaviour: Principles and Practice.* Blackwell Science, Oxford.

Redbo I, Redbo-Torstensson P, Odberg FO *et al.* (1998) Factors affecting behavioural disturbances in race-horses. *Anim Sci* **66**:475–481.

Waring G (2003) *Horse Behavior,* 2nd edn. Noyes Publications, William Andrew Publishing, Norwich.

Index

Note: Page numbers in **bold** refer to figures; those in *italic* refer to tables or boxes.

A

abdomen
    auscultation 516, 581
    palpation per rectum 516–17
    radiography 518
    trauma 591–2, 741–2
    ultrasonography **518**, 519
abdominal adhesions 533
abdominal hernia 594
abdominal muscles, rupture in broodmare 268–9
abdominocentesis 519–20, 542
    cecal rupture 560
    duodenitis/proximal jejunitis 547
    hemoperitoneum 590–1
    peritonitis 596
    splenic rupture 742
    uroperitoneum 665–6, 986
abducens nerve 749
abortion 277–9
    causes *272*
    clinical signs 277
    definition 277
    hydrocephalus 756, **757**
    incidence 277
    induction 268
    infectious causes 278–9
    mummified fetus 274, 275
    non-infectious causes 279
    prevention 265, 277
    twins 270, 274, 275, 279
abscesses
    clostridial muscle 232–3, **234**
    corneal 853–5
    foot 64–5
    intestinal wall 582
    liver 613
    lung, foals 993–4
    mediastinal 464
    perirectal 590
    R. equi pneumonia 458, 459
    skin/subcutis 903, 904–5
    strangles infection 454, **455**, 457
accessory carpal bones, fractures 120, 121, 123
accessory nerve 751
accessory sex glands 328, 329–30
    disorders 344, 364–5

acepromazine 19, 660
    behavioral problems 1000
    bladder dysfunction 660
    exertional rhabdomyolysis 230
    laminitis 71
    use in colic 520
Acer rubrum 721–2
acetate tape sampling 875
acetazolamide 226
acetyl-CoA 634
acetylcysteine, enema 980–1
'Achilles' tendon, injuries 221–3
acid–base disturbance
    chronic renal failure 649
    liver disease 600
    uroperitoneum 664, **665**, 986
acidosis, renal tubular 653–4
acne 905
actinic dermatosis 932
Actinobacillus spp. 460, 652, 772
Actinobacillus equuli 617, 652, 766, 794
Actinobacillus ligneri 504
Actinomyces spp. 907
activated charcoal 524, 668, 701, 785
acupuncture, back pain 177
acute renal failure 645–8
    diagnosis 645–6
    etiology/pathophysiology 645
    management 646–7
    specific etiologies 647
    urine biochemistry 641–2
acyclovir 617, 766
adactyly 46
adenoma, ovary 303–4
adenovirus infections 453
adhesions
    deep digital flexor tendon 217
    intestinal 533–4
    iris 856
    lateral digital flexor tendon 219
adipocytes, omental 632
adrenal gland 636
    tumors 636
adrenocorticotropic hormone 629, 630, 631
    premature foal 975
    resting plasma concentrations 630, 631
adrenocorticotropic hormone stimulation test 975
Aedes mosquito species 760, 761

aflatoxins 609–10
African horse sickness 453
agave 606, **607**
age, and breeding ability 247
agglutination 713, 720
aggressive behavior 342–3, 996, 1006
aging of horses 485–6
'Ahern' procedure 418
'air hunger' 440
airway obstruction 440–1
    recurrent (heaves) 465–7, *467*, *468*
    summer pasture-associated 467, *468*
alar fold disease 390
albinism, partial 832–3
albumin, serum 599, 642, 649
albumin/globulin ratio 599
albuterol *468*
alcohols, toxic plant 792
alfalfa 524, 667, 719
alkalemia *627*
alkaline phosphatase 599
    ejaculatory fluid 344, 363
alkaloids
    pyrrolizidine 604–6, 618
    Solanceae 791
    tropone 791
allantochorion 282
allantoic fluid 280
allantois 262
allergen-specific immunotherapy 893
allergy testing 876, 892–3
Allescheria boydii 315
allopurinol *800*
allyl-propyl disulfide 722
alopecia 893–902
    equine linear 924
alopecia areata 925
alpha-2 agonists 19, 364, 375, 512
    cerebral trauma 774
    colic 520
    urinary system 639
alpha-blockers 350, 351
alphavirus encephalitis 760–2
altrenogest 265, 1001
ameloblstoma 501
American Paint horse 226
amikacin *316*, 666, *960*, *968*, 992
    toxicity 647
amino acids, serum levels 599

aminoglycosides 547, 645, 669
   bladder rupture 666
   equine purpura hemorrhagica 732
   toxicity 647
aminophylline *468*
amitraz 891
amitriptyline 1000
ammonia
   blood 599, 618, 798
   liver failure 603, 604
ammonium, ingestion 784
ammonium chloride 670
ammonium sulfate 670
amniocentesis 264
amnion 280
amniotic fluid 280
   meconium contamination 976–7
amniotic membrane, dressing *949*
amphotericin B 908
ampicillin 461
   uterine infections *316*
ampicillin sodium trihydrate 603
ampullary glands 330, 333
   obstruction 344, 364
Amsinckia intermedia 604, **605**
amyloid A, serum 971, 992
amyloidosis
   cutaneous 911
   nasal 404
   renal 653
anabolic steroids, and male fertility *342*
anagen defluxion 901
analgesia
   castration 375
   colic 520, *521*
   exertional rhabdomyolysis 230
   eye examination 814–15
   opiates 228, 230
   regional/diagnostic 19–20, *20*, **21**
      back pain 176, 181, 184
      digital flexor tendon sheath 212
      foot 19, 63, 86, 88, 92, 94
      palmar digital nerve 19, 88, 92, 94
      tarsal joints 142
   synovial infections 961
   see also nonsteroidal anti-inflammatory drugs
Anaplasma phagocytophila 598, 770, 730–1
anemia 714
   aplastic 727–8
   chronic hemorrhage 717
   in chronic renal failure 649
   equine infectious 332, 723–4, 763

granulomatous enteritis 529
Heinz body 721, 722
immune-mediated hemolytic 719–20
   of inflammatory disease 725
   iron deficiency 726
   liver disease 603
   neonatal isoerythrolysis 973
   regenerative 714, **715**
   traumatic hemorrhage 715–17
anencephaly 781
anesthesia
   castration 375
   postanesthetic myopathy 227–8, 797
anestrus 242
   behavioral 322–3
   postpartum/lactational 323–4
aneurysm, sinus of Valsalva 706
angioedema 929
angiotensin converting enzyme inhibitors 698
Anglo-Arab horses 239
angular limb deformities 40–2, 163
   acquired 52–4
   shock-wave therapy 32, 54
anhidrosis 622, 900–1
aniridia 832
anisocoria 748–9
anisocytosis 973
anisognathism 499
ankylosis, tarsal joints 142
annular ligament, *see* palmar/plantar annular ligament
annular ligament syndrome **2**
anophthalmos 825
Anoplocephala perfoliata 524, 526, 563–4
anorectal lymphadenopathy 590
anorexia, in chronic renal failure 648, **649**
anovulatory hemorrhagic follicles 304
antacids 538
antebrachiocarpal joint, distension **121**
anterior chamber, paracentesis 819–20
anterior uveitis 853
anthelmintics 531, 770
   ascarids 549
   cyathostominosis 572–3, *572*
   gastric parasites 537
   large strongyles 577
   lungworm 469
   tapeworm 564

antibiotics
   aminoglycosides 547, 645, 669
   bacterial meningitis 767
   bacterial pneumonia 461, 462
      Rhodococcus equi 460, 994
   beta-lactam 652, 668
   borreliosis 768
   botulism 793
   canker 68
   causing diarrhea 565
   cerebral abscess 794–5
   clostridial myonecrosis 233
   colitis 568, 569
   corneal infections 850, 854
   cystitis 656
   duodenitis/proximal jejunitis 547
   foals
      diarrhea 989
      doses and metabolism 967, *968*
      pneumonia 460, 461, 462, 994
      septicemia 971
   foot infections 74, 89
   intraosseus *960*
   Lyme disease 162
   nephrotoxicity 647
   ocular disease 824
   otitis media/interna/temporohyoid osteoarthropathy 773
   pericarditis 702
   placentitis 265
   proliferative enteropathy 545
   septic arthritis/osteomyelitis 97, 98, *960*, 961, 991–2
   sulfonamides 668
   synovial infections 98, *960*, 961
   urinary tract disease 652, 663–4, 668–9
   see also named antibiotic agents
anticoagulants, toxicity 718–19
antidepressants 1000–1
antidiuretic hormone (vasopressin) 654
antifungal agents 317, 395, 850, 899, 908
antihistamines 863, 882, 929
antiproteinases, topical 850
antiprotozoal drugs 769
anuria *639*, 646, 647, 650
anus
   atresia 979–80
   squamous cell carcinoma **922**
   sphincter tone **754**, 755, 796
aortic arch, persistent right 509
aortic root disease 706–7
aortic valve, disease 698
aortoiliac thrombosis 707

apex beat 673
Apis mellifera 886
aplasia cutis congenita 936
aplastic anemia 727–8
Appaloosa horses 226, 837, 838
applanation tonometry 816
aqueous humor
    aspiration 819–20
    decreasing production/increasing
        outflow 872
Arabian fading syndrome (vitiligo)
    931
Arabian horses
    cerebellar abiotrophy 757–8
    occipitoatlantoaxial malformation
        758
arboviral diseases 760–3
arrhythmias 676, 677, 681–90
    sinus 687
arsenic poisoning **903**
arthritis, *see* osteoarthritis; septic
    arthritis
arthrocentesis,
    bog spavin 144–5
    see also synoviocentesis
arthrodesis
    chemical 143
    distal interphalangeal joint 97
    fetlock joint 108
    proximal interphalangeal joint 96,
        104, **104**, 105
    surgical 143–4
    tarsal joints 143–4
arthrogryposis 759
arthroscopy 30, 959, **960**
    fetlock joint 112
    septic arthritis **31**, 992
    sesamoid bone fracture 107
    stifle joint 152, **153**
    subchondral bone cysts 59
    synovial sepsis 959, **961**
    tarsal fractures 139
arthrotomy
    septic arthritis 992
    sesamoid bone fracture 107
artificial insemination 256–8
    advantages 256, 369
    chilled semen 339
    conception rates 256
    disadvantages 256
    frozen semen 257–8, 339
    mare preparation 258
    sex-sorting of sperm 340
    ultra-low-dose 340
aryepiglottic folds, axial deviation 432

arytenoid cartilages 384
    chondritis 426–7
    collapse 424
    hyperabduction after tie-back
        surgery **425**
    loss of abduction 435
arytenoidectomy 427
ascarid infection 549–50
ascites 704
ascorbic acid
    hypoxic–ischemic encephalopathy
        800
    red maple leaf toxicity 722
    urine acidification 658, 670
aspartate aminotransferase 28, 599
Aspergillus spp. 272, 279, 315, 464,
        608, 609, 772
Aspergillus fumigatus 394
asphyxia, perinatal 977–9
aspiration
    food material 508, 510
    meconium 976–7
    pneumonia 470–1
asthenia, cutaneous 936
Astragalus spp. 759, 790
ataxia 752
    alphavirus encephalitis 761
    equine degenerative myelo-
        encephalopathy 803–4
    hindlimbs 754, 803
    neurologic disorders 751, *753*
atheroma 391, 910, **911**
atlanto–occipital spinal tap 755
atlas, fracture **754**
atopy 892–3
atresia,
    choanal 393
    coli/recti/ani 979–80
atrial dilatation 705
atrial fibrillation 681–2, *683*, 684
atrial pacemaker, wandering 685
atrial premature contraction 685–6
atrial septal defect 692
atrial tachycardia 686
atrioventricular dissociation 686
atrioventricular valve disease
    left 695–6
    right 696–7
Atropa belladonna 791
atropine
    cardiovascular disease *683*, 684
    organophosphate poisoning 785
    topical
        adverse effects 851
        in eye disease 851, 858, 860

auriculopalpebral nerve block 814,
    824
auscultation
    abdomen 516, 581
    cardiac 674, *675*
    lung fields 384–5, 462
Australian noseband 417
Australian stringhalt 797
autogenous vaccines 916
autologous conditioned serum 96
autologous plasma infusions 317
avermectins 770
AW-3-LUDES 917
awareness, loss 746
azathioprine 720
    immune-mediated thrombo–
        cytopenia 729
azithromycin 460, 989, 994
azoospermia 355, 362–3, 364
azotemia *639*, 641
    acute renal failure 646, 647
    forms/etiologies 641
    hyperlipemia 634, 635
    uroperitoneum 664, 666

B
Babesia spp. 598, 724, 725
babesiosis 724–5
Bacillus Calmette–Guérin
immunomodulation 840, 916
back pain
    differential diagnosis 176
    osteoarthritis 183
    soft tissue injuries 175–7
bacterial cultures
    male reproductive system 335
    peritonitis 596
bacterial toxins
    gastrointestinal disease 547, 568,
        627
    metritis–laminitis–septicemia
        complex 295–6
Bacteroides fragilis 315
Bagby baskets 143
balanitis 369
balanoposthitis 352, 369
'ballerina' foal stance **43**
bandages
    abdominal support 269
    burns 957
    foot injuries 64
    Robert Jones 33, 115, 126, 950
    wound dressing 949–50, *949*
barbed-wire injuries **945**

barium enema 518
'barker' foals (perinatal) 977–9
basal cell carcinoma 917
Basidiobolus haptosporus 879
basisphenoid bone, fracture 776
basophils 712
bats, fruit 454
beclomethasone dipropionate *468*
bee stings 886
behavioral assessment 996–9
behavioral problems 996
   abnormal tongue movements
      1006, **1007**
   coprophagia 1001–2
   cribbing 1002–3
   drug treatment 1000–1
   foal rejection 1008
   hay dipping 1008–9
   head shaking 1004–5
   masculine after castration 380
   neurologic 746
   noise making 1003
   pawing 1009
   pica 1003–4
   psychogenic polydipsia 1009–10
   self-mutilation 1005–6
   and stable management 996
   stallion 342–3, 996, 1005–7
   stall walking 1010
   weaving 1004
   wood chewing 1010–11
Belgian draft foals 937
benzalkonium chloride 897
benzimidazoles 469
benzotropine mesylate 351
benzoyl peroxide 68
besnoitiosis 909
beta-2 adrenergic agonists 634
beta adrenergic blockers, topical 872
β-endorphin 629
beta-lactam antibiotics 652, 668
betamethazone 859
bethanecol chloride 510, *522*, 541,
   542, 544, 660, 670
bezoars 585
bicarbonate 228, 646, 648, 654, 670
biceps reflex 753
'big head disease' 625–7
bile acids 599, 603
bile duct, obstruction 612–13
bile ducts
   dilation 601
   stones (cholelithiasis) 612
bilirubin 599
bilirubin encephalopathy (kernicterus)
   617

biological dressings *949*
Biopty gun 358
bismuth subsalicylate 989
bisphosphonates 144
bites, insects 884–6
'bit seat' 491
bit sensitivity 491
bladder 656–60
   bacterial infections 656
   cystoliths 657–8
   eversion/prolapse 291
   irrigation 658
   paralysis/neurogenic incontinence
      659–60
   rupture 664–7, 985
      repair 666, **667**, 986
   tumors 656–7
   ultrasonography 643
bladder neck function 364
bleeding, *see* hemorrhage
bleeding disorders, inherited 718
blindness
   congenital 749
   equine recurrent uveitis 859, 860
   night, congenital stationary 837–8
   sudden-onset 810, 864
      differential diagnosis *811*
   unilateral (hemianopia) 748
blister beetle (cantharidin) toxicosis
   523–4, 627, 667–8, 701
blood–aqueous barrier 851, 859
blood cells 711–12
   enumeration 710
   see also red blood cells; white
   blood cells
blood culture 971
blood-gas analysis 389
blood group antigens 972
blood loss
   estimation 716
   splenic rupture 741
blood–ocular barrier 824
blood samples
   arterial 389
   collection 710
blood smear
   equine granulocytic ehrlichiosis
      731
   evaluation 711–12
   Heinz body anemia 722
   immune-mediated hemolytic
      anemia 720
   lead toxicity 733
   myelomonocytic leukemia 735
   neonatal isoerythrolysis 973
   regenerative anemia 714

thrombocytopenia 729
blood transfusion *716*, 717
   adverse reactions *716*
   foal 969, 973–4
   packed red cell 973–4
   splenic rupture 742
blood tubes 710
blood typing 713, 974
blood volume, foal 973
blow fly strike 887
blue-green algae 610
body condition 632, **633**
bone demineralization 625, 626
bone grafts 107
bone marrow
   aplastic anemia 727
   collection 712
   iron-deficiency anemia 726
   normal cellularity 728
   regenerative anemia 715
bone spavin **23**, 141–4
Boophilus microplus 891
borborygmi 516
Borna disease (North Eastern
   encephalitis) 760
Borrelia burgdorferi 29, 162, 767–8
botrymycosis 906
bots (*Gasterophilus* spp.) 504, 536–7
botulism 792–3
   antitoxin 793
bovine papillomavirus 913
'bowed tendon' 189
box walking 1010
brachial plexus injuries 782
brachygnathia (parrot mouth) 493–4
brachytherapy 840, 916, 922
bracken poisoning 791
bradycardia *683*
brainstem lesions 748–9, 753, 776
bran 625, *625*, 650
'bran disease' 625–7
'breaking of waters' 280
breakover point 72, 92, 96
breathing, coupling to locomotion
   421
breeding
   endometritis 314
   mare injuries 310
   minimal-contamination techniques
      255–6
   natural mating/covering 254–5
   stallion injuries 351–2, **354**, 355
breeding soundness examination
   broodmare 247–51
   stallion 330–5
brilliant green solution 897

brinzolamide 836, 872
broad ligament, hematoma 287, 288
bronchoalveolar lavage 388
    exercise-induced pulmonary
        hemorrhage 478, **479**
    heaves diagnosis 466
    inflammatory airway disease 472
bronchodilators 466, *468*, 472
bronchopneumonia 458–60, 993–4
bronchoscopy
    aspiration pneumonia 470, **471**
    exercise-induced pulmonary
        hemorrhage 478, **479**
    heaves 466
    inflammatory airway disease 471
    pleuropneumonia 462, **463**
broodmare
    blood tests 251
    breeding soundness examination
        247–51
    chromosomal abnormalities 301
    estrus abnormalities 322–5
    estrus manipulation 252–4
    fertility 247
        post-partum 254
    foal rejection 1008
    large-colon volvulus 576
    nutrition 162, 163, 237
    preparation for AI 258
    surrogate 258
    teasing 243–4, 254
    urethroplasty 664
    urovagina 308, 664
    vulvoplasty 298, 306–7, 310
    see also breeding; parturition
bruising 903, 940
    foot 66
bucked shins 116
bulbospongiosus muscle 328
bulbourethral glands 330
bullous pemphigoid 927
Burkholderia mallei 464–5, 906
Burkholderia pseudomallei 465
burns 956–7
    classification 956, *957*
bursitis
    intertubercular (bicipital) 135
    navicular bursa 97–9
    podotrochlear 216
bursoscopy 30
Buscopan 512, *521*, 989
buserelin 252, 323
butorphanol 283, 375, 520, *521*, 989
    foal *968*
N-butylscopolammonium bromide
    (Buscopan) 512, *521*, 989

C
caffeine *968*, 976
calcanean tendon, common
    ('Achilles') injuries 221–3
calcaneous
    fracture **137**, 138
    penetrating wound **958**
calcinosis circumscripta 155, 911
calcium
    administration 628, 785, 801
    diet 162–3, 235, 625
        requirements *626*, 628
        supplementation 626–7, 628
    fractional excretion *642*
    ionized serum 235, 627, 801
    mammary secretions 264, 265
    total serum 627–8, 801
calcium borogluconate 524, 547, 646,
    668, 801
calcium carbonate
    feeding 628
    urine crystals 641
calcium disodium EDTA 733, 788
calcium gluconate 226, 235, 628, 801
calcium:phosphorus balance 163,
    235, 625
calculi
    bladder 657–8
    renal pelvis 651
    salivary glands (sialoliths) 507
    ureteral 655
    urethral 662–3
calculus (dental) 498, 649, 805
Callitroga spp. 887
campylorrhinus lateralis (wry nose)
    46, **47**, 392, 494
Candida spp. 249, 315
    urethral infection 663–4
canine teeth 483
    disease 498
canker 68
cannon bone, *see* metacarpal bones,
    third; metatarsal bones, third
cantharidin toxicosis 523–4, 627,
    667–8, 701
capillary refill time 673
capped elbow 130
capped hock 140
carbamazepine 863
carbenicillin *316*
carbohydrate absorption testing 520,
    529, *548*
carbonic anhydrase inhibitors
    systemic 872
    topical 836, 872
carbon monoxide toxicity 474

carboxyhemoglobin 474
carboxypropeptides of type II
    collagen 28
cardiac auscultation 674, *675*
cardiac catheterization 680
cardiac cycle 677
cardiac impulse 673
cardiac tamponade 702
cardiac troponins 680
cardiomyopathies 700–1
cardiovascular disease
    acquired valvular disease 695–700
    arrhythmias 681–90
    cardiomyopathies 700
    congenital 690–4
    drugs used in management *683–4*
    general examination 673
    history 672
    hyperthyroidism 634
    laboratory evaluation 680
    myocardial 700–1
    pericardial 702–6
cardioversion, atrial fibrillation 682
carotid artery
    external 447–8
    inadvertent injection 775
    internal **443**, 445, 447, **747**
carpal canal syndrome 123
carpal flexion, foal, causing dystocia
    284
carpal flexion test 18
carpal sheath, distension 123
carpometacarpal joint, in splint bone
    fracture 118, 119
carpus (knee)
    conformation 120
    cuboidal bones
    collapse 224, 975, 990
    defective ossification 621–2, 624,
        975
    flexural deformity 44
    fractures 120–5
    hygroma 124
    infection **961**, 990, **991**
    lavage **961**
    luxation 124, 125
    osseous cyst-like lesions 124, 125
    osteoarthritis 124–5
    valgus/varus deformities 40–2
        acquired 52–4
cartilage, damage/loss in osteoarthritis
    38
cartilage oligomeric matrix protein
    28, 29
casein, iodinated *623*
Caslick score 306

Caslick's vulvoplasty 298, 306–7, 310
castration 374–80
  age of horse 374
  anesthesia and sedation 375
  complications 359, 378–80
  indications for 374
  preoperative considerations 374–5
  spermatic cord tumors 373
  surgical techniques 376–8
casts
  bivalved **951**, 962
  flexural deformities 43
  fractures 32–3, 34–5
  hoof injuries 77, 78
  pressure sores 35, 951
  tendon lacerations 962–3
  wound immobilization 950–1
casts (urine) 641
cataplexy 803
cataracts
  acquired 869–70
  causes 834, *835*, 869–70
  congenital 834–6, 868
  management 835–6, 870
  secondary to recurrent uveitis **835**,
    859, 860
catheterization, bladder 639
cauda equina, neuritis (polyneuritis
  equi) 795–6
cauda equina syndrome 178
cavernous spaces 328
cecum 560–4
  impaction 561–2
  infarction 560
  palpation per rectum 517
  rupture 276, 560, 562
  torsion 561
  trocarization *562*, *563*, 574
  tympany 562–3
ceftiofur
  liver disease 603
  Lyme disease 162
  purpura hemorrhagica 732
  synovial infections *960*
  uroperitoneum 666
  uterine infections 314, *316*
ceftriaxone, foal *968*
celiotomy 583
  midline 576, 579
cement, dental 484, 489
  hypoplasia 489–90
Centaurea melitensis 790
Centaurea solstitialis 790, **791**
central nervous system
  hypoxia–ischemia 799–800
  neoplasia 801

trauma 775–81
cephalosporins 461, 668, 971
ceratohyoidectomy 449
cerclage wiring 35, 168
cerebellum 746–7, 748
  abiotrophy 757–8
  hypoplasia 757
  trauma 776–7
cerebral abscess 794–5
cerebral edema 774–5, 794
  management 979
  perinatal asphyxia syndrome
    978–9
cerebral trauma 774–7
cerebrospinal fluid, collection and
  analysis 755
cervical spine
  malformations 758–9
  trauma 778
cervical vertebral instability/stenosis
  (wobbler syndrome) 806–8
cervix 247
  adhesions 320
  estrus 244, 245
  examination in pregnancy *261*
  injuries 294–5
Cesarean section 268, 284, 285–6
Cestrum diurnum 648
chasteberry 632
check ligament
  inferior
    desmitis 204–5
    desmotomy 56, 57, 205
  superior
    desmitis 123
    desmotomy 57, 123
cheek abscess 904–5
chelating agents 610, 733, 788
chemical agents
  pruritus 877
  scalding 895
chemical restraint, *see* sedation
chemotherapy
  melanoma 920–1
  sarcoids 840, 917
chest drain 388, 462–3
  air suction 476
  insertion 388
chewing, inability 749
'china eye' 830
chiropractic manipulation 177
chloramine solution 897
chloramphenicol 545, 824, 850
chlorhexidine 899, 905
  penile cleaning 366
chloride, excretion 642, *642*

chlorinated hydrocarbons 785
chlorulon 257
choanal atresia/stenosis 393
choke 470, 511–12
  treatment 512
'choking up' 416
cholangiohepatitis 602, 612–13
cholangitis 601, 612–13
choledocholithiasis 612
cholelithiasis 601, 612
cholesteatoma 796, **797**
chondroids 442, 444, 454
  management 444, 457
Chorioptes spp. 875, 888–9
chromium supplementation 632
chromosomal abnormalities
  mare 301
  see also karyotyping
chronic renal failure 648–50
  clinical presentation 648, **649**
  diagnosis 648–50
  etiology/pathophysiology 648, 651
  management 650
  prognosis 650
  urine biochemistry 641–2
chylothorax 476–7
cicutoxin 792
ciliary body, cyst 833
cimetidine 507, *538*, 920, 982
ciprofloxacin 850
cisapride *522*, 532
cisplatin
  melanoma 920–1
  sarcoid therapy 840, 917
clarithromycin 460, 994
cleft palate (palatoschiasis) 502
clenbuterol 265, 273, 283, 451, *468*
clindamycin 68
clitoral swab 248
clitorectomy 317
clitoris, enlargement 321, 345
cloprostenol 314
clostridial myonecrosis 232–3
Clostridium botulinum 531–2, 792
Clostridium chauvoei 232
Clostridium difficile infection 545,
  546, 565, 567, 987
Clostridium perfringens 232, 546, 565
  toxin production *565*
Clostridium piliformis 615
Clostridium septicum 232
Clostridium tetani 771
clotrimazole *316*
clotting factors 599, **713**, 718, 719
  deficiencies 718

clover
   alsike 608
   sweet 718, 719
'club foot' 55
coagulation
   evaluation 713
   pathways **713**
coagulation disorders 604, 718
coastal Bermuda grass hay 554, 786
coccidioidomycosis 473
coccygeal vertebrae, injuries 185
cocklebur 608
coffin bone, *see* distal phalanx
coffin joint, *see* distal interphalangeal
   joint
Coggins test 724
coital exanthema, equine 310–11,
   368, 895
'cold back' 176
cold therapy
   foot 66, 71
   paraphimosis 350
   tendon injuries 194
colic
   analgesia 520, *521*
   cecal impaction 561–2
   chronic/recurrent 530–1, 533
   colonic impaction 579–80
   gas (colonic tympany) 574–5
   intestinal parasites 524, 526, 531
   intussusception 526–7
   meconium impaction 980–1
   small-intestinal volvulus 552
   spasmodic 524–5
   strangulating lipoma 550–1
colitis 564–9
   Clostridial 566, 567
   idiopathic 565, 567
   right dorsal 570–1
   segmental eosinophilic 582
   see also enterocolitis
colitis X 565, 566–7
collagen fibers, tendons 189
collagen shields (eye) 823, 851
collateral cartilages, *see* ungual
   cartilages
collateral ligaments
   distal interphalangeal joint 27–8,
     100–1
   distal sesamoid 27–8, **91**
   elbow joint 130
   stifle joint 150, 153
colliculus seminalis 327–8
colloid dressings *949*
colobomas 828–9

colon
   examination per rectum 517
   large
     displacement 578–9
     impaction 579–80
     intramural lesions 582
     nephrosplenic entrapment 742
     sand enteropathy 569–70
     sand impaction 581
     volvulus 575–6
   small
     impaction 583
     obstruction 585
     segmental ischemic necrosis
       586
     strangulation 584
     stricture 523
     torsion 275–6
     tympany (gas colic) 574–5
Colorado artificial vagina 336
colostrum
   intake 967
   quality 967, 968–9
   red blood cell antibodies 972–3
coma 746, 978
comfrey 604, **605**
common calcanean ('Achilles') tendon
   injuries 221–3
companions 996, 999
compartment syndrome 964
compensatory inflammatory response
   syndrome 971
computed tomography 28, 188, 820
computer-assisted sperm motion
   analysis systems 337
conception rates
   artificial insemination 256
   foal heat 254
   natural covering 254
   see also fertility
conformation 13, 120
   broodmare 247–8
   foot 13–15, 80–2, 90, 91
   hock 141
congenital disorders
   atresia coli/ani/recti 979–80
   brachygnathia/prognathia 493–4
   cardiovascular 690–4
   choanal atresia/stenosis 393
   cleft palate (palatoschiasis) 502
   esophagus 509–11
   female reproductive tract 321
   hypothyroidism 621
   kidneys 651
   male reproductive tract 345–7

   musculoskeletal
     causing dystocia 284, 285
     limbs 40–9, 284, 285
     thoracolumbar/sacral spine
       174, **175**
   neurologic 756–60
   ocular 824–39, 869–70
   persistent/patent urachus 983–4
   scrotal/inguinal hernia 360, 361,
     558–9
   small intestine 554–6
   subepiglottic cyst 411–13
   umbilical hernia 984
   ureters 655
   wry nose 46, **47**, 392, 494
conjunctivae
   culture samples 818
   cytology samples 819
   drug injection 824
   normal flora 818
conjunctival grafts 851–3, 855
conjunctivitis 846–7
   common causes 846, *847*
consciousness, loss 774
contact dermatitis/hypersensitivity
   923–4, **933**
contact lenses, drug-releasing 823,
   851
contagious equine metritis 248, 366
contracted foal/limb syndrome 44,
   46, **47**
contusions 940
Coombs test 713, 720, 724, 973
copper deficiency 50, 162, 163
coprophagia 1001–2
corkwoods 791
cornea
   abscess 853–5
   melting (keratomalacia) 850
   perforation 868
   tissue samples 819, 849
corneal ulcers 848–53
   clinical presentation 848–9
   diagnosis 815–16, 849
   etiology/pathophysiology 848,
    848
   following cataract removal 836
   management 850–3
Cornell Collar 417
corneoconjunctival transpositions
   852–3
corn oil 571
corns 66
coronary band
   dystrophy 932
   injuries **15**, 76, 950, **951**

cor pulmonale 704
corpus luteum 243, 244, 263
   persistent 322, 323
   primary 260
   secondary 260
   ultrasonography 249
corticosteroids
   cardiac disease 700, 701
   cerebral trauma 775
   chronic diarrhea 574
   cyathostominosis 572
   endometritis 315
   equine purpura hemorrhagica 732
   facial nerve trauma 777
   habronemiasis 910
   immune-mediated hemolytic
anemia 720
   immune-mediated thrombo-
      cytopenia 729
   inflammatory airway disease and
heaves 466, *468*
   intra-articular 92, 96, 105, 142, 807
   liver disease 604
   and male fertility *342*
   newborn foal 975
   otitis media/interna 773
   parturition induction 282
   polyneuritis equi 796
   prenatal 975
   skin disorders 882, 911, 929
   uveitis 858, 859–60
   vasculitis 930
cortisol 630, 632
Corynebacterium spp. 652
Corynebacterium pseudotuberculosis
   234, 272, 905
cough 383
   induction 384
coumarin 718
covering 254–5, 335
coxofemoral joint, luxation 158–9
crackles, lung 385
'cramps' 235, 236
cranial nerves, examination 747–51
craniotomy 172
cranium
   fractures 171–2, 402–3, 776–7
   radiography 486–8, *486*
creatine kinase 524, 680
creatinine
   serum 646
   urine 641
creatinine phosphokinase 28
cremaster muscle 328
cribbing 1002–3

cromogens *468*
crossmatching 713, *716*
Crotalaria spectabilis 604, **605**
cruciate ligament injuries 150, 153
cryopreservation 339
cryotherapy
   glaucoma 836
   penile squamous cell carcinoma
      370
   sarcoids 840, 916
cryptorchid 331, 346–7, 380
   castration 374
Culex spp. 760, 761
Culicoides spp. 453, 763, 866, 881
   hypersensitivity (sweet itch) 881–3
Culiseta melanura 760
cunean tendon 225
   cutting 142–3
   tendonitis 225
curb 224–5
Cushing's disease, equine 622,
   629–32, 923
   clinical presentation 629–30, 923
   diagnosis 630–1
   etiology/pathophysiology 629
   management 631–2
Cushing's syndrome, peripheral
(equine metabolic) 632–4
cutaneous lupus erythematosus 924–5
cyanoacrylate adhesive 851
cyanobacteria 610
cyanosis 690
   after exercise 694
cyathostominosis 526, 560, 571–3
cyclocryoablation 836, 872
cyclophotoablation 872
cyclosporine A (CsA), intravitreal 860
Cynoglossum officinale 604, **605**
cypermethrin 883
cyproheptadine 632, 863, 1001
cystadenoma 303
cystitis 656, 660
cystogram, contrast 643
cystoliths 644, 657–8
cystoscopy 644, 658, 661
cystotomy, pararectal 658
cysts
   ciliary body 833
   paranasal sinuses 408–9
   subchondral bone 50, 58–9
   subepiglottic 411–13
   uveal 831–2

D

dacryocystitis 829, 830, 868
dacryocystorhinography 868
dantrolene sodium 228, 230, 240
Datura spp. 791
day length, and reproduction 242, 252
dazzle reflex 812
deep digital flexor tendon
   accessory ligament (inferior check
      ligament) 56
      desmitis 204–5
      desmotomy 56, 205
   distal
      adhesions 90, **90**
      injuries 100–1
   lacerations 962
   magnetic resonance imaging 27–8
   pastern 217
   tendonitis 123, 216–17
   tenotomy 72
deferoxamine 610
degenerative joint disease, *see*
osteoarthritis
degloving injuries 940, **941**
deglutition 423, 508
dehydration
   assessment 638
   colitis 566
   hemoconcentration 739
deltoid tuberosity, fractures 131–2
dementia 761
Demodex spp. (demodicosis) 875,
   909
densimeters 337
dental cement 484, 489
   hypoplasia 489–90
dental enamel 484
dental impactions 493
dental infections 495–7
   secondary sinusitis 399–400
dental mark 483, 485
dental radiography 486–8, *486*
dental star 483, 486
dentigerous cysts 490–1, 501, 910
dentine 484
   secondary 486
Dermacentor spp. 789, 892
dermal asthenia, hereditary 936
Dermanyssus gallinae 875, 889
dermatitis
   contact 923–4, **933**
   Malassezia 878
   parasites 880–1
   pastern 935
   scrotum 356
dermatome 954

dermatophilosis 896–7, 933
  young foal 938
Dermatophilus congolensis 896–7, 933
dermoid 829
dermoid cysts 910
descemetocele 849
Descemet's membrane 819, 849, 855
desmitis
  distal interphalangeal joint
    collateral ligaments 27–8, 100–1
  inferior check ligament 204–5
  patellar ligaments 150, 152
  suspensory ligament **15**, 118, 119, 195
    body 200–1
    branch 201–3
    proximal 196–9
desmopathy, distal sesamoidean
  ligaments 206
desmopressin acetate 643
desmotomy
  inferior check ligament 56, 57, 205
  medial patellar ligament 148, 149–50
  palmar/plantar annular ligament 216
  superior check ligament 123
detomidine 283, 375, 520, *521*, 639
  foal *968*
developmental orthopedic diseases 50, 162–4
  see also osteochondrosis; physitis
deworming 531
  ascarids 549
  cyathostomes 572–3, *572*
  foals 549, 576
  gastric parasites 537
  lungworm 469
  tapeworm 564
dew poisoning 608
dexamethasone
  endometritis 315
  equine purpura hemorrhagica 732
  facial nerve trauma 777
  foal *968*
  immune-mediated hemolytic
anemia 720
  immune-mediated thrombo-
    cytopenia 729
  inflammatory airway disease/
    heaves *468*
  otitis media/interna 773
  parturition induction 282
  polyneuritis equi 796

toxic myocarditis 701
  uveitis 858, 859–60
dexamethasone suppression test 630, *631*
dexamethasone 21-isonicotinate *468*
diabetes insipidus 654–5
  diagnosis 643
diabetes mellitus 632, 636
dialysis, peritoneal 647
diaphragmatic flutter 236–7, 801
diaphragmatic hernia 592–4
diarrhea
  antimicrobial-associated 565
  chronic 573–4
  Clostridium perfringens 565
  foals 545–6, 987–9
  lactose intolerance 548
  rotavirus enteritis 545–6
  salmonellosis 564
diastemata 493, 494–5
diazepam
  behavioral problems 1001
  bladder dysfunction 660
  cerebral trauma 774
  epilepsy 802
  foal *968*
  hypoxic–ischemic encephalopathy *800*
  perinatal asphyxia syndrome 978
  stallion sexual function *341*
diazinon 890
dibutyl phthalate 886
dichlorphenamide 872
diclazuril 769
diclofenac 858
diclofenac sodium 777
Dictyocaulus arnfieldi 468–9
Didelphis albiventris 768
Didelphis virginiana 768
diestrus 242, 245
  ovulation 324
  prolonged/persistent 322
diet
  and angular limb deformities 54
  and behavior 999
  calcium:phosphorus balance 163, 235, 625
  carbohydrate excess 807
  cecal tympany 562, 563
  chronic diarrhea 574
  and chronic/recurrent colic 531
  colitis 568, 571
  colon impaction 579, 580
  equine metabolic syndrome 633
  fat 571, 650

flexural limb deformities 57
  and gastric ulceration 538
  hyperlipemia/hyperlipidemia 635
  hypocalcemia prevention 628
  ileal impaction 554
  intestinal adhesions 533
  liver failure 603–4
  nutritional hyperparathyroidism 625, *625*
  osteochondrosis 50
  probiotics 568, 574
  pyloric stenosis 541–2
  renal disease 646–7, 650
  silage 792
  and thyroid hormones 621
  urolithiasis 656
  wobbler syndrome 807
  see also nutrition
dietary supplements
  calcium 626–7, 628
  equine Cushing's disease 632
  iron 726
  mare 163
  vitamin E 804, 805, 979
diethylcarbamazine 858
digital arteries, lacerations 942
digitalis glycosides 785
digital pulse 16, 673
digital tendon sheath
  tenosynovitis 192, *193*, 211–13
  wounds 210, 959
digoxin
  applications *683*, 686, 706
  contraindications 701
  dose *683*
  toxicity *683*
dimethyl sulfoxide 228, 339
  alphavirus encephalitis 762
  bacterial meningitis 767
  cerebral trauma 775
  equine herpes myencephalopathy 766
  foal
    dosages *968*
    perinatal asphyxia syndrome 979
  hypoxic–ischemic encephalopathy *800*
  laminitis 71
  uterine infections 317
  verminous meningo-
    encephalomyelitis 770
  West Nile virus 763
  wobbler syndrome 807
dinoprostone 268
di-n-propyl disulfide 722

dioctyl sodium succinate 522, 528, 541, 580

dioxins 785

dipyrone, use in colic *521*

discospondylitis 795

disseminated intravascular coagulation 560, 566, **568**, 569, 729–30
clinical presentation 730
diagnosis 730
etiology/pathophysiology 729
management 730

distal interphalangeal joint
collateral ligament desmitis 27–8, 100–1
distension **15**, **94**
flexural deformities 43, 55–6, 204, 205
magnetic resonance imaging 27–8
osteoarthritis 94–6
regional analgesia 86, 92, 94
septic arthritis 96–7

distal phalanx (coffin bone)
bone resorption 86
displacement in white line disease 73, **73**
displacement/remodeling in laminitis 70, **71**, 72
fracture 84–5
osteitis 86
septic osteitis 87

distal sesamoidean ligaments, injuries 100, 206

distal sesamoid (navicular) bone 90
changes in normal aging 90
fracture 93
imaging **26**, 28
pathology in navicular syndrome 90, 91–2

di-tri-octahedral smectite 568

diuretics
cantharidin toxicosis 524, 668
cardiovascular disease *683*, 689, 706
loop 669
raised intracranial pressure 172, 794
renal dysfunction 647, 650, 669

diverticula, esophageal 513–14

DNA testing, hyperkalemic periodic paralysis 226

dogs, rabies 764

'dog-sitting' behavior 276, 284

domperidone 252, 323, 630

donkeys 468–9, 725

dopamine, and renal function 669

dopamine agonists 631

dopamine antagonists 252, 1000

Doppler echocardiography 678–80, 691

dorsal displacement of the soft palate
epiglottic flaccidity 433
intermittent 415–18
permanent 419–20
subepiglottic cyst 411, 412

dorsal spinous processes
analgesia **21**
impingement 180–1
injuries 175, 178, 179
removal of tips 181
scintigraphy **26**, 175, 181

dorzolamide 836, 872

dourine 311, 366

doxapram *968*

doxycycline 162, 731, 768
foal *968*, 994

drainage
hygroma 140
joint infections 992
pleural fluids 388, 462–3, 464
wounds 948

Draschia spp. 536, 770, 909

dressings, *see* wound dressings

drinking, psychogenic 1009–10

dropped elbow 14, **15**

drug eruption 924

Dubosia spp. 791

ductus arteriosus
fibrous remnant 509
patent 693

'dummy' foals, *see* asphyxia, perinatal

duodenitis 546–7

duodenojejunostomy 523

duodenoscopy 543

duodenum
normal endoscopy **543**
stenosis, secondary to ulceration 981
stricture 523
ulceration 543–4

duplication cysts, esophagus 509–10

dynamic compression plates 37

dynamic condylar screw 37

dynamic hip score 37

dysgerminoma 303–4

dysphagia
after tie-back operation 425
botulism 792, **793**
causes 166, 169
esophageal disease 508
facial nerve paralysis 777
foal/young horse 412
neurologic disease 751, 761

oral-phase 166, 448, 493
pharyngeal-phase 445, 446
subepiglottic cyst 411, 412
yellow star thistle ingestion **791**

dyspnea 383

dystocia 283–6
advice to owner 283
cervical injuries 294–5
epidural anesthesia 283–4
incidence 283
preparation of mare prior to examination 283

dysuria *639*

E
ear
dentigerous cyst 490–1, 910
otitis media–interna 772–3
ticks 892

early embryonic death 274–5

'early pregnancy factor' 250

Eastern equine encephalitis 760, 761–2

'easy keepers' 622

Echidnophaga gallinacea 881

Echinococcus granulosus subsp. *equinus* 614–15

Echinococcus multilocularis 615

Echium vulgare 604, **605**

echocardiography 678–80
aortic valve disease 698
atrial fibrillation 682
atrial septal defect 692
contrast 680
Doppler 678–80
heart failure 705
indications 678
M-mode 678
patent ductus arteriosus 693
sedation 680
tetralogy of Fallot 694
ventricular septal defect 691

ectoparasites
fleas 881
Habronema spp. 370, 909–10
lice 887–8, 938
mites 875, 888–91, 909
skin examination 875
ticks 891–2

edema
cerebral 774–5, 794, 978–9
limbs 673
peripheral/ventral 704, **705**
pulmonary 689

EDTA-Tris *316*

egg-bar shoes **82**, 92
Ehrlichia equi, see Anaplasma phagocytophila
Ehrlichia risticii, see Neorickettsia risticii
ehrlichiosis
   equine 770
   equine granulocytic 730–1
Eisenmenger's complex 691
ejaculation 335
   dysfunction 344
   induction 343, 1001
ejaculatory fluid 344, 363
elbow
   dropped 14, **15**, **128**, 129
   hygroma 130
   osteoarthritis 130–1
electrocardiography 675–7
   atrial fibrillation 682
   atrial premature contraction 685
   atrioventricular dissociation 686
   electrode placement 676, **677**
   fetal 264, **265**
   heart block 685
   interpretation 677
   pre-excitation syndrome 688
   premature ventricular complex 688
   sinus arrest/block 687
   sinus arrhythmia 687
   torsade de pointes 689
   ventricular tachycardia 689
   wandering atrial pacemaker 685
electrocautery 916
electrochemotherapy 917
electroencephalography 756
electrolyte abnormalities 163
   burns 956
   colitis 568
   chronic renal failure 649, 650
   duodenitis 547
   hypocalcemia 627–8
   liver disease 600
   uroperitoneum 986
   see also named electrolytes
electrolytes
   fractional excretion 642, *642*
   loss in sweat *626*, 628
   mammary secretions 264–5
electromagnetic therapy 31
electromyography 29, 756
   hyperkalemic periodic paralysis 226
   myotonia 239
electroretinography 820

enzyme-linked immunosorbent
   assay tests
      alphaviruses 762
      pregnancy diagnosis 263
      West Nile virus 763
emasculators 376
embryo, ultrasound imaging 262
embryo transfer 258–9
emphysema, subcutaneous 436, **437**
enalapril *684*, 698
enamel, dental 484
enamel points 499
enanthotoxin 792
encephalitis
   alphavirus 760–2
   North Eastern (Borna disease) 760
   West Nile virus 762–3
encephalocele 781
encephalomalacia, nigropallidal 790–1
encephalopathy
   bilirubin (kernicterus) 617
   hepatic 602, 798–9
   hypoxic–ischemic 617, 799–800
   neonatal (perinatal asphyxia syndrome) 977–9
encephalosis, equine 763
endocarditis, bacterial 698–700
endocrine disease 620
   diagnostic work up 620
endometritis 295–6, 305, 313
   management 314–15, 316
   persistent breeding 314
   sexually-transmitted 317
endometrium
   biopsy 250, 315, 318
   cysts 319
   edema 244, 246
endometrosis, degenerative 318
endophytic fungal toxicosis 786
endoscopy
   female reproductive tract 245, 248, 251
   guttural pouches 170, 386, 442, **443**, 446–7
   navicular bursa 98–9
   respiratory tract 386
      choanal atresia 393
      dorsal displacement of the soft palate **415**, 416, **417**
      larynx 386, 423–4, 429, 432, 433
      nasal passage trauma 409
      sinuses 387, 402
      subepiglottic cyst 412

      treadmill/overground video 389, 416, **417**, 421, 424, 432, 435
   stomach 535, 538, **539**
   thoracic cavity 389
   urinary tract 335, 644, 658, 661
   uterus 251
   see also arthroscopy; bronchoscopy
endotoxemia
   colitis 568
   duodenitis/proximal jejunitis 547
   hypercalcemia 627
   laminitis 70–1
enemas 583, 980–1
   foal 980–1
enilconazole 395, 899
enophthalmitis 838
enrofloxacin 68, *316*, 367, 669
enteritis
   foals 987–9
   granulomatous 529
   rotavirus 545–6, 987
Enterobacter spp. 460, 652
enterocentesis 520
enterocolitis, eosinophilic 529–30
enterolith 527, **528**
enteropathy, proliferative 544–5
enterotomy
   ascarid impaction 550
   epiploic foramen entrapment 557
   foreign body 528
entheseopathy
   annular ligament insertion 214, **215**
   distal sesamoidean ligaments **91**, 206
   fetlock joint 113
   suspensory ligament branch insertion 202, **203**
entropion 826–7, 966
   causes 826, *826*
   correction 827
enucleation 810, 840, 853, 870
environment
   change and horses' behavior 996
   enrichment 999
   management in *R. equi* infections 460, 994
eosinophilic enterocolitis 529–30
eosinophilic granuloma 911
eosinophils 712
Epicauta spp. 523, 667
epidermoid cyst, false nostril (atheroma) 391, 910, **911**

epididymis 327
   sperm granuloma 362
epididymitis 356–7
epidural anesthesia, dystocia 283–4
epiglottis
   augmentation 433
   endoscopy 429
   entrapment 430–1
   flaccidity 433
   hypoplasia 434
   retroflexion 434–5
   swallowing 508
epiglottitis 429–30
epilepsy
   acquired 802
   juvenile idiopathic 802
epinephrine 226
epiphysitis 60–1, 163, 625
epiploic foramen entrapment 556–7
epistaxis 171, 172, 404, 405, 409
   exercise-induced pulmonary
     hemorrhage 478
   guttural pouch mycosis 445–6
epitheliogenesis imperfecta 936
epoxide 609
equine chorionic gonadatropin 260,
   263
equine degenerative myeloencephalopathy 803–4
equine herpesviruses 451–2
   clinical presentation 452
   diagnosis 452
   EHV-1 272, 273, 277, 451–2, 765–6
     abortion/stillbirth 278, 617
      diagnosis 278
      vaccination 277
   EHV-3 310–11, 368, 895
   EHV-4 272, 451
   management 452
   myeloencephalopathy 765–6
equine infectious anemia 332, 723–4,
   763
   acute/chronic forms 722
   diagnosis 724
   management 724
equine influenza 450–1
equine motor neuron disease 29,
   804–5
equine myotonic dystrophy 239
equine polysaccharide storage
   myopathy 229
equine protozoal myeloencephalitis
   749, 768–9, 803
equine purpura hemorrhagica 455,
   732–3, 934

equine recurrent uveitis (moonblindness) **835**, 858–60
equine viral arteritis (EVA) 272, 278,
   332, 452–3, 903
   clinical presentation 368, 453
   diagnosis 368–9, 453
   management 369, 453
   vaccination 277, 278, 453
Equisetum spp. 791
erectile dysfunction 343
erythema multiforme 928
erythromycin
   foals *968*
     diarrhea 545, 989
   R. equi pneumonia 460, 994
erythromycin estolate 545
erythromycin lactobionate *522*
erythromycin phosphate 545
Escherichia coli 249, 272, 296, 315,
   460, 652, 766
   foal diarrhea 987
esophageal sphincter
   cranial 508
   distal 508, 510, 511
esophagitis, reflux 510–11
esophago-cutaneous fistula 514
esophagoscopy 508
esophagostomy 515
esophagotomy 513
esophagus
   anatomy 508
   clinical signs of disease 508
   diagnosis of disease 508
   diverticula 513–14
   duplication cysts 509
   foreign body penetration 514
   neoplasia 515
   obstruction 470, 508, 511–12
     treatment 512
   perforation 508
   persistent dilatation (mega-
     esophagus) 510
   rupture 515
   stricture 512, 513
   surgery 515
   ulceration 512–13
esotropia 826
estradiol-17β 253
estradiol cypionate 660
estrogen 243
   exogenous 253
   and incontinence 660
   pregnancy 260, 263
   stallion 326, 357
estrone sulfate 260, 263
estrous behavior 261

estrous cycle 242–3
   anomalies and abnormalities 322–5
   hormonal changes 243
   identifying stage 243–5
   manipulation 252–4
   ovarian tumors 302
   records 245
estrus 242
   synchronization 253
ethmoidal hematoma 404–6
etisazole, in DMSO 908
eventration, after castration 379
excessive transverse ridges 500
exercise, controlled program 31, 194,
   195
exercise-induced pulmonary
   hemorrhage 478–80, 681
exercise testing
   muscle damage 28
   respiratory function 389, 416, **417**,
     421, 424, 432, 435
exertional rhabdomyolysis 163, 175,
   229
   diagnosis 28, 229–30
   management 164, 230
   recurrent 229
exhausted horse syndrome 236
exophthalmos 845
exostoses
   fluoride toxicosis 164
   hereditary 48
   osteoarthritis 94, **95**
   second/fourth metacarpal/
     metatarsal bones ('splints') 120
   supracarpal volar (osteo-
     chondroma) 129
exotropia 826
extension tests 18
extensor carpi radialis tendon
   injuries 207–11
   rupture 211
extensor tendons
   injuries 46, 207–11
     lacerations 208, 963
     ruptures 46, 211
external carotid artery 447–8
external skeletal fixator 35, 168
extracorporeal shock-wave therapy
   32, 54, 144, 199
eye
   anatomy 810–11
   examination 812–13
     dark 817–18
     lighted 816
     sedation 814
   imaging 820

medication methods 821–4
  intraocular 824
  parenteral 824
  subconjunctival 824
  subpalpebral lavage 821–3
  topical application 821
neoplasia 839–46, 922
nerve blocks 814–15
neurologic disorders 861–6
parasitic diseases 856, 858, 866–7,
  909
sample collection 818–19
topical anesthetic 814
eyelid
  entropion 826–7
  melanoma 843–4
  squamous cell carcinoma 841–3,
  922
eye movements 749

F

facet joints 183
facial artery 673
facial muscles, hypertonia/hyper
  reflexia 750
facial nerve 750
  damage 748, 772, **773**, 777
facial sensation 749
facial swelling
  dental infections 496
  sinusitis 396
facial trauma 171–2, 402–3, 777
factor VII 718–19
failure of passive transfer of immunity
  968–9, 971
fallopian tubes (oviducts), disease
  305
falls, head trauma 776–7, 864
false nostril, atheroma 391, 910, **911**
faradic stimulation 31
farcy (glanders) 464–5, 906
farriery, *see* foot trimming; shoeing
Fasciola hepatica 615
Fascioloides magna 615
fasciotomy 228
fat, dietary 571, 650
fatty liver syndrome 616–17, 634
fecal egg counts
  large strongyles 577
  small strongyles (cyathostomes)
  572, 573
  Strongyloides westeri 576
fecal flotation test 564, 577
feces
  eating 1001–2
  sand evaluation 569

feeding behavior 999, 1008–9
feeds
  low-residue 533
  pelleted 635
  see also diet; nutrition
Fell pony immunodeficiency
  syndrome 970
female reproductive hormones
  fetal health 264
  pregnancy 260, 263
female reproductive tract
  examination 247–51
  neoplasia 302–4, 312–13
  see also parts and disorders of tract
feminization, testicular 321
femoral nerve, injury 783
femoropatellar joint
  osteochondrosis 151, 153–4
  see also patella; stifle joint
femur, fractures 33, 150, 156–7, 783
fenbendazole 531, 549, 770
  chronic diarrhea 574
  cyathostominosis 572, *572*
  large strongyles 577
fenoterol *468*
fentanyl patches 961
fertility
  mare 247
    post-partum 254
  stallion 357–8
    drugs affecting *342*
  see also conception rates
fetal membranes, *see* placenta
'fetlock drop' 16
  suspensory ligament injury 962
fetlock (metacarpo/metatarso-
  phalangeal) joint 108–13
  arthrodesis 108
  chronic proliferative synovitis 109
  deformities 44, 52, 55–6, 57
  hyperextension 109, 118
  intrasynovial analgesia 19
  osteoarthritis 38, **39**, 110–13
  sepsis **21**, **25**, 990, **991**
  subluxation 108
  ultrasonography **25**
fetoplacental unit
  assessing health 260, 263–5
  hormone production 280
fetotomy 284
fetus
  anomalies 279
  electrocardiogram 264, **265**
  hypermotility 266
  hypothyroidism 163
  mummification 274

septicemia 272
  ultrasonography 264
  viability tests 251
fibrin
  abdominal 533, 596
  pleural cavity 461
fibroma 917–18
fibrosarcoma 917–18
fimbrial adhesions 305
fipronil 888, 889, 891
fires 474, 956–7
'firing' 194
first aid, fractures 32–7, 115
fistula
  esophageal 514
  rectovaginal/vestibular 296, 299
'fistulous withers' 175
fleas, stickfast 881
flecainide *684*
Flehmen response 326
flexion tests 18
  distal limb joints 18, 91
  hindlimb 148, 150
  tendon injuries 217
flexor reflex 754, 783
flexor tendons, *see* deep digital flexor
  tendon; lateral digital flexor
  tendon; superficial digital flexor
  tendon
flexural limb deformities
  acquired 55–7
  congenital 43–4
  distal interphalangeal joint 55, 56,
  204, 205
  fetlock joint 55–6, 57
Flieringa ring 820
flies
  black 885–6
  buffalo 882, 885
  horn 885
  horse 882, 884
  hypersensitivity 882
  stable 883, 884–5
fluconazole 850
fluid therapy
  abdominal blood loss 591
  acute renal failure 646
  cantharidin toxicosis 524, 668
  colitis 568
  colon impaction 580
  chronic renal failure 650
  duodenitis 547
  foal diarrhea 988–9
  hyperlipemia 635
  hyperproteinemia 739
  liver failure 603

shock rate 591
splenic rupture 742
uterine artery rupture 288
flunixin meglumine
'anti-endotoxin' 547, 568, 596
arboviral diseases 762, 763
equine protozoal meningitis 769
equine granulocytic ehrlichiosis 731
equine herpes myencephalopathy 766
exertional rhabdomyolysis 230
eye disorders 836, 851
facial nerve trauma 777
laminitis 71
otitis media/interna 773
penile/urethral trauma 661
septic peritonitis 596
use in colic 521
uveitis 858, 860
verminous meningo-encephalomyelitis 770
wobbler syndrome 807
fluorescein staining 815–16, 849
fluoride toxicosis 164
fluoroquinolones 68, 316, 367, 669
5-fluorouracil 840
fluphenazine 1000
flurbiprofen 858, 867
fluticasone propionate 468
foal heat 254, 286, 987
foaling, see parturition
foaling dates, early 323
foals
atresia coli/recti/ani 979–80
bacterial meningitis 766–7
bronchopneumonia 458–60, 993–4
chylothorax 476–7
colostrum intake 967
coprophagia 1001–2
developmental orthopedic disease 50, 112, 162–4
diarrhea 545–6, 987–9
drug metabolism and doses 967, 968
duodenal ulcers 543
dysphagia 412
examination of neonate 966–7
failure of passive transfer 968–9
fractures 36, 37
femur 156–7
radius 126–7
ribs 477, 966, 967
sesamoid bone 107
tibia 146
ulna 129

gastroduodenal ulceration 537, 538, 981–2
hypothyroidism 620, 621–2, 624
ileocolonic aganglionosis (lethal white syndrome) 525
immunodeficiency disorders 968–84
inguinal rupture 557–8
inguinal/scrotal hernia 360–1, 558–9
iron supplementation/toxicity 610, 726
juvenile idiopathic epilepsy 802
lactose intolerance 548
liver disease 615, 617–18
meconium aspiration 976–7
meconium impaction 518, 980–1
musculoskeletal abnormalities 40–9, 55–7, 174, 284, 285
myotonia 239
neonatal isoerythrolysis 617, 972–4
neonatal septicemia 838–9, 970–2, 989
nutritional myodegeneration 237
ocular disorders 824–39
parasites
intestinal 549, 576, 987
lungworms 468–9
patellar luxation 148, 149
perinatal asphyxia syndrome 977–9
physiologic differences from mature horse 967
prematurity/dysmaturity 974–6
presentation difficulties 284
proliferative enteropathy 544–5
respiratory distress syndrome 799–800
routine care 967
septic arthritis/osteomyelitis 96, 990–2
sex determination in utero 262
skin diseases 936–8
thyroid hormones 623
Tyzzer's disease 615
umbilical hernia 984
umbilical infections 982–3
uroperitoneum 664–7, 985–6
Foley catheter, guttural pouch 446, 447
follicle, see ovarian follicle
follicle-stimulating hormone
mare 242, 243
stallion 326, 335, 357

folliculitis 905
pastern 933, 935
staphylococcal 898
foot
abscesses 64–5
bruising 67
conformation 13–15, 80–2, 90, 91
dressings and casts 64, 77, 78
examination 62
imaging 23, 25–6, 27–8, 63
tendon and ligament injuries 100–1, 206, 216
wounds 63–4
coronary band 15, 76, 950, 951
heel-bulb laceration 76–7, 950, 951
sole/frog puncture 87, 97–9
see also hoof
foot–pastern axis 14, 15, 80, 81, 82, 83, 90, 91
foot trimming
as cause of lameness 83–4
hoof cracks 75
limb deformities 43, 45, 54
forage, endophytic fungal toxicosis 786
'forage poisoning' 792
foramen ovale 692
foreign bodies
biliary tract 612–13
esophagus 514
eye 846
ingestion 527
intestinal 527–8, 585
nasal 409, 414
oral 503
pharyngeal/oropharyngeal 414–15
trachea 438
formalin
buffered neutral 591
injection 391, 406, 411, 507
thrush 67
fourth branchial arch defect syndrome 428–9
fractures
carpus 120–5
cranium/facial bones 171–2, 402–3, 776–7
dental 498, 500
distal sesamoid bone 93
femur 33, 150, 156–7, 783
foals 36, 37, 126–7, 129, 146, 156–7
humerus 33, 131–2
mandible/maxilla 166–8

metacarpal/metatarsal bones 114–15, 120
    splint bones 118–19
pelvis 160–1
phalanges
    distal (coffin bone) 84–5
    proximal 32, 34, 102–4
radius 33, **36**, 126–7
sesamoid bones (proximal) 106–7
spinal 177–9, **754**, 778–81
stifle joint/patella **22**, 148, 150–3
stress
    humerus 131, 132
    metacarpal/metatarsal III bones 116–17
    scapula 132, 133
    tibia 146, **147**
    vertebral laminae 178, 179, 183
tibia 33, 146–7, 150, 151, 153
treatment
    complications 37
    conservative 34–5
    first-aid 32–7, 115
    surgical fixation 35–7, 114, 168
ulna 127–9, *127*
free fatty acids 616, 634
friction rub 385
frog
    puncture wounds 97–9
    thrush infection 67
frog pads 71
frontal bones, fracture 168, 171–2
fumonsins 608–10
fundus
    curvilinear lesions 833
    examination 810, **811**
    mosaic (reticulated) pattern 863
    subalbinotic **811**, 830
fungal infections
    causing abortion 279
    causing ptyalism 507
    cornea *848*, 849, 850
    guttural pouches 445–8
    paranasal sinuses 401–2
    placentitis 272
    rhinitis 394–5
    skin 858, 878–9, 899–900, 907–8
    uterine 317
fungal toxins 608–10, **784**, 785–7
fungicides, mercury-containing 784
funiculitis 359, 379–80
furosemide
    cantharidin toxicosis 524
    cardiovascular disease *683*, 689, 706

exercise-induced pulmonary hemorrhage 479
renal dysfunction 647, 650, 669
furunculosis 905
Fusarium spp. 608–9, **849**
Fusarium moniliformis 786
Fusarium tricinctum 786
Fusiformis infection 933

G
gag (full-mouth speculum) 482, 488, **489**
gait
    kinetic analysis 30
    observation 16, **17**
gait abnormalities
    bone spavin 141
    common calcanean tendon injuries 222
    equine protozoal meningitis 768
    laminitis 63
    neurologic disorders 751, 752–3, *753*, 783
    stringhalt 797–8
    upward fixated patella 148
gamma aminobutyric acid 1001
gamma-glutamyltransferase
    serum 599, 603, 613
    urinary 641, 647
gammopathy
    monoclonal 739, 740
    polyclonal 740
gangrene, superficial (set-fast) 893–4
garlic 722
Gasterophilus spp. (bots) 504, 536–7
gastric decompression 521–2, 540, 547, 554
gastric distension 540, 546, 547
gastric emptying, increasing 542, 544
gastric impaction 540–1
gastric lavage 541
gastric protectants 511, 982
gastric reflux 546, 547
gastric ulceration 522, 717
    causing pyloric stenosis 541–2
    etiology 537
    foals 981–2
    grading 538, **539**
    management 538, *538*
gastrocnemius muscle, tendons 221–3
gastroduodenostomy 523
gastroesophageal reflux syndrome 510–11
gastrointestinal tract
    components 516, **517**
    diagnostic tests 518–20

foreign bodies 527–8, 585
impaction 579–80, 581, 583
neoplasia 534–5
physical examination 516–17
transit time 516, 517, 851
see also parts and disorders of tract
gastroscopy 535, 538, **539**
gelding
    masculine behavior 380
    see also castration
genetic testing 28, 226
geniohyoideus muscle 751
genital tubercle 262
gentamicin
    cerebral abscess 795
    equine purpura hemorrhagica 732
    eye disease 850
    foal *968*
    liver disease 603
    penile infections 367
    septic arthritis/synovitis *960*, 992
    toxicity 647
    uroperitoneum 666
    uterine infections *316*
gestation, length 280, 285, 974
gestational age 974
gingivitis 494–5, 498
glanders (farcy) 464–5, 906
glaucoma 871–2
    acquired 871
    congenital 836, 871
    management 872
    secondary 844, 871
globulins, serum 642, 739
glomerular function 640
glomerulonephritis, immune-mediated 651
glosso-epiglottic duct 411
glossopharyngeal nerve 747, 751
glottis, failure to close 422
glucose, blood *548*, 600, 603–4, 799, 971
glucose absorption test 520, *548*
glucose tolerance test 633
glucosuria 640
glutamate dehydrogenase 599, 603
glutamine 976, 979
glycopyrrolate *683*
glycosides, cardiac 701
goiter, foals 620, 624
goitrogens 621
Gökel's operation 658
Gomen disease 796–7
gonadal dysgenesis (63XO syndrome) 301

gonadotropin-releasing hormone
    mare 242, 243
        injection/implants 252, 253
    stallion 326
        exogenous *341*
        vaccine *341*
goniosynechiae 834
goserelin 252
grafts
    bone 107
    conjunctival 851–3
    skin 954–6
granula iridica 810
    hypoplasia 833
granulation tissue 944
    exuberant (proud flesh) 943, **945**, 952
    heel-bulb laceration 77
    trimming 952, 955
granuloma
    arytenoid cartilage 427
    cholesterol (cholesteatoma) 796, **797**
    eosinophilic 911
    Habronema 663, 664
    sperm 362
granulomatous enteritis 529
granulomatous pneumonia 473
granulosa (thecal) cell tumors 251, 302–3
    rupture 590, **591**
grass, bear 606, **607**
grass sickness (equine dysautonomia) 531–2
grazing
    natural behavior 999
    tooth wear 498–9
'greasy heels' 896, 897, 932–4
griseofulvin 900
grove poisoning 791
growth factors, use in tendon injuries 194
'grunt to a stick test' 422
guttural pouches 442–9
    chondroids 442, 454
    clinical examination 384
    cranial nerves 747
    distension 420, 421
    empyema 442–4, 455
    endoscopy 170, 386
    lavage 444
    mycosis 445–8
    tympany 444–5

H

H7N7 viruses 450
Haab's striae 871
habronemiasis 234, 770, 909–10
    gastric 536
    male genitalia 370
    management 370, 536, 910
    ocular signs 867
    periocular 909
    skin 909–10
    urethral granuloma 663, 664
Haemaphysalis longicornis 891
Haematobia spp. (buffalo flies) 882, 885
Haematopinus asini 887–8
haircoat
    equine Cushing's disease 629, 631, 923
    sampling 875
Halamid disinfectant 897
Halicephalobus spp. 770
halothane 227, 797
hamartoma, vagina 312
hard palate, swelling (lampus) 504
Havemeyer system 423–4, *423*
hay
    alfalfa 524, 667
    coastal Bermuda grass 554, 786
    containing poisonous plants 790, 791
    feeding in inflammatory airway disease *467*
hay dipping 1008–9
head
    posture and movement 746–7, 750
    radiography 486–8, *486*
    trauma 774–5, 776–7, 864–5
head nod, lameness 16
head shaking
    behavioral 1004–5
    photic 169, 170, 862–3
head tilt 746
    temporohyoid osteoarthropathy 448
    vestibular disease/trauma 747, 750, 772, **773**
head tremor 746–7, 777
heart, interventricular septum **690**
heart-bar shoe **75**
heart block
    first-degree 684, **685**
    second-degree 684, **685**
    third-degree 684
heart failure *683*, 692, 704–6

heart murmurs 672, 674, *675*
    aortic regurgitation 698
    characterization *675*
    left atrioventricular valve disease 695
    'machinery' 693
    right atrioventricular valve disease 697
    types and causes *676*
    ventricular septal defect 691
heart rate
    fetal 264
    in gastrointestinal disorders 546
    neonatal foal *966*
heart sounds 674, *674*
heart valves 674
    acquired disease 695–700
    congenital deformities 693–4
    location 674
    vegetative lesions 699
heaves (recurrent airway obstruction) 465–7
    drugs used *468*
heels
    contracted 80
    dermatophilosis 896–7
    'greasy' 896, 897, 932–4
    lacerations 76–7, 942, **951**
    low heel/long toe conformation 14, **15**, 80
    sheared 80, 82
    staphylococcal infection **933**
    underrun 80, 91
Heinz bodies 721–2
Heliotropium spp. 604, **605**
hemangioma 918
hemangiosarcoma 918
hematology, endocrine disease 620
hematomas
    broad ligament 287, 288
    ethmoidal 404–6
    impact trauma **940**, 964
    muscle tear 156
    ovary 304
    penis 349, 351–2
    small colon wall 585
    vagina/vulva 300
hematuria 523, 640
hemianopia 748
hemoabdomen 741–2
hemoconcentration 739
hemocytometer, sperm concentration determination 337
hemoglobin products, bovine-source polymerized 742

hemoglobinuria 640
hemomelasma ilei 577
hemoperitoneum **518**, 519, 590–1, **716**
hemorrhage
    after castration 378
    blood loss estimation 716
    chronic 717
    intra-abdominal 741–2
    pulmonary 478–80
    trauma/wounds 715–17, 942
    uterine artery rupture 287–8
    vaginal varicosity 309
hemorrhages, petechial 730
hemosiderin, alveolar macrophages 478, **479**
hemospermia 363
hemostasis 941
hemostat, urethral calculus removal **662**, 663
hemothorax 477, 715
Hendra virus 454
heparin 617, 635, 730
hepatic encephalopathy 602, 603, 798–9
    diagnosis 798
    management 604, 799
hepatic fibrosis, congenital 618
hepatitis
    chronic active 611–12
    suppurative 600–1
hepatoblastoma 614
hepatocellular carcinoma 614
hepatotoxins 604–10
hereditary multiple exostosis 48
hermaphroditism 321, 345
hernia
    abdominal 594–5
    diaphragmatic 592–4
    incisional 594, 595
    scrotal/inguinal 360–1, 558–9
    umbilical 984
heterochromia iridis 830–1
heterotopic polydontia (dentigerous cysts) 490–1
high blowing 390, 421
hip abduction test 18
'hip hike' 16
hip joint, injuries and disease 158–9
hip score, dynamic 37
histamine 2 blockers 538, 920, 982
histiocytoma, malignant fibrous 918
histoplasmosis 908
Hobday operation 436

hock
    capped (tuber calcis hygroma) 140
    conformation 141
    cuboidal bones
        defective ossification 42
        fracture **137**
    dropped 138, 222
    fractures 136–9
    intertarsal synovitis/osteoarthritis **23**, 141–4
    radiography 23
    sepsis **31**
        foal 990, **991**
        wounds **958**
    solitary osteochondroma **49**
    tarsocrural synovitis (bog spavin) 144–5
    thoroughpin 218–20
hoof, structure 62
hoof balance 14, **15**, 80–2, 90, 92, 101
hoof pain, palmar 14, **15**, 19
hoof testers 16, 62, 66
hoof wall
    avulsion 78–9
    cracks **15**, 74–6
    resection 72
hormonal testing
    mare 251
    stallion 334–5
Horner's syndrome 861–2
    causes *861*
horsetail poisoning 791
Hotz–Celsus procedure 827
hound's tongue 604, **605**
human chorionic gonadatropin 252, 253, 258
    stimulation test 334–5, 346, 357
humerus, fractures 33, 131–2
Hyalomma anatolicum 760
hyaluronic acid
    intra-articular 92, 96, 105, 134, 142, 807
    tendon injection 194
    tendon sheath injection 210
hydatidosis 614–15
hydralazine *684*, 706
hydration status, assessment 638
hydrocele 360
    after castration 380
hydrocephalus 267, 756–7
    hypertensive 756
    normotensive 756
hydrochloric acid 367
hydrogel dressings *949*

hydrogen peroxide, uterine flushing *316*
hydronephrosis 653
hydrops, amnion/allantois 267–8
hydrothorax 478
11β-hydroxysteroid dehydrogenase 632
hydroxyzine 882, 929
hygiene
    breeding 255, 273
    dystocia 283
hygroma
    carpus 124
    elbow 130
    tuber calcis (capped hock) 140
hymen, persistent 308–9
hyoid apparatus 505–6
hypalgesia 754, **754**, 755, 783
hyperammonemia 603, 604, 618, 798
hyperbaric oxygen therapy 479, *800*
hyperbilirubinemia 598, 617
hypercalcemia 534
hypercapnia 389
hyperelastosis cutis 936
hyperextension
    congenital 45
    fetlock joint 109, 110
hyperglobulinemia 739–40
hyperglycemia 600, 640
hypericin 917
Hypericum perforatum 932
hyperkalemia 646
hyperkalemic periodic paralysis 226
hyperlipemia/hyperlipidemia 616–17, 634, **634**–5
hypermetria 752, 758
hypernatremia 646, 800–1
hyperparathyroidism, nutritional secondary 163–4, 625–7
hyperphosphatemia 163
hyperproteinemia 739–40
hypersensitivity
    contact 923–4
    insect 881–3
    type 1 (atopy) 892–3
    type 4 924
hyperthyroidism 624
    induced in equine metabolic syndrome 634
hypertrophic osteopathy 165
hypoalbuminemia 529, 530, 545, 599, 602, 649
    cyathostominosis 572
hypocalcemia 163, 235, 627–8, 801
    conditions associated with *627*

Hypochoeris radicata 797
hypocretins 803
Hypoderma spp. 770, 883
hypodermiasis 883
hypoglossal nerve 747, 751, 772
hypoglycemia 600, 603–4, 799, 971
hypometria 752
hyponatremia 642, 800
hypoproteinemia 529, 530, 534, 545, 591, 599
hypopyon 856
hyporeflexia 755, 804
hypothalamus 621
hypothermia, and wound healing 943
hypothyroidism 620–4
    adults 621, 622, 624
    fetus 163
    foals 620, 621–2, 624
hypotonia 755
hypoxia 389
    nervous tissue 799–800
hypoxic–ischemic injury, perinatal 977–9
hysteroscopy 251

I

icterus 598
ileocolonic aganglionosis (lethal white syndrome) 525
ileum
    impaction 554
    muscular hypertrophy 553
    stricture 523
ileus 521–2
ilial wing fracture 160–1
imidocarb 724–5
imipenem, foal *968*
imipramine *341*, 343, 364, 803
immune-mediated diseases
    failure of passive transfer 968–9, 971
    glomerulonephritis 651
    hemolytic anemia 719–20
    polysynovitis 161–2
    skin 874, 923–30
    thrombocytopenia 591, 728–9
    uveitis 856
immunity, immunodeficiency disorders 968–74
immunofluorescence testing 876
immunoglobulin G, foal serum levels 969
immunohematology 713
immunostimulants 452
immunosuppressive drugs 720, 729

incisional hernia 594, 595
incontinence, urinary 659–60, 894
Indigofera spp. 791
infarction, intestinal 560, 577
inflammatory airway disease 471–2
inflammatory bowel disease 529–30
inflammatory response 941, 971
influenza, *see* equine influenza
infrared thermography 26, 177
inguinal hernia 360–1, 558–9
inguinal rings, internal 333
inguinal rupture 557–8
inhalation therapy 472
inhibin 357
injection, carotid artery 775
injection abscess **25**
insecticides, causing dermatitis/pruritus 877
insect repellents 883
insects, causing pruritus 881–92
insulin
    administration 226, 617, 635
    fasting serum 630
    overdose 799
insulin-like growth factor-1 194
insulin resistance 616, 632, 633, 634, 635, 636
intensive care, foal 286
interferon alpha 763
interleukin receptor antagonist protein 96
interlocking nails 35
internal carotid artery **443**, 445, 447, **747**
intersex conditions 321, 345
intestinal adhesions 533–4
intestinal impaction, ascarid infestation 550
intestinal motility, assessment 516
intestinal stricture 522–3
intestines, *see also* colon; small intestines
intra-articular medication, *see* joint injections
intracranial pressure, raised 171, 172, 775, 794–5, 979
intracytoplasmic sperm injection 340
intradermal skin testing 876, 892–3
intraocular pressure
    control 872
    decreased 856
    elevation 836, 871
    measurement 816, 872
    normal range 872

intraspinatus muscle, atrophy 132, **133**
intussusception 526–7
iodine 620, 621
    poisoning 901
    thyroid function 621
iodine tincture 67, 878
ionophore toxicosis 701
ipratropium bromide *468*
iridectomy 869
iridocyclitis, recurrent, *see* uveitis, equine recurrent
iris
    coloboma 828–9
    color variation 830–1
    hypoplasia 832
    prolapse 848, **849**, 868–9
    synechiae 856, **857**
iron
    deficiency anemia 726
    supplementation 610, 726
    toxicity 600, 610
ischemia
    nervous tissue 799–800
    small colon 586
ischium, fracture 160
isoerythrolysis, neonatal 617, 972–4
isoflupredone acetate *468*
isothenuria *639*, 646, 649, 667
isoxsuprine 92
itraconazole 850
ivermectin
    ascarids 549
    cyathostominosis 572, *572*, 573
    gastric parasites 537
    habronemiasis 536, 867, 910
    large strongyles 577
    lice treatment 888
    lungworm 469
    mange 890
    onchocerciasis 858, 881
    tapeworm 564
Ixodes spp. ticks 162, 730, 767, 789, 892

J

jasmine, flowering 648
jaw closure, asymmetric 749
jejunitis 546–7
jejunocecal anastomosis 552
jejunojejunostomy 523
jimsonweed 791
joint effusion
    carpus 121
    stifle 150, **151**
    tarsocrural joint 144–5

joint infections
    distal interphalangeal joint 96–7
    foals 990–2
    open drainage 992
joint injections
    cervical spine 807
    elbow 130
    interphalangeal joints 92, 96, 105
    scapulohumeral joint 134
    subchondral bone cysts 58
    tarsal joints 142
joint lavage 96–7, 959, **961**, 992
joint markers 28
joints
    'high-motion' 38
    'low-motion' 38
    nerve blocks 20, **21**
    ultrasonography 24, **25**
    wounds involving 958–61
    see also named joints
joint space loss 38, **39**, **95**
jugular veins
    assessment 673
    thrombophlebitis 708
junctional epidermolysis bullosa 937

K

karyotype, normal mare 301
karyotyping
    mare 251
    stallion 340
keratectomy
    lamellar 851
    superficial 858
    therapeutic penetrating 855
keratitis
    fungal *848*, 849, 850
    ulcerative 848–53
keratoconjunctivitis sicca 847
keratoma 79
keratomalacia 850
keratopathy, band 858, 860
keratoplasty, posterior lamellar 855
keratosis, equine linear 926
kernicterus 617
ketanserin *949*
ketoconazole 317, 395, 908
ketoprofen *521*, 661
Kevlar 75–6
kicking, stable doors/walls 1003
kick injuries
    fractures 118, **133**
    hematoma 964
    joints 136–7, **958**

kidneys
    biopsy 644, 650
    changes in chronic renal failure 648–9
    congenital disorders 651
    enlargement **645**, 646
    imaging 643
    neoplasia 653
kinetic analysis 30
'kissing lesion' 427
kissing spines 180–1
Klebsiella spp. 249, 272, 279, 315, 460, 652, 766, 794
Klebsiella pneumoniae 255, 317, 365, 369
knapweed, Russian 790
knee, *see* carpus
'kunkers' 878, 879, 909
kyphosis 174, **175**

L

lactase 548
lactate 971
lactate dehydrogenase 28, 599, 680
lactation
    hypocalcemia 235
    nonpregnant mare 629, 1000, *1000*
lactational anestrus 323–4
lactose intolerance 548
lactulose 604, 635, 799
lag screw fixation **36**, 37, 114, 122
lameness
    clinical examination 13–18
    diagnostic analgesia 19–20, *20*, **21**, 86, 91–2
    and foot balance 80–2, 90, 92, 101
    gait analysis 30
    grading 16
    history 12–13
    imaging 22–8
    laboratory tests 28–9
    management/therapies 30–2
    muscle injuries 238
    shoeing/trimming as cause 83–4
laminitis 69–72
    acute 63, 70, 71
    chronic 70, 72
    clinical presentation 69–70
    diagnosis 70
    equine Cushing's disease 630, 631
    etiology/pathophysiology 69
    gastrointestinal disease 546
    management 70–2

    post foaling 295–6
        fetal membrane retention 294
    septic osteitis 87
lampus 504
lantana 606, **607**
laparoscopic surgery
    bladder repair 666, **667**
    cystolith removal 658
    retained testicle removal 347
laparotomy
    flank 266
    ovarian tumor removal 303
    uterine rupture 289
laryngeal neuropathy, *see* recurrent laryngeal neuropathy
laryngoplasty (tie-back procedure) 425–6
laryngotomy, scar 422, **422**
larynx
    clinical examination 384
    embryology 428
    endoscopy 386, 422–3, 429, 432, 433
    fourth branchial arch defect syndrome 428–9
    innervation 751
    palpation 422, **428**, 429
    paralysis 447, 602
    re-innervation 425–6
    sound 421, 751
    swallowing **423**, 508
lasalocid 701
laser therapy
    endometrial cysts 319
    glaucoma 872
    lameness 31
    periocular squamous cell carcinoma 843
    subepiglottic cyst 413
    uveal cysts 831
lateral cartilages, *see* ungual cartilages
lateral digital extensor tendon, injuries 207–10
lateral digital flexor tendon, injury 218, 219
Lawsonia intracellularis infection 544–5, 987
laxative diet 298
laxatives 522
lead acetate solution 897
lead toxicity 733, 788
legumes, feeding 650
leiomyoma 312–13
leiomyosarcoma 918

lens
  foldable intraocular 870
  opacity, see cataracts
  subluxation 834
leopard complex locus 837
Leptospira spp. 652, 856
Leptospira interrogens 858
Leptospira pomona 272, 279, 617, 856, 858
lethal white syndrome 525
Leucaena spp. 901
leukemias 735
  lymphocytic 736, **737**
leukocytes 711–12
  wound healing 941
leukocytoclastic vasculitis, pastern 934–5
leukoderma 930
leukoencephalomalacia 608, 786–7
leukotrichia 930–1
Leydig cells 326, 372
libido, stallion 332, 335, 340–1
lice 887–8, 938
  collection 875
licking behavior 1006, **1007**
lidocaine
  cardiovascular disease *683*, 689
  epidural anesthesia 283
  use in colic/ileus 520, *521, 522*
ligament injuries
  check ligaments 123, 204–5
  distal interphalangeal joint 27–8, 100–1
  palmar/plantar annular ligaments 214–16
  plantar ligaments 224–5
  stifle joint 150–3
  suspensory ligament 196–203
  thoracolumbar spine 176–7
lighting, estrous cycle manipulation 252, 323
lightning strike 774
limb deformities
  acquired 52–7
  congenital 40–5, 55–7
limestone 628
lime sulfur 891, 899
linear keratosis 926
lipemia 616
lipidosis, hepatic (fatty liver syndrome) 616–17
lipoma 919
  abdominal, strangulation 550–1
lipoprotein lipase 634, 635
Listeria monocytogenes 766
listeriosis 766

lithotripsy 655
liver
  biopsy 602, 603
  imaging 600–1
  palpation 598
liver disease
  abscesses 613
  cirrhosis 600
  clinical signs 598
  clinicopathologic abnormalities 598–9
  fatty syndrome 616–17, 634
  foals 615, 617–18
  neoplasia 614
  oral photosensitization 504–5
  parasites 601, 614–15
  prognosis 602
  toxic causes 604–8
liver enzymes 599
  cholelithiasis 612
  liver failure 603
  plant toxicoses 606
liver failure 602–4, 798–9
  clinical presentation 602, 798
  diagnosis 603
  differential diagnosis 603
  encephalopathy 602, 798–9
  etiology/pathophysiology 602
  management 603–4
  treatment 799
liver flukes 601, 615
liver function tests 599
'Llewellyn' procedure 417
loading problems 996
locking compression plates 115
'lockjaw' 771
locoweed intoxication 759, 790
longissimus dorsi muscle, spasm 238
long plantar ligament 224
  injuries 224, 225
loperamide 989
lordosis 174, **175**
lumbar spine
  trauma 779
  see also thoracolumbar spine
lumbrosacral spinal tap 755
lungs
  abscesses 458, **459**, 993–4
  auscultation 384–5, 462
  biopsy 389
  neoplasia 480
  percussion 385, 462
lungworms 468–9
lupus erythematosus, cutaneous 925–6

luteinizing hormone
  mare 242–3
  stallion 326
luxation
  carpus 124, 125
  elbow 130
  patella 148, 149
  superficial digital flexor tendon 220
  shoulder joint 134, 135
  temporomandibular joint 169
  see also subluxation
Lyme disease (borreliosis) 29, 162, 767–8
lymphadenitis 738
lymphadenopathy
  anorectal 590
  equine influenza 450
  lymphoma 736
  sinusitis 396
lymphangioma 919
lymphangitis
  C. pseudotuberculosis abscess 234
  epizootic (histoplasmosis) 908
  ulcerative 907
lymphedema 912
lymph nodes
  parotid 384
  'reactive' 738
  retropharangeal 384
  strangles abscess 454, **455**
  submandibular 384, 396
lymphocytes 712
lymphocytic hyperplasia 738
lymphoid hyperplasia, pharyngeal 413–14
lymphoma 736, 743, 801
lymphosarcoma 534, 919
  eye/adnexa 844–5

M

McConkey medium 249
magnesium, supplementation 668
magnesium sulfate
  cardiovascular disease 682, *683*, 689
  hypoxic–ischemic encephalopathy *800*
  laxative/cathartic 522, 580
magnetic resonance imaging
  eye 820
  musculoskeletal system 26–8, 63, 92, 188
magnetic therapy 31
malabsorption 529
Malassezia spp. dermatitis 878

malathion 883, 890
Maldison wash 883, 890, 891
male reproductive tract
    congenital abnormalities 345–7
    examination 330–5
    neoplasia 370–3
maleruption 493
mallein test 465
malocclusions 493
'mal seco', *see* grass sickness
mammary glands, mastitis 325
mammary secretions
    electrolytes 264–5
    see also colostrum
management practices
    behavioral problems 996, 999
    heaves/inflammatory airway
        disease 466, *467*
mandible, fractures 166–8
mandibular nerve 749
mange
    chorioptic 888–9
    psoroptic 890
    sarcoptic 890
manica flexoria 212, 213
mannitol
    adverse effects 669
    hypoxic–ischemic encephalopathy
        800
    raised intracranial pressure 172,
        775, 794, 979
    renal disease 647, 650, 669
    wobbler syndrome 807
mare, *see* broodmare
masculinization 302
massage 31
mast cell tumors 920
mastication 485
    tooth wear 498–9
masticatory muscles, atrophy 169,
    749, 768
mastitis 325
mastocytoma 920, **921**
masturbation 1007
maxilla, fracture 166–8
maze tests 816
mean cell volume 716
mean corpuscular hemoglobin
    concentration 716
Meckel's diverticulum 554–5
meconium aspiration 976–7
meconium impaction 518, 980–1
medial canthus, habronemiasis 909
medial palmar intercarpal ligament
    124–5

median nerve injury 783
medullary crest necrosis 647
megaesophagus 510
melanocytes 930
melanocytoma 920–1
melanoma 920–1
    causes 843
    central nervous system invasion
        801
    eyes/eyelid/adnexa 843–4
    lymph node metastasis 737
    management 920–1
    parotid gland 507, **921**
    penis/prepuce 372
    perineum 285, 312–13
α-melanophore-stimulating hormone
    629, 630, 631
melatonin 242, 863
Melilotus spp. 718, 719
melioidosis 464–5
meloxicam, use in colic *521*
menace response
    assessment 812, **813**
    decreased/absent 748, 758
    foal 812, 824
meningitis, bacterial 766–7
meningoencephalomyelitis
    bacterial 766–7
    verminous 770
meniscal injuries 150, 152
mental status, assessment 746
mepivacaine 19, 92
    epidural 283
mercury toxicity 784
mesenteric artery, cranial 516
mesenteric portography 602
mesh-expansion technique 946
mesodiverticular band 555–6
mesometrium, hematoma 287, 288
mesotherapy 177
metabolic syndrome, equine 632–4
metacarpal/metatarsal bones
    second/fourth
        exostosis ('splints') 120
        fractures 118–19
    third
        fractures 114–15
        physitis 61
        stress fractures 116–17
metacarpophalangeal joint, *see* fetlock
metaldehyde toxicosis 787
metalloproteinases 38, 69
methazolamide 872
methemoglobinemia 721–2

methylprednisolone
    eosinophilic granuloma 911
    intra-articular 105
    recurrent uveitis 859–60
metoclopramide 510, *522*, 542, 544
metritis, contagious equine 248
metritis–laminitis–septicemia complex
    295–6
metronidazole
    chronic diarrhea 574
    clostridial myonecrosis 233
    foal dosages *968*
    gastrointestinal infections 547, 568,
        574, 989
    liver failure 604
    topical 68
    white line disease 74
miconazole 395, 850, 899
microfilariae 866
microphthalmos 825
Microsporum spp. 900, 938
midazolam 978
midbrain syndrome 776
middle ear disorders 170, 750, 772–3,
    776
midges 881
Mimosa pudica 901
mineral oil
    gastrointestinal disorders 575, 541,
        522, 528, n 580
    liver failure 604
    toxicities 524, 668, 701, 785
misoprostol 538
Missouri artificial vagina 336
mites 888–91
    collection 875
    Demodex spp. 875, 909
    Psoroptes 875, 890
    red poultry 889
    Sarcoptes 890
    trombiculid 891
mitochondrial myopathy 229
mitral valve, dysplasia 693
molecular biology 28, 226
molluscum contagiosum 903
monensin 701, 785
monoclonal gammopathy 739, 740
monocytes 712, 941
monoiodoacetic acid 143
moonblindness (equine recurrent
    uveitis) 858–60
Morgan horses 618, 798, 832, 834,
    835
morphine 520, 961
mosquitoes 760, 761, 762, 886

motor neuron disease 863–4
mouth, *see* oral cavity
moxidectin 469, 549
    ascarids 549
    cyathostominosis 572, *572*
    gastric parasites 537
    habronemiasis 867
    large strongyles 577
    lungworm 469
    Onchocerca infection 881
mucocele, salivary 507
Mucor spp. 315
mucous membranes
    examination 673
    icterus 598
    petechial hemorrhages 730
müllerian ducts 345
multiple myeloma 739
multisystemic eosinophilic
    epitheliotropic disease 529–30
mummification, fetus 274
murmurs, *see* heart murmurs
muscle biopsy 29
muscle disorders 226–40
    abscess 232–4
    atypical myopathy 240
    clostridial myonecrosis 232–3
    Corynebacterium abscesses 234
    fibrotic and ossifying myopathy
        230–1
    hypocalcemia 235
    hyperkalemic periodic paralysis
        226
    myotonia 239
    myotonic dystrophy 239
    nutritional degeneration 163, 237
    postanesthetic myoneuropathy
        227–8, 797
    rhabdomyolysis 229–30
muscle enzymes 28, 163, 229
muscle ('faradic') stimulation 31
muscle fasciculations/cramps 235,
    236
muscle injuries 238
muscle tone, assessment 753, 754
musculocutaneous nerve 783
mustard 621
muzzle, deviation 773, 777
mycetoma 907–8, 934
mycosis
    guttural pouch 445–8
    skin/subcutaneous 907, 908
mycotoxicosis 608–10, **784**, 785–7
mydriatics 817, 860
myelodysplasias 781

myeloencephalitis, equine protozoal
    749, 768–9, 803
myeloencephalopathy, equine
    degenerative 803–4
myelography 756, 807
myeloproliferative disorders 735
myiasis (hypodermiasis) 887
myocarditis
    primary 700
    toxic 701
myodegeneration, nutritional 163, 237
myoglobinuria 237, 640, 646
    atypical 240
myoglobulinemia 648
myonecrosis, clostridial 232–3
myoneuropathy, postanesthesia
    227–8, 797
myopathy
    atypical 240
    equine polysaccharide storage 229,
        798
    fibrotic and ossifying 230–1
    mitochondrial 229
myorelaxants 228, 230
myotenectomy 231
myotonia 239
myotonic dystrophy 239

N

nail bind 83
nail prick 83
naloxone 591, 1001
    foal *968*
narcolepsy 803
nares, examination 383
nasal bleeding 718, **719**
nasal bones, fracture 168, 171
nasal discharge 383
    choanal atresia/stenosis 393
    fungal rhinitis 394–5
    guttural pouch infection 442
    nasal/sinus tumors 406
    sinusitis 396, 401
    strangles 454, **455**
nasal diverticulum, *see* false nostril
nasal passages 392–5
    amyloidosis 404
    foreign bodies 409, 414
    iatrogenic trauma 409
    neoplasia 399, 406–7
    wry nose deformity 46, **47**, 392,
        494
nasal septum, deformity 392
nasal strips 479
nasofrontal suture, periosteitis 173

nasogastric intubation 518
    colon impaction 580
    duodenitis/proximal jejunitis 547
    esophageal rupture 515
    force feeding 635
    gastric dilation 540
    gastric impaction 541
    ileus 521–2
    strangulating lipoma 550, 551
nasogastric reflux 551
nasolacrimal system
    atresia 829–30
    flushing 819, 823, 868
    obstruction 868
    patency assessment 816, 819
nasopharyngeal cicatrix 410
nasopharynx, collapse 420
nasotracheal catheter 388
natamycin 395, 850
navicular bone, *see* distal sesamoid
    bone
navicular bursa 90
    corticosteroid injection 92
    regional analgesia 20, **21**, 86, 92
    sepsis 97–9
navicular syndrome 14, **15**, 90–2
necrosis
    colon 586
    medullar crest 647
    muscle 232–3
    ungual cartilages 89–90
    wounds 940, **941**, 943
nedocromil sodium *468*
Negri bodies 764
neomycin
    liver failure 604
    uterine infections *316*
neomycin–polymixin–bacitracin 850
neonatal isoerythrolysis 617, 972–4
neoplasia
    adrenal gland 636
    bladder 656–7
    esophagus 515
    eye/orbit/adnexa 839–46
    female reproductive tract 302–4,
        312–13
    gastrointestinal 534–5
    hoof keratoma 79
    liver 614
    lower respiratory tract 480
    lymphatic tissue 736–7
    male reproductive tract 370–3
    myeloproliferative disorders 735
    nasal/sinuses 399, 400, 406–7
    nervous tissues 801
    oral cavity 501–2

1041

ovary 302–4
pericardial 703–4
renal 653
salivary glands 507
skin 892, 913–23
spleen 743
thyroid gland 621
Neorickettsia risticii (Potomac horse fever) 564, 565, 598
Neospora hughesi 768
neostigmine *522*, 791, 793
nephritis, interstitial 651
nephroliths 651
nephrotoxins 645, 647, 648
nerve blocks, *see* analgesia, regional/diagnostic
nervous tissue
    hypoxia/ischemia 799–800
    neoplasia 801
neurectomy
    bilateral infraorbital 863
    bone spavin 143
    palmar digital nerve 92, 93
neurofibroma 801, 921
neurofibrosarcoma 801
neurologic disease
    bladder dysfunction 659
    congenital and developmental 756–60, 781
    eye 861–6
    infections 760–73
    peripheral nerves 781–4
    toxin-associated 784–93
neurologic examination 746–55
    cranial nerves 747–51
    diagnostic tests 755–6
    gait and posture 751–3
    head posture and coordination 746–7
    mental status 746
    neck and forelimbs 753
    recumbent animal 753–4
    tail/anus 755
    trunk/hindlimbs 754
neuromuscular pedicle graft 425–6
neutrophils 712, 941
nictitans
    dermoid 829
    squamous cell carcinoma **842**
nightshade
    black 791
    deadly 791
nigropallidal encephalomalacia 790–1
nitazoxanide 769
nitrofurazone ointment 366

nitroglycerin 706
nitroprusside 706
Nocardia spp. 272, 907
noise making 1003
Nolina texana 606, **607**
nonsteroidal anti-inflammatory drugs
    adverse effects 537, 570, 647–8
    alternative drugs 648
    broodmare 265
    castration 375
    corneal abscess 854
    corneal ulceration 851
    ehrlichiosis 731
    exertional rhabdomyolysis 230
    eye disorders 836, 851
    facial nerve trauma 777
    foals
        respiratory infections 994
        septic arthritis 992
    laminitis 71
    navicular syndrome 92
    osteoarthritis 96
    synovial infections 961
    tendon injuries 194
    topical 777, 858
    use in renal disease 647–8, 669
    uveitis 858, 860
    see also named agents
nostrils 390–1, 910, **911**
nuclear imaging 25–6
nutrition
    broodmare 237
    epiphysitis 60, 61
    fatty liver syndrome 617
    foal diarrhea 989
    liver failure 603–4
    neonatal septicemia 972
    parenteral 542, 635
    perinatal asphyxia syndrome 979
    premature/dysmature foal 976
    see also diet
nutritional deficiencies 162–4
    copper 50
    diagnosis 163
    iron 726
    selenium 621, 700
    vitamin E 700, 803, 863, 912
nutritional hyperparathyroidism 163–4, 625, *625*
nutritional myodegeneration 237
nymphomania 302
nystagmus 749, 750
nystatin *316*, 447
nystatin powder 395

O

obesity 632
obstacle course 816
obturator nerve paralysis 784
occipital artery **447**
occipital bone, fracture 776
occipitoatlantoaxial malformation 758–9
oculomotor nerve 748–9
odontoblasts 486
odontomas 501–2
oils, dietary 571
olecranon, fracture 37
olfactory nerve 747
oligodontia 490
oligospermia 362–3
oliguria *639*, 646, 647, 650
omeprazole 538, 982
Onchocerca cervicalis infection
    ocular 856, 858, 866–7
    skin 356, 880–1
    treatment 858, 881
oncotic therapy 545
onions, ingestion 722
oocyte transfer 258
ophthalmoscopy 817–18
    direct 810, **811**, 817
    indirect 818
opiate blockers 1001
opiates 228, 230, 233, 375, 961
oppossum, Virginia 768
optic chiasm 748
optic disk 810
optic nerve 747–8
    hypoplasia 838
    trauma 776, 864–5
optic nerve head 810, 817
    edema 864
    exudates 865
optic neuritis 865, *865*
optic neuropathy
    benign exudative/proliferative 866
    traumatic 864–5
oral cavity
    examination 482–3, 488–9, 516
    neoplasia 501–2
    photosensitization of tissues 504–5
    wounds and foreign bodies 503
orbit, neoplasia 845–6
orchitis 356–7
orexins 803
organophosphates
    fly repellents 883
    poisoning 785
oro-antral fistula 400, **401**

oropharynx, foreign bodies 414–15
orthomyxoviruses, type A 450
osmotic agents
    colon impaction 580
    see also mannitol
osseous cyst-like lesions 58, **59**
    carpus 124, 125
    elbow 130
    fetlock joint/distal MC/MT III 110, 112
    phalanges 104, 105
    scapulohumeral joint 134, 135
ossifying myopathy 230–1
osteoarthritis, carpal bones 124–5
osteoarthritis 38–9, 94–6
    distal interphalangeal joint 84, 85, 94–6
    elbow 130–1
    fetlock 38, **39**, 110–13
    following distal phalanx fracture 84, 85
    hip 158–9
    intertarsal joints **23**, 141–4, 238
    joint markers 28
    pathogenesis 38
    proximal interphalangeal joint 94–6, 104–5
    stifle 154
    temporomandibular joint 169
    thoracolumbar spine 182–3
osteoarthropathy, temporohyoid 448–9
osteochondral fragments ('joint mice') 50, 110, *111*, 153
osteochondritis dissecans 50, **51**, 134
osteochondroma 129
    solitary 48, **49**
osteochondrosis 50–1
    cervical spine 806, **807**
    etiology 50
    fetlock joint 110–13
    foals 112
    interphalangeal joints 104, 105
    scapulohumeral joint 134–5
    stifle joint 50, **51**, 150, 151, 153–4
    tarsocrural joint 144, 145
osteomyelitis
    foals 990–2
    following fracture treatment 37
    vertebral 795
osteopathy, hypertrophic 165
osteophytes 38, **39**, 94, **95**, 110, **125**
otitis media/interna 772–3
Otobius megnini 892

ovarian follicle
    anovulatory 324–5
    assessment 245–6, 257
ovaries
    hematoma 304
    neoplasia 302–4
    palpation 242, 244
    ultrasonography 244, 249, 302, 303, 324
Overo lethal white syndrome 525
overreaching injuries 962
oviduct disease 305
ovulation 242, 243
    diestral 324
    foal heat 286
    induction 253
    prediction 243–5
    synchronization 253
Ovuplant™ 252, 253
oxalate intake 163, 625
oxidant compounds 722
oxidative injury 863
oxyfendazole *572*
oxygen demand, nervous tissue 799
oxygen therapy 479, *800*, 978, 994
oxytetracycline 545, 568, 731, 768, 770
    congenital limb deformities 43, 44
    foal *968*, 994
    uterine infections *316*
oxytocin 256, 268, 282
    endometritis management 314
    esophageal obstruction 512
    fetal membrane release 293
    parturition induction 282
    post partum 283
    uterine involution 290, 300
Oxytropis spp. 790
Oxyuris equi 875, 881

P

pacemaker implantation 687
packed cell volume 734, 973
palatine artery 448
palatopharyngeal arch, rostral displacement 428–9
palatopharyngoplasty 418
palatoplasty, thermal 418
palatoschiasis (cleft palate) 502
palmar digital artery, laceration 942
palmar digital nerve
    analgesia 19, 88, 92, 94
    neurectomy 92, 93
palmar/plantar annular ligament syndrome 214–16

palpebral responses 812, **813**
pampiniform plexus 328
Panicum virgatum 606
panniculitis 912
papillomatosis 903–4
    female reproductive tract 312, 313
    neonate 937
    penis/prepuce 372
papular dermatosis, unilateral 912
parafimbrial cysts 305
paralysis
    botulism 792, **793**
    peripheral nerve injuries 782–3
    post-foaling 784
paraphimosis 343, 349–50
    hydrotherapy 350
    spinal trauma **779**, 780
Parascaris equorum 469, 549–50, 614
parasites
    causing dermatitis/pruritus 880–1
    causing meningoencephalomyelitis 770
    eye/periocular 856, 858, 866–7, 909
    gastric 536–7
    intestinal
        ascarids 549–50
        causing colic 524, 526, 531
        causing infarction 560, 577
        cyathostomes (small strongyles) 526, 560, 571–3
        foals 549, 576, 987
        large strongyles 577, 615
        liver migration 614, **615**
        pasture management 550, 573, 577
        tapeworm 524, 526, 563–4
    liver flukes 615
    respiratory tract 468–9
    skin
        examination 875
        Habronema spp. 370, 909–10
        lice 887–8, 938
        mites 888–91, 909
        ticks 891–2
parathyroid hormone 163, 625
Parelaphastrongylus tenuis 770
parenteral nutrition 542, 635
parotid gland
    duct trauma 506
    neoplasia 507, **921**
paroxetine 1000
parrot mouth (brachygnathia) 493–4
partial thromboplastin time 599, 603, 713, 718–19

parturition
  complications
    bladder eversion/prolapse 291
    cervical injuries 294–5
    delayed uterine involution 300
    dystocia 283–6
    gastrointestinal 275–6, 586–8
    metritis–laminitis–septicemia
      complex 295–6
    obturator nerve paralysis 784
    perineal injuries 296–9
    premature placental separation
      291–2
    retained fetal membranes 292–4
    uterine artery rupture 287–8
    uterine rupture 288–9
    vaginal lacerations 310
  endocrinology 280
  induction 268, 282
  normal 280–2
  physical signs 280
  umbilicus management 281, 967,
    983
paspalum staggers 786
passive transfer of immunity 987
pastern
  deep digital flexor tendon injuries
    217
  dermatitis 935
  folliculitis 933, 935
  see also foot–pastern axis;
phalanges, proximal
pasture factors
  atypical myopathy/myoglobinuria
    240
  nutritional myodegeneration 237
Pasturella spp. 460, 794
pasture management
  intestinal parasite control 550, 573,
    577
  Rhodococcus equi infections 460
patella 148–50
  fracture 22, 148
  lateral luxation 48, 49, 148, 149
  upward fixation 148–50, 158
patellar ligament, medial, desmotomy
  148, 149–50
patellar reflex 754, 783
patent ductus arteriosus 693
pawing 1009
pectoral muscles, injuries 238
pectoral nerve 782
pedal bone, see distal phalanx
pedal osteitis 86
pediculosis (lice) 887–8, 938
Pelodera strongyloides 880, 938

pelvic flexure
  enterotomy 580, 585
  examination 516, 517
  stricture 523
'pelvic hike' 16
pelvis
  asymmetry 158, 160, 161
  fracture 33, 160–1, 783
pemphigoid, bullous 927
pemphigus foliaceus 926, 927
pemphigus vulgaris 927
penicillins
  duodenitis/proximal jejunitis 547
  foal dosages 968
  liver disease 603
  urinary tract disease 666, 668
  uterine infections 265, 316
penis
  amputation 370, 371
  anatomy 328–9
  bacterial colonization 367–8
  balanitis/balanoposthitis 369–70
  cleaning/disinfection 255, 352,
    367, 369
  deviations 353
  examination 332
  habronemiasis 370
  neoplasia 333, 370–2, 922
  paralysis 350
  paraphimosis 349–50, 779, 780
  phimosis 348
  priapism 351
  smegma accumulation 352, 353,
    370
  suspensory ligament rupture 353
  trauma 349, 351–2, 380, 660–1
Penrose drain 140, 948
pentobarbital 774
percussion
  cardiac 673
  gastrointestinal tract 516
  lung fields 385, 462
  paranasal sinuses 396
performance-altering drugs 342
performance records 672
pergolide 631
pericardiocentesis 702, 703
pericarditis 702
pericardium, neoplasia 703–4
perineal body transection (Pouret's
  operation) 307, 308
perineal reflex 755
perineum
  lacerations/bruising 296–300
  neoplasia 312–13

periodic ophthalmia, see equine
  recurrent uveitis
periodontal ligament complex 484
periodontal pocket 495
periodontitis 494–5
periosteal new bone 117, 165
periosteal stripping 54
periosteitis, nasofrontal suture 173
peripheral nerve disorders 781–4
peripheral vestibular disease 746,
  747, 750
peritoneal fluid 276, 518, 519–20
  bacterial culture 596
  cecal rupture 560
  granulocytic ehrlichiosis 731
  septic peritonitis 596
  uroperitoneum 665–6, 986
peritoneal wall 517
peritonitis
  after castration 379
  cecal rupture 276, 560
  post foaling 276
  septic 595–6
permethrin 883, 888
peroneal nerve injury 783
peroneus tertius muscle, contracture
  45
peroneus tertius tendon, rupture 221
petechiae 730
pethidine, reaction 924
petrosal bone, fracture 776
Peyer's patches 534
phacoemulsification 835–6, 870
phaeohypomycosis 908
phalanges, proximal
  fractures 32, 34, 102–4
    osseous cyst-like lesions 104, 105
    osteochondral fragments 110, 111
    unilateral hypoplasia 48, 49
  see also distal phalanx (pedal/coffin
    bone); proximal interphalangeal
    joint
phantom mount 335, 336, 351
pharyngeal collapse 420–1
pharyngeal lymphoid hyperplasia
  413–14
pharynx
  cysts 410–11
  innervation 751
phenobarbital
  cerebral trauma 774
  foal 968, 978
  hypoxic–ischemic encephalopathy
    800
  juvenile epilepsy 802

phenobarbitone, *see* phenobarbital
phenol 722
phenothiazines *342*, 350, 722
phenoxybenzamine 660, 670
phenylbutazone
    adverse effects 647–8
    corneal ulceration 851
    exertional rhabdomyolysis 230
    laminitis 71
    navicular syndrome 92
    otitis media/interna 773
    stallion sexual function *341*
    synovial infections 961
    use in colic *521*
    uveitis 858, 860
phenylephrine 579, 858
phenylpropanolamine 364
phenytoin 798, *968*, 978
pheochromocytoma 590, 636
phimosis 348
phlebotomy 734
phosphorus:calcium balance 163, 625
phosphorus
    dietary 162–3
    fractional excretion 626, *642*
photocautery, soft palate 418
photodynamic therapy 917
photoperiod 242, 252
photosensitivity
    dermatophilosis 896, 897
    oral 504–5
    plant toxicities 606, 608, 932
phrenic nerve, hyperexcitability 236, 801
phthisis bulbi 825, 856, 857, 859
phylloerythrin 505
physiotherapy 31, 177, 194, 238
physitis 60–1, 163, 625
physostigmine 791, 803
pica 1003–4
pigmentation disorders 930–2
pigment nephropathy 648
pigmenturia 640
pinch grafts 955–6
pineal gland 326
pinna, dentigerous cyst 490–1, 910
pin worm 875, 881
piroplasmosis (babesiosis) 724–5
pituitary gland dysfunction 622, 629–32
placenta
    expulsion 282
    premature separation 291–2
    retention 292–4
    villous atrophy 279

placentitis 265, 272–3, 279, 291
    causative organisms 272
    fetal death 274
plantar ligaments, injuries 224–5
plant toxicosis 604–8, 645, 790–2
    bracken 791
    causing alopecia 901–2
    grove poisoning 791
    hepatotoxins 604–10
    locoweed 790
    nephrotoxins 648
    nigropallidal encephalomalacia 790–1
    photosensitization 606, 608, 932
        oral 504–5
    pyrrolizidine alkaloids 604–6, 618
    red maple leaves 721–2
    saponins 606, **607**
    selenium poisoning 902
    Solanaceae 791
    stringhalt 797
    umbellifers 792
plaque reduction neutralization test 763
plasma transfusion 969
plasma volume, loss 739–40
platelets 711
    destruction in immune-mediated thrombocytopenia 729, 730
pleural cavity
    air (pneumothorax) 475–6
    blood (hemothorax) 477, 715
    chyle 476–7
    fibrin 461
    fluid/effusion 461, 462, 463, 464, 478
        drainage 388, 462–3, 464
pleuritis/pleuropneumonia, bacterial 461–3
pneumoconiosis, silicate 473
Pneumocystis jiroveci 464
pneumonia
    aspiration 470–1
    bacterial 458–61, 993–4
    foal 993–4
    granulomatous 473
    Pneumocystis jiroveci 464
pneumothorax 475–6
pneumovagina 306–7
podotrochlear bursitis 216
poll, trauma 776, 777
pollakiuria 523, *639*
polo injuries 102, 104
polycythemia 734–5

polydactyly 46, **47**
polydipsia 636, 643, 648
    psychogenic 1009–10
polyetrafluoroethylene (Teflon) paste 433
polymerase chain reaction 452, 615
polymixin B 568
polymorphonuclear cells, semen 365
polymyxin B 547
polyneuritis equi 795–6
polyps
    female reproductive tract 312, 313
    nasal 407
polysaccharide storage myopathy 229, 798
polysulfated glycosaminoglycans 58, 194
polysynovitis, immune-mediated 161–2
polyuria/polydipsia 636, 643, 648
ponazuril 769
portosystemic shunts 602, 618, 798
postanesthetic myoneuropathy 227–8, 797
posterior chamber, paracentesis 819–20
posterior lamellar keratoplasty 855
posterior synechiae 870, 871
potassium
    fractional excretion *642*
    mammary secretions 264, 265
    supplementation 547, 654
potassium bromide 802
potassium penicillin 795
potassium permanganate 897
potato 791
Potomac horse fever 564, 565, 566, 567
poultry red mite 889
Pouret's operation 307, 308
povidone–iodine solutions
    foot infections 67
    skin disease 897, 899, 905
    uterine infections *316*, 317
    wound lavage 947
pralidoxime chloride 785
praziquantel 564
prednisolone
    eosinophilic granuloma 911
    equine protozoal meningitis 732
    inflammatory airway disease *468*
    urticaria 929
    vasculitis 930
pre-excitation syndrome 688

pregnancy
  complications 266–76
    early embryonic death 274–5
    gastrointestinal 275–6
    placentitis 272–3
  diagnosis 261–3, *261*
  duration 280, 285
  endocrinology 260
  fetal assessment 263–5
  hypocalcemia *627*
  management of high-risk 265
  maternal recognition 260
  postpartum period 286–7
  twin 261, 270–1, 279
  see also abortion; parturition
prekallikrein deficiency 718
premature ventricular complexes 688
pre-pubic tendon, rupture 594–5
prepuce 328–9
  squamous cell carcinoma 370–1,
  922
prepurchase examination 810
pressure sores, cast application 35,
  951
priapism 343, 351
prilocaine 19
probiotics 568, 574, 989
procainamide *683*
procaine penicillin 265, 656, 732
progestagens
  estrus synchronization 253
  and male fertility *342*
progesterone
  assays 251
  estrous cycle 243, 245, 251, 252,
    323
  exogenous 252
    behavioral problems 1001
    high-risk pregnancy 265
    intravaginal devices 252
  pregnancy 260, 263
prognathia (sow mouth) 493–4, 621
prokinetic drugs *522*
prolactin 1000
prolapse
  bladder 291
  rectum 291, 588–9
  uterus 289–90
proliferative enteropathy 544–5
pro-opiomelanocortin 629
propanolol *683*
proprioceptive deficits 752
prostaglandin F$_2\alpha$ 243, 253, 254, 282

prostaglandins
  estrus manipulation 286, 322, 323
  and non-steroidal anti-
    inflammatory drugs 570, 647,
    858
  uveitis 858
prostate gland 329
protein
  dietary 163, 650
  impaired absorption 520
  total plasma determination 714
  see also hyperproteinemia;
    hypoproteinemia
proteinuria 640, 649
Proteus miralbilis 652
prothrombin time 599, 602, 713,
  718–19
proton-pump inhibitors 538, 982
proud flesh 943, **945**, 952
proximal interphalangeal joint
  arthrodesis 104, 105
  osteoarthritis 94–6, 104–5
  P2 fracture 102, 103
pruritus 877
  atopy 892–3
  chemical-induced 877
  fungal disease 878–9
  insect-induced 881–92
  parasitic disease 880–1
  physical 877
pseudarthroses 180
Pseudoallescheria boydii 394, 907
pseudohermaphrodites 321, 345
Pseudomonas spp. 272, 279, 315, 652
Pseudomonas aeruginosa 255, 317,
  320, 365, 369
Psorophora mosquito species 761
Psoroptes spp. mites 875, 890
psyllium 570, 571, 574, 581
Pteridium aquilinum 791
ptosis 750, 861
ptyalism 166, 507, 792, **793**
pubis, fracture 160
pulmonary edema 689
pulmonary function tests 389
pulmonary hemorrhage, exercise-
  induced 478–80
pulmonary hypertension 704
pulmonary valve, stenosis 693
pulp 484
pulpitis 484, 495–7
pulses
  assessment 673
  digital 16, 673
punch biopsy, testicles 358

punch grafts 955–6
puncture vine 606, **607**
puncture wounds 940
  foot 87, 97–9
pupil 748, 749
pupillary light response 748, 812, **813**
  abnormal *811*
  absence 869
  direct 812, **813**
  indirect 812, **813**
pure red cell aplasia 727–8
Purkinje–Sanson images 817
purpura hemorrhagica 455, 732–3,
  934
purse-string suture 589
pyelonephritis 652–3
pyometra 320
pyrantel 577
pyrantel pamoate 549, 564
pyrantel tartrate 549, 564, 572–3, *572*
pyrethrins 883
pyrimethamine 769
pyrrolizidine alkaloids 604–6, 618
Pythium spp. (pythosis) 410, 878–9
pyuria 640–1

Q

quarantine
  contagious equine metritis 366
  strangles 456, 457
quarter cracks **15**, 74
Quarter horses 90, 226, 229, 230, 239,
  838, 936
'Queensland itch' (sweet itch) 881–3
quidding 493
quinidine
  applications 682, *683*, 686, 689
  dose *683*
  toxicity 680, *683*
quinidine gluconate 682, *683*
quinidine sulfate 682, *683*
quittor 89–90

R

rabies 764
radial nerve paresis 14, **15**, 782
radioallergosorbent test 876
radiofrequency hyperthermia 840,
  917
radiography
  abdomen 518
  dental 486–8, *486*
  digital 23
  foot 63
  health and safety 24
  lameness investigation 22–4

neurologic disease 756
respiratory tract 386–7
spine **175**, 179
radiotherapy
sarcoids 840, 916
squamous cell carcinoma 922
radius
fractures 33, **36**, 126–7
physitis 60–1
ragwort 604, **605**
rain scald 896–7
ramps 499
ranitidine *538*, 982
rattlesnake bite 789
rebreathing bag 471
reciprocal apparatus 221
rectal examination
female reproductive tract 248
dystocia 283
fetal assessment 264
ovaries 242, 244
pregnancy diagnosis 261
gastrointestinal tract 516–17
male reproductive organs 333
rectal prolapse 291, 588–9
management 589
types/degrees 588, **589**
rectovaginal/rectovestibular fistula
296, 299
rectum, tears 586–8
recumbent animal
facial nerve damage 777
neurologic evaluation 753–4
recurrent airway obstruction (heaves)
465–7
drugs used *468*
recurrent laryngeal nerve 435
recurrent laryngeal neuropathy
421–6, 440
scoring system 423–4, *423*
'red bag' delivery 291–2
red blood cells 711
agglutination 720
basophilic stippling 733
rouleaux formation 711
red-cell antigens 972
red cell aplasia, pure 727–8
red cell distribution width 714
red maple leaf toxicosis 721–2
reflexes, evaluation 753–4
reflux esophagitis 510–11
refractometer 714, 967, 969
renal calculi 651
renal failure, *see* acute renal failure;
chronic renal failure
renal pharmacology 668–9

renal tubular acidosis 653–4
reperfusion, after anesthesia 227, 228
repin 790
reproductive hormones
mare 242–3, 251
stallion 326, 334–5
reserpine *342*
respiratory disease
classification 382
clinical examination 382, 383–5
diagnostic tests 386–9
history and signalment 382–3
lower tract 458–80
medical conditions 458–65
obstructive conditions 465–7,
468
parasitic conditions 468–9
upper tract
medical conditions 450–7
surgical conditions 390–449
respiratory distress
diaphragmatic hernia 593–4
neonate 799–800
respiratory noises
alar fold disease 390
axial deviation of aryepiglottic folds
432
epiglottic entrapment 430
foal 412
'high blowing' 390
recurrent laryngeal neuropathy
421–2
'roaring' 421, 751
'whistle' 421
respiratory rate 383
neonatal foal *966*
respiratory support 479, *800*, 978
retinal detachment 828, 837, 859
retinal dysplasia 837
retrobulbar nerve block 815
retropharyngeal lymph nodes
adenitis 738
strangles abscess 454, **455**, 457
reverse heel wedge 18
rhabdomyolysis
atypical myoglobinuria 240
exertional 28, 163, 164, 229–30
neonatal foal 800
pigment nephropathy 648
rhinitis, fungal 394–5
Rhizoctonia legumincola 507
Rhodococcus equi 161, 458–60, 795,
990, 993–4
antibiotics 460, 994
reducing incidence 460, 994

rib fracture 966, **967**
hemothorax 477, 715
rifampicin 989, 994
rifampin 460, 545
foal *968*
rima glottidis 421, 423
rim cast 78
ringworm 899–900
foal 938
microsporosis 900
trichophytosis 899
'roaring' 421, 751
Robert Jones bandage 33, 115, 126,
950
Rocky Mountain horses 832–3
rodenticides, anticoagulant 718–19
rolling
management of colon displacement
579
management of uterine torsion 266
romifidine 283
rostral displacement of the palatopharyngeal arch 428–9
rotavirus enteritis 545–6, 987
roughage, dietary 1010
round ligament, rupture 158, 159

S

sacral spine, injuries 177, 178, 179,
780, 781
sacrocaudalis dorsalis medialis, biopsy
805
sacroiliac joint 176, 184–5
saddles, ill-fitting 175
St John's wort 932
salinomycin 701
salivary glands 506–7
calculi 507
inflammation 507
neoplasia 507
sublingual 507
trauma 506–7
salivation, excessive 507
salmeterol *468*
Salmonella spp. 545, 546, 652
gastroenteritis 564–8, 987–9
meningitis 766
Salmonella abortus equi 272, 279
salmonellosis 564–8, 987–9
salpingitis 305
salt, addition to diet 656, 658
Salter–Harris fractures, type II 115,
146
salt poisoning 800–1
sand enteropathy 569–70

sand impaction 581
saponin-containing plants 606, **607**
Sarcocystis spp. 615, 768–9
sarcoidosis 927
sarcoids 913–17
    etiology 913
    fibroblastic 915, 943
    malevolent 915–16
    management 840, 916–17
    mixed 915
    nodular 839, 914
    occult 839, 914
    penis/prepuce 372
    periocular 839–41, **915**
    prognosis 840–1
    verrucous 839, 914
Sarcoptes scabei var. *equi* 890
saucer fractures 117
savaging 1006
saw-horse stance 771
scapula, fractures 33, 132–3
scapulohumeral joint, disease 134–5
scar 895
scar tissue, tendons 189, 192
Schirmer tear test 812, 815
schwannoma 921
sciatic nerve, injury 783
scintigraphy 25–6
    carpal fractures 121
    dental infections 400
    fetlock joint 112
    liver 601
    navicular bone 92
    sacroiliac region 184
    suspensory desmitis 199
    tarsal fractures 139
    thoracolumbar spine **26**, 175, 176, 181
    urinary disease 644
    vertebral fractures 179
scirrhous cord 359
scoliosis 754
    cervical 770
    lateral 174
scrotal hernia 360–1, 558–9
scrotum
    anatomy 326–7
    dermatitis 356
    edema 354
    total width measurement 332, 333, *347*
    trauma **354**, 355
sebaceous gland tumors 923
seborrheic disease 902

sedation
    castration 375
    cerebral injury 774
    dystocia 283
    echocardiography 680
    eye examination 814
    hepatic encephalopathy 604, 799
    hypoxic-ischemic encephalopathy *800*
    perineural nerve blocks 19
    per-rectum examination 516
Seidel test 869
seizures 746
    bacterial meningitis 766, **767**
    cerebral trauma 774
    epilepsy 802
    focal 746, 802
    generalized 746, 802
    hypoxic–ischemic encephalopathy 799
    perinatal asphyxia syndrome 978
selenium 163
    deficiency 621, 700
    dietary intake 237
    toxicity 74, 902
selenium sulfide shampoo 886, 888
self-mutilation 1005–6
semen
    blood (hemospermia) 363
    chilled 257, 339
    collection 334, 335, 336
    evaluation 334, 337–9
    fresh 257
    frozen 257–8, 339
    polymorphonuclear cells 365
    urine contamination 364
semen extenders 336, 364
seminal vesicles 333
seminoma 372
semitendinosus muscle, fibrotic and ossifying myopathy 230–1
Senecio jacobaea 604, **605**, 618
sensation
    facial 749
    trunk and limbs 754
septic arthritis 958–61
    antibiotic therapy 97, 98, *960*, 961, 991–2
    distal interphalangeal joint 96–7
    foals 96, 990–2
    temporomandibular joint 169
septicemia
    fetus 272
    foal 766, 970–2, 989
        ocular lesions 838–9

serology 29
seroma 954
serotonin 1000–1
    antagonists 632, 1001
    reuptake blockers 1000
Sertoli cells 345
Sertoli-cell tumors 372
sesamoid bones (proximal), fracture **35**, 106–7
sesamoiditis 113
Setaria spp. 770
set-fast 893–4
severe combined immunodeficiency **938**, 970
sex reversal, XY 321, 345
sexually-transmitted diseases, *see* venereal diseases
'shaker-foal' syndrome 792
Sharpie's fibers 484
shear mouth 498–9
shins, sore/bucked 116
shivers 798
shock
    hypovolemic 590, 591
    septic 595, 596
shock-wave therapy 32, 54, 144, 199
shoeing
    as cause of lameness 66, 83–4
    check ligament injury 205
    foot bruising/corns 66
    hoof cracks 75–6
    laminitis 71, 72
    limb deformities 43, 45, 54, 57
    navicular syndrome 92
    osteoarthritis 96
shoes
    egg-bar **82**, 92
    glue-on 54
    heart-bar **75**
    heel extension 45
    toe extension 57
    traction devices 84
shoulder, fractures 132–3
sialoadenitis 507
sialoliths 507
sidebone 88
silage, feeding 792
silastic intravaginal devices 252
'silent heat' 322–3
Silver Dapple locus 833
silver sulfadiazine *949*
Simulium spp. 885–6
single radial hemolysis 451
'sinker line **71**
sinus arrest/block 687
sinus arrhythmia 687

sinuscopy 387, 402
sinuses, paranasal 171, 395–403
  anatomy 395
  cysts 408–9
  examination 383, 387
  lavage 397–8
  neoplasia 406–7
  percutaneous centesis 387
  trauma 402–3
sinusitis
  fungal 401–2
  primary 395–9
  secondary 399–400, 496–7, 501
63XO syndrome 301
64XY syndrome 345
skin 874
  biopsy 875–6
  examination 874
  sampling 875
skin diseases
  bacterial 878–9, 896–8, 904–7
  causing alopecia 893–902
  causing pruritus 877–93
  congenital/developmental 910–11
  external genitalia 356, 369–70
  foals 936–8
  fungal 858, 878–9, 899–900, 907–8
  immune-mediated 874, 911–12,
    923–30
  insect-induced 881–93
  neoplasia 892, 913–23
  nodular 902–12
  parasitic 370, 875, 881, 887–92,
    909–10
  pigmentation disorders 930–2
  protozoal 909
  seborrheic 902
  viral 895, 903–4
skin grafting 954–6
skin tent 566
skull, see cranium
slab fractures
  carpal bones 120, 121, 122
  tarsal bones 138, **139**
slaframine toxicity 507
'slap test' 384, 751
sling
  cervical spine trauma 780
  stallion 348, 350
slug/snail bait poisoning 787
small intestines 543–9
  absorption tests 520, 529, *548*
  epiploic foramen entrapment
    556–7
  eventration following castration
    379

ileal hypertrophy 553
Meckel's diverticulum 554–5
mesodiverticular band 555–6
palpation per rectum 517
strangulating lipoma 550–1
stricture 523
ulceration 543–4
volvulus 552, 555
smegma 370
  accumulation 352, **353**
smoke inhalation 474, 956–7
smooth-muscle relaxants 512, *521,*
  989
snakebite 789
snare of Gigli 413
sodium
  excretion 642, *642*
  mammary secretions 264, 265
  serum 646, 800–1
sodium bicarbonate 228, 646, 648,
  654, 670
sodium cromoglycate *468*
sodium iodide 878, 879
sodium penicillin 666, 795
sodium sulfate 522, 580
soft palate
  'billowing' 418
  intermittent dorsal displacement
    415–18
  permanent dorsal displacement
    419–20
soil, eating 1003
Solanum nigram 791
sorbitol dehydrogenase 599, 602
sore shins 116
sow mouth (prognathia) 493–4, 621
spavin
  bog 144–5
  bone **23**, 141–4
spavin test 18, 141–2
speculum
  full-mouth (gag) 482, 488, **489**
  vaginal 245, 248
sperm
  concentration 337–8
  intracytoplasmic injection 340
  maturation 328
  morphology 338
  motility 337
  production and testis size 333
  recovery from deceased stallion
    339
  sexing 340
spermatic cord 328
  funiculitis 359, 379–80

neoplasia 373
torsion 358–9
spermatogenesis 355, 362
sperm granuloma 362
spherocytes 720
spina bifida 781
spinal cord
  computed tomography 28
  fibrocartilagenous emboli 781
  lesions causing gait abnormalities
    752–3
  myelodysplasias 781
  vascular abnormalities 760
spinal reflexes 753–4
spinal tap 755
spine
  dorsal spinous processes 175,
    180–1
  malformations
    cervical 758–9
    thoracolumbar/sacral 174, **175**
  osteoarthritis 182–3
  osteomyelitis 795
  soft-tissue lesions 175–7
  trauma 177–9, 778–81
    coccygeal 185
    sacrococcygeal 177, 178, 179,
      780–1
    thoracolumbar 177–9, 778–9
spleen
  neoplasia 743
  rupture 590, 741–2
  ultrasonography **601**, 741, 743
splenomegaly 742
splint bones, fractures 118–19
splints
  extensor tendon rupture 210
  fractures 32–3, 34, 115, 126
  tendon lacerations 962–3
  wound immobilization 949–50
'splints' (exostosis of MC/MT II/IV)
  120
split-thickness grafts 956
spondylitis 795
spondylosis 182
sporocysts 768
sporotrichosis 908, 909
squamous cell carcinoma 922
  esophagus 515
  female reproductive tract 312–13
  gastric 534, 535
  male genitalia 333, 370–1, **922**
  management 843, 922
  nasal passages 399
  periocular/cutaneous 841–3, 922

1049

SRY gene 345
stables
    insect proofing 883
    management and behavioral
        problems 996, 999
    management in inflammatory
        airway disease *467*
staggers, mycotoxicosis 786
stallion
    behavioral problems 342–3,
        1005–7
    breeding behavior 335
    breeding soundness examination
        330–5
    coital exanthema 310–11, 895
    ejaculatory dysfunction 344
    erectile dysfunction 343
    equine viral arteritis 278
    handling 330, 342–3
    libido 332, 335, 340–1
    management during covering 254,
        255
    scrotal hernia 558–9
stall walking 1010
stance of horse, lameness 14, **15**
staphylectomy 417
staphylococcal infections, heels 933
Staphylococcus spp. 249, 272, 325,
    365, 772
Staphylococcus aureus 315, 898
Staphylococcus hyicus 898
Staphylococcus intermedius 898
'Stars of Winslow' 810, **811**
stay apparatus
    forelimb 129
    hindlimb 148, 221, 222
Steinmann pins 35
stem cell therapy, tendonitis 194
step mouth 500
sternothyrohyoid ('strap') muscles,
myotomy 417, 418
stifle joint
    calcinosis circumscripta 155
    osteoarthritis 154
    osteochrondrosis 50, **51**, 151,
        153–4
    subchondral bone cyst **59**
    trauma **22**, 33, 150–2
stillbirth 272–3
    hydrocephalus 756
    occipitoatlantoaxial malformation
        758
stomach 517
    capacity 542
    decompression 521–2, 540
    dilation 540

impaction 540–1
mucosa 537
neoplasia 534–5
parasites 536–7
rupture 537, 542
ulceration 522, 537–8, **539**
see also entries beginning with
    gastric
stomatitis 504
Stomoxys spp. 882, 884–5
strabismus 749, 826
strangles 454–7, 738
    abscess 904
    'bastard' 454
    clinical presentation 454–7
    diagnosis 456
    lymphadenitis 738
    management 456–7
    purpura hemorrhagica 732
    vaccination 457
    vasculitis 929, **934**
    'Wyoming' 905
stranguria 523, *639*
'streetnail' procedure 98, **99**
Streptococcus spp. 272, 365, 369, 460,
    652, 772
    β-hemolytic 249, 315, 460
Streptococcus equi 454–7, 652, 794
    abscess 904
    skin infection 898
    subsp. *zooepidemicus* 279, 315,
        460, 794
    vasculitis 929, **934**
streptomycin 647
stress fractures
    humerus 131, 132
    metacarpal/metatarsal III bones
        116–17
    scapula 132, 133
    tibia 146, **147**
    vertebral laminae 178, 179, 183
stricture
    esophagus 512, 513
    intestinal 522–3
stringhalt 797–8
strongyles
    large 577
    small (cyathostomes) 526, 560,
        571–3
Strongyloides westerii 576, 880, 938
Strongylus edentatus 577, **615**
Strongylus equinus 577
Strongylus vulgaris 560, 577, 590, 770
stylohyoid bone 170, **443**, **747**
    fracture 448, 505, 506, 772
subchondral bone cysts 50, 58–9

subchondral bone sclerosis **60**, 110,
    117
subepiglottic cyst 411–13
subluxation
    fetlock joint 108
    proximal interphalangeal joint 104,
        105
submandibular lymph nodes 384, 396
    lymphoma **736**
    strangles abscess **455**
subpalpebral lavage systems 821–3,
    854
succinoxidase inhibitors 237
suckling, failure 967
sucralfate 511, 524, *538*, 982
Sudan pasture, hybrid 759
sudden collapse/death 690, 706–7
sulfamethoxazole 668, 773
sulfonamides 669, 769
    ocular disease 824
sulpiride 252, 1000
summer pasture-associated
    obstructive pulmonary disease
    467, *468*
'summer sores', *see* habronemiasis
sun blocks 897, 935
superficial digital flexor tendon
    accessory ligament (superior check
    ligament) 57
    desmitis 123
    hindlimb
        injuries 221–3, 224, 225
        luxation 220
    lacerations 962
    tendonitis 123, 188–95
    ultrasonography 190–3
superovulation 258
supraglenoid tubercle, fracture 132,
    133
supraorbital nerve block 814
suprascapular nerve, injury 782
supraspinatus muscle
    atrophy 132, **133**
    postanesthetic myopathy 227
supraspinous bursa 175
    infection (fistulous withers) 179
supraspinous ligament 175, 176, 177
suprofen 858
surrogate mare 258
suspensory ligament
    desmitis 118, 195
        body injury 24, 200–1
        branch injury 201–3
        proximal injury **15**, 196–9
    lacerations 962

sustenaculum tali
  defects/fragmentation 218, 219
  fracture 138
  fractures 138, 139
suture materials 947, *947*
sutures
  alar folds 390
  bolster 953
  mattress 390, 952–3
  rectal prolapse 589
  tension-relieving 140, 952–3
  wounds 947–8
swallowing 423, 508
swamp fever, *see* equine infectious
    anemia
sway reaction 754
sweat gland tumor 923
sweating
  electrolyte loss *626*, 628
  Horner's syndrome 861
  inability (anhidrosis) 622, 900–1
  localized 227, 754
'Sweeney' 782
sweet itch 881–3
swimming exercise 31
Swiss Freiberger horses 618
switchgrass 606
Symphytum officinale 604, **605**
synovial fluid
  collection and analysis 20–2, 958
  immune-mediated polysynovitis
      161
  normal parameters *22*
  viscosity 38
synovial sepsis 96–7, 210, 215, 958–61
synoviocentesis 20–2, 958
synoviocytes 38
synovitis
  chronic proliferative 109
  fetlock joint 110–13
  intertarsal joints 141–4
  tarsocrural joint (bog spavin)
      144–5
syringomyelia 781
systemic inflammatory response
syndrome 971

T
Tabanid spp. (horse flies) 882, 884
tachycardia
  atrial 686
  gastrointestinal disorders 546, 560
  ventricular 689
tail injuries 185, 781
tail pull (test) 752
tail tone 755, 796

tapeworm infection 524, 526, 563–4
  clinical presentation 564
  diagnosis 564
  management 564
tarsocrural joint
  osteochondrosis lesions 50, **51**
  synovitis (bog spavin) **13**, 144–5
tarsometatarsal joint, splint bone
fracture 118, 119
tarsus
  intra-articular analgesia 142
  sepsis **31**, 990, **991**
  synovitis/osteoarthritis (bone
      spavin) **23**, 141–4
  see also hock
tartar (dental) 498, 649, 805
tattoo, nonpigmented skin 843
Taylorella equigenitalis 248, 366, 369
teasing 243–4, 254
technetium⁹⁹ᴹTc 25
teeth
  abnormalities of wear 498–500
  age-related changes/aging of
      horses 485–6
  apical infections 399–400, 495–7
  calculus accumulation 498, 649,
      805
  canine 483, 498
  cheek
      cemental hypoplasia 489–90
      extraction 497
      focal overgrowths 498–9
      fractures 500–1
      loss 490
      normal wear 498–9
  composition 484
  discoloration in fluoride toxicosis
      164
  eruption *485*, 486
  examination 482–3
  extraction 491–2, 497
  imaging 486–8
  loss/absence (oligodontia) 490
  maleruption 493
  normal dentition 483–4
  retained deciduous 492
  routine prophylaxis 489, 499
  temporomandibular joint disease
      169
  trauma 168, 498, 500–1
  Triadan nomenclature 482, 484
  tumors 501–2
  wolf (vestigial premolar) 483,
      491–2
Teflon paste, subepiglottic mucosal
    injection 433

temperature, and wound healing 943
temperature, rectal, neonatal foal *966*
temporohyoid joint, osteoarthropathy
    170, 448–9, 505, 772–3
temporomandibular joint 169, 498
tendon injuries
  common calcanean tendon 221–3
  cunean tendon 225
  deep digital flexor tendonitis
      216–17
  diagnostic techniques 27, 186–8
  etiology and pathophysiology
      188–9, 216
  extensor tendons 207–10
  lacerations 208, 210, 962–3
  scar tissue formation 189, 192
  superficial digital flexor tendonitis
      123, 188–95
  ultrasonography 24
  within foot 100–1
tendon rupture
  extensor carpi radialis 211
  peroneus tendon 221
  superficial digital flexor tendon
      223
tendons
  'flaccid' 45
  imaging 186–8
tendon sheath markers 29
tendon sheaths
  digital 192, **193**, 211–13
  extensor tendons 207–10
  tarsal 218–20
  wounds involving 210, 959
tenography 186
tenorrhaphy 962, **963**
tenoscopy 30, 220
tenosynovitis 186
  annular ligament 214, **215**
  carpal canal 123
  digital flexor tendon sheath 192,
      193, 211–13
  extensor tendon sheaths 207–10
  idiopathic 211, 212
  primary/secondary traumatic 211
  septic 210, 215, 959
  sympathetic 211
  tarsal sheath (thoroughpin) 218–20
tenotomy knife 216
tenotomy ('tendon splitting') 72, 194,
    202
tension band wire fixation **128**, 129
teratoma 303

1051

testicles
  anatomy 327, 328
  biopsy 357–8
  descent 326
  hypoplasia 347
  neoplasia 372
  retained abdominal 346
  rotation 327
  size and measurement 332–3, 347, *347*
  trauma **354**, 355
  vascular supply 328
testicular degeneration 357–8
testicular feminization 321
testosterone 326, 335
  exogenous *341*, 1001
  ovarian tumors 304
tetanolysin 771
tetanospasmin 771
tetanus 771–2
  antitoxin 772
  vaccination 63, 772
tetany 235, 627–8, 801
tetracosactide acetate (Synacthen), foal *968*
tetracycline 162
tetralogy of Fallot 694
Theileria equi 724
Theiler's disease 611, 772
therapeutic penetrating keratectomy 855
thermal palatoplasty 418
thermography 26, 177
thiaminase 791
thiamine therapy 733, 788, *800*
thiocyanates 621
thistle
  Malta star 790
  yellow star 790, **791**
thoracic percussion 673
thoracocentesis 388, 462–3, 464, 476, 477
thoracolumbar spine
  congenital abnormalities 174, **175**
  soft tissue injuries 175–7, 238
  spondylosis 182
  trauma/fractures 177–9, 778–9
thoracoscopy 389
thornapple 791
thoroughpin 218–20
threadworm (*Strongyloides westeri*) 576, 938
thrombocytopenia, immune-mediated 591, 728–9
thrombophlebitis 708

thrombosis, aortoiliac 707
thrush 67
  differentiation from canker 68
thyroid cartilage 422
thyroid-function tests 622–3
thyroid gland disorders 620–4
thyroid hormones 621
  reference ranges *623*
  supplementation 624, *624*, 634
thyroid-stimulating hormone 621, 622, 623
  reference ranges *623*
thyrotropin-releasing hormone 621, 622
thyrotropin-releasing hormone stimulation test 623, *623*, 630
L-thyroxine *624*
thyroxine (T4) 621, *623*
tibia
  fractures 146–7
    first aid 33
    intercondylar eminence 150, **151**
    medial malleolus **136**
    tuberosity 150, 153
tibial nerve, paralysis 783
ticarcillin
  foals *968*
  uterine infections *316*
tick-borne disease
  Borna disease 760
  borreliosis 164, 767–8
  equine granulocytic ehrlichiosis 730–1
tick paralysis 789
ticks
  ears 892
  infestation 891–2
tie-back procedure (laryngoplasty) 425–6
'tie-forward' procedure 419
tiludronate 144
timolol maleate 836, 872
tissue glue 851
tissue necrosis 940, **941**, 943
tissue plasminogen activator 858
tocolytic drugs 265, 273
toe extension shoes 57
toltrazuril 769
tongue
  abnormal movements 1006, **1007**
  innervation 751
  lacerations 503
  tone 792, **793**
tongue-tie 417

tonometry 816, 872
Tonopen 872
torsade de pointes 682, 689
torsion
  cecum 561
  colon 275–6
  spermatic cord 358–9
  uterus 266
total scrotal width 332, 333, *347*
toxicities
  cantharadin 523–4, 627, 667–8, 701
  carbon monoxide 474
  causing myocarditis 701
  fluoride 164
  iron 600, 610
  hepatotoxins 604–10
  lead 733, 788
  mercury 784
  metaldehyde 787
  monensin 785
  nephrotoxins 645, 647, 648
  neurological disease 784–93
  organophosphates 785
  selenium 74, 902
  slaframine 507
  urea/non-protein nitrogen 784–5
  see also mycotoxicosis; plant toxicosis
trace minerals 50, 162–3, 621, 700
trachea
  clinical examination 384
  collapse 439–40
  foreign bodies 438
  stenosis 440
  trauma 436–7
tracheal lavage 388
tracheotomy 441, **441**, 474
transcutaneous electrical nerve stimulation 31
transphyseal bridging 54
trauma
  abdominal 591–2, 741–2
    spleen rupture 741–2
  eye 868
  facial 171–2, 402–3, 777
  foot/hoof 78–9, 87, 97–9, 950, **951**
  head 774–7, 864–5
  hematoma **940**, 964
  hemorrhage 715–17, 942
  osteoarthritis following 94
  oral cavity (soft tissue) 503
  penis 349, 351–2, 380, 660–1
  peripheral nerves 781–4
  salivary glands/ducts 506
  scrotal/testicular **354**, 355

spinal 177–9, 778–81
teeth 168, 498, 500–1
thoracic 475, 477
trachea 436–7
see also fractures; wounds
treadmill endoscopy 389
   aryepiglottic fold deviation 432
   dorsal displacement of the soft
      palate 416, **417**
   pharyngeal collapse 421
   recurrent laryngeal neuropathy 424
   vocal-cord collapse 435
tremors
   head 746–7
   mycotoxicosis 786
trephination
   hoof wall 89–90
   paranasal sinuses 397–8
Triadan system 482, 484
triamcinolone
   inflammatory airway disease *468*
   intra-articular 96, 142
Tribulus terrestris 606, **607**
triceps muscle, injuries 238
triceps reflex 753
trichobezoar 585
Trichophyton spp. 899, 938
Trichostrongylus axei 536–7
Tricide 68
tricuspid valve, deformity 693
tricyclic antidepressants 1001
trifoliosis 608
Trifolium hybridum 608
trigeminal nerve 749
triglycerides, serum 616, 617, 634, 635
tri-iodothyronine (T3) 621
   hypothyroidism *624*
   reference ranges *623*
trilostane 632
trimethoprim-sulfadiazine 461, 603,
      656, 660, 661, 668, 732, 850, 905
trimethoprim-sulfamethoxazole 615,
      668, 773
trocarization, cecum *562, 563, 574*
trochlear nerve 749
trombiculidiasis 891
tropicamide 817, 858, 860
troponins 680
trotting up 16, **17**
TRPM1 gene 837
Trypanosoma equiperdum 311, 366,
      369
trypanosomiasis 770
tubera sacrale, asymmetry 184

tuber calcis
   hygroma 140
   luxation of superficial digital flexor
      tendon 220
tuber coxae, fractures 160
tuber ischii, fracture 160–1
tubular necrosis 647
tunica albuginea 327, 355
tunica dartos 327
tunnel grafts 956
turnout 999
twin foals 261, 270–1
   abortion 270, 274, 275, 279
   diagnosis 262, 264, 265, 271
   incidence 270
   prematurity/dysmaturity 974–6
   reduction 270, 271
tympanic bulla, thickening 170
typhlectomy 563
typhlotomy 561, 562, 563
Tyzzer's disease 615

U

uasin gishu disease 903
ulceration
   duodenal 543–4
   esophagus 512–13
   gastric 522, 537–8, **539**, 541, 981–2
   skin 893
ulna, fractures 33, 127–9, *127*
ulnar nerve injury 783
ultrasonography
   abdominal
      hemoperitoneum **518**, 519, **716**
      intussusception 527
      liver 600–1, 603
      spleen **601**, 741, 743
      uroperitoneum 665, 987
   abdominal wall muscles 268, 269
   eye 820
   female reproductive tract 249
      air-filled vagina/uterus 306
      endometrial cysts 319
      endometritis 314
      estrous stage 244–5
      ovaries 249, 302, 303, 324
      placentitis 273
      pregnancy 249, 261–2, **263**, 264,
         270
      pyometra 320
   male reproductive tract 335, 355
      accessory sex glands 329, 330
      vesicular glands 365
   myonecrosis 232, 233

tendons/ligaments 24, **25**, 187
   choice of probe 187
   common calcanean tendon
      222–3
   deep digital flexor tendon
      injuries 217
   digital tendon sheath 212–13
   distal sesamoidean ligaments
      206, 207
   extensor tendon injuries 208–10
   inferior check ligament 205
   palmar annular ligament 214,
      215
   superficial digital flexor tendon
      190–3
   septic tenosynovitis 210
   stifle joint 152
   suspensory ligament injuries **24**,
      196–9, 200, **201**, 202, **203**
   tarsal sheath injuries 219
   therapeutic 31
   thoracic 387, 462, 476
   urinary tract 643, **646**, 649, 652
umbilical hernia 984
umbilical vein, abscessation 613
umbilicus 279
   infections 982–3
   management 280, **281**, 967, 983
ungual (collateral) cartilages
   lacerations 76, **77**
   ossification (sidebone) 88
   septic necrosis (quittor) 89–90
Unopette 337
urachus, patent/persistent 983–4
urea:creatinine ratio 641
urea, serum 599
urea poisoning 784–5
uremia, in chronic renal failure 648
ureterolithiasis 655
ureters, ectopic 655
urethra
   calculi 662–3
   endoscopy 335
   trauma 660–1
urethritis 660, **661**, 663–4
urethrogram, contrast 661
urethroplasty 664
urethrosphincterotomy 658
urethrotomy, subischial 658
urinalysis 639–41
   acute renal failure 646
   biochemistry 641–2
   endocrine disease 620
   pyelonephritis 652

urinary incontinence 659–60, 894
urinary tract
    endoscopy 335, 644, 658, 661
    physical examination 638
    radiography 643
    ultrasonography 643, **646**, 649, 652
urinary tract disease
    diagnostic tests 639–44
    drugs used 668–9
    terminology *639*
urination
    control 659
    output 638
urine
    acidification 658, 670
    alkalization 670
    collection 639
    physical and chemical properties
        640–1, *640*
        pH 640, 658, 670
        specific gravity 640, 642, 646,
            649
    sediment 640–1, 649
urine scalding 894
urobilinogen 600
urolithiasis 644, 657–8, 662–3
uroperitoneum 664–7, 985–6
urospermia 364
urovagina 308
urticaria 928–9
uterine artery rupture 287–8
uterine lavage 255–6
    clearance of membranes/infection
        293, 294, 296
    delayed involution 300
    embryo collection 258–9
    endometritis 314
uteroscopy (hysteroscopy) 251
uterus 313–20
    air-filled 306
    cytology 250
    delayed involution 300
    dorsoretroflexion 266
    fluid 257, 314
    infections 314–17
    prolapse 289–90
    rupture 288–9
    swab 249
    tone 244, *261*
    torsion 266
    tumors 312–13
    ultrasonography 244–5
uterus masculinus 330
uveal cysts 831–2

uveitis 851, 856–8
    anterior 853, 856
    cataracts **835**, 859, 860
    causes *856*
    equine recurrent **835**, 858–60
    posterior 856

V

vaccination
    alphavirus encephalitis 762
    botulism 793
    C. perfringens 569
    EHV-1 278
    equine herpes myencephalopathy
        766
    equine influenza 451
    equine viral arteritis 277, 278, 369,
        453
    leptospirosis 858
    rabies 765
    rotavirus enteritis 546
    sarcoids 916
    strangles 457
    tetanus 63, 772
    West Nile virus 763
vaccines, chimera 763
vagal tone 681
vagina
    air (pneumovagina) 306
    artificial 336
    cranial lacerations 310
    hematoma 300
    urine pooling 308, 664
    varicose veins 309
vaginal cavity 327
vaginal discharge 272, 273
vaginal examination 248, 261, *261*,
    264
vaginal tunic 327, 328
vaginoscopy 245, 248
vagus nerve 747, 751, 772
valgus deformities 40–2
vancomycin, synovial infections *960*
varicose veins, vaginal 309
variocele 359
varus deformities 40–2, 52, 53
vasculitis 929–30
    equine purpura hemorrhagica
        732–3
    pastern leukocytoclastic 934–5
    purpura hemorrhagica 934
    S. equi associated 929, **934**
vasopressin (antidiuretic hormone)
    654
    challenge test 643, 654

venereal diseases 366–70
    bacterial colonization of the penis
        367–8
    coital exanthema 310–11, 368, 895
    contagious equine metritis 248,
        366
    control 369
    dourine 311, 366
    endometritis 317
    equine viral arteritis 272, 278, 332,
        368–9, 452–3, 903
    examination of mare 248, 369
    examination of stallion 335, 369
Venezuelan equine encephalitis 761,
    762
venous catheter, thrombophlebitis
    708
ventral hernia 594–5
ventricular fibrillation 690
ventricular septal defects 680, 690–2,
    694
ventriculocordectomy 436
verminous meningoencephalomyelitis
    770
vertebral laminae, stress fractures 178,
    179, 183
very low density lipoproteins 616,
    634
vesicular glands 329, 365
vestibular disease 749, **751**, 772–3
    central 750
    peripheral 746, **747**, 750
vestibular sphincter 247, 248
vestibular trauma 776
vestibulocochlear nerve 750, 772, **773**
video endoscopy 416, **417**, 420, 424,
    432, 435
villous atrophy
    placenta 279
    small intestines 529
vinegar, uterine flushing *316*
viral papillomas, *see* papillomatosis
virulence-associated proteins (Vap)
    458
vision, evaluation 810, 816
vitamin C, urine acidification 658, 670
vitamin D 625, 648
vitamin E 237, 769, 770, 863
    administration 701
    deficiency 700, 803, 863, 912
    hypoxic–ischemic encephalopathy
        800
    supplementation 804, 805, 979
vitamin K 718
vitamin K1 604, 719
vitamin K3 719

vitiligo 931
  acquired 930
  lateral limbus **867**
vitrectomy 860
vitreocentesis 819–20
vitreous, protein accumulation **857**
vocal-cord collapse 435–6
voluntary effort, assessment 754
volvulus
  large colon 575–6
  small intestines 552, 555
vomeronasal glands 326
voriconazole 850
vulva
  conformation 247–8, 306, 308
  hematoma 300
vulvoplasty, Caslick's 306–7, 310

W

'wall eye' 830
warble fly 883
wasp stings 886
water-deprivation test 642, 654
water intake
  and colon impaction 579, 580
  encouraging 658
  and urine output 638
wave mouth 500
weakness, neurological disease 752,
  754
weaving 1000, 1004
weight bearing, fracture repair 37
weight reduction 633, 634
Werneckiella (Damalinia) equi 887–8
Western equine encephalitis 760–2
West Nile virus 762–3
wheat bran 163
wheeze 385
Whirl-Pak bag 339
'whistle' 421
white blood cells 711–12
  synovial fluid *22*, 161
  wound healing 941
white line disease 73–4
white muscle disease 163, 237
windgalls 211, 212
wire injuries **945**
withers
  injuries 175, 178
    fracture 179
wobbler syndrome 806–8
Wolff–Parkinson–White syndrome
  688
wolf teeth 483, 491
  extraction 491–2
wood chewing 1010–11

wound closure 947–8
  primary 944, **945**
  secondary 944, 946
wound dressings 949–50, *949*
  burns 957
  foot injuries 64
  semi-occlusive 950, *950*
wound healing
  complications 952–4
  factors affecting 942–3
  second-intention 942
  stages 941–2
wounds
  abdominal 591–2
  burns 956–7
  classification 940
  dehiscence **945**, 952–3
  drainage 948
  foot 63–4, 87, 97–9
  heel-bulb 76–7, 942, **951**
  immobilization 950–1
  infection 943
  involving synovial structures 96–7,
    210, 958–61
  lavage 947
  penis/urethra 661
  seroma formation 954
  skin grafting 954–6
  surgical debridement 947
wound scalding 895
wry nose 46, **47**, 392, 494

X

Xanthium spp. 608
xylazine 19, 520, *521*, 639
xylose absorption test 520
XY sex reversal syndrome 321, 345

Y

yeast infections
  skin 878
  uterus 317
yogurt 574
yolk sac 262

Z

zinc, deficiency 162–3
zinc sulfate 897